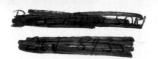

CURRENT SURGICAL DIAGNOSIS & TREATMENT

3RD EDITION

current
SURGICAL
DIAGNOSIS
& TREATMENT

By

J. ENGLEBERT DUNPHY, MD

Professor of Surgery Emeritus
University of California School of Medicine
(San Francisco)

LAWRENCE W. WAY, MD

Professor of Surgery
University of California School of Medicine
(San Francisco)

And Associate Authors

Illustrated by **LAUREL V. SCHAUBERT**

Lange Medical Publications

LOS ALTOS, CALIFORNIA

1977

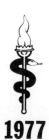

A Concise Medical Library for Practitioner and Student

Current Surgical Diagnosis & Treatment, 3rd ed. $18.00

Current Medical Diagnosis & Treatment 1977 (annual revision). Edited by M.A. Krupp and M.J. Chatton. 1066 pp. — 1977

Current Pediatric Diagnosis & Treatment, 4th ed. Edited by C.H. Kempe, H.K. Silver, and D. O'Brien. 1053 pp, *illus.* — 1976

Current Obstetric & Gynecologic Diagnosis & Treatment. Edited by R.C. Benson. 911 pp, *illus.* — 1976

Review of Physiological Chemistry, 16th ed. H.A. Harper, V.W. Rodwell, and P.A. Mayes. 681 pp, *illus.* — 1977

Review of Medical Physiology, 8th ed. W.F. Ganong. 599 pp, *illus.* — 1977

Review of Medical Microbiology, 12th ed. E. Jawetz, J.L. Melnick, and E.A. Adelberg. 542 pp, *illus.* — 1976

Review of Medical Pharmacology, 5th ed. F.H. Meyers, E. Jawetz, and A. Goldfien. 740 pp, *illus.* — 1976

Basic & Clinical Immunology. Edited by H.H. Fudenberg, D.P. Stites, J.L. Caldwell, and J.V. Wells. 653 pp, *illus.* — 1976

Basic Histology, 2nd ed. L.C. Junqueira, J. Carneiro, and A.N. Contopoulos. 453 pp, *illus.* — 1977

General Urology, 8th ed. D.R. Smith. 492 pp, *illus.* — 1975

General Ophthalmology, 8th ed. D. Vaughan and T. Asbury. 379 pp, *illus.* — 1977

Correlative Neuroanatomy & Functional Neurology, 16th ed. J.G. Chusid. 448 pp, *illus.* — 1976

Principles of Clinical Electrocardiography, 9th ed. M.J. Goldman. 412 pp, *illus.* — 1976

Handbook of Psychiatry, 3rd ed. Edited by P. Solomon and V.D. Patch. 706 pp. — 1974

Handbook of Obstetrics & Gynecology, 6th ed. R.C. Benson. 772 pp, *illus.* — 1977

Physician's Handbook, 18th ed. M.A. Krupp, N.J. Sweet, E. Jawetz, E.G. Biglieri, and R.L. Roe. 754 pp, *illus.* — 1976

Handbook of Pediatrics, 12th ed. H.K. Silver, C.H. Kempe, and H.B. Bruyn. About 710 pp, *illus.* — 1977

Handbook of Poisoning: Diagnosis & Treatment, 9th ed. R.H. Dreisbach. About 520 pp. — 1977

Table of Contents

Preface

The third edition of this surgical text makes available in concise form the basic information and the most recent developments in general surgery and each of the surgical specialties for medical students, residents, and practicing surgeons and physicians.

The chapters on surgical nutrition, burns, the thyroid, the spleen, and legal medicine have been completely rewritten. New information has been added to most chapters, and the bibliographies have been updated in all. New sections on tumor immunology and special diagnostic procedures have been added.

The editors acknowledge their appreciation for the cooperation of all the contributors in the numerous additions, alterations, and deletions which have been made in order to make each chapter an integrated part of the text. We wish to express our special thanks to Dr. Paul Ebert for his editorial supervision of the chapters on the heart and thoracic wall, pleura, lungs, and mediastinum.

We have recently become aware that our occasional use of the masculine pronoun to refer to both male and female physicians and patients is a cause of resentment on the part of some of our readers. In future editions we intend to make appropriate changes in wording in order to avoid giving this unintended offense.

Translations have been completed in Spanish, Serbo-Croatian, and Japanese and will soon be available in German, Portuguese, Italian, and Polish.

J. Englebert Dunphy, MD
Lawrence W. Way, MD

San Francisco
August, 1977

Authors

John E. Adams, MD
Guggenhime Professor of Neurological Surgery, University of California School of Medicine (San Francisco).

Robert E. Allen, Jr., MD
Associate Clinical Professor of Surgery, University of California School of Medicine (San Francisco).

Allen I. Arieff, MD
Chief, Nephrology Service, Veterans Administration Hospital; Associate Professor of Medicine, University of California School of Medicine (San Francisco).

Folkert O. Belzer, MD
Professor of Surgery and Chairman, Department of Surgery, University of Wisconsin Center for Health Sciences (Madison).

Walter Birnbaum, MD
Clinical Professor of Surgery Emeritus, University of California School of Medicine (San Francisco).

F. William Blaisdell, MD
Professor of Surgery, University of California School of Medicine (San Francisco).

Edwin B. Boldrey, MD
Professor of Neurological Surgery, University of California School of Medicine (San Francisco).

Barton A. Brown, MD
Assistant Clinical Professor of Neurological Surgery, University of California School of Medicine (San Francisco).

Jesse L. Carr, MD
Clinical Professor of Pathology & Forensic Medicine Emeritus, University of California School of Medicine (San Francisco).

Norman L. Chater, MD
Clinical Professor of Neurological Surgery, University of California School of Medicine (San Francisco).

Orlo H. Clark, MD
Assistant Professor of Surgery, University of California School of Medicine (San Francisco).

Edward S. Connolly, MD
Chief, Section of Neurosurgery, Ochsner Clinic (New Orleans).

Herbert H. Dedo, MD
Associate Professor of Otolaryngology, University of California School of Medicine (San Francisco).

Alfred A. deLorimier, MD
Associate Professor of Surgery, University of California School of Medicine (San Francisco).

J. Englebert Dunphy, MD
Professor of Surgery Emeritus, University of California School of Medicine (San Francisco).

L. Henry Edmunds, Jr., MD
W.M. Measey Professor of Cardiothoracic Surgery, University of Pennsylvania (Philadelphia).

William K. Ehrenfeld, MD
Associate Professor of Surgery, University of California School of Medicine (San Francisco).

Nicholas J. Feduska, MD
Assistant Professor of Surgery, University of California School of Medicine (San Francisco).

Roy A. Filly, MD
Assistant Professor of Radiology and Chief, Diagnostic Ultrasonography, University of California School of Medicine (San Francisco).

Peter H. Forsham, MD
Professor of Medicine & Pediatrics and Director of Metabolic Research Unit, University of California School of Medicine (San Francisco).

Karen K. Fu, MD
Associate Professor of Radiation Oncology, University of California School of Medicine (San Francisco).

Maurice Galante, MD
Associate Professor of Surgery, University of California School of Medicine (San Francisco).

Jerry Goldstone, MD
Assistant Professor of Surgery, University of California School of Medicine (San Francisco) and Chief of Vascular Surgery, Veterans Administration Hospital (San Francisco).

William P. Graham III, MD
Professor of Surgery and Chief, Division of Plastic and Reconstructive Surgery, The Milton S. Hershey Medical Center, The Pennsylvania State University College of Medicine, Hershey, Pennsylvania.

Orville F. Grimes, MD
Associate Professor of Surgery, University of California School of Medicine (San Francisco).

Neri P. Guadagni, MD
Associate Professor of Anesthesia, University of California School of Medicine (San Francisco).

Albert D. Hall, MD
Clinical Professor of Surgery, University of California School of Medicine (San Francisco).

Harold A. Harper, PhD
Professor of Biochemistry, Departments of Biochemistry & Surgery, University of California School of Medicine (San Francisco).

Edward C. Hill, MD
Professor of Obstetrics & Gynecology, University of California School of Medicine (San Francisco).

Julian T. Hoff, MD
Associate Professor of Neurological Surgery, University of California School of Medicine (San Francisco).

Yoshio Hosobuchi, MD
Associate Professor of Neurological Surgery, University of California School of Medicine (San Francisco).

Michael H. Humphreys, MD
Assistant Professor of Medicine, University of California School of Medicine (San Francisco) and Chief, Renal Service, San Francisco General Hospital.

Thomas K. Hunt, MD
Professor of Surgery, University of California School of Medicine (San Francisco).

Ernest Jawetz, PhD, MD
Professor of Microbiology and Chairman, Department of Microbiology, Professor of Medicine, and Lecturer in Pediatrics, University of California School of Medicine (San Francisco).

Floyd H. Jergesen, MD
Clinical Professor of Orthopedic Surgery, University of California School of Medicine (San Francisco).

Eugene S. Kilgore, MD
Clinical Professor of Surgery, University of California School of Medicine (San Francisco).

Melvyn T. Korobkin, MD
Associate Professor of Radiology, University of California School of Medicine (San Francisco).

Samuel L. Kountz, MD
Professor and Chairman, Department of Surgery, State University of New York, Downstate Medical Center (Brooklyn, New York).

Marcus A. Krupp, MD
Clinical Professor of Medicine, Stanford University School of Medicine (Stanford) and Director of Research, Palo Alto Medical Research Foundation.

Robert C. Lim, Jr., MD
Associate Professor of Surgery, University of California School of Medicine (San Francisco).

Harold H. Lindner, MD
Clinical Professor of Topographical & Regional Anatomy & Surgery, University of California School of Medicine (San Francisco).

Alexander R. Margulis, MD
Professor of Radiology and Chairman, Department of Radiology, University of California School of Medicine (San Francisco).

Carleton Mathewson, Jr., MD
Clinical Professor of Surgery Emeritus, University of California School of Medicine (San Francisco).

Wesley S. Moore, MD
Professor of Surgery and Head of Section of Vascular Surgery, University of Arizona Medical Center (Tucson).

William J. Morris, MD
Associate Clinical Professor of Surgery, University of California School of Medicine (San Francisco).

Jack Nagan, JD
Office of Veterans Administration General Counsel (San Francisco).

John Q. Owsley, Jr., MD
Associate Clinical Professor of Surgery, University of California School of Medicine (San Francisco).

Robert F. Palmer, MD
Assistant Clinical Professor of Neurological Surgery, University of California School of Medicine (San Francisco).

Steven N. Parks, MD
Clinical Instructor of Surgery, University of California School of Medicine (San Francisco).

Roland K. Perkins, MD
Associate Clinical Professor of Neurological Surgery, University of California School of Medicine (San Francisco).

Byron C. Pevehouse, MD
Clinical Professor of Neurological Surgery, University of California School of Medicine (San Francisco).

Theodore L. Phillips, MD
Professor of Radiation Oncology, University of California School of Medicine (San Francisco).

Lawrence Pitts, MD
Assistant Professor, Department of Neurosurgery, University of California School of Medicine (San Francisco).

Malcolm R. Powell, MD
Assistant Clinical Professor of Radiology and Medicine, University of California School of Medicine (San Francisco).

Howard A. Reber, MD
Assistant Professor of Surgery, University of California School of Medicine (San Francisco).

Benson B. Roe, MD
Professor of Surgery, University of California School of Medicine (San Francisco).

Oscar Salvatierra, Jr., MD
Associate Professor of Surgery and Urology and Director, Kidney Transplant Service, University of California School of Medicine (San Francisco).

Theodore R. Schrock, MD
Associate Professor of Surgery, University of California School of Medicine (San Francisco).

Robert J. Seymour, MD
Assistant Clinical Professor of Neurological Surgery, University of California School of Medicine (San Francisco).

George F. Sheldon, MD
Associate Professor of Surgery and Chief of Trauma Service, University of California School of Medicine (San Francisco).

Glenn E. Sheline, MD, PhD
Professor of Radiology, University of California School of Medicine (San Francisco).

Donald R. Smith, MD
Professor of Urology Emeritus, University of California School of Medicine (San Francisco) and Consulting Urologist, Project Hope (Egypt).

Maurice Sokolow, MD
Professor of Medicine, University of California School of Medicine (San Francisco).

Francis A. Sooy, MD
Professor of Otolaryngology, University of California School of Medicine (San Francisco).

Lynn E. Spitler, MD
Assistant Professor of Medicine, University of California School of Medicine (San Francisco) and Director of Research, Children's Hospital of San Francisco.

Samuel D. Spivack, MD
Associate Clinical Professor of Medicine and Radiology, University of California School of Medicine (San Francisco).

Muriel Steele, MD
Associate Clinical Professor of Surgery, University of California School of Medicine (San Francisco).

Emil A. Tanagho, MD
Professor of Urology and Chairman, Department of Urology, University of California School of Medicine (San Francisco).

Arthur N. Thomas, MD
Associate Professor of Surgery, University of California School of Medicine (San Francisco).

Donald D. Trunkey, MD
Associate Professor of Surgery, University of California School of Medicine (San Francisco) and Director of the Burn Unit, San Francisco General Hospital.

Kenneth Tuerk, MD
Clinical Instructor of Neurological Surgery, University of California School of Medicine (San Francisco).

Daniel J. Ullyot, MD
Associate Professor of Surgery, University of California School of Medicine (San Francisco).

Daniel G. Vaughan, MD
Clinical Professor of Ophthalmology, University of California School of Medicine (San Francisco).

Ralph O. Wallerstein, MD
Clinical Professor of Medicine, University of California School of Medicine (San Francisco).

Lawrence W. Way, MD
Professor of Surgery, University of California School of Medicine (San Francisco).

Phillip R. Weinstein, MD
Assistant Professor of Neurological Surgery, University of California School of Medicine (San Francisco).

Charles B. Wilson, MD
Professor of Neurosurgery and Chairman, Department of Neurosurgery, University of California School of Medicine (San Francisco).

John L. Wilson, MD
Professor of Surgery, Stanford University School of Medicine (Stanford).

Edwin J. Wylie, MD
Professor of Surgery, University of California School of Medicine (San Francisco).

1...
Approach to the Surgical Patient

J. Englebert Dunphy, MD

The successful management of surgical disorders requires (1) the effective application of a broad knowledge of the basic sciences to the problems of diagnosis and total care before, during, and after the operation; and (2) a genuine sympathy for, understanding of, and indeed love for the patient. The surgeon must be a doctor in the old-fashioned sense, an applied scientist, an engineer, an artist, and a minister to his fellow man. Because life or death often depends upon the validity of his decisions, his judgment must be matched by courage in action and by a high degree of technical proficiency.

THE HISTORY

The surgeon's first contact with the patient is crucial. This is the time to gain the patient's confidence and to convince him that help is available and will be given and—above all—that the surgeon is concerned about the patient as a person who needs help and not just as a "case" to be processed through the surgical ward. This is not always easy to do, and there are no rules of conduct except to be gentle and considerate. Most patients are eager to like and trust their doctors and respond gratefully to a sympathetic and understanding manner. Some surgeons are able to establish a confident relationship with their patients with the first few words of greeting; others can only do so by means of a stylized and carefully acquired bedside manner. It does not matter how it is done so long as an atmosphere of sympathy, personal interest, and understanding is created. Even in an emergency situation (unless the patient is unconscious), this subtle transmission of sympathetic concern can and does occur.

Eventually, all histories must be formally structured, but much can be learned about the patient by letting him ramble a little. Discrepancies and omissions in the history are often due as much to overstructuring and leading questions as to the unreliability of the patient. The enthusiastic novice asks leading questions; the cooperative patient gives the answer that seems to be wanted; and the interview concludes on a note of mutual satisfaction with the wrong answer thus derived.

BUILDING THE HISTORY

History-taking is detective work. Preconceived ideas, snap judgments, and hasty conclusions have no place in it. The diagnosis must be established by inductive reasoning. The interviewer must first determine the facts and then search for essential clues, realizing that the patient may conceal the most important symptom—eg, the passage of blood by rectum—in the hope (born of fear) that if it is not specifically inquired about or if nothing is found to account for it in the physical examination, it cannot be very serious.

Common symptoms of surgical conditions that require special emphasis in the history-taking are discussed in the following paragraphs.

Pain

A careful analysis of the nature of pain is one of the most important features of a surgical history. The examiner must first ascertain how the pain began. Was it explosive in onset, rapid, or gradual? What is the precise character of the pain? Is it so severe that it cannot be relieved by medication? Is it constant or intermittent? Are there classical associations, such as the rhythmic pattern of small bowel obstruction or the onset of pain preceding the limp of intermittent claudication?

The nature of abdominal pain is of particular importance and is dealt with in some detail in Chapter 24.

One of the most important aspects of pain is the patient's reaction to it. The overreactor's description of his pain is often obviously inappropriate. Smilingly he describes "excruciating" pain. If the patient shrieks and thrashes about, he is either grossly overreacting or suffering from renal or biliary colic. Very severe pain—due to infection, inflammation, or vascular disease—forces the patient to move as little as possible. He may writhe with pain, but he will not bounce around in the bed or climb the wall.

Moderate pain is made agonizing by fear and anxiety. Reassuring the patient and restoring his confidence are often a more effective analgesic than an injection of morphine.

Vomiting

What did the patient vomit? How much? How often? What did it look like? Was it projectile? It is especially helpful if the examiner can see the vomitus. There are many important clues which are described in detail in Chapter 24.

Change in Bowel Habits

A change in bowel habits is a common complaint that is often of no significance. However, when a person who has always had regular evacuations notices a distinct change, particularly toward intermittent constipation and diarrhea, he must be presumed to have a neoplasm of the colon. Too much emphasis is placed upon the size and shape of the stool—eg, many patients who normally have well-formed evacuations may complain of irregular small stools when their routine is disturbed by travel or a change in diet.

Passage of Blood

Bleeding from any orifice demands the most critical analysis and can never be dismissed as due to some immediately obvious cause. The most common error is to assume that bleeding from the rectum is attributable to hemorrhoids. The character of the blood can be of great significance. Does it clot? Is it bright red? Is it changed in any way, as in the coffee-ground vomitus of slow gastric bleeding or the dark, tarry stool of upper gastrointestinal hemorrhage? The full details and variations cannot be included here, but will be emphasized under separate headings elsewhere.

Trauma

Trauma occurs so commonly that it is often difficult to establish a relationship between the chief complaint and an episode of trauma. Children, in particular, are subject to all kinds of minor trauma, and the family may attribute the onset of an illness to a specific recent injury. On the other hand, children may be subjected to severe trauma and their parents be unaware of it. The possibility of trauma having been inflicted by the parent ("battered child syndrome") must not be overlooked.

When there is a history of trauma, the details must be established as precisely as possible. What was the position of the patient when the accident occurred? Did he lose consciousness? Retrograde amnesia (inability to remember events just preceding the accident) always indicates some degree of cerebral damage. If a patient can remember every detail of an accident, has not lost consciousness, and there is no evidence of external injury to the head, brain damage can be ruled out.

In the case of gunshot wounds and stab wounds, the nature of the weapon, its size and shape, the probable trajectory, and the position of the patient when hit may be very helpful in evaluating the probable nature of the resultant injury.

The possibility that an accident might have been caused by preexisting disease such as epilepsy, diabetes, coronary artery disease, or hypoglycemia must be carefully explored.

•   •   •

When all the facts and essential clues have been gathered, the examiner is in a position to complete his study of the present illness. By this time he may have been led inductively to consider only a few possible diagnoses. If asked the causes of shoulder pain, the novice will include ruptured ectopic pregnancy in his thinking. The experienced physician will automatically consider the age and sex of the patient and eliminate that possibility if the patient is male.

Family History

The family history is of great significance in a number of surgical conditions. Polyposis of the colon is a classic example, but diabetes, Peutz-Jeghers syndrome, chronic pancreatitis, multiglandular syndromes, other endocrine abnormalities, and cancer are often better understood and better evaluated in the light of a careful family history.

Past History

The details of the past history may illuminate obscure areas of the present illness. It has been said that patients who are well are almost never sick, and patients who are sick are almost never well. It is true that the patient who has a long and complicated history of diseases and injuries is likely to be a much poorer risk than even the aged patient experiencing his first major surgical illness.

In order to make certain that important details of the past history will not be overlooked, the "system review" must be formalized and thorough. By always reviewing the past history in the same way, the experienced examiner never omits a significant detail. Many skilled examiners find it easy to review the past history as they perform the physical examination, inquiring about each system as that part of the body is being examined.

In reviewing the past history, it is important to consider the nutritional background of the patient. There is an increasing awareness throughout the world that the underprivileged malnourished patient responds poorly to disease, injury, and operation. Indeed, there is some evidence that various lesions such as carcinoma may be more fulminating in malnourished patients. Malnourishment may not be obvious on physical examination and must be elicited by questioning.

Acute nutritional deficiencies, particularly fluid and electrolyte losses, can be understood only in the light of the total (including nutritional) history. For example, a low serum sodium may be due to the use of diuretics or a sodium-restricted diet rather than to acute loss. In this connection, the use of any medications must be carefully recorded and interpreted.

A detailed history of acute losses by vomiting and diarrhea—and the nature of the losses—is helpful in estimating the probable trends in serum electrolytes. Thus, the patient who has been vomiting persistently but shows no evidence of bile in his vomitus is likely to have acute pyloric stenosis associated with benign ulcer, and hypochloremic alkalosis is to be anticipated. Chronic vomiting without bile—and particularly with evidence of changed and previously digested food—is suggestive of chronic obstruction, and the possibility of carcinoma should be considered.

It is essential for the surgeon to think in terms of nutritional balance. It is often possible to begin therapy before the results of laboratory tests have been obtained because the specific nature and probable extent of fluid and electrolyte losses can often be estimated on the basis of the history and the physician's clinical experience. Laboratory data should be obtained as soon as possible, but a knowledge of the probable level of the obstruction and of the concentration of the electrolytes in the gastrointestinal fluids will provide sufficient grounds for the institution of appropriate immediate therapy.

The management of electrolyte imbalances is discussed fully in Chapter 12.

The Patient's Emotional Background

Psychiatric consultation is seldom required in the management of surgical patients, but there are times when it is of immense help. Emotionally and mentally disturbed patients require surgical operations as often as others, and full cooperation between the psychiatrist and the surgeon is essential. On occasion, however, either before or after a surgical operation, patients develop major psychotic disturbances which are beyond the ability of the surgeon to appraise or manage. Prognosis, drug therapy, and overall management require the participation of a psychiatrist.

On the other hand, there are many situations in which the surgeon himself can and should deal with the emotional aspects of his patient's illness rather than resorting to psychiatric assistance. Most psychiatrists prefer not to be called upon to deal with minor anxiety states. As long as the surgeon accepts the responsibility for the care of the whole patient, such services are superfluous.

This is particularly true in the care of patients with malignant disease or those who must undergo mutilating operations such as amputation of an extremity, ileostomy, or colostomy. In these situations the patient can be supported far more effectively by the surgeon and the surgical team than by a consulting psychiatrist.

Surgeons are becoming increasingly aware of the importance of psychosocial factors in surgical convalescence. Recovery from a major operation can be greatly enhanced by our awareness of the patient's ability to cope not only with the stresses of the immediate illness

but with a variety of emotional, social, and economic problems affecting his life.

Incorporation of these factors into the problem-oriented record (Weed) is contributing substantially to better total care of the surgical patient.

THE PHYSICAL EXAMINATION

The complete examination of the surgical patient includes the physical examination, certain special procedures such as gastroscopy and esophagoscopy, laboratory tests, x-ray examination, and follow-up examination. In some cases, all of these may be necessary; in others, special examinations and laboratory tests can be kept to a minimum. It is just as poor practice to insist on unnecessary "thoroughness" as it is to overlook those procedures that contribute to the diagnosis. Painful, inconvenient, and costly procedures should not be ordered unless there is a reasonable chance that the information gained will be useful in making clinical decisions.

THE ELECTIVE PHYSICAL EXAMINATION

The elective physical examination should be done in an orderly and detailed fashion. One should acquire the habit of performing a complete examination in exactly the same sequence so that no step is inadvertently omitted. When the routine must be modified, as in an emergency, the examiner recalls without conscious effort what must be done to complete the examination later. The regular performance of complete examinations has the added advantage of familiarizing the beginner with what is normal so that he can more readily recognize what is abnormal.

All patients are sensitive and somewhat embarrassed at being examined. It is both courteous and clinically useful to put the patient at his ease. The examining room and table should be comfortable, and drapes should be used if the patient is required to strip for the examination. Most patients will relax if they are allowed to talk a bit during the examination, and this is another reason why taking the past history while the examination is being done can be helpful.

A useful rule is to first observe the patient's general physique and habitus and then to carefully inspect his hands. Many systemic diseases show themselves in the hands (cirrhosis of the liver, hyperthyroidism, Raynaud's disease, pulmonary insufficiency, heart disease, and nutritional disorders).

Details of examination cannot be included here, and the beginner is urged to consult special texts.

Inspection, palpation, and auscultation are the time-honored essential steps in appraising both the normal and the abnormal. Comparison of the 2 sides of the body often suggests a specific abnormality. The slight droop of one eyelid that is characteristic of Horner's syndrome can only be recognized by careful comparison with the opposite side. Inspection of the female breasts, particularly as the patient raises and lowers her arms, will often reveal slight dimpling indicative of an infiltrating carcinoma which is barely detectable on palpation.

Successful palpation requires skill and gentleness. Spasm, tension, and anxiety caused by painful examination procedures may make an adequate examination almost impossible—particularly in children. Another important feature of palpation is the "laying on of hands" that has been called part of the "ministry of medicine." A disappointed and critical patient often will say of a doctor, "He hardly touched me—no wonder he made a mistake." Careful, precise, and gentle palpation not only gives the physician the information that he needs, but the manner in which he does it inspires confidence and trust.

When examining for areas of tenderness, it may be necessary to use only one finger in order to precisely localize the extent of the tenderness. This is of particular importance in examination of the acute abdomen. (See Chapter 24 for details.)

Auscultation, once thought to be the exclusive province of the physician, is now more important in surgery than it is in medicine. Radiologic examinations, including cardiac catheterization, have relegated auscultation of the heart and lungs to the status of preliminary scanning procedures in medicine. In surgery, however, auscultation of the abdomen and peripheral vessels has become absolutely essential. The nature of ileus and the presence of a variety of vascular lesions are revealed by auscultation. Bizarre abdominal pain in a young woman can easily be ascribed to hysteria or anxiety on the basis of "a negative physical examination and x-rays of the gastrointestinal tract." Auscultation of the epigastrium, however, may reveal a murmur due to severe obstruction of the celiac artery.

Examination of the Body Orifices

Complete examination of the ears, mouth, rectum, and pelvis is accepted as a part of a complete examination. Palpation of the mouth and tongue is as essential as inspection. Inspection of the rectum with a sigmoidoscope is now regarded as part of a complete physical examination. Every surgeon should acquire a familiarity with the use of the ophthalmoscope and sigmoidoscope and should use them regularly in doing complete physical examinations.

there may be no history if the patient is unconscious and there are no other informants. Although the details of an accident or injury may be very useful in the total appraisal of the patient, they must be left for later consideration. The primary considerations are the following: Is the patient breathing? Is the airway open? Is there a palpable pulse? Is his heart beating? Is he bleeding massively?

If the patient is not breathing, airway obstruction must be ruled out by thrusting the fingers into the mouth and pulling the tongue forward. If the patient is unconscious, the respiratory tract should be intubated and mouth-to-mouth respiration started. If there is no pulse or heartbeat, cardiac resuscitation must be started.

The details of establishing and maintaining artificial respiration and external cardiac massage are described in Chapter 22.

If there is serious external loss of blood from an extremity, it can be controlled by elevation and pressure. Tourniquets are rarely required.

Every victim of major blunt trauma should be suspected of having a vertebral injury capable of causing damage to the spinal cord if he is inappropriately manipulated.

Some injuries are so life-threatening that action must be taken before even a limited physical examination is done. Penetrating wounds of the heart, large open sucking wounds of the chest, massive crush injuries with flail chest, and massive external bleeding— all require emergency treatment before any further examination can be done.

In most emergencies, however, after it has been established that the airway is open, the heart is beating, and there is no massive external hemorrhage— and after antishock measures have been instituted if necessary—a rapid survey examination must be done. Failure to perform such an examination can lead to serious mistakes in the care of the patient. It takes no more than 2 or 3 minutes to carefully examine the head, thorax, abdomen, extremities, genitalia (particularly in females), and back. If cervical cord damage has been ruled out, it is essential to turn the injured patient and carefully inspect his back, buttocks, and perineum.

Tension pneumothorax and cardiac tamponade may easily be overlooked if there are multiple injuries.

Upon completion of the survey examination, control of pain, splinting of fractured limbs, suturing of lacerations, and other types of emergency treatment can be started.

THE EMERGENCY PHYSICAL EXAMINATION

In an emergency, the routine of the physical examination must be altered to fit the circumstances. The history may be limited to a single sentence, or

LABORATORY & OTHER EXAMINATIONS

Laboratory Examination

Laboratory examinations in surgical patients have

the following objectives: (1) screening for asymptomatic diseases that may affect the surgical result (eg, unsuspected anemia or diabetes); (2) appraisal of diseases that may contraindicate elective surgery or require treatment before surgery (eg, diabetes, heart failure); (3) diagnosis of disorders that require surgery (eg, hyperparathyroidism, pheochromocytoma); and (4) evaluation of the nature and extent of metabolic or septic complications.

Patients undergoing major surgery, even though they seem to be in excellent health except for their surgical disease, should have a complete blood and urine examination. A history of renal, hepatic, or heart disease requires detailed studies. Latent, asymptomatic renal insufficiency may be missed since many patients with chronic renal disease have varying degrees of nitrogen retention without proteinuria. A fixed urine specific gravity is easily overlooked, and preoperative determination of the BUN and creatinine is frequently required. Patients who have had hepatitis may have no jaundice but may have severe hepatic insufficiency that can be precipitated into acute failure by blood loss or shock.

Medical consultation is frequently required in the total preoperative appraisal of the surgical patient, and there is no more rewarding experience than the thorough evaluation of a patient with heart disease or gastrointestinal disease by a physician and a surgeon working together. It is essential, however, that the surgeon not become totally dependent upon his medical consultant for the preoperative evaluation and management of the patient. The total management must be his responsibility, and he cannot delegate it. Moreover, the surgeon is the only one with the experience and background to interpret the meaning of laboratory tests in the light of other features of the case—particularly the history and physical findings.

Radiologic Examination

Modern patient care calls for a variety of critical radiologic examinations. The closest cooperation between the radiologist and the surgeon is essential if serious mistakes are to be avoided. This means that the surgeon must not refer the patient to the radiologist, requesting a particular examination, without providing him with an adequate account of the history and physical findings. Particularly in emergency situations, review of the films and consultation are needed.

When the radiologic diagnosis is not definitive, the examinations must be repeated in the light of the history and physical examination. Despite the great accuracy of x-ray diagnosis, a negative gastrointestinal study still does not exclude either ulcer or a neoplasm; particularly in the right colon, small lesions are easily overlooked. At times the history and physical findings are so clearly diagnostic that an operation is justifiable despite negative x-ray findings.

Special Examinations

Special examinations such as cystoscopy, gastroscopy, esophagoscopy, colonoscopy, angiography, and bronchoscopy are often required in the diagnostic appraisal of surgical disorders. The surgeon must be familiar with the indications and limitations of these procedures and be prepared to consult with his colleagues in medicine and the surgical specialties as required. The place of special diagnostic procedures is discussed in Chapter 51.

• • •

THE PROBLEM-ORIENTED RECORD

The history, physical examination, laboratory studies, x-ray and other special diagnostic procedures provide the "data base" underlying the diagnosis and the surgeon's plan for the care of the patient.

The **problem-oriented record** is becoming the most accepted and reliable way in which to document and program management. It also lends itself to reliable peer review. According to this system, the word "problem" represents the most specific generalization that can be supported by the available clinical data. It may be the name of a disease but often is less specific, indicating the diagnostic uncertainty that still exists. Thus, the list of problems represents what is considered factual; speculation and hypotheses are recorded in the plans. Management focuses on the problems, which should either be further defined by obtaining more data if necessary or resolved by appropriate therapy. Progress notes relate to each specific problem and are recorded as narrative notes and on flow sheets. The problem-oriented record is an improved logical and chronologic documentation of the care of the patient.

• • •

General References

Dunphy JE: On caring for the patient with cancer. N Engl J Med 295:313, 1976.

Dunphy JE, Botsford TW: *Physical Examination of the Surgical Patient,* 4th ed. Saunders, 1975.

Johns MW, Dudley HAF, Masterton JP: Psychosocial problems in surgery. J R Coll Surg Edinb 18:91, 1973.

Morgan WL, Engel GL: *The Clinical Approach to the Patient.* Saunders, 1969.

Shackelford RT: *Diagnosis of Surgical Disease.* 3 vols. Saunders, 1968.

Weed LL: *Medical Records, Medical Education, and Patient Care.* Year Book, 1970.

2 . . .
Preoperative Care

John L. Wilson, MD

The care of the patient with a major surgical problem commonly involves distinct phases of management which occur in the following sequence:
(1) Preoperative care
    Diagnostic work-up
    Preoperative evaluation
    Preoperative preparation
(2) Anesthesia and operation
(3) Postoperative care
    Postanesthetic observation
    Intensive care
    Intermediate care
    Convalescent care

Preoperative Care

The **diagnostic work-up** is concerned primarily with determining the cause and extent of the present illness. **Preoperative evaluation** consists of an overall assessment of the patient's general health in order to identify significant abnormalities which might increase operative risk or adversely influence recovery. **Preoperative preparation** includes treatments and procedures dictated by the findings on diagnostic work-up and preoperative evaluation and by the nature of the expected operation.

Postoperative Care

The **postanesthetic observation** phase of management comprises the few hours immediately after operation during which the acute reaction to surgery and the residual effects of anesthesia are subsiding. A "recovery room" with special staff and equipment is usually provided for this purpose. Patients who have had severe operations or whose general condition is precarious for other reasons should be transferred from the operating room or the recovery room to an "intensive care unit." The duration of stay in an intensive care unit may vary from 1–2 days to many weeks depending upon the condition of the patient.

Large general hospitals now usually have a variety of specialized intensive care units adapted to the needs of medical, surgical, and pediatric patients. Intensive surgical care can of course be provided on a regular nursing unit by mobilizing the necessary personnel and equipment when needed by individual patients. If there is a constant census of 5–10 critically ill patients, it is more efficient and effective to establish an intensive care unit.

It should be noted that not all postoperative patients require intensive care. Uncomplicated operations for hernia, appendicitis, anal conditions, and other problems of similar magnitude ordinarily require only a few days of hospitalization and an intermediate level of care on a regular nursing unit.

Postoperative **intermediate care** can be described as that normally available on the regular nursing units of the hospital. This type of care, and the **convalescent care** provided to the ambulatory patient outside the hospital, will not be reviewed here because they pose no special problems not touched on in the following chapters on postanesthetic and intensive care or in Chapter 4.

The Continuum of Surgical Care

The continuum of surgical care has been represented above as progressing through a series of pre- and postoperative phases. In practice, these phases merge, overlap, and vary in relative importance from patient to patient. Morbidity, mortality, and therapeutic end result in the surgical patient depend upon the competence with which each succeeding phase is managed. The rapid progression and severe episodic stress of major surgical illness leave small margin for errors of management. The care immediately preceding and following operation, which includes preoperative evaluation and preparation and postanesthetic observation and intensive care, is especially critical. Improved surgical results in recent years are due chiefly to improvements in the management of these important phases of surgical care.

PREOPERATIVE EVALUATION

General Health Assessment

The initial diagnostic work-up of the surgical patient is concerned chiefly with determining the cause of the presenting complaints. Except in strictly minor surgical illness, this initial work-up should be supplemented by a complete assessment of the patient's general health. Such an evaluation, which should be completed prior to all major operations, seeks to identify abnormalities which may influence surgical risk or which may have a bearing on the patient's future well-being. Preoperative evaluation thus involves a comprehensive examination and should include at least a complete history and physical examination, urinalysis, complete blood count, serology, and posterior-anterior and lateral chest x-rays. In patients over 40, it is advisable also to obtain an electrocardiogram, stool test for occult blood, and blood chemistry screening battery. Open wounds and infections usually require culture and determination of antibiotic sensitivity.

In addition to the foregoing studies, all significant specific complaints and physical findings should be adequately evaluated by appropriate special tests, examinations, and consultations. Bleeding tendencies, medications currently being taken, and allergies and reactions to antibiotics and other agents should be noted and prominently displayed on the chart. Psychiatric consultation should be considered in patients with a past history of significant mental disorder which may be exacerbated by surgery and in patients whose complaints may have a psychoneurotic basis.

The physical examination should be thorough and must include neurologic examination and check of peripheral arterial pulses (carotid, radial, femoral, popliteal, posterior tibial, and dorsalis pedis). A rectal examination should always be done, and a pelvic examination should be performed unless contraindicated by age, marital status, or other valid reason. A Papanicolaou smear of the cervix should be obtained in women over 30 years of age. Sigmoidoscopy is required for completeness of evaluation when there are rectal or colonic complaints. This can usually be accomplished at the time of the physical examination; if necessary, the rectum and lower sigmoid can be rapidly cleared by administration of a hypertonic sodium phosphate enema.

In summary, the preoperative evaluation should be comprehensive in order to assess the patient's overall state of health, to determine the risk of the impending surgical treatment, and to guide the preoperative preparation.

Nonsurgical Diseases Affecting Operative Risk

Nonsurgical disorders frequently increase the risk of surgical procedures. An analysis of the causes of surgical mortality shows that fatal complications are often related to preexisting organic disease, particularly of the cardiovascular, respiratory, and genitourinary systems (see Chapter 5).

Other Factors Affecting Operative Risk

A. The Pediatric Patient: See Chapter 48.

B. The Elderly Patient: Operative risk should be judged on the basis of physiologic rather than chronologic age, and an elderly patient should not be denied a needed operation because of his age alone. The hazard of the average major operation for the patient over 60 is increased only slightly provided there is no cardiovascular, renal, or other serious systemic disease. Assume that every patient over 60—even in the absence

of symptoms and physical signs—has some generalized arteriosclerosis and potential limitation of myocardial and renal reserve. Accordingly, the preoperative evaluation should be comprehensive. Occult cancer is not infrequent in this age group; therefore, even minor gastrointestinal and other complaints should be thoroughly investigated.

Administer intravenous fluids with care not to overload the circulation in the elderly. Monitoring of intake, output, body weight, serum electrolytes, and central venous pressure is an important means of evaluating the cardiorenal response and tolerance in this age group.

Regarding medications, aged patients generally require smaller doses of strong narcotics and are frequently depressed by routine doses. Codeine is usually tolerated. Sedative and hypnotic drugs often cause restlessness, mental confusion, and uncooperative behavior in the elderly and should be used cautiously. Preanesthetic medications should be limited to atropine or scopolamine in the debilitated elderly patient, and anesthetic agents should be administered in minimal amounts.

C. The Obese Patient: Obese surgical patients have a greater than normal tendency to serious concomitant disease and a higher incidence of postoperative wound and thromboembolic complications. Obesity also usually increases the technical difficulty of surgery and anesthesia. For these reasons, it may at times be advisable to delay elective surgery until the patient loses weight by appropriate dietary measures.

D. The Pregnant Patient: See Chapter 5.

E. The Compromised or Altered Host: A patient may be considered a "compromised or altered host" if the capacity of his systems and tissues to respond normally to infection and trauma has been significantly impaired by some disease or agent. Preoperative recognition and special evaluation of these patients is obviously important.

1. Increased susceptibility to infection—Certain drugs may reduce the patient's resistance to infection by interfering with host defense mechanisms. Corticosteroids, immunosuppressive agents, cytotoxic drugs, and prolonged antibiotic therapy are associated with an increased incidence of invasion by fungi and other organisms not commonly encountered in infections. A combination of irradiation and corticosteroid therapy is found experimentally to produce lethal fungal infections. It is possible that the synergistic combination of irradiation, corticosteroids, and serious underlying disease may set the stage for clinical fungal infection. A high rate of wound, pulmonary, and other infections is seen in renal failure, presumably due to decreased host resistance. Granulocytopenia and diseases which may produce immunologic deficiency—eg, lymphomas, leukemias, and hypogammaglobulinemia—are frequently associated with septic complications. The uncontrolled diabetic is also observed clinically to be more susceptible to infection (see Chapter 5).

2. Delayed wound healing—This problem can be

anticipated in certain categories of patients whose tissue repair process may be compromised. Many factors have been alleged to influence wound healing. However, only a few are of possible clinical significance. These include protein depletion, ascorbic acid deficiency, marked dehydration or edema, and severe anemia. It has been shown experimentally that hypovolemia, vasoconstriction, increased blood viscosity, and increased intravascular aggregation and erythrostasis due to remote trauma will interfere with wound healing, probably by reducing oxygen tension and diffusion within the wound. Large doses of corticosteroids have been shown to depress wound healing in animals. This effect is apparently increased by mild starvation and protein depletion. Humans appear to react similarly to corticosteroid excess, and it is therefore reasonable to assume that wounds in patients who have received appreciable doses of corticosteroid preoperatively should be closed with special care to prevent disruption and managed postoperatively as though healing will be delayed.

Surgery may be required on a patient receiving cancer chemotherapy with cytotoxic drugs. These drugs usually interfere with cell proliferation and (theoretically at least) tend to decrease the tensile strength of the surgical wound. Although experimental evidence to support this assumption is equivocal, it is wise to manage wounds in patients receiving cytotoxic drugs as though healing will be slower than normal. Slow healing and decreased tensile strength during the healing stage are sometimes observed clinically in debilitated patients such as those with advanced cancer, renal failure, gastrointestinal fistulas, and chronic infection. Protein and other nutritional deficiencies are doubtless the chief cause of the sluggish wound repair. Preoperative assessment and correction of nutritional depletion may serve to minimize troublesome wound complications in such cases. On the whole, systemic factors are infrequently the cause of delayed wound healing because the healing wound receives high priority in the body economy of even the aged or depleted patient for the protein, catalysts, and other components which are required for collagen synthesis and deposition.

Decreased vascularity and other local changes occur after a few weeks or months in tissues which have been heavily irradiated. These are potential deterrents to wound healing, a point which should be kept in mind in planning surgical incisions in patients who have been irradiated. Radiation therapy at levels of 3000 R and above are injurious to the skin and to connective and vascular tissues. Chronic changes include scarring, damage to fibroblasts and collagen, and degenerative changes with subsequent hyalinization in the walls of blood vessels. Capillary budding in granulation tissue and collagen formation are inhibited when these changes are well established, so that surgical wounds in heavily irradiated tissues may heal slowly or may break down in the presence of infection. When therapeutic doses of radiation are used as a surgical adjunct, it is generally agreed that there is an optimal delay period (2–12 weeks) after completion of the radiation therapy to minimize wound complications. In general, technical problems in correctly timed operations for cancer are not increased by low-dosage (2000–4000 R) adjunctive radiotherapy. With radiation dosage in the therapeutic range (5000–6000 R), an increased incidence of wound complications can be expected although this can be minimized by careful surgical technic and proper timing.

F. Drug Effects: The surgical patient who is being evaluated and prepared for a major operation is about to face a formidable series of stresses in the course of which he will probably receive a variety of potent medications. Drug allergies, sensitivities, and incompatibilities and adverse drug effects which may be precipitated by surgery must be foreseen and, if possible, prevented. A history of skin or other untoward reaction or sickness after injection, oral administration, or other use of any of the following substances should be noted so that they may be avoided.

> Penicillin or other antibiotic
> Morphine, codeine, meperidine, or other narcotic
> Procaine or other anesthetic
> Aspirin or other analgesic
> Barbiturates
> Sulfonamides
> Tetanus antitoxin or other serums
> Iodine, thimerosal (Merthiolate), or other germicide
> Any other medication
> Any foods such as eggs, milk, or chocolate
> Adhesive tape

A personal or strong familial history of asthma, hay fever, or other allergic disorder should alert the surgeon to possible hypersensitivity to drugs.

Drugs currently or recently taken by the patient may require continuation, dosage adjustment, or discontinuance. Medications such as digitalis, insulin, and corticosteroids must usually be maintained and their dosage carefully regulated during the operative and postoperative periods. Prolonged use of corticosteroids such as cortisone (even though discontinued 1 month or more preoperatively) may be associated with hypofunction of the adrenal cortex, which impairs the physiologic responses to the stress of anesthesia and surgery. Such a patient should receive a corticosteroid immediately before, during, and after surgery. Anticoagulant drugs are an example of a medication to be strictly monitored or eliminated preoperatively.

The anesthesiologist is concerned with the long-term preoperative use of CNS depressants (eg, barbiturates, opiates, and alcohol), which may be associated with increased tolerance for anesthetic drugs; tranquilizers (eg, phenothiazine derivatives such as chlorpromazine); and antihypertensive agents (eg, rauwolfia derivatives such as reserpine), which may be associated with hypotension in response to anesthesia.

Consultations

The opinion of a qualified consultant should be obtained when it may be of benefit to the patient, when requested by the patient or his family, or when it may be of medicolegal importance. The physician should take the initiative in arranging consultation when the treatment proposed is controversial or exceptionally risky, when dangerous complications occur, or when he senses that the patient or his family is unduly apprehensive regarding the plan of management or the course of events. Consultation with cardiac or other medical or surgical specialists preoperatively is important if the patient has abnormal findings in their fields of competence. It is also beneficial for the specialist consultant to become acquainted with the patient and his condition preoperatively when the possibility exists that the consultant will be called upon for advice later in connection with a postoperative complication or development.

Anesthesia consultation is always requested prior to major surgery if an anesthesiologist is available. In poor-risk patients, this consultation should be requested several days in advance of operation if possible. The patient's prospects for a smooth and uncomplicated anesthesia are greatly improved by the anesthesiologist's preoperative evaluation and advice. Respiratory, cardiovascular, and other complications related to anesthesia are forestalled or minimized when the anesthesiologist has an opportunity to adapt the anesthesia to the patient's special circumstances. When an anesthesiologist is available for preoperative consultation, he will usually write the orders for premedication, for the withholding of oral intake, and for other measures which relate directly to the anesthesia. When an anesthesiologist is not available, preanesthetic orders are written by the surgeon in accordance with the principles discussed in Chapter 14.

Preoperative Note

When the diagnostic work-up and preoperative evaluation have been completed, all details should be reviewed and a "preoperative note" written in the chart. This is usually done on the day before the operation. The note summarizes the pertinent findings and decisions, gives the indications for the operation proposed, and attests that a discussion of these complications and the risks of operation has occurred between surgeon and patient (ie, informed consent). This constitutes a final check on the adequacy of the analysis of the patient's problem, his need for treatment, and his understanding of these facts.

PREOPERATIVE PREPARATION

Major operations create surgical wounds and cause severe stress, subjecting the patient to the hazard of infection and metabolic and other derangements. Appropriate preoperative preparation facilitates wound healing and systemic recovery by making certain that the patient's condition at operation is optimal. Surgery also results in psychic trauma to the patient and his family and has significant medicolegal implications, all of which deserve special consideration preoperatively to avoid postoperative repercussions. In emergency conditions, time for preparation is limited but is usually sufficient to permit the principles of good surgical preparation to be followed. In elective surgery, meticulous preoperative preparation is both possible and mandatory and includes the following steps.

Informing the Patient

Surgery is a frightening prospect for the patient and his family. Their psychologic preparation and reassurance should begin at the initial contact with the surgeon. Appropriate explanation of the nature and purpose of preoperative studies and treatments establishes confidence. When all pertinent information has been gathered, it is the surgeon's responsibility to describe the planned surgical procedure and its risks and possible consequences in understandable terms to the patient and usually also to his next of kin. Similarly, prompt postoperative interpretation of pertinent findings and prospects to the patient and his family contributes to rapport and to intelligent cooperation during the recovery period.

Operative Permit

The patient or his legal guardian must sign (in advance) a permit authorizing a major or minor operation or a procedure such as thoracentesis, lumbar puncture, or sigmoidoscopy. The nature, risk, and probable result of the operation or procedure must be made clear to the patient or a legally responsible relative or guardian so that the signed permit will constitute "informed consent." A signed consent is not ordinarily valid except for the specific operation or procedure for which it was obtained.

Therapeutic abortions and operations which adversely affect the sexual or childbearing functions should usually be undertaken only with the concurrence in writing of the marital partner. It may not be required in a particular state or jurisdiction that the husband give his consent, but it is generally desirable that he be informed of the procedure and its effects.

Emergency, lifesaving operations or procedures may have to be done without a permit. In such cases, every effort should be made to obtain adequate consultation, and the director of the hospital should be informed in advance if possible.

Legal and institutional requirements regarding permits vary. It is essential that the physician know and follow local specifications.

Preoperative Orders

On the day before surgery, orders are written which assure completion before operation of the final steps in the preparation of the patient. These orders will usually include the following:

A. Skin Preparation: See p 12.

B. Diet: Omit solid foods for 12 hours and fluids

for 8 hours preoperatively. Special orders are written for diabetics and for infants and children.

C. Enema: Enemas need not be given routinely. Patients with well-regulated bowel habits do not require a preoperative enema except in the case of operations on the colon, rectum, and anal regions or operations (chiefly abdominal) likely to be followed by paralytic ileus and delayed bowel function.

Constipated patients and those scheduled for the above types of operations should be given a flushing enema 8–12 hours preoperatively with 500–1500 ml of warm tap water or, preferably, physiologic saline, or with 120–150 ml of hypertonic sodium phosphate solution conveniently available in a commercial kit (Travad Enema, Fleet Enema). Tap water enemas are contraindicated in congenital megacolon because of the danger of excessive water absorption. When thorough cleansing of the bowel is not essential, satisfactory evacuation on the evening before operation can usually be accomplished by use of a 10 mg bisacodyl (Dulcolax) rectal suppository. A hypertonic sodium phosphate enema or bisacodyl rectal suppository is also effective in the rapid preparation of the colon and rectum for sigmoidoscopy.

D. Bedtime and Preanesthetic Medication: If the anesthesia is to be given by a physician anesthesiologist, he will usually examine the patient and write the premedication order. If not, follow the guidelines laid down in Chapter 14.

E. Special Orders: In addition to the above more or less routine preoperative orders required for most major operative procedures, additional special orders related to the type and severity of the operation should be written. Antibiotic prophylaxis is discussed in Chapter 11. Other examples are given below.

1. Blood transfusion—If blood transfusions may be needed during or after operation, have the patient typed and arrange for a sufficient number of units to be cross-matched and available prior to operation.

2. Nasogastric tube—A nasogastric tube on suction is usually advisable after operations on the gastrointestinal tract to prevent distention due to paralytic ileus. If the patient has gastrointestinal obstruction with possible gastric residual, a nasogastric tube is passed preoperatively and the stomach aspirated or placed on continuous suction to reduce the possibility of regurgitation and aspiration during induction of anesthesia. If an emergency operation is to be undertaken on a patient who has eaten within the past 8–12 hours, lavage of the stomach with a large-bore Ewald tube followed by insertion of a nasogastric tube should be considered. When there is no indication for nasogastric intubation prior to surgery and the patient is to be under general anesthesia, the anesthesiologist can pass the tube into the stomach after the patient is unconscious.

3. Bladder catheter—If urinary retention or a need for hourly monitoring of urinary output postoperatively is anticipated, a Foley catheter is inserted for constant bladder drainage. If bladder distention will interfere with exposure in the pelvis (eg, during abdominoperineal resection), a catheter should be placed preoperatively. Catheterization can be done on the nursing unit just before the patient leaves for the operating room or after he has been anesthetized.

4. Venous or arterial catheter—Operations associated with marked blood loss call for preoperative placement of one or two 14 or 16 gauge intravenous plastic catheters for rapid administration of blood, fluids, or medication. Percutaneous insertion is usually possible; if not, a cutdown should be done to expose a vein, usually the antecubital. Central venous pressure monitoring may be required for assessment of the circulation during certain procedures such as complicated cardiovascular and pulmonary operations. For central venous pressure determination, a catheter should be passed into the superior vena cava via the subclavian or internal jugular vein (see Chapter 51). Arterial catheterization or cannulation, usually of the radial or brachial artery, is done primarily for monitoring blood pressure and obtaining blood gas measurements during and after operation in selected patients in whom repeated, accurate measurement of these parameters is essential. Central venous and arterial catheterization can usually be deferred until the patient is anesthetized.

5. Continuing medications—Certain patients will be receiving continuing medications whose dosage or route of administration must be altered as the result of operation. Insulin and corticosteroids are examples of hormone preparations requiring special preoperative orders. Digitalis, other cardiac drugs, antibiotics, etc may require shift to parenteral route of administration and altered dosage in the immediate preoperative period and during operation. Foresight in the adjustment of medication orders will minimize the possibility of under- or overdosage of potent and essential drugs.

6. Prophylactic antibiotics—See Chapter 11.

Asepsis & Antisepsis in the Prevention of Wound Infection

The protection of the surgical patient from infection is a primary consideration throughout the preoperative, operative, and postoperative phases of care. The factor of host resistance that influences the individual patient's susceptibility to infection has been discussed above. The incidence and severity of infection, particularly wound sepsis, are related also to the bacteriologic status of the hospital environment and to the care with which basic principles of asepsis, antisepsis, and surgical technic are implemented. The entire hospital environment must be protected from undue bacterial contamination in order to avoid colonization and cross-infection of surgical patients with virulent strains of bacteria which will invade surgical wounds in the operating room in spite of aseptic precautions taken during surgery. Prevention of wound infection therefore involves both application of general concepts and technics of antisepsis and asepsis in the hospital at large, and the use of specific procedures in preparation for operation.

A. Sterilization: The only completely reliable methods of sterilization in wide current use for surgical instruments and supplies are steam under pressure (autoclaving), dry heat, and ethylene oxide gas.

1. Autoclaving—Saturated steam at a pressure of 750 mm Hg (14.5 lb/sq inch above atmospheric pressure) at a temperature of 120 C (248 F) destroys all vegetative bacteria and most resistant dry spores in 13 minutes. Additional time (usually a total of 30 minutes) must be allowed for the penetration of heat and moisture into the centers of packages. Sterilization time is markedly shortened by the high-vacuum or high-pressure autoclaves now widely used.

2. Dry heat—Exposure to continuous dry heat at 170 C (338 F) for 1 hour will sterilize articles which would be spoiled by moist heat or which are more conveniently kept dry. If grease or oil is present on instruments, safe sterilization calls for 4 hours' exposure at 160 C (320 F).

3. Gas sterilization—Liquid and gaseous ethylene oxide as a sterilizing agent will destroy bacteria, viruses, molds, pathogenic fungi, and spores. It is also flammable and toxic, and will cause severe burns if it comes in contact with the skin. Gas sterilization with ethylene oxide is an excellent method for sterilization of most heat-sensitive materials, including telescopic instruments, plastic and rubber goods, sharp and delicate instruments, and miscellaneous items such as electric cords and sealed ampules. It has largely replaced soaking in antiseptics as a means of sterilizing materials that cannot withstand autoclaving. Care must be exercised in selecting items for gas sterilization because chemical interaction may occur with ethylene oxide or the agent with which it is mixed. For example, some acrylic plastic materials, polystyrene, certain lensed instruments, and pharmaceuticals may be damaged by ethylene oxide. Gas sterilization is normally carried out in a pressure vessel (gas autoclave) at slightly elevated pressure and temperature. It requires 1¾ hours for sterilization in a gas autoclave utilizing a mixture of 12% ethylene oxide and 88% dichlorodifluoromethane (Freon 12) at a temperature of 55 C (131 F) and a pressure of 410 mm Hg (8 lb/sq inch above atmospheric pressure). Following sterilization, a variable period of time is required for dissipation of the gas from the materials sterilized. Solid metal or glass items such as knives, drills, and thermometers may be used immediately following sterilization. Lensed instruments and packs including cloth, paper, rubber, and other porous items must usually be kept on the shelf exposed to air for 24–48 hours before use. Certain types of materials or complex instruments, such as a cardiac pacemaker, may require 7 days of exposure to air before use.

4. Boiling—Instruments should be boiled only if autoclaving, dry heat, or gas sterilization is not available. The minimum period for sterilization in boiling water is 30 minutes at altitudes less than 300 meters. At higher altitudes, the period of sterilization must be increased. The addition of alkali to the sterilizer increases bactericidal efficiency by raising pH so that sterilization time can safely be decreased to 15 minutes.

5. Soaking in antiseptics—Sterilization by soaking is rarely indicated and should never be relied upon if steam autoclaving, dry heat, or gas sterilization is suitable and available. Under some circumstances, it may be necessary or more convenient to sterilize lensed or delicate cutting instruments by soaking in a liquid germicide. A wide variety of such germicides are available. The liquid disinfectant of current choice for lensed instruments and certain other critical items which should be sterile when used is glutaraldehyde in 2% aqueous alkaline concentration (Cidex). This solution is bactericidal and virucidal in 10 minutes and sporicidal within 3 hours.

B. Antiseptics: Antiseptics are chemical agents which kill bacteria or arrest their growth; they may or may not be sporicidal. Antiseptics should not be used in wounds since their toxicity to host cells far outweighs the possible advantages of their antibacterial effect. Many new and more versatile antiseptics have been developed in recent years. The most promising of these are discussed below.

1. Antiseptics for general utility purposes—Soap solution is one of the best all-purpose cleansing agents, but it is a weak antiseptic. A number of basic chemicals, more bactericidal than soap, are now in general use in hospitals and offices for cleaning floors, furniture, and operating room equipment and for soaking contaminated utensils and materials. The most valuable of these germicidal chemicals are (1) synthetic phenolics, (2) polybrominated salicylanilides, (3) iodophors, (4) alcohols, (5) quaternary ammonium compounds, (6) glutaraldehyde preparations, and (7) chlorhexidine gluconate. An increasing number of institutions are using the synthetic phenolics and polybrominated salicylanilides (**PBS**) as general purpose disinfectants because of their effectiveness under actual working conditions. These agents retain high potency in the presence of organic matter and are notable for their excellent residual activities on surfaces. This is probably a reflection of their stability, compatibility with ionic and alkaline agents, and marked resistance to deactivation by organic matter. Synthetic phenolics and PBS compounds are compatible with soaps, detergents, and numerous other anionic and alkaline agents broadly used in hospitals. Iodophors and quaternary ammonium compounds tend to be rapidly diminished in activity by anionic or alkaline materials and are subject to a degree of volatilization.

a. Phenol compounds—Phenol (carbolic acid) is one of the most potent bactericidal chemicals available, but it is too caustic for safe use. The same is true to a lesser degree of cresol (Lysol). These have been superseded by synthetic phenolic germicides such as Lamar SP-63, Vestal Vasphene, and Western Polyphene. They kill gram-positive and gram-negative bacteria (including tubercle bacilli) and fungi. Surfaces properly treated with these compounds have demonstrated antibacterial properties for periods of 10–14 days. However, residual antibacterial activity should not be relied upon as a substitute for adequate routine cleaning and disinfection.

b. Polybrominated salicylanilide (PBS)—This is the newest class of antibacterial chemical. The antimicrobial spectrum and residual surface action are similar to those of the phenolics. When PBS preparations are used in laundries, textiles take on a self-sanitizing antibacterial finish. A disadvantage of PBS preparations is the white powdery film which remains on metal and other surfaces when the cleaning solution dries. PBS is the essential ingredient in Lamar L-300.

c. Iodophors—These are chemicals in which iodine is combined with a detergent (Wescodyne, Surgidine) or with polyvinylpyrrolidone (Betadine, Isodine). The toxicity of the iodine is practically eliminated, but surface and skin disinfection is efficient.

d. Alcohols—Seventy percent ethyl alcohol is a powerful germicide. Isopropyl alcohol should be used as 70–90%. Neither of these alcohols is effective against spores.

e. Quaternary ammonium compounds—These are less effective than phenol, iodine, and alcohol and are inactivated by soap and adsorbed by fibers. Benzalkonium chloride is the prototype.

f. Formaldehyde and glutaraldehyde—Aqueous solutions of formaldehyde are known as formalin, which, when purchased commercially, is approximately 40% formaldehyde in water. The high-level germicidal activity of formaldehyde is increased by adding alcohol; a combination of 8% formaldehyde (20% formalin) in 70% alcohol is rapidly bactericidal and is sporicidal within 3 hours. Irritating fumes and tissue toxicity limit the usefulness of formaldehyde preparations. Glutaraldehyde is chemically related to formaldehyde, but it has a low tissue toxicity and does not have an irritating odor. Glutaraldehyde in 2% aqueous alkaline concentration (Cidex) is approximately equivalent to 8% formaldehyde in alcohol. Glutaraldehyde is a good chemical sterilizing agent for soaking of instruments, cleaning of anesthesia equipment, and decontamination of operating room items such as basins, bottles, tubing, rubber goods, etc after exposure to septic fields.

g. Chlorhexidine gluconate—This agent is a hexamethylene bis (biguanidine), distinctly different chemically from hexachlorophene and other commonly used antimicrobials. It is marketed as Hibiclens, a sudsing skin cleanser containing 4% weight per volume of chlorhexidine gluconate; and as Hibitane tinted tincture, a 0.5% solution of chlorhexidine gluconate in 70% isopropanol. These preparations have rapid, potent, and persistent antimicrobial activity against both gram-positive and gram-negative organisms, with only a negligible tendency to cause skin reactions. As a result of these properties, Hibiclens is highly effective as a general skin cleanser and for the hand scrub of the surgical team; Hibitane is equivalent to an iodophor in preparation of the operative field.

h. Other chemicals—Hypochlorites, chloramine, mercury salts, and solutions of azo dyes have been largely replaced by more reliable compounds.

2. Skin antiseptics—The most important applications of skin antisepsis are the hand scrub of the operating team and the preparation of the operative field. Hexachlorophene is widely used in skin disinfection, usually in combination with a detergent (eg, pHisoHex) or with liquid or bar soap (eg, Septisol, Gamophen, Dial). Daily use of hexachlorophene in surgical scrubs produces a sustained lowering of the bacterial count on the skin, and absorption through the skin is insufficient to cause toxicity. Sporadic or one-time use of hexachlorophene in soap or other preparation has no special value. Alcohol dissolves hexachlorophene and should not be applied if a prolonged surface effect is desired.

a. Hand scrub routine—Always scrub for 10 minutes except when changing gloves and gown aseptically between clean cases; in these circumstances, scrub for 5 minutes.

(1) Wash hands and forearms thoroughly with soap or a hexachlorophene or other preparation.

(2) Clean fingernails.

(3) Scrub for 5 minutes with a sterile brush or sponge, covering the entire surface of the hands and forearms repeatedly with soap, a hexachlorophene or chlorhexidine preparation, or an iodophor.

(4) Scrub for another 5 minutes with a second sterile brush or sponge (a total of 10 minutes by the clock) unless operating daily.

(5) Wash with 70% ethyl alcohol for 1 minute while rubbing the skin surface with a gauze sponge and allow to dry. This optional step in the scrub routine will improve its effectiveness. Omit alcohol rinse if hexachlorophene preparation is used regularly for prolonged effect.

b. Preparation of the operative field—

(1) On the day before operation—Initial preparation of the skin is usually done the afternoon or evening before operation. Designate the specific area to be prepared in the preoperative orders. The area should be washed with soap and water, making sure that it is grossly quite clean. A shower or tub bath is satisfactory. The type of soap used makes little difference. Soap is a weak antiseptic and it is useful because of its nonirritating detergent action, especially when washing is combined with mechanical friction.

Shaving is usually but not always required as part of the ward preparation. Shaving may be omitted where no hairs are present, as on the abdomen of a child. Where coarse hairs are present, shaving is necessary. Shaving must be skillfully done with a new blade and adequate soap lather. Slight nicks and scratches of the skin may be followed in a few hours by an abnormal increase in bacterial flora of the skin. For this reason, it is sometimes preferred—eg, in preparation for a craniotomy—to have the patient shaved just prior to surgery. It is not necessary to apply antiseptics such as alcohol or other germicides to the skin or to cover the prepared area with a sterile dressing.

For elective operations involving areas with high levels of resident bacteria (eg, hands, feet) or likely to be irritated by strong antiseptics (eg, face, genitalia), preoperative degerming of the skin can be improved by repeated use of chlorhexidine gluconate (Hibiclens) or hexachlorophene soap or solution. Instruct the patient to wash the area several times daily for 3—5 days before operation exclusively with one of these preparations.

(2) In the operating room—Use aseptic technic and prepare the operative field as follows:

(a) Wash for 5—10 minutes with gauze and soap solution, or, preferably, a detergent preparation containing iodophor, chlorhexidine gluconate, or hexachlorophene. Blot the field dry by applying a sterile towel to the surface.

(b) Apply one of the following antiseptics to the operative field:

(i) Iodophor solution (Betadine, SeptoDyne).

(ii) Chlorhexidine gluconate tincture (Hibitane).

(iii) 1% iodine in 70% (by weight) ethyl alcohol. Iodine is one of the most efficient skin antiseptics available. It rarely causes skin reactions in this concentration. Avoid streaming of iodine outside of operative field. Do not use iodine on the perineum, genitalia, or face; on irritated or delicate skin (eg, small children); or when the patient gives a history of iodine sensitivity.

(iv) 80% isopropyl or 70% ethyl alcohol. Apply to the skin with a gauze swab for 3 minutes and allow to dry before draping. Alternatively, tinted tincture of benzalkonium (1:750) may be used.

(v) For sensitive areas (perineum, around the eyes, etc), apply iodophor, chlorhexidine, or 1:1000 aqueous benzalkonium solution.

C. Control of Hospital Environment: Hospital cross-infection with hemolytic, coagulase-positive *Staphylococcus aureus* and other organisms is always a potential problem. Strains endemic in hospitals are often resistant to many antimicrobial drugs as a consequence of the widespread use of these agents. Relaxation of aseptic precautions in the operating theater and wards and an unwarranted reliance on "prophylactic" antibiotics contribute to the development of resistant strains. The result may be a significant increase in the incidence of hospital-acquired wound infection, pneumonitis, and septicemia, the latter 2 complications especially affecting infants, the aged, and the debilitated.

Although the pyogenic cocci are the major offenders, the enteric gram-negative bacteria (particularly the coliform and proteus groups and *Pseudomonas aeruginosa*) are increasingly prominent in hospital-acquired infections.

1. Hospital administration—

a. The surgical infection control program should be coordinated closely with that of other services through a Hospital Infection Committee set up to promulgate and enforce regulations.

b. All significant infections should be reported immediately. A clean wound infection rate of more than 1—2% indicates a need for more effective control measures. The wound infection rate should be continuously monitored on the surgical services.

2. Cultures—

a. Obtain culture and antibiotic sensitivity studies on all wounds, ulcerations, and significant infections.

b. Phage typing of staphylococci and detailed identification of other organisms may be useful.

3. Isolation—Isolate every patient with a significant source of communicable bacteria; every case of suspected communicable infection until the diagnosis has been ruled out; and every patient in whom cross-infection will be serious.

4. Aseptic technic—

a. **Operating room**—The operating room should be considered an isolation zone which may be entered only by persons wearing clean operating attire (which may not be worn elsewhere).

b. **Ward procedures**—All open wounds should be aseptically dressed to protect them from cross-infection and to prevent heavy contamination of the environment. Eliminate dressing carts containing supplies and equipment for multiple bedside dressings.

c. **Hand washing**, preferably with hexachlorophene soap, before and after each contact with a patient is a simple but important routine measure in control of infection.

5. Housekeeping—

a. Bedding must be laundered, and mattresses, furniture, and cubicles cleaned with a general utility antiseptic after a patient is discharged.

b. Housekeeping procedures throughout the hospital must be thorough. Wet mopping and cleaning are required in order to prevent accumulation or raising of dust.

6. Antibiotics—Prophylactic use of antibiotics should be minimized. When possible, antibiotic therapy should be based on sensitivity studies. Antibiotics should be given in adequate doses and discontinued as soon as possible.

7. Epidemiology—

a. Personnel with active staphylococcal infections should be excluded from patient contact until they have recovered. Personnel carrying staphylococci in their nasal passages or gastrointestinal tracts must observe personal hygiene, but need not be removed from duty unless they prove to be a focus of infection. The advisability of treatment of the carrier is uncertain since the carrier state is frequently transient or recurrent in spite of treatment.

b. Every significant infection acquired in the hospital should be investigated to determine its origin and spread, possible contacts and carriers, and whether improper technics may have been responsible.

• • •

3...
Postoperative Care

John L. Wilson, MD

General Considerations

The postoperative care of patients who are seriously ill after a major surgical procedure usually progresses through several fairly well defined phases. The management of such patients is improved when appropriate facilities are available. The phases of progressive care and the optimum facilities are as follows:

Phases	Facilities
Postanesthetic observation	Recovery Room
Intensive care	Intensive Care Unit
Intermediate care	General Nursing Unit
Convalescent care	Home or Extended Care Unit

Postanesthetic observation and intensive care are discussed in some detail in this chapter because of their special features and because of their importance to the end results of major surgery. During these phases of postoperative care, attention is directed specifically to the prevention, early detection, and prompt treatment of the severe, life-threatening complications that are liable to occur in the hours and days immediately following operation. Such complications are chiefly responsible for prolonged morbidity and mortality in the postoperative period.

Patients who have received general anesthesia should be observed in the Recovery Room until they are conscious and vital signs are stable. Upon recovery from anesthesia, patients without complications who are relatively self-sufficient can be well managed in the General Nursing Unit of a general hospital. Patients who are poor risks or who have been severely stressed by extensive surgery require close observation and meticulous management postoperatively. It is possible to achieve this level of care in the General Nursing Unit by arranging for special nursing and other supportive services. Experience has shown, however, that intensive care is most effectively provided in an Intensive Care Unit which is designed and staffed for the specific purpose of managing critically ill patients. The Recovery Room and the Intensive Care Unit are such important adjuncts to postoperative care that their functions will be reviewed.

Specialized Facilities for Postoperative Care; the Recovery Room & Intensive Care Unit

Intensive care concepts have gained increasingly wide acceptance since World War II. This trend has been encouraged by favorable experience in postanesthesia recovery rooms, in centralized respiratory care of bulbar poliomyelitis during the 1950 epidemic, and, more recently, in coronary care units. Hospitals are rarely designed today without provision for special units in which seriously ill patients can receive close observation, intensive 24-hour nursing care, and emergency resuscitation and other complex treatment. In small hospitals, a single unit may serve for all types of intensive care. Large medical centers commonly have a variety of units such as Recovery Room, Intensive Care Unit, Coronary Care Unit, Respiratory Care Unit, Renal Dialysis Unit, Burn Unit, Pediatric Intensive Care Unit, Premature Nursery, etc.

The Recovery Room and surgical Intensive Care Unit provide environments in which qualified personnel and special equipment can be concentrated for the most effective surveillance and treatment of postoperative patients. The ready availability and frequent attendance of the anesthesiologist and surgeon are essential to the proper function of these units, which are more efficient when adjacent to each other. Also indispensable is the continuous presence of nurses experienced in identifying and interpreting the symptoms and signs of postoperative complications and in taking the necessary emergency action independently.

A. Recovery Room: The Recovery Room should be connected directly to the operating suite. Its dimensions are determined by the fact that one or 2 beds are generally required for each operating room. Most recovery rooms are open-style, with beds located so that all patients can be seen by the nurse. Following regional or local anesthesia, the patient is kept in the Recovery Room until the danger of adverse circulatory, respiratory, or other immediate postoperative complication has passed. Patients who have had general anesthesia are kept in the Recovery Room until there is no longer a possibility of asphyxia, shock, or other complications requiring respiratory or circulatory resuscitation. The stay in the Recovery Room is usually a few hours at most; the patient is then transferred to either a general nursing unit of the hospital or, if continued close observation is needed, to an Intensive Care Unit.

B. Intensive Care Unit: The design and organization of an Intensive Care Unit (ICU) serving postoperative patients in a specific hospital will depend upon such factors as the number of acute medical and surgical beds and the characteristics of the patients being treated. As a general rule, a hospital with 300–500 acute beds will need an ICU of 10–15 beds, but requirements are quite variable. Ample space around each ICU bed is essential for treatment procedures and equipment. Ideally, each bed should be in a separate cubicle with a glass wall to assure quiet, isolation when necessary, and privacy while allowing continuous observation. Many ICUs have been created by remodeling existing space and present a distinct compromise in terms of location and layout. As new hospitals are built, joint planning by architects, physicians, nurses, and biomedical engineers is creating a new generation of facilities based on progressive care principles which emphasize the relationship of structure to function. Serious acute surgical and medical illnesses and severe trauma make up an increasing proportion of patients in general hospitals—hence the growing importance of intensive care services.

The staffing and equipment requirements of an ICU are dictated by the conditions and complications that must be treated. Almost all critically ill patients have severe involvement of one or more of the following systems: respiratory, cardiovascular, or renal. The major postoperative complications seen in an ICU are cardiac arrhythmias and failure, respiratory failure, shock; fluid, electrolyte, and acid-base imbalance; renal failure, invasive sepsis, and coagulation problems. The chief causes of death in postoperative patients in the ICU are cardiac, respiratory, septic, and hemorrhagic complications. Critically ill patients tend to deteriorate rapidly and may be impossible to evaluate without frequent or even continuous determination of physiologic variables not ordinarily crucial during the postoperative period. As a result, extensive effort is being made to develop monitoring technics that are sufficiently reliable and practicable for general use in the intensive care setting.

The purpose of the ICU is to care for patients who require the following types of life support services.

1. Continuous attendance by a registered nurse.
2. Continuous monitoring of vital signs, ECG, and fluid balance.
3. Continuous ventilatory support with maintenance and protection of the airway.
4. Management of shock, cardiovascular instability, and acute respiratory or renal failure.
5. Management of overwhelming infection or toxemia.
6. Management of severe metabolic, thermal, and other life-threatening disorders.

Monitoring

Continuous observation of the patient by an alert and competent team of nurses and physicians is the cornerstone of high-quality intensive care. However, future improvement in this care will be influenced significantly by technologic progress in monitoring. The term monitoring is used here in its broadest sense to mean close surveillance of the patient, using all available methods to obtain necessary data, either continuously or intermittently, regarding his changing condition. Monitoring of the critically ill patient is facilitated by a number of electronic devices now in general or experimental use and by repeated laboratory tests and bedside measurements. Assessment of data obtained in this manner informs the intensive care team of developments and trends that cannot be followed by the usual methods of examination. For example, continuous monitoring of the ECG can warn of dangerous arrhythmia or change in pulse rate which, if undetected, might lead to cardiac failure or arrest. Intermittent monitoring of the arterial pH, P_{O_2}, and P_{CO_2} provides invaluable and frequently unexpected evidence of respiratory insufficiency, permitting corrective measures before serious deterioration occurs.

A. Parameters Monitored: The following is a partial list of the observations and examinations which may be needed in the monitoring of difficult postoperative problems in the Recovery Room and ICU:

1. **Cardiovascular system—**
   Pulse rate
   Electrocardiogram
   Arterial blood pressure
   Central venous pressure
   Pulmonary arterial pressure
   Cardiac output (or index)
   Total peripheral resistance
2. **Respiratory system—**
   Respiratory rate
   Respiratory volume
   Respiratory flow rate
   Respiratory pressure
   Respiratory compliance
   Respiratory gases (P_{O_2}, P_{CO_2})
   Blood gases (pH, P_{aO_2}, P_{aCO_2})
   Chest tube drainage
   Chest roentgenography
3. **Central nervous system—**
   Electroencephalogram
   Ventricular pressure
4. **Gastrointestinal system—**
   Fluid intake by mouth
   Nasogastric or intestinal tube drainage and electrolyte analysis of recovered fluid
   Fistula drainage and electrolyte analysis of fluid
   Abdominal roentgenography
5. **Hematopoietic system—**
   Complete blood count
   Hematocrit
   Coagulation studies
   Platelet count
   Blood volume (red cell, plasma, total)
6. **Urinary system—**
   Urine output, hourly
   Urinalysis (routine and microscopic)
   Blood urea nitrogen (BUN)
   Serum creatinine
   Creatinine clearance
   Urine/plasma osmolality ratio

Urine electrolytes (Na⁺/K⁺ ratio)

7. **Metabolism—**
   Temperature
   Body weight
   Intravenous fluid volume (electrolyte,
     colloid, blood)

B. Electronic Aids to Monitoring: Electronic instruments make possible the continuous visual display—and permanent recording when required—of physiologic variables such as pulse rate, ECG, and blood pressure. An automatic feature can be incorporated so that variation in pulse rate or electrocardiographic complex beyond a predetermined range will activate an alarm and start a permanent recording. The commonest type of electronic monitoring equipment now in use is the electrocardiographic monitor, which is standard in operating theaters, recovery rooms, and intensive care units.

Electronic devices are no substitute for direct observation by trained personnel but do provide a convenient and accurate means of obtaining certain information. Biomedical engineering research will undoubtedly provide many new and improved electronic instruments and systems for the continuous monitoring of patients and for the rapid performance of tests and calculations that are too time-consuming and costly by current methods. In view of the present frequent use of electronic instrumentation in postoperative care and the certainty that this will increase, some of the principles involved will be discussed.

A basic electronic monitoring system has 3 parts: transducer, signal conditioner, and readout device.

1. Transducer—The function of the transducer is to interface with the patient, pick up the energy to be measured, and transmit it as an electrical signal. A few of the commoner types of transducers will be briefly described:

If the energy is electrical, as in the case of the ECG and EEG, the **bioelectric electrodes** applied to the skin or elsewhere serve as transducers. **Pressure transducers** convert pressure change into electrical energy. They are widely employed to measure blood pressure via an indwelling needle or catheter. The device consists of a rigid chamber fitted at one end with a flexible diaphragm. The chamber is filled with liquid or gas and connected by tubing to the pressure source. Small motions of the diaphragm due to pressure changes are transmitted mechanically to electrical elements attached to the diaphragm. Resistance in these elements is altered when they are deformed, with the result that the output voltage of the transducer varies proportionately to the pressure change. This produces an electrical signal analogous to pressure. Since the electrical signal is proportionate or analogous to the mechanical variable, it is termed an analog signal. The transducer does not measure absolute pressure and therefore requires calibration. **Temperature transducers** or thermistors are simple, reliable, and very satisfactory for monitoring body temperature. They operate on the principle that the electrical resistance of certain materials varies widely with temperature change. Special probes are available for easy insertion into the rectum or esophagus or for application to the skin. **Electrochemical transducers** are available to measure pH, P_{O_2}, P_{CO_2}, Na⁺, Cl⁻, K⁺, and certain other ions and compounds. **Electromagnetic transducers** and **ultrasonic transducers** can measure blood flow. **Photosensitive transducers** react to changes in dilution of exogenous dyes injected intravascularly in the determination of cardiac output.

The design of improved transducers for sensing biologic signals is a promising field of research.

2. Signal conditioning—The signal-conditioning section of the monitoring system receives the electrical signal generated or transmitted by the transducer. It is the function of this section to amplify, integrate, and otherwise modify the signal so that it is of appropriate energy level and quality for activation of the readout device on which the signal will be displayed or recorded. Intensive care personnel are often called upon to manipulate the controls of the signal-conditioning equipment in order to calibrate the instrument or to adjust the amplitude or other characteristics of the displayed tracing.

3. Readout device—The standard readout instrument in operating theaters and intensive care areas is the cathode ray oscilloscope. The commonest display is the continuous electrocardiographic tracing. Pressure pulse wave, arterial and venous blood pressure, EEG, and other dynamic variables may be displayed when required. Permanent records can be obtained by direct writing methods employing hot styluses, ink pens, or light beams. Information may also be stored on tapes or disks for later replay. The analog signal or tracing of biologic variables can be converted to digital form by a digital computer with the result that numerical values for pulse rate, blood pressure, etc can be presented on a television screen. Because analog to digital conversion is a continuous process and takes place in a fraction of a second, the numerical values are precise and current.

C. Practical Application of Continuous Electronic Monitoring: Electronic monitoring systems which record and analyze multiple physiologic variables are in experimental use in many medical centers (Lewis FJ & others: Surg Gynecol Obstet 130:333, 1970). Clinical application of the full range of currently available monitoring technics is limited by a number of factors, including cumbersome and invasive methods of interfacing with the patient and complexity and cost of equipment. In an individual patient, it is important to decide whether there is need to obtain a continuous record of vital signs and other variables or whether intermittent observations and tests will serve equally well. In most patients, the latter will be the case. Experience has shown that, except in the research setting, it is feasible and useful to monitor only a few parameters on a continuous basis and that this is required in only a selected group of critically ill patients. In the majority of postoperative patients, necessary information can be satisfactorily obtained by clinical observation supplemented by repeated laboratory tests. The following are the physiologic variables that can be monitored continuously in the usual well-staffed and well-equipped ICU:

Physiologic Variable	Transduction
ECG and pulse rate	Chest wall electrodes.
Respiratory rate	Transthoracic electrical impedence from electrocardiographic electrodes.
Body temperature	Thermistor in the rectum, esophagus, or ear or on the skin.
Blood pressure	Pressure transducer connected to arterial catheter (an automatic blood pressure cuff device will provide intermittent blood pressure readings but is inaccurate when blood pressure drops significantly).

For practical purposes, the above is the scope of continuous monitoring available for routine clinical application in most hospitals. Monitoring of the other parameters listed on p 15 is on an intermittent basis.

Postoperative Orders

Postsurgical patients should be accompanied by a physician or other qualified attendant while en route to the Recovery Room, ICU, or General Nursing Unit. Detailed written orders should be sent with each postoperative patient, and the nurse receiving him should be given a verbal report of his condition. The postoperative orders should provide for appropriate observations and treatments which, in the case of the patient requiring intensive care, may include many of the procedures listed above under the parameters to be monitored. As a guide to the preparation of an inclusive set of postoperative orders, each of the following categories should be considered:

A. Special Observations:

1. Vital signs—Blood pressure, pulse, and respiration should be recorded at regular intervals after all major operations (eg, every 15–30 minutes until stable, and then hourly). A significant drop in blood pressure should be reported to the surgeon immediately. (Specify the level to be reported.)

2. Continuous monitoring of ECG—This is indicated in many critically ill patients. Other parameters to be monitored continuously will depend upon the patient's needs and the equipment available.

3. Central venous pressure—This requires percutaneous placement of an inlying catheter in the superior vena cava or right atrium via the internal jugular or subclavian vein or an antecubital vein (see Chapter 51). Record central venous pressure at stated intervals in patients in shock, those with a borderline cardiac or respiratory status, those who require large fluid volume replacement, or those with oliguria.

4. Miscellaneous—Orders should be given as indicated to observe closely for such developments as

cardiac arrhythmias, respiratory distress, wound bleeding or drainage, impaired circulation in an extremity (eg, distal to a cast or vascular procedure), etc.

B. Position in Bed: Designate specifically, eg, flat or on side, sitting, or foot of bed elevated.

C. Mobilization: Prescribe bed rest, standing to void, up in chair, or ambulation. While recovering from general anesthesia, the patient should be turned from side to side every 30 minutes until conscious and then hourly for the first 8–12 hours. Require active position change and active motion of the feet and legs every 1–2 hours while awake until ambulated. Order elastic bandages or antiemboli stockings for the legs for elderly patients or when ambulation is delayed.

D. Respiratory Care: Hyperventilation, coughing, tracheal suction, and respiratory therapy should be ordered as required. Percutaneous placement of a small catheter in the trachea may be needed for injection of saline or water to stimulate cough (see p 30).

E. Oxygen Therapy: See p 31.

F. Intake and Output: Order either nothing by mouth or a specific diet. Record the fluid intake and output for as long after surgery as required for control of fluid balance. Prescribe the parenteral fluids to be administered during the first 24 hours. Continuous catheter drainage of the bladder may be required to follow urine output closely in suspected renal impairment due to shock or other cause. If the patient is on catheter drainage, specify intervals for measurement of urine volume (eg, hourly).

G. Voiding: Place an order for notification of the surgeon if the patient is unable to pass urine within a specified period (usually 6–8 hours) after operation.

H. Body Weight: Patients with fluid balance problems should be weighed daily.

I. Drainage Tubes: If a nasogastric or intestinal tube is in place, it should be connected to suction and irrigated every 1–2 hours with 15–30 ml of saline. Urethral, chest, biliary, and other drainage catheters call for specific orders.

J. Medications: A narcotic for pain relief is usually required. Other drugs frequently used include sedatives, antibiotics, and antiemetic drugs. Resume essential preoperative medications such as digitalis, insulin, and corticosteroids.

K. Special Laboratory Examinations: During the first 24 hours, it may be necessary to determine the hematocrit, complete blood count, arterial blood pH, P_{O_2}, and P_{CO_2}; to order urinalyses and blood chemistries; and to obtain portable x-rays.

Special Postoperative Problems

Certain life-threatening complications occur with relative frequency in the early period after major surgery or trauma. The most important of these are the acute pulmonary, cardiovascular, and renal/electrolyte derangements which are chief causes of prolonged morbidity and increased mortality rates after severe operation or injury. Many of these patients have preexisting diseases or are elderly, and these factors compound the difficulty of their treatment.

An ICU environment is essential to the most effective management of these complications. Study of ICU activity in a major medical center will usually show that there has been a striking increase in the incidence of surgical patients with respiratory insufficiency and failure in recent years. There are many reasons for this. Blood gas and other respiratory tests are now widely used and have served to disclose marked deficits in function which were previously unrecognized. Older patients and those with multiple organ disease are being operated on more often. With improved management of cardiovascular, renal, and other complications, failure of the respiratory system is becoming a chief limiting element in recovery. Faster transportation and better resuscitation of trauma victims in military and civilian practice have resulted in survival of individuals whose lungs subsequently develop progressive posttraumatic changes.

Technical improvements in mechanical ventilatory support have accompanied significant advances in knowledge of the pathophysiology of pulmonary insufficiency. As a result, the ICU team is alert to the possibility of occult respiratory deficits and is more aggressive in the use of intubation and artificial ventilation in both prevention and treatment. Because management of respiratory failure has become one of the most demanding aspects of postoperative care, this condition has been selected for detailed discussion in this chapter. Various other serious postoperative complications such as cardiac arrhythmias and acute renal failure are discussed elsewhere in this text.

ACUTE RESPIRATORY FAILURE IN THE SURGICAL PATIENT

Essentials of Diagnosis

- Precipitating cause such as operation, trauma, or sepsis.
- Predisposing condition such as chronic obstructive pulmonary disease (frequently present).
- Dyspnea, tachycardia, and cyanosis are typical findings, but acute respiratory failure may be present without pathognomonic physical signs.
- Late signs include transient hypertension followed by hypotension, mental confusion or stupor progressing to coma, respiratory and cardiac irregularity, and cardiac arrest.
- Arterial blood gases show decreased oxygen tension or increased CO_2 tension (or both). A blood gas abnormality may be the only diagnostic sign of early respiratory failure.

General Considerations

Respiratory failure is the result of inability of the pulmonary system to maintain normal arterial oxygen or CO_2 tension. Acute respiratory failure is character-

ized by an arterial P_{O_2} of less than 60 mm Hg (normal, 75–100 mm Hg) or an arterial P_{CO_2} of more than 50 mm Hg (normal, 35–45 mm Hg) while the patient is breathing room air at rest—particularly if repeated arterial samples show the P_{O_2} to be falling and the P_{CO_2} to be rising (and not due to respiratory compensation for metabolic alkalemia). In interpreting blood gas determinations, it is important to bear in mind that arterial P_{O_2} is normally decreased with age (Sorbin & others: Respiration 25:3, 1968) and that patients with long-standing lung disease may have chronic respiratory insufficiency with continuously abnormal blood gases.

From the standpoint of management, 2 groups of patients with acute respiratory failure may be identified. One group consists chiefly of medical patients whose acute respiratory failure is often due to an exacerbation of severe chronic obstructive pulmonary disease and in whom treatment usually involves carefully controlled oxygen therapy with delay in use of artificial ventilation. The other group consists chiefly of surgical patients in whom acute respiratory failure is precipitated by trauma, operation, or sepsis. Artificial ventilation is more frequently indicated in the latter group, who usually have slight or no preexisting lung disease. Patients who have severe chronic lung disease such as emphysema and chronic bronchitis are especially prone to develop acute respiratory failure after surgical stress.

Acute respiratory failure is commonly associated with certain major physiologic disturbances which occur singly or together. These include (1) increased physiologic shunting (most often due to atelectasis); (2) increased physiologic dead space (which may be caused by hypotension, pulmonary embolism, or atelectasis); (3) increased work of breathing (frequently due to decreased compliance associated with interstitial pulmonary edema); and (4) decreased oxygen transport (usually related to diminished cardiac output). The conditions predisposing to these physiologic disturbances will be discussed and their clinical manifestations described.

Predisposing Conditions

Numerous factors predispose to pulmonary insufficiency and contribute to the development of acute respiratory failure in surgical patients.

A. Pain: After operation or trauma, pain involving the chest or abdomen has a restrictive influence on respiratory function. Thoracic and abdominal incisions—particularly upper abdominal—are known to reduce vital capacity significantly in the immediate postoperative period with resulting decreased effectiveness of cough and increased incidence of retained secretions, atelectasis, and pulmonary infection. Statistics on the frequency of clinically important atelectasis and pneumonitis after major thoracic and abdominal operations are difficult to interpret because of variability among the reports in the literature, but it is reasonable to assume that the incidence is at least 15–20%.

B. Abdominal Distention: This is a frequent contributing cause of respiratory insufficiency and failure. Increased intra-abdominal pressure reduces lung volumes and capacities by raising the diaphragm and reducing diaphragmatic excursion.

C. Restrictive Binders and Dressings: These inhibit pulmonary expansion and function.

D. Anesthetic Drugs and Narcotics: Ventilation is reduced and cough and other respiratory reflexes are suppressed by depressant drugs. Hypoxia and hypercapnia due to hypoventilation in the immediate postoperative period may become severe unless the patient's respiration is assisted until the effects of anesthetics and relaxants have subsided. Narcotics such as morphine must be used judiciously in the postoperative period in order to avoid ventilatory depression, hypercapnia, and atelectasis. Doses of narcotic which are normally well tolerated may have a marked depressant effect on pulmonary function in the very ill, debilitated, or elderly patient.

E. Thoracic Conditions: Decreased lung volume and impaired ventilatory efficiency due to acute thoracic conditions have a direct effect on respiratory function. Flail chest, extensive pulmonary resection, large accumulations of pleural air or fluid, and other severe chest abnormalities create circumstances under which respiratory failure may develop rapidly.

F. Extrathoracic Trauma, Surgery, and Sepsis: When severe, these conditions often have an indirect but seriously adverse effect on the respiratory system. Pulmonary insufficiency, related in most cases to pulmonary vascular congestion and interstitial edema, is a leading cause of death in fatal cases of shock, trauma, and infection. Intravenous fluid overload during treatment may be a contributing factor. Accordingly, patients suffering from these conditions should be observed with special care so that early evidence of failing lung function (eg, arterial blood gas derangement) will be discovered. Acute respiratory failure secondary to severe trauma or extensive operations has been variously termed posttraumatic pulmonary insufficiency, postoperative lung syndrome, shock lung, pump lung, wet lung, and adult respiratory distress syndrome (see p 28).

G. Chronic Conditions: A variety of preexisting conditions have a significant influence on the incidence of respiratory problems after major surgery or trauma.

1. Chronic obstructive pulmonary disease is an increasingly common finding in surgical patients and is associated with an exceptionally high incidence of postoperative complications. Stein & others (JAMA 181:765, 1962) found that 70% of all patients with emphysema and chronic bronchitis developed atelectasis and pneumonia following operation, whereas the incidence was only 3% in patients with normal preoperative lung function. Chronic pulmonary disease, even though not severe, predisposes strongly to respiratory complications after trauma or operation.

2. Smoking is associated with an increased incidence of emphysema, chronic bronchitis, and postoperative respiratory difficulty. Morton (Lancet 1:368, 1944) found that the incidence of postoperative pulmonary complications was 3 times higher among heavy smokers than among nonsmokers.

3. Old age is related to a higher rate of postoperative complications in general, including respiratory.

4. Severe obesity decreases vital capacity and the efficiency of respiratory muscles and increases the work of breathing. Markedly obese patients have a higher than normal oxygen uptake and CO_2 production. They are known to be especially susceptible to hypoventilation and to postoperative pulmonary complications.

5. Neurologic diseases and lesions such as poliomyelitis, multiple sclerosis, polyneuritis, and brain and spinal cord injuries may severely compromise the patient's pulmonary function and make him vulnerable to respiratory failure following trauma or surgery.

Clinical Findings

A. Symptoms and Signs: Pulmonary complications usually develop gradually over hours or days following surgery, trauma, or severe sepsis. Where predisposing conditions such as those described above are present, the patient must be evaluated with special care and arterial blood gas determinations performed if any suspicion of deteriorating pulmonary function arises even though definite evidence of acute respiratory failure is lacking. Mild to severe grades of respiratory failure may occur insidiously in the absence of pathognomonic symptoms or physical signs.

1. Hypoxia—The clinical findings in acute respiratory failure vary widely depending upon the cause and the patient's general condition. Dyspnea, tachycardia, and cyanosis form a classic triad of signs indicative of hypoxia of pulmonary or cardiac origin. A minimum of 5 g of reduced hemoglobin per 100 ml of blood must be present before cyanosis is clinically apparent. Although cyanosis is a manifestation of hypoxia, it ordinarily is not perceptible until the arterial oxygen saturation is below 80–85%, and severe tissue hypoxia can occur in the absence of detectable cyanosis. Stridor, wheezing, and retraction of supraclavicular and intercostal spaces are clear evidences of airway obstruction, respiratory insufficiency, and probable hypoxia. Decreased respiratory effort resulting in hypoventilation is also associated with hypoxia as well as CO_2 retention and is much more difficult to recognize and evaluate. Mild hypoxia usually causes an increase in heart rate, respiratory rate, cardiac output, peripheral resistance (vasoconstriction), and blood pressure. Tachycardia, tachypnea, and hypertension are thus common early signs of mild hypoxia. Late and severe hypoxia produces bradycardia, arrhythmias, and hypotension which may be followed by cardiac arrest. Old or debilitated patients often pass very rapidly into the late or terminal stage of hypoxia and circulatory failure.

2. Hypercapnia—Certain manifestations of acute respiratory failure may be due to CO_2 retention or hypercapnia. An early circulatory sign of CO_2 retention is vasodilatation with increased cutaneous blood flow and sweating. There is also stimulation of sympathetic activity with increased circulating catecholamines (epinephrine and norepinephrine), resulting in increased cardiac output, heart rate, and blood pressure. This reaction occurs only in those patients still able to respond to sympathetic activation. Increase of CO_2 content has a direct action on the respiratory center, leading to hyperventilation. However, the CNS depression and muscular weakness produced by hypercapnia may prevent hyperventilation. The degree of central depression caused by elevated blood levels of CO_2 is quite variable and ranges from mild sedation to deep coma. Respiratory arrest may occur. Other possible manifestations of hypercapnia are mental confusion, muscle twitching, visual defects, and cardiac arrhythmias. The combined depressant and stimulant effects of CO_2 retention, frequently accompanied by hypoxia, tend to produce a variable clinical picture.

3. Physical examination of the chest—Valuable clues to the presence of respiratory failure are usually found on chest examination. Increased tracheobronchial secretions and signs of atelectasis, pneumonitis, or pulmonary edema are common findings in respiratory failure. On the other hand, percussion and auscultation may occasionally disclose no significant changes. Physical examination of the chest must be integrated with other observations in order to develop a composite clinical impression of pulmonary status.

4. General evaluation—Certain categories of patients are known to be highly susceptible to respiratory failure and should be followed with special care. For example, the elderly patient with a long history of heavy smoking and of chronic obstructive lung disease is a likely candidate for respiratory failure after severe trauma or extensive surgery, particularly if conditions such as abdominal distention, obesity, and respiratory limitation by pain or narcotic are also present. Such patients require intensive preventive management and should be evaluated by appropriate laboratory studies before significant respiratory distress appears. In some patients, respiratory failure develops occultly in the absence of impressive symptoms and signs, and in such cases it is necessary to measure arterial blood gases to confirm or dispel the suspicion of respiratory failure. Usually, however, respiratory failure is associated with definite symptoms and signs, including at least dyspnea and tachycardia. Chest examination shows signs of atelectasis, pneumonitis, or pulmonary congestion when these conditions are overtly present. Depending upon the severity of failure and other factors, there may also be cyanosis, stupor, or hypertension. Restlessness in the postoperative period is a common sign of hypoxia which should be ruled out before sedation is ordered. Marked hypoxia is also an important cause of hypotension and indicates a late stage of respiratory failure in which bradycardia, arrhythmia, and cardiac arrest are imminent.

B. X-Ray Findings: A baseline chest film should be taken prior to all major operations and as soon as possible after severe trauma. Chest x-ray is an important adjunct to physical examination in patients suspected of respiratory failure and will frequently disclose evidence of atelectasis, pulmonary congestion, chest fluid, and other abnormalities not otherwise detectable. Portable films are taken during the immediate postoperative or posttraumatic period if transport of the patient to the radiology department is impracticable. Patients with severe chronic lung disease usually require early and repeated chest films after major surgery or trauma. Chest x-ray during the first few hours following thoracotomy and periodically thereafter enables accurate assessment of lung expansion and of air and fluid accumulations.

There are no pathognomonic radiologic signs of acute respiratory failure, and there is frequently no correlation between x-ray findings and the blood gas

Table 3—1. Tests for assessing respiratory function in critically ill patients.*

Oxygenation
Inspired oxygen concentration ($F_{I_{O_2}}$)
$P_{a_{O_2}}$ on controlled and spontaneous ventilation
$P_{(A-aD_{O_2})}^{1.0}$† or $P_{(A-aD_{O_2})}^{0.5}$†
Hematocrit or hemoglobin concentration
Arterial oxygen content ($C_{a_{O_2}}$)‡
Right-to-left shunt ($\dot{Q}_S/\dot{Q}_T$)‡

Ventilation
Tidal volume (V_T); frequency (f)
Minute ventilation ($\dot{V}_E$)
$P_{a_{CO_2}}$
Dead space to tidal volume ratio (V_D/V_T)
Carbon dioxide production ($\dot{V}_{CO_2}$)
Ventilator dead space and compression volume

Ventilatory reserve and mechanics
Total vital capacity
Forced expiratory volume in 1 second (FEV_1)
Maximum expiratory flow rate (MEFR)
Inspiratory force
Effective compliance
Dynamic compliance‡
Functional residual capacity (FRC)
Check for ventilatory discoordination‡

Related diagnostic procedures
Chest x-ray and fluoroscopy
Sputum smear and culture; antibiotic sensitivity
Body weight
Water balance
Serum and urine electrolytes
Serum protein concentration
Central venous pressure‡
Mixed venous oxygen content‡
Cardiac output‡
Pulmonary artery and capillary wedge pressures‡

*Revised slightly and reproduced, with permission, from Pontoppidan H, Geffin B, Lowenstein E: N Engl J Med 287:743, 1972.

†Difference in alveolar-arterial oxygen tension measured during ventilation with 100% and 50% oxygen, respectively.

‡Tests performed under special circumstances in the critically ill, unstable patient with respiratory or circulatory failure or both; facilities and technics are now available for doing these more complex tests at the bedside when indicated.

values. However, chest x-ray is the only method of identifying many subtle parenchymal and other changes such as vascular congestion which accompany or contribute to respiratory failure. Serial films are usually the only means available for following these changes.

Pulmonary Function Tests

Pulmonary function tests are essential in patients with respiratory failure for diagnosis, for evaluating responses to treatment, and as an aid in deciding whether or not to start or to discontinue tracheal intubation and artificial ventilation. The most useful tests are listed in Table 3–1. Most of these tests can be performed at the bedside during both spontaneous and controlled respiration. Some of them are particularly helpful in determining when a patient in acute respiratory failure should receive ventilatory support by tracheal intubation and assisted respiration (Table 3–2). Predicted values for pulmonary function tests have been tabulated by Bates & others (*Respiratory Function in Disease,* 2nd ed. Saunders, 1971; pp 93–94). These tables of predicted norms provide useful baseline information with which to compare the findings in patients with respiratory problems.

Selected pulmonary function tests from Table 3–1 and the physiologic principles involved in their interpretation will be discussed in order to show how they may be used in the management of patients with acute respiratory failure. Preliminary to this discussion, it is advisable to review some of the standard symbols and abbreviations used in pulmonary physiology and testing to facilitate the recording of data and the calculation of results. The accompanying display (Table 3–3) of primary and secondary symbols can be arranged in various combinations to designate the blood and gas phases of physiologic variables. (See Federation Proceedings, Report Fed Proc 9:602, 1950.)

A. Tests of Oxygenation:

1. **Measurement of inspired oxygen concentration** (F_{IO_2})—In complex respiratory problems, particularly those requiring assisted or controlled ventilation, it is essential to be able to monitor and to adjust the concentration of inspired oxygen. The concentration of inspired oxygen can be measured by the Scholander technic or with the oxygen electrode. At the bedside, oxygen concentration being delivered to the patient can be determined by sampling the inspired gas line with the portable paramagnetic oxygen analyzer. In calculating the alveolar-arterial oxygen gradient ($A-aD_{O_2}$), it is necessary to be certain that all the nitrogen has been washed out during 100% oxygen breathing ($F_{IO_2} = 1.0$). Ten to 20 minutes of breathing 100% oxygen have been found to be sufficient for this purpose unless severe chronic obstructive pulmonary disease is present. This can be checked by attaching a nitrogen analyzer to the expired gas line if such an instrument is available. When expired nitrogen levels fall below 1%, inspired oxygen has replaced all alveolar gas except CO_2 and water vapor. When nitrogen has been thoroughly washed out by breathing 100% oxygen, the Pa_{O_2} will reflect the alveolar-arterial gradient ($A-aD_{O_2}$) and the pulmonary shunt ($\dot{Q}s/\dot{Q}_T$).

2. **Measurement of arterial oxygen tension (Pa_{O_2})**—Arterial blood samples may be obtained from a peripheral artery, preferably the radial, with a fine needle and heparinized syringe. For repeated samples, an indwelling plastic catheter may be inserted into the artery. Pa_{O_2} and other measurements listed below can be performed rapidly and accurately in the laboratory. All of the following examinations are usually done on each arterial blood sample obtained from the patient with a respiratory problem:

Table 3–2. Guidelines for ventilatory support in adults with acute respiratory failure.[*][†]

	Normal Range	Tracheal Intubation & Ventilation Indicated
Mechanics		
Respiratory rate	12–20	>35
Vital capacity (ml/kg body wt‡)	65–75	<15
FEV$_1$ (ml/kg body wt‡)	50–60	<10
Inspiratory force (cm water)	75–100	<25
Oxygenation		
Pa_{O_2} (mm Hg)	75–100 (air)	<70 (on mask O$_2$)
$P_{(A-aD_{O_2})}^{1.0}$ § (mm Hg)[**]	25–65	>450
Ventilation		
Pa_{CO_2} (mm Hg)	35–45	>55††
V_D/V_T	0.25–0.40	>0.60

[*]Reproduced, with permission, from Pontoppidan H, Geffin B, Lowenstein E: N Engl J Med 287:743, 1972.

[†]The trend of values is of utmost importance. The numerical guidelines should obviously not be adopted to the exclusion of clinical judgment. For example, a vital capacity below 15 ml/kg may prove sufficient provided the patient can still cough "effectively," if hypoxemia is prevented, and if hypercapnia is not progressive. However, such a patient needs frequent blood gas analyses and must be closely observed in a well-equipped, adequately staffed recovery room or intensive care unit.

[‡]"Ideal" weight is used if weight appears grossly abnormal.

[§]See Table 3–1, note (†).

[**]After 10 minutes of 100% oxygen.

[††]Except in patients with chronic hypercapnia.

	Normal Range
Pa_{O_2}	On air: 75–100 mm Hg
	On 100% oxygen: 610–670 mm Hg
Percentage saturation	>95%
Pa_{CO_2}	35–45 mm Hg
HCO_3^-	23–25 mEq/liter
pH	7.36–7.44

Facilities for performing the above panel of tests should be available around the clock in proximity to the operating theater, recovery room, and ICU. All blood gas determinations should be carried out immediately after the sample is drawn, especially if the arterial oxy-

Table 3–3. Standard symbols in pulmonary physiology.

SYMBOLS FOR GAS PHASE

Primary symbols

V	Volume of gas
$\dot{V}$	Volume flow of gas per unit time
P	Pressure of gas
F	Fractional concentration of gas
R	Respiratory exchange ratio (volume CO_2/volume O_2)
D	Diffusion capacity (volume per unit time per unit pressure difference)
f	Respiratory frequency (breaths per minute)

Secondary symbols (subscripts)

I	Inspired gas
E	Expired gas
A	Alveolar gas
T	Tidal gas
D	Dead space gas
B	Barometric

SYMBOLS FOR BLOOD PHASE

Primary symbols

Q	Volume of blood
$\dot{Q}$	Volume flow of blood per unit time
C	Concentration of gas in blood
S	Percent saturation of hemoglobin with oxygen

Secondary symbols (subscripts)

b	Blood in general
a	Arterial blood
v	Venous blood
c	Capillary blood

GENERAL SYMBOLS

$\bar{X}$	Dash (—) over any symbol indicates a mean value
$\dot{X}$	Dot (·) over any symbol indicates a time derivative
s	Subscript to denote steady state
STPD	Standard temperature, pressure, dry (0 C, 760 torr*)

*One torr = 1 atm/760, almost exactly equivalent to 1 mm Hg.

FREQUENTLY USED COMBINATIONS OF SYMBOLS
(See also Table 3–1.)

V_T	Tidal volume (ml)
V_D	Dead space volume (ml)
V_D/V_T	Dead space to tidal volume ratio
$\dot{V}_A$	Alveolar ventilation (liters/min)
$\dot{V}_{O_2}$	Oxygen consumption (ml/min, STPD)
$\dot{V}_{CO_2}$	Carbon dioxide production (ml/min, STPD)
$F_{I_{O_2}}$	Fractional concentration of oxygen in inspired gas
$\dot{Q}_T$	Cardiac output, total (liters/min)
$\dot{Q}_S$	Blood flow "shunted" through pulmonary capillaries exposed to nonventilated alveoli (liters/min)
$\dot{Q}_S/\dot{Q}_T \times 100$	Percentage of cardiac output perfusing nonventilated areas of the lung. The $\dot{Q}_S/\dot{Q}_T$ ratio in normal lungs measured while breathing 100% oxygen defines the anatomic intrapulmonary right-to-left shunt.
$P_{a_{O_2}}$	Partial pressure of arterial oxygen
$P_{a_{CO_2}}$	Partial pressure of arterial carbon dioxide
$P_{A_{O_2}}$	Partial pressure of alveolar oxygen
$P_{A_{CO_2}}$	Partial pressure of alveolar carbon dioxide
$P_{(A-a_{D_{O_2}})}$	Alveolar to arterial oxygen difference or gradient
P_B	Barometric pressure 760 mm Hg

ABBREVIATIONS

The following abbreviations are among many in common use:

VC	Vital capacity (total)
FEV	Forced expiratory volume
FEV_1	First-second vital capacity
MVV	Maximal voluntary ventilation; same as MBC, maximal breathing capacity
MEFR	Maximal expiratory flow rate
MMFR	Maximal midexpiratory flow rate
FRC	Functional residual capacity
CPPB	Continuous positive pressure breathing
IPPV	Intermittent positive pressure ventilation
PEEP	Positive end-expiratory pressure

gen tension is high. If delay is inevitable, the syringe containing the arterial sample should be kept in ice.

Measurement of $P_{a_{O_2}}$ serves as an index of the adequacy of arterial oxygenation when the hemoglobin content is known. Also, if inspired oxygen concentration ($F_{I_{O_2}}$) is known, alveolar-arterial oxygen difference ($A-a_{D_{O_2}}$) provides an estimate of the magnitude of the physiologic shunt (see below). $P_{a_{O_2}}$ normally must be high enough to maintain full oxygenation of the blood as measured by the arterial oxygen content ($C_{a_{O_2}}$). The arterial oxygen content depends upon the arterial oxygen tension, on the hemoglobin content, and, to a lesser extent, on arterial CO_2 tension and pH. The total content of oxygen in arterial blood is made up of 2 components: (1) oxygen combined with hemoglobin to form oxyhemoglobin, and (2) a very small amount of oxygen physically dissolved in plasma. The normal value for arterial oxygen content when breathing air and assuming a hemoglobin content of 15 g/100

ml is about 20 ml/100 ml. On 100% oxygen, the arterial oxygen content rises slightly in normal individuals to about 22 ml/100 ml due mainly to an increase in O_2 dissolved in plasma at high $P_{a_{O_2}}$. Hemoglobin saturation also goes from 97.5% to 100%, thus contributing slightly to the rise in O_2 content.

Transport to the tissues of an adequate supply of oxygen depends not only on arterial oxygen content but also on volume and distribution of cardiac output (normal cardiac output = 5–6 liters/min). Assuming an arterial-venous oxygen content difference of 6 ml/100 ml and a cardiac output of 5 liters, oxygen consumption is 300 ml/min at rest in a normal individual. When arterial oxygen content is decreased as a result either of low $P_{a_{O_2}}$ or low hemoglobin content, there must be a compensatory increase in cardiac output to maintain adequate tissue oxygenation.

Maintenance of normal blood gases depends upon the relationship of effective alveolar ventilation ($\dot{V}_A$)

to pulmonary blood flow or perfusion ($\dot{Q}$). The normal ventilation-perfusion ratio ($\dot{V}_A/\dot{Q}$) is about 0.80, based on normal values for $\dot{V}_A$ of 4 liters/min and for $\dot{Q}$ of 5 liters/min. *The most important cause of decreased Pa_{O_2} is abnormality of the ventilation-perfusion relationship ($\dot{V}_A/\dot{Q}$) in the lung.* Inspired oxygen concentration (F_{IO_2}) is the other major factor related to pulmonary function which determines arterial oxygen tension (Pa_{O_2}). When there is a significant increase in physiologic shunt with resultant decrease in Pa_{O_2} due to abnormal $\dot{V}_A/\dot{Q}$, the administration of oxygen increases Pa_{O_2} and decreases the effect of the shunt on arterial oxygen content.

3. Estimation of physiologic shunt by measurement of alveolar-arterial oxygen tension difference ($P_{[A-aD_{O_2}]}$)—The physiologic shunt is that portion of the cardiac output that does not participate in pulmonary blood gas exchange but returns to the left heart as unoxygenated venous admixture to arterial blood. The total physiologic shunt has 2 components: (1) the **anatomic shunt** through bronchial, pleural, and thebesian veins (approximately 2% of cardiac output); and (2) the **capillary shunt** via the pulmonary capillaries. The capillary shunt is normally minimal but may be markedly increased by conditions that prevent ventilation of alveoli which continue to be perfused with blood. The following are the major causes of increased physiologic shunting in surgical patients:

a. Atelectasis (massive or patchy) is a common postoperative problem in which unventilated alveoli may be perfused by a significant portion of the cardiac output. The arterial Po_2 may be quite low. The arterial Pco_2 may remain normal or may even be decreased by hyperventilation.

b. Emphysema, pulmonary fibrosis, obesity, and mitral valvular disease may be associated with marked shunting as a result of *uneven distribution* of ventilation and perfusion. The shunt effect is caused by incomplete mixing of inspired air and its unequal distribution to alveoli.

c. A number of miscellaneous conditions associated with respiratory failure in the surgical patient are characterized by increased physiologic shunting. These conditions have been variously termed wet lung, respirator lung, postoperative lung, shock lung, pump lung, posttraumatic pulmonary insufficiency, and adult respiratory distress syndrome (see p 28). They are complex syndromes, and it is possible that some of them are separate entities. Precipitating circumstances vary as indicated by the descriptive titles. Pulmonary vascular congestion is a prominent component. Interstitial edema, alveolar exudate, and widening of alveolar-capillary septa are commonly present. Veno-arterial shunting occurs within the lung, which usually shows decreased compliance and either normal or increased respiratory resistance. Arterial blood gas studies when the patient is breathing room air frequently show low Pco_2 and low Po_2 accompanied by a base deficit secondary to hypoxia. Loss of normal alveolar surfactant, fat emboli, microembolism from intravascular coagulation, and oxygen toxicity are among the possible contributing factors.

d. Diffusion or alveolar-capillary block, presumably due to thickening of the alveolar-capillary membrane, is probably rarely responsible for significant physiologic shunting. Severe disturbance of the ventilation-perfusion ratio is usually the actual cause of what appears to be a diffusion block.

When cardiac output and arterial-venous oxygen content difference are relatively normal, the measurement of $P_{(A-aD_{O_2})}$ provides a convenient and reasonably accurate indication of the magnitude of physiologic shunting. The procedure consists of determining Pa_{O_2} and Pa_{CO_2} after the patient has been breathing 100% oxygen (F_{IO_2} = 1.0) for 15—20 minutes. Alveolar oxygen tension (PA_{O_2}) is calculated by subtracting water vapor pressure (47 mm Hg at 37 C) and Pa_{CO_2} (eg, 40 mm Hg) from the barometric pressure:

$$PA_{O_2} = 760 - (47 + 40) = 673 \text{ mm Hg (normal)}$$

Actual values for Pa_{O_2} in healthy subjects breathing 100% oxygen at sea level range from 610–670 mm Hg. Therefore, if Pa_{O_2} after breathing 100% oxygen is normal (eg, 640 mm Hg), then

$$P_{(A-aD_{O_2})}^{1.0} = PA_{O_2} - Pa_{O_2} = 673 - 640 = 33 \text{ mm Hg}$$

Under normal circumstances, the range for $P_{(A-aD_{O_2})}^{1.0}$ is 25–65 mm Hg. The alveolar-arterial oxygen difference rises when blood is shunted through unventilated alveoli. Values of $P_{(A-aD_{O_2})}$ greater than 450 mm Hg indicate severe ventilation-perfusion disturbance and are usually an indication for tracheal intubation and ventilatory support in patients with acute respiratory failure (see Table 3—2).

When $P_{(A-aD_{O_2})}$ is determined after breathing 100% oxygen, the shunt that is measured is caused chiefly by (1) the fixed anatomic shunt (2–3% of cardiac output) and (2) atelectasis. The shunt that occurs as a result of pulmonary congestion and interstitial edema in posttraumatic pulmonary insufficiency is also included in the measurement. In certain conditions such as obesity and chronic obstructive lung disease, significant shunting may occur as a result of uneven distribution of ventilation to perfusion when the patient is breathing room air. In such cases, it may be useful to determine $P_{(A-aD_{O_2})}$ when the patient is breathing room air (or 50% oxygen if ambient air is not tolerated).

When F_{IO_2} is substantially less than 100%, it is necessary for precise calculation of PA_{O_2} to use the alveolar gas equation (Nunn JF: *Applied Respiratory Physiology With Special Reference to Anesthesia.* Appleton-Century-Crofts, 1969; p 108) and either to measure the ventilation-perfusion ratio ($\dot{V}_A/\dot{Q}$) or to assume it to be 0.8. For rough calculation of PA_{O_2} when F_{IO_2} is less than 100%, the following formula can be used:

$$PA_{O_2} = F_{IO_2} \times (P_B - P_{H_2O}) - Pa_{CO_2}$$

Although measurement of $P_{(A-aDO_2)}$ during temporary ventilation with 100% oxygen is a useful guide to the magnitude of right-to-left shunt under most circumstances, actual determination of the shunt ($\dot{Q}_S/\dot{Q}_T$) is necessary for accurate data. Oxygen content of arterial, mixed venous, and pulmonary end-capillary blood must be measured or calculated and substituted in the following "shunt equation":

$$\dot{Q}_S/\dot{Q}_T = \frac{CcO_2 - CaO_2}{CcO_2 - CvO_2}$$

where $\dot{Q}_S$ = portion of cardiac output perfusing nonventilated areas (ie, right-to-left shunt flow in liters/min),

$\dot{Q}_T$ = total cardiac output,

Cc_{O_2}, Ca_{O_2}, and Cv_{O_2} = oxygen content (ml/100 ml STPD) of pulmonary end-capillary, arterial, and mixed venous blood, respectively, and

$\dot{Q}_S/\dot{Q}_T \times 100$ = % right-to-left shunt.

Precise calculation of the percentage of shunt by the above formula requires cardiac catheterization to obtain samples of mixed venous blood from the pulmonary artery. This is usually not feasible in acutely ill patients—hence the frequent reliance on $P_{(A-aDO_2)}$ as a practical indicator of the magnitude of right-to-left shunting.

The relationship of $P_{(A-aDO_2)}$ to percentage of shunt ($\dot{Q}_S/\dot{Q}_T \times 100$) can be estimated by use of a set of curves calculated from the shunt equation and published by Pontoppidan & others (Adv Surg 4:173, 1970). It is also possible to calculate the percentage of shunt from a simplified version of the shunt equation which is reliable only when the Pa_{O_2} is high enough to ensure full saturation of hemoglobin (ie, Pa_{O_2} above 150 mm Hg):

$$\dot{Q}_S/\dot{Q}_T = \frac{P_{(A-aDO_2)} \times 0.0031}{P_{(A-aDO_2)} \times 0.0031 + C_{(a-vDO_2)}}$$

where 0.0031 is the factor for conversion of partial pressure into oxygen content at 37 C. By making the assumption that the arterial-venous oxygen content difference ($C_{[a-vDO_2]}$) is normal (6 ml/100 ml) and thus avoiding the necessity for obtaining a mixed venous oxygen content on a pulmonary artery sample, the formula for determining the percentage of shunt can be further simplified as follows:

$$\dot{Q}_S/\dot{Q}_T = \frac{P_{(A-aDO_2)} \times 0.0031}{P_{(A-aDO_2)} \times 0.0031 + 6}$$

According to this formula, the percentage of shunt when $P_{(A-aDO_2)}$ is 450 mm Hg may be calculated as follows:

$$\dot{Q}_S/\dot{Q}_T = \frac{450 \times 0.0031}{450 \times 0.0031 + 6} = 0.19$$

$$\dot{Q}_S/\dot{Q}_T \times 100 = 19\% \text{ shunt}$$

The limitations of $P_{(A-aDO_2)}$ as a measure of shunting must be kept in mind. Changes in cardiac output and arterial-venous oxygen difference may alter the values of both $P_{(A-aDO_2)}$ and $\dot{Q}_S/\dot{Q}_T$. On the other hand, the agreement of alveolar-arterial oxygen difference with percentage of shunt is good when the cardiac output and the arterial-venous oxygen difference are within fairly normal limits.

Physiologic shunting of 10–15% due to atelectasis and other factors occurs in almost all patients after major trauma and may even be present after uncomplicated upper abdominal surgery. Wilson & others (Curr Top Surg Res 1:361, 1969) found that patients with posttraumatic pulmonary failure with physiologic shunt fractions below 40% will generally survive when provided with intensive supportive care whereas few patients survive with shunts of greater than 50%. If the shunt fraction approaches 30–35% in any patient, some form of ventilatory assistance is usually indicated.

B. Tests of Ventilation:

1. Tidal volume (V_T)—Tidal volume (V_T) is the volume of gas inspired or expired during each respiratory cycle. It is easily measured at the bedside and is controlled at a prescribed level during ventilatory assistance. Tidal volume is usually 400–500 ml (7 ml/kg) in a healthy young adult. It varies with age and state of health. A nomogram is available from which the normal basal tidal volume can be predicted from the breathing frequency, body weight, and sex (Radford & others: N Engl J Med 251:877, 1954). This nomogram applies only to patients with normal lungs.

2. Minute expired volume ($\dot{V}_E$)—Minute expired volume ($\dot{V}_E$) is tidal volume multiplied by respiratory frequency ($\dot{V}_E = V_T \times f$). Normal ventilation is the minute expired volume required in a normal person to maintain normal arterial CO_2 tension (Pa_{CO_2}). Because physiologic dead space (V_D) is frequently increased in patients with pulmonary disease and in acute respiratory failure, the "normal" minute ventilation as predicted from the above-mentioned nomogram is often grossly inadequate to prevent retention of CO_2 (hypercapnia). It is important to emphasize that adequacy of ventilation in the very sick patient cannot be determined simply by measuring the volume of ventilation. In a specific patient, adequate ventilation is defined as the minute expired volume which is in fact needed to maintain normal arterial CO_2 tension. Accordingly, when a patient is receiving respiratory assistance, the minute expired volume is adjusted upward or downward depending upon the arterial CO_2 values.

3. Measurement of arterial CO_2 tension (Pa_{CO_2})—*Arterial CO_2 tension is the only valid measure of the adequacy of ventilation.* CO_2 tension in arterial blood is usually measured directly by means of a Severinghaus glass electrode. CO_2 tension can also be obtained from the Henderson-Hasselbalch equation when the CO_2 content and the pH of plasma are known. Normal ventilation is the minute volume of ventilation ($\dot{V}_E$) required to maintain normal arterial CO_2 tension in a normal person. In patients with respiratory disease and failure, there is frequently an increase in physiologic dead space (see below). Under these circumstances, the predicted volume of ventilation is grossly inadequate to eliminate CO_2, so that arterial CO_2 tension increases and hypercapnia results. Voluntary overbreathing and excessive ventilation—due, for example, to a brain lesion or to a poorly adjusted mechanical ventilator—are among the causes of hyperventilation and hypocapnia seen clinically.

In summary, where there is a steady state, the condition of alveolar ventilation is defined by the CO_2 tension in arterial blood (P_{aCO_2}). The average normal value of P_{aCO_2} is 40 mm Hg, and the normal range is 35–45 mm Hg. A higher than normal value indicates alveolar hypoventilation and hypercapnia.

4. Dead space to tidal volume ratio (V_D/V_T)—Physiologic dead space (V_D) is that portion of each tidal volume which does not exchange gas and is a calculated quantity rather than an actual physical space. It consists of 2 components: anatomic and alveolar dead space. **Anatomic dead space** comprises the volume of the conducting airway (nose, mouth, pharynx, larynx, trachea, bronchi, and bronchioles down to the functional bronchiolar-alveolar junction). The anatomic dead space in an adult in milliliters is about equal to his ideal weight in pounds. Tracheostomy reduces the anatomic dead space by about 33%. At large tidal volumes, the anatomic dead space may be increased by as much as 50%, and at low tidal volumes it falls below predicted values.

Alveolar dead space is the difference between the calculated physiologic dead space and the anatomic dead space. Alveolar dead space is small in normal humans at rest, so that under these conditions anatomic dead space is approximately equal to physiologic dead space, ie, about 30% of tidal volume.

The ratio of dead space to tidal volume (V_D/V_T) is a measure of the efficiency of CO_2 elimination and thus of ventilation. It represents that portion of the tidal volume that is not effective in the removal of CO_2 from the blood. The actual determination of the V_D/V_T ratio involves collection of expired gas in a balloon or chamber and simultaneous collection of an arterial blood sample. The pressure of CO_2 is measured in the expired air (P_{ECO_2}) and in the arterial blood (P_{aCO_2}), and the values are substituted in the following formula:

$$V_D/V_T = \frac{P_{aCO_2} - P_{ECO_2}}{P_{aCO_2}}$$

The test can be performed at the bedside on patients with artificial ventilation or spontaneous respiration. The normal range for V_D/V_T is 0.25–0.40 (see Table 3–2).

An increase in the V_D/V_T ratio results in alveolar hypoventilation and reduced elimination of CO_2. The arterial CO_2 level (P_{aCO_2}) rises and remains high unless compensation is achieved by an increase in tidal volume and alveolar ventilation. In acute respiratory failure, the patient may be unable to compensate without artificial ventilation. Table 3–2 indicates that respiratory support should be considered when V_D/V_T exceeds 0.6. In most such patients, the ventilatory requirements are substantially greater than those predicted for normal individuals. The objective in the patient who is receiving respiratory support for respiratory failure is to adjust the minute volume of respiration to the level required to maintain normal arterial CO_2 tension. This requires measurement of P_{aCO_2}, which is used as a guide to adjustment of tidal volume and breathing frequency. Ventilation requirements in such patients change from day to day or even from hour to hour, so that it may be necessary to determine P_{aCO_2} and to adjust the minute volume several times a day. Each time the P_{aCO_2} is measured in the patient on artificial ventilation, it is advisable also to measure tidal volume and minute ventilation (by attaching a ventilation meter to the exhalation part of the respirator) and to record the peak airway pressure (see p 27).

The following conditions are commonly associated with increased physiologic dead space (V_D) and increased dead space to tidal volume ratio (V_D/V_T): **(1) Pulmonary embolism** interrupts alveolar capillary blood flow, resulting in nonperfusion of ventilated alveoli and thus increasing V_D/V_T. **(2) Hypotension** due to hemorrhage and other causes lowers pulmonary arterial pressure so that blood flow is redistributed by gravity to the dependent portions of the lung. Perfusion of ventilated alveoli in the remainder of the lung is diminished, and V_D/V_T is increased. **(3) Atelectasis** is characterized by nonventilation of perfused atelectatic alveoli, which results in shunting (see p 23). When these atelectatic alveoli resist inflation during constant volume artificial ventilation, ventilation is redistributed to air spaces in other parts of the lung without a matching redistribution of perfusion. The net effect is an increase in V_D/V_T. It is also observed that increase in V_D/V_T may correlate with radiographic evidence of atelectasis, pneumonia, and pulmonary edema and that a substantial drop in abnormally elevated V_D/V_T may be accompanied by concomitant improvement in the chest x-ray. **(4) High mean airway pressure** during artificial ventilation, particularly in the hypotensive patient, may inhibit capillary perfusion of ventilated alveoli and thus raise the V_D/V_T.

C. Tests of Ventilatory Reserve and Mechanics: The following tests of ventilatory reserve and mechanics are useful (1) to disclose respiratory insufficiency which has not progressed to the point of decreased alveolar ventilation, and (2) to evaluate the progress of patients in whom spontaneous breathing is capable of providing adequate alveolar ventilation:

1. Vital capacity (VC)—Total vital capacity (VC) is the simplest and most frequently used lung volume measurement. It is the maximum volume which can be expelled after a maximum inspiration without limit of time. It is a gross index of the ventilatory reserve for inspiratory effort in the conscious and cooperative patient. For adequate reserve, the vital capacity should be at least 3 times the tidal volume. In other words, the patient's ventilatory reserve may be considered inadequate if his vital capacity is less than 3 times his average tidal volume. Adequate reserve is necessary for effective deep breathing and coughing and in order to permit an appropriate increase in minute ventilation when the ventilation requirement becomes greater as a result of enlarged dead space or increased metabolic demand. The normal range of vital capacity is 65–75 ml/kg body weight. For adequate sustained spontaneous ventilation, most patients require a total vital capacity of 20–25% of predicted normal or at least 15 ml/kg body weight. Vital capacity of less than 15 ml/kg suggests the need for ventilatory support (see Table 3–2).

2. First-second vital capacity (FEV$_1$)–The forced expiratory volume (FEV) is also known as the "timed vital capacity." It consists of the maximum volume which can be expelled in a timed interval by a maximally fast expiration starting from a full inspiration. The volume expelled may be measured at 0.50, 0.75, 1, and 3 seconds. The volume expelled in 1 second (FEV$_1$) is normally about 85% of actual vital capacity, and the volume expelled in 3 seconds (FEV$_3$) is normally about 95% of actual vital capacity. FEV$_{0.75}$ multiplied by 40, or FEV$_1$ multiplied by 30, is usually approximately equal to the maximal voluntary ventilation (MVV) in liters per minute.

A reduced FEV usually but not always indicates increased airway resistance due to obstructive bronchopulmonary disease. Improvement in FEV after administration of a bronchodilator is consistent with some degree of reversibility. The FEV$_1$ is more informative than the VC in acute or chronic obstruction to air flow because decreased volume expelled per unit of time usually indicates not only resistance to air flow but also reduced capacity to cough and to generate the work of breathing. The normal range of FEV$_1$ is 50–60 ml/kg body weight, or 3–4 liters in the adult male. For sustained, adequate spontaneous ventilation, the FEV$_1$ should exceed 10 ml/kg. Values below 10 ml/kg suggest the need for ventilatory support (see Table 3–2).

3. Maximal voluntary ventilation (MVV)–The maximal voluntary ventilation is also termed the maximal breathing capacity (MBC). This test is performed by having the patient breathe in and out as rapidly and as deeply as possible, usually at a rate of 60–90 times per minute, for 15 seconds. The total volume breathed in or out during this period is expressed in liters per minute. Full cooperation by a well-coordinated patient is necessary for the successful performance of this test, which may be too strenuous for a chronically or acutely ill patient. There is also considerable variation in the results of this test, so that a healthy person may deviate as much as 25–35% from the predicted normal value. The indirect MVV calculated from the FEV$_{0.75}$ or FEV$_1$ (as noted above) has been found useful in those patients who are too ill to undertake the MVV test. The MVV is another of the methods used to assess airway resistance and obstructive bronchopulmonary disease. The range of normal values for young and middle-aged adult males is 100–150 liters/min.

The "match test" is a simple bedside test which correlates grossly with the results of the FEV$_1$ and the MVV. It may rarely be useful in circumstances where more accurate tests are unavailable. The test consists of determining the ability of the patient to blow out a burning match held 4–6 inches from his mouth. Inability to do so constitutes a positive result. After inhaling as deeply as possible, the patient is instructed to exhale forcibly with his mouth kept widely open. To assure maximal patient effort, the test is repeated several times. If the match test is positive, it is advisable to obtain FEV$_1$ and, if possible, MVV. Snider & others (JAMA 170:1631, 1959) found that 80% of patients with MVV greater than 60 liters/min could extinguish the match, whereas 80% of those with MVV of less than 60 liters/min could not. Eighty-five percent of those with FEV$_1$ greater than 1.6 liters/sec could extinguish the match, whereas 85% with FEV$_1$ less than 1.6 liters/sec could not.

The prognostic value of MVV was studied by Anderson & others (JAMA 186:763, 1963). They found a 2½ times greater incidence of postoperative pulmonary complications in patients with MVV less than 60% of predicted than in a comparable group of patients with MVV greater than 60% of predicted.

4. Maximal expiratory flow rate (MEFR)–This test is also a method of quantitating airway resistance and the severity of obstructive lung disease. The patient takes a maximal inspiration and, after a short pause, expires as fast and as forcefully as possible into a spirometer with a rapidly rotating drum. The MEFR is the flow between the first 200 ml and 1200 ml expressed in liters/min (normal for adult male: 350–550 liters/min). The maximal midexpiratory flow rate (MMFR) is the flow between the first 25% and 75% of the total forced expiratory volume (FEV) and is expressed in liters/sec. A reduced flow rate has the same significance as a reduced FEV$_1$ and is typical of increased airway resistance and obstructive lung disease. Normal MMFR is 2–4 liters/sec. Patients with significant chronic obstructive lung disease usually have an MMFR below 1 liter/sec and often below 0.5 liters/sec.

5. Inspiratory force–Inspiratory force is measured by simple equipment consisting of a face mask (or connector to an endotracheal tube) fitted with a manometer capable of registering below atmospheric pressure. Inspiratory force is the maximum inspiratory pressure below atmospheric which the patient can exert during a period of 10–20 seconds against a completely occluded airway. The method does not depend upon the patient's cooperation and is particularly useful in the comatose or anesthetized patient. The normal range of inspiratory force is 75–100 cm water below atmospheric. CNS depression or muscular weakness may cause low values. When lung compliance is decreased, greater inspiratory force is required to achieve adequate tidal ventilation. Experience has shown that artificial ventilation is usually required in patients with acute respiratory failure when inspiratory force is less than 25 cm water (see Table 3–2). It has also been found that successful weaning from intermittent positive pressure ventilation requires an inspiratory force exceeding 30–40 cm water.

6. Effective compliance—Lung compliance is defined as the volume change per unit pressure change:

$$\text{Compliance} = \frac{\text{Volume change}}{\text{Pressure change}} = \text{ml/cm water}$$

It is a measure of the elastic resistance (or distensibility) of the lungs and chest wall, either separately or together. Compliance of the lungs plus that of the chest wall can be measured in a spontaneously breathing patient by analyzing continuous recordings of airway pressure, gas flow, and tidal volume. In a patient with no spontaneous respiratory effort, total static compliance can be measured by using a large syringe to inject a predetermined volume of air (within the normal range of the patient's tidal volume) into the lungs while reading the airway pressure on a manometer.

In the patient on assisted ventilation, it is simple to determine the "effective compliance," which is defined as the ratio of tidal volume to peak airway pressure:

$$\text{Effective compliance} = \frac{\text{Tidal volume}}{\text{Peak airway pressure}} = \text{ml/cm water}$$

Average values for effective compliance are 40–50 ml/cm water for adult males and 35–45 ml/cm water for adult females with normal lungs. This measure may be misleading in the presence of high airway resistance.

A fall in effective compliance in the patient on assisted ventilation may be an early sign of atelectasis, pneumonia, or interstitial pulmonary edema (as in posttraumatic pulmonary insufficiency or "shock lung") before auscultative or radiographic evidence appears. These complications require prompt treatment. They are often associated with increased physiologic shunting. Decrease in effective compliance therefore indicates a need to determine arterial blood gases and possibly to readjust the pattern of ventilation and the concentration of inspired oxygen. Pontoppidan & others (N Engl J Med 273:401, 1965) found that decrease in effective compliance is significantly related to an increase in the dead space to tidal volume (V_D/V_T) ratio and indicates the need for reassessment of ventilation requirements. Finally, if an undetected fall in compliance occurs in a patient on a pressure-limited respirator, tidal volume will decrease, with possible rapid development of hypoxia and hypercapnia, unless the respirator is properly readjusted. Relatively high airway pressures may be necessary to provide required alveolar ventilation.

Differential Diagnosis

The etiologic differential diagnosis of acute respiratory failure after operation or trauma can usually be made by means of the history and physical examination and by taking special note of predisposing condi-

tions (see p 18). However, it is again emphasized that laboratory studies—particularly blood gases—are essential to the evaluation of patients with complex problems and to the identification of occult cases of respiratory failure when there are minimal or no physical findings. Acute respiratory failure is usually due either to hypoventilation or to ventilation-perfusion disproportion—or, more frequently, to a combination of the two. Pulmonary function tests and blood gas analysis are especially helpful in following the patient's progress, in deciding when respiratory assistance should be started and discontinued, and in determining the pathogenesis (Tables 3–1 and 3–2). Tidal and minute volumes of ventilation are decreased in hypoventilation but are often increased in severe ventilation-perfusion defects. If the cause of respiratory failure is primarily hypoventilation, the usual finding is decreased arterial P_{O_2} and increased arterial P_{CO_2}. If the problem is due to ventilation-perfusion defect, the arterial P_{O_2} will be low whereas the arterial P_{CO_2} may be elevated but is frequently normal or low.

Hypoventilation and ventilation-perfusion disproportion will be discussed below in more detail. As an important example of ventilation-perfusion abnormality, posttraumatic pulmonary insufficiency will be specifically reviewed.

A. Hypoventilation: Simply stated, hypoventilation results from failure to move sufficient air in and out of the lungs with the result that respiratory exchange is inadequate to remove CO_2 and to oxygenate the blood. Hypoventilation is associated with low tidal and minute volumes, resulting in deficient alveolar ventilation. The patient's respirations are either too shallow or too slow to maintain a normal partial pressure of oxygen in the alveoli and to remove accumulating CO_2. On room air, arterial P_{O_2} tends to fall and arterial P_{CO_2} to rise. These blood gas changes are frequently the only indication of the seriousness of the ventilatory deficiency. When the $P_{a_{CO_2}}$ exceeds the normal range, there is respiratory acidosis. Severe and prolonged hypoxia (low $P_{a_{O_2}}$) produces metabolic acidosis characterized by a base deficit due to anaerobic glycolysis in the tissues with release of lactic acid. Such diverse signs as restlessness, depressed sensorium, hypertension, and hypotension may be manifestations of serious hypoventilation.

Hypoventilation is the commonest cause of respiratory failure in the immediate postanesthetic period. It is important to be alert to its insidious development caused by the residual effects of anesthetic agents and muscle relaxants, prolonged hyperventilation during anesthesia, narcotic administration, or ventilatory inhibition by wound pain. Hypoxemia secondary to hypoventilation in the postanesthesia recovery room may result in cardiac arrhythmias and death, and depressed ventilation may predispose to the development of atelectasis and other pulmonary complications later in the postoperative period. In a series of patients with abdominal operations, Thompson & Eason (Am J Surg 120:649, 1970) found $P_{a_{O_2}}$ levels as low as 60 mm Hg in the immediate postanesthetic period in some patients and observed that the longer the operation, the lower the Pa_{O_2}. From the clinical point of view, these patients all seemed to be ventilating adequately as indicated by absence of cyanosis and apparently good chest wall excursion. Marshall & Millar (Anesthesia 20:408, 1965) found that low arterial oxygen tensions in the immediate postanesthetic period persisted for up to 3 hours. Reduction in Pa_{O_2} was greatest in older patients, after mechanical overventilation, and when there was preexisting lung disease.

During the early postoperative days and after complete recovery from anesthesia, the danger of hypoventilation and its sequelae persists. Such a problem is particularly common after thoracic and upper abdominal operations; less common after lower abdominal procedures; and still less likely to occur after surgery on the extremities. The duration of operation is again noted to be a significant factor. As an example of postoperative inhibition of ventilation, Anscombe (*Pulmonary Complications of Abdominal Surgery,* Year Book, 1957) observed a 50–60% reduction in vital capacity and in expiratory and inspiratory flow rates for several days after gastrectomy. The adverse effects of hypoventilation may be accentuated by higher tissue needs for gas exchange, which may increase to 120% of normal in the postoperative period and, in the presence of severe infection, may increase to 140%.

In summary, hypoventilation occurs frequently in the postanesthetic and early postoperative period and following severe trauma. It is characterized by decreased tidal and minute volumes, decreased Pa_{O_2}, and increased Pa_{CO_2}. Because it may exist to a marked degree even in the absence of physical signs, alertness to the possibility of hypoventilation is vital to its recognition. The causes of hypoventilation include the residual effects of anesthetic drugs, postoperative pain, narcotics given to relieve pain, mechanical restrictions such as abdominal and chest binders, pleural effusion, hemothorax, pneumothorax, abdominal distention, obesity, neuromuscular conditions causing paralysis or weakness of the muscles of respiration, and traumatic flail chest. Fortunately, hypoventilation can usually be corrected promptly if the diagnosis is suspected and, when necessary, confirmed by pulmonary function and blood gas measurements.

B. Ventilation-Perfusion ($\dot{V}_A/\dot{Q}$) Disproportion: Even though tidal volume and minute volume may be normal or increased, CO_2 elimination and oxygenation may be inadequate due to uneven distribution of ventilation and perfusion to the alveoli. This abnormality is common after major operations or severe trauma and may lead to acute respiratory failure. There are 2 main types of ventilation-perfusion defect, and they frequently occur simultaneously. In one type, some alveoli are well ventilated and poorly perfused. (*Examples:* hypotension, pulmonary embolism). The result is an increase in physiologic dead space, V_D/V_T ratio, and Pa_{CO_2}. Under these circumstances, high Pa_{CO_2} usually responds to increase in tidal volume and alveolar ventilation. Oxygen administration may also be neces-

sary (see p 31). Nonperfusion of ventilated lung may occur during mechanical ventilation if mean airway pressure is elevated sufficiently in some alveoli to cause redistribution of blood flow to the remainder of the lung (Werko L: Acta Med Scand, Suppl 193:1, 1947). If atelectasis is present and resists inflation by high mean airway pressure, the blood flow which is redistributed from the hyperinflated alveoli elsewhere in the lung will go to the atelectatic areas. Under these circumstances, there is both an increase in dead space to tidal volume ratio (V_D/V_T) and an increase in the physiologic shunt (Finley TN, Hill TR, Bonica JJ: Am J Physiol 205:1187, 1963). High mean airway pressure is more likely to produce these redistribution effects on perfusion and ventilation when hypotension or hypovolemia is present.

In the other type of ventilation-perfusion defect, some alveoli are well perfused but poorly ventilated. (*Examples:* atelectasis, pulmonary fibrosis, and posttraumatic pulmonary insufficiency.) The result is a large veno-arterial shunt associated with low arterial Po_2 and increased alveolar-arterial oxygen difference ($P_{[A-a}D_{O_2}]$). The arterial P_{CO_2} is usually relatively normal or below normal. If the shunt is extensive enough to require treatment, hypoxemia may be relieved by oxygen administration, and assisted or controlled respiration may also be necessary (see p 34). Identification and relief of the underlying cause of the ventilation-perfusion defect are, of course, a primary concern in every case.

C. Posttraumatic Pulmonary Insufficiency: Progressive pulmonary insufficiency (adult respiratory distress syndrome) culminating in acute respiratory failure may occur after severe trauma, extensive surgery, shock, cardiopulmonary bypass, and profound sepsis. There are thus a number of precipitating causes which result in similar pathophysiologic changes. The condition has a variety of synonyms such as posttraumatic pulmonary insufficiency, postoperative lung syndrome, shock lung, pump lung, and wet lung. Preexisting chronic lung disease is a predisposing factor.

Moore & others (*Post-Traumatic Pulmonary Insufficiency.* Saunders, 1969) have described 4 progressive phases of the posttraumatic pulmonary insufficiency syndrome: (1) an initial phase, occurring immediately after injury and resuscitation, usually characterized by high cardiac output, lowered peripheral resistance, hyperventilation, and mild hypoxemia and hypocapnia; followed by (2) a period of early respiratory difficulty with stable circulation; followed by (3) continued progression of pulmonary failure; and, finally, (4) severe hypoxia, hypercapnia, lactic acidosis, and cardiac arrest. The pathophysiology of this syndrome is discussed on p 23, where it was noted that pulmonary vascular congestion and interstitial edema are characteristic features of the acute pulmonary insufficiency that follows a number of different types of nonthoracic trauma and certain other severe stresses. Most of the functional abnormalities observed have been attributed to disturbances in ventilation and perfusion. The role, if any, of diminished diffusion capacity or "alveolar-capillary block" in acute respiratory failure in general and posttraumatic pulmonary insufficiency in particular has not been established.

Posttraumatic pulmonary insufficiency has been recognized in recent years as a frequent and often fatal condition, especially in military and civilian hospitals that treat major trauma victims. It was reported to be the commonest cause of death following initial resuscitation of combat casualties in the Vietnam war. Early diagnosis depends upon anticipation of this type of pulmonary complication. Blood gas determinations and other respiratory tests are indicated on suspicion of developing respiratory failure. Factors which contribute to the pulmonary changes include fluid overload; pulmonary edema secondary to fluid retention associated with prolonged mechanical ventilation, head injury, and renal failure; aspiration of gastric contents; fat embolism; transfusion microembolism from debris in banked blood; and, very importantly, the low-flow states associated with hemorrhagic and septic shock.

Diagnostic & Monitoring Procedures

The onset of acute respiratory failure may be insidious. Early diagnosis requires not only alertness to premonitory physical signs but also the ready availability of test equipment in the postanesthetic and intensive care areas. Table 3–1 lists the examinations which are useful in diagnosis and in monitoring. The following basic pieces of apparatus will make it possible to perform the most frequently needed of the diagnostic and monitoring procedures: blood gas and pH analyzer, paramagnetic oxygen analyzer, low-resistance nonrebreathing and expired gas collection system, Wright respirometer for bedside determination of expired respiratory volumes, and a Collins spirometer for recording of measurements such as FEV_1 and MEFR. Improved results in recent years in the treatment of patients with respiratory failure are attributable to aggressive management based on physiologic principles and guided by objective data from respiratory function studies.

The indications for ventilatory support in patients with acute respiratory failure are summarized in Table 3–2. In Table 3–4, Pontoppidan & others (Adv Surg 4:163, 1970) have proposed a set of guidelines for the identification of patients who require preventive measures (see below) and close monitoring because of borderline respiratory compensation.

Prevention

Acute respiratory failure is largely preventable, and moderate pulmonary insufficiency can frequently be corrected promptly by relatively simple measures. A prime consideration in postoperative and traumatized patients is the prevention of atelectasis, which commonly sets the stage for a series of changes, including progressive collapse and pneumonitis, which may lead to respiratory failure. Avoidance of excess body fluid is another preventive measure which is of special importance in patients with borderline or failing

Table 3–4. Indications for preventive measures and close monitoring.

	Acceptable Range	Preventive Measures and Monitoring Required
Mechanics		
Respiratory rate	12–25	25–35
Vital capacity (ml/kg)	70–30	30–15
Inspiratory force (cm water)	100–50	50–25
Oxygenation		
$P_{a_{O_2}}$ (mm Hg)	100–75 (air)	200–70 (on mask O_2)
$P_{(A-a_{DO_2})}{}^{1.0}$ (mm Hg)	50–200	200–350
Ventilation		
$P_{a_{CO_2}}$ (mm Hg)	35–45	45–60
V_D/V_T	0.3–0.4	0.4–0.6

pulmonary function—particularly those who are likely candidates for the development of posttraumatic pulmonary insufficiency. The prophylaxis of atelectasis and fluid overload can be briefly outlined as follows:

A. Atelectasis: The frequency with which atelectasis occurs in the postoperative period and its deleterious effects on pulmonary function have already been described. The aim of preventive measures is to minimize the occurrence of alveolar collapse, which may occur as a result of depressed respiratory excursions, small airway obstruction by secretions, or both.

1. Preoperative preparation—Chronic obstructive lung disease, chronic bronchitis, and acute respiratory infections should be brought under control by preoperative inhalation therapy, mist bronchodilator drugs, antibiotics, chest physical therapy, and other indicated methods of treatment so that secretions and respiratory obstruction will be minimized in the postoperative period. Smoking should be stopped. These measures should be continued postoperatively as required. Cooperation in deep breathing and coughing after operation is improved by preoperative instruction and practice.

2. Anesthesia and postanesthesia management—Endotracheal suction and frequent sighing and overexpansion of the lungs during and immediately after operation are indispensable procedures. Frequent turning of the patient and insistence on deep breathing and coughing in the recovery room (and throughout the early postoperative period) are essential. Laver & Bendixen (Prog Surg 5:1, 1966) noted that atelectasis is the commonest cause of hypoxia in the postoperative period and that the atelectasis is most frequently due to perpetuation of the periodic collapse of alveoli which is part of the normal pattern of ventilation. This is prevented by intermittent hyperventilation or deep breathing. Postanesthetic hypoventilation can usually be avoided by retaining the orotracheal or nasotracheal tube until spontaneous ventilation is well established.

The tube not only facilitates tracheobronchial suction but also makes it possible to inflate the lungs several times every 15 minutes by hand compression of a self-inflating bag. When significant postoperative hypoventilation cannot be corrected by these simple means, continued intubation and ventilatory assistance are necessary.

3. Postoperative endotracheal intubation and artificial ventilation—The preventive value of continued controlled or assisted ventilation in selected patients after major surgery or severe trauma is firmly established. Some degree of respiratory failure can be predicted and often forestalled in patients with extensive injuries and operations, particularly if complicated by shock, sepsis, heart disease, obesity, muscular weakness, general debility, or chronic lung disease. The orotracheal tube can be left in place after operation, or a cuffed nasotracheal tube can be substituted for it. Mechanical ventilation, usually volume controlled, can then be continued for 24 hours—and several additional days if necessary—without undue hazard when proper equipment and experienced personnel are available. For example, mechanical ventilation for 24–48 hours after cardiac surgery is common practice and makes it possible to control the ventilatory pattern, lung expansion, and Pa_{CO_2}; to provide optimum oxygen intake ($F_{I_{O_2}}$) and oxygenation (Pa_{O_2}); to remove secretions and prevent atelectasis by endotracheal suction; to reduce the work of breathing; and to facilitate accurate monitoring and control of the major parameters of pulmonary function.

4. Oxygen therapy—Warm humidified oxygen prevents drying of the tracheobronchial mucosa and aids in mobilization of secretions, thus helping in the prevention of atelectasis. If hypoxia is suspected—or confirmed by a finding of Pa_{O_2} below 75 mm Hg—humidified oxygen may be delivered at a rate of 10 liters/min by a face tent which will provide about 40% inspired oxygen, which may be adequate; or by a snug mask which will raise inspired oxygen to 60–80%. A nasal catheter or cannula is simpler but provides less humidification; a flow of 100% oxygen at a rate of 5–10 liters/min results in inspired oxygen of 30–40%. Flow of oxygen through a nasal catheter should be limited to about 5 liters/min. A nasal cannula is more comfortable than a catheter and permits oxygen flow of up to 10 liters/min.

5. Nasotracheal suction—Introduction of a sterile 14F catheter into the tracheobronchial tree via the nose is an effective means of stimulating cough and aspirating sputum when the patient is unable or unwilling to cough up his secretions. This procedure should be performed early and as often as necessary in the postoperative period. Bronchoscopy may on rare occasion be required.

6. Transtracheal catheter—Some patients require stimulation of cough and can then raise sputum without tracheal aspiration. Under these circumstances, transtracheal catheterization may occasionally be a useful procedure (Radigan LR, King RD: Surgery 47:184, 1960; Sizer JS, Frederick PL, Osborne MP:

Surg Gynecol Obstet 123:336, 1966). A standard No. 14 Intracath (Bard) is inserted percutaneously under local anesthesia into the trachea just below the cricoid cartilage. Alternatively, a plastic catheter can be passed through a No. 18 needle. Injection of 2–3 ml of sterile saline (or distilled water if necessary for stimulation) through the catheter will excite cough. The injection may be repeated as often as required to mobilize secretions and clear the airway. The catheter is too small to permit effective aspiration of secretions but may permit obtaining a specimen for culture.

7. Chest physical therapy—Encouragement of the patient to hyperventilate, cough vigorously, and raise secretions is a normal feature of good postoperative nursing care and, if done assiduously, will often obviate the need for mechanical aids. Blow bottles are a useful means of obtaining the cooperation of the patient in deep breathing, the achievement of maximal voluntary inhalation being the objective. This is more effectively accomplished by a simple device called an "incentive respirometer," which requires sustained full inspiration for its operation (Bartlett RH, Gazzaniga AB, Geraghty TR: JAMA 224:1017, 1973). Inhalation of mist from an ultrasonic device or heated nebulizer is a useful adjunct to chest physical therapy when secretions are thick and difficult to raise. Intermittent positive pressure breathing has its advocates, but its value is uncertain and it is generally overrated as a postoperative measure. IPPB is a useful means of delivering a mist of bronchodilator drug when bronchospasm is present. Postural drainage, percussion, and vibration under the direction of an experienced nurse or respiratory therapist may encourage cough and the raising of secretions.

8. Guides to prevention—Atelectasis should be anticipated and the above measures utilized appropriately in patients who are at risk by virtue of their circumstances. By the time physical signs and x-ray changes have occurred, atelectasis is an established and advanced process. Widespread patchy atelectasis due to alveolar collapse is a common early development that may be detected only by determination of blood gases which show decreased Pa_{O_2} and increased $P(A-a_{D_{O_2}})$.

B. Fluid Overload: Positive water balance should be avoided in postoperative and posttraumatic patients who are at risk of respiratory failure either because of the severity of their injury or the presence of chronic pulmonary disease. In shock or sepsis, water and protein may enter the interstitial space of the lung as a result of loss of integrity of the capillary endothelium. Under these circumstances, edema fluid accumulates primarily in the dependent portions of the lung even in the absence of increased capillary hydrostatic pressure (Cottrell & others: Circulation Res 21:783, 1967). For unknown reasons, patients on prolonged artificial ventilation also tend to retain water.

It is therefore important to maintain correct water and electrolyte balance in patients with impending or actual respiratory deficiency. This is usually accomplished through monitoring of intake and output, blood electrolytes, and body weight. Limitation of fluid intake and diuretic therapy may be necessary to maintain equilibrium. In the absence of damage to pulmonary capillaries, diuretic therapy and restriction of water lead to improvement of respiratory function. Colloid is administered only if there is circulatory evidence of hypovolemia or if hypoalbuminemia is present.

In patients with hemorrhagic or septic shock or drug intoxication, left-sided heart failure may exist in the presence of a low central venous pressure. If blood, albumin, or electrolyte solution is infused until arterial pressure and central venous pressure are normal, interstitial pulmonary edema and increased shunting (rising $A-aDO_2$) will almost invariably occur. In such patients, replacement should be considered adequate when urine output is satisfactory in spite of subnormal systemic arterial and venous pressure. If decreased urinary output is secondary to inadequate cardiac output and renal blood flow in the presence of adequate blood volume, it is frequently necessary to improve cardiac output by intravenous infusion of isoproterenol, epinephrine, or dopamine or possibly transvenous cardiac pacing. Under these circumstances also, the best end point in terms of systemic blood pressure is the return of urinary flow (Pontoppidan & others: N Engl J Med 287:690, 1972). Balloon flotation catheterization of the central circulation with a Swan-Ganz catheter permits repeated measurement of cardiac output, filling pressures of right and left ventricles, and other important variables in those critically ill patients who are impossible to evaluate and manage without such information (Swan HJC: Crit Care Med 3:83, 1975).

Positive water balance in patients with impending or established respiratory failure should be recognized as a potentially serious problem and should be avoided. Prevention may involve limitation of fluid intake to 25–30 ml/kg/day. Body weight should decline by 350–500 g daily in patients with no caloric intake, and failure of such patients to lose weight means water retention. It should be remembered that the contribution of the nebulizer to body fluid may amount to 300–500 ml a day. Management by fluid restriction—and diuretics if necessary—is usually effective in reversing the trends toward fluid overload (Pontoppidan H: J Trauma 8:938, 1968).

Treatment

There are 2 major aspects to the treatment of respiratory failure. The first consists of measures for relief of conditions in the chest and elsewhere which are primarily responsible for the decrease in pulmonary function. These conditions include respiratory depression, thoracic disease or injury, atelectasis, and fluid overload, which have been discussed above. Measures to correct these conditions are essential in both prevention and treatment of respiratory failure.

The second aspect of treatment consists of procedures to maintain adequate oxygenation and ventilation while the patient recovers from the underlying causes of respiratory failure. These procedures consist chiefly of oxygen therapy and mechanical ventilation.

A. Oxygen Therapy: Oxygen, like any other therapeutic agent, has specific indications, dosages, methods of administration, hazards, and toxicity.

1. Indications—Any circumstances in which cellular oxygenation is impaired may be an indication for oxygen therapy. One cause of impaired cellular oxygenation is a decreased arterial oxygen tension (Pa_{O_2}). The Pa_{O_2} is normally 80–100 mm Hg when inspiring ambient air at sea level, and decreases gradually with age so that at age 70 a Pa_{O_2} of 70 mm Hg may be regarded as normal. Hypoventilation or mismatching of ventilation and perfusion in the lung may result in a reduced Pa_{O_2}.

Tolerance to hypoxemia varies with the patient's age, hemoglobin concentration, the rate of onset, the presence of coronary or cerebrovascular disease, cardiac output, body temperature, and many other factors. Since tolerance is not predictable, it is generally wise to administer oxygen to hospitalized patients with an acute decrease in Pa_{O_2} to less than 55–60 mm Hg.

Cellular oxygenation may be impaired without significant decrease in Pa_{O_2}: low cardiac output, anemia, abnormal hemoglobin, shifts in the oxyhemoglobin dissociation curve, impaired cellular uptake of oxygen, and increased metabolic requirements of the cell are just a few examples. It may be appropriate or necessary to administer oxygen in these circumstances, but consideration of oxygen transport in the blood demonstrates the limitations. Each gram of normal hemoglobin can carry 1.36 ml of O_2 when fully saturated (Pa_{O_2} = 150 mm Hg). Raising the Pa_{O_2} above this level adds very little oxygen to the blood—0.3 ml dissolved O_2 per 100 ml of blood for each 100 mm Hg rise in Pa_{O_2}. It is evident that, whereas administering O_2 is appropriate, a greater effect on O_2 transport might be achieved by controlling hemoglobin concentration and cardiac output or reducing tissue requirements when feasible.

The clinical signs of tissue hypoxemia are variable. The brain and the myocardium have relatively high O_2 consumptions, and the initial manifestations of inadequate oxygenation may be cerebral or myocardial dysfunction rather than signs of respiratory distress. Arterial blood gas values should be checked in any patient with unexplained deterioration of CNS or cardiac function. Cyanosis is a late sign of severe hypoxemia, and absence of cyanosis does not exclude significant hypoxemia.

2. Dosages and methods of administration—In addition to the dose of oxygen required, patient comfort, economy, convenience of administration, and reliability must all be considered.

Nasal cannulas or plastic face masks are adequate for the vast majority of patients. Other methods of oxygen administration are also described below.

Oxygen from a cylinder or wall supply is completely dry and must be passed through a humidifier to prevent drying of the airway mucosa.

a. Nasal cannulas and catheters—The nasal cannula is the best method of oxygen delivery for general use. Flow rates of 6–8 liters/min deliver 30–40% inspired oxygen. Higher rates are uncomfortable and cause local irritation. Mouth breathing does not significantly affect the inspired concentration, but bilateral nasal obstruction obviously will.

Nasal catheters deliver similar concentrations. They are inserted to the nasopharynx (half the distance from nose to ear), and care must be taken to prevent accidental intubation of the esophagus.

b. Plastic face masks—Loose-fitting plastic face masks deliver 30–50% O_2 at a flow rate of 8–10 liters/min. A reservoir bag may slightly increase the O_2 concentration delivered, but a more important factor is the mask fit. It is important to keep in mind that, should the mask be removed for eating, coughing, suctioning, or other purposes, the patient is deprived of any supplemental oxygen.

c. Rubber face masks—The Boothby, Lovelace, Bulbulian (BLB) mask and the Barach and Eckman meter mask (OEM) are tighter-fitting masks which are capable of delivering high concentrations of oxygen (80%) but are too hot, heavy, and uncomfortable to use for more than 10–15 minutes.

d. Face hood—The face hood is an unreliable method of administering oxygen since it is difficult to keep in place. It is appropriate to use for the delivery of high humidity from mist generators.

e. Oxygen tent—The oxygen tent is essentially obsolete for adults because of its bulk and inconvenience, the fire hazard involved, separation of the patient from nursing personnel and family, and inability to achieve high concentrations of oxygen. It is occasionally useful for small children. A minimum flow of 12 liters/min is required to achieve O_2 concentrations of 40%, and opening the tent lowers the concentration.

f. Venturi masks—These are designed to deliver inspired oxygen concentrations not exceeding 24%, 28%, 35%, or 40%. They are for use in patients with chronic hypercapnia when it is necessary to avoid raising the Pa_{O_2} to greater than 60 mm Hg (see below).

g. Plastic head box—A rigid clear plastic box with a cutout for the neck may be used for infants, usually up to 1 year of age. Oxygen flow of 5–10 liters/min can provide up to 100% inspired O_2 concentration; the inspired O_2 must therefore be monitored frequently.

h. T-piece—A T-piece is often used for delivery of oxygen and humidity to patients with endotracheal tubes or tracheostomies. It provides a simple and safe system without valves. The inspired O_2 concentration will vary with the concentration and flow of oxygen delivered, the length of the connections, and the inspiratory flow rate and respiratory frequency.

3. Hazards and complications—

a. Infection—The water in the humidifier can serve as a culture medium and source of infection. The humidifier should be changed every 24 hours to prevent this.

b. Retrolental fibroplasia—Elevated *arterial* oxygen levels may produce blindness in premature infants. No premature infant should be in an environment of more than 40% oxygen unless specifically prescribed

for cyanosis or sustained tachypnea, as in respiratory distress syndrome. In case higher concentrations of oxygen are used, incubator oxygen concentration should be monitored and adjusted so that the infant's Pa_{O_2} is in the range of 60–80 mm Hg in the radial or temporal artery (umbilical artery sample may be diluted by a patent ductus arteriosus).

c. Ventilatory depression—This is of concern *only* in patients with chronic hypercapnia. This does not mean that O_2 should not be administered when necessary but that it must be carefully titrated so that the Pa_{O_2} does not exceed 60 mm Hg. This can be done with a nasal cannula at flow rates of 1–2 liters/min or a Venturi mask. In either case, frequent monitoring of arterial blood gas values is essential.

d. Pulmonary oxygen toxicity—Pulmonary toxicity from O_2 probably does not occur with inspired concentrations of less than 50%. Since it is difficult or impossible to achieve higher concentrations for a significant length of time unless a tracheostomy or endotracheal tube is in place, pulmonary toxicity is not a concern with the standard methods of oxygen administration.

e. Fire—Flames and sparks must be kept away from high oxygen atmospheres.

B. Mechanical Ventilation:

1. Indications for mechanical ventilation—Mild cases of hypoventilation and ventilation-perfusion disproportion usually respond to supplementary oxygen and other preventive measures (see above). When adequate ventilation and oxygenation cannot be maintained by these methods, respiratory support by mechanical ventilation is needed. The criteria for respiratory support are summarized in Table 3–2 and the criteria for monitoring in Table 3–4. The decision to provide an airway and begin mechanical ventilation should not be delayed until the patient's condition deteriorates. The preventive value of respiratory support in selected patients at high risk of respiratory failure has already been emphasized. Respiratory support is probably indicated if a patient who is receiving oxygen at 10 liters/min by face tent or mask has a Pa_{O_2} of 70 mm Hg or a Pa_{CO_2} of 55 mm Hg and the trend in these values is worsening, or if a poorly oxygenated patient has rapid, shallow respirations and is tiring (see Table 3–2). By the time the patient is gasping for breath and developing ventricular arrhythmias, there has been too much delay.

Once the diagnosis of acute respiratory failure and the need for respiratory support are established, treatment by mechanical ventilation is required to increase alveolar ventilation and to deliver greater amounts of oxygen to the arterial blood. The procedures involved are tracheal intubation and operation of a mechanical ventilator. Positive pressure ventilation by way of a tight-fitting face mask is useful in emergency resuscitation, but this technic is not efficient nor is it tolerated by the patient for very long. Therefore, tracheal intubation is necessary if mechanical support of respiration is required in respiratory failure.

2. Tracheal intubation—A cuffed endotracheal

tube is passed through the mouth if the situation is urgent. If feasible, intubation through the nose is more comfortable for the patient. However, tube size is limited by the nostrils and turbinates, and nasotracheal tubes are longer, narrower, offer greater resistance to gas flow, are harder to keep patent, and have a greater tendency to kink than orotracheal tubes. The tube can be left in place for 2 weeks if properly cared for. Once the tube is inserted and mechanical ventilation begun, it is possible to decide at leisure whether tracheostomy should be done. There is thus rarely a need for emergency tracheostomy.

3. Indications for tracheostomy—Elective tracheostomy is performed for the following reasons: (1) anatomic or traumatic abnormality precludes intubation from above; (2) obvious long-term need (ie, more than 2 weeks) for tracheal intubation; (3) failure to tolerate oral or nasal intubation; or (4) inability to cope with excessive secretions or other problems without tracheostomy. Placement of an endotracheal tube prior to tracheostomy is of great advantage because it permits good ventilation and oxygenation during tracheostomy and makes the procedure technically easier. Emergency tracheostomy is required when intubation from above is technically impossible or inadequate in such conditions as acute upper airway obstruction, massive aspiration, pulmonary hemorrhage, head and neck wounds, respiratory burns, and severe respiratory failure.

4. Management of the intubated patient—A competent attendant must *always* be present when an intubated patient is on mechanical ventilation. Disconnection or failure of the equipment can be rapidly lethal. Aseptic technic should be observed in handling the connections and during aspiration of the tube. The trachea should be suctioned as often as necessary to avoid accumulation of secretions and to prevent atelectasis. The patient should be well oxygenated prior to suctioning, and ventilation should be interrupted for no more than 15 seconds. In order to avoid drying of secretions in the airway, the respiratory gas mixture should be humidified by passage through heated water and delivered at 39 C. Mist should be visible but not densely so. Excessive volume of tracheal secretions suggests excessive humidification.

5. Complications of intubation—Laryngeal or tracheal ulceration and stenosis are common sequelae of intubation when great care is not taken to prevent these serious complications. Prolonged use of orotracheal or nasotracheal tubes may cause severe damage to the larynx, resulting in hoarseness, difficulty in swallowing, impaired laryngeal activity, and varying degrees of respiratory obstruction. By taking care to reduce trauma due to the tube, the safe period of prolonged endotracheal intubation can in some cases be extended up to 2 weeks. Maximal damage to the trachea from endotracheal or tracheostomy tubes typically develops at the level of the inflatable cuff. Tracheoesophageal fistula or erosion into a major artery may rarely occur, but the most frequent complication is fibrosis and stenosis of the trachea. By using low-pressure pliable cuffs on endotracheal and tracheos-

tomy tubes, the incidence of these complications can be greatly reduced (Grillo & others: J Thorac Cardiovasc Surg 62:898, 1971). Inflation of the endotracheal or tracheal tube cuff should be just sufficient to prevent air leakage into the mouth during positive pressure ventilation. The cuff can be deflated for about 5 minutes every hour if the patient can tolerate being off mechanical ventilation for that length of time. It may otherwise be necessary to deflate the cuff only briefly at hourly intervals. Suctioning of the oropharynx prior to letting the balloon down may prevent aspiration of material into the trachea.

6. Use of mechanical ventilators—

a. Types of ventilators—A wide variety of ventilators are available, and there is frequent misunderstanding of their relative capabilities. Ventilators are commonly classified, by the mechanism producing cessation of inspiration, into pressure-cycled (Bird) and time-volume cycled (Ohio 560, Bennett PR-4, Bennett MA-1, Emerson, Engstrom). In the former, the operator determines a preset pressure, and the tidal volume delivered by the machine varies with the compliance of the lung-thorax and the airway resistance. If the compliance of the lung-thorax system decreases (from patient contraction of chest and abdominal muscles, airway secretions, atelectasis, pneumothorax, etc), the tidal volume delivered by the ventilator will decrease and the respiratory rate will increase. The time-volume cycled ventilator in this circumstance will generate higher pressures and deliver a more constant tidal volume with little or no change in respiratory rate. It seems obvious, therefore, that with use of pressure-cycled ventilators the tidal volume must be monitored and with time-volume cycled ventilators the inflation pressure must be monitored.

Another major difference between the 2 classes of ventilators is their response to leaks in the patient-ventilator system. The pressure-cycled machine will compensate for small leaks, taking a longer time to deliver the same volume, and will "stick" in the inspiratory phase if the leak is so large that the preset pressure cannot be achieved. The time-volume ventilator will not compensate for leaks, and the tidal volume will be decreased proportionate to the leak. (The tidal volume is *not* constant.) It is therefore essential to have an alarm system when the patient is dependent on the ventilator.

A third difference is that most of the presently available time-volume cycled ventilators are capable of generating higher inspiratory flow rates and inflation pressures than the pressure-cycled ventilators and are more effective in the presence of severely decreased compliance or increased airway resistance. Most models of pressure-cycled ventilators can generate peak pressures of approximately 50 cm water, whereas many time-volume cycled ventilators can double this value.

Thus, in the presence of severely decreased compliance, elevated airway resistance, or rapidly changing compliance or airway resistance, time-volume cycled ventilators are more effective. Many other considerations enter into the selection of a ventilator: cost, size, power source, ease of sterilization, ability to control inspired O_2 concentration, ability to apply positive end-expiratory pressure, reliability, performance of the humidifier, etc. It should be borne in mind that the cost of time-volume cycled ventilators is approximately 10 times that of pressure-cycled machines. The success of ventilator care depends more on the quality and performance of the medical and nursing personnel involved than on the specific ventilator utilized.

It is axiomatic that a patient dependent on a ventilator must be cared for in an environment where continuous observation is possible. Management of these patients consists of a multitude of measures aimed at preventing the complications of therapy, and the chances of success are improved if the patient is in an intensive care unit manned by highly skilled nursing and medical personnel.

b. Assisted vs controlled ventilation—Assisted ventilation is a form of respiratory support triggered by the patient's spontaneous respiratory effort in response to which a mechanical ventilator inflates the patient's lungs until a preset pressure has been reached, at which point the inspiratory phase stops and expiration begins. With the use of a pressure-limited ventilator, tidal volume is a function of airway resistance and pulmonary compliance. These parameters tend to change from time to time in acute respiratory failure, so that expired minute volume and tidal volume must be monitored frequently to assure adequate alveolar ventilation when a pressure-limited ventilator is used for ventilatory assistance.

Controlled ventilation is respiratory support provided by a mechanical ventilator which delivers a constant preset minute and tidal volume regardless of changes in airway resistance and pulmonary compliance. Respiratory rate is determined by the setting on the ventilator. In controlled ventilation, the patient's spontaneous respiratory effort must be completely overridden and not allowed to become asynchronous with the ventilator; otherwise, the patient will fight the respirator and respiratory insufficiency will be increased. If lung compliance is severely reduced, the volume-controlled or volume-limited ventilator may be the only means of providing adequate alveolar ventilation. In controlled ventilation, the patient's respiratory effort must be eliminated so that the ventilator can completely take over the rhythm and depth of respiration. If sedation is necessary to depress the patient's respiratory drive or to prevent coughing or bucking on the endotracheal tube, small intravenous doses of morphine (2–3 mg) or meperidine (10–20 mg) should be given. It may occasionally be necessary to paralyze the patient with tubocurarine in repeated doses of 5–10 mg IV or, preferably, pancuronium bromide (Pavulon), 2–6 mg IV, until the desired effect is obtained.

Assisted ventilation is indicated when impending or frank respiratory failure is associated with decreased tidal volume and an increased respiratory rate. If the patient has normal respiratory drive, it is generally safer to assist rather than control respiration, so that the patient's respiratory center "sets" the respiratory frequency and the arterial CO_2 tension (Pa_{CO_2}). Controlled ventilation is indicated when ventilation or oxygenation is inadequate on assisted ventilation at acceptable oxygen tensions. Flail chest and marked tachypnea are other indications. The energy cost of breathing is reduced by either assisted or controlled ventilation, but maximum reduction is achieved by controlled ventilation. It is often advisable to use controlled ventilation initially in very ill patients.

c. Ventilation—On controlled or assisted ventilation, the magnitude of the patient's ventilation is determined by adjustment of tidal volume and respiratory frequency. These are regulated to maintain a normal Pa_{CO_2} of 35–40 mm Hg. Pa_{CO_2} is thus the guide to the minute volume of ventilation required by the patient. Hyperventilation resulting in a Pa_{CO_2} of 30–35 mm Hg is tolerable, but lower levels of Pa_{CO_2} should be avoided.

d. Oxygenation and oxygen toxicity—Oxygenation of the blood is maintained if possible at a minimum Pa_{O_2} of 80–90 mm Hg. This is accomplished by increasing the fraction of oxygen in inspired air ($F_{I_{O_2}}$) as required to raise the Pa_{O_2}. It is usually appropriate to begin with 40% humidified oxygen. It is not useful to raise the Pa_{O_2} above 130 mm Hg. Clinical experience suggests that oxygen concentrations of 50% or higher are likely to produce serious pulmonary damage due to "oxygen toxicity" when used for more than 2 days. The higher the $F_{I_{O_2}}$, the more rapid the onset of damage (Clark & others: Pharmacol Rev 23:37, 1971). The morphologic changes presumably caused by oxygen toxicity include interstitial and intra-alveolar edema, hemorrhage, and hyaline membranes. These are nonspecific responses to a variety of injuries of which oxygen toxicity is only one. Except in chronically hypoxemic patients, it is generally advisable to select an $F_{I_{O_2}}$ that will result in a Pa_{O_2} in the normal range. However, if the arteriovenous shunt is so large (marked elevation of $P_{[A-aD_{O_2}]}$ and $\dot{Q}_S/\dot{Q}_T$) due to atelectasis or other cause that an $F_{I_{O_2}}$ above 50% is necessary to maintain a normal Pa_{O_2}, it may be preferable to accept a Pa_{O_2} in the slightly hypoxemic range.

e. Tidal volume adjustment—Certain alterations in the ventilatory pattern have been found to improve oxygenation. Patients on controlled ventilation at normal tidal volumes of 7 ml/kg complain of dyspnea and inadequate chest expansion even though Pa_{O_2} and Pa_{CO_2} are normal. Larger tidal volumes (10–15 ml/kg) are therefore advised and are well tolerated. Excessive hypocapnia can be corrected by introduction of mechanical dead space (Suwa & others: Anesthesiology 29:1206, 1968). It has also been noted that the larger tidal volumes are associated with a reduction in $P_{(A-aD_{O_2})}$, whereas normal tidal volumes may be associated with a rise in $P_{(A-aD_{O_2})}$ indicative of progressive atelectasis.

f. Positive end-expiratory pressure (PEEP)—Other variations in ventilatory pattern which may improve the efficiency of oxygenation are continuous positive pressure breathing (CPPB) and positive end-expiratory pressure (PEEP). On controlled ventilation with intermittent positive pressure ventilations (IPPV), airway pressure falls to zero during expiration, whereas normally the expiration is slowed by the continued action of the inspiratory muscles. In mechanically ventilated patients with stiff lungs due to decreased compliance, expiration is completed more quickly; with the ventilator pressure falling to zero during expiration, there is a greater tendency to alveolar collapse. It is possible that IPPV may in this way contribute to atelectasis. It has been observed clinically that CPPB with PEEP of 7–10 cm water is valuable in the treatment of hypoxemia and large $P_{(A-aDO_2)}$ in patients with severe respiratory failure not responding to other means of therapy (Ashbaugh & others: J Thorac Cardiovasc Surg 57:31, 1969). The chief mechanism by which PEEP (or CPPB) relieves hypoxemia is probably through prevention of alveolar collapse and shunting during the expiratory phase of respiration. Criteria for instituting PEEP include failure to maintain a P_{aO_2} of 70 mm Hg with an F_{IO_2} of 50% or more during IPPV; failure to reduce the shunt ($\dot{Q}_S/\dot{Q}_T$) by other measures such as treatment of cardiac failure, fluid overload, retained secretions, atelectasis, and pneumonitis. Blood volume should be adequate in order to avoid an adverse circulatory response to PEEP (Kumar & others: N Engl J Med 283:1430, 1970). The hazards of PEEP (as compared to IPPV) are an increased rate of complications such as subcutaneous and mediastinal emphysema and tension pneumothorax.

g. Surfactant depletion—Pulmonary surfactant, a lipoprotein which lines the walls of the alveoli, has the unique property of reducing alveolar surface tension, thus offsetting the inherent instability of air spaces. It lowers the interfacial tension in the alveoli as they become smaller and tends to prevent alveolar collapse at low transpulmonary pressure. Impairment of surfactant function results in progressive closure of air spaces with shunting, particularly at end-expiration when lung volume and alveolar size are least. It has been suggested that high oxygen concentrations, mechanical ventilation, and excessively large tidal volumes may all cause surfactant depletion, but there is no convincing evidence in man that a primary defect in the surfactant system is an etiologic factor in pulmonary disease, including acute respiratory failure (Clements JA: Am Rev Resp Dis 101:984, 1970; Scarpelli EM: *The Surfactant System of the Lung.* Lea & Febiger, 1968). Morgan (N Engl J Med 284:1185, 1971) has recently summarized experimental data that suggest that alveolar ventilation is sufficient to preserve surfactant synthesis following loss of perfusion, whereas loss of both ventilation and perfusion results in rapid depletion of the surfactant system. In spite of continuing uncertainty regarding the role of surfactant deficiency in acute respiratory failure, it is appropriate to minimize the conditions which may possibly deplete surfactant, eg, high F_{IO_2} and continuous hyperinflation or collapse of alveoli.

h. Circulatory and other effects—It should be kept in mind that positive pressure breathing may decrease the venous return to the heart and the cardiac output. The central venous pressure will be elevated. The extent of these changes and the degree of circulatory support required to cope with them will be related to respiratory pressures and to the status of the lungs and circulation. Gastric distention is a common occurrence in patients on ventilators, and intubation of the stomach is frequently necessary. Positive pressure ventilation may cause pneumothorax and mediastinal and subcutaneous emphysema, as noted above. Patients with thoracic injuries are particularly prone to develop pneumothorax, and insertion of a chest tube at the outset of mechanical ventilation may be advisable to prevent development of a severe acute pneumothorax.

i. Weaning from the ventilator—The transition from mechanical to spontaneous ventilation should be attempted only when there is objective evidence that pulmonary function is adequate. Sustained spontaneous ventilation requires a minimal vital capacity of 10 ml/kg, or a volume essentially twice as large as the normal tidal volume. Ventilatory support can usually be permanently discontinued and the endotracheal or tracheostomy tube removed when the vital capacity exceeds 15–20 ml/kg. Although vital capacity has been found to be a more reliable guide to weaning than $P_{(A-aDO_2)}$ and V_D/V_T, it has been observed that weaning is rarely successful when $P_{(A-aDO_2)}$ is greater than 350 mm Hg and V_D/V_T is above 0.6 (see Table 3–2). Arterial P_{O_2} is also a valuable indicator of readiness for weaning. If P_{aO_2} is maintained at 200 mm Hg or above on the ventilator with F_{IO_2} of 40%, it is probable that the patient will tolerate a short trial period off the ventilator. On the other hand, if the patient can barely maintain a normal P_{aO_2} while on the ventilator and receiving a high F_{IO_2}, he cannot be expected to tolerate weaning.

Weaning should be approached cautiously when chest wall trauma has been the primary indication for controlled ventilation and paradoxic motion of the chest wall is still present. The average time for stabilization of the rib cage is usually at least 10 days for patients under 30 and 20 days for patients over 50. This will vary with the extent of injury.

The process of weaning must usually be gradual if the patient has had acute respiratory failure. The longer the period of mechanical ventilation, the more difficult will be the weaning. Weaning can begin with 5–15 minutes per hour or half-hour of spontaneous respiration off the ventilator but with a T connector to the tracheal tube delivering 60–80% humidified oxygen. The ECG, the depth and rate of respirations, and the patient's general reactions are observed for signs of distress. Periods of spontaneous respiration are lengthened and oxygen administration decreased as tolerated. If possible, the patient should be out of bed and ambulatory during this time. Blood gas determinations are often needed to evaluate the respiratory status at this stage. It may be advisable to return the patient to mechanical ventilation at night during the early weaning period so that he may sleep under good control. Weaning may take several days if mechanical ventilation has been used for a week or more.

Intermittent mandatory ventilation (IMV) has been proposed as an aid to weaning (Downs JB & others: Chest 64:331, 1973). This technic enables the patient to breathe spontaneously through a one-way valve but also provides a preset number of mechanical ventilations per minute. As the patient improves, the preset number of mechanical breaths is progressively reduced until breathing is completely unassisted. Although IMV is being used in a number of centers, its true value to the weaning process is yet to be determined by controlled studies (Sahn SA, Lakshminarayan S, Petty TL: JAMA 235:2208, 1976).

Prognosis

Preventive measures and therapy based on physiologic principles have greatly improved the outlook for surgical patients with progressive pulmonary insufficiency or acute respiratory failure. Because many more patients are now receiving mechanical ventilatory support on a prophylactic basis than was formerly the case, it is difficult to quantitate the improvement in prognosis of acute respiratory failure which has taken place over the past 5–10 years. Reports from the Respiratory Unit at Massachusetts General Hospital are among the most specific in this regard. The majority of patients admitted to that unit are postoperative or posttraumatic, and most patients require tracheal intubation or tracheostomy and artificial ventilation for a large part of their stay. The average length of stay is 18 days. The mortality rate on the unit was 35–40% during the period 1961–1965 and fell to 11% in 1970 (Bendixen & others: *Respiratory Care.* Mosby, 1965; Pontoppidan & others: N Engl J Med 287:690, 1972). Other institutions have observed similar improvement in prognosis of patients with acute respiratory failure (O'Donahue & others: Chest 58:603, 1970). The decreased mortality rates can be ascribed to the fact that substantial progress has been made over the past decade in almost all aspects of management of pulmonary insufficiency.

●   ●   ●

General References

Ballinger WF, Drapanas T: Pages 157–174 in: *Practice of Surgery, Current Review.* Vol 1. Mosby, 1971.

Barnes RW, Merendino KA: Post-traumatic pulmonary insufficiency syndrome. Surg Clin North Am 52:625, 1972.

Bates DV, Macklem PT, Christie RV: *Respiratory Function in Disease,* 2nd ed. Saunders, 1971.

Bendixen HH & others: *Respiratory Care.* Mosby, 1965.

Berk JL & others: *Handbook of Critical Care.* Little, Brown, 1976.

Blaisdell FW, Lewis FR Jr: *Respiratory Distress Syndrome of Shock and Trauma.* Saunders, 1977.

Boyd DR: Monitoring patients with posttraumatic pulmonary insufficiency. Surg Clin North Am 52:31, 1972.

Cambell GS: Respiratory failure in surgical patients. Curr Probl Surg 13:5, Feb 1976.

Committee on Pre- and Postoperative Care, American College of Surgeons: *Manual of Preoperative and Postoperative Care,* 2nd ed. Kinney JM, Egdahl RH, Zuidema GD (editorial subcommittee). Saunders, 1971.

Hedley-Whyte J & others: *Applied Physiology of Respiratory Care.* Little, Brown, 1976.

Hirsch EF & others: The lung: Responses to trauma, surgery and sepsis. Surg Clin North Am 56:909, 1976.

Kumar A & others: Continuous positive-pressure ventilation in acute respiratory failure: Effects on hemodynamics and lung function. N Engl J Med 283:1430, 1970.

Lewis FJ & others: Automatic monitoring in the postoperative recovery room. Surg Gynecol Obstet 130:333, 1970.

Moore FD & others: *Post-Traumatic Pulmonary Insufficiency.* Saunders, 1969.

Pontoppidan H, Geffin B, Lowenstein E: Acute respiratory failure in the adult. (3 parts.) N Engl J Med 287:690, 743, 799, 1972.

Pontoppidan H, Laver MB, Geffin B: Acute respiratory failure in the surgical patient. Adv Surg 4:163, 1970.

Seeley TW, Hedley-Whyte J: Weaning from intermittent positive-pressure ventilation. N Engl J Med 292:903, 1975.

Skillman JJ: *Intensive Care.* Little, Brown, 1975.

Teplitz C: The core pathobiology and integrated medical science of adult acute respiratory insufficiency. Surg Clin North Am 56:1091, 1976.

4...
Postoperative Complications

Muriel Steele, MD, & F. William Blaisdell, MD

After successful surgery, the postoperative course should consist of rapid return to health. Anesthesia and surgery both have unavoidable temporary ill effects on normal physiology. A simple operation performed under local anesthesia causes minimal systemic effects. A major abdominal dissection such as that required for removal of a malignant retroperitoneal sarcoma can be expected to alter normal physiology markedly.

Incisional discomfort may be acute for 24–48 hours and should gradually subside over 3–4 days. During the period of acute discomfort, splinting of abdominal muscles may interfere with deep breathing and coughing. Intra-abdominal dissection and irritation of the peritoneum during the operation result in temporary paralysis of the peristaltic activity of the bowel (paralytic ileus). Some degree of ileus is normal following any intra-abdominal procedure. If the field of the operation is limited—eg, as in simple appendectomy—ileus may not persist longer than 12–24 hours. After major abdominal procedures associated with mechanical trauma to the bowel or peritoneum, paralysis of intestinal motility may continue for 3–4 days.

In addition to local changes which result from surgical trauma, a systemic ("stress") reaction is inevitable following major surgery. This reaction is proportionate to the magnitude of the surgical trauma and the extent of loss of blood, fluids, and electrolytes. The response to any injury is catabolic as the body mobilizes protein, fat, and carbohydrate to provide energy and repair damaged tissues. This mechanism is activated by certain metabolic and endocrine factors. After a few days to several weeks, an anabolic response follows. Caloric intake is increased, and nitrogen balance switches from negative to positive (see Chapter 13).

Increased metabolic activity is associated with the "stress response." Unless complications develop, body temperature rarely exceeds 37.8 C (100 F) even after major operations. The pulse and respiratory rates are only slightly above those recorded preoperatively. Cardiac output and oxygen utilization increase proportionately. A temperature elevation above 37.8 C or a marked elevation of the pulse or respiratory rate signifies a postoperative complication.

PREVENTION OF POSTOPERATIVE COMPLICATIONS

In order to avoid high morbidity and possible mortality from the operation, every effort must be made to prevent postoperative complications. It is far easier to prevent these complications than to treat specific problems once they develop. There is no substitute for good operative technic, and the principles of Halsted are just as applicable today as they were 50 years ago: meticulous hemostasis, gentle handling of tissues, careful approximation of wounds to avoid dead space, and rigid asepsis. Other important aspects of good operative technic are selection of the proper anesthetic, adequate preparation of the skin, good lighting, proper placement of incisions, adequate exposure, careful wound closure, care to avoid leaving foreign materials in the wound or body cavities, and team discipline and training.

The respiratory system should be evaluated at the completion of the operation.* Mucus plugs and accumulated secretions may obstruct bronchi, and respiration may remain depressed following major anesthesia. The conscious patient should be encouraged to breathe deeply and to cough; if he is not cooperative or has a depressed sensorium, nasotracheal aspiration should be instituted to remove retained secretions and stimulate the cough reflex. The patient's position should be changed frequently by encouraging him to sit up every 3 or 4 hours or by rolling him from side to side or changing the inclination of the bed.

The adequacy of peripheral perfusion should be assessed immediately after surgery by noting the skin color and warmth. Urine output and other fluid losses should be recorded. A patient in unstable condition should have an indwelling urethral catheter to allow for hourly measurements of urinary output. In addition, in the critically ill patient, a central venous pressure line will facilitate vascular volume assessment, permit early recognition of congestive failure, and help prevent inadvertent fluid overload. Any blood volume deficits which are identified should be promptly corrected.

Overhydration may be manifested by rales in the

*Acute respiratory failure is discussed in the preceding chapter.

dependent portions of the lung, excessive gain in weight, urine output over 100 ml/hour, dependent or sacral edema, or fullness of the neck veins. If overhydration is evident, fluids should be restricted and sodium withheld. If the fluid overload threatens cardiopulmonary function, diuretics may be required.

Antibiotic therapy should be given only as necessary to treat specific infections and known contamination. Cultures should be taken at surgery whenever contamination is present; a smear should be made simultaneously, stained with Gram's stain, and examined microscopically so that antibiotics can be selected on the basis of the general nature of the organism while culture and sensitivity tests are being completed. Prophylactic antibiotics are rarely indicated in clean surgical operations, and the incidence of wound infections is not affected by their use. They have the disadvantage of encouraging the emergence of resistant strains, so organisms which do infect the patient are more virulent. If gross contamination has occurred during surgery or if the field is grossly infected, antibiotics may be advisable. When contamination is likely to be unavoidable, antibiotics should be started 12 hours before the operation so that high concentrations will be present in the blood and in the wound.

Overdistention of the bladder may develop in the anesthetized or sedated patient—particularly one who has been overhydrated during the operation—and the physician must be alert to this possibility. The lower abdomen should be percussed for bladder dullness in the immediate postoperative period; if a suprapubic mass is detected and the patient cannot void, immediate bladder catheter drainage is indicated. If the patient voids frequent small amounts (50 ml) postoperatively, overdistention should also be suspected. The patient is likely to be voiding small amounts from a grossly distended bladder.

As soon as possible in the postoperative course, the patient should be encouraged to sit up, cough and breathe deeply, and, if possible, to walk. The upright position permits expansion of basilar lung segments, which may be collapsed as a result of diaphragm elevation due to abdominal distention or splinting of the posterior aspects of the chest wall. Walking increases the circulation of the lower extremities and thus helps to prevent venous stasis and lessens the danger of venous thromboembolism.

Oral intake should be restricted postoperatively to prevent air swallowing and aggravation of abdominal distention. Return of function of the gastrointestinal tract after abdominal surgery is verified by the passing of flatus, spontaneous bowel movement, and normal peristalsis on auscultation. At this point, liquids can be instituted safely and the diet advanced as seems appropriate.

Cutdowns utilized for intravenous fluids should be discontinued at 24–48 hours to minimize the risk of thrombophlebitis. It is preferable to switch the intravenous catheter every 1–2 days rather than to accept the risk of septic thrombophlebitis, which almost always occurs when prolonged intravenous

catheterization is utilized. (See Chapter 51 for further details.)

COMMON POSTOPERATIVE COMPLICATIONS

A postoperative complication is arbitrarily defined as any untoward event that occurs within 30 days after the operation. It may seem that myocardial infarction 2 weeks following an uneventful operation should not be listed as a surgical complication. However, the incidence of myocardial infarction in the postoperative period is higher than in similar groups of patients who have not had an operation, and the surgeon must assume that this complication was related to the surgery.

Any interruption in the smooth postoperative course must raise the question of whether a complication has developed. Careful observation of the patient and his vital signs should make it possible to determine the nature of any given postoperative complication.

Postoperative complications can be manifested by temperature, pulse, or respiratory changes. The most common abnormality in the postoperative vital signs is fever. Any rectal temperature over 37.8 C (100 F) is abnormal, and a temperature over 38.3 C (101 F) indicates that a major problem is present. Tachypnea, tachycardia, hypertension, and hypotension are also frequent manifestations of surgical complications. Any change in one or more of these vital signs should be investigated and the cause determined.

Complications can occur in the wound, in any body cavity, or in organs adjacent to or far removed from the site of operation. Complications may be immediate or delayed and may be either a direct result of the surgery or of the disease being treated (eg, peritonitis following surgery for a ruptured appendix). Complications may occur as a result of immobilization (venous thrombosis) or exposure to an infectious agent in the hospital ("hospital acquired infections"). Complications can result from aggravation of some underlying condition such as an unsuspected bleeding disorder or from stress to a marginal psychiatric patient.

Atelectasis, wound infection, ileus, urinary retention, and lower extremity venous thrombosis are the most common complications and will be discussed separately. Some complications are particularly common following catastrophic illness or secondary to other postoperative complications. These include respiratory distress syndrome, stress ulcer, gastric dilatation, renal failure, and hepatic failure. Most of the cardiovascular complications (eg, cerebrovascular accidents, myocardial infarction, and pulmonary embolism) and almost all of the serious infections (eg, peritonitis) follow some grave complication such as anastomotic disruption, postoperative hemorrhage, or shock.

Altemeier WA & others: Infections: Prophylaxis and management: A symposium. Surgery 67:369, 1970.

Bartlett RH & others: Studies on the pathogenesis and prevention of postoperative pulmonary complications. Surg Gynecol Obstet 137:925, 1973.

Bolagny BL & others: The hazards of intravenous polyethylene catheters in surgical patients. Surg Gynecol Obstet 130:342, 1970.

Cole WH: Operability in the young and aged. Ann Surg 138:145, 1953.

Cullen DJ, Cullen BL: Post-anesthetic complications. Surg Clin North Am 55:987, 1975.

Finland M, McGowan JE Jr: Nosocomial infections in surgical patients. Arch Surg 111:143, 1976.

Hamilton WK & others: Postoperative respiratory complications. Anesthesiology 25:607, 1964.

Johnstone FRC: Infection on a surgical service. Am J Surg 120:192, 1970.

Owens WD & others: Development of two indices of postoperative morbidity. Surgery 77:586, 1975.

Sheiner NM & others: Assessment of pulmonary function in postoperative patients. Am J Surg 120:714, 1970.

Subcommittee on Aseptic Methods: Aseptic methods in the operating room suite. Lancet 1:705, 763, 831, 1968.

Tera H, Aberg C: Mortality after laparotomy: A ten-year series. Acta Chir Scand 142:67, 1976.

PULMONARY COMPLICATIONS*

Most postoperative complications occur in the lungs. The incidence of those complications varies with the preoperative status of the patient, the quality of the anesthesia, the duration and type of operation, and the quality of the postoperative care. Patients with obstructive pulmonary airway disease—eg, chronic bronchitis with excessive tracheobronchial secretions—are particularly prone to develop respiratory difficulty postoperatively. Heavy smokers invariably have chronic bronchitis and fall into the high-risk group. During anesthesia, failure to aspirate secretions, faulty placement of the endotracheal tube, or failure to expand the lung fully predisposes the patient to postoperative difficulty, as does extubation in a still heavily sedated patient also. The longer the operation, the more vulnerable the patient becomes to minor omissions of these procedures.

Certain operations—particularly thoracic and upper abdominal operations—cause discomfort with respiration and impair the patient's ability to breathe deeply and to cough. As a result, pulmonary complications are much more frequent than in operative procedures carried out on the lower abdomen, perineum, neck, or extremities. Prolonged immobility in bed, abdominal pain, and abdominal distention all predispose to respiratory difficulty in postoperative patients; postoperative procedures such as encouraging deep breathing and coughing and, in selected patients, nasotracheal aspiration of the tracheobronchial tree are direct measures used to prevent respiratory complica-

*Acute respiratory failure is discussed in Chapter 3.

tions. Appropriate use of analgesic agents, early mobilization of patients, and positional changes are of value in all patients and will lessen the incidence of postoperative pulmonary complications.

Atelectasis (Collapse of a Lung Segment or Lobe)

Atelectasis is the most common of all postoperative complications. It is thought to be due to inadequate ventilation during anesthesia, with collapse of lung segments or the accumulation of pulmonary secretions during or just after the operation. Accumulation of secretions results in obstruction of small bronchi, absorption of air, and collapse of the segment supplied by the occluded bronchus.

Atelectasis is the most common cause of postoperative fever. It usually develops within the first 48 hours following surgery. The first clinical sign of atelectasis may be present the evening after an operation. The patient may develop fever to 39 C (102 F), tachypnea (24–30/minute), and moderate tachycardia. Physical examination may reveal elevation or splinting of the diaphragm, scattered rales, and diminished breath sounds with bronchial breathing over the affected area—most commonly at the lung bases or at the posterior lung segments. There may be a shift of cardiac dullness to the affected side.

Studies in asymptomatic postoperative patients have demonstrated that arterial oxygen tensions are frequently much lower than expected. This is due to intrapulmonary shunting because it does not respond to the administration of 100% oxygen. This is presumably caused by miliary atelectasis because chest x-ray may be normal and physical signs absent.

The principal impact of atelectasis is its effect on oxygenation of the blood. The healthy patient usually has considerable reserve, and minor degrees of atelectasis are well tolerated. In patients with marginal reserve or cardiovascular disease, the consequences of atelectasis can be great, and hypoxia is the precipitating cause of many cases of cardiac arrhythmia and cardiac arrest.

Atelectasis is aggravated by a painful abdominal or thoracic incision with sufficient splinting of the chest wall or diaphragm to impair ventilation. Inability to breathe deeply and to cough results in progression of the process.

Treatment consists of stimulating the patient to cough and to breathe deeply. Frequent change in position of the bedridden patient facilitates ventilation of all portions of the lung. The patient should be moved from side to side and encouraged to sit up. If he cannot be moved easily or is uncooperative, endotracheal aspiration should be performed using a plastic catheter passed nasotracheally. This can be done by pulling the tongue forward with a sponge and asking the patient to inhale as the catheter is passed nasally. Analgesic drugs in small amounts may diminish incisional pain and improve the depth of spontaneous ventilation. Humidification of inspired air will assist in liquefying and mobilizing bronchial secretions. When the atelectasis involves an entire lung or lobe and is resistant to treatment, bronchoscopy may be indicated to remove secretions or mucus plugs.

Respiratory Distress Syndrome

Respiratory distress syndrome has been recognized only in the past few years. It has many names, eg, pump lung, shock lung, posttraumatic lung, fat embolism, and congestive atelectasis. This complication was at first thought to result only from cardiopulmonary bypass. Similar lesions are now being recognized in patients who have been in septic, hypovolemic, or cardiogenic shock or other types of catastrophic illness such as massive trauma or major burns.

Careful monitoring of postoperative patients with major illnesses has permitted definition of the clinical syndrome. Within 24 hours of clinical insult, the patient develops evidence of respiratory distress characterized by tachypnea and increased effort in breathing. Arterial blood gas measurements done at this time may show arterial desaturation. Chest x-ray shows diffuse, cloudy infiltrates in the lung, but—in contrast to pulmonary edema—there is no cardiac enlargement or increase in vascular markings. The compliance of the lungs is decreased, and increased pressures are often required to maintain adequate tidal volume. If the arterial P_{O_2} is below 60 mm Hg, an endotracheal tube should be inserted and positive pressure ventilation instituted with sufficient oxygen to maintain an arterial P_{O_2} of 70–100 mm Hg. With prompt institution of positive pressure ventilation, the lesion is usually reversible, and gradual recovery can be expected in 3–7 days. If the insult is severe and the patient's underlying disease is not fully reversible, a progressive downhill course may result until oxygen arterial desaturation occurs and the patient dies. On gross examination, the lung is hemorrhagic and resembles liver. If autopsy is done within the first 24 hours, histopathologic examination reveals platelet and fibrin emboli filling the microcirculation of the lung. This is followed by congestion and then intra-alveolar hemorrhage at 24–72 hours. When death occurs between 3 and 5 days, intra-alveolar hemorrhage and hyaline membranes are the predominant lesions. If the patient is carried successfully through this insult, pneumonitis develops, so that when death occurs more than 5–7 days following onset the principal changes are those of pneumonia.

Aspiration

Aspiration is a relatively common pulmonary complication. It usually occurs in the postanesthetic period when the patient's sensorium is depressed and vital reflexes such as swallowing and coughing are absent. Aspiration of oral secretions may precipitate pneumonia, usually mild, which can be managed by vigorous therapy similar to that described for atelectasis.

A far more lethal type of aspiration is that secondary to vomiting and inhalation of gastric contents. This can occur during induction of anesthesia in any patient who has recently eaten or one who has ileus

and a stomach distended with intestinal contents. Aspiration of gastric contents produces a severe, often lethal pneumonitis. For this reason, access to the airway should be obtained immediately with an endotracheal tube or bronchoscope. This permits suctioning of aspirated material from the tracheobronchial tree and thorough cleansing with saline irrigations. Nonetheless, severe tracheobronchitis may result from breakdown of the mucosa and secondary infection.

Positive pressure ventilation and specific antibiotics directed against cultured organisms offer the most effective treatment.

Pneumonia

Pneumonia may follow atelectasis or aspiration. Aspiration of nasopharyngeal secretions during or immediately following anesthesia or atelectasis may set the stage for the development of frank pneumonia. Abundant tracheobronchial secretions from preexisting bronchitis also predispose to this complication.

Atelectasis produces moderate fever in the first few postoperative days. If this is followed by higher temperatures, systemic toxicity, and respiratory difficulty, a presumptive diagnosis of pneumonia is justified.

As pneumonia develops, secretions become progressively more abundant and the cough becomes productive. Physical examination may reveal evidence of pulmonary consolidation, and numerous coarse rales are often present. Chest x-ray usually shows diffuse patchy infiltrates or lobar consolidation.

The treatment of pneumonia includes deep breathing and coughing. The patient should be encouraged to change position and move about as much as possible. Nasotracheal suction may be used to stimulate the cough reflex. Specific antibiotic therapy should be instituted on the basis of sputum smears and revised as dictated by subsequent cultures and sensitivity tests. In weak or debilitated patients with a poor cough reflex, endotracheal intubation or tracheostomy may be indicated to permit adequate ventilation. Positive pressure ventilation may improve the depth of respiration and eliminate the work of breathing in weak or extremely ill patients.

Pulmonary Embolism & Infarction*

Pulmonary embolism and infarction are most apt to occur late in the postoperative course—on the seventh to tenth postoperative days. The diagnosis of pulmonary embolism can only be made by maintaining a high index of clinical suspicion. The early manifestations are rising respiratory and pulse rates out of proportion to the degree of fever.

It is probable that only about 10% of pulmonary emboli are recognized clinically. The remainder do not produce symptoms except for minor changes in respiratory rate. The patient may be assumed to have atelectasis or some other minor pulmonary condition.

---

*See Chapters 21 and 39 for detailed discussions of the causes, prevention, diagnosis, and treatment of pulmonary emboli.

Fewer than 10% of emboli produce pulmonary infarction with the classical manifestations: hemoptysis, pleuritic pain, and a wedge-shaped density on chest x-ray.

Bartlett JG: Treatment of postoperative pulmonary infections. Surg Clin North Am 55:1355, 1975.

Blaisdell FW: Pathophysiology of the respiratory distress syndrome. Arch Surg 108:44, 1974.

Blaisdell FW, Lewis FR: *The Respiratory Distress Syndrome of Shock and Trauma.* Saunders, 1977.

Crane C & others: The management of major pulmonary embolism. Surg Gynecol Obstet 128:27, 1969.

Craven JL & others: The evaluation of the incentive spirometer in the management of postoperative pulmonary complications. Br J Surg 61:793, 1974.

Cullen DJ, Cullen BL: Postanesthetic complications. Surg Clin North Am 55:987, 1975.

Harbord RP, Bosworth PP: Therapy for atelectasis. Anesth Analg 45:684, 1966.

Hirsch EF & others: The lung: Responses to trauma, surgery, and sepsis. Surg Clin North Am 56:909, 1976.

Jones RH, Sabiston DC Jr: Pulmonary embolism. Surg Clin North Am 56:891, 1976.

Spray SB, Zuidema GD, Cameron JL: Aspiration pneumonia. Am J Surg 131:701, 1976.

Tarhan S & others: Risk of anesthesia and surgery in patients with chronic bronchitis and chronic obstructive pulmonary disease. Surgery 74:720, 1973.

Teplitz C: The core pathobiology and integrated medical science of adult acute respiratory insufficiency. Surg Clin North Am 56:1091, 1976.

Zikria BA & others: Alterations in ventilatory function: Breathing patterns following surgical trauma. Ann Surg 179:1, 1974.

WOUND COMPLICATIONS

Wound complications include hematoma, seroma, infection, dehiscence, evisceration, and hernia.

Hematoma

Hematoma formation is the initial wound complication as it is manifested in the immediate postoperative period. Bleeding usually starts at the time of wound closure, and the hematoma presents within the first 24 hours. If the bleeding is in the deeper portions of a large wound, the presence of a hematoma may not be recognized until secondary infection occurs. The presence of blood in the wound increases local vascularity, and bleeding is potentiated by the presence of the hematoma. When the hematoma produces swelling and discomfort, the wound should be reexplored under sterile conditions, the hematoma evacuated, and the bleeding site controlled. When the hematoma is superficial, it may be possible to remove 1–2 sutures from the wound and express the blood. If bleeding continues despite local evacuation, wound reexploration is mandatory. Much morbidity can be averted by prompt definitive reoperation in such cases.

Seroma

Collection of serum in a wound is most apt to occur in incisions where it is difficult to avoid dead space, as in operations on the groin and breast where large flaps of skin are necessarily undermined. Meticulous closure of the wound in layers is the best way to avoid these collections. When a seroma is recognized, needle aspiration of the fluid and firm pressure may prevent recurrence. It is preferable not to open the wound because contamination of the tissue may lead to infection. When the seroma is large, it is appropriate to explore the wound in the operating room under sterile conditions. Operations on the groin, particularly along the course of the femoral artery and veins, are not only associated with a high incidence of seroma formation; but because the lymphatics of the lower extremities are often divided, a frank leak of lymph with the formation of a lymphocele may occur. Careful ligation of divided lymphatics will reduce the incidence of this complication.

Some of the apparent accumulations of serum may be due to traumatized fat. Seromas in wounds which cross very few lymphatics such as longitudinal abdominal incisions are most apt to be due to traumatic fat necrosis.

Infection*

Infection is the most common wound complication and may be due to poor surgical technic or gross contamination during the operation. The contribution of poor technic to the incidence of postoperative wound infection would be minimal if all surgeons mastered the fundamental surgical principles of gentle handling of tissue, careful hemostasis, meticulous approximation of tissues, and avoidance of dead space. Almost all wounds are contaminated to some degree; good aseptic technic ensures that wound contamination will be minimal. Given a fixed degree of contamination, the incidence of wound infection will vary from one surgeon to the next because wound infection is related to the presence or absence of dead space, which gives rise to collections of blood or serum—both ideal culture media for bacteria. Infection may be due to excessive trauma to the tissues or abuse of the electrocautery or ligatures. Another factor related to the incidence of wound infection is vascularity: the better the blood supply to a wound, the lower the incidence of infection. (See Chapter 10.)

A **clean wound** is an operative wound which has not become contaminated at any point in the operation. Herniorrhaphy and blood vessel surgery are examples of operations where the wound is clean. Infection is uncommon in these wounds; the incidence should not exceed 2%.

Contaminated operations are those in which gross contamination of the operative field has occurred. Appendectomy for rupture of the appendix and delayed laparotomy for perforated ulcer are typical examples. If the skin were closed, these wounds would

*Other aspects of wound infection are discussed in Chapter 11.

be expected to become infected. Therefore, the skin and subcutaneous tissue should be left open whenever possible. Once wound defenses have been mobilized (4–5 days), delayed primary closure of the skin and subcutaneous tissue can be carried out or the wound can be left open to close secondarily.

Contamination of the wound is most likely at the time of surgery, yet wound infections usually appear about the fifth to the seventh postoperative day. The principal exception is streptococcal infection, when erythema, fever, and systemic toxicity develop within 24–48 hours of contamination. Since streptococcal infections are nonnecrotizing, specific systemic antibiotic therapy is all that is needed and the wound does not require drainage. Wound infections which appear 5–7 days after surgery are invariably necrotizing and are due to staphylococci or gram-negative rods. These infections produce collections of pus in the wound, and treatment requires adequate drainage. This usually consists of opening the wound widely. These infections almost always occur in subcutaneous tissue and only rarely involve the fascial or muscle layers, so that opening the superficial layers of the wound establishes adequate drainage and permits the natural defense mechanisms of the body to become operative. This results in rapid control of the infection with or without specific antibiotics. The wound can sometimes be closed secondarily several days later.

When the wound is opened and infection seems to be coming from fascia or deep to the fascia, one should suspect an intraperitoneal source (see next section).

Dehiscence, Evisceration, & Hernia

Partial wound **dehiscence** implies disruption of several layers of the wound, such as peritoneum and fascia, but not all layers. Without treatment, fascial dehiscence is usually followed by complete dehiscence of the skin closure and escape of viscera from the abdominal or thoracic cavity **(evisceration)**.

Wound dehiscence and evisceration usually begin in the first few days after operation, when coughing or straining disrupts the peritoneum and fascial layers and a loop of bowel or omentum is pushed into the wound. However, it does not generally become clinically evident until the fifth to tenth days, often just after the skin sutures are removed. A sudden discharge of serosanguineous fluid heralds fascial and peritoneal dehiscence, and evisceration will follow unless the wound is opened and repaired.

The patient may describe a popping sensation during an episode of coughing. Once wound dehiscence starts, the wound usually opens like a zipper as additional strain is exerted on the remaining sutures. Prompt reoperation is imperative when dehiscence is recognized; evisceration requires reoperation to return abdominal contents to the peritoneal cavity. In rare cases in obese, poor-risk patients, dehiscence may be controlled by scultetus type binders, but this is inevitably followed by incisional hernia (see below).

Wound dehiscence or evisceration should not occur. Wound closure should be adapted to the requirements of the situation. For example, one would use a different closure for an emergency operation on an alcoholic who may have delirium tremens postoperatively than on a patient undergoing an elective cholecystectomy. Although retention sutures do not prevent the complications of dehiscence and evisceration, they can give considerable support to the wound and decrease the chances of a major disruption.

Incisional **herniation** occurs principally in abdominal incisions. It is the result of an unrecognized, unrepaired wound dehiscence, where the fascial layers have separated and the skin closure remains intact. Although the opening in the fascia may be small initially, progressive enlargement of a ventral hernia is inevitable. Therefore, unless some serious medical contraindication exists, all ventral incisional hernias should be repaired when recognized. Delaying repair always results in a larger, more complicated hernia. If major contraindications to surgery exist, it may be appropriate to control the ventral hernia with binders or girdles. (See Chapter 36.)

Alexander HC, Prudden JF: The causes of abdominal wound disruption. Surg Gynecol Obstet 122:1223, 1966.

Brote L, Gillquist R, Tarnvik A: Wound infections in general surgery. Acta Chir Scand 142:99, 1976.

Cruse PJE, Foord R: A five-year prospective study of 23,649 surgical wounds. Arch Surg 107:206, 1973.

Grace RH, Cox S: Incidence of incisional hernia after dehiscence of the abdominal wound. Am J Surg 131:210, 1976.

Polk HC Jr: Diminished surgical infection by systemic antibiotic administration in potentially contaminated operations. (Editorial.) Surgery 75:312, 1974.

Polk HC Jr, Fry D, Flint LM Jr: Dissemination and causes of infection. Surg Clin North Am 56:817, 1976.

Stone HH, Hester TR Jr: Incisional and peritoneal infection after emergency celiotomy. Ann Surg 177:669, 1973.

Stone HH & others: Antibiotic prophylaxis in gastric, biliary and colonic surgery. Ann Surg 184:443, 1976.

Walker PE: Surgical infection rates: What should they be? Bull Am Coll Surg 46:7, 1961.

PERITONEAL COMPLICATIONS

Following laparotomy—particularly one carried out for some type of septic condition such as a ruptured appendix, perforated ulcer, or perforated diverticulum—contamination may spread throughout the peritoneal cavity and cause generalized peritonitis or abscesses. Peritonitis and intraperitoneal abscess formation are rare complications after clean elective operations. The peritoneum is capable of withstanding large amounts of contamination, and infection usually occurs only when contamination is overwhelming. Overlooked collections of pus after rupture of a hollow viscus, contamination of the peritoneal cavity with intestinal contents or blood, and serum or lymph collections which provide culture media for bacteria are the usual sources of intraperitoneal infection. When laparotomy is done for a perforated viscus, careful cleaning of the abdominal cavity is mandatory; all foreign material and abscesses should be carefully aspirated. Undrained pockets of contamination set the stage for infection.

The complications which occur within the peritoneal cavity are generalized peritonitis and localized infection (intraperitoneal abscess).

Whenever a patient develops unexplained fever or localized abdominal pain after laparotomy, particularly from the fourth to seventh days, the wound should be inspected. If no wound infection is present, digital examination of the rectum should be done to rule out the possibility of pelvic abscess. The presence of cul-de-sac fullness and tenderness is diagnostic. The abdomen and flanks should be carefully palpated. Absence of local tenderness suggests that the abscess is not within the portion of the peritoneal cavity below the costal margins. Because intra-abdominal abscesses are frequently in the subphrenic and subhepatic spaces, these areas are the most likely possibilities if no other site is found.

Chest x-ray is often helpful because abscesses under the diaphragm may be associated with fluid in the sulcus and atelectasis of the lower lobes of the lung. The pulmonary changes may confuse the picture and suggest an intrapleural process, but primary pulmonary disease, for all practical purposes, rarely develops after the first few postoperative days unless some other complication supervenes. Inspiratory-expiratory films or fluoroscopy may reveal impaired motion of the diaphragm. Abnormal gas collections or air-fluid levels may also help localize the infection when gas-forming organisms are present. Collections along the undersurface of the liver (the subhepatic space) are difficult to diagnose because there may be little evidence on the chest film to help localize the collection. Careful observation will usually reveal splinting on the appropriate side and a high diaphragm. The diagnosis and treatment of intraperitoneal abscess and peritonitis are discussed in Chapter 11.

Altemeier WA & others: Intra-abdominal abscesses. Am J Surg 125:70, 1973.

DeCosse JJ & others: Subphrenic abscess. Surg Gynecol Obstet 138:841, 1974.

Golovsky D, Connolly WB: Observations on wound drainage with review of the literature. Med J Aust 1:289, 1976.

Konvolinka CW, Olearczyk A: Subphrenic abscess. Curr Probl Surg, Jan 1972.

CARDIAC COMPLICATIONS

Cardiac complications following major surgery are rare unless other major complications develop. Although any cardiac disability occurring during the postoperative period has been considered as being due to the "stress" of operation, most cardiac complications are secondary to some other major complication.

If the patient's hydration is adequate and the operation is competently and cleanly done, the incidence of cardiac complications is low even in patients with advanced cardiac impairment. Patients with valvular heart disease and old myocardial infarctions tolerate surgery quite well. Myocardial infarction does present an increased risk if the operation is undertaken sooner than 6 months after the ischemic episode. Whenever possible, surgery should be delayed in patients who have had a recent infarction or who have ischemic changes on ECG.

Pulmonary Edema

In older patients with cardiac disease, excessive administration of fluids or blood during surgery or in the immediate postoperative period may precipitate pulmonary edema. This can be combated by administering digitalis and diuretics and by restricting fluids. Positive pressure ventilation may also be of great help if congestive failure does not respond promptly to conventional medical management.

Cardiac Arrhythmias

Cardiac arrhythmias may complicate the postoperative course. Many are secondary to anoxia caused by atelectasis or pneumonia. If the patient is on digitalis, hypokalemia may produce an arrhythmia. Other cases may be related to electrolyte imbalance, particularly hypokalemia; myocardial infarction; or pulmonary embolism.

Treatment consists of management of congestive failure. Paroxysmal atrial tachycardia may respond to carotid artery compression. Other arrhythmias may be reversed by cardioversion.

Myocardial Infarctions

Myocardial infarction is a serious complication of major surgery. If the patient is conscious, he may complain of chest pain. It is important to recognize myocardial infarction as such and not assume that the patient is complaining about incisional pain. If cardiovascular instability or an arrhythmia develops in any postoperative patient, an ECG should be obtained. Careful monitoring should be started once the signs of myocardial infarction are evident. Blood gas studies should be obtained, and oxygen and respiratory support administered as indicated. Careful fluid management is necessary. Anticoagulation should be considered in the postoperative patient with a massive myocardial infarct, particularly if low cardiac output and shock result, since there is a high incidence of thromboembolic complications in these patients.

Dack S: Postoperative myocardial infarction. Am J Cardiol 12: 423, 1963.

Hechtman HB: Adequate circulatory responses or cardiovascular failure. Surg Clin North Am 56:929, 1976.

Merideth J: Cardiac arrhythmias in the postoperative patient. Surg Clin North Am 49:1083, 1969.

Perlroth MG, Hultgren HN: The cardiac patient and general surgery. JAMA 232:1279, 1975.

GASTROINTESTINAL COMPLICATIONS

Gastrointestinal complications are most apt to occur after abdominal operations, but they may complicate other types of surgery also. In fact, any serious illness may cause malfunction of the gastrointestinal tract.

Gastric Distention

Gastric distention is a common postoperative complication. It is caused by accumulation of air and, to a lesser extent, gastric juices in the stomach. Most patients with nausea or paralytic ileus will swallow air. If intestinal peristalsis is depressed, the swallowed gas accumulates in the stomach. As gastric distention increases, the movement of the diaphragm may be inhibited. When the patient develops hyperpnea and appears to be splinting his diaphragm, a nasogastric tube should be passed immediately and gastric aspiration continued as long as ileus persists.

Gastric Dilatation

Gastric dilatation, as opposed to gastric distention, is a grave postoperative complication that has been associated with a mortality rate as high as 50%. Gastric dilatation is defined as distention of the stomach with fluid to such a degree that secondary hemorrhage occurs. The gastric juice becomes brown or black from the contained hemoglobin. Gastric dilatation may follow untreated gastric distention, but it often is a complication of very serious illnesses of the type associated with low cardiac output. The cause may be extra-abdominal and may be associated with such procedures as open heart surgery.

Vomiting of brown or black material means gastric dilatation or intestinal obstruction. A nasogastric tube should be passed immediately. Decompression of the stomach reverses the gastric distention and secondary bleeding and prevents aspiration. Large quantities of fluid and electrolytes usually have been lost. Shock is often present, and correction of hypovolemia is an intrinsic part of therapy.

Postoperative Ileus (Paralytic Ileus)

Paralytic ileus consists of paralysis of intestinal peristalsis or lack of effective coordinated peristalsis. It usually follows an intraperitoneal irritative process such as laparotomy or intraperitoneal sepsis. It may result from low cardiac output and may occasionally be due to extra-abdominal causes such as pneumonia. The abdomen is distended and quiet. Faint or irregular bursts of peristalsis may be heard. An abdominal x-ray will demonstrate distended loops of bowel, but gas is typically distributed throughout both large and small bowel.

Air is often swallowed reflexly, and this accounts for many cases of gastric and bowel distention. When ileus is advanced, secretions may be "sequestered" in the bowel, adding to the distention.

Abdominal distention in the postoperative period is usually the result of ileus, and, if moderate or severe, should be treated by nasogastric decompression. Gastric aspiration usually reveals green to yellow fluid—as opposed to that seen with bowel obstruction or gastric dilatation, when the fluid is dark brown or black. The quantity aspirated is usually not more than 1–2 liters/24 hours; if larger quantities are obtained, bowel obstruction should be suspected. Once the nasogastric tube has been inserted, it should be kept on suction until intestinal peristalsis resumes and the patient begins to pass flatus.

Postoperative Intestinal Obstruction

Bowel obstruction may occur as a complication of any abdominal operation. It is most apt to occur as a consequence of peritonitis or generalized irritation of the peritoneal surface. These disorders produce varying degrees of adhesions. Obstruction results when these adhesions trap or kink a segment of intestine. Adhesions which form within the first few weeks after surgery are rubbery and seldom result in compromise of the circulation of the bowel. Dense, fibrous adhesions develop over 8–12 weeks or more, and these are more likely to entrap bowel and cause strangulation. For this reason, it is possible to treat early postoperative bowel obstruction conservatively by nasogastric intubation or by the use of long intestinal tubes. Tube decompression will often result in realignment of the bowel and relief of the obstruction, or adhesions may give enough to allow spontaneous decompression. When conservative management is elected, an arbitrary period of tube decompression should be decided upon in advance; if the obstruction does not respond within that period (eg, 48–72 hours), reoperation is necessary. Intestinal obstruction is discussed in detail in Chapter 34.

Pancreatitis

Pancreatitis is an infrequent complication of surgery. It is seen just often enough to be considered in the differential diagnosis of postoperative fever or severe ileus, particularly when the surgery involved the biliary tract or when the dissection was carried out in the duodenal or pancreatic area. It can follow any type of surgery and has been described as a complication of appendectomy.

Postoperative pancreatitis causes symptoms in the first 48 hours following surgery. It can vary in severity from mild edematous to full-blown hemorrhagic pancreatitis. Pain may be negligible or may be thought to be incisional. The temperature may go as high as 40 C (104 F). Epigastric tenderness and ileus are consistent findings, although the epigastric tenderness may be confused with incisional tenderness.

Postoperative pancreatitis and its management are discussed further in Chapter 30.

Stress Ulcer

This complication is most apt to occur in the patient who has developed some other grave complication. For this reason, the mortality rate is high. The principal manifestation is gastrointestinal bleeding. A more detailed consideration of stress ulcer may be found in Chapter 26.

Pseudomembranous Enterocolitis

Pseudomembranous enterocolitis is diffuse ulceration with fibromembrane formation involving colon or small bowel. There is usually an overgrowth of staphylococci, and indeed it was once thought that this lesion was the result of administration of broad-spectrum antibiotics. Another explanation is mucosal damage of the gut following decreased circulation in unrecognized shock or low flow states. It is a toxic, depleting lesion, requiring urgent administration of intravenous fluids and electrolytes and specific antibiotics.

Fecal Impaction

Fecal impaction is a common cause of diarrhea in the postoperative patient. Whenever the patient develops diarrhea, digital rectal examination should be done immediately. If hard stool is encountered in the ampulla, the diagnosis of fecal impaction is verified. The condition is due to limitation of oral fluids and is especially prone to occur in elderly patients and others confined to bed. It may be aggravated by previous gastrointestinal series or barium enema with accumulation of barium in the colon.

The treatment of fecal impaction is digital disimpaction of the firm fecal masses after an oil retention enema.

Parotitis

Postoperative parotitis occurs mainly in elderly and debilitated patients. As is true of pancreatitis also, dehydration leading to parotid duct obstruction by viscous secretions may set the stage for parotitis. Poor oral hygiene with overgrowth of mouth organisms favors infection of the gland. Parotitis usually develops late in the postoperative course. Fever may be moderate or high, with a septic swing. On inspection, the parotid gland is enlarged and swollen. Inflammation of the orifice of Stensen's duct or purulent discharge from the duct is conclusive evidence of parotitis. The usual causative organism is *Staphylococcus aureus*.

Therapy consists of hydration, stimulation of parotid secretions by encouraging the patient to suck on hard candies, and specific antibiotics.

Feiner H: Pancreatitis after cardiac surgery: A morphologic study. Am J Surg 131:684, 1976.

Flowers RS, Kyle K, Hoerr SO: Postoperative hemorrhage from stress ulceration of the stomach and duodenum. Am J Surg 119:632, 1970.

Krippaehne WW, Hunt TK, Dunphy JE: Acute suppurative parotitis: A study of 161 cases. Ann Surg 156:251, 1962.

Silen W, Skillman JJ: Gastrointestinal responses to injury and infection. Surg Clin North Am 56:945, 1976.

White TT, Morgan A, Hopton D: Postoperative pancreatitis: A study of 70 cases. Am J Surg 120:132, 1970.

HEPATIC COMPLICATIONS

Hepatic problems are rare but potentially lethal complications of surgery.

Liver Abscess

Intrahepatic abscess can occur as a complication of intra-abdominal sepsis and has the same causes as other intraperitoneal infections. Hepatic abscess may develop as a result of cholangitis secondary to biliary obstruction or septic thrombophlebitis of the portal vein (pylephlebitis) (see Chapter 32).

Hepatic abscess is difficult to recognize and is rarely diagnosed early. When it is suspected, hepatic radioisotope scanning should be done. Demonstration of an intrahepatic filling defect confirms the diagnosis, and drainage should be instituted.

Serum Hepatitis

Administration of blood or plasma carries the risk of serum hepatitis. This is usually a late postoperative complication; it rarely occurs earlier than 4 weeks and seldom later than 12 weeks following blood transfusion. This virulent infection is transmitted in the serum of donors, and the hepatitis which occurs following serum injection is far more lethal than infectious hepatitis. Its incidence varies with the quality of banked blood but is probably 0.1–0.5% of all patients who receive blood. It is fatal in about 10% of cases. Conservatism in the administration of blood or blood products and careful selection of blood donors can decrease the incidence of this complication.

Postoperative Jaundice

Postoperative jaundice may develop from various causes other than the above. Serum hepatitis can be ruled out if enzyme studies are normal. Halothane (Fluothane) anesthesia has been held responsible for postoperative liver necrosis and may account for occasional jaundice, particularly if the patient has been anesthetized repeatedly with halothane.

Hemolysis due to transfusion reaction should always be considered in the differential diagnosis of jaundice, and the Coombs test should be done to establish the presence or absence of transfusion antibodies.

Shock produces a characteristic lesion (centrilobular necrosis) that may simulate obstructive jaundice. The jaundice presumably results partially as a result of liver damage plus an increased bilirubin load, which follows blood transfusion. Most of the serum enzyme studies are normal, although the alkaline phosphatase is elevated.

Drug-induced cholestasis should always be considered and the drug history reviewed for drugs which can produce jaundice.

Allen JG: Commercially obtained blood and serum hepatitis. Surg Gynecol Obstet 131:277, 1970.

Howard JH, Simmons RL: Viral infections and the surgical patient. Surg Gynecol Obstet 137:1029, 1973.

Klion FM & others: Hepatitis after exposure to halothane. Ann Intern Med 71:467, 1969.

Lim RC Jr, Lau G, Steele M: Prevention of complications after liver trauma. Am J Surg 132:156, 1976.

Norton L & others: Liver failure in the postoperative patient. Surgery 78:6, 1975.

Nunes G, Blaisdell FW, Margaretten W: Mechanism of hepatic dysfunction following shock and trauma. Arch Surg 100:546, 1970.

Strasberg SM, Silver MD: Postoperative hepatogenic jaundice. Surg Gynecol Obstet 132:81, 1971.

Tompkins RK: The hepatorenal syndrome. Surg Gynecol Obstet 143:297, 1976.

URINARY COMPLICATIONS

Urinary complications are common after surgery. Prompt diagnosis and treatment are essential to prevent serious residual disability.

Urinary Retention

Urinary retention is a frequent postoperative complication. It is most apt to occur after simple rectal operations such as hemorrhoidectomy, although it may occur after any type of surgery. It tends to occur in bedridden patients and in elderly males with prostatic disease. Excessive administration of fluids during operation may result in distention of the bladder, causing bladder decompensation and urinary retention.

All sets of postoperative orders should include a request to record urine output. The patient should be examined immediately after operation and the suprapubic area percussed to determine bladder size. If the patient has not voided by the evening of the day of surgery and fluid therapy has been adequate, bladder distention should be suspected and confirmed by palpation or percussion.

The normal capacity of the urinary bladder is 500 ml. If this capacity is exceeded, permanent damage to the urinary tract may result. Therefore, if his condition permits, the patient should be encouraged to get out of bed to void on the evening after his operation. If the patient is unable to void, a catheter should be passed into the bladder using sterile precautions. If less than 300 ml of urine are found, the catheter should be removed. If more than 500 ml are released from the bladder, the catheter should be left in place until acute abdominal pain has subsided or until the patient is able to move around or stand to void. Inadequate decompression of the bladder or unskilled catheterization may lead to urinary tract infection.

Urinary Tract Infection

Urinary tract infection may develop immediately in the postoperative period in a patient with preexisting contamination of the urinary tract. This is due to the urinary retention that follows surgery, anesthesia, or immobilization. The normal bladder is uncontaminated before surgery and remains so unless bacteria are introduced by instrumentation or catheterization. The systemic manifestations of urinary tract infection usually develop within 48 hours after removal of the urinary catheter. Fever due to urinary tract infections is usually high and may reach 40 C (104 F). Infection may be suspected when, despite high fever, the patient is not as toxic as would be expected with most other conditions that cause high fever. Flank tenderness may be present, suggesting pyelonephritis. Pus or bacteria are seen in the urine sediment. Residual urine, which is usually present, tends to perpetuate the infection and predisposes to ascending infection and pyelonephritis.

Treatment includes forcing fluids and encouraging activity to facilitate complete emptying of the bladder. After urine specimens are obtained for culture, appropriate antibiotic therapy should be instituted based on the appearance of the organisms on a gram-stained smear. Reinstitution of catheter drainage may be necessary in patients with residual urine of 100 ml or more. Older patients with preexisting prostatic hypertrophy may require prostatic resection to permit complete emptying of the bladder. (See Chapter 43.)

Renal Failure

Renal failure is a relatively rare but serious complication of surgery. Oliguria is present when hourly urinary output drops below 30 ml/hour—the amount required to excrete metabolic wastes—and may reflect renal failure. It tends to occur in patients with other serious postoperative complications. With better fluid management and prompt treatment of shock, renal failure occurs much less frequently now than in the past. In patients with catastrophic illness, renal failure may occur as a terminal event.

Renal failure can often be prevented by careful monitoring of the postoperative urinary output in all patients undergoing major surgery or in patients with major surgical illnesses. If urinary output falls below 30 ml/hour, careful monitoring of cardiovascular function should be instituted. Using the central venous pressure as a guide to prevent fluid overload, plasma or blood should be added to restore vascular volume. With correction of hypovolemia, renal output usually returns promptly and renal tubular damage is avoided. Occasionally, drug reactions or prolonged shock may result in renal tubular necrosis, and the kidneys may not respond to the initial fluid load. If this is the case, fluid should be restricted to the amount required to replace insensible losses and fluid and electrolytes carefully monitored. A rising serum potassium which approaches 7 mEq/liter should be treated promptly.

Baek S-M & others: Clinical determinants of survival from postoperative renal failure. Surg Gynecol Obstet 140:685, 1975.

Danielson R: Differential diagnosis and treatment of oliguria in post-traumatic and post-operative patients. Surg Clin North Am 55:697, 1975.

Hinman F: Postoperative overdistention of the bladder. Surg Gynecol Obstet 142:901, 1976.

Lucas CE: The renal response to acute injury and sepsis. Surg Clin North Am 56:953, 1976.

Ray JF & others: Post-operative renal failure in the 1970s: A continuing challenge. Arch Surg 108:526, 1974.

Thornton GF, Andriole VT: Bacteriuria during indwelling catheter drainage. II. Effect of a closed sterile drainage system. JAMA 214:339, 1970.

CEREBRAL COMPLICATIONS

Cerebral changes occur relatively rarely in the postoperative period.

Cerebrovascular Accident

An older patient with underlying cerebrovascular disease may develop thrombosis of a cerebral vessel and suffer a cerebrovascular accident. This seems to occur more frequently after other serious complications, particularly those associated with shock.

Treatment is conservative and supportive. Hypertension should be treated to lessen the risk of secondary hemorrhage into the ischemic infarct, a lethal complication. The airway should be kept clear and oxygen administered as necessary to maintain normal arterial oxygenation.

Cerebral Fat Embolism

Cerebral fat embolism is a syndrome which has been thought to be a complication of long bone fracture in which there is release of medullary fat into the blood stream. However, fat embolism is far more complicated than this, for many of the fat droplets noted in the blood streams of patients following trauma are derived from the plasma. Fat embolism can occur in patients who have had a major episode of shock in which there has been no trauma. Fat embolism is most common in patients with the combination of extensive soft tissue injury and hypovolemic shock.

In many cases, fat droplets can be found simultaneously in urine and sputum. However, fat droplets can be seen in many patients who never develop the full-fledged syndrome. If these patients are monitored carefully, it is apparent that the primary lesion is not cerebral but pulmonary and that cerebral symptoms do not occur if anoxia is prevented. Fat embolism results when tissue damage has been extensive. The presence of gross fat and marrow droplets in the blood stream demonstrates that tissue thromboplastin release has been massive. Thromboplastin initiates intravascular clotting as the primary event which produces the organ damage in the fat embolism syndrome. The greatest impact is on the lung, and treatment is as described for respiratory distress syndrome.

POSTOPERATIVE PSYCHOSIS

Psychosis may occur in any postoperative patient, particularly if the patient is apprehensive about the operation or his ability to recover fully. It is most apt to occur in a previously marginally adjusted patient. Psychosis can also be toxic in origin or drug-induced. In addition, hypoxia is always a possibility in the confused or agitated patient, so that assessment of blood gases ($P_{O_2} + P_{CO_2}$) should be carried out immediately and before assuming that a psychiatric problem exists.

Postoperative psychosis is usually self-limited. With support and sedation, the patient usually recovers without residual emotional disability.

VENOUS COMPLICATIONS

The venous complications following surgery are due to clot formation, usually in the lower extremities, accompanied by varying degrees of local reaction and obstruction. Significant clinical sequelae are pulmonary embolism and deep venous incompetence in the lower extremities. This topic is discussed in detail in Chapter 39.

● ● ●

General References

Alexander JW: Emerging concepts in the control of surgical infections. Surgery 75:934, 1974.

Altemeier WA & others: Changing patterns in surgical infections. Ann Surg 178:436, 1973.

Bartlett RH, Gazzinaga AB, Geraghty TR: Respiratory maneuvers to prevent postoperative pulmonary complications: A critical review. JAMA 224:1017, 1973.

Byrne JJ & others: Symposium on postoperative complications. Am J Surg 116:325, 1968.

Committee on Pre and Postoperative Care, American College of Surgeons: *Manual of Preoperative and Postoperative Care,* 2nd ed. Kinney JM, Egdahl RH, Zuidema GD (editorial subcommittee). Saunders, 1971.

Doromal NM, Canter JW: Hyperosmolar hyperglycemic nonketotic coma complicating intravenous hyperalimentation. Surg Gynecol Obstet 136:729, 1973.

Feller I, Richards KE, Pierson CL: Prevention of postoperative infections. Surg Clin North Am 52:1361, 1972.

LaMont JT, Isselbacher KJ: Postoperative jaundice. N Engl J Med 288:305, 1973.

Noe JM: Mechanism of capillarity in surgical dressings. Surg Gynecol Obstet 143:454, 1976.

Strode JE (editor): Symposium on unexpected complications of surgery. Surg Clin North Am 50:289, 1970.

Walters MB, Stanger HAD, Rotem CE: Complications with percutaneous central venous catheters. JAMA 220:1455, 1972.

Webb WR (editor): Pulmonary problems in surgery. Surg Clin North Am 54:5, 1974.

Zarem HA: The management of complications in head and neck surgery. Surg Clin North Am 53:191, 1973.

5...
Special Medical Problems in Surgical Patients

ENDOCRINE DISEASE & THE SURGICAL PATIENT
Peter H. Forsham, MD

Surgery on the endocrine glands is covered elsewhere in this text. General surgery performed on patients with endocrine diseases is the subject of this section. In any patient with endocrine disease, surgery carries the usual surgical hazards with some added risks. Endocrine abnormalities must be recognized and treated preoperatively if mishaps during and after surgery are to be prevented.

Blood Pressure & Circulatory Competence

These are endangered in patients with diminished blood volume as in adrenocortical insufficiency, pheochromocytoma, and diabetes insipidus.

In **adrenocortical insufficiency**, fluid depletion is due to sodium and water loss from the kidneys and from the intestinal tract. The preoperative management must include administration of saline and fludrocortisone 0.1–0.2 mg orally, for at least 2 days preoperatively. Soluble hydrocortisone phosphate or hemisuccinate, 50 mg IM every 6 hours, should be given on the day of surgery. When blood volume is adequately restored, one rarely has to use vasoconstrictors.

In a patient with **pheochromocytoma** whose plasma volume is decreased preoperatively, administration of human albumin and, on occasion, blood transfusion are indicated to prevent postoperative hypotension. This may prove lifesaving in view of the usual postoperative tendency to hypotension. Alphablocking agents such as phenoxybenzamine (Dibenzyline) may also be used preoperatively for a few days for gradual restoration of blood volume.

In patients with **diabetes insipidus** and increased free water clearance, there is marked hemoconcentration and a low plasma volume. Administration of vasopressin (Pitressin), 10–20 units IM every 4 hours or an infusion of 5 units in 1000 ml of 5% dextrose in water, is indicated preoperatively until the elevated osmolality returns to normal.

Respiratory Exchange

Adequate respiratory exchange is severely reduced in patients with advanced **myxedema**. Surgery should be postponed until the patient has been made euthyroid with thyroid therapy. If surgery must be done within a week, give triiodothyronine (T_3), 50–100 μg/day orally. If it is possible to delay surgery for a month, sodium thyroxine (T_4), 0.1–0.4 mg/day orally, is used. In both instances, the dosage must be reduced if angina pectoris or cardiac irregularities appear.

Very **obese** subjects should be placed on assisted ventilation during and after surgery to guarantee adequate oxygenation.

Anesthesia

Anesthesia may be life-threatening in patients with untreated **adrenocortical** or **pituitary insufficiency** or a lack of **hypothalamic corticotropin releasing** factors. The cortisol response to stress is absent, and the anesthesia, with its accompanying vasodilatation, may lead to vascular collapse. There is little point in pretesting for such a possible collapse. Adrenocortical response with either metyrapone or insulin hypoglycemia shows an inadequate correlation with vascular collapse at surgery. Most surgeons and anesthesiologists prefer to give hydrocortisone phosphate preoperatively whenever there is a possibility that hypotension due to adrenocortical insufficiency may occur during or after surgery. The dosage is 100 mg or more IM.

Hemostasis

Hemostasis may be particularly difficult in patients with excessive glucocorticoid activity, as in **Cushing's disease**, when their ability to constrict arteriolar and larger vessels is severely diminished. Severed blood vessels will thus produce increased bleeding in the surgical field unless one ties vessels with care.

Infections

Wound infection must be guarded against in **Cushing's disease**. The intrinsic protective mechanisms are markedly diminished in this condition because of excess glucocorticoid secretion. Phagocytosis and antibody formation are inadequate.

In uncontrolled **diabetes mellitus**, phagocytosis is markedly diminished and there is thus an increased danger of wound infection.

In both diseases, the use of bactericidal rather than bacteriostatic antibiotics is preferable.

Wound Healing

Wound healing is definitely impaired in **Cushing's disease** because of impaired fibroplasia and enhanced tissue breakdown, in part as a result of increased lysosomal membrane instability. Uncontrolled **diabetes mellitus** impairs wound healing by reducing protein synthesis. Marked **hyperthyroidism** leads to a negative nitrogen balance. **Hypogonadism** definitely slows wound healing because of a lack of anabolic steroids.

Bowel & Bladder Functions

Abnormal bowel function may be related to endocrinopathies. Diarrhea is found in far-advanced **diabetic autonomic neuropathy** and at times in the presence of **hyperthyroidism**. Constipation is seen with excess calcium levels in **hyperparathyroidism** and with **hypothyroidism** or **myxedema**. Simple remedial treatment should precede surgery.

Bladder function may be inadequate in advanced long-standing **diabetes mellitus** because of impairment of the parasympathetic system.

Nutrition

Alimentation calls for specific management in several instances of endocrine disease before and after surgery. In patients with **hyperthyroidism**, a caloric intake as high as 4000 Cal/day may be required during the acute stages of the disease, together with water-soluble vitamin supplementation since these vitamins are used up excessively in this condition. A high-protein diet with at least 120 g of protein and 2 g of calcium should be given to patients with **Cushing's disease** in order to affect the negative nitrogen balance and osteoporosis to some extent. A diet low in sodium and high in potassium must precede surgery in patients with **primary aldosteronism** in order to overcome the dangerously low serum potassium with its tendency to cause ascending paralysis of the extremities. Preoperative **anemia** calls for iron supplementation and, more importantly, appropriate endocrine substitution therapy for many weeks preoperatively if the anemia is due to **myxedema**, **Addison's disease**, male **hypogonadism**, or **diabetes mellitus** associated with renal insufficiency.

Management of Surgery in the Diabetic Patient

Well-controlled diabetes mellitus probably does not increase operative risk. However, the uncontrolled diabetic must be properly treated and controlled before elective surgery. In emergency situations, constant vigilance is necessary to prevent complications. In all major surgical procedures, the patient must be under constant care to prevent ketosis or hypoglycemic reactions.

A clear distinction must be drawn between a diabetic controlled on **diet** and perhaps **oral medications** and one who is **insulin-dependent**. In the former group, an attempt should be made to minimize the period of overnight starvation so that it does not exceed 6–8 hours. After surgery, blood or urinary glucose levels should be determined. If possible, oral treatment should be maintained and, in addition, 10% glucose in water should be infused slowly intravenously up to 2000 ml/day. This will furnish the carbohydrate necessary to minimize ketoacidosis.

There are 2 alternative ways to manage an insulin-dependent diabetic after an overnight fast.

The traditional method is to give subcutaneously two-thirds of the short-acting (regular) insulin and one-third of the intermediate-acting (lente or NPH) insulin, U-100, on the morning of surgery. This is immediately followed by an infusion of 10% dextrose in water at 100 ml/hour (ie, 5 g of glucose per hour) up to 2000 ml during and after surgery.

Alternatively, the level of fasting blood sugar obtained on the morning of surgery should be divided by 150; this gives approximately the units of regular insulin per hour needed for blood sugar control during the operation. Regular insulin (U-100) should be added to 1000 ml of 5% dextrose in 0.25 N saline solution in amounts to yield the calculated units per hour in each 100 ml. *Example:* Fasting blood sugar 300 mg/100 ml; 300 divided by 150 equals 2 units of regular insulin per hour. Add 20 units of regular insulin to 1000 ml of dextrose in 0.25 N saline and infuse at 100 ml/hour. To correct for the adsorption of insulin to the equipment, add an extra 5 units to the container. Continue the intravenous infusion for 2–8 hours and then resume subcutaneous insulin while following either blood glucose or freshly voided urine glucose. At no time should either insulin or carbohydrates be withheld before, during, or after major surgery.

Because diabetics are especially vulnerable to urinary tract infections, urinary catheters should not be used unless they are absolutely required. If so, the patient should be given prophylactic antibiotics.

Ambulation

Early ambulation after surgery is imperative in patients who undergo **total adrenalectomy** or removal of an **active adrenal adenoma** for Cushing's disease to minimize thromboembolic phenomena. Sudden reduction in cortisol apparently predisposes to thromboembolism, and adequate hydration and early ambulation are therefore necessary.

Sedation

With **Cushing's disease**, where wakefulness and anxiety are extreme, one must use high doses of hypnotics. Unless **Addison's disease** is well treated, sedatives and cholinergics (eg, bethanechol [Urecholine]) have increased potency and must be used with care. In **hyperthyroidism**, because of the rapid metabolic rate, doses of hypnotics and analgesics must be markedly increased to be effective. This is true also in **hypoparathyroidism**, with its increased neuromuscular irritability. The reverse is true in **hypothyroidism** and in **hyperparathyroidism**.

CARDIAC DISEASE &
THE SURGICAL PATIENT
Maurice Sokolow, MD

Anesthesia and general surgery are a hazard to any patient, but the risk in the cardiac patient is increased. Acidosis, arterial hypoxemia, hypercapnia, decreased systemic vascular resistance, decreased cardiac contractility and conduction, and hypotension with or without decreased blood volume, which may result from bleeding—all are deleterious to cardiovascular function. Other important hazards are arrhythmias due to release of catecholamines, bradycardia due to the muscle-relaxing drugs, and impaired coronary perfusion as a result of decreased systemic flow. Postoperative problems that must be considered include thromboembolism, myocardial ischemia, and atelectasis. Because of these hazards, the physician is often asked to evaluate a surgical patient with heart disease preoperatively and judge whether the risk is warranted.

Key questions that must be answered are the following: (1) Is the operation urgent or elective? (2) If elective, does the patient have cardiac disease? (3) What is the risk of the underlying surgical disease if surgery is not performed? (4) What additional risk does the heart disease impose on the surgical procedure? (5) Is the surgical diagnosis correct, or could the symptoms, such as abdominal pain, be a manifestation of cardiac disease and not of surgical disease? The physician must distinguish between elective and emergency procedures and judge when the risk of surgery exceeds the risk of the underlying disease or vice versa.

Urgent operations must be done regardless of the underlying cardiac disease in such conditions as gross hemorrhage, strangulated hernia, perforation of the bowel or gallbladder, bowel obstruction, dissecting or ruptured aortic aneurysm, or removal of large arterial emboli which threaten life or limb.

The presence of heart disease does not mean that the patient will not tolerate the surgical procedure; one should not withhold a lifesaving procedure merely because of the presence of heart disease.

Cardiac Conditions Masquerading as Surgical Illnesses

Gastrointestinal symptoms, including acute abdominal pain, may so dominate the clinical picture that heart disease is not recognized or, if recognized, is thought not to be responsible for the symptoms. Early evidence of cardiac failure is often overlooked because it is overshadowed by the gastrointestinal symptoms. The most common causes of diagnostic confusion are the following:

(1) Angina pectoris or myocardial infarction presenting with epigastric pain.

(2) Fairly abrupt right heart failure presenting with right upper quadrant pain simulating gallbladder disease. This is particularly apt to occur in patients with tight mitral valve disease who develop atrial fibrillation or following exercise in patients with mild right heart failure.

(3) Slowly developing right heart failure, which may present with nonspecific gastrointestinal symptoms of anorexia, nausea, a sensation of heaviness and fullness after meals, and perhaps vomiting. These lead to weight loss and may seem to justify a diagnosis of carcinoma of the upper gastrointestinal tract. If there are no murmurs, the diagnosis of heart disease is often missed.

(4) Pulmonary infarction presenting as jaundice, leading to a diagnosis of biliary tract disease.

(5) Right heart failure or constrictive pericarditis presenting as ascites.

(6) Dysphagia, which may be the presenting symptom in a variety of heart diseases, eg, mitral stenosis with a large left atrium, pericarditis, aortic aneurysm, dissecting aneurysm, or anomalies of the aortic arch.

(7) Acute rheumatic fever, which may present with acute abdominal pain, especially in children.

(8) Acute abdominal pain, which may result from emboli to the splenic, renal, or mesenteric arteries in infective endocarditis or atrial fibrillation.

(9) Nausea and vomiting, which may occur in cardiac failure, especially as a result of digitalis therapy.

Space does not permit a differential diagnosis of these conditions, but one should search for positive diagnostic evidence of heart disease: (1) A history of angina pectoris, dyspnea on effort, orthopnea, or previous ventricular arrhythmias or atrial fibrillation or flutter. (2) Cardiac enlargement with a left ventricular heave, with or without characteristic murmurs. (3) Evidence of right heart failure, with increased venous pressure, enlarged and tender liver, and edema or ascites. Orthopnea, decreased vital capacity, and rales and gallop rhythm may be present in left ventricular failure. (4) Signs of myocardial necrosis with fever, tachycardia, or enzyme changes. (5) Typical serial ECG changes of ischemia, infarction, hypertrophy, pericarditis, etc. (6) Radiologic evidence of cardiac enlargement or pulmonary venous congestion.

Considering the possibility of heart disease often leads to an adequate examination and appropriate therapy.

Preoperative Evaluation of the Surgical Patient
With Cardiovascular Disease

The presence of heart disease is recognized on the basis of symptoms, significant murmurs, an enlarged heart or evidence of cardiac failure, hypertension, conduction defects, and atrial fibrillation or flutter and ventricular arrhythmias. A history of angina pectoris or previous myocardial infarction, Stokes-Adams attacks, cardiac failure, intermittent claudication, or cerebral ischemic attacks may alert the physician to the possibility of cardiac disease. A history of antihypertensive treatment or treatment for cardiac failure may be obtained.

Preoperative ECGs are often valuable but may be

difficult to interpret. A patient with known previous myocardial infarction may have a normal ECG; even more importantly, a patient with "unstable angina" may have a normal ECG. Conversely, grossly abnormal changes may be due to an old healed infarct and are therefore of less importance in deciding whether or not elective surgery should be performed. A baseline ECG is advisable to interpret postoperative changes. An ECG may also show evidence of digitalis therapy, electrolyte disturbances, conduction defects, or arrhythmias. In general, a stable abnormality in the ECG in the absence of cardiac failure or a change in the pattern of angina pectoris indicates that the patient will probably tolerate surgery almost as well as a normal individual. Such a patient with a healed previous myocardial infarction has an added mortality risk of about 3–5%.

The most important conditions which should contraindicate elective surgery are recent angina pectoris, a crescendo change in the pattern of angina pectoris in recent weeks or months, unstable angina, acute myocardial infarction, severe aortic stenosis, a high degree of atrioventricular block, untreated cardiac failure, and severe hypertension.

Specific Disease Problems

A. Coronary Heart Disease: The usual patient seen for preoperative evaluation is an older individual with possible coronary heart disease. One searches for a history of recent crescendo in the character of the anginal pain, pain at rest, unstable angina, or the possibility of recent myocardial infarction. If known coronary disease is stable, without change in the pattern of pain or in serial ECGs; if there are no symptoms or signs of cardiac failure; and if at least 6 months have elapsed since myocardial infarction, the surgeon can proceed if the indications for surgery are clear and definite.

Emergency surgery must often be done despite a recent myocardial infarction, but the mortality rate is high. Important but not lifesaving surgery is best delayed at least 3 weeks if possible. Purely elective surgery should be postponed for 3–6 months whenever possible.

B. Hypertension: Patients with uncomplicated chronic hypertension, even with left ventricular hypertrophy and an abnormal ECG, tolerate surgery without significantly increased mortality if there are no evidences of coronary heart disease or cardiac failure and if renal function is normal. Unless the diastolic pressure exceeds 110 mm Hg, it is best to decrease or even stop antihypertensive medication for a week prior to surgery and to be certain, if thiazides have been used, that the body potassium has been replenished. The catechol depletion that follows the administration of reserpine, methyldopa, and guanethidine can be managed satisfactorily if the anesthesiologist is forewarned and prepared to give vasopressors in the event of hypotension.

C. Arrhythmias: Chronic atrial fibrillation with a well-controlled ventricular rate does not increase the risk of surgery, nor does an asymptomatic isolated right or left bundle branch block. Second or third degree atrioventricular block is a warning sign, especially if associated with left ventricular conduction defects; a transvenous electrode catheter should be inserted into the right ventricle prior to the surgical procedure and the patient monitored with a pacemaker available in case ventricular standstill occurs. Infrequent atrial or ventricular premature beats usually do not require special treatment and can often be relieved with phenobarbital. If ventricular premature beats are frequent and from multiple foci, they are best depressed with drugs such as quinidine, 200–400 mg orally 2–4 times daily, or procainamide, 250–500 mg orally 3 or 4 times daily. They can be quickly abolished with lidocaine, 2% solution (20 mg/ml), 50 mg IV, followed by an intravenous infusion of 1–2 mg/minute.

D. Valvular Heart Disease: Severe aortic stenosis, tight mitral stenosis, and severe coronary ostial involvement due to syphilitic aortitis are the 3 major "valvular" conditions in which general surgery presents a considerably increased hazard. An aortic systolic murmur not associated with evidence of severe aortic valvular disease or significant left ventricular hypertrophy does not increase the mortality. Mitral insufficiency is usually tolerated well, but tight mitral stenosis, especially if the patient has sinus rhythm, may result in acute pulmonary edema if the patient abruptly fibrillates during surgery.

E. Congenital Heart Disease: In the absence of cardiac failure, ventricular septal defect and atrial septal defect usually pose no particular problems or extra hazard. Pulmonary hypertension with Eisenmenger's syndrome carries a significantly increased mortality risk, and surgery should be performed only upon urgent indications. Patients with coarctation of the aorta and patent ductus arteriosus should have their congenital lesions repaired before undergoing elective general surgical procedures. Mild pulmonic stenosis is not a contraindication to elective surgery, but severe pulmonic stenosis is a contraindication because of the hazard of acute right heart failure and a reversed shunt through the foramen ovale or a small atrial septal defect. Patients with tetralogy of Fallot are relatively poor surgical risks because of the polycythemia and because of the possibility of contraction of the infundibulum of the right ventricle with resulting poor cardiac output.

F. Cardiac Failure: Patients with mild cardiac failure whose symptoms and signs are controlled with digitalis and diuretics have only a slightly increased risk from general surgery provided ordinary activity does not cause symptoms. Patients with dyspnea on walking on level ground, orthopnea or nocturnal dyspnea, and signs of cardiac failure such as gallop rhythm, increased venous pressure, and rales are at a significantly increased risk, and surgery should be delayed if possible. Cardiac failure should be treated adequately before surgery. It is desirable to have the patient stabilized for at least a month before surgery, avoiding digitalis toxicity and potassium depletion by diuretics. Diuretics and digitalis can then be withheld for a few days before surgery. Digitalization of a patient with cardiac hypertrophy but no heart failure is probably unwise because of the hazard of digitalis toxicity, including arrhythmias. Although digitalis has a positive inotropic action even in normal hearts, clinical evidence of benefit from the drug has not been demonstrated when it has been given to patients with hypertrophy but no failure. If there is a question about whether or not heart failure is present preoperatively, a period of bed rest and restricted dietary sodium may be adequate treatment.

Special Precautions

With the emphasis on the surgical condition, one may overlook certain special precautions such as stopping anticoagulants, continuing corticosteroids, and inquiring about antihypertensive or insulin therapy and the patient's hypersensitivities to drugs, especially antibiotics or sedatives. Particular care should be taken to control the speed and volume of sodium-containing infusions used in preoperative preparation. Red cell mass rather than whole blood should be given to the cardiac patient if there is substantial blood loss or severe anemia preoperatively. The infusion should be given while the patient is supine so that he can be placed in the Fowler position if dyspnea or rales develop. The surgeon should examine the patient frequently during the infusion and should be alert for dyspnea, orthopnea, rales, or elevation of venous pressure.

If urgent surgery is required in the patient with severe coronary disease, aortic stenosis, or atrioventricular block, the patient should be monitored with an arterial catheter, pulmonary artery pressure determinations, periodic blood gas measurements, and an electrode transvenous catheter in case ventricular standstill or arrhythmia occurs. Isoproterenol, pressor agents, lidocaine, and facilities for defibrillation should be readily available.

The choice and details of anesthesia are left to the anesthesiologist, but it is well to alert him to any possible problems he might expect.

Aberman A, Fulop M: The metabolic and respiratory acidosis of acute pulmonary edema. Ann Intern Med 76:173, 1972.

Angelini P & others: Cardiac arrhythmias during and after heart surgery. Prog Cardiovasc Dis 16:469, 1974.

Ayres SM, Grace WJ: Inappropriate ventilation and hypoxemia as causes of cardiac arrhythmias: The control of arrhythmias without antiarrhythmic drugs. Am J Med 46:495, 1969.

Bigger JT Jr, Heissenbuttel RH: Clinical use of antiarrhythmic drugs. Postgrad Med 47:No. 1, 119, 1970.

Byyny R: Withdrawal from glucocorticoid therapy. N Engl J Med 295:30, 1976.

Fisch C: Relation of electrolyte disturbances to cardiac arrhythmias. Circulation 47:408, 1973.

Giardina EV, Heissenbuttel RH, Bigger JT Jr: Intermittent intravenous procaine amide to treat ventricular arrhythmias. Ann Intern Med 78:183, 1973.

Hurst JW, Logue RB: The Heart, Arteries and Veins, 3rd ed. McGraw-Hill, 1974.

Hurst JW & others: Management of patients with atrial fibrillation. Am J Med 37:728, 1964.

Katz RL, Epstein RG: The interaction of anesthetic agents and adrenergic drugs to produce cardiac arrhythmias. Anesthesiology 29:763, 1968.

Lindsay J, Hurst JW: Drug therapy of dissecting aortic aneurysms. Circulation 37:216, 1968.

Marriott HJL: Differential diagnosis of supraventricular and ventricular tachycardia. Geriatrics 25:91, 1970.

Monahan JP, Denes P, Rosen KM: Portable electrocardiographic monitoring. Arch Intern Med 135:1188, 1975.

Moss AJ, Davis RJ: Brady-tachy syndrome. Prog Cardiovasc Dis 16:439, 1974.

Perlroth MG, Hultgren HN: The cardiac patient and general surgery. JAMA 232:1279, 1975.

Raftery EB: Diagnosis and management of myocardial infarction during anesthesia. Proc R Soc Med 66:1209, 1973.

Sagar S & others: Efficacy of low-dose heparin in prevention of extensive deep-vein thrombosis in patients undergoing total-hip replacement. Lancet 1:1151, 1976.

Salem MR & others: Cardiac arrest related to anesthesia: Contributing factors in infants and children. JAMA 233:238, 1975.

Samet P: Cardiac arrhythmias: Hemodynamic sequelae of cardiac arrhythmias. Circulation 47:399, 1973.

Schamroth L: How to approach an arrhythmia. Circulation 47:420, 1973.

Shubin H, Weil MH: Bacterial shock. JAMA 235:421, 1976.

Williams JF Jr, Morrow AG, Braunwald E: The incidence and management of "medical" complications following cardiac operations. Circulation 32:608, 1975.

RESPIRATORY DISEASE & THE SURGICAL PATIENT
John L. Wilson, MD

Operative morbidity and mortality are increased by acute or chronic respiratory tract diseases.

Specific Diseases & Problems

A. Acute Conditions: Acute respiratory tract infections (colds, pharyngitis, tonsillitis, bronchitis, or pneumonitis) are contraindications to elective surgery because they are associated with an increased postoperative incidence of atelectasis and pneumonitis. The patient should be completely recovered from an acute respiratory tract infection for 1–2 weeks before operation. If emergency operation must be undertaken in the presence of acute respiratory tract infection, avoid inhalation anesthesia, if possible; employ prophylactic measures for atelectasis postoperatively; and administer an antibiotic (after obtaining throat or sputum culture) if the infection is marked or progressive. Penicillin G is usually given until the antibiotic sensitivity report on throat or sputum culture is obtained.

B. Chronic Bronchopulmonary Infection: Chronic

bronchitis, bronchiectasis, emphysema, asthma, pulmonary fibrosis, and tuberculosis are among the disorders commonly associated with chronic bronchial or pulmonary infection in surgical patients. Many of these patients are elderly, and smoking is often an aggravating factor. Any patient who has smoked over 20 cigarettes a day for 10 years can be assumed to have chronic bronchopulmonary inflammation. Heavy smokers should abstain for at least 2 weeks before elective major surgery. The major hazard in the patient with chronic bronchopulmonary infection is excessive bronchial secretions during and after operation with a marked tendency to postoperative atelectasis and pneumonitis. Preoperative evaluation of these patients includes sputum culture and sensitivity with preoperative control of infection by administration of the appropriate antibiotic. When bronchospasm is present as determined by physical examination and pulmonary function tests, it is treated pre- and postoperatively with a mist bronchodilator.

C. Chronic Pulmonary Insufficiency: Diminished pulmonary reserve is caused by a wide variety of disorders, particularly those mentioned above as associated with bronchopulmonary infection. When there is clinical evidence of chronically reduced lung function such as significant shortness of breath not due to extrapulmonary causes, pulmonary function tests are indicated in connection with preoperative evaluation. Reevaluation of lung function after treatment for infection and bronchospasm will frequently show improvement. During operation, the patient with chronic pulmonary insufficiency can usually be well oxygenated by the anesthesiologist. Problems begin to arise during the immediate postoperative period when atelectasis, hypoxia, and hypercapnia are the imminent dangers. These may be foreseen and minimized by careful preoperative evaluation and preparation and by intensive postoperative care. Consequently, with the exception of those thoracic resections which reduce pulmonary reserves to an intolerable level, pulmonary insufficiency is rarely severe enough to contraindicate necessary surgery.

D. Preoperative Evaluation of Pulmonary Function: Preoperative pulmonary function tests are useful in selected patients to assess the risk of postoperative pulmonary complications and to determine the need for preoperative treatment of existing pulmonary conditions. Not all patients require pulmonary function tests preoperatively. Indications for testing include exertional dyspnea, chronic cough, sputum production, wheezing or asthma, and a history of heavy smoking. Individuals in vigorous health with good exercise tolerance and no pulmonary symptoms have good pulmonary reserve, and tests are generally superfluous. Operations on the thorax and abdomen cause the greatest temporary reduction in pulmonary function and are associated with the highest morbidity and mortality rates from pulmonary complications. Therefore, pulmonary function tests prior to such procedures should be considered in the presence of even slight symptoms and signs, particularly in older pa-

Table 5–1. Indicators of high risk of postoperative pulmonary complications.

Test	Normal Value*	High Risk
VC	4.8 liters	< 1.0 liters
FEV_1	4.0 liters	< 0.5 liters
MEFR	400 liters/min	< 100 liters/min
MVV	150 liters/min	< 50 liters/min
Pa_{O_2}	75–100 mm Hg	< 55 mm Hg
Pa_{CO_2}	35–45 mm Hg	> 45 mm Hg

*These normal values are for healthy, resting young men. A detailed description of symbols and tests may be found in Chapter 3.

tients in whom chronic obstructive lung disease, emphysema, and other pulmonary abnormalities are common findings.

Pulmonary function can usually be adequately evaluated by an appropriate combination of the following examinations: history, physical examination, posteroanterior and lateral chest x-ray, electrocardiography, spirometry, maximum voluntary ventilation (MVV), and arterial blood gases. Radioisotope ventilation-perfusion scan of the lung is a noninvasive method for determining the functional state of various anatomic portions of the lung when major pulmonary resection is anticipated.

Numerous investigators have attempted to correlate various pulmonary function tests with the risk of postoperative pulmonary complications. As a result, minimal levels of function have been identified below which the incidence of pulmonary complications and even death tends to increase sharply. Such data, summarized in Table 5–1, are useful but must be combined with sound clinical judgment in order to reach valid conclusions regarding individual patients.

The risk of postoperative pulmonary complications can be reduced significantly by preoperative treatment in patients with partially correctable problems such as chronic bronchitis from smoking or infection and chronic obstructive lung disease with bronchospasm. Helpful measures are cessation of smoking for several weeks before surgery, sputum culture and specific or empiric antibiotic therapy, inhalation therapy with heated or ultrasonic mist with or without bronchodilator drugs, and chest physical therapy.

Auchincloss JH: Preoperative evaluation of pulmonary function. Surg Clin North Am 54:1015, 1974.

Hodgkin JE: Evaluation before thoracotomy. West J Med 122:104, 1975.

Miller RD: Preoperative pulmonary evaluation of the dyspneic surgical candidate. Surg Clin North Am 53:805, 1973.

Schwaber JR: Evaluation of respiratory status in surgical patients. Surg Clin North Am 50:637, 1970.

Stein M, Cassara EL: Preoperative pulmonary evaluation and therapy for surgical patients. JAMA 211:787, 1970.

RENAL DISEASE & THE SURGICAL PATIENT
Allen I. Arieff, MD

More patients with renal disease are undergoing surgery now than in the past, largely because of new technics for the management of patients with acute or chronic renal failure. Because of these advances, elective surgery is not usually deferred because of renal disease. In most cases, a simple work-up will suffice to screen patients for the presence of unsuspected renal disease. A complete urinalysis and measurement of serum creatinine, albumin, and BUN, when combined with the history and physical examination, will disclose impaired renal function. Suggestive findings include hematuria, proteinuria, hypoalbuminemia, and elevated BUN or serum creatinine.

If potential complications are anticipated, renal disease per se is rarely a contraindication to surgery. In patients with chronic renal failure who do not require maintenance dialysis (GFR usually exceeds 15 ml/min, with serum creatinine less than 9 mg/100 ml), preoperative hydration and blood transfusion to raise the hematocrit above 32% are usually required. During surgery, strict attention to fluid balance is essential, since dehydration will often precipitate acute renal failure.

In patients maintained by intermittent dialysis therapy (GFR below 5 ml/min), transfusion to a hematocrit above 32% is usually necessary preoperatively. These patients are more susceptible to infection, and, because they are anephric, fluid and electrolyte management is more difficult. Patients on dialysis tend to be hypercatabolic and malnourished, and this tendency will be accentuated by surgery. Excessive accumulation of toxic metabolites can be minimized by performing dialysis the day before surgery and as soon postoperatively as allowed by considerations of hemostasis.

Certain renal diseases often present unique hazards. In particular, patients with renal insufficiency due to diabetes mellitus are more susceptible to infection and cardiovascular complications such as stroke and acute myocardial infarction and demonstrate poorer wound healing. Diagnostic procedures which would be benign to most patients can be disastrous to the diabetic. Acute renal failure has been frequently reported after intravenous urography and other intravenous dye studies. Patients with macroglobulinemia, multiple myeloma, and amyloid renal disease also show a propensity to develop acute renal failure after intravenous contrast procedures. Patients with obstructive jaundice have a higher than expected incidence of postoperative renal failure.

Drugs & the Kidney

Many drugs are toxic to the kidney. Therapeutic agents whose dosage should be modified in patients with renal disease include antibiotics, antituberculosis agents, anti-inflammatory agents, hypoglycemic agents, analgesics and anesthetics, hypnotics, and antineoplas-

tic drugs. The number of drugs is too vast to list here, and the reader is referred to the nearly complete list (with recommended dosage modifications) in the chapter by Anderson and others cited in the references below. The worst offenders are antibiotics such as gentamicin, kanamycin, methicillin, tetracyclines, and amphotericin B, gold salts, analgesics such as phenacetin, hypoglycemic drugs such as phenformin, and anesthetic drugs, including methoxyflurane. These drugs are potentially even more toxic when used in combination. For example, the cephalosporin antibiotics are usually not nephrotoxic when used alone, but the combination of cephalothin and gentamicin commonly leads to acute renal failure.

Digitalis preparations deserve special mention because they are used so frequently in elderly patients who may require surgery. Although these drugs are largely protein-bound, excretion (with the exception of digitoxin) is mainly (85%) by the renal route, and dosage must be modified accordingly in patients with renal insufficiency. A number of technics for dosage modification have been devised, based on the patient's creatinine clearance and body weight. With normal renal function, about 20% of body digoxin stores are lost daily, while with a 50% reduction in renal function only 10% will be lost each day. Thus, maintenance digoxin dosage is reduced in proportion to the decline in GFR. Digitoxin, unlike digoxin, is not significantly excreted by the kidneys.

Acute Oliguria & Acute Renal Failure

Acute oliguria (urine output less than 20 ml/hour) in the surgical patient can be of either intrinsic (renal) or extrinsic origin. The more common extrinsic causes include reduced effective blood volume (prerenal), which may be due to actual external fluid loss, as with hemorrhage, dehydration, and gastrointestinal fluid loss, or to internal "third space" accumulation of fluid, as may occur with bowel obstruction, pancreatitis, and trauma to a limb. Postrenal extrinsic causes of oliguria include prostatic hypertrophy, retroperitoneal tumor, and unilateral stone or tumor in a solitary kidney. Oliguria due to intrinsic renal damage is commonly called **acute tubular necrosis**. Acute tubular necrosis with *normal* 24-hour urine volume is an uncommon variant called polyuric acute tubular necrosis.

There are several simple tests that should enable the physician to distinguish between extrinsic causes of oliguria versus acute renal failure (ARF). In patients with ARF, the urine sediment usually contains renal tubular cells and renal tubular cell casts. The urine sodium concentration usually exceeds 40 mEq/liter in patients with ARF and is below 20 mEq/liter in patients with prerenal azotemia. In most patients with prerenal azotemia, the 1-hour phenolsulfonphthalein (PSP) excretion test exceeds 5%; the urine/plasma (U/P) creatinine ratio exceeds 40:1; and the U/P osmolar ratio exceeds 1.1:1. Additional diagnostic procedures include evaluating the response to intravenous mannitol (12.5 g) or furosemide (80 mg). An increase of urine volume to over 40 ml/hour within 2 hours is strong evidence that oliguria is due to extrinsic causes.

If it is determined that the patient has ARF, he should be put in readiness for dialysis as soon as possible. This will involve preparation of an arteriovenous shunt or fistula for vascular access if hemodialysis is to be done, or insertion of a peritoneal cannula if peritoneal dialysis is selected. The decision between peritoneal dialysis versus hemodialysis in patients with ARF is not resolved at present, with certain advantages claimed for each procedure. Relative contraindications to the use of peritoneal dialysis include an abdominal vascular prosthesis (as in repair of an aortic aneurysm) and systemic hypotension (because of reduced peritoneal blood flow), whereas a pronounced bleeding tendency constitutes a relative contraindication to the use of hemodialysis. Although the use of dialysis has markedly altered the treatment of patients with ARF, the physician should not let the assembled gadgetry cause him to forget other fundamental principles of treatment. These include prevention and treatment of infection, maintenance of fluid and electrolyte balance, and adequate nutrition. Hyperalimentation involving administration of essential amino acids may reverse the negative nitrogen balance often associated with ARF and improve survival. (See Chapter 12.)

Over the past decade there has been a reappraisal of the use of dialysis therapy for patients with ARF. Whereas such patients had previously been dialyzed only as a means of managing symptoms (hyperkalemia, pericardial effusion, obtundation), the trend now is toward early dialysis regardless of symptoms or the results of blood chemical analyses. In addition, dialysis is usually performed every 2–3 days—again, regardless of the blood chemical tests. Such prophylactic dialysis has been found to significantly reduce both the mortality rate and the occurrence of such complications as gastrointestinal bleeding and sepsis.

Abel RM & others: Improved survival from acute renal failure after treatment with intravenous essential L-amino acids and glucose: Results of a prospective double blind study. N Engl J Med 288:695, 1973.

Anderson RJ & others: Fate of drugs in renal failure. Pages 1911–1948 in: *The Kidney*. Brenner BM, Rector FC (editors). Saunders, 1976.

Blagg CR: Visual and vascular problems in dialyzed diabetic patients. Kidney Int 6 (Suppl 1):27, 1974.

Diaz-Buxo JA & others: Acute renal failure after excretory urography in diabetic patients. Ann Intern Med 83:155, 1975.

Harrington JT, Cohen JJ: Acute oliguria. N Engl J Med 292:89, 1975.

Kleinknecht D & others: Uremic and nonuremic complications in acute renal failure: Evaluation of early and frequent dialysis on prognosis. Kidney Int 1:190, 1972.

Maher JF: Toxic nephropathy. Pages 1355–1395 in: *The Kidney*. Brenner BM, Rector FC (editors). Saunders, 1976.

Silberman H: Renal failure and the surgeon. Surg Gynecol Obstet 144:775, 1977.

HEMATOLOGIC DISEASE & THE SURGICAL PATIENT

Ralph O. Wallerstein, MD

SURGERY IN PATIENTS WITH CHRONIC ANEMIA

In general, moderate anemia does not increase the hazard of surgery. If time permits, deficiencies of iron, folic acid, and vitamin B_{12} should be repaired before surgery. In an emergency, chronic anemia can be corrected by transfusion of red cells before surgery. If possible, surgery should be deferred for a day after transfusion to permit readjustment of blood volume and to give the transfused red cells a chance to accumulate a normal level of 2,3-diphosphoglycerate (2,3-DPG), which is necessary for efficient delivery of oxygen to tissues.

Patients with iron deficiency anemia and the various congenital and acquired hemolytic anemias do not ordinarily present any unusual risk at surgery provided their blood volumes and hemoglobin levels are adequate. In the case of megaloblastic anemias (pernicious anemia and folic acid deficiency), surgery should be deferred if possible until specific therapy (vitamin B_{12} or folic acid) has repaired the generalized tissue defect, because in these 2 conditions all the cells of the body are affected by the vitamin deficiency, and transfusions alone do not render surgery safe. It probably takes 1–2 weeks to reach adequate tissue levels.

Patients with sickle cell disease have a higher than normal incidence of thromboses, particularly pulmonary. Normally, only a few cells in the circulation are sickled; under the stressful conditions of surgery, excessive sickling, which leads to thrombosis, may be precipitated by anoxia and acidosis. The risk is greatest in a patient with sickle cell anemia, but it is appreciable also in hemoglobin S-C disease and in sickle cell thalassemia. If these patients must go to surgery, they should be transfused with whole blood to normal hemoglobin levels; this creates a relative dilution of their own sickled cells and prevents sickling of large columns of abnormal cells in the smaller blood vessels. A patient with sickle cell trait has an increased risk during surgery if the oxygen saturation falls to critically low levels.

A few hematologic disorders may simulate acute abdominal surgical conditions.

Sickle Cell Anemia

Painful abdominal crises in sickle cell anemia may suggest appendicitis, cholecystitis, a ruptured viscus, or other acute abdominal conditions. In a patient with this kind of pain, helpful diagnostic points are the following: (1) In sickle cell anemia, while the abdomen may be rigid and tender, peristalsis is usually normal. (2) The leukocytosis in sickle cell anemia has a relatively normal differential count—eg, with a white count of 20,000/µl, only 65% granulocytes. (3) Leukocyte counts above 20,000/µl are seen in many patients with sickle cell anemia who are not acutely ill.

Henoch-Schönlein or Nonthrombocytopenic Purpura

These conditions are usually associated with obvious skin lesions or perhaps hematuria but may on occasion present with acute abdominal pain. The symptoms are apparently due to bleeding into the bowel wall. Intussusception may occur and may require surgical intervention. No reliably effective treatment is available to prevent or treat abnormal bleeding, although prednisone may be tried.

Lead Poisoning

Lead poisoning may cause acute abdominal pain. A history of possible exposure to lead may be of great importance. Laboratory clues are moderate anemia with striking stippling and a marked elevation of urinary coproporphyrin. The diagnosis is established by finding elevated lead levels in blood and urine.

Abdominal Wall Hemorrhage

Hemorrhage into the abdominal wall may simulate acute appendicitis in patients with thrombocytopenia, hemophilia, or other severe coagulation disorders.

SURGERY IN PATIENTS WITH HEMATOLOGIC MALIGNANCIES

Occasionally it is necessary to operate on patients who have leukemia, lymphoma, myeloma, or related disorders. Such patients can always undergo surgery without increased risk if they are in hematologic remission, and surgery may be relatively safe in partial remission. In acute leukemia, the risk of surgery is low if the white count is not excessive, the hemoglobin is over 10 g/100 ml, and the platelet count is near 100,000/µl. Other coagulation factors are not usually disturbed in acute leukemia. If surgery must be done in spite of very abnormal blood counts and excessive bleeding develops, transfusions and platelet packs are used.

In patients with chronic myelocytic leukemia with platelet counts in excess of 1 million/µl or white counts above 100,000/µl, bleeding may be a problem. In patients with chronic lymphatic leukemia and a normal platelet count, even white counts in excess of 100,000/µl are no contraindication to surgery.

Patients with polycythemia vera have a greatly increased incidence of bleeding and thromboses. A qualitative platelet defect can be detected when the red cell count and the platelet count are high. In patients with very high packed cell volumes (over 60%), prothrombin time and partial thromboplastin time will appear falsely prolonged unless allowance is made for the relatively small plasma volume by reducing the

amount of citrate in the test tube. Similarly, fibrinogen may be too low for the volume of whole blood. When blood counts have become normal (after phlebotomy, radiotherapy, or chemotherapy), surgery is safer, but the incidence of complications is still increased.

Patients with multiple myeloma or macroglobulinemia may bleed excessively in surgery because their elevated abnormal globulin may interfere with the coagulation process. Plasmapheresis before surgery should be considered.

Patients with all of the above have no increased difficulty with wound healing or postoperative infections as long as their total granulocyte count is at least 1500/µl. The common anticancer chemotherapeutic agents—mercaptopurine (Purinethol), busulfan (Myleran), melphalan (Alkeran), methotrexate, and cyclophosphamide (Cytoxan)—do not interfere with wound healing.

SURGERY IN PATIENTS RECEIVING ANTICOAGULANTS

Heparin

Since the average dose of heparin (5000 units IV) maintains the whole blood clotting time at twice the control value for only 3–4 hours, a short wait will let the coagulation time return to normal. If a large dose has been administered, it may be necessary to neutralize its effect in a patient who suddenly becomes a candidate for emergency surgery.

Immediately after an intravenous dose of heparin, the amount of protamine sulfate required (in milligrams) is equal to 1/100 the last dose of heparin (in units). The biologic half-life of heparin is less than 1 hour. The dose of protamine is reduced if some time has elapsed since the last dose of heparin: In 30 minutes, only about half the amount of protamine is required; in 4–6 hours, there is seldom need for neutralization. After the subcutaneous administration of heparin, the dose of protamine should be only 50–75% (in mg) × 1/100 of the last heparin dose (in units), but repeated doses of protamine may be required because of the continued absorption of heparin.

Protamine should always be given by slow intravenous injection. Rapid injection may cause thrombocytopenia. If given in excessive amounts, protamine may act as a weak anticoagulant.

During open heart surgery and extracorporeal circulation, large doses of heparin are required to prevent coagulation in the pump oxygenator and the patient's circulatory system; at the end of the procedure, the heparin must be neutralized. The dose of protamine should be based on the amount of heparin used. Heparin neutralization is not required in some vascular operations if the protamine dosage is calculated and timed so as to lose its effect at the end of the operation.

Coumarin Anticoagulants

Surgery in patients given coumarin derivatives for anticoagulation is relatively safe when the prothrombin time is 25% or greater. In patients with lower values prophylactic measures are in order if surgery is necessary. Vitamin K, 5 mg IV, will return the prothrombin time to safe levels (40% or better) in approximately 4 hours and to normal levels in 24—48 hours. However, its administration may render the patient refractory to all coumarin therapy for a week or more. For immediate, transient (a few hours') restoration of normal prothrombin values, one may infuse 250—500 ml of plasma. Factors II, VII, IX, and X—the factors lowered by coumarin therapy—are quite stable in banked plasma. As an alternative, one may give the commercially available factor IX concentrate Proplex (Hyland), which also contains factors II, VII, and X. The dosage is 500 units, or 1 ampule.

Abbreviations Used in This Section	
ACD	Acid-citrate-dextrose
ACT	Activated coagulation time
AHF	Antihemophilic factor
CPD	Citrate-phosphate-dextrose
DIC	Disseminated intravascular coagulation
FDP	Fibrin degradation products
HBAg	Hepatitis B-associated antigen
PC	Platelet concentrate
PRP	Platelet-rich plasma
PT	Prothrombin time
PTC	Plasma thromboplastin component (factor IX)
PTT	Partial thromboplastin time

SPECIAL PROBLEMS IN PATIENTS WITH LIVER DISEASE

Bleeding from the gastrointestinal tract in patients with cirrhosis of the liver is not usually due to abnormal coagulation but to esophageal varices, gastritis, or hemorrhoids. Factors II (prothrombin), V, VII, and X may be reduced and prolong the prothrombin time, but rarely to clinically important levels (below 20%). Factors IX and XI also may be reduced somewhat but do not constitute a bleeding hazard. Factor VIII is not lowered by liver disease.

Platelets may be severely reduced, below 30,000/μl, in acute alcoholism and may be responsible for bleeding problems, but they rise spontaneously to normal levels in a few days when alcohol is withdrawn. Moderate thrombocytopenia (50—100 thousand/μl) that does not remit spontaneously may be a sign of hypersplenism secondary to cirrhosis; the spleen can either be felt, or its enlargement can be demonstrated by scanning with [99m]technetium colloid.

A rare hemorrhagic complication of liver disease is acute generalized oozing. It may be caused by (1) disseminated intravascular coagulation (DIC), characterized by prolonged PT and thrombin time, greatly prolonged PTT, low plasma fibrinogen, a low platelet count, a poor clot, the presence of fibrin degradation products (FDP), and fibrin monomer; or (2) primary fibrinolysis, where the necrotic liver fails to clear plasminogen activators. In general, platelets and factors V and VIII are less strikingly reduced than in DIC. Elevated levels of FDP are not diagnostic; their clearance may be impaired by severe liver disease without bleeding.

Clotting factor deficiency resulting from liver damage does not respond to vitamin K even when given parenterally in large doses. Vitamin K can only repair those deficiencies that result from impaired vitamin K absorption due to obstructive jaundice, as

reflected in a prolonged prothrombin time.

Platelet deficiency may become a problem if more than 10 units of whole blood are given in rapid succession (see next section on transfusions). Factors V and VIII, the only factors that deteriorate significantly on storage, do not present an unusual problem in liver disease even with multiple transfusions. Factor V requires a minimum level of only 5—10% of normal for hemostasis, and factor VIII is usually elevated in liver disease.

TRANSFUSION OF BLOOD, BLOOD COMPONENTS, & PLASMA SUBSTITUTES

Transfusion of blood, blood components, and plasma substitutes for surgical patients may be required for one or more of the following reasons: (1) to restore and maintain normal blood volume, (2) to correct severe anemia, or (3) to correct bleeding and coagulation disorders. Certain other blood abnormalities such as granulocytopenia or hypoalbuminemia cannot be satisfactorily corrected by blood transfusion.

Decisions about the need for transfusion and selection of the proper type and amount of transfusion material must be based upon careful evaluation of the individual patient. Urgency of need and the availability of diagnostic and therapeutic resources are obviously the determining factors. Attention must be given to the total clinical picture:

(1) History of hemorrhage, bleeding tendencies, treatment with anticoagulant drugs, or systemic disease predisposing to blood loss.

(2) Determination of the presence and severity of anemia based on blood count.

(3) Estimation of effective circulating blood vol-

ume by monitoring blood pressure, central venous pressure, and rate of urine formation.

(4) Evaluation of bleeding time, clotting studies, prothrombin time (PT), partial thromboplastin time (PTT), or activated coagulation time (ACT).

Choice of Transfusion Material

The routine use of whole blood to meet all transfusion requirements is not desirable since in most cases only one element of the blood is required for therapy. Most urban centers have blood bank facilities for collection and fractionation of whole blood into components.

Freshly drawn blood (ie, the same day's procurement) is seldom required, since most clinical situations can be treated optimally with blood components or relatively fresh stored blood ($< 4-7$ days old). Fresh blood is required only if functioning donor platelets are needed. The age of the blood (within the expiration period) is relatively unimportant if the need is only for correction of volume deficits or anemia.

Plasma substitutes may be administered (1) on an emergency basis for the treatment of hypovolemic shock, or (2) to provide necessary fluid, electrolytes, and nutrients.

WHOLE BLOOD

Patients with presumably normal bone marrow activity who need blood transfusions because of acute blood loss may receive stored (bank) blood of any age up to the expiration date (usually 21 days). Hemolysis during storage is almost negligible (less than 1% at 21 days). The increased content of lactic acid, inorganic phosphate, ammonia, and potassium in stored blood is usually clinically insignificant. Except for patients with severe hepatic or renal impairment or extreme debility, the use of acceptable aged blood imposes no significant metabolic burden on the recipient.

Most coagulation factors are stable in stored blood, but platelets, factor V (proaccelerin), and factor VIII (antihemophilic globulin) deteriorate. Bank blood which has been stored in the refrigerator for more than 2 days is essentially devoid of viable platelets. Massive replacement with this blood (eg, giving 10−15 units in rapid succession) may result in thrombocytopenia. Loss of other clotting factors is usually less important. For factor V, only 5−10% of normal levels is adequate for hemostasis; reductions to this level rarely result from multiple transfusions, even of older blood. Factor VIII deficiency (hemophilia A) is better treated with cryoprecipitate (see below).

Serologic Considerations (Blood Typing)

The antigens for which routine testing should always be performed in donors and recipients are A, B, and D (Rh_0) for administration of group-specific blood. Pretransfusion compatibility tests use the serum

of the recipient and the cells of the donor (major cross-match). To ensure a maximal margin of safety, each transfusion should be preceded (if possible) by a 3-part compatibility procedure: (1) at room temperature in saline; (2) at 37 C fortified by the addition of albumin; and (3) at 37 C followed by an antiglobulin test. It usually takes about 1½ hours to complete these procedures.

(1) ABO System Groups: Whenever possible, use type-specific blood, even in an emergency when the patient must be transfused before the routine cross-matching tests can be completed. The older approach to this situation—giving low-titer type O ("universal donor") Rh-negative blood to A, B, or AB recipients—is rarely justified since this can lead to late complications which can be avoided by giving type-specific blood. Plasma of type O blood containing high titers of anti-A or anti-B isoagglutinins may cause hemolysis of the recipient's blood. If only 2 or 3 units of group O blood have been given successfully to a patient who is not group O, it is safe to return to group-specific blood, but the infusion set must be changed before specific blood is started.

After the uneventful transfusion of 4 or more units of group O to an adult who is not group O, the administration of group O blood is usually continued even though group-specific blood becomes available. The decision to change back to group-specific blood (if more transfusions are needed) is best based upon the presence or absence of anti-A or anti-B in subsequent samples of the recipient's blood as determined on the cross-match. If an AB recipient has received either group A or group B blood, his plasma will contain anti-A or anti-B. The decision to change to yet another blood group must be based upon consideration of the antibodies concerned.

(2) Rh System Groups: A few units of Rh-positive blood can be administered with relative safety to Rh-negative recipients if compatible on a Coombs cross-match. This substitution, however, must not be made in girls or in women of childbearing age.

Rh-negative blood may be administered to Rh-positive patients.

Amount of Blood for Transfusion

A. Adults: Two units (1000 ml) of whole blood will raise the hemoglobin by 2−3 g/100 ml in the average adult (70 kg). The red blood cell count will rise by 0.8−1 million/μl, and the hematocrit by 8−9%. Ten ml of whole blood per kg body weight will produce a 10% hemoglobin rise.

B. Children:

1. Over 25 kg—Give 500 ml of whole blood.
2. Under 25 kg—Give 20 ml/kg of whole blood.
3. Premature infants—Give 10 ml/kg of whole blood.

Rate of Transfusion

Blood is normally given at a rate of 80−100 drops per minute, or 500 ml in 1½−2 hours. In patients with heart disease, one should allow 2−3 hours for the transfusion. For rapid transfusions in emergencies, it is best to use a 15-gauge plastic cannula and allow the blood to run freely. The use of added pressure to increase flow is dangerous unless it can be applied by gentle compression of collapsible plastic blood containers. Central venous pressure monitoring is a safeguard against overtransfusion; it is a measure of the heart's ability to handle venous return.

Massive Transfusions

An actively bleeding patient receiving over 10 units of bank blood in a few hours may have some difficulty with adequate oxygenation of his tissues because blood collected in acid-citrate-dextrose (ACD) gradually becomes more acid and loses some of its 2,3-diphosphoglycerate (DPG); the hemoglobin's affinity for oxygen increases ("hemoglobin dissociation curve shifts to left"), resulting in a fall of central venous oxygen tension. This process is reversible, and all values return spontaneously to normal after 1–2 days. In these clinical situations, blood only 1–3 days old—or blood collected with citrate-phosphate-dextrose (CPD) as an anticoagulant—is more desirable. Massive transfusions may also lead to thrombocytopenia and bleeding. (See Platelet Transfusion, below.) Whenever possible, fresh whole blood should be used for massive replacement, as in the patient with multiple severe injuries.

Complications of Blood Transfusion

Although some of the following complications of blood transfusion are not preventable, most of the fatal complications can be avoided by careful selection of donors, proper cross-matching of blood, and careful collection, storage, labeling, patient identification, and administration of blood:

(1) Hemolytic reactions are a serious complication of blood transfusion. The most severe reactions are due to ABO incompatibility, but serious hemolytic reactions may also be due to antibodies resulting from isoimmunization following previous transfusion or pregnancy. Symptoms may include apprehension, headache, fever, chills, pain at the injection site or in the back, chest, and abdomen, and shock; but in the anesthetized patient spontaneous bleeding from different areas and changes in vital signs may be the only clinical evidence of transfusion reactions. Posttransfusion blood counts fail to show the anticipated rise in hemoglobin. Free hemoglobin can be detected in the plasma within a few minutes. Hemoglobinuria and oliguria may occur. Exact identification of the offending antibody should be made, and this is usually possible when the Coombs test is positive.

(2) Other conditions in which clots fail to form in vitro are circulating anticoagulant and heparin administration. In vitro clotting may be greatly prolonged to 1 hour or more in the hemophilias and in factor XII deficiency.

(3) Allergic reactions occur in about 1% of transfusions. They are usually mild and associated with itching, urticaria, and bronchospasm, but they may be severe or even fatal. (The reaction results from an antigen-antibody reaction between a protein in the donor plasma and a corresponding antibody in the patient. Some of these reactions are caused by an antibody to IgA.) If reactions are mild, the transfusion may be cautiously continued. Antihistamines, epinephrine, and corticosteroids may be required.

(4) Too rapid transfusions of large quantities of blood may result in circulatory complications (eg, cardiac or respiratory failure). This is particularly true of elderly or debilitated patients. Careful monitoring should help prevent this complication.

(5) Abnormal bleeding—ie, massive oozing of blood—may follow transfusion of large amounts of stored blood, which contains few platelets. Fresh blood is often needed, especially with massive transfusions. Here again, citrate-phosphate-dextrose is preferable to acid-citrate-dextrose as an anticoagulant.

(6) Transfer of viral, bacterial, spirochetal, or protozoal disease by blood from an infected donor can occur. Infectious hepatitis of the long incubation type (serum hepatitis) is the most common (0.5%) blood-transmitted infection in the USA. Testing of the prospective donor's blood for hepatitis B-associated antigen (HBAg) reduces the incidence and the severity of this complication. Other transmitted diseases include rubella, syphilis, malaria, and brucellosis.

(7) Bacterial contamination of blood may occur through improper collection, storage, and administration. Reactions—noted early in the course of transfusions—are serious and may be fatal. Treat as for septic shock (see Chapter 15). Prevention is obviously the most important consideration.

(8) Unknown pyrogens may cause "nonspecific" febrile reactions which usually subside with symptomatic treatment within 24 hours. Other causes should be ruled out.

After antibody screening of the patient's serum, transfusions with compatible blood may be advisable. If no compatible blood can be found, plasma expanders (eg, dextran) and plasma may have to be used instead of whole blood. Pressor agents may be necessary.

Some studies suggest that osmotic diuretics such as mannitol can prevent renal failure following a hemolytic transfusion reaction. After an apparent reaction and in oliguric patients, a test dose of 12.5 g of mannitol (supplied as 25% solution in 50 ml ampules) is administered IV over a period of 3–5 minutes; this dose may be repeated if no signs of circulatory overload develop. A satisfactory urinary output following the use of mannitol is 60 ml/hour or more. Mannitol can be safely administered as a continuous intravenous infusion; each liter of 5–10% mannitol should be alternated with 1 liter of normal saline to which 40 mEq of KCl have been added to prevent serious salt depletion. If oliguria develops despite these efforts, treat as for acute renal failure.

PACKED RED BLOOD CELLS

Packed red cells have a storage (shelf) life of 21 days and a hematocrit of 70%. They are the treatment of choice for anemia without hypovolemia. Most blood transfusions can be given as packed red cells, even in patients with moderate degrees of blood loss. The use of packed red cells instead of whole blood not only conserves a precious and limited resource of plasma but reduces the potential hazard of (1) circulatory overload; (2) excessive electrolyte and metabolic loads (eg, increased potassium and ammonium of stored blood); (3) exposure to certain antigens (eg, granulocytes and plasma proteins, and food or drug allergens in donor blood); and (4) transmission of infectious agents. It is possible to concurrently administer balanced salt solutions.

PLATELET TRANSFUSION

For the treatment of thrombocytopenia and thrombasthenia, freshly drawn whole blood, fresh platelet-rich plasma (PRP), or platelet concentrate (PC) may be needed. Enough must be given to raise the platelet count to 100,000 /μl.

Platelets cannot be preserved for long periods, but survival may extend to several days if platelet-rich plasma is not refrigerated but stored at room temperature after collection. Compatibility tests are not mandatory for platelet concentrate or PRP if the recipient's blood has been screened for antibodies; it need not be type-specific, but A platelets should not be given to O recipients. Many blood banks usually stock type O, Rh-positive platelets. PC made from the blood of more than one donor carries a higher risk of transmitting hepatitis.

Administration of platelets is indicated for uncontrollable bleeding due to temporary thrombocytopenia following surgery; for purpura or bleeding in thrombocytopenic patients who require surgery; and for bleeding in patients who have developed thrombocytopenia after transfusion with 10 or more units of blood in a period of a few hours.

Platelets should not be administered to patients with conditions associated with a very short life span of transfused platelets—eg, most cases of idiopathic thrombocytopenic purpura or disseminated intravascular coagulation. Platelets should not be transfused unless absolutely necessary lest isoantibody formation prevent their being effective at a time when they are critically needed.

Sources of platelets are as follows:

(1) Fresh whole blood: If transfused within 24 hours of collection, the number of viable platelets will be sufficient to maintain the platelet count at a safe level during massive transfusion. Correction of thrombocytopenia, however, cannot be accomplished with whole blood since it does not contain enough platelets per unit volume.

(2) Platelet-rich plasma: PRP has the advantage that it is easier to prepare than platelet concentrate and damages the platelets less. Its volume is only 50% of the original whole blood, yet it contains most of the platelets. Even so, its relatively large volume still limits the number of platelets that can be administered at one time.

(3) Platelet concentrate: PC is prepared by centrifugation of PRP at high gravitational force. The platelets are deposited in a small mass and plasma is then removed, leaving 25–30 ml in which the platelets are resuspended before transfusion. Platelet concentrate should be transfused within 4 hours of collection. Platelets may be administered in any quantity required. It usually takes 6–8 units of the concentrate to raise the platelet count to 100,000/μl. Platelet viability is approximately 50% of that in PRP. In general, one can expect only 30% of the platelets in the original unit to survive in the recipient. This form of replacement therapy is very expensive because of the many units required. The platelet mass must be resuspended in the remaining plasma by manual compression of the bag. Before transfusion, the suspension should be homogeneous (without visible clumps).

Platelets are usually transfused through a standard set containing a filter.

FIBRINOGEN

Hypofibrinogenemia, either congenital or acquired, is associated with faulty or absent clot formation. Prothrombin time, PTT, and thrombin time are prolonged. The administration of 4–5 g of fibrinogen should promptly raise the plasma fibrinogen level by 100–150 mg/ml. The fibrinogen deficiency must be demonstrated before administering this material. The commercial preparations are expensive and are associated with a high (5%) incidence of infectious hepatitis.

COAGULATION FACTOR CONCENTRATES

Stored blood or plasma provides all coagulation factors except factor V (proaccelerin) and factor VIII (AHF, antihemophilic factor). Frozen plasma preserves factors V and VIII. A concentrate prepared from fresh-frozen plasma (cryoprecipitate) contains 15–20 times the AHF concentration of fresh whole plasma and is very effective in the treatment of factor VIII deficiency (hemophilia A or "classic" hemophilia) and von Willebrand's disease (pseudohemophilia). One unit of the cryoprecipitate for each 6 kg body weight raises the AHF level to 50%—enough for most surgical procedures. For difficult cases, it may have to be followed by half that amount every 12 hours given as long as necessary.

Proplex (Hyland) is a concentrate in powder form which contains the vitamin K-dependent coagulation factors (II, VII, IX, and X) and is used for the treatment of bleeding due to the deficiency of these factors. The commonest deficiency of these 3 is that of factor IX (PTC) deficiency, which causes so-called Christmas disease (hemophilia B).

PLASMA

Any of the various plasma preparations such as fresh plasma, fresh-frozen plasma, or lyophilized or reconstituted plasma may be employed for the treatment of acute hypovolemia (shock), for the correction of plasma loss (eg, due to extensive burns), or for the correction of coagulation disorders. Pooled plasma is usually readily procurable, may be rapidly set up for administration, and does not require preliminary blood typing. However, pooled plasma carries a high risk of transmission of infectious hepatitis regardless of aging or processing with ultraviolet light. Although pooled plasma is still used on an emergency basis for the treatment of hypovolemic shock, its use has decreased in favor of more specific treatment with blood. Obviously, plasma cannot be substituted for whole blood if red cells are essential. Most centers now use lactated Ringer's injection until blood arrives.

Fresh plasma and fresh-frozen plasma are used to correct coagulation defects due to deficiency of certain of the blood coagulation factors (see above).

PLASMA SUBSTITUTES

Dextrans

Dextrans are fairly effective plasma "substitutes" for the emergency treatment of shock. These water-soluble biosynthetic polysaccharides have high molecular weights, high oncotic pressures, and the necessary viscosity, but they have not proved to be as useful as plasma, and their use is not without hazard because it is usually not safe to give more than 15 ml/kg/24 hours. They have the advantages of ready availability, of compatibility with other preparations used in intravenous solutions, and of not causing infectious hepatitis. They may also help prevent thrombosis by interfering with platelet aggregation.

Dextran 40 (Rheomacrodex, Gentran), a low molecular weight (40,000) dextran, is available as a 10% solution in either isotonic saline or 5% dextrose in water for intravenous use. It decreases blood viscosity and appears to assist the microcirculation. Rapid initial infusion of approximately 100–150 ml within the first hour is followed by slow maintenance for a total of 10–15 ml/kg/24 hours (preferably less than 1 liter/day). This preparation may also reduce the risk of intravascular coagulation in the severely injured or septic patient.

Dextrans must be used cautiously in patients with cardiac disease, renal insufficiency, or marked dehydration to avoid pulmonary edema, congestive heart failure, or renal shutdown, and patients must be observed for possible anaphylactoid reactions. Dextran 40 has considerably less antigenicity than high molecular weight dextran 75. Prolongations of bleeding time have been reported, and dextran should probably not be used in thrombocytopenic patients. Blood for typing and cross-matching must be obtained before dextran therapy since dextran may interfere with these tests.

Electrolyte & Dextrose Solutions

Experimental and clinical studies have shown that substantial blood losses can be effectively replaced or augmented with appropriate balanced salt solutions. With careful monitoring of central venous pressure, vital signs, urinary output, and serum electrolyte determinations, specific fluid and electrolyte abnormalities may be corrected and apparently normal blood volume maintained.

Balanced salt solutions may be augmented with specific electrolytes, vitamins, dextrose, and special protein nutriments to provide successful intravenous alimentation for prolonged periods. (See Chapters 12 and 13.)

PREGNANCY & THE SURGICAL PATIENT
Edward C. Hill, MD

The incidence of surgical illness is the same in pregnant women as in nonpregnant women of the same age group. Pregnancy may alter or mask the signs and symptoms of the disease, so that recognition is more difficult. Furthermore, the fetus must be considered in planning a surgical procedure, and pregnancy may modify the timing of a semi-elective operation or the surgical approach of an emergency abdominal procedure. Purely elective surgery should be deferred until the postpartum period. Any major operation represents a risk not only to the mother but to the fetus as well. During the first trimester, congenital anomalies may be induced in the developing fetus by hypoxia. It is preferable to avoid surgical intervention during this period; if surgery does become necessary, the greatest precautions must be taken to prevent hypoxia and hypotension. The second trimester is usually the optimum time for operative procedures.

Diagnostic radiologic examinations of the lower abdomen and pelvis should be avoided during pregnancy, if possible, especially during the first 6 weeks of gestation when the fetus is particularly susceptible to irradiation. There is statistical evidence that mothers of leukemic children had a higher incidence of abdominal radiologic studies during pregnancy. The use of radioactive isotopes poses a particular hazard to the fetus when used in the pregnant patient. Radioactive iodine or pertechnetate for thyroid scanning, selenomethionine for imaging of the pancreas, and bone scanning with radioactive strontium or calcium are contraindicated during pregnancy because they all cross the placenta and are taken up by the fetal tissues. Sonography has proved to be a useful diagnostic method in many circumstances and avoids the pitfalls of x-ray exposure. At present, it is considered safe for use during pregnancy.

The following surgical problems which may occur in pregnant women are discussed briefly in the following paragraphs: acute appendicitis, cholecystitis and cholelithiasis, intestinal obstruction, hernias, breast cancer, and ovarian tumors.

Saunders P, Milton PJD: Laparotomy during pregnancy: An assessment of diagnostic accuracy and fetal wastage. Br Med J 3:165, 1973.
Sternberg J: Radiation and pregnancy. Can Med Assoc J 109:51, 1973.
Stocker J & others: Ultrasonography: Its usefulness and reliability in early pregnancy: Review of 210 cases. Am J Obstet Gynecol 121:1084, 1975.

Appendicitis

Acute appendicitis occurs about once in every 2000 pregnancies. The signs and symptoms are the same as those that occur in nonpregnant women, but they may be considerably modified. Because of the nausea and vomiting and lower abdominal discomfort which are seen frequently in the first and second trimesters of normal pregnancy, as well as the moderate leukocytosis and elevated sedimentation rate, errors in diagnosis are more frequently made. Moreover, the enlarging uterus often carries the appendix higher in the abdomen, so that McBurney's point can no longer be used as a point of reference, and maximal tenderness is proportionately higher. For the same reason, the presence of the gravid uterus may effectively block off the omentum and loops of small intestine and thus hinder the walling-off process, particularly in the third trimester. Therefore, rupture of the appendix is more often associated with widespread dissemination of infection, generalized peritonitis, and a high mortality rate. If an abscess does form following perforation, the gravid uterus forms the medial wall of the abscess. The intense inflammatory process often initiates uterine contractions, with premature labor and the loss of the fetus. With evacuation, there is a sudden reduction in the size of the uterus; the abscess then ruptures into the free peritoneal cavity.

Because of the flaccidity of the anterior abdominal wall during the last trimester, there may be relatively little rigidity associated with inflammation of

the appendix, and rebound tenderness may be difficult to define, so that one cannot rely upon these physical findings.

The treatment of acute appendicitis during pregnancy is immediate operation. Because of the extreme seriousness of perforation when it occurs, it is better to remove a normal appendix when the diagnosis is in doubt than to wait for typical signs or symptoms and risk the consequences.

Regional anesthesia is preferred, and the transverse or oblique muscle-splitting incision should be placed somewhat higher than in the nonpregnant individual. In fact, late in the third trimester the appendix may be in the right upper quadrant of the abdomen. Premature labor is not common following an uncomplicated appendectomy.

Cunningham FG, McCubbin JH: Appendicitis complicating pregnancy. Obstet Gynecol 45:415, 1975.

Cholecystitis & Cholelithiasis

Normal pregnancy may contribute to the formation of gallstones by encouraging bile stasis, increasing the concentration of cholesterol in the bile, and fostering changes in the solubility of the bile salts. Thus, cholelithiasis is more common in women who have borne children.

Acute cholecystitis in pregnancy occurs less often than acute appendicitis, the prevalence being about one in 3500–6500 pregnancies. It is associated with gallstones in the vast majority of instances.

The symptoms are the same as in the nonpregnant patient, with an abrupt onset of colicky right upper quadrant abdominal pain radiating to the right scapula, low-grade fever, and nausea and vomiting. Cholecystitis may be difficult to distinguish from acute appendicitis, with the high position of the appendix associated with the third trimester of pregnancy.

Unlike appendicitis, however, acute cholecystitis in pregnancy is best managed conservatively with hospitalization, parenteral fluids, nasogastric suction, antispasmodics, analgesics, and broad-spectrum antibiotics. In 3 out of 4 patients thus treated, there will be a definite improvement within 2 days, and a definitive surgical procedure can be deferred until the postpartum period. Surgery should be done whenever there is doubt regarding the differentiation from acute appendicitis or if there is no response to conservative therapy as manifested by an enlarging mass (empyema), jaundice (common duct obstruction), evidence of rupture, or associated pancreatitis. Cholecystectomy is the procedure of choice, but cholecystostomy may be performed if technical difficulties warrant it, the excision of the gallbladder being delayed until the puerperium.

Intestinal Obstruction

Intestinal obstruction occurs infrequently during pregnancy, but it should be considered in the differential diagnosis of any pregnant patient with an abdominal scar who develops abdominal pain and vomiting.

Adhesive bands are the most common cause of intestinal obstruction, and displacement of the intestine is most likely to occur when uterine growth carries the pregnancy into the abdomen around the fourth or fifth month of gestation; near term, when lightening occurs; or postpartum, with sudden reduction in the size of the uterus. Other causes of intestinal obstruction during pregnancy are volvulus, intussusception, and large bowel malignancy.

The symptoms and signs of intestinal obstruction are the same as those that occur in the nonpregnant woman, although the clinical picture may be obscured by the nausea and vomiting of early pregnancy, round ligament pain, and the abdominal distention already produced by the pregnancy.

When surgical intervention is indicated, it should be performed without delay, ignoring the pregnancy. Near term, a cesarean section may be required in order to obtain necessary exposure.

Hernias

Hiatal hernias are common during pregnancy; perhaps 15–20% of pregnant women develop this condition as a result of pressure against the stomach by the enlarging uterus. The principal symptom is reflux esophagitis with severe heartburn, aggravated by recumbency or by the ingestion of a large meal and relieved by assuming an upright position or by taking antacids. Hematemesis may occur due to ulceration of the esophageal mucosa.

Elevation of the upper half of the body while reclining; frequent, small, bland meals; and antacids given liberally are usually effective treatment. Most hiatal hernias disappear following the pregnancy. Surgical correction is required only for those that persist and remain symptomatic.

Umbilical, inguinal, and ventral hernias usually are unaffected by pregnancy. Repair can be carried out electively after delivery. Surgery during pregnancy is indicated only in the rare event of an incarcerated or strangulated hernia.

Cancer of the Breast

Cancer of the breast occurs infrequently during pregnancy, but it is a significant complication when it does occur. The breast changes which occur during gestation make detection of early breast carcinoma much more difficult. The disease is more malignant during pregnancy, perhaps as a consequence of hormonal changes. Most cases are advanced by the time they are diagnosed. Biopsy and appropriate surgical treatment should be undertaken as soon as the cancer is suspected. If the malignancy is confined to the breast, the prognosis is good; if the axillary nodes are involved, the outlook is poor. Statistically, the overall cure rate for cancer of the breast developing during pregnancy is about half of that of nonpregnant women of comparable age.

Therapeutic abortion is not indicated in the patient with localized disease of a favorable microscopic type. Interruption of an early pregnancy may be of some palliative benefit to the woman with advanced disease, but if the pregnancy has progressed beyond the 20th week, the life of the fetus should take precedence.

Applewhite RR & others: Carcinoma of the breast associated with pregnancy and lactation. Am Surg 39:101, 1973.

Haagensen CD: Cancer of the breast in pregnancy and during lactation. Am J Obstet Gynecol 98:141, 1967.

Ovarian Tumors

A cystic corpus luteum is the most frequent cause of ovarian enlargement during pregnancy. This structure rarely exceeds 6 cm in diameter and gradually diminishes in size as the pregnancy progresses. It is usually asymptomatic, and only careful observation is required to distinguish it from a proliferative type of cystic enlargement.

True ovarian neoplasms are encountered in 1:1000 pregnancies, the majority being detected during the first trimester. Some are not found until the immediate postpartum period, when the uterine size no longer masks its presence and the abdominal wall is flaccid. Most ovarian neoplasms are cystic; solid tumors are quite rare. Frequently they are silent, producing few symptoms unless there is hemorrhage into the tumor, rupture of the cyst, or torsion of the pedicle—complications which are definitely increased during pregnancy (see Chapter 44).

The cystic neoplasms most often seen during pregnancy are benign cystic teratomas (about 40% are of this variety), serous and mucinous cystadenomas, and endometrial cysts. Dysgerminoma is the most frequently encountered solid tumor. Malignant ovarian neoplasms rarely complicate pregnancy, constituting only 2–3% of ovarian neoplasms. Serous and mucinous cystadenocarcinomas and endometrioid carcinomas are the most common histologic types.

Because of the danger of inducing an abortion during the first trimester, surgical removal of a suspected true neoplasm should be deferred until the fourth month of gestation except in the event of an acute abdominal emergency caused by torsion, rupture, or hemorrhage. When discovered during the immediate postpartum period, removal should be done as soon as possible in order to avoid the complications of infection, hemorrhage, rupture, and torsion.

White KC: Ovarian tumors in pregnancy. Am J Obstet Gynecol 116:544, 1973.

• • •

6...
Legal Medicine for the Surgeon

Jack Nagan, JD, & Jesse L. Carr, MD

Historically, the civil and criminal legal restraints on the practice of medicine have developed in parallel with the profession's own attempts at peer control by means of licensing procedures, accreditation of hospitals, and other means. The function of these forces has been to define and defend the rights and responsibilities of the 3 parties to every medical contract, written or otherwise: the patient, the physician or surgeon, and "society."

Common law, inherited largely from England and frequently augmented by statutory provision, comprises most of our legal code. A steady progression of precedent-setting court decisions continually establishes new legal principles that in turn are either confirmed or overruled by subsequent judicial decisions. Legislatures passing new statutes will have them declared constitutional or unconstitutional by the courts, while the several State Supreme Courts and the United States Supreme Court continually add crucial new laws by edict, and these may be altered by subsequent Supreme Court decisions, constitutional amendment, or legislation.

OVERVIEW: CIVIL & CRIMINAL LAW

There are 2 kinds of law: civil and criminal. Medical malpractice belongs in the former category. When laymen discuss medical negligence, however, the 2 areas are often confused. For example, one is not guilty of negligence but liable for negligence; guilt is a criminal finding, and negligence is a civil wrong. Other essential distinctions between civil and criminal law should also be kept in mind. For example, the party who brings the complaint is always the plaintiff, but the civil complainant is a person or entity seeking redress for his own injury whereas in criminal law "the people" bring the action against the defendant. That is why criminal cases bear titles such as "People versus Smith" and civil cases "Jones versus Smith." The victim in a criminal case is said to be the state, ie, even though a particular individual may have been murdered or raped, the crime is, in theory, one against society.

The purpose of the criminal suit is punishment and deterrence of crime; the object of civil litigation is generally to remedy a wrong so as to place the plaintiff in the same position he would have occupied if the wrong had not occurred. The idea is to make him whole. Thus, civil redress is usually seen in terms of compensation, although there are certain narrowly restricted situations in which punishment is allowed in the form of exemplary damages (discussed below).

The scale used to judge the plaintiff's allegations differs in criminal and civil law. In both criminal and civil law, of course, the plaintiff bears the burden of proving each element of his case. Every cause of action, whether it be a complaint for murder, robbery, negligence, or breach of contract, is composed of certain required elements which, taken as a whole, are known as the prima facie case for that cause of action. Both the civil and the criminal plaintiff bear the burden of establishing their prima facie case, but the standard by which the plaintiff's case is judged is different in civil and criminal proceedings. In a criminal case the defendant is assumed to be innocent until and unless the state can prove each element of its prima facie case beyond a reasonable doubt. In a civil action, the defendant remains blameless and free of liability until and unless the plaintiff can establish each element of his prima facie case by a preponderance of the evidence. Obviously, there is a significant difference between the 2 standards, although an exact definition of reasonable doubt remains elusive. It is quite clear that "beyond a reasonable doubt" is meant to be very close to certainty, as opposed to a "preponderance of the evidence," which requires only that a fact be established as more likely to be true than not to be true.

The sanctions imposed for criminal guilt and civil liability are also different. Criminal guilt may be punished by death, imprisonment, or fine, whereas civil liability in most cases is imposed in terms of a judgment for money damages.

It is possible that the same act may involve both a criminal and a civil wrong, as, for instance, in the case of rape. That act may be prosecuted in a criminal court as rape and may also be the subject of a civil action for the intentional tort of battery. Where an act results in the possibility of both criminal and civil actions, the 2 cases must be tried separately, and, given the difference in the required levels of proof, might well result in a judgment for damages but a verdict of not guilty on the criminal charge.

LITIGATION

The legal process in the USA is characterized by the adversary system. The adversary system does not guarantee justice, just as the physician practicing medicine does not guarantee a cure. Both the legal and medical systems employ sets of procedures which have been tested and found by experience to be sound. All of these procedures are constantly under review and are continually being refined in an attempt to improve the result. In the adversary system, the assumption is that a contest between 2 equally knowledgeable and equally well prepared adversaries, judged by an impartial third party, affords a thorough airing of each issue of fact and law, which in most cases leads to a finding or reconstruction of what actually happened. It is this process that is the immediate goal of the legal system, with "justice" generally appearing as the ultimate product. It is well to remember that in law the result depends on what is *proved* rather than what *is*.

The roles of the participants in a civil trial are easily explained. Each attorney presents evidence of facts most favorable to his client, minimizing by deletion or explanation any unfavorable evidence and rebutting damaging evidence produced by opposing counsel. Testimonial evidence is presented by witnesses to fact, who relate their first-hand experience of relevant subjects within lay comprehension. As to matters outside lay understanding, testimony is limited to the expert witness (eg, physicians) who alone can offer opinions as evidence. Where there is a judge and a jury, the judge sits as the trier of law only; it is not his task to decide which evidence presented, whether testimonial or physical, is true and which is not true. That decision is reserved for the jury, which sits as the trier of fact. After all of the evidence has been presented, the jury decides which are the facts based on the evidence. It disbelieves some evidence, believes other evidence, and weighs every piece of evidence according to each juror's knowledge, experience, and understanding.

The judge, as trier of law, controls the conduct of the trial and, most importantly, determines the admissibility of evidence sought to be presented to the jury by counsel for each side. If, at the completion of the plaintiff's presentation of his case, the judge finds that the plaintiff has not met his burden of proof in establishing the prima facie case, he may direct a nonsuit against the plaintiff, which terminates the action in favor of the defendant. He may also find that, although the plaintiff in his presentation met his burden of proof, the defendant's presentation substantially rebutted the plaintiff's evidence, and he may thus direct a verdict in favor of the defendant. The defendant may fail so completely to rebut the plaintiff's case that a directed verdict is entered by the judge in favor of the plaintiff. The judge also has the option of allowing the jury to reach its own verdict, but even then, if he believes that there is no rational basis for the jury's decision, he may direct a judgment "notwithstanding the verdict" in favor of either party.

When the plaintiff and defendant have concluded their presentations and the judge has decided to let the case go to the jury, he will instruct the jury on matters of law relevant to the case. These instructions are generally framed to indicate that certain findings of fact by the jury require certain conclusions of law. The judge even has the power to reduce the amount of the jury's money verdict (remittitur) or to increase it (additur). Although there must be agreement by the plaintiff to remittitur and agreement by the defendant to additur, the judge can "jaw-bone" the agreement of either party by indicating that unless agreement is reached, a motion for a new trial will be granted and the judgment of the jury set aside. There are, of course, numerous other decisions of law that must be made by the judge, such as matters of jurisdiction, venue, and appropriateness of parties to the action, which can greatly affect the initiation, location, and outcome of the litigation.

In cases where there is no jury, the judge acts as finder of fact as well as trier of law.

The physician's defense counsel in a medical negligence action may prefer to present his case to a judge sitting as trier of fact as well as of law. A trial to the judge alone is conducted with a great deal more flexibility than a trial before a judge and jury because the judge is not concerned so much about evidence that may be prejudicial. That is, a jury of lay people may be somewhat dumbfounded by emotionally charged or complex evidence. The evidence may be so technical, as in many medical malpractice cases, that it is hopelessly beyond lay understanding (perhaps even with the assistance of expert witnesses). The judge is probably better informed than the average juror and may be familiar with medical terminology as a result of other cases he has tried. He is much less likely to be influenced by emotional testimony or information that might be otherwise prejudicial to laymen. As a result, questions of admissibility before a judge alone are more likely to be resolved in favor of admission, whereas a judge might hesitate to admit the same evidence in a jury trial because of the possibility of an effect on the jury out of proportion to the real weight of the evidence.

The matter of appeal is sometimes misunderstood by those unfamiliar with the legal process. When a case is appealed, the facts are no longer in dispute. The trier of fact has already heard all of the evidence and made its decision, and the facts are as found. Unless it can be said that there was no rational basis for the finding of fact, which is an exceedingly difficult standard to meet, the findings as to facts will stand on appeal. The issues being contested by an appeal are questions of law decided by the judge during the trial. Any of the trial judge's decisions referred to above may become the basis for an appeal to a higher court. It then becomes a question of the opinion of an appellate judge, or panel of appellate judges, against that of the trial judge. Trial judges do not like to be overruled on appeal, so they try to keep their decisions and instructions on law to acceptable, frequently used standards.

Although criminal law in the USA is almost exclusively governed by the state penal codes, American civil law is still largely based on the common law system, which began with decisions of English courts and acts of Parliament and was adopted by the American states at the time of the Revolution. This inherited body of common law has since been augmented by decisions of appellate courts at both the state and federal levels. The key to understanding the common law system is the doctrine of stare decisis, which is the rule of legal precedent requiring lower courts to adopt decisions of higher courts. When the issue is "on all fours" with an earlier decided appellate court decision, the earlier decision will control the present case.

CONTRACT BASIS OF THE PHYSICIAN-PATIENT RELATIONSHIP

Civil law obligations are of 3 types: contract, quasi-contract, and tort. A basic understanding of these areas is useful to physicians because the doctor-patient relationship is a complex that may involve all of them. The essence of a contractual relationship is voluntary agreement between the parties, expressed orally or in writing, or implied by conduct. A quasi-contractual relationship is the result of a voluntary commitment of only one of the parties and the imposition of an agreement on the other party to avoid his unjust enrichment. The ordinary purchase of goods or services is the simplest example of a contractual relationship, where one party agrees to furnish the goods or services and the other party agrees to pay for them. An example of a quasi-contractual situation is providing essential medical care for a patient who is incapable of contractual assent, such as an unconscious person, a minor, or an incompetent. The law will impose a quasi-contractual obligation on the patient or his legal representative (eg, parent or guardian) to pay for the medical care (Greenspan v Slate, 97 A2d 390, New Jersey 1957).

If the doctor and patient enter into a written contract for treatment, or if a verbal exchange takes place in which the patient promises to pay and the physician promises to treat, or if there is conduct in place of a promise (patient comes to doctor's office, doctor treats), the doctor-patient relationship is contractual. Subsequent failure of the patient to pay would amount to a breach of contract. Once having undertaken the obligation to treat the patient, a physician who fails to do so commits a particular type of breach known as abandonment.

The relationship that is formed is one of fiduciary trust, based on the unavoidable reliance of the layman on the professional. This means that, unlike the usual "arm's length" sales transaction, there is a special obligation on the part of the physician: a duty of affirmative disclosure. Physicians deal with patients at all times in the context of this special trust. The relationship continues in the ordinary course of events until the treatment is completed. However, there may be situations where the patient wishes to terminate earlier. The patient can terminate at any time without notice. He may decide at any time for any reason that he is not going to see that doctor any more, and that is the end of it.

There is, however, the possibility that a patient who demonstrates his intent to terminate unilaterally might change his mind later and claim abandonment by the physician when, for example, an incision is slow in healing or the doctor's bill is higher than he expected. To guard against this situation, the physician should confirm the patient's intent to terminate by written notification to the patient with a return receipt to document the change in relationship for his office file.

The physician can also terminate the relationship unilaterally, but special conditions apply. He must first give notice to the patient and then provide information on past treatment to the new physician. In one case, a patient was brought to an emergency room with a gunshot wound in the neck. He was examined, admitted, and sent up to the ward by his surgeon, who then went home. The surgeon was called shortly thereafter and told that his patient was having difficulty breathing and needed a tracheostomy. The admitting physician failed to return, and by the time another surgeon got the patient to the operating room it was too late. The patient died 4 hours after admission. Even though only a few hours had passed and there had been no formed intent on the part of the admitting doctor to permanently discontinue treatment, the court nevertheless ruled that the doctor had abandoned the patient (Johnson v Vaughn, 370 SW2d 591, Kentucky 1963). So the definition of abandonment is highly flexible. For instance, if a fracture has been set by an orthopedic surgeon, it might be appropriate for him to check the patient every few months until healing and rehabilitation are complete. Even though there is no contact between doctor and patient for months, the relationship remains intact. Thus, for a doctor to protect himself in terminating the physician-patient relationship, he must first give the patient notice. How much notice is required varies with the case. In general, the courts have held that 30 days is sufficient.

Of course, there are difficult situations, like the doctor who is working in a small community, where there is literally no other doctor available, in which case he may be unable to terminate. The period of reasonable notice is based in large part on the availability of adequate medical coverage; it is the responsibility of the terminating physician not only to give the patient enough notice to find another physician but also to furnish information to his successor fast enough so that there is no delay in treatment. What constitutes unreasonable delay may also vary with the details of the illness. In the average case, a routine mailing of the records to the new physician and being available for telephone consultation would be sufficient.

Occasionally a physician who does not intend to

terminate treatment delays it too long. In this case, the legal issue concerns a possible breach of the standard of care. There are situations where abandonment may result in both contractual liability and tort liability, and damages may be recovered for either.

Once the doctor-patient relationship is formed, the obligation of the physician is defined as the possession and application of care, skill, and knowledge common to other physicians of good standing. However, a physician may increase the level of this obligation by expressly promising or "warranting" a particular result or a cure, in which event the failure to achieve the promised result will render the physician liable in contract for breach of warranty. The prima facie case for breach of contract is simple since it only requires proof of the contract and that the physician made a particular promise which he failed to substantially perform. Thus, there is a considerable legal difference between the obstetrician who promises to perform a tubal ligation and one who promises to sterilize the patient. However successful a given procedure has been in the hands of a surgeon, he is well advised to limit his discussion of results to the expected and hoped for, the statistical probabilities, and the sincere promise that he will do his best.

Money judgments for breach of contract in most states are limited to the value of the patient's "loss of the bargain" (which assumes that the promised treatment was obtained elsewhere at a greater cost) or "out of pocket" cost to the patient for securing the treatment elsewhere. A minority of jurisdictions do, however, allow recovery of money damages for pain and suffering where it was foreseeable at the time of the breach that failure of the doctor to perform his promise, or delay in performance, would result in such pain and suffering for the patient. Actions for breach of contract against physicians are not often seen today. They are encountered where the patient wishes to "punish" the physician for a bad result although he knows that the physician was not negligent, and in instances where a negligence action is barred by the shorter statute of limitations for tort and the only option still available is a breach of warranty suit because the longer statute of limitations for contract actions has not yet run.

INTENTIONAL TORTS

The third—and by far the most important—area of civil law for the physician is tort law. There are 2 kinds of tort: intentional and negligent. Although some categories of torts involve invasions of property rights, our concern here will be solely with invasions of personal rights, ie, those of the patient.

The category of intentional torts includes assault, battery, false imprisonment, defamation, invasion of privacy, infliction of emotional distress, and intentional misrepresentation. The prima facie case for the intentional torts is established by proving that the defendant's conduct was deliberate. If the conduct results in actual injury to the plaintiff, it is compensable in money damages. If conduct is established but injury is not, the damages will be limited to a nominal sum. But if the act (or omission) was particularly outrageous, punitive damages may be awarded in addition to compensatory or nominal damages. It should be emphasized that the only intent required for the commission of an intentional tort is the intent to commit the act, not an intent to bring about the ultimate injury. Another way of saying this is that the intention to bring about the ultimate injury is presumed from the commission of the act.

The act required to establish an **assault** is that which places another in immediate apprehension of harm. Traditionally, words alone without supporting gestures do not establish a cause of action for assault. A **battery** is simply an unauthorized touching of another. Of course, the authorization or consent for contact may not always be expressed. For instance, the fact that a patient has presented himself to a physician for treatment implies consent to reasonable physical contact necessary for the examination. However, when the physician's treatment entails more than such customary contact, as in surgery, invasive diagnostic procedures, and drug treatment involving the risk of special harm, the consent of the patient to the specific procedures must first be obtained. In the absence of such consent, treatment by the physician would be a battery, as would also be the case where consent was obtained to operate on a specific site and the consent was exceeded by operating on a different site, either instead of or in addition to the area of original consent. In situations where the issue is not whether **any** consent was obtained from the patient but rather whether the physician disclosed **enough** information for a reasonable patient to make an intelligent choice, the trend of the courts is to view the lack of so-called "informed consent" as a form of negligence in the disclosure of information by the physician. The matter of informed consent has been the subject of so much attention recently that it will be discussed below under its own heading.

The intentional tort of **false imprisonment** consists of an invasion of the personal interest in freedom from restraint of movement. Thus, a physician who orders a patient placed in restraints or drugged to the point of immobility by mistake or without a good medical reason may be liable for damages for false imprisonment. The physician most often involved in false imprisonment actions is the psychiatrist who orders involuntary commitment.

The intentional tort of **defamation** consists of injury to reputation by means of slanderous (verbal) or libelous (written) statements to another person that diminish the respect in which the plaintiff is held by others and lessen his standing in the community. The extent of the injury caused by verbal defamation must be proved by the plaintiff except in the case of slander involving an accusation of criminal conduct, loathsome disease (eg, syphilis, leprosy), acts incompatible with one's business, trade, or profession, or unchastity of a woman. These are the 4 categories of slander per se from which general damages are presumed to result without need of proof.

Special (actual) damages need not be proved in the case of libel inherent on the face of a publication, but where reference to extrinsic information is needed to create the libelous meaning (known as libel per quod), general damages will be presumed only in the same 4 areas as above. Otherwise, special injury must be proved to establish the prima facie case of libel. The defendant may avoid liability for defamation by establishing a privilege of immunity that covers the statement or by establishing that the statement was true.

Invasion of privacy is a new and still developing area of tort law dating in broad acceptance from the 1930s. The types of invasion recognized in this category are public use for profit of personal information about another or some type of intrusion on one's physical solitude. The most common defenses to an action for invasion of privacy are the privileges that exist for publication of information of public interest or concerning public figures. Specific state statutes define exceptions to the restrictions of defamation and invasion of privacy law. Such statutes commonly include infectious diseases, gunshot and stab wounds, seizure disorders, and child abuse (*Examples:* California Penal Code 11160, 11161, 11161.5, California Health and Safety Code 410, 3125.) Giving out details of medical treatment concerning patients (eg, celebrities), even if the information is truly newsworthy, can exceed the privilege. Without a signed release from the patient, caution is the rule: "If in doubt, don't give it out." The same caution extends to identifying a patient if a description of his case is published. Also, no outsiders are allowed in the operating room without the patient's advance consent. (Standard consent forms usually allow observers to view surgery for educational purposes.)

Infliction of mental distress as a cause of action independent of contemporaneous physical injury has only recently achieved judicial recognition. The conduct or language must be outrageous and extreme and the emotional upset apparent (most successful suits have involved resulting physical illness). The law requires an individual to be somewhat tough-skinned, and annoyance or insult alone is not actionable. Nevertheless, the special closeness and reliance which characterize the fiduciary relationship between doctor and patient add weight to possible liability for ill-considered conduct by physicians, who have a duty to protect and comfort their patients.

Intentional torts are not covered by professional insurance and are not included in the protection afforded by governmental immunity statutes. Where liability for an intentional tort is established, the judgment comes out of the doctor's own pocket.

NEGLIGENT TORTS

Although few physicians will ever have to face a suit for intentional tort, fewer still will complete a career without some involvement in a medical negligence action, whether as defendant, factual witness, expert witness, or forensic consultant. A basic understanding of negligence law lessens the physician's chances of becoming a defendant and increases his prospects for making an effective, rational response if he does become involved.

The prima facie case for negligence consists of 4 elements: duty, breach, causation, and damages. Each of these elements must be proved by the plaintiff by a preponderance of the evidence, and failure to do so will be fatal to the plaintiff's cause of action. In the case of a medical negligence action, the duty owed is coextensive with the doctor-patient relationship. It consists of the obligation on the doctor's part to acquire and maintain the same level of skill, care, and knowledge possessed by other members of the profession in good standing and to exercise that skill, care, and knowledge in treating his patients. There is no duty to accept a patient for treatment, and the physician may refuse to accept any person as a patient for any reason or for no reason at all.

There is one situation in which a physician may undertake treatment of an individual without creating a doctor-patient relationship and thus without incurring the obligation to treat, ie, by rendering emergency treatment outside the normal scope of the physician's practice. Public policy in favor of physicians stopping to aid accident victims is so strong that the states have enacted special statutes, known generally as Good Samaritan Acts, which provide immunity for liability arising out of ordinary negligence in treatment of such victims and often even for injury due to gross negligence. In addition, some states have enacted special statutes that provide for immunity of medical specialists who are called in emergencies as consultants to "bail out" another physician whose patient has deteriorated despite (or as a result of) earlier treatment. The following statutes enacted in California are typical examples: Section 2144 of the Business and Professions Code is entitled "Exemptions; Emergency Care; Liability for Acts or Omissions" and contains the following wording: "No person licensed under this Chapter, who in good faith renders emergency care at the scene of the emergency, shall be liable for any civil damages as result of any acts or omissions by such person in rendering the emergency care."

Section 2144.5 of the Business and Professions Code, entitled "Emergency Care for Complication Arising From Prior Care by Another; Exemption from Liability," reads as follows: "No person licensed under this Chapter, who in good faith upon the request of another person so licensed, renders emergency medical care to a person for a medical complication arising from prior care by another person so licensed, shall be liable for any civil damages as a result of any acts or omissions by such licensed person in rendering such emergency medical care."

One problem under the general heading of the physician's duty is the **unintentional** formation of a physician-patient relationship. This situation usually arises where a doctor is consulted very briefly and usually very casually by an individual seeking a quick (and free) "curbstone opinion." Where such an opinion is rendered by a physician in surroundings which quite clearly indicate that no professional relationship was intended, such as a social gathering, the courts have not found the existence of a doctor-patient relationship. The findings may be otherwise, however, where the doctor is consulted in the hospital, and—for example—instead of telling the questioner to come to his office for a regular appointment or referring him to another source for medical advice, or even saying nothing at all, he gives an opinion on which the "patient" relies. Even late-at-night advice by telephone to call another doctor in the morning may be held to constitute treatment, since it assumes that the patient can afford to wait until the morning before seeking care. The best course to follow when confronted with such a request, unless the doctor does intend to treat the patient, is to offer no advice at all other than an immediate referral to another source of medical treatment (eg, a hospital emergency room).

The physician's duty to the patient is performed within the "standard of care," and it is the failure of a physician to meet the standard of care in a given case that constitutes the "breach" element of the prima facie case for negligence. In the great majority of medical negligence cases, determining what the specific standard of care should be is beyond the comprehension of the laymen on the jury. In these cases, the law requires that the standard be established by expert medical testimony. This method of setting the standard requires a physician to take the witness stand and testify about the treatment required in the particular case. Although technically any physician may testify as an expert on any medical specialty, in practice, the medical expert will be of the particular specialty appropriate to the facts of the case.

At one time the standard of care was established by comparison with good medical practice in the same community in which the defendant was practicing. This so-called **locality rule** has undergone extensive change, until today most jurisdictions have broadened the standard to include treatment by physicians in good standing **under similar circumstances**—one of those circumstances being similarity of locale in terms of proximity to major medical centers and accessibility of medical information generally. Some states have gone so far as to abolish the locality rule entirely, holding that dissemination of medical advances, especially in the newer specialties, is so effective today that there is, in effect, a national standard of care for those fields of medicine. The well-established trend is away from the narrow confines of the locality rule and toward a national standard (and perhaps, eventually, an international standard of care, beginning with English-speak-

ing countries). Obviously, it is the efficacy of the treatment that is important in setting the standard of care and not the country or city that is the source of the treatment. The courts have increasingly recognized that geographic isolation should not offer protection for the use of modes of treatment that have been discredited and discarded by physicians in general.

Even in situations where one mode of therapy is preferred by the majority of specialists in the field, the law does not require that this particular form of treatment be adopted as the standard of care by which all physicians in that field shall be judged. It is sufficient that the treatment actually rendered be approved by a "respected minority of medical thought" in order for it to come within the standard of care.

The requirement of expert medical testimony to establish the standard of care has one well-established exception, ie, where the alleged negligence is within the lay understanding of the jury. In such cases, which include the "foreign object" cases, the judge must decide as a matter of law whether a medical expert will be required to establish the prima facie case in any particular respect. The judge may let the jury decide whether leaving a sponge, needle, clamp, or other object inside of the patient is negligent (ie, a breach of the standard of care) but may require medical expert testimony on the element of causation.

The standard of care based on the modes of treatment employed by members of the medical specialty group in good standing is a **minimum standard**. There are 2 situations in which that minimum standard can be raised to require a higher level of treatment by a medical defendant. The first is that a physician will be bound by his own representations to the patient of greater skill or experience than he actually has. In other words, a generalist who holds himself out to the patient as possessing the skill and experience of a specialist (or, if a specialist, that of a subspecialist) will be bound as a matter of law by the higher standard of care whether he possesses it or not. The second situation rarely arises and occurs when the court itself determines that the standard of treatment in current use is simply not high enough to protect society. The likelihood of such a finding by a court is increased in cases where the added burden on the physician in meeting the higher standard proposed is very slight and the benefit to patients is very great. Where the existing standard of care is not adequate to protect the patient, the court may impose a stricter standard. This type of reasoning has been demonstrated in recent years by the "glaucoma test case," Helling v Carey, 519 P2d 981, Washington 1974, and the "informed consent case" of Cobbs v Grant, 502 P2d 1, California 1972.

It is plain from the decisions on standard of care that the law requires every physician to know his own limitations. The physician who overreaches his abilities in a nonemergent case is risking liability for failure to consult or refer.

The element of causation has been the source of considerable confusion in the law. The plaintiff's case must include 2 types of causation: causation in fact and proximate cause. The test used most often in determining the presence of factual causation is simply that the defendant's conduct must be a substantial factor in bringing about the injury complained of. A minority of jurisdictions approach factual causation somewhat differently and require that the defendant's conduct be an indispensable antecedent to the plaintiff's injury, but in most cases the result is the same whichever test is used. Under either of these tests, the substance of the factual causation element is the same: proof of a sequence of events that connects breach of duty to conform to the standard of care with injury to the plaintiff.

The importance of the factual causation element is demonstrated by cases in which the treatment rendered is palliative and does not affect the course of the underlying disease process. In such cases, where the patient dies as a result of the disease, a breach of the standard of care by the physician in administering the palliative treatment does not as a matter of law lead to liability for the death because the treatment was not a cause in fact of the patient's death.

For the purposes of this discussion, it is best to think of the second type of causation, known either as proximate cause or legal cause, as a set of limitations on causation in fact. Having established causation in fact, the court may nevertheless fail to find liability if the injury is too far removed from the physician's conduct or where some abnormal force intervenes to break the chain of events connecting the conduct with the result. The effect of the proximate cause requirement is that, in addition to proving the chain of events connecting the conduct and the result, the plaintiff must also establish a close and direct relationship between the conduct and the result.

RES IPSA LOQUITUR

The 3 elements of duty, breach, and causation are commonly referred to collectively as the liability aspect of a negligence case. With 2 basic exceptions, the plaintiff must establish the defendant's liability by a preponderance of the evidence in order to recover. The first of these exceptions is the doctrine of **res ipsa loquitur** ("the thing speaks for itself"). Considering the reams of print and judicial contention that have been generated by this doctrine, its origin was rather prosaic. The term was first applied by Baron Pollack in the 1863 case of Byrne v Boadle (2 H & C 772, 159 Eng Rep 299 [1863]), tried on appeal before the English Court of Exchequer. In the words of Pollack: "There are certain cases of which it may be said res ipsa loquitur, and this seems one of them." In some cases the courts have held that the mere fact of the accident having occurred is evidence of negligence . . . . "The present case upon the evidence comes to this, a man is passing in front of the premises of a dealer in flour, and there falls down upon him a barrel of flour. I think

it apparent that the barrel was in the custody of the defendant who occupied the premises, and who is responsible for the acts of his servants who had the control of it; and in my opinion the fact of its falling is prima facie evidence of negligence."

The doctrine evolved steadily from that case down to the landmark decision of the California Supreme Court in Ybarra v Spangard (154 P2d 687, California 1944), a 1944 case applying the doctrine of res ipsa loquitur to medical negligence. The holding of the court in *Ybarra* was that "where a plaintiff receives unusual injuries while unconscious and in the course of medical treatment, all those defendants who had any control over his body or the instrumentalities which might have caused the injuries may properly be called upon to meet the inference of negligence by giving an explanation of their conduct."

The doctrine itself serves as a substitute for the elements of breach and causation, although the plaintiff must still establish the existence of the duty element and must show damages. In order to gain the benefit of this substitution, the plaintiff must establish, first, that the accident is of a kind that ordinarily does not occur in the absence of someone's negligence; second, that it must be caused by an instrumentality within the exclusive control of the defendant; and third, that it must not have been due to any voluntary action on his own part. If the court finds as a matter of law that these requirements have been met by the plaintiff, the court will instruct the jury that it may infer breach and causation by the defendant unless the inference is successfully rebutted by defendant's proof. As an inference of negligence, the doctrine of res ipsa loquitur operates as a substitute for evidence that would be especially difficult for the plaintiff to produce. The threshold issue—whether the injury is of a type that ordinarily does not occur in the absence of negligence—may itself call for expert medical testimony. If such testimony establishes that the injury occurs as an inherent risk in a documented percentage of cases not involving negligence, the doctrine will not be applied.

VICARIOUS LIABILITY

The other method of bypassing the prima facie case for negligence against a particular defendant is by imputed negligence. This method relies on the rule of law known as respondeat superior that holds the principal responsible for the acts of his agents. This doctrine is manifested in the operating room in the form of the so-called "captain of the ship" doctrine. As the captain of the ship, the surgeon is held responsible for negligent injury to the patient while the surgeon is directing the operation. It is the exercise of control over others by the surgeon that is the key to the application of the doctrine. For this reason, the actions of the anesthesiologist are generally not imputed to the surgeon. Of course, to the extent that the surgeon issues specific orders to the anesthesiologist, he assumes secondary liability if the anesthesiologist is negligent in carrying out the orders. In addition, in a medical partnership, the negligence of one partner is imputed to the other partners, and all partners become equally liable for damages which ensue. These instances of vicarious liability are exceptions to the general rule requiring that the elements of the prima facie case be established against the particular defendant only in the sense that once they are established as to one defendant they may fix liability on another defendant as well, based on the legal relationship of the parties.

DAMAGES

Of course, even when the plaintiff has established the elements of duty, breach, and causation by a preponderance of the evidence as to each, he still faces the requirement of proving the last element of his prima facie case: damages. Considering that the average cost today of bringing a medical malpractice case through trial is over $10,000, it is plainly impractical for a plaintiff's attorney to bring a case to trial unless the alleged injury to the plaintiff has been substantial and offers a potential money judgment well in excess of expenses incurred.

The 2 categories of compensatory damages in personal injury cases are general damages, which include such intangible elements as pain and suffering, and special damages, which include documented economic loss from costs of medical care and diminished income. In a wrongful death action, the general damages exclude pain and suffering but include the family's loss of "comfort and society," and the special damages include loss of economic support along with funeral expenses. In both personal injury and wrongful death actions, proof of gross negligence or especially outrageous conduct may result in exemplary (punitive) damages, which are fixed in relation to the wealth of the defendant.

DEFENSES

Common defenses to medical negligence actions are the statutes of limitations and contributory or comparative negligence. The purpose of **statutes of limitations** is to avoid litigation over stale claims by requiring a plaintiff to initiate suit within a fixed number of years after the negligent act or omission. Although the number of years varies from state to state, the effect of the running of the statutory period is the same everywhere—the plaintiff is forever barred from instituting suit based on that particular act or omis-

sion. The period begins to run on the date of the occurrence of the alleged negligence unless the negligence results in an injury that the plaintiff would typically be unaware of, such as the foreign body type of case. To cover this situation, most states and all federal jurisdictions apply the "discovery rule" under which the statutory period does not begin to run until the plaintiff knows, or in the exercise of reasonable diligence should have known, that the injury he suffered was the result of his treatment. Also, in many states the statutory period is tolled (suspended) by a legal disability on the part of the plaintiff such as minority or incompetency, by misrepresentation of the facts surrounding the treatment by the defendant physician, or by the "continuing care rule" which tolls the statute until the physician-patient relationship is terminated. The importance of a detailed medical record to the maintenance of a statute of limitations defense cannot be overemphasized.

The defense of **contributory negligence** operates in a minority of jurisdictions as a complete bar to the maintenance of the plaintiff's action when it is established that his injury was *in any way* the result of his own negligence. Thus, even if it were found that the surgeon was 75% responsible for the injury and the plaintiff only 25% responsible, a verdict for the defendant must result. A bare majority of states now employ the **comparative negligence** approach, which apportions the total amount of damages according to the relative negligence of the plaintiff and the defendant. Thus, in comparative negligence jurisdictions, if it is found that the plaintiff has been injured to the extent of $100,000 in damages but that he was 25% negligent himself, the defendant would be assessed $75,000 in damages.

INFORMED CONSENT

Much attention has been paid to the topic of informed consent in recent years, but, for all the reams of analysis, the new case law on consent does not actually affect the basic process of securing consent for medical treatment. The big question has always been, "How much should the patient be told?"

The new cases on consent, founded on the Canterbury v Spence (464 F2d 772, District of Columbia Cir 1972) and Cobbs v Grant (502 P2d 1, California 1972) decisions of 1972, do not change the priority of the question; neither do they answer it. Common sense is still the best guideline. The exchange between physician and patient in securing consent need be no different for any given treatment now than it was 5 years ago. The requirements are a description of the procedure, its chances of success, the risks, and the alternatives. The physician has always compared risks and benefits in deciding what mode of treatment to recommend. Explaining them to the patient in language he can understand is all that was ever required and is as sound in law today as it has always been good medical practice.

Traditionally, American courts have used the "customary practice" standard to determine whether enough information was presented to the patient for him to make a rational decision. The new line of cases, which now constitutes a growing minority trend, holds that reliance on the custom of doctors in good standing is an illusory standard. These courts have substituted a standard of materiality to the patient. Under this minority approach, the test becomes whether a reasonable man would have refused the treatment if he had known of the complication that occurred.

The effect of this materiality test is that the more important the procedure is to the patient's health, the less likely that he will be heard later to say that he would not have agreed to it had he known about the risk of the complication in question. Also, the less important the procedure to his health, the more credible is a later complaint that he would not have allowed it had he fully known its risks.

Put in its simplest form, a fully detailed informed consent is less crucial where the procedure may save life or limb and more important where the treatment objective is cosmetic. This principle finds its ultimate expression in the long-established rule that consent is implied in a medical emergency.

The signed consent form is merely evidence that the consent process occurred. It should always be backed up by the physician's own brief entry in the progress notes, with date and time. If the need to alter an entry arises, there is only one safe method: Line out the error (without obliterating it), initial and date the deletion, and enter the correct information.

MEDICAL INSURANCE

Discussions of the present status of the availability of medical malpractice insurance are usually phrased in terms of crisis. For the physician approaching private practice, it is imperative that he have sufficient understanding of the basics of professional insurance so he can at least ask the right questions.

The insurance crisis was generated by the loss of profitability of medical liability insurance. This resulted from reduction of surpluses owing to investment losses by the insurance companies, large increases in the cost to the primary insurer of reinsurance (beginning in 1970), and the combination of unpredictability of occurrence claims and the small physician base from which to generate the premium pool. Of the many proposals to remedy the problem, several have found nationwide application. First, there has been a direct shift in the type of policy written from "occurrence" to "claims made."

Briefly, an occurrence policy provides coverage for events that become the basis for claims in the year that the event occurs, while the claims made policy provides coverage only for the year in which a claim is presented to the insurer, regardless of when the underlying event took place. The practical effect of the change from occurrence to claims made policies is that the physician is only secure so long as he continues to buy coverage every year without lapse. For claims made policies, therefore, it is imperative that the insurance contract include provision for purchase by the doctor of the "tail" of his coverage. In other words, there must be liability coverage for the years following the doctor's retirement or change in practice from patient care to nonpatient care. Care should also be taken that "presentation" of a claim under a claims made policy be defined, since some contracts allow presentation only by a third party (plaintiff or attorney) and not by the physician himself. Attention must also be given to exclusions from coverage, which may place certain high-risk operations outside the scope of the policy.

The purposes of medical liability insurance are protection against costs of defending a suit (commonly as high as $15,000) and payment of adverse judgments. Any physician considering "going bare" (practicing without liability coverage) must weigh the potential impact on himself of these costs. As difficult to achieve as it is, attaining "judgment-proof" status (eg, irrevocable transfer of assets to another person prior to threat of suit) only protects against payment of a judgment. The only way to avoid litigation costs as well would be to submit to default judgment. The hazards of going bare thus make the cost of insurance more palatable.

Progress has been made recently in the formation of doctor-owned insurance companies and state no-fault medical liability systems. The long-term resolution of the insurance problem is most likely to be found in alternatives to litigation. The most promising alternative is compulsory binding arbitration. State programs establishing arbitration procedures are appearing with more frequency. The most recent decision in the area was by the Florida Supreme Court, upholding the compulsory arbitration law of the state (Carter v Sparkman, 335 So2d 802, Florida 1976; cert den January 11, 1977, 45 LW 3463). The United States Supreme Court refused to accept the patient's appeal in January 1977. Although federal action in this area has been discussed, such a course is highly unlikely because too few states are involved in the medical litigation explosion to justify a uniform national remedy.

FEES FOR THE MEDICAL WITNESS

The physician who performs services as a medical expert or a medical witness is entitled to compensation. Although requests for such services are made by an attorney, they are not performed for him even though he could not function as an attorney without them. The physician who testifies as a witness to fact (ie, one who actually treated the patient) is entitled only to the standard witness fee—currently $35.00 in federal courts. The medical expert hired to analyze the treatment rendered should agree in advance to a reasonable charge for his time. The patient has the same obligation to pay for medicolegal services as for hospital services necessary to enable a surgeon to perform his duties. An attorney may advance the money as a matter of convenience, but the client must pay the fees of a medical witness as a proper cost of litigation.

Under the principles of medical ethics of the American Medical Association, it is unethical for a physician to enter into any arrangement in which the amount of his fee for medicolegal services is contingent upon the outcome of the litigation. However, there is no objection if a physician contributes his medicolegal services without charge, just as he may contribute other professional services.

Excessive charges for medicolegal services give the medical profession a bad image, but the physician should not suffer financial loss because of time spent in preparing or giving medical evaluations or expert testimony. He should be compensated on a roughly computed hourly basis depending upon his hourly income from medical practice. While most physicians consider medicolegal services burdensome and disagreeable, excessive compensation is not justified as an inducement to accept this burden. With the growing trend toward liability litigation, it is essential that all physicians cooperate in the solution of medicolegal problems on a reasonable fee basis.

Many medical societies have drawn up agreements with bar associations whereby they provide a panel of experts which may be consulted by all lawyers. Members of the panel may confer with attorneys on either side and give them an unbiased, impartial evaluation. This arrangement, together with a relative fee schedule worked out between the bar association and the medical society on an hourly rate, promises to make medicolegal evaluations available to the lawyer and to be less stigmatizing to the physician.

THE ANATOMY OF MALPRACTICE

Wherever there is practice there is malpractice, and every physician commits malpractice at some time during his career. If good rapport has been established between the physician and his patient, legal actions for malpractice are rare. If there is bad feeling between the physician and patient, even a successful result may be regarded as unsatisfactory and cause a patient to think in terms of charges, litigation, and damages.

Physicians who are sued often do not realize that they have contributed to their difficulty because they lack tact, sensitivity, a good personality, or "bedside manner." They may be distracted by illness, overwork, or personal problems, or they may actually be negligent or unsympathetic.

Every physician must at least seem to like his patients, and he will have to understand them—otherwise, he will be prone to damage suits. Any physician who feels recurring antagonism or who has recurring episodes of tension between himself and his patients is perhaps ill-suited to his specialty, his profession, or his environs. Introspection and, if indicated, medical assistance in such instances may forestall disastrous litigation.

A strong contributing factor to the decision to sue is family prodding. A patient may respect the physician and appreciate his care, but the spouse, a relative, or even a neighbor may provoke an attitude of discontent. Surgeons in particular must pay careful attention to the patient's family and associates both before and after surgery, since they will have a major impact on his relationship with the patient. He must also extend this respect, courtesy, and cordiality to his peers, since one of the major reasons for the increased frequency of malpractice suits is careless conversation and criticism by physicians of the work of their colleagues. Such practices breed and encourage an awareness of the benefits of malpractice suits, as do the news media which make the public malpractice conscious. All scripts and articles written by physicians for nonprofessional audiences should be carefully screened for possible ill effects on the patient-physician relationship which may lead to unwarranted malpractice actions.

Second to bad rapport as a cause of malpractice action is the litigious patient. Some people are habitually alert for grievances—not only when they go to the doctor but always and everywhere in their lives. Such people are hard to recognize on an initial visit, but every physician should develop a habit of evaluating new patients for their suit-prone possibilities. If such an attitude is suspected, extra effort and caution are indicated in developing effective and cordial communication. If it becomes apparent at any time during the relationship that the physician and his patient are simply not getting along, the patient should be told in a polite and kindly manner that he would do better with another doctor. The patient who is suit-prone or antagonistic in his dealings with one physician may get along quite well with another. Good medicine requires a continuing close relationship characterized by strong mutual confidence on both sides.

The third major cause of malpractice is money. The physician must charge fairly and within the patient's circumstances, have a complete understanding of insurance coverage, handle insurance forms efficiently, and carefully evaluate extra charges. A preliminary or preoperative discussion of all medical and hospital costs is most important. Any unsettled dispute over fees may generate malpractice action.

Before a bill for medical services is turned over to a collection agency or a threat is made to sue the patient for an unpaid bill, the physician should check the medical records and think back over his conduct of the case. Could the patient think he has been negligent or careless? Routine business collection methods cannot always be used in medicine, and a threat of suit is often followed by a threat of countersuit. It may be better to forego a fee than to get involved in what may be an unwarranted but defensible malpractice action. Malpractice suits are always traumatic and embarrassing even though successfully defended.

If a malpractice action is instituted, the physician's position is always better if he has limited his practice to his competence, has called in consultants when indicated, has kept the patient and his family informed about the seriousness of the illness, and has kept meticulous records.

The physician who does not keep accurate, up-to-date records invites multiple hazards in court. It may be that he was sued in the first place because he relied on his memory and forgot something essential. He may not only have forgotten essential matters during the course of therapy, but without good records he is almost sure to forget significant facts when he appears in court. In the minds of a jury he is not primarily a medical witness but a doctor and an accused person, and the jurors feel that when they themselves go to a doctor they are putting their lives in his hands. All juries react adversely when a physician's records are inadequate, sloppy, and incomplete. Records that have been altered after a claim has been made constitute irrefutable damaging evidence against the physician and the hospital.

The most infrequent but most costly of all occasions for malpractice claims is the major bad result, and bad results are usually worse than the patient's original problem. The toxicity of potent new drugs, the hazard of new anesthetic procedures, and the risks of radical surgical procedures have begun to contribute materially to morbidity and mortality statistics. New procedures are often less safe than time-tested ones and may bring the patient closer to the threshold of death. In the past, the patient usually died if the result was bad and a successful suit for wrongful death ended with the payment of a suitable death award. With current anesthetics, resuscitative methods, and artificial support mechanisms, the patient may not die but live on as a vegetative organism, incurring high costs for custodial care. He may be wheeled into the courtroom staring vacantly at the doctor and being stared at by a sympathetic jury. Awards in such cases are high, for the current verdicts include compensation for projected loss of companionship, services, and income to the family as well as provision for prolonged and expensive support and medical care.

Of paramount importance is honesty. The physician who has committed an error in treatment should explain what happened in plain language to the patient. Such explanations should stick to the facts and avoid opinions and conclusions of law (such as admissions of negligence). Documentation of the discussion is essential.

Malpractice litigation is a problem area of medical practice in great need of medicolegal reform. The best hope for the future is that the disciplinary review boards of the state boards of medical examiners, the plaintiff's panels of county medical societies, peer control, and the development of arbitration agreements between doctor and patient established before treatment may lead to fewer actions for alleged malpractice and to the settlement of justifiable malpractice action without litigation.

●　　●　　●

General References

The Best of Law and Medicine. American Medical Association, 1966–1968, 1968–1970, and 1970–1973.

The Citation: A Medicolegal Digest for Physicians. American Medical Association.

Harney DM: *Medical Malpractice.* Allen Smith Co. (Indianapolis), 1973.

Holder AR: *Medical Malpractice Law.* Wiley, 1975.

Journal of Legal Medicine. GMT Medical Information Systems, Inc. (New York).

Louisell DW, Williams H: *Medical Malpractice.* Mathew Bender Co. (New York), 1960. [Annual supplements.]

Prosser WL: *Handbook of the Law of Torts,* 4th ed. West Publishing Co., 1971.

Report of the Secretary's Commission of Medical Malpractice: *Medical Malpractice.* Publication No. (05) 73-88, U.S. Department of Health, Education & Welfare.

Waltz JR, Inbau FE: *Medical Jurisprudence.* Macmillan, 1971.

7...
Radiation Therapy: Basic Principles & Clinical Applications

Karen K. Fu, MD, Glenn E. Sheline, PhD, MD, & Theodore L. Phillips, MD

BASIC RADIATION THERAPY

Radiation therapy deals with the treatment of disease using ionizing radiations. Since most diseases treated by radiation therapy are malignant, radiation therapy is actually a branch of oncology. Radiation therapy is the treatment of choice for the control of cancer in many sites. In other situations it is used, with curative intent, in conjunction with surgery or chemotherapy. It is also used for the relief of symptoms resulting from cancer. In order to know when and how to apply radiation therapy, the radiotherapist must be familiar with the biologic behavior of various forms of cancer and with the results obtainable by all treatment methods available. The realization that cancer is the second most common cause of death and that over 60% of cancer patients will require radiation therapy during the course of their disease underscores the importance of this branch of medical science.

PHYSICAL PRINCIPLES & RADIATION SOURCES

The radiations commonly used in radiotherapy include x-rays, gamma (γ) rays, electrons, and beta (β) rays. X-rays and γ rays are identical in properties but are produced by different sources. Electrons and β rays also differ only in the source from which they are derived. The efficacy of other types of radiation—eg, neutrons, protons, alpha (a) particles, and pi mesons—is presently under investigation. All have the common property of producing ionization within tissue. Ionization and other effects, such as excitation and free radical formation, cause chemical changes in cellular components. The total amounts of energy absorbed are exceedingly small, and the biologic effects are caused by the sensitivity to ionization of certain portions of cells.

X-rays and γ rays are electromagnetic radiations with neither mass nor charge; electrons and β rays are charged particles. X-rays are derived from the interaction between moving electrons and matter, whereas γ

rays are emitted during the decay of radioactive isotopes (radium, cobalt 60, etc). In biologic material, these rays give up energy by ejecting electrons from atomic orbits; in turn, the ejected electrons deposit energy in creating charged ions (ionization) within the target material. Most of the total ionization is caused by these secondary electrons. The distribution of the absorbed energy is related both to the absorption pattern of the primary radiation and the distance the secondary electrons travel within the tissue. When a beam of x-rays enters tissue, the energy absorption at first increases because the secondary electrons are building to a maximum. The depth of this maximum point beneath the surface increases with the energy of the x-rays. After a maximum, the energy absorption decreases in an exponential fashion.

In the case of electron beams, the ionization within tissue is due in large part to the primary electrons. The energy is deposited fairly uniformly along the pathway of the electron. Such electrons travel a finite distance and then stop. With a monoenergetic electron beam, energy absorption in soft tissue is thus relatively

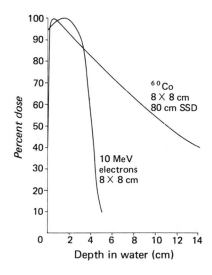

Figure 7–1. Comparison of the depth dose distribution for a γ ray beam and an electron beam. Dose is expressed as a percentage of the maximum and plotted against depth for an 8 × 8 cm ^{60}Co beam and an 8 × 8 cm 10 MeV electron beam. SSD = source-skin distance.

constant from the surface to near the end of the electron's path, at which point the deposition of energy rises slightly and then falls abruptly to zero. The different absorption characteristics—exponential after an initial build-up interval for x-ray photons and approximately linear with rapid drop-off for electrons—can be adapted to fit various clinical situations (Fig 7–1).

In modern radiotherapy, 2 or more radiation beams are often combined to produce a more desirable distribution of absorbed energy than would result from a single beam. Furthermore, compensating or wedge-shaped filters are frequently used to compensate for body contour or to alter the shape of the absorption curve (Fig 7–2).

During the last 2 or 3 decades there has been an increasing trend to megavoltage (greater than 1 million volt) x-rays or γ rays for radiotherapy of deeply situated lesions. The advantages of the higher energy radiations are (1) "skin sparing," (2) less absorption in bone, (3) decreased energy absorption by healthy tissue, and (4) greater penetration. "Skin sparing" derives from the fact that the absorbed energy or dose at any depth depends largely on the secondary electrons. With x-rays generated by a 250 kilovolt peak (kVp) x-ray machine, the secondary electrons travel such short distances that the maximum energy absorption is essentially at the surface. With higher energies, the secondaries travel many millimeters or even centimeters; therefore, energy absorption builds up and does not reach its maximum until a considerable depth has been reached. In the case of ^{60}Co gamma rays, the maximum energy deposition is at 5 mm; for x-rays from a 25 million electron volt (MeV) betatron, the maximum is at 5 cm beneath the surface (Fig 7–3). Decreased absorption of megavoltage irradiation in bone compared to soft tissues is due to the difference in atomic

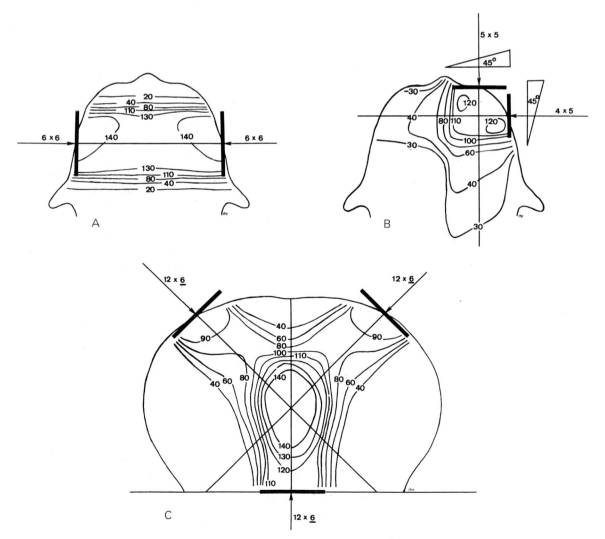

Figure 7–2. Isodose curves for several combinations of external radiation beams from ^{60}Co. *A:* Two 6 × 6 cm beams with opposed central axes. *B:* Two beams, 4 × 5 cm and 5 × 5 cm, with central axes at right angles utilizing 45 degree wedge filters. *C:* Three 12 × 6 cm beams with central axes at 120 degree angles to each other.

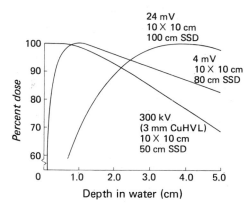

Figure 7—3. Comparison of the depth doses for x-ray beams of different energies. SSD = source-skin distance; CuHVL = copper half value layer.

number of the atoms within these 2 types of tissue. The fact that higher energy radiations undergo less side-scatter and hence have a more sharply defined beam contributes to a decrease in radiation dose to healthy tissue surrounding the target volume.

A detailed discussion of the sources of external beam therapy is beyond the scope of this book, but a few broad statements about presently available equipment may be useful.

Conventional x-ray machines produce x-rays with energies up to 300 kVp. This is known as "kilovoltage" or "orthovoltage." The ^{137}Cs (cesium 137) therapy machine gives radiation approximately equivalent to an 800 kVp x-ray generator. At present, the most common source for deep therapy is the artificial radioisotope ^{60}Co (cobalt 60), which yields gamma rays of 1.17 and 1.33 MeV. Electron linear accelerators producing x-rays or electron beams with energies up to 18 MeV are also widely used. Less common but available in some centers are linear accelerators and betatrons capable of energies of 25, 35, or even 45 MeV. All photon or x-ray beams above 1 MeV are known as "megavoltage" beams.

Short distance radiotherapy (brachytherapy) takes advantage of the rapid decrease in dose with distance from a radiation source. For this purpose, the radiation source may be placed within a cavity (intracavitary) or inserted directly into tissue (interstitial). One or more sources may be used, with the geometric arrangement dictated by the clinical circumstances of the particular lesion. After a prescribed period of time, the sources are usually removed. They may be in the form of needles, narrow tubes, wires, or small seeds. While the most commonly used radioactive material is radium, interstitial and intracavitary sources may contain radon gas or artificially produced radioactive cesium, cobalt, gold, yttrium, or iridium. Beta ray applicators, such as the ^{90}Sr-loaded eye applicator, are used for the treatment of thin superficial lesions.

Two units for describing radiation dosages are in common usage. One relates to the amount of radiation

needed to produce a certain amount of ionization per unit volume of air; the other relates to the energy absorbed per unit mass. The roentgen (R), a unit of exposure, is defined only for x-ray and γ ray photons; it is the amount of radiation which will produce ionization equivalent to a charge of 1 electrostatic unit in 1 ml of air at standard temperature and pressure. Since different tissues will actually absorb different amounts of energy when exposed to the same beam of radiation, the concept of **absorbed dose** has been developed. The unit of absorbed dose is the rad, and represents the absorption of 100 ergs (energy units) per gram of matter. Ionizing radiation of all types can be measured in rads. For x-rays or gamma rays with energies of a few MeV, exposure of soft tissue to 1 R will result in the absorption of 0.96 rad. The ratio of rads to roentgens varies according to the energy of the x-ray and γ radiation and the composition of the substance irradiated. With low-energy x and γ rays and material of higher atomic number, such as bone, the ratio may be as high as 4:1.

BIOLOGIC BASIS OF RADIATION THERAPY

In radiobiology, cell death is usually defined as loss of reproductive integrity. Following radiation, a cell may appear physically intact and may be able to make protein or synthesize DNA or even undergo several mitoses, but if it has lost the ability to divide indefinitely it is considered dead. This definition of cell death, in terms of loss of reproductive integrity, is particularly relevant to the radiotherapy of tumors since one of the most important characteristics of a tumor is its ability to divide indefinitely. The basic aim in the radiotherapy of tumors is either to destroy them or to render them unable to divide and cause further growth and spread of cancer.

The mechanism of radiation-induced cell death is not fully understood. However, the great bulk of radiobiologic data suggests that the most sensitive site of radiation injury in the cell is in the nucleus. Experiments on mammalian cells using a microbeam technic in which either the nucleus or cytoplasm could be selectively irradiated indicate that the nucleus is 100–1000 times more sensitive than the cytoplasm. There is strong circumstantial evidence that the DNA of the chromosomes constitutes the primary target for radiation-induced cell lethality. Some studies have shown that radiation can cause breaks in one or both DNA strands and that the number of double strand breaks as well as the number of chromosomal aberrations corresponds to the fraction of cells killed.

In vitro studies of cell cultures have shown that cell death following irradiation appears to be a complex exponential function of dose, ie, a specified radiation dose kills a constant fraction of irradiated cells. Thus, the dose required to kill a given number of tumor cells depends on the number of tumor cells initially present and is related to the tumor size. Fig 7—4 shows typical survival curves for mammalian cells exposed to radiation plotted on a semilogarithmic scale. For densely ionizing radiation such as neutrons, the dose-response curve is a straight line. For sparsely ionizing radiation such as x-rays, the dose-response curve may have an initial shoulder followed by a portion which is straight, or almost straight. The slope of the final straight portion of the survival curve is usually related to the D_0 or the dose required to reduce the

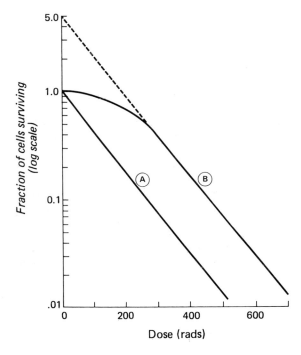

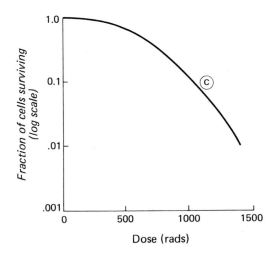

surviving fractions to 37%. The D_0 increases directly with cellular radioresistance. With the exception of lymphocytes and germinal cells, the D_0 levels for most mammalian cells irradiated in vitro lie within the range of 110—240 rads.

The survival curve for sparsely ionizing radiation shown in Fig 7—4 curve B is often referred to as a multi-target single-hit survival curve which assumes that all cells in the population contain a number of targets (N) of uniform size; a target is inactivated by single hit, and cell death occurs only when N targets have been hit. The multi-target survival curve can be described by the following equation:

$$S/S_0 = 1 - [1 - e^{-D/D_0}]^N$$

The multi-target equation often gives a poor fit to survival data in the very low dose and very high dose regions for some cell lines and culture conditions. Recently, a 2-component cell survival model has been proposed to describe radiation cell inactivation by a linear-quadratic equation;

$$S/S_0 = e^{[-aD-\beta D^2]}$$

According to this model, cell inactivation by radiation can result from single hit (a) or double hit (β) events. This 2-component model appears to give a better fit for most mammalian cell survival data than the multi-target equation (curve C). This model was developed from molecular and microdosimetric theories and equates the cellular surviving fraction with the product of 2 exponential terms depending upon the first and second order of the dose, respectively.

In vivo, other factors affect the end results of irradiation, and the situation is far more complex than in a cell culture. Apparent growth or shrinkage of any normal tissue or tumor will depend upon the balance between new cell production and the natural cell death rate as well as upon cell killing by an outside agent. Two tumors with equal cellular sensitivity and equal numbers of cells but different cell growth and cell loss rates may show the effect of irradiation at different times; one may be misled if a judgment on sensitivity is made too soon. Comparison of cell survival after doses given as single exposure vs the same dose given in multiple exposures separated by various time intervals has shown that in most cell systems cellular repair and increased survival follow divided doses. With such fractionation it may require a total dose 2—5 times greater than that given as a single dose to produce an equal effect (Fig 7—5). Ways of improving the therapeutic ratio* using various dose fractionation patterns are under study.

The radiation response of mammalian cells is influenced by many different chemical, biologic, and physical factors. One of the most important chemical factors which influence radiosensitivity is oxygen.

Figure 7—4. Cell survival curves following irradiation of cell cultures. *Curve A:* Survival curve for densely ionizing radiation. *Curve B:* Survival curve for sparsely ionizing radiation—multi-target single-hit model. *Curve C:* Survival curve for sparsely ionizing radiation—2-component linear-quadratic model.

*Therapeutic ratio = $\dfrac{\text{Damage to tumor}}{\text{Damage to normal tissue}}$

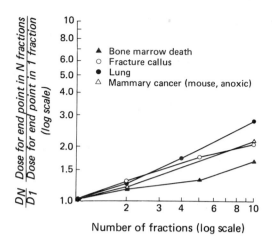

Figure 7–5. A demonstration of the effect of recovery between doses on radiation tolerance. The ratio of the dose for a given end point in N fractions to the dose for the same end point in one fraction is plotted against the number of fractions. Both are on logarithmic scales.

Well-oxygenated cells are 2½–3 times as sensitive as anoxic cells. With few exceptions, normal tissues have an adequate oxygen supply. In animal tumors, up to 30% of cells are severely hypoxic, and the same presumably applies to human tumors. If it were not for the phenomenon called reoxygenation, hypoxia would tend to protect tumor cells. With fractionated radiation exposures, the death and subsequent loss of oxygenated cells permit hypoxic ones to come into position nearer a capillary and thus regain sensitivity. The effectiveness of fractionated clinical radiation therapy is probably due in large part to reoxygenation. Failure of reoxygenation may account for the resistance of some tumors. Certain compounds such as metronidazole (Flagyl) and a 2-nitroimidazole derivative, Ro 07–0582, appear to selectively radiosensitize hypoxic cells and are currently under clinical investigation for potential improvement of the therapeutic ratio. Other compounds such as cysteine and the thiophosphate WR2721 which contain sulfhydryl groups appear to offer preferential radioprotection to normal tissues. In addition, some chemotherapeutic agents such as dactinomycin, doxorubicin (Adriamycin), and bleomycin are known to enhance radiation effects on normal tissues as well as tumors.

The radiosensitivity of mammalian cells also varies with the position in the cell cycle (cell age). This variation of radiosensitivity with cell cycle phase appears to be different for different cell lines.

Neutrons, helium ions, heavy ions, and pi mesons cause dense ionizations in tissues and are referred to as high LET (linear energy transfer) radiation. The sensitivity of mammalian cells exposed to these types of radiation appears to be less dependent on the oxygen concentration and position in the cell cycle. These particles are currently under clinical investigation.

Many interrelated factors play a role in clinical application of radiation therapy. They are: (1) the inherent sensitivity of normal cells and tumor cells in the volume treated, (2) the total number of various types of cells present, (3) the ability of normal cells to migrate and tumor cells to metastasize, (4) the capability of repopulation of tumor vs normal tissue, (5) rearrangement of cells in the cell cycle, (6) repair of sublethal damage in tumor and normal cells, and (7) oxygen tension and reoxygenation. The extent to which these factors affect the sparing of normal tissue cells and the killing of tumor cells forms the basis of radiation therapy.

NORMAL TISSUE REACTIONS & INJURY

Any cancer can be locally destroyed by radiation if the dose is sufficient. In clinical practice, the dose-limiting factor is the damage unavoidably received by nearby normal tissues. When radiation therapy was done with medium-voltage radiation and by incompletely trained physicians, complication rates were understandably high; with fully trained radiotherapists and modern equipment, the incidence of clinically significant complications is very low.

The reactions in rapidly renewing cell systems which appear within days after exposure and heal early should be distinguished from the delayed late reactions that may be progressive and mean permanent damage. The extent of late radiation effects in all tissues is influenced by the degree of injury to the supporting structures, particularly the vascular system, where prevention of proliferation of endothelial cells, endarteritis, and obliteration of capillary lumens may occur. If the vascular injury is excessive, late damage appears in the form of atrophy, fibrosis, and even ulceration. Such changes due to the action of radiation on the vascular and connective tissue systems may appear many months or years after completion of treatment.

In tissues with rapid cell turnover—eg, the epithelium of gut and skin—injury reactions appear within a matter of days and, if the dose is not excessive, healing is equally rapid. In other tissues, such as brain, slow cell reproduction means that the damage will become evident only after many months or years. Permanent suppression of osteocyte production may contribute to the failure of a fracture to heal. Alteration in saliva may result in late severe changes in dental structures, even outside of irradiated areas, and this may in turn permit introduction of infection into devitalized bone. Since these late reactions appear only after long intervals of time, they are of no value in judging the conduct of a particular course of radiation therapy. Knowledge of them and of the frequency and severity with which they occur under various circumstances is essential in treatment planning.

Late reactions in the CNS may cause focal brain necrosis or radiation myelitis and spinal cord transection. Late changes in the thorax include pericarditis and radiation pneumonitis. Radiation nephritis can occur after abdominal irradiation. The total dose that leads to these late complications varies according to the organ included in the radiation beam. In general, the organs most sensitive to clinically significant late damage are the kidneys, liver, lungs, and lenses. Somewhat less sensitive are the bowel, spinal cord, brain, pericardium, cornea, and retina. Among structures least likely to show clinically significant late injury are skeletal muscle, subcutaneous connective tissue, and other supportive tissues in the body, including bone. The limiting doses when the weekly treatment is given as 5 fractions of 200 rads each (1000 rads per week) are 2000 rads for the kidneys and lungs, 2500 rads for the liver, and 4500 rads for structures of intermediate sensitivity such as spinal cord. The other tissues usually withstand 6000 rads or more. These doses can be increased if the treated volume is small or the fractionation used involves smaller individual doses.

PRE- & POSTOPERATIVE RADIATION THERAPY

The rationale for combining radiation therapy and surgery in the treatment of cancer is that each method may compensate for deficiencies of the other. Irradiation may be used to sterilize the margins of a lesion; surgical resection may then be relied upon to remove the less radiosensitive central portion or extensions into bone and cartilage. Irradiation may, by killing the majority of cancer cells prior to resection, reduce the probability of seeding or dissemination of viable cancer cells during surgery. The use of such combined therapy is rational for highly invasive, poorly differentiated cancers with a high risk of spread and in situations where adequate surgical resection is impossible for anatomic reasons.

Pre- or postoperative radiation therapy may also be given to regional lymph nodes. This is not combination therapy in the sense that both methods are applied to the same area; rather, the radiation is used to extend the definitive therapy beyond the limits of the surgical excision. An example of such combination therapy is the irradiation of supraclavicular and internal mammary lymph nodes following radical mastectomy for breast cancer.

SELECTION & MANAGEMENT OF RADIATION THERAPY PATIENTS

Specific indications for the selection of patients for curative radiation therapy will be given below in the discussion of specific diseases. In general, the smaller, superficial, exophytic lesions are most amenable to radiation therapy; large, avascular, necrotic tumors and those with bone involvement are less likely to be controlled permanently by radiation therapy alone. Radiation should be used when it offers either a higher cure rate or the same cure rate as surgery with a lower morbidity or better functional result. Radiation therapy may occasionally be used instead of surgery if the patient's general condition contraindicates a radical operation.

Palliation involves the relief of symptoms by the use of a specific treatment method. Patients selected for palliative treatment with radiation should have a local problem, present or impending, that can be relieved or significantly delayed in onset by treatment. Palliative radiotherapy may be employed for pain due to local invasion or bone involvement, obstruction of hollow organs, involvement of functioning areas in the brain or spinal cord, irritation or ulceration of mucosal surfaces such as those of the bronchi or bladder, or local ulcerating, infected tumor masses. In certain cancers, such as those arising in the oral or pharyngeal mucosa, the dosage required for palliation is essentially the same as that used for cure. Palliation of obstructive or brain lesions also requires large doses. Lasting palliation of bone pain can often be achieved with substantially lower doses.

The proper selection of patients for radiation therapy requires close cooperation between the surgeon, radiotherapist, and chemotherapist. A combined plan, involving 2 or 3 methods of treatment, may offer the best chance of cure or palliation. It is usually best if the patient is seen jointly by all members of the oncology team and the treatment planned as a joint effort from the beginning.

A patient being considered for radiation therapy should have a thorough medical evaluation, including history, physical examination, and laboratory tests. Significant medical problems should be attended to and housing and transportation problems solved before treatment is undertaken. The most frequent problem arising during radiation therapy is the maintenance of adequate food and fluid intake. Patients irradiated around the head and neck often lose their appetite because of changes in saliva and impaired taste sensation. Specially prepared foods and suitable encouragement may be of value. Special diets may be needed for patients with bowel problems. Changes in diet or use of medication for the control of symptoms resulting from radiation should never be undertaken without first consulting the radiotherapist since he will be using the severity of the reaction as a guide to treatment.

Cancer patients are often ill and subject to numerous concomitant medical problems. Acute myocardial infarction, serum hepatitis, acute appendicitis, perforation of a peptic ulcer, and many other unrelated major medical or surgical problems may occur in patients undergoing radiation therapy. The tendency to ascribe such problems to the irradiation should be resisted so that definitive therapy will not be delayed.

RADIATION THERAPY
OF SPECIFIC DISEASES

This discussion of the radiation therapy of specific diseases is intended only to outline the place of radiation therapy, with enough comment to give the reader a general understanding of the levels of dose used, the areas or volumes treated, and the results obtainable. It is not intended for use as a manual of radiation therapy. In clinical practice, treatment planning is varied for each patient and each disease. Treatment plans, including the daily and total dose to be delivered, are often altered during the course of treatment depending upon the response of the lesion and the effects on the patient. A discussion sufficiently detailed to permit conduct of treatment for a specific patient is beyond the scope of this book.

Before proceeding to the discussion of specific diseases, a final word of caution may be appropriate. The physician or physicians who are to be responsible for the management of a cancer patient should be consulted before any act, even biopsy, is performed. Seeing the intact, untouched lesion can be of immense help in planning the definitive treatment, whether it be surgery, radiation therapy, or a combination of the two. To excise the evidence and then refer the patient elsewhere for treatment imposes a severe handicap upon the therapist and the patient.

SKIN MALIGNANCIES

Basal Cell & Squamous Cell Carcinomas

Basal cell and squamous cell carcinomas are the most common malignancies of the skin. Basal cell carcinomas tend to invade slowly but they rarely metastasize. Metastases from squamous cell carcinomas, although more frequent than from basal cell lesions, are also rare. Both types are sufficiently radiosensitive to be controllable by radiation doses well within the limits of skin tolerance. While locally advanced carcinomas with infiltration into bone are more difficult to control, radiation therapy of the smaller lesions yields a cure rate of greater than 95%. Since surgical excision gives approximately equal control rates, the choice of treatment in a specific situation depends on the complexity of the surgical procedure and the resulting functional or cosmetic deficiency. In the absence of infection, radiation is the treatment of choice for lesions of the eyelids and over cartilage. Small carcinomas of the lip (eg, 1 cm) can be either excised or irradiated. Larger lip lesions which require a more complex surgical procedure are better treated by radiation, which provides a better functional result. Carcinomas of the trunk where there is adequate skin for closure are best treated surgically. Surgery is the preferred treatment for lesions on the backs of the hands. Surgi-

cal resection is preferred for the rare case of lymph node metastasis.

Carcinomas of the skin up to 2–3 cm in size may be treated with orthovoltage x-ray radiation delivering skin doses of about 4500 rads in 15 fractions over 3 weeks. The fields are shaped by lead sheeting to include a generous margin around the lesion. The details of treatment (energy, filtration, etc) depend upon the particular situation. Larger lesions are treated more slowly and to higher doses. Deeply infiltrating ones are treated with higher energy and more heavily filtered radiation. Protective lead shields are used under eyelids and behind the lips. Treatment over cartilage is not contraindicated but requires greater fractionation.

Malignant Melanomas

Most malignant melanomas respond to radiation, but the doses required are high and the control less certain than for skin carcinomas. In most situations, surgical resection is the treatment of choice, with radiation therapy reserved for patients who refuse surgery, for those in whom the disease is so extensive that surgery is not feasible, and for those with symptomatic metastases. Radiation therapy of fixed nodes or of extensive local recurrence has sometimes resulted in local control for several years.

BREAST CANCER

Current opinions regarding the proper treatment for carcinoma of the breast vary widely. The primary goal of surgery and radiotherapy in the management of carcinoma of the breast is control of the primary and regional disease. As chemotherapeutic agents become increasingly effective in controlling microscopic metastasis, it is even more important to obtain local control.

The role of radiotherapy in the management of breast carcinoma depends on the extent of disease. In patients with early (T_1, T_2) disease, results of conservative surgery such as tumorectomy or wedge or quadrant resection combined with radiotherapy are similar to those of radical mastectomy and can be offered to patients with early disease as an alternative to more radical surgery. Usually, the chest wall and regional lymph nodes including the axillary, supraclavicular, and internal mammary lymph nodes are irradiated with 5000 rads in 5½ weeks. An additional 1500–3000 rads are delivered to the primary lesion through reduced field with external radiotherapy or an interstitial implant. When there are clinically positive axillary lymph nodes, an additional 1000–1500 rads are delivered to the axilla.

Although there is no proof that postoperative radiotherapy following radical mastectomy improves survival, there are substantial data to support the view that modern megavoltage radiotherapy in moderate dosage can reduce the overall incidence of chest wall or regional lymph node recurrence from about 10–20%

without postoperative radiotherapy to approximately 5% with postoperative radiotherapy. When the axillary lymph nodes are negative for metastasis, postoperative radiotherapy with 5000 rads in 5½ weeks delivered to the ipsilateral internal mammary and supraclavicular lymph nodes may be indicated, but only for patients with medial or central lesions. When several axillary lymph nodes are positive, when the primary is large or invading the skin, or when a simple mastectomy was done, the chest wall as well as regional lymph nodes are irradiated with 5000 rads in 5½ weeks. No postoperative radiotherapy should be given for patients with outer quadrant lesions and negative axillary nodes. The axilla is also given full doses of irradiation when only a simple mastectomy is performed or when more than 50% of the axillary lymph nodes are positive following modified radical or radical mastectomy. No convincing evidence exists that postoperative radiotherapy is harmful to the patient.

For patients with locally advanced inoperable carcinoma of the breast, long-term local control and sometimes cure can be achieved with vigorous radiotherapy to the primary disease and regional lymph nodes.

Radiotherapy also plays an important and undisputed role in the treatment of local recurrence or metastases from breast carcinoma. Its use must be carefully coordinated with systemic therapy with hormones or chemotherapeutic agents. With judicious use of radiotherapy, soft tissue and bone metastases can often be controlled for years. Radiotherapy remains one of the most effective means of palliation of painful bone metastases. When there is impending fracture in weight-bearing bones or the long bones of the upper extremities, orthopedic stabilization with internal fixation is usually done prior to radiotherapy. Radiation castration, while slower than surgical castration, is apparently as effective and may be accomplished by doses of 2000 rads in 2–3 weeks. Radiation castration is utilized when there is a contraindication to oophorectomy or when other pelvic structures require radiation therapy at the same time.

BONE TUMORS

Reticulum Cell Sarcoma

Radiation therapy is highly effective in the local control of primary reticulum cell sarcoma (histiocytic lymphoma) of the bone. Because of the tendency for these tumors to extend throughout the marrow cavity, the entire bone is irradiated with a dose of 4000–4500 rads in 4–5 weeks and an additional 1000 rads in 1 week to the primary lesion. The 5-year survival rate is about 50%. Metastases may be irradiated in conjunction with combination chemotherapy.

Ewing's Sarcoma

In Ewing's sarcoma, radiotherapy is used for the control of the primary tumor. Usually the entire bone with a generous margin of soft tissue is irradiated with 4000–4500 rads in 4–5 weeks and an additional 1500–2000 rads in 1½–2½ weeks is delivered to reduced fields encompassing only the clinically and radiographically evident lesion. Because subclinical metastases are probably present at the time of diagnosis in the majority of the patients, combination chemotherapy using drugs such as cyclophosphamide, vincristine, dactinomycin, and doxorubicin is given in conjunction with radiotherapy for 1–2 years. This approach has resulted in a marked prolongation of disease-free survival times, and improved cure rates may be expected.

In patients presenting with metastatic disease, radiotherapy is delivered to the primary tumor and to areas where large metastases are located concurrently with combination chemotherapy. When the entire lungs are irradiated concurrently with dactinomycin or doxorubicin, the total dose should not exceed 1350 rads in 2 weeks. Small areas of the lung may be treated to higher doses.

Osteosarcoma

Local control of osteosarcoma by radiation alone is rare even with large doses exceeding normal tissue tolerance. Amputation is the treatment of choice. Recent results suggest that adjuvant chemotherapy using high-dose methotrexate with citrovorum rescue or doxorubicin delays the appearance of pulmonary metastases and may lead to improved survival. Radiotherapy is of value in the treatment of osteosarcoma in nonresectable locations and in conjunction with combination chemotherapy in providing symptomatic relief for patients with metastatic disease.

Chondrosarcoma & Fibrosarcoma

As is the case with osteosarcoma, these tumors are primarily treated by surgery. Radiotherapy is used for nonresectable tumors and for the occasional patient who refuses surgery.

Multiple Myeloma

The primary treatment of multiple myeloma is chemotherapy. Radiotherapy is highly effective in providing pain relief for lesions unresponsive to chemotherapy. Solitary plasmacytoma of the bone is rare, although permanent control has been achieved with radiotherapy in the dose range of 3500–4000 rads in 4 weeks.

Benign Bone Tumors

Certain benign bone tumors such as benign giant cell tumors and aneurysmal bone cysts are controllable with radiation therapy with doses in the range of 3000–4000 rads in 3–4 weeks. In giant cell tumors it is exceedingly important to obtain adequate biopsy to rule out malignancy. Eosinophilic granuloma is highly radiosensitive, and local control can be achieved with 1000–2000 rads in 1–2 weeks.

SOFT TISSUE TUMORS

During the past decade, substantial evidence has been accumulated to show that small to moderate-sized soft tissue sarcomas can be treated effectively by conservative surgery combined with high-dose radiotherapy using modern equipment and sophisticated technics. Furthermore, some medically or technically inoperable lesions can be successfully controlled by high-dose megavoltage radiotherapy alone. Usually 5000 rads per 5–6 weeks are delivered to all areas of potential microscopic involvement. An additional 1500–2000 rads are delivered to a reduced volume encompassing the primary site using external radiotherapy, electron beam, or interstitial implants. With this approach, local control rates of 90% have been achieved. For lesions of the extremities, useful limbs can be retained in most patients and amputation is reserved for occasional failures. In addition to the size of the lesion, the histologic grade appears to be an important indicator of prognosis; 2-year disease-free survival rates of 86%, 51%, and 17% for grades I, II, and III have been reported.

Low-grade nonmetastasizing tumors such as desmoids, infiltrating neurofibromas, and infiltrating myxomas, which are inaccessible or too extensive for surgical extirpation, can often be treated successfully with high doses of radiotherapy. Many months to years may be required before the complete response to therapy becomes evident.

In childhood rhabdomyosarcomas, the prognosis has been significantly improved by using a multimodality approach with limited surgery combined with high-dose radiotherapy and chemotherapy using vincristine, dactinomycin, and cyclophosphamide. For tumors in the head and neck area, a 70% 3-year survival and 90% local control rate have been achieved using this approach.

CNS TUMORS

Radiation, after biopsy and decompression, is the treatment of choice for the radiosensitive medulloblastomas, ependymomas, and certain lesions of the pineal gland. In conjunction with decompressive shunt, radiation is the accepted therapy for tumors in areas such as the pons, medulla, and brain stem, where attempts at biopsy carry prohibitively high mortality and morbidity rates. For most gliomas, postoperative radiation often prolongs useful survival and increases survival rates. The totally resected cystic cerebellar astrocytoma has a high cure rate with surgery alone. For glioblastoma multiforme, radiotherapy in conjunction with carmustine can prolong survival. Meningiomas are primarily a surgical problem, but radiation contributes to control in the incompletely resected lesion and, as a preoperative measure, may significantly reduce vascularity.

Ependymomas and pinealomas should be treated with large local fields, including the adjacent ventricular system. While intracranial ependymomas occasionally seed down the spinal canal, in our experience this has been evident clinically in less than 5% of patients. Treatment of the local area with doses of about 5000 rads in 5½ weeks has produced a 5-year survival rate of 85%; the failures usually have been at the primary site.

Unbiopsied tumors of the brain stem and most of the differentiated gliomas are treated with doses of 5000–5500 rads in 6–7 weeks. With these doses, complications from the radiation are few. In one well-documented series, use of radiation yielded a 5-year survival rate of 25% for unbiopsied intrinsic brain stem tumors. For glioblastoma multiforme, all of the brain is treated to a dose of 6000 rads in 6½ weeks.

Radiation treatment of intracranial metastases from carcinomas and lymphomas is often rewarding. Lymphomas are usually controlled by relatively small doses, and many patients with metastatic carcinoma can be maintained in a functional state for long periods with 4500–5000 rads in 5–6 weeks. Because of the frequency of multiple lesions, both of these entities require therapy to the entire intracranial volume. With lymphomas, it may be necessary to treat the spinal canal either at the same time or later.

NEUROBLASTOMA

Neuroblastomas are radiosensitive tumors of childhood. They may arise in the adrenal gland or any sympathetic ganglion and commonly metastasize to bone. The primary treatment is surgery if the tumor is resectable. Radiotherapy is given postoperatively to patients with residual disease or unresectable tumors and is particularly beneficial in patients with stage III disease. In patients with disseminated disease, radiotherapy is of value in the palliation of symptomatic metastases. Occasionally, radiotherapy is used to reduce the size of a nonresectable lesion prior to a second operation. Doses in the range of 1500–4000 rads given at 150–200 rads/day have been used depending on the age of the patient. Lower doses are used for metastatic lesions. Spontaneous regression or maturation into ganglioneuromas sometimes occurs in very young children even with advanced disease.

The value of adjuvant chemotherapy in combination with surgery or radiotherapy is currently under investigation. Although the overall survival rate for neuroblastoma has not changed during the past 20 years, preliminary reports of combined drug therapy are encouraging.

CARCINOMA OF THE THYROID

Papillary and follicular carcinomas are primarily surgical problems. Even in the presence of multiple bilateral cervical metastases cure is obtained in a substantial percentage of cases by thyroidectomy and neck dissection. Local invasion or inoperable recurrence and isolated distant metastases are treated with external irradiation, and control lasting many years may be achieved. In the case of widespread (especially pulmonary) metastases, radioactive iodine (^{131}I) may prove effective. Administration of thyroid hormone may control or at least retard the growth of metastases from some papillary and follicular carcinomas.

Undifferentiated adenocarcinomas with local invasion and lymphosarcomas of the thyroid are treated primarily with radiation. Radiation therapy should be offered for spindle cell and giant cell carcinomas, but these lesions have an exceedingly poor prognosis irrespective of the therapy applied.

OCULAR & INTRAORBITAL TUMORS

The tumors of importance to radiotherapy in this anatomic area include retinoblastoma, embryonal rhabdomyosarcoma of the eye muscles, adenocarcinoma of the lacrimal gland, and the squamous cell carcinoma and melanoma of the conjunctiva. All are relatively rare. Retinoblastomas and embryonal rhabdomyosarcomas occur in childhood and are quite sensitive to radiation. These lesions spread along the optic nerve or metastasize via the blood stream, but regional lymph node metastases are rare. Because of the regional nature and radiosensitivity, both retinoblastoma and rhabdomyosarcoma are best treated by radiation therapy.

The control rate for retinoblastoma may be as high as 80% depending upon the size of the lesion. It is important to use a well-defined megavoltage radiation beam and a special shield to protect the lens. The optic nerve should be included. The dose to the retina is 5000 rads in 25 fractions over about 6 weeks. Enucleation is used for radiation failure.

Rhabdomyosarcomas are treated by irradiation of the entire orbit, with corneal shielding whenever possible. The dose is carried to 5000–6000 rads in 6–7 weeks. Local control can be achieved in 80% of cases.

Superficial conjunctival lesions may be treated with ^{90}Sr applicators. Lacrimal gland carcinomas are irradiated postoperatively when surgical margins are not clear or surgical failure has occurred, or as primary treatment if the lesion is inoperable. Doses of at least 6000 rads to the entire orbit are required.

Possible complications of radiation include cataract, dry eye, corneal ulceration, and retinal damage. Depending upon the location and nature of the tumor, these can usually be prevented by careful beam placement and shielding, but surgical removal of a cataract or enucleation is an occasional unavoidable consequence of successful therapy.

MALIGNANT LESIONS OF THE HEAD & NECK

The great majority of malignant neoplasms of the mucosa of the head and neck are squamous cell carcinomas of various degrees of differentiation and moderate radiosensitivity. Adenocarcinomas of salivary and mucous glands are relatively rare. Radiotherapy and surgery have been the primary methods of treatment in the management of carcinomas of the head and neck. The choice of treatment depends on the site of the primary lesion and the extent of disease. In general, for early lesions, radiotherapy and surgery have about equal local control rates. Radiotherapy is often the preferred treatment because of better functional and cosmetic results. For moderately advanced lesions, surgery combined with pre- or postoperative radiotherapy results in a higher local control rate than either radiotherapy or surgery alone. In advanced surgically incurable lesions, radiotherapy usually offers worthwhile palliation and occasionally a chance of cure. The value of combination chemotherapy and radiotherapy for advanced surgically incurable head and neck cancers is currently under investigation.

Radiotherapy is generally the treatment of choice for carcinomas arising in the nasopharynx, tonsils, the floor of the mouth, the soft palate, the epiglottis, the false vocal cords, the laryngeal ventricle, and the true vocal cords. Early carcinomas of the tongue or tonsillar pillars are equally well controlled by radiation (interstitial implant or peroral cone) or surgery, but radiotherapy usually offers better functional results. A hard, deeply infiltrating carcinoma of the tongue or pillar is less likely to be controlled by radiotherapy alone. Laryngeal carcinoma with extension into the preepiglottic space with or without fixation of the cords, lesions involving bone, carcinomas of the piriform sinus, and carcinomas of the subglottic area are rarely controlled by radiotherapy alone and are usually managed with combined radiotherapy and surgery. Carcinomas of the gingival ridge and salivary glands are usually treated primarily by operation. Most carcinomas arising from the mucosa of the maxillary antrums are treated by radiotherapy alone or postoperatively following surgical debulking of the tumor and establishment of adequate drainage. Smaller lesions are managed by preoperative irradiation.

The control of cervical lymph node metastases from primary squamous cell carcinomas of the head and neck depends on the size, the number of nodes involved, the site of origin of the tumor, and the mobility of the metastatic lymph node. Nodes less than 3 cm in diameter are often controlled with radiotherapy alone. When the metastatic cervical lymph node is greater than 3 cm in diameter, when multiple lymph nodes are involved, or when the site of origin is the oral cavity, radical neck dissection in combination with pre- or postoperative radiotherapy is the treatment of choice. Even large nodes from a tonsil or nasopharyngeal primary may be controlled with irradiation alone. Moderate doses of radiotherapy (5000 rads in 5½ weeks) control occult cervical lymph node metastases in greater than 90% of cases.

The 5-year local control rates by radiotherapy vary according to the primary site, the size and extent of the primary lesions, and the distribution and character of the involved lymph nodes. The control rate for stage I carcinoma of the vocal cords is 90–95%. Early carcinomas of the oral tongue, the free portion of the epiglottis, the floor of the mouth, the soft palate, the nasopharynx, the tonsils, the hypopharynx, the false vocal cords, and the laryngeal ventricle can be controlled by radiotherapy in about 80–90% of cases. More advanced lesions and those associated with lymph node metastases have lower cure rates.

CARCINOMA OF THE LUNG

Histologically, carcinoma of the lung may be classified as adenocarcinoma, squamous cell carcinoma, large cell undifferentiated carcinoma, and oat cell carcinoma. For the localized operable adenocarcinomas and squamous cell carcinomas, surgery is the treatment of choice. Few cases of oat cell carcinoma are thought to be curable after clinical evaluation, and for this reason this tumor is treated mostly by radiation. This is because treatment can be directed to tissues beyond the lung and because these carcinomas are sensitive to radiation.

Unfortunately, most bronchogenic carcinomas are inoperable, and less than 10% are curable at the time of diagnosis. Factors that preclude surgical resection are involvement of the parietal pleura, extensively involved or fixed mediastinal lymph nodes, recurrent or vagus nerve paralysis, bronchial extension approaching the carina, invasion of major vessels, pericardium, or trachea, and distant metastases. If the lesion is inoperable but still localized, an attempt at radiation cure is justified. Limited peripheral lesions involving the chest wall (as in some superior sulcus tumors) or lesions of the carina contribute a few radiation cures. Squamous cell carcinomas are treated with relatively small fields, usually including the primary and hilus; in the case of undifferentiated and oat cell carcinomas, lymph node regions of the mediastinum and the supraclavicular area are included also. With conventional fractionation schemes, the differentiated and large cell carcinomas require doses of 6000–6500 rads, whereas 5000 rads is usually an adequate dose for oat cell carcinomas. Survival rates up to 5–10% have been reported. The value of adjuvant chemotherapy in the management of oat cell carcinoma is being investigated.

THYMUS

Tumors arising in the thymus may be malignant in that they invade locally and seed over the pleural surfaces. Histologically, it is difficult to recognize malignancy in the epithelial tumors. The sites of local invasion include the pericardium, heart, great vessels, nerves, and other structures in the mediastinum. Distant metastases are rare in the early stages.

Encapsulated thymic tumors should be totally resected surgically, since rupture of the capsule may lead to seeding. It is questionable whether any surgery other than biopsy is indicated for tumors that invade important mediastinal structures. Many can be controlled by radiation. There is no place for surgery in the management of lymphosarcomas, Hodgkin's disease (including the so-called granulomatous thymomas), and seminomas that occur in the thymus. These lesions are treated with radiation therapy, utilizing large treatment fields and modest radiation doses.

About 40% of patients with thymomas have myasthenia gravis. On the other hand, approximately 15% of patients with myasthenia gravis have a thymoma. Thymic irradiation may be useful for symptomatic control of patients with myasthenia without a demonstrable thymoma. To lessen the possibility of myasthenic crisis, all patients scheduled for surgery for thymic tumors should receive preoperative irradiation; in these cases it is important to begin with small daily doses and limit the total dose to about 2500 rads.

GASTROINTESTINAL TRACT

Esophagus

With rare exceptions, malignant lesions of the esophagus are squamous cell carcinomas. Esophageal neoplasms give rise to symptoms only when deeply penetrating or when obstruction, which occurs late because of the inherent distensibility of the organ, is imminent. Because of the rich lymphatic supply and absence of serosal covering, these carcinomas tend to extend long distances up and down the esophagus and frequently infiltrate surrounding mediastinal structures by the time of diagnosis. For these reasons, radiation therapy must include long segments of the esophagus and adjacent soft tissues.

In the proximal third of the esophagus, surgical access and reconstruction are difficult and results with radiation therapy are at least as good as with excision. Therefore, radiation is the treatment of choice. Special tissue compensating filters are used, and a dose of 6500–7000 rads in 7–8 weeks is recommended. Care must be taken to avoid excessive radiation to the spinal cord.

In the middle third, the best results appear to be with a combination of preoperative radiation therapy followed, in resectable cases, by esophagectomy. The entire esophagus receives up to about 5000 rads in 6 weeks; 5–6 weeks later, esophagectomy is performed.

Primary surgery is probably preferable for lesions arising in the distal esophagus.

Even though cure rates of 25% or higher have

been reported for well-selected series of patients, the overall cure rate is probably no better than 5%. Radiation therapy alone will reopen the esophagus and control local symptoms in 70–75% of patients. Thus, gastrostomy for feeding purposes is rarely indicated.

Stomach & Bowel

Adenocarcinomas are moderately radiosensitive, but the radiation doses required are not well tolerated by the abdominal organs and surgery is usually the treatment of choice.

The lymphomas which occur in stomach or bowel should be treated by radiation following surgical resection. An effort is made to treat the entire abdomen with doses as high as 3000–4000 rads, with shielding of the kidneys after 2000 rads and of the liver after 2500 rads. Such large fields are not well tolerated, and the daily dose to the midplane of the abdomen is often limited to 150 rads or less.

Rectum & Anus

During the past decade, a randomized study by the Veterans Administration Surgical Adjuvant Group has demonstrated that for cancer of the rectum, preoperative irradiation with 2500 rads given in 10 fractions over 12 days is beneficial to irradiated patients who undergo abdominal perineal resection when compared with nonirradiated controls. This advantage is reflected in improved 5-year survival rates (40.8% vs 28.4%), reduction of lymph node metastases (24% vs 38%), fewer local recurrences (29% vs 40%), and fewer distant metastases (47% vs 63%). With higher doses of preoperative radiotherapy (5000 rads in 5 weeks), local recurrences can be almost completely eliminated. The value of postoperative radiotherapy for stage B2 and stage C1 and C2 carcinoma of the rectosigmoid colon and rectum is currently under investigation.

In advanced inoperable or recurrent carcinoma of the rectum and rectosigmoid colon, radiotherapy is often of value for palliation and relief of obstruction.

Excellent local control rates can be achieved with intracavitary irradiation for small, fairly well differentiated tumors in the lower third of the rectum. This is an acceptable alternative treatment to radical surgery for elderly or poor-risk patients and those who refuse colostomy. A 5-year survival rate of 78% has been reported.

Squamous cell carcinoma is the most common type of anal malignancy. Lesions originating in or extending above the pectinate line tend to spread upward along the rectal wall and into the rectal lymphatics and are primarily surgical problems. Those below the line behave like ordinary squamous cell carcinomas of the skin and can be controlled by radiation with preservation of the anus and anal sphincter.

FEMALE GENITAL TRACT

Ovaries

Most ovarian carcinomas are of epithelial origin and are primarily managed surgically with salpingo-oophorectomy, hysterectomy, or omentectomy, singly or in combination. Postoperative radiotherapy can increase the local control rate when there is residual disease confined to the pelvis. However, ovarian carcinoma commonly spreads to the peritoneal cavity and periaortic lymph nodes. Recent studies have shown a high incidence of previously unappreciated lymph node and subdiaphragmatic metastases even in patients with apparently stage I and stage II disease. Whole abdominal irradiation to encompass all the common sites of potential spread is limited by the tolerance of the kidneys, liver, and spinal cord. Clinical trials to define the optimal use of radiotherapy either alone or in combination with chemotherapy following surgery for early disease and for palliation of advanced inoperable disease are in progress.

Dysgerminoma of the ovary—the counterpart of testicular seminoma—is highly radiosensitive. With rare exceptions, postoperative irradiation of the pelvis and abdominal lymph nodes should be done routinely. Pelvic irradiation should include the entire pelvis with the dose carried to 3000–3500 rads in 3–4 weeks. If abdominal lymph nodes are involved, the treatment fields should be extended to include the mediastinum and supraclavicular areas. When peritoneal implants are present, the entire pelvis and abdomen receive 2500–3000 rads in 5–6 weeks with kidney shielding after 2000 rads. Control may still be achieved in the presence of distant metastases.

Uterus

Adenocarcinoma of the endometrium is primarily treated by operation. Most well-differentiated adenocarcinomas of the endometrium are cured by surgery alone. In grade II tumors, preoperative intracavitary radium insertion decreases the incidence of pelvic and vaginal recurrence. External radiotherapy of the whole pelvis is indicated when the tumor is poorly differentiated or when there is cervical involvement, deep myometrial invasion, enlargement of the uterus to greater than 8 cm, pelvic lymph node metastases, or known extension of the disease outside of the uterus. Radiotherapy may aid in the local control of mixed mesodermal sarcomas and carcinosarcomas but adds little to the treatment of leiomyosarcomas, which are primarily surgical problems.

Cervix

Ninety-five percent of cervical malignancies are squamous cell carcinomas; most of the remainder are adenocarcinomas. Although adenocarcinomas tend to respond more slowly, both are about equally radiosensitive and their control rates by radiotherapy are similar. Because of the great tolerance of the cervical and vaginal mucosa to radiation and the accessibility of the vagina and uterus for brachytherapy insertions, radiotherapy plays a major role in the treatment of cervical carcinoma. Metastases in pelvic lymph nodes may also be controlled by external beam radiotherapy.

For in situ carcinoma, total hysterectomy is an

adequate prodecure, has a low morbidity rate, and is generally the treatment of choice. Lesser surgical procedures may be done when the patient is desirous of retaining her uterus and can be kept under close observation (see Chapter 44).

With invasive carcinoma clinically limited to the cervix (stage I), there is a 10–20% chance that pelvic node metastases are present. Radical surgical procedures or radiotherapy for stage I lesions yields about equal 5-year survival rates (80–90%). Because of the low rate of major complications (bowel damage or fistula formation in 2% of cases following radiotherapy), radiotherapy is the treatment of choice except in young patients. Radical surgical procedures are reserved for radiation failures. Radiotherapy typically includes 2 brachytherapy insertions into the uterus and vaginal fornices supplemented with external irradiation to raise the dose delivered to the lymph nodes in the lateral pelvis.

For advanced cervical carcinomas, radiotherapy is even more strongly preferred to surgery. Greater use is made of external irradiation, with a corresponding reduction of the emphasis on intracavitary radium. The value of periaortic lymph node irradiation in patients with periaortic lymph node metastasis demonstrated by biopsy or lymphangiogram is under investigation.

Vagina

Vaginal carcinomas are chiefly squamous cell in type. Carcinoma of the proximal vagina tends to spread along the same lymphatic channels as carcinoma from the cervix; carcinoma of the distal vagina tends to metastasize to the inguinal lymph nodes.

In general, radiotherapy is the treatment of choice. It utilizes a combination of external radiation and intravaginal sources or an interstitial implant with radium needles or iridium with the relative emphasis determined by the extent and location of the lesion. External radiation is usually given first, with the entire vaginal canal and adjacent tissue carried to a dose of 4000–5000 rads in 4½–5½ weeks. For lesions of the proximal vagina, treatment is extended to the whole pelvis. Radioactive sources are then inserted into the vagina in such fashion that the entire vaginal and cervical mucosa receives another 3000–4000 rads. Lesions of the vaginal vault and introitus are best treated by interstitial radiotherapy alone or in combination with external radiotherapy.

Five-year absolute survival rates of 70% for stage I and stage II disease and 30% for stage III disease have been reported.

Vulva

Because of the poor tolerance of the vulva to large doses of radiation, vulvar carcinomas are primarily surgical problems. Inoperable lesions have been controlled by electron beam, implants, and external beam therapy, and preoperative irradiation has been of value.

MALE GENITAL TRACT

Testis

Testicular tumors arising from the germinal epithelium include seminoma, embryonal carcinoma, teratocarcinoma, choriocarcinoma, and mixtures of these types. Seminomas are very sensitive to radiation, and the others exhibit variable degrees of radiosensitivity. The initial spread is usually via lymphatics to the periaortic and renal hilar lymph nodes.

When a tumor of the testis is suspected, orchiectomy should be done through an inguinal incision with ligation at the internal inguinal ring. Seminomas are then treated by radiation to the ipsilateral pelvic, renal hilar, and periaortic lymphatics up to the diaphragm with doses of about 3000 rads in 4 weeks. If abdominal lymph node metastases have been demonstrated at surgery or by intravenous urogram or lymphangiography, the mediastinum and supraclavicular fossa should also be treated with 2500–3000 rads.

In the case of embryonal carcinomas and teratocarcinomas, treatment of the abdominal lymph nodes is controversial. Similar results have been obtained with radiotherapy alone with doses of 4500–5000 rads or various combinations of periaortic node dissection alone or with radiotherapy. In any case, radiotherapy of the mediastinum and supraclavicular lymphatics with 4500 rads is advised. In patients with advanced testicular carcinomas, radiotherapy is often used in conjunction with combination chemotherapy.

Choriocarcinomas have a high tendency to disseminate via the blood stream, and prophylactic radiotherapy of lymph nodes is of questionable value.

The 5-year survival rate for seminomas is over 90%. Even with distant spread, seminomas are curable by radiation therapy. The overall cure rate for other types of testicular carcinomas (except choriocarcinoma) treated by orchiectomy and radiation is approximately 70–90% for stage I, 40–60% for stage II, and less than 10% for stage III disease.

Prostate

Carcinoma of the prostate is locally controlled in 80–90% of patients by megavoltage radiotherapy. In stage A disease, 6500–7000 rads in 7–8 weeks is usually delivered to the prostate using a rotation technic. In stage B and stage C disease, the entire pelvis is irradiated with a 4-field technic delivering 4500–5000 rads in 5–6 weeks with an additional 1500–2000 rads in 2–2½ weeks through reduced fields to the prostate using a rotation technic. Five- and 10-year disease-free survival rates of 70% and 42% have been achieved for patients with disease limited to the prostate and rates of 37% (5-year) and 20% (10-year) for those with extracapsular extension.

Potency is maintained by about 60% of patients. Whether significant benefits can be achieved by extension of radiotherapy to encompass the periaortic lymph node involvement as shown by biopsy or lymphangiography is being investigated.

TUMORS OF THE URINARY TRACT

Renal Parenchyma

Wilms's tumor is a radiosensitive tumor of childhood. At present, radiotherapy is usually given in combination with surgery and drugs such as dactinomycin and vincristine in the following situations: (1) to the postoperative renal bed crossing the midline when there is capsular invasion or local lymph node involvement; (2) to the whole abdomen when there is tumor rupture or gross residual disease within the peritoneal cavity; (3) to metastases; (4) to recurrent disease; and (5) to tumors in the contralateral kidney when there is bilateral involvement. In rare situations, radiotherapy is given preoperatively to reduce the size of a massive tumor and render it amenable to surgery. Using a combined approach with surgery, radiotherapy, and chemotherapy, 2-year disease-free survival rates of 80% for localized Wilms's tumor and 50% for children with metastatic disease have been achieved.

Adenocarcinomas of the renal parenchyma are generally regarded as radioincurable. Surgery is the primary treatment of choice. Postoperative radiotherapy may be beneficial when there is known residual disease, capsule invasion, or regional lymph node metastasis. Preoperative radiotherapy has no proved value but may be used in cases of borderline operability.

Bladder

The majority of bladder carcinomas are transitional cell in type. Superficial grade I papillary tumors may be cured by transurethral resection. Grade I papillary tumors have a tendency to recur and become less well differentiated with time. Higher grade carcinomas spread through the lymphatics of the bladder wall as well as to the adjacent pelvic lymphatics and require treatment of the entire bladder as well as the pelvic lymph nodes. In stage I (0, A) and stage II (B1) disease, the results of megavoltage radiotherapy are as good as with total cystectomy alone, and the functional results are better. In stage I low grade tumors, only the bladder is irradiated. The usual dose is 6000–6500 rads in 6–7 weeks. For more advanced high-grade tumors, because of the high incidence of pelvic lymph node metastases, the entire pelvis is irradiated to 5000–6500 rads in 5½–6 weeks with an additional 1000–1500 rads in 1–2 weeks through reduced fields to the bladder using a rotation technic.

With radiotherapy alone, 5-year survival rates are approximately 50% for stage I and II disease, 15–25% for stage III, and 5–10% for stage IV. Preoperative irradiation followed by cystectomy gives better results than radiotherapy alone for T_3 lesions but no improvement over radiotherapy alone for T_1 and T_2 lesions. An actuarial survival rate of 50% for stage III disease has been reported using this combined approach.

Urethra

Carcinomas of the urethra are often treated with radiation. External irradiation, radium implants, or a combination of the 2 is used, depending upon the anatomic distribution of the involvement.

MALIGNANT LYMPHOMAS & LEUKEMIAS

Hodgkin's Disease

During the past decade there has been a dramatic improvement in the prognosis of Hodgkin's disease. This largely results from better understanding of the natural history of the disease, the use of surgical staging, extended field and total nodal megavoltage radiotherapy, and combination chemotherapy with MOPP (mechlorethamine, Oncovin [vincristine], procarbazine, and prednisone) and other agents. Staging laparotomy entails splenectomy, biopsy of suspicious periaortic, perihepatic, splenic hilar, or celiac lymph nodes, needle and wedge biopsy of the liver and open biopsy of the iliac crest bone marrow, and ovariopexy in young female patients. A dose of 3500–4500 rads is usually delivered in 4–5 weeks to each treatment volume. In stage I and stage IIA disease, a 5-year survival rate of 96% has been achieved with subtotal nodal irradiation. In stages I, IIB, and IIIA, 5-year actuarial survival rates of 80–90% can be achieved with total nodal irradiation alone or in combination with chemotherapy. In stages IIIB and IV, 5-year survival of greater than 60% has been achieved with low-dose radiotherapy (1500–2500 rads) to sites of bulky disease following combination chemotherapy.

Non-Hodgkin's Lymphoma

Although lymphomas are extremely radiosensitive, the role of radiotherapy in non-Hodgkin's lymphomas is less well defined than in Hodgkin's disease. Radiotherapy is curative in over 50% of patients with stage I and II non-Hodgkin's lymphomas. However, most patients have stage III and IV disease on presentation. Total body irradiation in a dosage of 15 rads twice a week to a total dose of 150 rads appears to be effective therapy in stage III and IV nodular lymphocytic lymphomas. Chemotherapy is more frequently used in patients with stage III and IV diffuse lymphomas and histiocytic lymphomas. Radiotherapy is sometimes given to areas of bulky disease in conjunction with chemotherapy in stage III and IV disease.

Leukemias

In children with acute lymphoblastic leukemia (ALL) who have achieved complete remission induced by intensive chemotherapy, cranial irradiation with 2400 rads in 3 weeks given in conjunction with intrathecal methotrexate has been successful in reducing the incidence of CNS relapse from 62% to 4.4%. With this combined approach, 5-year leukemia-free survival rates of over 50% can now be achieved.

In chronic lymphocytic leukemia, total body irradiation with 100–400 rads delivered in small (10–25 rad) fractions in several weeks to several months is sometimes effective in inducing complete clinical and hematologic remissions. Radiotherapy even with low doses (several hundred rads) can often provide rapid palliation of pain or other symptoms arising from leukemia infiltration of bones, joints, soft tissues, and spleen. During splenic irradiation, blood counts must be followed closely since a precipitous drop in the white count or platelet count can occur following doses of less than 100 rads.

NONNEOPLASTIC DISEASES

In a few situations, radiation therapy is of value in the treatment of benign disease. Local inflammatory lesions such as acute parotitis and resistant staphylococcal infections often respond to a few hundred rads in fractionated doses. For acute parotitis in elderly debilitated patients, radiation may be lifesaving. Subacute thyroiditis usually responds favorably to similar treatment. The pain arising from ankylosing spondylitis of the spine is relieved in most patients by radiation, but the course of the disease is unaltered.

Overgrowth of fibrous tissue, as in keloid formation, may be prevented or subsequent symptoms relieved by low-dosage superficial radiotherapy. In already developed keloids, treatment usually consists of excision followed within 3 days by a single dose of 600–1000 rads or 5 daily fractions of 300 rads of superficial radiotherapy.

After excision, 2000–3000 rads of very superficial β-ray irradiation may prevent recurrences of pterygium.

External radiation to the retrobulbar orbital tissues is helpful in reducing or preventing progression of the changes in severe progressing infiltrative exophthalmos associated with Graves' disease. Both orbits are treated with doses of about 200 rads daily for a total of 10 treatments. Care must be taken to avoid the lens. The treatment of hyperthyroidism with parenteral radioiodine has replaced thyroidectomy in selected patients, but a discussion of the advantages and disadvantages of such treatment is beyond the scope of this presentation.

Radiation is also used for prevention of a threatened rejection of transplanted tissues. The usual dose is 150 rads given 3 times on 3 successive days. If necessary, the course of therapy may be repeated twice.

Radiation therapy is often of value in treating peptic ulcer. The treatment is 1800 rads in 2 weeks to the entire acid-secreting portion of the stomach.

* * *

General References

Ackerman LV, del Regato J: *Cancer: Diagnosis, Treatment, and Prognosis*, 4th ed. Mosby, 1970.

Bagshaw MA & others: External beam radiation therapy of primary carcinoma of the prostate. Cancer 36:723, 1975.

Buschke F, Parker R: *Radiation Therapy in Cancer Management*. Grune & Stratton, 1972.

Casaret AP: *Radiation Biology*. Prentice-Hall, 1968.

Fabrikant J: *Radiobiology*. Year Book, 1972.

Fisher B & others: Effect of radiotherapy following radical mastectomy. Ann Surg 172:711, 1970.

Fletcher GH: *Textbook of Radiotherapy*, 2nd ed. Lea & Febiger, 1973.

Hall EJ: *Radiobiology for the Radiologist*. Harper & Row, 1973.

Hendee WR: *Medical Radiation Physics*. Year Book, 1970.

Holland JF, Frei E: *Cancer Medicine*. Lea & Febiger, 1973.

Hustu HO & others: Prevention of central nervous system leukemia by irradiation. Cancer 32:585, 1973.

Johns HE, Cunningham JR: *Physics of Radiology*. Thomas, 1971.

Johnson RE: Total body irradiation (TBI) as primary therapy for advanced lymphosarcoma. Cancer 35:242, 1975.

Kaplan HS, Rosenberg SA: Hodgkin's disease: Current recommendations for management. CA 25:306, 1975.

Moss WT, Brand WN, Battitor H: *Radiation Oncology: Rationale, Technique, Results*, 4th ed. Mosby, 1973.

Papillon J: *Conservative Treatment of Early Breast Cancer by Tumorectomy and Irradiation. Current Concepts in Breast Cancer and Tumor Immunology*. Proceedings of San Francisco Cancer Symposium of 1973. Castro J & others (editors). Medical Examination Publishing Co., 1974.

Papillon J: Intracavitary irradiation of early rectal cancer for cure: A series of 186 cases. Cancer 36:696, 1975.

Pizzarello DJ, Witcofski RL: *Medical Radiation Biology*. Lea & Febiger, 1972.

Pomeroy TC, Johnson RE: Combined modality therapy of Ewing's sarcoma. Cancer 35:36, 1975.

Roswit B, Higgins GA, Keehn RJ: Preoperative irradiation for carcinoma of the rectum and rectosigmoid colon: Report of a national Veterans Administration randomized study. Cancer 35:1597, 1975.

Rubin P, Casaret AP: *Clinical Radiation Pathology*. 2 vols. Saunders, 1968.

Selman J: *The Basic Physics of Radiation Therapy*. Thomas, 1973.

Sheline GE: Radiation therapy of primary tumors. Semin Oncol 2:29, 1975.

Suit HD: Adenocarcinoma of colon and rectum: Role of radiation therapy. Surg Clin North Am 54:733, 1974.

Suit HD: Role of therapeutic radiology in cancer of bone. Cancer 35:930, 1975.

Suit HD, Russell WO: Radiation therapy of soft tissue sarcomas. Cancer 36:759, 1975.

Van Der Werf-Messen B: Radiotherapeutic treatment of testicular tumors. Int J Radiat Oncol Biol Phys 1:235, 1976.

Weichselbaum RR, Marck A, Hellman S: The role of postoperative irradiation in carcinoma of the breast. Cancer 37:2682, 1976.

8...
Nuclear Medicine in Surgical Diagnosis

Malcolm R. Powell, MD

Nuclear medicine is a medical specialty that uses radionuclides in medical diagnosis and treatment. Radionuclide tracers provide methods of studying the structure and function of internal organs. Tracer procedures differ from conventional x-ray studies in several fundamental respects. Radioactive tracers are physiologically insignificant and do not impose the chemical, osmolal, or volume stresses that occur when x-ray contrast materials are used. The emission images obtained with radiotracers are of lower resolution than roentgenograms, but many of the organs imaged are not as readily susceptible to x-ray examination. Unlike the tomographic sections that are imaged by sonography or computerized tomography, radionuclide images show the entire organ or tissue that concentrates the radiopharmaceutical. Radionuclide distribution is readily quantified, providing the basis for testing of physiologic function. Although nuclear medicine tests are sensitive in detecting pathologic conditions and defining their location, they do not usually provide a specific diagnosis. Nuclear medicine procedures are free of morbidity and can be readily performed on outpatients.

PRINCIPLES OF RADIOACTIVITY DETECTION & INFORMATION PRESENTATION IN NUCLEAR MEDICINE

Radioactivity

Radioisotopes are unstable forms of elements which have the same chemical properties (atomic number) as the stable isotope but a different atomic mass. They decay to other isotopes, emitting particles and electromagnetic radiation with each radioactive decay. Individual radioisotopes have characteristic half-lives (the time at which 50% of the original number of atoms of the radioisotope will have undergone decay to another isotope). Ideally, each isotope used in nuclear medicine would have a half-life similar to the time required for the test and would emit only useful types of radiation, thus limiting radiation exposure of the patient. If an isotope is given for a test that entails in vivo counting, the radiation should have a relatively low absorption in the patient, since it must escape to

be counted. If a radioisotope is administered for therapy, it would be ideal if the emitted radiation were entirely absorbed within the target tissue.

Diagnostic tests such as thyroid uptake tests, radioisotope renograms, and organ imaging are generally performed by detecting gamma rays. The gamma ray is electromagnetic radiation with no charge or mass, properties which allow it to pass through tissue without absorption. Gamma radiation is readily located and counted with external detectors.

The radioactive emissions used for therapy in nuclear medicine are beta particles. These have sufficient mass and charge that they penetrate only short distances through tissue and usually deliver their entire energy after traveling less than 1 mm.

Instrumentation

Knowledge of the instruments used in nuclear medicine is important to utilize these tests efficiently. Fig 8–1 shows the simplest form of detector for gamma rays. A sodium iodide crystal is used to absorb gamma rays and convert their energy to bursts of light (scintillations). The scintillations are detected by the photo-cathode of the multiplier photo tube. The photo-cathode converts each scintillation to a pulse of electrons which is multiplied in the tube. After amplification, the pulse voltage is proportionate to the original gamma photon energy and may be identified as specific for the isotope. This allows detection of one isotope in the presence of others.

Radioisotope imaging devices provide planar projections of the radioactivity distribution "seen" by the instrument. Radioisotope scanners do this by systematically moving a detector back and forth over the surface of the patient, detecting radioactive count rate and recording it as a pattern on paper or by exposing x-ray film proportionate to the radioactivity. Scanning devices detect radioactivity through a "focused" collimator which is most sensitive to radiation originating from a focal point 3–5 inches from the surface of the collimator. Thus, as this type of detector moves across a patient, the image corresponds to a plane within the patient, and the rectilinear scan image is largely tomographic.

The scintillation camera employs a stationary detector containing a sodium iodide crystal 12–16 inches wide and ½ inch thick. An array of multiplier photo

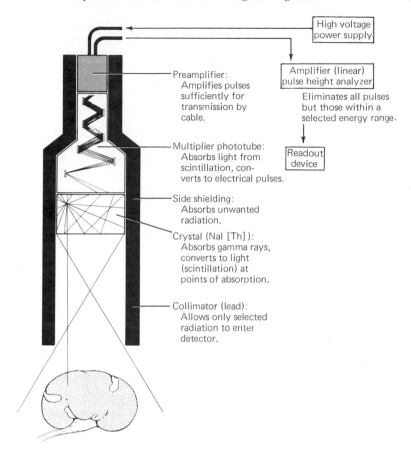

High voltage power supply

Preamplifier: Amplifies pulses sufficiently for transmission by cable.

Amplifier (linear) pulse height analyzer

Eliminates all pulses but those within a selected energy range.

Multiplier phototube: Absorbs light from scintillation, converts to electrical pulses.

Readout device

Side shielding: Absorbs unwanted radiation.

Crystal (NaI [Th]): Absorbs gamma rays, converts to light (scintillation) at points of absorption.

Collimator (lead): Allows only selected radiation to enter detector.

Figure 8—1. Detector. NaI(Th) = thallium-activated sodium iodide crystal.

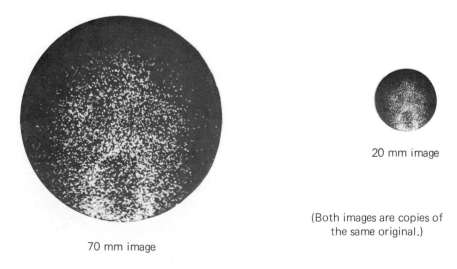

70 mm image

20 mm image

(Both images are copies of the same original.)

Figure 8—2. Image size and pattern recognition. Despite the minified nature of scintiphotographs, the small images are somewhat larger than ideal for viewing at arm's length. For comparison, 2 copies of the same image are shown here, one more than twice the usual scintiphotograph size and the other reduced to approximately 40% of the usual size. Most interpreters will find it easier to recognize the pathology in the smaller image (or in the larger image at a distance of 5—10 feet). This is an illustration of the anterior view of a patient's head during the arterial phase of a brain blood flow study after the peripheral intravenous injection of ^{99m}Tc pertechnetate. Two curvilinear defects of arterial filling are seen laterally over each hemisphere with medial displacement of the middle cerebral artery arborizations. These defects are large subdural hematomas. This test is often a valuable aid in the diagnosis of acute neurosurgical problems.

Table 8—1. Comparison of scans and scintiphotos.

	Scans	Scintiphotos
Speed of image formation	Slow (static studies)	Fast (static or dynamic studies)
Data density; resolution	Lower	Higher
Image depth	Tomographic	Images as deeply as permitted by absorption of gamma photons in the subject
Image size	Usually 1:1, 1:2, or 1:5	Approximately 1:7
Image media	Paper print, x-ray film	Polaroid film, 35 or 70 mm film, x-ray film (multiple images)
Field of view	Larger (14 × 17 inches or more)	Smaller (10—14 inch circle)*

*With parallel hole collimator; larger with other collimators, but at expense of speed or image resolution.

tubes is used to locate the position of scintillations within the crystal, and this information is displayed on an oscilloscope. The oscilloscope is photographed to collect the image information. Collimators for scintillation cameras are analogous to lenses in photographic cameras since they allow gamma rays to interact with the detector crystal in a pattern corresponding to radioactivity distribution in the subject. Gamma rays from meaningless orientations are absorbed in the lead collimator. Since the scintillation camera detector is stationary, rapidly changing radioisotope distributions may be recorded as "stop motion" photographs. Scintillation camera data may also be recorded by computer for numerical data analysis.

Table 8—1 compares rectilinear scans and scintiphotographs. The principal difference between scans and scintiphotos is that the scintiphotos are usually miniaturized. This is appropriate for the limited information density produced by nuclear medicine images. Fig 8—2 demonstrates the value of image minification: "life-size" or 1:1 scan is larger than desirable for the information density.

Scintiphotos are best used for primary acquisition of data on radioisotope distribution. In addition to obtaining images, scintillation cameras are increasingly used to obtain quantitative regional data for evaluation of physiologic processes such as pulmonary perfusion, ventilation, renal cortical function, and cardiac function.

Rectilinear scans are useful to provide 1:1 images for exact correlation with topical or palpable anatomy (eg, a renal scan in the biopsy position for kidney localization; or a thyroid scan for correlation with a palpable nodule [Fig 8—3]) or to image large areas (eg, whole body scan), as used for bone, bone marrow, or tumor imaging (Fig 8—4).

Radiopharmaceuticals

Nuclear medicine procedures require preferential localization of a radiopharmaceutical in the organ or tissue which is to be studied. If a physiologic function is to be quantified, then the radiopharmaceutical must specifically label the process measured. When an imaging study is used to detect abnormal tissue within an organ, the abnormality may be detected either by (1) localization of the radiopharmaceutical in the lesion or (2) by less radiotracer in the lesion compared to the surrounding organ. Examples of increased localization in abnormal tissue include the labeling of

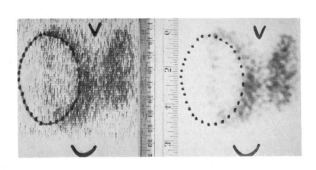

Scanning time, 15 minutes

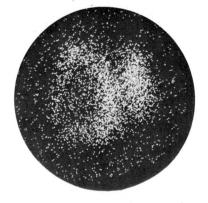

Scintiphotography time, 4 minutes

Figure 8—3. Comparison of scans and scintiphotograph. A large defect is easily recognized in the lateral right lobe of the thyroid. This large adenoma has displaced the right lobe of the thyroid gland to rotate it forward around the trachea. This illustration compares the presentation of information in scans and scintiphotographs after photographic copying at the same size. Scans show the linear pattern caused by detector motion and generally are obtained on x-ray film, although the simultaneously obtained "tap scan" (on left) may also be useful. Exact outlines of palpable findings can be drawn directly on scan images, a direct comparison of anatomic findings which is more difficult on scintiphotographs. Markers are conventionally shown on scans at the thyroid cartilage notch and at the suprasternal notch. The scintillation camera, in contrast, provides an image more rapidly and often shows more effective resolution of abnormalities than the spatial resolution available in scans.

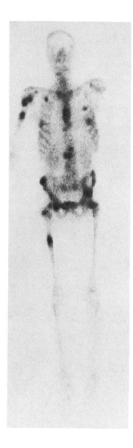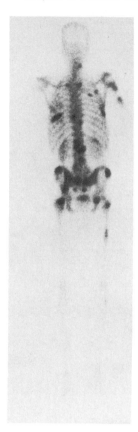

Figure 8—4. The anterior and posterior views shown here are of a patient with multiple bone metastases from carcinoma of the colon. The intensity of uptake of the ^{99m}technetium-pyrophosphate tracer is such that there is less left for accumulation in normal bones. Therefore, normal bone detail is not as well demonstrated in this scan as is usual in a normal individual. Since this agent is excreted in the urine, some visualization of the kidneys and the bladder is seen in the scan. The patient was instructed to void just prior to scanning. The lesions shown here were not definitely recognizable on current roentgenograms. Scanning has been shown to be a more sensitive way of detecting bone metastases early in the course of their development than x-ray bone surveys. Increased retention of the bone-seeking tracer in the scan demonstrates increased bone blood flow and reactive bone formation due to multiple causes including neoplastic disease, infection, arthritis, Paget's disease, and many other abnormalities.

brain or bone lesions. Examples of diminished localization in abnormal tissue include abnormal areas in lung, liver, spleen, kidney, and pancreas images.

Many radiopharmaceuticals are prepared in the nuclear medicine laboratories where they are used. This is particularly convenient for radioisotopes with short half-lives such as technetium-99m (6 hours), which is obtained by separation from its longer-lived parent, molybdenum-99 (2.7 days).

The common radiopharmaceuticals for static radionuclide imaging are listed in Table 8–2. Technetium-99m is especially useful because its radiopharmaceuticals will label so many organs and tissues. It has a

short half-life and emits only a single gamma ray; furthermore, because of the absence of beta radiation, the radiation exposure to the patient is extremely low.

In addition to the static procedures tabulated in Table 8–2, a number of dynamic procedures are commonly performed using technetiated albumin or red cells for rapid imaging of vascular spaces and the heart, radioxenon gas and solution for pulmonary studies, radioiodinated rose bengal for hepatobiliary studies, radioiodinated hippurate for kidney function studies, and a variety of radioactive compounds to study CSF pathways.

PRINCIPLES OF RADIOISOTOPE IMAGING PROCEDURES

The size of the smallest lesion that can be detected in a scan or scintiphotograph varies depending upon whether it actively takes up the radiopharmaceutical or whether it appears as a "cold area" in a labeled organ. With sufficiently active uptake of the radiopharmaceutical, an infinitely small lesion can be seen. "Cold" lesions are more difficult to identify. They are seen most easily when on the surface or edge of a solid organ and least easily when located centrally. A central lesion in the liver 2.5 cm in diameter should be detectable, whereas a peripheral one half that size should be seen. Generally speaking, scintillation cameras provide better resolution of small detail than rectilinear scanners. The speed of the scintillation camera also allows more photographs, providing better opportunity to detect minimal abnormalities.

Brain

Brain imaging procedures are widely used as screening tests for CNS disease. Scintiphotography provides a cine study of arterial and venous distributions of the tracer immediately after intravenous injection. This permits determination of vascularity in any lesion that is later identified in the static scintiphotographs and also provides an angiographic evaluation which can identify displacement by subdural hematomas (Fig 8–2), lack of perfusion after a stroke, and prolonged transit time, such as occurs with brain ischemia. Abnormal capillary permeability is detected by static views an hour or more after tracer injection and reveals about 90% of primary brain tumors and approximately 75% of metastatic brain lesions, but also accompanies a variety of other diseases such as inflammation, ischemia, infection, and vasculitis. Brain imaging should precede elective craniotomy. The extent of a lesion or the multiplicity of lesions is often appreciated only in the scintiphotographs. Fig 8–5 shows the typical appearance of an abnormal focus of brain labeling in both dynamic and static scintiphotographs.

Thyroid

Thyroid scanning provides a regional evaluation

Table 8—2. Radiopharmaceuticals for common static imaging procedures.

Organ or Tissue Imaged	Radionuclide	Chemical Form	Labeling Mechanism
Brain	6-hour ^{99m}Tc	Technetium pertechnetate or DTPA	Increased capillary permeability in abnormal brain (normal brain unlabeled).
Thyroid	8-day ^{131}I 13-hour ^{123}I	Iodide Iodide	Incorporated in thyroid iodide metabolism.
Lung	6-hour ^{99m}Tc 8-day ^{131}I	Macroaggregates (various) Macroaggregated albumin	Particles (average diameter, 30 μm) lodge for 2—8 hours in one of every 10,000 pulmonary arterioles.
Liver, spleen, marrow	6-hour ^{99m}Tc	Colloid	Phagocytosis by reticuloendothelial cells of liver (85%), spleen (10%), marrow (5%).
Pancreas	120-day ^{75}Se	Selenomethionine	Participates in pancreas (and liver) amino acid metabolism.
Kidney	6-hour ^{99m}Tc	Glucoheptonate or dimer-captosuccinic acid	Uptake in renal tubular cells proportionate to renal blood flow. Partial excretion.
Bone	6-hour ^{99m}Tc	Technetium pyrophosphate, polyphosphate, or diphosphonate	Accumulates in regions of active bone deposition; increased labeling of most abnormal areas.
Vascular spaces	6-hour ^{99m}Tc	Technetium albumin or red blood cells	Label vascular spaces in placenta, heart, great vessels.
Tumor or abscess	3.2-day ^{67}Ga	Gallium citrate	Labels neoplasms and abscesses by uptake in tumor cells and leukocytes.
Myocardial infarct	6-hour ^{99m}Tc	Technetium pyrophosphate	Accumulates in damaged myocardium 8 hours to 1 week after onset of infarct.

Dynamic scintiphotos after intravenous injection of a bolus of ^{99m}Tc pertechnetate

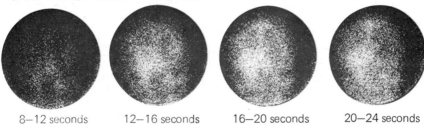

| 8—12 seconds | 12—16 seconds | 16—20 seconds | 20—24 seconds |

Static scintiphotos 90 minutes postinjection

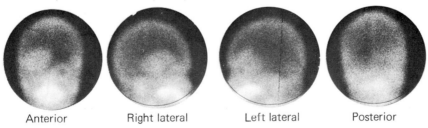

| Anterior | Right lateral | Left lateral | Posterior |

Figure 8—5. Sphenoid ridge meningioma. Scintiphotographic examinations allow both dynamic studies of brain blood flow patterns and static photographs of later localization of the radiopharmaceutical. A right sphenoid ridge meningioma is illustrated here which shows rapid filling during the arterial phase of brain vascular filling. There is actually some slight delay of filling of the right hemisphere—seen in the 8- to 12-second scintiphotograph, followed in the next scintiphotograph by a rapid "blooming" of the entire region of the meningioma which persists in its brightly labeled appearance through the 20- to 24-second picture. The static scintiphotographs show the bright frontotemporal abnormality in all projections, but the 2 projections that show it best are the anterior and the right lateral views, where the tumor is closest to the detector. This highly vascular appearance is typical of a meningioma.

of thyroid function. The functional status of a palpable nodule may be determined, and if the nodule is cold the scan provides supportive evidence for excisional biopsy. If a nodule is hot, with evidence of suppression of the remainder of the gland, an autonomous nodule is the likely diagnosis. This may be confirmed by administering thyroid hormone (25 μg of triiodothyronine 3 or 4 times daily for 7 days in adults) and repeating the neck ^{131}I uptake and scan to determine whether the nodule has been suppressed. Autonomously functioning nodules are benign lesions and may be managed in a variety of ways, including long-term observation. Radioiodide ablation of autonomous nodules never leads to hypothyroidism when the normal tissue is suppressed and does not take up the ^{131}I. Nodules with limited function detected by scan are almost always benign since thyroid cancer does not take up radioiodide when thyrotropic hormone (TSH) levels are normal. Care must be exercised in interpretation of a thyroid scan so that a cold nodule superimposed over functioning tissue will not be misinterpreted as a functioning nodule. Other uses of the thyroid scan include evaluation of goiters too large for accurate palpation, determination of the extent of a substernal goiter, and detection of carcinoma and ectopic thyroid tissue. Before it will concentrate radioiodide, thyroid cancer must be stimulated by elevated levels of TSH. The author prefers endogenous TSH in a state of temporary hypothyroidism and iodide depletion. Most follicular and papillary thyroid carcinomas show radioiodide uptake with adequate patient preparation. Fig 8—6 shows examples of radioiodide concentration in thyroid carcinoma.

Lung

The lung is most commonly imaged for diagnosis of suspected thromboemboli. Labeling of the lung with macroaggregates 30 μm in diameter shows the distribution of pulmonary arterial flow by lodging a tracer microembolus in approximately one of every 10,000

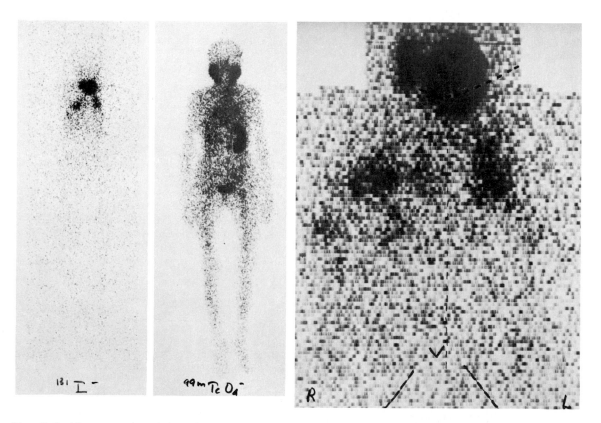

Figure 8—6. After preparation of the patient to induce a high endogenous secretion of TSH, metastatic thyroid carcinoma will usually show sufficient radioiodide uptake to allow radioiodide therapy. These scans show radioiodide retention in tumor metastases 72 hours after administration of a large tracer dose of radioiodide-131 and a comparison whole body scan with the patient in the same position using another isotope, technetium-99m pertechnetate, to show body outlines and the relative position of lesions shown in the radioiodide scan. The 2 scans showing the whole body are made with a whole body imaging adaptation of the scintillation camera. On the right is a conventional rectilinear scan using a single probe scanner which shows with somewhat better definition the distribution of individual lesions in the chest and neck. The most prominent area of radioiodide retention is in cervical lymph nodes. Below this are seen several areas of retention in each lung. Other body areas were largely cleared of radioiodide by the time this scan was taken. This amount of radioiodide uptake is often sufficient to allow complete radioiodide ablation of thyroid carcinoma metastases, although successful treatment often requires several doses of radioiodide and always requires meticulous attention to the details of patient preparation for radionuclide treatment.

patent pulmonary arterioles. Only partial and temporary arterial obstruction results from the particle localization. The image, therefore, shows blood flow distribution in smaller vessels than those seen in angiograms. There are many other causes of defects of pulmonary perfusion, eg, bronchospasm, atelectasis, inflammation, and bronchogenic carcinoma. Comparison of regional ventilation using radioxenon gas with a perfusion study may help to differentiate the specific cause of decreased perfusion. Preoperative lung perfusion imaging is good practice for comparison purposes in patients who are prone to pulmonary emboli. Perfusion and ventilation studies also often contribute unique information in the work-up of a patient before thoracotomy.

Heart

The heart may be imaged in a variety of ways. Scintiangiography following peripheral intravenous injection of a technetium tracer can be used, by identification of abnormal heart anatomy, for diagnosis of congenital and acquired heart disease. It also provides numerical data that when properly analyzed can provide useful information on cardiac function. Pulmonary transit of the tracer can be analyzed to detect left-to-right shunts and to calibrate their size. The first transit of the tracer through the heart can be used to estimate the size of the heart chambers, ejection fraction, and cardiac output. If an intravascular tracer such as technetiated albumin is used, electrocardiographic gating may be used to accumulate images representing only systole or diastole. Gated images may also be used to estimate chamber volume and ejection fraction. Using agents that localize in the normal myocardium proportionate to heart blood flow (eg, thallium-201), static images of the left ventricular wall may be obtained that show myocardial perfusion defects caused either by myocardial infarctions or by coronary insufficiency due to exercise stress at the time of injection. Fresh myocardial infarcts may be imaged directly be-

tween 8 hours and 1 week after onset using technetium Tc 99m pyrophosphate, which localizes in the damaged tissue. These various noninvasive tracer tests have become increasingly important in the management of heart disease.

Liver

Liver scintiphotography may be performed using colloids that localize in the reticuloendothelial tissue or using rose bengal dye, which is extracted from blood by hepatocytes and excreted into the bile. Technetium sulfur colloid defines liver anatomy and also the spleen and bone marrow. Irregularly decreased uptake of colloid is a sensitive indicator of parenchymal liver diseases. Space-occupying liver lesions produce focal defects with discrete margins. Although the spleen and bone marrow most frequently demonstrate abnormality secondary to liver disease, the colloid scan may demonstrate intrinsic lesions in both, and spleen and marrow imaging are important adjuncts to liver imaging. Fig 8–7 illustrates echinococcal cysts in the liver. Rose bengal I 131 dye provides information about hepatocyte function and the cause of jaundice. Since the dye is secreted into bile and only small amounts are needed for identification of biliary structures, this test may be particularly useful in distinguishing between intrahepatic and extrahepatic causes of jaundice.

Kidney

Renal structure is best evaluated by an agent which labels the cortex and is retained long enough to obtain a high-resolution image. Several newer technetium compounds are used for this purpose. Kidney function may be imaged during excretion of radioiodinated hippurate, and renal blood flow may be photographed after rapid peripheral intravenous injection of any ^{99m}Tc-radiopharmaceutical. Renal carcinoma causes a cold defect in the cortex which shows both displacement of the normal cortex by the neo-

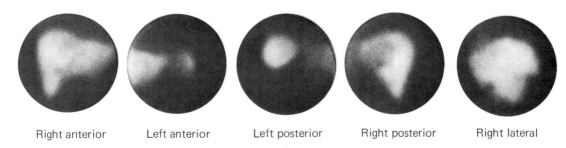

Right anterior   Left anterior   Left posterior   Right posterior   Right lateral

Figure 8–7. Echinococcal disease. Any mass lesion in the liver or spleen will show as a defect in the uniform uptake of colloid within these organs. In addition to demonstrating involvement by cancer, isotope scanning is useful in the diagnosis of many nonneoplastic lesions which are of interest to the surgeon, such as this grossly abnormal liver involved by echinococcal cysts. Small defects are appreciated at the inferior margin of the anterior segment of the right lobe in the right anterior view; in the posterior inferior margin of the posterior segment of the right lobe in the right lateral view; and in several other locations. There is a much larger defect approximately 6.5–7.5 cm in diameter occupying the medial and superior aspects of the posterior segment of the right lobe, as best visualized in the right posterior view. The spleen is normal in size, shape, and position in this illustration, and the vertebral bone marrow is not visible at these photographic settings, indicating that the amount of colloid uptake in the marrow is not increased. The presence of mass lesions within this liver does not appear to have greatly influenced either its normal functions or its size, since the amount of colloid uptake in unaffected areas of the liver is normal and liver size is not increased.

plasm and the influence of the carcinoma on perfusion of the remainder of the kidney. The degree of vascularity in perfusion studies may also be used to detect renal ischemia responsible for hypertension. In addition to diminished perfusion of the ischemic kidney or portion of the kidney, the rate of accumulation of hippurate will be diminished and transit time prolonged, causing late retention of the radiotracer in the ischemic tissue. Renal imaging may also be used for evaluation of kidney trauma, differentiation of cysts from neoplasms, study of transplants for competency of vascular and ureteral anastomoses, and for the evaluation of renal failure. Valuable information may be obtained by hippurate imaging studies even in the presence of severe degrees of renal failure.

Bone

Bone scanning is principally of value in the detection of asymptomatic foci of metastatic carcinoma before there is sufficient loss of mineral to show in roentgenograms. Abnormalities appear in bone scans weeks to months before roentgenograms are positive. Carcinoma, infections, trauma, arthritis, and neurotrophic changes may cause focal abnormalities of bone labeling with any of several tracers. Abnormal bone labeling is usually recognized as an area of increased uptake of the tracer as illustrated in Fig 8–4.

Miscellaneous

Many other organs, tissues, or spaces may be imaged: adrenals, joints, parathyroid adenomas, pancreas, placenta, brain ventricles and cisterns, other CSF spaces (and leaks), salivary glands, urinary bladder, and any abnormal space (such as pericardial effusion). Gallium-67 tumor and abscess scans are coming into wide use. Tumor scans are performed 48 or more hours after intravenous administration, but abscess scans are often strongly positive in only 4 hours. Gallium localizes in the liver and to a limited extent in the bones and spleen. Bowel preparation is required prior to scanning except in the first few hours. It appears to be useful in staging various malignant diseases as well as in detection of occult primary neoplasms. With sufficient attention to technical details, these less frequently utilized tests often provide valuable diagnostic information.

In Vivo Counting Procedures

In vivo counting refers to tests such as the thyroid radioiodide uptake where the amount of isotope in an area is counted. In general, these tests require far less tracer than imaging tests since a more sensitive lead cylinder collimator is used that allows more exposure of the detector crystal than do imaging collimators.

The thyroid uptake test measures radioiodide uptake in the neck. The number of radioiodide counts detected in the thigh is subtracted from those detected simultaneously in the neck (assuming equal tissue volumes), and the difference is the content of radioiodide in the thyroid. Exposure to exogenous iodides will cause the radioiodide tracer to represent less of a fraction of the available iodide atoms and result in a decrease of measured percentage uptake in the thyroid. Conversely, a decreased iodide pool will cause elevation of measured percentage thyroid uptakes. Fortunately, iodide pool sizes are relatively constant in most populations. Common sources of increased plasma inorganic iodide are radiographic dyes, tincture of iodine, seafood, and various drugs. Decreased plasma inorganic iodide is most commonly due to diuretic therapy.

If thyroid uptake is in the upper normal range, euthyroid patients should respond to suppressive therapy with triiodothyronine by reduction of the neck uptake ("suppression test"). Similarly, patients with low radioiodide uptake may be restudied after administration of TSH. Response of a low uptake to TSH suggests a diagnosis of secondary hypothyroidism due to pituitary disease; the thyroid does not respond to exogenous TSH stimulation in primary hypothyroidism. The interpretation of these tests is discussed in detail in Chapter 19.

In vivo counting is also used for estimating radioiodide uptake by functioning metastases from thyroid carcinoma to determine whether ^{131}I therapy will be effective.

Regional in vivo counting is used elsewhere to help decide whether to treat hemolytic anemia or thrombocytopenia by splenectomy. Red blood cells or platelets tagged with ^{51}Cr are used to study survival and sequestration by the spleen. Splenectomy usually relieves hemolysis when spleen to liver count ratios are greater than 3:1. Since the counts obtained depend on spleen and liver size and position in addition to the extent of splenic sequestration, this test should be performed in laboratories with considerable hematologic experience.

The radioisotope renogram measures the rate (counts per minute) at which hippurate I 131 is excreted by the kidneys. No image of the kidney is obtained unless the test is performed during scintiphotography. The renogram is sensitive to renal abnormalities and is used for screening and sequential studies of renal function in disease.

In Vitro Counting Procedures

Radiotracer technics allow precise and specific measurement of minute amounts of a wide variety of molecules. Displacement assays measure the displacement of a labeled molecule from binding sites in an equilibrium mixture after addition of an unknown amount of an unlabeled molecule of the same type. In radioimmunoassays, a specific antibody to the unknown molecule is employed to react with it and allow its measurement.

The most widely used radiotracer assays are the serum thyroxine and "T_3 uptake," a measure of available thyroxine binding capacity, by displacement assay technics. Measurement of T_3 by radioimmunoassay has been found to confirm thyroid toxicity with surprising frequency in patients with normal serum thyroxines and even normal radioiodide uptakes. These are usually patients with nodular goiter, prior thyroid surgery, or prior ^{131}I therapy. The number of other radiotracer assays and their modes of use in surgical diagnosis are large and growing rapidly, as is evident from other chapters. A few diverse examples include cervical vein sampling for parathormone assays to locate parathyroid adenomas; monitoring gastrointestinal cancer patients with carcinoembryonic antigen assays to detect recurrence; surveying families with medullary thyroid carcinoma for calcitonin to detect occult neoplasm; and measurement of plasma aldosterone after desoxycorticosterone injections to confirm lack of suppressibility in primary aldosteronism.

Plasma volume can be determined by injecting radioiodinated human serum albumin (RISA) intravenously and then measuring its dilution after mixing but before protein loss. Extravascular loss of protein in edematous states, nephrosis, burns, and similar conditions will cause falsely high results.

Red cell mass is determined by tagging the patient's own red cells with chromium-51. The tagged cells are injected intravenously and whole blood, obtained after mixing, is counted to obtain the blood volume. The patient's hematocrit is used to determine the red cell mass and, indirectly, the plasma volume. Similarly, the red cell mass may be determined indirectly from the RISA plasma volume and hematocrit. Tagged red cells may also be used to quantitatively estimate gastrointestinal loss of blood since no reabsorption of the ^{51}Cr occurs from the gut.

The **Schilling test** estimates ileal absorption of vitamin B_{12}. Radioactive vitamin B_{12} tracer is given orally, and the amount excreted in the urine is measured after a "flushing" dose (1 mg) of unlabeled vitamin B_{12} given parenterally 1 hour later. Reduced excretion in the urine is interpreted to mean reduced intestinal absorption. If, in a repeat test, the addition of intrinsic factor to the vitamin B_{12} tracer raises urinary excretion to normal, the faulty absorption may be due to intrinsic factor deficiency. Strictures or diverticulosis of the small intestine, or other types of blind loop syndrome with bacterial overgrowth, may produce vitamin B_{12} malabsorption correctable with antibiotic therapy. Since vitamin B_{12} absorption is confined to the terminal ileum, ileal resection or disease (regional enteritis) may also lower its absorption. Occasionally, severe neurologic sequelae of vitamin B_{12} deficiency are seen in diseases other than classic pernicious anemia and could be avoided or treated after detection of the absorption defect. Displacement assays may also be used to estimate serum vitamin B_{12}, intrinsic factor concentrations in gastric juice, and anti-intrinsic factor antibodies in the serum. Direct in vitro assay of vitamin B_{12} does not require the administration of large "flushing doses" of vitamin B_{12} as in the Schilling test.

Other tests entailing stool counting include measurement of intestinal loss of serum protein in exudative enteropathy by ^{51}Cr albumin, rose bengal I 131 excretion in neonatal jaundice, and fat absorption using radioiodinated fats.

Radioisotope Therapy

With the exception of limited use of agents such as ^{32}P colloid for therapy of effusions and of soluble ^{32}P phosphate for suppression of bone metastases in hematopoietic and reticuloendothelial malignancies, radioisotope therapy in nuclear medicine is limited to treatment of thyroid tissue with ^{131}I. This isotope emits several beta particles which deliver most of the therapeutic energy. Since beta particles penetrate tissue to a maximum of a few millimeters, over 90% of the dose of radiation from ^{131}I is restricted to the thyroid. Radioiodide therapy is used in the following circumstances: (1) Thyrotoxicosis in adults (diffuse or nodular goiters) and in juveniles when surgery is contraindicated. (2) Autonomous adenomas with toxicity or symptoms from local pressure. (3) Goiters with local symptoms if surgery is contraindicated (uncommon). (4) Thyroid ablation. (5) Thyroid cancer.

Radioiodide therapy is never used during pregnancy or in nursing mothers. The average course of therapy for Graves' disease delivers an ovarian radiation dose as high as a sacral roentgenographic examination. The radiation dose to the testicles is lower. Ophthalmopathy is not aggravated by radioiodide therapy, and there are no local effects (eg, hypoparathyroidism or recurrent laryngeal nerve injury). Large numbers of patients treated with radioiodide have been followed for many years without observation of an increase in incidence of leukemia or thyroid carcinomas. Most clinics have dropped the minimal age for therapy to the postadolescent age group.

Even skilled therapists find a 45–55% incidence of hypothyroidism 10 years after radioiodide therapy, but similar incidences of hypothyroidism were observed after surgery in the same studies. However, it is unusual to have a complete loss of thyroid function after surgery as is sometimes seen after radioiodide therapy.

After proper patient preparation, radioiodide therapy is often curative for thyroid carcinoma metastatic to the lungs, frequently shows complete suppression of radioiodide uptake in metastatic lymph nodes, and is usually only palliative for metastatic bone lesions. Few follicular or papillary carcinomas show enough function for evaluation by ^{131}I iodide until normal thyroid tissue is removed and the patient becomes clinically hypothyroid. The thyroidectomized patient should be prepared by withdrawing long-acting thyroid hormone preparations. Exposure to exogenous iodide should be avoided for at least 3 months. Maintenance therapy with triiodothyronine for 3 weeks will allow metabolism of most previously administered tetraiodothyronine. All replacement therapy is then stopped for a further 3 weeks before evaluation with radioiodide. After discontinuing triiodothyronine, the hypothyroid patient will secrete endogenous TSH and stimulate ^{131}I uptake by the tumor. Sites of uptake are detected by whole body scanning, and uptake can be quantitated. Decisions about when to use ^{131}I therapy, its palliative or curative objectives in the individual case, the desirability of further surgical removal of metastatic deposits, and the possibility of radiation teletherapy should be made in conference between the surgeon, nuclear medicine physician, and radiation therapist. If radioiodide therapy is elected, the best results are obtained when it is given in repeated courses to a hypothyroid and iodide-deprived patient until no further localization is detected.

•   •   •

General References

Blahd WH: *Nuclear Medicine,* 2nd ed. McGraw-Hill, 1971.

Blumhardt R, Nusynowitz ML: A guide to bone scanning. Am Fam Physician 9:153, Jan 1974.

DeLand FH, Wagner HN Jr: *Atlas of Nuclear Medicine.* Vol 3: *Reticuloendothelial System, Liver, Spleen and Thyroid.* Saunders, 1972.

Freeman LM, Blaufox MD (editors): Seminars in Nuclear Medicine. [Since 1971.]

Gottschalk A, Potchen EJ: *Diagnostic Nuclear Medicine.* Williams & Wilkins, 1976.

Gumerman LW: Nuclear medicine studies in the diagnosis of diseases of the liver, pancreas, and spleen. Surg Clin North Am 55:427, 1975.

Hoffer PB, Gottschalk A: Tumor scanning agents. Semin Nucl Med 4:305, 1974.

Matin P: *Handbook of Clinical Nuclear Medicine.* Medical Examination Publishing Co., 1977.

Maynard CD: *Clinical Nuclear Medicine.* Lea & Febiger, 1969.

Quinn JL, Henkin RE: Scanning techniques to assess thyroid nodules. Annu Rev Med 26:193, 1975.

Sodee B, Early PJ: *Technology and Interpretation of Nuclear Medicine Procedures.* Mosby, 1972.

Werner SC, Ingbar JH (editors): *The Thyroid,* 3rd ed. Harper & Row, 1971.

9...
Special Diagnostic Procedures

Alexander R. Margulis, MD, Melvyn T. Korobkin, MD, & Roy A. Filly, MD

Radiologic procedures have played an important role in diagnosis since the turn of the century. In the last few years, technologic advances have greatly extended the importance and scope of special diagnostic procedures, performed for the most part in departments of radiology.

ULTRASOUND
(Figs 9–1 to 9–4)

Echocardiography has assumed an important role in the evaluation of heart disease involving the valves and the septum and in determining the presence and extent of pericardial effusion. B mode (spatial reconstruction imaging of reflected ultrasound waves) and real time echography (rapid spatial reconstruction of reflected ultrasound waves capable of demonstrating motion but lacking in fine detail) have become important in obstetric practice. B mode gray scale ultrasonography (gray scale uses television display and reconstruction of images demonstrating a broad scale of amplitude differences and better resolution) has been a significant advance. It is noninvasive except when used to guide and control needle biopsies.

Ultrasonography uses no ionizing radiation; in the energy range applied diagnostically, it has no demon-

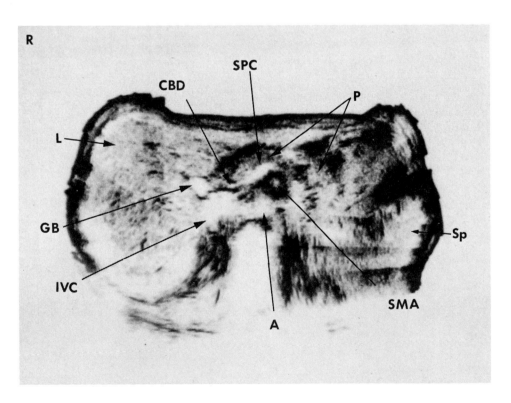

Figure 9—1. High-resolution cross-sectional gray scale ultrasonogram demonstrating the body of the pancreas (P). If the patient is obese and bowel gas is minimal, transducers of higher frequency can be used to demonstrate small structures such as the distal common bile duct (CBD) and the superior mesenteric artery (SMA). (R, right; L, liver; GB, neck of gallbladder; SPC, confluence of splenic and portal veins; IVC, inferior vena cava; A, aorta; Sp, spleen.)

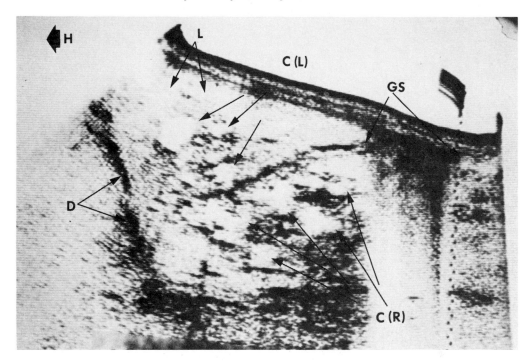

Figure 9–2. Parasagittal gray scale ultrasonogram obtained 5 cm to the right of midline demonstrates a grossly enlarged right kidney elevating the right hepatic lobe (L) and extending to the diaphragm (D). The kidney contains numerous cysts (C) in a disorganized pattern typical of polycystic disease. Associated cysts within the liver (C) are visible. However, bowel gas casts an acoustic shadow (GS) that obscures the lower pole of the kidney. (H, head.)

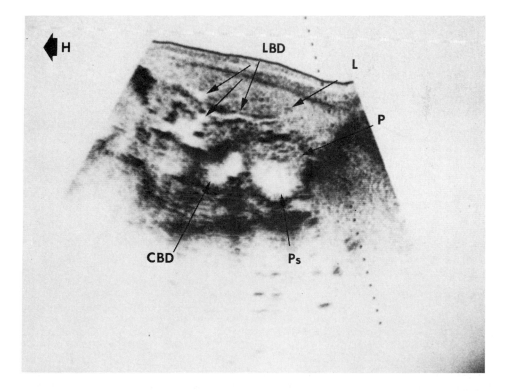

Figure 9–3. Parasagittal gray scale ultrasonogram obtained slightly to the right of the abdominal midline. The left hepatic lobe (L) contains multiple dilated bile ducts (LBD); the common bile duct (CBD) is enlarged; and a pseudocyst (Ps) elevates the pancreatic head (P). (H, head.)

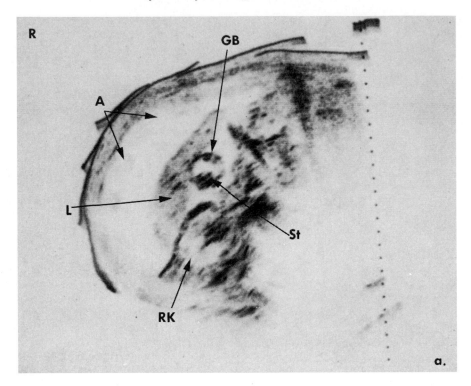

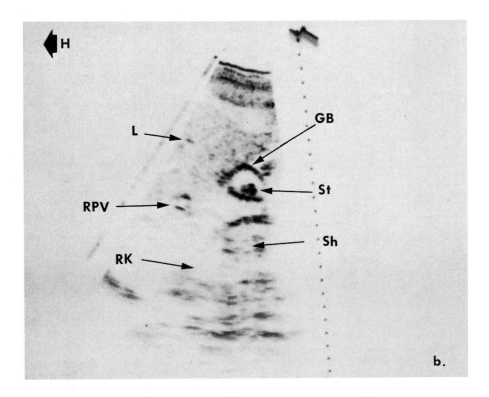

Figure 9—4 a. Partial cross-sectional gray scale ultrasonogram of the right (R) side of the abdomen. The caudal portion of the right hepatic lobe (L) is surrounded by echo-free ascites (A). The gallbladder (GB), partially surrounded by ascites, contains stones (St) in its dependent portion. (RK, right kidney.) b: A limited single sector sweep of the gallbladder (GB) in a longitudinal plane demonstrates 2 stones (St). Each stone casts an acoustic shadow (Sh). (H, head; RPV, segment of right portal vein.)

strable biologic side-effects and causes no somatic or genetic damage. Ultrasonography has the advantage of spatial reproduction in transverse and longitudinal directions, thus giving data in 3 dimensions. Since information is obtained from reflections at interfaces between media of differing acoustic impedance, image detail is not dependent on fat for contrast (Fig 9–1). Thus, even cachectic individuals can be successfully studied. In fact, obese patients may be difficult to study with ultrasonography because of the limited range of high-frequency sound beams.

The disadvantages of ultrasonography are as follows:

(1) Contrast media have not been developed to widen the applicability of the method.

(2) Ultrasound is not well transmitted through gas, eg, one cannot adequately study the abdomen when the intestine is full of gas. Therefore, many acutely ill patients are poor subjects. Study of the lungs is not possible for the same reason.

(3) Most ultrasound equipment is not automated, and great skill is required of the operator.

A special advantage of ultrasonography is that the equipment is relatively inexpensive and the examinations can be performed at a lower cost than CT scans or arteriograms. This factor plus the great variety of information that can be obtained without radiation exposure makes ultrasonography a valuable and useful diagnostic method.

Abdomen

In the abdomen, ultrasonography is useful to study the liver, pancreas, spleen, gallbladder, and retroperitoneal tissues. Examination of the kidneys can differentiate cystic from solid lesions and demonstrate hydronephrosis, polycystic kidneys, perinephric fluid collections, and other morphologic alterations.

In the liver, solid lesions can be distinguished from fluid-filled ones such as cysts or abscesses. The technic may also detect bile ducts distended by distal obstruction. Metastatic lesions can also be demonstrated. Ultrasonography can demonstrate the size of the gallbladder and may identify stones as small as 2–3 mm in diameter. However, stones are not always seen by ultrasonography.

Ultrasonography can demonstrate pancreatic cysts and pseudocysts and enlargement of the pancreas. As yet, it cannot show small tumors of the pancreas. Large tumors are poorly differentiated from other causes of pancreatic enlargement such as inflammatory edema. Calcifications are occasionally demonstrated. If the patient has large amounts of intestinal gas, as is often the case in acute pancreatitis, ultrasonography may be useless.

Ultrasonography may detect postoperative abscesses and other fluid collections, but associated ileus may interfere with the procedure because of excessive bowel gas.

Masses in the female reproductive organs can be examined and uterine enlargement distinguished from adnexal masses. The cystic or solid nature of ovarian masses can be determined.

Ultrasound can detect and differentiate renal cysts and tumors if the lesions are at least 1 cm in diameter. Ultrasonography has proved valuable in verifying the diagnosis of abdominal aortic aneurysms and in accurately determining their diameter.

CT SCANNING

CT scanning was first used to diagnose intracranial lesions. The method depends on computerizing and reconstructing data of density differences from tiny cubes of tissue traversed by an extremely narrow x-ray beam. The density difference data are obtained from sensitive detectors, much more efficient than silver halide film, which utilize only a small fraction of the energy that traverses them. The computer reconstructs a transverse cross-section of the body and displays the image on a television monitor. The ability of the detectors to distinguish small differences in density results in detailed images of abdominal and soft tissues previously unavailable.

The value of CT body scanning can be enhanced by intravascular injection of iodine-containing contrast media or instillation of diluted water-soluble contrast media into the gut. Gas and barium in the bowel do not invalidate the examination but do produce annoying artifacts (less pronounced on the rotating type of scanner).

In the abdomen, the greatest indications for CT scanning are diseases of the liver, spleen, retroperitoneal tissues, kidney, pancreas, and pelvic organs. The potential of CT scanning has not yet been fully realized. As new contrast media are developed, new areas of application will undoubtedly appear. The use of CT scanning for the mediastinum, chest, and bones is just beginning.

The disadvantages of CT scanning, particularly when compared with ultrasonography, are as follows:

(1) Inability to obtain longitudinal sections.

(2) Radiation doses, although in the permissible range of other gastrointestinal examinations, are nevertheless appreciable (ie, about 0.5–1.5 rad/slice).

(3) In the abdomen, good delineation of detail by CT depends heavily on the presence of fat. In cachectic individuals, the images and details are poor.

(4) Motion artifacts. The shortest body scanning time at present is approximately 5 seconds. While most individuals can hold their breath for this long, slight motion still occurs from heartbeats, involuntary twitching, etc—all of which produce artifacts. Machines with a fan beam and linear motion are subject to artifacts from dense radiopaque structures. Because of the longer scanning time (about 18 seconds) of these instruments, breathing artifacts occur in dyspneic individuals.

Abdomen

In the liver, cysts, abscesses, and primary and

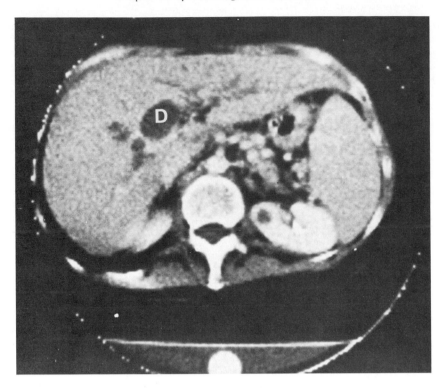

Figure 9–5. CT scan in a jaundiced patient after the intravenous injection of contrast material shows dilated intrahepatic bile ducts (D) as linear and oval low-density structures. A tumor of the common bile duct produced the obstructive jaundice. Note the incidental finding of a small left renal cyst.

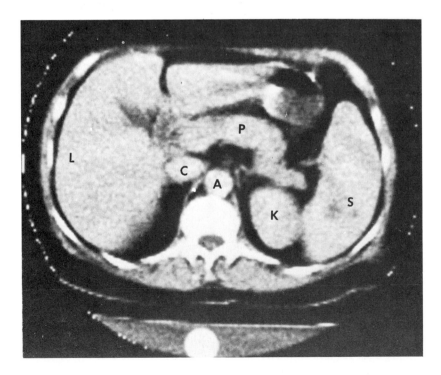

Figure 9–6. CT scan through the upper abdomen shows a normal tail, body, and portion of the head of the pancreas (P). The liver (L), spleen (S), aorta (A), inferior vena cava (C), and upper pole of the left kidney (K) are also demonstrated.

metastatic tumors can be clearly outlined. After the CT scan has been performed, it may be repeated following intravenous injection of radiopaque water-soluble contrast media. The contrast medium increases the density of normal parenchyma and accentuates the abnormal lesions (eg, neoplasms, cysts). Dilatation of biliary ducts can usually be distinguished from the portal venous system following intravenous injection of contrast medium (Fig 9–5). The finding of widened biliary ducts may lead to percutaneous transhepatic cholangiography (injection of contrast medium directly into the biliary ducts) and more precise demonstration of the site, appearance, and, frequently, the cause of extrahepatic biliary obstruction.

CT scans show the gallbladder but are not as useful for detecting stones as ultrasonography. Stones can be missed if they lie between levels of CT sections.

CT scans of the spleen are performed first without and then with injection of intravenous contrast material. Subcapsular hematomas, parenchymal rupture, abscesses, cysts, and neoplasms are readily diagnosed.

Although the spatial resolution of CT scanning does not approach that of conventional excretory urography, cysts can be differentiated from tumors. After injection of contrast medium, renal calyces are clearly shown, although the resolution is less than with urography.

CT scanning can demonstrate retroperitoneal masses such as lymphomas or metastatic lesions. For this reason, CT scans are of great value to radiation therapists. The outline of the mass can be coordinated with isodose curves. The radiation treatment fields; which will cover the entire lesion, can be accurately mapped. Tumor invasion of vertebrae and displacement of the aorta or other major vessels are easily demonstrable.

CT scanning has failed to detect pancreatic tumors too small to alter the contour of the organ. Nevertheless, cysts, pseudocysts, large tumors, and phlegmons due to pancreatitis can be easily shown. If diluted water-soluble iodine-containing contrast medium is ingested, the pancreas can be differentiated from adjacent bowel. CT scanning of the pancreas has stimulated interest in devising contrast media that would be excreted by this organ. With computer enhancement, contrast medium excreted in exocrine secretions even in small concentrations may be of substantial diagnostic value.

Head

CT is now the procedure of choice in the diagnosis of a vast array of known or suspected structural abnormalities of the brain and cranial vault. Where CT scanners are available, there has been a marked reduction in the number of pneumoencephalograms performed and a similar but lesser decrease in the number of cerebral arteriograms. Tumors, cysts, abscesses, infarcts, and hematomas of the brain are reliably and accurately imaged by CT, and a normal CT examina-

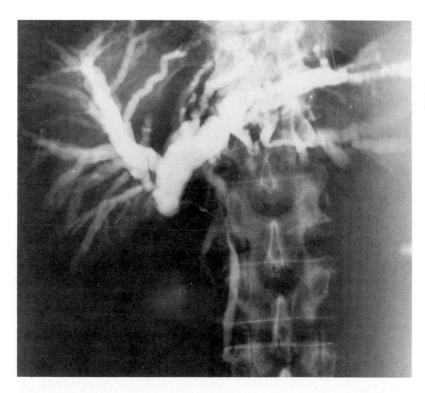

Figure 9–7. Percutaneous transhepatic cholangiogram showing greatly dilated obstructed biliary radicles from carcinoma of the gallbladder. The mass has invaded and almost completely occluded the common hepatic duct, which is reduced to a thin strand.

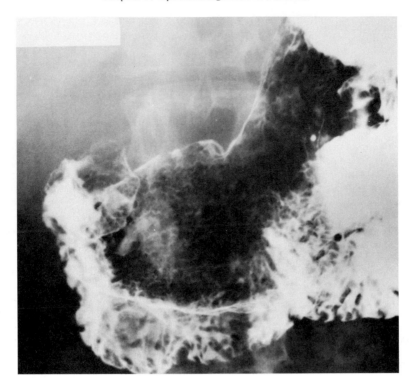

Figure 9—8. Double contrast study of the stomach demonstrating the grossly irregular surface of the gastric mucosa, confirmed endoscopically to represent gastritis.

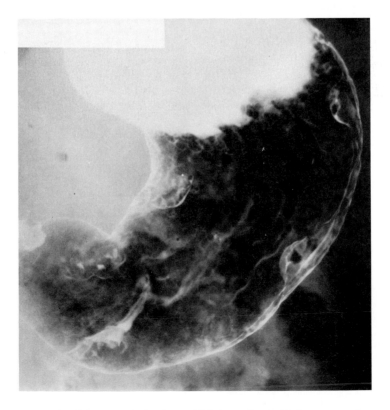

Figure 9—9. Double contrast study of the stomach showing multiple large ulcerated lesions representing mucosal metastases from malignant melanoma.

tion usually terminates the diagnostic evaluation of a suspected mass lesion.

Pelvis

CT of the pelvis provides important diagnostic information that cannot be obtained in any other way. The presence of abundant amounts of perivisceral fat allows one to determine the presence and degree of tumor extension to the pelvic side walls in many cases of genitourinary tract tumor. Such information is useful in clinical staging of pelvic neoplasms and in planning radiation therapy. In patients with mass lesions of the bony pelvis or adjacent soft tissues, the transaxial view of CT scans and the ability to display both bony and soft tissue detail on a single image provide surgeons with unique information to help guide the appropriate surgical approach. CT often shows both the presence and extent of pedicle attachment of soft tissue tumors to the bony pelvis as well as the extent of pedicle attachment of primary bone tumors to the pelvis. Such information is often difficult and usually impossible to extract from conventional radiographic examinations.

DOUBLE CONTRAST EXAMINATIONS OF THE UPPER GASTROINTESTINAL TRACT

Double contrast studies of the esophagus and stomach, which may demonstrate early superficial neoplasms, have significantly reduced the mortality rate from carcinoma of the stomach in Japan. The method involves giving a thick barium suspension to outline the wall of the stomach followed by tablets that release CO_2 in the presence of water; simethicone is given to reduce bubbles. This technic can also show fine linear ulcers in the stomach (Fig 9—8), erosive gastritis, and the surface details of neoplastic lesions (Fig 9—9). Small esophageal carcinomas that involve only one wall can be detected. Further control is obtained by administering intravenous glucagon to decrease gastric and duodenal peristalsis. With the gut thus paralyzed, excellent morphologic detail can be displayed. The duodenum can be selectively studied by passing a peroral tube into its lumen and instilling barium followed by air; glucagon, 2 mg, is given intravenously and x-rays made. This technic provides superb mucosal detail, and the absence of barium in the stomach simplifies examination of the duodenum.

• • •

General References

Chornich SM & others: Hypotonic duodenography with the use of glucagon. Gastroenterology 63:392, 1972.

Felson B (editor): A primer on sonography. Semin Roentgenol 10:247, Oct 1975. [Entire issue.]

Haaga JR & others: Computed tomography of the pancreas. Radiology 120:589, 1976.

Leopold GR, Asher WM (editors): *Fundamentals of Abdominal and Pelvic Ultrasonography*. Saunders, 1975.

Sanders RC (editor): Ultrasound. Radiol Clin North Am 13:389, Dec 1975.

Sheedy PF & others: Computed tomography of the body: Initial clinical trial with the EMI prototype. Am J Roentgenol Radium Ther Nucl Med 127:23, 1976.

Shirakabe H (editor): Double contrast studies of the stomach. Bunkodo Co., Ltd, Tokyo, Japan, 1971.

Stanley RJ & others: Computed tomography of the body: Early trends in application and accuracy of the method. Am J Roentgenol Radium Ther Nucl Med 127:53, 1976.

10 . . .
Wound Healing

Thomas K. Hunt, MD

Without the capacity for repair and regeneration, no organism could survive the trauma of surgery. Only a century ago, complicated and incomplete healing after injury was the rule rather than the exception. Surgeons had little choice but to accept infected, draining wounds. Lister's first application of antisepsis changed surgery as dramatically as the discovery of anesthesia had 30 years before. Today, surgeons tend to ignore the healing process since it usually proceeds without obvious incident. Even so, poor healing and excessive healing continue to be leading causes of disability and death.

In the last 100 years, knowledge of the basic mechanisms of healing has grown rapidly. For the first time in history, surgeons who have a detailed knowledge of these mechanisms can influence healing and are able to anticipate and often prevent problems of incomplete or excessive repair.

FORMS OF HEALING

Surgeons customarily divide the types of wound healing into first, second, and third intention healing (Fig 10–1). **First intention** healing occurs when tissue is cleanly incised and reapproximated, and repair occurs without complication. **Second intention** healing is the healing of an open wound (or a closed [dead] space) through formation of granulation tissue* and eventual coverage of the defect by spontaneous migration of epithelial cells. Most infected wounds and burns heal in this manner. One can easily see that primary (first intention) healing is simpler and requires less time and material than secondary healing, in which the defect must be filled with new tissue before coverage can take place. It sometimes happens that primary healing is possible but insufficient reserve is present to allow secondary healing. For example, an ischemic limb may heal primarily, but if the wound opens or becomes infected, the wound might not heal. Amputation may then become necessary.

*Granulation tissue is the red, granular, moist tissue which appears during healing of open wounds. Microscopically, it contains new collagen, blood vessels, fibroblasts, and inflammatory cells, especially macrophages.

Healing by **third intention,** clinically called delayed primary closure, occurs when a wound is left to accomplish the first phases of healing while open and is then closed to finish healing as if by first intention. Wound infection in contaminated wounds can often be avoided by leaving the wound open for 4 days and then closing it. The wound is less likely to become infected while open than the wound closed primarily. The closed wound is most susceptible to infection in the first 4 days. Closure of a wound by skin graft is also an example of third intention healing.

RESPONSE TO INJURY

When tissue is divided or otherwise injured, the extracellular matrix responds to injury by activating the complement cascade. Injured vessels bleed and then contract. Platelets, which are released into the surrounding tissue, bind to exposed collagen. As a result, phospholipids are released, activating both the extrinsic and the intrinsic coagulation mechanisms. The complement cascade, which is a series of enzymes, each activated by the product of its predecessor enzyme, acts as an amplifier of the injury signal. Eventually, the injury is converted to a chemical signal which calls forth an invasion of inflammatory cells.

Within a few hours, the area is heavily populated by polymorphonuclear neutrophils (PMNs) and lymphocytes. At the same time, however, the vasculature has thrombosed back to the nearest functioning vascular arcades. The circulation which was once adequate to maintain the uninjured tissue has now been diminished by the injury and is even less adequate in view of the added number of metabolizing inflammatory cells. A local energy crisis is inevitable, and the area rather quickly becomes acidotic due to accumulation of hydrogen ion, carbon dioxide, and lactate. Oxygen tensions fall to the neighborhood of 10 mm Hg with some areas demonstrated to be at zero. Local hypoxia and acidosis are properties of all the examples of wounds which have been tested (Fig 10–2).

Within a few days after injury, the PMNs and lymphocytes become less prominent and the wandering tissue monocyte becomes the dominant white cell. By this time, fibroblasts, which have been appearing

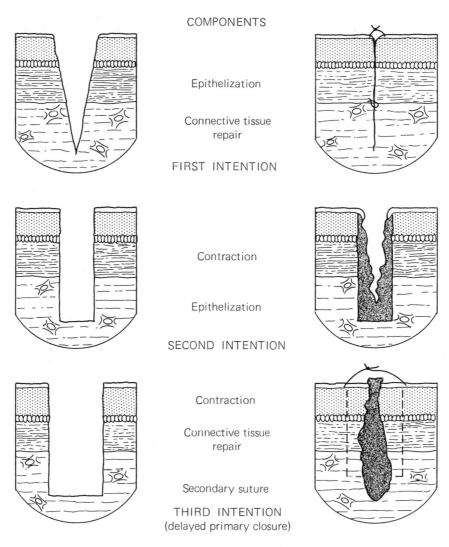

COMPONENTS

Epithelization

Connective tissue repair

FIRST INTENTION

Contraction

Epithelization

SECOND INTENTION

Contraction

Connective tissue repair

Secondary suture

THIRD INTENTION
(delayed primary closure)

Figure 10–1. Schematic illustration of healing by first, second, and third intention.

since about the second day after wounding, have become the other dominant cell, and this partnership between monocyte and fibroblast continues until the wound is healed. If the wound is cut and precisely reapproximated, as in a small corneal incision, the functioning vasculature can be seen to circulate red cells across the wound as early as the third day. Thus, the fibrinolytic mechanism must be at work to clear up the intravascular clotting which has occurred. Very little new vasculature may develop if the old vasculature reconnects promptly and in quantity. However, most wounds are not closed as precisely as those in corneas. By the fourth or fifth day, a host of new small vessels has formed, usually in greatest concentration near sutures. These vessels bring nutrition to the ischemic portion of the wound. They are found near sutures partly because of the inflammatory potential of suture material but more often because of the strangulating action of the suture. The tighter the suture, the greater the vascular proliferation near it.

The response to injury, therefore, involves the PMN, the lymphocyte, the macrophage, the fibroblast, and the capillary endothelial cell. These cells comprise a unit or module of a circulatory loop which is supported by new collagen made by the fibroblast. The new vessels bring new nutrition and allow fibroblasts to migrate forward. The macrophage seems to signal and govern the advance, while the PMNs and lymphocytes constitute the defense against infection and debridement of damaged tissue and foreign body.

CELLULAR COMPONENTS OF THE WOUND

Polymorphonuclear Leukocytes & Lymphocytes

Studies of the function of leukocytes show that their basic functions are largely unimpaired by their

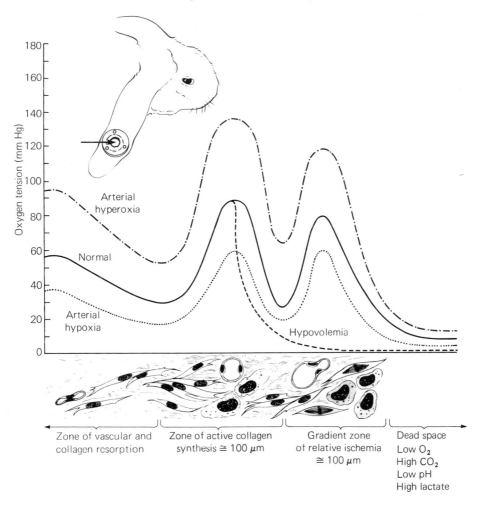

Figure 10—2. Schematic plot of oxygen tension as measured in a healing wound in a rabbit ear chamber. The gradient zone advances into the dead space, and behind it the neovasculature resorbs as the reparative tissue advances. The oxygen tension plot illustrates the effects of hyperoxia, hypoxia, and hypovolemia. Since oxygen is required for repair, little progress can be expected during hypovolemia.

translocation from the local circulation into the wound. Measures that eliminate these cells from the wound expose the wound to infection but do not influence the type or quality of repair of the clean, primarily closed wound. Presumably, the various types of lymphocytes act in conjunction with the macrophage to mount an immune response to foreign materials, bacteria, and possibly viruses. Wound fluid contains specific immune substances of obscure origin.

PMNs phagocytose and kill bacteria. Attachment of PMNs to bacteria preparatory to phagocytosis is facilitated by opsonins, a group of substances which includes complement, antibodies, and other naturally occurring plasma factors. Wound fluid contains opsonins for staphylococci but seems to be deficient in opsonins for coliforms. As the white cell contracts and surrounds the bacterium, its cytoplasmic granules begin to fuse with the developing phagosome. In this process, the granular enzymes may leak into the extracellular fluid. Many of these enzymes are bacteriostatic

or bactericidal and pass on this property to the extracellular fluid.

Mammalian leukocytes have developed an important oxidative killing mechanism involving a membrane-bound oxidase that reduces oxygen to superoxide anion, O_2^-. This anion then undergoes dismutation to form hydrogen peroxide. Subsequently, hydrogen peroxide reacts within the primary phagocytic vacuole to form aldehydes, hypohalides, and other microbicidal compounds. Many of these substances are antibacterial. This system is an important component of natural immunity, and when the leukocyte enters the wound, with its poor circulation and its low oxygen tension, the leukocyte's ability to kill bacteria is greatly impaired. Even in the normal wound the leukocyte is hampered, but in the pathologically hypoxic wound its killing capacity is even further diminished. Fortunately, even mild increases in local oxygen tension will restore and even increase the antibacterial capacity of the white cell.

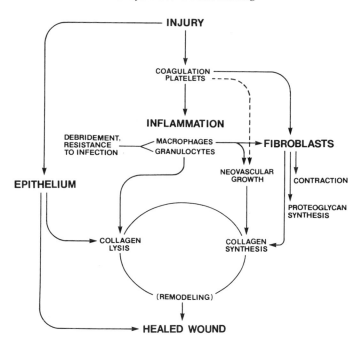

Figure 10–3. Schematic diagram of wound healing. (Reproduced, with permission, from Hunt TK, Van Winkle W Jr: *Fundamentals of Wound Management,* Vol 1. Chirurgecom Press, 1976.)

Platelets & Macrophages

In addition to their role in coagulation, platelets seem to be important in healing. For instance, platelets activated by thrombin produce a substance that stimulates fibroblasts to multiply in culture. When thrombin-stimulated platelets are injected into the cornea of the eye, capillary endothelial cells begin to proliferate and new vessels are seen migrating toward the site of infection. Macrophages seem even more important. When wound macrophages are injected into the cornea, fibroblasts multiply, collagen synthesis is stimulated, and capillary endothelial proliferation becomes prominent. The end result is a vascularized scar which eventually remodels itself and loses its vasculature (Fig 10–3). If macrophages are inactivated by an antimacrophage serum, even primary wound healing suffers. Macrophages activated by substances such as killed fungus spores or bacterial endotoxin increase the quantity of collagen synthesized by host tissue. If macrophages are injected into tissue which is then incised, the wound heals faster than one in tissue injected with culture media free of macrophages. Macrophages also seem to ingest and hydrolyze macromolecules and release amino acids, which can be picked up by fibroblasts and synthesized into collagen and proteoglycans.

The Capillary Endothelial Cell

The neovascularity of wounds facilitates continued supply of nutrients to tissue with an injured vasculature. There are 2 principal observations: First, new vessels originate from existing vessels; and second, whatever their ultimate size or function, all new vessels begin as capillary buds. Angiogenesis in wounds exhib-

its 3 major patterns. The first is the generation of a whole new vascular network. This mechanism is used when a tissue defect must be filled, as in healing by second intention. The second is joining of wound vessels with an unused circulation, as when the host bed provides circulation to a skin graft. The third is the joining of vessels across a primarily healing wound.

Regeneration of a whole new vascular network is secondary healing, in which a space in tissue is obliterated or healed. Sprouts of endothelial cells grow out toward the wound edge, apparently in response to unknown signals from platelets and macrophages. The capillary buds join with other similar buds to form new capillary loops. Blood flow is reestablished from high pressure zones to low pressure zones, and the pressure in the vessel is balanced by a collagenous gel formed by the local fibroblasts. Capillary endothelial cells make collagenase and seem to burrow their way through the new gel-like collagen. The basement membrane is incomplete in the newest vessels. Therefore, for a while the new endothelial cells fit loosely and the vessels are fragile and leaky.

In primary repair—in which the edges of the wound are accurately coapted and soon fused—both old and new vessels reconnect across the wound space. For this purpose, the endothelial bud seems to have a fibrinolytic enzyme which allows red cells to pass through the fibrin that glues the 2 edges together.

The surgeon has a unique chance to observe one form of neovascularization in the healing of skin grafts. When a skin graft is applied, it is bloodless and cadaveric. Within 2 days, the graft shows prominent purple spots. These look like hematomas but will blanch when pressure is applied. As time passes, the purple areas become pink and blanch more obviously on direct pressure. Gradually these areas of reestablished circulation enlarge and coalesce. Experimental studies leave no doubt that the old vessels of the graft first passively fill with red cells and then reestablish a functioning circulation.

Lymphatics also regenerate, but little is known of the process.

The Fibroblast

The fibroblast is a large cell, well endowed with protein-synthesizing endoplasmic reticulum, which synthesizes collagen and mucopolysaccharide. The fibroblast synthesizes the basic molecule—the monomer—of the polymeric collagen fiber, a long, thin, triple helix approximately 289 × 1.4 nm. These molecules are secreted into the extracellular space, where they slowly polymerize to form large, strong, insoluble fibers (Fig 10–4). The joining of the sides of a wound with collagen fibers is similar to building a bridge across a chasm. As each steel beam is locked into place, the bridge gains strength and span.

Wound fibroblasts appear to originate in the injured area. Most of them probably come from cells surrounding blood vessels. The nature of the signal to transform resting cells to fibroblasts is unknown except that its source is in the inflammatory reaction. Smooth muscle cells and fibroblasts are very similar. It seems possible that smooth muscle cells could have the genetic mechanism for collagen synthesis which becomes active under the proper stimulus. This seems to occur in healing arteries, and a so-called myofibroblast is seen in developing atheromas. The myofibroblast is also found in contracting wounds, as discussed below.

What is the signal for collagen synthesis? Experi-

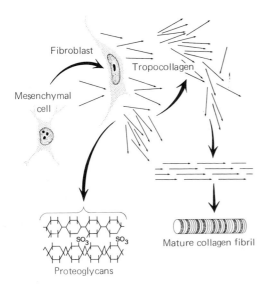

Figure 10–4. Schematic representation of collagen synthesis, deposition, and polymerization. The molecules polymerize with a "three-fourths stagger" overlap, which accounts for the crossbanding visible on electron microscopy.

ments in cultured fibroblasts indicate that a low oxidation-reduction potential coupled with a high lactate concentration or a high ascorbic acid concentration (which is possible only in the presence of a low oxidation-reduction potential) actually activates at least some of the collagen-synthesizing enzymes. This is an attractive hypothesis because a high concentration of lactate—10 times that of blood—is uniformly found in the extracellular fluid of wounds. Wounds made periodically hypoxic at simulated high altitudes and then brought to normal pressure heal somewhat faster than normal. If moderate arterial hyperoxia is maintained, the rate of collagen synthesis increases; but the lactate concentration of the extracellular fluid does not fall. Therefore, the thesis that lactate stimulates collagen synthesis fits the few experimental facts that are available.

During collagen synthesis, proline is incorporated into the growing peptide chain. Proline molecules are subsequently converted to hydroxyproline by the action of prolyl hydroxylase and molecular oxygen. Lysine is incorporated and hydroxylated similarly. These vital reactions require iron, molecular (dissolved) oxygen, ascorbic acid, and α-ketoglutarate. If proline is not hydroxylated, collagen transport from the cell is hindered. Without hydroxylation of lysine, intramolecular and intermolecular bonding is diminished and a structurally poor collagen results. This suggests that healing would be impaired by severe iron and ascorbic acid deficiencies and local or systemic hypoxia. In practice, iron deficiency does not seem to impair healing. Ascorbic acid and oxygen deficiencies, however, are well known for their deleterious effects on healing.

Hydroxylysine molecules are oxidized to the aldehyde form and condense with other such lysine groups to form covalent cross-links within and between molecules. This step adds rigidity to the molecule and fiber. The reaction can be inhibited by β-aminopropionitrile (BAPN) and by penicillamine. A disease known as lathyrism, which occurs naturally in animals fed peas containing BAPN, is of great interest to surgeons because it may offer a clue to the control of the physical properties of scar tissue. This disease is characterized by weak connective tissues and poor healing as a result of inadequate formation of lysine-lysine bonds.

In the differentiation phase of healing, a slow tightening of collagen fibers apparently occurs, which is why tensile strength increases despite a net loss of collagen. This remodeling may be due to a number of processes, including turnover of collagen, fiber shrinkage, and increasing intermolecular bonding. Remodeling is affected by mechanical stress, which partly determines the amount, form, and architecture of the final product (Figs 10–5 and 10–6).

The extracellular environment must be favorable for alignment and approximation of the collagen monomers. It is presumed that the ground substance, which is composed of sulfated and nonsulfated mucopolysaccharides of high molecular weight (also synthesized by fibroblasts), provides this environment. These

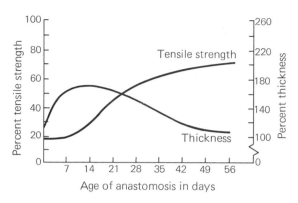

Figure 10–5. The strength of an anastomosis increases while its thickness or mass decreases during the resorptive phase.

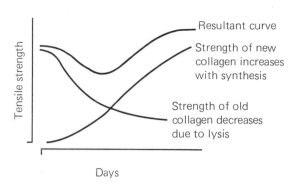

Figure 10–7. Tensile strength is the resultant between the strength of old collagen as affected by lysis and new collagen as affected by synthesis and lysis.

substances give the wound its characteristic metachromatic staining properties. A small amount of mucopolysaccharide is incorporated into the collagen fiber.

In the early proliferative phase, synthesis of new and lysis of old collagen take place simultaneously, and the bridging of the tissue discontinuity becomes a struggle between the lysis and the synthesis of collagen. Any exaggeration of lysis of old collagen or delay or diminution of synthesis may cause dehiscence of the wound or leakage of an anastomosis (Fig 10–7). In the section on factors affecting healing (see below), this important concept is expanded. Collagenolytic enzymes have been identified and characterized.

If all goes well for the primarily closed wound,

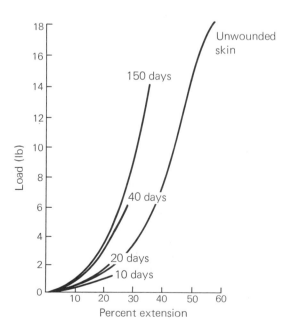

Figure 10–6. Tensile strength increases for at least 150 days after injury and suture. Extensibility also increases. Collagen remodeling must be occurring or the wound tissue would not become more pliable. (See Fig 17–3.)

tensile strength increases rapidly after a few days. Wounds in warm, highly vascular tissue such as the head and neck may be secure enough so that skin sutures can be removed by the third day. Wounds of the abdomen heal more slowly but are usually secure enough so that skin sutures can be removed by the seventh day, although they have now gained only about 20% of the original strength of the tissue. Wounds of the extremities heal even more slowly. The intense cellular activity of the wound during active collagen synthesis causes a ridge of induration about 1 cm wide around the wound. In a wound healing primarily this is called the "healing ridge" and can easily be felt. If this ridge is complete along the length of the wound, it implies good healing, and dehiscence will not occur. If it is absent by 7–9 days, dehiscence becomes a definite risk but is not inevitable.

Eventually, the individuality of the wound is slowly lost, and it begins to resemble normal tissue more and more closely. Fibroblasts and macrophages disappear, and excessive collagen is removed. Collagen is still synthesized more rapidly in the wound than in normal tissue even after many months, but a net resorption occurs during the late phases of repair. In fact, at about the 21st day for a primarily healing wound in skin, the net accumulation of collagen ceases and net collagen loss begins. As a consequence of turnover of collagen in this phase, the collagenous mass in the wound is remodeled. The amorphous mass of collagen seen in the early wound gradually becomes an interlocking network of small collagen fibers joining the more normal-appearing, larger collagen fibers at the edge of the wound. The edges of the wound are knit by a sort of welding of new collagen fibers between the cut ends of the old collagen fibers and an intertwining of new collagen through the spaces that separate the collagen fibers of the normal tissue. Presumably as a consequence of remodeling, the breaking strength of a skin or fascial wound increases up to 6 months, even though the total amount of collagen in the area decreases.

Unfortunately, remodeling does not proceed to

the point of normality. Skin and fascia, for example, eventually achieve only about 80% of their normal strength, and their other mechanical properties such as elasticity and capacity for energy absorption probably never return to normal. The end result is a serviceable but somewhat weak and brittle tissue—a scar.

CONTRACTION

Contraction is a mysterious process by which open skin wounds spontaneously shrink and close. The phenomenon in open wounds in man was recognized and described by John Hunter. It is perhaps better termed "intussusceptive" healing since normal tissue is pulled into the open area to achieve coverage. Huge defects on the back of the neck and other areas of loose skin will completely close by contraction, but in other areas of the body, where the skin is tight, the process is not as reliable. Contraction should be distinguished from contracture, or loss of joint motion from shrinking scar tissue.

The contractile force has been measured and is roughly equivalent to forces exerted by known cellular systems. It apparently depends on a contractile system in the fibroblast since it is independent of collagen content and other measurable biochemical components of the wound. Many reparative fibroblasts contain microfibrils indistinguishable from those of smooth muscle cells. Smooth muscle stimulators and inhibitors influence contraction of these cells. This similarity of function and appearance of fibroblasts and smooth muscle cells has also been noted in arterial injuries and atheromas. Cortisone and vinblastine stop contraction, and the process is not restored by vitamin A.

Experienced clinicians often remain patient and rely on contraction to close wounds in favorable areas. Thin skin grafts do not slow contraction, but thick ones or flaps can prevent or limit it. Large skin graft scars may remain where previously the wound was destined to be covered by normal skin.

EPITHELIZATION

Within a few days following injury, epithelial cells at the edge of the wound become rounded and mitoses appear in the basal layers. Cells begin to migrate across the wound, remaining always in contact with (and partly controlled by) mesenchymal tissues. They advance in a sort of leapfrog fashion. When the layer is complete, the cells again begin to divide and form a thicker epithelium. However, the epithelium never returns to normal. It is usually thinner and less pigmented, and it lacks the usual rete pegs.

Squamous cells will advance deep to dead tissue, using a collagenase to cleave the tissue ahead of the advancing cells. A tissue defect which is allowed to dry will form an eschar and epithelium will form below the eschar, presumably at a point where the local nutrition is sufficient to support the squamous cells. If the wound is kept moist and protected from exposure, the epithelial cells will advance on top of the wound, a faster and more economical process.

Epithelial repair in special tissues, such as the gastrointestinal tract, is, in general, about the same as that in squamous cells. There are unusual features, however, which are beyond the scope of this chapter.

HEALING OF SPECIALIZED TISSUES

Nerve

Brain heals largely through connective tissue scar formation in which glial and perivascular cells seem to differentiate to fibroblasts. When a peripheral nerve is severed, the distal nerve degenerates, leaving the axon sheaths to heal together by inosculation. The axon then regenerates from the nerve cell through the reconstituted sheaths, advancing as much as 1 mm/day. Unfortunately, because individual neural sheaths have no means of seeking out their original distal ends, the axon sheaths reconnect randomly, and motor nerve axons may regenerate in vain into a sensory distal sheath and end organ. The functional result of neural regeneration, therefore, is more satisfactory in the "purer" peripheral nerves.

Intestine

The intestine has received little attention from students of healing. The rate of healing apparently varies from one portion of the intestine to the other. Anastomoses of the colon and esophagus are quite precarious and likely to leak, whereas leakage of stomach or small intestinal anastomoses is rare. The intestinal anastomosis usually regains strength so rapidly that by 1 week it resists bursting more strongly than the more normal surrounding tissue. One reason for this is that the surrounding intestine participates in the reaction to injury, loses a large portion of its collagen by lysis, and consequently loses strength. For this reason, perforation is about as likely to occur a few millimeters from the anastomosis as it is in the anastomosis itself. The development of linear strength in intestine occurs at about the same rate as in skin, although the stomach and small bowel are somewhat quicker to heal. Bursting strength is greatly enhanced early after injury because edema and induration in the wound limit distention of the segment and hence protect against bursting.

Any event which delays collagen synthesis or exaggerates collagen lysis is likely to increase the risk of perforation and leakage. The danger of leakage is greatest from the fourth to seventh days, when tensile strength is normally expected to rise rapidly. Local infection promotes lysis and delays synthesis; it often occurs near esophageal and colonic anastomoses, thus increasing the likelihood of perforation.

Bone

Healing in bone depends largely on connective tissue synthesis. Bone healing, however, also depends on a unique process, the condensation of hydroxyapatite crystals on specific points on the collagen fiber with an end result analogous to reinforced concrete. The long time required for attainment of full strength in healing fractures is well known, but it is not really much longer than that required for development of full strength in soft tissue wounds. Full calcification is so important clinically that the impression is given that bone healing is protracted. Bone healing also graphically illustrates the process of remodeling described above for soft tissue. The large callus seen after a month or so in a healing fracture often remodels until x-ray films must be examined quite carefully to see where the fracture was. The effect of mechanical stress on connective tissue healing is also well illustrated by the fact that even though bone ends may be poorly aligned, the result after months of remodeling shows that the bone has healed along normal lines of stress.

Skin Grafts

The healing of skin grafts is unique in that their vascular supply has been completely interrupted. In the critical 3–4 days after a graft is placed, there is a remarkable inosculation of small vessels of the host to those of the graft. If enough vessels can be joined, the graft lives. We can now understand why immobilization of a skin graft is so important to its survival since very little collagen can be synthesized in these first few days and the graft is anchored only by the adhesiveness of fibrin. Immune mechanisms can attack a skin homograft only after circulation has been established. A second-set rejection usually occurs by 7 days, indicating that circulation is usually competent by then.

SUTURE MATERIALS

The ideal suture material has not been designed. The ideal suture must be flexible and strong and must tie easily and securely. It should excite little tissue reaction and should not be a nidus for infection. Monofilament suture is less likely to harbor bacteria, but it is also more likely to break and to tie poorly.

Stainless steel wire is inert and maintains strength for a long time. However, wire is difficult to tie, often causes the patient undue pain, and, being brittle, eventually fragments. It does not harbor bacteria, and it can be left in granulating wounds, when necessary, with the expectation that it will be covered by granulation tissue without causing abscesses.

Plastic sutures are generally inert and retain strength even longer than wire. However, they must usually be knotted at least 4 times, resulting in large amounts of retained foreign body. Contrary to popular opinion, most multifilament plastic sutures are just as apt to become infected and migrate to the surface as silk sutures. Monofilament plastic, in common with wire, will not harbor bacteria. Nylon monofilament is extremely nonreactive and is a good suture material for skin and cornea, although it is difficult to tie. Polyethylene suture has a tendency to break. Monofilament polypropylene seems a satisfactory suture and ties well but is slightly more reactive than nylon. Plastic sutures, because of their inertness, are best for cardiovascular work.

Silk is an animal protein but is nearly inert in human tissue. It ties easily and is commonly used. Since it does lose its strength over a long period, it is unsuitable for suturing arteries to plastic implants or for insertion of prosthetic cardiac valves. Because fibrous tissue cannot securely anchor many of the plastic prostheses to tissue, the sutures must maintain strength indefinitely. Silk sutures are multifilament and are a haven for bacteria, although even contaminated wounds sutured with silk will usually heal without infection. Occasionally, silk sutures form a focus for small abscesses which migrate and "spit" through the skin, forming small sinuses which will not heal until the offending silk is removed.

Catgut (made from the submucosa of sheep intestine) will eventually resorb, but the resorption time is highly variable. Catgut excites considerable inflammatory reaction, which is the means of resorption. Catgut suture is prepared in 2 ways: (1) Plain catgut is simply twisted and dried before sterilization; (2) chromic catgut is tanned like leather in a strong solution of chromate ion. The chromic catgut causes less inflammation and absorbs slowly (20 days or more). Plain catgut causes more inflammation and is absorbed more rapidly. Unfortunately, the more reactive a suture, the more likely it is to be the site of infection. Contrary to popular opinion, catgut is used in contaminated wounds simply because it will resorb if it becomes the site of infection and will not "spit" to the surface. If a wound sutured with catgut becomes infected, the catgut is likely to resorb quickly and break before the wound is secure.

Another technic in the manufacture of absorbable sutures involves the ultrafine division of bovine tendon and its reconstitution into so-called **collagen suture**. This material, almost pure collagen, appears to cause less inflammation and has a somewhat more constant resorption time than catgut.

Synthetic absorbable polyester sutures, introduced in the past few years, are strong, have predictable rates of loss of tensile strength, incite a minimal inflammatory reaction, and may have special usefulness in gastrointestinal surgery. Polyglycolic acid (Dexon) is a polyester of glycolic acid; polyglactin 910 (Vicryl) is a copolymer of glycolic acid on lactide. Compared with catgut, polyglycolic acid has been shown to retain tensile strength longer in gastrointestinal anastomoses, a manifestation of the invulnerability of polyglycolic acid to the proteolytic action of luminal enzymes.

Skin tapes are the skin closure of choice for so-called clean contaminated wounds because they minimize the probability of subcutaneous infection. They are somewhat harder to use than skin sutures and cannot be used on actively bleeding wounds or wounds with complex surfaces, such as the perineum. They minimize infection by avoiding the presence of a foreign body in the form of a skin suture which connects the skin surface to the wound dead space.

Sutures are foreign bodies which strangulate tissue and cause inflammation. They are at best a necessary evil, and needless sutures should be avoided. Postlethwaite and his associates have published extensive investigations into the properties of suture materials.

IMPLANTS

New prosthetic materials are constantly being introduced. Among the metals, titanium, and among the alloys, Vitallium, have shown the least tendency to corrode and wear. Solid implants such as joint replacements have worked well, but mesh implants have eventually fragmented.

Plastic implants are long-lasting and are well tolerated by tissue. Teflon, nylon, and Silastic are the most inert. Teflon has a nonwettable surface, and connective tissue will not penetrate fine Teflon mesh. As a result, the neo-intima in Teflon arterial prostheses tends to break off and embolize. High-density polyethylene has even been used for weight-bearing joint prostheses. Artificial joints made of a combination of plastic and metal are now being widely used to replace hips, knees, and even digital articular surfaces damaged by disease or injury. The plastic mesh commonly used for repair of hernias is made of polypropylene. Silastic seems to be the current material of choice for solid implants for plastic surgery since it can be easily molded and sutured in place.

Dacron has a wettable surface, and connective tissue will penetrate and envelop Dacron mesh. It is the current material of choice for vascular implants.

Even the best plastic is still a foreign body. Infection around plastic prostheses of all sorts remains a major problem. Polyethylene or polypropylene mesh of standard pore size will usually be incorporated even by granulation tissue of an infected wound. However, autologous tissue is mandatory for vascular grafting into a contaminated area.

CONTROLLABLE FACTORS AFFECTING HEALING
(Table 10–1)

Nutrition

Mild to moderate nutritional deficiencies do not affect healing, which seems to have a high priority in

Table 10–1. Controllable factors affecting healing.

Factors that decrease collagen synthesis. (All are active both before and after operation.)
  Preoperative
  Starvation (protein depletion)
  Steroids
  Infection
  Associated injuries
  Hypoxia
  Radiation injury
  Uremia
  Diabetes
  Advanced age
  Operative
  Tissue injury
  Poor blood supply
  Poor apposition of surrounding tissues (pelvic anastomosis, unreduced fracture, unclosed dead space)
  Postoperative
  Starvation
  Hypovolemia
  Hypoxia
  Drugs—actinomycin, fluorouracil, methotrexate, etc
Factors that increase collagen lysis
  Starvation
  Severe trauma
  Inflammation
  Infection
  Steroids

the body economy. However, major nutritional depletion does retard healing.

Protein depletion (as opposed to protein starvation) inhibits healing if recent weight loss exceeds 20% of original body weight. Dehiscence occurs more often in patients who have quickly lost large amounts of weight and have a low serum albumin concentration.

The first nutritional substance discovered to be important to wound healing was ascorbic acid. In scurvy, wound healing is arrested in early fibroplasia. Many fibroblasts appear in the wound, but synthesis of collagen is grossly impaired. The scorbutic wound responds rapidly to ascorbic acid treatment. Ascorbic acid is essential in the formation of collagen because it is required for the hydroxylation of proline. It has other less well defined functions also.

Zinc deficiency also retards wound healing. An indolent open wound with atrophic granulations and a prominent yellow-gray exudate suggests zinc deficiency. Serum zinc levels below 100 μg/100 ml have been associated with poor healing. Zinc sulfate, 220 mg 3 times daily, is an effective and safe treatment. The actual mechanism of action is not known. There is no evidence that supplemental zinc will accelerate the healing of wounds in nutritionally normal persons.

Despite the emphasis on a few substances which are known to affect repair, the surgeon should be aware that good nutrition in general is important to repair. Undoubtedly, many nutritional substances affect repair either directly or indirectly.

Diabetes

Healing is often retarded in diabetics. Several mechanisms are probably operative. Diabetic vascular disease probably leads to oxygen deficiency, which retards healing. Poor circulation also lowers tissue temperature, and this too can retard healing. Intermediary carbohydrate metabolism is prominent in healing tissue and is necessary to fulfill energy requirements for protein synthesis. Any impairment due to insulin deficiency would be expected to impair healing. Certainly, the susceptibility to infection which occurs in diabetes presents a hazard to primary healing.

Temperature

The rate of healing in poikilothermic animals is directly dependent upon body temperature. It is assumed that this is why cutaneous wounds of the cooler extremities heal less rapidly than those in the normally warmer skin of the trunk.

Oxygen

Wounds in ischemic tissue heal poorly or not at all. Recent research has shown that oxygen deficiency is a prominent feature common to most wounds. Any decrease in oxygen supply to the wound impairs healing, and increased oxygen supply can accelerate healing above the accepted normal rate. The place for supplemental oxygen in accelerating healing is not yet well defined, but it seems to be effective in open, poorly healing, nonnecrotic wounds where impaired blood supply is the major reason for inadequate healing. Extra oxygen appears to increase the take of skin grafts. On the other hand, oxygen supply can be impaired even when vascular disease is not present. Hypovolemia and vasoconstriction can rob a wound of its oxygen supply and virtually stop healing. Overly tight sutures can do the same. It is impossible to give enough oxygen to obliterate the essentially hypoxic nature of the zone of relative ischemia (Fig 10–2).

One might expect that anemia would also exaggerate hypoxia in wounds. In fact, this is not true. Studies on wound healing and anemia are of 2 types: (1) those in which anemia was produced by inducing hypovolemia and (2) those in which blood volume was kept normal. In the first group, all investigators have reported impaired healing. In the second group, healing has been normal. The P_{O_2} of arterial blood rather than the oxygen content of blood reaching the wound seems to be the principal determinant of oxygen supply to the wound since oxygen tensions and collagen synthesis are essentially normal in wounds in anemic but normovolemic animals. Furthermore, increasing arterial P_{O_2} above the hemoglobin-oxygen dissociation curve enhances collagen synthesis far beyond the effect to be expected on the basis of increased oxygen volume delivered.

Corticosteroids

Exogenous corticosteroids impair healing. In the primarily closed wound, these drugs interfere with healing most profoundly when given in the first 3 days after injury. After 3 days, the effect is much reduced. They reduce the inflammatory reaction and impair subsequent collagen synthesis. On the other hand, corticosteroids impair contraction of open wounds no matter when they are given. Their effect on collagen synthesis and inflammation does not readily explain the effect on contraction.

Vitamin A & Cartilage Powder

Under certain circumstances, vitamin A can restore corticosteroid-retarded healing toward normal. The effect is clinically useful. It occurs both with systemic and local application of vitamin A. Systemic use of vitamin A for patients who are receiving corticosteroids for control of inflammatory disease must be undertaken cautiously since, if the vitamin can counteract the effects of the corticosteroid on the wound, it presumably may counteract other anti-inflammatory effects of the drug.

Vitamin A is probably important to repair since severely hypovitaminotic animals synthesize collagen poorly. Less extensive human studies indicate but do not prove a role for vitamin A in human repair.

Cartilage powder will accelerate normal healing slightly in the first 7–10 days and will also antagonize the effect of corticosteroids. The mechanism is not known, but the active agent apparently is chitin.

INFECTION & RESISTANCE

The closed wound would seem an ideal site for bacterial growth. It is moist, dark, filled with serum, and the P_{CO_2} is high and the P_{O_2} low. However, although all wounds are contaminated, relatively few become infected. Resistance to infection is a property of the well-healing wound. Numerous studies have pointed out 3 major prerequisites for infection: (1) a receptive host, (2) contamination by microorganisms, and (3) some particular reason for susceptibility in the wound. All 3 are variable and act independently. The susceptible host is one who is debilitated, has a disease which is reducing the immune or inflammatory response, is taking corticosteroids, or is providing poor wound nutrition. The more bacteria contaminating the wound, the more likely is an infection. However, conditions in the wound are also extremely important. Clostridial infections will not occur unless dead tissue is present within the wound. Suture materials increase susceptibility. Trauma to the wound is as important a contributing factor in postoperative infection as the introduction of bacteria.

The hypoxic nature of wounds also probably makes them susceptible to certain types of infection. Many bacteria are killed or inactivated by antibodies and white cells provided only that the white cells are viable. Certain bacteria, however, are killed only when the white cell has an oxygen supply. Phagocytosis occurs even in the total absence of oxygen with anaer-

obic glycolysis as an energy source. The act of phagocytosis, however, stimulates a burst of oxygen consumption (when oxygen is available), and the oxygen is
converted to peroxide, probably superoxide, and finally to hypochlorite or hypoiodite, which attack the
bacterial cell wall and contribute to enzymatic breakdown. The local hypoxia of injury seems to be an
important factor in the development of infection since
deficient oxygenation of white cells favors the growth
of many bacteria, including *Staphylococcus aureus,*
some strains of streptococci, *Serratia marcescens,* and
some types of pseudomonas. These bacteria, of course,
in addition to clostridia, anaerobic streptococci, and
bacteroides—all of which are aided by hypoxia in
another manner—make up the majority of human
wound infections.

Antibiotics reach the wound in effective concentrations. Antibiotics given in such a manner that effective concentrations exist at the time of wounding will
prevent wound infection if the contaminating bacteria
are sensitive to the antibiotic used. Antibiotic prophylaxis, to be effective, depends on the coincidence of
the right antibiotic and the sensitive organism.
Obviously, prophylaxis is unlikely to be effective in
the vast majority of instances where the contaminants
may be multiple and unpredictable. However, a few
situations can be defined in which prophylaxis is useful. Penicillin should be given when streptococcal or
clostridial infections are a definite risk (rheumatic
heart disease, severe burns, severe tissue damage, and
contamination with dirt). It now appears that prophylaxis has value in the high-risk infection situation of
colon surgery, for instance. In prescribing prophylactic
antibiotics, one must always balance the risks of side-
effects and the emergence of resistant strains of bacteria against the probability of usefulness of the antibiotic. To be effective, antibiotics must be given long
enough before operation to ensure high tissue concentrations when the wound is open and exposed. In most
cases, less than one hour is required. For the clean
surgical operation, antibiotic prophylaxis has no value
and may be dangerous. The antibiotic is effective for
only a few hours after operation. After a "one time"
contamination, preventive antibiotics should be
stopped within 24 hours of operation.

There is increasing evidence that topical antibiotics and such antiseptics as povidone-iodine reduce
the incidence of infection in moderately contaminated
wounds.

The technic of wound closure can also be modified to reduce the risk of infection. Wounds have been
divided into 4 categories according to their propensity
to become infected. The first is the "clean" category,
in which the wound is not traumatic, no body cavity is
entered, and there is no break in surgical technic. Infection rates should be less than 2%, and in some
centers rates of less than 1% have been achieved for
many years. There are very few indications for the use
of prophylactic antibiotics in this group, and they
should be restricted only to patients in whom the
immune response is suppressed for any reason. These
wounds ordinarily will be closed primarily.

The second category is the "clean contaminated"
wound. In this case, the wound may be traumatic but
clean. There may be a minor break in technic, or a well-
prepared body cavity may be entered without major
bacterial contamination. Infection rates traditionally
range from about 5% to 15% in this category of
wound, but some centers are reporting rates as low as
2–3%. The surgeon should consider using some method to cleanse these wounds. He may elect, in some
cases, to use perioperative prophylactic antibiotics
starting immediately before and ending within 3–24
hours of completion of the operation; topical antibiotics or delayed primary closure may also be considered.

Delayed primary closure is a technic by which
the wound is gently propped open with a sterile gauze
dressing. The environs of the wound are then inspected
daily to be sure that no active invasive infection is
occurring. If there is no need to disturb the dressing, it
is left in place until the fourth or fifth day, when,
under sterile conditions, the dressing is removed and
the wound is closed with tapes or sutures. This is a
time-honored method which has served the military
surgeon well for many years. Its success depends on
the surgeon's skill in detecting signs that the wound is
not doing well and refusing to close those wounds.
Merely leaving the wound open for 4 days does not
guarantee that it will not become infected, and not all
wounds should be closed even on the fourth, fifth, or
sixth day. A skillful surgeon should expect 80–90% of
wounds he has managed by delayed primary closure to
heal without infection.

The third category of wound is the heavily contaminated wound that occurs in contaminating trauma
and when a heavily contaminated body cavity such as
the colon is entered. There may have been a major
break in technic such as an opening of the chest for
cardiac arrest without aseptic precautions. In this case,
antibiotics should be used and should be chosen for
their known effectiveness against the most likely contaminating organism. Once again, however, the effectiveness of the antibiotics is diminished by the third or
fourth hour after the wound has been made, and further use of antibiotics is probably unavailing. In this
category, serious consideration should be given to
leaving the wound open either in anticipation of delayed primary closure or with the intent to leave it
open and allow it to heal secondarily. Wound irrigation
by jet propulsion has been shown to be an effective
method of debridement.

The fourth category is the infected wound. In
this case, the wound is either infected to begin with or
made for the purpose of draining an infected area of
the body. These wounds should never be closed, and
antibiotics are used as treatment instead of prophylaxis. Simple drainage is sufficient to cure most abscesses, and antibiotics are not necessarily important
aspects of treatment.

DECUBITUS ULCERS

Decubitus ulcers are disastrous complications of immobilization either in bed or in casts. They result from prolonged pressure which robs tissue of its blood supply. However, in practice, irritative or contaminated injections and prolonged contact with moisture, urine, and feces also play a prominent role. Most patients who contract decubitus ulcers are also poorly nourished. Pressure ulcers are common in drug addicts who take overdoses and lie immobile for many hours. The ulcers vary in depth and often extend from skin to a bony pressure point such as the greater trochanter or the sacrum.

Most decubitus ulcers are preventable. Hospital-acquired ulcers represent inadequate nursing care.

Treatment is difficult and usually prolonged. The first important step is to incise and drain any infected necrotic spaces. Dead tissue is then debrided until the exposed surfaces are all viable and granulating. Many will then heal spontaneously. However, deep ulcers may require closure, sometimes with removal of underlying protuberant bone. The defect is closed by judicious cutting of flaps and movement of thick tissue over the susceptible area.

SURGICAL TECHNIC

Good surgical technic remains the most important means of achieving optimal healing. Most cases of healing failure are due to technical failures. Tissue should be protected from drying and from internal or external contamination. Fine instruments, sharp dissection, minimal and skillful use of the electrocautery, and minimal and skillful use of ligatures and sutures with the avoidance of strangulation of tissues are essential. All of these contribute to one of the greatest assets of a surgeon—gentleness in handling tissue. Even the best ligature or suture remains a foreign body which is tied tightly and may strangulate tissue. The skillful operator who uses sutures minimally and gently will be rewarded with the best results. Perfect hemostasis is a laudable objective, but with patience, gentleness, and skill, it can be obtained by securing a minimal number of bleeding points. Too much sponging and electrocautery and tying of small vessels is traumatic and invites infection.

In common with many other points of surgical technic, the exact method of wound closure may be less important than how well it is performed. The tearing strength of sutures from fascia is no greater than 3—4 kg. There is little reason for use of sutures of greater strength than this. Tight closure strangulates tissue and leads to hernia formation and infection.

Wound Closure

If surgeons could foresee the future, dehiscence would not occur since technics to prevent dehiscence are well known. The surgeon can choose his technics to meet the needs and risks of the individual wound (Figs 10—8 to 10—10).

The ideal closure for small wounds in healthy patients is done with fine, interrupted sutures placed loosely and conveniently close to the wound edge. In abdominal wounds, the peritoneum is usually closed with a running mattress of 0 or 00 catgut.

Unfortunately, the surgeon is often required to operate on patients who represent a major wound healing risk. In these cases, closures must be more secure in order to avoid dehiscence. A more secure closure usually begins with a chromic catgut running or mattress suture in the peritoneum (or joint capsule or submucosa). The closure is continued with vertical mattress buried retention sutures through fascia and peritoneum in which the farthest point of penetration is at least 1 cm from the wound edge. By placing the tension this far back, one avoids depending on the fascial fibers which become weakened by postinjury collagen lysis. The lytic effect extends for about 5 mm to each side of the wound edge. Fascial sutures can be placed in far-far, near-near fashion, or simply as widely placed sutures alternating with single narrower sutures. Subcutaneous layers can be approximated by a few subcuticular sutures. The skin is preferably closed with adhesive strips unless bleeding from the wound or an uneven surface makes the adherence of the strips precarious. This technic is secure and with it the skin of

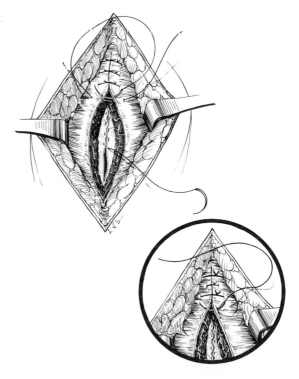

Figure 10—8. Closure of peritoneum with continuous suture. Fascia closure with figure-of-eight *(top)* and simple interrupted sutures *(bottom)* are illustrated.

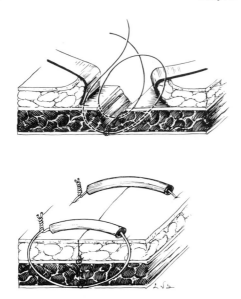

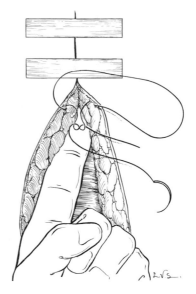

Figure 10—9. Types of retention sutures. Figure-of-eight suture is illustrated above and through-and-through retention sutures below.

Figure 10—10. Skin closure with interrupted subdermal sutures and Steri-Strips.

severely contaminated wounds can easily be left open for delayed primary or secondary closure.

Another very secure closure used in difficult wounds consists of through-and-through mattress sutures of No. 22—26 steel wire placed through all layers, including skin and peritoneum. They are placed about 2.5 cm away from the wound and 2.5 cm apart. With these sutures held on tension to approximate the wound edges, the peritoneum can be closed with a running chromic catgut suture, and the fascia—if possible or desirable—can be closed with a few "catgut" sutures. The heavy retention sutures are twisted together at the side of the wound to coapt the wound edges. Wound edema will make these sutures too tight within the next few days, and the twisted wires can be partly untwisted to prevent strangulation of tissue and cutting through of sutures. For this reason, plastic sutures are not recommended for this closure since they cannot be twisted to tighten or loosen as required. Sutures strung across an open wound edge act as bowstrings and can cut through bowel, resulting in fistula formation. This through-and-through retention closure with very strong wire is obviously rather painful to the patient and should be used only when necessary. It is excellent for closing the abdomen rapidly, and it is the best method for secondary closure of a wound dehiscence.

In all closures, sutures should be placed as far apart as possible consistent with approximation of tissue. Too close sutures obstruct blood supply to the wound. The 2 most common iatrogenic causes of dehiscence are infection and too tight sutures. In the vast majority of dehiscences, the suture material has cut through tissue and has not broken or become untied.

It is a useful exercise to assess the patient's "wound risk" in advance so that the proper choice of closure can be made easily at the end of the operation (see Table 10—1).

CARE OF THE WOUND

Postoperative care of the wound involves cleanliness, protection from trauma, and maximal support of the patient. Even closed wounds can be infected by surface contamination of bacteria, particularly within the first 2–3 days, as the classical experiments of DuMortier show. The bacteria gain entrance through the suture tracts and the wound. If a wound is likely to be traumatized or contaminated, it should be protected during this time. Such protection may require special dressings such as occlusive sprays or repeated cleansings as well as dressings.

The ideal care of the wound begins in the preoperative period and ends only months later. One must prepare the patient so that optimal conditions exist when the wound is made. One must be clean, gentle, and skillful in surgical technic and thoughtful and ingenious in protecting the postoperative wound. Postoperatively, wound care includes maintenance of nutrition, blood volume, and oxygenation. Although wound healing is in many ways a local phenomenon, the ideal care of the wound is essentially the ideal care of the patient.

•   •   •

General References

Branemark PI: Capillary form and function: The microcirculation of granulation tissue. Bibl Anat 7:9, 1965.

Brunius U: Wound healing impairment from sutures. Acta Chir Scand [Suppl] 395, 1968.

Conolly WB & others: Clinical comparison of surgical wounds closed by suture and adhesive tapes. Am J Surg 117:318, 1969.

Converse JM, Rapaport FT: The vascularization of skin autografts and homografts: An experimental study in man. Ann Surg 143:306, 1956.

Deveney K, Way L: Effect of different absorbable sutures on healing of gastrointestinal anastomoses. Am J Surg 133:86, 1977.

DuMortier JJ: The resistance of healing wounds to infection. Surg Gynecol Obstet 56:762, 1933.

Dunphy JE: The fibroblast: A ubiquitous ally for the surgeon. N Engl J Med 268:1367, 1963.

Edlich RD & others: Studies in the management of the contaminated wound (I and II). Am J Surg 117:323, 1969.

Ehrlich HP, Hunt TK: Effects of cortisone and vitamin A on wound healing. Ann Surg 167:324, 1968.

Forrester JC & others: Mechanical, biochemical, and architectural features of repair. In: *Repair and Regeneration.* Dunphy JE, Van Winkle W Jr (editors). McGraw-Hill, 1969.

Gillman T, Penn J: Studies on repair of cutaneous wounds. Med Proc 2:121, 1956.

Grant MP, Prockop DJ: The biosynthesis of collagen. N Engl J Med 286:194, 1972.

Gross J, Lapierce CM, Tanzer ML: Organization and disorganization of extracellular substances: The collagen system. Page 175 in: *Cytodifferentiation and Macromolecular Synthesis.* Locke M (editor). Academic Press, 1963.

Hawley P, Hunt TK, Dunphy JE: Etiology of colonic anastomotic leaks. Proc R Soc Med 63 (Suppl):28, 1970.

Hunt TK, Hawley P: Surgical judgment and colonic anastomoses. Dis Colon Rectum 12:167, 1969.

Jepsen OB, Larsen SO, Thomsen VF: Post-operative wound sepsis in general surgery. Acta Chir Scand [Suppl] 396:73, 1969.

Madden JW, Peacock EE Jr: Studies on the biology of collagen during wound healing. 1. Role of collagen synthesis and deposition in cutaneous wounds in the rat. Surgery 64:288, 1968.

Majno G & others: Contraction of granulation tissue in vitro: Similarity to smooth muscle. Science 173:548, 1971.

McMinn RMH: *Tissue Repair.* Academic Press, 1969.

Menkin V: *Newer Concepts of Inflammation.* Thomas, 1950.

Niinikoski J, Hunt TK, Dunphy JE: Oxygen supply in healing tissue. Am J Surg 123:247, 1972.

Pareira MD, Serkes KD: Prediction of wound disruption by use of the healing ridge. Surg Gynecol Obstet 115:72, 1962.

Peacock EE Jr: Dynamic aspects of collagen biology. 1. Synthesis and assembly. 2. Degradation and metabolism. J Surg Res 7:433, 481, 1967.

Peacock EE Jr, Van Winkle W Jr: *Surgery and Biology of Wound Repair.* Saunders, 1970.

Polk HC Jr, Lopez-Mayor JF: Postoperative wound infection: A prospective study of determinant factors and prevention. Surgery 66:97, 1969.

Pories WJ & others: Zinc deficiency as a cause for delayed wound healing. Curr Top Surg Res 1:315, 1969.

Postlethwaite RW & others: Wound healing. 2. An evaluation of surgical suture material. Surg Gynecol Obstet 108:555, 1959.

Schilling JA: Wound healing. Physiol Rev 48:374, 1968.

Trueblood HW, Nelson TS, Oberhelman HA: The effect of acute anemia and iron deficiency anemia on wound healing. Arch Surg 99:113, 1969.

Van Winkle W Jr: Wound contraction. Surg Gynecol Obstet 125:131, 1967.

11...
Inflammation, Infection, & Antibiotics

Thomas K. Hunt, MD, & Ernest Jawetz, PhD, MD

A surgical infection is a localized suppuration which is not likely to resolve without operation and can be either surgically excised or incised and drained. Common examples are appendicitis, cholecystitis, diverticulitis, cutaneous or perianal abscesses, wound infections, osteomyelitis, empyema, peritonitis, ascending cholangitis, cavitating tuberculosis, hepatic, pulmonary, subphrenic, or pelvic abscesses, clostridial infections, and necrotizing fasciitis.

PATHOGENESIS OF SURGICAL INFECTIONS

Three elements are common to surgical infections: (1) a closed space in the tissues, (2) an infectious agent, and (3) a susceptible host.

The Closed Space

Any wound—especially one that has been severely traumatized or poorly closed—contains at least a potential space which is separated from the circulation by hemostasis in small vessels surrounding the area of injury. Antibacterial defenses are impaired, and infectious organisms can multiply in these protected conditions. Dead tissue following trauma (eg, chips of bone in a fracture) or infarction (eg, from infected emboli) and pockets of extravasated blood (hematoma) all predispose to infection.

Some natural spaces with narrow outlets such as the appendix, gallbladder, and intestinal diverticula are particularly prone to become closed and infected.

The peritoneal and pleural cavities are not normally "spaces." Contaminating bacteria are usually spread over a wide area by movement of the viscera, so that natural defenses are more effective. Foreign bodies and dead tissue interfere with this spreading action and greatly potentiate peritoneal or pleural infections. When infection becomes established, inflammation may bind the moving surfaces, thus establishing a closed space in which an abscess may form.

Foreign bodies in tissue produce closed spaces and carry their own bacteria as well. Wood slivers are the most common example, and foreign bodies from plant material are in general the most susceptible to infection. Vascular grafts, metallic objects, etc all have a similar effect.

No matter what its origin, the space behaves essentially like a wound (see Chapter 10). Its internal environment is characterized by hypoxia, high P_{CO_2}, and low pH, conditions which favor bacterial growth. White cells require oxygen to kill bacteria, and the P_{O_2} within the dead spaces of most wounds is below the optimum for killing the types of bacteria which most commonly cause surgical infections.

The Infectious Agent

Almost any infectious agent can contaminate the closed space and cause infection. Streptococci invade even minor breaks of the skin and spread through connective tissue planes and lymphatics. Pseudomonas and serratia are seen most frequently as opportunistic invaders. Many fungi (histoplasma, coccidioides, actinomyces) and even parasites (amebas, echinococci) may cause abscesses or sinuses. Other rare diseases such as psittacosis, cat-scratch fever, and tularemia may become surgical infections when they cause abscesses in lymph nodes. The multiplicity of organisms found in surgical infections underscores the need for the surgeon to smear and culture the contents and the tissue wall of an abscess whenever he drains or excises one. The surgeon must inform the bacteriologist of the conditions under which he took the samples so that optimal conditions to isolate and characterize the offending organisms can be chosen. Anaerobes are now being found more frequently because of improvements in culture technics.

The Susceptible Host

Resistance to infection is impaired in patients with multiple infections, severe malnutrition, low cardiac output, or poor tissue perfusion. Malnutrition interferes with both T and B cell function. Patients with immature or depressed immune systems and those receiving anti-inflammatory steroids are also particularly susceptible. Alcoholism increases susceptibility by inhibiting leukocyte migration, ciliary motion, and the cough reflex. Streptococcal infections of the extremities are particularly common in alcoholics, and the organisms multiply rapidly because of poor hygiene, poor nutrition, dehydration, and exposure. Severe trauma, even remote from the infection, may increase susceptibility by causing hypoperfusion, hypoxia, and hypercapnia of the tissues. Extensive operations, hypovolemia, and multiple transfusions also impose a high risk of infection. Indeed, any condition that interferes with tissue perfusion reduces resistance to local infection.

In burned or severely injured patients, white cell function is impaired. Such patients are highly susceptible to opportunistic infections. Rarely, patients may have genetic deficiencies of the enzyme systems that participate in bacterial killing. Granulomatous disease of childhood is the best known example. Others are Job's syndrome and lazy leukocyte syndrome.

Cline MJ: Drug potentiation of macrophage function. Infect Immun 2:601, 1970.

Hunt TK & others: Oxygen tension and wound infection. Surg Forum 23:47, 1972.

Meakins JL: Pathophysiologic determinants and prediction of sepsis. Surg Clin North Am 56:847, 1976.

Ryan GB: Inflammation and localization of infection. Surg Clin North Am 56:831, 1976.

COMPLICATIONS & SPREAD OF INFECTIONS

An established infection may spread locally or to distant sites or may exert secondary effects on the host.

Toxicity

Toxicity is one of the most obvious but least well understood effects of serious infection. In its clinical application, the word toxic denotes the appearance of a patient with severe infection and refers to lethargy or restlessness, weakness, or delirium in addition to fever, tachycardia, and leukocytosis. Toxemia is a broad term which refers to the spread via the blood stream of bacterial substances injurious to tissue. "Surgical scarlet fever" from streptococcal erythrogenic toxins is an example. The clostridia of gas gangrene produce a number of toxic enzymes, including a lecithinase which causes hemolytic anemia and jaundice. *Cl tetani* infection disseminates a potent neurotoxin. Septic shock may be associated with endotoxins released by bacteria. Ulcerative colitis with toxic megacolon is another example of a surgical infection in which toxemia plays an important part.

Bacteremia

Bacteremia with chills and fever signifies intermittent presence of bacteria in the blood stream (ie, positive blood cultures). Systemic bacteremia may lead to bacterial endocarditis or other metastatic abscesses (brain, lungs, etc). Portal vein bacteremia may produce liver abscesses or suppurative portal phlebitis (pylephlebitis). Colonic infections such as amebic colitis may also spread to the liver through the portal vein.

Extension of Infection

Bacteria tend to spread along susceptible tissue planes. Streptococcal cellulitis which spreads in subcutaneous tissue and dermis is a common example. Invasive clostridial myositis spreads rapidly along muscle and may require amputation for control. Clostridial cellulitis, on the other hand, extends in the subcutaneous plane.

The lymphatics also serve as routes of spread of infection. Lymphangitis—the so-called blood poisoning of the preantibiotic era—is spectacular when seen in the skin but may also occur where it is not seen, as in the pelvis or retroperitoneum.

Infections may spread along surfaces such as the peritoneum or pleura or even the skin to form satellite abscesses in the region of the original one.

In summary, the main dangers of surgical infection are (1) the spread to new sites and (2) toxicity, which threatens the function of other tissues and organs.

Polk HC Jr & others: Dissemination and causes of infection. Surg Clin North Am 56:817, 1976.

GENERAL PRINCIPLES OF TREATMENT

Treatment is directed at control or containment of the infection.

Incision & Drainage

The simplest and often the most effective procedure for an abscess is merely to open it and drain it to the outside. Bacteria, necrotic tissue, and toxins are thereby removed. The pressure and number of bacteria in the infected space are lowered, thus decreasing the tendency of toxins and bacteria to spread and cause further damage to the local microcirculation.

An abscess with systemic manifestations is a surgical emergency. Fluctuation is a late sign of abscess. Even huge abscesses in the parotid or perianal area may never become fluctuant, and if the surgeon temporizes, waiting for this sign, serious sepsis may result. Localized perianal "cellulitis" of a few days' duration will always be an abscess. Drainage creates an open wound, but the tissue will heal by second intention with remarkably little scarring.

Excision

A more definitive approach is to excise the infection, as is done in removing an infected appendix or gallbladder. In these cases, no further drainage may be necessary and the patient is cured on the operating table. On the other hand, excision of clostridial myositis may require amputation of the infected limb. The cure of cavitating pulmonary tuberculosis may require lobectomy. Surgical cure of bacterial endocarditis may require excision of an infected valve and replacement of the valve with a prosthesis. The success of such operations is greatly facilitated by intensive specific antimicrobial therapy.

Ancillary Measures

On occasion, the cure of surgical infection may involve operation in another area. Stubborn infections in ischemic extremities may be best cured by restoring blood flow to the infected area. Surgery may be performed to diminish the bacterial contamination of an infected area, as in a colostomy proximal to an area of diverticulitis. For complicated diverticulitis, excision of the affected segment and construction of a colostomy proximally allow the inflammation to resolve and the tissues to heal before the colon is reconnected.

A well-drained abscess with no systemic effects needs no antibiotic therapy. The uncomplicated case of appendicitis without peritonitis needs only appendectomy. An invasive infection, however, should be treated with antibiotics as well as surgery. One must obtain cultures at the earliest possible time and start specifically effective antibiotics as soon as possible. If antibiotics must be chosen empirically, start cultures before drugs are given and use laboratory results in a possible change in therapy.

DIAGNOSTIC AIDS

Physical examination is the simplest effective means of detecting the site of surgical infection. When a surgical infection is suspected but cannot be found initially, repeated examination will finally reveal subtle warmth, erythema, induration, tenderness, or splinting due to a developing abscess. Failure to repeat the physical examination is the most common reason for delayed diagnosis and therapy.

The most important diagnostic aids are smear and culture of pus or other infected material. The most common reason for inappropriate treatment of surgical infections is the failure to examine a gram-stained smear of the pus as an immediate guide to antibacterial and surgical therapy.

Radiologic examination is frequently helpful, particularly for the diagnosis of pulmonary infections. An elevated and immobile diaphragm is a clue to the presence of subphrenic abscess. Obliteration of the psoas shadow frequently indicates an appendiceal abscess. Whenever infection is close to bone, radiologic examination is indicated to detect early signs of osteomyelitis which might require aggressive surgical therapy. Scanning—particularly of the liver or brain—is useful for the detection of abscesses in these organs. On rare occasions, thermography can locate a hidden abscess. Computer-assisted tomography (CT) and ultrasound scanning are becoming particularly useful.

SPECIFIC TYPES OF SURGICAL INFECTION

FURUNCLE, CARBUNCLE, & HIDRADENITIS

Furuncles and carbuncles are cutaneous abscesses. Furuncles are the most common surgical infections, but carbuncles are rare.

Furuncles can be serious when multiple and recurrent (furunculosis). Furunculosis usually occurs in young adults and is associated with hormonal changes resulting in impaired skin function. The commonest organisms are staphylococci and anaerobic diphtheroids.

Hidradenitis suppurativa is a serious skin infection of the axillas or groins consisting of multiple abscesses of the apocrine sweat glands. The condition often becomes chronic and disabling.

Furuncles usually start in infected hair follicles, although some are caused by retained foreign bodies and other injuries. Hair follicles normally contain bacteria. If the pilosebaceous apparatus becomes occluded by skin disease or bacterial inflammation, the stage is set for development of a furuncle. Because the base of the hair follicle may lie in subcutaneous tissue, the infection can spread as a cellulitis or it can form a subcutaneous abscess. If a furuncle results from confluent infection of several hair follicles, a central core of skin may become necrotic and will slough when the abscess is drained.

A furuncle which extends in the subcutaneous tissue, forming a long, flat abscess, is called a phlegmon. This name may be applied also to such abscesses in other organs.

Clinical Findings

Furuncles are usually readily apparent because of the pain and itching they produce. The skin first becomes red and then turns white and necrotic over the top of the abscess. There is usually some surrounding erythema and induration. Regional nodes may become enlarged. Systemic symptoms are rare.

A carbuncle usually starts as a furuncle, but the infection dissects through the dermis and subcutaneous tissue in a myriad of connecting tunnels. Many of these small extensions open to the surface, giving the appearance of a large furuncle with many pustular openings. As the carbuncle enlarges, the blood supply to its center is destroyed and the central tissue becomes necrotic. A carbuncle on the back of the neck is seen most often in diabetic patients. The patient is usually febrile and mildly toxic. This is a serious problem that demands immediate surgical attention. Diabetes must be suspected and treated.

Simple furuncles should not be treated with antibiotics. Invasive carbuncles must be treated with antibiotics as well as operation. Between these 2 extremes, in many infections, the use of antibiotics depends on the location of the abscess and the degree of sepsis. Large abscesses near the nose and face are best treated with antibiotics in addition to surgical drainage. However, surgical drainage is the mainstay of treatment.

Differential Diagnosis

On occasion, the surgeon may be confronted with a localized area of erythema and induration without obvious suppuration. The majority of such lesions will go on to central suppuration and become an obvious furuncle. On the other hand, when these lesions are located near joints or over the tibia or when they are widely distributed, one must consider such differential diagnoses as rheumatoid nodules, gout, bursitis, synovitis, erythema nodosum, fungal infections, some benign or malignant skin tumors, and inflamed sebaceous or epithelial inclusion cysts.

Hidradenitis is differentiated from furunculosis by skin biopsy, which shows typical involvement of the apocrine sweat glands. One also suspects hidradenitis when abscesses are concentrated in the apocrine gland areas, ie, the axillas, groins, and perineum. Carbuncles usually present a typical picture.

Complications

Any of these infections may cause suppurative phlebitis when located near major veins. This is particularly important when the infection is located near the nose or eyes. Central venous thrombosis in the brain is a serious complication, and abscesses on the face usually must be treated with antibiotics as well as prompt incision and drainage.

Hidradenitis may disable the patient but rarely has systemic manifestations. Carbuncles on the back of the neck may go on to epidural abscess and meningitis.

Treatment

The classic therapy for furuncle is incision and drainage; antibiotics can only reduce the infection around the abscess. Patients with recurrent furunculosis should be checked for diabetes or immune deficiencies. Frequent washing with soaps containing hexachlorophene or other disinfectants is advisable. It may also be necessary to advise extensive laundering of all personal clothing and disinfection of the patient's living quarters in order to reduce the reservoirs of bacteria. Furunculosis associated with severe acne may benefit from tetracycline, 250 mg orally daily.

Infection associated with primary immune deficiency requires specific therapy with antibiotics and gamma globulin.

A **collar-button abscess** is a small infected blister under the epidermis which is contiguous through a small opening with a deeper and larger subcutaneous abscess. In cross-section, it is shaped like a collar button with the narrow point at the dermis. Removal of the top of the infected blister is inadequate treatment. When an abscess fails to resolve after a superficial incision, the surgeon must look for collar-button abscess.

Hidradenitis is usually treated by drainage of the individual abscess followed by good hygiene. The patient must avoid astringent antiperspirants and deodorants. Painting with mild disinfectants is sometimes helpful. Fungal infections should be searched for if healing after drainage does not occur promptly. If none of these measures are successful, the apocrine sweat-bearing skin must be excised and the deficit filled with a skin graft.

Carbuncles are often more extensive than the external appearance indicates. Incision alone is usually inadequate, and excision with the electrocautery is required. Excision is continued until the many sinus tracts are removed—usually far beyond the cutaneous evidence of suppuration. It is sometimes necessary to produce a large open wound. This may appear to be drastic treatment, but it achieves rapid cure and prevents further spread. The large wound usually contracts to a small scar and does not usually require skin grafting.

CELLULITIS

Cellulitis is a common invasive nonsuppurative infection of connective tissue. The term is loosely used and often misapplied. The microscopic picture is one of severe inflammation of the dermal and subcutaneous tissues. Although PMNs predominate, there is no gross suppuration except perhaps at the portal of entry.

Clinical Findings

Cellulitis usually appears on an extremity as a brawny red or reddish-brown area of edematous skin. It advances rapidly from its starting point, and the advancing edge may be vague or sharply defined (eg, in erysipelas). A surgical wound, puncture, skin ulcer, or patch of dermatitis is usually identifiable as a portal of entry. The disease often occurs in susceptible patients, eg, alcoholics with postphlebitic leg ulcers. Most cases are caused by streptococci, but other bacteria have been involved. A moderate or high fever is almost always present.

Lymphangitis arising from cellulitis produces red, warm, tender streaks 3 or 4 mm wide leading from the infection along lymphatic vessels to the regional lymph nodes. There is no suppuration. Bacteria are difficult to obtain for culture, but blood culture is often positive.

Differential Diagnosis

Since the visible features of cellulitis are all due to inflammation, the word cellulitis has come to be associated with visible signs of inflammation. This is unfortunate since cellulitis implies lack of suppuration and therefore is not an indication for incision and drainage. When the word is carelessly used it may lead to the inference that no suppuration is present when in fact incision and drainage are urgently required.

Thrombophlebitis is often difficult to differentiate from cellulitis, but swelling is usually greater with phlebitis, and tenderness may localize over a vein. Homans' sign does not always make the differentiation—nor does lymphadenopathy. Fever is usually greater with cellulitis, and pulmonary embolization does not occur in cellulitis.

Severe contact allergy, such as poison oak, may be indistinguishable from cellulitis in its early phase, but dense nonhemorrhagic vesiculation soon discloses the allergic cause.

Chemical inflammation due to drug injection may also mimic streptococcal cellulitis.

The appearance of hemorrhagic bullae and skin necrosis suggests necrotizing fasciitis as the correct diagnosis.

Treatment

Therapy should entail rest, elevation, massive hot wet packs, and penicillin, 2.4 million units per day IM (600,000 units every 6 hours). If a clear response has not occurred in 12−24 hours, one should suspect an abscess or consider the possibility that the causative agent is a staphylococcus or other resistant organism. The patient must be examined one or more times daily to detect a hidden abscess masquerading as cellulitis.

POSTOPERATIVE WOUND INFECTION

Postoperative wound infection results from bacterial contamination during or after a surgical procedure. The infection usually involves the subcutaneous tissues.

Despite every effort to maintain asepsis, most surgical wounds are contaminated with bacteria. If contamination is minimal, if the wound has been made without undue tissue injury, and if there is no dead space, infection rarely develops. In clean surgical wounds—as in hernia or thyroid operations—the incidence of infection should be no more than 1%. In "clean-contaminated" wounds—eg, biliary or gastric surgery—infection rates as high as 5−10% are experienced. Rates higher than this for these types of operation indicate poor asepsis or poor operative technic. Severely contaminated wounds such as in operations on the unprepared colon or emergency operations for intestinal bleeding or perforation may have an infection risk of 15−30%. To confine these rates to an acceptable range, one must make liberal use of isolation technics and delayed primary closure.

Unnecessary trauma from retractors, inappropriate use of electrocoagulation, gross ligation of bleeding points, foreign bodies, and dead space contribute heavily to postoperative wound infection. Whenever gross contamination of the wound cannot be avoided, the skin and subcutaneous tissues should be left open (see Prevention, below). Since even a minor postoperative wound infection prolongs hospitalization and

occasions economic loss, every effort must be made to keep the infection rate low.

Operative wounds can be divided into 4 categories: (1) clean (no contamination from exogenous or endogenous sources), (2) lightly contaminated, (3) heavily contaminated, and (4) infected (in which obvious infection has been encountered in the operation). Current University of California Medical Center rates are as follows: clean cases, 1.5% infection rate; lightly contaminated, 2.5%; heavily contaminated, 4%. The values in "infected" cases depend upon the extent of use of delayed primary closure. These rates are lower than those reported from most hospitals.

Clinical Findings

Wound infections usually appear between the fifth and tenth days after surgery, but they may appear as early as the first postoperative day or even years later. The first sign is usually fever, and postoperative fever requires inspection of the wound. The patient may complain of wound pain. The wound rarely appears severely inflamed, but edema may be obvious because the skin sutures appear tight.

Palpation of the wound may detect abscess. A safe and rewarding method is to pour surgical soap on the wound and, using it as a lubricant, palpate gently with the gloved hand. Firm or fluctuant areas, crepitus, or tenderness can be detected in this way with minimal pain and contamination. The rare infection deep to the fascia may be difficult to recognize. In doubtful cases when a decision must be made, one can carefully open the wound in the suspicious area. If no pus is present, the wound can be closed immediately with skin tapes.

The bacteriology of wound infection goes through cycles. Before the antibiotics became available, streptococcal and staphylococcal infections were the most feared. When antibiotics appeared, many surgeons felt the problem of surgical infection would disappear. Unfortunately, the problem of emerging resistance was not anticipated. Antibiotics were overused and were substituted for careful surgical technic. Severe problems with staphylococcal infections developed, requiring greater attention to housekeeping, preparation of the skin, surgical technic, and isolation. Soaps and antibiotics effective against resistant staphylococci were developed, and infections with gram-negative bacteria are now the major problem. Furthermore, the individual hospital or ward may have periodic outbreaks of infections due to one or another resistant organism. Currently, cycles of anaerobic infections are occurring.

Differential Diagnosis

Differential diagnosis includes all other causes of postoperative fever, wound dehiscence, and wound herniation (see Chapter 4).

Prevention

External bacterial contamination can be almost entirely eliminated by extraordinary precautions such as operating through ports in sterilized plastic chambers; but even then the patient contributes bacteria from deep in his skin and from his gastrointestinal, urinary, or respiratory tracts. As surgery is done today, one can assume that all wounds are contaminated to some slight extent. Nevertheless, prevention is still the most important aspect of wound infection.

There are 4 main aspects to prevention of infection: (1) careful, gentle, clean surgery; (2) reduction of contamination; (3) support of the patient's defenses; and (4) antibiotics. The first 2 are by far the most important.

The surgeon who traumatizes tissue, leaves foreign bodies or hematomas in wounds, uses too many ligatures, and exposes the wound to drying or pressure from retractors is exposing his patients to needless risk of infection.

Many technics are directed at reducing contamination. They include housekeeping in the operating theater, hand scrubbing, skin preparation, wound protectors, dressings, isolation chambers, and special ventilating systems.

Closure technics also influence infection rates. The purpose of sutures is to approximate tissues and hold them securely, and the right number to use is as few as possible to accomplish this aim. Since sutures strangulate tissue, they should be tied as loosely as the requirements of approximation permit. Subcutaneous sutures should be used rarely and only when dead space is sure to result if they are omitted. Using skin tapes when possible instead of skin sutures lowers infection rates, especially in contaminated wounds.

Severely contaminated wounds in which infection is likely to develop are best left open initially and managed by delayed primary closure. In the abdomen, chest, or skull this means that the deep layers are closed while skin and subcutaneous tissues are left open, sterilely dressed, inspected on the fourth day, and then closed (preferably with skin tapes) if no sign of infection is seen. A clean granulating open wound is superior to a wound infection. Scarring from secondary healing is usually minimal.

Postoperative care is also important since wound infections can originate on the ward as well as in the operating room. The patient himself is the most common source of contamination. Wounds are most susceptible to surface contamination for the first 24–48 hours. If contamination is likely, protective dressings should be used.

The patient has many defense mechanisms which the surgeon can support. Adequate blood volume, arterial oxygenation, nutrition, and immune defenses all help prevent infection.

ANTIMICROBIAL CHEMOPROPHYLAXIS

Antimicrobial drugs can prevent bacteremia and wound infection in selected surgical patients, but at a risk. Harmful effects include bacterial or fungal super-

infections, toxic or allergic reactions, and accumulation of bacterial strains resistant to antibiotics in the hospital environment. However, controlled studies have shown that the overall incidence of postoperative infections in "clean" operations is not diminished by administration of antimicrobials. Therefore, only highly selective use of chemoprophylaxis is defensible.

On rare occasions, the benefits of prophylactic antimicrobials may outweigh the risks even in clean operations. Such occasions may arise when a prosthetic device (eg, hip replacement, vascular graft) is implanted or when the life of a patient with seriously depressed immunity may be jeopardized if infection should occur.

As the probability of infection rises, the value of prophylactic or preventive antibiotics also rises. The probability of efficacy depends on choosing an antimicrobial agent that is effective against the potential contaminant. However, the antimicrobial need not be active against all potential pathogens. Drugs that decrease the total number of pathogens may permit host defenses to resist infection. Obviously, the chance of preventing infection after random contamination is slight. If one wishes to prevent a specific infection, eg, staphylococcal endocarditis after placement of a prosthetic cardiac valve, high doses of a penicillinase-resistant antimicrobial drug have demonstrated effectiveness. However, the risk of penicillin-resistant gramnegative infection remains.

In colon operations, systemic antibiotics (cephalosporins) have been shown to lower but not eliminate the risk of infection. In this example, if the risk of infection approximates 10%, the risk can be halved by using antimicrobials. Therefore, the risk of allergic or toxic complications (roughly 5%) is worth taking.

On the other hand, every instance of antibiotic administration increases the risk of establishing resistant organisms in the hospital environment where the risk to other patients is major. For example, deaths in the newborn nursery have been traced to neomycin given as bowel preparation on the surgical wards.

The timing of administration is critical. Prophylactic antimicrobials are vastly more effective when therapeutic drug levels are reached before the contamination occurs. When possible, administration should begin 1 or 2 hours before operation; starting the chemoprophylaxis after operation is useless in most cases. If the contamination is restricted to the operative period, the effectiveness of antimicrobials lasts only about 3 hours. Many surgeons give only 2 or 3 doses beginning just before operation. Currently, our recommendation is to stop antimicrobials within 24 hours after operation unless they are being used to treat an established infection.

After the wound is made, bolus doses of intravenous antibiotic will cause wound antibiotic concentration to rise rapidly to equal blood concentration about an hour after injection. The antibiotic is then trapped in the wound and remains there for a number of hours in higher concentrations than in serum until a new serum dose is given. The notable exceptions to

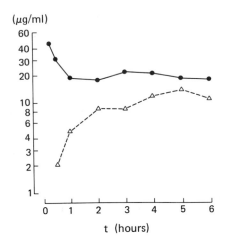

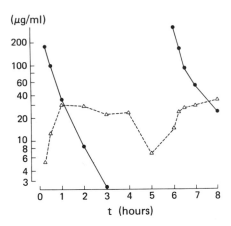

Figure 11–1. Antibiotic levels (cephaloridine in μg/ml wound interstitial fluid) after constant intravenous infusion with a small loading dose. Blood level is 10–20 μg/ml at 4–6 hours. Solid line = blood; dotted line = wound.

Figure 11–2. Antibiotic levels (cephaloridine in μg/ml wound interstitial fluid) after intravenous bolus dose of 8 mg/kg. Levels of 30 μg/ml are reached temporarily. Average level is 10–20 μg/ml. Solid line = blood; dotted line = wound.

this rule are the tetracyclines, whose wound levels (for unknown reasons) are always below blood levels; and gentamicin, whose wound levels are extremely low.

Among those antibiotics having excellent access to the wound are penicillin, ampicillin, and the cephalosporins. Clindamycin reaches intermediate concentrations, and carbenicillin, nafcillin, oxacillin, gentamicin, erythromycin, and polymyxin reach the lowest concentration. In general, all of these antibiotics—except clindamycin, tetracycline, and polymyxin—equilibrate with blood levels at about 90 minutes after bolus intravenous doses.

During constant infusion of antibiotic, with a low blood level which has reached a plateau, wound concentration rises slowly to equal blood concentration at about 6 hours. Although the net amount of antibiotic reaching the wound is the same for equal doses regardless of manner of injection, the appearance rate and peak concentrations are far greater after bolus injection (Figs 11–1 and 11–2).

There is a growing body of evidence that the local use of antibiotics for irrigating peritoneum and wounds may reduce the rate of infection in selected contaminated wounds (eg, after colon surgery and renal transplantation). Certain well-tolerated antiseptics such as povidone-iodine solution may also be effective.

Treatment

The basic treatment is to open the wound and allow it to drain. This is so effective that antibiotics are not necessary unless the infection is invasive. Culture is essential for several reasons: (1) to help locate the source and prevent further infection in other patients; (2) as a preview of the bacteriology in case other infections, such as pelvic abscess, develop deep to the wound; (3) for selection of preoperative antibiotics in case the wound must be entered again; and (4) in case the infection should become invasive.

As the wound granulates, a loose secondary closure with tapes can be used to shorten the time to complete closure.

Prognosis

Most wound infections increase morbidity. Wound infection correlates positively with mortality rates but is not often the cause of death. It is often the added factor that tips the scales against the success of an operation.

Alexander JW & others: Concentration of selected intravenously administered antibiotics in experimental surgical wounds. J Trauma 13:423, 1973.

Anderson B, Korner B, Östergaard AH: Topical ampicillin against wound infection after colorectal surgery. Ann Surg 176:129, 1972.

Burke JF: Wound infection and early inflammation. Monogr Surg Sci 1:301, 1964.

Conolly WB, Hunt TK, Dunphy JE: Management of contaminated surgical wounds. Surg Gynecol Obstet 129:593, 1969.

Edlich RF & others: Studies in the management of the contaminated wound. Am J Surg 117:323, 1969.

Ehrlich HP, Licko V, Hunt TK: Kinetics of cephaloridine in experimental wounds. Am J Med Sci 265:33, 1973.

Griffiths DA & others: Single-dose preoperative antibiotic prophylaxis in gastrointestinal surgery. Lancet 2:325, 1976.

Jepsen OB, Larsen SO, Thomsen VF: Post-operative wound sepsis in general surgery. Acta Chir Scand [Suppl] 396:73, 1969.

Stone HH & others: Antibiotic prophylaxis in gastric, biliary and colonic surgery. Ann Surg 184:443, 1976.

CLOSTRIDIAL INFECTIONS

1. CLOSTRIDIAL INFECTIONS OTHER THAN TETANUS

Gas gangrene is generally associated with grossly contaminated war injuries. However, it is an important problem in civilian surgical practice also. The rising civilian accident rate and the appreciable incidence of clostridial infection after elective surgery, especially after biliary and colon operations, make the prevention and treatment of gas gangrene a matter of major concern to the surgeon.

Clinically, a broad spectrum of disease is caused by these organisms, ranging from negligible surface contamination through invasive "cellulitis" of connective tissue to invasive anaerobic infection of muscle with massive tissue necrosis and profound toxemia.

Six species cause infection in man. Several species may be found in the same lesion. *Clostridium perfringens (Cl welchii)* is recovered in about 80%, *Cl novyi* in 40%, and *Cl septicum* in 20%.

Pathophysiology & Bacteriology

Clostridia are saprophytes. Vegetative and spore forms are widespread in soil, sand, clothing, and feces. They are, generally, fastidious anaerobes requiring a low redox potential to grow and to initiate conversion of the spores to vegetative, toxin-producing forms.

There are several means by which tissue redox potentials are diminished: impaired blood supply, muscle injury, pressure from casts, severe local edema, foreign bodies, or the presence of oxygen-consuming organisms. Clostridial infections frequently occur in the presence of other bacteria, especially gram-negative bacilli. Cancer patients are particularly susceptible.

Clostridia proliferate and produce toxins which diffuse into the surrounding tissue. The toxins devitalize cells and destroy the local microcirculation. This allows further invasion which can advance at an astonishing rate. The alpha toxin, a necrotizing lecithinase, is thought to be particularly important in this sequence, but other toxins, including collagenase, hyaluronidase, leukocidin, protease, lipase, and hemolysin, also contribute. When the disease has advanced sufficiently, toxins enter the systemic circulation, causing the systemic features of pallor, anxiety, restlessness, delirium, severe tachycardia, jaundice, and ultimately shock and death. The progress of the local lesion can often be judged fairly accurately by the general state of the patient as well as by the local signs.

Clinical Findings

Clostridial infections are classified, in ascending order of lethal potential, as simple contamination, gas abscess, clostridial cellulitis, localized clostridial myositis, diffuse clostridial myositis, and edematous gangrene. The term gas gangrene is reserved to describe clostridial myositis.

A. Simple Contamination: Many open wounds are superficially infected or contaminated with clostridia but there is no significant local or systemic disease. There is often a brown seropurulent exudate. The condition is not invasive because the surrounding tissue is basically healthy, and the clostridia are confined to necrotic surface tissue. Debridement of dead surface tissue is usually the only treatment necessary, but this condition can develop into invasive gangrene if a severe hemodynamic abnormality or further injury decreases the oxidation-reduction potential of the surrounding tissue.

B. Gas Abscess (Welch's Abscess): Gas abscess is a localized infection not usually thought of as invasive. In this case, muscle has not been injured and is not involved in the infection. The incubation period is usually a week or more. There is usually little pain; the edema is moderate; and the patient does not appear toxic, although he may have fever and tachycardia. The wound, however, has the characteristic brown seropurulent exudate and the characteristic autopsy room odor, and gas may be found diffused through the connective tissues. Except for the involved area, the limb appears well perfused. Treatment usually consists of incision and penicillin.

C. Crepitant Clostridial Cellulitis: This type ("anaerobic cellulitis") is an invasive infection of subcutaneous tissue which has been made susceptible by injury or ischemia. The dissection occurs above the deep fascia and may spread at an exceptionally rapid rate, often producing discoloration of the skin and edema as well as crepitus. The systemic symptoms and signs are remarkably less than the surface appearance and extent of gas production might indicate, and this distinguishes "cellulitis" from "myositis." This differentiation is important since adequate therapy for "cellulitis" is far less aggressive than that appropriate for "myositis."

D. Localized Clostridial Myositis: Localized clostridial myositis occurs occasionally. The injury and infection involve muscle, but the infection is not invasive. The wound has the characteristic odor, edema, crepitation, and appearance, but the findings are localized and the limb appears well perfused, with intact pulses. The systemic reaction may include fever and tachycardia but not severe prostration, delirium, and other signs of toxemia.

E. Diffuse Clostridial Myositis (Gas Gangrene): Diffuse clostridial myositis usually begins less than 3 days after the injury, with rapid increase of pain in the wound, edema, and a brown seropurulent exudate, often containing bubbles. There is marked tachycardia, but fever is variable. Crepitus may or may not be present. Profound toxemia often appears early and progresses to delirium and hemolytic jaundice. The surface edema, necrosis, and discoloration are usually less extensive than the underlying muscle necrosis. The disease characteristically progresses rapidly with loss of blood supply to the infected muscle. The swelling and edema may produce ischemia, especially under tight dressings or plaster casts. Following injury with vascular damage, delay in debridement or inadequate debridement furnishes the same critical factor—dead tissue. Since gas gangrene often develops under plaster casts, a sudden deterioration within 3 or 4 days of injury coupled with a muscle injury, an autopsy room odor, and a brown exudate require removal or windowing of the cast.

F. Edematous Gangrene: Edematous gangrene is a variant caused by *Cl novyi (oedematiens)*. No gas is produced, but edema of muscle is prominent. This is a particularly aggressive and often fatal infection requiring rapid and radical surgical debridement.

Differential Diagnosis

Diffuse clostridial myositis ("gas gangrene") is most often confused with other gas-producing infections, which are usually due to mixtures of gram-negative bacilli and gram-positive cocci. These mixed infections are not usually as virulent as gas gangrene and respond well to incision and drainage. Crepitant cellulitis should not be confused with clostridial gangrene since it, too, is well treated by lesser means (see below). Gas in the tissues is not a good differentiating point since some species (eg, *Cl novyi*) do not produce gas, nonclostridial organisms (eg, *Escherichia coli*) often produce gas, and air can enter tissues through a penetrating wound or from the chest or joint areas.

The diagnosis must be made early. The cornerstones of diagnosis are the clinical appearance of the wound and presence of large gram-positive rods on smears of exudate or tissue. *Cl perfringens* in tissue is not sporulated, but other common invasive forms contain spores.

Prevention

Almost all clostridial infections are preventable. The keystone of prevention is early debridement of dead tissue and support of the circulation.

Suspicion should be directed at any wound received out of doors and contaminated with a foreign body, soil, or feces and any wound in which tissue (particularly muscle) has been extensively injured. This type of wound should be carefully examined under sufficient anesthesia to permit full inspection and debridement. The minimum criteria for tissue viability are that the tissue bleeds freely when it is cut and that muscle contracts when gently pinched.

Antibiotic prophylaxis is valuable. Penicillin is most often used, although many antibiotics have prevented gas gangrene in laboratory animals. However, *no antibiotic can prevent gas gangrene without adequate surgical debridement.*

Polyvalent gas gangrene antitoxin has been advocated for both prevention and treatment, but its effectiveness is unproved.

Treatment

The major emphasis in treatment is inevitably surgical. Antibiotics are often essential but are ineffective without surgical control of the disease.

A. Surgical Treatment: The wound must be opened, and dead and severely damaged tissue must be excised. Tight fascial compartments must be decompressed. Immediate amputation is necessary when there is diffuse myositis with complete loss of blood supply or when adequate debridement would have to be so extensive that a useless limb would result.

Surgical treatment for clostridial cellulitis must be aggressive, *but amputation is not necessary.* Extensive debridement, with excision of necrotic skin and wide-open drainage, is essential. One must be careful to determine whether muscle is involved, because myositis and cellulitis may coexist. This will usually determine whether amputation should be done or whether extensive debridement of skin is all that is necessary. Multiple debridements may be required. Localized gas gangrene requires only local debridement.

When clostridial infections follow penetrating injuries of the colon and rectum, diverting proximal colostomy is required with wide drainage of the flanks, buttocks, or perineum. On occasion, clostridial infections involve tissues which cannot be extensively debrided such as spinal cord, brain, or retroperitoneal tissues. Surgical drainage is required in such cases, but major reliance is placed on antibiotics and hyperbaric oxygenation.

B. Hyperbaric Oxygenation: Hyperbaric oxygenation is beneficial in treating clostridial infections, but it cannot replace surgical therapy since no amount of increased arterial P_{O_2} can force oxygen into dead tissue. Hyperbaric oxygen may inhibit bacterial invasion, but it cannot eliminate the focus of infection. It probably prevents production of alpha toxin by bacteria in environments where P_{O_2} is above 90 mm Hg. Treatment for 1 or 2 hours at 3 atmospheres repeated every 6—12 hours is recommended, and only 3—5 exposures are usually necessary. Where large hyperbaric chambers are available, surgery and hyperbaric oxygenation can be accomplished simultaneously. Early use of hyperbaric oxygen can reduce tissue losses.

Because even hyperbarically administered oxygen will fail to reach the tissues in hypovolemic patients, vigorous support of blood volume is necessary. Many patients with gas gangrene and extensive injuries require multiple blood transfusions. In this case, reduced 2,3-diphosphoglycerate stores in red cells diminish tissue oxygenation. Fresh blood must be given early, and serum phosphate must be measured and kept within the normal range. Depressed serum phosphate also leads to rigidity of the red cells, which probably diminishes tissue oxygenation.

C. Antibiotics: Penicillin (20—40 million units per day) should be given intravenously. If the patient is allergic to penicillin, tetracyclines or other antibiotics are given.

D. Gas Gangrene Antitoxin: Antitoxins are available against the toxins of *Cl perfringens, Cl novyi, Cl histolyticum,* and *Cl septicum,* usually in the form of concentrated immune globulins. Polyvalent antitoxin (containing antibodies to several toxins) is usually used. While such antitoxin is often administered to individuals with contaminated wounds containing much devitalized tissue, the effectiveness of the antitoxin is uncertain. Certainly, surgical management and antibiotics are more effective.

Prognosis

Without treatment, clostridial cellulitis and myositis are fatal diseases. With adequate treatment, deaths are rare and should occur only when treatment is delayed, in patients who are already severely ill with other diseases, or in patients with advanced invasion of vital structures. The overall mortality rate is approximately 20%.

The prognosis for salvage of functioning limbs is not so favorable. When clostridial myonecrosis is added to injury, affected limbs often become useless and must be amputated to save life.

Altemeier WA, Fullen WD: Prevention and treatment of gas gangrene. JAMA 217:806, 1971.

Demello FJ, Haglin JJ, Hitchcock CR: Comparative study of experimental *Clostridium perfringens* infection in dogs treated with antibiotics, surgery, and hyperbaric oxygen. Surgery 73:936, 1973.

Weinstein L, Barza MA: Gas gangrene. N Engl J Med 289:1129, 1973.

2. TETANUS

Essentials of Diagnosis

- Limitation of movements of the jaw, with painful muscle spasm and spasm of the facial muscles (risus sardonicus).
- Stiffness of the neck and laryngospasm.
- Tonic spasms and generalized convulsions.
- Presence of penetrating wounds which have not been debrided.

General Considerations

Tetanus is a specific anaerobic infection mediated by the neurotoxin of *Clostridium tetani* which leads to nervous irritability and tetanic muscular contractions. The causative organism enters and flourishes in hypoxic wounds contaminated with soil or feces. The tetanus-prone wound is usually a puncture wound or one containing devitalized tissue or foreign body.

The incubation period of tetanus varies from 1–54 days, with an average of 8 days. The greater the delay before debridement and antitoxin therapy, the shorter the incubation period is likely to be. The longer the delay from injury to the onset of symptoms, the better the prognosis.

Clinical Findings

A. Symptoms and Signs: The first symptom is usually pain or tingling in the area of injury and limitation of movements of the jaw (lockjaw) and spasms of the facial muscles (risus sardonicus). This is followed by stiffness of the neck, difficulty in swallowing, and laryngospasm. Hesitancy in micturition due to sphinc-

ter spasm is also seen. In the more acute cases, severe spasms of the muscles of the back produce opisthotonos. Spasms become increasingly frequent and involve more and more muscle groups. As chest and diaphragm spasms occur, longer and longer periods of apnea follow. The temperature is normal or slightly elevated. Sweating tends to be profuse. Marked elevation of the pulse rate is a grave sign. The severity of cases varies widely; some are very mild and barely recognizable.

B. Laboratory Findings: Polymorphonuclear leukocytosis may be present.

Prevention

Specific preventive measures for patients with wounds are outlined as follows by the Committee on Trauma of the American College of Surgeons (1972 Revision).

A. Previously Immunized Individuals:

1. Immunized within the past 10 years—Give 0.5 ml IM of refined tetanus toxoid as a booster unless it is certain that the patient has received a booster within the previous 3–5 years.

2. Immunized more than 10 years previously—Give 0.5 ml IM of adsorbed tetanus toxoid. To those with severe, neglected, or old (more than 24 hours) tetanus-prone wounds, give, in addition, 250 units of tetanus immune globulin (human), and consider the use of penicillin.

3. Caution—The following is quoted from Furste W: The Fourth International Conference on Tetanus. J Trauma 16:755, 1976: "Booster toxoid treatment of previously completely immunized individuals without simultaneous use of antitoxin proved successful in the U.S. Army during World War II. Of 2,734,819 hospital admissions for wounds and injuries, only 4 cases of tetanus occurred in completely, actively immunized individuals. However, tetanus toxoid is a sensitizing agent which can give rise to many types of reactions, and these increase in intensity and frequency with greater numbers of injections. Reactions range from mild local inflammation to edematous local reactions, urticaria (sometimes persisting for weeks), arthralgia, nephrosis, and anaphylactic shock. Therefore, the dosage and frequency of injection must be balanced against the chances of undesired reactions. The goal is optimal protection with minimal complications."

B. Individuals Not Previously Immunized:

1. Clean minor wounds (tetanus unlikely)—Give 0.5 ml of adsorbed tetanus toxoid as initial immunizing dose. Then give the patient a written record and instruct him to complete the immunization schedule. Basic immunization with precipitated toxoid requires 3 injections: one initially, one at 4–6 weeks, and one in 6 months to 1 year.

2. All other wounds—Give 0.5 ml IM of adsorbed tetanus toxoid as initial immunizing dose plus 250 units IM of tetanus immune globulin (human)—in a different syringe and at a different site—and consider the use of antibiotics. Plan to complete the toxoid series.

C. Use of Tetanus Antitoxins: Equine antitoxin

should never be used prophylactically unless tetanus immune globulin (human) is not available, and then only if the possibility of tetanus outweighs the considerable danger of allergic reaction to the equine antitoxin. Question the patient and test for sensitivity to horse serum. If the patient is not sensitive to equine tetanus antitoxin, give 3000–6000 units IM. If the patient is sensitive, give large doses of penicillin and no antitoxin; the danger of anaphylaxis and other complications probably outweighs the danger of tetanus.

Caution: Human tetanus antitoxin is gamma globulin. It should *never* be given intravenously. Tetanus toxoid may not be effective in immunosuppressed patients.

Treatment

Intensive treatment should be started as soon as the diagnosis is made, since the respiratory paralysis may advance rapidly. Treatment often becomes extremely complicated and requires the combined efforts of a surgeon, an anesthesiologist, and an internist or clinical pharmacologist.

Treatment of tetanus is usually arranged in a sequence of priorities:

A. Fix toxin with human tetanus immune globulin. The usual dose of human immune globulin is 3000–6000 units IM, given preferably in the proximal portion of the wounded extremity or in the vicinity of the wound. Repeated doses may be necessary since the half-life of the antibody is about 3 weeks. The total dose is still under controversy. Lesser amounts may be as effective.

B. Excise and debride the suspected wound under anesthesia appropriate to a complete and unhurried excision. Ordinarily, surgery should be done approximately an hour after the systemic serotherapy has begun. The wound must be left open and may be treated with peroxide.

C. Medical control of the nervous system disorder should begin whenever necessary. The patient should be isolated from sudden stimuli and should be spared unnecessary movement and excitement. Barbiturates or other sedatives may be employed, but overdoses often cause cardiorespiratory failure. Diazepam (Valium) is also useful to help lower the amount of barbiturate necessary to control spasms. Curarization is preferable to cardiodepressant doses of barbiturates even though curarization necessitates the use of mechanical ventilation. Cardiac arrhythmias, pyrexia, peripheral vasoconstriction, and increased catecholamine excretion have been notable features in certain cases. When these manifestations of intense sympathetic nervous system activity occur, they can be successfully reversed with peripheral blocking agents such as propranolol.

D. The patient with respiratory problems usually requires tracheostomy since mechanical ventilation, once it becomes necessary, must be continued for weeks. The patient should be intubated as soon as respiratory problems appear. All modern technics for proper control of respiration and prevention of pneumonia are required. Tracheal stenosis is common after prolonged intubation for tetanus.

E. Aqueous penicillin G, 10–40 million units a day by intermittent intravenous bolus injection. The penicillin is given to kill clostridial organisms and prevent the release of more neurotoxin. Penicillin has no effect on the already liberated toxin.

Prognosis

For the established case of tetanus with respiratory insufficiency, mortality rates are 30–60%. The mortality rate is inversely proportionate to the length of the incubation period and directly proportionate to the severity of symptoms. An attack of tetanus does not confer lasting immunity, and such patients after recovery require active immunization according to the usual recommended schedules.

Blake PA & others: Serologic therapy of tetanus in the United States, 1965–1971. JAMA 235:42, 1976.

Faust RA & others: Tetanus: 2,449 cases in 68 years at Charity Hospital. J Trauma 16:704, 1976.

Smith JWG & others: Prevention of tetanus in the wounded. Br Med J 3:453, 1975.

Tsueda K, Oliver PB, Richter RW: Cardiovascular manifestations of tetanus. Anesthesiology 40:588, 1974.

NECROTIZING FASCIITIS

Necrotizing fasciitis is an invasive infection of fascia, usually due to multiple pathogens. It is characterized by thrombosis of vessels passing between the skin and deep circulation, producing skin necrosis superficially resembling ischemic vascular or clostridial gangrene.

Clinical Findings

Fasciitis usually begins in a localized area such as a puncture wound or leg ulcer. The infection spreads along the relatively ischemic fascial planes, meanwhile causing the penetrating vessels to thrombose. The skin is thus devascularized, whereas the muscle and bone are usually unaffected. Externally, hemorrhagic bullae are usually the first sign of skin death. The fascial necrosis is usually wider than the skin appearance indicates. The bullae and skin necrosis are surrounded by edema and inflammation. Crepitus is occasionally present, and the skin may be anesthetic. The patient often seems alert and unconcerned, although he appears toxic and has fever and tachycardia.

Bacteriologic cultures and gram-stained smears are helpful for diagnosis and treatment. The infection is usually a mixed one with microaerophilic streptococci, staphylococci, or both, commonly in conjunction with gram-negative bacilli. Penicillin should be given empirically, but the sensitivities of the gram-negative bacilli are not predictable. Clostridia are sometimes seen, and the disease has many clinical features in common with clostridial cellulitis. Bacteroides may also be a part of the mixed flora. At surgery, the findings of edematous and dull-gray and necrotic fascia and subcutaneous tissue confirm the diagnosis. Thrombi in penetrating veins are often visible.

One may encounter related infections in which severe fascial or muscle gangrene may occur with relatively little evidence that such a severe process is occurring. Muscle necrosis may be encountered and should always be suspected. It can usually be removed with limited excision.

Differential Diagnosis

Although it is essential to avoid underestimating the severity of the disease and confusing it with cellulitis, localized abscess, and phlebitis, it is also necessary not to confuse necrotizing fasciitis with clostridial cellulitis or myositis or vascular gangrene. Fasciitis advances rapidly; Meleney's ulcer (chronic progressive cutaneous gangrene) advances very slowly.

Treatment

No preventive measures are available. Treatment consists of surgical debridement, antibiotics, and support of the local and general circulation.

A. Surgical Treatment: Debridement, under general or spinal anesthesia, must be thorough, with removal of all avascular skin and fascia. This may require extensive denudation of an extremity. Where necrotic fascia undermines viable skin, longitudinal skin incisions (not too close together) aid debridement of fascia without sacrificing excessive amounts of skin. It is essential to avoid confusing fasciitis with deep gangrene. It is a tragic error to amputate an extremity when removal of dead skin and fascia will suffice. A functional extremity can usually be salvaged in fasciitis; if not, amputation can be safely performed later. If debridement is adequate, antibiotic irrigation of the wound should not be necessary.

It is often difficult to distinguish necrotic from edematous tissue. Careful daily inspections of the wound will demonstrate whether repeated debridements will be necessary. If possible, all obviously necrotic tissue should be removed the first time. When viability of the remaining tissue is assured and the infection has been controlled, homografting is sometimes useful until autografting can be performed.

B. Antibiotics: Penicillin, 20–40 million units IV daily, is begun as soon as material has been taken for smear and culture. Because gram-negative bacteria are so often seen in this disease, another appropriate antibiotic (eg, kanamycin, 15 mg/kg/day, or gentamicin, 5 mg/kg/day) should be added and changed if indicated by reports of antibiotic sensitivity.

C. Circulatory Support: Blood volume must be maintained by transfusions of blood or plasma. Debridement often leaves a large raw surface which may bleed extensively. Since tissue oxygenation is critical, early transfusion with fresh blood is a rational procedure. Diabetes mellitus, if present, should be treated appropriately.

Prognosis

Reliable data on prognosis are not available since the proper diagnosis is so often missed. Death often results, especially in elderly patients.

Rea WJ, Wyrick WJ: Necrotizing fasciitis. Ann Surg 172:957, 1970.
Stone HH, Martin JD Jr: Synergistic necrotizing cellulitis. Ann Surg 175:702, 1972.

OTHER ANAEROBIC INFECTIONS

A number of bacteria can cause the typical features of anaerobic infection. Microaerophilic streptococci, gram-negative bacilli, and, more frequently, bacteroides *(B fragilis)* are being seen. Some of these are gas-producing and others are not. In general, they are less aggressive than clostridia, but they are also less easily treated. These bacteria may invade alone or in combination.

LUDWIG'S ANGINA

Ludwig's angina is an acute invasive infection which causes severe edema in the upper neck that may cause airway obstruction. It is usually caused by streptococci or staphylococci, but other organisms, including anaerobes, may play a role. It is a cellulitis involving the deeper structures of the neck and usually remains localized to the upper neck and the floor of the mouth. Constitutional symptoms may be severe, however, and respiratory difficulty is common.

The disease usually begins in some form of oral lesion such as an alveolar abscess which spreads into the floor of the mouth and soft tissues of the neck. At times, the origin is obscure. Edema and swelling often increase rapidly, but there may be no fluctuation. Redness of the skin is a late sign. Edema of the glottis, respiratory obstruction, and bronchopneumonia with rapid demise of the patient occur unless treatment is instituted promptly.

The disease is now rare, but failure to recognize its lethal potential still results in fatalities.

The diagnosis is based largely on the clinical findings, with confirmation by smear and culture if pus can be found. Treatment should be started with penicillin, 10–20 million units daily IV, if gram-positive cocci in chains are found on smear. If staphylococci are found, a penicillinase-resistant penicillin should be used.

The response to antibiotics is usually rapid, but because the infection produces tension in the deeper structures of the neck with respiratory insufficiency, radical incision and drainage are often indicated. Although a large amount of pus may not be released by drainage, improvement is usually prompt.

Tracheostomy may be lifesaving and should

always be considered early if the response is not dramatically favorable to antibiotics—and drainage. General anesthesia must be given with tracheostomy or intubation done before invasion is attenuated since respiratory obstruction may be imminent and pus is easily inhaled if the airway is not controlled.

VINCENT'S ANGINA

Vincent's angina—also called trench mouth, ulceromembranous stomatitis, and necrotizing ulcero-gingivostomatitis—usually presents as an acute inflammatory disease of the mouth or pharynx which starts as a red edematous area in which a grayish-white pseudomembrane develops over an ulcer. The etiologic agents are a spirochete and a fusiform bacillus. The ulcers are shallow, tender, and painful and rarely larger than 0.5 cm in diameter. The disease usually lasts 8—16 days and rarely causes systemic symptoms.

Penicillin is effective treatment.

NOMA

Noma is a rapidly advancing gangrenous infection of mucous membranes and skin usually occurring in the gingival and facial tissues of undernourished or debilitated small children. It can advance rapidly and is often extremely destructive. Tissue is first destroyed by vascular necrosis, with black gangrenous areas of skin appearing especially about the mouth and nose.

The actual pathogen of noma has not been identified, but anaerobes seem important. Penicillin effectively arrests the gangrenous advancement. However, surgical debridement and, in many cases, extensive plastic surgery are required. It is not unusual for a child with noma to lose most of his lower face.

This disease was once seen almost worldwide. It has disappeared from most industrialized nations and is associated with malnutrition.

RABIES

Rabies is a viral encephalitis transmitted through the saliva of an infected animal. Humans are usually inoculated by the bite of a rabid bat, skunk, raccoon, fox, wolf, dog, cat, or other animal. Since the established disease is almost invariably fatal, early preventive treatment is essential.

The incubation period varies in humans from 10 days to several months. Clinical symptoms begin with pain and numbness around the site of the wound followed by fever, irritability, malaise, and spasms of the face and muscles of swallowing. Paralysis and convulsions occur terminally.

Rabies and tetanus have many features in common. The history is the most useful differentiating point.

Prevention

The wound should be flushed immediately and cleaned repeatedly with soap and water. Tetanus prophylaxis should be given. For severe exposure, the area around the wound should be infiltrated with antirabies serum.

If the animal has escaped, try to determine if the bite was provoked. If so, treatment with vaccine and serum becomes less urgent. Consultation with local health authorities about prevalence of rabies may facilitate the decision whether to use serum or vaccine.

If the animal can be captured, do not kill it but confine it under veterinary observation for 10 days. If it becomes rabid, the animal should be sacrificed and its brain examined for rabies antigen by immunofluorescence. If the animal dies of any cause, or if it is inadvertently killed before 10 days have passed, the head should be sent to the nearest public health or other competent laboratory for examination. Consult local health authorities to determine if any animal rabies has been reported recently.

A single postexposure injection of hyperimmune

Table 11—1. Postexposure treatment of rabies.*

These recommendations are only a guide. They should be used in conjunction with knowledge of the animal species involved, circumstances of the bite or other exposure, the vaccination status of the animal, and the presence of rabies in the region.

If antiserum is given, up to 50% of the dose should be used to infiltrate the wound and the rest should be given intramuscularly.

V = rabies vaccine   S = antirabies serum

Animal	Condition of Animal at Time of Attack	Treatment Bite†	Treatment Nonbite†
Wild			
Skunk, fox, raccoon, bat	Regard as rabid	S + V‡	S + V‡
Domestic			
Dog, cat	Healthy	None§	None§
	Escaped (unknown)	S + V	V**
	Rabid	S + V‡	S + V‡
Other	Consider individually		

*Reproduced, with permission, from *Report of the Committee on Infectious Diseases,* 17th ed. American Academy of Pediatrics, 1974.

†Bite = any penetration of skin by teeth. Nonbite = scratches, open wounds, or abrasions contaminated with saliva.

‡Discontinue vaccine if fluorescent antibody tests of animal killed at time of attack are negative.

§Begin S + V at first sign of rabies in biting dog or cat during holding period (10 days).

**Begin 14 doses of duck embryo vaccine.

serum plus 5 immunizing injections of a new rabies vaccine produced in cultures of human diploid cells has been reported to provide complete protection against the development of clinical rabies. The indications for vaccine and serum are summarized in Table 11—1.

Bahmanyar M & others: Successful protection of humans exposed to rabies infection: Postexposure treatment with the new human diploid cell rabies vaccine and antirabies serum. JAMA 236:2751, 1976.

Corey L, Hattwick MAW: Treatment of persons exposed to rabies. JAMA 232:272, 1975.

Gode GR & others: Intensive care in rabies therapy: Clinical observations. Lancet 2:6, 1976.

Public Health Service Advisory Committee on Immunization Practices: Risk, management, prophylaxis, and immunization. Ann Intern Med 86:452, 1977.

Wilson JM & others: Presenting features and diagnosis of rabies. Lancet 2:1139, 1975.

ANTHRAX

Anthrax (woolsorter's disease, malignant pustule) was once a common disease, particularly in Europe, but is now rare. The causative organism is *Bacillus anthracis,* a gram-positive spore-forming bacillus which is found in long chains on the smear. The infection is usually acquired by handling the wool or hides of infected animals. The reservoir includes sheep, cattle, horses, guinea pigs, hogs, and rabbits.

The disease is usually divided into 3 types: (1) The cutaneous type is most common and has a very low mortality rate. It usually begins as a furuncle which then develops a black, necrotic center. (2) The pulmonary form of the disease is presumably the result of inhalation of spores. The patient becomes rapidly ill, with chills, fever, tachycardia, cough, and pulmonary edema. This form is usually fatal because the diagnosis is made too late for effective treatment. (3) The intestinal infection causes chills, fever, diarrhea, and vomiting. This form also has a high mortality rate.

All forms of the disease respond to parenteral penicillin, 2—5 million units per day. Tetracycline is a somewhat less effective second choice.

TYPHOID FEVER

Typhoid fever is now much less common than formerly. Its initial manifestations are protean and are best described in textbooks of infectious diseases.

Typhoid fever is discussed here because of its surgical complications. It often causes necrosis of lymphoid tissue of the intestine. This develops into ulcers, usually of the ileum, which occasionally perforate. The signs of typhoid perforation may be occult but often are obvious, with abdominal pain and signs of spreading peritonitis. The diagnosis is confirmed by the discovery of free air on x-ray of the abdomen. Significant hemorrhage sometimes results from the mucosal ulcer and may require emergency operation. Small perforations can be simply closed if bacteriologic control has been achieved. Larger lesions may require resection or exteriorization of the intestinal segment.

Although cholecystitis due to typhoid is rarely diagnosed, it is a fairly common cause of the carrier state. When patients continue to excrete *Salmonella typhi* in the stool despite adequate treatment, cholecystectomy may be indicated.

The other common surgical complications of typhoid are osteomyelitis and chondritis.

Either chloramphenicol (2—3 g/day orally), ampicillin, or co-trimoxazole (trimethoprim with sulfamethoxazole) may be effective.

In Asia, recrudescence of typhoid fever is a fairly common complication of abdominal surgery.

Kim JP & others: Management of ileal perforation due to typhoid fever. Ann Surg 181:88, 1975.

Welch TP, Martin NC: Surgical treatment of typhoid perforation. Lancet 1:1078, 1975.

ECHINOCOCCOSIS
(Hydatid Disease)

Echinococcosis is caused by a tapeworm, *Echinococcus granulosus,* which forms larval cysts in human tissue. Dogs and, in some areas, foxes are the definitive hosts which harbor adult worms in their intestines. Ova are passed in the feces and are ingested by intermediate hosts such as cattle, man, rodents, and particularly sheep. Dogs become infected by eating uncooked sheep carcasses which contain hydatid cysts.

Most human infection occurs in childhood following ingestion of materials contaminated with dog feces. The ova penetrate the intestine and pass via the portal vein to the liver and then to the lung or other tissues. In the tissue, the ovum develops into a cyst filled with clear fluid. Brood capsules containing scoleces bud into the cyst lumen. Such "endocysts" may cause secondary intraperitoneal cyst formation if spilled into the peritoneal cavity.

The disease may cause systemic allergic manifestations or local symptoms due to pressure by the cyst. The patient may complain of hives, or, if the cyst ruptures, he may go into anaphylactic shock. Eosinophilia is present in about 40% of infected patients. Sixty percent of patients have one cyst; the remainder have 2 or more. About 50% are located in the liver, 30% in the lung, and 20% in other organs. Forty percent of patients with a lung cyst have a liver cyst, and 25% of those with a liver cyst have one in the lung. In 25% of patients, the parasite dies, the cyst wall calcifies, and therapy is not required.

Diagnosis may be substantiated by serologic tests.

The Casoni skin test is 80–90% accurate. Hemagglutination inhibition and complement fixation tests are accurate and useful since they become negative if treatment eradicates the parasite. The overall mortality rate is about 15%, but it is only 4% in surgically treated cases.

Hydatid Disease of the Liver

Hydatid disease of the liver usually presents with hepatomegaly and chronic right upper quadrant pain in a past resident of an endemic area. Many cases are first seen after the cyst has ruptured into the bile ducts, in which case biliary colic and jaundice are present. Liver scan will outline the cyst or cysts, usually in the right lobe. In about 15% of cases, there are 2 cysts. Selective hepatic arteriography should also be obtained.

The only effective treatment is surgical. Because of the dangers of anaphylaxis or implantation, great care must be taken to avoid rupturing the cyst and spilling its contents into the peritoneal cavity. In some cases, the cyst fluid can be aspirated and replaced by a scolicidal agent such as hypertonic (20–30%) sodium chloride solution or 0.5% sodium hypochlorite solution. More often, this is impossible because debris repeatedly plugs the needle as attempts are made to apply suction. Formalin and phenol have been used in the past but should not be injected into the cyst because they can severely damage the bile ducts if a communication exists.

The cyst can usually be shelled out intact by developing a cleavage plane between the endocyst and ectocyst layers. The resulting cavity can be drained, but it is simpler to fill it with normal saline solution and close it with catgut sutures. Hepatic lobectomy may be required for especially large cysts. If the cyst communicates with intrahepatic bile ducts, the common duct should be explored to remove debris, scoleces, and daughter cysts.

Hydatid Disease of the Lungs

Hydatid cysts of the lung cause chest pain and dyspnea. They may secondarily communicate with bronchioles and become infected. Oral expulsion of the cyst fluid may follow rupture into a bronchus, after which an air-fluid level can be seen on chest x-ray.

Removal of pulmonary cysts presents fewer technical difficulties than those in the liver. The lung is incised over the cyst, and, while the anesthesiologist inflates the lung, the cyst can be slowly delivered intact. Large cysts may be managed by lobectomy, but pneumonectomy is rarely necessary. Secondary bacterial infection and abscess formation should be treated as for pulmonary abscess in general.

Amir-Jahed AK & others: Clinical echinococcosis. Ann Surg 182:541, 1975.
Heslop JH: An assessment of the efficacy of hydatid scolicidal agents used locally in surgery. Aust NZ J Surg 37:205, 1967.
Lewis JW Jr & others: A review of echinococcal disease. Ann Surg 181:390, 1975.
Lichter I: Surgery of pulmonary hydatid cyst: The Barrett technique. Thorax 27:529, 1972.
Pissiotis CA & others: Surgical treatment of hydatid disease. Arch Surg 104:454, 1972.
Saidi F: *Surgery of Hydatid Disease.* Saunders, 1976.
Schiller CF: Complications of Echinococcus cyst rupture. JAMA 195:220, 1966.
Testing for hydatid disease. (Editorial.) Lancet 2:553, 1976.

AMEBIASIS

Amebiasis is caused by the protozoal parasite *Entamoeba histolytica.* Ten percent of the world's population is infected. The active vegetative form—the trophozoites—often inhabit the colon where they subsist on bacteria, usually without causing symptoms. The trophozoites may develop into more resistant cystic forms which are passed in stools. The infection is transmitted by oral-fecal contact. Invasion by trophozoites produces disease principally in the colon and liver. Skin, brain, vagina, etc are involved rarely. Active disease is accompanied by elevated antibody titers, best detected by the indirect hemagglutination test. Titers tend to remain high after the disease is eradicated.

Clinical Findings

A. Intestinal Amebiasis: When the amebas invade the colon, they burrow through the colonic mucosa, producing ulcers by undermining the mucosa. The resulting colitis may vary in severity from chronic and indolent to acute and fulminating.

1. Amebic dysentery—The average case begins with intermittent cramps. After weeks to months, mild diarrhea with blood-stained mucus develops. Fever is usually less than 38.5 C (101.3 F), and the patient is rarely seriously ill. Tenderness is present to palpation in both lower quadrants, and the liver is often slightly enlarged.

Trophozoites can be demonstrated in stools examined in the fresh warm state. It may be necessary to examine 3 or 4 (or more) specimens obtained on different days without purgatives.

2. Severe amebic colitis—This form of the disease may progress to colonic perforation and peritonitis. It may begin suddenly with severe diarrhea of blood and mucus. Abdominal pain, cramps, tenesmus, and dehydration are severe. The patient is toxic, with fever from 39–40 C (102.2–104 F) and leukocytosis in the range of 25,000/μl. The stools often contain sloughs of colonic mucosa.

Sigmoidoscopy demonstrates the typical small, white-capped amebic ulcers, but the examination must be performed gently to avoid perforation. Stool or mucosa obtained by sigmoidoscopy may reveal the trophozoites. Colonic dilatation may resemble acute ulcerative colitis. This distinction is critical because administration of corticosteroid drugs severely aggravates amebic colitis and colectomy is usually fatal, whereas amebicides and tetracycline usually control the disease. Very rarely, operation may be necessary for perforation.

3. Localized intestinal disease—Amebas may invade only a short segment—usually the cecum and sigmoid colon—and may lead to stricture formation or a granulomatous mass called **ameboma**. The typical patient presents with pain in the right lower quadrant and an enlarged and tender cecum and ascending colon. A history of dysentery is usually obtained, and trophozoites may be demonstrated in stool specimens. Barium enema shows concentric narrowing of the affected bowel. Resection may be indicated for intestinal obstruction, but in most cases drug therapy is curative.

Amebic rectal strictures may be confused with neoplasms or lymphogranuloma venereum.

B. Hepatic Amebiasis: Hepatic involvement results from seeding of the liver via the portal vein and is usually a single abscess. In less than 10% of cases, liver abscess develops, with right upper quadrant pain, fever, and tenderness. In 50%, the amebic abscess appears with no history of dysentery. The right lobe is involved 90% of the time. The abscess contains sterile pus ("anchovy paste") which varies from pink to chocolate-brown in color. Trophozoites are found only at the active periphery of the abscess. Even there, they are difficult to identify.

Fever usually ranges from 38–39 C (100.4–102.2 F), and the white count is elevated to 15,000–25,000/μl. There is tenderness in the right upper quadrant, maximal over the abscess. Motion makes the pain worse. Serum bilirubin is usually normal unless secondary pyogenic infection occurs. The serum alkaline phosphatase is often increased. X-rays show an elevated right diaphragm and pleural fluid in the right hemithorax. Radioactive hepatic scan shows the location of the abscess and helps in selecting the site for percutaneous aspiration.

The distinction from pyogenic abscess may be difficult. In fact, secondary pyogenic infection is common. The presence of infection elsewhere in the abdomen in a severely toxic patient suggests a bacterial abscess. The presence of trophozoites in the stool, sterile pus in the abscess, and serologic tests are the major differential features.

The abscess may burst into the peritoneal cavity, the pleural space, or the peritoneum.

Treatment

Metronidazole (Flagyl), 750 mg orally 3 times daily for 10 days, is usually sufficient for hepatic abscess or amebic dysentery. When the patient cannot take metronidazole orally, it can be given once daily as a retention enema (2 g/200 ml of normal saline). This technic has been shown to produce therapeutic blood levels of the drug in addition to having a topical effect in the colon. Especially large hepatic abscesses should be aspirated percutaneously one or more times to

hasten their resolution and prevent rupture. Aspiration of left lobe abscesses is more urgent since they may penetrate the pericardium.

Where metronidazole is unavailable or too expensive, use the following:

A. Intestinal Amebiasis: For mild intestinal infections, give tetracycline (250 mg orally or IM 4 times daily) or paromomycin (same dose) for 10 days, plus diiodohydroxyquin (Diodoquin), 650 mg orally 3 times daily for 20 days. For severe intestinal infections, add dehydroemetine to above, 1–1.5 mg/kg IM daily (maximal total dose, 1 g), until the severe symptoms are controlled.

B. Hepatic Abscess: The combination of dehydroemetine (10 days) with or without chloroquine, 500 mg orally daily for 10 weeks, plus diiodohydroxyquin according to the above dosage schedules or with metronidazole will cure most abscesses and intestinal infections.

Balikian JR & others: Intestinal amebiasis. Am J Roentgenol Radium Ther Nucl Med 122:245, 1974.

Cohen HG, Reynolds TB: Comparison of metronidazole and chloroquine for the treatment of amebic liver abscess: A controlled trial. Gastroenterology 69:35, 1975.

Datta DV & others: The clinical pattern and prognosis of patients with amebic liver abscess and jaundice. Am J Dig Dis 18:887, 1973.

Everett ED: Metronidazole and amebiasis. Am J Dig Dis 19:626, 1974.

Judy KL: Amebiasis presenting as an acute abdomen. Am J Surg 127:275, 1974.

Lenczner EM & others: Surgical aspects of amebiasis. Can J Surg 17:323, 1974.

Pittman FE & others: Studies of human amebiasis: Clinical and laboratory findings in eight cases of acute amebic colitis. Gastroenterology 65:581, 1973.

Pittman FE & others: Studies of human amebiasis. 3. Ameboma: A radiologic manifestation of amebic colitis. Am J Dig Dis 18:1025, 1973.

Ramachandran S, Goonatillake HD: Amoebic liver abscess: Syndromes of "pre-rupture" and intraperitoneal rupture. Br J Surg 61:353, 1974.

Stamm WP: Amoebic aphorisms. Lancet 2:1355, 1970.

Wilmot AJ: *Clinical Amoebiasis.* Blackwell, 1962.

TULAREMIA

Tularemia is caused by *Francisella (Pasteurella) tularensis,* which is endemic in many rodents and other animals. The organism can be transmitted by ticks or biting flies. Most human infections, however, result from handling or dressing infected animals. Cooking usually destroys the bacteria.

The patient usually gives a history of hunting or handling wild animals and minor injury of the hands. The incubation period varies from 4–30 days, and asymptomatic infections are common.

A. Symptoms and Signs:

1. Ulceroglandular type (most common)—The

onset is sudden, with fever, chills, headache, muscle pains, and occasionally delirium. At the site of inoculation, a superficial ulcer forms. Occasionally, the primary lesion is not apparent. The lymph nodes draining the area of inoculation become enlarged, discrete, and slightly tender. The surgeon is called because the initial ulcer fails to heal and the lymph nodes suppurate.

2. Other forms—The primary lesion is inapparent or the adenopathy is not prominent. These forms are rarely seen by the surgeon. They occur when the organism primarily involves the gastrointestinal tract, the lungs, or the eyes.

B. Laboratory Findings: The diagnosis is usually made from smear and culture of the primary lesion or a suppurating lymph node. Blood cultures may be positive.

The suppurative nodes may require incision and drainage or occasionally excision, but the mainstay of treatment is the use of tetracyclines or streptomycin. Sites of incision and drainage are characteristically slow to heal. With early treatment, the mortality rate is 1–2%.

ACTINOMYCOSIS & NOCARDIOSIS

These are chronic, slowly progressive infections which may involve many tissues, resulting in the formation of granulomas and abscesses which drain through sinuses and fistulas. The lesions resemble those produced by fungi, but the organisms are true bacteria.

Actinomycetes are gram-positive nonacid-fast filamentous organisms which usually show branching and may break up into short bacterial forms. They are strict anaerobes which form part of the normal flora of the human pharynx and tonsils. They are generally susceptible to penicillin. Inflammatory nodular masses, abscesses, and draining sinuses occur most commonly on the head and neck. One-fifth of the cases have primary lesions in the chest and an equal proportion in the abdomen, most commonly involving the appendix and cecum. Multiple sinuses are commonly formed, and the discharging pus may contain "sulfur granules," yellow granules of tangled bacterial chains. The inflammatory lesions are often hard and relatively painless and nontender. Systemic symptoms, including fever, are inconstantly present. The discharging sinus tracts or fistulas usually become secondarily infected with other bacteria.

Abdominal actinomycosis may simulate appendicitis, and early appendectomy may be curative. If the appendix perforates, multiple lesions and sinuses of the abdominal wall form. Thoracic actinomycosis may give rise to cough, pleural pain, fever, and weight loss simulating mycobacterial or mycotic infection. Later in the course of the disease, the sinuses perforate the pleural cavity and the chest wall, often involving ribs or vertebrae.

All forms of actinomycosis are treated with penicillin (5–20 million units daily) for many weeks. In addition, surgical extirpation or drainage of lesions—or repair of defects—may be required for cure.

Nocardiae are gram-positive, branching, filamentous organisms which may be acid-fast. The filaments often fragment into bacillary forms. Nocardiae are aerobes which are sometimes found in the normal flora of the respiratory tract. Nocardiae are not susceptible to penicillin but are often inhibited by sulfonamides.

Nocardiosis may present in 2 forms: One is localized, chronic granuloma, with suppuration, abscess, and sinus tract formation resembling actinomycosis. A specialized disorder occurs in the extremities as "Madura foot" (mycetoma), with extensive bone destruction but little systemic illness.

A second form is a systemic infection, beginning as pneumonitis with suppuration and progressing via the blood stream to involvement of other organs, eg, meninges or brain. Systemic nocardiosis produces fever, cough, and weight loss and resembles mycobacterial or mycotic infections. It is particularly apt to occur as a complication of immunodeficiency in lymphoma or drug-induced immunosuppression.

Nocardiosis is best treated with sulfonamides (eg, sulfisoxazole, 6–8 g daily orally) for many weeks. The simultaneous administration of minocycline (200–400 mg daily orally) may be advantageous. Surgical drainage of abscesses, excision of fistulas, and repair of defects is an essential part of management.

Brewer NS & others: Primary anorectal actinomycosis. JAMA 228:1397, 1974.

Hathaway BM, Mason KN: Nocardiosis: Study of 14 cases. Am J Med 32:903, 1962.

Hart PD & others: The compromised host and infection. 2. Deep fungal infection. J Infect Dis 120:169, 1969.

INFECTIONS RESULTING FROM DRUG ABUSE

The recent increase of drug abuse has resulted in a number of atypical infections which demand unusual expertise on the part of the surgeon.

Clinical Findings

Infections associated with drug abuse commonly result from intravascular or extravascular injection of drugs with irritating or even necrotizing foreign substances which may contain bacteria. In a high percentage of cases, the local lesion is complicated by large areas of necrosis, bacteremia, and inflammation. The needle may penetrate the fascia, causing deep space infections in which fluctuation or other external signs of abscess may be absent. The patient is often debilitated and may be highly susceptible to infection.

Bacterial contamination occurs through use of unsterile syringes, needles, and drugs. Drugs are often mixed with methamphetamine, talcum powder, lighter fluid, barbiturates, or milk, all of which kill tissue and provide an ideal medium for bacterial growth. The addict may give an inaccurate history and may use drugs even while under treatment.

A typical problem is a grossly swollen, tense, immobile forearm which is acutely tender but shows no localizing signs of infection. Fever and tachycardia are usually not severe. Many such acute, possibly sterile reactions will subside with rest, elevation, and hot packs. On the other hand, if sepsis is suspected on the basis of the systemic effects, surgical drainage is mandatory even though localization may be difficult. Unfortunately, addicts have many reasons for fever, including other drug-related problems such as withdrawal, pneumonia, empyema, hepatitis, or endocarditis.

Complications

Infections complicating drug abuse are multiple. The most important are pneumonia (from aspiration), hepatitis, endocarditis, meningitis, tetanus, suppurative phlebitis, and empyema.

Treatment

Drainage of abscesses is essential, but they are often difficult to find. When the abscess is not found in the subcutaneous tissue, the deep fascia and muscle compartments must be opened. Neurologic findings may help, eg, median nerve paresis is an indication for extensive deep exploration if the injection was in the antecubital fossa. Infection may spread along the vein and necessitate its removal, often up to the next major tributary. Necrotic skin indicates extensive deeper damage requiring extensive excision. Fever that does not respond to drainage within 24 hours indicates additional sites of infection or inflammation.

Prolonged use of amphetamines may lead to arterial aneurysms, often in the visceral arteries. Concomitant bacteremia may result in mycotic endarteritis. Arteriograms followed by excision during specific antibiotic therapy may be required. Coexisting endocarditis (bacterial or candidal) must be considered. Drug-related cardiac valvulitis may require emergency excision and replacement. Early diagnosis and aggressive therapy are extremely important.

Tetanus is also prevalent in addicts, and immunization is imperative.

Intra-arterial injection of barbiturates or methamphetamine may cause acute vascular obstruction which may at first mimic cellulitis or abscess. Heroin is often diluted with barbiturates, and inadvertent arterial injection of heroin may cause a serious reaction. Pentazocine injections produce a severe, local sterile inflammation which can destroy muscles, nerves, and tendons. There is no known cure or prevention.

Prognosis

The prognosis for long-term survival is poor in heroin or methamphetamine addicts who have destroyed their veins to the point where extravasation occurs or they are reduced to "skin popping" (subcu-

taneous injection). Many limbs have been crippled or lost as a result of this pattern of abuse.

Butterfield WC: Surgical complications of narcotic addiction. Surg Gynecol Obstet 134:237, 1972.

VENEREAL DISEASES

Venereal diseases are now treated principally by medical means, but their complications may require surgery.

Syphilis

Syphilis is rarely a surgical disease, but the cutaneous lesions of syphilis may masquerade as skin tumors or as stubborn infectious lesions. The primary ulcer (chancre) occurs most often on the genitalia, face, or anus and is self-limited. Secondary lesions usually begin as indurated nodules which break down to form punched-out ulcers with sharp epidermal edges. They may occur anywhere but are particularly common on the legs. Recently, oval ulcers have become more common.

Syphilis is known as "the great imitator." It produces gummas (tumorous granulomas specific to syphilis) which may involve the gastrointestinal tract, skin, bones, joints, or nose and throat. They may invade tissues such as the nasal septum, where perforations occur, and may cause masses in liver or in bone.

The diagnosis is made by darkfield or immunofluorescent examination of smears or exudates and by serologic tests. Treatment is with penicillin.

Yaws

Yaws (frambesia) is not a venereal disease but is closely related to syphilis since it is caused by *Treponema pertenue*. It causes ulcerating papules resembling those of syphilis. The disease is endemic, particularly among children, in hot tropical countries.

Diagnosis and treatment are as for syphilis.

Gonorrhea

Although gonorrhea usually begins with urethritis, producing a creamy exudate, it may also cause a painful proctitis—now commonly seen both in women and in homosexual males. It may also cause epididymitis and prostatitis; may involve the joints or even the meninges; and can cause serious systemic symptoms. Surgery is rarely needed except for gonococcal strictures of the urinary tract or for excision of tubo-ovarian abscess.

The diagnosis is made by finding gram-negative intracellular diplococci on smear. Culture revealing *Neisseria gonorrhoeae* is also usually necessary. Treatment is with penicillin or tetracyclines.

Chancroid

Chancroid is not a surgical disease. In its primary

phase, it can be differentiated from syphilis on the basis of its angular, very shallow genital ulceration, with purulent discharge and pain—as opposed to the usually painless chancre, with raised edges, of syphilis. Chancroid does not give a positive serologic test for syphilis, but patients with chancroid may have or have had syphilis. Darkfield examination is negative. Smear reveals a mixed flora including gram-negative rods in chains. The major organism is *Haemophilus ducreyi.*

Treatment usually consists of tetracyclines or sulfonamides.

Lymphogranuloma Venereum

Lymphogranuloma venereum (esthiomene, tropical bubo, lymphopathia venereum) can produce serious surgical lesions. It is caused by an organism (Chlamydia) similar to that which causes psittacosis. The disease may manifest itself in 2 major ways. In men, the most common feature is inguinal adenopathy progressing to suppuration and nonhealing sinuses. In women and homosexual males, the most common presentation is ulcerative proctitis. The proctitis, if improperly treated, frequently results in stricture of the anus and rectum and multiple perianal infections. The infections may form multiple anal fistulas which in turn cause the so-called "watering pot perineum." This complication may require colostomy and multiple plastic surgical procedures of the anus. Occasionally, condylomatous lesions about the anus occur. Elephantiasis of the genitalia may result from chronic lymphatic obstruction.

The diagnosis is confirmed by serologic tests. Treatment usually consists of tetracycline, chloramphenicol, or sulfonamides.

Granuloma Inguinale

Granuloma inguinale is a relatively uncommon infection caused by *Donovania (Calymmatobacterium) granulomatis.* The lesion usually begins as a pustule in or around the genitalia. It soon ulcerates, produces a milky secretion, and slowly invades the adjacent skin. Although it is an infectious disease, it can behave in almost a malignant fashion when not treated. It rarely causes pain or tenderness and usually advances radially from the genitalia or from the anus.

Diagnosis is best made by finding "Donovan bodies" in biopsy material. Treatment is usually with tetracyclines. Streptomycin and ampicillin are second-choice drugs.

Condylomata Acuminata (Venereal Warts)

Venereal warts are a common surgical problem. They are usually seen around the genitalia and anus as painful cauliflower-like papillomas with a rough papillated surface. The etiologic agent is a virus related to or identical with that of molluscum contagiosum. Rarely, these warts invade the urethra and bladder or rectum. When this occurs, extensive operative procedures may be needed to eradicate the warts and their obstructive effects.

The differential diagnosis includes syphilitic or lymphogranulomatous condylomas, hemorrhoids, and skin cancer. All warts which fail to respond to podophyllum resin should be cultured and biopsied.

The vast majority of external venereal warts are best treated by painting with tincture of podophyllum resin. This is extremely effective, but the podophyllum resin can cause pain, and extensive cases should be treated in segments. Warts within the urethra, bladder, anal canal, or rectum usually require fulguration. In stubborn cases, other antiviral agents may be useful.

Brown WJ (editor): *Syphilis and Other Venereal Diseases.* Harvard Univ Press, 1970.

Medical Letter Handbook of Antimicrobial Therapy, Vol 14, No. 3, January 21, 1972.

SNAKEBITE

Although venomous snakes are found in greatest numbers in tropical and subtropical countries, significant numbers may be found in temperate regions also. Only 4 poisonous snakes are indigenous to the USA. Three are pit vipers: the rattlesnake, the cottonmouth, and the copperhead. The coral snake is a member of the Elapid family (cobra-like) and has a venom unrelated to that of the pit vipers. Pit vipers can be distinguished from nonvenomous snakes by a rounded mouth with a pit between the eyes and the nares on each side.

Snake venom contains proteolytic enzymes and other substances which, when injected through the hollow teeth of the snake, can cause local tissue destruction and necrosis of blood vessels as well as profound neurotoxic or hemotoxic systemic reactions. Secondary edema spreads rapidly and may contribute to ischemia of an extremity. Bites on the fingers or toes may cause widespread destruction of digits, muscle compartments, and subcutaneous tissues. When intravascular injection occurs, bleeding secondary to low fibrinogen and platelet levels may ensue. Hemorrhage into tissue will exacerbate local pressure effects. Hemolysis of red cells may occur and produce acute tubular necrosis.

Treatment

A. First Aid Measures: There is much disagreement on the best way to treat snakebite. Physicians in snake-infested areas should be familiar with the types of snakes that may cause envenomation and be prepared to give advice or treatment based on their understanding of the most responsible current practice.

1. Assess the extent of envenomation—A bite by a poisonous snake results in envenomation in only 50–70% of cases. Envenomation may be **mild** (scratch followed by a minimal swelling and not much pain); **moderate** (fang marks and local swelling and definite pain); or **severe** (fang marks, severe and progressive swelling, and severe pain).

2. Restrict activity—Provide reassurance and prevent exertion. The patient should be carried to a vehicle and transported to the nearest hospital.

3. Tourniquet—Apply a flat tourniquet proximal to the bite, just tight enough to interrupt venous and lymphatic flow without affecting the arterial supply. Loosen every 30 minutes to avoid local tissue necrosis.

4. Local treatment of the wound—Incision and suction are recommended by some authorities and interdicted by others. After the tourniquet is in place, venom may be digitally expressed through the fang marks or after making a linear or cruciate incision through both fang marks and about 8 mm beyond. Mechanical suction may retrieve a significant amount of venom; mouth suction may be used but imposes a hazard of infection. Local treatment with ice has been said to increase the danger of necrosis, but some authorities feel that the risk of necrosis is outweighed by the advantages of holding the venom in situ until antivenin can be administered.

5. Antivenin—If envenomation has occurred and a commercial antivenin kit is available, administer the antivenin according to the instructions that accompany the kit after testing for horse serum sensitivity.

B. Hospital Treatment: Blood should be drawn for emergency determination of prothrombin time, plasma fibrinogen level, fibrin split products, hematocrit, and platelet count. Emergency hospital treatment consists of administering antivenin by intravenous drip as well as locally around the bite, plus fluids or blood as required. Antivenin should not be injected into a closed compartment such as a finger. Coagulation defects should be treated with appropriate component therapy or fresh blood.

The local injury should be assessed with a view toward further debridement. It is usually best to debride the nearby fascia and subcutaneous tissue under general anesthesia to prevent increasing edema and tissue destruction. If the underlying muscle is grossly edematous, hemorrhagic, or necrotic, the fascia should be opened widely and debridement performed.

High doses of corticosteroids are recommended for 48–72 hours by some authorities.

Prognosis

The death rate following snakebite should be no more than 7% if adequate supportive care and specific antivenin are given. Significant morbidity may occur as a result of failure to perform early debridement and improper use of tourniquets.

Glass TG Jr: Early debridement in pit viper bites. JAMA 235:2513, 1976.

Lockwood WE: Pitfalls in rattlesnake bite. Tex Med 66:23, 1970.

Minton SA (editor): *Snake Venoms and Envenomation.* Dekker, 1971.

Reid HA: Snake bite. 1. Clinical features. 2. Treatment. Trop Doct 2:155, 1972.

ARTHROPOD BITES

Stings and bites of arthropods are most often merely a nuisance. Some arthropods, however, can produce death by direct toxicity or by hypersensitivity reactions. Because of their prevalence and widespread distribution, bees and wasps kill more people than any other venomous animal, including snakes.

Bees & Wasps

When a bee stings, it becomes anchored by the 2 barbed lancets so that withdrawal is impossible. In the struggle, a bee will usually avulse its stinging apparatus and die. After being stung by a bee, one should scrape the exuded poison sac with a sharp knife. Any attempt to pull the poison apparatus out will simply cause more venom to be squeezed into the tissue. The stinger, once imbedded, remains present. If this has occurred in an eyelid, it may irritate the globe of the eye months after the sting.

The stinging lancets of the wasp are not barbed and can easily be withdrawn by the insect to allow it to reinsert or to escape. It is unusual, therefore, to find a stinger left in place after a wasp sting. The females of the variety called yellow jackets are very aggressive. These insects sometimes bite prior to stinging.

The venom of bees and wasps contains histamine, basic protein components of high molecular weight, free amino acids, hyaluronidase, and acetylcholine. Antigenic proteins are species-specific and may lead to cross-reactivity between insects. Symptoms of arthropod stings may vary from minimal erythema to a marked local reaction or severe systemic toxicity (especially from multiple stings). Infection may occur. A generalized allergic reaction has been described which resembles serum sickness.

Early application of ice packs to reduce swelling is indicated. Elevation of the extremity is also useful. Oral antihistimines may be of some use in reducing urticaria. Parenteral corticosteroids may reduce delayed inflammation. If infection occurs, treatment consists of local debridement and antibiotics. Moderately severe reactions will present as generalized syncope or urticarial reactions. If an anaphylactic reaction or severe reaction is present, aqueous epinephrine, 0.5–1 ml of 1:1000 solution, should be given IM. A repeat dose may be given in 5–10 minutes, followed by 5–20 mg of diphenhydramine slowly IV. Administration of corticosteroids and general supportive measures such as oxygen administration, plasma expanders, and pressor agents may be required in case of shock. Previously sensitized patients should carry identifying tags and a kit for emergency intramuscular injection of epinephrine.

Spiders

The black widow spider (*Latrodectus mactans*) and the brown recluse spider (violin spider; *Loxosceles reclusa*) are most commonly incriminated as dangerous to man.

A. Black Widow Spider: The female black widow spider is characterized by a shiny black body with a red hourglass design on the under side of the abdomen. The male is smaller, less dark, and does not bite. The bite is usually followed by pain and muscular rigidity. Within 24 hours, the pain becomes severe, and a board-like abdomen is often present. A variety of symptoms such as convulsions, shock, and delirium may follow. Acute symptoms usually subside within 48 hours. Mortality may be as high as 5%.

Symptoms are usually self-limited. Initial treatment with debridement or tourniquet is to be condemned as the effect of black widow spider venom is instantaneous. Ice packs will reduce the pain. Intravenous injections of 10% calcium gluconate will relieve the muscle pain and spasm. A specific antivenin (horse serum) is available which is packaged with sterile water. Horse serum sensitivity testing and, if necessary, desensitization must precede use. The usual dose is 2.5 ml of reconstituted serum given IM.

B. Brown Recluse Spider: The brown spider is dark tan in color and has 3 pairs of eyes on the anterior part of the cephalothorax. After biting, there is little local pain. At the puncture site, an erythematous bulla is present surrounded by a patch of ischemia. Within 8–10 hours after biting, this becomes dark, firm, and necrotic. An ulcer may form which may become indolent. A variety of severe systemic symptoms varying from hemoglobinuria to jaundice have been reported.

Corticosteroids should be given immediately to avert or alleviate systemic reactions. Treatment is with antibiotics, antihistamines, and often local debridement.

Denny WF & others: Hemotoxic effect of *Loxosceles reclusus* venom: In vivo and in vitro studies. J Lab Clin Med 64:291, 1964.

Frazier CA: Diagnosis and treatment of insect bites. Ciba 20:75, 1968.

Hershey FB, Aulenbacher CE: Surgical treatment of brown spider bites. Ann Surg 170:300, 1969.

Russell FE: Injuries by venomous animals. Am J Nurs 66:1322, 1966.

ANTIMICROBIAL CHEMOTHERAPY

Microbial infection has always been an accompaniment of surgical procedures, has either delayed or prevented successful results, and has often resulted in death of the patient. Conversely, localized infections of many types—ranging from simple pus collections to infected prosthetic heart valves—have required surgery for cure. The first major step in the control of infectious complications of surgery was the concept of antisepsis, sterilization of instruments, and asepsis. The second was the development of effective antimicrobial drugs which could be used for the control of systemic microbial infections.

Frequent reference is made to the use of antimicrobial drugs in surgery elsewhere in this book, and the cardinal principle often stated is that these drugs are effective adjuncts but not panaceas. Antimicrobial drugs never are a substitute for sound surgical technic, but they can be of help in the management of local infections and may be lifesaving in systemic disseminated infections. Improper application of antimicrobials not only fails to cure the patient but may contribute significantly to patient morbidity and mortality. Widespread improper administration of antimicrobials favors the emergence of drug-resistant organisms, enhances the risk of hospital infections, produces dangerous sensitization of the population, and carries the risk of serious direct toxic effects.

This section summarizes simple principles for the selection of antimicrobials and describes briefly the characteristics and clinical uses of the more important classes of drugs employed in the treatment of microbial infections.

PRINCIPLES OF SELECTION OF ANTIMICROBIAL DRUGS

Selection of an Antimicrobial Drug on Clinical Grounds

For optimal treatment of an infectious process, a suitable antimicrobial must be administered as early as possible. This involves a series of decisions: (1) The surgeon decides, on the basis of a clinical impression, that a microbial infection probably exists. (2) Analyzing the symptoms and signs, the surgeon makes a guess at the most likely microorganism causing the suspected infection; he attempts an etiologic diagnosis on clinical grounds. (3) The surgeon selects the drug most likely to be effective against the suspected organism, ie, he aims a specific drug at a specific organism. (4) Before ordering the drug, the surgeon must secure specimens which are likely to reveal the etiologic agent by laboratory examination. (5) He observes the clinical response to the prescribed antimicrobial. Upon receipt

Table 11–2. Drug selections, 1976–1977.

Suspected or Proved Etiologic Agent	Drug(s) of First Choice	Alternative Drug(s)
Gram-negative cocci		
Gonococcus	Penicillin[1], ampicillin	Tetracycline[2], spectinomycin
Meningococcus	Penicillin[1]	Chloramphenicol
Gram-positive cocci		
Pneumococcus	Penicillin[1]	Erythromycin[3], cephalosporin[4]
Streptococcus, hemolytic groups A,B,C,G	Penicillin[1]	Erythromycin[3]
Streptococcus viridans	Penicillin[1]	Cephalosporin, vancomycin
Staphylococcus, nonpenicillinase-producing	Penicillin[1]	Cephalosporin, vancomycin
Staphylococcus, penicillinase-producing	Penicillinase-resistant penicillin[5]	Cephalosporin, vancomycin, lincomycin
Streptococcus faecalis (enterococcus)	Ampicillin plus aminoglycoside	Vancomycin
Gram-negative rods		
Enterobacter (Aerobacter)	Kanamycin or gentamicin	Chloramphenicol
Bacteroides (except *B fragilis*)	Penicillin[1] or chloramphenicol	Clindamycin
B fragilis	Clindamycin	Chloramphenicol
Brucella	Tetracycline plus streptomycin	Streptomycin plus sulfonamide[6]
Escherichia		
E coli sepsis	Kanamycin or gentamicin	Cephalosporin, ampicillin
E coli urinary tract infection (first attack)	Sulfonamide[7] or co-trimoxazole	Ampicillin, cephalexin
Haemophilus (meningitis, respiratory infections)	Chloramphenicol	Ampicillin, co-trimoxazole
Klebsiella	Cephalosporin or kanamycin	Gentamicin, chloramphenicol
Mima-Herellea (Acinetobacter)	Kanamycin	Tetracycline, gentamicin
Pasteurella (plague, tularemia)	Streptomycin plus tetracycline	Sulfonamide[6]
Proteus		
P mirabilis	Penicillin or ampicillin	Kanamycin, gentamicin
P vulgaris and other species	Gentamicin or kanamycin	Chloramphenicol
Pseudomonas		
Ps aeruginosa	Gentamicin or polymyxin	Carbenicillin, amikacin
Ps pseudomallei (melioidosis)	Tetracycline	Chloramphenicol
Ps mallei (glanders)	Streptomycin plus tetracycline	
Salmonella	Chloramphenicol or ampicillin	Co-trimoxazole[8]
Serratia	Gentamicin, amikacin	Co-trimoxazole[8] plus polymyxin
Shigella	Ampicillin or chloramphenicol	Tetracycline, co-trimoxazole
Vibrio (cholera)	Tetracycline	Co-trimoxazole
Gram-positive rods		
Actinomyces	Penicillin[1]	Tetracycline, sulfonamide
Bacillus (eg, anthrax)	Penicillin[1]	Erythromycin
Clostridium (eg, gas gangrene, tetanus)	Penicillin[1]	Tetracycline, erythromycin
Corynebacterium	Erythromycin	Penicillin, cephalosporin
Listeria	Ampicillin plus aminoglycoside	Tetracycline
Acid-fast rods		
Mycobacterium tuberculosis	INH plus rifampin or ethambutol[9]	Other antituberculosis drugs
Mycobacterium leprae	Dapsone or sulfoxone	Other sulfones, amithiozone
Mycobacteria, atypical	INH plus ethambutol	Rifampin
Nocardia	Sulfonamide[6]	Minocycline
Spirochetes		
Borrelia (relapsing fever)	Tetracycline	Penicillin
Leptospira	Penicillin	Tetracycline
Treponema (syphilis, yaws)	Penicillin	Erythromycin, tetracycline
Mycoplasma	Tetracycline	Erythromycin
Chlamydiae (agents of psittacosis, LGV, and trachoma)	Tetracycline, sulfonamide[6]	Erythromycin, chloramphenicol
Rickettsiae	Tetracycline	Chloramphenicol

[1] Penicillin G is preferred for parenteral injection; penicillin G (buffered) or penicillin V for oral administration. Only highly sensitive microorganisms should be treated with oral penicillin.

[2] All tetracyclines have the same activity against microorganisms and all have comparable therapeutic activity and toxicity. Dosage is determined by the rates of absorption and excretion of different preparations.

[3] Erythromycin estolate and troleandomycin are the best absorbed oral forms.

[4] Cephalothin and cefazolin are the best accepted parenteral cephalosporins, cephalexin or cephradine the best oral forms.

[5] Parenteral methicillin, nafcillin, or oxacillin. Oral dicloxacillin or other isoxazolylpenicillin.

[6] Trisulfapyrimidines have the advantage of greater solubility in urine over sulfadiazine for oral administration; sodium sulfadiazine is suitable for intravenous injection in severely ill persons.

[7] For previously untreated urinary tract infection, a highly soluble sulfonamide such as sulfisoxazole or trisulfapyrimidines is the first choice.

[8] Co-trimoxazole is a mixture of 1 part trimethoprim plus 5 parts sulfamethoxazole.

[9] Either or both.

of laboratory identification of a possibly important microorganism, he weighs this new information against his original "best guess" of etiologic organism and drug. (6) The surgeon may choose to change his drug regimen then or upon receipt of further laboratory information on drug susceptibility of the isolated organism. However, laboratory data need not always overrule a decision based on clinical and empiric grounds, especially when the clinical response supports the initial etiologic diagnosis and drug selection.

Selection of an Antimicrobial by Laboratory Tests

When an etiologic pathogen has been isolated from a meaningful specimen, it is often possible to select the drug of choice on the basis of current clinical experience. Such a listing of drug choices is given in Table 11—2. At other times, laboratory tests for antimicrobial drug susceptibility are necessary, particularly if the isolated organism is of a type which varies greatly in response to different drugs. The most common laboratory test for antimicrobial susceptibility is the disk test. This test measures the ability of a drug that diffuses through agar to inhibit the growth of an isolated microorganism. The size of the zone of inhibition cannot be directly related to the in vivo activity of the drug. The zone of microbial growth inhibition by a given drug must be compared to a standard for this drug to estimate microbial susceptibility. Zone sizes are not comparable from one drug to another. The disk test determines only growth inhibition and therefore provides no direct guidance when bactericidal activity is required for cure, eg, in bacterial endocarditis, acute hematogenous osteomyelitis, or infection in severely debilitated or immunosuppressed individuals.

In general, disk tests give valuable results. At times, however, there is a marked discrepancy between the results of the test and the clinical response of the patient treated with the chosen drug. Some possible explanations for such discrepancies are listed below.

(1) The organism isolated from the specimen may not be the one responsible for the infectious process. The usual cause for this is failure to culture *tissue* instead of pus.

(2) Failure to drain a collection of pus, debride necrotic tissue, or remove a foreign body. Antimicrobials can never take the place of surgical drainage and removal.

(3) Superinfection occurs fairly often in the course of prolonged chemotherapy. New microorganisms may have replaced the original infectious agent. This is particularly common with open wounds or sinus tracts.

(4) The drug may not reach the site of active infection in adequate concentration. The pharmacologic properties of antimicrobials determine their absorption and distribution. Certain drugs penetrate poorly into phagocytic cells and thus may not reach intracellular organisms. Some drugs may diffuse poorly into the eye, CNS or pleural space unless injected directly into the area.

Table 11—3. Use of antibiotics in patients with renal failure.

	Principal Mode of Excretion or Detoxification	Approximate Half-Life in Serum		Proposed Dosage Regimen in Renal Failure		Significant Removal of Drug by Dialysis (H = Hemodialysis; P = Peritoneal Dialysis)
		Normal	Renal Failure*	Initial Dose†	Give Half of Initial Dose at Interval of	
Penicillin G	Tubular secretion	0.5 hour	6 hours	6 g IV	8—12 hours	H, P no
Ampicillin	Tubular secretion	1 hour	8 hours	6 g IV	8—12 hours	H yes, P no
Carbenicillin	Tubular secretion	1.5 hours	16 hours	4 g IV	12—18 hours	H yes, P no
Methicillin	Tubular secretion	0.5 hour	6 hours	6 g IV	8—12 hours	H, P no
Cephalothin	Tubular secretion	0.8 hour	8 hours	4 g IV	18 hours	H, P yes
Cephalexin	Tubular secretion and	2 hours	15 hours	2 g orally	8—12 hours	H, P yes
Cefazolin	glomerular filtration	2 hours	30 hours	2 g IM	24 hours	H, P yes
Streptomycin	Glomerular filtration	2.5 hours	3—4 days	1 g IM	3—4 days	H, P yes‡
Kanamycin	Glomerular filtration	3 hours	3—4 days	1 g IM	3—4 days	H, P yes‡
Gentamicin	Glomerular filtration	2.5 hours	2—4 days	3 mg/kg IM	2—3 days	H, P yes‡
Vancomycin	Glomerular filtration	6 hours	6—9 days	1 g IV	5—8 days	H, P no
Polymyxin B	Glomerular filtration	6 hours	2—3 days	2.5 mg/kg IV	3—4 days	P yes, H no
Colistimethate	Glomerular filtration	4 hours	2—3 days	5 mg/kg IM	3—4 days	P yes, H no
Tetracycline	Glomerular filtration	8 hours	3 days	1 g orally or 0.5 g IV	3 days	H, P no
Chloramphenicol	Mainly liver	3 hours	4 hours	1 g orally or IV	8 hours	H, P poorly
Erythromycin	Mainly liver	1.5 hours	5 hours	1 g orally or IV	8 hours	H, P poorly
Clindamycin	Glomerular filtration and liver	2.5 hours	4 hours	600 mg IV or IM	8 hours	H, P no

*Considered here to be marked by creatinine clearance of 10 ml/minute or less.

†For a 60 kg adult with a serious systemic infection. The "initial dose" listed is administered as an intravenous infusion over a period of 1—8 hours, or as 2 intramuscular injections during an 8-hour period, or as 2—3 oral doses during the same period.

‡Aminoglycosides are removed irregularly in peritoneal dialysis. Gentamicin is removed 60% in hemodialysis.

(5) Rarely, 2 or more microorganisms participate in an infectious process but only one may have been isolated from the specimen. The antimicrobial being used may be effective only against the less virulent organism.

(6) In the course of drug administration, resistant microorganisms may have been selected from a mixed population, and these drug-resistant organisms continue to grow in the presence of the drug.

Assessment of Drug & Dosage

An adequate therapeutic response is an important but not always sufficient indication that the right drug is being given in the right dosage. Proof of drug activity in serum or urine against the original infecting organisms may provide important support for a selected drug regimen even if fever or other signs of infection are continuing. If drug therapy is adequate, the patient's serum will be markedly bactericidal in vitro against the organism isolated from that patient prior to therapy. In infections limited to the urinary tract, the patient's urine must exhibit marked activity against the organism originally isolated from the patient's urine.

Determining Duration of Therapy

The duration of drug therapy is determined in part by clinical response and past experience and in part by laboratory indications of suppression or elimination of infection. Ultimate recovery must be verified by careful follow-up. In evaluating the patient's clinical response, the possibility of adverse reactions to antimicrobial drugs must be kept in mind. Such reactions may mimic continuing activity of the infectious process by causing fever, skin rashes, CNS disturbances, and changes in blood and urine. In the case of many drugs, it is desirable to examine specimens of blood and urine and to assess liver and kidney function at intervals. Abnormal findings may force the surgeon to reduce the dose or even discontinue a given drug.

Oliguria, Impaired Renal Function, & Uremia

Oliguria, impaired renal function, and uremia have an important influence on antimicrobial drug dosage since most of these drugs are excreted—to a greater or lesser extent—by the kidneys. Only minor adjustment in dosage or frequency of administration is necessary with relatively nontoxic drugs (eg, penicillins) or with drugs that are detoxified or excreted mainly by the liver (eg, erythromycins or chloramphenicol). On the other hand, aminoglycosides (streptomycin, kanamycin, gentamicin), polymyxins, tetracyclines, and vancomycin must be drastically reduced in dosage or frequency of administration if toxicity is to be avoided in the presence of nitrogen retention. Some general guidelines for the administration of such drugs to patients with renal failure are given in Table 11–3. The administration of particularly nephrotoxic antimicrobials such as aminoglycosides to patients in renal failure may have to be guided by direct, frequent assay of drug concentration in serum.

In the newborn or premature infant, excretory mechanisms for some antimicrobials are poorly developed and for this reason special dosage schedules must be used in order to avoid toxic accumulation of drugs.

Intravenous Antibiotics

When an antibiotic must be administered intravenously (eg, for life-threatening infection or for maintenance of very high blood levels), the following cautions should be observed:

(1) Give in neutral solution (pH 7.0–7.2) of isotonic sodium chloride (0.9%) or dextrose (5%) in water.

(2) Give alone without admixture of any other drug in order to avoid chemical and physical incompatibilities (which can occur frequently).

(3) Administer by intermittent (every 2–6 hours) addition to the intravenous infusion to avoid inactivation (by temperature, changing pH, etc) and prolonged vein irritation from high drug concentration, which favors thrombophlebitis.

(4) The infusion site must be changed every 48 hours to reduce the chance of superinfection.

ANTIMICROBIAL DRUGS USED IN COMBINATION

Indications

Possible reasons for employing 2 or more antimicrobials simultaneously instead of a single drug are as follows:

(1) Prompt treatment in desperately ill patients suspected of having a serious microbial infection. A good guess about the most probable 2 or 3 pathogens is made, and drugs are aimed at those organisms. Before such treatment is started, it is essential that adequate specimens be obtained for identifying the etiologic agent in the laboratory. Gram-negative sepsis is the most important disease in this category at present.

(2) To delay the emergence of microbial mutants resistant to one drug in chronic infections by the use of a second or third non-cross-reacting drug. The most prominent example is active tuberculosis of any organ with large microbial populations.

(3) Mixed infections, particularly those following massive trauma. Each drug is aimed at an important pathogenic microorganism likely to cause bacteremia.

(4) To achieve bactericidal synergism (see below). In a few infections, eg, enterococcal sepsis, a combination of drugs is more likely to eradicate the infection than either drug used alone. Unfortunately, such synergism is unpredictable, and a given drug pair may be synergistic for only a single microbial strain.

Disadvantages

The following disadvantages of using antimicrobial drugs in combinations must always be considered:

(1) The surgeon may feel that since he is already giving several drugs he has done all he can for the patient. This attitude leads to relaxation of the effort to establish a specific diagnosis. It may also give the surgeon a false sense of security.

(2) The more drugs are administered, the greater the chance for drug reactions to occur or for the patient to become sensitized to drugs.

(3) Unnecessarily high cost.

(4) Antimicrobial combinations usually accomplish no more than an effective single drug.

(5) On very rare occasions, one drug may antagonize a second drug given simultaneously. Antagonism resulting in increased morbidity and mortality has been observed mainly in bacterial meningitis when a bacteriostatic drug (eg, tetracycline or chloramphenicol) was given with a bactericidal drug (eg, penicillin or ampicillin). However, antagonism can usually be overcome by giving a larger dose of one of the drugs in the pair and is therefore a very infrequent problem in clinical therapy.

Synergism

Antimicrobial synergism can occur in several situations. Synergistic drug combinations must be selected by complex laboratory procedures.

(1) Sequential block of a microbial metabolic pathway by 2 drugs. Sulfonamides inhibit the use of extracellular para-aminobenzoic acid by some microbes for the synthesis of folic acid. Trimethoprim or pyrimethamine inhibits the next metabolic step, the reduction of dihydro- to tetrahydrofolic acid. The simultaneous use of a sulfonamide plus trimethoprim is effective in some bacterial infections (eg, urinary tract, enteric) and in malaria. Pyrimethamine plus a sulfonamide is used in toxoplasmosis.

(2) One drug may greatly enhance the uptake of a second drug and thereby greatly increase the overall bactericidal effect. Penicillins enhance the uptake of aminoglycosides by enterococci. Thus, a penicillin plus an aminoglycoside may be essential for the eradication of enterococcal (*Streptococcus faecalis*) infections, particularly sepsis or endocarditis. Similarly, carbenicillin plus gentamicin may be synergistic against some strains of pseudomonas.

●　　●　　●

General References

Altemeier WA & others: *Manual on Control of Infection in Surgical Patients.* Lippincott, 1976.

Andersen B, Korner B, Östergaard AH: Topical ampicillin against wound infections after colorectal surgery. Ann Surg 176:129, 1972.

Ballinger WF, Rutherford RB, Zuidema GD (editors): *The Management of Trauma,* 2nd ed. Saunders, 1973.

Bauer AW & others: Antibiotic susceptibility testing by a standardized single disc method. Am J Clin Pathol 45:493, 1966.

Bennett WM & others: A guide to drug therapy in renal failure. JAMA 230:1544, 1974.

Cave EF, Burke JF, Boyd RJ (editors): *Trauma Management.* Year Book, 1974.

Ericsson HM, Sherris JC: Antibiotic sensitivity testing. Acta Pathol Microbiol Scand, Suppl 217, 1971.

Feller I (editor): Symposium on surgical infections. Surg Clin North Am 52:1359, 1972.

Florey L (editor): *General Pathology,* 4th ed. Saunders, 1970.

Garibaldi RA & others: Factors predisposing to bacteriuria during indwelling urethral catheterization. N Engl J Med 291:215, 1974.

Garrod LP, O'Grady F: *Antibiotics and Chemotherapy,* 4th ed. Livingstone, 1973.

Gorbach SL, Bartlett JG: Anaerobic infections. (3 parts.) N Engl J Med 290:1177, 1237, 1289, 1974.

Hendren WH III (editor): Symposium on pediatric surgery. Surg Clin North Am, April 1976. [Entire issue.]

Hunt TK & others: Antibiotics in surgery. Arch Surg 110:148, 1975.

Johnstone FRC: Infection on a surgical service. Am J Surg 120:192, 1970.

Kagan BM (editor): *Antimicrobial Therapy,* 2nd ed. Saunders, 1974.

Kunin CM (chairman): Veterans Administration Ad Hoc Interdisciplinary Advisory Committee on Antimicrobial Drug Usage: 1. Prophylaxis in surgery. JAMA 237:1003, 1977.

Levin HS, Kagan BM: Antimicrobial agents: Pediatric dosages, routes of administration, and preparation procedures for parenteral therapy. Pediatr Clin North Am 15:275, 1968.

Meakins JL: Pathophysiologic determinants and prediction of sepsis. Surg Clin North Am 56:847, 1976.

Meyers FH, Jawetz E, Goldfien A: *Review of Medical Pharmacology,* 5th ed. Lange, 1976.

Miller ME: Enhanced susceptibility to infection. Med Clin North Am 54:713, 1970.

Polk HC Jr & others: Dissemination and causes of infection. Surg Clin North Am 56:817, 1976.

Ryan GB: Inflammation and localization of infection. Surg Clin North Am 56:831, 1976.

Shubin H, Weil MH: Bacterial shock. JAMA 235:421, 1976.

Weinstein L: Common sense (clinical judgment) in the antibiotic therapy of etiologically undefined infections. Pediatr Clin North Am 15:141, 1968.

Weinstein L, Dalton AC: Host determinants of response to antimicrobial agents. (3 parts.) N Engl J Med 279:467, 524, 580, 1968.

Zweifach BW, Grant L, McCluskey RT (editors): *The Inflammatory Process,* 2nd ed. Vol 3. Academic Press, 1974.

12 . . .
Fluid & Electrolyte Management

Michael H. Humphreys, MD, George F. Sheldon, MD, & Donald D. Trunkey, MD

The surgical patient is liable to develop numerous disorders of body fluid volume and composition, some of which may be iatrogenic. Understanding the physiologic mechanisms that regulate the composition and volume of the body fluids and the principles of fluid and electrolyte therapy is therefore essential for patient management.

BODY WATER & ITS DISTRIBUTION

Total body water comprises 45–60% of body weight; the percentage in any individual is influenced by age and the lean body mass, but in health it remains remarkably constant from day to day. Table 12–1 lists the average values of total body water as a percentage of body weight for men and women of different ages. Total body water is divided into intracellular (ICF) and extracellular (ECF) compartments. Intracellular water represents about two-thirds of total body water, or 40% of body weight. The remaining one-third of body water is extracellular; ECF is divided into 2 compartments: (1) plasma water, comprising approximately 25% of ECF, or 5% of body weight, and (2) interstitial fluid, comprising 75% of ECF, or 15% of body weight.

The composition of solids in intracellular and extracellular fluid compartments differs markedly (Fig 12–1). ECF contains principally sodium, chloride, and bicarbonate, with other ions in much lower concentrations. ICF contains mainly potassium, organic phosphate, sulfate, and various other ions in lower concentrations.

Even though plasma water and interstitial fluid have similar electrolyte compositions, plasma water contains more protein than interstitial fluid. This re-sults in slight differences in electrolyte concentrations, as governed by the Gibbs-Donnan equilibrium. The plasma proteins, chiefly albumin, account for the high colloid osmotic pressure of plasma, which is an important determinant of the distribution of fluid between vascular and interstitial compartments, as defined by the Starling relationships.

The kidneys maintain the volume and composition of body fluids constant by 2 distinct but related mechanisms: (1) filtration and reabsorption of sodium, which adjust urinary sodium excretion to match changes in dietary intake; and (2) regulation of water excretion in response to changes in secretion of antidiuretic hormone. These 2 mechanisms allow the kidneys to maintain the volume and osmolality of body fluid constant within a few percentage points despite wide variations in intake of salt and water. A corollary is that analysis of the composition and volume of the urine usually provides valuable clues in the diagnosis of disorders of body fluid volume and composition.

Although the movement of certain ions and proteins between the various body fluid compartments is restricted, water is freely diffusible. Consequently, the osmolality (total solute concentration) of all the body compartments is identical—normally, about 290 mOsm/kg H_2O. The solutes dissolved in body fluids contribute to total osmolality in proportion to their molar concentration: In ECF, sodium and its salts account for most of the osmolality, while in ICF salts of potassium are chiefly responsible. Control of osmolality occurs through regulation of water intake (thirst) and water excretion (urine volume, insensible loss, and stool water), with the kidneys being the chief regulator. If water intake is low, the kidneys can reduce urine volume and raise urine solute concentration 4-fold above plasma (ie, to 1200–1400 mOsm/kg H_2O). If water intake is high, the kidneys can excrete a large volume of dilute (50 mOsm/kg H_2O) urine.

Concentrations of electrolytes are usually expressed as equivalent weights: a 1 molar solution contains 1 atomic weight of a compound dissolved in 1 liter of fluid; 1 equivalent (Eq) of an ion is equal to 1 mole multiplied by the valence of the ion. For example, in the case of the monovalent sodium ion, 1 equivalent is equal to 1 mole. In the case of calcium, which is divalent, 1 equivalent is equal to 0.5 mole. In

Table 12–1. Total body water (as percentage of body weight) in relation to age and sex.

Age	Male	Female
10–18	59	57
18–40	61	51
40–60	55	47
Over 60	52	46

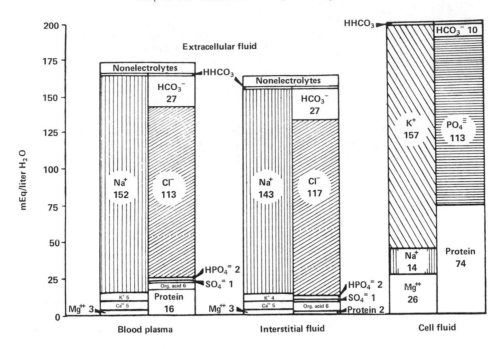

Figure 12–1. Electrolyte composition of human body fluids. Note that the values are in mEq/liter of water, not of body fluid. (Reproduced, with permission, from Leaf & Newburgh: *Significance of Body Fluids in Clinical Medicine,* 2nd ed. Thomas, 1955.)

the relatively dilute conditions of body fluids, the sum of the molar concentrations of ions is approximately equal to total fluid osmolality. However, because the chemical activities of these solutes differ, it is usually more accurate to estimate osmolality by multiplying the serum sodium concentration by 2.

The sensitive regulation of salt and water excretion by the kidney produces an intimate relationship between body fluid osmolality and volume. Edelman and his coworkers showed that the osmolality of plasma or any other body fluid can be closely approximated by the sum of exchangeable sodium (Na_e^+) and its anions (A^-) plus exchangeable potassium (K_e^+) and its anions divided by total body water (TBW):

$$osmolality = \frac{(Na_e^+ + A^-) + (K_e^+ + A^-)}{TBW} \quad \dots Eq\,(1)$$

The plasma sodium concentration (P_{Na}) can be determined by the expression shown in equation 2:

$$P_{Na} = \frac{(Na_e^+) + (K_e^+)}{TBW} \quad \dots Eq\,(2)$$

Although it is neither practical nor necessary to measure exchangeable sodium, exchangeable potassium, or total body water routinely, equation 2 illustrates the major factors that affect the serum sodium concentration and helps one understand the cause and therapy of many fluid and electrolyte disturbances.

In a steady state, the volume and composition of the urine depend upon the intake of water and dietary solutes. An average Western diet generates about 600

mOsm of solute daily that must be excreted by the kidneys. Most people ingest more than 5 g/day of sodium chloride, equivalent to about 85 mEq Na^+ (1 g NaCl = 17 mEq Na^+). Potassium excretion averages 40–60 mEq/day. Water intake is more variable but usually amounts to about 2 liters/day; an additional 400 ml H_2O/day is generated from cellular metabolism. Extrarenal (insensible) water loss amounts to 10 ml/kg body weight/24 hours equally divided among losses from the lungs, the skin, and in the stool. Losses from the lungs and skin may vary under physiologic conditions, but stool water rarely exceeds 200 ml/day in health. Thus, a typical 24-hour urine volume is 1500 ml and has the approximate solute concentrations shown in Table 12–2.

Table 12–2. Typical daily solute balances in normal subjects.

	Concentration	Total Amount
Intake		
Water		
Ingested	. . .	2 liters
Cell metabolism	. . .	0.4 liters
Total solute	. . .	600 mOsm
Sodium	. . .	100 mEq
Potassium	. . .	60 mEq
Urinary excretion		
Water	. . .	1.5 liters
Total solute	400 mOsm/kg H_2O	600 mOsm
Sodium	60 mEq/liter	90 mEq[*]
Potassium	36 mEq/liter	54 mEq[*]

[*]Small amounts of sodium and potassium are lost extrarenally (stool, sweat).

VOLUME DISORDERS

RECOGNITION & TREATMENT OF VOLUME DEPLETION

Since volume depletion is common in surgical patients, a general approach to the diagnosis and treatment of volume depletion should be developed and applied to each patient systematically. The clinical manifestations of volume depletion are low blood pressure, narrow pulse pressure, tachycardia, poor skin turgor, and dry mucous membranes. The history may suggest the reason for volume depletion. Records of intake and output, changes in body weight, urine specific gravity, and analysis of the chemical composition of the urine should confirm the clinical impression and be useful when devising a treatment plan. Therapy must aim to correct the volume deficit and associated aberrations in electrolyte concentrations.

VOLUME DEPLETION

The simplest form of volume depletion is water deficit without accompanying solute deficit. However, in surgical patients, water and solute deficits more often occur together. Pure volume deficits occur in patients who are unable to regulate intake. They may be debilitated or comatose, or have increased insensible water loss from fever. Patients given tube feedings without adequate water supplementation and those with diabetes insipidus may also develop this syndrome. Pure water deficit is reflected biochemically by hypernatremia; the magnitude of the deficit can be estimated from the serum $[Na^+]$ (Equations 2, 3).

Associated findings are an increase in the plasma osmolality, concentrated urine, and a low urine sodium concentration (less than 15 mEq/liter) despite the hypernatremia. The clinical manifestations are chiefly caused by the hypernatremia, which can depress the CNS, resulting in lethargy or coma. Muscle rigidity, tremors, spasticity, and seizures may occur. Since many patients suffering from water deficit have primary neurologic disease, it is often difficult to tell if the symptoms were caused by hypernatremia or by the underlying disease.

Treatment involves replacement of enough water to restore the plasma sodium (P_{Na}) concentration to normal. The excess sodium for which water must be provided can be estimated from the following expression:

$$\Delta Na = (140 - P_{Na}) \times TBW \qquad \dots Eq~(3)$$

The Δ Na represents the total milliequivalents of sodium in excess of water. Divide Δ Na by 140 to obtain the amount of water required to return the serum sodium concentration to 140 mEq/liter. Because of the dehydration, an estimate of total body water (TBW) should be used that is somewhat lower than the normal values listed in Table 12–1. In addition to correcting the existing water deficit, ongoing obligatory water losses (due to diabetes insipidus, fever, etc) must be satisfied. Treat the patient with 5% dextrose in water unless hypotension has developed, in which case hypotonic saline should be used. Rarely, isotonic saline may be indicated to treat shock from dehydration even though the patient is hypernatremic.

VOLUME & ELECTROLYTE DEPLETION

Combined water and electrolyte depletion may occur from gastrointestinal losses due to nasogastric suction, enteric fistulas, enterostomies, or diarrhea. Other causes are excessive diuretic therapy, adrenal insufficiency, profuse sweating, burns, and body fluid sequestration following trauma or surgery. Diagnosis of combined volume and electrolyte deficiency can be made from the history, physical signs, and records of intake and output. The clinical findings are similar to those of pure volume depletion. However, the urine Na^+ concentration is often less than 10 mEq/liter, a manifestation of renal sodium conservation resulting from the action of aldosterone on the renal tubule. The urine is usually hypertonic (sp gr > 1.020), with an osmolality $> 450–500$ mOsm/kg. The decreased blood volume diminishes renal perfusion and often produces prerenal azotemia, reflected by elevated BUN and serum creatinine. Prerenal azotemia is characterized by a disproportionate rise of BUN compared to creatinine; the normal BUN/creatinine ratio of 10:1 is exceeded and may go as high as 20–25:1. This relationship helps differentiate prerenal azotemia from acute tubular necrosis, in which the BUN/creatinine ratio remains close to normal as the serum levels of both substances rise.

Combined water-electrolyte deficits are corrected by restoring volume and the deficient electrolytes. The magnitude of the volume deficit can be estimated by serial measurements of body weight, since acute changes in body weight primarily reflect changes in body fluid. Central venous or pulmonary artery pressure may be low in blood volume deficits and may be useful to monitor replacement.

The composition of the replacement fluid should take into account the plasma sodium concentration: If the $[P_{Na}^+]$ is normal, fluid and electrolyte losses are probably isotonic, and the replacement fluid should be isotonic saline or its equivalent. Hyponatremia may result from salt loss exceeding water loss (ie, the decrease in Na_e^+ will be greater than the decrease in TBW, Equation 2) or from previous administration of hypotonic solutions. In this situation, the magnitude of the salt deficit can be calculated from Equation 3.

Replacement therapy should be planned in 2 steps: First, the sodium deficit should be calculated; second, the volume deficit should be estimated from clinical signs and changes in body weight. From these calculations, a hypothetical replacement solution can be devised in which the sodium deficit is administered as NaCl and the volume deficit as isotonic NaCl solution. Then administer isotonic NaCl solutions containing appropriate amounts of additional NaCl and monitor the patient's response (ie, urine volume and composition, serum electrolytes, and clinical signs). When replacement is adequate, renal function and serum Na^+ and Cl^- concentrations will return to normal.

VOLUME OVERLOAD

Hormonal and circulatory responses to surgery result in postoperative conservation of sodium and water by the kidneys independent of the status of the ECF volume. Antidiuretic hormone, released during anesthesia and surgical stress, promotes water conservation by the kidneys. Renal vasoconstriction and increased aldosterone activity reduce sodium excretion. Consequently, if fluid intake is excessive in the immediate postoperative period, circulatory overload may occur. The tendency for water retention may be exaggerated if heart failure, liver disease, renal disease, or hypoalbuminemia is present. Clinical manifestations of volume overload include edema of the sacrum and extremities, jugular venous distention, tachypnea (if pulmonary edema develops), increased body weight, and elevated pulmonary artery and central venous pressure. A gallop rhythm would indicate cardiac failure.

Volume overload may precipitate prerenal azotemia and oliguria. Examination of the urine usually shows low sodium and high potassium concentrations consistent with enhanced tubular reabsorption of Na^+ and water.

Management of volume overload depends upon its severity. For mild overload, sodium restriction will usually be adequate. If hyponatremia is present, water restriction will also be necessary. Diuretics must be used for severe volume overload. If cardiac failure is present, digitalis must be given.

Inappropriate secretion of antidiuretic hormone (which may occur with head injury, some cancers, and burns) will produce a syndrome characterized by hyponatremia, concentrated urine, elevated urine sodium concentration, and a normal or mildly expanded ECF volume. The serum Na^+ values may drop below 110 mEq/liter and produce confusion and lethargy. In most cases, restriction of water intake alone will be sufficient to correct the abnormality. Occasionally, a potent diuretic (eg, furosemide) should be given and intravenous isotonic saline infused at a rate equal to the urine output; this will rapidly correct the hyponatremia.

SPECIFIC ELECTROLYTE DISORDERS

SODIUM

Regulation of the sodium concentration in plasma or urine is intimately associated with regulation of total body water (Equation 2) and clinically reflects the balance between total body solute and TBW.

Hypernatremia represents chiefly loss of water; this condition has been discussed above.

In addition to dilutional hyponatremia and isotonic dehydration, apparent hyponatremia may develop in patients with marked hyperlipidemia or hyperproteinemia, because fat and protein contribute to plasma bulk even though they are not dissolved in plasma water. The sodium concentration of plasma water in this situation is usually normal.

Hyponatremia in severe hyperglycemia results from the osmotic effects of the elevated glucose concentration, which draws water from the intracellular space to dilute ECF sodium. In hyperglycemia, the magnitude of this effect can be estimated by multiplying the blood glucose concentration in mg/100 ml by 0.016 and adding the result to the existing serum sodium concentration. The sum represents the predicted serum sodium concentration if the hyperglycemia were corrected.

In most cases, hyponatremia can be successfully treated by administering the calculated sodium needs in isotonic solutions. Infusion of hypertonic saline solutions is rarely indicated and could precipitate circulatory overload. Only when severe hyponatremia (usually with P_{Na^+} <110 mEq/liter) produces mental obtundation and seizures should the patient be treated with hypertonic sodium solutions. Hyponatremia with volume overload usually indicates impaired renal ability to excrete sodium.

POTASSIUM

The potassium in extracellular fluids constitutes only 2% of total body potassium (Fig 12–1); the remaining 98% is within body cells.

The serum potassium concentration $[K^+]$ is determined primarily by the pH of extracellular fluid and the size of the intracellular K^+ pool (Fig 12–2). With extracellular acidosis, a large proportion of the excess hydrogen is buffered intracellularly by an exchange of intracellular K^+ for extracellular H^+; this movement of K^+ may produce dangerous hyperkalemia. Alkalosis has an opposite effect: As the pH rises, K^+ moves into cells.

In the absence of an acid-base disturbance, serum K^+ reflects the total body pool of potassium (Fig 12–2). With excessive external losses of potassium (eg,

Table 12—3. Volume and electrolyte content of gastrointestinal fluid losses.*

	Na^+ (mEq/liter)	K^+ (mEq/liter)	Cl^- (mEq/liter)	HCO_3^- (mEq/liter)	Volume (ml)
Gastric juice, high in acid	20 (10—30)	10 (5—40)	120 (80—150)	0	1000—9000
Gastric juice, low in acid	80 (70—140)	15 (5—40)	90 (40—120)	5—25	1000—2500
Pancreatic juice	140 (115—180)	5 (3—8)	75 (55—95)	80 (60—110)	500—1000
Bile	148 (130—160)	5 (3—12)	100 (90—120)	35 (30—40)	300—1000
Small bowel drainage	110 (80—150)	5 (2—8)	105 (60—125)	30 (20—40)	1000—3000
Distal ileum and cecum drainage	80 (40—135)	8 (5—30)	45 (20—90)	30 (20—40)	1000—3000
Diarrheal stools	120 (20—160)	25 (10—40)	90 (30—120)	45 (30—50)	500—17,000

*Average values/24 hours with range in parentheses.

from the gastrointestinal tract) (Table 12—3), the serum [K⁺] falls: A loss of 10% of total body K⁺ drops the serum [K⁺] from 4 to 3 mEq/liter at a normal pH.

Although pH and body composition influence potassium metabolism, measurement of potassium intake and urinary potassium excretion allows the clinician to control potassium balance. Renal excretion of potassium is regulated by mineralocorticoid (aldosterone) levels. Renal failure, particularly acute oliguric renal failure, results in potassium retention and hyperkalemia. Adrenal insufficiency may produce hyperkalemia through impaired renal excretion. Hypokalemia from excessive renal excretion may follow administration of diuretics, adrenal steroid excess, and certain renal tubular disorders associated with potassium wasting. Rarely, potassium deficiency can arise from deficient dietary potassium intake, as in alcoholic patients or in those receiving total parenteral nutrition with inadequate potassium replacement.

1. HYPERKALEMIA

Hyperkalemia is a treatable problem that may prove fatal if undiagnosed. Blood potassium levels must be closely monitored in susceptible patients such as those with severe trauma, burns, crush injuries, renal insufficiency, or marked catabolism from other causes. Hyperkalemia may also be due to Addison's disease. Clinical evidence of significant hyperkalemia is usually not present. Nausea, vomiting, colicky abdominal pain, and diarrhea may occur. The ECG changes are the most helpful indicators of the severity of the disorder: Early changes include peaking of the T waves, widening of the QRS complex, and depression of the S—T segment. With further elevation of the blood potassium level, the QRS widens to such a degree that the tracing resembles a sine wave, a finding that portends imminent cardiac standstill.

A number of factors must be rapidly considered in assessing the hyperkalemic patient. First, is the serum potassium level a true metabolic abnormality or has it been elevated by hemolysis, marked leukocytosis, or thrombocytosis? Platelet counts greater than 1 million/μl may elevate the serum potassium, since the ion is liberated from platelets as they are consumed during clotting. Second, the acid-base status should be assessed to ascertain its influence (Fig 12—2). Finally, the rapidity with which the elevated serum potassium should be corrected must be determined.

There are 3 general approaches to the treatment of hyperkalemia. Initially, an intravenous infusion of 100 ml of 50% dextrose solution containing 20 units

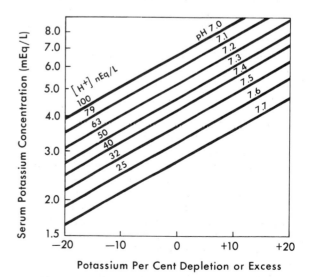

Figure 12—2. Relationship of serum potassium to total body potassium stores at different blood pH levels. (Reprinted, with permission, from: *University of Washington Teaching Syllabus Course on Fluid and Electrolyte Balance.* Edited by Belding Scribner, MD.)

of regular insulin will lower extracellular K^+ by promoting its intracellular transport in association with glucose. Intravenous $NaHCO_3$ solutions will lower serum K^+ as acidosis is corrected. Calcium antagonizes the tissue effects of potassium; an infusion of calcium gluconate will transiently reverse cardiac depression from hyperkalemia without changing the serum potassium concentration. A slower method of controlling hyperkalemia is to administer the cation exchange resin sodium polystyrene sulfonate (Kayexalate) orally or by enema at a rate of 40–80 g/day. This drug binds potassium in the intestine in exchange for sodium. It is often given with sorbitol to induce osmotic diarrhea and enhance the rate of potassium removal. Finally, when hyperkalemia is a manifestation of renal failure, peritoneal or hemodialysis is often necessary.

2. HYPOKALEMIA

Hypokalemia may be associated with alkalosis through either of 2 mechanisms: (1) intracellular shift of potassium in exchange for hydrogen or (2) renal wasting of potassium. The clinical manifestations of hypokalemia relate to neuromuscular function: Decreased muscle contractility and muscle cell potential develop, and, in extreme cases, death may result from paralysis of the muscles of respiration.

When assessing hypokalemia, the initial goal is to identify the cause. If alkalosis is the cause of hypokalemia, the K^+ needs can be determined from the nomogram in Fig 12–2. If there is no acid-base imbalance, or if hypokalemia persists after alkalosis is corrected, renal losses are probably excessive. Urine potassium excretion of more than 30 mEq/24 hours associated with a serum $[K^+] < 3.5$ mEq/liter indicates renal potassium wasting. The primary problem in this situation is usually diuretic therapy, alkalosis, or increased aldosterone activity. If renal potassium excretion is less than 30 mEq/24 hours, the kidneys are conserving potassium appropriately, and hypokalemia reflects a total body deficit.

Treatment consists of correcting the cause of hypokalemia and administering potassium. If the patient is able to eat, potassium should be given orally; otherwise, it should be given intravenously. Usually, potassium concentrations in intravenous solutions should not exceed 40 mEq/liter. In moderate to severe hypokalemia ($[K^+] < 3$ mEq/liter), potassium may be administered at a rate of 20–30 mEq/hour. With mild hypokalemia ($[K^+]$ 3–3.5 mEq/liter), potassium should be replaced slowly to avoid hyperkalemia. Potassium should usually be administered intravenously as the chloride salt; in metabolic alkalosis, potassium chloride is specific, since it helps to correct the acid-base abnormality as well as the hypokalemia.

CALCIUM

Calcium is an important mediator of neuromuscular function and cellular enzyme processes even though most of the body calcium is contained in the skeleton. The usual dietary intake of calcium is 1–3 g/day, most of which is excreted unabsorbed in the feces.

The normal serum calcium concentration (8.5–10.5 mg/100 ml, 4.25–5.25 mEq/liter) is maintained by humoral factors, mainly vitamin D, parathyroid hormone, and calcitonin. Acidemia increases and alkalemia decreases the serum ionized calcium concentration. Approximately half of the total serum calcium is bound to plasma proteins, chiefly albumin; a small amount is complexed to plasma anions, such as citrate; and the remainder (approximately 40%) of the total serum calcium is free or ionized calcium, which is the fraction responsible for the biologic effects. The ionized calcium usually remains constant when the total serum calcium concentration changes with different serum albumin concentrations. Unless the ionized calcium is measured, the serum calcium can only be reliably assessed if accompanied by measurement of the serum albumin concentration.

Severe disturbances of calcium concentration are uncommon in surgical patients, although transient asymptomatic hypocalcemia is common. After operations on the thyroid or parathyroids, the serum calcium concentration should be measured at regular intervals to detect hypocalcemia early if it appears.

1. HYPOCALCEMIA

Hypocalcemia occurs in hypoparathyroidism, hypomagnesemia, severe pancreatitis, chronic or acute renal failure, severe trauma, crush injuries, and necrotizing fasciitis. The clinical manifestations are neuromuscular: hyperactive deep tendon reflexes, a positive Chvostek sign, muscle and abdominal cramps, carpopedal spasm, and, rarely, convulsions. Hypocalcemia is reflected in the ECG by a prolonged Q–T interval.

The initial step is to check the whole blood pH; if alkalosis is present, it should be treated. Intravenous calcium, as calcium gluconate or calcium chloride, may be needed for the acute problem (eg, after parathyroidectomy). Chronic hypoparathyroidism requires vitamin D, oral calcium supplements, and often aluminum hydroxide gels to bind phosphate in the intestine.

2. HYPERCALCEMIA

Hypercalcemia most frequently is caused by hyperparathyroidism, cancer with bony metastases, ectopic production of parathyroid hormone, vitamin D intoxication, hyperthyroidism, sarcoidosis, milk-alkali syndrome, or prolonged immobilization (especially in young patients or those with Paget's disease). It is also a rare complication of thiazide diuretics.

The symptoms of hypercalcemia are fatigability, muscle weakness, depression, anorexia, nausea, and constipation. Long-standing hypercalcemia may impair renal concentrating mechanisms, resulting in polyuria and polydipsia and in metastatic deposition of calcium. Severe hypercalcemia can cause coma and death; a serum concentration above 12 mg/100 ml should be regarded as a medical emergency.

With severe hypercalcemia ($Ca^{++} > 14.5$ mg/100 ml), intravenous isotonic saline should be given to expand the ECF, increase urine flow, enhance calcium excretion, and reduce the serum level.

Furosemide and intravenous sodium sulfate are other methods to increase renal calcium excretion. Mithramycin is particularly useful for hypercalcemia associated with metastatic cancer. Adrenal corticosteroids are useful for hypercalcemia associated with sarcoidosis, vitamin D intoxication, and Addison's disease. Calcitonin is indicated in patients with impaired renal and cardiovascular function. When renal failure is present, hemodialysis may be required.

MAGNESIUM

Magnesium is largely present in bone and cells, where it serves an important role in cellular energy metabolism. The normal plasma magnesium concentration is 1.5–2.5 mEq/liter. Magnesium is excreted primarily by the kidneys. The serum magnesium concentration reflects total body magnesium. Serum magnesium levels may be elevated in hypovolemic shock as magnesium is liberated from cells.

1. HYPOMAGNESEMIA

Hypomagnesemia occurs with poor dietary intake, intestinal malabsorption of ingested magnesium, or excessive losses from the gut (eg, severe diarrhea, enteric fistulas, use of purgatives, or nasogastric suction). It may also be caused by excessive urinary losses (eg, from diuretics), chronic alcohol abuse, hyperaldosteronism, and hypercalcemia. Hypomagnesemia occasionally develops in acute pancreatitis, diabetic acidosis, in burned patients, or after prolonged total parenteral nutrition with insufficient magnesium supplementation. The clinical manifestations resemble those of hypocalcemia: hyperactive tendon reflexes, a positive Chvostek sign, and tremors which may progress to delirium and convulsions.

The diagnosis of hypomagnesemia depends on clinical suspicion with confirmation by measurement

of the serum magnesium. Treatment consists of administering magnesium, usually as the sulfate or chloride. In moderate magnesium deficiency, oral replacement is adequate. In more severe deficits, parenteral magnesium must be administered intravenously (40–80 mEq of $MgSO_4$ per liter of intravenous fluid). When large doses are infused intravenously, there is a risk of producing hypermagnesemia, with tachycardia and hypotension. The ECG should be inspected for prolongation of the Q–T interval. Magnesium should be administered cautiously to oliguric patients or those with renal failure and only after magnesium deficiency has been unequivocally documented.

2. HYPERMAGNESEMIA

Hypermagnesemia usually occurs in patients with renal disease; it is rare in surgical patients. Patients with renal insufficiency should have their serum magnesium levels monitored closely. Strict attention must be paid to excess magnesium intake, which can occur from a variety of commonly administered antacids and laxatives and which may produce severe and even fatal hypermagnesemia in renal insufficiency.

The initial signs and symptoms of hypermagnesemia are lethargy and weakness. ECG changes resemble those in hyperkalemia (widened QRS complex, S–T segment depression, and peaked T waves). When the serum level reaches 6 mEq/liter, deep tendon reflexes are lost; with levels above 10 mEq/liter, somnolence, coma, and death may ensue.

Treatment of hypermagnesemia consists of giving intravenous isotonic saline to increase the rate of renal magnesium excretion. This may be accompanied by a slow intravenous infusion of calcium since calcium antagonizes some of the neuromuscular actions of magnesium. Patients with hypermagnesemia and severe renal failure may need dialysis.

PHOSPHORUS

Phosphorus is primarily a constituent of bone, but it is also an important intracellular ion with a role in energy metabolism. The serum phosphorus level is only an approximate indicator of total body phosphorus and can be influenced by a number of factors, including the serum calcium concentration and the pH of blood. Phosphorus is an important buffer in urine, which facilitates the excretion of acids formed by intermediary metabolism. Urine phosphate buffer is reflected by the excretion of titratable acid.

1. HYPOPHOSPHATEMIA

Clinically important hypophosphatemia may follow poor dietary intake (especially in alcoholics), hyperparathyroidism, and antacid administration (antacids bind phosphate in the intestine). Hypophosphatemia was at one time a frequent complication of total parenteral nutrition until phosphate supplementation became routine. Clinical manifestations appear when the serum phosphorus level falls to 1 mg/100 ml or less. Neuromuscular manifestations include lassitude, fatigue, weakness, convulsions, and death. Red blood cells hemolyze, oxygen delivery is impaired, and white cell phagocytosis is depressed. Chronic phosphate depletion has been implicated in the development of osteomalacia.

Treatment of hypophosphatemia principally involves oral phosphorus replacement. In patients receiving total parenteral nutrition, 20 mEq of potassium dihydrogen phosphate should be given for every 1000 Cal infused (see Chapter 13).

2. HYPERPHOSPHATEMIA

Hyperphosphatemia most often develops in severe renal disease, after trauma, or with marked tissue catabolism. It is rarely caused by excessive dietary intake. Hyperphosphatemia is usually asymptomatic. Because it raises the calcium-phosphorus product, the serum calcium concentration is depressed. A high calcium-phosphate product predisposes to metastatic calcification of soft tissues. Treatment of hyperphosphatemia is by diuresis to increase the rate of urinary phosphorus excretion. Administration of phosphate-binding antacids, such as aluminum hydroxide gels, will diminish the gastrointestinal absorption of phosphorus and lower the serum phosphorus concentration. In patients with renal disease, dialysis may be required.

ACID-BASE BALANCE

NORMAL PHYSIOLOGY

During the course of daily metabolism of protein and carbohydrate, approximately 70 mEq (or 1 mEq/kg of body weight) of hydrogen ion are generated and delivered into the body fluids. In addition, a large amount of carbon dioxide is formed which combines with water to form carbonic acid (H_2CO_3). If efficient mechanisms for buffering and eliminating these acids were not available, the pH of body fluids would fall rapidly. Although mammals have a highly developed system for handling daily acid production, disturbances of acid-base balance are common in disease.

Hydrogen ions generated from metabolism are buffered through 2 major systems. The first involves intracellular protein, eg, the hemoglobin in red blood cells. More important is the bicarbonate/carbonic acid system, which can be understood from the Henderson-Hasselbalch equation:

$$pH = pK + \log \frac{[HCO_3^-]}{0.03 \times P_{CO_2}} \qquad \ldots Eq\ (4)$$

where pK for the HCO_3^-/H_2CO_3 system is 6.1.

Hydrogen ion concentration is related to pH in an inverse logarithmic manner. The following transformation of equation 4 is easier to use because it eliminates the logarithms:

$$[H^+] = \frac{24 \times P_{CO_2}}{[HCO_3^-]} \qquad \ldots Eq\ (5)$$

There is an approximately linear inverse relationship between pH and hydrogen ion concentration over the pH range of 7.1–7.5: for each 0.01 decrease in pH, the hydrogen ion concentration increases 1 nmol. Remembering that a normal blood pH of 7.40 is equal to a hydrogen ion concentration of 40 nmol/liter, one can calculate the approximate hydrogen ion concentration for any pH between 7.1 and 7.5. For example, a pH of 7.30 is equal to a hydrogen ion concentration of 50 nmol/liter. This estimation introduces an error of approximately 10% at the extremes of this pH range.

A consideration of the right-hand side of equation 5 demonstrates that hydrogen ion concentration is determined by the ratio of the P_{CO_2} to the plasma bicarbonate concentration. In body fluid, CO_2 is dissolved and combines with water to form carbonic acid, the acid part of the acid-base pair. If any 2 of these 3 variables are known, the third can be calculated using this expression.

Equation 5 also illustrates how the body excretes acid produced from metabolism. Blood P_{CO_2} is normally controlled within narrow limits by pulmonary ventilation. The plasma bicarbonate concentration is regulated by the renal tubules by 3 major processes: (1) Filtered bicarbonate is reabsorbed, mostly in the proximal tubule, to prevent excessive bicarbonate loss in the urine; (2) hydrogen ions are secreted as titratable acid to regenerate the bicarbonate that was buffered when these hydrogen ions were initially produced and to provide a vehicle for excretion of about one-third of the daily acid production; and (3) the kidneys also excrete hydrogen ion in the form of ammonium ion by a process which regenerates bicarbonate initially consumed in the production of these hydrogen ions. Volume depletion, increased P_{CO_2}, and hypokalemia all favor enhanced tubular reabsorption of HCO_3.

ACID-BASE ABNORMALITIES

The management of clinical acid base disturbances is facilitated by the use of a nomogram (Fig 12–3) which relates the 3 variables in equation 5.

Primary respiratory disturbances cause changes in the blood P_{CO_2} (the numerator in equation 5) and produce corresponding effects on the blood hydrogen ion concentration. Metabolic disturbances primarily affect the plasma bicarbonate concentration (the denominator in equation 5). Whether the disturbance is primarily respiratory or metabolic, some degree of compensatory change occurs in the reciprocal factor in equation 5 to limit or nullify the magnitude of perturbation of acid-base balance. Thus, changes in blood P_{CO_2} from respiratory disturbances are compensated for by changes in the renal handling of bicarbonate. Conversely, changes in plasma bicarbonate concentration are blunted by appropriate respiratory changes.

Because acute changes allow insufficient time for compensatory mechanisms to respond, the resulting pH disturbances are often great and the abnormalities may be present in pure form. By contrast, chronic disturbances allow the full range of compensatory mechanisms to come into play, so that blood pH may remain near normal despite wide variations in the plasma bicarbonate or blood P_{CO_2}.

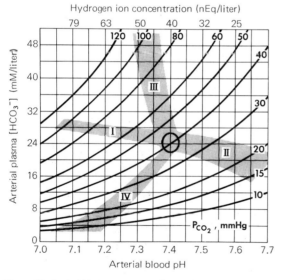

Figure 12–3. Acid-base nomogram for use in evaluation of clinical acid-base disorders. (Courtesy of Anthony Sebastian, MD, University of California Medical Center, San Francisco.) Hydrogen ion concentration *(top)* or blood pH *(bottom)* is plotted against plasma HCO_3^- concentration; curved lines are isopleths of CO_2 tension (P_{CO_2}, mm Hg). Knowing any 2 of these variables permits estimation of the third. The circle in the center represents the range of normal values; the shaded bands represent the 95% confidence limits of 4 common acid-base disturbances: I, acute respiratory acidosis; II, acute respiratory alkalosis; III, chronic respiratory acidosis; IV, sustained metabolic acidosis. Points lying outside these shaded areas are mixed disturbances and indicate 2 primary acid-base disorders.

1. RESPIRATORY ACIDOSIS

Acute respiratory acidosis occurs when respiration is suddenly inadequate. CO_2 accumulates in the blood (the numerator in equation 5 increases), and hydrogen ion concentration increases. This occurs most often in acute airway obstruction, aspiration, respiratory arrest, certain pulmonary infections, and pulmonary edema with impaired gas exchange. There is acidemia and an elevated blood P_{CO_2} but little change in the plasma bicarbonate concentration. Over 80% of the carbonic acid resulting from the increased P_{CO_2} is buffered by intracellular mechanisms: about 50% by intracellular protein and another 30% by hemoglobin. Because relatively little is buffered by bicarbonate ion, the plasma bicarbonate concentration may be normal. An acute increase in the P_{CO_2} from 40 to 80 mm Hg will increase the plasma bicarbonate by only 3 mEq/liter. This is why the 95% confidence band for acute respiratory acidosis (I in Fig 12–3) is nearly horizontal, ie, increases in P_{CO_2} directly decrease pH with little change in plasma bicarbonate concentration. Treatment involves restoration of adequate ventilation. If necessary, tracheal intubation and assisted ventilation or controlled ventilation with morphine sedation should be employed.

Chronic respiratory acidosis arises from chronic respiratory failure in which impaired ventilation gives a sustained elevation of blood P_{CO_2}. Renal compensation raises plasma bicarbonate to the extent illustrated by the 95% confidence limits in Fig 12–3 (the area marked by III). Rather marked elevations of P_{CO_2} produce small changes in blood pH because of the increase in plasma bicarbonate concentration. This is achieved primarily by increased renal excretion of ammonium ion, which enhances acid excretion and regenerates bicarbonate, which is returned to the blood. Chronic respiratory acidosis is generally well tolerated until severe pulmonary insufficiency leads to hypoxia. At this point, the long-term prognosis is very poor. Paradoxically, the patient with chronic respiratory acidosis appears better able to tolerate additional acute increases in blood P_{CO_2}.

Treatment of chronic respiratory acidosis depends largely on attention to pulmonary toilet and ventilatory status. Rapid correction of chronic respiratory acidosis, as may occur if the patient is placed on controlled ventilation, can be dangerous since the P_{CO_2} is lowered rapidly and the compensated respiratory acidosis may be converted to a severe metabolic alkalosis.

2. RESPIRATORY ALKALOSIS

Acute hyperventilation lowers the P_{CO_2} without concomitant changes in the plasma bicarbonate concentration and thereby lowers the hydrogen ion concentration (II in Fig 12–3). The clinical manifestations are paresthesias in the extremities, carpopedal spasm, and a positive Chvostek sign. Acute hyperventilation with respiratory alkalosis may be an early sign of bacterial sepsis.

Chronic respiratory alkalosis occurs in pulmonary and liver disease. The renal response to chronic hypocapnia is to decrease the tubular reabsorption of filtered bicarbonate, increasing bicarbonate excretion with a consequent lowering of plasma bicarbonate concentration. As the bicarbonate concentration falls, the chloride concentration rises. This is the same pattern seen in hyperchloremic acidosis, and the 2 can only be distinguished by blood gas and pH measurements. Generally, chronic respiratory alkalosis does not require treatment.

3. METABOLIC ACIDOSIS

Metabolic acidosis is caused by increased production of hydrogen ion from metabolic or other causes or from excessive bicarbonate losses. In either case, the plasma bicarbonate concentration is decreased, producing an increase in hydrogen ion concentration (see equation 5). With excessive bicarbonate loss (eg, severe diarrhea, diuretic treatment with acetazolamide or other carbonic anhydrase inhibitors, certain forms of renal tubular disease, and in patients with ureterosigmoidostomies), the decrease in plasma bicarbonate concentration is matched by an increase in the serum chloride, so that the anion gap (the sum of chloride and bicarbonate concentrations subtracted from the serum sodium concentration) remains at the normal level, below 15 mEq/liter. On the other hand, metabolic acidosis from increased acid production is associated with an anion gap exceeding 15 mEq/liter. Conditions in which this occurs are renal failure, diabetic ketoacidosis, lactic acidosis, methanol ingestion, salicylate intoxication, and ethylene glycol ingestion. The lungs compensate by hyperventilation, which returns the hydrogen ion concentration toward normal by lowering the blood P_{CO_2}. In long-standing metabolic acidosis, minute ventilation may increase sufficiently to drop the P_{CO_2} to as low as 10–15 mm Hg. The shaded area, marked IV on the nomogram (Fig 12–3), represents the confidence limits for sustained metabolic acidosis.

Treatment of metabolic acidosis depends on identifying the underlying cause and correcting it. Often, this is sufficient. In some conditions, particularly when there is an increased anion gap, alkali administration is required. The amount of sodium bicarbonate required to restore the plasma bicarbonate concentration to normal can be estimated by subtracting the existing plasma bicarbonate concentration from the normal value of 24 mEq/liter and multiplying the resulting number by half the estimated total body water. This is a useful empirical formula. In practice, it is not usually wise to administer enough bicarbonate to return the

plasma bicarbonate completely to normal. It is better to raise the plasma bicarbonate concentration by 5 mEq/liter initially and then reassess the clinical situation. The administration of sodium bicarbonate may cause fluid overload from the large quantity of sodium and may overcorrect the acidosis. The long-term management of patients with metabolic acidosis entails providing adequate alkali, either as supplemental sodium bicarbonate tablets or by dietary manipulation. In all cases, attempts should be made to minimize the magnitude of bicarbonate loss in patients with chronic metabolic acidosis.

4. METABOLIC ALKALOSIS

Metabolic alkalosis is probably the most common acid-base disturbance in surgical patients. In this condition, the blood hydrogen ion concentration is decreased as a result of accumulation of bicarbonate in plasma. The pathogenesis is complex but involves at least 3 separate factors: (1) loss of hydrogen ion, usually as a result of loss of gastric secretions rich in hydrochloric acid; (2) volume depletion, which is often severe; and (3) potassium depletion, which almost always is present.

HCl secretion by the gastric mucosa returns bicarbonate ion to the blood. Gastric acid, after mixing with ingested food, is subsequently reabsorbed in the small intestine, so that there is no net gain or loss of hydrogen ion in this process. If secreted hydrogen ion is lost through vomiting or drainage, the result is a net delivery of bicarbonate into the circulation. Normally, the kidneys are easily able to excrete the excess bicarbonate load. However, if volume depletion accompanies the loss of hydrogen ion, the kidneys work to preserve volume by increasing tubular reabsorption of sodium and whatever anions are also filtered. Consequently, because of the increased sodium reabsorption, the excess bicarbonate cannot be completely excreted. This perpetuates the metabolic alkalosis. At first, some of the filtered bicarbonate escapes reabsorption in the proximal tubule and reaches the distal tubule. Here it promotes potassium secretion and enhanced potassium loss in the urine. The urine pH will be either neutral or alkaline because of the presence of bicarbonate. Later, as volume depletion becomes more severe, the reabsorption of filtered bicarbonate in the proximal tubule becomes virtually complete. Now, only small amounts of sodium, with little bicarbonate, reach the distal tubule. If potassium depletion is severe, sodium is now reabsorbed in exchange for hydrogen ion. This results in the paradoxically acid urine sometimes observed in patients with advanced metabolic alkalosis.

Assessment should involve examination of the urine electrolytes and urine pH. In the early stages, bicarbonate excretion will obligate excretion of sodium as well as potassium, so the urine sodium concentration will be relatively high for a volume-depleted patient and the urine pH will be alkaline. In this circumstance, the urine chloride will reveal the extent of the volume depletion: A urine chloride of less than 10 mEq/liter is diagnostic of volume depletion and chloride deficiency. Later, when bicarbonate reabsorption becomes virtually complete, the urine pH will be acid, and urine sodium, potassium, and chloride concentrations will all be low. The ventilatory compensation in metabolic alkalosis is variable, but the maximal extent of compensation can only raise the blood P_{CO_2} to about 55 mm Hg. A P_{CO_2} greater than 60 mm Hg in metabolic alkalosis suggests a mixed disturbance also involving respiratory acidosis.

To treat metabolic alkalosis, fluid must be given, usually as sodium chloride. With adequate volume repletion, the stimulus to tubular sodium reabsorption is diminished, and the kidneys can then excrete the excess bicarbonate. Most of these patients are also substantially potassium-depleted and will require potassium supplementation. This should be administered as KCl, since chloride depletion is another hallmark of this condition and potassium given as citrate or lactate will not correct the potassium deficit.

5. MIXED ACID-BASE DISORDERS

In many situations, mixed disorders of acid-base balance develop. The most common example in surgical patients is metabolic acidosis superimposed on respiratory alkalosis. This problem can arise in patients with septic shock or hepatorenal syndrome. Since the two acid-base disorders tend to cancel each other, the disturbance in hydrogen ion concentration is usually small. The reverse situation, ie, respiratory acidosis combined with metabolic alkalosis, is less common. Combined metabolic and respiratory acidosis occurs in cardiorespiratory arrest and obviously constitutes a medical emergency. Circumstances involving both metabolic and respiratory alkalosis are rare. The clue to the presence of a mixed acid-base disorder can come from plotting the patient's acid-base data on the nomogram in Fig 12−3. If the set of data falls outside one of the confidence bands, then by definition the patient has a mixed disorder. On the other hand, if the acid-base data fall within one of the confidence bands, it suggests (but does not prove) that the acid-base disturbance is pure or uncomplicated.

PRINCIPLES OF FLUID & ELECTROLYTE THERAPY

The development of a rational plan of fluid and electrolyte therapy requires an understanding of the principles developed earlier in this chapter. First, maintenance fluid requirements must be determined. Second, existing deficits of volume or composition should be calculated. This involves the analysis of 4 aspects of the patient's fluid and electrolyte status based on weight changes, serum electrolyte concentrations, and blood pH and P_{CO_2}: (1) the magnitude of the volume deficit present, (2) the pathogenesis and treatment of abnormal sodium concentration, (3) assessment of any potassium requirement, and (4) management of any coexistent acid-base disturbance. Finally, therapy must also recognize the presence of ongoing obligatory fluid losses and include these losses in the daily plan of treatment.

Normal maintenance requirements can be determined using the guidelines in Table 12−2. Fever or elevated ambient temperature will increase insensible losses and thereby increase these requirements. The normal response to the stress of surgery is to conserve water and electrolytes, so maintenance requirements are decreased in the immediate postoperative period. In addition, increased catabolism will deliver more potassium to the circulation, so that this ion can be omitted from maintenance solutions for several days postoperatively.

Correction of preexisting deficits must be based on the 4 decisions listed above. Volume deficit is best estimated on the basis of acute changes in weight or from clinical estimates, remembering that deficits less than 5% of body water will not be detectable and that loss of 15% of body water will be associated with severe circulatory compromise. The relationship of net sodium to net fluid deficit is given by the serum sodium concentration according to equation 3. If the serum sodium concentration is normal, fluid losses have been isotonic; if hyponatremia is present, more sodium than water has been lost. In either case, initial replacement should be with isotonic saline solutions. Any potassium excess or deficit must be assessed in the light of the blood pH according to Fig 12−2. If hypokalemia exists at normal pH, the magnitude of the total body potassium deficit can also be estimated using Fig 12−2. For example, a serum potassium concentration of 2.5 mEq/liter at pH 7.40 suggests a 20% depletion of total body potassium. A normal human has a potassium capacity of 45 mEq/kg body weight; a moderately wasted patient, 35 mEq/kg. For a normal 70 kg man, total potassium capacity is 45 × 70 or 3150 mEq; the deficit is 20% of this, or 630 mEq, and this amount must be considered in therapy calculations. Principles of acid-base therapy have already been outlined.

Two rules of thumb should be applied in prescribing parenteral therapy for fluid and electrolyte deficits. The first is that for most problems, half of the calculated deficits should be replaced in a 24-hour period, with subsequent reassessment of the clinical situation. The second is that a fluid or electrolyte abnormality should take as long to correct as it took to develop. By adherence to these guidelines, overly vigorous replacement will be avoided and, along with it, the production of a different (iatrogenic) electrolyte abnormality.

Ongoing losses must be considered also in the daily fluid therapy plan, with regard to both volume and composition. Characteristic measurements for fluids removed from different segments of the gastrointestinal tract are shown in Table 12–3.

ILLUSTRATIVE EXAMPLE

A 40-year-old man whose normal weight is 70 kg is admitted to the hospital after 5 days' protracted vomiting, during which time he has been able to ingest nothing but an occasional glass of water. Physical examination shows evidence of dehydration, and diagnostic studies confirm the admitting impression of a duodenal ulcer with pyloric obstruction. Weight on admission is 65 kg. Initial laboratory studies include the following: serum Na^+ 122 mEq/liter, K^+ 2 mEq/liter, Cl^- 80 mEq/liter; HCO_3^- 35 mEq/liter; arterial blood pH 7.5, P_{CO_2} 44 mm Hg; BUN 42 mg/100 ml, creatinine 1.7 mg/100 ml; urine Na^+ 27 mEq/liter, Cl^- 8 mEq/liter, K^+ 64 mEq/liter, pH 7.0.

Discussion

Volume depletion is suggested by weight loss of 5 kg, evidence of volume depletion, elevation of BUN and creatinine, and urine Cl^- less than 10 mEq/liter. The underlying abnormality is metabolic alkalosis and chloride depletion from loss of gastric juice. Hyponatremia results from loss of sodium (gastric juice and urine) with ingestion only of water. Urine pH is neutral because of bicarbonate excretion, obligating sodium excretion, and the high urine potassium is reflective of the potassium wasting occurring in metabolic alkalosis despite hypokalemia.

Parenteral fluid therapy for the first 24 hours should consider the following:

Maintenance requirements will be unchanged from the normal in the absence of fever. Based on weight, the volume deficit is about 5 liters. The sodium deficit, calculated from equation 3, is 585 mEq; this amount is required to restore the serum sodium concentration to 140 mEq/liter. To this must be added the amount of sodium in 5 liters of isotonic replacement fluid, or 700 mEq, for a total sodium deficit of 1285 mEq. The serum potassium, when corrected to normal pH, would be about 2.4 mEq/liter, consistent with a 20% deficit, or about 630 mEq. The alkalosis in this setting will be responsive merely to volume replacement and requires no special therapy; sodium and potassium replacements, however, must be with chloride as the anion. If gastric losses via nasogastric suction continue in the hospital, they should be included in the plan (Table 12–3). These considerations result in the following:

	Volume (liters)	Na^+ mEq	K^+ mEq
Maintenance	2	100	60
Correction of deficit	5	1285	630
Ongoing losses (estimated)	2	40	20

Using the rule of thumb that half of deficits should be replaced in 24 hours, initial orders for intravenous therapy should consist of about 6.5 liters of fluid, 780 mEq of sodium, and 260 mEq of potassium; this last figure is not sufficient to replace half of the potassium deficit but limits the potassium concentration in intravenous fluid to 40 mEq/liter, the highest concentration routinely advisable. This combination can be approximated with 4 liters of 5% dextrose in isotonic sodium chloride and 2.5 liters of 5% dextrose in 0.5 N saline, with potassium added to each bottle to achieve a concentration of 40 mEq/liter. These fluids should then be administered at a rate of 250 ml/hour and the situation then reassessed after 24 hours.

• • •

General References

General

Chapman WH & others: *The Urinary System: An Integrated Approach.* Saunders, 1973.

Deane N: *Kidney and Electrolytes: Foundation of Clinical Diagnosis and Physiologic Therapy.* Prentice-Hall, 1966.

Maxwell MH, Kleeman CR (editors): *Clinical Disorders of Fluid and Electrolyte Metabolism,* 2nd ed. McGraw-Hill, 1972.

Pitts RF: *Physiology of the Kidney and Body Fluids,* 3rd ed. Year Book, 1974.

Scribner BH (editor): *Teaching Syllabus for the Course on Fluid and Electrolyte Balance,* 7th ed. Univ of Washington Book Store, 1969.

Sunderman FW, Sunderman FW Jr (editors): *Clinical Pathology of the Serum Electrolytes.* Thomas, 1966.

Fluid Volume

Bricker NS, Klahr S: The physiologic basis of sodium excretion and diuresis. Adv Intern Med 16:17, 1970.

Earley LE, Daugharty TM: Sodium metabolism. N Engl J Med 281:72, 1969.

Githers JH: Hypernatremic dehydration. Clin Pediatr (Phila) 2:453, 1963.

Hantman D & others: Rapid correction of hyponatremia in the syndrome of inappropriate secretion of antidiuretic hormone. Ann Intern Med 78:870, 1973.

Katz M: Hyperglycemia-induced hyponatremia: Calculations of expected serum sodium depression. N Engl J Med 289:843, 1973.

Kleeman CR, Fichman MP: The clinical physiology of water metabolism. N Engl J Med 277:1300, 1967.

Loeb JN: The hyperosmolar state. N Engl J Med 290:1184, 1974.

Nolph KD & others: Sodium, potassium and water metabolism in the syndrome of inappropriate antidiuretic hormone secretion. Am J Med 49:534, 1970.

Schrier RW (editor): Symposium on water metabolism. Kidney Int, Vol 9, June 1976.

Hydrogen Ion

Albert MS, Dell RB, Winters RB: Quantitative displacement of acid-base equilibrium in metabolic acidosis. Ann Intern Med 66:312, 1967.

Davenport HW: *The ABC of Acid-Base Chemistry,* 2nd ed. Univ of Chicago Press, 1974.

Diarrhea and acid-base disturbances. (Leading article.) Lancet 1:1305, 1966.

Garella S & others: Severity of metabolic acidosis as a determinant of bicarbonate requirements. N Engl J Med 289:121, 1973.

Kassirer JP: Serious acid-base disorders. N Engl J Med 291:773, 1974.

Kassirer JP, Schwartz WB: The response of normal man to selective depletion of hydrochloric acid: Correction of metabolic alkalosis in man without repair of potassium deficiency. Am J Med 40:10, 1966.

Manfredi F: Effects of hypocapnia and hypercapnia on intracellular acid-base equilibrium in man. J Lab Clin Med 69:304, 1967.

Pitts RF: The role of ammonia production and excretion in the regulation of acid-base balance. N Engl J Med 284:32, 1971.

Seldin DW, Rector FC Jr: The generation and maintenance of metabolic alkalosis. Kidney Int 1:306, 1972.

Simpson DP: Control of hydrogen ion homeostasis and renal acidosis. Medicine 50:503, 1971.

Statement of acid-base terminology. Ann Intern Med 63:885, 1965; Anesthesiology 27:7, 1966; Ann NY Acad Sci 133:251, 1966.

Steinmetz PR: Excretion of acid by the kidney: Functional organization and cellular aspects of acidification. N Engl J Med 278:1102, 1968.

Tranquada RE, Grant WJ, Peterson CR: Lactic acidosis. Arch Intern Med 117:192, 1966.

Van Ypersele de Strihou C, Brasseur L, McConinck J: The "carbon-dioxide response curve" for chronic hypercapnia in man. N Engl J Med 275:117, 1966.

Potassium

Kassirer JP & others: The critical role of chloride in the correction of hypokalemic alkalosis in man. Am J Med 38:172, 1965.

Katsikas JL & others: Disorders of potassium metabolism. Med Clin North Am 55:503, 1971.

Papper S, Whang R: *Hyperkalemia and Hypokalemia.* Disease-A-Month. Year Book, June 1964.

Rovner DR: Use of pharmacologic agents in the treatment of hypokalemia and hyperkalemia. Ration Drug Ther 6:1, Feb 1972.

Surawicz B: Relationship between electrocardiogram and electrolytes. Am Heart J 73:814, 1967.

Weatherall M: Ions and the actions of digitalis. Br Heart J 28:497, 1966.

Calcium

Breuer RI, LeBauer J: Caution in the use of phosphates in the treatment of severe hypercalcemia. J Clin Endocrinol Metab 27:695, 1967.

Foster GV: Calcitonin (thyrocalcitonin). N Engl J Med 279:349, 1968.

Goldsmith RS, Ingbar SH: Inorganic phosphate treatment of hypercalcemia of diverse etiologies. (2 parts.) N Engl J Med 274:1, 284, 1966.

Kleeman CR & others: The clinical physiology of calcium homeostasis, parathyroid hormone, and calcitonin. (2 parts.) Calif Med 114:16 (March), 19 (April), 1971.

Perlia CP & others: Mithramycin treatment of hypercalcemia. Cancer 25:389, 1970.

Rasmussen H: Ionic and hormonal control of calcium homeostasis. Am J Med 50:567, 1971.

Singer FR & others: Mithramycin treatment of intractable hypercalcemia due to parathyroid carcinoma. N Engl J Med 283:634, 1970.

Suki WN & others: Acute treatment of hypercalcemia with furosemide. N Engl J Med 283:836, 1970.

Magnesium

Gitelman HJ, Welt LG: Magnesium deficiency. Annu Rev Med 20:233, 1969.

Hall RCW, Joffe JR: Hypomagnesemia: Physical and psychiatric symptoms. JAMA 224:1749, 1973.

MacIntyre I: Magnesium metabolism. Adv Intern Med 13:143, 1967.

Wacker WEC, Parisi AF: Magnesium metabolism. N Engl J Med 278:772, 1968.

13...
Surgical Metabolism & Nutrition

George F. Sheldon, MD, Harold A. Harper, PhD, & Lawrence W. Way, MD

METABOLISM DURING HOMEOSTASIS, STARVATION, & DISEASE

Energy Requirements

A primary nutritional requirement is the provision of energy to support metabolic processes. Carbohydrate, fat, and protein of the diet are the energy-yielding components. The daily requirement for calories is the sum of what is required to maintain life (so-called basal energy demand) plus that required for activity. Under normal circumstances, the caloric demand is increased during growth or in pregnancy. In disease, the convalescent period requires extra energy to support the repair process. Metabolism requiring extra energy will be accelerated in hyperthyroidism or as a result of fever. In the latter instance, there is an increase of approximately 12% over the basal caloric requirement for each degree Celsius (7% per degree Fahrenheit) by which the temperature exceeds normal. The current recommended daily allowances for various nutrients in healthy individuals of varying ages and weights are given in Table 13–1. Twenty-five to 30 Cal/kg/day are required for maintenance. The daily requirements for calories in adult patients may increase during disease as indicated below:

Afebrile, minor injury or illness, at bed rest	2000 Cal
Severe injury or illness	2500–4000 Cal
Previously depleted	3500 Cal
Severe sepsis, fever	5000 Cal

When oral feeding is not possible and feeding must be by the intravenous route, provision of adequate calories is extremely important, particularly in abnormal states characterized by heavy caloric demand. Inability to supply adequate exogenous energy from the diet often ranks as the principal problem in the care of surgical patients.

Protein Requirements

In surgical patients, the problem of supplying adequate protein is almost as great as the problem of meeting caloric requirements. Protein is a unique dietary constituent in that it cannot be replaced by any other food. The recommended daily intakes of protein for healthy individuals are shown in Table 13–1; however, the quantity of protein required by surgical patients may be only slightly above normal or may be considerably increased—up to 200 or 300 g/day or more, as in severe burns.

If possible, at least 100 g of protein per day should be given to sick or injured persons. Patients with severe hepatic or renal disease and those who have had portacaval anastomoses are exceptions. The liver is the principal organ involved in the metabolism of protein. The action of intestinal bacteria on ingested protein produces ammonia, which normally is absorbed in the portal blood and carried directly to the liver, where it is detoxified by conversion to urea. In liver disease, the liver may perform this function inadequately; and after portacaval anastomosis, the ammonia bypasses the liver. In both instances, ammonia may rise to toxic levels in the peripheral blood. In these situations the oral intake of protein must be restricted even though a high-protein diet may otherwise be desirable. When giving high-protein diets, one must be certain to provide enough fluid to permit renal excretion of the increased amounts of urea produced from protein breakdown. Renal function must also be adequate.

Following trauma, some depletion of body protein inevitably occurs, first because labile reserves are limited but mainly because skeletal muscle is catabolized. Depletion of the body protein prolongs convalescence, impairs wound healing, increases susceptibility to infection, and results in skeletal muscle weakness, edema, anemia, impaired gastrointestinal motility, and a number of postoperative complications.

Dietary protein, although not primarily useful because it supplies energy, will be utilized for this purpose unless adequate amounts of nonprotein calories are simultaneously supplied. Efficient incorporation of dietary protein into tissue protoplasm requires 150 or more nonprotein calories per gram of nitrogen. In the immediate posttraumatic period, a negative nitrogen balance is difficult to prevent regardless of the amounts of protein and calories supplied. However, after a variable period of time—usually only a few days after moderate stress—protein anabolism returns, and if adequate calories are also provided the body utilizes administered protein more efficiently. Nonetheless, during the postoperative period, an intake of as much

Table 13–1. Recommended daily dietary allowances.[1] (Revised 1974.)

	Age (years)	Weight (kg)	Weight (lbs)	Height (cm)	Height (in)	Energy (kcal)[2]	Protein (g)	Fat-Soluble Vitamins Vitamin A Activity (RE)[3]	Vitamin A Activity (IU)	Vitamin D (IU)	Vitamin E Activity[4] (IU)	Water-Soluble Vitamins Ascorbic Acid (mg)	Folacin[5] (μg)	Niacin[6] (mg)	Riboflavin (mg)	Thiamine (mg)	Vitamin B_6 (mg)	Vitamin B_{12} (μg)	Minerals Calcium (mg)	Phosphorus (mg)	Iodine (μg)	Iron (mg)	Magnesium (mg)	Zinc (mg)
Infants	0.0–0.5	6	14	60	24	kg × 117	kg × 2.2	420[7]	1400	400	4	35	50	5	0.4	0.3	0.3	0.3	360	240	35	10	60	3
	0.5–1.0	9	20	71	28	kg × 108	kg × 2.0	400	2000	400	5	35	50	8	0.6	0.5	0.4	0.3	540	400	45	15	70	5
Children	1–3	13	28	86	34	1300	23	400	2000	400	7	40	100	9	0.8	0.7	0.6	1.0	800	800	60	15	150	10
	4–6	20	44	110	44	1800	30	500	2500	400	9	40	200	12	1.1	0.9	0.9	1.5	800	800	80	10	200	10
	7–10	30	66	135	54	2400	36	700	3300	400	10	40	300	16	1.2	1.2	1.2	2.0	800	800	110	10	250	10
Males	11–14	44	97	158	63	2800	44	1000	5000	400	12	45	400	18	1.5	1.4	1.6	3.0	1200	1200	130	18	350	15
	15–18	61	134	172	69	3000	54	1000	5000	400	15	45	400	20	1.8	1.5	2.0	3.0	1200	1200	150	18	400	15
	19–22	67	147	172	69	3000	54	1000	5000	400	15	45	400	20	1.8	1.5	2.0	3.0	800	800	140	10	350	15
	23–50	70	154	172	69	2700	56	1000	5000		15	45	400	18	1.6	1.4	2.0	3.0	800	800	130	10	350	15
	51+	70	154	172	69	2400	56	1000	5000		15	45	400	16	1.5	1.2	2.0	3.0	800	800	110	10	350	15
Females	11–14	44	97	155	62	2400	44	800	4000	400	12	45	400	16	1.3	1.2	1.6	3.0	1200	1200	115	18	300	15
	15–18	54	119	162	65	2100	48	800	4000	400	12	45	400	14	1.4	1.1	2.0	3.0	1200	1200	115	18	300	15
	19–22	58	128	162	65	2100	46	800	4000	400	12	45	400	14	1.4	1.1	2.0	3.0	800	800	100	18	300	15
	23–50	58	128	162	65	2000	46	800	4000		12	45	400	13	1.2	1.0	2.0	3.0	800	800	100	18	300	15
	51+	58	128	162	65	1800	46	800	4000		12	45	400	12	1.1	1.0	2.0	3.0	800	800	80	10	300	15
Pregnant						+300	+30	1000	5000	400	15	60	800	+2	+0.3	+0.3	2.5	4.0	1200	1200	125	18+[8]	450	20
Lactating						+500	+20	1200	6000	400	15	80	600	+4	+0.5	+0.3	2.5	4.0	1200	1200	150	18	450	25

Reference: *Recommended Dietary Allowances,* 8th rev ed. Food and Nutrition Board, National Research Council–National Academy of Sciences, 1974.

[1] The allowances are intended to provide for individual variations among most normal persons as they live in the USA under usual environmental stresses. Diets should be based on a variety of common foods in order to provide other nutrients for which human requirements have been less well defined. See text for more detailed discussion of allowances and of nutrients not tabulated.

[2] Kilojoules (kJ) = 4.2 × kcal.

[3] RE = Retinol equivalents.

[4] Total vitamin E activity, estimated to be 80% as α-tocopherol and 20% other tocopherols. See text for variation in allowances.

[5] The folacin allowances refer to dietary sources as determined by *Lactobacillus casei* assay. Pure forms of folacin may be effective in doses less than one-fourth of the recommended dietary allowance.

[6] Although allowances are expressed as niacin, it is recognized that on the average 1 mg of niacin is derived from each 60 mg of dietary tryptophan.

[7] Vitamin A activity is assumed to be all as retinol in milk during the first 6 months of life. All subsequent intakes are assumed to be half as retinol and half as β-carotene when calculated from international units. As retinol equivalents, three-fourths are as retinol and one-fourth as β-carotene.

[8] This increased requirement cannot be met by ordinary diets; therefore, the use of supplemental iron is recommended.

Table 13–2. Some numerical constants useful in estimates of metabolic changes.

Protein catabolized = urinary nitrogen $\times$ 6.25

Wet lean tissue broken down = urinary nitrogen $\times$ 30 or protein $\times$ 4.75

Wet lean tissue is assumed to be 73% water and 27% protein

In muscle tissue:

Extracellular potassium = 3.8–4.3 mEq/liter

Intracellular potassium = 148–155 mEq/liter

Potassium content = 100 mEq/kg wet weight

Energy considerations:

Caloric equivalents of nutrients:

Carbohydrate	= 4 Cal/g
Fat (triglycerides)	= 9 Cal/g
Protein	= 4 Cal/g
Ethyl alcohol	= 7 Cal/g

Respiratory quotient (RQ) = CO_2/O_2 ratio

RQ for oxidation of carbohydrate = 1.00

RQ for oxidation of fat = 0.70

When carbohydrate is being converted to fat, RQ is > 1.00

On the usual mixed diet, RQ = 0.75–0.85

Basal Metabolic Rate (adults) = 36–41 Cal/sq m/hour (approximately 1600–1800 Cal/day)

For 1800 Cal energy expenditure, oxygen consumption = 250 ml/min

Carbohydrate consumption	= 400 Cal (100 g)
Fat consumption	= 1160 Cal (130 g)
Protein consumption	= 240 Cal (60 g)
Total	= 1800 Cal/day

as 0.5 g/kg of nitrogen (1 g of nitrogen equals 6.25 g of protein) and 45 Cal/kg will be necessary to restore positive nitrogen balance in a previously depleted patient.

Carbohydrate & Fat Requirements

Carbohydrate—particularly glucose—has long been regarded as the main source of calories. Only recently has the importance of endogenous fat stores as sources of energy been fully appreciated. The utilization of glucose as a source of energy is so characteristic of some tissues that this fuel may be regarded as virtually an obligatory metabolite. Examples are the brain, erythrocytes, bone marrow, peripheral nerves, and adrenal medulla. In addition, fibroblasts and phagocytes, which are essential to wound healing, use glucose as their principal energy source. However, other tissues can also catabolize fatty acids and their metabolic products (ketones) for energy, and do so to an increasing extent as carbohydrate becomes less available. This may occur even after brief fasting. For example, skeletal muscle, heart muscle, renal cortex, and brain can adapt to the use of lipid substrates for virtually all their energy needs.

For a fasting adult man, approximately 100 g of glucose per day seems sufficient to ensure maximal protein sparing for brief periods. This conclusion is based on measurement of the conversion of protein to carbohydrate (gluconeogenesis), as determined by the excretion of nitrogen in the urine. The caloric deficit (100 g of glucose provides only 400 Cal) is met by utilization of stored fat. Glucose generated by hepatic gluconeogenesis and that given parenterally are diverted to tissues that are unable to use lipid substrates. Consequently, at the start of a total fast, total urinary nitrogen per 24 hours may be as high as 12 g (equivalent to 75 g of tissue protein broken down). But the normal adaptive response to fasting will quickly produce energy by mobilizing increasing amounts of lipid, and protein catabolism will be reduced to 20 g of protein per day (or less). If this did not occur, and the initial rate of protein loss persisted, a critical reduction in body protein would result. Because the only significant source of this protein is muscle, muscle weakness and skeletal muscle atrophy are characteristic of prolonged undernutrition. Humans cannot usually survive a loss of more than one-third to one-half of total body protein.

During starvation, increasing amounts of fatty acids, derived from lipolysis of adipose tissue, are present in the blood and tissues. The metabolism of fatty acids in the liver produces ketones, which can be measured in the blood and quantitatively reflect the extent of lipid catabolism.

Even the brain can adapt to the use of ketones for up to 70% of its total energy requirement, and other tissues, notably muscle, may derive practically all of their energy from ketones during starvation. In the liver, the oxidation of fatty acids to ketones may substitute for the energy the liver otherwise obtains from amino acid oxidation through gluconeogenesis. Obviously, this also spares protein breakdown.

These observations on the role of lipid as a metabolite during starvation suggest that ketogenesis is not only normal; it is essential in the metabolic adaptation to starvation. Only with maximal utilization of lipid reserves will endogenous nitrogen (protein) catabolism be reduced to a minimum.

In a normal human subject, lipolysis of the total lipid reserves may produce as much as 100–150 thousand Cal. At normal rates of energy consumption, the amount of stored fat in adipose tissues of a previously healthy individual is adequate to supply energy for 2–3 months. Loss of half of this total or more is not harmful.

Insulin plays a key role in regulating the balance between lipolysis and lipogenesis. Therefore, elevating the blood sugar (eg, by infusing glucose) evokes in nondiabetic individuals a prompt increase in insulin secretion which favors lipogenesis. This reduces the levels of fatty acids and ketones in the blood by fostering their conversion to triglyceride, which is stored in adipose tissue. This action of insulin may also be thought of as inhibiting lipolysis and reducing the availability of lipid as an energy source. However, as noted above, lipid mobilization is an essential metabolic response to caloric undernutrition.

Vitamins

Utilization of nutrients requires other nutritional factors such as vitamins, minerals, and water. When a normal individual is consuming a balanced diet, all of the required vitamins, minerals, and water can be secured from dietary sources; supplementation must be considered in various abnormal states or when digestion or absorption is impaired. The recommended daily allowances for normal persons for various vitamins are given in Table 13–1. It is likely, however, that increases in these recommended allowances will be necessary in many disease states.

A. Vitamin B Complex: The water-soluble vitamins of the B complex are directly involved as cofactors in important metabolic processes. Since metabolism may be increased in disease, it is desirable to increase the intake of these vitamins. The recommended therapeutic daily doses of the most important of these vitamins are as follows:

Thiamine (B₁)	5–10 mg
Riboflavin (B₂)	5–10 mg
Niacinamide	100 mg
Pantothenic acid	20 mg
Pyridoxine (B₆)	2 mg
Folic acid (folacin)	1 mg
Vitamin B₁₂	4 μg

B. Vitamin C: Vitamin C helps to maintain the normal intercellular material of cartilage, dentine, and bone and participates in collagen synthesis. This involves the vitamin specifically in wound healing. There are large amounts of vitamin C in the adrenal cortex which are rapidly depleted when the adrenal gland is stimulated (as by stress). Increased losses of vitamin C accompany fever and infection. These observations suggest the need for increased amounts of vitamin C after trauma, and a minimum of 500 mg/day is recommended.

C. Fat-Soluble Vitamins: Vitamins A, D, and K are the fat-soluble vitamins generally considered to be important in human nutrition, although a requirement in adult humans for vitamin D is questionable since it can by synthesized within the body. Vitamin A is important for wound healing, and vitamin K is essential for the production of prothrombin by the liver. Under normal circumstances, vitamin A is present in adequate amounts in a balanced diet; the synthesis of vitamin K by intestinal bacteria assures production of adequate amounts of this vitamin. However, these fat-soluble vitamins are not adequately absorbed from the intestinal tract if fat digestion or absorption is impaired, as may occur in obstructive jaundice, biliary fistula, pancreatic disease, or any disease that extensively involves the gastrointestinal tract. For surgical patients, a deficiency of vitamin K may be especially significant because of its effects on blood coagulation. If the patient is deficient, vitamin K should be given parenterally until the prothrombin level is at least 60–70% of normal. The required dose of the water-soluble vitamin K preparation menadione sodium bisulfite is 2–5 mg IV or IM. Lack of a prompt rise in serum prothrombin following the injection suggests that the liver is severely damaged.

Nutritional Importance of Potassium

Although the mineral elements are present in the tissues in relatively small amounts, they are essential to many body processes. In surgical patients the importance of certain of these elements, such as sodium and potassium, relates mainly to regulation of water and acid-base balance. The significance of potassium must be stressed. Potassium deficiency is likely to develop in any protracted illness when patients are maintained on intravenous fluids without potassium. Potassium deficiencies are also common in chronic wasting diseases, malnutrition, prolonged negative nitrogen balance, gastrointestinal losses (including those incurred in all types of diarrhea, gastrointestinal fistulas, and continuous suction), and metabolic alkalosis.

In muscle, the proportion of potassium to nitrogen is 3 mmol K⁺ per gram of nitrogen. Storage of nitrogen as muscle protein during protein repletion requires that the diet contain both protein and potassium. For example, synthesis of 5 kg of muscle protein requires 600 mEq of potassium in addition to the protein nitrogen.

Although potassium can be given parenterally, severe deficiencies are best corrected with orally administered salts. In the long-term nutrition of surgical patients who may incur potassium deficits, foods rich in potassium should be prescribed. Foods with a high content of potassium (300–600 mg/serving) are meats, fish, and poultry, dried apricots, dried peaches, bananas, raisins, prunes, figs, dates, and certain fruit juices (eg, prune, tomato, orange, and pineapple). Among the vegetables, yams, squash, potatoes, brussels sprouts, cauliflower, lentils, and broccoli are high in potassium. Certain foods that are rich in potassium may also contain considerable sodium, which in some cases may not be desired. Examples are ham, bacon, milk, and tomato juice.

METABOLIC EFFECTS OF TRAUMA

General Considerations

The concept of injury (accidental or as a planned surgical procedure) as an event affecting the entire body is relatively new to medicine. A wound or infection in an extremity calls forth a series of responses that are concerned with preservation of oxygen delivery, acid-base regulation, cardiac output, and overall homeostasis. Following the initial phase of compensation, sequential steps occur that deplete body fuel sources and may cause progressive deterioration of cell mass.

Moore has described a system for quantifying injury on a scale of 1–10 in which various operations were graded according to the severity of their effect on the total organism. Some operations that were "external" and seemingly innocuous nonetheless had a high metabolic "price." Some "major" operations, on the other hand, demanded less from body energy stores.

Convalescence from injury was divided by Moore into 4 clinical phases: (1) the injury phase, (2) the turning point, (3) the muscle rebuilding or anabolic phase, and (4) the weight gain phase. This categorization correlates clinically with various changes in hormone levels, energy production, nutritional status, and water and electrolyte balance. The duration of each phase is variable, depending to a considerable degree on the magnitude of the initial wounding incident.

During the initial phase after injury, pain ordinarily limits motion of the injured part. Hyperventilation from pain or blood loss produces a low partial pressure of CO_2 and respiratory alkalosis. As a response to blood volume loss, depletion injury, or anesthetic agents, an outpouring of adrenocortical steroid hormones will occur. Afferent stimuli reaching the CNS through large neurons cause the hypothalamus to secrete corticotropin-releasing factor (CRF). The resulting stimulation of the anterior pituitary releases adrenocorticotropic hormone (ACTH). ACTH stimulates the adrenal cortex to secrete glucocorticoids (cortisol and corticosterone), which accelerate gluconeogenesis and increase deposition of liver glycogen. In addition, mobilization of stored fat from adipose tissue elevates serum levels of free fatty acids. The net effect is to increase carbohydrate and lipid intermediates to produce the so-called "diabetes of injury."

Perhaps more significant for the maintenance of an adequate blood volume is the release of mineralocorticoids from the zona glomerulosa of the adrenal cortex. After trauma—and particularly following acute loss of blood—aldosterone secretion may be increased as much as 30-fold. Diminished renal blood flow may also liberate renin, which converts plasma angiotensinogen into angiotensin, producing vasoconstriction and elevation of the blood pressure. Aldosterone enhances renal tubular reabsorption of sodium while increasing excretion of hydrogen ion and potassium.

Following blood loss or trauma, antidiuretic hormone (vasopressin) is released from the posterior pituitary, and this substance conserves water by increasing renal tubular permeability and reabsorption. The net effect is to reduce urine volume and to increase urine osmolality. Sodium is retained, and extracellular water volume is restored by transcapillary refill within 24 hours after a hemorrhage.

Following stabilization after injury, the complex interaction between body composition, foodstuffs, parenterally administered nutrients, and incompletely understood endocrine mechanisms determine whether a patient heals his wounds or succumbs.

Moore regards the body components as the total functioning energy source. Body fat, the richest source of potential energy, may comprise as much as 50% of body mass in an obese individual. A trim athlete, on the other hand, may have less than 10% of his body mass in the form of fat. At puberty, women gain mostly fat whereas men gain more protein.

The skeleton is devoid of fat and potassium. However, 10% of the fat-free weight of an individual is present in the skeleton. During starvation, nutritional

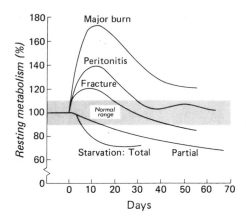

Figure 13–1. Starvation and injury are related but evoke different metabolic responses. Total energy expenditure decreases in starvation but not in injury. Nitrogen loss, particularly when at its maximum, tends to parallel the magnitude of trauma. (Redrawn and reproduced, with permission, from Kinney JA: Energy deficits in acute illness and injury. *Proceedings of a Conference on Energy Metabolism and Body Fuel Utilization,* pp 167–177, Harvard University Printing Office, 1966.)

deficiency may stunt bone growth and repair.

Kinney has demonstrated that in the normal pre- and postoperative period little change occurs in the respiratory quotient or interaction of foodstuffs. However, significant changes occur after major fractures or burns (Fig 13–1).

For convenient reference, Table 13–2 lists some numerical data that may be useful in making estimates of changes in various metabolic parameters.

Protein Catabolic Response to Trauma

It has often been observed that the rate of excretion of nitrogen is increased after trauma or the stress of an operation. This is not due simply to starvation. Under normal circumstances, an individual receiving no protein nitrogen maintains urinary nitrogen excretion at a normal or reduced rate (4–6 g/day) for a time, after which excretion gradually declines. In contrast, after major trauma and with no protein intake, urinary nitrogen may increase to as much as 7–15 g/day for 2–5 days. With more extensive trauma, nitrogen excretion may reach 20 g/day, and major injury complicated by infection can be associated with loss of as much as 30 g/day, equivalent to the loss of 180 g of protein per day derived from about 1 kg (wet weight) of lean tissue, largely skeletal muscle.

In the first 5 days after major trauma, the average patient loses a total of about 50 g of nitrogen (equivalent to 312 g protein; 1500 g wet weight lean tissue). Most of the lost protein is derived from skeletal muscle. No other tissue could support such large losses of protein as have been observed in these catabolic states. After severe trauma and prolonged infection, a decrease in skeletal muscle mass of 30% has been observed.

Through gluconeogenesis, the metabolic breakdown of protein produces carbohydrate, which can be utilized for energy. For example, when enough muscle is sacrificed to give a daily urinary excretion of 20 g of nitrogen, about 125 g of glucose (500 Cal of energy) are produced.

The oxidation of 1 kg of fat produces slightly more than 100 ml of water of oxidation. One kilogram of lean tissue produces 730 ml of cellular water plus another 250 ml of water of oxidation from protein breakdown. All of this additional "endogenous" water contributes to overhydration of patients in the immediate posttrauma period.

Extensive losses of nitrogen constitute a serious nutritional problem after extensive burns. After soft tissue trauma with uncomplicated convalescence and healing, the period of increased nitrogen excretion persists for only 2–5 days. However, nitrogen catabolism is prolonged after burns of even moderate severity. The excretion of nitrogen tends toward a maximum of 25–35 g of nitrogen per day at the end of the first postburn week. Beginning about 7–10 days after the burn, the nitrogen loss diminishes slowly, but positive nitrogen balance is not attained until 30–40 days after injury and only when the burn wound is healed or grafted.

In the burned patient, nitrogen is also lost in the protein-rich exudate that escapes from the burned surface. For example, one man with a 33% burn was found to lose 7.8 g/day of nitrogen (equivalent to 49 g of protein) in this way. Plasma protein may also pass from the circulation directly into the injured tissues.

The nitrogen losses of the early postburn period undoubtedly result from extensive tissue catabolism. During the first 10 days after a severe burn, if the mean nitrogen loss is 18 g/day, the whole tissue loss would be as much as 540 g/day. In one study, burn patients lost a total of 8.2–11.7 kg of lean body tissue during the catabolic period.

Only when large amounts of readily utilized calories and protein are provided during the catabolic period can the net nitrogen loss be halted. This indicates that the metabolic effects of trauma on protein nutrition are mainly attributable to factors other than starvation. The severe stimulus for protein catabolism during the period early after trauma is quite difficult to overcome by providing exogenous nutrients. For example, during the early postburn period (7–10 days), ambitious attempts at feeding often result in nausea, vomiting, and diarrhea, which worsen the nutritional status of the patient.

The hormonal trigger for the catabolism of trauma appears to be release of catecholamines from the adrenal medulla. The serum levels and duration of catecholamine secretion are determined by the type and severity of the injury and associated events, such as shock and hypoxia. ACTH, released in response to catecholamine stimulation, liberates adrenal corticosteroids. Adrenal mineralocorticoids and the renal hormones renin and angiotensin evoke retention of sodium and water by the kidney. The relative resistance to insulin characteristic of the posttraumatic state is most likely due to direct peripheral effects of catecholamines plus indirect effects from glucagon released from the pancreas.

Potassium Metabolism in Trauma

Potassium losses are substantial whenever there is tissue breakdown and nitrogen loss. In the first day after moderately severe trauma, 2.7–3.5 g (38–50 mEq) of potassium may be excreted. A negative potassium balance of 2–5 g/day occurs immediately after a burn. In contrast to nitrogen, posttraumatic potassium losses tend to decrease rapidly, so that if adequate amounts of potassium are provided, positive balance is regained in 3–6 days.

Caloric Deficits in Trauma

Inadequate caloric intake follows severe injury or extensive surgery, particularly if the peritoneal cavity is opened. Patients usually lose weight during the immediate postoperative period. If not, overloading with water and salt should be suspected.

The caloric deficit requires that energy sources within the body be mobilized to meet minimal energy needs. Carbohydrate—mostly as liver and muscle glycogen and glucose in the extracellular fluid—will be quickly utilized. The total available carbohydrate in these forms is no more than 300–500 g, equivalent to 1200–2000 Cal of energy. Within 8–16 hours after any significant surgical procedure, these readily available carbohydrate stores will be exhausted.

PARENTERAL NUTRITION

When the gastrointestinal tract cannot be used for nutritional purposes and only the intravenous route is available, specific nutrients can be added to the intravenous fluids. The principal problem under these circumstances is to provide sufficient calories.

Nutrients added to peripheral intravenous solutions given to the average postoperative patient who will be eating again within a week significantly reduce protein catabolism by inhibiting gluconeogenesis, but they fail to meet the entire caloric expenditure. In most cases this is acceptable. However, when caloric or protein needs are especially urgent, the patient must be considered as a candidate for total parenteral nutrition as described in the next section. The following comments deal with the nutritional management of the ordinary postoperative patient, who experiences a short period of incomplete caloric replacement.

Carbohydrates

A. Glucose: One liter of 5% dextrose (glucose) provides less than 200 Cal. With an average total fluid intake of 3 liters/day in adults, 5% dextrose solutions provide a maximum of 510 Cal/day. The minimum caloric expenditure of a patient confined to bed is 1800 Cal/day. Thus, a substantial caloric deficit from exogenous sources always exists during postoperative parenteral nutrition. Although more concentrated glucose solutions yield more calories, they are hypertonic and must be given through a central venous catheter.

B. Fructose: When administered intravenously, fructose disappears from the blood faster than dextrose. It therefore can be administered more rapidly than dextrose and with less loss into the urine. For this reason, fructose has been studied for use as a possible substitute for dextrose in intravenous nutrition. The caloric value of fructose is the same as that of dextrose; however, the advantages of fructose are not significant enough to recommend its general use as a substitute for dextrose in parenteral fluids. There is evidence that considerable energy is required for the liver to convert fructose to glucose, a step required for utilization of fructose by most tissues.

Fat

The addition of fat to an intravenous regimen would minimize the caloric deficit which is otherwise inevitable under these circumstances. Emulsions of 10% soybean oil (Intralipid 10%) for intravenous use serve as an effective source of calories. For short-term use as a caloric supplement in the average patient, this preparation is too expensive. However, it does have an increasing role in regimens for total parenteral nutrition (see next section).

Protein

To administer protein parenterally, amino acid mixtures may be used. These 5% protein solutions in dextrose are generally well tolerated if given at rates not exceeding 300 ml/hour. It has been shown that 5% amino acid solutions are slightly more effective than 5% dextrose for protein sparing in postoperative patients. However, they are more expensive than 5% dextrose and cannot be justified for routine postoperative use. It is in regimens for total parenteral nutrition, where protein anabolism is the objective, that the amino acid solutions are so important (see next section).

Plasma or purified fractions of plasma such as albumin, when given intravenously, are used in part for nutritional purposes; however, as a source of protein nitrogen, albumin is uneconomical compared with amino acids. Consequently, these proteins should not be administered solely for nutritional purposes.

TOTAL PARENTERAL NUTRITION (TPN)*
(Hyperalimentation)

Anatomic or functional loss of the gut is no longer inevitably followed by malnutrition since it is now possible to supply enough calories and amino acids intravenously to maintain homeostasis for months. High-caloric nutrition can also be given intravenously to supplement oral feeding when caloric demands exceed what can be absorbed through the gastrointestinal tract. The gastrointestinal tract should be used to the extent possible with oral or tube feeding. If the gut is unavailable, TPN is employed.

Indications & Results of Total Parenteral Nutrition

The indications for TPN are difficult to define precisely. In general, TPN is most useful for patients with severe protein-calorie malnutrition, for patients who will be unable to take adequate nourishment orally for 2 weeks or more, and for patients with especially high metabolic expenditure from disease or injury. The most common indications are for patients with postoperative enterocutaneous fistulas, prolonged intestinal obstruction, abdominal or thoracic infection, burns, major trauma, short bowel syndrome, uremia, severe ulcerative colitis, and Crohn's disease and for preoperative replenishment of malnourished patients with cancer. A recent loss of 10% or more of body weight or a serum albumin level below 3 g/100 ml is a clinical manifestation of severe malnutrition and suggests that a 2- to 3-week period of TPN might be useful if elective surgery is being contemplated.

Preliminary reports suggest that TPN may have a specific rather than just a supportive role in the treatment of patients with inflammatory bowel disease. Especially in regional enteritis confined to the small intestine, prompt remissions have followed a 2- to 3-week period of TPN in conjunction with other therapy. With Crohn's disease of the colon or ulcerative colitis, the results have been less striking.

The use of TPN in the treatment of patients with cancer is controversial. If the malignancy is preterminal, TPN is meddlesome. On the other hand, if prolonged palliation can be realistically anticipated with radiation or chemotherapy, TPN may offset the complications of diarrhea, nausea, and weight loss that so frequently accompany such treatment.

First, an attempt is made to estimate the caloric requirements. Assume that for adults the basal caloric expenditure is approximately 1800 Cal/day; that 1 degree F of fever will cause a 7% rise in caloric need; and that bed rest alone will account for 30% of the total caloric need of the patient. In the absence of special considerations, approximately 2500–3000 Cal/day will meet caloric requirements. However, more than 45 Cal/kg/day must be administered to malnourished patients to make them anabolic. The most severely injured patients with uncontrolled infection may need as much as 5000–6000 Cal/day.

Nitrogen balance is in part dependent on the carbohydrate content of infusions, since carbohydrate promotes incorporation of plasma amino acid into muscle protein. The optimal calorie:nitrogen ratio may vary. The normal adult diet contains 150 to 200 nonprotein calories per gram of nitrogen. From 150 to 250 nonprotein calories per gram of nitrogen are usually

---

*The acronym TPN will be used throughout this section to denote high-caloric intravenous feeding, and will be considered loosely synonomous with the terms "total parenteral nutrition" and "hyperalimentation."

optimal for TPN solutions. However, there is a linear relationship between the percentage of nitrogen incorporated into protoplasm and the amount of carbohydrate administered until a level of approximately 425 nonprotein calories per gram of nitrogen is reached. In disorders contributing to urea retention (eg, renal failure), a calorie to nitrogen ratio of 200–300:1 is needed to depress urea formation.

Anabolic storage of nitrogen (as protoplasm) requires positive balances of phosphorus and potassium and is strongly influenced by the availability of sodium and chloride. Balance data from patients receiving TPN show that each new protoplasmic unit requires a specific amount of intracellular and extracellular fluid with their characteristic ionic compositions. Administered carbohydrate that cannot participate in protein anabolism because of insufficient inorganic salt is stored as fat, a relatively undesirable end point. In one study, when patients were given amino acids as a nitrogen source (2.5 g amino acid/kg ideal body weight/day), inorganic salts, and about 4500 Cal/day, weight gain consisted of 35–50% as protoplasm, 35–50% as extracellular fluid, 5–25% as adipose tissue, and less than 1% as bone.

Protein Base Solutions for TPN

The currently available protein base solutions are either crystalline synthetic L-amino acids or hydrolysates of fibrin or casein. The protein hydrolysates are supplied as 10% solutions and the amino acids as 3.5–8.5% solutions. These base solutions should be diluted with concentrated dextrose to half of the original protein concentration before they are administered.

Protein hydrolysate solutions were the only available source of protein when TPN was first introduced and are still frequently used. However, a variable amount—up to 40% in some preparations—of the nitrogen in the protein hydrolysates exists as polypeptides and cannot participate in protein anabolism. Free ammonia is also present and may be undesirable under certain circumstances (eg, in infants or patients with hepatic disease). The amino acid solutions have neither of these drawbacks. Although the protein hydrolysates are acceptable and effective, it seems probable that over the next few years they will gradually be replaced by amino acid solutions for routine use in TPN.

The amino acid solutions contain essential and nonessential amino acids as acetate salts (eg, Freamine II). The original preparations, in which the amino acids existed as chloride salts, have been withdrawn from the market because hyperchloremic acidosis occasionally developed from the high chloride load.

A preparation containing only essential amino acids (known as Freamine E or Nephramine), currently available for experimental use only, may have special application in the treatment of patients with renal failure in whom maximal anabolism with minimal urea production is the therapeutic objective.

Other specially designed solutions emphasizing certain amino acids or groups of amino acids are certain to become available as research defines the peculiar metabolic needs in specific diseases. For example, there is accumulating evidence that patients with hepatic decompensation should receive larger amounts of branched chain amino acids and less aromatic amino acids than patients with normal liver function.

Preparation of Solutions

Originally, the dextrose/amino acid solutions were prepared by mixing anhydrous dextrose with protein hydrolysate and 5% dextrose solutions. Now, 500 ml bottles of 50% or 70% dextrose are available for combining with the 500 ml bottles of 8.5% crystalline amino acids or 10% protein hydrolysate. Preparation of the solutions must be performed by a trained pharmacy technician under a laminar flow hood with the utmost precautions to avoid contamination. The protein base is diluted 1:1 with one of the concentrated glucose solutions (and water if necessary) to achieve any desired final glucose concentration between 15% and 35%. Electrolyte concentrates are then added in amounts tailored to the patient's needs as reflected by his recent serum values. Unless contraindicated, 50 mEq of Na^+, 40 mEq of K^+, and 15–25 mEq of phosphate (as KH_2PO_4) should be added per 1000 Cal (ie, per liter), using concentrated solutions of the electrolytes.

Fortification with vitamins should be accomplished by equally dividing among the 3 bottles 10 ml of a preparation of fat- and water-soluble vitamins (MVI). Magnesium (4–8 mEq/day) may also be added as magnesium sulfate. Intramuscular injections of vitamin B_{12}, K, and folic acid should be given intermittently during prolonged TPN. If plasma analysis suggests the need, calcium gluconate should also be supplied. Unless there has been a preexisting iron deficiency or extensive hemorrhage, or both, iron is not required. Transfusions of whole blood will supply iron, as will intramuscular administration of iron dextran injection (Imferon). Trace mineral elements such as zinc, copper, manganese, cobalt, and iodine may be added if TPN is prolonged beyond 1 month.

Table 13–3 summarizes the average nutrient composition of 2500–3000 ml of solution prepared as described above for TPN in adults. Solutions intended for use in children requiring long-term TPN are prepared as for adults with minor modifications. This subject is discussed further in Chapter 48.

Technic of Administration

Because they are hypertonic, the solutions described above for TPN must be infused into a vein with rapid blood flow. The preferred site for inserting the catheter is the subclavian vein, a relatively fixed structure beneath the clavicle. With the catheter in this location, the patients can be ambulatory and use their upper extremities. In certain cases, one may elect to administer the solution through an arteriovenous fistula (eg, Scribner shunt; see Chapter 51). For use at home, the Broviac right atrial catheter ("artificial gut") has been successful.

Since the ability of the endocrine pancreas to re-

Table 13–3. Average daily composition of adult TPN solution.*

Water	2500–3000 ml
Protein hydrolysate (amino acids)	100–130 g
Nitrogen	12–18 g
Carbohydrate (dextrose)	525–625 g
Calories	2500–3000
Sodium	125–150 mEq
Potassium	75–120 mEq
Phosphorus	20–25 mEq/1000 Cal
Magnesium	4–8 mEq

*Calcium is added to the solution when indicated. Iron is added to the solution, or given intramuscularly in depot form as iron dextran injection, or given as blood transfusion if indicated. Vitamin B_{12}, vitamin K, and folic acid are given intramuscularly or added for intravenous administration as indicated. Trace elements such as zinc, copper, manganese, cobalt, and iodine are added only after total intravenous therapy exceeds 1 month.

spond with adequate insulin increases with the duration of the demand, the quantity of glucose infused must be increased gradually over several days or the sugar may not be completely utilized. This can be accomplished either by gradually increasing the concentration of glucose, keeping the fluid volume constant, or by gradually increasing the volume of solution, keeping the concentration of glucose constant.

With the former method, therapy should be initiated with 2500–3000 ml of 15% glucose and 4.25% amino acid (or protein hydrolysate) solution, increasing the concentration of glucose by 5% each day. The usual end point is a final concentration of 25–30%. The advantage of this approach is that from the start, the volume of solution will usually satisfy the total daily fluid requirement.

If it is decided to start with a 25 or 30% concentration of glucose, the total fluid requirement (3000 ml in the average patient) will not be provided through the nutrient solution for several days. The first day's fluids are given as 1000 ml of 30% glucose per 4.25% amino acids over 24 hours. The additional fluid (about 2000 ml) is given in the usual way through a peripheral vein. Each succeeding day an additional 1000 ml of TPN solution is given with the rate adjusted so that the total volume is administered at a constant rate over 24 hours. By the third or fourth day, the patient is receiving about 3000 ml of TPN solution and no peripheral fluid supplementation is usually required.

The amount of available nitrogen varies with the different protein base solutions. For example, 5% Travamin provides 6.5 g of nitrogen per liter and, in 30% glucose, a calorie:nitrogen ratio of 157:1. If Freamine II is used, a glucose concentration of 30% provides a ratio of 163:1. With 30% glucose, 5.5% Travasol provides a ratio of 220:1.

With the institution of TPN, the plasma glucose should be monitored daily and the urine glucose every 6 hours. The blood sugar should stabilize below 200 mg/100 ml. A urine sugar of 1+ or 2+ does not require

treatment; larger amounts of glycosuria require insulin, which should be added to the TPN solution (10–20 units of regular insulin per liter will usually suffice). The occurrence of severe hyperglycemia or excessive glycosuria in the first few days of therapy may require a slower schedule for building up to the maximum glucose load. Glycosuria should be stringently avoided by all available means. Consistent 2–3+ glycosuria means that 30% of the infused calories are being excreted in the urine. Some patients are best maintained at final glucose concentrations lower than 25 or 30 mg/100 ml. Although diabetics usually require supplementary insulin, they can be managed with little difficulty in most cases. Once the glucose tolerance has been determined, it remains quite stable in most patients. Sudden decreased tolerance to glucose during the course of established therapy suggests infection and demands immediate attention.

For efficient utilization of calories and nitrogen, the rate of administration must be constant. A microdrip regulator can be used, but a calibrated infusion pump (eg, IVAC pump) is much better. Excessive amounts infused over short periods will result in loss of glucose in the urine and may precipitate hyperosmotic coma as a result of the osmotic diuresis. Hyperosmotic coma is the most significant early complication and carries a 60% mortality rate. For this reason, the nursing staff should be cautioned not to increase the rate of administration to catch up if the volume infused lags behind schedule.

When therapy is discontinued suddenly, serum levels of insulin may remain high enough to cause hypoglycemia. Therefore, it is usually best to taper the therapy by gradually cutting back on the amount of glucose over 48 hours before withdrawing it completely.

After the infusion is begun, careful monitoring is required (see insert protocol). Signs of success are weight gain, increased levels of serum proteins, and a fall in BUN. The BUN drops (sometimes to low levels, eg, 3–5 mg/100 ml) because the glucose inhibits gluconeogenesis.

Measurement of nitrogen balance is the simplest and most useful way to assess the adequacy of therapy. Approximately 90% of nitrogen lost from the body each day is excreted in the urine, and urea nitrogen comprises 70% of the total urinary nitrogen. Therefore, a reasonable estimate of the total nitrogen excretion per day (in grams) can be obtained by measuring the urea nitrogen concentration in an aliquot of urine and multiplying this number by the 24-hour urine volume. Add 2 g to account for the other sources of urinary nitrogen (ammonia, uric acid, amino acids, etc) and the result is nitrogen excretion. To estimate nitrogen balance, calculate nitrogen intake from the concentration of amino acid nitrogen and volume of TPN fluid being given per 24 hours and subtract the nitrogen excretion.

To determine more directly if caloric needs are being satisfied, oxygen consumption can be measured using any of several technics generally available (eg,

---

Monitoring Protocol for Total Parenteral Nutrition

1. Baseline studies to be obtained before starting TPN:

Hemoglobin	Fasting blood sugar	SGOT
Hematocrit	BUN	Alkaline phosphatase
Red blood cell indices	Creatinine	
Platelet count	Uric acid	Cholesterol
Na^+ Ca^{++}	Total protein	Triglycerides
K^+ $PO_4^{\equiv}$	Albumin	Serum osmolality
Cl^- Mg^{++}	Prothrombin time	
CO_2	Bilirubin	Urinalysis
Serum iron and iron-binding		Chest x-ray
capacity		ECG

2. Studies to be obtained daily until the patient is stabilized (5–7 days):

   Fractional urine for glucose every 6 hours (with simultaneous blood glucose determinations for the first 24–48 hours)
   Blood glucose
   Serum electrolytes
   Accurate records of intake and output
   Body weight
   Nitrogen balance

3. Routine studies after the patient is stabilized:

   Daily: Intake and output, body weight, fractional urines for glucose 2–3 times weekly: Electrolytes (Na^+, K^+, Cl^-, CO_2)
   Once weekly: Complete platelet count, prothrombin time, BUN, serum creatinine, calcium, phosphorus, red blood cell indices
   Once monthly: Repeat baseline studies and also measure serum vitamin B_{12} and folate.

4. Measurement of nitrogen balance indicates whether anabolism has been achieved. If the patient is not gaining weight, oxygen consumption may be measured to calculate caloric needs.

Douglas bag). The oxygen consumption in liters per 24 hours multiplied by 4.825 gives a reasonable estimate of caloric expenditure.

If the patient is not responding to therapy as expected, remember that to stimulate anabolism 1.75–2 times the basal energy expenditure in calories (over 45 Cal/kg/day in a patient with a normal metabolic rate) must be provided and the solutions must contain a nonprotein calorie:gram of nitrogen ratio of 150:1 or greater.

Intravenous Fat Emulsion

A 10% soybean oil emulsion (Intralipid 10%) is available as a caloric source for intravenous administration. The emulsified fat particles are about 0.5 μm in diameter, and, because the solution is isotonic, it can be infused through a peripheral vein. The exact composition is 10% soybean oil, 1.2% egg yolk phospholipids, and 2.25% glycerol in water.

The preparation is not associated with allergic reactions such as those that occurred with use of older fat preparations (eg, Lipomul) designed for intravenous use. The fat is metabolized as an energy source, but, because of limitations on the rate of utilization and continued requirements for carbohydrate and protein, it cannot be given alone. The fraction of calories from fat should not exceed 70% of the total daily caloric intake; the remainder should be derived from glucose and amino acids.

Although fat has the theoretic advantage of a higher caloric content (9 Cal/g) than dextrose (4 Cal/g), a 500 ml unit of 10% Intralipid contains only 550 Calories. Intravenous fat costs approximately 3 times more than dextrose for an equivalent amount of calories. Moreover, it is not yet clear whether fat is as effective as carbohydrate for inducing protein sparing and anabolism.

The most clearly defined indication for intravenous fat is in the treatment or prevention of essential fatty acid (EFA) deficiency, which appears with diets that chronically supply less than 2% of calories as linoleic acid. Patients treated with standard TPN solutions devoid of lipid will develop biochemical evidence of EFA deficiency within 3 days of treatment and may show clinical signs of the deficiency within 10 days. EFA deficiency is characterized biochemically by low serum or red cell levels of essential polyunsaturated fatty acids and a compensatory increase in saturated fatty acids. Fatty acid alterations may be expressed in absolute terms or as a ratio of the trienoic to tetraenoic acids. This ratio, which rises during EFA deficiency, may be used as a guide to follow the response to fatty acid replacement. Additionally, the specific fatty acid $\Delta^{5,8}$-eicosatrienoic acid, is virtually absent from normal serum but is elevated during EFA deficiency; its presence in serum is diagnostic of EFA deficiency.

Clinical signs of EFA deficiency are most apparent in the skin as a flat, scaly, erythematous dermatitis, especially in the groin or axilla. In advanced cases, elephantine folds are present.

Essential fatty acid deficiency may be prevented (or treated) by administering 500 ml of intravenous soybean emulsion (Intralipid 10%) on alternate days to patients who are receiving hypertonic dextrose/amino acid solutions.

The 10% soybean oil emulsion may also be used to achieve total parenteral nutrition through a peripheral vein, but less than 3000 Calories per day can be given this way. Because of this limitation and the others cited above, most workers currently feel that a hypertonic dextrose regimen via a central venous line is preferable for most patients who need TPN.

A technic for TPN through a peripheral vein is as follows:

To provide 2000 Cal in 3100 ml of fluid per 24 hours:

  5% glucose in 4.25% amino acid solution given at a rate of 87 ml/hour, plus—
  10% Intralipid given at a rate of 42 ml/hour.

The glucose/amino acid solution should be infused simultaneously with the 10% soybean oil emulsion, either into a separate vein or through a Y connector. All electrolytes, vitamins, and micronutrients should be added to the glucose/amino acid solution; anything added to the fat solution endangers the stability of the emulsion. The initial infusion rate of fat solution in adults should be 1 ml per minute for the first 30 minutes. If no adverse reactions are apparent (dyspnea, cyanosis, allergic reactions, nausea, etc—see product literature for complete list), increase the infusion rate so that 500 ml are infused on the first day. Subsequently, up to 1500 ml may be infused over a 24-hour period.

Each 1000 ml of glucose/amino acid mixture should contain at least 20 mEq of NaCl and 20 mEq of KCl. For protein anabolism, the electrolyte requirements are similar to those with hypertonic glucose and amino acid solutions. The amounts of electrolytes must be varied according to the clinical and laboratory findings in the individual patient. One ampule of multivitamins should be given daily in portions divided among the infusion bottles.

The patient's capacity to clear the infused fat from the circulation must be monitored by measuring serum lipid concentrations; 4 hours after the end of fat infusion, the lipemia should have cleared. During continuous fat infusion, the serum triglyceride levels rise to 2–3 times normal, but deleterious effects have not been seen. In patients who deviate from these parameters, the fat emulsion should probably be stopped.

Complications of TPN

Mechanical complications related to inserting a subclavian catheter are discussed in Chapter 51. An insidious complication, which probably will be reported with increasing frequency, is thrombosis of the subclavian vein and superior vena cava. In children, the catheter is inserted by a cutdown into the facial vein and is threaded into the superior vena cava through the internal jugular vein. For long-term use in children, some protection from infection will be provided if the line is tunneled subcutaneously into the neck through a scalp incision.

A. Sepsis: Sepsis is a serious complication of TPN, in part because the high-caloric, high-protein solution serves as an ideal culture medium. Infection rates as high as 30% were reported in a survey by the Center for Disease Control, but by using strict precautions it is possible to reduce the incidence to about 3%. The risk of catheter sepsis is greater in patients with intermittent bacteremia. Such patients can be given TPN safely if the subclavian catheter is removed whenever fever develops. In such circumstances, the tip of the catheter, the filter, and the tubing should be cultured as well as the solution itself. The septicemia usually clears if the catheter is promptly removed. The indications for removal of the TPN catheter are listed in Table 13–4.

Avoidance of septic complications begins when the catheter line is first placed. Cap, gown, and mask should be worn, and sterile technic should be followed. The tubing from the bottle of TPN fluid as well as the filter should be changed daily. On alternate days, the dressing should be removed, the incision site defatted with acetone, cleaned, and sealed, and a sterile occlusive dressing applied.

Contamination of the intravenous solution itself should be rare even though the low pH (5.5) of most of these solutions provides an ideal environment for growth of candida. The solutions must be freshly prepared by a pharmacist under a laminar air flow hood and cultures should be obtained regularly from the prepared solution.

B. Metabolic Complications:

1. Hyperosmolar nonketotic dehydration—This is a direct consequence of administering glucose faster than it can be metabolized, with the production of an osmotic diuresis by prolonged severe glycosuria. If coma occurs, death is common. Prevention entails regularly monitoring the urine specific gravity and glucose content, the blood sugar, and the serum osmolarity. In uremic patients or those with low creatinine

---

Table 13–4. Indications for removal of TPN catheter.

Relative Indications

  Fever.

  Glycosuria.

  Persistent sepsis after apparently adequate treatment for an infection unrelated to the TPN.

  Appearance of candida infections at sites unrelated to the TPN catheter.

  Contamination of the TPN line.

Absolute

  Septicemia or septic shock.

  Proved or suspected infection at the catheter insertion site.

clearance, urine sugar will not accurately reflect blood sugar. Since both glucose and urea are osmotically active, the serum osmolality must be measured frequently when giving TPN to patients in renal failure. If hyperosmolality occurs, the patients must be hydrated and given insulin to drive glucose into the cells. Exogenous potassium is also required because potassium enters the cells as the glucose is converted to glycogen.

2. Hyperchloremic metabolic acidosis—Because the amino acids in Freamine existed as chloride salts, hyperchloremic metabolic acidosis was an occasional complication of the high chloride load. To obviate this problem, Freamine II was marketed with acetate as the anion and the earlier preparation was withdrawn.

3. Azotemia—The protein hydrolysate solutions contain free ammonia, which is poorly tolerated by patients with hepatic and renal dysfunction. Azotemic patients must be observed carefully while receiving any of the amino acid or protein hydrolysate solutions. Freamine E, which contains only essential amino acids, is metabolized more efficiently than hydrolysates or amino acid solutions which have a 1:1 ratio of essential to nonessential amino acids. Freamine E is optimal for the uremic patient, who has excess circulating nitrogen compounds, which can participate in anabolism if adequate substrate in the form of hypertonic dextrose and essential amino acids is administered. TPN in uremia is an intravenous form of the Giordano-Giovanetti treatment, which may control potassium and BUN levels, thus delaying the need for dialysis. Improved survival has been reported with this therapy compared to the use of hypertonic dextrose alone in patients with acute tubular necrosis.

4. Hypophosphatemia—Some of the available base solutions do not contain adequate amounts of phosphate, and, unless phosphate is added as a supplement, hypophosphatemia will develop within 48 hours after starting TPN therapy. If 20 mEq of potassium dihydrogen phosphate are given per 1000 Cal, hypophosphatemia can be prevented. The hypophosphatemia results from intracellular accretion of phosphate from the serum and is accompanied by a drop in urinary phosphate excretion. Hypophosphatemia produces a decline in red cell adenosine triphosphate (ATP) and 2,3-diphosphoglycerate (2,3-DPG) which results in impairment of the capacity of the blood to deliver oxygen to the tissues. If hypophosphatemia develops, serum inorganic phosphate levels will return to normal within 12 hours of discontinuing the TPN solution. TPN-associated phosphate debt is cumulative. If hypophosphatemia occurs, more than 20 mEq of phosphate per 1000 Calories must be given to correct the deficiency.

Ambulatory Parenteral Nutrition

Technics have recently been devised to administer chronic TPN ("artificial gut") at home for ambulatory patients afflicted with short bowel or severe malabsorption syndromes. The nutrient solution is administered most satisfactorily through a right atrial catheter (Broviac shunt) which is tunneled beneath the chest wall, maintained with a heparin lock, and capped. Depending on the amount of caloric support required, the patient can connect the catheter to a pump and receive the solution at night while asleep. For patients who require total parenteral nutrition, infusions can be administered around the clock, using a battery-driven pump worn around the waist like a belt. This therapy, which is somewhat similar to home renal dialysis, has provided new hope for a relatively normal life for patients with short bowel syndrome.

TUBE FEEDING

Tube feeding is often the best way to nourish patients with complete or partially intact gastrointestinal tracts, who nonetheless cannot take food orally. For example, tube feeding is frequently indicated for comatose patients, patients with lesions of the mouth, pharynx, or esophagus, patients with enterocutaneous fistulas, and sometimes as a dietary supplement that can be administered while the patient is asleep. In general, if nutritional needs can be satisfied in this way, tube feeding is preferable to TPN, but the eventual objective is to resume oral intake of a normal diet as soon as possible.

Most formulas for tube feeding are designed to provide about 1 Cal/ml. Higher concentrations are not well tolerated, producing bloating, cramps, flatulence, and diarrhea. In addition, the daily caloric load cannot usually be pushed much beyond 3000 Cal with these solutions before diarrhea and other side-effects appear. Consequently, tube feeding may have to be supplemented by high-caloric intravenous fluids in patients with especially great caloric requirements (eg, burns, multiple fractures, major sepsis).

Tube Feeding Formulas

The types of liquid diets for tube feeding include the following: (1) commercially available balanced liquid formulas, (2) commercially available low-residue balanced formulas, (3) elemental diets, requiring no endogenous digestion, (4) hospital-prepared milk and sugar formulas, and (5) blenderized food. Because these diets offer excellent support for bacterial growth after they are prepared for infusion, they must be used within 24 hours. In most hospitals, the ease of handling the commercially available products will more than outweigh their greater expense compared with locally prepared solutions.

When choosing a liquid diet for tube feeding, consider if the patient has special requirements that might indicate the need for a low-residue or elemental diet. If he does not, use one of the less specialized balanced formulas. Some characteristics of the tube feeding solutions marketed in the USA are given in Table 13–5.

A. Balanced Liquid Formulas: These preparations are designed to provide a complete range of required

Table 13—5. Commercial preparations for tube-feeding a balanced diet.

| Preparation | Percent by Weight | | | Cal/g N | Na+/K+ (mEq/liter) | Cal/ml | Osmolality (mOsm/kg) | Remarks* |
	Carbo-hydrate	Fat	Protein					
Balanced tube feeding formulas								
Complete-B	60	20	20	156	60/37	1	468	Blenderized meat, vegetable and milk base.
Ensure	66	17	17	168	32/32	1	450	No lactose. Carbohydrate as sucrose. Fat as corn oil. Soy and casein protein.
Isocal	63	21	16	192	22/32	1.04	350	No lactose. Fat as MCT and soy oil. Soy and casein protein.
Nutri-1000	54	28	17.6	181	23/31	1.06	500	Skim milk, casein, corn oil, sucrose.
Portagen	58	24	17.7	178	22/32	1	236	No lactose. Fat as MCT.
Low-residue formulas								
Precision LR	84	0.3	9.1	263	27/20	1.08	600	Protein as egg albumin. Fat as soy-
Precision HN	75	0.2	16.6	150	41/22	1	580	bean oil. Carbohydrate as maltodex-
Precision MN	64	13.2	15.2	192	37/19	1.12	475	trin (44%) and sucrose (6%).
Elemental diets								
Vivonex Std	85	0.54	(20.4)	300	37/30	1	500	Carbohydrate as glucose. Nitrogen as
Vivonex HN	79	0.33	(41.7)	150	34/18	1	844	synthetic essential and nonessential amino acids.
Flexical	78	15	22.5	277	15/32	1	724	Fat as soy oil and MCT. Protein as casein hydrolysate plus L-Met, L-Trp, L-Tyr.

*MCT = medium chain triglycerides.

nutrients in physiologic quantities and proportions, suitable for prolonged use as the sole source of nourishment. Several of these products have little or no lactose, a sugar which is poorly tolerated by many adults. Medium chain triglycerides are included in 2 of the preparations.

B. Low-Residue Formulas: These preparations include egg albumin as the source of protein. They are more palatable than the elemental diets.

C. Elemental Diets: Vivonex and Flexical contain nitrogen in the form of amino acids instead of intact protein. Vivonex is manufactured with synthetic amino acids; Flexical is a casein hydrolysate with 3 amino acids added. Despite the addition of flavoring, these preparations are relatively unpalatable, a consequence of their amino acid content. The principal advantage of elemental diets is that they can be absorbed over relatively short (100–150 cm) lengths of intestine and do not require digestion by pancreatic and biliary secretions. Their major uses are in the management of patients with gastrointestinal fistulas or short bowel syndromes. Because its pH is low, Vivonex can be particularly irritating if it is aspirated into the tracheobronchial tree.

The addition of flavoring to elemental diets does not improve palatability to the extent that they become acceptable in large volumes to the average patient. Furthermore, the high osmolality of these solutions may cause diarrhea if the rate of administration is not smooth. Therefore, elemental diets are not particularly useful as dietary supplements and should be regarded as formulas with limited special usefulness when tube feeding is indicated.

When it is planned to administer 2000–3000 Cal/day of an elemental diet preparation, the full amount cannot be given at the start. The preparation should be diluted to half the ordinary strength and instilled at a rate of 50 ml/hour. Gradually, the concentration and rate of administration are increased over 5–7 days while the intestine adapts. Because it is rarely possible to accelerate this schedule, elemental diets are not a practical consideration unless tube feeding will be required for more than a week.

D. Hospital-Prepared Liquid Formulas: In preparing formulas for tube feeding, simple sugars such as dextrose and large amounts of fat such as cream should be avoided because they cause diarrhea. The preferred source of carbohydrate is a dextrinized starch such as Dextri-Maltose. A simple formula for tube feeding is as follows:

Homogenized milk	2200 ml
Eggs	600 ml
Dextri-Maltose	7 tbsp

(In a total volume of 3000 ml, this mixture contains 120 g protein and 3000 Cal.)

Homogenized milk alone is often the simplest substance to use at the beginning of a tube feeding regimen. It contains 3.5 g of protein and about 70 Cal/100 ml.

E. Blenderized Diets and Purees: More concentrated mixtures can be a problem with gastrostomy tubes. A simple formula that utilizes commercially available pureed infant foods is as follows:

	Protein (g)	Calories
3½ oz strained beef	14.6	103
4½ oz beets	1.5	51
3 raw eggs	18.0	225
Homogenized milk (640 ml)	23.3	466
Totals	57.4	845

Other meats and vegetables can be used to vary the formula.

Administration of Tube Feedings

The infusion should begin with about half the volume and concentration eventually desired and should build up gradually over 24–48 hours.

The best nasogastric tube for prolonged feeding is 8F or less in diameter. The flaccid tube can be placed by wedging the tip inside a gelatin capsule alongside the tip of a 16F nasogastric tube. The 2 tubes are passed as a unit. Two hours later, water is flushed down the larger tube to wash away the remnants of the capsule and the large tube is withdrawn, leaving the feeding tube in position. The position of nasogastric feeding tubes should usually be verified radiographically before starting the infusion.

When instillation of the formula is begun, check every 2 hours during the first day to make certain that the feeding is leaving the stomach. Always be alert to the possibility of gastric distention if new events occur in the clinical course (eg, operation, sepsis) that might produce ileus. Gastric retention is common in the kinds of patients who require tube feeding, and aspiration can be a lethal complication.

Bolus feeding through tubes is usually less satisfactory than a continuous infusion. Intermittent instillation of 200–300 ml may be satisfactory for gastrostomy feedings, but most patients requiring temporary tube feeding tolerate it better if a constant rate of infusion is provided (eg, IVAC pump).

None of the tube feeding formulas supply enough free water to meet metabolic needs. A liter or more of water must be given daily in addition to the formula to prevent hypernatremia and hyperosmolar coma. It can be given by further diluting the formula or as 5% dextrose in water through a peripheral vein.

Dietary Supplements

Dietary supplements are similar to tube feeding formulas, but these products emphasize palatability over a completely balanced formulation. Their principal role is as an adjunct to the main dietary regimen. For example, dietary supplements might be prescribed for burned patients who need far more than the 2500 Cal provided by the regular hospital diet. Examples of commercially available dietary supplements are Carnation Instant Breakfast, Citrotein, Meritene, Nutramigen, Sustacal, and Sustagen.

DIETS

An **optimal diet** should have the following distribution of energy sources: carbohydrate 55–60%, fat 30%, protein 10–15%. Refined sugar should comprise no more than 15% of dietary energy and saturated fats no more than 10%, the latter balanced by 10% monounsaturated and 10% polyunsaturated fats. Cholesterol intake should be limited to about 300 mg/day (one egg yolk contains 250 mg of cholesterol). The amount of salt in the average American diet, 10–18 g, far exceeds the recommended 3 g. For Western societies to meet these criteria for an optimal diet, consumption of fat would have to decrease (from 40%) and carbohydrate (principally complex carbohydrates such as potatoes and bread) would have to increase. As a source of protein, meat is presently overemphasized at the expense of grain, legumes, and nuts.

The following describes the therapeutic diets most commonly prescribed in clinical practice:

Regular diets have an unrestricted spectrum of foods and are most attractive to the patient. An average regular hospital diet for one day contains 230–275 g of carbohydrate, 95–110 g of fat, and 70–75 g of protein, with a total caloric content of 2000–2500. This composition reflects the nutritional needs of well persons of average height and weight and will not meet the increased demands imposed by malnutrition or disease.

A **soft diet** is nutritionally the same as a regular diet, but high-fiber vegetables and meats or shellfish with a tough texture are omitted.

In a **bland diet,** caffeine, spices, alcohol, and hot or cold foods are eliminated from the regular diet to make it bland. In many cases bland diets contain large amounts of milk and cream, making them high in fat content. The potential for accelerating atherosclerosis has led most workers to abandon the use of bland diets for long periods. Contrary to previous belief, a bland diet has no specific therapeutic usefulness in peptic ulcer disease.

Low residue diets are restricted in the amounts of fibrous vegetables, fruits, nuts, and milk. They emphasize lean meat, starchy vegetables, refined cereals, and carbohydrate. Low residue diets are expensive because of the large amounts of meat. Constipation may require stool softeners, bulk-forming agents such as Metamucil, or cathartics.

High bulk diets are now thought to protect against the development of diverticulosis and its complications. Bulk can be increased in the regular (relatively low bulk) diet typical of Western cultures by adding bran (60 g daily).

Clear liquid diets contain easily digestible sugars, small amounts of protein, and a caloric concentration of about 600 Cal per 2000 ml. A clear liquid diet is often prescribed for a day or 2 after an abdominal operation before the patient can resume a less restricted diet.

Full liquid diets include a wide spectrum of juices and other foods that remain liquid at body temperature. Caloric content is about 1700 Cal per 2500 ml, with 45 g of protein, 60 g of fat, and 240 g of carbohydrates.

Sodium restricted diets are often indicated for

Table 13—6. Composition of sodium-restricted diets.

Food Substance	2400—4500 mg Sodium	1000 mg Sodium	500 mg Sodium	250 mg Sodium
Milk	1 pint	1 pint	1 pint	Low-sodium ad lib.
Egg	One	One	One	One
Salt-free meat, fish, poultry	Ad lib.	6 oz	5 oz	5 oz
Bread	Ad lib.	Two slices plus low-sodium bread ad lib.	Low-sodium bread ad lib.	Low-sodium bread ad lib.
Butter, margarine, mayonnaise	Ad lib.	Two tsp regular; sweet ad lib.	Sweet ad lib.	Sweet ad lib.
Cream	Ad lib.	2 oz	2 oz	2 oz
Vegetables	Ad lib.	Low-sodium ad lib.	Low-sodium ad lib.	Low-sodium ad lib.
Fruit and juices	Ad lib.	Ad lib.	Ad lib.	Ad lib.
Desserts	One serving: cake, gelatin, ice cream, pie, pudding, sherbet	Special low-sodium only.	Special low-sodium only.	Special low-sodium only.
Cereals and starches	Ad lib.	Low-sodium only.	Low-sodium only.	Low-sodium only.

patients with cardiovascular or renal disease. Daily sodium intake in an unrestricted diet ranges from 4—6 g (174—261 mEq Na$^+$). In general, a 1000 mg sodium diet is enough restriction for most patients; more severe restriction is indicated for refractory cases.

Lactose intolerance and lactose-free diets. A variable amount of intolerance to lactose is present in many adults and is manifested by diarrhea, bloating, and flatulence after ingesting milk or milk products. Lactose intolerance is genetically determined and in adults is found in 5—10% of European Caucasians, 60% of Ashkenazic Jews, 70% of blacks, and 100% of Orientals. A previously subclinical lactose intolerance commonly becomes unmasked by an unrelated disease or operation on the gastrointestinal tract. For example, following gastrectomy, symptomatic relief from non-specific complaints may be obtained by interdicting lactose-containing foods. Similar advice is often useful in managing patients with Crohn's disease or ulcerative colitis. The frequency of lactose intolerance is high enough in the general population that it should be considered as a possible cause of flatulence and diarrhea in many clinical circumstances. The efficiency of lactose digestion and absorption can be measured by giving 100 g of lactose orally and measuring the blood glucose concentration at 30-minute intervals for 2 hours. Patients with lactose intolerance exhibit a rise in blood glucose of 20 mg/100 ml or less. However, unpredictable variations in gastric emptying interfere with its reliability, so in most cases it is better to observe the results of eliminating lactose from the diet than to perform a lactose tolerance test.

●   ●   ●

General References

Abel RM & others: Improved survival from acute renal failure after treatment with intravenous essential L-amino acid and glucose. N Engl J Med 288:695, 1973.

Ballinger W (editor): *Manual of Surgical Nutrition.* Saunders, 1975.

Blackburn GL, Bistrian BR: Nutritional care of the injured and/or septic patient. Surg Clin North Am 56:1195, 1976.

Blackburn GL & others: Peripheral intravenous feeding with isotonic amino acid solutions. Am J Surg 125:447, 1973.

Bistrian BR & others: Protein status of general surgical patients. JAMA 230:858, 1974.

Border JR & others: Multiple systems organ failure: Muscle fuel deficit with visceral protein malnutrition. Surg Clin North Am 56:1147, 1976.

Cahill GF Jr: Starvation in man. N Engl J Med 282:668, 1970.

Clowes GHA Jr & others: Energy metabolism and proteolysis in traumatized and septic man. Surg Clin North Am 56:1169, 1976.

Copeland EM III & others: Intravenous hyperalimentation as an adjunct to cancer chemotherapy. Am J Surg 129:167, 1975.

Davidson S & others: *Human Nutrition and Dietetics.* Churchill, 1975.

Dudrick SJ & others: Parenteral hyperalimentation: Metabolic problems and solutions. Ann Surg 176:259, 1972.

Fischer JE (editor): *Total Parenteral Nutrition.* Little, Brown, 1976.

Freeman JB & others: The elemental diet. Surg Gynecol Obstet 142:925, 1976.

Greenberg GR & others: Protein-sparing therapy in postoperative patients. N Engl J Med 294:1411, 1976.

Gump FE & others: Oxygen consumption and caloric expenditure in surgical patients. Surg Gynecol Obstet 137:499, 1973.

Hansen LM & others: Fat emulsion for intravenous administration: Clinical experience with Intralipid 10%. Ann Surg 184:80, 1976.

Jeejeebhoy KN & others: Metabolic studies in total parenteral nutrition with lipid in man. J Clin Invest 57:125, 1976.

Jeejeebhoy KN & others: Total parenteral nutrition at home: Studies in patients surviving 4 months to 5 years. Gastroenterology 71:943, 1976.

Moore FD: La maladie post-operatoire: Is there order in variety? The six stimulus-response sequences. Surg Clin North Am 56:803, 1976.

Reilly J & others: Hyperalimentation in inflammatory bowel disease. Am J Surg 131:192, 1976.

Riella MC, Scribner BH: Five years' experience with a right atrial catheter for prolonged parenteral nutrition at home. Surg Gynecol Obstet 143:205, 1976.

Riella MC & others: Essential fatty acid deficiency in human adults during total parenteral nutrition. Ann Intern Med 83:786, 1975.

Ryan NT: Metabolic adaptations for energy production during trauma and sepsis. Surg Clin North Am 56:1073, 1976.

Sheldon GF & others: Phosphate depletion and repletion: Relation to parenteral nutrition and oxygen transport. Ann Surg 182:683, 1975.

Viteri FE & others: Gastrointestinal alterations in protein-calorie malnutrition. Med Clin North Am 58:1487, 1974.

Wilmore DW: Hormonal responses and their effect on metabolism. Surg Clin North Am 56:999, 1976.

Wilmore DW & others: Clinical evaluation of 10% intravenous fat emulsion for parenteral nutrition in thermally injured patients. Ann Surg 178:503, 1973.

14 . . .
Anesthesiology

Neri P. Guadagni, MD

Every surgeon should have a thorough knowledge of the regional anesthetic procedures he performs himself but need not know the details and technicalities of general anesthesia conducted by a physician specialist in that field. The surgeon must understand the potentials, limitations, and hazards of all anesthetic technics and should be able to recognize good anesthesia or what is as good as a particular clinical situation permits. This chapter offers principles and guidelines for the conduct of anesthetic procedures performed by the surgeon and discusses basic concepts of the management of anesthetic procedures performed by others. The emphasis accorded to various aspects is not proportionate to their importance in anesthesiology as a branch of medical science.

Most surgical procedures cause a degree of pain or discomfort that neither the patient nor modern society will accept. Advances in methods of relieving pain and sustaining life during surgery now embody an art and science which has broadened to a discipline concerned with more than relief of pain. It serves both patient and surgeon, offering the patient freedom from pain during surgery with or without awareness and with maximum safety and provides the surgeon with a "quiet field," often in otherwise inaccessible areas, for as long as required. The methods used to achieve these goals vary with the age, size, personality, and physical condition of the patient and with the location, duration, and technical intricacies of the operation. The same technics and skills essential to these goals also have application in the emergency room, recovery room, and the intensive care ward. In the form of "nerve blocks," they have both diagnostic and therapeutic uses.

Administration of anesthesia by the operating surgeon is a practical and safe expedient limited only by his knowledge and experience and by the magnitude of the surgical or anesthetic procedure. The limitations are obvious if either surgery or anesthesia requires the undivided attention of one person. General anesthesia, even when used for minor surgery, requires continuous attention and monitoring. No surgeon should attempt to give general anesthesia and also perform the surgery except in unavoidable emergency circumstances. He may have to assume the responsibility for anesthetic management when administered by a technician such as a nurse anesthetist who

is not supervised by a qualified physician. In such a situation, the use of technicians of proved skill and reliability is of paramount importance, but the surgeon should have enough personal experience with general anesthesia to be able to help when necessary.

REGIONAL ANESTHESIA

Regional anesthesia is adequate for many procedures. It is particularly indicated for procedures performed on ambulatory patients, and is also useful for many operations done on hospitalized patients. A partial list of these operations includes surface surgery such as plastic procedures, biopsies, excision of moles and cysts, hernia repairs, many eye, ear, nose, and throat operations, and endoscopies of the respiratory, urinary, and gastrointestinal tracts.

Tissue infiltration of a small amount of local anesthetic for a minor procedure such as suturing a wound carries minimal risks. The risks increase with the amount of drug used and the extent of the procedure. The safety and practicality of regional anesthesia depend on the proper selection and preparation of the patient, the knowledge and skill of the surgeon, and his ability to diagnose and treat the complications of anesthesia as they arise.

Selection of Patient

In general, young or emotionally unstable patients are poor candidates for regional anesthesia. However, hand lacerations can be sutured and wrist fractures can be manipulated following a brachial plexus block achieved with a fine needle by the axillary approach in a mildly sedated preschool child, whereas it is unreasonable to expect an older child to remain motionless under surgical drapes during a longer procedure done with regional anesthesia. Common sense and rapport with the child offer the best guidelines for the decision to use regional anesthesia. Emotionally unstable adults usually demand general anesthesia, and experienced surgeons seldom try to talk them out of it except for very minor operations.

The patient with severe cardiac or pulmonary disease presents a special problem that calls for sound clinical judgment. Such patients face a higher risk from general anesthesia than from regional anesthesia if the surgery is minor or limited to a small field or if it is of brief duration (eg, cataract extraction). If the procedure is extensive or prolonged, general anesthesia may be less hazardous. The systemic toxicity of local anesthetics used in large amounts becomes a factor, and the anxiety and discomfort of the patient during the administration of the local anesthetic and during surgery increase epinephrine release, oxygen consumption, and carbon dioxide production, imposing a greater burden on a decompensating cardiorespiratory system than a well-conducted general anesthetic procedure. Obvious exceptions include situations such as the amputation of a gangrenous leg using low spinal anesthesia which requires a simple injection of a small amount of drug and causes little discomfort.

Preparation of the Patient

The well-informed patient with whom the surgeon has established good rapport is a calmer, more cooperative subject for regional anesthesia. Anxiety can be reduced by sedatives such as barbiturates, which have the added advantage of reducing the incidence of convulsions caused by local anesthetics. However, if the barbiturate dose is excessive or if the patient is particularly susceptible, he may become confused or excited by painful stimuli and exhibit unpredictable and unmanageable behavior. Cautious dosage and the addition of a small amount of a narcotic usually prevent these problems and produce a mild euphoria which most patients find agreeable. Increments can be administered intravenously to achieve the desired effect before and during the procedure. Barbiturates are contraindicated if the patient is confused or experiencing pain. They increase the confusion and reduce pain tolerance. Tables 14–4 and 14–5 list some of the drugs and dosages used for premedication in adults and children. Table 14–6 offers a guide to which drugs should be used with various types of anesthetics.

The patient's stomach should be empty. During regional anesthetic procedures on a conscious patient in good physical condition, vomiting is not a serious matter; if the patient is debilitated or heavily sedated, vomitus may be aspirated into the lungs with disastrous results.

Local Anesthetic Agents

Local anesthetic agents block the transmission of nerve impulses because the segment of a nerve axon exposed to the drug becomes incapable of generating the necessary action potential. The exact mechanism is not known, but it is proposed that these drugs act by altering the permeability of the cell membrane to the passage of ions, thus stabilizing the resting potential.

Susceptibility of individual nerve fibers is inversely proportionate to the cross-sectional diameter of the fibers: the smaller the fiber, the more susceptible it is to local anesthetics. Therefore, during regional anesthesia, perception of light touch, pain, and temperature and vasomotor control are abolished sooner and with less of the agent than are perception of pressure or the motor activity of striated muscles.

Many chemical substances are capable of interrupting nerve conduction, but only those that are completely reversible, nonirritating, and cause minimal systemic toxicity are used clinically. Rapidity of onset, predictability of duration, and ease of sterilization are other desirable properties.

Table 14–1 summarizes the uses and doses of the commonly used local anesthetics. When absorbed into the systemic circulation, all local anesthetics have dose-related side-effects which are discussed in detail on p 182.

The oldest local anesthetic, cocaine, has properties not shared by the others. The long-acting CNS stimulation that it produces gives a feeling of euphoria that can lead to addiction. Cocaine also possesses norepinephrine-like effects such as local vasoconstriction, pupillary dilatation, and potentiation of injected sympathomimetics. Its local vasoconstriction and excellent topical effectiveness make it ideal for "shrinking" and anesthetizing the mucosa of the nasal passages. Cocaine is not stable at the temperatures required for autoclaving, which is a minor disadvantage since it is only used as a topical agent.

Technics

Pharmacologic interruption of nerve conduction is known as regional anesthesia, local anesthesia, or conduction anesthesia. The technics used to apply the drugs to the nerves include topical, infiltration, nerve and plexus block, and subarachnoid and epidural spinal anesthesia.

A. Topical Anesthesia: Topical anesthesia is achieved by absorption of the agent through the surface of an intact membrane. Skin is an effective barrier to such absorption, but the conjunctiva of the eye and the mucosa of the mouth, nose, throat, respiratory tract, urethra, and urinary bladder can be rendered insensitive by this method.

All local anesthetics are not equally effective when used topically. The agents, dosages, and concentrations are given in Table 14–1. Systemic absorption of topical anesthetics leading to toxic blood concentrations may be very rapid, particularly if the solution is swallowed. Application to the surface to be anesthetized can be done by spraying, gargling, applying soaked pledgets or packs, or direct injection. When expertly performed, topical anesthesia is ideal for bronchoscopy and laryngoscopy.

B. Local Infiltration: Local infiltration, with a hypodermic needle, of tissues to be incised or of tissues surrounding an operative site (field block) requires little description or discussion. Obviously, the solutions and equipment must be sterile. Dilute solutions yield satisfactory results because fine nerve fibers are the targets.

The hazards of systemic toxicity from overdosage must be kept in mind when large areas are anesthetized. This is best done by calculating in advance the number of milligrams of drug in the volume of solution

Table 14—1. Drugs used for local anesthesia.*

	Cocaine	Procaine (Novocain, Neocaine)	Tetracaine (Pontocaine)	Lidocaine (Xylocaine)	Bupivacaine (Marcaine)	Mepivacaine (Carbocaine)
Potency (compared to procaine)	3	1	10	2–3	9–12	1.5–2
Toxicity (compared to procaine)	4	1	10	1–1.5	4–6	1–1.5
Stability at sterilizing temperature	Unstable	Stable	Stable	Stable	Stable	Stable
Total maximum dose	100–200 mg	1 g	50–100 mg	500 mg	175 mg	500 mg
Topical						
Concentration	Eye, 1%; other, 4–10%	Not effective	Eye, 0.5%; other, 1–2%	Eye, 0.5%; other, 4%	. . .	Eye, 0.5%; other, 1–2%
Onset of action	Immediate	. . .	10–20 minutes	3–5 minutes	. . .	10–20 minutes
Duration	30–60 minutes	. . .	1–2 hours	30–60 minutes	. . .	1–2 hours
Infiltration						
Concentration	. . .	0.25–1%	0.05–0.1%	0.5–1%	0.25%	0.5%
Onset of action	. . .	5–15 minutes	10–20 minutes	3–5 minutes	5–10 minutes	5–10 minutes
Duration	. . .	45–60 minutes	1½–3 hours	30–60 minutes	90–120 minutes	1¼–2½ hours
Nerve block and epidural						
Concentration	. . .	1–2%	0.1–0.2%	1–2%	0.5%	1–2%
Onset of action	. . .	5–15 minutes	10–20 minutes	5–10 minutes	7–21 minutes	5–10 minutes
Duration	. . .	45–60 minutes	1½–3 hours	1–1½ hours	2–6 hours	1¼–2½ hours
Subarachnoid						
Concentration	. . .	3–5%	0.1–0.5%	5%	. . .	. . .
Dose	. . .	50–200 mg	5–20 mg	40–100 mg	. . .	. . .
Onset of action	. . .	3–5 minutes	5–10 minutes	1–3 minutes	. . .	. . .
Duration	. . .	45–60 minutes	1½–2 hours	1–1½ hours	. . .	. . .

*Addition of vasopressor prolongs durations by 25–50% but not used topically.

that may be required and keeping to a limit below the toxic dose.

Infiltration of tissues that are inflamed or are close to an inflamed area should be avoided if possible. Such injections lower local tissue resistance to infection, may result in rapid systemic absorption because of the increased vascularity of inflamed tissues, and may also be ineffective if the local tissue pH is low enough to reduce the anesthetic agent's ionic dissociation, which is essential for anesthetic activity.

C. Nerve and Plexus Blocks: Peripheral nerves are accessible for blocking by one who is familiar with the anatomy of nerve distribution, the relation of nerves to surface or palpable landmarks, the tissue compartments and fascial planes that influence the spread of anesthetic solutions, and the surrounding structures that might be traumatized by the needle. To avoid intravascular injection, always aspirate before injecting the anesthetic agent. The need for sterility is again emphasized.

Figs 14—1 to 14—8 illustrate some common nerve blocks that are easily mastered.

D. Regional Anesthesia by the Intravenous Method: This technic has gained some popularity in recent years. It is accomplished by the intravenous injection of a dilute solution of a local anesthetic into the vein of an extremity kept ischemic by a tourniquet. It is particularly useful for the closed reduction of fractures.

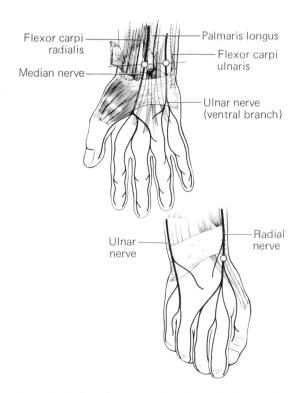

Figure 14—1. Nerve blocks at wrist. *Above:* Median and ulnar nerve block. *Below:* Radial nerve block.

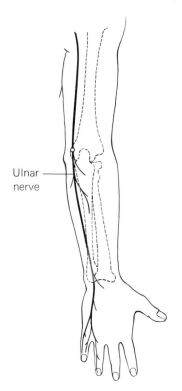

Figure 14–2. Ulnar nerve block at elbow.

A pneumatic tourniquet (eg, blood pressure cuff) is applied to the arm or thigh of the extremity to be anesthetized but left uninflated. A vein in the distal portion of the limb is cannulated, preferably with a pliable plastic needle. The limb is then elevated and drained of blood with the aid of an elastic bandage wrapped from distal to proximal. The tourniquet is then inflated rapidly to a pressure above systolic and kept inflated. Thirty to 50 ml of 0.5% lidocaine (Xylocaine) are then instilled into the vein. Excellent anesthesia below the tourniquet is achieved immediately and lasts 30–60 minutes.

After the procedure, the tourniquet is deflated momentarily and then reinflated. This is done 3 or 4 times at intervals of a few minutes so that small amounts of the anesthetic are released intermittently into the systemic circulation. Sudden complete release of the tourniquet may result in toxicity and immediate disappearance of anesthesia. Anyone using this technic must be prepared to cope with these problems.

E. Spinal Anesthesia: Spinal anesthesia is a safe method of providing excellent anesthesia for many procedures. It is somewhat unpopular with patients who desire total unawareness or who are misinformed about the incidence of complications. The technics consist of blocking the spinal nerves between their emergence from the spinal cord and their exit from the spinal canal through the intervertebral foramens. In the spinal canal, the spinal nerves course through the subarachnoid space where they are bathed in spinal fluid and then traverse the epidural space. They may be blocked in either location. Table 14–1 gives the dosages of drugs used in spinal anesthesia.

To obtain **subarachnoid spinal anesthesia**, a lumbar puncture is performed and the anesthetic agent is injected. Ampules of drugs used must be autoclaved and not stored in disinfectant solutions that might chemically contaminate the ampule contents through minute undetectable cracks. The lumbar puncture may be done in the sitting or lateral decubitus position at any level between L1 and S1. The anesthetic blocks all spinal nerves below the site of injection as well as those reached by the cephalad spread of the anesthetic solution. This cephalad spread can be controlled by positioning the patient to allow the anesthetic solution to "sink" or "float" in the desired direction. For this purpose, the anesthetic solutions are either made heavier than the CSF (hyperbaric) by the addition of 10% dextrose or lighter than the CSF (hypobaric) by dissolving the anesthetic drug in distilled water to make a dilute solution (eg, 1 mg tetracaine per 1 ml distilled water). The effective spread is limited as dilution by the CSF occurs. After 20 minutes, the solution is "fixed" and further spread is unlikely.

Duration of anesthesia depends on the agent selected; larger doses than those given in Table 14–1 increase the duration of anesthesia only slightly. Addition of 0.2–0.4 ml of 1:1000 epinephrine or 3 mg phenylephrine (Neo-Synephrine) increases the duration 30–50%.

To obtain **epidural spinal anesthesia** a needle is introduced into the epidural space at any level of the spinal canal. It is easiest at the lumbar interspaces or through the sacral hiatus. In the lumbar area the space is recognized by advancing a blunt needle in the same manner as for a lumbar puncture but stopping when resistance to injection is no longer felt but no CSF can

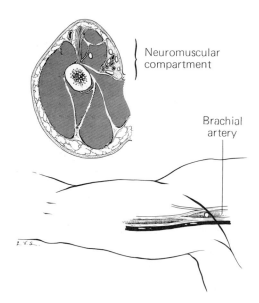

Figure 14–3. Brachial plexus block in axilla. *Above:* Cross-section of the arm at the axilla. *Below:* Surface landmarks for axillary block.

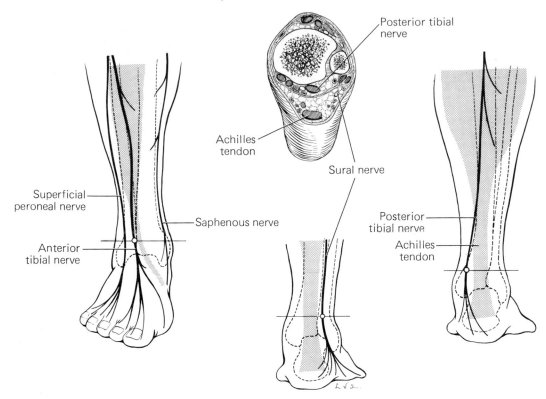

Figure 14–4. Nerve blocks at ankle. *Left:* Anterior tibial nerve block. *Right:* Posterior tibial nerve block. *Center, above:* Cross-section showing relationship of nerves to skin and bone. *Center, below:* Sural nerve block.

be aspirated. A test dose that would achieve subarachnoid spinal anesthesia but is insufficient for epidural anesthesia is used for proof that the subarachnoid space has or has not been entered.

A catheter may be inserted through the needle for continuous epidural anesthesia with repeated injections. The needle is withdrawn, leaving the catheter in position. Catheters should never be withdrawn through the needle for fear of cutting the catheter in the spinal canal.

The concentrations of local anesthetics used and the rate of onset of anesthesia are the same as for peripheral nerve blocks. The area anesthetized depends on the spread of the injected solution in the spinal canal and is therefore dependent on the volume, although considerable individual variation occurs. The dangers of toxicity must be kept in mind because the total dose required may be large.

Subarachnoid and epidural anesthesia produce excellent analgesia and loss of motor function in the area of distribution of the spinal nerves affected. This can include the motor nerves to the diaphragm and cessation of respiration if the level reaches the fourth cervical vertebra. The minute volume of respiration is not diminished by loss of intercostal muscle acitivity.

1. Side-effects of spinal anesthesia—Most of the side-effects of spinal anesthesia are related to block of the nerve fibers of the sympathetic nervous system as they accompany the anterior roots of the spinal nerves

from the first thoracic to the second lumbar vertebrae (thoracolumbar outflow). This sympathetic block upsets many physiologic regulating mechanisms. Interruption of central vasomotor control to the affected areas leads to vasodilatation or at least to a loss of tone of both arterioles and veins. The loss of resistance and the peripheral venous pooling (if not compensated by position) contribute to a fall in blood pressure. Moreover, cardiac rate and action are deprived of the stimulation of the cardiac sympathetic innervation and of the epinephrine normally released by sympathetic stimulation of the adrenal medulla. Meanwhile, the vagus has an unopposed parasympathetic effect of cardiac slowing. The hypovolemic or hypotensive patient reacts poorly to this situation. The arteriosclerotic hypertensive patient may have a precipitous blood pressure drop. The other effects of sympathetic loss such as increased intestinal peristalsis caused by unopposed vagal activity and the loss of sweating are of lesser consequence. Nausea and vomiting during spinal anesthesia may be related to the sympathetic blockade, but the mechanism is not entirely clear. They are frequently associated with hypotension.

The general management of the patient under spinal anesthesia includes maintenance of good ventilation and oxygenation, positioning to favor good venous return, and the use of vasopressors if necessary. An intravenous infusion should be started before high spinal anesthetics are administered.

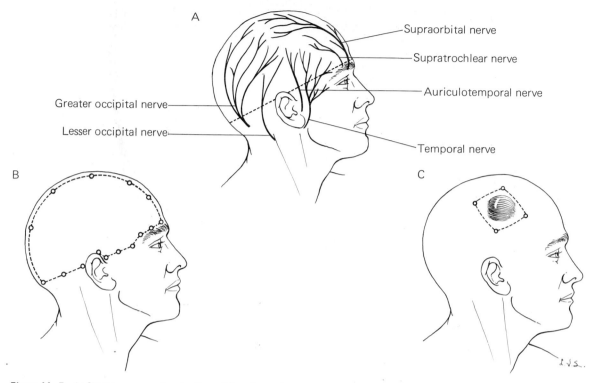

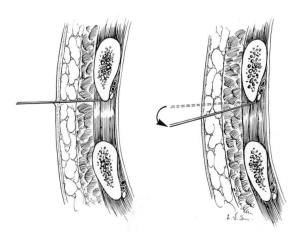

Figure 14—5. *A:* Sensory nerves of scalp. Dotted line shows sites of injection. *B:* Field block of scalp. *C:* Field block for excision of scalp lesion.

2. Subarachnoid versus epidural blocks—The subarachnoid spinal is technically easier to accomplish, uses a much smaller amount of drug, and has a more rapid onset than the epidural. The epidural method avoids "spinal headaches" due to CSF leakage through the arachnoid puncture site and lends itself to a continuous technic for many hours by repeated injections through an epidurally placed catheter. A continuous catheter technic for subarachnoid spinal anesthesia has so many complications that it is infrequently warranted.

3. Complications of spinal anesthesia—Headache, lasting for up to a week, develops in about 15% of patients following spinal anesthesia. It usually begins 24—48 hours postoperatively and characteristically is worse in the erect position and better in the supine. It is believed to be due to spinal fluid leak at the puncture site. Large caliber needles increase the incidence.

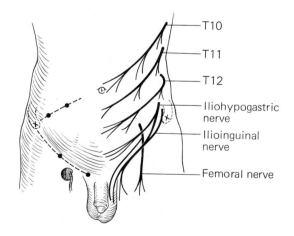

Figure 14—6. Intercostal nerve block. *Left:* Needle locating lower edge of rib. *Right:* Needle under edge of rib for injection of anesthetic agent.

Figure 14—7. Nerves and sites for inguinal nerve block.

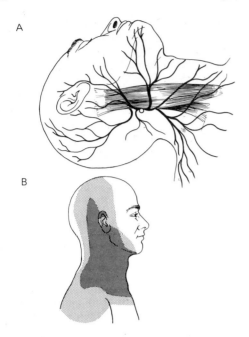

Figure 14—8. *A:* Site of injection for superficial cervical block. *B:* Total (dark area) and partial (light area) anesthesia after block. The latter is due to overlapping innervation by other nerves.

Treatment consists of the recumbent position, hydration, sedation, and, in severe cases, epidural injection of 10 ml of the patient's blood, which is thought to work by plugging the leak.

Nerve injuries and transverse myelitis have followed spinal anesthetics, resulting in transient or permanent disabilities ranging from minor paresthesias to complete paraplegia. Their incidence is much lower than the incidence of cardiac arrest during general anesthesia, but their tragic impact gives them a notoriety out of proportion to their frequency. Contaminants, drug sensitivity, and excessive drug concentration have been implicated in individual cases. They have followed epidural as well as subarachnoid spinal anesthesia.

Winnie AP: Regional anesthesia. Surg Clin North Am 55:861, 1975.

ADVERSE REACTIONS TO LOCAL ANESTHETICS

Clinical Manifestations

Allergic reactions to local anesthetics are rare. Vasovagal syncope may occur when the patient is very apprehensive or imaginative. Tachycardia and palpitations may be caused by the sympathomimetic vasoconstrictors added to the anesthetic solution.

Overdosage toxicity is the most serious and frequent adverse reaction to the local anesthetics. Table 14—1 gives the recommended maximum dosage for each of the commonly used agents when injected into tissues or used topically. Ten to 20% of this amount can produce overdosage symptoms if injected intravenously. The amount employed for dental anesthesia, suturing of minor lacerations, and most biopsies is usually less than the intravenously dangerous dose.

Overdosage toxicity is manifested by CNS stimulation followed by CNS and cardiovascular depression. The latter may appear without prior CNS stimulation. Excitement, apprehension, and nausea are the first symptoms, but they may be masked by sedative premedication. They may be accompanied by cardiovascular and respiratory changes. In most cases, the physician is first alerted by minor twitches of the muscles around the mouth and eyes. These spread and progress to full generalized convulsions whose duration varies with the amount of drug absorbed and the continuing absorption. A period of depression ensues which is characterized by a loss of consciousness, at times to the point of areflexia, coma, and a shock-like state. During the convulsive phase, the coordinated, rhythmic pattern of contraction and relaxation of the muscles of respiration is disrupted by random uncoordinated spasmodic contractions. If the abdominal muscles contract simultaneously with the diaphragm or with the adduction of the vocal cords, the increased intra-abdominal pressure causes evacuation of the bladder and rectum. Pulmonary ventilation ceases or is reduced, and oxygen consumption is increased. It is the resulting hypoxia, not the neuronal discharges or muscular movements, that constitutes the threat to life. If the patient progresses to the stage of depression, this hypoxia contributes to a more profound CNS and cardiovascular depression.

Prevention of Local Anesthetic Overdosage

Premedication with barbiturates or diazepam (Valium) offers some protection from convulsions (Table 14—4).

The ideal dosage of local anesthetics is the smallest amount of drug in the most dilute solution that will provide adequate anesthesia. The total maximum doses shown in Table 14—1 represent average safe limits. Obviously, the total safe dose for a big, young, healthy patient is not the same as for a small, elderly, and debilitated patient. The site of injection or application must also influence the calculation of a maximum single dose. Rapid systemic absorption occurs from highly vascularized tissues or from the stomach, which often receives much of the anesthetic used topically in the mouth, throat, and larynx unless the patient is encouraged to spit it out.

Epinephrine should be added to the anesthetic solution to a final concentration of 1:200,000 whenever near toxic amounts are injected. This produces local vasoconstriction that slows the rate of absorption and prolongs the anesthetic effect. However, the cardiac effects of epinephrine must be kept in mind if the patient has increased cardiac irritability.

Table 14–2. Physical status classification of the American Board of Anesthesiologists. Although this scheme is sometimes used in evaluating a patient's risk for anesthesia, the true risk involves so many other factors that physical status alone correlates poorly with the anesthetic mortality rate.*

Class 1	No organic, physiologic, biochemical, systemic, or psychiatric disturbance in a patient scheduled for a localized operation, eg, elective tonsillectomy in a healthy patient.
Class 2	Mild to moderate systemic disturbance, eg, mild, well-controlled diabetes or hypertension.
Class 3	Severe systemic disturbance, eg, severe organic heart disease or diabetes with vascular complications.
Class 4	Severe systemic disorder that is life-threatening, eg, severe angina, advanced renal or hepatic diseases.
Class 5	Moribund patient not expected to survive, eg, ruptured abdominal aneurysm with shock or massive pulmonary embolus with shock.
Emergency operation	The letter **E** is appended to any of the above 5 categories to indicate that the contemplated operation is an emergency.

*For a detailed analysis of this complicated subject, see Goldstein A Jr, Keats AS: The risk of anesthesia. Anesthesiology 33:130, 1970.

Treatment of Local Anesthetic Overdosage

A. Oxygen and Assisted Respiration: Treatment must be initiated with the first sign of overdosage reaction. Oxygen by mask may be all that is necessary if it maintains adequate alveolar oxygen concentrations in compensation for the reduced ventilation. Assisted respiration by positive pressure is seldom necessary if oxygen is given promptly, but it may be lifesaving if oxygen is not immediately available. If there is evidence of hypoxia (eg, cyanosis), it is better to perform artificial ventilation with a bag and mask or by means of mouth-to-mask or mouth-to-mouth breathing than to leave the patient for the purpose of obtaining oxygen equipment. Hypoxia can be prevented or treated by good pulmonary ventilation with air. The addition of oxygen is desirable but not essential.

B. Drugs: Intravenous barbiturates can control or terminate convulsions by a central action. Small doses (eg, 25–50 mg of thiopental or pentobarbital) are sufficient. However, oxygen therapy or artificial ventilation must not be delayed while the barbiturates are obtained, drawn into a syringe, and injected. Moreover, barbiturates, particularly in too large doses, add further depression to the postconvulsion depression. Other CNS depressants can be used to control convulsions, but all have the same efficacy and hazards as the barbiturates.

Muscle relaxants such as succinylcholine can stop the gross muscular contractions, although their neurogenic cause persists. They do not add to the postconvulsion depression but should be used only by physicians who have the experience and equipment to perform artificial respiration.

Convulsions caused by local anesthetic overdosage can be managed with ease and safety by ensuring ventilation with or without drugs. Indecision, panic, and overtreatment are the real hazards.

C. Antishock Measures: The depression or shock stage requires treatment. Hypoxia must be prevented. The Trendelenburg position or elevation of the legs seems beneficial. The value of vasopressors is not firmly established. (See Chapter 15 for a full discussion of shock and its treatment.)

GENERAL ANESTHESIA

The patient should be visited by the anesthesiologist* before the day of surgery. Whenever possible, the surgeon should consult with the anesthesiologist several days before the operation if he anticipates any problem related to anesthesia; better preparation of the patient and fewer last-minute cancellations can be achieved in this way. Any discussion of anesthesia between the surgeon and the patient should avoid committing the anesthesiologist to any particular agent or technic until he has been consulted or has seen the patient. This does not prevent the surgeon from listening to the patient's views concerning anesthesia and discussing with him what anesthetic technics are usually used in similar cases while at the same time stressing that every patient must be individually evaluated by whoever administers the anesthetic. The best rapport between the patient and his physicians occurs when the patient senses an agreement of opinion and mutual confidence between the surgeon, the anesthesiologist, and any other consultant. Faced by this united front, doubts and indecision usually disappear.

THE PREANESTHETIC VISIT

The preanesthetic visit by the anesthesiologist has several purposes. The patient gets to know the anesthesiologist, learns what to expect and how he can cooperate, can ask questions about anesthesia, and can have misconceptions corrected. The anesthesiologist gets to know the patient, evaluates his condition (Table 14–2), institutes treatments, and plans the anesthetic management.

It is useful to review the patient's hospital record before the visit. This review may duplicate much of the information obtainable directly from the patient but may uncover details that the patient has forgotten or of which he is unaware. The anesthesiologist then obtains a history and does a physical examination (usually limiting himself to information relevant to

*A person administering an anesthetic is an anesthetist. In the USA the physician anesthetist is called an anesthesiologist.

anesthetic management), and discusses the anesthetic with the patient. The most important inquiries concern previous anesthetic experiences, past or chronic illnesses, habits such as smoking or alcohol consumption, drugs used, allergies and sensitivities, and extent of physical activity. Previous anesthetics that posed technical difficulties and were associated with undesirable drug responses or complications should suggest using different agents and methods.

A myocardial infarction within 3 months of an elective operation is associated with a 35% incidence of reinfarction; during the period 3–6 months after an infarction, the reinfarction rate is 15%; with longer intervals, the risk remains steady at 5%. The mortality rate of postoperative infarction is about 50%. Thus, whenever possible, elective surgery should be postponed to more than 6 months after a myocardial infarction.

Asthma, hay fever, and other allergic conditions, neurologic disease, and a history of productive cough all influence the choice of anesthetic management. Heavy cigarette smoking should alert the anesthesiologist to expect a very active cough reflex. Barbiturate habituation or narcotic addiction suggests tolerance to these agents.

Many commonly used medications have implications for anesthetic management and the points mentioned in Table 14–3 must be considered preoperatively.

Lastly, the patient's limit of physical activity is a remarkably good indication of the ability of his cardiorespiratory system to withstand the stresses of an anesthetic. The patient should be asked about his or her ability to do housework, climb stairs, play golf or tennis, etc to assess general physical status.

The physical examination is directed toward finding variations and anomalies that have implications related to anesthetic management. Signs of diseases of the circulatory or respiratory system are most important, but certain minor findings have particular interest for the anesthesiologist. Bad teeth and fragile dental prostheses should be noted, and the patient should be warned that they may be damaged in spite of all precautions during general anesthesia. Conditions that might lead to technical problems of airway maintenance are looked for. The patient with inspiratory stridor should be told that he will undergo endotracheal intubation under local anesthesia before he can be put to sleep safely. The site of injection for regional anesthesia is examined for anatomic deformities or signs of infection.

A complete urinalysis and hemoglobin or hematocrit determination are the minimal preanesthetic laboratory requirements. The preoperative examination by the anesthesiologist may turn up indications for chest x-rays, serum electrolyte determinations, ECGs, and other tests that were not necessary for the surgical diagnosis but whose findings influence anesthetic management, suggest pre- or postanesthetic therapy, or simply establish baselines. Tests frequently obtained to determine the status of the cardiac or respiratory sys-

Table 14–3. Commonly used drugs with significant effects during anesthesia and surgery.

Drug	Comment
Anticoagulants	Usually should be discontinued or dosage reduced before surgery.
Tetracycline	Predisposes to renal insufficiency when given with methoxyflurane anesthesia.
Aminoglycoside antibiotics (kanamycin, gentamicin, streptomycin, neomycin)	May enhance neuromuscular blockage following tubocurarine, etc.
Propranolol	During anesthesia may enhance myocardial depression, induce bronchospasm, and inhibit circulatory response to blood loss.
Quinidine, procainamide, lidocaine	May enhance myocardial depression, impair conduction, cause peripheral vasodilatation, and potentiate neuromuscular blockade.
Antihypertensives	May aggravate hypotension.
Corticosteroids	Increased demand during surgery usually requires increased dosage.
Anticonvulsants (eg, phenobarbital, phenytoin)	By inducing hepatic microsomal enzymes, may increase metabolism of anesthetic drugs.
MAO inhibitors (eg, tranylcypromine, pargyline)	May cause hypertensive crises when given in conjunction with sympathomimetic agents.
Phenothiazines	May enhance hypotensive effects of other drugs.
Neostigmine	May predispose to respiratory failure postoperatively in patients with myasthenia gravis.
Levodopa	May cause hypotension and occasionally arrhythmias.
Glaucoma medication	These drugs should usually be discontinued preoperatively.
Insulin	Dosage should be reduced during surgery (see p 49).

tems include pulse rate changes with minor exercise, analysis of arterial blood for P_{O_2}, P_{CO_2}, and pH, and measurements of respiratory rates, tidal volume, vital capacity, and forced expiratory volume during 1 second.

PREPARATION OF THE PATIENT FOR ANESTHESIA

The patient should be in the best physical condition possible within the limits of what medical treatment can accomplish and the urgency of the surgery. Shock, hypovolemia, electrolyte imbalances, cardiac decompensation, diabetic acidosis, and fever are some of the conditions that require treatment before anesthesia if possible. The stomach should be emptied by suction or allowed to empty, remembering that pain

Table 14–4. Common drugs and average doses of drugs for premedication (adults).

Drug	Dosage	Route and Time
Barbiturates*		
Pentobarbital	50–200 mg	Give orally, 2–4 hours before induction; or IM, 30 minutes before induction; or IV, 15 minutes before induction.
Secobarbital	50–200 mg	
Amobarbital	50–200 mg	
Diazepam (Valium)	10 mg	Give orally or IM 1–2 hours before surgery.
Narcotics*		
Morphine	5–15 mg	Give subcutaneously, 1 hour before induction; or IM, 30–45 minutes before induction; or IV, 5–15 minutes before induction.
Meperidine (Demerol)	50–150 mg	
Alphaprodine (Nisentil)	30–60 mg	
Belladonna alkaloids		
Atropine	0.2–0.6 mg	Give subcutaneously, 30–60 minutes before induction. (Can be combined with narcotic.)
Scopolamine†	0.2–0.6 mg	

*Dosages of barbiturates and narcotics should be reduced if premedication includes phenothiazines.

†Reduce or eliminate scopolamine dose in the elderly.

Table 14–6. Selection of premedication for various anesthetic agents.

Anesthetic Agent	Barbiturates	Narcotics	Atropine or Scopolamine
Ether	++	+	+++
Cyclopropane	++	+	++
Thiopental with N_2O	++	+++	++
Enflurane	++	+	+++
Halothane	++	+	++
Methoxyflurane	++	+	++
Local anesthetic Less than 200 mg procaine or lidocaine or 20 mg tetracaine	++	++	+
More than 200 mg procaine or lidocaine or 20 mg tetracaine	+++	++	+

Legend: + None or reduced dosage
          ++ Desirable
          +++ Indicated

and apprehension retard emptying time. Aspiration of vomitus is one of the most dangerous complications of general anesthesia for emergency surgery.

The pharmacologic preparation of the patient for anesthesia varies with the age and condition of the patient and the anesthetic technic planned. For this reason it should be ordered by the anesthesiologist. Most patients prefer some sedation before surgery, and some demand to be made totally unaware of their surroundings before reaching the operating room. Since anesthetic management is easier if the patient is cooperative and oriented, a compromise must be reached. Respiratory depression must be avoided unless the anesthesiologist is in continuous attendance from the time the sedative drugs are administered. It may be desirable to reduce the secretions of the mouth and respiratory tract or to depress vagal reflexes with parasympatholytic drugs. Tables 14–4, 14–5, and

14–6 list some of the drugs used for anesthetic premedication and suggest which ones to use with different types of anesthesia. As a rule, infirmity and age diminish the need for and increase the hazards of premedication. These hazards include confusion, restlessness, respiratory depression, hypotension (with or without a postural component), nausea and vomiting, and delayed awakening.

SELECTION OF ANESTHETIC AGENTS & TECHNICS

General anesthesia is a drug-induced depression of the CNS that is reversible by the body's elimination or destruction of the drug. It is a state of analgesia,

Table 14–5. Anesthetic premedication for infants and children.*†

	Average Weight (lb)	Pentobarbital or Secobarbital	Atropine or Scopolamine	Morphine or	Meperidine or (Demerol)	Alphaprodine (Nisentil)
Newborn	7	. . .	0.1 mg	. . .	. . .	. . .
6 months	16	30 mg	0.2 mg	. . .	. . .	. . .
1 year	21	50 mg	0.2 mg	1 mg	10 mg	4 mg
2 years	27	60 mg	0.3 mg	1.5 mg	20 mg	8 mg
4 years	35	90 mg	0.3 mg	3 mg	30 mg	12 mg
6 years	45	100 mg	0.4 mg	4 mg	40 mg	15 mg
8 years	55	120 mg	0.4 mg	5 mg	50 mg	20 mg
10 years	65	150 mg	0.4 mg	6 mg	60 mg	25 mg
12 years	85	150 mg	0.6 mg	8 mg	80 mg	30 mg

*Modified and reproduced, with permission, from Smith: *Anesthesia for Infants and Children.* Mosby, 1959.

†Reductions must be made for underweight or poorly developed patients. Barbiturates are given rectally at least 90 minutes before induction, or IM (with two-thirds above dosage), 30 minutes before induction. Morphine and atropine or scopolamine are given subcutaneously 45 minutes before induction.

amnesia, and unconsciousness, with loss of reflexes and muscle tone. The drugs used must produce no permanent tissue damage and must not interfere with respiratory or vascular functions to the point of tissue hypoxia. The physical and chemical properties of the drugs should allow convenient, controllable, and predictable methods of introducing them into the circulation for transport to the CNS. Rapid onset of action is a desirable property not usually provided by absorption from tissues or from the gastrointestinal tract. Either the direct intravenous injection or the introduction into the respiratory tract for absorption from the lungs is the usual method.

Most surgical procedures can be performed with anesthesia provided by a variety of agents and technics. There are few absolute indications or contraindications, as shown by the comparable success of competent anesthesiologists who differ in their selection of methods. Each makes a decision based on the requirements of the surgery, the condition of the patient, and his skill and experience with the methods at his disposal. He is influenced by patient preference (eg, intravenous induction), the site of the surgery, the use of electrocautery, the need for muscular relaxation, etc. If ideal conditions for the surgery are not compatible with safe anesthesia, this should be discussed with the surgeon. Other physicians who consult on the case may render invaluable advice but must not dictate the anesthetic management unless they are prepared to carry it out themselves.

INHALATION ANESTHESIA

Inhalation anesthetics diffuse from the lung alveoli to the blood, which transports them to the CNS. If the drug is a compressed gas provided in cylinders (nitrous oxide, cyclopropane, ethylene), it can be administered in any inhaled concentration up to 100% by an anesthetic machine (see below). If it is a liquid at room temperature (ethyl ether, halothane, enflurane, etc), it requires vaporization before it can be inhaled by the patient. Vaporization may be achieved by dripping the liquid on a gauze mask held over the patient's mouth and nose. This open drop technic has been the method used in millions of ether administrations for over a century. It has been largely supplanted by methods of vaporization that flow other gases over the surface of the volatile liquid or that bubble other gases through the volatile liquid. If the system is efficient, the gas exposed to the volatile liquid by either method becomes saturated with the vapor of the liquid. The concentration of the agent so vaporized is a function of the agent's vapor pressure, which varies with its temperature as a liquid at the time of vaporization. At the usual operating room temperatures (20 C), halothane has a vapor pressure of 240 mm Hg. If 100 ml of oxygen are passed through an efficient halothane vaporizer, the oxygen becomes saturated with halothane vapor, which exerts a pressure of 240 mm Hg, or approximately one-third of an ambient atmospheric pressure of 760 mm Hg. Therefore, the mixture that emerges from the vaporizer will consist of 100 ml of oxygen and 50 ml of halothane, making the mixture two-thirds oxygen and one-third halothane (240 mm Hg). If a 150 ml/minute flow of halothane is desired, 300 ml of oxygen must be put through the vaporizer. Efficient vaporizers deliver approximately 33% halothane, 60% ethyl ether (vapor pressure 450 mm Hg), or 3% methoxyflurane (vapor pressure 27 mm Hg). The desired inhaled concentration is achieved by dilution, but many anesthetic vaporizers (eg, Fluotec) are calibrated to deliver desired concentrations and relieve the anesthesiologist of having to calculate the dilutions necessary.

The transport of an inhalation anesthetic to the lung alveoli and from lung capillaries to the brain is passive. Its molecules are carried by the flow of gas in the airways and of blood in the vascular system. Passage of the agent from alveoli to blood and from blood to brain is accomplished by diffusion. This mechanism is the same for all gases in solution, including oxygen and CO_2. Each gas seeks equilibration of tension independent of other gases in solution in the same medium. Gas tensions must not be confused with number of molecules in solution, although for an individual gas the 2 are interdependent. The solubility of any gas in a particular liquid determines the number of molecules in solution at any chosen tension. For example, the solubility of ethyl ether in blood is so much greater than that of nitrous oxide that at equal tensions more than 30 molecules of the ether are held in solution for every molecule of nitrous oxide. For anesthetic purposes, solubility is best expressed as the **blood-gas partition coefficient,** which tells us the proportionate distribution of a sample of gas added to a volume of air exposed to an equal volume of blood at 37.5 C. This coefficient for ethyl ether is 12.5, which means that 12.5 as many molecules of ether will dissolve in blood for every molecule that remains in air when the volume of air and blood are equal.

Uptake, Distribution, & Elimination of Inhalation Anesthetics

The depth of anesthesia is dependent on the gaseous tension of the anesthetic in the brain. This is established by equilibration of tension with the arterial blood perfusing the brain. In turn, the tension of the agent in the arterial blood represents an equilibration with alveolar tension. It follows that controlling the alveolar tension of an inhalation agent will control the depth of anesthesia. Venous-arterial shunts that bypass the lungs or ventilation-perfusion anomalies that act as shunts interfere with alveolar-arterial equilibration of inhalation agents just as they do for oxygen.

Building and maintaining a desired alveolar tension of an inhalation agent depends on the inspired concentration, the pulmonary ventilation, the blood-gas partition coefficient (solubility), and the cardiac output. The first 2 require little explanation. A

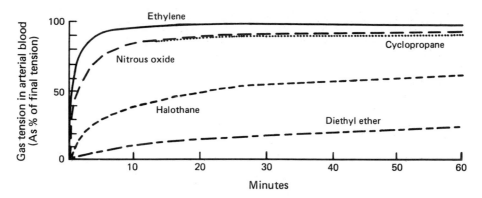

Figure 14—9. The rate of rise of tension of anesthetic in arterial blood with different agents administered at a constant inspired tension. (Reproduced, with permission, from Dripps, Eckenhoff, & Vandam: *Introduction to Anesthesia,* 3rd ed. Saunders, 1967.)

high inspired concentration and an active transport mechanism (pulmonary ventilation) obviously deliver more anesthetic agent to the alveoli than lesser inspired concentrations or lesser minute volumes of alveolar ventilation. If the gas is very soluble (eg, ethyl ether), it will diffuse into the blood in such quantities that the alveolar tension and subsequent arterial blood tension rise slowly. Fig 14—9 plots the gas tension in arterial blood of several agents during induction under normal conditions.

During recovery, the soluble agents are "held" by the tissues and blood. Only a small portion of a highly soluble gas diffuses to the alveoli during the passage of any volume of blood through the lungs. The agents with low solubility are cleared from tissues and blood as rapidly as pulmonary ventilation clears them from the alveoli.

The distribution of cardiac output and its effect on anesthesia are worth noting here. About 70% of cardiac output goes to the brain, heart, kidneys, and liver. These organs are saturated rapidly with an anesthetic tension equal to that in arterial blood and in alveolar gases. During shock, the vasoconstriction of all organs except the brain and heart diverts an even greater share of cardiac output to the brain and heart, causing their rapid and potentially dangerous saturation with anesthetic. Uptake from alveoli or redistribution continues until gas tensions in all tissues approach equality. Failure to provide for this continuing uptake after the desired depth of anesthesia is reached results in diminishing depth as redistribution of the agent removes it from the brain.

When inhalation anesthesia is administered clinically, the depth is evaluated by observing the response of the patient and not by analysis of gas tensions. Progressive administration of an anesthetic agent depresses physiologic functions such as respiration, cardiac action, vasomotor tone, striated muscle tone, and reflexes. Changes in these functions are the signs of anesthesia. They are depressed by agents to different degrees and possibly in different sequences. For example, at the same level of respiratory depression, the muscle relaxant and circulatory effects of

ether, cyclopropane, chloroform, and halothane are different. The clinical signs at various stages and planes of ether anesthesia (as classically described by Guedel) are still useful signs for monitoring the patient's response to any agent, but their significance in determining the depth of anesthesia varies with the agent. By observing these signs, one strives to provide optimal surgical conditions commensurate with minimal depression of vital functions. Increases in the inspired concentration deepen the anesthetic level, and decreases in the inspired concentration lighten it.

The Anesthetic Machine

Most inhalation anesthetics are administered with an anesthetic machine that permits the administration of inhaled gases in known and controlled mixtures. The mixtures are prepared by accurately measuring flows of gases which may be available by piping from a central hospital source or from high-pressure tanks attached to the machine. In either instance, there must be foolproof safeguards against delivery of any but the desired gas or mixture, ie, it must be impossible to attach a nitrous oxide tank or hose to an oxygen inlet, or any other gas source to any but its own properly labeled flow system. Most anesthetic machines also have one or more vaporizers for the delivery of accurately measured concentrations of volatile liquid anesthetic agents such as ether, halothane, and enflurane. If the anesthetic is administered by insufflation into the patient's mouth or throat, allowances must be made for dilution with room air. More commonly, the gases are administered by methods that exclude room air and contain the gas mixture in a system made continuous with the respiratory tract via a face mask or endotracheal tube. Such a system is a circle arrangement of a reservoir bag, a CO_2 absorber, a one-way overflow ("pop-off") valve, and 2 conducting tubes to the face mask with valves that allow circulation in one direction only. The reservoir bag allows the patient to breathe gases at flow rates which even during quiet respiration are greater (25—35 liters/minute) than the flowmeters of most machines can deliver. When manually compressed, the bag exerts a positive pressure on

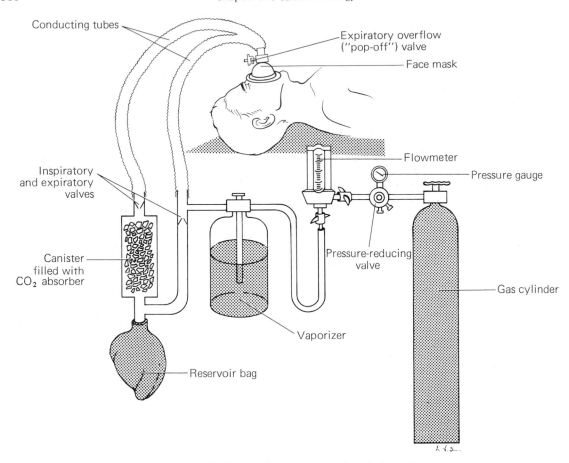

Figure 14—10. The essential components of anesthetic machine.

the contained gases, which is the usual method for applying positive airway pressure for controlled or assisted pulmonary ventilation during anesthesia. During spontaneous respiration, the bag gives visual evidence of rate and volume of respiration.

The CO_2 absorber is essential whenever the flow of gas from the machine to the system is not sufficient to exhaust all of the patient's exhaled CO_2 from the system through the overflow ("pop-off") valve. The absorber contains granules of the hydroxides of sodium, calcium, barium, or mixtures of these substances. In the presence of moisture, CO_2 dissolves and forms carbonic acid (H_2CO_3), which reacts with the hydroxides to form carbonates and water. The freshness of the granules can be verified by indicators that change color when hydroxide is spent and the surface of the granules becomes acid. The conducting tubes ("elephant hoses") connect the mask or endotracheal tube to the reservoir bag. Unidirectional valves restrict one tube to inhalation only and the other to exhalation only. This arrangement prevents the rebreathing of exhaled gas until it has gone "around the circle" to the other tube, has had its CO_2 content removed by the CO_2 absorber or by overflow, and fresh gas has been added. In other words, dead space is not increased by a circular absorber system.

Fig 14–10 illustrates the essentials of an anesthetic machine. All physicians, nurses, and technicians who work in operating rooms should know how to use an anesthetic machine for the administration of oxygen and artificial ventilation.

The Inhalation Anesthetics

The commonly used inhalation anesthetics are listed below. The brief description of each covers only those properties and clinical uses of interest to the surgeon.

A. Nitrous Oxide: Nitrous oxide (N_2O), one of the oldest inhalation anesthetics, is an inorganic gas that compresses to a liquid at about 50 atmospheres and is available in that state in cylinders. It is noncombustible (although it supports combustion by liberating oxygen) and has minimal side-effects outside the CNS. Its low solubility in blood permits rapid induction and recovery. The main drawback of nitrous oxide is its weak potency. It can be administered in concentrations up to 80% if the remaining 20% of the mixture is oxygen. Even at these concentrations (which allow normal inspired oxygen), the addition of more potent inhalation agents or of narcotics or barbiturates is necessary to achieve surgical anesthesia. The patient in shock may be adequately anesthetized with a concentration of nitrous oxide as low as 50%. Nitrous oxide reduces by approximately 50% the required concentration for adequate anesthesia of other inhalation agents given simultaneously. The potential for hypoxia is naturally greater with N_2O than with more potent agents that can be administered with higher oxygen concentrations.

B. Ethylene: Ethylene (CH_2CH_2) is available as a compressed gas in cylinders. It is more potent than nitrous oxide, with no greater toxicity. Its explosiveness and unpleasant odor have limited its popularity.

C. Cyclopropane: Cyclopropane (C_3H_6) is a highly explosive gas that liquefies at only 5 atmospheres at room temperature and consequently can be made available in light tanks. It offers smooth, rapid induction, minimal irritation of the respiratory passages, a wide margin of safety between anesthetic (5–25%) and toxic (40%) concentrations, and increased cardiac output with concentrations used clinically. It is well tolerated by the patient in shock. The circulatory effects of cyclopropane are not direct actions of the drug but responses to endogenous epinephrine released by it.

Cyclopropane is a potent respiratory depressant that leads to hypercapnia if pulmonary ventilation is not augmented. If hypercapnia is allowed to occur, arrhythmias are frequent and hypotension ("cyclo shock") may occur in the postoperative period. The latter is probably caused by the sudden cessation of epinephrine release by the cyclopropane plus the hypercapnia. During anesthesia, ventricular fibrillation can result from catecholamine injections (epinephrine, levarterenol, etc). Noncatechol vasoconstrictors such as phenylephrine (Neo-Synephrine) are preferable during cyclopropane anesthesia.

D. Diethyl Ether: Diethyl ether ($CH_3CH_2OCH_2$-CH_3), usually referred to as ethyl ether or just ether, vies with nitrous oxide as the oldest anesthetic and is still one of the safest. It is the safest anesthetic in unskilled hands, with a wide margin between the concentration adequate for surgery and the concentration causing severe depression of the respiratory and cardiovascular systems. Ether is a liquid at room temperature and can be administered with a minimum of equipment, which, combined with low cost, is an attractive feature in many parts of the world. It provides excellent muscular relaxation.

The main disadvantages of ether are explosiveness; irritation of the respiratory passages, which can cause excessive secretions (blocked by parasympatholytic drugs); induction of laryngospasm and breathholding; slowness of induction and recovery (high solubility); and frequent postanesthesia nausea and vomiting.

E. Vinyl Ether (Vinethene): Vinyl ether ($CH_2CHOCHCH_2$) is a potent volatile liquid anesthetic whose principal advantage is rapidity of induction and recovery. It is as explosive as diethyl ether and more toxic, but it is useful for open drop inductions or for short procedures (less than 15 minutes) because it is rapid acting and less irritating to respiratory passages.

F. Ethyl Chloride: Ethyl chloride (CH_3CH_2Cl) is a gas at room temperature but is provided as a liquid in well-stoppered bottles (boiling point, 12.3 C). Its low cost has encouraged its use as an induction agent in many countries, but its great potency, rapidity of action, and tendency to cause myocardial depression or irritability make it a hazardous agent except for induction by open drop administered by someone experienced in using it.

G. Trichloroethylene (Trilene): Trichloroethylene ($CHClCCl_2$) is a noncombustible volatile liquid anesthetic that has been used as an adjunct to nitrous oxide. It decomposes to toxic products when exposed to the heat and alkalies of CO_2 absorbers. It does not produce good muscular relaxation. It causes tachypnea which is believed to be due to sensitization of lung stretch receptors. In recent years it has been almost entirely supplanted by halothane.

H. Chloroform: Chloroform ($CHCl_3$) is the oldest of the halogenated liquid anesthetics. Its advantages are minimal irritation of the respiratory passages, rapidity of induction and recovery, low cost, ease of administration, and excellent muscular relaxation. Because it produces dose-related liver damage which may progress to hepatic failure, this otherwise excellent anesthetic has been almost completely abandoned.

I. Halothane (Fluothane): Halothane ($BrClHCCF_3$) is a nonexplosive volatile liquid. It provides smooth induction, almost no irritation of the respiratory tract, and moderate muscular relaxation which is adequate for surgery in infants and children. It causes minimal postanesthetic nausea.

Halothane depresses the circulation both by a direct action on the myocardium and by loss of vasomotor tone. It predisposes the myocardium to arrhythmias if epinephrine is injected or if the release of endogenous catecholamines is raised by hypercapnia. Cases of hepatitis severe enough to cause death have been traced to halothane, although the full explanation is not yet clear; case finding and proof of relationship to halothane are complicated by other causes of hepatitis such as viruses and other drugs. There is evidence that about one in 10,000 patients breaks down the halothane molecule to a product that causes liver damage, with increasing sensitization with each exposure. An otherwise unexplainable fever in the first 48 hours after halothane anesthesia suggests sensitivity and contraindicates future use. Other agents should be used when there is a possibility of jaundice due to other causes in order not to complicate the differential diagnosis in the postoperative period.

Many patients have had numerous uneventful halothane anesthesias. The many excellent characteristics of this drug have been amply demonstrated in millions of administrations; on balance, halothane has probably prevented more morbidity and mortality than have been caused by its potential for liver toxicity.

J. Enflurane (Ethrane): Enflurane, a halogenated ether with the formula $CHClFCF_2OCHF_2$, is a volatile liquid with many properties resembling halothane, such as smooth induction, better muscular relaxation, minimal postanesthetic nausea, and nonflammability. High concentrations combined with hypocapnia may cause easily reversed CNS seizure activity without sequelae. It provides anesthesia without arrhythmias in the presence of high endogenous (from elevated P_{CO_2}) or exogenous (by injection) catecholamine levels.

K. Methoxyflurane (Penthrane): Methoxyflurane ($CHCl_2CF_2OCH_3$) is a halogenated ether that is a liquid with a very low vapor pressure at room temperature. It provides good analgesia that lasts into the postoperative period. A dose-related high output renal failure limits the duration and depth of anesthesia and patient selection.

Research continues in the field, and new halogenated anesthetics may replace those discussed above.

Anesthetic Explosions

Several of the inhalation anesthetics discussed above are explosive in their effective concentrations. Explosions occur when a source of ignition (spark, flame, or heat) comes in contact with a highly combustible substance in the presence of oxygen. Anesthetic explosions may kill or injure not only the patient but others in the immediate vicinity. They can only be prevented by unremitting vigilance when explosive anesthetic mixtures are used. Spark-producing equipment such as electrocautery units and other electrical apparatus not declared spark-proof by the National Board of Fire Underwriters should not be used in the operating room when an explosive anesthetic is in use. To minimize sparks from static electricity, the relative humidity in operating rooms should be above 50% and all equipment and personnel should be grounded to a conductive floor. Drapes and external wearing apparel should not create static charges by friction. Floor conductivity, although sufficient to drain static charges, ought not be so great as to constitute an electrocution hazard for the personnel in the operating room.

INTRAVENOUS ANESTHESIA

Intravenous anesthesia has the advantage of ease of administration and great popularity with patients who desire general anesthesia but dislike the anesthetic mask and the slowness of induction of inhalation anesthesia. Intravenous anesthesia is also fatally easy to administer by the untrained or unskilled. Once injected into a vein, the agent cannot be removed at will, whereas inhalation agents can be eliminated by ventilation of the lungs.

Intravenous Barbiturates

Thiopental (Pentothal) and thiamylal (Surital) are the most frequently used barbiturates for anesthesia. They are marketed as powders consisting of the sodium salts and are easily dissolved in water to make an alkaline solution. They are so similar in action that what is said here about thiopental applies also to thiamylal.

Thiopental is administered in a 0.2–2.5% solution. Accidental intra-arterial injections of higher concentrations can cause severe damage to peripheral tissues by arterial spasm, endothelial injury, and clotting. An intravenously injected dose of thiopental is distributed to all tissues, but the richly perfused organs such as the brain, heart, and kidneys receive a higher share of the dose. If the injected amount is sufficient (100–300 mg), loss of consciousness ensues. Awakening from a single dose is not due to destruction or excretion of the drug but is the result of a diminishing concentration of thiopental in the brain as distribution to other tissues takes place. Repeated or continued administration to maintain unconsciousness will eventually saturate all body tissues to the same concentration as the brain. When that point is reached, awakening will be dependent on the metabolism of the barbiturate by the liver during the subsequent 24–48 hours. This is one of the reasons why thiopental is not a good choice as the sole agent for anesthesia of more than a few minutes' duration.

Thiopental is ideal for induction and as a basal anesthetic or adjunct to nitrous oxide anesthesia.

Thiopental induces a CNS depression that is characterized by better hypnosis than analgesia. Its failure to block afferent pathways except at great depth can lead to laryngospasm if the larynx is stimulated, overt movement following surgical stimulation, and retention of many other reflexes.

Hypotension frequently follows the administration of thiopental. The degree of hypotension depends on the amount and rate of injection and the physical condition of the patient. It is probably caused by a combination of central vasomotor depression, sympathetic ganglionic blockade, and direct myocardial depression. *Caution:* This hypotension can be disastrous in shock and hypovolemic states.

Intravenous Narcotics

Morphine, meperidine (Demerol), and other narcotics can be used intravenously for anesthesia; in contrast to the barbiturates, they provide excellent analgesia with little hypnosis. Increasing respiratory depression progresses in step with the analgesic effect. Narcotics are well tolerated in very large doses by poor-risk patients, causing minimal circulatory depression if the patient's pulmonary ventilation is maintained artificially during and after surgery.

A narcotic antagonist such as naloxone hydrochloride (Narcan) can reverse the depressant actions of the narcotics.

Narcotics are not used as the sole agents for anesthesia but only in combination with nitrous oxide or barbiturates. A mixture of a narcotic (fentanyl) and a tranquilizer (droperidol), marketed as Innovar, has some popularity as an intravenous anesthetic. It produces sedation, reduced muscular activity, and profound analgesia, sometimes called neuroleptanalgesia. The droperidol has a longer duration than fentanyl, which can be administered alone if supplementation of analgesia is necessary. Clinically, Innovar is combined with nitrous oxide anesthesia. Good postoperative analgesia and absence of nausea are important advantages. Severe respiratory depression may occur and requires surveillance and treatment.

Ketamine (Ketalar)

Ketamine is an intravenous agent that is almost as rapidly effective when administered intramuscularly. It causes an almost immediate trance-like analgesic state with no respiratory depression and no loss of muscle tone. Circulation is not depressed and blood pressure is raised, which contraindicates its administration to hypertensive patients. Pharyngeal and laryngeal muscle tone and reflexes are not lost, so that the airway remains patent even in awkward positions. Although the duration of anesthesia is only 5—10 minutes, repeated injections can be given to maintain analgesia for over an hour.

Ketamine analgesia is associated with unpleasant hallucinations during recovery in some patients (usually adults), which limits its usefulness.

Neuromuscular Blocking Agents

Neuromuscular blockers or muscle relaxants are a group of drugs that prevent striated muscles from contracting when their motor nerves are stimulated. They do not affect the sensorium. Their mode of action is by one of 2 mechanisms. Tubocurarine (curare) and gallamine triethiodide (Flaxedil) are competitive inhibitors of acetylcholine at the neuromuscular junction but do not cause a depolarization of the end plate that initiates contraction. A reversal of effect occurs if sufficient acetylcholine can accumulate at the neuromuscular junction for successful competition with the drugs. This can be produced clinically by the administration of neostigmine (Prostigmin), which inhibits cholinesterase, the enzyme responsible for the breakdown of acetylcholine. Neostigmine is therefore an effective antagonist to curare. Neostigmine has muscarinic effects (bradycardia, excessive salivation, etc) that must in turn be blocked by giving atropine before or simultaneously with the neostigmine used for curare reversal. Clinically, a mixture of 2.5 mg of neostigmine and 1 mg of atropine per 5 ml of solution is injected slowly over a period of minutes to reverse curare. The maximum useful dose is 10 ml of the solution, but less that half of that is usually sufficient.

Succinylcholine chloride (Anectine) and decamethonium bromide (Syncurine) produce a neuromuscular block by acting like acetylcholine to depolarize the membrane of the motor end plate. However, unlike acetylcholine, they do not permit the immediate repolarization necessary for another contraction. This type of neuromuscular block does not respond to neostigmine initially; however, when sustained by large doses over a period of time, it becomes curare-like and responds to neostigmine. This so-called phase II block

is not fully understood. An occasional patient whose plasma is deficient in pseudocholinesterase will be unable to deactivate succinylcholine and may develop prolonged paralysis with a small dose. Mechanical ventilation and time are the antidotes.

The clinical use of the neuromuscular blocking agents has been one of the major advances in anesthesia of this century. Usually given intravenously, these drugs provide all degrees of muscular relaxation with minimal side-effects, thus diminishing the required dosage of general anesthetics with their many undesirable properties. Because they do not cross the placental barrier in effective concentrations, they are useful for cesarean sections. They should never be used by anyone without the means and experience to carry out mechanical ventilation.

Tubocurarine is the oldest and most commonly used muscle relaxant. It is partly excreted in the urine and partly metabolized. After a peak effect at about 10 minutes, its clinical action diminishes during the next hour, largely because of distribution away from the neuromuscular junctions. Therefore, prolongation of the neuromuscular block can be achieved with subsequent smaller doses. The degree of effectiveness of the block can be assessed objectively in clinical situations by observing the absence or fading strength of muscle twitches upon electrical stimulation of nerves. For example, the absence of contraction or the diminished strength of contraction of hand muscles in response to ulnar nerve stimulation can be observed.

A fall in blood pressure due to ganglionic blocking action and bronchospasm caused by histamine release are very rare adverse reactions to curare. A fall in blood pressure may also be due to the preservatives in some curare preparations. Ether anesthesia, quinidine, lidocaine, and a number of antibiotics (neomycin, kanamycin) intensify the effect of curare.

The paralyzing dose of curare is 15—30 mg IV.

Gallamine triethiodide (Flaxedil) has a curare-like action at the neuromuscular junction, a slightly shorter duration of action, does not liberate histamine, causes tachycardia by its vagolytic action, and is dependent on renal function for its elimination. The paralyzing dose is 100—200 mg IV.

Succinylcholine chloride (Anectine) has a duration of action of 3—5 minutes after a paralyzing dose of 20—50 mg. It is frequently administered by continuous intravenous drip of a solution containing 1—2 mg/ml.

MANAGEMENT OF GENERAL ANESTHESIA

Endotracheal intubation is performed routinely as part of the management of general anesthesia for the majority of extensive surgical procedures. The technics of inserting the tube into the larynx are many and can only be mastered by practice. They are facilitated by deep anesthesia or muscle relaxants. During anesthesia, intubation provides better control of the upper airway, removes the anesthetic mask from the surgical field in oral and facial surgery, facilitates assisted or controlled ventilation, and prevents aspiration of foreign materials into the lungs.

Balanced anesthesia is a term applied to anesthesia produced by the combination of 2 or more drugs. Ideally, each agent contributes its most desirable property, and none is given in toxic amounts. The combined effect is tailored to suit the condition of the patient and the requirements of the operation by variations in the dosages of the component agents. An example is the use of thiopental for a rapid, pleasant induction, nitrous oxide for its nontoxic, nonexplosive properties, a narcotic or potent inhalation agent to deepen the anesthetic level, and curare to provide muscular relaxation.

The desired depth of anesthesia for surgery is not difficult to achieve. Pushing the plunger of a syringe or turning the flow valve of an anesthetic machine to deepen anesthesia requires little knowledge. The experience and skill of the anesthesiologist are called into play in keeping the patient alive, safe, and relatively unharmed in spite of the necessary trauma of the operation and the anesthetic drugs used to facilitate it. During general anesthesia, the unconscious patient loses many protective reflexes, and vital respiratory and circulatory functions may be depressed. Corneal ulcers, pressure sores, nerve palsies caused by prolonged unphysiologic positioning, and injuries to joints and to intervertebral disks are examples of the damage the patient may sustain without complaint during anesthesia. Although protecting the patient from such trauma is important, the primary function of the anesthesiologist is the prevention of tissue hypoxia by maintaining adequate arterial blood oxygen tension and tissue perfusion. The signs of insufficient arterial blood oxygen tension progress from cyanosis (which is not reliable) and initial tachycardia to bradycardia, hypotension, dilated pupils, and cardiac arrest. The ventilatory causes of arterial oxygen desaturation are insufficient oxygen tension in the respired gases, insufficient pulmonary ventilation, or maldistribution of the ventilation in the lungs. A hypoxic inhaled mixture must be suspected immediately regardless of the contrary evidence of the flowmeters of the anesthetic machine whenever cyanosis develops in spite of good pulmonary ventilation and good circulation. Believing the machine instead of the clinical evidence has caused many fatalities.

Insufficient pulmonary ventilation may be due to central depression by the anesthetic drugs; to weakness or paralysis of the respiratory muscles caused by neuromuscular blockers or deep anesthesia; or, most commonly, to obstruction of the air passages. Although insidious, the first 2 are easily prevented or treated by assisted or controlled respiration. The signs of obstruction are absence of air movement (total obstruction) or noisy respiration (partial obstruction); noticeably increased muscular effort during inspiration; and indrawing of the soft tissues of the thoracic

wall (suprasternal notch, supraclavicular fossas, and intercostal spaces) during inspiration. Deep anesthesia and muscle relaxants obscure the signs related to muscular efforts. Partial obstruction is diagnosed by auscultation of the air movement with an ear or stethoscope over the trachea, the mouth, or the rebreathing tubes of the anesthetic machine. Total or partial obstruction of the paralyzed patient is diagnosed by noting the duration and degree of pressure required to inflate the lungs and also by listening for adventitious sounds. Obstruction of the airway may occur anywhere from the nose and lips to the alveoli. The possible causes are numerous and include tongue obstruction, laryngospasm, inflammatory disorders, foreign bodies, and neoplasms. The anesthetic state itself causes some types of airway obstruction. During anesthesia, the tone of the lingual and mandibular muscles may be so diminished as to allow the tongue of the supine patient to drop back into the pharynx and obstruct air flow. This is the most frequent form of obstruction in anesthesia. It can be prevented or corrected by extending the patient's head and neck and drawing the mandible forward. Mechanical devices such as oropharyngeal and nasopharyngeal airways or endotracheal tubes may be required also.

Obstruction of the airway by laryngospasm occurs during light anesthesia. It can be corrected by deepening the anesthesia or by positive airway pressure. The expert anesthesiologist seldom resorts to paralysis with succinylcholine to relieve laryngospasm.

Airway obstruction may also be due to vomitus. Aspiration of vomitus may lead to severe postoperative pneumonitis. It is best avoided by withholding anesthesia until the stomach is empty or, if that is impossible, by intubating the trachea with the patient awake or following a rapid induction. General anesthesia should never be induced unless an efficient suction apparatus is available. The decision whether a tracheostomy should be done under local anesthesia before general anesthesia is administered to a patient with upper airway obstruction is a matter of clinical judgment.

One impediment to respiration that does not involve obstruction of the airway is interference with lung expansion, the most common form of which is pneumothorax. It can occur during surgery of the neck or of the subdiaphragmatic area. It behaves like an airway obstruction except that adventitious sounds during respiration are absent. If it is caused by leakage of air from the lung, it can develop into a tension pneumothorax which embarrasses circulation. Treatment consists of removal of air from the pleural cavity. This is discussed in Chapter 21.

The circulatory deficiencies that interfere with tissue oxygenation are outlined in Chapter 15. Anesthesia contributes to circulatory failure by causing myocardial and vasomotor depression. The anesthesiologist's role in its management is to maintain minimal anesthesia compatible with surgery, to replace fluid and blood, to maintain a good arterial oxygen tension, and to position the patient to assist venous return.

Vasopressor drugs are useful in the treatment of hypotension during spinal anesthesia or simple syncope but are only stopgap measures in hypovolemia.

. . .

MONITORING DURING ANESTHESIA

There are many technics for monitoring patients. The experienced observer's senses and his ability to integrate the information obtained with them can be aided but not replaced by sophisticated electronic devices. Observations of the movements of the chest and of the reservoir bag together with continuous auscultation of breath sounds with a chest or esophageal stethoscope are the best monitors of pulmonary ventilation. Changes in volume and rhythm of breathing as well as the signs of airway obstruction are readily detected. Tissue color, bleeding (and the color of arterial blood in the wound), the quality of the pulse, the arterial blood pressure, the quality of the heart sounds (obtained with a precordial or esophageal stethoscope), the filling of neck veins and central venous pressure, the size and reactivity of the pupils, and urine outflow are all observable in most cases. The status of the heart, circulation, and tissue perfusion can thus be followed in a continuous manner. An earpiece molded to fit the observer's external ear canal is more comfortable than the binaural stethoscope during prolonged procedures. Continuous ECG and EEG tracings, arterial pressures obtained by intra-arterial catheters connected to pressure transducers, continuous analysis of expired CO_2 tension, and frequent sampling of arterial blood for determinations of P_{O_2}, P_{CO_2}, and pH provide critically important information in selected cases. The diagnosis of certain cardiac arrhythmias, hypercapnia, and acidosis cannot be made without them.

POSTANESTHETIC MANAGEMENT

The anesthetic state cannot be terminated and the patient returned to his preanesthetic condition in an instant at the end of the surgical procedure. The central depressant drugs, the neuromuscular blockers, and the physiologic trespasses of regional anesthesia continue to act for variable periods of time. The trauma of the surgery, hemorrhage, and loss of circulating volume to the extravascular compartments are all additive to the residual anesthetic state. This situation may last many hours, during which time the patient requires the same monitoring and the same support of his vital functions as he did during the operation.

The stage is still set for failure of any of the links of the oxygen transport mechanism. The cardinal sin in managing postoperative patients is to administer sedatives to control restlessness since this is so often a manifestation of hypoxemia. Restlessness calls for increased inspired oxygen or assisted ventilation and measurement of arterial oxygen tension.

Pulmonary atelectasis of patchy areas or entire lobes is the most common postoperative complication. The causes include impediments to good expansion of the lungs such as central sedation, neuromuscular weakness, airway obstruction of any kind, excessive secretions in the airways, pain from respiratory movements, and tight dressings. Treatment consists of removal of the cause if possible and reexpansion of the lungs by encouraging the patient to cough and to breathe deeply. Artificial means include tracheal suction, stimulation by administration of 5% CO_2 or by increasing the dead space, and assisted ventilation with respirators. Bronchoscopic removal of bronchial obstruction is occasionally necessary. The use of a high inspired oxygen tension to compensate for shunting or inadequate ventilation neither prevents nor cures atelectasis.

. . .

General References

Bertrand CA & others: Disturbances of cardiac rhythm during anesthesia and surgery. JAMA 216:1615, 1971.

Collins VJ: *Principles of Anesthesia,* 2nd ed. Lea & Febiger, 1976.

Covino BG, Vassallo HG: *Local Anesthetics: Mechanisms of Action and Clinical Use.* Grune & Stratton, 1976.

Cullen DJ & others: Clinical signs of anesthesia. Anesthesiology 36:21, 1972.

Cullen SC, Larson CP Jr: *Essentials of Anesthetic Practice.* Year Book, 1974.

Dodson ME, Richards TG: A prospective study of changes in liver function after operation under two forms of general anesthesia. Br J Anaesth 44:47, 1972.

Dripps RD & others: *Introduction to Anesthesia,* 4th ed. Saunders, 1972.

Eyring H & others: A molecular mechanism of general anesthesia. Anesthesiology 38:415, 1973.

Goldstein A Jr, Keats AS: The risk of anesthesia. Anesthesiology 33:130, 1970.

Grogono AW, Lee P: Danger lists for the anesthetist. Anesthesia 25:518, 1970.

Hedley-Whyte J & others: *Applied Physiology of Respiratory Care.* Little, Brown, 1976.

Hill DW: *Physics Applied to Anesthesia,* 3rd ed. Butterworth, 1976.

Kaufman RD: Biophysical mechanisms of anesthesia action. Anesthesiology 46:49, 1977.

Keszler H: The anesthetist and coronary artery disease. Anesthetist 21:381, 1972.

Lee TA, Atkinson RS: *A Synopsis of Anesthesia,* 7th ed. Year Book, 1973.

Milledge JS, Nunn JF: Criteria of fitness for anesthesia in patients with chronic obstructive lung disease. Br Med J 3:670, 1975.

Miller KW & others: Physicochemical approaches to the mode of action of general anesthetics. Anesthesiology 36:339, 1972.

Phillips OC, Capizzi LS: Anesthesia mortality. Clin Anesth 10(3):220, 1974.

Quimby CW Jr & others: Anesthesia and the infarcted heart. Anesth Analg 53:394, 1974.

Ravin MB: Comparison of spinal and general anesthesia for lower abdominal surgery in patients with chronic obstructive pulmonary disease. Anesthesiology 35:319, 1971.

Scurr C, Feldman S: *Scientific Foundations of Anesthesia,* 2nd ed. Year Book, 1974.

Siegel JH, Chodoff P (editors): *The Surgical Management of the Aged and High Risk Patient.* Grune & Stratton, 1976.

Tarhan S, Moffitt EA: Anesthesia and supportive care during and after cardiac surgery. Ann Thorac Surg 11:64, 1971.

Tarhan S & others: Myocardial infarction after general anesthesia. JAMA 220:1451, 1972.

Tarhan S & others: Risk of anesthesia and surgery in patients with chronic bronchitis and chronic obstructive pulmonary disease. Surgery 74:720, 1973.

Wollman H, Greenhow DE (editors): Symposium on recent developments in anesthesia. Surg Clin North Am 55:757, 1975. [Entire issue.]

Wylie WD, Churchill-Davidson HC: *A Practice of Anesthesia,* 3rd ed. Lloyd-Luke Ltd, 1972.

15 . . .
Shock

Donald D. Trunkey, MD, & F. William Blaisdell, MD

Shock is a breakdown of effective circulation at the cellular level. It occurs in association with many types of major illness such as trauma, hemorrhage, burns, infection, and cardiac disease and is the final event in most terminal illnesses.

CIRCULATORY PHYSIOLOGY

The circulatory system is composed of the heart, the blood vessels (arteries, capillaries, and veins), and the blood. The arteries conduct blood to the tissues. Their terminal branches, the arterioles, provide resistance, control the blood pressure, and determine the perfusion of individual vascular beds. The veins act as the reservoir (capacitance) system, store more than half of the blood volume, and, by providing the priming pressure of the heart, help to determine cardiac output.

The normal blood volume averages about 8% of body weight and consists of 5–6 liters in the average adult. At any one moment, 10% of this volume will be in the arterial system, 20% in the capillaries, and 70% in the venous reservoir and heart. Measuring the pressure in the venous system (central venous pressure, CVP) provides a rough estimate of the blood volume.

In a resting subject, the heart ejects 70–90 ml of blood with each beat; this stroke volume correlates roughly with the blood volume and produces a systolic pressure of about 120 mm Hg. Stroke volume is determined by the effects of preload, afterload, and the contractile state of the myocardium. Preload is the resting force per unit area of muscle which stretches the sarcomeres, and the force of contraction is directly related to it. Preload will be affected by the amount of venous return to the heart and pulmonary vascular resistance. The force of contraction is inversely related to afterload, the force resisting shortening per unit area of muscle. Provided there are no anatomic abnormalities of the heart, afterload is a function of peripheral vascular resistance largely provided by the arterioles. Contractility is the inherent capacity of the myocardium to create a force independent of preload and afterload. The balance between cardiac output and peripheral resistance maintains pressure between car-

diac contractions of roughly 80 mm Hg. This results in a mean pressure in the large arteries of about 95 mm Hg and in the arterioles of about 35 mm Hg. Under normal circumstances, the blood vessels have the capacity for autoregulation—ie, through local reflexes which determine arteriolar tone, flow can be adjusted in accordance with tissue needs through a wide range of heart rates and blood pressures.

The pressure in the capillaries averages about 25 mm Hg at the arterial end and 15 mm Hg at the venous end. The higher pressure at the arterial end drives fluid out of the vessel into the interstitial space (filtration pressure). This is opposed by the oncotic pressure inside the capillary provided by the plasma proteins. Oncotic pressure exceeds filtration pressure at the venous end of the capillary and pulls fluid back into the vascular system. At any one moment, an average of 20% of the capillaries are open. This is all that is required to provide for normal cell nutrition and remove metabolic waste. Local accumulation of metabolites brings about dilatation of precapillary sphincters and increased perfusion of individual vascular beds.

Although the exact anatomic pathways are not well defined, arteriovenous shunts capable of diverting blood from the arterial to the venous system are present in almost all vascular beds. They open in response to certain stimuli (eg, heat), usually in circumstances in which precapillary sphincters are closed.

On the venous side, pressure decreases progressively from the venules (15 mm Hg) to the large central veins (4–5 mm Hg). Within physiologic limits, the higher the venous pressure, the greater the priming pressure of the heart, the greater the ventricular filling, and the greater the resulting stroke volume and cardiac output.

Responses to Volume Loss

The vascular system acts to maintain tissue perfusion so that fluctuations in blood volume elicit reflexes which tend to restore flow to normal. Decreases in pressure or volume activate sympathetic and renal responses. Baroreceptors in the carotid sinus and the large thoracic arteries sense changes in tension in the arterial wall. Decreased tension activates the sympathetic nervous system and the adrenal medulla. These stimulate the strength (inotropic effect) and the rate (chronotropic effect) of cardiac contraction and increase cardiac output with increasing volume deficit. Vasoconstriction is produced successively in the skin and subcutaneous tissue, in skeletal muscle, and in the splanchnic circulation. The splanchnic reservoir is emptied into systemic veins. The lowered filtration pressure in the capillaries favors oncotic attraction of fluid into the vessels, and this tends to restore vascular volume. The only vascular systems not constricted by the sympathetic nerves and catecholamines are the coronary and cerebral arteries, as the body's defense mechanism preserves flow to these organs at the expense of all others.

A drop in renal artery pressure and flow produces renal artery vasoconstriction and results in decreased glomerular filtration and decreased urine output. Renin secretion is increased and evokes aldosterone secretion by the adrenal cortex, which promotes salt and water retention. Renin release results in the production of angiotensin II, another potent vasoconstrictor which raises blood pressure.

Loss of blood volume also activates a generalized venous reflex; this produces venous constriction, which increases venous return to the heart and cardiac filling pressure and improves cardiac output.

In addition to these acute changes from loss of vascular volume, other long-term compensatory mechanisms are activated. The liver is stimulated, and increased protein synthesis results in a rapid rise in serum fibrinogen and other clotting factors. Albumin synthesis is increased; within 24 hours, serum proteins return to normal. Erythropoietin appears in the circulation to stimulate red blood cell synthesis. Red cell volume returns to normal over a period of several weeks.

Aviado DM: Hypotension and the autonomic nervous system. Ann NY Acad Sci 66:998, 1957.

Bassin R & others: Rapid and slow hemorrhage in man: 1. Sequential hemodynamic responses. Ann Surg 173:325, 1971.

Moore FD: Effects of hemorrhage on body composition. N Engl J Med 273:567, 1965.

TYPES OF SHOCK

Shock can be defined as peripheral circulatory failure such that tissue perfusion is inadequate to meet the nutritional requirements of the cells and remove the waste products of metabolism.

Various types of shock result from failure in one or more of the 3 major components of the circulatory system: pump, peripheral resistance, or blood volume. The major types are hypovolemic, cardiogenic, neurogenic, and septic shock. Table 15–1 summarizes the circulatory changes that occur in each.

Hypovolemic Shock

(Due to hemorrhage, burns, bowel obstruction, etc.)

Table 15–1. Major changes in the principal types of shock.

Type of Shock	Cardiac Function	Arteriolar Resistance	Venous Reservoir
Hypovolemic	↑	↑	↓↓
Cardiogenic	↓↓	↑	↑
Neurogenic	↑	↓↓	↑
Septic	↓	↓	↓

Hypovolemic shock results from decreased blood volume due to loss of blood, plasma, or body water and electrolytes. The characteristic changes in hypovolemic shock are decreased venous pressure, increased peripheral resistance, and tachycardia.

Cardiogenic Shock

(Due to myocardial infarction, cardiac arrhythmias, congestive heart failure, etc.)

The principal problem in cardiogenic shock is pump failure with a reduction in cardiac output. Blood backs up behind the heart, so that there is an increase in venous pressure. Peripheral resistance increases and directs the remaining flow to critical vascular beds. In chronic heart failure, complex intracellular compensatory mechanisms from reduced tissue oxygen levels allow the organism to survive chronically reduced cardiac output, but these cannot be activated in time to meet the needs of an acute reduction of similar magnitude.

Neurogenic Shock

(Due to quadriplegia, spinal anesthesia, etc.)

Neurogenic shock is due to a failure of arterial resistance with pooling of blood in dilated capacitance vessels. Cardiac activity increases to maintain a normal stroke volume in an attempt to preserve perfusion pressure.

Septic Shock

(Due to infection, peritonitis, meningitis, etc.)

Septic shock is most often due to gram-negative septicemia. Hypovolemia develops as a result of pooling of blood in the microcirculation and loss of fluid from the vascular space as a result of a generalized increase in capillary permeability. There may also be a direct toxic effect on the heart, with depressed cardiac function. Peripheral resistance is usually decreased as a result of the opening of arteriovenous shunts. Gram-positive sepsis occasionally produces hypovolemia, but in these instances loss of fluid is limited to the area of infection.

Miscellaneous Types of Shock

These include otherwise unclassified types of shock. Pulmonary embolism produces right heart failure when the pulmonary vasculature is filled by thrombus, with obstruction to flow. Shock can occur secondary to inadequate cardiopulmonary bypass during heart surgery. Other types of shock include anaphylaxis and insulin shock.

Carey LC: Hemorrhagic shock. Curr Probl Surg, Jan 1971.

Christy JH: Pathophysiology of gram-negative shock. Am Heart J 81:694, 1971.

Lillehei RC & others: Hemodynamic changes in endotoxin shock. Pages 442–462 in: *Shock and Hypotension.* Mills LJ, Moyer JH (editors). Grune & Stratton, 1965.

MacLean LD & others: The patient in shock. Can Med Assoc J 103:853, 1970.

McCabe WR: Gram negative bacteremia. Adv Intern Med 19:135, 1974.

Rutherford RB, Trow RS: The pathophysiology of irreversible hemorrhagic shock in monkeys. J Surg Res 14:538, 1973.

Scheidt S & others: Shock after myocardial infarction: A clinical and hemodynamic profile. Am J Cardiol 26:556, 1970.

Siegel JH & others: The surgical implications of physiologic patterns in myocardial infarction shock. Surgery 72:126, 1972.

Thal AP, Kinney JM: On the definition and classification of shock. Prog Cardiovasc Dis 9:527, 1967.

PATHOPHYSIOLOGY OF SHOCK

In shock there is depression of cell metabolism, and all metabolism ultimately ceases as death approaches. Before total collapse and death, individual metabolic factors are variably affected by shock.

(1) Protein metabolism is altered, for there is increased catabolism with cell breakdown and a rise in blood urea, serum creatinine, and serum uric acid.

(2) Changes in **fat metabolism** result as catechol amines initiate lipolysis. Tissue lipids and serum triglycerides are converted to free fatty acids. These changes are reflected in increased free fatty acids in the blood.

(3) Carbohydrate metabolism. Elevated catecholamine levels produce increased liver glycogenolysis with an increase in blood glucose. The metabolic pathway for glucose is compromised by the switch from aerobic to anaerobic metabolism in cells with inadequate perfusion. The ordinary metabolic pathway of glucose consists of breakdown into the 3-carbon pyruvate and then acetyl-CoA. Further metabolism (the citric acid [Krebs] cycle) releases large quantities of high-energy ATP with CO_2 and water. When oxygen is not available, the standard metabolic pathway cannot proceed beyond pyruvate. During anaerobic metabolism, glucose is converted to pyruvate and then lactate with release of small quantities of high-energy ATP, a much less efficient metabolic pathway but one that is capable of energy production in the absence of oxygen. As shock continues, there is a build-up of lactate in the blood. If liver perfusion is sufficient, the lactate load can be further metabolized there; otherwise, acidosis increases as lactate accumulates. This adds to the acidosis already produced by the changes in fat metabolism.

Energy is required to maintain an ionic differential between the cell and the surrounding interstitial fluid. This maintains the high intracellular potassium and extracellular sodium concentrations. Decreased nutrition of the cell results in decreased cell energy. Cell work diminishes, and cell membranes are thereby damaged by shock. Sodium moves into the cell and potassium moves out. Body water follows the sodium ion—so that, as sodium moves into the cell, obligatory cell edema occurs. The serum sodium falls and the serum potassium rises (Fig 15–1).

The mechanisms theoretically accountable for these changes include a direct membrane effect altering permeability. This could be secondary to disruption of the bilipid layer with rearrangement of the fatty acids. A second possibility is that toxic substances within the circulating plasma act as ionophores (ion carriers), thus increasing membrane transport. A third possibility is reduction of energy phosphates within the cell, thus shutting down ATP-dependent systems such as active transport of sodium.

Depending on the severity of shock, mitochondrial and lysosomal membranes swell and eventually burst. Once the lysosomal membranes disrupt, acid phosphatases and dehydrogenases enter the cytosol, causing further damage to organelles. Some of these acid phosphatases may cause systemic toxic symptoms. Disruption of mitochondria causes an inhibition of stage 3 respiratory activity (ADP-dependent), de-

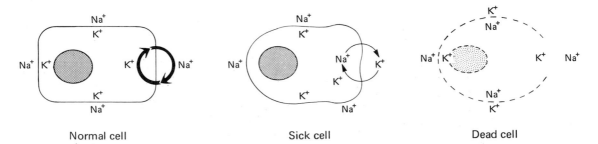

Figure 15–1. Progressive cell damage and cell death in shock. In the normal cell, energy is required to keep the membrane sodium-potassium pump functioning and to maintain the gradient between high intracellular potassium and high extracellular sodium concentrations. As shock progresses, adequate energy stores are no longer available, the pump breaks down, and sodium chloride and water enter the cell, leading to swelling.

creased ATPase activity, and decreased energy-dependent calcium transport. There is an inhibition of oxidative phosphorylation reflected in decreased cytochrome activity. Additional membrane changes are seen in endoplasmic and sarcoplasmic reticulum. In excitable cells—particularly cardiac muscle—changes in these structures can impair contractile mechanisms. As the low perfusion state progresses, alterations in excitation-contraction coupling may then take place, leading to arrhythmias and decreased contractile force.

Anoxia of cells in the CNS results in hyperventilation with respiratory alkalosis. Later, there is anaerobic metabolism and lactate accumulation. As the renal compensatory mechanism fails, there is progressive metabolic acidosis. Many vicious cycles are set in motion simultaneously (Fig 15–2).

The principal result of all types of shock is insufficient microcirculatory flow. The changes in the microcirculation progress in several phases (Fig 15–3). The following is a general description, not necessarily applicable to all organs.

Compensation Phase (Fig 15–3A)

The first response of the circulation to hypovolemia is contraction of precapillary arterial sphincters. This causes the filtration pressure in the capillary to fall, and, since osmotic pressure remains the same, fluid moves into the vascular space with a corresponding increase in blood volume. If this compensatory mechanism is adequate to return blood volume to normal, the precapillary sphincter relaxes and microcirculatory flow returns to normal. If shock is prolonged and profound, the next phase is entered.

Cell Distress Phase (Fig 15–3B)

If the precapillary sphincter contraction does not restore the volume and flow to normal, the precapillary sphincter remains closed. Arteriovenous shunts may open and divert arterial flow directly into the venous system. The cells in the bypassed segment of the microcirculation must rely on anaerobic metabolism for energy. This decreases the glucose and oxygen available for the cells and results in accumulation of metabolic waste products such as lactate. An inadequate supply of energy substrate results in a form of cell distress. Histamine is released, producing closure of the postcapillary sphincter. This serves to slow the remaining capillary flow and hold the red blood cells and nutrients in the capillaries longer. The empty capillary bed in this phase of shock totally constricts, and very few patent capillaries remain.

Decompensation Phase (Fig 15–3C)

In the agonal phase, just before cell death, local reflexes (perhaps due to accumulation of metabolites and local acidosis) result in reopening of the precapillary sphincter while the postcapillary sphincter remains closed. Prolonged vasoconstriction of the capillary bed damages endothelial cells and results in increased capillary permeability. When the capillary reopens, fluid and protein are lost into the interstitial space and the capillary distends with red blood cells which pile up on one another and agglutinate (sludge). White cell and platelet aggregates accumulate in the venules, where acidosis is most profound. Cell membranes may also have increased permeability, and because of profound energy deficits active transport is reduced. Sodium, cal-

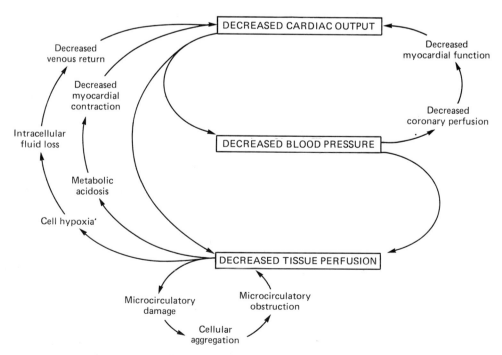

Figure 15–2. Vicious cycles in shock. The problem can be initiated at numerous points in any cycle: decreased tissue perfusion, decreased coronary perfusion, metabolic acidosis.

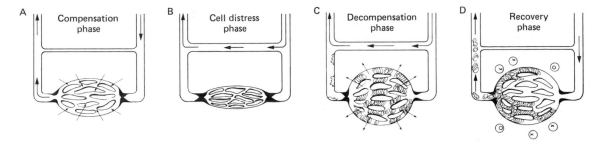

Figure 15—3. Microcirculatory changes in shock. *A:* Compensation phase. The precapillary sphincter closes, filtration pressure in the capillary drops, and fluid is drawn back into the vascular system by osmotic attraction. *B:* Cell distress phase. Arteriovenous shunts open, the postcapillary sphincter closes, and no fluid moves in or out of the capillary. *C:* Decompensation phase. The precapillary sphincter opens and the postcapillary sphincter remains closed. Fluid is lost from the damaged capillary bed with sludging of red blood cells in the capillary. *D:* Recovery phase. Normal volume has been restored. The precapillary and postcapillary sphincters are open. Sludged red cells and aggregates of platelets and white cells are washed into the systemic circulation.

cium, and water shift into the cell and potassium and magnesium leave the cell. The swollen cells reduce the size of the interstitial space and ultimately the extracellular volume, thus compounding the shock state. Arteriovenous communications which opened during the cellular distress phase remain open during the decompensation phase, so that peripheral arteriolar flow is diverted directly back into the venous system for recirculation to vital areas such as the heart and brain.

Recovery Phase (Fig 15—3D)

If blood volume is restored at some point in the decompensation phase, while the effects on the microcirculation are still reversible, many of the badly damaged cells are capable of recovery. As the cell membrane regains its integrity, water is lost over a period of 2—3 days and cation and anion homeostasis is restored. Following severe shock, return of complete homeostasis—particularly potassium homeostasis—may require several days. Capillary integrity may be regained as the sludge is washed into the venules, where red blood cell masses break up and return to the circulation. Some cell aggregates may be filtered out by the lungs or other microcirculatory beds. Platelet and white cell aggregates which form in the venules during the decompensation phase are also washed into the systemic circulation. If microcirculatory damage has been profound, large amounts of procoagulants from dead or dying cells, red cell sludge, and platelet aggregates may be released into the circulation and cause serious secondary morbidity (see Morbidity & Mortality, p 204). Other capillaries may be so badly damaged and filled with sludge that they remain permanently closed. Cells dependent upon these capillaries die.

Baue AE: Metabolic abnormalities of shock. Surg Clin North Am 56:1059, 1976.

Hechtman HB: Adequate circulatory responses or cardiovascular failure. Surg Clin North Am 56:929, 1976.

Levy MN: The cardiovascular physiology of the critically ill patient. Surg Clin North Am 55:483, 1975.

CLINICAL FINDINGS IN SHOCK

If the clinician fails to recognize the clinical signs of shock, proper treatment is delayed and the patient's chances of recovery may be compromised. Shock can be classified as mild, moderate, or severe (Table 15—2).

Mild shock (loss of 10—20% of the blood volume) is manifested by poor perfusion of the skin, a result of increased sympathetic activity. The patient appears pale and the skin is cool and moist, starting first in the extremities and progressing to involve the trunk. The patient usually complains of feeling cold and is often thirsty. Tachycardia may or may not be present. A low (physiologic) urine volume and increased specific gravity reflect renal responses aimed at restoring blood volume to normal.

Moderate shock occurs when 20—40% of the blood volume has been lost. Physiologic responses attempt to preserve the remaining blood flow to the heart and brain at the expense of other viscera. The key to monitoring of this stage of shock is the urinary output. For this reason, all patients who show signs of

Table 15—2. Clinical classification of hemorrhagic shock.

Mild shock (up to 20% blood volume loss)
  Pathophysiology: Decreased perfusion of nonvital organs and tissues (skin, fat, skeletal muscle, and bone).
  Manifestations: Pale, cool skin. Patient complains of feeling cold. Urine is concentrated.

Moderate shock (20—40% blood volume loss)
  Pathophysiology: Decreased perfusion of vital organs (liver, gut, kidneys).
  Manifestations: Oliguria to anuria and slight to significant drop in blood pressure.

Severe shock (40% or more blood volume loss)
  Pathophysiology: Decreased perfusion of heart and brain.
  Manifestations: Restlessness, agitation, coma, cardiac irregularities, ECG abnormalities, and cardiac arrest.

---

mild shock should be catheterized and hourly urinary output measured. If urinary output drops below 0.5 ml/kg/hour—the amount needed to excrete metabolic waste—it can be assumed that the patient has marked hypovolemia and poor renal blood flow and that at least 20% of the blood volume is depleted.

Severe shock occurs when more than 40% of the blood volume has been lost. By clinical definition, severe shock means inadequate perfusion of the 2 most critical organs: the heart and the brain. The cardinal cerebral symptoms are restlessness and agitation, progressive deterioration into stupor and coma, and finally death. Unfortunately, if the patient has been drinking and has the odor of alcohol on his breath, the restlessness and agitation may be ascribed to the alcohol and the significance of the symptoms may not be recognized until coma or cardiac arrest occurs. The inexperienced clinician may attribute the cause to a head injury. Cardiac manifestations at this time may include arrhythmias and evidence of myocardial ischemia on ECG. This classification of shock must be modified for the older patient who may have an arteriosclerotic vascular system with a fixed peripheral vascular resistance or a low cardiac index and cannot activate protective coagulation mechanisms. In these patients, as little as 10–20% blood volume loss may cause symptoms of moderate or severe shock.

MONITORING THE SHOCK PATIENT

Although treatment should be instituted promptly, accuracy requires precise monitoring of the patient to avoid complications related to overenthusiastic therapy (overtreatment) or suboptimal resuscitation of the vascular system (undertreatment).

Pulse & Blood Pressure

These are generally not reliable guides to the severity of shock. All patients with major illnesses, particularly at the time of initial presentation at the hospital, are apprehensive and have increased pulse rates whether or not actual shock is present. Decreased blood pressure is always significant, but the blood pressure may be normal—or nearly normal—until marked depletion of vascular volume occurs. This is particularly true in young patients, who by intense vascular constriction are able to maintain systolic pressure. In older, arteriosclerotic patients, a progressive drop in blood pressure usually parallels volume loss, but too much reliance on blood pressure in the past has resulted in gross undertreatment of shock. Arterial pressure results from the balance between the cardiac output and peripheral resistance. The diastolic pressure is a reflection of the status of the peripheral resistance; the pulse pressure (ie, the difference between the systolic and diastolic pressures) is related to the force and volume of cardiac systole and elasticity of the arterial vessels.

Warm skin with normal color indicates that peripheral perfusion is good. Since vasoconstriction is manifested first in the skin and subcutaneous tissues, good peripheral perfusion indicates normal peripheral resistance. A red, warmer than normal skin indicates a decrease in arteriolar resistance and is seen early in some cases of septic shock and in neurogenic shock. A cold, pale, moist skin signifies vasoconstriction with increased arteriolar resistance.

Urine Output

Urinary output is the most sensitive index of the adequacy of vital organ perfusion, and an indwelling urinary catheter is indicated for any patient in shock or in whom shock is likely to develop. Unless the patient has a history of renal disease, oliguria or anuria should be assumed to be due to inadequate perfusion resulting from myocardial failure or inadequate volume replacement. Vigorous treatment should be continued until the urine output exceeds 0.5 ml/kg/hour.

Central Venous Pressure

Central venous pressure (CVP) is a valuable guide to vascular volume replacement, especially when colloids are given (blood, plasma, or plasma substitutes). Because colloids remain in the vascular system, CVP assesses restoration of blood volume fairly accurately and usually can be relied upon to prevent overtreatment.

In order to accurately determine the status of the venous reservoir, a catheter should be threaded into a major vein (eg, the superior or inferior vena cava) and the CVP measured directly using a saline manometer. High CVP is reflected accurately in the peripheral veins of the extremities, but when vasoconstriction occurs, the peripheral venous pressure may be falsely high as an index of blood volume.

Normal CVP is 5 cm water. Any venous pressure under 15 cm water with the patient supine is considered within the clinically optimal range. Even more reliable than absolute values for clinical purposes are changes in the CVP level, eg, a rising CVP indicates filling of the venous reservoir either from restoration of total intravascular volume or from cardiac failure. The zero point for venous pressure measurement in the supine patient is 5 cm below the sternal angle—roughly at the level of the anterior axillary line.

Cardiac Output & Oxygen Transport

Generally, shock is associated with low cardiac output, and the clinical findings described above accurately reflect the output. In certain states such as septic shock, cardiac output may be high and actual measurements may be necessary. During resuscitation, other indices are probably more helpful. These include pulmonary artery pressure and pulmonary artery wedge pressure, measured with the Swan-Ganz balloon catheter (see Chapter 51). Insertion of this catheter through a peripheral vein cutdown can be done without difficulty in most modern critical care units, and the catheter can be floated through the right heart into the pulmonary artery.

The Swan-Ganz catheter also allows one to obtain mixed venous blood from the pulmonary artery, which is an index of the mean oxygen levels in the capillaries and tissues being perfused. It does not give an index of individual organ perfusion and may be misleading in that it reveals nothing about tissue oxygen levels in nonperfused areas. Nonetheless, a mixed venous oxygen level below 25 mm Hg is indicative of serious tissue hypoxia.

Another useful index of oxygen transport is total oxygen consumption, which is again dependent on the right heart catheter. Cardiac output is measured (eg, by the thermodilution technic), converted to cardiac index (liters per minute per square meter), and multiplied by the arteriovenous oxygen difference (obtained by subtracting the mixed venous oxygen from the arterial oxygen). An oxygen consumption less than 115 ml/minute/sq m is grossly abnormal (normal is 150 ml/minute/sq m).

Arterial Blood Gases*

The partial pressures of oxygen (Pa_{O_2}) and CO_2 (Pa_{CO_2}) have become indispensable therapeutic guides. Using the Astrup nomogram, it is possible to calculate the base deficit and titrate it with appropriate amounts of bicarbonate solution. An arterial oxygen tension (Pa_{O_2}) of 80−100 mm Hg is normal; a tension below 60 mm Hg indicates a marginal respiratory reserve. If the patient's Pa_{O_2} when breathing room air falls below 60 mm Hg, increased concentrations of oxygen in the inspired air (FI_{O_2}) are indicated.

The Pa_{CO_2} should be monitored frequently and should be kept under 40 mm Hg. A Pa_{CO_2} over 45 mm Hg indicates that serious hypoventilation is present. In shock, unless there is underlying pulmonary disease, Pa_{CO_2} (as opposed to Pa_{O_2}) is usually low or within normal limits. A Pa_{CO_2} rising above 45 or 50 mm Hg with good ventilatory exchange is an ominous indication of severe pulmonary insufficiency.

The arterial pH is also an indispensable blood measurement during resuscitation of shock. From the pH, bicarbonate and base deficit may be calculated and adequacy of resuscitation inferred. As perfusion improves, metabolic acidosis should diminish, reflected by a reduction of the base deficit. Determination of arterial blood pH is performed easily and much more rapidly than measurement of the serum lactate level.

Serum Lactate Levels (Normal = 0.44−1.8 mM/liter.)

Serum lactate determination is often used as a prognostic guide. Prolonged, severe shock results in a switch to anaerobic metabolism. Initial lactate levels correlate well with mortality rates: Levels of 2 mM/liter have been found to be associated with a mortality rate of 15%; 5 mM/liter or greater, a mortality rate of 75%; and 10 mM/liter or greater, a mortality rate of 95%. In shock, the initial lactate level may serve as a guide to the duration of preexisting shock and to the

*See also Chapter 3.

magnitude of the circulatory deficit. More effective therapy has reduced the number of deaths, so that initial lactate levels are of less prognostic value than suggested by the above figures.

Blood Volume

Blood volume can be assessed by giving radioiodinated serum albumin and calculating plasma volume or by giving chromium-51 red blood cells and determining red cell mass. Using the hematocrit of blood from the vena cava, the blood volume can be computed independently from either plasma volume or red cell volume.

A major disadvantage of the use of blood volume determinations as a guide to therapy is that red cells are trapped in the microcirculation and effective blood volume tends to be overestimated. In addition, increased permeability of the microcirculation results in transcapillary loss of albumin, leading to errors in the estimation of plasma volume. For these reasons, blood volume measurements are not useful for monitoring or treating patients in shock.

Packed Cell Volume (PCV, Hematocrit) & Hemoglobin

These clinical indices should be monitored serially. An abnormally high PCV indicates plasma loss in excess of red cell loss, as seen in septic shock and some types of cardiogenic shock. When the hematocrit is used to monitor hemorrhagic shock, there is considerable lag before it reflects the true loss of red cell mass. Studies performed during the first hour after massive hemorrhage may provide no clue whatever to the magnitude of the volume deficit; PCV may remain relatively normal, and only with appropriate hydration and support and 4−6 hours' observation will the hematocrit fall and correctly reflect the amount of blood loss. In the average adult, PCV falls 3−4% for every 500 ml of blood lost.

DelGuercio LRM, Cohn JD: Monitoring: Methods and significance. Surg Clin North Am 56:977, 1976.

Lehninger A: Ca^{2+} transport by mitochondria and its possible role in the cardiac contraction-relaxation cycle. Circ Res (Suppl 3) 35:83, 1974.

Swan HJC, Ganz W: Use of balloon flotation catheters in critically ill patients. Surg Clin North Am 55:501, 1975.

Weil MH, Afifi AA: Experimental and clinical studies on lactate and pyruvate as indicators of the severity of acute circulatory failure (shock). Circulation 41:989, 1970.

TREATMENT OF SHOCK

Ensure Airway

The first principle in resuscitation of the patient in shock is to ensure adequacy of the airway. No resuscitation will be successful if the patient is not ventilating adequately. Clinical evaluation alone is insufficient in the critically ill patient. Arterial blood gas (P_{aO_2} and P_{aCO_2}) and blood pH determinations should be done in any seriously ill patient, and oxygen should be administered by nasal catheter or by endotracheal tube depending upon the severity of the abnormality.

Restore Blood Volume

Following resuscitation from shock, there is dilatation of most capillary beds, which now can accommodate much of the blood volume. Sludging and anoxic damage result in increased permeability of the microcirculation and produce loss of red blood cells and plasma from the circulation and cellular edema. If a bleeding patient has his blood volume replaced as rapidly as it is lost and is never permitted to go into shock, volume for volume replacement is sufficient. If, on the other hand, the patient has been in shock for several hours, optimal circulatory resuscitation may require fluid replacement which exceeds by several times the calculated loss. The longer shock persists, the greater the obligatory fluid deficit, so that there is no arbitrary rule which permits ready calculation of the volume required for adequate treatment. In general, frequent clinical assessment of peripheral perfusion, maintenance of the central venous pressure between 5 and 15 mm Hg, and a urine output above 0.5 ml/kg/hour are indices of adequate treatment.

Two types of fluids are used to resuscitate patients in shock: crystalloids and colloids.

A. Crystalloids: The crystalloids are electrolyte solutions such as 0.9% sodium chloride solution ("normal saline") or the so-called balanced salt solutions, eg, lactated Ringer's injection.* One liter of lactated Ringer's injection contains 130 mEq of sodium, 4 mEq of potassium, 3 mEq of calcium, 109 mEq of chloride, and 28 mEq of lactate. This is a buffering solution, for, as the lactate is metabolized, excess H^+ can be neutralized. It should be pointed out that in lactated Ringer's the lactate exists in the racemic form and the D form may be incompletely metabolized. For this reason, some clinicians prefer to use Ringer's acetate, which is completely metabolized to bicarbonate. Acetate has another advantage in that it enters the citric acid cycle at a level below that of lactate. It should be remembered that when crystalloid is used for resuscitation, 3 parts of crystalloid are lost to the extravascular space for every part that remains in the vascular system. Therefore, 2000 ml are required to increase the vascular volume by 500 ml. If the patient has been in shock for a matter of hours, the effective therapeutic ratio is even less and may approach 8:1 or 10:1.

In the treatment of hemorrhagic shock, initial resuscitation with crystalloids is favored because the solutions are readily available and they effectively

*Often called Ringer's solution in common hospital parlance. However, the NF XIII monograph on Ringer's solution contains the following caution: "Do not use Ringer's Solution for parenteral administration or in preparations to be used parenterally. For such purposes use Ringer's Injection, USP XVIII."

restore vascular volume for short periods. They lower blood viscosity and enhance resuscitation of the microcirculation. Time is thus gained for definitive typing and cross-matching of blood, and, if the patient continues to bleed during the period of resuscitation, the infused crystalloid solution is expendable—ie, blood bank reserves are not wasted and are available for restoration of blood volume after bleeding has been controlled. Provided the oxygen-carrying capacity of the blood is supplemented by increased oxygen in the airway, it is almost impossible to dilute the blood sufficiently to prevent adequate tissue oxygenation. However, as salt and water are lost from the circulation into the tissues, continued resuscitation with crystalloids promotes both pulmonary and tissue edema. Ideally, initial resuscitation with crystalloids should be promptly followed by blood replacement.

B. Colloids: The colloids used to treat hypovolemic shock consist of blood, plasma, serum albumin, and plasma substitutes such as dextran. Although type O Rh-negative blood was at one time routinely used for resuscitation, major injury requires massive transfusion; the minor mismatch which often results from transfusion of type O Rh-negative blood may thus be magnified and result in serious morbidity or even fatal reactions. Thus, type-specific blood should be used, even if it is not cross-matched. When possible, it is preferable to treat with crystalloid solutions while awaiting complete cross-match.

Plasma fractions, including albumin and albumin-containing solutions (Plasmanate), are contraindicated during resuscitation of deep sustained hypovolemic shock. Because of alteration in endothelial permeability or microvascular forces, particles below MW 125,000 will leak into the interstitial space, thus increasing tissue oncotic pressure and causing edema. These plasma proteins are mobilized by tissue lymphatics, a process which may take as long as 3–4 weeks. This prolonged interstitial edema may be deleterious in such organs as the lungs and brain. In contrast, the interstitial edema that results from crystalloid administration is transitory since the fluid is mobilized back into the vascular space and excreted by the kidneys, usually on the second or third postinjury day. Plasma fractions are not contraindicated following chronic or subacute blood loss when endothelial membranes have not lost their integrity.

Burn shock, which produces a greater deficit of plasma volume than of red cell volume, is the principal form of shock which still requires large quantities of colloid for treatment. It is prudent to withhold colloid administration during the first 24 hours of resuscitation in cases of severe burns. Using radioiodinated serum albumin, it has been demonstrated that, in patients who sustained full thickness burns over more than 30% of the body, an endothelial membrane leak is present for the first 18–24 hours. Administration of albumin during this time is not effective and may result in more tissue edema. For this reason, it is better to base resuscitation primarily on crystalloid solution during the first 24 hours, with addition of colloid later as the membranes regain their integrity.

Dextran is the most widely used plasma substitute at present. Two types are available in the USA: clinical dextran, with a molecular weight of 70,000; and low molecular weight dextran, with a molecular weight of 40,000. Clinical dextran is the most effective colloid since it stays in the vascular system for up to 24 hours. Its disadvantage in hemorrhagic shock is that it interferes with blood typing and may impair the coagulation mechanism. Low molecular weight dextran (LMWD) is a relatively short-acting colloid, staying in the vascular system approximately 8 hours. It interferes much less with blood typing and does not usually depress the coagulation mechanism in doses under 1.5 g/kg/24 hours. Above this amount, LMWD decreases platelet adhesiveness, reducing hemostasis.

Improve Cardiac Function

Shock may be the result of primary cardiac malfunction such as arrhythmias, infarcts, or pericardial tamponade. Conversely, shock may adversely alter myocardial performance, and it may be difficult to separate cause and effect. If decreased cardiac performance is documented or suspected, it is important to eliminate easily correctable causes such as hemorrhage (external and internal) and to replace volume. Pericardial tamponade should be promptly evacuated even if this requires immediate thoracotomy. Tension pneumothorax, which causes a shift of the mediastinum, kinking of the great veins, and decreased venous return to the heart, is easily correctable with a tube thoracostomy. Lesions that are less easy to correct include pulmonary embolus, decreased peripheral resistance (following head injury), and hypermetabolic states.

Cardiac reserve may be manipulated by optimizing heart rate, preload, afterload, and contractility. If cardiac output is low and the heart rate is below 100 beats per minute, increased stroke volume can be achieved by increasing the heart rate to 105–110 beats per minute. This is best accomplished with isoproterenol. The filling pressure of the atria is optimal at about 15 mm Hg provided there is no pericardial tamponade. These pressures are easily measured with the central venous pressure (right atrium) or the Swan-Ganz catheter. The Swan-Ganz catheter (see Chapter 51) allows one to follow both atrial filling pressures since the pulmonary diastolic pressure is approximately the same as the right atrial pressure and the pulmonary artery wedge pressure is assumed to be the same as the left atrial pressure.

It is sometimes advantageous to manipulate the afterload in shock due to myocardial infarction or head injury, and occasionally when there is systemic hypertension despite decreased cardiac output. It may also be necessary to decrease afterload when the thoracic aorta is clamped, as in aneurysmectomy. Afterload can be quickly reduced with agents such as nitroprusside, trimethaphan, phentolamine, and phenoxybenzamine which decrease peripheral resistance. Chlorpromazine may also be effective in less severe shock.

If preload is adequate—and in the absence of increased afterload and pericardial tamponade—a primary defect in myocardial contractility may be assumed. Stroke volume may be increased by a continuous infusion of dopamine in a dose of 2–9 μg/kg/min. Epinephrine and isoproterenol are not as effective. The clinician must also be aware of calcium depletion states such as those which follow severe hypovolemic shock, cardiopulmonary bypass, and massive blood replacement with citrated blood. In these instances, hypocalcemia will interfere with the normal excitation-contraction coupling and alter contractility. Therapy consists of administration of 10 ml of calcium chloride over 1–5 minutes.

The oxygen transport capacity of the blood must be kept optimal by keeping hemoglobin levels between 12 and 15 g/100 ml. The ability of red cells to function effectively should be ensured by maintaining the oxyhemoglobin dissociation curve in the optimal position. This is done by preventing inorganic phosphate depletion, treating hypothermia, and avoiding alkalosis. Blood pH should be carefully monitored and metabolic acidosis corrected, since pH levels below 7.2 or 7.3 depress myocardial contractility.

Modify the Microcirculatory Lesion

Sludging of blood, platelet aggregation, and intravascular coagulation all follow microcirculatory damage and cell death. Increased attention is now being directed toward definitive treatment of inadequate microcirculatory perfusion. Low molecular weight dextran has been used to decrease blood viscosity and the tendency toward red cell sludging and platelet aggregation. It also decreases platelet adhesiveness. One to 2 units (500 ml each) are usually given in the initial resuscitation of shock. The maximal dose following initial priming by 2 units of dextran consists of 1 unit of dextran daily.

Heparin is being used to treat certain shock states, particularly shock due to gram-negative sepsis, where intravascular coagulation has been demonstrated to develop from gram-negative endotoxemia. Intravascular coagulation is also a factor in shock due to trauma associated with extensive tissue damage or necrosis. When heparin can be administered early in such cases, it may prevent or modify many of the secondary effects due to intravascular coagulation. The dosage varies, but as a rule 2500–5000 units are given IV every 4–6 hours.

The secondary effects of blood cell aggregation and intravascular clotting are principally on the lung. Pulmonary function may be improved and pulmonary lesions modified by early institution of mechanical ventilation. Therefore, endotracheal intubation and positive pressure ventilation are of value in profound shock.

Adrenal Corticosteroids

Massive doses of adrenocorticosteroids may modify some of the adverse effects of gram-negative sepsis and lessen the morbidity following shock. This effect is presumably due to the ability of these drugs to stabilize cell membranes. The amounts used are 10–20 times the usual clinical doses. The dose advocated for dexamethasone is 1 gm IV every 6–8 hours.

However, the experimental evidence to support the effectiveness of these agents suggests that therapy must be initiated before shock occurs. In addition, corticosteroids block the immune mechanism and render the patient vulnerable to infection. For these reasons, corticosteroids are rarely indicated in the primary treatment of shock unless there is a question of adrenocorticosteroid depletion. In the latter circumstance, unless shock does not respond to other standard treatment methods, physiologic doses (such as 100 mg of hydrocortisone) may be tried.

Berk JL: Use of vasoactive drugs in the treatment of shock. Surg Clin North Am 55:721, 1975.

Carrico CJ & others: Fluid resuscitation following injury: Rationale for the use of balanced salt solutions. Crit Care Med 4:46, 1976.

Christy JH: Treatment of gram-negative shock. Am J Med 50:77, 1971.

Drop LJ, Laver MB: Low plasma ionized calcium and response to calcium therapy in critically ill man. Anesthesiology 43:300, 1975.

Forrester JS & others: Peripheral vasodilators in low cardiac output states. Surg Clin North Am 55:531, 1975.

Holcroft J, Trunkey DD: Extravascular lung water following hemorrhagic shock in the baboon. Ann Surg 180:408, 1974.

Schumer W: Steroids in the treatment of clinical septic shock. Ann Surg 184:333, 1976.

Shoemaker WC: Algorithm for resuscitation: A systematic plan for immediate care of the injured or postoperative patient. Crit Care Med 3:127, 1976.

Shoemaker WC: Comparison of the effectiveness of whole blood transfusions and various types of fluid therapy in resuscitation. Crit Care Med 4:71, 1976.

Skillman JJ: The role of albumin and oncotically active fluids in shock. Crit Care Med 4:55, 1976.

Walt AJ, Wilson RF: The treatment of shock. Adv Surg 9:1, 1975.

Weil MH & others: Treatment of circulatory shock: Use of sympathomimetic and related vasoactive agents. JAMA 231:1280, 1975.

MORBIDITY & MORTALITY IN SHOCK

As understanding of the pathogenesis of shock increases and therapy becomes more effective, "irreversible shock" is seen with decreasing frequency. Even so, patients still die of shock, principally as a result of irreversible damage to the brain or heart, because of respiratory failure from lung damage, or because of uncontrolled infection following profound shock. Hemorrhagic shock should be reversible if the patient responds initially to resuscitation and if cerebral damage has not occurred. Despite a favorable response to resuscitation, patients still die days or weeks following an episode of shock, and investigations are being conducted to identify the causes.

Organs that may at times be so badly damaged in shock as to cause death are discussed in the following paragraphs.

Brain

It is commonly stated that 4 minutes of total circulatory arrest at normothermia results in permanent cerebral damage. Death occurs when brain damage is irreversible. However, many patients who have apparently had circulatory arrest for more than 10 minutes have been successfully resuscitated without irreversible brain damage.

Recent evidence suggests that injury to the microcirculation within the brain may itself be the major factor responsible for CNS damage. Brain cells in tissue culture can withstand 10–15 minutes of total ischemia, whereas clinical experience has documented that 4–5 minutes of circulatory arrest may produce irreversible cerebral ischemia at normothermia. It should be noted that few patients have a "pure" cardiac arrest. Usually there is antecedent hypovolemia, hypoxemia, or both, and 4–5 minutes is an extremely dangerous time lag in terms of cerebral perfusion.

Heart

In experimental animals, the heart can be resuscitated 30–60 minutes after circulatory arrest. Cardiac transplantation has also demonstrated that, unless there is a myocardial lesion, cardiac resuscitation should be possible for most patients, and myocardial factors should rarely be a cause of irreversible shock except in the case of primary cardiogenic shock. Despite these observations, it is sometimes impossible to resuscitate the heart after short periods of profound ischemia. Part of the problem may be brain stem damage with secondary depression of respiration and resulting anoxic compromise of myocardial function. Another factor may be related to microcirculatory damage. One investigator has demonstrated that ADP-induced platelet aggregation, although only transiently obstructive to the microcirculation, can produce myocardial infarction. This may explain the absence of vascular lesions in many of the patients who die.

Lungs

In general hospitals where large numbers of trauma victims are treated, most of the late deaths after initial successful resuscitation have been due to pulmonary damage and respiratory failure. Many patients in intensive care units are receiving mechanical respiratory support, and anesthesiologists have taken an active interest in ICU care principally because of the high incidence of pulmonary complications in major illness.

Many types of respiratory insufficiency are seen following shock, including aspiration of gastric contents, airway obstruction by plugs of mucus or blood, pulmonary edema resulting from overenthusiastic fluid therapy, atelectasis, oxygen toxicity, pulmonary contusion, pneumonia, and pulmonary embolism and infarction.

Respiratory distress syndrome (shock lung, hemorrhagic lung) usually becomes evident within the first 24 hours following an episode of shock. The early clinical signs are tachypnea and increased respiratory effort. Evaluation reveals a progressive decrease in pulmonary compliance, decreased Pa_{O_2}, and increased pulmonary arteriovenous shunting. The lungs sound dry to auscultation, and pulmonary secretions are minimal. Chest x-ray shows diffuse alveolar infiltrates which may progress to complete consolidation. As the pulmonary lesion progresses, increasing inspiratory pressures are needed to maintain normal tidal volume. Greater inspiratory oxygen concentrations are required to provide adequate arterial oxygen tensions. With intensive support and meticulous respiratory care, the patient may recover gradually over 3–5 days. If he does not, respiratory insufficiency progresses so that inflation pressures of 50–60 cm of water are required and—despite the administration of 100% oxygen—oxygen tensions in the blood drop to critical levels and the patient dies. Autopsy reveals lungs which grossly resemble liver owing to intense hemorrhagic consolidation.

The lesion principally responsible for pulmonary insufficiency in shock is pulmonary microembolism. Emboli also develop from sludging of red cells and from white cell and platelet aggregations which occur in the microcirculatory beds damaged by shock. Resuscitation washes the products of coagulation into the systemic circulation, where they are filtered out by the lung. The normal lung is capable of clearing a surprisingly large volume of such material. If the patient has underlying pulmonary insufficiency or the load is massive, the microcirculation of the lung may be overwhelmed. Overgrowth of organisms in damaged stiff lungs results in death due to pulmonary infection, or progressive pulmonary damage produces irreversible diffuse pulmonary fibrosis.

Hirsch EF & others: The lung: Responses to trauma, surgery, and sepsis. Surg Clin North Am 56:909, 1976.

Kidneys

Better fluid resuscitation has made renal failure a rare complication, and the artificial kidney provides support until ultimate renal recovery occurs in patients who do develop renal failure.

Lucas CE: The renal response to acute injury and sepsis. Surg Clin North Am 56:953, 1976.

Liver

Because only 15% of its parenchyma is needed for survival, the liver can be severely compromised before clinical catastrophe occurs. Jaundice occurs in 2–5% of patients with massive and prolonged shock. The derangement simulates obstructive jaundice because alkaline phosphatase and bilirubin rise in excess of the SGOT and SGPT. Pathologic studies reveal centrilobular necrosis. Some degree of hemolysis occurs after massive transfusion, and an increased load of hemoglobin is presented to marginally damaged liver cells.

Champion HR & others: A clinicopathologic study of hepatic dysfunction following shock. Surg Gynecol Obstet 142:657, 1976.

Intestines

Circulation to the gut is compromised early in hypovolemia by intense splanchnic vasoconstriction. Since the mucosa is the most active tissue metabolically, the impact of decreased circulation is principally on the mucosa. If shock is prolonged, mucosal necrosis may occur. The bowel may be responsible for much of the liver damage seen following shock; when the portal circulation has been diverted away from the liver, or when the bowel is isolated and perfused during experimental shock in dogs, liver damage rarely occurs.

Silen W, Skillman JJ: Gastrointestinal responses to injury and infection. Surg Clin North Am 56:945, 1976.

Adrenals

Adrenal hemorrhage and insufficiency may result following profound shock, and in refractory cases small doses of corticosteroids should be administered to rule out the possibility of adrenocortical failure as the primary factor in irreversibility.

● ● ●

General References

Baue AE & others: Cellular alterations with shock and ischemia. Angiology 25:31, 1974.

Blaisdell FW, Lewis FR Jr: *Respiratory Distress Syndrome of Shock and Trauma.* Saunders, 1977.

Clowes GHA Jr (editor): Symposium on response to infection and injury. 1. Physiology. Surg Clin North Am 56(4), Aug 1976. [Entire issue.]

Committee on Trauma, American College of Surgeons: *Early Care of the Injured Patient,* 2nd ed. Saunders, 1976.

Freeark R, Davis J: Shock. West J Med 124:510, 1976.

Harken A: Lactic acidosis. Surg Gynecol Obstet 142:593, 1976.

Kirklin JW, Archie JP Jr: The cardiovascular subsystem in surgical patients. Surg Gynecol Obstet 139:17, 1974.

Malinin TI & others (editors): *Acute Fluid Replacement in the Therapy of Shock.* Intercontinental Medical Book Corp, 1974.

McArdle CS, Fisher WD: Cardiac sequelae of hemorrhagic shock. Br J Surg 60:803, 1973.

Scheidt S & others: Intra-aortic balloon counterpulsation in cardiogenic shock. N Engl J Med 288:979, 1973.

Shoemaker WC, Reinhard J: Tissue perfusion defects in shock and trauma states. Surg Gynecol Obstet 137:980, 1973.

Skillman JJ (editor): *Intensive Care.* Little, Brown, 1976.

Trunkey DD: Assessment and resuscitation of the injured patient. West J Med 121:153, 1974.

16 . . .

Management
of the Injured Patient

GENERAL PRINCIPLES
Carleton Mathewson, Jr., MD

Each year, the public pays a frightful price in lives, pain, and money for accidents. In the USA, 102,000 people died in 1975 from trauma. Statistics for 1974 indicate that 10.6 million people were temporarily disabled and 370,000 permanently disabled. The cost in hospital care is astronomical: 19 million hospital days a year—more than required for heart or cancer patients.

Some progress has been made through better design of motor vehicles, the wearing of seat belts, and the nationwide 55 mile-per-hour speed limit. In 1975, the death rate for 100 million vehicle miles was the lowest on record: 3.5%.

Although significant progress has been made, lack of proper emergency treatment at the scene of the accident, during transportation, and in the hospital emergency room still remains a serious contributing factor to death and disability. Areawide organized cooperative plans to assure civilians the same quality of emergency care provided the Armed Forces in war are essential. Important contributions are being made in this area by a number of agencies, including various medical societies and especially the American College of Surgeons, federal agencies, and the American Trauma Society.

Multiple injuries involving several body systems constitute a significant factor in mortality and prolonged or permanent disability. Yet our present knowledge of the management of multiple severe injuries is such that, if it were properly applied, many lives could be saved and residual disabilities avoided. The important steps in emergency care which should be familiar to every physician and surgeon are presented in the following pages.

IMMEDIATE MEASURES AT
THE SCENE OF AN ACCIDENT

When first seen, the victim of an accident may not appear to be badly injured. There may be little or no gross external evidence of trauma. Therefore, when the mechanism of trauma has been such that severe injury might be expected, it is important that the victim be handled as if severe injury has occurred.

The injured person must be protected from further trauma. First aid at the scene of an accident should be administered by trained personnel whenever possible. Inexperienced persons should not move a victim of trauma. The simple act of moving an accident victim from one position to another, if done improperly, may compound a fracture, compress or lacerate the spinal cord, puncture a lung, or sever a major vessel—thereby converting a simple injury into a major surgical problem.

Wherever the patient is first seen—on the battlefield, beside a road, in the emergency ward, or in the hospital—the basic principles of initial management are the same:

(1) Is he breathing? If not, provide an airway and maintain respiratory exchange.

(2) Is there a pulse or heartbeat? If not, begin external cardiac massage.

(3) Is there gross external bleeding? If so, elevate the part if possible and apply external pressure over the major artery to the part. A tourniquet is rarely needed.

(4) Is there any question of injury to the spine? If so, protect before moving the patient.

(5) Splint obvious fractures.

As soon as these steps have been taken, the patient can be safely transported. In the emergency ward, shock is treated even as the emergency survey examination is performed, followed by definitive treatment.

The details of each step in management are as follows:

Asphyxia

A. Airway Obstruction: (Fig 16–1.) An open airway is essential to life and must be provided at once. This can often be done by simple manipulation of the mandible or traction on the tongue, particularly in unconscious or semiconscious patients. After the mouth is forced open, the tongue can be grasped between the thumb and forefinger covered with a handkerchief or gauze bandage. The tip of the tongue should be pulled forward beyond the front teeth. The

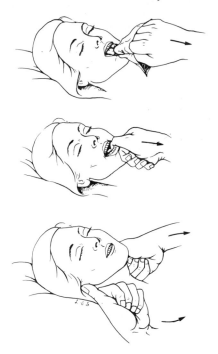

Figure 16—1. Relief of airway obstruction.

mandible should be manipulated either by pulling forward the angles of the lower jaw or by inserting the thumb between the teeth, grasping the mandible in the midline, and drawing it forward until the lower teeth are leading. Often, however—particularly in the presence of severe facial injury—it may be necessary to introduce an artificial airway (Fig 16—2). This requires the immediate availability of trained attendants with the proper instruments. Tracheostomy should not be

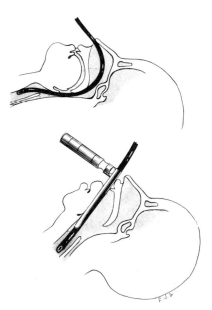

Figure 16—2. *Top:* Nasotracheal intubation. *Bottom:* Orotracheal intubation.

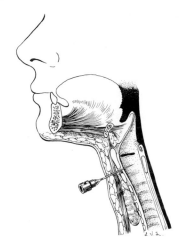

Figure 16—3. Needle in trachea to establish temporary airway.

attempted at the scene of an accident. On rare occasions, the introduction of a large-bore needle (eg, 13 gauge) into the trachea may provide an adequate temporary airway (Fig 16—3).

Suctioning of the mouth and pharynx may clear them sufficiently of blood, mucus, or vomitus to permit normal respiration. Repeated suctioning may be required to maintain an adequate airway at the scene of the accident and during transit to a medical facility. Aspiration of vomitus is a frequent cause of sudden death and must be prevented at all costs. A lateral and slightly head-down position is best for patients who are liable to vomit. In respiratory arrest, a clear airway must be provided and mouth-to-mouth breathing instituted if other means of ventilation are not available (Fig 16—4).

B. Sucking Wound: An open or sucking wound of the chest must be closed as soon as it is recognized. This is best done at the scene of an accident by strapping or holding a sterile or clean dressing over the open wound. In desperate situations with marked respiratory distress, one should not hesitate to close the wound as nearly airtight as possible with any material available (towel, scarf, shirt, etc).

C. Tension Pneumothorax: Tension pneumothorax is a common cause of asphyxiation which is usually not recognized until a physician examines the patient. Increasing dyspnea and cyanosis are the principal features. Absent breath sounds, hyperresonance, cardiac displacement, pallor, and a rapid, feeble pulse are other clinical signs. If untreated, tension pneumothorax can be fatal because the collapse of one lung is soon followed by a shift of the mediastinum to the opposite side and interference with cardiac filling and function of the opposite lung. Aspiration of air from the pleural cavity with a needle and syringe may be sufficient as a temporary measure to relieve the intrathoracic tension (Fig 16—5).

Cardiac Arrest (See also Chapter 22 part I.)

Cardiac arrest, when encountered at the scene of

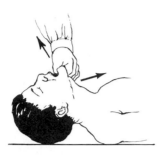
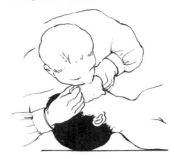

Method A: Clear mouth and throat. Place patient supine. Insert left thumb between patient's teeth, grasp mandible firmly in midline, and draw it forward (upward) so that the lower teeth are leading. Close patient's nose with right hand. Gauze (as shown) or airway may be used but is not necessary.

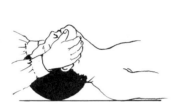
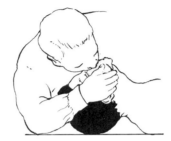

Method B: Clear mouth and throat. Place patient supine. Pull strongly forward at angle of mandible. Close patient's nose with your cheek. Gauze (as shown) or airway may be used but is not necessary.

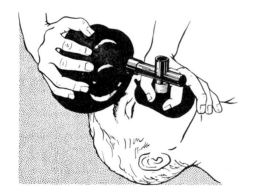

Instructions for Use of Manual Resuscitator

1. Lift the victim's neck with one hand.
2. Tilt head backward into maximum neck extension. Remove secretions and debris from mouth and throat, and pull the tongue and mandible forward as required to clear the airway.
3. Hold the mask snugly over the nose and mouth, holding the chin forward and the neck in extension as shown in diagram.
4. Squeeze the bag, noting inflation of the lungs by the rise of the chest wall.
5. Release the bag, which will expand spontaneously. The patient will exhale and the chest will fall.
6. Repeat steps 4 and 5 approximately 12 times per minute.

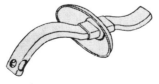

Airway for Use in Mouth-to-Mouth Insufflation. The larger airway is for adults. The guard is flexible and may be inverted from the position shown for use with infants and children.

Figure 16–4. Technic of mouth-to-mouth resuscitation and assisted ventilation with a bag and face mask.

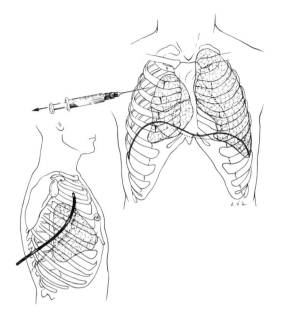

Figure 16–5. Relief of pneumothorax. Tension pneumothorax must be immediately decompressed by a needle introduced through the second anterior intercostal space. A chest tube is usually inserted through the second or third anterior intercostal space in the midclavicular line and directed toward the apex of the thorax. The tube is attached to the suction device, and the rate of escape of air is indicated by the appearance of bubbles in the second of the 3 bottles. When bubbling ceases, this suggests that the air leak has become sealed.

an accident, is usually fatal because it is not recognized as such by lay personnel. Absence of heart sounds and pulse means cardiac arrest. Lives may be saved by immediate action. Blood flow to the brain must be reestablished within 4 minutes if permanent cerebral damage or death is to be avoided. Begin the following 2 procedures immediately: (1) Establish ventilation by mouth-to-mouth breathing. (2) Start closed chest cardiac massage (see Chapter 22 part I).

Hemorrhage

Gross hemorrhage from accessible surface wounds is usually obvious and can be controlled in the great majority of cases by local pressure and elevation of the part. Firm pressure on the major artery in the axilla, antecubital space, wrist, groin, and popliteal space or at the ankle may suffice for temporary control of arterial hemorrhage distal to these points. When other measures have failed, a tourniquet may rarely be necessary to control major hemorrhage from extensive wounds or major vessels in an extremity. However, failure to release a tourniquet periodically may cause irreparable vascular or neurologic damage, and the tourniquet must therefore be kept exposed and loosened at least every 20 minutes for 1 or 2 minutes while the patient is in transit and permanently as soon as definitive care is given. It is wise to write the letters TK on the patient's forehead with skin-marking pencil or adhesive tape.

Restoration of blood volume at the scene of an accident and during transit to a hospital by the intravenous administration of lactated Ringer's injection or normal saline solution is at times a lifesaving measure and emphasizes the importance of the availability of proper equipment and personnel for immediate care.

Shock (See also Chapter 15.)

Some degree of shock accompanies most severe injuries and is manifested initially by pallor, cold sweat, weakness, lightheadedness, hypotension, tachycardia, thirst, air hunger, and eventual loss of consciousness.

A. Primary or Neurogenic Shock (Syncope or Fainting): Primary shock is due to the rapid pooling of blood in the splanchnic bed and voluntary muscles and is usually caused by psychic or nervous stimuli such as fright, sudden pain, or anxiety. It is self-limited and can be relieved by rest in the recumbent or Trendelenburg position. If the patient does not improve quickly, other types of shock must be considered.

B. Hypovolemic or Oligemic Shock: Hypovolemic shock is due to loss of whole blood or plasma. Blood pressure may be maintained initially by vasoconstriction. As hypotension ensues, tissue hypoxia increases; if prolonged, it may cause irreparable damage to the vital centers and shock becomes irreversible. Massive or prolonged hemorrhage, severe crushing injuries, major fractures, and extensive burns are the most common causes. The presence of any of these conditions is an indication for prompt institution of fluid replacement.

The patient must be kept recumbent and given reassurance and analgesics as necessary. Opiates, if necessary for relief of pain, are best administered intravenously in small doses. Subcutaneous injections are poorly absorbed in these circumstances and, if repeated, may accumulate and cause respiratory depression as circulating blood volume is restored.

Fractures

The recognition and splinting of major fractures and the immobilization of all injured parts before transportation are essential features of early management. Improper handling of the injured may increase or prolong shock and aggravate existing trauma beyond the possibility of definitive repair. "Splint 'em where they lie" is a time-honored rule of emergency care of fractures that has only a few exceptions—eg, when it is necessary to remove an injured patient from imminent danger of fire, explosion, escaping gas, etc. Improvised splints can be fashioned with boards, pillows, blankets, or other materials, but some sort of immobilization must be provided even at the cost of a delay in transporting the patient to a hospital (Figs 16–6 to 16–9).

Transportation

Transportation by ground or air ambulance is preferable when feasible. A station wagon or truck is preferable to a passenger car. The manipulation necessary to load a seriously injured person into a passenger car may be most harmful. Patients with internal

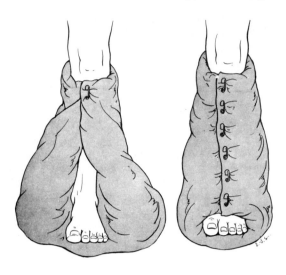

Figure 16—6. Pillow splint.

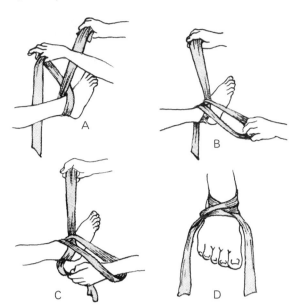

Figure 16—8. Method of tying Collins hitch.

injuries, head injuries, spinal, pelvic, and lower extremity injuries, patients in shock, and patients with major soft tissue wounds should be transported in the supine position. The time lost in waiting for proper transportation is rarely as harmful as the added trauma of improper transportation. Resuscitation of the seriously injured should be maintained during transportation, and a constant effort must be made to avoid airway obstruction and aspiration if the patient is vomiting.

EMERGENCY ROOM CARE

Temporary measures to control the immediate effects of trauma have usually been taken before the patient arrives in the emergency room. More definitive measures must be initiated as soon as he is delivered to a hospital. All clothing should be removed at once (cut off, if necessary) from the seriously injured patient, taking great care to avoid unnecessary movement. Immediate steps must be taken to correct life-endangering asphyxia, hemorrhage, and shock.

A rapid and complete history and physical examination (with a written record of the findings) is imperative in patients with serious or multiple injuries. Progressive changes in signs and symptoms are often the key to correct diagnosis, and negative findings which change to positive may be of great importance in revising an initial clinical evaluation. This is particularly true in intra-abdominal, intrathoracic, and head injuries, which frequently do not become manifest until hours after the initial trauma.

Everyone who may have information about the circumstances of the injury should be questioned. Knowing the mechanism of the injury often gives a clue to concealed trauma. Unfortunately, obvious injuries may absorb the attention of the examiner and cause him to overlook less obvious but more serious head, spinal, abdominal, or thoracic lesions. Serious underlying medical problems may be overlooked in the

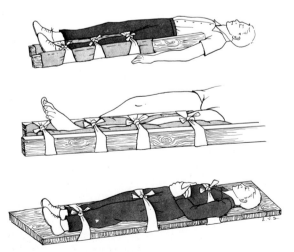

Figure 16—7. Fracture of femur. Emergency immobilization.

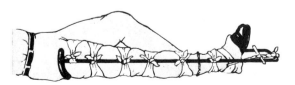

Figure 16—9. Keller-Blake half-ring splint for transportation of patient with fracture of thigh or leg. Spanish windlass on a Collins hitch.

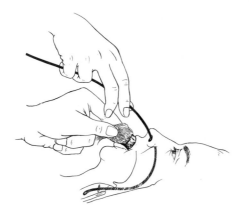

Figure 16–10. Tracheal aspiration.

absence of an accurate history. Distorted extremity fractures, bleeding lacerations, and head injuries are usually obvious and attract almost immediate attention. Too frequently, patients with these injuries are sent for prolonged x-ray studies while less apparent but more serious internal injuries go undetected.

Certain types of trauma are apt to cause more than one injury. Fractures of the calcaneus resulting from a fall from a great height are often associated with central dislocation of the hip and with fractures of the spine and the base of the skull. A crushed pelvis is often combined with rupture of the posterior urethra or bladder. Crush injuries of the chest are often associated with lacerations or rupture of the spleen, liver, or diaphragm. Penetrating wounds of the chest may involve not only the thoracic contents but also the abdominal viscera. These combinations of injuries occur frequently and should always be suspected.

Laboratory Studies

At the same time that intravenous needles or catheters are inserted for the treatment of shock, blood should be drawn for laboratory studies. If there is any indication that the injury is major or complex, the following should be obtained: hematocrit, P_{O_2}, P_{CO_2}, BUN, serum creatinine, serum electrolytes, and serum amylase. Arterial pH should be determined in critical cases. The urine should be examined for specific gravity, red and white cells, protein, and sugar. Catheterization may be necessary. If the patient is in critical condition, the catheter should be left in place for continuous recording of urinary output.

These determinations are a guide to the severity of the injuries and provide an essential baseline for continuing management.

X-Ray Examination

Films of the chest and abdomen are required in all cases of major injury. An intravenous urogram is of critical importance in abdominal injuries and pelvic fractures. It should not be done while the patient is in shock.

X-rays of the skull and long bones can usually be

deferred until the more critical injuries of the thorax and abdomen have been cared for.

Coma

Various stages of coma due to a variety of causes may accompany injury and will require treatment while initial steps are being taken to diagnose and treat the associated trauma.

Coma may be due to many causes. The most common are alcoholic intoxication, cerebrovascular accidents, diabetic acidosis, barbiturate poisoning, narcotic overdosage, and hypovolemic shock. Less common causes are epilepsy, eclampsia, and electrolyte imbalances associated with metabolic and systemic diseases. Other causes include anaphylaxis, heavy metal poisoning, electric shock, tumors, severe systemic infections, hypercalcemia, asphyxia, heat stroke, severe heart failure, and hysteria.

The differential diagnosis of unconsciousness depends upon (1) a careful history from available informants; (2) a careful and complete physical examination, with particular attention to the neurologic examination; and (3) laboratory tests such as urinalysis, blood counts, blood cultures, blood glucose, urea, ammonia, electrolytes, and alcohol, and CSF examination; and (4) skull x-rays. One should also search the patient for a medical card or medallion indicating known preexisting disease.

A. Immediate Care: If the injuries are extensive and there are signs of hypovolemic shock, coma is very likely due to cerebral ischemia. Resuscitation and blood volume replacement have first priority. If there are no signs of shock, head injury and other causes of coma are likely (see Chapter 40).

Early gastric lavage with activated charcoal may be helpful in preventing further absorption of alcohol or ingested drugs. Care must be taken to prevent aspiration. Deepening stupor in patients under observation should arouse suspicion of an expanding intracranial lesion requiring repeated thorough neurologic examinations. Too often one accepts obvious acute alcoholism as the cause of the unconscious state only to learn that increasing treatable intracranial hemorrhage has been overlooked.

B. Laboratory Studies in the Emergency Evaluation of Coma: When coma is present, laboratory studies may be helpful in ruling out the following diseases: blood alcohol levels in acute alcoholism; blood and urine glucose levels in diabetic coma and hypoglycemic shock; and serum potassium, BUN, and creatinine in uremia.

Treatment Priorities

Certain injuries are so critical that operative treatment must be undertaken as soon as the diagnosis is made. In these cases, resuscitation is continued as the patient is being operated on. At times the situation is so urgent that anesthesia is induced after the operation has begun rather than beforehand. Profound shock may render the patient unconscious from cerebral ischemia. For example, with certain penetrating wounds of the heart, the chest should be opened in the emergency ward and the hole in the heart plugged with a finger. Resuscitation, induction of anesthesia, and a formal thoracotomy are then carried out simultaneously. Many abdominal wounds involving the aorta and vena cava cause such massive hemorrhage that shock cannot be corrected until the bleeding is controlled and surgical repair must become a part of resuscitation. Rarely, wounds near the hilus of the lung may produce the same type of exsanguinating hemorrhage. Usually, however, the life-threatening complications of chest injuries such as tension pneumothorax, open sucking wounds, or flail chest can be corrected immediately without operation as described above.

Cerebral injuries take precedence in care only when there is rapidly deepening coma. Extradural bleeding is a critical emergency requiring operation for its control and cerebral decompression. Subdural bleeding may produce a similar emergency. If the condition of the patient permits, arteriography should be performed for localization of the bleeding. In many cases of combined cerebral and abdominal injury with massive bleeding, laparotomy and craniotomy are carried out simultaneously.

On the other hand, fractures of the skull have a low priority and usually can be dealt with after the treatment of more critical abdominal or thoracic injuries.

Most urologic injuries are managed simultaneously with associated intra-abdominal injury. Pelvic fractures present special problems discussed in Chapters 43 and 45.

Unless there is associated vascular injury with threatened ischemia of the limb, fractures of the long bones can be splinted and treated on a semi-emergency basis. On the other hand, open contaminated wounds should be cleansed and debrided as soon as possible.

Injuries of the hand often present the critical problem of potential infection which, if not treated early, may result in lifelong handicap to the patient. Early treatment of the hand at the same time as the life-threatening injuries avoids infection and preserves the patient's means of livelihood as well as his life.

In all cases of multiple injury, there must be a "captain of the team" who directs the resuscitation, decides which x-rays or special diagnostic tests should be obtained, and establishes priority for care by continuous consultation with other surgical specialists and anesthesiologists. A general surgeon with extensive experience in the care of the injured patient usually has this role.

Details of definitive management of injuries are discussed in the sections on trauma that follow and in the various organ system chapters.

Tetanus prophylaxis (see Chapter 11) should be given in all instances of open contaminated wounds, puncture wounds, and burns. No single prophylaxis plan can be applied to all patients.

Artz CP: Trauma can be conquered. J Trauma 14:819, 1974.

Baker SP: The injury severity score: A method for describing patients with multiple injuries and evaluating emergency care. J Trauma 14:187, 1974.

Baker SP, O'Neill B: The injury severity score: An update. J Trauma 16:882, 1976.

Cleveland HC & others: A civilian air emergency service. J Trauma 16:452, 1976.

Cowley RA & others: A prognostic index for severe trauma. J Trauma 14:1029, 1974.

Hampton OP Jr: Categorization of hospital emergency capabilities. J Trauma 16:21, 1976.

Hampton OP Jr: The epidemiology of trauma. Bull Am Coll Surg 61:18, July 1976.

PRINCIPLES OF MANAGEMENT OF SPECIFIC TYPES OF INJURIES

NECK INJURIES
Robert E. Allen, Jr., MD

All injuries to the neck are potentially life-threatening because of the many vital structures in this area. Injuries to the neck are classified as blunt or penetrating, and the treatment is different for each.

Penetrating trauma to the posterior neck may injure the vertebral column, the cervical spinal cord, the interosseous portion of the vertebral artery, and the neck musculature. Penetrating trauma to the anterior and lateral neck may injure the larynx, trachea, esophagus, thyroid, carotid arteries, subclavian arteries, jugular vein, and subclavian veins.

Blunt cervical trauma may cause fracture or dislocation of the cervical vertebrae (with the risk of spinal cord injury), traumatic occlusion of the carotid arteries, CSF cysts, or laryngeal and tracheal injuries complicated by hemorrhage and airway obstruction.

The patient must be examined closely for associated head and chest injuries. The initial level of consciousness is of paramount importance; progressive depression of the sensorium signifies intracranial bleeding and requires craniotomy. Injuries of the base of the neck may lacerate major blood vessels. Hemorrhage into the pleural cavity may occur suddenly as contained hematomas rupture.

Clinical Findings

Injuries to the larynx and trachea may be asymptomatic or may cause hoarseness, laryngeal stridor, or dyspnea secondary to airway compression or aspiration of blood. Subcutaneous emphysema may appear if the wall of the larynx or trachea has been disrupted.

Esophageal injuries are rarely isolated and alone may not cause immediate symptoms. Severe chest pain and dysphagia are characteristic of esophageal perforation. Hours later, as mediastinitis develops, progressive sepsis may become manifest. Mediastinitis results because the deep cervical space is in direct continuity with the mediastinum. Esophageal injuries can be recognized promptly if the physician is alert to the possibility. Exploration of the neck or radiographic examination of the esophagus with contrast medium confirms the diagnosis.

Cervical spine and cord injuries should always be suspected in deceleration injuries or following direct trauma to the neck. If the patient complains of cervical pain or tenderness or if the level of consciousness is depressed, the head and neck should be immobilized (eg, with sandbags) until cervical x-rays can be taken to rule out cervical fracture.

Injury to the great vessels (subclavian, common carotid, internal carotid, and external carotid arteries; subclavian, internal jugular, and external jugular veins) may follow penetrating trauma. Fractures of the clavicle or first rib may lacerate the subclavian artery and vein. With vascular injuries, the patient typically presents with visible external blood loss and hematoma formation and in varying degrees of shock. Occasionally, bleeding may be contained and the injury temporarily undetected. Auscultation may reveal bruits which suggest arterial injury.

Diagnosis

With any penetrating cervical trauma, the likelihood of significant injury is high because there are so many vital structures in such a small space. The location of the trauma suggests which structures may be involved. Vascular injuries at the base of the neck require thoracotomy to obtain proximal and distal control of injured blood vessels before exposing the site of probable injury. Arteriography should be performed, if possible, before exploration of any injury in which blood vessels may be damaged below the level of the cricoid cartilage or above a line connecting the mastoid process with the angle of the jaw. Arterial injuries above this line are practically inaccessible. If injury to the carotid artery at the base of the skull is confirmed by arteriography, repair may not be possible and ligation may be required to control bleeding. In addition, injured carotid arteries which have produced a neurologic deficit should be ligated.

Vertebral artery injuries should be suspected when bleeding from a posterior or lateral neck wound cannot be controlled by pressure on the carotid artery or when there is bleeding from a posterolateral wound associated with fracture of a cervical transverse process.

X-rays of the soft tissues and cervical spine should be taken routinely. Fractures of the cervical spine can be confirmed by x-ray. X-rays of the soft tissues can locate opaque foreign bodies if present and help determine the route of the missile.

The most important injuries resulting from blunt cervical trauma are (1) cervical fracture, (2) cervical spinal cord injury, (3) vascular injury, and (4) laryngeal and tracheal injury. X-rays of the cervical spine and soft tissues are essential. Careful neurologic examination can differentiate between injuries to the cord, brachial plexus, and brain.

Complications

The complications of untreated neck injuries are related to the individual structures injured. Injuries to the larynx and trachea can result in acute airway obstruction, late tracheal stenosis, and sepsis. Cervicomediastinal sepsis can result from esophageal injuries. Carotid artery injuries can produce death from hemorrhage, brain damage, and arteriovenous fistula with cardiac decompensation. Major venous injury can result in exsanguination, air embolism, and arteriovenous fistula if there is concomitant arterial injury. Cervical fracture can result in paraplegia, quadriplegia, or death.

Prevention of these complications depends upon immediate resuscitation by intubation of the airway; prompt control of external hemorrhage and blood replacement; protection of the head and neck when cervical fracture is possible; accurate and rapid diagnosis; and prompt operative treatment when indicated.

Treatment

Any wound of the neck which penetrates the platysma requires prompt surgical exploration to rule out major vascular injury. If the patient presents with a neurologic deficit that is clearly not due to head injury, primary repair of the artery and reestablishment of blood flow to the brain will make the neurologic deficit worse since an ischemic area of infarction in the brain is thus converted into a more lethal hemorrhagic infarction; in such cases, the carotid artery should be ligated. Arteries damaged by high-velocity missiles require debridement. End-to-end anastomosis of the mobilized vessels is preferred, but if a significant segment is lost an autogenous vein graft can be used. Vertebral artery injury presents formidable technical problems because of the interosseous course of the artery shortly after it arises from the subclavian artery. It is best to ligate the vertebral artery rather than to attempt repair. Unilateral vertebral artery ligation has been followed by fatal midbrain or cerebellar necrosis because of inadequate communication to the basilar artery. However, only about 3% of patients with left vertebral ligation and 2% of patients with right vertebral ligation develop these complications. In the face of massive hemorrhage from a partially severed vertebral artery, the risks of immediate ligation must be accepted.

Subclavian artery injuries are best approached through a combined cervicothoracic incision. Proper exposure is the key to success in the management of these difficult and too often fatal injuries. Ligation of the subclavian artery is relatively safe, but primary repair is preferable.

Venous injuries are best managed by ligation. The possibility of air embolism must be kept constantly in mind. A simple means of preventing this complication is to lower the patient's head until bleeding is controlled.

Esophageal injuries should be sutured and drained. Drainage is the hallmark of treatment. Extensive injury to the esophagus is often immediately fatal because of associated injuries to the spinal cord. Systemic antibiotics should be administered routinely in esophageal injuries.

Minor laryngeal and tracheal injuries do not require treatment, but immediate tracheostomy should be performed when airway obstruction exists. If there has been significant injury to the thyroid cartilage, a temporary laryngeal stent (Silastic) should be employed to provide support. Mucosal lacerations should be approximated before insertion of the stent. Conveniently located small perforations of the trachea can be utilized for tracheostomy. Otherwise, the wounds can be closed after they are debrided and a distal tracheostomy performed. Extensive circumferential tracheal injuries may require resection and anastomosis or reconstruction using synthetic materials.

Primary neurorrhaphy should be attempted for nerve injury. Bilateral vagal nerve injury results in hoarseness and dysphagia. Cervical spinal cord injury should be managed in such a way as to prevent further damage. When there is cervical cord compression—from hematoma formation, vertebral fractures, or foreign bodies—decompression laminectomy is necessary.

Blunt trauma to the neck rarely requires direct surgical treatment. More commonly, the soft tissues are contused, and hematomas develop which may cause tracheal compression and respiratory insufficiency. Tracheostomy is indicated in this instance. Cervical fractures are managed with skull tongs and traction. Surgical stabilization of cervical fractures is rarely indicated before 3 weeks after injury unless there is progressive paraplegia. The common or internal carotid arteries can be torn or can undergo disruption of the intima and require vascular reconstruction. Carotid arteriograms are essential to the diagnosis.

Prognosis

The prognosis after neck trauma varies with the extent of injury and the structures involved. Severance of the cervical spinal cord results in paralysis. Injuries to the soft tissues of the neck, trachea, and esophagus have a good to excellent prognosis if promptly treated. Major vascular injuries have a good prognosis if promptly treated before the onset of irreversible shock or neurologic deficit. The overall mortality rate for cervical injuries is about 10%.

Bricker DL & others: Vascular injuries of the thoracic outlet. J Trauma 10:1, 1970.

Hunt TK & others: Vascular injuries of the base of the neck. Arch Surg 98:586, 1969.

Knightly JJ & others: Management of penetrating wounds of the neck. Am J Surg 126:575, 1973.

Marks RL, Freed MM: Nonpenetrating injuries of the neck and cerebrovascular accident. Arch Neurol 28:412, 1973.

McInnis WD & others: Penetrating injuries to the neck. Am J Surg 130:416, 1975.

Monson DO & others: Carotid vertebral trauma. J Trauma 9:987, 1969.

Penn I: Penetrating injuries of the neck. Surg Clin North Am 53:1469, 1973.

Saletta JD & others: Penetrating trauma of the neck. J Trauma 16:579, 1976.

Saletta JD & others: Trauma to the neck region. Surg Clin North Am 53:73, 1973.

Sheely CH & others: Management of acute cervical tracheal trauma. Am J Surg 128:805, 1974.

Silvernail WJ & others: Carotid artery injury produced by blunt neck trauma. South Med J 68:310, 1975.

Teal JS & others: Aneurysms of the cervical portion of the internal carotid artery associated with nonpenetrating neck trauma. Radiology 105:353, 1972.

Work WP, McDoy EG: Surgical repair of the cervical trachea following trauma. Ann Otol Rhinol Laryngol 65:573, 1956.

THORACIC INJURIES
Arthur N. Thomas, MD

Most thoracic injuries are from blunt or penetrating trauma. Eighty percent of blunt traumatic injuries are caused by automobile accidents. Penetrating chest injuries from knives, bullets, etc are almost as frequent as those from blunt trauma and increase annually as the level of civilian violence escalates. The mortality rate in hospitalized patients with isolated chest injuries is 4–8%; it is 10–15% when one other organ system is involved and rises to 35% if multiple additional organs are injured.

Combined injuries of multiple intrathoracic structures are usual. Frequently there are other injuries to the abdomen, head, or skeletal system. Ninety percent of chest injuries do not require open thoracotomy, but immediate use of lifesaving measures is often necessary and should be within the competence of all physicians. The most common chest injuries requiring immediate treatment are (1) airway obstruction, (2) massive hemothorax, (3) cardiac tamponade, (4) tension pneumothorax, (5) flail chest, (6) open pneumothorax, and (7) massive tracheobronchial air leak.

When the physician is confronted with an injured patient, a rapid estimate of cardiorespiratory status and possible associated injuries gives a valuable overview. For example, patients with upper airway obstruction appear cyanotic, ashen, or gray; there are strident crowing or gurgling sounds, ineffective respiratory excursion, constriction of cervical muscles, and retraction of the suprasternal, supraclavicular, intercostal, or epigastric regions. The character of chest wall excursions and the presence or absence of penetrating wounds can be observed. If respiratory excursions are not visible, ventilation is probably inadequate. Severe parodoxical chest wall movement in flail chest is usually located anteriorly and can be seen immediately. Sucking chest wounds of the chest wall should be obvious. A large hemothorax can usually be detected by percussion, and subcutaneous emphysema is easily detected. Both massive hemothorax and tension pneumothorax may produce absent or diminished breath sounds and a shift of the trachea to the opposite side, but in massive hemothorax the neck veins are usually collapsed. If the patient has a thready or absent pulse and distended neck veins, the main differential diagnosis is between cardiac tamponade and tension pneumothorax. In moribund patients, diagnosis must be immediate and treatment may require chest tube placement, pericardiocentesis, or thoractomy in the emergency room. The first priority of management should be to provide an airway and restore circulation. Then one can reassess the patient and outline definitive measures. A cuffed endotracheal tube and assisted ventilation are required for apnea, ineffectual breathing, severe shock, deep coma, airway obstruction, flail chest, or open sucking chest wounds. Persistent shock or hypoxia may be due to massive hemorrhage, cardiac tamponade, or tension pneumothorax. Shock due to thoracic trauma may be caused by any of the following: massive hemopneumothorax, cardiac tamponade, tension pneumothorax or massive air leak, or air embolism. If hemorrhagic shock is not explained readily by findings on chest x-ray or external losses, it is almost certainly due to intra-abdominal bleeding.

Types of Injuries

A. Chest Wall: Rib fracture, the commonest chest injury, varies from simple fracture to those with hemopneumothorax to severe multiple fractures with flail chest and internal injuries. With simple fractures, pain on inspiration is the principal symptom. Treatment consists of strapping the chest wall with adhesive tape, intercostal nerve block, and analgesics. Particularly in the elderly, multiple fractures may be associated with voluntarily decreased ventilation and subsequent pneumonitis.

Flail chest (Fig 16-11) occurs when a portion of the chest wall becomes isolated by multiple fractures and moves in and out with inspiration and expiration with a potentially severe reduction in ventilatory efficiency. The magnitude of the effect is determined by the size of the flail segment and the amount of pain with breathing. Usually the rib fractures are anterior

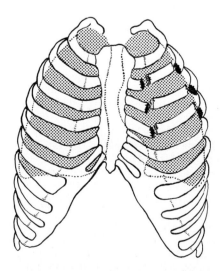

Figure 16-11. Flail chest.

and there are at least 2 fractures of the same rib. Bilateral costochondral separations and the sternal fractures can also cause a flail segment. These injuries are often underestimated when first seen because in only half is the flail apparent at the time of admission. Often an associated lung contusion is present which 24-48 hours later produces a drop in lung compliance. Increased negative intrapleural pressure is then required for ventilation, and chest wall instability becomes apparent. If ventilation becomes inadequate, atelectasis, hypercapnia, hypoxia, accumulation of secretions, and ineffective cough occur. Arterial P_{O_2} is often low before clinical findings appear. Serial blood gas determination is the best way to determine if a treatment regimen is adequate. For minor cases, intercostal nerve block and analgesics may be adequate treatment. However, most cases require ventilatory assistance for 2-3 weeks with a cuffed endotracheal tube and a mechanical ventilator. External fixation of the chest wall is less reliable than positive pressure ventilation for the average case but may be useful for severe sternal flail or other extensive injuries with chest wall instability.

B. Pleural Space: Hemothorax, or blood within the pleural cavity, is classified, according to the amount of blood, as minimal, 350 ml; moderate, 350-1500 ml; or massive, 1500 ml or more. The rate of bleeding after evacuation of the hemothorax is clinically even more important. If air is also present, the condition is called **hemopneumothorax.**

Hemothorax should be suspected with penetrating or severe blunt thoracic injury. There may be decreased breath sounds and dullness to percussion, but a chest x-ray (upright or semiupright, if possible) should be promptly obtained (Fig 16-12). Tube thoracostomy using one or 2 large-bore pleural catheters should be promptly performed. Needle aspiration is never adequate. In 85% of cases, tube thoracostomy is the only treatment required. If bleeding is persistent, as noted by continued output from the chest tubes, it is more likely to be from a systemic (eg, intercostal) than a pulmonary artery. When the rate of bleeding is 100-200 ml/hour or the total hemorrhagic output exceeds 1000 ml, thoracotomy should usually be performed. In most cases, the chest wall is the source of hemorrhage, but the lung, heart, pericardium, and great vessels account for 15-25%.

Pneumothorax* occurs in lacerations of the lung or chest wall following penetrating or blunt chest trauma. Hyperinflation (eg, blast injuries, diving accidents) can also rupture the lungs. After penetrating injury, 80% of patients with penumothorax also have blood in the pleural cavity. **Tension pneumothorax** develops when a flap-valve leak allows air to enter the pleural space but prevents its escape; intrapleural pressure rises, causing total collapse of the lung and a shift of the mediastinal viscera to the opposite side. It must be relieved immediately to avoid interference with ventilation in the opposite lung and impairment of cardiac function. Sucking chest wounds, which allow air to

*Spontaneous pneumothorax is discussed in Chapter 21.

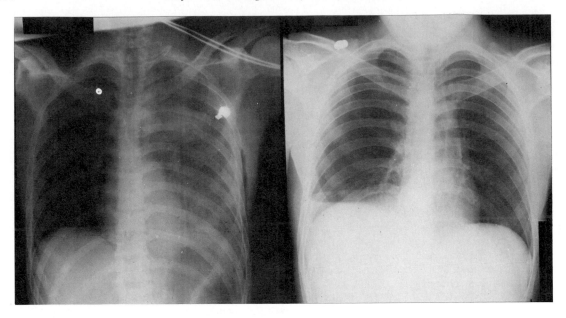

Figure 16—12. Hemopneumothorax. Upright *(left)* and supine films (on different patients).

pass in and out of the pleural cavity, should be promptly treated by an occlusive dressing and tube thoracostomy. The pathologic physiology resembles flail chest except that the extent of associated lung injury is usually less. After emergency measures have been instituted, traumatic pneumothorax should be treated by tube thoracostomy.

C. Lung Injury: Pulmonary contusion due to sudden parenchymal concussion occurs after blunt trauma or wounding with a high-velocity missile. Pulmonary contusion occurs in 75% of patients with flail chest but can also occur following blunt trauma without rib fracture. Alveolar rupture with fluid transudation and extravasation of blood are early findings. Fluid and blood from ruptured alveoli enter alveolar spaces and bronchi and produce localized airway obstruction and atelectasis. Increased mucous secretions and overzealous intravenous fluid therapy may combine to produce copious secretions (wet lung) and further atelectasis. The patient's ability to cough and clear secretions effectively is weakened because of chest wall pain or mechanical inefficiency from fractures. Elasticity of the lungs is decreased, resistance to air flow increases, and, as the work of breathing increases, blood oxygenation and pH drop and P_{CO_2} rises. The cardiac compensatory response may be compromised because as many as 35% of these patients have an associated myocardial contusion.

Treatment is often delayed because clinical and x-ray findings often do not appear until 12—24 hours after injury. The clinical findings are loose, copious, blood-tinged secretions, chest pain, restlessness and apprehensiveness, and labored respirations. Eventually, dyspnea, cyanosis, tachypnea, and tachycardia develop. X-ray changes are patchy parenchymal opacification or diffuse linear peribronchial densities which

may progress to diffuse opacification ("white-out").

Mechanical ventilatory support permits adequate alveolar ventilation and the use of enriched oxygen mixtures and thus reduces the work of breathing. Blood gases should be monitored frequently and arterial saturation adequately maintained. There is some controversy over the best regimen for fluid management, but excessive hydration or blood transfusion should be avoided. Optimal management requires placement of a Swan-Ganz catheter in the pulmonary artery, preferably with a thermistor tip for measurement of cardiac output by thermodilution. Serial measurement of central venous pressure, pulmonary arterial pressure, wedge pressures, mixed venous oxygen saturation, and cardiac output help to avoid either under- or overtransfusion. Despite optimal therapy, about 15% of patients with pulmonary contusion die.

Most **lung lacerations** are caused by penetrating injuries, and hemopneumothorax is usually present. Tube thoracostomy is indicated to evacuate pleural air or blood and to monitor continuing leaks. Since expansion of the lung tamponades the laceration, most lung lacerations do not produce massive hemorrhage or persistent air leaks.

Lung hematomas are the result of local parenchymal destruction and hemorrhage. The x-ray appearance is initially a poorly defined density which becomes more circumscribed a few days to 2 weeks after injury. Cystic cavities occasionally develop if damage is extensive. Most hematomas resolve adequately with expectant treatment.

D. Trachea and Bronchus: Blunt tracheobronchial injuries are often due to compression of the airway between the sternum and the vertebral column in decelerating steering wheel accidents. The distal trachea or main stem bronchi are usually involved. Penetrating tracheobronchial injuries may occur anywhere. Most patients have hemopneumothorax, subcutaneous emphysema, pneumomediastinum, and hemoptysis. Cervicofacial emphysema may be dramatic. Hilar injuries should be suspected when there is a massive air leak. In penetrating injuries of the trachea or main bronchi, there is usually massive hemorrhage and hemoptysis. In blunt injuries, the tracheobronchial injury may not be obvious and may be suspected only after major atelectasis develops several days later. Diagnosis may require tracheobronchoscopy.

Suture closure is indicated for tracheobronchial lacerations.

E. Heart and Pericardium: Blunt injury to the heart occurs most often from compression by a steering wheel in auto accidents. The injury varies from localized contusion to cardiac rupture. Autopsy studies of victims of immediately fatal accidents show that as many as 65% have rupture of one or more cardiac chambers and 45% have pericardial lacerations. The incidence of myocardial contusion in patients who reach the hospital is unknown but is probably higher than generally suspected.

The early clinical findings include friction rubs, chest pain, tachycardia, murmurs, arrhythmias, or evidence of low cardiac output. Electrocardiograms show nonspecific RS–T and T wave changes. Serial tracings should be obtained since abnormalities may not appear for 24 hours after injury. Serum enzyme determinations such as SGOT, LDH, or CPK are not valuable since elevations can be due to associated musculoskeletal injury.

Management of myocardial contusion should be the same as for acute myocardial infarction. Hemopericardium may occur without tamponade and can be treated by pericardiocentesis. Tamponade in blunt cardiac trauma is often due to myocardial rupture or coronary artery laceration. Tamponade produces distended neck veins, shock, and cyanosis. Emergency treatment consists of pericardiocentesis (Fig 16–13), which also proves the clinical diagnosis. Immediate thoracotomy and control of the injury is indicated. Treatment of injuries to valves, papillary muscles, and septum must be individualized; when tolerated, delayed repair is usually recommended.

Pericardial lacerations from stab wounds tend to seal and cause tamponade, whereas gunshot wounds leave a sufficient pericardial opening for drainage. Gunshot wounds produce more extensive myocardial damage, multiple perforations, and massive bleeding into the pleural space. Hemothorax, shock, and exsanguination occur in nearly all cases of cardiac gunshot wounds. The clinical findings are those of tamponade or blood loss.

Treatment of penetrating cardiac injuries has gradually changed from initial management by pericardiocentesis to prompt thoracotomy and pericardial decompression. Pericardiocentesis is reserved for selected cases when the diagnosis is uncertain or in preparation for thoracotomy. The myocardial laceration is closed with sutures placed to avoid injury to coronary

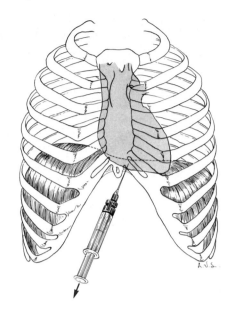

Figure 16–13. Aspiration of pericardial tamponade.

arteries. Most patients do not require cardiopulmonary bypass. In 90% of cases of stab wounds and 50–60% of cases of gunshot cardiac wounds, the patient survives the operation. However, it is estimated that 80–90% of patients with gunshot wounds of the heart do not reach the hospital.

F. Esophagus*: Anatomically, the esophagus is well protected, and perforation from external penetrating trauma is relatively infrequent. Blunt injuries are very rare. The most common symptom of esophageal perforation is pain; fever develops within hours in most patients. Regurgitation of blood, hoarseness, dysphagia, or respiratory distress may also be present. Physical findings include shock, local tenderness, subcutaneous emphysema, or Hamman's sign (ie, pericardial or mediastinal "crunch" synchronous with cardiac sounds). Leukocytosis occurs soon after injury. X-ray findings on plain chest films include evidence of a foreign body or missile and mediastinal air or widening. Pleural effusion or hydropneumothorax is frequently seen, usually on the left side. Contrast x-rays of the esophagus should be performed but are positive in only about 70% of proved perforations.

A nasogastric tube should be passed to evacuate gastric contents. If recognized within 24–48 hours of injury, the esophageal perforation should be closed and pleural drainage instituted with large-bore catheters. Long-standing perforations require special technics which include buttressing of the esophageal closure with pleural or pericardial flaps; pedicles of intercostal, diaphragmatic, or cervical strap muscles; and serosal patches from stomach or jejunum. Morbidity and mortality are due to mediastinal and pleural infection.

*Instrumental perforation of the esophagus and injuries from ingestion of corrosives are covered in Chapter 23.

G. Thoracic Duct: Chylothorax and chylopericardium are rare complications of trauma but, when they occur, are difficult to manage. Penetrating injuries of the neck, thorax, or upper abdomen can injure the thoracic duct or its major tributaries. The occurrence of chylothorax after a trivial injury should lead one to suspect underlying malignancy.

Symptoms are due to mechanical effects of the accumulations, eg, shortness of breath from lung collapse or low cardiac output from tamponade. The diagnosis is established when the fluid is shown to have characteristics of chyle, or by special tests such as feeding the patient fat and a lipophilic dye.

The patient should be maintained on a fat-free, high-carbohydrate, high-protein diet and the effusion aspirated. Chest tube drainage should be instituted if the effusion recurs. Intravenous hyperalimentation with no oral intake may be effective in persistent leaks. Three or 4 weeks of conservative treatment usually are curative. If daily chyle loss exceeds 1500 ml for 5 successive days or persists after 2–3 weeks of conservative treatment, the thoracic duct should be ligated via a right thoracotomy. Intraoperative identification of the leak may be facilitated by preoperative administration of fat containing a lipophilic dye.

H. Diaphragm: Penetrating injuries of the diaphragm outnumber blunt diaphragmatic injuries at least 4:1. Wounds of the diaphragm must not be overlooked because they rarely heal spontaneously and because herniation of abdominal viscera into the chest can occur either immediately or years after the injury.

Associated injuries are usually present, and as many as 25% of patients are in shock when first seen. There may be abdominal tenderness, dyspnea, shoulder pain, or unilateral breath sounds. The diagnosis is often missed since chest x-rays are entirely normal in about 30% of cases. The most common finding is ipsilateral hemothorax. Pneumothorax is often present and occasionally is confused with a distended herniated stomach. Passage of a nasogastric tube before x-ray examination will help identify an intrathoracic stomach.

Once the diagnosis is made, the diaphragm should be sutured with closely placed heavy nonabsorbable sutures. Because pulmonary complications are frequent, when there is no other injury requiring thoracotomy the diaphragmatic one should be approached through the abdomen.

Beal AC Jr: Penetrating wounds of the heart and great vessels. Resident and Staff Physician 102:11s, 1975.

Bertelsen S, Howitz P: Injuries of the trachea and bronchi. Thorax 27:188, 1972.

Borja AR, Randsdell HT: Treatment of penetrating gunshot wounds of the chest: Experience with one hundred forty-five cases. Am J Surg 122:81, 1971.

Fleming WH, Bowen MC: The use of diuretics in the treatment of early wet lung syndrome. Ann Surg 175:505, 1972.

Hewitt RL & others: Penetrating cardiac injuries: Current trends in management. Arch Surg 101:683, 1970.

Kish G & others: Indications of early thoracotomy in the management of chest trauma. Ann Thorac Surg 22:23, 1976.

Madoff IM, Desforges G: Cardiac injuries due to nonpenetrating

thoracic trauma. Ann Thorac Surg 14:505, 1972.

McInnis WD, Cruz AB, Aust JB: Penetrating injuries to the neck. Am J Surg 130:416, 1975.

Moore BP: Operative stabilization of nonpenetrating chest injuries. J Thorac Cardiovasc Surg 70:619, 1976.

Naclerio EA: *Chest Injuries: Physiologic Principles and Emergency Management.* Grune & Stratton, 1971.

Neugebauer MK, Fine JB, Hoyt TW: Traumatic rupture of the trachea and right mainstem bronchus. J Trauma 14:265, 1974.

Pearce W, Blair E: Significance of the electrocardiogram in heart contusion due to blunt trauma. J Trauma 16:136, 1976.

Popovsky J, Lee YC, Berk JL: Gunshot wounds of the esophagus. J Thorac Cardiovasc Surg 72:609, 1976.

Relihan M, Litwin MS: Morbidity and mortality associated with flail chest injury: A review of 85 cases. J Trauma 18:663, 1973.

Reul GJ Jr & others: Recent advances in the operative management of massive chest trauma. Ann Thorac Surg 16:52, 1973.

Richardson DJ: First rib fracture: A hallmark of severe trauma. Ann Surg 181:251, 1975.

Sankaran S, Wilson RF: Factors affecting prognosis in patients with flail chest. J Thorac Cardiovasc Surg 60:402, 1970.

Selle JG, Snyder WH III, Schreiber JT: Chylothorax: Indications for surgery. Ann Surg 177:245, 1973.

Sheely CH II & others: Penetrating wounds of the cervical esophagus. Am J Surg 130:707, 1975.

Shoemaker WC & others: Hemodynamic monitoring for physiological evaluation, diagnosis and therapy of acute hemopericardial tamponade from penetrating wounds. J Trauma 13:36, 1973.

Thomas AN: Penetrating thoracic trauma. West J Med 121:510, 1974.

Thomas AN, Stephens BG: Air embolism: A cause of morbidity and death after penetrating chest trauma. J Trauma 14:633, 1974.

Wise L & others: Traumatic injuries to the diaphragm. J Trauma 13:946, 1973.

ABDOMINAL INJURIES
Donald D. Trunkey, MD

Abdominal trauma is classified as either blunt or penetrating. Blunt trauma tends to injure solid viscera such as spleen, kidneys, liver, and pancreas. Particularly if it is distended, blunt trauma may also injure a hollow viscus such as the bladder or, less frequently, a segment of the gut. Deceleration forces, particularly from motor vehicle accidents and falls, may tear organs from their points of fixation. For example, the liver may be torn from the diaphragm and inferior vena cava, the bladder from the bladder neck, and the gut from the mesentery. A steering wheel or other solid object, in striking the abdomen, may disrupt any of the organs that cross the vertebral column (eg, pancreas, duodenum, or vena cava). Injuries from blunt trauma are more common than those from penetrating missiles and are more difficult to assess. Associated fractures of ribs, pelvis, or transverse processes are of significance because they indicate the patient has been subjected to substantial forces. If intra-abdominal injury seems likely, diagnostic laparotomy should be performed.

Penetrating wounds from bullets, knives, etc which enter the abdomen are indications for exploration. Because of the nearby blast effect, bullet wounds that pass close to abdominal structures require laparotomy even if the peritoneal cavity was not traversed. This is particularly true with high-velocity missiles. Knife wounds that appear to be superficial should be explored under local anesthesia by extending the wound if necessary to determine the extent of penetration. If the wound extends to or below the posterior rectus sheath or if it cannot be determined where it extends, exploratory laparotomy should be undertaken. Isolated abdominal injuries with blunt trauma are rare, and associated injuries (eg, head, pelvis, chest) are the rule. If a patient arrives in the Emergency Department in extremis and his condition remains unstable after initial resuscitation, the only diagnostic test necessary is a chest x-ray. If the chest film is normal and there is no obvious source of blood loss, hypovolemia must be due to intra-abdominal bleeding and exploratory laparotomy must be performed immediately. In stable patients, other clues may point to an intra-abdominal injury.

A history of the mechanism of injury is often helpful, particularly if a direct blow to the abdomen can be ascertained. Abdominal pain and tenderness, the most common manifestations of visceral injury, may be difficult to differentiate from pain of associated injuries such as fractures of vertebral bodies, ribs, or pelvis. Distention may or may not be present; involuntary guarding is the most reliable indication that laparotomy should be performed.

The following signs in patients with blunt trauma are often associated with the specific injuries indicated: posterior lateral rib fractures on the left or left shoulder pain, and splenic rupture; fracture of right lower ribs or right shoulder pain, and liver injuries; ecchymosis of the flanks or muscular spasm, and visceral injury; gross blood from the urethra or hematuria, and injury of the genitourinary tract.

Some patients with intraperitoneal injury have few manifestations. Splenic rupture can be asymptomatic since blood does not always irritate the peritoneum. Bowel lacerations with minimal leakage may be nearly painless. In certain cases (eg, comatose patients, infants), physical findings may either be lacking or difficult to detect. In these types of situations, diagnostic laparotomy or peritoneal lavage may be indicated. (See Chapter 51 for the technic and interpretation of results.)

Laboratory tests should include serial hematocrits, white blood count, urinalysis, and other special studies as indicated. A urethrogram, cystogram, or intravenous urogram is indicated for gross or microscopic hematuria, the specific test depending on the nature of the injury.

Plain films of the abdomen should be obtained but are diagnostic in less than one-third of cases. Free intraperitoneal air is pathognomonic of viscus rupture and mandates laparotomy. Other findings on plain film may include obliteration of the properitoneal fat line or the psoas margin and displacement of the gastric air bubble. Occasionally, a duodenal cutoff sign indicative of duodenal injury may be seen. Emergency upper gastrointestinal series with water-soluble contrast media may be indicated to reveal a suspected but otherwise occult injury of the gut. A serum amylase determination should be obtained in all patients with blunt trauma to the upper abdomen and epigastric tenderness. A high amylase level suggests that pancreatic injury has occurred. If it has been more than a few hours since injury, urine amylase determination may be more helpful. It is usually advisable during the initial resuscitation to draw extra blood and keep the serum for other laboratory tests if they become indicated (eg, electrolytes, creatinine, toxic substances).

Angiography may occasionally be useful, particularly in patients with multiple injuries or possible vascular injuries. Angiograms can demonstrate pancreatic, hepatic, or splenic injuries when the clinical presentation is puzzling. When a need for intra-operative angiograms is anticipated, the patient should be placed on an x-ray cassette holder before the laparotomy is begun.

Treatment

A. General: The first treatment priority is the airway; the second is circulatory resuscitation, based on assessment of cardiac function and functional blood volume. If the patient stabilizes with initial resuscitating efforts, further diagnostic studies can be performed as mentioned above. If the patient does not stabilize or deteriorates, it must be assumed that there is continued blood loss and further delay is dangerous. If chest x-ray is normal, continued circulatory instability means intra-abdominal bleeding.

At laparotomy, control of hemorrhage is usually possible with packs and pressure, but in extreme cases arterial bleeding may require thoracotomy and clamping the descending aorta or abdominal aorta as it passes through the diaphragm. In general, packs will stop venous hemorrhage or hemorrhage from viscera. Further contamination from lacerations of the gut should be halted as quickly as possible with intestinal clamps. At this point, careful exploration should be performed, inspecting the retroperitoneal duodenum and pancreas, particularly if there is staining of blood in these areas. A retroperitoneal hematoma about the kidney or in the pelvis need not be opened unless it expands while being observed or pulsates. Attention should then be turned to the treatment of specific injuries.

B. Specific Injuries:

1. Hepatic injury—Most liver injuries can be treated by simple evacuation of intraperitoneal blood and clots and drainage of the laceration. A detailed discussion of the management of hepatic injuries is presented in Chapter 27.

2. Splenic injury—Usually there is no justification for conservative treatment of splenic injuries, and splenectomy is the only accepted surgical treatment. In young children where decreased immunocompetence may follow splenectomy, attempts to repair very minor lacerations are warranted. See Chapter 31 for a complete discussion of splenic injuries.

3. Gallbladder and extrahepatic biliary injury—Cholecystectomy is the treatment of choice for injuries of the gallbladder. The appropriate procedure for disruption of the common bile duct varies according to the extent of the injury. If the laceration is small and the location is suitable, a T tube should be inserted into the duct. If the injury is more severe but still focal, an end-to-end anastomosis over a T tube is advisable. If part of the duct must be resected, it may be necessary to perform a Roux-en-Y anastomosis of the duct to the jejunum. Extensive injuries involving the ampulla of Vater may require pancreaticoduodenectomy.

4. Pancreatic injuries—Careful exploration and examination of the pancreas is mandatory when the capsule is blood-stained or if a peripancreatic hematoma is present. Complete disruption often occurs where the body of the gland crosses the vertebral column, an injury which is best treated by distal pancreatectomy and splenectomy. For mild contusions, drainage alone is sufficient. Injuries to the head of the pancreas have a high mortality rate with either conservative or radical surgical treatment. If the injury is severe but the blood supply to the duodenum is intact, a 90–95% pancreatectomy is probably best. If the duodenal blood supply has been compromised, pancreaticoduodenectomy is required. Thorough drainage is important regardless of the extent of injury or resection.

5. Stomach and duodenal injury—The stomach is rarely injured by blunt trauma, but penetrating injuries are common and are usually found in pairs. Treatment consists of debridement and suture closure.

Duodenal injuries may follow blunt or penetrating trauma. For a simple laceration, transverse closure is sufficient provided it does not compromise the lumen. In more extensive injuries, resection and end-to-end anastomosis may be required. Pancreaticoduodenectomy is rarely necessary for extensive injuries since they can usually be managed by primary repair, use of an onlay serosal patch, or diversion. In all but minor duodenal injuries, drainage is a useful adjunct; duodenostomy with a No. 10 Foley catheter may help decompress the injury.

6. Small bowel injuries—The appropriate treatment for penetrating small bowel injuries depends on the velocity of the missile and the amount of surrounding damage. Simple lacerations and those from low-velocity missiles can usually be treated by transverse closure. More extensive wounds or those involving the mesenteric blood vessels may require resection and end-to-end anastomosis. Blunt injuries severe enough to cause disruption of the small bowel almost always require resection.

7. Large bowel injuries—Injuries to the large bowel are potentially more serious than those of the small bowel because its intraluminal contents are more virulent and blood supply less abundant. Injury to the large bowel is a definite indication for broad-spectrum antibiotics, preferably started preoperatively or during operation. Depending on the velocity of the missile, surrounding damage, the amount of fecal contamination, and the location of the injury, treatment may be simple or complex. Clean lacerations of the right or left colon with no fecal contamination or loss of blood supply may, on occasions, be closed primarily. More extensive injuries require either exteriorization of the injured portion or resection and diverting end colostomy. Those of the right colon require a right colectomy and diverting ileostomy and end mucous fistula. In most cases, the best approach is to resect the damaged bowel and construct temporary stomas of the open ends rather than take a chance with primary anastomosis. A loop colostomy proximal to the site of injury is rarely useful since it is an inefficient means of fecal diversion.

The 3 principles of management for rectal injuries are to (1) completely divert the fecal stream, (2) irrigate all fecal material from the distal segment, and (3) insert presacral or retrorectal drains from the perineum. There is never an indication for primary closure of a rectal injury.

8. Urogenital tract injuries—If hematuria is present, an intravenous urogram and cystogram should be obtained. For injuries to the kidney, unless there is gross extravasation or complete nonfilling of the renal parenchyma—and provided there are no other indications for abdominal exploration—nonoperative management is indicated. If the abdomen has been explored for other reasons and a retroperitoneal hematoma over the kidney is found, it should be left undisturbed unless it is expanding or pulsating. Bleeding from the kidney is often tamponaded adequately by an intact retroperitoneum. If the renal injury requires exploration, the following principles must be observed: (1) establish that the patient has a normal contralateral kidney by exploration or intravenous urogram; and (2) in general, conserve as much renal tissue as possible but perform nephrectomy instead of more time-consuming repairs if the operation must be expedited because of associated injuries.

For ureteral injuries, simple transverse suture repair may be possible for small lacerations or defects. Resection and end-to-end anastomosis are appropriate when more extensive damage exists. When a substantial segment of the ureter has been lost, ureteroureterostomy or ureteroneocystostomy must be considered. Rarely, autotransplantation of the kidney into the pelvis is indicated. Ureteral anastomosis is best accomplished with fine technic, using vascular suture material and avoiding intraluminal stents.

Disruption of the bladder is often seen with pelvic fractures. Peritoneal and extraperitoneal rupture require suprapubic cystostomy and suprapubic drainage of the paravesical space. Lacerations of the bladder should be sutured and a Foley catheter inserted. For disruption of the bladder neck, a No. 20—22 Foley catheter with a 30 ml balloon should be placed transurethrally and connected to traction (0.5—1 lb) for 5—7 days. The Foley is then allowed to remain for an additional 1—2 weeks.

If a urethral injury has been demonstrated by urethrogram, an indwelling urethral catheter is the treatment of choice. If difficulty is encountered in passing the urethral catheter, the bladder should be explored, concomitant transvesical and transurethral passage performed, and suprapubic cystostomy and perivesical drains inserted.

Injuries of the female reproductive organs are infrequent except in combination with genitourinary or rectal trauma. Minor injuries to the uterus and adnexa can usually be repaired by chromic catgut sutures, and drainage is not necessary. In more extensive injuries, hysterectomy may be preferable. The vaginal cuff may be left open for drainage, particularly if there is an associated genitourinary or rectal injury.

Injuries involving the pregnant uterus are associated with a low rate of fetal salvage. Bleeding may be massive in such patients, particularly in women near parturition. Cesarean section and hysterectomy may be the only alternative.

Banowski LH, Wolfel DA, Lackner HL: Considerations in diagnosis and management of renal trauma. J Trauma 10:587, 1970.

Bull JC Jr, Mathewson C Jr: Exploratory laparotomy in patients with penetrating wounds of the abdomen. Am J Surg 116:223, 1968.

Cass AS, Ireland GW: Comparison of the conservative and surgical management of the more severe degrees of renal trauma in multiple injured patients. J Urol 109:8, 1973.

Cerise E, Scully JH: Blunt trauma to small intestine. J Trauma 10:46, 1970.

Freeark RJ, Love L, Baker RJ: An active diagnostic approach to blunt abdominal trauma. Surg Clin North Am 48:97, 1968.

Ganchrow M, Lavenson G, McNamara J: Surgical management of traumatic injuries of the colon and rectum. Arch Surg 100:515, 1970.

Gibbs BF, Crow JL, Rupnick EG: Pancreatoduodenectomy for pancreatoduodenal injuries. J Trauma 10:702, 1970.

Hawkins L, Pomerantz M, Eiseman B: Laparotomy at the time of pelvic fracture. J Trauma 10:619, 1970.

Hawkins M, Mullen JT: Duodenal perforation from blunt abdominal trauma. J Trauma 14:290, 1974.

Holcroft JW & others: Renal trauma and retroperitoneal hematomas: Indications for exploration. J Trauma 15:1045, 1975.

Howell HS & others: Blunt trauma involving the colon and rectum. J Trauma 16:624, 1976.

Jones RC, Shires GT: Management of pancreatic injuries. Arch Surg 90:502, 1965.

Kazarian KK & others: Stab wounds of the abdomen: An analysis of 500 patients. Arch Surg 102:465, 1971.

Lavenson G, Cohen A: Management of rectal injuries. Am J Surg 122:226, 1971.

Nelson JF: The roentgenologic evaluation of abdominal trauma. Radiol Clin North Am 4:415, 1966.

Persley L, Hock W: Renal trauma. Curr Probl Surg, Sept 1972.

Root HD, Keizer PJ, Perry JF: Peritoneal trauma: Experimental and clinical studies. Surgery 62:679, 1967.

Root HD & others: Diagnostic peritoneal lavage. Surgery 57:633, 1965.

Schrock TR: Injuries to the colon and rectum. West J Med 123:236, 1975.

Sheldon GF, Cohn LH, Blaisdell FW: Surgical treatment of pancreatic injuries. J Trauma 10:795, 1970.

Thompson IM, Johnson EL, Ross G Jr: The acute abdomen of unrecognized bladder rupture. Arch Surg 90:371, 1965.

Trunkey D, Hays R, Shires GT: Management of rectal trauma. J Trauma 13:411, 1973.

Trunkey D & others: Management of pelvic fractures in blunt trauma injuries. J Trauma 14:912, 1974.

ARTERIAL INJURIES
Albert D. Hall, MD

The repair of injured blood vessels to preserve normal circulation is an essential immediate extension of primary resuscitation. Until experience in the Korean conflict demonstrated the feasibility of repairing acute vascular injuries even under combat conditions, it was standard procedure to ligate disrupted arteries to control hemorrhage and accept the resulting 50% amputation rate recorded in World War II. This figure was reduced to 13% in the Korean experience largely because of more expeditious evacuation of casualties, the availability of blood for prompt resuscitation, a better understanding of blood vessel repair and bypass technics, the use of operative angiography, the appropriate use of heparin, and the more effective control of infections with the use of wound debridement, secondary closure, and antibiotics. Further improvement of survival and limb salvage rates has been achieved in recent years by more effective means of managing shock, the use of hemodialysis units, and the introduction of the Fogarty balloon catheter for extraction of peripheral thrombi. When managed well, the casualty with major vascular injuries can have an uncomplicated course. Without proper assessment and optimum treatment, a reversible condition becomes irreversible.

Types of Injuries

A. Incisions and Lacerations: Incisions or lacerations, commonly caused by knives or glass, may or may not produce overt hemorrhage depending upon the extent of the injury and the location of the vessel. A completely divided artery can retract and constrict, so that bleeding is minimal; or an artery with a gaping lateral defect can bleed massively. If an adjacent vein has been incised simultaneously, an acute **arteriovenous fistula** is formed. Sharply lacerated arteries are readily treated by simple closure or anastomosis, and injured veins repaired or ligated.

B. Perforations: Perforations due to small, high-velocity missiles (bullets) or sharp instruments (ice picks, pointed knives) can produce life-threatening—

even though initially occult–vascular injuries. External evidence of injury may be minimal and the significance of a wound not appreciated until hemorrhagic shock occurs or a pulsating hematoma, false aneurysm, or delayed arteriovenous fistula develops. Whenever a penetrating wound is located anywhere near the site of a major vessel, an important vascular injury may be present. Normal pulses do not rule out such injuries.

C. Puncture Wounds: Puncture wounds such as those produced by percutaneous catheterization of peripheral arteries during diagnostic procedures can cause defects in the arterial wall that bleed and form false aneurysms or pulsating hematomas. When a needle or catheter dislodges an arteriosclerotic plaque or elevates the intima, a vessel will thrombose, leading to acute ischemia of a limb. In either case, such an injury must be recognized promptly by careful observation of the patient after such a procedure. Restoration of blood flow is accomplished at emergency exploration.

D. Contusions or Crushing Injuries: These produce either transmural or partial disruption of arteries, resulting in elevation of the intima and formation of intramural hematomas which lead to occlusion of the lumen. Repair of these vessels may require replacement of the segment or a bypass graft. Contused arteries are seen with fractures, dislocations, or damage to muscles, nerves, and skin, leading to a less favorable prognosis for limb salvage. These complex problems–common in both military and some civilian casualties–may involve any vessel, including the extracranial cerebral arteries and the vasculature leading to any of the viscera. The brachial and popliteal arteries, coursing across joints and exposed to direct trauma, are particularly susceptible to injuries associated with fractures and dislocations.

E. Arterial Spasm: Segments of arteries, frequently within musculofascial compartments–and especially the muscular arteries (brachial, popliteal)–may become narrowed by intense constriction of smooth muscle evoked by the injury. Such vessels may also be compressed by hematoma and edema. Although the involved artery may not be injured, it frequently supplies tissues that have been rendered ischemic by trauma, and a vicious cycle is created. Vasospasm alone is rarely sufficiently intense or persistent to produce numbness or paralysis of the distal extremity. When this occurs, objective evidence of patency of the system should be obtained since unnecessary delay in restoring perfusion may jeopardize the limb. An arteriogram can be performed when it is not clear whether an occlusion exists. A Doppler ultrasonic flow probe is a useful adjunct for detecting pulsatile flow.

F. Disruption of Thoracic Aorta or Brachiocephalic Vessels: Crushing blows to the chest or abrupt deceleration from high speed can disrupt the thoracic aorta, most often just distal to the ligamentum arteriosum. Forces are dissipated through points of fixation in a manner that disrupts the intima and media. This usually leads to fatal hemorrhage, but occasionally the adventitia and pleura contain the extravasated blood and a false aneurysm is formed. Such a lesion must be suspected when the upper ribs are fractured and the chest x-ray shows widening of the mediastinum. The diagnosis can be confirmed by arteriography and operative repair performed–usually with the aid of left heart bypass. The innominate, subclavian, and carotid arteries are subject to similar disruption by direct blows to the sternum.

G. Chemical Injury: Inadvertent intra-arterial injection of hypnotics (eg, thiopental) and other agents produces occlusion of small peripheral vessels which may be so severe that all or part of a limb may be lost. This can occur when the ulnar artery is superficial at the elbow in cases of high bifurcation of the brachial artery and is a hazard that must be avoided by anesthesiologists in the operating room. Severe pain in the hand is associated with intense vasoconstriction, which may gradually subside after a few hours. When a high dose of the agent has been injected, thrombosis may progress to involve major vessels of the hand and forearm, ultimately requiring amputation. When such an injection is recognized, the needle should be left in place and 15,000 units of heparin injected through it. Reserpine (0.5 mg) has been recommended, although its only effect experimentally has been to protect against the release of catecholamines from the vessel walls when it is given before the injection of thiopental. Brachial plexus block or exploration of the vessel may be of some value in reducing the vasospasm.

Manifestations of Arterial Injury

A. Hemorrhage: Although the diagnosis of arterial injury is obvious when there is pulsatile external hemorrhage, a bleeding site may not be readily identified when blood is accumulating in deep tissues or draining freely into the thorax, abdomen, or retroperitoneum. In these cases, the primary presenting manifestation is hemorrhagic shock. The peripheral vasoconstriction that accompanies such shock makes it difficult to evaluate peripheral pulses until the blood volume is restored. Recognition of arterial contusions and thromboses associated with multiple injuries is delayed by the difficulty in differentiating local from systemic factors. These effects of arterial injury are reciprocal, since ischemic tissue prolongs acidosis, venous stasis, and microembolization to the lungs, the latter compromising pulmonary function.

B. Ischemia: Until proved otherwise, ischemia of a part–whether of an extremity or a visceral organ–must be treated as though it were due to primary vascular injury. When an extremity is involved, paralysis or anesthesia rapidly develops, indicating anoxia of the peripheral nerves. It may not be possible to predict whether a given degree of ischemia will be tolerated by the part. For example, sudden occlusion of the carotid artery will result in brain damage within minutes unless collateral circulation provides a near physiologic perfusion pressure. Injury to a renal artery may produce a nonfunctioning kidney that can be restored by an arterial repair even several hours after the injury. An ischemic extremity may have sufficient perfusion to preserve some but not all muscle, the most susceptible to necrosis being those without major collateral arterial supply and located within nondistensible fascial compartments. Although 6 or 8 hours of ischemia may be tolerated by skeletal muscle, any delay in restoring perfusion risks the appearance of a vicious cycle consisting of subfascial edema, venous occlusion, propagation of thrombi within vascular spaces, and disruption of arterioles and capillaries which upon reperfusion will bleed and produce progressive swelling and necrosis. Time is a critical factor in the management of all vascular injuries to preserve life and organ function.

C. False Aneurysm: A false aneurysm may be formed by the outer layers of a partially disrupted artery or by the encapsulation of a **pulsating hematoma.** These may develop without interrupting distal blood flow, and in the acute phase are prone to rupture without warning. Although frequently tolerated for a time, they expand to produce symptoms either by compression of adjacent nerves or collateral circulation, and ultimately rupture.

D. Arteriovenous Fistula: Arteriovenous fistulas occur after simultaneous injury to adjacent arteries and veins, usually due to stab wounds or missiles. There may be little bleeding because the arterial pressure is decompressed into the vein. Fistulas are also produced by operative injuries—when a common ligature is applied to an artery and a vein (nephrectomy, thyroidectomy)—or by inadvertent injury of the vena cava or iliac veins and the aorta (removal of herniated intervertebral disks). Delayed arteriovenous fistulas are seen when infected hematomas erode into adjacent veins.

E. Venous Injury and Obstruction: When major venous drainage of a part is interrupted, tissue perfusion is compromised by the sequence of edema and compression of tissues in closed compartments. Propagation of thrombus from these veins can lead to pulmonary embolism. Venous injury should be suspected when peripheral veins in the extremity are abnormally prominent.

Principles of Diagnosis

(1) Vascular injury must be suspected in any wound in the vicinity of major blood vessels.

(2) Search for evidence of hemorrhage into body cavities.

(3) Suspect primary vascular injury whenever tissue perfusion or organ function is impaired (fractures, dislocations, penetrating wounds, direct trauma).

(4) Differentiate between the effects of hemorrhagic shock and vascular occlusion (monitor responses to blood volume restoration by observing urinary output and peripheral pulses).

(5) Search for physical signs of vascular injury (expanding or pulsating hematomas, to-and-fro murmurs of false aneurysms, continuous murmurs of arteriovenous fistulas, loss of pulses, progressive swelling of the part, unexplained ischemia or dysfunction).

(6) Differentiate between arterial injury and vaso-

spasm (sympathetic block, topical or intra-arterial papaverine, ultrasonic Doppler flow probe, arteriogram).

(7) **Arteriography,** although of great value in elective cases, may unduly delay emergency operations (control of hemorrhage), and it is not always performed preoperatively unless definitive information concerning the injury is required to determine the operative approach (injuries at base of neck, thoracic aorta) or if confirmation of the clinical diagnosis of arterial injury is needed.

Treatment

A. Primary Care: The clinical assessment of the severity of acute injuries is accomplished without delay. The patient is immediately moved to the operating room if massive hemorrhage precludes resuscitation in the emergency room.

Restoration of blood volume and control of hemorrhage are carried out simultaneously. External bleeding is best controlled by continuous pressure or packing. Tourniquets—which may jeopardize the success of future arterial reconstruction—are avoided. Atraumatic vascular clamps are applied to bleeding vessels when they are accessible. Large-bore intravenous cannulas are inserted (superior or inferior vena cava), and blood is drawn for cross-matching. Blood volume is restored with lactated Ringer's injection, plasma, and type-specific blood. Cross-matched blood is given as soon as it is available. Resuscitation is not continued in the emergency room when the patient ought to be in the operating room, since surgical exposure of inaccessible bleeding vessels (thorax, abdomen, neck) must be accomplished without delay.

B. Associated Measures: Endotracheal intubation may be required to control ventilation or to prevent aspiration of blood from nasopharyngeal injuries. One or more thoracostomy tubes are inserted under local anesthesia and attached to underwater suction when hemothorax or hemopneumothorax is diagnosed. Symptoms and signs of pericardial tamponade can be relieved by pericardiocentesis done from the perixiphoid approach using a long, thin-walled No. 17 needle.

If the clinical signs of intra-abdominal bleeding are not diagnostic (as in comatose patients), abdominal paracentesis may be used to detect free blood in the peritoneal cavity. An indwelling urinary catheter is used to assess the adequacy of renal perfusion and to detect possible urinary tract injuries.

Fractures are reduced and stabilized before arterial repair is accomplished in the extremities. Antibiotics are started, and tetanus prophylaxis (see Chapter 11) is administered preoperatively.

C. Operative Repair of Arterial Injuries: The feasibility of repairing injured vessels is determined by the magnitude of the wound. Extensive contamination and destruction of soft tissues, bones, blood vessels, and nerves—common in military casualties—preclude primary repair because thrombosis, gangrene, or delayed hemorrhage from infection will develop.

Proximal arterial ligation and amputation are usually required as lifesaving procedures for these massive injuries.

Most vascular injuries seen in civilian practice and in certain military casualties are reparable because there is minimal contamination and tissue damage. When operated upon under optimal aseptic conditions with adequate anesthesia, qualified personnel, and proper instrumentation, such injured vessels are usually restored to normal function.

Adequate exposure of the involved vessel is required for control of bleeding and subsequent repair. In the extremities, incisions are placed parallel to the course of the vessel far enough above and below the lesion so that the damaged area is not disturbed. Control of the vessel is obtained proximal and distal to the injury by passing umbilical tapes around the vessel so that the lumen can be occluded with atraumatic clamps at these points. The injured area may then be dissected free without further bleeding in preparation for repair.

Proximal and distal thrombi are removed by flushing the proximal limb and backbleeding the distal limb. A Fogarty balloon catheter is then passed into the distal tributaries where thrombus is extracted. After completion of these maneuvers, a catheter the size of the artery lumen is inserted into the distal limb for injection of heparin solution (1000–2000 units). If there is concern about the adequacy of the distal thrombectomy and the status of a preexisting diseased arterial bed, an **operative arteriogram** is performed by injecting contrast media through the distal catheter.

Devitalized tissue is debrided from the wound and hematomas evacuated. Except in children or when a smaller vessel seems to be critical for limb survival, vessels under 5 mm in diameter are usually not repaired.

Simple lateral repair is permissible when a large artery has a small incision and closure does not produce narrowing. To avoid narrowing the vessel, a lateral vein patch may be used if the vessel is not contused. When there are multiple defects in a segment or the vessel is contused, excision and end-to-end anastomosis gives the best results. If this produces tension, a replacement or bypass graft is used. The latter is less desirable because it requires that dissection be performed in normal tissues where collaterals may be interrupted.

When possible, autogenous tissue is used for grafting. The saphenous vein is used most commonly and the cephalic vein occasionally. Segments from the hypogastric or external iliac artery are sometimes used as autografts in visceral artery repairs. The iliac artery is then replaced by a prosthetic graft. Prosthetic grafts, although satisfactory when vein grafts are unavailable, are not favored in trauma cases because they are more prone to infection and thrombosis and disruption when used in a contaminated wound.

Cohen AC & others: Carotid artery injuries: An analysis of eighty-five cases. Am J Surg 120:210, 1970.

Connolly J: Management of fractures associated with arterial injuries. Am J Surg 120:33, 1970.
DeBakey ME, Simeone FA: Battle injuries of the arteries in World War II: An analysis of 2471 cases. Ann Surg 123:534, 1946.
Drapanas T & others: Civilian vascular injuries: A critical appraisal of three decades of management. Ann Surg 172:351, 1970.
Eastcott HHG: Arterial injuries. Page 236 in: *Arterial Surgery.* Lippincott, 1973.
Hunt TK, Blaisdell FW, Okimoto J: Vascular injuries at the base of the neck. Arch Surg 98:586, 1969.
Hunt TK & others: Arteriovenous fistulas of major vessels in the abdomen. J Trauma 11:483, 1971.
Hewitt RL, Smith AD, Drapanas T: Acute traumatic arteriovenous fistulas. J Trauma 13:901, 1973.
Perry MO & others: Management of arterial injuries. Ann Surg 173:403, 1971.
Reul GJ Jr & others: The early operative management of injuries to great vessels. Surgery 74:862, 1973.
Rich NM & others: Acute arterial injuries in Viet Nam: 1000 cases. J Trauma 10:359, 1970.
Rich NM & others: Repair of lower extremity venous trauma: A more aggressive approach required. J Trauma 14:639, 1974.
Shaker IJ & others: Special problems of vascular injuries in children. J Trauma 16:863, 1976.

BLAST INJURY
Arthur N. Thomas, MD

Blast injuries in civilian populations occur as a result of fireworks or household explosions or industrial accidents. Urban guerrilla tactics may take the form of letter bombs, car bombs, or satchel-suitcase bombs. Injuries occur from the effects of the blast itself, propelled foreign bodies, or in large blasts, from objects falling from buildings. Military blast injuries may also involve personnel submerged in water. Water increases energy transmission and the possibility of injury to the viscera of the thorax or abdomen.

Clinical Findings

A. Symptoms and Signs: The injury is dependent upon proximity to the blast, space confinement, and detonation size. Large explosions cause multiple foreign body impregnations, bruises, abrasions, and lacerations. Gross soilage of wounds from clothing, flying debris, or explosive powder is usual. About 10% of all casualties have deep injuries to the chest or abdomen. Lung damage usually involves rupture of the alveolus with hemorrhage. Air embolism from bronchovenous fistula may cause sudden death. The mechanisms of lung injury are thought to be due to spalling effects (splintering forces produced when a pressure wave hits a fluid-air interface), implosion effects, and pressure differentials.

Letter bombs cause predominantly hand, face, eye, and ear injuries. Energy transmission within the fluid media of the eye can cause globe rupture, dialysis of the iris, hyphema of the anterior chamber, lens capsule tears, retinal rupture, or macular pucker. Blindness or permanent impairment of vision can occur. Ear injuries may be drum rupture or cochlear damage. There may be nerve or conduction hearing deficit or deafness. Tinnitus, vertigo, and anosmia are also seen in letter bomb casualties.

B. Laboratory Findings: The chest roentgenogram may initially be normal or may show pneumothorax, pneumomediastinum, or parenchymal infiltrates.

Treatment

Severe injuries with shock from blood loss or hypoxia require resuscitative measures to restore perfusion and oxygenation. Surgical treatment of extremity injuries requires wide debridement of devitalized muscle, thorough cleansing of wounds, and removal of foreign materials. The usual criteria for exploring penetrating wounds of the thorax or abdomen are employed. Eye injuries may require immediate repair. Ear injuries are usually treated expectantly. Respiratory insufficiency may result from pulmonary injury or may be secondary to shock, fat embolism, or other causes. Tracheal intubation and prolonged respiratory care with mechanical ventilation may be necessary.

Complications

Minor complications include tattooing of exposed skin. The possibility of gas gangrene in grossly contaminated extensive muscle injuries may warrant open treatment.

Results & Prognosis

Permanent loss of extremities or their function may require extensive reconstruction or rehabilitation. Permanent deficits of vision or hearing are common in letter bomb injuries. Patients with pulmonary injury may die despite intensive respiratory support.

Jamra FA, Halasa A, Salman S: Letter bomb injuries: A report of three cases. J Trauma 14:275, 1974.

Kennedy TL, Johnston GW: Civilian bomb injuries. Br Med J 1:382, 1975.

McCaughey W, Coppel DL, Dundee JW: Blast injuries to the lungs: A report of two cases. Anaesthesia 28:2, 1973.

● ● ●

General References

American College of Surgeons Committee on Trauma: Essential equipment list for ambulances. Bull Am Coll Surg 55:7, May 1970.

Borrie J: *Management of Emergencies in Thoracic Surgery.* Appleton-Century-Crofts, 1972.

Boswick JA Jr (editor): Symposium on trauma. Surg Clin North Am 53:6, 1973.

Deaver RM, Ritchett RH: Motorcycle trauma. J Trauma 15:678, 1975.

DeMuth WE Jr: Ballistic characteristics of "magnum" sidearm bullets. J Trauma 14:227, 1974.

DeMuth WE Jr: The mechanism of shotgun wounds. J Trauma 11:219, 1971.

Drysdale WF & others: Injury patterns in motorcycle collisions. J Trauma 15:90, 1975.

Gurdjian ES: Prevention and mitigation of head injury from antiquity to the present. J Trauma 13:931, 1973.

Levitt S: Fatal road accidents: Injuries, complications, and causes of death in 250 subjects. Br J Surg 55:481, 1968.

Lim R, Trunkey D, Blaisdell FW: Acute abdominal aortic injury: An analysis of operative and postoperative management. Arch Surg 109:706, 1974.

Lucas CE, Ledgerwood AM: Prospective evaluation of hemostatic techniques for liver injuries. J Trauma 16:442, 1976.

Lucas CE, Walt A: Analysis of randomized biliary drainage for liver trauma in 189 patients. J Trauma 12:925, 1972.

MacArthur JD, Moore FD: Epidemiology of burns: The burn-prone patient. JAMA 231:259, 1975.

Mathewson C Jr: Early management of trauma patient. Surg Clin North Am 52:531, 1972.

May PRA & others: Woodpeckers and head injury. Lancet 1:454, 1976.

Mays T: Lobar dearteriolization for exsanguinating wounds of the liver. J Trauma 12:397, 1972.

McNair TJ (editor): *Hamilton Bailey's Emergency Surgery,* 9th ed. Williams & Wilkins, 1972.

Schimpff SC: Infection in the severely traumatized patient. Ann Surg 179:352, 1974.

Shires GT, Jones RC: Initial management of the severely injured patient. JAMA 213:1872, 1970.

Shires GT & others: Principles in treatment of severely injured patients. Adv Surg 4:255, 1970.

Shires T: Initial care of the injured patient. J Trauma 10:940, 1970.

Spencer JH: *The Hospital Emergency Department.* Thomas, 1972.

Walt AJ (editor): Symposium on trauma. Surg Clin North Am 57:1, 1977. [Entire issue.]

Walt AJ, Wilson R: *Management of Trauma.* Lea & Febiger, 1974.

17 . . .
Burns & Other Thermal Injuries

Donald D. Trunkey, MD, Steven Parks, MD, Thomas K. Hunt, MD, & Lawrence W. Way, MD

A severe thermal injury can be one of the most devastating physical and psychologic injuries a person can suffer. Recent statistics indicate that over 12,000 lives are lost annually in the USA from burns, and in 50–75% of cases the primary cause of death was smoke inhalation. Every year, 300,000 Americans are injured by fire, and 50,000 of these remain in hospitals from 6 weeks to 2 years. The fire death rate in the USA (57.1 deaths per million population) is the second highest in the world and the highest of all industrialized countries–almost twice that of second ranking Canada (29.7 deaths per million).

Anatomy & Physiology of the Skin

The skin is the largest organ of the body, ranging from 0.25 sq m in the newborn to 1.8 sq m in the adult. It consists of 2 layers, epidermis and dermis or corium. The outermost cells of the epidermis are dead cornified cells which act as a tough protective barrier against the environment. The second, thicker layer, the corium (0.06–0.12 mm), is composed chiefly of fibrous connective tissue. The corium contains the blood vessels and nerves to the skin and the epithelial appendages of specialized function. Since the nerve endings that mediate pain are found only in the corium, partial thickness injuries may be extremely painful whereas full thickness burns are usually anesthetic. The corium is a barrier that prevents loss of body fluids by evaporation.

Sweat glands help maintain body temperature by controlling the amount of water of evaporation. They also excrete small amounts of sodium chloride and cholesterol and traces of albumin and urea. The corium is interlaced with sensory nerve endings that identify the sensations of touch, pressure, pain, heat, and cold. This is a protective mechanism which allows an individual to adapt to changes in the physical environment. Lastly, the skin manufactures vitamin D, which is synthesized by the action of sunlight on certain intradermal cholesterol compounds.

Depth of Burns (Fig 17–1)

The depth of the burn significantly affects all subsequent clinical events. The depth may be difficult to determine and in some cases is not known until after spontaneous healing has occurred or when the eschar is removed and granulation tissue is seen.

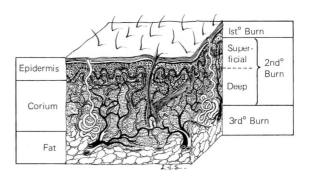

Figure 17–1. Layers of the skin showing depth of first, second, and third degree burns.

Traditionally, burns have been classified as first, second, and third degree, but the current emphasis on burn healing has led to classification as partial thickness burns, which heal spontaneously, and full thickness burns, which require skin grafting.

A **first degree burn** involves only the epidermis and is characterized by erythema and minor microscopic changes; tissue damage is minimal, protective functions of the skin are intact, skin edema is minimal, and systemic effects are rare. Pain, the chief symptom, usually resolves in 48–72 hours, and healing takes place uneventfully. In 5–10 days the damaged epithelium peels off in small scales, leaving no residual scarring. The most common causes of first degree burns are overexposure to sunlight and brief scalding.

Second degree burns are deeper, involving all of the epidermis and some of the corium. The systemic severity of the burn and the quality of subsequent healing are directly related to the amount of undamaged corium. Redness and blisters are characteristic. The deeper the burn, the more common are the blisters, which increase in size during the hours immediately following the injury. Complications are rare from superficial second degree burns, which usually heal with minimal scarring in 10–14 days unless they become infected.

In deep dermal burns, injured skin may resemble the skin lying over third degree burns except that it is usually red or pink. These wounds heal over a period of 25–35 days with a fragile epithelial covering that arises from the residual uninjured epithelium of the

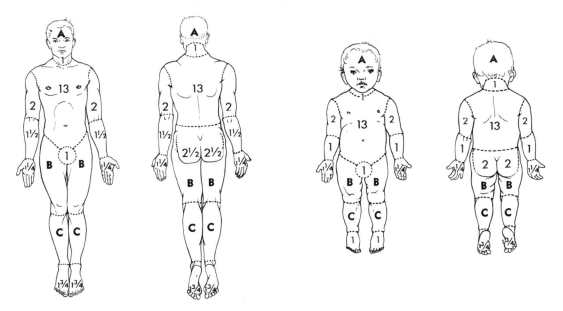

Relative Percentages of Areas Affected by Growth

Area	Age		
	10	15	Adult
A = half of head	5½	4½	3½
B = half of one thigh	4¼	4½	4¾
C = half of one leg	3	3¼	3½

Relative Percentages of Areas Affected by Growth

Area	Age		
	0	1	5
A = half of head	9½	8½	6½
B = half of one thigh	2¾	3¼	4
C = half of one leg	2½	2½	2¾

Figure 17—2. Table for estimating extent of burns. In adults, a reasonable system for calculating the percentage of body surface burned is the "rule of nines": each arm equals 9%, the head equals 9%, the anterior and posterior trunk each equal 18%, and each leg equals 18%; the sum of these percentages is 99%.

deep dermal sweat glands and hair follicles. Dense scarring is common with this injury, and it frequently develops into a third degree (full thickness) burn if it becomes infected. Fluid losses and metabolic effects of deep dermal burns are the same as for third degree burns.

Full thickness or **third degree burns** have a tough leathery surface that may be brown, tan, black, white, or even red. They are anesthetic because the entire thickness of the skin, including the pain receptors, has been destroyed. If pressure is applied to the burn eschar, the surface will not blanch and refill because the blood vessels have been destroyed or thrombosed. The tissue is dead.

Determination of Severity of Injury

Morbidity and mortality are related to the size (surface area) and depth of the burn, the age of the victim and his prior state of health, the location of the burn wound, and the severity of associated injuries (if any).

The total body surface area involved in the burn is most accurately determined by using the age-related charts designed by Lund and Browder (Fig 17—2). A set of these charts should be filled out for every

burned patient as soon as he is admitted and resuscitation is begun.

A careful calculation of the percentage of total body burn is useful for several reasons. First, there is a general tendency to underestimate the size of the burn and thus its severity. The American Burn Association has recently adopted a severity index for burn injury (Table 17—1). Second, prognosis is directly related to the extent of injury. Third, the decision about who should be treated in a specialized burn facility or managed as an outpatient is based in part on the estimate of burn size. Finally, early estimates of fluid requirements are related to burn size.

Patients under age 2 and over 60 have a significantly higher mortality rate for any given extent of burn. The higher mortality rate in infants is presumably due to greater susceptibility to infection from incompletely developed immune competence. Associated conditions such as cardiac disease, diabetes, or chronic obstructive pulmonary disease significantly worsen the prognosis.

Other factors such as the location of the burn (eg, whether on the hands, face, or perineum) also affect the outcome. All patients with certain kinds of burns (eg, electrical, chemical, or those involving the respira-

Table 17—1. Summary of American Burn Association patient severity categorization.

Major burn injury
  Second degree burn of > 25% body surface area in adults.
  Second degree burn of > 20% body surface area in children.
  Third degree burn of > 10% of body surface area.
  All burns involving hands, face, eyes, ears, feet, or perineum.
  All patients with the following:
    Inhalation injury.
    Electrical injury.
    Burn injury complicated by other major trauma.
  Poor risk patients with burns.
Moderate uncomplicated burn injury
  Second degree burn of 15—25% body surface area in adults.
  Second degree burn of 10—20% body surface area in children.
  Third degree burn of < 10% body surface area.
Minor burn injury
  Second degree burn of < 15% body surface area in adults.
  Second degree burn of < 10% body surface area in children.
  Third degree burn of < 2% body surface area.

tory tract) should be admitted to the hospital because the injury often appears deceptively insignificant on initial evaluation.

Pathology & Pathophysiology

The microscopic pathologic feature of the burn wound is principally coagulation necrosis. Beneath any obviously charred tissue there are 3 distinct zones. The first is the zone of "coagulation," with permanently irreversible coagulation and no capillary blood flow. The depth of this most severely damaged zone is determined by the temperature and duration of exposure. Beneath this is a zone of stasis, characterized by sluggish capillary blood flow. Although damaged, the tissue has not been coagulated. Stasis can occur early or late. Avoiding additional injury from rubbing or dehydration may prevent stasis changes from developing and thereby prevent extension of the depth of the burn. Prevention of venous occlusion is important because it may lead to thrombosis and infarction in this zone. The third zone is that of "hyperemia," which is the usual inflammatory response of healthy tissue to nonlethal injury.

Metabolic Response to Burns & Metabolic Support

In the hours immediately after the burn has occurred, the metabolically active zones of the wound are flooded with fluid, plasma proteins, and PMNs.

The systemic impairment of capillary membrane integrity produces additional loss of fluid from the intravascular compartment as reflected by the fact that with burns of more than 40% of total body surface, at least 4.4 ml/kg/hour are required to maintain a constant circulating blood volume no matter what kind of solution is infused. However, by 6—8 hours, if resuscitation is appropriate, capillary integrity begins to return, and by 18—24 hours has stabilized. As with any major injury, the body increases the secretion of catecholamines, cortisol, renin-angiotensin, antidiuretic

hormone, and aldosterone. The consequence is a tendency toward retention of sodium and water and excretion of potassium by the kidneys. Early in the response, energy is supplied by the breakdown of stored glycogen. In the burned patient, instead of the acute stress response ending at the conclusion of adequate resuscitation, it continues for days or even months until the wound is closed. As the stored glycogen is used up, new sources of energy must be utilized. The magnitude of late hypermetabolic events is related to the surface area of burn in the relatively smaller (eg, 10—40%) burns. It is accentuated by the presence of associated injuries and by the operations required to care for the wound. The metabolic response reaches a maximal level with burns of 40% of total body surface.

During the first postburn week, the metabolic rate (or heat production) and oxygen consumption rise progressively from the normal level present during resuscitation and remain elevated until the wound is covered. The reasons for the sustained hypermetabolism are thought to be the increased catecholamine secretion, evaporative heat loss from the wound, and elevated glucagon levels.

The evaporative water loss from the wound may reach 300 ml/sq m/hour (normal is about 15 ml/sq m/hour), which produces a heat loss of about 580 Cal/liter. Experimentally, when evaporative loss has been eliminated by covering the burn with an impermeable membrane, the hypermetabolism continues although at a slightly reduced rate. Similarly, placing the burned patient in a warm environment, where convection and radiant loss of heat are minimized, reduces the metabolic rate to nearly normal.

For some reason, catecholamine secretion remains persistently high throughout convalescence until the wound has been covered. Although it is of no value in patient management, the administration of adrenergic blocking agents to patients with large burns lowers the metabolic rate to nearly normal.

Associated with the catabolic state induced by catecholamines are elevated glucagon levels even in the presence of hyperglycemia. The resulting high glucagon-insulin ratio stimulates gluconeogenesis and fosters muscle breakdown, urea production, and loss of lean body weight.

Immunologic Factors in Burns

The predisposition of burned victims to infections is believed to result largely from associated immunologic abnormalities. Serum immunoglobulins A, M, and G are significantly decreased, reflecting depressed B cell function. Plasma levels reach a nadir 2—5 days after the injury, and in younger patients the deficiency may persist for 60 days. Cell-mediated immunity, or T cell function, is also impaired as demonstrated by prolonged survival of homografts and xenografts. Experimentally, depressed phagocytic activity of the A cells has been demonstrated to affect liver, spleen, and alveolar macrophages. Abnormal A cell function is of special significance because T cell and B cell function are A cell dependent.

Treatment

A. Acute Resuscitation: After admission to the hospital, the patient should be assessed and treated as any patient with major trauma. The first priority is to ensure an adequate airway. If there is a possibility that smoke inhalation has occurred, as suggested by exposure to a fire in an enclosed space or burns of the face, nares, or upper torso, arterial blood gases, including carboxyhemoglobin, should be determined immediately and oxygen should be administered. If the patient has extreme air hunger or is otherwise critically ill, endotracheal intubation is indicated. Intubation should be done early in all doubtful cases because delayed intubation may be difficult to achieve in cases associated with pharyngeal edema or upper airway injury, and an emergency tracheostomy may become necessary later in difficult circumstances. If the burn is severe, a Foley catheter should be inserted into the bladder to monitor urine output. A large-bore intravenous catheter should be inserted, preferably into a central vein.

After intravenous fluids are started and an adequate urine flow obtained, the wound should be debrided and cleansed with cool or tepid balanced salt solution and the patient should be wrapped in a sterile or clean sheet. External cooling is beneficial as long as 45 minutes after the injury. The optimal temperature of the water is 22–25 C (71.6–77 F), approximately that of household cold faucet water. Colder temperatures may damage tissues and cause systemic hypothermia, which may interfere with oxyhemoglobin dissociation.

Tetanus toxoid, 0.5 ml, should be administered; if the wound is greater than 50% of the body surface area, 250 units of human tetanus antitoxin should be given.

Severe burns are characterized by large losses of extracellular fluids, which are greatest during the first 12 hours. Fluid loss is partly due to increased permeability at the site of the burn, where transudation may be copious. In addition, with the onset of burn shock, the vascular endothelium becomes more permeable, resulting in interstitial sequestration of water and protein from the vascular space. Protein concentrations in the extravascular space may reach 3 g/100 ml, altering fluid equilibrium through changes in oncotic pressure. With adequate volume replacement, the endothelium regains its integrity, usually within 8–24 hours following the burn. Colloid administration is least effective during the first 24 hours because it crosses the endothelium and augments extravascular fluid retention. This effect can be critical in the lung, where fluid accumulation may produce pulmonary insufficiency and other pulmonary complications. Accumulation of extravascular water can also be critical in the brain, since cerebral edema may result in this closed space.

The amount of crystalloid solution administered during the first 24 hours varies depending on the individual patient and his injury (Tables 17–2 and 17–3). It should not be rigidly governed by a formula, though formulas are useful for planning. The best indicator of

Table 17–2. Evans, Brooke, and Baxter formulas for intravenous fluid maintenance in burns.

Evans

First 24 hours:
Colloid: 1 ml/kg/% burn
Saline: 1 ml/kg/% burn
5% dextrose in water: 2000 ml maintenance

Second 24 hours:
Colloid: 0.5 ml/kg/% burn
Saline: 0.5 ml/kg/% burn
5% dextrose in water: 2000 ml maintenance

Brooke

First 24 hours:
Colloid: 0.5 ml/kg/% burn
Lactated Ringer's injection: 1.5 ml/kg/% burn
5% dextrose in water: 2000 ml maintenance

Second 24 hours:
Colloid: 0.25 ml/kg/% burn
Lactated Ringer's injection: 0.75 ml/kg/% burn
5% dextrose in water: 2000 ml maintenance

Baxter

First 24 hours:
Lactated Ringer's injection: 4 ml/kg/% burn

Second 24 hours:
5% dextrose in water: 2000 ml maintenance
Plasma in sufficient volume to restore plasma volume

adequate fluid resuscitation is the left ventricular end-diastolic filling pressure. However, this measurement is sometimes impractical to obtain, and central venous pressure is usually sufficient. Urine output, another critical indicator of volume replacement, should be kept at 0.5–1 ml/kg/hour. Other parameters such as peripheral perfusion and sensorium should also be assessed.

It is especially important to avoid administering excessive amounts of fluid to patients with inhalation burns. On the other hand, fluid should not be restricted to the point that renal function is compromised, since inhalation injury when combined with renal shutdown is usually lethal. Balanced salt solutions such as lactated Ringer's injection should be administered with care because they are slightly hypotonic and can produce an undesirable alkalosis. Frequent determination of serum pH will avoid the latter problem.

Restoration of plasma volume is most successful with electrolyte solutions during the first 24 hours, but in the second 24 hours colloid solutions are better,

Table 17–3. Comparison of formula recommendations for intravenous fluids in a 70 kg man with 40% burn—first 24 hours.

Water administered	
Evans	12,400 ml
Brooke	12,400 ml
Baxter	13,400 ml
Sodium administered	
Evans	1736 mEq
Brooke	1694 mEq
Baxter	1716 mEq

particularly in patients with greater than 40% burns. Thus, fluid therapy during the second 24 hours should consist of enough free water to maintain the serum sodium near 140 mEq/liter and enough plasma to keep the plasma volume normal.

Hypertonic salt solution has been advocated by some for use in fluid resuscitation on the assumption that, compared with standard crystalloid solutions, it inhibits weight gain and wound edema. Patients given hypertonic saline demonstrate a marked natriuresis and do not develop pulmonary edema; in addition, ileus is uncommon. In general, however, studies comparing resuscitation with hypertonic and hypotonic fluids have failed to demonstrate a superiority of either. In addition, surgeons at the Surgical Research Institute, Brooke Army Hospital, have shown that when patients are allowed to drink fluids ad lib, the postinjury obligatory edema is just delayed, not avoided, by hypertonic solutions.

Fluid balance may continue to be a problem throughout the patient's course, particularly during the stages of debridement and grafting. Evaporative water loss can be considerable, and the best indices of water and electrolyte balance to follow are serum osmolality and serum sodium. Urine output may increase as a result of increased water intake from nebulizers and vaporizers on respirators, or from the osmotic diuresis that follows studies such as an intravenous urogram. Optimal fluid therapy is achieved by examining the patient frequently and performing repeated laboratory studies and not by relying on predicted losses or on formulas.

Treatment should aim to decrease catecholamine stimulation and provide enough calories to offset the effects of the hypermetabolism. Hypovolemia should be prevented by giving enough fluid to make up for the body losses. After the initial resuscitation, this can usually be done orally. To help reduce adrenergic responses, raising the room temperature or applying external radiant heat will reduce the heat loss to convection and radiation and will diminish the hypermetabolism. Painful stimuli should be minimized by the judicious use of analgesics during debridement and dressing changes.

Many patients can eat the required number of calories, but caloric expenditure sometimes reaches 4 times normal basal levels (4 $\times$ 1800 = 7200 Cal/day). If the nutritional status is in doubt, nitrogen balance can be measured and intake adjusted upward if the patient is in a catabolic state. Supplemental calories beyond what the patient is taking spontaneously can usually be provided through a feeding tube using balanced liquid diets, but high-calorie total parenteral nutrition is occasionally required. Strict attention to the nutritional needs is critical to the recovery of patients with the most severe burns. The reader should consult Chapter 13 for detailed information on this subject.

The use of antibiotics (eg, penicillin) during the first few days following the occurrence of a burn is a controversial subject. We feel it is better to treat strep-

tococcal infections in the few patients who acquire them than to cover all patients prophylactically. Broad-spectrum antibiotics should never be given for prophylaxis.

Vitamin A supplementation should be begun within the first 24–48 hours. The use of heparin in the postburn period is controversial. The rationale for heparin is that it (1) prevents thrombosis in the microcirculation, decreasing the chances of converting a partial thickness to a full thickness burn, (2) prevents thromboembolic phenomena, particularly in patients who may be bedridden for long periods, and (3) prevents disseminated intravascular clotting, a common complication of burns.

B. Care of the Burn Wound: In the management of first and second degree burns, one must provide as aseptic an environment as possible to prevent infection. Occlusive dressings to minimize exposure to air may reduce pain. If there is no infection, the burns will heal spontaneously. The goals in managing full thickness (third degree) burns are to prevent invasive infection (ie, burn wound sepsis), to remove dead tissue, and to cover the wound with skin as soon as possible.

There are 3 principal methods of therapy for the burn wound: exposure, occlusive dressings, and primary excision. The aim of all methods of treatment is to prevent invasive infection, and the end result of each is to remove dead tissue and allow coverage with skin grafts.

Exposure therapy is indicated for surfaces that are easily left exposed, such as the face. The burn is initially cleansed and then is allowed to dry. A second degree burn will form a crust which after 2 or 3 weeks will fall off, revealing minimally scarred skin beneath.

Full thickness burns will not form a crust because of the overlying dead eschar. The goal of exposure therapy is to soften the eschar and to remove it. Exposure allows the eschar to dry. After the eschar dries, saline soaks will soften it and hasten spontaneous separation from the underlying tissues. The advantage of this kind of treatment is that the patient is not immobilized in bulky dressings. It is particularly useful in burns that cover less than 20% of the body surface area. The disadvantage is that the protection against infection afforded by sterile dressings is absent. Exposure therapy is usually combined with the use of antibacterial creams such as mafenide acetate, silver sulfadiazine, or povidone-iodine ointment. Silver nitrate cannot be used with exposure therapy.

Occlusive dressings, usually combined with topical antibacterial agents, are more commonly used in the treatment of extensive burns. The ointment or cream may be applied to the patient or to the gauze. The bandages must be absorptive as well as occlusive and thus are usually bulky and restrictive. The older method of leaving occlusive dressings on for several days has been discarded in favor of dressing changes every 8–24 hours.

In both of the above methods of wound treatment the patient should be immersed daily in a Hubbard tank where remaining dressings and cream are washed off and loose tissue debrided. The patients are encouraged to move about to reduce contracture formation. The tub should contain a plastic liner to minimize bacterial contamination.

Operative debridement is stressful to the patient. Hypovolemia develops quickly, and preoperative blood transfusions are often necessary. During the operation, heat, water, and blood are lost rapidly. A warming blanket should be used to restore heat, and fluids and blood should be given as soon as the debridement is begun. Some surgeons limit the debridement by stopping as soon as the patient's temperature drops below about 35 C (95 F) or when blood loss exceeds 4 units.

Lastly, the physician can wait for spontaneous separation of the eschar, but this takes much more time, and during the wait the dense layer of connective tissue under the granulation thickens and contracts, and scarring is greater.

Primary excision of the burn, which is gaining in popularity, removes the necrotic eschar immediately, allowing the burn site to be grafted early, and produces the earliest closure of burn wounds and least chance of infection. The disadvantages are that it is difficult to differentiate between deep partial thickness and full thickness injury early in the postburn period, and operative blood loss is often great. The need for transfusions can be reduced by combining hypotensive anesthesia with newer surgical technics such as tangential excision, cautery, and use of the laser scalpel. Primary excision is particularly worthwhile for full thickness and deep burns of the hands. Occasionally, primary skin grafting is delayed for 24–48 hours while the wound is covered with a porcine xenograft.

Topical antibacterial agents have definitely advanced the care of burn patients. Although burn wound sepsis is still a major problem, the incidence is lower and the mortality rate has been reduced, particularly in burns of less than 50% of body surface area. Silver sulfadiazine is the most widely used preparation today. Povidone-iodine ointment is gaining popularity because it is fungicidal; with the reduction of bacterial contamination, candida infection has become more common. Gentamicin ointment was used at one time, but approximately 40% of pseudomonas organisms have become resistant to it, and this preparation should only be used now for specific indications.

Topical agents are not without problems. Many patients are allergic to mafenide. Mafenide can also be extremely painful, especially on partial thickness burns, because of its hydroscopic effects, although the pain is usually tolerated when analgesics are given concomitantly. Mafenide is absorbed through the burn and acts on the kidney as a carbonic anhydrase inhibitor. Renal tubular bicarbonate production is blocked, which may result in metabolic acidosis. The patient can usually eliminate excess CO_2 through the lungs provided respiratory complications do not supervene, but patients with pulmonary insufficiency may not be able to tolerate mafenide.

Silver nitrate is difficult to use. The dressings must be soaked frequently because the silver ion is inactivated on contact with protein. The markedly hypotonic solution leaches Na^+, K^+, and Cl^- from the burn surface, and water toxicity may develop. Sodium, chloride, potassium, and calcium need to be replaced frequently. In the presence of light, the silver nitrate blackens, giving the patient, linen, nurses, and the room an unappealing dirty appearance.

Povidone-iodine tends to "tan" (stiffen) the eschar, which, although not a major problem, does make debridement more difficult and may accentuate deformities over the skin of the face and joints. Absorbed iodine raises the PBI but has no effect on thyroid function.

Renewed interest in debridement with proteolytic enzymes has followed the introduction of sutilains (Travase), an effective nonallergenic, nontoxic product that appears not to affect normal tissue. Obviously, a nonsurgical, atraumatic method of removing the eschar would have great usefulness. Unfortunately, this enzyme predisposes to burn wound sepsis, allowing rapid entry of bacteria. Incorporating mafenide or silver sulfadiazine 1% with sutilains has not solved this problem. At present, use of this agent is best restricted to small full thickness burns.

White cells and bacteria contain collagenases which make an eschar separate more rapidly when infected. Unfortunately, infection also deepens the burn by destroying residual epithelium. New connective tissue regenerates as the eschar begins to separate, and it is revealed as the eschar comes off.

Circumferential burns of an extremity or of the trunk pose special problems. Swelling beneath the unyielding eschar may act as a tourniquet to blood and lymph flow, and the distal extremity may become swollen and tense. More extensive swelling may compromise the arterial supply. Longitudinal escharotomy, or excision of the eschar, may be required. To avoid permanent damage, escharotomy must be performed before arterial ischemia develops. Constriction involving the chest or abdomen may severely restrict ventilation and may require longitudinal escharotomies. When an escharotomy is performed on the chest or abdomen, at least 3 long incisions should be made. Anesthetics are rarely required, and the procedure can usually be performed in the patient's room.

Split thickness porcine xenografts are commercially available and have recently gained popularity as a biologic dressing that can be applied to clean burn wounds. If the xenografts are changed daily, the underlying granulation tissue often becomes ready for grafting much more rapidly. Porcine xenografts can also be used to cover primarily excised areas when grafting must be delayed or when autografts are not available. Homografts (human skin) work better for this purpose but are difficult to obtain.

Xenografts and homografts are particularly effective on second degree burns, especially in children. After the initial cleansing and removal of blisters, immediate application of pigskin prevents fluid loss, protects against infection, and stops pain. The patient can walk about in comfort immediately. The temporary grafts should be changed every 3–4 days so that the "take" is minimal. The resultant healing has minimal scarring.

The maintenance of functional motion during evolution of the burn wound is especially desirable to avoid loss of motion at joints. Wound contraction, a normal event during healing, may result in extremity contracture. Immobilization may produce joint stiffness, which at one time was thought to be caused by edema but probably is more a result of pain, disuse, or immobilizing dressings. Contracture of the scar, muscles, and tendons across a joint also causes loss of motion and can be diminished by traction, early motion, and pressure distributed directly over the wound to decrease the hypertrophic scar formation.

The scar is a metabolically active tissue, continually undergoing reorganization. The extensive scarring that frequently occurs after burns can lead to disfiguring and disabling contractures, but it may be avoided by the use of splints and elevation to maintain a functional position before grafting. Following application of the skin graft, either traction and exposure of the new skin or dressings with splints are indicated. In the convalescent period, pressure and isoprene splints will result in less hypertrophic scarring and contracture. The pressure should be maintained with elastic garments for at least 6 months and in some cases may be necessary for as long as a year.

Contracture tends to be balanced to some degree by the remodeling of scar that occurs during the first 6 months. Early burn contractures can usually be stretched by constant light force.

If reinjury does not occur, the amount of collagen in the scar tends to decrease with time. Stiff collagen becomes softer, and on flat surfaces of the body, where reinjury and inflammation are prevented, remodeling may totally eliminate contracture. However, around joints or the neck, contractures usually persist and plastic surgical reconstruction is often necessary. The sooner granulation tissue can be covered with skin grafts, the less likely is contracture.

Skin grafting is the final method of coverage for most full thickness injuries. Split thickness skin is obtained from unburned areas using a dermatome. The face, neck, and surfaces around joints are the first priority for grafting. For best cosmetic and functional results, nonmeshed skin should be used in these areas. When possible, the grafts are left open for inspection and to evacuate the small pockets of serum that collect under the graft. For grafts in other areas we prefer a 3:1 mesh graft which takes and heals readily. The graft may be left open or covered with occlusive dressings, which are left undisturbed for 48 hours. Mesh grafts have the advantage of covering large areas with a small amount of donor skin. The mesh may be applied without being opened to its fullest stretch, which results in rapid healing and a good cosmetic result.

Constant pressure on biologically evolving scars may cause a hypertrophic scar to recede. Reddened, inflamed tissue is biologically active, ie, it is vascular and is rapidly turning over collagen. It can be stretched and will lose collagen if direct pressure reduces its blood supply. Heat-malleable plastic, Silastic foams, and other materials are available from which tailored splints can be fashioned. Skeletal traction may be necessary in special instances. Sleeves, stockings, body jackets, etc are other ways to maintain pressure.

COMPLICATIONS

Infection remains a critical problem in burns, although the incidence has been reduced by modern therapy with topical antibacterial agents. Sequential quantitative cultures of the burn will show when a concentration of 10^5 organisms–the level defining invasive infection–are present. The cultures also show the sensitivity of the bacteria, and when the bacterial concentration passes 10^5 organisms/g specific antibiotics should be infiltrated beneath the eschar.

Disorientation of the patient heralds overwhelming sepsis. Spiking fever and paralytic ileus usually develop and become progressively more severe over 2–3 days. The temperature may fall below normal, the appearance of the wound may deteriorate, and the white count may fall, ending finally with septic shock. Aggressive antibiotic therapy must be initiated and an attempt made to identify the source of the infection. Pneumonitis, urinary tract infection, and intravenous catheter sepsis should be considered in the differential diagnosis. If other causes are not found, the wound is usually the septic focus and will have to be debrided. Blood volume, nutrition, and oxygenation must be assessed. Steroids should *not* be given because they depress already weakened immune defenses.

Acute gastroduodenal ulcers (Curling's ulcer), another frequent complication, appear as small circumscribed duodenal or gastric lesions that usually present clinically by bleeding. Routine endoscopy of burned patients has shown that subclinical ulceration of the duodenum develops in about 75% of burned patients, although only a few bleed. Antacids should be given routinely to all burned patients during their first few weeks in the hospital, a practice that will reduce the incidence of serious hemorrhage. Management of Curling's ulcers is covered in Chapter 26.

A complication unique to children is seizures, which may result from electrolyte imbalance, hypoxemia, infection, or drugs; in one-third of cases, the cause is unknown. Hyponatremia, the most frequent cause, is becoming less common with the diminishing use of topical silver nitrate. Drugs that have been implicated include penicillin, phenothiazine, diphenhydramine, and aminophylline.

Acute gastric dilatation, which occurs in the first week after injury, should be suspected when the patient repeatedly vomits small quantities of food. Fecal impaction resulting from immobilization, dehydration, and narcotic analgesics is a fairly common occurrence.

RESPIRATORY TRACT INJURY IN BURNS

Today the major cause of death after burns is injury or complications in the respiratory tract. The problems include inhalation injury, aspiration in unconscious patients, bacterial pneumonia, pulmonary edema, pulmonary embolism, and posttraumatic pulmonary insufficiency.

Direct inhalation injuries, which predispose to other complications, are divided into 3 categories: carbon monoxide poisoning (Table 17–4), heat injury to the airway, and inhalation of noxious gases (Table 17–5).

Direct inhalation of dry heat is a rare cause of damage below the vocal cords, because in most cases the upper airway effectively cools the inspired gases before they reach the trachea and reflex closure of the cords and laryngeal spasm halt full inhalation of the hot gas. Direct burns to the upper airway are associated with burns of the face, lips, nasal hairs, and necrosis or swelling of the pharyngeal mucosa. Acute edema of the upper tract may cause airway obstruction and asphyxiation without lung damage. If there are any signs of actual or impending laryngeal obstruction, the trachea should be intubated or tracheostomy performed immediately. We feel that with good nursing care, better endotracheal tubes, and improved experience, intubation is preferable to tracheostomy in the average case, especially if the neck has been burned. If airway management is inadequate with the endotracheal tube, a tracheostomy may be required.

Inhalation of droplets, another cause of direct lower airway injury, is characterized by damage to the epithelial lining cells and mucous membranes, resulting in pulmonary edema and pneumonitis. Treatment is primarily supportive, including maintenance of pulmonary toilet, mechanical ventilation (when indicated), and antibiotics for pneumonia.

Carbon monoxide poisoning must be considered in every patient suspected of having inhalation injury on the basis of having been burned in a closed space, physical evidence of inhalation, or dyspnea. Arterial blood gases and carboxyhemoglobin level must be determined. Levels of carboxyhemoglobin above 5% in nonsmokers and above 10% in smokers indicate carbon monoxide poisoning. Carbon monoxide has an affinity

Table 17–5. Sources of noxious chemicals in smoke.

Polyethylene, polypropylene	Clean burning combustion to CO_2 and H_2O
Polystyrene	Copious black smoke and soot— CO_2, H_2O, some CO
Wood, cotton	Aldehydes (acrolein)
Polyvinylchloride	Hydrochloric acid
Acrylonitrile, polyurethane, nitrogenous compounds	Hydrogen cyanide
Fire retardants may produce toxic fumes	Halogens (F_2, Cl_2, Br_2), ammonia

for hemoglobin 200 times that of oxygen, displaces oxygen, and produces a leftward shift in the oxyhemoglobin dissociation curve (P-50, the oxygen tension at which half the hemoglobin is saturated with oxygen, is lowered). Measurements of oxyhemoglobin saturation may be misleading because the hemoglobin combined with carbon monoxide is not detected and the percentage saturation of oxyhemoglobin may appear normal.

Mild carbon monoxide poisoning (less than 20% carboxyhemoglobin) is manifested by headache, slight dyspnea, mild confusion, and diminished visual acuity. Moderate poisoning (20–40% carboxyhemoglobin) leads to irritability, impairment of judgment, dim vision, nausea, and fatigability. Severe poisoning (40–60% carboxyhemoglobin) produces hallucinations, confusion, ataxia, collapse, and coma. Levels in excess of 60% carboxyhemoglobin are usually fatal.

Various toxic chemicals in inspired smoke produce specific respiratory injuries. Inhalation of kerosene smoke, for example, is relatively innocuous. Smoke from a wood fire is extremely irritating because it contains aldehyde gases, particularly acrolein. Direct inhalation of acrolein, even in low concentrations, irritates mucous membranes and produces an outpouring of fluid. A concentration of 10 ppm will cause pulmonary edema. Smoke from some of the newer plastic compounds, such as polyurethane, is the most serious type of toxic irritant. Poisonous gases such as chlorine, sulfuric acid, or cyanides are given off and can be lethal if absorbed.

Inhalation injury causes severe mucosal edema followed soon by sloughing of the mucosa. Almost immediately, peribronchiolar and perivascular edema develop. The destroyed mucosa in the larger airways is replaced by a mucopurulent membrane. The edema fluid enters the airway and, when mixed with the pus in the lumen, may form casts and plugs in the smaller bronchioles. Terminal bronchioles and alveoli may contain carbonaceous material. The interstitial lung tissue also becomes edematous and may obstruct the bronchioles. Acute bronchiolitis and bronchopneumonia commonly develop within a few days.

When inhalation injury is suspected, early endoscopic examination of the airway with either fiberoptic or standard bronchoscopy is indicated to determine the extent of injury (upper or lower airway). Aspiration may be diagnosed and the aspirated material removed.

Table 17–4. Carbon monoxide poisoning.

Carboxyhemoglobin Level	Severity	Symptoms
20%	Mild	Headache, mild dyspnea, visual changes, confusion
20–40%	Moderate	Irritability, diminished judgment, dim vision, nausea, easy fatigability
40–60%	Severe	Hallucinations, confusion, ataxia, collapse, coma
60%	Fatal	

Uncommon causes of respiratory failure are pulmonary embolus and "overload" pulmonary edema. Emboli usually occur later in the course of treatment after prolonged bed rest and should be suspected if respiratory function suddenly deteriorates. Since heparin has been included in the primary treatment regimen in many burn centers, emboli are less common. When a pulmonary embolus is diagnosed, heparin anticoagulation is indicated (see Chapter 39).

Pulmonary edema from fluid overload during resuscitation usually occurs in patients with preexisting heart disease. The treatment is diuresis and digitalis. When pulmonary edema is seen in association with renal failure, phlebotomy and dialysis are urgently required.

Probably the most common cause of respiratory failure is bacterial pneumonia from inhalation injury, contamination of the lungs through a tracheostomy or endotracheal tube, airborne infection, or hematogenous spread of bacteria from the burn wound.

Pulmonary insufficiency may develop following severe trauma and is usually associated with sepsis and disseminated intravascular clotting. Differentiating this condition from bacterial pneumonia may be difficult. There is damage to the pulmonary capillaries and leakage of fluid and protein into the interstitial spaces of the lung. Loss of compliance and difficulty in oxygenating the blood are progressive. Modern methods of ventilatory support and vigorous pulmonary toilet have significantly reduced the mortality rate in recent years.

Atelectasis due to chest wall restriction may occur when a large area of the chest wall is burned. Complete circumferential burns are worst, but restriction occurs when as little as half of the circumference is burned. In these cases, the eschar acts as a vise, restricting motion of the chest wall. Multiple longitudinal escharotomies are usually required to permit adequate ventilation.

Treatment

Management of a burned patient should include frequent evaluation of the lungs throughout the hospital course. All patients who initially have evidence of smoke inhalation should receive humidified oxygen in high concentrations. If carbon monoxide poisoning has occurred, 100% oxygen should be given until the carboxyhemoglobin saturation drops below 20%, which may take 2–3 hours. The administration of lower oxygen concentrations (30–40% oxygen) is advisable for the next few hours.

The use of corticosteroids for inhalation injuries is controversial. In the absence of proved efficacy in controlled studies, these drugs should probably be avoided because of their adverse effects on immunologic defenses.

Bronchodilators such as isoproterenol by aerosol or aminophylline intravenously may help if wheezing is due to reflex bronchospasm. Mist may liquefy tracheobronchial secretions, and chest physical therapy with postural drainage is also indicated.

When endotracheal intubation is used without mechanical ventilation (eg, for upper airway obstruction), mist and continuous positive pressure ventilatory assistance should be included. The humidity will help loosen the secretions and prevent drying of the airway; the continuous positive pressure will help prevent atelectasis and closure of lung units distal to the swollen airways.

An automatic respirator should be used when the patient cannot adequately ventilate and oxygenate his blood. In general, the following are the indications for mechanical ventilation: (1) inability to oxygenate arterial blood, as shown by an oxygen tension of less than 60 mm Hg at room air or an alveolar arterial oxygen difference of 300 mm Hg on 100% inspired oxygen, (2) arterial P_{CO_2} greater than 50 mm Hg, or (3) vital capacity less than 10 ml/kg body weight, or less than 3 times normal tidal volume.

Once a patient is placed on a ventilator, large tidal volumes (10–14 ml/kg) are used to prevent atelectasis and reexpand collapsed lung. Controlled ventilation and sedation are used initially because burned patients usually have greatly increased energy expenditures.

A detailed discussion of ventilatory support can be found in Chapter 3.

REHABILITATION

Plastic surgical revisions of scars are often necessary after the initial grafting, particularly to release contractures over joints and for cosmetic reasons. The physician must be realistic in defining an acceptable result, and the patient should be told that it may require years to achieve. Burn scars are often unsightly, and although hope should be extended that improvement can be made, total resolution is not possible in many cases.

The patient must take special care of the skin of the burn scar. Exposure to sunlight should be avoided, and, when the wound involves areas such as the face and hands which are frequently exposed to the sun, ultraviolet screening agents should be used. Hypertrophic scars and keloids are particularly bothersome, and may be reduced with the use of pressure dressings in the first 6 months after the injury. Topical agents such as steroid creams may also help reduce the amount of scar but should be confined to small areas. Since the skin appendages are often destroyed by full thickness burns, use of creams and lotions may be required to prevent drying and cracking and to reduce itching. Substances such as lanolin, A and D ointment, and Eucerin cream have all proved effective.

Achauer BM & others: Pulmonary complications of burns: The major threat to the burn patient. Ann Surg 177:311, 1973.

America Burning: The Report of the National Commission on Fire Prevention and Control. Superintendent of Documents, US Government Printing Office, Washington, DC.

Arturson G & others: Changes in immunoglobulin levels in severely burned patients. Lancet 1:546, 1969.

Artz CP, Moncrief JA: *The Treatment of Burns.* Saunders, 1969.

Baxter CB: Crystalloid resuscitation in burn shock. Pages 7–32 in: *Contemporary Burn Management.* Polk HC Jr, Stone HH (editors). Little, Brown, 1971.

Burke JF, Bondoc CC, Quinby WC: Primary burn excision and immediate grafting: A method of shortening illness. J Trauma 14:389, 1974.

Burke JF & others: Temporary skin transplantation and immunosuppression for extensive burns. N Engl J Med 290:264, 1974.

Dressler D, Shornik WA: Alveolar macrophage in the burned rat. J Trauma 14:1036, 1974.

Howard R, Simmons R: Acquired immunologic deficiencies after trauma and surgical procedures. Surg Gynecol Obstet 139:771, 1974.

Larson DL & others: Techniques for decreasing scar formation and contractures in the burned patient. J Trauma 11:807, 1971.

Loebl EC & others: The use of quantitative biopsy cultures in bacteriologic monitoring of burn patients. J Surg Res 16:1, 1974.

Monafo WW, Aulenbacher CE, Pappalardo C: Early tangential excision of the eschars of major burns. Arch Surg 104:503, 1972.

Moncrief JA: Burn formulae. J Trauma 12:538, 1972.

Moncrief JA: Burns. N Engl J Med 288:444, 1973.

Nance F & others: Aggressive outpatient care of burns. J Trauma 12:144, 1972.

Ofeigsson OJ, Mitchell R, Patrick RS: Observations of the cold water treatment of cutaneous burns. J Pathol 108:145, 1972.

Polk HC Jr: Prolongation of xenograft survival in patients with pseudomonas sepsis: A clarification. Surg Forum 19:514, 1968.

Polk HC Jr, Stone HH: *Contemporary Burn Management.* Little, Brown, 1971.

Pruitt BA, Erickson DR, Morris A: Progressive pulmonary insufficiency and other pulmonary complications of thermal injury. J Trauma 15:369, 1975.

Pruitt BA & others: Pulmonary complications in burn patients: A comparative study of 697 patients. J Thorac Cardiovasc Surg 59:7, 1970.

Rudowski W & others: *Burn Therapy and Research.* Johns Hopkins Univ Press, 1976.

Trunkey D, Parks S: Burns in children. Curr Probl Pediatr 6:3, Jan 1976.

Wilmore DW & others: Catecholamines: Mediator of the hypermetabolic response to thermal injury. Ann Surg 180:653, 1974.

Wilmore DW & others: Effect of ambient temperature on heat production and heat loss in burn patients. J Appl Physiol 10:593, 1975.

Wilmore DW & others: Alterations in hypothalamic function following thermal injury. J Trauma 15:697, 1975.

Zawacki BE: Reversal of capillary stasis and prevention of necrosis in burns. Ann Surg 180:98, 1974.

Zikria BA, Ferrer JM, Flock HF: The chemical factors contributing to pulmonary damage in "smoke poisoning." Surgery 71:704, 1972.

·   ·   ·

ELECTRICAL INJURY

There are 3 kinds of electrical injuries: electrical current injury, electrothermal burns from arcing current, and flame burns caused by ignition of clothing. Occasionally, all 3 will be present in the same victim.

Flash or arc burns are thermal injuries to the skin caused by a high-tension electrical current reaching the skin from the conductor. The thermal injury to the skin is intense and deep because the electrical arc has a temperature of about 2500 C (high enough to melt bone). Flame burns from ignited clothing are often the most serious part of the injury. Treatment is the same as for any thermal injury.

The damage from electrical current is directly proportionate to its intensity as governed by Ohm's law:

$$\text{Amperage (intensity of current)} = \frac{\text{Voltage (tension or potential)}}{\text{Resistance}}$$

Thus, the amperage depends on the voltage and on the resistance provided by various parts of the body. Voltages above 40 V are considered dangerous.

Once current has entered the body, its pathway depends on the resistances it encounters in the various organs. The following are listed in descending order of resistance: bone, fat, tendon, skin, muscle, blood, and nerve. The pathway of the current determines immediate survival; for example, if it passes through the heart or the brain stem, death may be immediate from ventricular fibrillation or apnea. Current passing through muscles may cause spasms severe enough to produce long bone fractures or dislocations.

The type of current is also related to the severity of injury. The usual 60-cycle alternating current that causes most injuries in the home is particularly severe. Alternating current causes tetanic contractions, and the patient may find himself "locked" to the contact. Cardiac arrest is common from contact with house current.

Electrical current injuries are more than just burns. Focal burns occur at the points of entrance and exit through the skin. Once inside the body, the current travels through muscles, causing an injury more like a crush than a thermal burn. Thrombosis frequently occurs in vessels deep in an extremity, causing a greater depth of tissue necrosis than is evident at the initial examination. The treatment of electrical injuries depends on the extent of deep muscle and nerve destruction more than any other factor.

Myoglobinuria may develop with the risk of acute tubular necrosis. The urine output must be kept 2–3 times normal with intravenous fluids. Alkalinization of the urine and osmotic diuretics may be indicated if myoglobinuria is present.

A rapid drop in hematocrit sometimes follows sudden destruction of red blood cells by the electrical energy. Bleeding into deep tissues may occur as a result of disruption of blood vessels and tissue planes. In some cases, thrombosed vessels disintegrate later and cause massive interstitial hemorrhage.

The skin burn at the entrance and exit sites is usually a depressed gray or yellow area of full thickness destruction surrounded by a sharply defined zone of hyperemia. Charring may be present if an arc burn coexists. The lesion should be debrided to underlying healthy tissue. Frequently there is deep destruction not initially evident. This dead and devitalized tissue must also be excised. A second debridement is usually indicated 24–48 hours after the injury because the necrosis is found to be more extensive than originally thought. The strategy of obtaining skin covering for these burns can tax ingenuity because of the extent and depth of the wounds.

In general, the treatment of electrical injuries is complex at every step, and after the initial resuscitation these patients should be referred to specialized centers.

Artz CP: Changing concepts of electrical injury. Am J Surg 128:600, 1974.

Starium HS: The treatment of electrical injuries. J Trauma 11:959, 1971.

HEAT STROKE

Heat stroke occurs when core body temperature exceeds 40 C (104 F) and produces severe CNS dysfunction. Two other related syndromes induced by exposure to heat are heat cramps and heat exhaustion.

Heat cramps, painful muscles after exertion in a hot environment, have usually been attributed to salt deficit. It is probable, however, that many cases are really examples of **exertional rhabdomyolysis.** The latter condition, which may also be a complicating factor in heat stroke, involves acute muscle injury due to severe exertional efforts beyond the limits for which the individual has trained. It often produces myoglobinuria, which rarely affects kidney function except when it occurs in patients also suffering from heat stroke. Complete recovery is the rule after uncomplicated heat cramps.

Heat exhaustion consists of fatigue, muscular weakness, tachycardia, postural syncope, nausea, vomiting, and an urge to defecate caused by dehydration from heat stress. Although body temperature is normal in heat exhaustion, there is a continuum between this syndrome and heat stroke.

Heat stroke kills about 4000 persons yearly in the USA. It is the result of imbalance between heat production and heat dissipation. Exercise-induced heat stroke most often affects young people (eg, athletes, military recruits, laborers) who are exercising strenuously in a hot environment, usually without adequate training. Sedentary heat stroke is a disease of elderly or infirm people whose cardiovascular systems are unable to adapt to the stress of a hot environment. Epidemics

of heat stroke in elderly people can be predicted when the ambient temperature surpasses 32.2 C (90 F) and the relative humidity reaches 50–75%.

In humans, heat is dissipated from the skin by radiation, conduction, convection, and evaporation. When the ambient temperature rises, heat loss by the first 3 is impaired; loss by evaporation is hindered by a high relative humidity. Predisposing factors to heat accumulation are dermatitis, use of diuretic or anticholinergic drugs, intercurrent fever from other disease, obesity, and alcoholism.

The mechanism of injury is direct damage by heat to the parenchyma and vasculature of the organs. The CNS is particularly vulnerable, and cellular necrosis is found in the brains of those who die of heat stroke. Hepatocellular and renal tubular damage are apparent in severe cases. Subendocardial damage and occasionally transmural infarcts are discovered in fatal cases even in young persons without previous cardiac disease. Disseminated intravascular coagulation may develop, aggravating injury in all organ systems and predisposing to bleeding complications.

Prevention

For the most part, heat stroke in military recruits and athletes in training is preventable by adhering to a graduated schedule of increasing performance requirements that allows acclimatization over 2–3 weeks. Heat produced by exercise is dissipated by increased cardiac output, vasodilatation in the skin, and increased sweating. With acclimatization there is increased efficiency for muscular work, increased myocardial performance, expanded extracellular fluid volume, greater output of sweat for a given amount of work, and a lower salt content of sweat.

Access to drinking water should be unrestricted during vigorous physical activity in a hot environment. Most training regimens should not include the use of supplemental salt tablets since enough salt (10–15 g/day) will be consumed with food to meet the losses in sweat, and hypernatremia can develop if ingested salt tablets are not taken with sufficient water. Clothing and protective gear should be lightened as heat production and air temperature rise, and heavy exercise should not be scheduled at the hottest times of day, especially at the beginning of a training schedule.

Clinical Findings

A. Symptoms and Signs: Heat stroke should be suspected in anyone who develops sudden coma in a hot environment. If the patient's temperature is above 40 C (104 F) (range: 40–43 C [104–109.4 F]), the diagnosis of heat stroke is definite. In less than half of cases, a syndrome consisting of confusion, belligerent behavior, or stupor precedes coma. Convulsions may occur after admission to the hospital.

The skin is pink or ashen and often, paradoxically, dry and hot; dry skin, which is not invariably present, is virtually pathognomonic in the presence of hyperpyrexia. The heart rate ranges from 140–170, central venous or pulmonary wedge pressure is high, and in some cases the blood pressure is low. Hyperventilation may reach 60/min and may give rise to a respiratory alkalosis. Pulmonary edema and bloody sputum may develop in severe cases. Jaundice is frequent within the first few days after onset of symptoms.

Dehydration, which may produce the same CNS symptoms as heat stroke, is an aggravating factor in about 15% of cases.

B. Laboratory Findings: There is no characteristic pattern to the electrolyte changes: The serum sodium concentration may be normal or high; the potassium concentration may be low, normal, or high. In the first few days the SGOT, LDH, and CPK may be elevated, especially in exertional heat stroke. Alkalosis may follow hyperventilation; acidosis can result from lactic acidosis or acute renal failure. Proteinuria and granular and red cell casts are seen in urine specimens collected immediately after diagnosis. If the urine is dark red or brown, it probably contains myoglobin. The BUN and serum creatinine rise transiently in most patients, and they continue to climb if renal failure develops. The hematologic findings may be normal or may be typical of disseminated intravascular coagulation (ie, low fibrinogen, increased fibrin split products, low prothrombin and partial thromboplastin times, and decreased platelet count).

Treatment

The patient must be cooled rapidly, preferably in an ice bath or with wet towels, bags of ice, and fans. Monitor the rectal temperature frequently. To avoid overshooting the end point, vigorous cooling should be stopped when the temperature reaches 38.9 C (102 F). Shivering should be controlled with parenteral phenothiazines. Oxygen should be administered, and if the Pa_{O_2} drops below 65 mm Hg, tracheal intubation should be performed to control ventilation. Fluid, electrolyte, and acid-base balance must be controlled by frequent monitoring. Fluid administration must avoid overhydration and should be based on the central venous or pulmonary artery wedge pressure, blood pressure, and urine output. On the average, about 1400 ml of fluid are required in the first 4 hours of resuscitation. Intravenous mannitol (12.5 g) may be given early if myoglobinuria is present. Renal failure may require hemodialysis. Disseminated intravascular coagulation may require treatment with heparin. Digitalis and occasionally inotropic agents (eg, isoproterenol, dopamine) may be indicated in the management of cardiac insufficiency.

Prognosis

The following are bad prognostic signs: a temperature of 42.2 C (108 F) or more, coma lasting over 2 hours, shock, hyperkalemia, and an SGOT greater than 1000 Karman units during the first 24 hours. The mortality rate is about 10% in patients who are correctly diagnosed and treated promptly. Deaths in the first few days are usually due to cerebral damage; later deaths may be from bleeding or cardiac, renal, or hepatic failure.

Clowes GHA Jr, O'Donnell TF Jr: Heat stroke. N Engl J Med 291:564, 1975.

Knochel JP: Dog days and siriasis: How to kill a football player. JAMA 233:513, 1975.

Medical Staff Conference, University of California, San Francisco: Heat stroke. West J Med 121:305, Oct 1974.

O'Donnell TF Jr: Acute heat stroke. JAMA 234:824, 1975.

Vertel RM, Knochel JP: Acute renal failure due to heat injury. Am J Med 43:435, 1967.

Wheeler M: Heat stroke in the elderly. Med Clin North Am 60:1289, 1976.

FROSTBITE

Frostbite involves freezing of tissues. Ice crystals form between the cells and grow at the expense of intracellular water. The resulting cellular dehydration coupled with ischemia due to vasoconstriction and increased blood viscosity are the mechanisms of tissue injury. Skin and muscle are considerably more susceptible to freezing damage than tendons and bones, which explains why the patient may still be able to move severely frostbitten digits.

Frostbite is caused by cold exposure, the effects of which can be magnified by moisture or wind. For example, the chilling effects on skin are the same with an air temperature of +6.7 C (+20 F) and a 40 mile-per-hour wind as with an air temperature of −40 C (−40 F) and only a 2 mile-per-hour wind. Contact with metal or gasoline in very cold weather can cause virtually instantaneous freezing; skin will often stick to metal and be lost. The risk of frostbite is increased by generalized hypothermia, which produces peripheral vasoconstriction as the organism attempts to preserve the core body temperature.

Two related injuries, **trenchfoot** and **immersion foot**, involve prolonged exposure to wet cold above freezing (eg, 10 C [50 F]). The resulting tissue damage is produced by ischemia.

Clinical Findings

Frostnip, a minor variant of this syndrome, is a transient blanching and numbness of exposed parts that may progress to frostbite if not immediately detected and treated. It often appears on the tips of fingers, ears, nose, chin, or cheeks and should be managed by rewarming through contact with warm parts of the body or warm air.

Frostbitten parts are numb, painless, and of a white or waxy appearance. With **superficial frostbite**, only the skin and subcutaneous tissues are frozen, so the tissues beneath are still compressable with pressure. **Deep frostbite** involves freezing of underlying tissues, which imparts a wooden consistency to the extremity.

After rewarming, the frostbitten area becomes mottled blue or purple and painful and tender. Blisters appear that may take several weeks to resolve. The part becomes edematous and to a varying degree painful.

Treatment

The frostbitten part should be rewarmed (thawed) in a water bath at 40–42.2 C (104–108 F) for 20–30 minutes. Thawing should not be attempted until the victim can be kept permanently warm and at rest. It is far better to continue walking on frostbitten feet even for many hours than to thaw them in a remote cold area where definitive care cannot be provided. If a thermometer is unavailable, the temperature of the water should be adjusted to be warm but not hot to a normal hand. Never use the frozen part to test the water temperature or expose it to a source of direct heat such as a fire. The risk of seriously compounding the injury is great with any method of thawing other than immersion in warm water.

After thawing has been completed, the patient should be kept recumbent and the injured part left open to the air, protected from direct contact with sheets, clothing, etc. Blisters should be left intact and the skin gently debrided by immersing the part in a whirlpool bath for about 20 minutes twice daily. No scrubbing or massaging of the injured part should be allowed, and topical ointments, antiseptics, etc are of no value. Vasodilating agents and surgical sympathectomy do not appear to improve healing.

The tissues will heal gradually, and any dead tissue will become demarcated and will usually slough spontaneously. Early in the course it is nearly impossible, even for someone with considerable experience in the treatment of frostbite, to judge the depth of injury; most early assessments tend to overestimate the extent of permanent damage. Therefore, expectant treatment is the rule and surgical debridement should be avoided even if evolution of the injury requires many months. Surgery may be indicated to release constricting circumferential eschars, but rarely should the process of spontaneous separation of gangrenous tissue be surgically facilitated. Even in severe injuries, amputation is rarely indicated before 2 months.

Concomitant fractures or dislocations create challenging and complex problems. Dislocations should be reduced immediately after thawing. Open fractures require operative reduction, but closed fractures should be managed with a posterior plastic splint. An anterior tibial compartment syndrome, which may develop in patients with associated fractures, may be diagnosed by arteriography and treated by fasciotomy.

After the eschar separates, the skin is noted to be thin, shiny, tender, and sensitive to cold; occasionally it exhibits a tendency to perspire more readily. Gradually it returns toward normal, but pain on reexposure to cold may persist indefinitely.

Prognosis

The prognosis for normal function is excellent if treatment is appropriate. Individuals who have recovered from frostbite have increased susceptibility to another frostbite injury on exposure to cold.

Ward M: Frostbite. Br Med J 1:67, 1974.
Washburn B: Frostbite. N Engl J Med 266:974, 1962.

ACCIDENTAL HYPOTHERMIA

Accidental hypothermia (in contrast with deliberate iatrogenic hypothermia used as an adjunct to anesthesia, etc) consists of the uncontrolled lowering of core body temperature below 35 C (95 F) by exposure to cold. In Britain, hypothermia largely affects elderly people living alone in inadequately heated homes. In the USA, most patients are alcoholics who have experienced excessive cold exposure during a binge. Alcohol facilitates the induction of hypothermia by producing sedation (inhibiting shivering) and cutaneous dilatation. Other sedatives, tranquilizers, and antidepressants are occasionally implicated. Diseases that predispose to hypothermia are myxedema, hypopituitarism, cerebral vascular insufficiency, mental impairment, and cardiovascular disorders.

Accidental hypothermia differs from controlled hypothermia principally by its longer duration. The heart is the organ most sensitive to cooling and is subject to ventricular fibrillation or asystole when the temperature drops to between 21–23.9 C (70–75 F). Cardiac standstill may cause death in less than 1 hour in shipwreck victims immersed in cold (< 6.7 C [< 20 F]) water. Increased capillary permeability, manifested by generalized edema and pulmonary, hepatic, and renal dysfunction, may develop as the patient is rewarmed. Disseminated intravascular coagulation is seen occasionally. Pancreatitis and acute renal failure are common in patients whose temperature on admission is below 32.2 C (90 F).

Clinical Findings

A. Symptoms and Signs: The patient is mentally depressed (somnolent, stuporous, or comatose), cold, and pale to cyanotic. The core temperature ranges from 21–35 C (70–95 F). Shivering is absent when the temperature is below 32 C (90 F). Respirations are slow and shallow. Many patients have bronchopneumonia. The blood pressure is usually normal and the heart rate slow.

B. Laboratory Findings: Dehydration may increase the concentrations of various blood constituents. The serum amylase is elevated in about half of cases, but autopsy studies show that it does not always reflect pancreatitis. Diabetic ketoacidosis becomes a management problem in some of the patients whose amylase values are elevated on entry. The SGOT, LDH, and CPK enzymes are usually elevated but are of no predictive significance. The ECG shows lengthening of the P–R interval, delay in interventricular conduction, and a pathognomonic J wave at the junction of the QRS complex and ST segment.

Treatment

For severe cases, rewarming should be performed with hyperthermic blankets or a warm 40–42 C (104–108 F) water bath at a rate of 1–2° per hour. Mild cases (body temperature 32.2–35 C [90–95 F]) may need nothing more than wool blankets (passive rewarming) for a few hours. The patient's temperature should be constantly monitored with a rectal or esophageal probe until normal body temperature has been reached.

In severe cases, endotracheal intubation should be used for better management of ventilation and protection against aspiration, a common lethal complication. Antibiotics are often indicated for coexisting pneumonitis. Fluid administration must be gauged by central venous or pulmonary artery wedge pressures, urine output, and other circulatory parameters. Increased capillary permeability following rewarming predisposes to the development of pulmonary edema. To avoid this complication, the CVP or wedge pressure should be kept below 12–14 cm water.

As rewarming proceeds, the patient should be continually reassessed for signs of other concomitant diseases which may have been masked by hypothermia. Myxedema and hypoglycemia must be sought in all patients.

Prognosis

Survival can be expected in only 50% of patients whose core temperature drops below 32.2 C (90 F). Coexisting diseases (eg, stroke, neoplasm, myocardial infarction) are common and increase the mortality rate to 75% or more. Survival does not correlate closely with the lowest absolute temperature reached. Death may result from pneumonitis, heart failure, or renal insufficiency.

Exton-Smith AN: Accidental hypothermia. Br Med J 4:727, 1973.

Maclean D & others: Acute pancreatitis and diabetic ketoacidosis in accidental hypothermia and hypothermic myxoedema. Br Med J 4:757, 1973.

Weyman AE & others: Accidental hypothermia in an alcoholic population. Am J Med 56:13, 1974.

• • •

18 . . .
Tumors of the Head & Neck

Maurice Galante, MD

Cancers of the lips, tongue, floor of the mouth, hard and soft palate, alveolar mucosa, and pharynx account for 5% of all malignant neoplasms recorded, or about 30,000 cases in the USA each year.

Death rates from cancer around the world suggest that the incidence of head and neck cancer is related to ethnic and environmental factors (Table 18–1). The cause of oral cancer is not known, but the disease is associated with exposure to various biologic, chemical, and physical agents. An association between the use of tobacco and oral cancer was suspected as long ago as the early 18th century, when cancer of the lip was noted among smokers. A report to the Surgeon General (1964) based upon retrospective studies showed a significant association of oral cancer with smoking or chewing of tobacco or the use of snuff. The mortality rate from oral cancer is 4.2 times as high in cigarette smokers as in nonsmokers. For cigar and pipe smokers (compared with nonsmokers), oral cancer has the highest mortality ratio (3.3) of all causes of death, exceeding cancer of the esophagus, pharynx, and lungs.

No virus has been isolated that will induce oral cancer in humans, but an unusual type of oral cancer (Burkitt's lymphoma), perhaps caused by a virus, occurs in a narrow zone across Central Africa. This tumor affects children as well as adults of different racial backgrounds—European, Asian, and Indian— provided they live in an area with an elevation less than 5000 feet, an annual rainfall of more than 200 inches, and a temperature that does not fall below 15.5 C (60 F). These prerequisites suggest that the tumor may be transmitted by a vector such as a mosquito, and virus-like particles have been identified in cell cultures of Burkitt's tumor. Tumors similar to Burkitt's lymphoma have been identified in various countries.

Diagnosis

Even though tumors of the head and neck and of the oral cavity are readily accessible to inspection, one frequently encounters examples that are enormous and far-advanced when first seen by a physician. Most tumors of the head and neck are relatively asymptomatic early and are therefore ignored or overlooked by the patient even when readily accessible.

The diagnosis of head and neck tumors depends on 2 steps: (1) **Careful inspection of all structures.** The proper examination of the patient requires a thorough inspection of all the recesses of the oral and nasal cavities, nasopharynx, oropharynx, and hypopharynx. This requires proper lighting and a head lamp or a head mirror. Palpation should be utilized whenever possible. All triangles of the neck should be thoroughly inspected and palpated in the search for metastases or margins of direct spread. Direct or indirect endoscopy is necessary for areas that are not readily accessible to visual inspection. Diagnostic technics include indirect laryngoscopy, direct laryngoscopy, nasopharyngoscopy, roentgenography, arteriography, and laminography.

(2) **Histologic diagnosis by biopsy.** The biopsy should always be obtained from a representative area of the tumor. Regardless of the method utilized (incisional or excisional biopsy, punch biopsy, needle biopsy), it should always provide the pathologist with enough tissue to adequately examine the lesion.

Cytologic examination is particularly helpful in detection of small lesions that are not readily seen by direct inspection and in follow-up care after treatment. In general, definitive treatment should not be started on the basis of a cytologic diagnosis alone.

Cawson RA: Premalignant lesions in the mouth. Br Med Bull 31:164, 1975.

Table 18–1. Incidence of oral cancer, 1970–1971. (Age-adjusted death rate per 100,000 population, 15 countries.)

	Males	Females
Canada	4.3	1.2
Denmark	2.3	0.8
England, Wales	3.0	1.4
France	12.0	1.0
Germany	2.0	0.6
Hong Kong	18.4	6.8
Ireland	4.2	1.8
Israel	1.1	0.8
Italy	6.0	0.9
Japan	1.6	0.6
Philippines	3.5	2.7
Portugal	4.8	1.1
Singapore	13.5	4.8
Switzerland	5.8	0.9
USA	4.7	1.5

Chandler JR & others: Clinical staging of cancer of the head and neck. Am J Surg 132:525, 1976.

El-Domeiri AA, Chandhuri P: Management of oral and pharyngeal cancer. Surg Clin North Am 55:107, 1975.

Gilbert H, Kagan AR: Recurrence patterns in squamous cell carcinoma of the oral cavity, pharynx, and larynx. J Surg Oncol 6:357, 1974.

Moore C: Cigarette smoking and cancer of the mouth, pharynx, and larynx. JAMA 218:553, 1971.

Rubin P: Cancer of the head and neck: General aspects. JAMA 215:450, 1971.

Spiro RH & others: Cervical node metastasis from epidermoid carcinoma of the oral cavity and oropharynx. Am J Surg 128:562, 1974.

TUMORS OF THE SKIN

Both benign and malignant lesions of the skin are common on the head and neck. The incidence is much higher in sunny climates (5% of all cancers in England but 50% of all cancers in Australia) and in fair-skinned individuals (seldom seen in blacks).

Benign Tumors

Senile keratosis is the most common benign skin lesion. It appears grossly as an irregular gray area covered with fine scales. It is generally considered precancerous, and malignant change occurs in 1 out of 25 lesions. When excessive amounts of keratin are produced, a cutaneous horn results.

All premalignant lesions need definitive treatment. The skin of the face and neck should be carefully examined, and all suspicious areas excised and examined histologically.

Malignant Tumors

Malignant lesions occurring on the skin of the head and neck are as follows: basal cell carcinoma, squamous cell carcinoma, adenocarcinoma (arising in sweat or sebaceous glands), melanoma, mycosis fungoides, Kaposi's disease, lymphomas, and metastatic lesions.

Basal cell and squamous cell carcinomas—the most frequent skin malignancies—occur principally in elderly individuals (60s and 70s) and infrequently in patients under 40. They may present as small nodular or superficial plaques with or without ulceration and with or without deep infiltration into underlying soft tissues and cartilage.

It is occasionally difficult to distinguish clinically between basal cell and squamous cell carcinomas. Histologic diagnosis should be established before treatment is started. Both of these lesions may become large and invade vital structures.

Preventive measures for skin cancer consist of the following: (1) Avoidance of prolonged exposure to sunlight by susceptible individuals. (2) Careful observation of the skin to facilitate early diagnosis. (3) Use of protective skin creams. (4) Excision of precancerous

lesions such as isolated keratoses. (5) Surgical planing of skin with multiple areas of involvement too numerous for individual excision.

Malignant lesions are curable if discovered early because they are accessible, grow slowly, and metastasize late. Some lesions may develop over a period of 10–20 years and present as an extensive, disfiguring, infected ulcerations. Metastases to lymph nodes from basal cell lesions are almost unknown. Particularly on the head and neck, squamous cell carcinoma of the skin metastasizes infrequently (5%).

Both radiation therapy and surgery are effective in the management of skin cancers. The selection of one method or the other depends upon the location and extent of the lesion, the feasibility of protection of vital structures (eye, middle ear, brain, cartilage, etc), previous treatment, the number of surgical procedures required for repair of the resulting defect, and patient factors such as availability for treatment and occupational hazards.

In most cases, surgical excision is preferred when it can be done simply. Primary closure of the surgical defect is more expeditious and results in a more satisfactory cosmetic effect. Larger surgical defects may require coverage with skin grafts or with flaps.

Although relatively advanced lesions can be successfully handled by radical surgery, radiation therapy, and plastic reconstructive procedures, some neglected lesions may be uncontrollable by the most radical surgery or radiation therapy.

CANCER OF THE ORAL CAVITY

The oral cavity extends from the vermilion border of the lips to and including the anterior faucial pillars which separate it from the oropharynx.

The important biologic differences between tumors of the mucosa lining the oral cavity and that lining the oropharynx are based on different degrees of cellular differentiation, tendency to infiltrate the adjacent tissues, and rate of spread to regional lymphatics.

Ninety percent of all tumors of the oral cavity are squamous cell carcinomas. They are usually better differentiated, more locally invasive, and less likely to metastasize to regional lymph nodes than malignant tumors of the oropharynx. One group of tumors—mucoepidermoid carcinomas—may be difficult to differentiate from epidermoid carcinoma because of epithelial metaplasia.

Salivary gland adenocarcinomas occur in 8% of cases and constitute the next most frequent type of tumor. Along with mucoepidermoid carcinomas, they have a tendency to grow slowly, invade locally, and metastasize late to lymph nodes.

The remaining lesions are rare tumors originating

in practically any tissue that is present in the oral cavity: muscle, blood vessels, nerves, connective tissue, etc.

Oral cancer usually occurs between the ages of 45 and 85 in individuals with associated vascular diseases, leukoplakia, heavy smoking and alcohol intake, and poor oral hygiene. Syphilis is not a significant contributing factor today.

Delay in diagnosis may be due to failure of the patient to seek medical help or to failure of the physician to appreciate the importance of early pathologic changes. The recent emphasis on oral cancer in the education of dentists has resulted in earlier detection of many lesions.

Although most lesions can be identified by their gross appearance, the diagnosis of intraoral cancer is established principally by biopsy. The physician who will provide definitive treatment should be the one who performs the biopsy so he can see the lesion before it is surgically altered. This is especially important for small lesions that could be totally removed by an excisional biopsy. Difficult problems of management may arise later if the physician responsible for definitive treatment cannot detect a residual lesion or even find the site of biopsy.

Biopsies should be obtained with a scalpel or biopsy forceps to avoid destruction or alteration of cellular detail and should be repeated if there is a suspicion of malignancy.

There is usually no need to biopsy palpable lymph nodes in the presence of a recognizable primary cancer. It may occasionally be necessary to do an aspiration biopsy of an involved cervical lymph node and, if negative, to do an excisional biopsy. Incisional biopsies should be avoided unless it is impossible to remove an intact lymph node because of its large size or infiltration into deeper structures.

Although cytology is never a substitute for an adequate biopsy, cytologic examination of exfoliated buccal cells is of great value in the early detection of cancer in the oral cavity.

Cady B: Carcinoma of the oral cavity. Surg Clin North Am 51:537, 1971.

Clinical staging system for carcinoma of the oral cavity. Cancer 18:163, 1968.

Jesse RH & others: Cancer of the oral cavity: Is elective neck dissection beneficial? Am J Surg 120:505, 1970.

Jimenez JR: Roentgen examination of the oropharynx and oral cavity. Radiol Clin North Am 8:413, 1970.

Millard J: Oral exfoliative cytology as an aid to diagnosis. J Am Dent Assoc 69:547, 1964.

Rubin P: Cancer of the head and neck. Oral cavity: Neck nodes. JAMA 217:451, 1971.

Rubin P: Head and neck cancer. Oral cavity: Primary lesion. JAMA 215:943, 1971.

Shah JP: Carcinoma of the oral cavity: Factors affecting treatment failure at the primary site and neck. Am J Surg 132:504, 1976.

Trodahl JN, Sprague WG: Benign and malignant melanocytic lesions of the oral mucosa. Cancer 25:812, 1970.

CARCINOMA OF THE LIP

Carcinoma of the vermilion border of the lip is an entity distinct from cancer of the skin and is the most frequent of all intraoral malignant cancers (20–30%). Most cancers of the lip are squamous cell carcinomas; fewer than 3% are basal cell lesions.

Cancer of the lip has the same relationship to exposure to actinic rays as cancer of the skin and is therefore more frequent in farmers, sailors, and individuals who are exposed to sunlight over long periods of time. Carcinoma of the lip is also more frequent in males than in females and occurs primarily in the sixth and seventh decades of life; although it usually occurs on the lower lip, an occasional cancer may occur on the upper lip—more often in women than in men.

Carcinoma of the lip is usually a well-differentiated lesion presenting as an infiltrating or an ulcerating or exophytic tumor. It is small initially but may eventually become quite large, involve the entire lip from commissure to commissure, and destroy the soft tissues of the chin.

Metastases occur via the lymphatics in an orderly manner to the regional lymph nodes. First the submental, then the submaxillary, and eventually the cervical lymph nodes are involved. Distant metastases occur rarely. Carcinoma of the upper lip metastasizes to the facial and submaxillary lymph nodes—occasionally to the preauricular and parotid nodes. Metastases occur in 10–25% of cases depending on the size of the primary lesion and its histologic differentiation.

Treatment

Both surgery and radiation therapy are most effective in the control of carcinoma of the lip. The choice of treatment depends on the size of the lesion, the facilities available, occupational hazards of the patient, recurrence of the lesion following previous treatment, the presence of regional metastases, the presence of underlying bone involvement, and the condition of the skin (leukoplakia, atrophy, etc).

Small lesions are ordinarily best treated by localized surgical excision—a method which is simple, expeditious, and cosmetically satisfactory. Larger lesions can be managed most effectively with radiation therapy, avoiding unneccessary wide resections and multiple plastic procedures. Recurrence of disease in scar or in previously irradiated areas or involvement of bone ordinarily precludes the use of radiation therapy.

Cervical lymphadenectomy (radical neck dissection) is effective in the control of disease that involves the lymph nodes. The slow and orderly progression of metastases in the cervical chain of lymph nodes and their accessibility to frequent examination and evaluation make it possible to withhold surgery until the lymph nodes become clinically palpable (therapeutic neck dissection). Most patients who develop palpable nodes do so within 2 years after discovery of the primary tumor. Whereas 25% are found to have microscopically involved lymph nodes when the adenectomy is elective, tumor is found in 85% of patients undergoing therapeutic neck dissection.

Prognosis

The prognosis depends on the size of the tumor, the location of the lesion, the degree of differentiation, and the presence or absence of metastatic disease. Surgery and radiation therapy are about equally effective for comparable "curable" lesions.

The reported 5-year survival rates for cancer of the lip treated by surgery or by radiation therapy vary between 85 and 95% for lesions up to 2 cm in size. The cure rates are lower for larger lesions. The presence of metastases to the regional lymph nodes reduces the cure rate by 50% regardless of whether the neck dissection is elective or therapeutic.

Brown RG & others: Advanced and recurrent squamous carcinoma of the lower lip. Am J Surg 132:492, 1976.

Wurman LH & others: Carcinoma of the lip. Am J Surg 130:470, 1975.

CARCINOMA OF THE BUCCAL MUCOSA

The buccal mucosa lines the inner side of the cheek from the anterior commissure of the lip to the ascending ramus of the mandible and from the upper to the lower gingiva. This epithelium gives rise to carcinomas that are usually well differentiated and locally infiltrating. Larger lesions may extend from the superior to the inferior gingivobuccal sulci and gingivae, anteriorly to the commissure, and posteriorly to the "retromolar trigone"; they may infiltrate deeply through the buccinator muscle and be confused with tumors arising primarily in these regions.

Carcinoma of the buccal mucosa rarely metastasizes to the regional lymph nodes. When metastases do occur they do so in the form of isolated involvement of one or 2 lymph nodes (superficial facial, submaxillary, upper cervical nodes).

Treatment

Smaller lesions, particularly those surrounded by leukoplakia, can be excised surgically and closed primarily. Larger excisions require coverage of the resulting defect with skin grafts. Deeply infiltrating lesions may require excision of full thickness of cheek and repair of the resulting defect with mobilization of flaps previously prepared for that purpose.

Radiation therapy has been found to be as effective as surgery in the management of carcinoma of the buccal mucosa. It appears, however, that for highly differentiated tumors surgical extirpation is the treatment of choice.

Metastases to the cervical lymph nodes are best managed surgically.

The reported 5-year survival rates for both methods of treatment vary from 50–68%. Histologic

involvement of the lymph nodes reduces the prospect of curability by about two-thirds.

Krishnamurthi S & others: Combined therapy in buccal mucosal cancers. Radiology 99:409, 1971.

Skolnik EM & others: Carcinoma of the buccal mucosa and retromolar area. Otolaryngol Clin North Am 5:327, 1972.

CANCER OF THE ORAL TONGUE

For purposes of discussion the tongue should be considered as composed of an oral portion (mobile anterior two-thirds) and a pharyngeal portion (posterior third). The circumvallate papillae constitute the line of demarcation between the 2 segments.

Carcinoma of the oral tongue occurs from the fourth to the eighth decades of life, usually in males, in association with heavy smoking and alcohol intake and poor oral hygiene. The lesion is usually well differentiated and frequently arises along the lateral margin, although it may also occur on the tip, the dorsum, or the undersurface. Multiple primary carcinomas of the tongue are uncommon (3%). The lesion may progress in any direction and extend into the floor of the mouth to involve laterally the dental alveoli or posteriorly the anterior tonsillar pillar. Some lesions may be so large that it is impossible to determine the primary site of origin.

Metastases to the regional lymph nodes are frequent and may first appear on the contralateral side. At the time of initial diagnosis, 40–45% of patients have palpable lymph nodes. Another 20% will develop metastases to the cervical lymph nodes within a short time after control of the primary lesion.

Treatment

The location and size of the lesion, the condition of the adjacent tissues, the availability of treatment, and the general health of the patient determine the selection of treatment. In general, surgery and radiation therapy appear to be equally effective. However, radiation therapy has the advantage of permitting preservation of tissue, which results in better function than after resection.

Surgical excision is the treatment of choice for small lesions, particularly those located at the tip of the tongue, because it is expeditious, effective, and produces negligible impairment of function.

Interstitial implantation of radium needles is indicated for lesions of moderate or larger size. This is a major surgical procedure requiring a general anesthetic, hospitalization, specialized training in the manipulation of radium needles, and expert nursing care for several days. The procedure may cause great discomfort, and its use in debilitated patients requires careful consideration.

If their location permits, smaller lesions can be treated by means of peroral irradiation.

In selecting the initial mode of treatment for the primary lesion, one should appreciate that surgery can still be utilized if radiation fails. Many experienced clinicians advocate prophylactic cervical lymphadenectomy because the lymph nodes are involved in 40–45% of cases before the disease is clinically apparent.

Prognosis

The rate of local control of the tumor depends on its location and size. Whereas the 5-year survival rate for lesions of the tip of the tongue is 75–80%, it decreases to 55% for those at the lateral margins and to 40% for those on the dorsum. The 5-year survival rate is 78% for patients without metastases but drops to 14% for those with involved lymph nodes.

Ange DW & others: Management of squamous cell carcinoma of the oral tongue and floor of mouth after excisional biopsy. Radiology 116:143, 1975.

Fu KK & others: External and interstitial radiation therapy of carcinoma of the oral tongue. Am J Roentgenol Radium Ther Nucl Med 126:107, 1976.

Gilbert EH & others: Carcinoma of the oral tongue and floor of mouth: Fifteen years' experience with linear acceleratory therapy. Cancer 35:1517, 1975.

Spiro RH, Strong EW: Surgical treatment of cancer of the tongue. Surg Clin North Am 54:759, 1974.

CARCINOMA OF THE FLOOR OF THE MOUTH

The anterior and the 2 lateral gingivolingual sulci constitute the floor of the mouth. They are continuous posteriorly with the glossopharyngeal sulci and the piriform sinuses. The mucosa of the floor of the mouth has important anatomic relationships to the underlying musculature, the submaxillary gland, the lingual nerve, and the lingual artery.

Carcinoma of the floor of the mouth constitutes 15–20% of all intraoral malignant lesions. The tumor is usually a squamous cell carcinoma which is usually less well differentiated than tumors occurring on the oral tongue. It may extend medially to involve the undersurface of the tongue, laterally to involve the gingivae, the underlying periosteum, or the mandible itself to produce bone destruction. Inferior extension may involve the submaxillary duct, the lingual nerve, and the lingual artery, or the tumor may spread between muscle planes.

Most of these cancers arise in the anterior floor of the mouth. Invasion of lymphatics occurs early; 50–60% of patients have palpable lymph nodes at first examination. In some series, lymph node involvement has been reported in 90% of patients within 12 months after diagnosis. Metastases occur to the submaxillary, subdigastric, and upper deep cervical lymph nodes. Metastases to the contralateral side occur in 10–15% of cases.

Treatment

The propensity for carcinoma of the floor of the mouth to extend to the tongue and gingivae and to infiltrate deeply into the musculature of the submental and submaxillary regions makes most of these lesions unsuitable for local surgical or radiotherapeutic management as the primary treatment method.

The selection of treatment depends to a great extent on the size of the lesion and the presence or absence of involvement of the adjacent structures. Occasionally, a small lesion can be controlled by wide local excision or by peroral roentgen therapy or interstitial irradiation. Larger lesions may require either (1) wide excision in continuity or (2) external irradiation over the entire floor of the mouth and adjacent regional lymphatics, followed by a radical neck dissection. Extensive lesions of the floor of the mouth have been successfully treated using preoperative irradiation followed by radical surgery through tissues whose margins have been sterilized of tumor.

The treatment of choice of involved lymph nodes is therapeutic radical neck dissection.

Prognosis

Five-year survival rates between 40–75% have been reported, depending upon the size of the lesion and the presence or absence of cervical lymphadenopathy at the time of primary treatment.

Campos JL & others: Radiotherapy of carcinoma of the floor of the mouth. Radiology 99:677, 1971.

Fayos JV: Management of squamous cell carcinoma of the floor of the mouth. Am J Surg 123:706, 1972.

Flynn MB, Mullins FX, Moore C: Selection of treatment in squamous carcinoma of the floor of the mouth. Am J Surg 126:477, 1973.

CANCER OF THE SOFT PALATE & ANTERIOR FAUCIAL PILLARS

The most frequent malignant tumors arising in these structures are squamous cell carcinomas. They are usually well-differentiated tumors with various degrees of local infiltration of the underlying musculature. They remain localized for a long time and metastasize late to regional lymph nodes. The presence of extensive adenopathy renders the prognosis grave.

The long period of localization of these tumors renders them amenable to wide surgical excision. Radiation therapy is frequently utilized as definitive treatment for superficial lesions or as preoperative treatment for those too extensive to be treated by surgery or radiation therapy alone. Planned preoperative irradiation of an extensive tumor may reduce its size significantly and permit its resection through margins sterilized of tumor cells.

Adenocarcinomas of salivary gland origin may occasionally arise in the soft palate. They are locally invasive and are best treated by surgical resection.

Lindberg RD & others: Evolution of the clinically negative neck in patients with squamous cell carcinoma of the faucial arch. Am J Roentgenol Radium Ther Nucl Med 111:60, 1971.

CARCINOMA OF THE "RETROMOLAR TRIGONE"

Lesions originating in the mucosa behind the last molar teeth constitute a special class of tumors presenting serious problems of management. Epidermoid carcinoma arising in this site is particularly radioresistant. It has a tendency to involve bone early, to infiltrate adjacent musculature, and to travel along nerve structures such as the mandibular and the lingual nerves. It may extend early along the pterygoid plate to the base of the skull. All of these features frequently make primary surgery of these tumors a futile effort. During the past 10 years, these tumors have been managed by intensive preoperative irradiation followed by radical surgical resection.

Skolnik EM & others: Carcinoma of the buccal mucosa and retromolar area. Otolaryngol Clin North Am 5:327, 1972.

CARCINOMA OF THE LOWER GINGIVAE

It is important to distinguish between carcinoma of the gingivae and cancer of the jaw. The first is an epidermoid carcinoma arising in the epithelium covering the alveolus, whereas the latter signifies bone tumor arising in the mandible.

Epidermoid carcinoma of the mucosa of the lower gingivae is usually well differentiated and infiltrates underlying bone early and frequently (40–50%). It may first become apparent as a small ulceration adjacent to a tooth that was extracted after failure to recognize the true cause of local symptoms. The open socket then constitutes an avenue for invasion of bone by the cancer. The tumor may extend laterally to involve the buccal mucosa or medially to involve the floor of the mouth.

Metastases to the regional lymph nodes occur frequently (35–40% of cases). Extensive tumors involving the floor of the mouth to the midline may metastasize to the contralateral side.

Small superficial verrucous lesions of the gingivae can be controlled with radiation therapy.

Resection of the primary lesion (mandibulectomy) in continuity with radical lymphadenectomy is the treatment of choice for moderate-sized lesions of the alveolus with or without palpable lymph nodes.

For more extensive lesions, planned preoperative irradiation followed by combined resection yields the best results.

The overall 5-year survival rate is 35–45%.

CARCINOMA OF THE UPPER GINGIVAE & HARD PALATE

Cancers arising in the mucosa of the upper gingivae and the hard palate are usually well-differentiated epidermoid carcinomas which metastasize late. They frequently are confused with cancers that arise in the antrum and spread inferiorly. X-rays are necessary to distinguish between the 2 entities. Bone involvement may be extensive. The rare metastases are found in retropharyngeal, submaxillary, or subdigastric lymph nodes.

Wide surgical resection of the involved tissues is the treatment of choice. The resulting extensive surgical defects can be easily covered by prosthetic appliances. Five-year survival rates are about 60%.

CANCER OF THE OROPHARYNX

The oropharynx extends from the soft palate to the level of the hyoid bone and is delineated anteriorly by the lingual circumvallate papillae and the anterior faucial pillars. Epidermoid carcinomas, lymphoepitheliomas, and lymphosarcomas are the most common malignancies found in this region.

The epidermoid tumors are poorly differentiated, bulky lesions which metastasize early to both sides of the neck. They tend to be noninvasive but produce local symptoms by compression. Surgery is unsuccessful, but both primary and metastatic tumors usually respond to radiotherapy. Death often results from distant metastases.

Al-Saleem T & others: Malignant lymphomas of the pharynx. Cancer 26:1383, 1970.
Banfi A & others: Malignant lymphomas of Waldeyer's ring. Br Med J 3:140, 1972.
Jesse RH, Sugarbaker EV: Squamous cell carcinoma of the oropharynx: Why we fail. Am J Surg 132:435, 1976.
Rubin P: Cancer of the head and neck: Oropharynx. JAMA 217:940, 1973.
Silva N: Pattern of lymphatic spread in pharyngeal cancer. J Surg Oncol 3:415, 1971.
Weller SA & others: Carcinoma of the oropharynx. Am J Roentgenol Radium Ther Nucl Med 126:236, 1976.

CANCER OF THE BASE OF THE TONGUE
(Pharyngeal or Posterior Third)

The pharyngeal tongue originates from a different anlage than the anterior two-thirds and is covered by a squamous epithelium that is less well differentiated. The base of the tongue is infiltrated with lymphoid tissue and has abundant lymphatics that drain directly to the subdigastric lymph nodes. Because they are initially silent, tumors of the base of the tongue are usually detected late, after extensive infiltration has occurred into the deep musculature. The extent of infiltration is difficult to delineate clinically, and examination under general anesthesia is occasionally necessary to judge the size of the lesion and the extent of local spread. Pain, dysphagia, and voice changes may occur but are often preceded by unilateral or bilateral cervical lymphadenopathy. Lymph node involvement ranges from 40—90% depending on the stage of the lesion.

The treatment of choice for carcinoma of the pharyngeal tongue is external radiation to the primary lesion and to the cervical lymph nodes on both sides. Curative surgical excision would necessitate such an extensive resection that swallowing would be impossible without aspiration. The location of the primary tumor makes the use of interstitial radium needles very difficult.

The overall 5-year survival for treated carcinoma of the pharyngeal tongue is about 10%.

Spanos WJ Jr & others: Time, dose, and tumor volume relationships in irradiation of squamous cell carcinomas of the base of the tongue. Cancer 37:2591, 1976.

CARCINOMA OF THE VALLECULA

Lesions originating in the vallecula are often difficult to detect by inspection. Palpation and a lateral soft tissue x-ray film of the area may be necessary to establish the diagnosis. The characteristic roentgenographic finding is a pocket of air in the musculature of the tongue.

Lesions of this area are usually superficial rather than deeply infiltrating, and they spread in all directions to involve the pharyngeal wall and the tongue. They metastasize early to the cervical lymph nodes. The primary mode of treatment is external radiation therapy.

CARCINOMA OF THE TONSIL

Malignancies of the tonsil are often mistaken for inflammatory lesions until incontrovertible proof of tumor slowly appears. Both the anterior and posterior faucial pillars may be involved, and the tumor may spread into the soft palate and the uvula. Inferiorly, the tumor may extend into the glossopharyngeal sulcus and into the base of the tongue. Trismus may result from invasion of the pterygoid muscles. The tumor may spread to the base of the skull along nerve channels.

Histologically, malignant tumors of the tonsil are poorly differentiated epidermoid carcinomas (75%), lymphosarcomas (15%), and lymphoepitheliomas (10%).

It is most important to separate malignant lesions arising in the tonsil and tonsillar bed from those arising in the anterior tonsillar pillar since the 2 have entirely different biologic characteristics. This differentiation is not always possible because of the tendency of tonsillar carcinomas to spread widely into adjacent structures in all directions. In cancer of the tonsil, massive involvement of the ipsilateral lymph nodes is often the first clinical manifestation of the disease. Three-fourths of patients have palpable lymph nodes at the time of first examination. Distant metastases to bone, lungs, and liver occur frequently, particularly with lymphoepitheliomas.

Metastatic disease is occasionally found in a cervical lymph node even when the most meticulous examination has failed to detect a primary lesion. Histologic survey of a previously removed tonsil may reveal a small "occult" carcinoma.

Radiation therapy is the treatment of choice both for the primary lesions and the cervical metastases. Supervoltage external irradiation is given to large areas which include the primary and the neck to the level of the clavicle. Combined preoperative irradiation and surgery may be utilized in exceptional cases, but the exact place of this method of treatment is still under evaluation. Combined resection and radiation is better reserved for residual or recurrent disease.

Survival following treatment varies according to the extent of the primary lesion and the presence and extent of metastatic disease in the neck. Reported 5-year survival rates are 62% for patients without cervical adenopathy and 26% for patients with cervical adenopathy. The overall survival rate varies between 30—35%.

Fleming PM & others: Carcinoma of the tonsil. Surg Clin North Am 56:125, 1976.
Perez CA & others: Nonrandomized comparison of preoperative irradiation and surgery versus irradiation alone in the management of carcinoma of the tonsil. Am J Roentgenol Radium Ther Nucl Med 126:248, 1976.

CARCINOMA OF THE OROPHARYNGEAL WALLS

Lesions arising in the walls of the oropharynx are usually poorly differentiated carcinomas presenting a central ulceration surrounded by wide infiltration of the adjacent walls. They arise in the lateral or the posterior pharyngeal walls and have a tendency to metastasize early to the regional lymph nodes. They may extend to the nasopharynx superiorly or the hypopharynx inferiorly. Lesions arising in the lateral pharyngeal wall frequently extend to the epiglottis and piriform fossa and may exhibit an almost continuous induration with the involved midcervical lymph nodes. The deep prespinal fascia is rarely involved and is penetrated only late in the disease. Tumor may involve the ninth cranial nerve and extend to the base of the skull.

Exophytic lesions of the pharyngeal wall that are noninfiltrative and present discrete borders can be treated either by radiation therapy or by surgery if laryngectomy is not necessary for complete eradication of the tumor.

Infiltrating lesions are best treated by radiation therapy, which has the advantage of sparing the larynx. This is particularly true in patients with bilateral involvement of the cervical lymph nodes.

Larger lesions with wide involvement of the adjacent structures are treated surgically by means of laryngopharyngectomy and neck dissection, unilateral or bilateral as indicated.

No end results from large series have been reported. A 5-year survival rate of 32% has been reported in one series of 48 patients.

Wilkins SA: Carcinoma of the posterior pharyngeal wall. Am J Surg 122:477, 1972.

CANCER OF THE EPIGLOTTIS

Malignant lesions of the epiglottis are usually ulcerating or bulky tumors that may completely destroy the epiglottis. The lesions are usually well-differentiated epidermoid carcinomas and have a tendency to metastasize late.

Treatment of the primary lesion is usually by radiation therapy. Metastatic lymph nodes are treated by radical neck dissection.

.   .   .

TUMORS OF THE NASOPHARYNX

The nasopharynx has been called a "blind spot" because tumors occurring in this area usually are diagnosed late and in an advanced stage. There is usually a delay of 8–10 months from the onset of signs to the time when the diagnosis is established. The initial signs and symptoms may vary depending on involvement by tumor of one or more of the following: cranial nerves III–VII and IX–XII, the mandibular and the auriculo-temporal nerves, the levator muscle of the soft palate, the pterygoid muscles, the foramen lacerum and the carotid canal, and the eustachian tubes. No other tumor of the head and neck can present with such a variety of symptoms: nasal (obstruction), aural (hypoacusia, deafness, earache, tinnitus, pain, and headache), ocular (proptosis, diplopia, even blindness), neurologic (diplopia, facial paresthesias, Horner's syndrome), and olfactory.

Cervical adenopathy is the presenting symptom in over one-third of cases, and well over three-fourths may have lymphadenopathy at the time of the initial examination. The nasopharyngeal mucosa and submucosa are richly supplied by lymphatics which drain into the jugulodigastric chain (70%) and the upper deep cervical lymph nodes (65%). Lymph nodes in the spinal accessory and inferior cervical areas may also be involved. Lymphadenopathy—particularly if bilateral—in the absence of an obvious primary tumor should direct the search to the nasopharynx.

Epidermoid carcinoma, transitional cell carcinoma, and lymphoepithelioma are the most common nasopharyngeal tumors. Lymphosarcoma, adenocarcinoma, plasmacytoma, miscellaneous sarcomas, malignant melanomas, and other types also occur. Although the principal route of metastasis is via the lymphatics to the lymph nodes, regional or even distant hematogenous spread may occur with lymphomas and lymphoepitheliomas.

Treatment

The nasopharynx is surgically inaccessible except for biopsy, and the distribution of cervical metastases makes effective neck dissection impossible. Fortunately, these tumors are radiosensitive; treatment of the primary and its metastases consists of radiation. The entire nasopharynx is treated with fields that cover all possible areas of extension and the 2 sides of the neck down to the level of the clavicles.

Complications of treatment may include dry mouth, pharyngitis, epidermatitis, and bone necrosis. A dread but infrequent complication is myelitis of the cervical spinal cord, which can occasionally result in death.

Curability depends on the stage of the lesion and the extent of tumor at the time of treatment. The overall 5-year survival in major centers in the USA is 30–35%. Lymphosarcomas have the best survival rate. Bilateral involvement of the cervical lymph nodes and of bone or nerves makes the prognosis poor. Local reappearance of the tumor may occur several years after the initial treatment and can sometimes be controlled with intracavitary radiation.

Fu KK & others: Treatment of locally recurrent carcinoma of the nasopharynx. Radiology 117:425, 1975.
Hoppe RT & others: Carcinoma of the nasopharynx. Cancer 37:2605, 1976.

CANCER OF THE HYPOPHARYNX*

The hypopharynx is directly behind the larynx and is composed of the piriform sinuses, the aryepi-

*Carcinoma of the larynx is discussed in Chapter 41.

glottic folds, the lateral and posterior pharyngeal walls, and the postcricoid mucosa.

Malignant lesions of the hypopharynx comprise approximately 4% of all malignant oropharyngeal tumors in man. Cancer of the hypopharynx is more frequent in men than in women but shows a peculiar geographic distribution in that it is more frequent in Scandinavian women in association with the Plummer-Vinson syndrome.

Unlike carcinomas occurring in the oral cavity, tumors of the hypopharynx have a tendency to be highly undifferentiated. Metastases occur to the regional lymph nodes along lymphatics that exit between the hyoid bone and the upper edge of the thyroid cartilage to the upper deep cervical lymph nodes.

Lesions arising in the hypopharynx are ordinarily silent in the early stages and may reach considerable size before they cause symptoms. Cervical adenopathy is occasionally the first clinical manifestation of the disease. Disturbances of the swallowing mechanism usually precede impairment of respiration or speech, the latter being symptoms of advanced lesions.

Malignant lesions of the hypopharynx can be divided into 2 groups: (1) carcinomas arising in the aryepiglottic folds and the upper lateral and posterior hypopharynx (prognostically more favorable); and (2) lesions which arise in the piriform sinus, the post-cricoid and postarytenoid areas, and the lower reaches of the hypopharynx (prognosis is poor).

Attempts to control lesions arising in the hypopharynx by surgery or radiation therapy usually meet with little success. Survival rates have greatly improved since the advent of radical surgery, whereby laryngectomy, hypopharyngectomy, and radical neck dissection are performed in continuity at one stage. When these tumors are treated by radiation, surgery can be performed later in the event of radiation failure.

As for other lesions arising in the upper respiratory and digestive tracts, the combination of preoperative irradiation and surgery offers considerable promise for some of these lesions, but its exact value is yet to be established.

Futrell JW & others: Predicting survival in cancer of the larynx or hypopharynx. Am J Surg 122:451, 1971.

Jing B-S: Roentgen examination of the larynx and hypopharynx. Radiol Clin North Am 8:361, 1970.

Ogura JH & others: Elective neck dissection for pharyngeal and laryngeal cancers. Ann Otol Rhinol Laryngol 80:646, 1971.

Rubin P: Cancer of the head and neck. 1. Hypopharynx and larynx. JAMA 221:68, 1972.

Shah JP & others: Carcinoma of the hypopharynx. Am J Surg 132:439, 1976.

CANCER OF THE NASAL FOSSA

Although cancers of the nasal fossa represent only 1% or less of tumors of the head and neck, the mortal-

ity and morbidity they can produce is great. They present individual problems according to the areas in which they arise.

Primary tumors arising in the nasal fossa must be distinguished from those arising in adjacent sinuses, the nasopharynx, the oral cavity, and the skin and those extending into the nasal fossa because of uncontrolled growth.

According to the stage of the lesion, the symptoms vary from abnormal nasal discharge to bleeding, obstruction, and eventually pain.

Most are squamous cell tumors which are either bulky, obstructive, and exophytic tumors or deeply infiltrating and painful. Other types of tumors are lymphosarcomas, malignant melanomas, olfactory neuroblastomas (esthesioneuroepitheliomas) arising in the olfactory mucosa, plasmacytomas, sarcomas, and adenocarcinomas of salivary gland origin.

Malignant lesions of the nasal fossa chiefly present problems of local invasion, although they do sometimes metastasize to the regional lymph nodes and occasionally to distant sites via the blood stream.

Epidermoid carcinomas and lymphosarcomas of the nasal fossa are usually managed with radiation therapy, which is more successful here than for tumors arising in the paranasal sinuses or those invading the nasal fossa.

Radical surgery is the treatment of choice for mucous or salivary gland adenocarcinomas and malignant melanomas of the nasal cavity.

Considerable palliation can frequently be achieved with radiation therapy for nonresectable tumors.

Boone MLM & others: Malignant disease of the paranasal sinuses and nasal cavity: Importance of precise localization of extent of disease. Am J Roentgenol Radium Ther Nucl Med 102:627, 1968.

Jesse RH: Preoperative versus postoperative radiation in treatment of squamous carcinoma of the paranasal sinuses. Am J Surg 110:552, 1965.

Paulus DD Jr, Dodd GD: The roentgen diagnosis of tumors of the nasal cavity and accessory paranasal sinuses. Radiol Clin North Am 8:343, 1970.

CANCER OF THE PARANASAL SINUSES

Tumors of the paranasal sinuses are more frequent in men than in women and constitute less than 1% of all head and neck tumors.

Histologically, most of these tumors are of the epidermoid squamous cell type. However, other types of tumors such as transitional cell carcinoma, lymphoepithelioma, adenocarcinoma, and lymphosarcoma may occur. These tumors spread by local invasion to adjacent areas and metastasize to the cervical lymph nodes and eventually to distant sites.

Most of these tumors arise in the maxillary sinus; an occasional tumor arises in the ethmoid sinus.

Tumors arising in the frontal and sphenoid sinuses are extremely rare.

The symptoms of pain, nasal obstruction, and nasal discharge occur only when the tumor is relatively locally advanced and has destroyed surrounding structures. Radiologic findings usually are not conclusive until bone destruction has taken place. Early diagnosis is important since death is usually due to local growth. Often the patient has been treated for a long time with antibiotics for sinusitis while the underlying cause of symptoms is carcinoma.

Local spread causes the following symptoms: (1) Anterior extension: bone erosion and swelling. (2) Posterolateral extension into the infratemporal fossa: trismus and swelling. (3) Posterior extension into the pterygopalatine fossa: erosion of the base of the skull. (4) Medial extension into the ethmoid sinuses superiorly and into the nasal fossa medially: obstruction and bleeding. (5) Direct extension superiorly: erosion of the floor of the orbit, resulting in ocular signs. (6) Inferior extension: may involve the upper canines and molars, producing toothache, loosening of the teeth, and eventual protrusion into the gingivobuccal sulcus.

Treatment

Surgical excision is the major treatment for carcinoma of the maxillary sinuses, but it is utilized primarily for well-differentiated squamous cell carcinomas and adenocarcinomas. Radiation therapy rarely controls these tumors and is usually utilized only for palliation. The trend in recent years has been to treat patients with maxillary sinus carcinoma by radical surgery after preoperative irradiation.

Orbital exenteration is sometimes necessary when tumors arising in the superior portion of the maxillary sinus invade the floor of the orbit.

Because these tumors metastasize late, prophylactic neck dissection is not indicated. However, therapeutic neck dissections are indicated for clinically involved lymph nodes. Radiation therapy to the cervical region is used only for palliation.

The role of radiation therapy in palliation cannot be underestimated in a disease where a significant number of patients die of uncontrollable local tumor. It is most effective in controlling pain, discharge, proptosis, bleeding, etc. Preservation of the eye by protection of the cornea is feasible when management is by palliative radiation therapy.

Prognosis

Preoperative irradiation and radical surgery yields 5-year survivals of about 40–45%.

Boone MLM & others: Malignant disease of the paranasal sinuses and nasal cavity: Importance of precise localization of extent of disease. Am J Roentgenol Radium Ther Nucl Med 102:627, 1968.

Jesse RH: Preoperative versus postoperative radiation in treatment of squamous carcinoma of the paranasal sinuses. Am J Surg 110:552, 1965.

Kurohara SS & others: Role of radiation therapy and of surgery in the management of localized epidermoid carcinoma of the maxillary sinus. Am J Roentgenol Radium Ther Nucl Med 114:35, 1972.

Paulus DD Jr, Dodd GD: The roentgen diagnosis of tumors of the nasal cavity and accessory paranasal sinuses. Radiol Clin North Am 8:343, 1970.

CANCER OF THE SALIVARY GLANDS

Salivary gland tissue is both ectodermal and entodermal in origin and is divided into 2 groups: (1) major salivary glands (parotid, submaxillary, sublingual) and (2) minor salivary glands (small deposits of salivary tissue scattered throughout the mucosa of the oral cavity, maxilla, and nasopharynx). About 80% of tumors occurring in major salivary glands are found in the parotid. Considering all salivary gland tumors, the parotid is the site of 50%.

The mixed tumor is a benign lesion that has the potentiality of malignant transformation even after many years.

Benign tumors may become large without invasion of the adjacent areas. Malignant tumors grow by local invasion of facial muscles, facial nerve, mandible, pterygoid muscles, or the base of the skull. They may enter the skull along the facial nerve or the mandibular branch of the trigeminal nerve.

Parotid carcinomas, especially epidermoid and mucoepidermoid lesions, tend to metastasize to the cervical lymph nodes. Hematogenous metastases may occur, particularly to lungs and bones. Peculiar cases have been reported where lung metastases progress slowly for 10–20 years.

MAJOR SALIVARY GLANDS

Classification

A. Parotid Gland: The parotid gland is the largest of the 3 major salivary glands. It is bounded by the masseter muscle, the ascending ramus of the mandible, and the pterygoid muscles. Inferiorly, the parotid may extend along the posterior belly of the digastric muscle. The gland is divided into 2 major portions, a superficial and a deep lobe joined by a bridge of tissue called the isthmus. The structure most closely related to the parotid gland is the facial nerve. In its course between the 2 lobes, it subdivides into 2 trunks, the zygomaticofacial and the cervicofacial. These in turn subdivide at the periphery of the gland into branches that supply the temporal, zygomatic, buccal, maxillary, and mandibular areas. The plane in which the main trunks of the facial nerve lie is not always easy to identify, and dissection of the nerve may be difficult.

The main lymphatics of the parotid gland drain first into the deep and superficial parotid lymph nodes and then into the superficial posterior cervical chain. The deep parotid lymph nodes drain to the subparotid node located below the angle of the mandible and ultimately into lymph nodes along the spinal accessory nerve or the deep jugular chain.

B. Submaxillary Gland: The submaxillary gland is located in the submaxillary triangle between the anterior and posterior bellies of the digastric muscle. The submaxillary duct lies close to the lingual and hypoglossal nerves, and tumor may spread along perineural spaces into the cranial cavity. The marginal mandibular nerve also lies close to the submaxillary gland and must be avoided during resection of the gland.

C. Sublingual Gland: This smallest of the 3 major salivary glands is located in the floor of the mouth beneath the deep buccal mucosa. It is rarely the site of a malignant process.

Types of Tumors

A. Mixed Tumors: "Mixed tumors," the most frequent neoplasm of salivary glands, comprise 85% of benign parotid tumors. The epithelial cells may be spindle-shaped or stellate and arranged in sheets or in glandular patterns. The stroma may be myxoid, hyalinized, and even cartilaginous. Areas of necrosis can often be observed. Metaplasia of the epithelium into well-differentiated squamous cells occasionally occurs. The distinction between histologically benign and malignant tumors is often difficult, in which case the diagnosis can only be established by the clinical course.

B. Mucoepidermoid Carcinoma: The division of these tumors into low-grade and high-grade malignancy depends on the relative amounts of mucoid material secreted by the ductal cells and on the squamous cell component, which predominates in the more highly malignant lesions.

C. Squamous Cell or Epidermoid Carcinoma: These tumors evolve from squamous metaplasia of the ductal epithelium. Occasionally, the diagnostic dilemma arises of distinguishing a primary epidermoid carcinoma of the parotid gland from metastatic squamous cell carcinoma to an intraparotid lymph node.

D. Papillary Cystadenoma Lymphomatosum (Warthin's Tumor): This is the second most common benign tumor and is found only in the parotid. It is composed of proliferating salivary gland cells in lymphoid tissue and grossly appears as cysts with multiple papillary projections from the wall within the parotid gland. It is often multicentric and tends to recur postoperatively. It is 9 times more common in men than in women, is bilateral in 10% of cases, and is uncommon in blacks. This tumor may be identified preoperatively by ^{99m}Tc since it is the only parotid lesion that concentrates this isotope. On clinical examination, the mass may seem to be separate from the parotid, in which case it may not be recognized as a parotid tumor.

E. Adenocarcinoma:

1. Adenoid cystic carcinoma (cylindroma)—This tumor consists of small nests or strands of epithelial cells with relatively large nuclei and poorly defined cytoplasm. Mucicarmine stains are usually positive, and hyalin is often present.

2. Acinic cell carcinoma—This uncommon tumor resembles the acinic cells of the parotid gland. The cells are usually polygonal, with large eccentric nuclei, arranged in alveolar groups. They may metastasize to local lymph nodes and distant sites.

3. Miscellaneous adenocarcinomas varying according to the histologic pattern of the tumor—A small group of malignant lesions have been classified as trabecular, anaplastic, mucus carcinomas, etc. They are highly malignant tumors with great propensity for local and distant metastases.

F. Oxyphil Adenoma (Oncocytoma): These lesions are composed of pleomorphic eosinophilic cells, arranged in small groups separated by thin fibrovascular septa.

G. Benign Lymphoepithelial Tumors (Godwin's Tumor): These tumors consist essentially of an enlargement of the parotid gland containing a mixture of inflammatory cells such as plasma cells and lymphocytes containing scattered reticulum cells. Islands of epithelial cells are found with zones of hyalinization.

Clinical Findings

The diagnosis of parotid tumors depends on the ability to differentiate inflammatory lesions from primary and metastatic neoplasms. Viral or bacterial parotitis and sialolithiasis are characterized by recurrent fever, pain, tenderness, and other symptoms which are not present with malignant lesions. Unless nerve structures are invaded, malignant lesions are asymptomatic.

The possibility of metastatic spread to the parotid lymph nodes from primary tumors located elsewhere in the head and neck should always be recognized.

The definitive diagnosis is established by histologic examination of the specimen. Needle or incisional biopsies must be performed with the utmost care to avoid seeding of malignant cells and eventual local recurrence. Biopsies should be planned so as not to interfere with the definitive cancer operation.

Treatment

Treatment of benign or malignant salivary gland tumors is surgical. Enucleation, particularly with mixed tumors, leads to a high rate of local recurrence.

A. Surgical Treatment: The entire parotid gland is exposed, the superficial lobe elevated, the facial nerve dissected, and the lobe excised en bloc with the intraglandular and paraglandular lymphatics and lymph nodes.

Occasionally, a tumor may be located deeply within the deep lobe and appear in the tonsillar fossa. In such cases it is always possible to preserve the facial nerve while removing the deeply located tumor. The facial nerve should never be sacrificed unless it is directly involved with malignant tissue.

Radical cervical lymphadenectomy is indicated

whenever a malignant tumor of the parotid gland is accompanied by enlarged cervical lymph nodes. The yield of positive lymph nodes with prophylactic neck dissection is low, so that one may defer this operation until nodes become palpable.

B. Radiotherapy: Radiotherapy is indicated (1) when the primary tumor is not resectable, (2) for recurrent tumors not amenable to surgical extirpation, (3) when tumor is present at the surgical margins, and (4) for control of residual tumor in the surgical bed.

Complications of Surgery

The most frequent complications following surgery of the parotid gland are those resulting from temporary or permanent injury to the facial nerve and a peculiar set of symptoms grouped under the name of auriculotemporal nerve syndrome (Frey's syndrome).

Dysfunction of facial muscles may occur following extensive manipulation of the facial nerve even when the latter is not sectioned and may last from a few weeks to a few months. Function can be satisfactorily restored after accidental section of the facial nerve by immediate direct anastomosis. Function following the intentional sacrifice of the facial nerve can occasionally be reestablished by grafting from the greater auricular nerve.

Following parotidectomy, a few patients develop flushing and increased sweating in the parotid region at mealtime **(Frey's syndrome).** There is no satisfactory explanation for the symptoms, but it has been postulated that it is due to injury of the auriculotemporal nerve followed by abnormal regeneration of parasympathetic fibers which are carried in this nerve. It may appear from a few weeks to a year or more after operation.

A special feature of malignant tumors of the submaxillary gland is the 3–4 times higher incidence of metastases to the regional lymph nodes than for similar lesions occurring in the parotid. Radical neck dissection is therefore indicated whenever the submaxillary gland is removed for a malignant lesion.

Beahrs OH, Chong GC: Management of the facial nerve in parotid gland surgery. Am J Surg 124:473, 1972.

Dunn EJ & others: Parotid neoplasms: A report of 250 cases and review of the literature. Ann Surg 184:500, 1976.

Hanna DC: Management of recurrent salivary gland tumors. Am J Surg 132:453, 1976.

Kagan AR & others: Recurrences from malignant parotid salivary gland tumors. Cancer 37:2600, 1976.

Meine JF, Woloshin HJ: Radiologic diagnosis of salivary gland tumors. Radiol Clin North Am 8:475, 1970.

Rossman KJ: The role of radiation therapy in the treatment of parotid carcinomas. Am J Roentgenol Radium Ther Nucl Med 123:492, 1975.

Spiro RH, Huvos AG, Strong EW: Adenoid cystic carcinoma of salivary origin. Am J Surg 128:512, 1974.

Spiro RH & others: Carcinoma of the parotid gland. Am J Surg 130:452, 1975.

Spiro RH & others: Tumors of the submaxillary gland. Am J Surg 132:463, 1976.

Ward CM: Injury of the facial nerve during surgery of the parotid gland. Br J Surg 62:401, 1975.

Woods JE & others: Experience with 1,360 primary parotid tumors. Am J Surg 130:460, 1975.

MINOR SALIVARY GLANDS

The 2 most frequent sites of origin of minor salivary gland carcinomas are the hard palate and the sinuses. These tumors may also occur at the base of the tongue, in the gums, the buccal mucosa, the larynx, the inner surface of the lip, the pharynx, the floor of the mouth, the nasopharynx, the soft palate, etc. Histologically, these tumors may be (in order of frequency) adenoid cystic carcinomas, mucoepidermoid carcinomas, benign mixed tumors, malignant mixed tumors, or various types of adenocarcinomas. Most tumors of minor salivary glands are malignant.

If left untreated, these tumors spread locally by invasion of muscle, bone, and nerves to areas inaccessible to surgical extirpation.

Contrary to common belief, a significant number of tumors arising in minor salivary glands metastasize to the cervical lymph nodes—an occurrence of grave portent. Hematogenous spread to lung and bones is frequent.

The tumors consist usually of a bulky mass covered by an overlying intact mucosa of firm, rubbery consistency. They are diagnosed by direct or indirect visualization and occasionally in the case of the paranasal sinuses—by x-ray examination. Radiologic examination may also help detect enlargement of the respective foramens when tumors extend to the cranial cavity along the mandibular or the maxillary nerves.

Treatment

The treatment of choice for minor salivary gland tumors, whether benign or malignant, is surgical excision. For malignant tumors, the excision should be radical and should include removal of adjacent nerves and tissues. Examination of the cut ends of nerves and the surgical margins is of paramount importance.

Radical cervical lymphadenectomy is indicated when there is lymphadenopathy.

Radiotherapy is reserved for postoperative management of lesions that are suspected to have been incompletely removed; recurrent tumors when surgery is no longer feasible; and for palliation of bulky tumors considered unresectable. The role of radiotherapy is thus limited to an adjuvant or palliative function.

Coates HLC & others: Glandular tumors of the palate. Surg Gynecol Obstet 140:589, 1975.

Frable WJ, Elzay RP: Tumors of minor salivary glands. Cancer 25:932, 1970.

Kadish SP & others: Treatment of minor salivary gland malignancies of upper food and air passage epithelium. Cancer 29:1021, 1972.

BENIGN TUMORS

Benign tumors of the head and neck are comparatively common. **Pigmented nevi, hemangiomas, dermoid cysts, inclusion cysts (nevi),** and **keratoses** are particularly apt to be seen on the skin of the face, neck, and scalp. Surgical excision, often under local anesthesia, is usually appropriate (see Chapter 46).

Dermoid cysts occur frequently at the angle of the jaw, and particular care should be taken not to mistake an early parotid tumor for a dermoid cyst. In fact, a "dermoid cyst" at the angle of the jaw should be regarded as a parotid tumor until proved otherwise. Excisional biopsy should be done under circumstances permitting resection of the parotid gland if necessary.

A variety of **benign tumors and cysts** occur in the neck. Congenital cysts, branchial cleft cysts, and cystic hygromas are discussed in Chapter 48.

Benign peripheral nerve tumors are fairly common. Excision is usually required to establish the diagnosis and exclude other lesions, including lymph node metastasis from unknown sites.

Carotid body tumor is a painless neck mass attached to the carotid bifurcation. It is diagnosed by palpation and carotid arteriography (vascular "blush" and separation of internal and external carotid arteries by the mass). Its treatment is discussed in Chapter 38.

MALIGNANT NECK TUMORS WITH UNKNOWN PRIMARY

Because the cure rate is very low if metastatic carcinoma in the neck is treated without locating and controlling the primary lesion, patients with lumps in the neck must be examined very thoroughly. A thorough ear, nose, and throat examination must be done, including examination of the nasopharynx, nose, sinuses, pharynx, hypopharynx, larynx, and neck. If the primary tumor is not detected with diagnostic biopsies of the nasopharynx, the tonsillar fossa, the base of the tongue, and the area of the aryepiglottic fold, treatment is controversial. The best treatment is probably excisional biopsy of the mass to obtain a specimen for frozen section analysis, planning the incision appropriately for a radical neck dissection. If the lesion is a squamous cell carcinoma (metastatic to the lymph node), the incision should be extended and radical neck dissection done followed by full-course radiation therapy to the nasopharynx, the tonsillar fossa, the base of the tongue, and the piriform sinus.

Barrie JR & others: Cervical nodal metastases of unknown origin. Am J Surg 120:467, 1970.
Pico J & others: Cervical lymph node metastases from carcinoma of undetermined origin. Am J Roentgenol Radium Ther Nucl Med 111:95, 1971.

OPERATIONS ON THE HEAD & NECK

A multitude of operations are performed on the head and neck for the control of tumors. Although the description of the procedures is beyond the scope of this chapter, 2 operations deserve special mention: radical neck dissection and combined resection.

RADICAL NECK DISSECTION
(Radical Cervical Lymphadenectomy)

This operation was originally standardized by Crile in 1906 and was designed for the removal and control of metastatic deposits to the cervical lymph nodes from various primaries occurring in the head and neck. The deep cervical lymphatics and the cervical lymph nodes are removed from the level of the mandible superiorly to the level of the clavicle inferiorly, and from the midline anteriorly to the anterior border of the trapezius muscle posteriorly. The specimen usually includes the sternocleidomastoid muscle, the omohyoid muscle, the internal jugular vein, and frequently the spinal accessory nerve. The contents of the submental and submaxillary triangle are removed, along with the submaxillary gland and the tip of the parotid gland. The carotid vessels, the vagus and phrenic nerves, the sympathetic chain, the brachial plexus, the hypoglossal nerve, and the digastric muscle are preserved. Occasionally, the thoracic duct must be transected and ligated.

Modified types of neck dissection done with the intention of preserving one or more structures listed above usually fail except when used for the control of papillary carcinoma of the thyroid gland.

When radical neck dissection is performed alone, control of the primary lesion by surgery or radiation therapy is a necessary prerequisite. The operation is not performed when there is extension of disease below the level of the clavicles or to more distant sites.

For midline lesions, bilateral neck dissection is occasionally indicated. The morbidity and mortality rates are higher for this operation, and the postoperative course is marked by profound facial edema. Sparing the jugular vein on one side or staging the operation by delaying the procedure on the second side for a period of several weeks reduces the morbidity and the mortality rate significantly.

COMBINED RESECTION

The removal of the primary tumor in continuity with a radical neck dissection constitutes a combined resection (also called "composite operation," "commando operation"). The principle underlying the combined resection is one of in-continuity removal of the primary lesion and the areas of lymphatic drainage. The mandible is frequently removed for lesions involving the floor of the mouth and the tonsillar fossa. For tumors involving the larynx, the latter is removed in continuity with the contents of the neck. The deformity resulting from mandibular resection depends on the extent and location of the resection: the more anteriorly the mandible is resected, the greater the resulting deformity. A temporary tracheostomy is usually indicated in combined operations.

For lesions that are too extensive to be safely removed with the combined operation, planned preoperative radiation therapy has been found to be most useful in reducing the size of the lesion and permitting resection through tumor-free margins. The advent of supervoltage and modern technics of irradiation permit major operative procedures with morbidity rates that are no greater than those following surgery through nonirradiated tissues.

● ● ●

General References

Ackerman LV, DelRegato JA: *Cancer,* 4th ed. Mosby, 1970.

Ansfield FJ & others: Treatment of advanced cancer of the head and neck. Cancer 25:78, 1970.

Bakamijian VY & others: The concept of cure and palliation by surgery in advanced cancer of the head and neck. Am J Surg 126:482, 1973.

Cruz AB, McInnis WD, Aust JB: Triple drug intra-arterial infusion combined with x-ray therapy and surgery for head and neck cancer. Am J Surg 128:573, 1974.

Fitzpatrick PJ, Brown TC, Reid MA: Malignant melanoma of the head and neck, a clinico-pathological study. Can J Surg 15:90, 1972.

Fletcher GH: Elective irradiation of subclinical disease in cancers of the head and neck. Cancer 29:1450, 1972.

Gollin FF & others: Combined therapy in advanced head and neck cancer: A randomized study. Am J Roentgenol Radium Ther Nucl Med 114:83, 1972.

Jesse RH, Lindberg RD: The efficacy of combining radiation therapy with a surgical procedure in patients with cervical metastases from squamous cell cancer of the oropharynx and hypopharynx. Cancer 35:1163, 1975.

Kerth JD, Sisson GA, Becker GD: Radical neck dissection in carcinoma of the head and neck. Surg Clin North Am 53:179, 1973.

Kogelnik HD & others: Clinical course of patients with squamous cell carcinoma of the upper respiratory and digestive tract with evidence of disease 5 years after initial treatment. Radiology 115:423, 1975.

Lindberg R: Distribution of cervical lymph node metastases from squamous cell carcinoma of the upper respiratory and digestive tracts. Cancer 29:1446, 1972.

Lo TC & others: Combined radiation therapy and 5-fluorouracil for advanced squamous cell carcinoma of the oral cavity and oropharynx: A randomized study. Am J Roentgenol Radium Ther Nucl Med 126:229, 1976.

Marchetta FC, Sako K: Preoperative irradiation for squamous cell carcinoma of the head and neck: Does it improve five year survival or control figures? Am J Surg 130:487, 1975.

O'Brien PH & others: Metastasis in epidermoid carcinoma of the head and neck. Cancer 27:304, 1971.

Probert JC, Thompson RW, Bagshaw MA: Patterns of spread of distant metastasis in head and neck cancer. Cancer 33:127, 1974.

Regezi JA & others: Dental management of patients irradiated for oral cancer. Cancer 38:994, 1976.

Rubin P & others: Cancer of the head and neck: Nose, paranasal sinuses. JAMA 219:336, 1972.

Rush BF & others: Integrated radiation and operation in the treatment of carcinoma of the head and neck. J Surg Oncol 3:151, 1971.

Schneider JJ & others: Control by irradiation alone of nonfixed clinically positive lymph nodes from squamous cell carcinoma of the oral cavity, oropharynx, supraglottic larynx, and hypopharynx. Am J Roentgenol Radium Ther Nucl Med 123:42, 1975.

Shedd DP: Rehabilitation problems of head and neck cancer patients. J Surg Oncol 8:11, 1976.

Spiro RH & others: Cervical node metastasis from epidermoid carcinoma of the oral cavity and oropharynx. Am J Surg 128:562, 1974.

Waldron CA, Shafer WG: Leukoplakia revisited. Cancer 36:1386, 1975.

Williams RG: Recurrent head and neck cancer: The results of treatment. Br J Surg 61:691, 1974.

Woods JE: Current status of chemotherapy in the treatment of head and neck cancer. Arch Surg 111:1055, 1976.

Wynder EL: Etiological aspects of squamous cancers of the head and neck. JAMA 215:452, 1971.

Zarem HA: Current concepts in reconstructive surgery in patients with cancer of the head and neck. Surg Clin North Am 51:149, 1971.

19 . . .
Thyroid & Parathyroid

Orlo H. Clark, MD

I. THE THYROID GLAND

EMBRYOLOGY & ANATOMY

The main anlage of the thyroid gland develops as a median entodermal downgrowth from the first and second pharyngeal pouches. During its migration caudally, it contacts the ultimobranchial bodies developing from the fourth pharyngeal pouches. When it reaches the position it occupies in the adult, just below the cricoid cartilage, the thyroid divides into 2 lobes. The site from which it originated persists as the foramen cecum at the base of the tongue. The path the gland follows may result in thyroglossal remnants (cysts) or ectopic thyroid tissue (lingual thyroid). A pyramidal lobe is frequently present. Agenesis of one thyroid lobe may occur.

The normal thyroid weighs 15–25 g and is attached to the trachea by loose connective tissue. It is a highly vascularized organ that derives its blood supply principally from the superior and inferior thyroid arteries. A thyroid ima artery may also be present.

PHYSIOLOGY

The function of the thyroid gland is to synthesize, store, and secrete the hormones thyroxine (T_4) and triiodothyronine (T_3). Iodide is absorbed from the gastrointestinal tract and actively trapped by the acinar cells of the thyroid gland. It is then oxidized and combined with tyrosine in thyroglobulin to form monoiodotyrosine (MIT) and diiodotyrosine (DIT). These are coupled to form the active hormones T_4 and T_3, which initially are stored in the colloid of the gland. Following hydrolysis of the thyroglobulin, T_4 and T_3 are secreted into the plasma, becoming almost instantaneously bound to plasma proteins. T_3 is also produced by extrathyroidal conversion of T_4 to T_3.

The function of the thyroid gland is regulated by a feedback mechanism which involves the hypothalamus and pituitary. Thyrotropin-releasing factor (TRF), a tripeptide amide, is formed in the hypothalamus and stimulates the release of thyrotropin (TSH), a glyco-

protein, from the pituitary. Thyrotropin binds to TSH receptors on the thyroid plasma membrane, stimulating increased adenylate cyclase activity; this increases cyclic AMP production and thyroid cellular function.

Brown J & others: Thyroid physiology in health and disease. Ann Intern Med 81:68, 1974.

Greer MA: Factors regulating triiodothyronine (T_3) and thyroxine (T_4) in blood. Mayo Clin Proc 47:944, 1972.

Ingbar SH: Autoregulation of the thyroid: Response to iodide and depletion. Mayo Clin Proc 47:814, 1972.

Vagenakis AG & others: Recovery of pituitary thyrotropic function after withdrawal of prolonged thyroid-suppression therapy. N Engl J Med 293:681, 1975.

EVALUATION OF THE THYROID

In a patient with enlargement of the thyroid (goiter), the history and examination of the gland are most important and are complemented by the selective use of thyroid function tests. The surgeon must develop a systematic method of palpating the gland to determine its size, contour, consistency, nodularity, and fixation and to examine for displacement of the trachea and the presence of palpable cervical lymph nodes.

Thyroid function tests (Table 19–1) should be interpreted in light of the clinical situation. One test alone may be insufficient. Serum T_3, T_4, and TSH can be accurately measured by radioimmunoassay; serum T_4 can also be measured by a competitive protein binding method. These tests have replaced PBI and BEI in the evaluation of thyroid function because they are more reliable and unaffected by exogenous iodine. The T_3 resin uptake is an in vitro measurement that indirectly measures the concentration of unsaturated thyroxine-binding globulin in the serum. Thyroid uptake of radioiodine is useful in the assessment of thyroid function and also for thyroid scanning.

Britton KE & others: A strategy for thyroid function tests. Br Med J 3:350, 1975.

Vagenakis AG, Braverman LE: Thyroid function tests–which one? Ann Intern Med 84:607, 1976.

Table 19–1. Thyroid function tests.

Test	Normal Values	Value	Increased	Decreased
Serum thyroxine competitive protein binding (T_4 CPB) or radioimmunoassay (T_4 RIA)	3.0–7.0 µg/100 ml (varies with laboratory)	Simple; unaltered by iodide. Excellent screening test for hyperthyroidism and hypothyroidism. 90% accurate.	(1) Hyperthyroidism. (2) Acute thyroiditis. (3) Early hepatitis. (4) Elevated thyroid-binding globulin: pregnancy; estrogen administration. (5) Exogenous T_4.	(1) Hypothyroidism. (2) Decreased thyroid-binding globulin: anabolic steroids; androgens; nephrosis. (3) Abnormal binding or conversion: salicylates; sulfonamides; phenytoin (Dilantin). (4) Exogenous T_3.
Triiodothyronine radioimmunoassay (T_3 RIA)	60–190 ng/100 ml (varies with laboratory)	Measures circulating T_3 concentration; unaltered by iodide.	(1) Hyperthyroidism. (2) T_3 toxicosis. (3) Exogenous T_4 (more than 300 mg daily).	Advancing age.
Thyrotropin radioimmunoassay (TSH RIA)	10 µU/ml (varies with laboratory)	Best for primary hypothyroidism.	Primary hypothyroidism.	(1) Hyperthyroidism. (2) After pyrogens. (3) After large doses of glucocorticoids. (4) Secondary hypothyroidism.
Triiodothyronine resin uptake (T_3 RU)	Varies with laboratory	Indirectly measures the concentration of unsaturated thyroid-binding globulin. When used with T_4, corrects for abnormal concentration of serum proteins. Unaffected by exogenous iodine compounds.	(1) Hyperthyroidism. (2) Phenytoin (Dilantin), salicylates, phenylbutazone, anticoagulants, cortisone, androgens, anabolic steroids, large doses of penicillin.	(1) Hypothyroidism. (2) Pregnancy. (3) Estrogens. (4) Lipemia.
Radioactive iodine uptake (RAI) and scan	10–30% (at 24 hours)	Simple index of iodide clearance from plasma by the thyroid gland.	(1) Hyperthyroidism. (2) Glandular hormone depletion. (3) Iodine depletion. (4) Excessive hormonal losses.	(1) Primary and secondary hypothyroidism. (2) Increased iodine intake, including contrast media. (3) Exogenous thyroid hormones. (4) Subacute thyroiditis.

DISEASES OF THE THYROID

HYPERTHYROIDISM
(Thyrotoxicosis)

Essentials of Diagnosis

- Nervousness, weight loss with increased appetite, heat intolerance, increased sweating, muscular weakness and fatigue, increased bowel frequency, polyuria, menstrual irregularities, infertility.
- Goiter, tachycardia, warm moist skin, thyroid thrill and bruit, cardiac flow murmur; gynecomastia.
- Eye signs: staring, lid lag, exophthalmos.
- Iodine uptake, T_3, T_4, T_3 resin uptake all increased. TSH absent. T_3 suppression test abnormal.

General Considerations

Hyperthyroidism can be due to a hypersecreting solitary or multinodular toxic goiter (**Plummer's disease**) or a diffusely hypersecreting goiter (**Graves' dis-** ease). In all forms, the symptoms of hyperthyroidism are due to increased levels of thyroid hormone in the blood stream. The clinical manifestations of thyrotoxicosis may be subtle or marked and tend to go through periods of exacerbation and remission. Some patients ultimately develop hypothyroidism spontaneously or as a result of treatment. The cause of Graves' disease remains unknown, although there are indications that it may be an autoimmune disease. Many cases are easily diagnosed on the basis of the signs and symptoms; others (eg, mild or apathetic hyperthyroidism) may be recognized only with difficulty.

Recently, thyrotoxicosis has been described with a normal T_4 concentration, normal or elevated radioiodine uptake, and normal protein binding but with increased serum T_3 by RIA (**T_3 toxicosis**). Thyrotoxicosis associated with toxic nodular goiter is usually less severe than that associated with Graves' disease and is only rarely if ever associated with the extrathyroidal manifestations of Graves' disease such as exophthalmos and pretibial myxedema.

If left untreated, thyrotoxicosis causes progressive and profound catabolic disturbances and cardiac damage. Death may occur in thyroid storm or because of heart failure or severe cachexia.

Table 19–2. Clinical findings in thyrotoxicosis.*

Clinical Manifestations	Percent	Clinical Manifestations	Percent
Tachycardia	100	Weakness	70
Goiter	98	Increased appetite	65
Nervousness	99	Eye complaints	54
Skin changes	97	Leg swelling	35
Tremor	97	Hyperdefecation (without diarrhea)	33
Increased sweating	91		
Hypersensitivity to heat	89	Diarrhea	23
		Atrial fibrillation	10
Palpitations	89	Splenomegaly	10
Fatigue	88	Gynecomastia	10
Weight loss	85	Anorexia	9
Bruit over thyroid	77	Liver palms	8
Dyspnea	75	Constipation	4
Eye signs	71	Weight gain	2

*Data from Williams RH: J Clin Endocrinol Metab 6:1, 1946.

Clinical Findings

A. Symptoms and Signs: The clinical findings are those of hyperthyroidism as well as those related to the underlying cause (Table 19–2). Nervousness, increased diaphoresis, heat intolerance, tachycardia, palpitations, fatigue, and weight loss in association with a nodular, multinodular, or diffuse goiter are the classical findings in hyperthyroidism. The patient may have a flushed and staring appearance.

The skin is warm, thin, and moist and the hair is fine. In Graves' disease, there may be exophthalmos, pretibial myxedema, or vitiligo, usually not seen in single or multinodular toxic goiter. The Achilles reflex time is shortened in hyperthyroidism and prolonged in hypothyroidism. The patient on the verge of thyroid storm has accentuated symptoms and signs of thyrotoxicosis, with hyperpyrexia, tachycardia, cardiac failure, neuromuscular excitation, delirium, or jaundice.

B. Laboratory Findings: Laboratory tests reveal elevation of the T_4, T_3, T_3 RU, and RAI (Table 19–1). A history of medications is important since certain drugs and organic iodinated compounds affect some thyroid function tests, and iodide excess may result in either iodide-induced hypothyroidism or iodine-induced hyperthyroidism (**jodbasedow***). In mild forms of hyperthyroidism, the usual diagnostic laboratory tests are likely to be only slightly abnormal. In these difficult-to-diagnose cases, 2 additional tests are helpful: the thyroid suppression test and the thyrotropin-releasing hormone (TRH) test. In the thyroid suppression test, hyperthyroid patients fail to suppress the thyroidal uptake of radioiodine when given exogenous thyroid hormone. In the TRH test, the normal increase in TSH after parenteral administration of TRH is absent in hyperthyroidism.

Other findings include low serum cholesterol, lymphocytosis, and occasionally hypercalcemia, hypercalciuria, or glycosuria.

*Jodbasedow = Ger. *Jod* (iodine) + Basedow's disease, ie, iodine-induced hyperthyroidism or Graves' disease.

Differential Diagnosis

Anxiety neurosis, heart disease, anemia, gastrointestinal disease, cirrhosis, tuberculosis, myasthenia and other muscular disorders, menopausal syndrome, pheochromocytoma, primary ophthalmopathy, and thyrotoxicosis factitia may be clinically difficult to differentiate from hyperthyroidism. Differentiation is especially difficult when the thyrotoxic patient presents with minimal or no thyroid enlargement.

Anxiety neurosis is perhaps the condition most frequently confused with hyperthyroidism. Anxiety is characterized by persistent fatigue usually unrelieved by rest, clammy palms, a normal sleeping pulse rate, and normal laboratory tests of thyroid function. The fatigue of hyperthyroidism is often relieved by rest, the palms are warm and moist, tachycardia persists during sleep, and thyroid function tests are abnormal.

Organic disease of nonthyroidal origin which may be confused with hyperthyroidism must be differentiated largely on the basis of evidence of specific organ system involvement and normal thyroid function tests.

Other causes of exophthalmos (eg, orbital tumors) or ophthalmoplegia (eg, myasthenia) must be ruled out by ophthalmologic, ultrasonographic, and neurologic examinations.

Treatment

Hyperthyroidism may be effectively treated by antithyroid drugs, radioactive iodine, or thyroidectomy. Treatment must be individualized and depends on the patient's age and general state of health, the size of the goiter, the underlying pathologic process, and the patient's ability to obtain follow-up care.

A. Antithyroid Drugs: The principal antithyroid drugs used in the USA are propylthiouracil (PTU), 300–1000 mg orally daily, and methimazole (Tapazole), 30–100 mg orally daily. These agents interfere with organic binding of iodine and prevent coupling of iodotyrosines in the thyroid gland. One advantage over thyroidectomy and radioiodine in the treatment of Graves' disease is that they inhibit the function of the gland without destroying tissue; therefore, there is a lower incidence of subsequent hypothyroidism. This form of treatment may be used either as definitive treatment or in preparation for surgery or radioactive iodine treatment. When propylthiouracil is given as definitive treatment, the goal is to maintain the patient in a euthyroid state until a natural remission occurs. Reliable patients with small goiters are good candidates for this regimen. A prolonged remission after 18 months of treatment occurs in 50% of patients. Side-effects include rashes and fever (3–4%) and agranulocytosis (0.1–0.4%). Patients must be warned to stop the drug and see the physician if sore throat or fever develops.

B. Radioiodine: Radioiodine (^{131}I) is safe, is less expensive than operative treatment, and is effective. It is indicated for patients who are elderly or are poor risks for surgery and for patients with recurrent hyperthyroidism. To date radioiodine treatment has not been associated with an increase in leukemia, thyroid malignancy, or the induction of congenital anomalies. However, an increased incidence of benign thyroid tumors has recently been noted to follow treatment of hyperthyroidism with radioiodine. Although malignancy was not more common, when it did occur, the tumors were more often of the undifferentiated type with a poor prognosis. In young patients, the radiation hazard is certainly increased and the chance of developing hypothyroidism is greater: After the first year of treatment with radioiodine the incidence of hypothyroidism increases 2–3 percent per year.

Hyperthyroid children and pregnant women should not be treated with radioiodine.

C. Surgery:

1. Indications for subtotal thyroidectomy—The main advantages of subtotal thyroidectomy are rapid control of the disease and a lower incidence of hypothyroidism than can be achieved with radioiodine treatment. Associated conditions in which surgery is recommended are as follows: (1) presence of a large goiter, (2) presence of a thyroid nodule that may be cancer, (3) treatment of a pregnant patient, and (4) treatment of psychologically or mentally incompetent patients or patients who are for any reason unable to maintain adequate long-term follow-up evaluation.

2. Preparation for surgery—The risk of thyroidectomy for toxic goiter has become negligible since the introduction of the combined preoperative use of iodides and antithyroid drugs. Propylthiouracil or one of its derivatives is administered until the patient becomes euthyroid and is continued until the time of operation. Two to 5 drops of potassium iodide solution or Lugol's iodine solution are then given for 10–15 days before surgery in conjunction with the propylthiouracil to decrease the friability and vascularity of the thyroid, thereby technically facilitating its removal.

An occasional untreated or inadequately treated hyperthyroid patient may require an emergency operation for some unrelated problem such as acute appendicitis and thus require immediate control of the hyperthyroidism. Such a patient should be treated in a manner similar to one in **thyroid storm** since thyroid storm or hyperthyroid crises may be precipitated by surgical stress or trauma. Treatment of hyperthyroid patients requiring emergency operation or those in thyroid storm is as follows: Prevent release of preformed thyroid hormone by administration of Lugol's iodine solution; give the beta-adrenergic blocking agent propranolol to antagonize the peripheral manifestations of thyrotoxicosis; and decrease thyroid hormone production and extrathyroidal conversion of T_4 to T_3 by giving propylthiouracil. Other important considerations are to treat precipitating causes (eg, infection, drug reactions); to support vital functions by giving oxygen, sedatives, intravenous fluids, and corticosteroids; and to reduce fever. Reserpine may be useful in the patient in whom nervousness is a prominent symptom, and a cooling blanket should be used in patients requiring operation.

3. Subtotal thyroidectomy—The treatment of hyperthyroidism by subtotal thyroidectomy eliminates both the hyperthyroidism and the goiter. As a rule, all but 3–10 g of thyroid are removed (depending on the size of the goiter and the severity of the hyperthyroidism before preoperative preparation), sparing the parathyroid glands and the recurrent laryngeal nerves.

The mortality rate associated with the procedure is extremely low—less than 0.1% in a recent collected review. Subtotal thyroidectomy thus provides safe and rapid correction of the thyrotoxic state. The frequency of recurrent hyperthyroidism and hypothyroidism depends on the amount of thyroid removed and on the natural history of the hyperthyroidism. Given an accomplished surgeon and good preoperative preparation, injuries to the recurrent laryngeal nerves and parathyroid glands occur in less than 2% of cases. Adequate exposure and precise identification of the vasculature, recurrent laryngeal nerves, and parathyroid glands are essential.

Ocular Manifestations of Graves' Disease

The pathogenesis of the ocular problems in Graves' disease remains unclear. Evidence originally supporting the role of either long-acting thyroid stimulator (LATS) or exophthalmos-producing substance (EPS) has not been authenticated.

The eye complications of Graves' disease may begin before there is any evidence of thyroid dysfunction or after the hyperthyroidism has been appropriately treated. Usually, however, the ocular manifestations develop concomitantly with the hyperthyroidism. Relief of the eye problems is often difficult to accomplish until coexisting hyperthyroidism or hypothyroidism is controlled.

The eye changes of Graves' disease vary from no signs or symptoms to loss of sight. Mild cases are characterized by upper lid retraction and stare with or without lid lag or proptosis. These cases present only minor cosmetic problems and require no treatment. When moderate to severe eye changes occur, there is soft tissue involvement with proptosis, extraocular muscle involvement, and finally optic nerve involvement. Some cases may have marked chemosis, periorbital edema, conjunctivitis, keratitis, diplopia, ophthalmoplegia, and impaired vision. Ophthalmologic consultation is required.

Treatment of the ocular problems of Graves' disease includes maintaining the patient in a euthyroid state without increase in TSH secretion, protecting the eyes from light and dust with dark glasses and eye shields, elevating the head of the bed, using diuretics to decrease periorbital and retrobulbar edema, and giving methycellulose or guanethidine eyedrops. High doses of glucocorticoids are beneficial in certain patients, but their effectiveness is variable and unpredictable. If exophthalmos progresses despite medical treatment, lateral tarsorrhaphy, surgical decompression of the orbit, or retrobulbar irradiation may be necessary. Total thyroid ablation has been recommended, but whether it has a beneficial effect is controversial. In treating a patient with ophthalmopathy, it is important that the patient be made aware of the natural history of the disease and also that he be euthyroid since hyper- and hypothyroidism may produce visual deterioration. Operations to correct diplopia should only be performed after the ophthalmopathy has stabilized.

Das G, Krieger M: Treatment of thyrotoxic storm with intravenous administration of propranolol. Ann Intern Med 70:935, 1969.

Dobyns BM & others: Malignant and benign neoplasm of the thyroid in patients treated for hyperthyroidism: A report of the cooperative thyrotoxicosis therapy follow-up. J Clin Endocrinol Metab 38:976, 1974.

Georges P & others: Metabolic effects of propanolol in thyrotoxicosis. Metabolism 24:11, 1975.

Green M, Wilson GM: Thyrotoxicosis treated by surgery or iodine-131 with special reference to development of hypothyroidism. Br Med J 1:1005, 1964.

Grove AS Jr: Evaluation of exophthalmos. N Engl J Med 292:1005, 1975.

Harrison TS: The treatment of thyroid storm. Surg Gynecol Obstet 121:837, 1965.

Heimann P, Martinson J: Surgical treatment of thyrotoxicosis. Br J Surg 62:683, 1975.

Ingbar SH: When to hospitalize the patient with thyrotoxicosis. Hosp Pract 10:45, Jan 1975.

Kriss JP: Graves' ophthalmopathy: Etiology and treatment. Hosp Pract 10:125, March 1975.

Livadas D & others: Malignant cold thyroid nodules in hyperthyroidism. Br J Surg 63:726, 1976.

McDougall IR & others: Radioactive iodine (^{125}I) therapy for thyrotoxicosis. N Engl J Med 285:1099, 1971.

Michie W: Whither thyrotoxicosis. Br J Surg 62:673, 1975.

Mukhtar ED & others: Relation of thyroid-stimulating immunoglobulins to thyroid function and effects of surgery, radioiodine and antithyroid drugs. Lancet 1:713, 1975.

Nofal MM, Beierwaltes WH, Patno ME: Treatment of hyperthyroidism with I 131. JAMA 197:605, 1966.

EVALUATION OF THYROID NODULES & GOITERS

Thyroid Nodules

The problems facing the clinician when confronted by a patient with a nodular goiter or thyroid nodule are whether the lesion is symptomatic and whether it is benign or malignant. The differential diagnosis includes benign goiter, intrathyroidal cysts, thyroiditis, and benign and malignant tumors. The history should specifically emphasize the duration of swelling, recent growth, local symptoms (dysphagia, pain, or voice changes), and systemic symptoms (hyperthyroidism, hypothyroidism, or those from possible tumors metastatic to the thyroid). The patient's age, sex, place of birth, family history, and history of radiation to the neck are most important. Radiation in infancy or childhood is associated with an increased incidence of thyroid cancer in later life. A thyroid nodule is more likely to be a cancer in a man than in a woman and in a young patient than in an old one. In certain geographic areas, endemic goiter is common,

making benign nodules more common. Thyroid cancer has also been described in families and in identical twins.

The clinician must systematically palpate the thyroid to determine whether there is a solitary thyroid nodule or if it is a multinodular gland and whether there are palpable lymph nodes. A solitary thyroid nodule is more likely to be malignant than a multinodular goiter.

The radioiodine scan is helpful in determining whether the lesion is single or multiple and whether it is functioning (warm or hot) or nonfunctioning (cold). Hot solitary thyroid nodules may cause hyperthyroidism but are rarely malignant, whereas cold solitary thyroid nodules have an incidence of malignancy of about 25% and should be removed. Thyroid carcinoma is found in about 20% of multinodular goiters and 25% of solitary nodular goiters referred for thyroidectomy. Patients with thyroid nodules who received x-ray treatments to the head and neck in infancy and childhood have a 35—50% chance of the nodule being malignant. Thyroid malignancy occurs in more than half of children with solitary cold thyroid nodules; therefore, thyroidectomy is indicated.

In many patients, the possibility of malignancy is difficult to exclude short of microscopic examination of the gland itself. The recent use of thermography and ultrasound (echography) for differentiating solid and cystic lesions is encouraging since purely cystic lesions less than 4 cm in diameter are almost never cancer. Unfortunately, only 10—20% of cold solitary lesions are cystic. Fluorescent scanning using a collimated source of radiation is now being used to differentiate benign from malignant thyroid nodules. This procedure has the advantage that no radioactive materials are introduced into the body and total radiation to the neck is only 50 mrads. Soft tissue x-rays of the thyroid region, or xerography, and a chest x-ray should be performed since some papillary carcinomas are finely stippled with calcium and some benign adenomatous goiters and medullary carcinomas may be heavily calcified. Needle biopsy of thyroid nodules has been advocated, but tissue obtained in this way is often unrepresentative of the true histologic status of the lesion.

The principal indications for surgical removal of a nodular goiter are (1) suspicion of malignancy, (2) symptoms of pressure, (3) hyperthyroidism, (4) substernal extension, and (5) cosmetic deformity. Solitary thyroid nodules that are cold on radioiodine scan and solid by ultrasound should be removed. Nonoperative treatment is indicated in patients with multinodular goiters unless there is a clinically suspicious area which is growing or if the patient was exposed to radiation or has a family history of medullary carcinoma.

Simple or Nontoxic Goiter
(Diffuse & Multinodular Goiter)

Simple goiter may be physiologic, occurring during puberty or the menses or during pregnancy; or it may occur in patients from endemic (iodine-poor) regions or as a result of prolonged exposure to goitrogenic foods or drugs. As the goiter persists, there may be a tendency to form lobulations. Goiter may also occur early in life as a consequence of a congenital defect in thyroid hormone production. It is generally assumed that nontoxic goiter represents a compensatory response to inadequate thyroid hormone production. Nontoxic diffuse goiter usually responds favorably to thyroid hormone administration. Without medical treatment, this type of goiter may develop into a multinodular goiter with or without toxicity in later years.

Symptoms are usually awareness of a neck mass and dyspnea, dysphagia, or symptoms caused by interference with venous return. In diffuse goiter, the thyroid is symmetrically enlarged and has a smooth surface without areas of encapsulation. However, most patients have multinodular glands by the time they seek medical care. The T_4, T_3, and T_3 RU measurements (Table 19–1) may all be within normal limits, although radioiodine uptake may be increased. Surgery is indicated to relieve the pressure symptoms of a large goiter or to rule out malignancy when there are localized areas of hardness or rapid growth.

Astwood EB, Cassidy CE, Aurbach GD: Treatment of goiter and thyroid nodules with thyroid. JAMA 174:459, 1960.

Clark OH: Evaluation of thyroid nodules. West J Med 124:232, 1976.

Clark OH & others: Evaluation of solitary cold thyroid nodules by echography and thermography. Am J Surg 130:206, 1975.

Greenspan FS: Thyroid nodules and thyroid cancer. West J Med 121:359, 1974

Patton JA & others: Differentiation between malignant and benign solitary thyroid nodules by fluorescent scanning. J Nucl Med 17:17, 1976.

Shimaoka K, Sokal JE: Suppressive therapy of nontoxic goiter. Am J Med 57:576, 1974.

INFLAMMATORY THYROID DISEASE

The inflammatory diseases of the thyroid are termed acute, subacute, or chronic thyroiditis, which can be either suppurative or nonsuppurative.

Acute suppurative thyroiditis is uncommon and is characterized by the sudden onset of severe neck pain accompanied by dysphagia, fever, and chills. It usually follows an acute upper respiratory tract infection and is treated by surgical drainage. The organisms are most often streptococci, staphylococci, pneumococcus, or coliforms.

Subacute thyroiditis, a nonbacterial condition, is characterized by thyroid swelling, head and chest pain, fever, weakness, malaise, and weight loss. The erythrocyte sedimentation rate and serum gamma globulin are almost always elevated and RAI uptake is very low or absent. Corticotropin and the corticosteroids relieve symptoms but have no effect on the disease.

Hashimoto's thyroiditis, the most common form

of chronic thyroiditis, is characterized by enlargement of the neck with pain and tenderness in the region of the thyroid. It usually occurs in women and may cause difficulty in breathing and swallowing as a result of compression of the trachea and esophagus.

Hashimoto's thyroiditis is believed to be an autoimmune disease in which the patient becomes sensitized against his own thyroid tissue and forms antithyroid antibodies. The high serum titers of antimicrosomal and antithyroglobulin antibodies are helpful in making the diagnosis. The appropriate treatment for most patients consists of suppressive doses of thyroid hormone. Operation is indicated for marked pressure symptoms, suspected malignant tumor, and for cosmetic reasons. In patients with pressure or choking symptoms, surgical division of the isthmus may provide relief. If the thyroid is large or asymmetrical, subtotal thyroidectomy and subsequent thyroid hormone replacement are indicated. Needle biopsy has been recommended by some thyroidologists to confirm the diagnosis of Hashimoto's disease.

Riedel's thyroiditis is a rare condition that presents as a hard woody mass in the thyroid region with marked fibrosis and chronic inflammation in and around the gland. The inflammatory process infiltrates muscles and causes symptoms of tracheal compression. Hypothyroidism is usually present, and surgical treatment is required to relieve tracheal or esophageal obstruction.

Colcock PB, Pena O: Diagnosis and treatment of thyroiditis. Postgrad Med 44:83, Aug 1968.

Doniach D: Thyroid autoimmune disease. J Clin Pathol 20:285, 1967.

Greene JN: Subacute thyroiditis. Am J Med 71:97, 1971.

Hall R, Stanbury JB: Familial studies of autoimmune thyroiditis. Clin Exp Immunol 2:719, 1967.

Hirabayashi RN, Lindsay S: The relation of thyroid carcinoma and chronic thyroiditis. Surg Gynecol Obstet 121:243, 1965.

Thomas WC Jr & others: Clinical studies in thyroiditis. Ann Intern Med 63:808, 1965.

BENIGN TUMORS OF THE THYROID

Benign thyroid tumors are adenomas, involutionary nodules, cysts, or localized thyroiditis. Most adenomas are of the follicular type. Adenomas are usually solitary and encapsulated and compress the adjacent thyroid. The major reasons for removal are a suspicion of malignancy; functional overactivity producing hyperthyroidism; and cosmetic disfigurement.

MALIGNANT TUMORS OF THE THYROID

Essentials of Diagnosis

- History of irradiation to the neck in some patients.
- Painless or enlarging nodule, dysphagia, or hoarseness.
- Firm or hard, fixed thyroid nodule; cervical lymphadenopathy.
- Normal thyroid function; nodule stippled with calcium (x-ray), cold (radioiodine scan), solid (ultrasound).

General Considerations

An appreciation of the classification of malignant tumors of the thyroid is important because thyroid tumors demonstrate a wide range of growth and malignant behavior. At one end of the spectrum is **papillary adenocarcinoma,** which usually occurs in young adults, grows very slowly, metastasizes late through lymphatics, and is compatible with long life even in the presence of metastases (Table 19—3). At the other extreme is **undifferentiated carcinoma,** which appears late in life and is nonencapsulated and invasive, forming large infiltrating tumors composed of small or large anaplastic cells. The prognosis of this type is poor; the patient usually succumbs as a consequence of local recurrence, pulmonary metastasis, or both. Between these 2 extremes are follicular and medullary carcinomas, sarcomas, lymphomas, and metastatic tumors. The prognosis depends on the histologic pattern and the extent of tumor spread at the time of diagnosis.

The cause of most cases of thyroid carcinoma is unknown, but patients who received therapeutic radiation to the thymus, tonsils, scalp, and skin in infancy, childhood, and adolescence have an increased risk of developing thyroid cancer. The latent period before developing clinically evident thyroid carcinoma after therapeutic radiation may be as long as 30 years. Both children and adults up to 50 years of age who were exposed to the atomic blast at Hiroshima had an increased incidence of thyroid cancer.

Types of Thyroid Cancer

A. Papillary Adenocarcinoma: Papillary adenocarcinomas account for 60—70% of malignancies of the thyroid gland. The neoplasm often appears in childhood or early adult life, remains localized, and eventually metastasizes to the pericapsular and paratracheal lymph nodes, then along the internal jugular veins and into the lateral triangles of the neck, appearing later in the anterior superior mediastinum, lungs, and bones. Microscopically, the tumor is composed of papillary projections of columnar epithelium, and the sections may show a pure papillary pattern with psammoma bodies or may contain a mixed papillary and follicular pattern. Occasionally, the primary tumor may become anaplastic, or the metastases may be follicular or anaplastic though the primary tumor is papillary. Papillary carcinoma presenting as a solitary nodule spreads by way of the intraglandular lymphatics to other parts of the same lobe, the isthmus, or the opposite lobe and then to the subcapsular and pericapsular lymph nodes. The rate of growth may be stimulated by TSH.

B. Follicular Adenocarcinoma: Follicular adenocarcinoma accounts for approximately 20% of malignant thyroid tumors. It appears later in life than the papillary form and may be elastic or rubbery or even soft on palpation. It may appear to be encapsulated and to contain colloid on gross examination. Microscopically, follicular carcinoma may be difficult to distinguish from normal thyroid tissue. Capsular and vascular invasion are important findings. Although it may metastasize to the regional lymph nodes, it has a greater tendency to spread by the hematogenous route to the lungs, skeleton, and liver. Metastases from this neoplasm often demonstrate an avidity for radioactive iodine after total thyroidectomy. Skeletal metastases from follicular carcinomas may appear 10—20 years after resection of the primary lesion and may follow a relatively benign course, although in general the prognosis is not as good as with the papillary type (Table 19—3).

C. Medullary Carcinoma: Medullary carcinoma accounts for approximately 2—5% of malignant tumors of the thyroid. It contains amyloid and is a solid, hard, nodular tumor which takes up radioiodine poorly. It is felt that medullary carcinomas arise from cells of the ultimobranchial bodies, which also secrete calcitonin. Familial occurrence of medullary carcinoma associated with bilateral pheochromocytoma and hyperparathyroidism is known as **Sipple's syndrome** or **type II multiple endocrine adenomatosis.**

Medullary thyroid cancer in relatives of patients with medullary carcinoma may be diagnosed by determining serum calcitonin concentrations both basally and after calcium or pentagastrin stimulation. Hyperplasia of the parafollicular cells (presumably a precancerous condition) has been demonstrated in relatives of patients with Sipple's syndrome.

D. Undifferentiated Carcinoma: This rapidly growing tumor occurs principally in women beyond middle life and accounts for 5% of all thyroid malignancies. On occasion, this lesion evolves from a papillary or follicular neoplasm. It is a solid, quickly enlarging, hard, irregular mass diffusely involving the gland and invading the trachea, muscles, and neurovascular structures early. The tumor may be painful and somewhat tender, may be fixed on swallowing, and may cause laryngeal or esophageal obstructive symptoms. Microscopically, the cells are anaplastic, varying from

Table 19—3. Survival rates after surgical treatment for papillary, follicular, and undifferentiated thyroid cancer in 390 patients (Hirabayashi and Lindsay).

	10 years	20 years	30 years
Papillary	83.8%	62.6%	58.5%
Follicular	57.2%	36.6%	36.2%
Undifferentiated	14.3%	14.3%	...

small to large or multinucleated, and undergo frequent mitoses. Cervical lymphadenopathy is occasionally present, but pulmonary metastases are more common. Local recurrence after surgical treatment is the rule. External radiation therapy is helpful in controlling the local process. The prognosis is poor, and radioiodine therapy is ineffective (Table 19–3).

Treatment

The treatment of differentiated thyroid carcinoma is operative removal. For papillary carcinoma either total lobectomy with isthmectomy or total thyroidectomy is followed by a 10-year survival rate of over 80% (Table 19–3). Subtotal or partial lobectomy is contraindicated because the incidence of tumor recurrence is greater and survival is shorter. Total thyroidectomy is recommended by the authors for papillary, follicular, and medullary carcinomas if the operation can be done without producing permanent hypoparathyroidism or injury to the recurrent laryngeal nerves. Total is preferred over subtotal thyroidectomy because of the high incidence of multifocal tumor within the gland, a clinical recurrence rate of about 7% in the contralateral lobe if it is spared, and the ease of assessment for recurrence during follow-up examinations.

A conservative neck dissection preserving the sternocleidomastoid muscle is performed if lymph nodes are grossly involved. If extensive infiltrating tumor is present, a more radical neck dissection may be necessary. All thyroid tumors must be studied by frozen section during the operation to help plan the best procedure.

Medullary carcinoma has such a high incidence of nodal involvement that concomitant or interval prophylactic neck dissection is usually justified, especially if serum calcitonin levels remain elevated after thyroidectomy.

Metastatic deposits of follicular and papillary carcinoma should be treated with ^{131}I after total thyroidectomy or thyroid ablation with radioactive iodine. All patients with thyroid cancer should be maintained indefinitely on suppressive doses of thyroid hormone. Measurement of serum thyroglobin levels helps in the postoperative assessment of patients who have had differentiated thyroid cancer.

For **undifferentiated carcinoma, malignant lymphoma,** or **sarcoma,** the tumor should be excised as completely as possible and then treated by radiation and chemotherapy. Doxorubicin (adriamycin), vincristine, and chlorambucil are the most effective agents. Carcinomas of the kidney, breast, and lung and other tumors sometimes metastasize to the thyroid, but they rarely present as a solitary nodule.

Block GE: A modified neck dissection for carcinoma of the thyroid. Surg Clin North Am 51:139, 1971.

Block MA: Management of carcinoma of the thyroid. Ann Surg 185:133, 1977.

Cady B & others: Changing clinical, pathologic, therapeutic, and survival patterns in differentiated thyroid carcinoma. Ann Surg 184:541, 1976.

Clark RL & others: What constitutes an adequate operation for carcinoma of the thyroid? Arch Surg 92:23, 1966.

Crile G Jr: The endocrine dependency of certain thyroid cancers and danger that hypothyroidism may stimulate their growth. Cancer 10:1119, 1957.

DeGroot L, Paloyan E: Thyroid carcinoma and radiation. JAMA 255:487, 1973.

Favus MJ & others: Thyroid cancer occurring as a late consequence of head-and-neck irradiation. N Engl J Med 294:1019, 1976.

Gottlieb JA, Hill CS: Chemotherapy of thyroid cancer with adriamycin. N Engl J Med 290:193, 1974.

Heitz P & others: Thyroid cancer. Cancer 37:2329, 1976.

Noguchi S & others: Papillary carcinoma of the thyroid. Cancer 26:1053, 1970.

Parker LN & others: Thyroid carcinoma after exposure to atomic radiation. Ann Intern Med 80:600, 1974.

Refetoff S & others: Continuing occurrence of thyroid carcinoma after radiation of the neck in infancy and childhood. N Engl J Med 292:171, 1975.

Staunton MD, Greening WP: Treatment of thyroid cancer in 293 patients. Br J Surg 63:253, 1976.

Thomas CG Jr, Buckwater JA: Poorly differentiated neoplasms of the thyroid gland. Ann Surg 177:632, 1973.

Tollefsen HR & others: Papillary carcinoma of the thyroid. Am J Surg 124:468, 1972.

Van Herle AJ, Uller RP: Elevated serum thyroglobulin, a marker of metastases in differentiated thyroid carcinomas. J Clin Invest 56:272, 1975.

Wolff HJ & others: C cell hyperplasia preceding medullary thyroid carcinoma. N Engl J Med 289:437, 1973.

II. THE PARATHYROID GLANDS

EMBRYOLOGY & ANATOMY

Phylogenetically, the parathyroids appear rather late, being first seen in amphibia. They arise from branchial pouches III and IV and may be arrested as high as the level of the hyoid bone during their descent to the posterior capsule of the thyroid gland. Four parathyroid glands are present in 90% of the population. Occasionally, one or more may be incorporated into the thyroid gland or thymus and hence are intrathyroidal or mediastinal in location. Parathyroid III, which normally assumes the inferior position, may be found overlying or alongside the trachea in the suprasternal area, behind the clavicles, the upper sternum or esophagus, or in the anterior or posterior mediastinum. The upper parathyroids (parathyroid IV) usually remain in close association with the upper portion of the lateral thyroid lobes but may be loosely attached by a long vascular pedicle. The parathyroid glands may be separated from the thyroid gland, lying in front of or behind the internal jugular vein and common carotid artery.

The normal parathyroid gland has a distinct yellowish-brown color, is ovoid, tongue-shaped, polypoid, or spherical, and varies in size from 2–5 mm to 3–8 mm. The total mean weight of 4 normal parathyroids is about 140 mg. These encapsulated glands are usually supplied by a branch of the inferior thyroid artery but may be supplied by the superior thyroid or, rarely, the thyroid ima arteries. The vessels can be seen entering a hilus-like structure, a feature which differentiates parathyroid glands from fat.

Alveryd DA: Parathyroid glands in thyroid surgery. Acta Chir Scand (Suppl) 389:1, 1968.

Wang CA: The anatomic basis of parathyroid surgery. Ann Surg 183:271, 1976.

PHYSIOLOGY

Parathyroid hormone (PTH), vitamin D, and probably calcitonin play vital roles in calcium and phosphorus metabolism in bone, kidney, and gut. Specific radioimmunoassays are available to measure PTH, vitamin D, and calcitonin. Ionized calcium, the physiologically important fraction, can now be measured, but most laboratories are only equipped at present to measure total serum calcium concentration, which is composed of approximately 48% ionized calcium, 46% protein-bound calcium, and 6% calcium complexed to organic anions. Total serum calcium varies directly with plasma protein concentrations, but calcium ion concentrations are unaffected.

PTH and calcitonin work in concert to modulate fluctuations in plasma levels of ionized calcium. When the ionized calcium level falls, the parathyroids secrete more PTH and the parafollicular cells within the thyroid secrete less calcitonin. The rise in PTH and fall in calcitonin produce increased bone resorption and tubular resorption of calcium in the kidneys. More calcium enters the blood and ionized calcium levels are returned to normal.

In the circulation, immunoreactive PTH is heterogeneous, consisting of the intact hormone and several hormonal fragments. The amino terminal fragment (N-terminal fragment) is biologically active whereas the carboxyl terminal fragment (C-terminal fragment) is biologically inert. Certain antisera to PTH are specific for the N-terminal or the C-terminal fragments. This probably explains why some patients with histologically proved hyperparathyroidism have been reported to have normal PTH determinations. Measurement of the C-terminal fragment is best for screening for hyperparathyroidism. Because it is cleared rapidly from the circulation, measurement of the N-terminal fragment has some advantages in selective venous catheterization to localize the source of PTH production.

Because PTH levels rise in normal subjects if ionized calcium levels are low, calcium and PTH must be determined from samples drawn simultaneously to diagnose hyperparathyroidism. The combination of increased PTH and hypercalcemia is almost pathognomonic of hyperparathyroidism.

Arnaud CD & others: Native human parathyroid: An immunochemical investigation. Proc Natl Acad Sci USA 67:415, 1970.

Sherwood LW & others: Evaluation by radioimmunoassay of factors controlling the secretion of parathyroid hormone. Nature 209:52, 1966.

Silverman R, Yalow RS: Heterogenicity of parathyroid hormone: Clinical and physiological implications. J Clin Invest 52:1958, 1973.

DISEASES OF THE PARATHYROIDS

PRIMARY HYPERPARATHYROIDISM

Essentials of Diagnosis

- Increased muscular fatigability, nausea, vomiting, constipation, polydipsia, polyuria, psychiatric disturbances, renal colic, bone and joint pain; "stones, bones, and abdominal groans."
- Hypertension, kyphosis, clubbing, band keratopathy.
- Serum calcium, PTH, chloride increased; serum phosphate low or normal; urine calcium increased, normal, or decreased; urine phosphate increased; TRP decreased.
- X-rays: subperiosteal resorption of phalanges, demineralization of the skeleton, bone cysts, and nephrocalcinosis or nephrolithiasis.

General Considerations

Primary hyperparathyroidism is due to excess PTH secretion from a single parathyroid adenoma, multiple adenomas, hyperplasia, carcinoma, or a nonparathyroid malignant tumor producing a parathormone-like substance. Once thought to be rare, primary hyperparathyroidism is now found in 0.1–0.5% of the general population. It is uncommon before puberty; its peak incidence is between the third and fifth decades, and it is 2–3 times more common in women than in men.

Overproduction of parathyroid hormone results in mobilization of calcium from bone and inhibition of the renal reabsorption of phosphate, thereby producing hypercalcemia and hypophosphatemia. This causes a wasting of calcium and phosphorus, with osseous mineral loss. **Osteitis fibrosa cystica** may result in cases of sufficient severity or long duration. Other associated or related conditions which offer clues to the diagnosis of hyperparathyroidism are nephrolithiasis, nephrocalcinosis, bone disease, peptic ulcer, pancreatitis, hypertension, and gout or pseudogout. Hyperparathyroidism also occurs in both type I and type II multiple endocrine adenomatosis (MEA)—known as **Wermer's syndrome** and **Sipple's syndrome,** respectively. The former is characterized by hyperparathyroidism, Zollinger-Ellison syndrome, pituitary tumor, adrenocortical tumor, and insulinoma; the latter consists of hyperparathyroidism in association with medullary carcinoma of the thyroid and pheochromocytoma.

At the University of California Medical Center in San Francisco, the morphologic findings in more than 380 patients with primary hyperparathyroidism were single adenoma in 92%, multiple parathyroid adenomas in 4%, primary parathyroid hyperplasia in 3%, and less than 1% parathyroid carcinoma. Adenomas may be single or multiple and are always accompanied by one or more normal parathyroids. The tumors range in weight from 35 mg to over 35 g, and the size usually parallels the degree of hypercalcemia. Microscopically, these tumors may be of chief cell, water cell, or, rarely, oxyphil cell type.

Primary parathyroid hyperplasia involves all of the parathyroid glands. Microscopically, there are 2 types: chief cell hyperplasia and water-clear cell (wasserhelle) hyperplasia. Hyperplastic glands are almost always larger than normal, but in any one patient there may be a wide variation in size of the glands.

Parathyroid carcinoma is rare and cannot always be diagnosed by its architectural or cytologic features since the histologic findings may be identical with those found in benign parathyroid tumors. Malignancy can be diagnosed with greatest certainty when there is evidence of invasion into adjacent tissues or when metastases are demonstrated.

Clinical Findings

A. Symptoms and Signs: Historically, the clinical manifestations of hyperparathyroidism have changed. Thirty years ago, the diagnosis was based on bone pain and deformity (osteitis fibrosa cystica), and in later years on the renal complications (nephrolithiasis and nephrocalcinosis). At present, over two-thirds of patients have apparently asymptomatic hypercalcemia which is detected by routine screening. After successful surgical treatment, many of these patients become aware of improvement in unrecognized preoperative symptoms such as muscle fatigability, weakness, psychiatric disturbances, constipation, polydipsia and polyuria, and bone and joint pain. Hyperparathyroidism should be suspected in all patients with hypercalcemia and the above symptoms, especially if associated with nephrolithiasis, nephrocalcinosis, hypertension, peptic ulcer, pancreatitis, or gout.

B. Laboratory and X-Ray Findings and Differential Diagnosis (Approach to the Hypercalcemic Patient): (Table 19–4.)

1. Laboratory findings—Hyperparathyroidism and malignancy are responsible for about 80% of cases of hypercalcemia. However, in the evaluation of a hypercalcemic patient, all possible causes should be considered, including laboratory error, a tight tourniquet, and the numerous other clinical conditions listed in Table 19–5. In many patients the diagnosis is obvious,

Table 19–4. Laboratory evaluation of moderate hypercalcemia. With few exceptions, every patient with hypercalcemia should receive the entire battery of tests before one attempts to make a final diagnosis. If the diagnosis is still unclear at this point, special tests described in the text may be indicated.

Blood tests	X-rays
Calcium	Chest x-ray
Phosphorus	Abdominal plain films
Chloride	
Protein; albumin/globulin	
Parathyroid hormone	
Alkaline phosphatase	
Creatinine and BUN	
pH	
Uric acid	

while in others it may be exceedingly difficult. At times, more than one reason for hypercalcemia may exist in the same patient, such as cancer or sarcoidosis plus hyperparathyroidism. A careful history must be obtained documenting (1) the duration of any symptoms possibly related to hypercalcemia, (2) symptoms related to malignant disease, (3) conditions associated with hyperparathyroidism, such as renal colic, peptic ulcer disease, pancreatitis, hypertension, or gout, or (4) possible excess use of milk products, antacids, baking soda, or vitamins. In patients with a recent cough, wheeze, or hemoptysis, epidermoid carcinoma of the lung should be considered. Hematuria might suggest hypernephroma, bladder tumor, or renal lithiasis. Chest roentgenograms and intravenous urograms should be performed as appropriate. A long history of

Table 19–5. Causes of hypercalcemia.

Condition	Approximate Frequency (%)
Malignancy	35
Breast cancer	
Metastatic tumor	
PTH-secreting tumor (lung, kidney, others)	
Multiple myeloma	
Acute and chronic leukemia	
Hyperparathyroidism	28
Artifact (eg, laboratory error, dirty glassware, cork stopper contamination, tight tourniquet)	10
Vitamin D overdose	8
Thiazide diuretics	4
Hyperthyroidism	3
Milk-alkali syndrome	3
Sarcoidosis	3
Other causes	6
Immobilization	
Paget's disease	
Addison's disease	
Idiopathic hypercalcemia of infancy	
Dysproteinemias	
Vitamin A overdosage	
Myxedema	
Pancreatic cholera (WDHA) syndrome	

renal stones or peptic ulcer disease suggests that hyperparathyroidism is likely.

The most important blood tests for the evaluation of hypercalcemia are serum calcium, phosphate, chloride, parathyroid hormone, serum protein electrophoretic pattern, and alkaline phosphatase activity. Occasionally useful tests include serum magnesium, uric acid, and creatinine, erythrocyte sedimentation rate, blood urea nitrogen, urinary calcium, and tubular resorption of phosphate (TRP).

A high serum calcium and a low serum phosphate suggest hyperparathyroidism, but about half of patients with hyperparathyroidism have normal serum phosphate concentrations. Patients with vitamin D intoxication, sarcoidosis, malignant disease without metastasis, and hyperthyroidism may also be hypophosphatemic, but patients with breast cancer and hypercalcemia are only rarely so. In fact, if hypophosphatemia and hypercalcemia are present in association with breast cancer, concomitant hyperparathyroidism is probable. Measurement of **serum parathyroid hormone** has its greatest value in this situation since the PTH level is low or nil in patients with hypercalcemia due to *all* causes other than primary or ectopic hyperparathyroidism. In general, serum PTH levels should be measured in all cases of persistent hypercalcemia without an obvious cause other than hyperparathyroidism, and in normocalcemic patients who are suspected of having hyperparathyroidism. Determination of serum PTH levels is indicated on this basis in approximately half of patients being evaluated for hypercalcemia and in all patients scheduled for parathyroidectomy.

Patients with hyperparathyroidism and normal renal function have hyperphosphaturia due to low **tubular resorption of phosphate (TRP):**

$$\text{TRP (in \%)} = 100 \times \left(1 - \frac{\text{Urinary P} \times \text{Serum creatinine}}{\text{Urinary creatinine} \times \text{Serum P}}\right)$$

This test is of value only when renal function is normal. A high phosphate diet (3 g daily for 3 days) will lower the TRP to below 70% in patients with hyperparathyroidism.

An elevated serum chloride concentration is a useful diagnostic clue found in about 40% of hyperparathyroid patients. PTH acts directly on the proximal renal tubule to decrease the resorption of bicarbonate, which leads to increased resorption of chloride and a mild hyperchloremic renal tubular acidosis. Other causes of hypercalcemia do not give increased serum chloride concentrations. Calculation of the **serum chloride to phosphate ratio** takes advantage of slight increases in serum chloride and slight decreases in serum phosphate concentrations. A ratio above 33 suggests hyperparathyroidism.

Serum protein electrophoretic patterns should always be measured to exclude multiple myeloma and sarcoidosis. Hypergammaglobulinemia is rare in hyperparathyroidism but is not uncommon in patients with multiple myeloma and sarcoidosis. Roentgenograms of the skull will often reveal typical "punched out" bony

lesions, and the diagnosis of myeloma can be firmly established by bone marrow examination. Sarcoidosis can be difficult to diagnose because it may exist for several years with few clinical findings. A chest x-ray revealing a diffuse fibronodular infiltrate and prominent hilar adenopathy is suggestive, and the demonstration of noncaseating granuloma in lymph nodes is diagnostic. The **hydrocortisone suppression test** (150 mg of hydrocortisone per day for 10 days) reduces the serum calcium concentration in most cases of sarcoidosis and vitamin D intoxication and in many patients with carcinoma and multiple myeloma, but only rarely in hyperparathyroidism. It is therefore a useful diagnostic maneuver if these conditions are considered. Hydrocortisone suppression is used to treat the hypercalcemic crises that may occur with these disorders.

Serum alkaline phosphate levels are elevated in about 20% of patients with primary hyperparathyroidism and may also be increased in patients with Paget's disease and cancer. When the serum alkaline phosphatase level is elevated, serum 5'-nucleotidase, which parallels liver alkaline phosphatase, should be measured to determine if the increase is from bone or liver.

2. X-ray findings—Radiographic examination of bone may aid in the diagnosis, but overt skeletal changes are found in only 10% of patients with hyperparathyroidism. Bone changes are rare on x-ray unless the serum alkaline phosphatase concentration is increased. Primary and secondary hyperparathyroidism produce subperiosteal resorption of the phalanges and bone cysts (Fig 19–1). A ground glass appearance of the skull with loss of definition of the tables and demineralization of the outer aspects of the clavicles are less frequently seen. In patients with markedly elevated serum alkaline phosphatase levels without subperiosteal resorption on x-ray, Paget's disease or cancer must be suspected.

3. Differential diagnosis—The differentiation be-

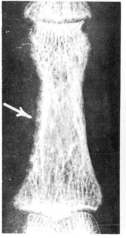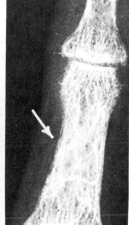

Figure 19–1. Subperiosteal resorption of radial side of second phalanges.

tween hyperparathyroidism due to primary parathyroid disease and that due to ectopic hyperparathyroidism or nonparathyroid cancer is often difficult. The most common tumors causing ectopic hyperparathyroidism are squamous cell carcinoma of the lung, hypernephroma, and bladder cancer. Less commonly it is due to hepatoma or to cancer of the ovary, stomach, pancreas, parotid gland, or colon. Recent onset of symptoms, increased sedimentation rate, anemia, serum calcium greater than 14 mg/100 ml, and increased alkaline phosphatase activity without osteitis fibrosa cystica suggest ectopic hyperparathyroidism; mild hypercalcemia with a long history of nephrolithiasis or peptic ulcer suggests primary hyperthyroidism. Specific radioimmunoassays for tumor PTH have been developed and should prove helpful in differentiating between primary and ectopic hyperparathyroidism.

In milk-alkali syndrome, a history of excessive ingestion of milk products, calcium-containing antacids, and baking soda is often obtained. These patients become normocalcemic after discontinuing these habits. Patients with milk-alkali syndrome usually have renal insufficiency and low urinary calcium concentrations and are usually alkalotic rather than acidotic. Because of the high incidence of ulcer disease in hyperparathyroidism, it should be kept in mind that milk-alkali syndrome may coexist with hyperparathyroidism.

Hyperthyroidism, another cause of hypercalcemia and hypercalciuria, can usually be differentiated because manifestations of thyrotoxicosis rather than hypercalcemia bring the patient to the physician. Occasionally an elderly patient with apathetic hyperthyroidism may be hypercalcemic, so that thyroid function tests should be evaluated in all hypercalcemic patients. Treatment of hyperthyroidism with antithyroid medications causes serum calcium to return to normal levels within 8 weeks.

Normal subjects who are given thiazides may develop a transient increase in serum calcium levels, usually less than 1 mg/100 ml. Larger rises in serum calcium induced by thiazides have been reported in patients with primary hyperparathyroidism and idiopathic juvenile osteoporosis. The best way to evaluate these patients is to switch them to another antihypertensive agent or diuretic and to measure the PTH level. Thiazide-induced hypercalcemia is not associated with increased serum PTH in patients without hyperparathyroidism.

Other miscellaneous causes of hypercalcemia are Paget's disease, immobilization (especially in Paget's disease or in young patients), adrenal insufficiency, myxedema, dysproteinemias, idiopathic hypercalcemia of infancy, vitamin A intoxication, and the pancreatic cholera syndrome (Table 19–5).

Other tests include bone biopsy, urinary cyclic AMP and hydroxyproline determinations, calcium infusion tests, and radioactive calcium turnover studies, but they are seldom necessary.

C. Approach to the Normocalcemic Patient With Possible Hyperparathyroidism: The incidence of normocalcemic hyperparathyroidism in patients with hypercalciuria and recurrent nephrolithiasis (idiopathic hypercalciuria) is not known. If these patients had primary hyperparathyroidism rather than hyperabsorption of calcium from the intestine (absorptive hypercalciuria) or a primary leak of calcium from the renal tubule (renal hypercalciuria), they would obviously benefit from parathyroidectomy. Because the serum calcium concentration may fluctuate, it should be measured on more than 3 separate occasions. The serum should be analyzed the day it is obtained because the calcium level decreases with refrigeration or freezing. If available, determination of serum ionized calcium is also useful, since it may be increased in patients with normal total serum calcium levels.

If a patient has elevated serum levels of ionized calcium and PTH, the diagnosis of normocalcemic hyperparathyroidism has been confirmed. About half of patients with idiopathic hypercalciuria have increased serum PTH and a normal serum calcium. The increase in PTH in many of these patients appears to be a physiologic response to the renal loss of calcium. By treating these patients for several months with benzothiazide diuretics, which decrease urinary calcium loss, and then repeating the serum PTH measurement, it is possible to distinguish between idiopathic hypercalciuria and normocalcemic hyperparathyroidism. In the former condition, serum PTH levels become normal because the thiazide corrects the excessive loss of calcium, whereas in the latter, increased serum PTH levels persist.

The **phosphate deprivation test** is also useful in differentiating between normocalcemic hyperparathyroidism and idiopathic hypercalciuria. For 3 days the patient is given (1) a diet normal in calories and calcium content but restricted to less than 350 mg of phosphate, and (2) aluminum hydroxide gel, 60 ml 4 times a day. Calcium, phosphate, and protein levels are determined for 4 days, starting the first day of the test. If the serum calcium goes above normal, this suggests hyperparathyroidism. Deficiencies of magnesium or vitamin D probably are factors in some cases of normocalcemic hyperparathyroidism. Correction of these deficiencies may give the expected hypercalcemia if hyperparathyroidism is truly present.

Treatment

The only successful treatment of symptomatic hyperparathyroidism is by operation. The authors feel that surgery should also be performed for asymptomatic patients with hyperparathyroidism unless there are contraindications to operation or the diagnosis is uncertain. About 20% of asymptomatic hyperparathyroid patients develop clinical manifestations within 5 years, and correction of the metabolic disorder at the time it is discovered seems advisable. Borderline cases should be followed until a definitive diagnosis can be made.

A. Marked Hypercalcemia (Hypercalcemic Crisis): The initial treatment in patients with marked hypercalcemia and acute symptoms is hydration and correction of hypokalemia and hyponatremia. While the patient is being hydrated, assessment of the underlying problem is essential so that more specific therapy may be started. Milk and alkaline products, estrogens, thiazides, and vitamins A and D should be immediately discontinued. Furosemide is useful to increase calcium excretion in the rehydrated patient. Calcitonin, mithramycin, and phosphate are usually effective for short periods in treating hypercalcemia regardless of cause. Glucocorticoids are very effective in vitamin D intoxication and sarcoidosis and in many patients with cancer, including those with peptide-secreting tumors, but are less effective when there is extensive bone disease. As mentioned previously, hyperparathyroid patients only occasionally respond to glucocorticoid administration.

In patients with marked hypercalcemia, once the diagnosis of hyperparathyroidism is established, cervical exploration and parathyroidectomy should be performed since this is the most rapid and effective method of reducing serum calcium.

B. Localization: Localization of parathyroid tumors is best done at operation by an experienced surgeon who is familiar with the normal and aberrant sites of the parathyroid glands. Numerous preoperative technics have been used, including arteriography, selenomethionine and ^{131}I scanning, cine-esophagograms, thyroid lymphography, thermography, and selective and highly selective venous catheterization with parathyroid hormone immunoassay. The most reliable localizing technics are highly selective venous catheterization with parathyroid hormone immunoassay and arteriography. These studies are usually recommended only after a previous unsuccessful exploration since an experienced surgeon can nearly always locate the tumor at operation. The success rate in persistent and recurrent hyperparathyroidism is lower because of obliteration of tissue planes by adhesions from the pre-

Table 19–6. Highly selective venous catheterization and parathyroid hormone immunoassay in patients requiring reoperation.

	Patients	Localized	Accuracy
O'Riordan (London) 1971	8	5	62%
Powell (Massachusetts General Hospital) 1972	6	6	100%
Wells (National Institutes of Health) 1973	8	8*	100%
Eisenberg (cooperative group) 1974	20	17†	85%

*In 2 patients, adenomas were removed but the serum calcium levels only fell transiently.

†Combined use of venous sampling and limited arteriography.

vious operation and because the tumor may be in an ectopic location. (See Fig 19–2 and Table 19–6.)

C. Operation: The approach is similar to that for thyroidectomy. In over 80% of cases, the parathyroid tumor is found attached to the posterior capsule of the thyroid gland (Fig 19–3). The parathyroid glands are usually symmetrically placed, and parathyroid tumors often overlie the recurrent laryngeal nerve. Parathyroid tumors may also lie cephalad to the superior pole of the thyroid gland, along the great vessels of the neck in the tracheoesophageal area, in thymic tissue, in the substance of the thyroid gland itself, or in the mediastinum. Care must be taken not to traumatize the tumor or tumors since color is useful in distinguishing them from surrounding thyroid, thymus, lymph node, and fat. Two maneuvers that are helpful in localizing parathyroid tumors at operation are following the course of a branch of the inferior thyroid artery and gently palpating for the parathyroid tumor. One should attempt to identify 4 parathyroid glands, although there may be more or fewer than 4. Parathy-

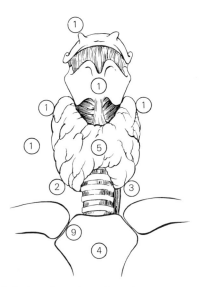

Figure 19–2. Locations of parathyroid adenomas in 28 patients who had previous cervical explorations before admission.

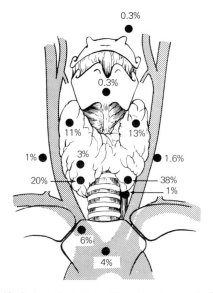

Figure 19–3. Locations of parathyroid adenomas in 300 consecutive operated cases.

roid cancers are hard and are palpable clinically in 50% of cases.

If a probable parathyroid adenoma is found, it is removed and the diagnosis confirmed by frozen section. If 2 adenomas are found, they are removed. It seems unwise to remove a grossly normal parathyroid gland intentionally, both because this has no beneficial effect and because the gland may be needed to maintain normal function after all the hyperfunctioning tissue is removed.

The presence of a normal parathyroid gland at operation indicates that the tumor removed is an adenoma rather than parathyroid hyperplasia, since in hyperplasia all the parathyroid glands are involved. A compressed rim of normal parathyroid tissue is also suggestive of an adenoma. When all parathyroid glands are hyperplastic, all but one should be removed and the remaining gland subtotally extirpated, leaving approximately 50 mg.

If exploration fails to reveal a parathyroid tumor, a conservative subtotal thyroidectomy is performed since tumors may be found intrathyroidally. If thyroid nodules are present, they should be treated as nodular goiter and removed. The incidence of differentiated thyroid carcinoma in patients with hyperparathyroidism at the University of California Medical Center in San Francisco is 7%.

Exploration of the mediastinum via a sternal split is necessary in only 1–2% of cases. If cervical exploration was nonproductive or if arteriography or highly selective venous catheterization and parathyroid immunoassay suggests a mediastinal tumor, the patient should be allowed to recover from his initial operation and return in 6–8 weeks for mediastinal exploration.

D. Postoperative Care: Following removal of a parathyroid adenoma or hyperplastic glands, the serum calcium concentration falls to normal in 24–48 hours. Patients with severe skeletal depletion ("hungry bones"), long-standing hyperparathyroidism, or high calcium levels may develop paresthesias, carpopedal spasm, or even seizures. If the symptoms are mild and serum calcium falls slowly, oral supplementation with calcium is all that is required. When marked symptoms develop, it is necessary to give intravenous calcium chloride slowly. If the response is not rapid, magnesium should also be given. (See section on hypoparathyroidism, below.)

E. Reoperation: Reexploration for persistent or recurrent hyperparathyroidism or after a previous thyroidectomy presents formidable problems and an increased risk of complications. Selective arteriography and highly selective venous catheterization with parathyroid hormone immunoassay are useful for localization in these cases. As seen in Fig 19–2, most such patients have a parathyroid tumor that can be found through a cervical incision, making mediastinal exploration unnecessary.

The recurrence rate of hyperparathyroidism after the removal of a single adenoma in most medical centers is 5% or less, so that the removal of normal-appearing parathyroid glands is unwarranted. In patients with multiple endocrine adenopathy and familial hyperparathyroidism, recurrent hyperparathyroidism is more common; therefore, extra care should be taken to remove all abnormal parathyroid tissue and to mark the normal glands at operation. If there is a role for subtotal parathyroidectomy in primary hyperparathyroidism, these are the patients in whom it should be used.

Albright F: A page out of the history of hyperparathyroidism. J Clin Endocrinol Metab 8:637, 1948.

Avioli LV: The diagnosis of primary hyperparathyroidism. Med Clin North Am 52:451, 1968.

Benson RC & others: Immunoreactive forms of circulating parathyroid hormone in primary and ectopic hyperparathyroidism. J Clin Invest 54:175, 1974.

Black WC III, Utley JR: The differential diagnosis of parathyroid adenoma and chief cell hyperplasia. Am J Clin Pathol 49:761, 1968.

Block MA & others: Primary diffuse microscopical hyperplasia of the parathyroid glands. Arch Surg 111:348, 1976.

Clark OH, Taylor S: Persistent and recurrent hyperparathyroidism. Br J Surg 59:555, 1972.

Clark OH & others: Recurrent hyperparathyroidism. Ann Surg 184:391, 1976.

Coe FL & others: Evidence for secondary hyperparathyroidism in idiopathic hypercalciuria. J Clin Invest 52:134, 1973.

Cope O & others: Primary chief-cell hyperplasia of the parathyroid glands: A new entity in the surgery of hyperparathyroidism. Ann Surg 148:375, 1958.

Cope O & others: Vicissitudes of parathyroid surgery: Trials of diagnosis and management in 51 patients with a variety of disorders. Ann Surg 154:491, 1961.

Egdahl RH & others: Measurement of circulating parathyroid hormone concentration before and after parathyroid surgery for adenoma or hyperplasia. Ann Surg 168:714, 1968.

Eisenberg H & others: Selective arteriography, venography and venous hormone assay in diagnosis and localization of parathyroid lesions. Am J Med 56:810, 1974.

Holmes EC & others: Parathyroid carcinoma: Collective review. Ann Surg 169:631, 1969.

Johansson H & others: Normocalcemic hyperparathyroidism, kidney stones, and idiopathic hypercalciuria. Surgery 77:691, 1975.

Kaplan RA & others: Metabolic effects of parathyroidectomy in asymptomatic primary hyperparathyroidism. J Clin Endocrinol Metab 42:415, 1976.

Lafferty FW: Pseudohyperparathyroidism. Medicine 45:247, 1966.

Lemann JL Jr, Donatelli AA: Calcium intoxication due to primary hyperparathyroidism: A medical and surgical emergency. Ann Intern Med 60:447, 1964.

Lloyd HM: Primary hyperparathyroidism: An analysis of the role of the parathyroid tumor. Medicine 47:53, 1968.

O'Riordan JL & others: Preoperative localization of parathyroid tumours. Lancet 2:1172, 1971.

Powell D & others: Primary hyperparathyroidism: Preoperative tumor localization and differentiation between adenoma and hyperplasia. N Engl J Med 286:1169, 1972.

Purnell DC & others: Treatment of primary hyperparathyroidism. Am J Med 56:800, 1974.

Raisz LG: The diagnosis of hyperparathyroidism (or what to do until the immunoassay comes). N Engl J Med 285:1006, 1971.

Reinhoff WF & others: The surgical treatment of hyperparathyroidism. Ann Surg 168:1061, 1968.

Steinbach HL & others: Primary hyperparathyroidism: A correlation of roentgen, clinical and pathologic features. Am J Roentgenol Radium Ther Nucl Med 86:329, 1961.

Wells SA & others: Preoperative localization of hyperfunctioning parathyroid tissue. Ann Surg 177:93, 1973.

Wilson RE & others: Hyperparathyroidism: The problems of acute parathyroid intoxication. Ann Surg 159:79, 1964.

Yendt ER, Gagne RJA: Detection of primary hyperparathyroidism with special reference to its occurrence in hypercalcemic females with "normal" or borderline serum calcium. Can Med Assoc J 98:331, 1968.

SECONDARY & TERTIARY HYPERPARATHYROIDISM

In secondary hyperparathyroidism, there is an increase in parathyroid hormone secretion in response to low plasma concentrations of ionized calcium, usually owing to renal disease and malabsorption. This results in chief cell hyperplasia. When secondary hyperparathyroidism occurs as a complication of renal disease, the serum phosphorus is usually high whereas in malabsorption, osteomalacia, or rickets it is frequently low or normal. Secondary hyperparathyroidism with renal osteodystrophy is a frequent if not universal complication of hemodialysis. Factors which play a role in renal osteodystrophy are (1) phosphate retention secondary to a decrease in the number of nephrons; (2) failure of the diseased or absent kidneys to hydroxylate 25-hydroxyvitamin D to the biologically active metabolite 1,25-dihydroxyvitamin D, with defective regulation of the intestinal absorption of calcium; (3) resistance of the bone to the action of parathyroid hormone; and (4) increased serum calcitonin concentrations. The resulting skeletal changes are identical with those of primary hyperparathyroidism.

Most patients with secondary hyperparathyroidism may be treated medically. Maintaining relatively normal serum concentrations of calcium and phosphorus during hemodialysis has decreased the incidence of bone disease dramatically.

Occasionally, a patient with secondary hyperparathyroidism develops relatively autonomous hyperplastic parathyroid glands (tertiary hyperparathyroidism). Some cases are identified after renal transplantation. Most often, the serum calcium concentration returns to normal spontaneously following renal transplantation, and one should wait at least 6 months after surgery before considering parathyroidectomy for persistent hypercalcemia. It is sometimes hard to know whether the patient has primary hyperparathyroidism with subsequent renal failure or whether he has tertiary hyperparathyroidism. In essence, surgical therapy for so-called tertiary hyperparathyroidism should be withheld until all medical approaches, including treatment with vitamin D, calcium supplementation, and phosphate binders, have been exhausted. In the rare patient in whom subtotal parathyroidectomy is indicated, all but about 50 mg of parathyroid tissue should be removed. These patients usually respond with dramatic relief of symptoms. Profound hypocalcemia frequently results following subtotal parathyroidectomy for renal osteodystrophy, both because of "hungry bones" and because of decreased parathyroid hormone secretion.

Arnaud CD: Hyperparathyroidism and renal failure. Kidney Int 4:89, 1973.

David DS: Calcium metabolism in renal failure. Am J Med 58:48, 1975.

Johnson WJ & others: Prevention and reversal of progressive secondary hyperparathyroidism in patients maintained by hemodialysis. Am J Med 56:827, 1974.

Massey SG & others: Skeletal resistance to parathyroid hormone in renal failure: Studies in 105 human subjects. Ann Intern Med 78:357, 1973.

Ogg CS: Parathyroidectomy in the treatment of secondary renal hyperparathyroidism. Kidney Int 4:168, 1973.

Slatopolsky E, Bricker NS: The role of phosphorus restriction in the prevention of secondary hyperparathyroidism in chronic renal disease. Kidney Int 4:141, 1973.

HYPOPARATHYROIDISM

Essentials of Diagnosis

- Paresthesias, muscle cramps, carpopedal spasm, laryngeal stridor, convulsions, malaise, muscle and abdominal cramps, tetany, urinary frequency, lethargy, anxiety, psychoneurosis, depression, and psychosis.
- Surgical neck scar. Positive Chvostek and Trousseau signs.
- Brittle and atrophied nails, defective teeth, cataracts.
- Hypocalcemia and hyperphosphatemia, low or absent urinary calcium, low or absent circulating parathyroid hormone.
- Calcification of basal ganglia, cartilage, and arteries on x-ray.

General Considerations

Hypoparathyroidism occurs most commonly as a complication of thyroidectomy, especially when performed for carcinoma or recurrent goiter. Hypoparathyroidism occurs only rarely as a complication of a first operation for goiter and is even less common after surgery for hyperparathyroidism unless 3 or more normal adenomatous or hyperplastic parathyroids are removed. Clinical hypoparathyroidism has been reported in a rare patient after ^{131}I therapy of Graves' disease. In idiopathic hypoparathyroidism, an autoimmune process is suspected because of its association with autoimmune adrenocortical insufficiency. Neonatal tetany may be associated with maternal hyperparathyroidism.

Clinical Findings

A. Symptoms and Signs: The manifestations of acute hypoparathyroidism are due to hypocalcemia. Low serum calcium levels precipitate tetany. Latent tetany may be indicated by mild or moderate paresthesias with a positive Chvostek or Trousseau sign. The initial manifestations are paresthesias, circumoral numbness, muscle cramps, irritability, carpopedal spasm, convulsions, opisthotonos, and marked anxiety. Dry skin, brittleness of the nails, and spotty alopecia including loss of the eyebrows are common. Since primary hypoparathyroidism is rare, a history of thyroidectomy is almost always present. Generally speaking, the sooner the clinical manifestations appear postoperatively, the more serious the prognosis. After many years, some patients become adapted to a low serum calcium concentration so that tetany is no longer evident.

B. Laboratory Findings: Hypocalcemia and hyperphosphatemia are demonstrable. The urine phosphate is low or absent, tubular resorption of phosphate is high, and the urine calcium is low.

C. X-Ray Findings: In chronic hypoparathyroidism, x-rays may show calcification of the basal ganglia, arteries, and the external ear.

Differential Diagnosis

A good history is most important in the differential diagnosis of hypocalcemic tetany. Occasionally, tetany occurs with alkalosis and hyperventilation. Symptomatic hypocalcemia occurring after thyroid or parathyroid surgery is due to parathyroid removal or injury by trauma or devascularization or is secondary to "hungry bones." Other major causes of hypocalcemic tetany are intestinal malabsorption and renal insufficiency. These conditions may also be suggested by a history of diarrhea, pancreatitis, steatorrhea, or renal disease. Laboratory abnormalities include decreased concentrations of serum proteins, cholesterol, and carotene and increased concentrations of stool fat in malabsorption and an increased BUN and creatinine in renal failure. Serum PTH concentrations are low in hypocalcemia secondary to idiopathic or iatrogenic hypoparathyroidism. Consequently, serum calcium concentrations and urinary calcium, phosphorus, and hydroxyproline levels are decreased, whereas serum phosphate concentrations are increased. In hypocalcemia secondary to malabsorption and renal failure, serum PTH concentrations are elevated and the serum alkaline phosphatase concentration is normal or increased.

Treatment

The aim of treatment is to raise the serum calcium concentration, to bring the patient out of tetany, and to lower the serum phosphate level so as to prevent metastatic calcification. Most postoperative hypocalcemia is transient; if it persists longer than 2–3 weeks, it is apt to require chronic treatment.

A. Acute Hypoparathyroid Tetany: Acute hypoparathyroid tetany requires emergency treatment. Make certain an adequate airway exists. Reassure the anxious patient to avoid hyperventilation and resulting alkalosis. Give calcium chloride, 10–20 ml of 10% solution slowly IV, until tetany disappears. Ten to 50 ml of 10% calcium chloride may then be added to 1 liter of saline or 5% dextrose solution and administered by slow IV drip. Adjust the rate of infusion so that hourly determinations of serum calcium are normal. Occasionally, hypomagnesemia may be found in some cases of tetany not responding to calcium treatment. In such cases, magnesium (as magnesium sulfate) should be given in a dosage of 4–8 g/day IM or 2–4 g/day IV.

B. Chronic Hypoparathyroidism: Once tetany has responded to intravenous calcium, change to oral calcium (gluconate, lactate, or carbonate) 3 times daily. The management of the hypoparathyroid patient is difficult because the difference between the controlling and intoxicating dose of vitamin D may be quite small. Episodes of hypercalcemia in treated patients are often unpredictable and may occur in the absence of symptoms. Vitamin D intoxication may develop after months or years of good control on a given therapeutic regimen. Dihydrotachysterol is useful in the exceptional case when the usual measures fail to control the hypercalcemia. Frequent serum calcium determinations are necessary to regulate the proper dosage of vitamin D and to avoid vitamin D intoxication. The dose of vitamin D required to correct hypocalcemia may vary from 25,000–200,000 IU/day. Phosphorus should also be limited in the diet; in most patients, simple elimination of dairy products is sufficient. In some patients, aluminum hydroxide gel may be necessary to bind phosphorus in the gut to increase fecal losses.

PSEUDOHYPOPARATHYROIDISM & PSEUDOPSEUDOHYPOPARATHYROIDISM

Pseudohypoparathyroidism is an X-linked autosomal syndrome due to a defective renal adenylate cyclase system. It is characterized by the clinical and chemical features of hypoparathyroidism associated with a round face, a short, thick body, stubby fingers, short metacarpal and metatarsal bones, mental deficiency, and x-ray evidence of calcification. There is evidence of increased bone resorption and osteitis fibrosa cystica despite the hypocalcemia that accompanies the syndrome. Patients with pseudohypoparathyroidism do not respond to intravenous administration of 200 units of parathyroid hormone with phosphaturia (Ellsworth-Howard test) and have increased serum concentrations of PTH. This condition is usually controlled with smaller amounts of vitamin D than idiopathic hypoparathyroidism, and resistance to therapy is uncommon.

Pseudopseudohypoparathyroidism is also a genetically transmitted disease with the same physical findings as pseudohypoparathyroidism but with normal serum calcium and phosphorus concentrations. Patients with this condition may become hypocalcemic during periods of stress such as pregnancy and rapid growth, thus suggesting a genetic defect in common with pseudohypoparathyroidism.

Avioli LV: The therapeutic approach to hypoparathyroidism. Am J Med 57:34, 1974.

Bronsky D & others: Idiopathic hypoparathyroidism and pseudohypoparathyroidism: Case reports and review of the literature. Medicine 37:317, 1958.

Kolb FO, Steinbach HL: Pseudohypoparathyroidism with secondary hyperparathyroidism and osteitis fibrosa. J Clin Endocrinol Metab 22:59, 1962.

Kooh SW & others: Treatment of hypoparathyroidism and pseu-dohypoparathyroidism with metabolites of vitamin D: Evidence for impaired conversion of 25-hydroxyvitamin D to 1α,25-dihydroxyvitamin D. N Engl J Med 293:840, 1975.

Parfitt AM: The spectrum of hypoparathyroidism. J Clin Endocrinol Metab 34:152, 1972.

●　●　●

General References

Bondy PK, Rosenberg CG (editors): *Duncan's Diseases of Metabolism,* 7th ed. Saunders, 1974.

DeGroot LJ, Stanbury JB: *The Thyroid and Its Diseases,* 4th ed. Wiley, 1975.

Dillon RS: *Handbook of Endocrinology.* Lea & Febiger, 1973.

Edis AJ, Ayala LA, Egdahl RH: *Manual of Endocrine Surgery.* Springer-Verlag, 1975.

Goldman L, Gordan GS, Roof BS: The parathyroids: Progress, problems and practice. Curr Probl Surg, Aug 1971.

Hellstrom J, Ivemark BI: Primary hyperparathyroidism: Clinical and structural findings in 138 cases. Acta Chir Scand (Suppl) 294:1, 1962.

Pittman JA Jr (editor): Symposium on the treatment of thyroid disease. Mod Treat 6:441, 1969.

Schneider AB, Sherwood LM: Calcium homeostasis and the pathogenesis and management of hypercalcemic disorders. Metabolism 23:975, 1974.

Sedgwick CI: *Surgery of the Thyroid Gland.* Saunders, 1974.

Wermer SC, Ingbar SH (editors): *The Thyroid: A Fundamental and Clinical Text,* 3rd ed. Harper & Row, 1971.

Williams RH (editor): *Textbook of Endocrinology,* 5th ed. Saunders, 1974.

20 . . .
Breast

John L. Wilson, MD

CARCINOMA OF THE FEMALE BREAST

Essentials of Diagnosis

- Higher incidence in women who have never borne children, those with a family history of breast cancer, and those with a personal history of breast cancer or dysplasia.
- Early findings: Single, nontender, firm to hard mass with ill-defined margins; nipple erosion, with or without a mass; mammography may detect cancer before development of a palpable mass.
- Later findings: Skin or nipple retraction; axillary lymphadenopathy; breast enlargement, redness, edema, pain, fixation of mass to skin or chest wall.
- Late findings: Ulceration; supraclavicular lymphadenopathy; edema of arm; bone, lung, liver, brain, or other distant metastases.

General Considerations

A. Incidence and Mortality Rate: The breast is the commonest site of cancer in women, and cancer of the breast is the leading cause of death from cancer among women in the USA. Breast cancer is the leading cause of death due to all causes in women age 40–44 and is frequent in women at all ages past 30. The probability of developing the disease increases throughout life. The mean and the median age of women with breast cancer is 60–61. Breast cancer occurs 100 times more frequently in women than in men.

The American Cancer Society estimates that 88,000 new cases of breast cancer will occur in women in the USA in 1976 (Fig 20–1). At the present rates of incidence, one of every 13 American women will develop breast cancer during her lifetime. Data from the Connecticut State Department of Health indicate that the annual age-adjusted incidence rate for breast cancer in that state increased from 55 per 100,000 in 1940–1944 to 72 per 100,000 in 1965–1968. This is similar to a nationwide incidence of 72.2 per 100,000 women reported by the Third National Cancer Survey for cases diagnosed in 1969. Thus, for reasons which are not understood, the incidence of female breast cancer appears to be increasing in the USA.

According to the annual report of vital statistics from the USPHS there were 32,850 deaths in women from breast cancer in the USA in 1974. The American Cancer Society estimates that the number of deaths will be 33,000 in 1976 (Fig 20–1). Despite all efforts to date, including the achievement of an 80–85% 5-year survival rate when treatment is instituted early, there has been no great reduction in the overall annual mortality rate from breast cancer in the past 45 years. When death rates are age-adjusted to permit valid comparisons from year to year, it is found that the annual death rate from breast cancer among American women has remained at approximately 22 per 100,000 since 1930.

B. Etiology and Risk Factors:

1. Heredity–The cause of breast cancer is not known, but a predisposition to breast cancer can be inherited. The mechanism of inheritance is not clear. Numerous investigations have shown that female relatives of women with mammary carcinoma have a higher rate of disease than the general population. There is evidence that a woman has at least twice the risk of breast cancer (as compared to the general population) if her family history includes breast cancer in her mother, grandmother, aunt, or sister (Macklin MT: J Natl Cancer Inst 22:927, 1959.) Reports of symmetric mammary cancer in monozygotic twins support the conclusion that inheritance plays a role in some cases.

2. Marital status, parity, and lactation–Marital status and parity also influence the incidence of breast cancer. Single and nulliparous women have a slightly higher incidence of breast cancer than married and parous women. Women with 3 or more children have a lower incidence than women with fewer children. Menarche after age 15 and artificial menopause are also associated with a lower incidence of breast cancer, whereas early menarche (under age 12) and late natural menopause (after age 50) are associated with a slight increase in risk of developing breast cancer. These observations regarding fertility and ovarian function suggest that hormonal factors have some influence on the incidence of breast cancer. Lactation probably does not protect from breast cancer, as formerly thought. Breast cancer patients do not differ from unaffected women with respect to a history of lactation if account is taken of the fact that breast cancer patients tend to be of low parity.

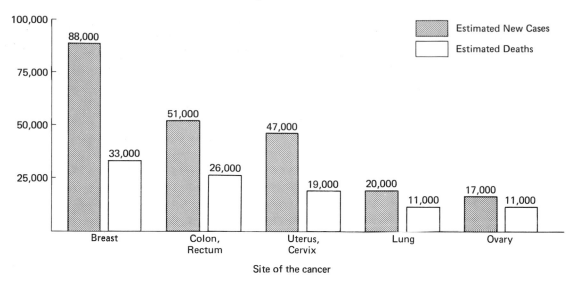

Figure 20–1. Estimated new cases of cancer (shaded bars) and deaths from cancer (open bars) in women in the USA in 1976. (American Cancer Society data.)

3. Mammary dysplasia—Mammary dysplasia (cystic disease of the breast), particularly when accompanied by proliferative changes, papillomatosis, or solid hyperplasia, is associated with an increased incidence of cancer. The apparent relationship between cancer and mammary dysplasia again raises the question of hormonal factors in the causation of breast cancer. Although the pathogenesis of mammary dysplasia is not known, this disorder is believed to result either from a relative or absolute increase in estrogen or a relative or absolute decrease in progesterone. The inference is inescapable that the variations in hormonal environment which cause the pathologic changes of mammary dysplasia may under certain conditions also induce neoplasia.

4. Cancer of uterus and ovary—Women with cancer of the uterine corpus have a breast cancer risk almost double that of the general population, and women with breast cancer have a comparably increased endometrial cancer risk. The association between cancer of the breast and cancer of the ovary is less well documented, but familial occurrence of both neoplasms together has been reported. The explanation for the association of breast cancer with cancer of the endometrium or ovary is unknown. The common causal factors are possibly endocrine, but this has not been established.

5. Endogenous hormones—Many studies have been done in an attempt to determine whether women with breast cancer or with a predisposition to the disease show an abnormal pattern of excretion of estrogens, androgens, hydroxycorticosteroids, or prolactin. These studies have proved very difficult to conduct, control, and interpret. As a result, evidence based on hormonal assays is conflicting, and it is not now possible to identify by these means those women with a high risk of developing breast cancer. It is suspected,

however, that a significant percentage of women with breast cancer may have an abnormal hormonal environment which will be of diagnostic importance when better understood.

6. Trauma—Both breast trauma and cancer are common, and there is no evidence that trauma to the breast causes cancer.

7. Environmental and ethnic factors—Age-adjusted female cancer death rates show that, in general, rates reported from developing countries are low whereas rates are high in developed countries, with the notable exception of Japan. Some of the variability may be due to underdiagnosis and underreporting in the developing countries or to differences in reporting practices, but undoubtedly there are environmental, dietary, hormonal, fertility, genetic, or other factors yet to be determined. There has been great interest in the low breast cancer rate in Japanese women, which is well illustrated by statistics from California. Although their breast cancer rates remain relatively low, Japanese women who have migrated to the USA and their daughters born in the USA show some increase in rates over those who stay in Japan. Changing reproductive patterns (ie, trend toward later initial pregnancy and more nulliparous individuals) probably contribute to the increased incidence of breast cancer in Japanese women in the USA as compared with those in Japan. However, this does not adequately account for the marked difference in incidence that exists or the increasing rate among Japanese-American women. Other causes must be sought among the dietary and environmental factors to which they are exposed (Buell P: J Natl Cancer Inst 51:1479, 1973).

8. Oral contraceptives and menopausal estrogens—Contraceptives containing estrogens and progestins may produce proliferation of epithelial elements within the breast and stimulation of the intralobular and interlobar connective tissues. The reaction in the ductal epithelium is particularly noticeable. Tenderness of the breasts, nodularity, galactorrhea, and fibroadenomas are among the rare gross breast changes that can occur. Although there is no definite evidence that oral contraceptives are related to human breast cancer, these agents may cause both gross and microscopic changes in the breast, and further information on their long-term effects must be accumulated before the possibility of a carcinogenic potential can be ruled out. Recent evidence presented by Hoover and associates (N Engl J Med 295:401, 1976) suggests that the administration of estrogens to menopausal women may result in an increased risk of breast cancer after 10–12 years. Definitive assessment of the possible carcinogenic effect of exogenous estrogenic hormones such as oral contraceptives and menopausal estrogens will require prolonged controlled studies involving large numbers of women. Until the issue has been settled by such studies, physicians who prescribe these agents and women who take them should keep in mind that potentially carcinogenic substances not uncommonly have long latent periods, sometimes measured in decades, during which risk cannot be determined.

9. Reserpine—Routine scanning of data from a multipurpose survey of inpatients in hospitals in the Boston area revealed an association between reserpine use and breast cancer (Boston Collaborative Drug Surveillance Program; Lancet 2:669, 1974). Similar findings were reported from England and Finland (Lancet 2:672, 1974; Lancet 2:675, 1974). More recent surveys by O'Fallon WM & others (Lancet 2:292, 1975), Laska EM & others (Lancet 2:296, 1975), and Mack TM & others (N Engl J Med 292:1366, 1975) have failed to confirm the relationship between chronic reserpine administration and breast cancer. An editorial by Jick H (JAMA 233:896, 1975) points out the difficulty of disproving the hypothesis that there is an association between reserpine and breast cancer. Pending further study of this question, individual physicians and their patients must decide for themselves what credence should be given to reports of cancer risk associated with the use of reserpine.

10. Summary of risk factors—Women who are at greater than normal risk of developing breast cancer should be identified by their physicians and followed appropriately. Screening programs involving periodic physical examination and mammography of asymptomatic women will be most productive when applied to individuals at increased risk. The summary of characteristics in Table 20–1 will aid in the selection of such individuals for special attention.

C. Host-Tumor Relationship: The growth rate of breast cancer and the capacity to metastasize are determined by the balance between the biologic behavior of the neoplasm and the immunologic response of the host. Growth potential of tumor and resistance of host vary over a wide range from patient to patient and may be altered during the course of the disease. The differing growth rates of breast cancers are well illustrated by the observation that the doubling time of breast

Table 20–1. Risk factors associated with increased incidence of breast cancer.*

	Characteristics
Race	Caucasian vs black or Oriental
Age	Over 50
Family history	Breast cancer in grandmother, aunt, mother, sister
Previous medical history	Endometrial cancer
	Mammary dysplasia
	Cancer in other breast
Menstrual history	Early menarche (under age 12)
	Late menopause (after age 50)
	Aggregate years of menstrual activity greater than 30
Marital history	Never married vs married
Pregnancy	Never pregnant
	One or 2 pregnancies vs 3 or more
	First child born after age 30

*Normal lifetime risk in Caucasian women = 1 in 13.

cancer cells ranges from 23 days in a rapidly growing lesion to 309 days in a slowly growing one. Assuming that the rate of doubling is constant and that the neoplasm originates in one cell, a slowly growing carcinoma may not reach a clinically detectable size (1 cm) for 8 years. On the other hand, rapidly growing cancers have a much shorter preclinical course and a greater tendency to metastasize to regional nodes or more distant sites by the time a breast mass is discovered.

Because of differing patterns of cancer growth and host resistance, the clinical manifestations of breast cancer are variable and often unpredictable. Although the mean duration of life in untreated carcinoma of the breast is about 3 years, some untreated patients succumb within a few months after diagnosis, others live 4 or 5 years, and a few survive as long as 15–30 years. Treatment plans, evaluation of various forms of treatment, and estimates of prognosis should take this diversity of behavior into account.

Clinical Findings

The patient with breast cancer usually presents with a lump in the breast. Clinical evaluation begins with the history and physical examination, the latter including special attention to the characteristics of the local lesion and to a search for evidence of metastases in regional nodes or distant sites. After the diagnosis of breast cancer has been confirmed histologically on tissue obtained by biopsy, additional laboratory studies are often needed to complete the search for distant metastases or an occult primary in the other breast. Then, prior to a decision on treatment, all the available clinical data are used to determine the extent or "stage" of the patient's disease. Initial therapy should always be preceded by careful clinical staging in order to avoid inappropriate measures such as, for example, radical mastectomy in a patient with distant metastases (see p 279).

A. Symptoms: Evaluation of the patient with a breast complaint includes a careful history and a com-

Table 20–2. Initial symptoms of mammary carcinoma.*

Symptom	Percentage of All Cases
Painless breast mass	66
Painful breast mass	11
Nipple discharge	9
Local edema	4
Nipple retraction	3
Nipple crusting	2
Miscellaneous symptoms	5

*Adapted from report of initial symptoms in 774 patients treated for breast cancer at Ellis Fischel State Cancer Hospital, Columbia, Missouri. Reproduced, with permission, from Spratt JS Jr, Donegan WL: *Cancer of the Breast.* Saunders, 1967.

plete physical examination. In the history, special note should be made of menarche, pregnancies, parity, artificial or natural menopause, date of last menstrual period, previous breast lesions, and a family history of breast cancer. Back or other bone pain may be the result of osseous metastases. Systemic complaints or weight loss should raise the question of metastases, which may involve any organ but most frequently the bones, liver, and lungs. The more advanced the cancer in terms of size of primary and extent of regional node involvement, the higher the incidence of metastatic spread to distant sites.

The presenting complaint in about 80% of patients with breast cancer is a lump (usually painless) in the breast (Table 20–2). About 90% of breast masses are discovered by the patient herself. Less frequent symptoms are breast pain; nipple discharge; erosion, retraction, enlargement, or itching of the nipple; and redness, generalized hardness, enlargement, or shrinking of the breast. Rarely, an axillary mass, swelling of the arm, or bone pain (from metastases) may be the first symptom.

B. **Examination of the Breast:** This should be meticulous, methodical, and gentle. Inspection is the first step and should be carried out with the patient sitting, arms at sides and then overhead (Fig 20–2). Abnormal variations in breast size and contour, minimal nipple retraction, and slight edema, redness, or retraction of the skin are best identified by careful observation in good light. Asymmetry of the breasts and retraction or dimpling of the skin can often be accentuated by having the patient raise her arms overhead or press her hands on her hips in order to contract the pectoralis muscles. Axillary and supraclavicular areas should be thoroughly palpated for enlarged nodes with the patient sitting (Fig 20–3). Palpation of the breast for masses or other changes is best performed with the patient supine and arm abducted (Fig 20–4). In some series, 5–10% of cases of breast carcinoma have been discovered during physical examination done for other purposes. The location, size, consistency, and other physical features of all mammary lesions should be recorded on a drawing of the breast for future reference.

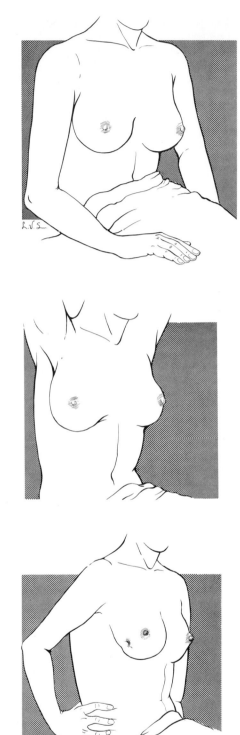

Figure 20–2. Inspection of breasts. Observe breasts with patient sitting, arms at sides and overhead, for presence of asymmetry and nipple or skin retraction. These signs may be accentuated by having the patient raise her arms overhead. Skin retraction or dimpling may be demonstrated by having the patient press her hand on her hip in order to contract the pectoralis muscles.

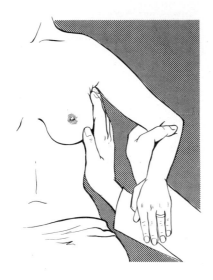
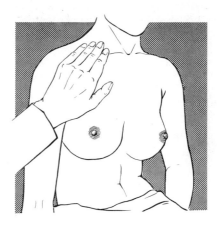

Figure 20—3. Palpation of axillary and supraclavicular regions for enlarged lymph nodes.

Breast cancer usually consists of a nontender, firm, or hard lump with poorly delimited margins (caused by local infiltration). Slight skin or nipple retraction is an important sign. Minimal asymmetry of the breast may be noted. Very small (1–2 mm) erosions of the nipple epithelium may be the only manifestation of carcinoma of the Paget type. Watery, serous, or bloody discharge from the nipple is an occasional early sign.

A lesion smaller than 1 cm in diameter may be difficult or impossible for the examiner to feel and yet may be discovered by the patient. She should always be asked to demonstrate the location of the mass; if the physician fails to confirm the patient's supicions, the examination should be repeated in 1 month. During the premenstrual phase of the cycle, increased innocuous nodularity may suggest neoplasm or may obscure an underlying lesion. If there is any question regarding the nature of an abnormality under these circumstances, the patient should be asked to return after her period.

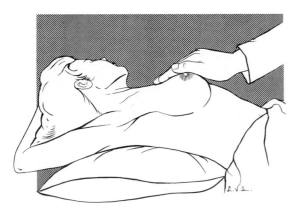

Figure 20—4. Palpation of breasts. Palpation is performed with the patient supine and arm abducted.

The following are characteristic of advanced carcinoma: edema, redness, nodularity, or ulceration of the skin; the presence of a large primary tumor; fixation to the chest wall; enlargement, shrinkage, or retraction of the breast; marked axillary lymphadenopathy; supraclavicular lymphadenopathy; edema of the ipsilateral arm; and distant metastases.

C. Examination of the Regional Nodes: Evaluation of the axillary and supraclavicular nodes is an essential feature of the breast examination. A clinical opinion regarding the presence or absence of metastases in these nodes is required in order to determine the stage of breast cancer for treatment purposes.

With regard to the axilla, one or 2 movable, nontender, not particularly firm lymph nodes 5 mm or less in diameter are frequently present and are generally of no significance. Firm or hard nodes larger than 5 mm in diameter must be assumed to contain metastases until proved otherwise. Axillary nodes which are matted or fixed to skin or deep structures indicate an advanced stage of the disease (at least stage III). Unfortunately, assessment of the axillary nodes by palpation is not always accurate. Histologic studies show that microscopic metastases are present in up to 30% of patients with clinically negative nodes. On the other hand, if the examiner thinks that the axillary nodes are involved, this will prove on histologic section to be correct in about 85% of cases. The incidence of positive axillary nodes increases with the size of the primary tumor and with the invasiveness of the neoplasm according to pathologic type.

Usually no nodes are palpable in the supraclavicular fossa. Firm or hard nodes of any size in this location, or just beneath the clavicle (infraclavicular nodes), are suggestive of metastatic cancer and should be considered for biopsy. Ipsilateral supraclavicular or infraclavicular nodes containing cancer indicate that the patient is in an advanced stage of the disease (at least stage III). Edema of the ipsilateral arm, commonly caused by metastatic infiltration of regional lymphatics, is also a sign of advanced cancer.

D. Special Clinical Forms of Breast Carcinoma:

1. Paget's carcinoma—The basic lesion is intraductal carcinoma, usually well differentiated and multicentric in the nipple and breast ducts. The nipple epithelium is infiltrated, but gross nipple changes are often minimal and a tumor mass may not be palpable. The first symptom is often itching or burning of the nipple with a superficial erosion or ulceration. The diagnosis is established by biopsy of the erosion.

Paget's carcinoma is not common (about 3% of all breast cancers), but it is important because it appears innocuous. It is frequently diagnosed and treated as dermatitis or bacterial infection, leading to unfortunate delay in detection. When the lesion consists of nipple changes only, the incidence of axillary metastases is about 5%. When a breast tumor is also present, the incidence of axillary metastases rises to about 67% with an associated marked decrease in prospects for cure by surgical or other treatment.

2. Inflammatory carcinoma—This is the most malignant form of breast cancer and comprises about 3% of all cases. The clinical findings consist of a rapidly growing, sometimes painful mass which enlarges the breast. The overlying skin becomes erythematous, edematous, and warm. The diagnosis should be made clinically only when the redness involves more than one-third of the skin over the breast. The inflammatory changes, often mistaken for an infectious process, are caused by carcinomatous invasion of the dermal lymphatics with resulting edema and hyperemia (Ellis DL, Teitelbaum SL: Cancer 33:1045, 1974; Saltzstein SL: Cancer 34:82, 1974). These tumors may be caused by a variety of histologic types. Metastases tend to occur early and widely, and for this reason inflammatory carcinoma is rarely curable. Radical mastectomy is seldom, if ever, indicated. Radiation and hormone therapy and anticancer chemotherapy are the measures most likely to be of value.

3. Occurrence during pregnancy or lactation— Only 1–2% of breast cancers occur during pregnancy or lactation. This overall low incidence in part reflects the fact that only 15% of mammary carcinomas occur during the reproductive years. When breast cancer occurs in women under age 35, it is concurrent with pregnancy in about 10–15% of cases. The diagnosis of breast cancer is frequently delayed during pregnancy or lactation because physiologic changes in the breast may obscure the true nature of the lesion. This results in a tendency of both patients and physicians to misinterpret the findings and to procrastinate in deciding on biopsy. When the neoplasm is confined to the breast, the 5-year survival rate after radical mastectomy is about 60%; therefore, the former extreme pessimism regarding prognosis was not justified. On the other hand, axillary metastases are already present in 60–70% of patients with breast cancer during lactation or pregnancy and are a grave prognostic sign. When they are present, the 5-year survival rate after radical mastectomy is only 5–10%. Pregnancy (or lactation) is not a contraindication to radical or modified radical mastectomy, and treatment should be based on the stage of the disease as in the nonpregnant (or nonlactating) woman.

4. Bilateral breast cancer—It is not surprising that mammary cancer is often bilateral since both breasts are subject to the same genetic and hormonal influences. The literature shows an incidence of simultaneous bilateral breast cancer of about 1%, but there is a 5–8% incidence of later occurrence of cancer in the second breast. Robbins and Berg (Cancer 17:1501, 1964), in a 20-year retrospective study, found that the risk increased about 10 times for the second breast; that bilaterality occurred more often in women under 50 years of age; and that it was more frequent when the tumor in the primary breast was multicentric or of comedo or lobular type.

Mammography and biopsy of the opposite breast are beginning to provide additional information on the simultaneous or later development of bilateral breast cancer. Mammography will occasionally show evidence of occult carcinoma preoperatively in the clinically uninvolved breast and is especially useful as a follow-up examination. Routine biopsy of the opposite breast has been debated for the past 2 decades and is of proved value in lobular carcinoma. According to reports in the literature, the incidence of bilateral involvement by lobular carcinoma ranges from 35–59% in the patients biopsied (Donegan WL, Perez-Mesa LM: Ann Surg 176:178, 1972).

E. Laboratory Findings: Carcinoma localized to the breast and axillary nodes causes no abnormalities detectable by clinical laboratory examinations. Certain tests may be useful as clues to the presence of more widespread disease. A consistently elevated sedimentation rate may be the result of disseminated cancer. Liver metastases may be associated with elevation of alkaline phosphatase. Hypercalcemia is an occasional important finding in advanced malignancy of the breast.

F. X-Ray Findings: Because of the frequency of metastases to the lungs, preparation for a radical mastectomy and initial evaluation of every patient with known breast cancer should include posteroanterior and lateral chest films.

G. Radionuclide Scanning: Bone scans utilizing a bone-seeking nuclide such as technetium Tc 99m-labeled phosphates or phosphonates and a rectilinear scanner or gamma camera are more sensitive than skeletal x-rays in detecting metastatic breast cancer. Therefore, bone scan may be useful in the diagnostic evaluation of patients with breast cancer before radical surgery even in the absence of symptoms or of findings on roentgenography (Hoffman HC, Marty R: Am J Surg 124:194, 1972). Unexpected bony metastases, even in early breast cancer, have been discovered on bone scans with sufficient frequency to warrant giving serious consideration to this relatively simple procedure before performing mastectomy for cancer. X-rays should be obtained of bony areas suggestive of metastatic involvement on scan.

Radionuclide scanning or computerized tomography of liver and brain is of value when metastases are suspected in these areas.

H. Mammography: A mammogram is a soft tissue radiologic examination of the breast. The 2 methods in common use for obtaining mammograms are ordinary film radiography and xeroradiography. In the latter method, in lieu of a roentgen film, an aluminum plate with an electrically charged selenium layer is exposed to x-rays and the electrostatic image is transferred to paper by a special process. From the standpoint of diagnosing breast cancer, radiography and xeroradiography give comparable results. Xeromammography has the advantage of lower radiation exposure for the patient except where low-dose film mammography is available.

Mammography is the only reliable means of detecting breast cancer before a mass can be palpated in the breast. Some breast cancers can be identified by mammography as long as 2 years before reaching a size detectable by palpation. A number of other methods have been used experimentally to search for breast cancer in a preclinical stage. The methods include thermography, ultrasonography, isotope scanning, and angiography. None of these technics—including thermography, which has been extensively studied—is sufficiently reliable to warrant general use.

Indications for mammography are as follows: (1) to evaluate the opposite breast when a diagnosis of breast cancer is made and periodically thereafter; (2) to evaluate questionable or ill-defined breast masses, nipple discharge, erosion, or retraction, skin dimpling or other suspicious change, or breast pain; (3) to search for occult breast cancer in women with metastatic disease from an unknown primary; and (4) to screen asymptomatic women at regular intervals for the early diagnosis of breast cancer.

Indications for mammography are continuously under review because of the possibility that repeated mammograms may result in exposure of the breast to a hazardous level of ionizing radiation. Bailar (Ann Intern Med 84:77, 1976) has summarized evidence which suggests that ionizing radiation in the amount delivered within a few years by annual screening mammography may be carcinogenic and thus associated with an increased incidence of breast cancer. The potential value of periodic mammography in patients at increased risk has led others to emphasize the importance of continuing screening programs under proper guidelines (see below).

Although false-positive and false-negative results are occasionally obtained with mammography, the experienced radiologist can interpret mammograms correctly in about 90% of cases. Where mammography is employed proficiently, the yield of malignant lesions on biopsy remains around 35%. This is in spite of the fact that more biopsies are done.

I. Biopsy: The diagnosis of breast cancer depends ultimately upon examination of tissue removed by biopsy. Treatment should never be undertaken without an unequivocal histologic diagnosis of cancer. The safest course is to biopsy all suspicious masses found on physical examination and, in the absence of a mass, suspicious lesions demonstrated by mammography. About 30% of lesions thought to be definitely cancer prove on biopsy to be benign, and about 15% of lesions believed to be benign are found to be malignant. These findings clearly demonstrate the fallibility of clinical judgment and the necessity for biopsy to settle the issue in most cases.

Specific indications for biopsy of the breast include the following: (1) persistent mass, (2) bloody nipple discharge, (3) eczematoid nipple, and (4) positive mammogram. Unexplained axillary adenopathy in the absence of a breast mass calls for mammography and, if negative, biopsy of the axillary node. Biopsy of the opposite breast is practiced in some centers when the diagnosis of operable breast cancer has been established. This procedure is most clearly justified in lobular carcinoma, which is frequently bilateral. The preferred biopsy site, provided there are no physical or mammographic indications of a lesion elsewhere, is the upper outer quadrant of the breast since this is the commonest site of breast cancer.

Various methods are used to perform breast biopsy, the procedure chosen depending upon the nature of the lesion and the preference of the operator.

The simplest method is needle biopsy, either by aspiration of tumor cells or by obtaining a small core of tissue with a Vim-Silverman or other special needle. This is an office procedure especially suitable for easily accessible lesions larger than a few centimeters in diameter. A negative needle biopsy should be verified by open biopsy. The experience of the pathologist is an important consideration when deciding whether to use needle biopsy.

Open biopsy in an operating room under local or general anesthesia without admitting the patient to the hospital is a procedure now widely favored. Decisions on additional work-up for metastatic disease and on definitive therapy can be made and discussed with the patient after the histologic diagnosis of cancer has been established. This approach has the advantage of avoiding unnecessary hospitalization and diagnostic procedures in many patients since cancer is found in only about 35% of patients who require biopsy for differential diagnosis of a breast lump. The biopsy procedure and the delay of definitive treatment for a few days do not adversely affect the course of the disease.

As an alternative in potentially operable lesions, the patient may be admitted directly to the hospital where the diagnosis is made on frozen section of tissue obtained by open biopsy under general anesthesia. If the frozen section is positive, proceed immediately with mastectomy.

J. Cytology: Cytologic examination of nipple discharge or cyst fluid may be helpful, but breast biopsy is usually required when nipple discharge or cyst fluid is bloody or cytologically questionable.

Early Detection

A. Screening Programs: A number of mass screening programs consisting of physical and mammographic examination of the breasts of asymptomatic women have been conducted in the past with encouraging results. Currently, the National Cancer Institute has joined with the American Cancer Society in establishing 27 Breast Cancer Detection Demonstration Projects across the USA to determine the value of available technology in finding early breast cancer in asymptomatic women. The objective is to screen 300,000 women age 35 and older over a 5-year period. The projects are discovering more than 6 cancers per 1000 women. They are finding that 79% of these women have negative axillary lymph nodes at the time of surgery whereas, by contrast, only 45% of patients found in the course of usual medical practice have uninvolved axillary nodes. Detecting breast cancer before it has spread to the axillary nodes greatly increases the chance of survival, and about 84% of such women will survive at least 5 years.

The most impressive finding of the ACS/NCI Demonstration Projects is that at least 45% of breast cancers have been detected by mammography alone. These lesions were not palpable on physical examination. For such minimal tumors without axillary metastases, 5-year survival rates of 95% have been reported compared to only about 45% when axillary nodes are involved.

Both physical examination and mammography are necessary for maximum yield in screening programs since about 45% of early breast cancers can be discovered only by mammography and about 40% can be detected only by palpation.

As noted above, questions have been raised regarding the possible carcinogenic effect of ionizing radiation on the breasts of women subjected to repeated mammography for screening purposes. Consideration is therefore being given to the advisability of restricting mammographic screening of asymptomatic women to those age 50 and older. Women at high risk of developing breast cancer because of family history, mammary dysplasia, or previous breast cancer may be appropriate candidates for periodic mammography after age 35 (Table 20–1). According to Sadowsky and associates (N Engl J Med 294:370, 1976), the correct interval between mammographic examinations in this group of high-risk patients is uncertain. The current recommendation is once a year.

In summary, mammography is a valuable adjunct to physical examination in the early diagnosis of breast cancer. However, the relative benefits and hazards of repeated mammography for screening purposes in asymptomatic women are as yet undetermined. It is expected that the Breast Cancer Detection Demonstration Projects will settle this issue. Until then, monthly self-examination by the patient and annual physical examination by a qualified examiner can do much to achieve the goal of early diagnosis of breast cancer.

B. Self-Examination: All women over 35 should be advised to examine their breasts monthly—in premenopausal women, just after the menstrual period.

The breasts should be inspected initially while standing before a mirror with the hands at the sides, overhead, and pressed firmly on the hips to contract the pectoralis muscles. Masses, asymmetry of breasts, and slight dimpling of the skin may become apparent as a result of these maneuvers. Next, in a supine position, each breast should be carefully palpated with the fingers of the opposite hand. Physicians should instruct their women patients in the technic of self-examination and advise them to report at once for medical evaluation if a mass or other abnormality is noted.

Differential Diagnosis

A. Benign Lesions: The following benign lesions must be distinguished from breast cancer. The differentiation is usually made by biopsy.

1. Mammary dysplasia—This condition, also called chronic cystic disease of the breast, is common in premenopausal women age 30–50. It occurs as single or multiple masses or thickenings of one or both breasts, often associated with tenderness in the mass or in the breast. There is a tendency to premenstrual increase in discomfort or size of the mass. Lesions tend to fluctuate in size and may appear rapidly and subside spontaneously. Mammary dysplasia is the condition most frequently confused with carcinoma of the breast, and biopsy is often required to establish the diagnosis. Carcinoma and mammary dysplasia are both common and may coexist in the breast.

2. Mammary duct ectasia—This rare lesion (also called comedomastitis or plasma cell mastitis) is characterized by dilatation of the ducts, inspissation of breast secretions, intraductal inflammation, and periductal and interstitial chronic inflammation in which plasma cells are prominent. Inspissation of secretions within the duct is the probable cause. This view is supported by the fact that about half of patients have inverted or cracked nipples or difficulty in nursing. The disorder tends to occur in the fifth decade and is of special clinical significance because it may produce a mass or induration, occasionally with skin or nipple retraction. Axillary node enlargement may further heighten the suspicion of cancer. Unlike cancer, however, the onset of mammary duct ectasia is usually associated with pain, tenderness, and redness, which suggest the inflammatory nature of the process. Biopsy may be required to establish the diagnosis.

3. Fibroadenoma—This benign neoplasm usually occurs in young women within 20 years after puberty. Fibroadenoma is characteristically a firm, round, discrete, nontender, fairly mobile lesion 1–5 cm in size. Occasionally it may be multiple. Excisional biopsy is advisable to confirm the diagnosis, which can be strongly suspected from the clinical appearance.

4. Intraductal papilloma—Papillomatosis is the most frequent cause of serous or bloody nipple discharge. The lesions are usually small and may not be palpable. The subareolar or para-areolar region is the usual tumor site; it is best localized by pressure directly over it so that a discharge from the nipple is expressed from the obstructed duct. Mammary dys-

Table 20—3. TNM staging system for carcinoma of the breast. Mutual classification of UICC and AJCCS (1973).

THE DEFINITIONS OF T, N, AND M CATEGORIES FOR CARCINOMA OF THE BREAST

T PRIMARY TUMORS

TIS Preinvasive carcinoma (carcinoma in situ), noninfiltrating intraductal carcinoma, or Paget's disease of the nipple with no demonstrable tumor.

> *Note:* Paget's disease associated with a demonstrable tumor is classified according to the size of the tumor.

T0 No demonstrable tumor in the breast.

T1* Tumor 2 cm or less in its greatest dimension.
    T1a With no fixation to underlying pectoral fascia and/or muscle.
    T1b With fixation to underlying pectoral fascia or muscle.

T2* Tumor more than 2 cm but not more than 5 cm in its greatest dimension.
    T2a With no fixation to underlying pectoral fascia and/or muscle.
    T2b With fixation to underlying pectoral fascia and/or muscle.

T3* Tumor more than 5 cm in its greatest dimension.
    T3a With no fixation to underlying pectoral fascia and/or muscle.
    T3b With fixation to underlying pectoral fascia and/or muscle.

T4 Tumor of any size with direct extension to chest wall or skin.

> *Note:* Chest wall includes ribs, intercostal muscles, and serratus anterior muscle but not pectoral muscle.

    T4a With fixation to chest wall.
    T4b With edema (including peau d'orange), ulceration of the skin of the breast, or satellite skin nodules confined to the same breast.
    T4c Both of above.

N REGIONAL LYMPH NODES

N0 No palpable homolateral axillary nodes.

N1 Movable homolateral axillary nodes.
    N1$_a$ Nodes not considered to contain growth.
    N1$_b$ Nodes considered to contain growth.

N2 Homolateral axillary nodes considered to contain growth and fixed to one another or to other structures.

N3 Homolateral supraclavicular or infraclavicular nodes considered to contain growth or edema of the arm.†

> *Note:* Edema of the arm may be caused by lymphatic obstruction; lymph nodes may not then be palpable.

M DISTANT METASTASES

M0 No evidence of distant metastases.

M1 Distant metastases present, including skin involvement beyond the breast area.

CLINICAL STAGE GROUPING IN CARCINOMA OF THE BREAST

TIS Carcinoma in situ.

Invasive carcinoma

Stage I	T1a N0 or N1$_a$	
	T1b N0 or N1$_a$	} M0

Stage II	T0 N1$_b$	
	T1a N1$_b$	
	T1b N1$_b$	} M0
	T2a or T2b N0, N1$_a$ or N1$_b$	

Stage III	Any T3 with any N	
	Any T4 with any N	
	Any T with N2	} M0
	Any T with N3	

Stage IV Any T any N with M1

---

*Dimpling of the skin, nipple retraction, or any other skin changes except those in T4b may occur in T1, T2, or T3 without affecting the classification.

†Homolateral internal mammary nodes considered to contain growth are included in N3 for surgical evaluation classification and postsurgical treatment classification.

plasia and carcinoma may also cause nipple discharge, which, if bloody, suggests malignancy. Biopsy or excision of the obstructed duct is usually required to settle the issue. Both ductal papilloma and cancer are capable of producing nipple discharge when too small to be palpable.

5. Fat necrosis—This is a rare condition which is usually indistinguishable from carcinoma without biopsy. The patient may or may not present with tenderness or with a history of trauma. Nipple or skin retraction may occur in fat necrosis, and this contributes further to its similarity in appearance to breast cancer.

B. Occult Carcinoma: Rarely, the first manifestation of breast cancer will be axillary node enlargement or distant metastases. No mass may be palpable in the breast. The mammary carcinoma in these circumstances is occult and only discovered by sectioning of excised breast tissue. Mammography may be useful in selecting the site for biopsy or may be used as a screening procedure to detect breast cancer.

Prevention

Breast cancer cannot be "prevented," but a diagnosis can be made in an earlier stage provided certain procedures are followed. The most important of these are discussed under Early Detection, above.

Clinical Staging

Patients with breast cancer can be grouped into stages according to characteristics of the primary tumor (T), regional lymph nodes (N), and distant metastases (M). Physical, radiologic, and other clinical examinations, usually including biopsy of the primary lesion, are used in determining the stage, which is based on all information available before therapy. Staging is useful in estimating the prognosis and deciding on the type of treatment to be advised. The International Union Against Cancer (UICC) and the American Joint Committee on Cancer Staging (AJCCS) formerly each recommended a slightly different TNM system. In 1973, a revised TNM staging system for breast carcinoma was developed jointly by UICC and AJCCS so that there is now a single system approved by both organizations (Table 20–3). When comparing series of breast cancer patients published in past literature, the reader should be aware of the staging system used and of the slight differences between UICC and AJCCS standards in the T and N categories.

Before treatment, all new cases of breast cancer should be staged in accordance with the 1973 revision of the TNM staging system.

The revised TNM classification was developed following a retrospective study of the medical records of 2500 patients with breast cancer diagnosed and initially treated before 1957 (Surg Gynecol Obstet 131:41, 1970; J Natl Cancer Inst 36:53, 1966). The data obtained in this study, showing 5-year survival rates in accordance with the revised staging system, are summarized in Table 20–4.

The Columbia Clinical Classification (Table 20–5) was devised in 1951 by C.D. Haagensen at

Table 20–4. Survival of patients with breast cancer according to 1973 revision of TNM system.[*]

Stage	Number of Cases	Percentage of Total	Five-Year Survival (%)
I	402	17	85
II	1287	53	66
III	673	28	41
IV	62	2	10

[*]Except for those in stage IV, all patients were treated by radical mastectomy.

Columbia-Presbyterian Medical Center in New York and has been widely used in the clinical staging of breast cancer. Stages A, B, C, and D of the Columbia Classification are broadly equivalent to stages I, II, III, and IV of the TNM system. Since many of the published reports of treatment of breast cancer are based on the Columbia Classification, it is reproduced here for reference.

Many British and European and some American reports of treatment of breast cancer use the Manchester System of clinical staging. This was developed in 1940 at Christie Hospital and Holt Radium Institute in Manchester, England (Table 20–6).

Location & Size of Primary Lesion

The relative frequency of carcinoma in various

Table 20–5. The Columbia Clinical Classification of breast cancer.

Stage	Clinical Criteria
A	No skin edema, ulceration, or solid fixation of tumor to chest wall; axillary nodes not clinically involved.
B	No skin edema, ulceration, or solid fixation of tumor to chest wall; clinically involved axillary nodes, but less than 2.5 cm in transverse diameter and not fixed to overlying skin or deeper structures of axilla.
C	Any one of 5 grave signs of advanced breast carcinoma: 1. Edema of skin of limited extent (involving less than one-third of the skin over the breast). 2. Skin ulceration. 3. Solid fixation of tumor to chest wall. 4. Massive involvement of axillary lymph nodes; a single node, or group of fused nodes, measuring 2.5 cm or more in transverse diameter. 5. Fixation of the axillary nodes to overlying skin or deeper structures of the axilla.
D	More advanced breast carcinoma, including— 1. A combination of any 2 or more of the 5 grave signs listed in stage C. 2. Extensive edema of skin (involving more than one-third of the skin over the breast). 3. Satellite skin nodules. 4. The inflammatory type of carcinoma. 5. Clinically involved supraclavicular lymph nodes. 6. Internal mammary metastases as evidenced by a parasternal tumor. 7. Edema of the arm. 8. Distant metastases.

Table 20—6. The Manchester System of clinical staging of breast cancer.

Stage	Criteria
I	The growth is confined to the breast. Involvement of the skin directly over and in continuity with the tumor does not affect staging provided that the area involved is small in relation to the size of the breast.
II	As in stage I, but there are palpable mobile nodes in the axilla.
III	The growth is extending beyond the corpus mammae, as shown by— (a) invasion of the skin, or fixation over an area large in relation to the size of the breast, or skin ulceration; (b) fixation of the tumor to the underlying muscle or fascia. Axillary nodes may or may not be palpable, but if nodes are present they must be mobile.
IV	The growth has extended beyond the breast area as shown by— (a) fixation or matting of the axillary nodes; (b) complete fixation of tumor to chest wall; (c) secondaries in supraclavicular nodes; (d) secondaries in opposite breast; (e) secondaries in the skin wide of tumor; (f) distant metastases, eg, bone, liver, lung.

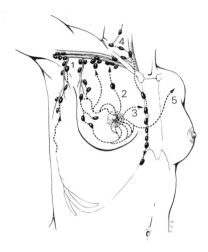

Figure 20—6. Lymphatic drainage of the breast to regional node groups. *1.* Main axillary group. *2.* Interpectoral node leading to apex of axilla. *3.* Internal mammary group. *4.* Supraclavicular group. *5.* Lymphatic channels to opposite axilla. (Modified from Ackerman LV, Del Regato JA: *Cancer,* 3rd ed. Mosby, 1962.)

anatomic sites in the breast is approximately as shown in Fig 20—5.

Almost half of cancers of the breast begin in the upper outer quadrant, probably because this quadrant contains the largest volume of breast tissue. The high percentage in the central portion is due to the inclusion of cancers that spread to the subareolar region from neighboring quadrants.

Cancer occurs 5—10% more frequently in the left breast than in the right; there is no satisfactory explanation for this difference.

Tumor size at the time of surgery gives some indi-

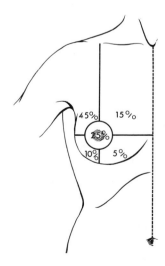

Figure 20—5. Frequency of breast carcinoma at various anatomic sites.

cation of the alertness of both patients and physicians to the presence of breast cancer. In the series of 2578 patients treated surgically in the National Surgical Adjuvant Breast Project, about half of the tumors were larger than 3 cm and about 5% were smaller than 1 cm (Fisher & others: Cancer 24:1071, 1969). Inasmuch as a 1 cm lesion should be readily identifiable by palpation if sought, it is clear that greater effort to discover small lesions is needed.

Metastases to Regional Lymph Nodes

The axillary and the internal mammary lymph node chains are the major (but not the only) routes of primary lymphatic spread of breast cancer (Fig 20—6). Treatment and prognosis depend upon clinical and pathologic assessment of the status of the regional nodes with respect to metastases. The supraclavicular nodes are in direct continuity with the axillary chain and are usually involved secondarily only after the axillary nodes have been infiltrated. Involvement of the supraclavicular nodes almost invariably means that distant spread of the cancer has already occurred and that attempts at curative surgical treatment are futile. Involvement of the axillary or internal mammary nodes is also an extremely serious prognostic finding and calls for detailed discussion.

The axillary and internal mammary lymph node chains may be involved independently of each other, or both may be involved. Metastases occur more frequently in axillary than in internal mammary nodes in patients with operable breast cancer. Location in the breast of the primary lesion has relatively little effect on the incidence of axillary lymph node involvement as determined by pathologic examination of the nodes after radical mastectomy. About half of the lesions located in any quadrant or centrally in the breast are associated with positive axillary lymph nodes on histologic examination. On the other hand, the incidence of spread to the internal mammary nodes is influenced by the location of the primary tumor. Cancers in the central and medial portions of the breast metastasize to internal mammary nodes more frequently than lateral lesions (Fig 20–7).

A. Axillary Lymph Node Metastases: Evaluation of the axillary nodes is a significant feature of the physical examination in breast cancer. A clinical opinion based on palpation of the axilla should be formed regarding the presence or absence of metastases in the nodes. One or 2 movable, not particularly firm lymph nodes 5 mm or less in diameter can frequently be palpated in the normal axilla, but firm or hard nodes larger than 5 mm in diameter must be assumed to contain metastases until proved otherwise. As shown in Table 20–3, the presence of clinically positive axillary nodes places the patient at least in stage II. Unfortunately, evaluation of the axillary nodes by palpation is not always accurate. Histologic studies show that microscopic metastases are present in up to 30% of patients considered by the clinician to have "negative nodes." On the other hand, if the clinician thinks that the axillary nodes are involved, he will prove to be correct about 85% of the time. Thus, the examiner is frequently unable to detect early metastatic involvement of the axillary nodes and should recognize his limitations in this regard.

The relationship between primary tumor size and axillary node involvement is of interest. According to data obtained in the National Surgical Adjuvant Breast Project (Fisher & others: Cancer 24:1071, 1969), the incidence of axillary node metastases varied with tumor size as shown in Table 20–7.

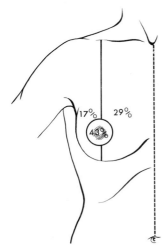

Figure 20–7. Percentage of internal mammary node metastases according to lateral, medial, or subareolar location of the primary tumor. The high percentage of metastases from central tumors is because large tumors originating laterally or medially and extending to the subareolar area are classified as central. (Haagensen CD & others: Ann Surg 169:174, 1969.)

Table 20–7. Relationship of size of breast tumor to incidence of axillary node metastases.

Size of Primary Tumor	Percentage With Positive Axillary Lymph Nodes
< 1 cm	22%
1–1.9 cm	38%
2–2.9 cm	41%
3–3.9 cm	53%
6+ cm	63%

It is of special importance that 22% of the patients with the smallest tumors (< 1 cm) had positive lymph nodes. When the extent of node involvement was studied for the entire series, patients with negative nodes were found to have significantly smaller tumors than those with 1–3 positive nodes. They in turn had smaller tumors than did patients with 4 or more positive lymph nodes. The proportion of patients with 4 or more positive nodes increased with increasing tumor size.

Stage of disease and initial therapy are decided on the basis of the clinical examination. Prognosis and subsequent therapy are influenced by histologic findings regarding the number and locations of involved axillary nodes when these are resected. Three anatomic levels of axillary nodes have been identified by Adair (Ann R Coll Surg Engl 4:36, 1949) as relevant to prognosis if involved by metastases in primarily operable cases treated by radical mastectomy (Table 20–8).

The surgeon who wishes to obtain the maximum amount of information from examination of the axillary contents should tag these 3 levels of nodes during operation as a guide to the pathologist.

B. Internal Mammary Lymph Node Metastases: As shown in Fig 20–7, medial or central lesions in the breast are associated with a higher incidence of internal mammary invasion than lateral tumors. The incidence of internal node metastases also increases in relation to the size of the primary tumor. Haagensen & others (Ann Surg 169:174, 1969) performed internal mammary node biopsies on 1007 patients with tumors of different sizes and obtained the results shown in Table 20–9.

Table 20–8. Influence of anatomic location of involved axillary nodes on survival in breast cancer treated by radical mastectomy.

Level	Anatomic Location	Five-Year Survival if Nodes Positive
I	Nodes in low axilla up to the inferior border of the pectoralis minor muscle	65%
II	Nodes posterior to insertion of pectoralis minor muscle	45%
III	Nodes above superior border of pectoralis minor muscle	28%

Table 20–9. Relationship of size of breast tumor to incidence of metastases in internal mammary nodes.

Size of Primary Carcinoma	Percentage With Internal Mammary Metastases
3 cm	16%
3–5 cm	20%
5–8 cm	39%
7–8 cm	57%
All cases	33%

When the axillary nodes are involved, the incidence of metastases to the internal mammary nodes is increased. Urban & Farrow (Acta; Univ Int contra Cancrum 19:1551, 1963) reported on 248 cases of primary operable breast cancer treated by extended radical mastectomy which involved resection of both axillary and internal mammary nodes. When axillary nodes were negative histologically, the incidence of internal mammary node involvement ranged from zero to 22%, depending upon whether the cancer was in the lateral or medial portion of the breast. When axillary nodes were positive, the internal mammary nodes were positive in 33–67% of cases, with the higher incidence related to tumors in the medial portion of the breast.

The frequency of involvement of the internal mammary nodes in operable breast cancer (stages I and II) was first determined by Handley & Thackray (Lancet 2:276, 1949), who found that the internal mammary nodes were already invaded in about one-fourth of these cases and that radical mastectomy

Table 20–10. Classification of mammary carcinoma according to the cellular growth pattern. (Kouchoukos & others: Cancer 20:948, 1967.)

Type I: Rarely metastasizing (not invasive)
1. Intraductal or comedocarcinoma without stromal invasion. Paget's disease of the breast may exist if the epithelium of the nipple is involved.
2. Papillary carcinoma confined to the ducts.
3. Lobular carcinoma in situ.

Type II: Rarely metastasizing (always invasive)
1. Well-differentiated adenocarcinoma.
2. Medullary carcinoma with lymphocytic infiltration.
3. Pure colloid or mucinous carcinoma.
4. Papillary carcinoma.

Type III: Moderately metastasizing (always invasive)
1. Infiltrating adenocarcinoma.
2. Intraductal carcinoma with stromal invasion.
3. Infiltrating lobular carcinoma.*
4. All tumors not classified as types I, II, or IV.

Type IV: Highly metastasizing (always invasive)
1. Undifferentiated carcinoma having cells without ductal or tubular arrangement.
2. All types of tumors indisputably invading blood vessels.

*Infiltrating lobular carcinoma has been moved from type II to type III because of growing experience with its metastasizing potential.

would consequently fail to remove all of the disease. As a result of this observation, Haagensen and his co-workers formerly performed internal mammary node biopsies in selected patients and refrained from radical mastectomy in those with positive internal mammary nodes. Haagensen now relies on clinical criteria in deciding on radical mastectomy and has abandoned internal mammary node biopsy on the ground that it is helpful only in a few selected cases of borderline operability.

Other surgeons have advocated extended radical mastectomy which includes resection of the internal mammary chain of nodes. Kaae & Johansen (pages 93–102 in: *Prognostic Factors in Breast Cancer.* Livingstone, 1968) compared extended radical mastectomy with simple mastectomy plus radiotherapy in a controlled study of randomized patients and concluded that the results were virtually identical up to 10 years after treatment.

Pathologic Types

The behavior of breast cancer can be correlated with the histologic appearance of the lesion. Information on the microscopic characteristics of the neoplasm is therefore helpful in deciding on management and in estimating the prognosis. The pathologist can distinguish 4 types of mammary carcinoma on the basis of cellular differentiation and invasiveness, as shown in Table 20–10.

A. Relative Frequency of Pathologic Types: Kouchoukos and his associates studied specimens from 432 radical mastectomies. It can be estimated from their data that the relative frequency of the various pathologic types in surgically treated patients is approximately as shown in Table 20–11.

B. Incidence of Axillary Metastases: Axillary metastases occur more frequently in patients with tumors of types III and IV, an indication of their greater metastasizing potential. Table 20–12 shows the approximate incidence of axillary spread by type in patients undergoing radical mastectomy (Kouchoukos & others).

C. Survival in Relation to Type: As expected, survival rates after radical mastectomy vary inversely with local invasiveness and a tendency to metastasize to regional nodes. The 5-year survival rate after radical mastectomy in patients with the 4 pathologic types of tumors is approximately as shown in Table 20–13.

Table 20–11. Relative frequency of pathologic types of breast cancer.

Type	Characteristics	Percentage of Total Cases
I	Rarely metastasizing (not invasive)	5%
II	Rarely metastasizing (always invasive)	15%
III	Moderately metastasizing (always invasive)	65%
IV	Highly metastasizing (always invasive)	15%
		100%

Table 20—12. Relationship of pathologic type of breast cancer to incidence of axillary node metastases.

Type	Percentage With Positive Nodes
I	13%
II	34%
III	58%
IV	57%

D. Bilateral Occurrence of Type I Tumors: Type I noninfiltrating neoplasms, particularly those of the intraductal and the lobular in situ varieties, are of special interest because of their tendency to occur bilaterally. At the time of initial operation for breast cancer, Urban performed random biopsies of the opposite breast on 73% of 488 patients in his series. When an infiltrating type of carcinoma was present in the primarily involved breast, the overall rate of bilateral cancer was 12%—approximately 8% simultaneous and 4% asynchronous. However, when noninfiltrating cancer was found in the primary breast, the overall rate of bilateral involvement was 20–30% simultaneous and 10% asynchronous. Bilaterality is particularly likely to occur in patients with in situ lobular carcinoma, which should be recognized as a preinvasive form of breast cancer and treated accordingly. Lobular carcinoma may progress in time from an in situ to an infiltrating stage. It may be in situ in one breast and infiltrating in the other. Periods of 1–20 years may elapse between the diagnosis of in situ lobular carcinoma and the development of invasive cancer in the same or opposite breast.

In addition to physical examination and mammography, there is a need to develop ways of diagnosing breast cancer during what may be, especially in type I tumors, a prolonged preclinical or "silent" stage. Biopsy of the opposite "negative" breast at the time of mastectomy for cancer is an approach to the problem of early diagnosis worthy of consideration in patients with lobular and intraductal carcinoma.

E. Implications of Pathologic Typing: In most statistical studies of survival after treatment for carcinoma of the breast, the various pathologic types are not separately identified. As a result, the influence of pathologic type on response to therapy is usually obscured. Those few studies which do correlate clinical stage and pathologic type reveal that stage I lesions less

Table 20—13. Relationship of pathologic type of breast cancer to survival.

Type	Five-Year Survival Rate		All Cases
	Axillary Nodes		
	Negative	Positive	
I	95%	95%	95%
II	85%	70%	80%
III	80%	50%	60%
IV	80%	40%	55%

than 5 cm in size and of pathologic type I or II rarely metastasize beyond the nodes in the lower axilla. Such lesions, therefore, are in a particularly favorable category from the standpoint of such a surgical procedure as modified radical mastectomy. Studies of treatment methods for breast cancer should be based on both clinical stage and pathologic type of the tumor. Otherwise it is impossible to be sure of the comparability of the cases involved no matter how carefully they are matched for other variables.

Hormone Receptor Sites

In addition to determining the pathologic type of a breast carcinoma, it is often useful to know whether the cancer cells contain estrogen receptor sites. When estrogen receptor is present in the neoplastic cells, there is a 60% probability that they will regress in response to hormone manipulation such as ovariectomy, adrenalectomy, hypophysectomy, or administration of hormones. Such treatment is rarely successful when estrogen receptor is absent.

This behavior is currently explained by the following theory of hormone dependence in breast cancer. Normal mammary cells contain cytoplasmic or membrane receptor sites for each of the hormones known to influence the growth and function of the mammary gland, including estrogen, progesterone, prolactin, and testosterone. The initial reaction between the hormone and the cell takes place at the receptor site, and this triggers within the cell the biochemical chain of events characteristic of the particular hormone. When a mammary cell undergoes malignant transformation, it may retain all or only part of the normal complement of receptor sites. If the cell retains the receptor sites, its growth and function are potentially susceptible to regulation by the hormonal environment, as in a normal cell; however, if the receptors are lost in consequence of malignant transformation, the cell is no longer affected by circulating hormones and endocrine control is absent. This theoretically accounts for the usual failure of a breast cancer to respond to endocrine therapy if its cells lack estrogen receptor (McGuire WL, Carbone PP, Vollmer EP [editors]: *Estrogen Receptors in Human Breast Cancer.* Raven Press, 1975, pp 17–30).

It is now possible to assay breast cancer tissue either from the primary tumor or from metastases for the presence of estrogen receptor. In view of the importance of this information as a guide to future treatment, it is advisable, if possible, to obtain an estrogen receptor assay on every breast cancer at the time of initial diagnosis (McGuire WL: Cancer [Suppl] 36:638, 1975). The tissue requires special handling, and the laboratory should be consulted for instructions.

Curative Treatment

Treatment may be curative or palliative. Curative treatment is advised for clinical stage I and II disease and for selected patients in stage III. Palliative treatment (discussed below) by irradiation, hormones, endocrine ablation, or chemotherapy is recommended for patients in stage IV (distant metastases), for stage III patients unsuitable for curative efforts, and for previously treated patients who develop distant metastases or ineradicable local recurrence.

A. Radical Mastectomy: This operation involves en bloc removal of breast, pectoral muscles, and axillary nodes and has been the standard curative procedure for breast cancer since the turn of the century, when W.S. Halsted and Willy Meyer independently described their versions of the technic. Experience with radical mastectomy is extensive, and, in properly selected patients, no other form of therapy has produced better results. Radical mastectomy removes the local lesion and the axillary nodes with a wide safety margin of surrounding tissue. Various breast incisions are used depending upon the location of the primary tumor and the preference of the surgeon. If the disease has already spread to the internal mammary or supraclavicular nodes or to more distant sites, radical mastectomy alone will not cure the patient.

B. Extended Radical Mastectomy: This procedure involves, in addition to standard radical mastectomy, removal of the internal mammary nodes. The extended operation has been recommended by a few surgeons for medially or centrally placed breast lesions and for tumors associated with positive axillary nodes because of the known frequency of internal mammary node metastases under these circumstances. Retrospective clinical comparisons suggest that the 5-year survival and incidence of chest wall recurrence may be slightly better after extended radical mastectomy than after standard radical mastectomy in selected patients, but a controlled prospective clinical trial is required to settle the issue. It does not appear that extended radical mastectomy is significantly more effective than irradiation in preventing recurrence from internal mammary metastases. For this reason, extended radical mastectomy has few advocates at this time.

C. Modified Radical Mastectomy: This terminology has been applied to many different technics. All include removal of the breast and preservation of the pectoralis major muscle, but the extent of axillary dissection varies and the pectoralis minor muscle may or may not be excised. The procedure most appropriately referred to as modified radical mastectomy is that described by Patey (Br J Cancer 2:71, 1948) and used extensively by Handley (Breast 2:16, 1976). The operation consists of en bloc removal of the breast with the underlying pectoralis major fascia and including excision of the pectoralis minor muscle and all axillary lymph nodes. Except for preservation of the pectoralis major muscle, this procedure is of the same extent as the standard radical mastectomy.

Auchincloss (Ann Surg 158:37, 1963) has described a lesser procedure which is frequently performed and may be referred to as a modified radical mastectomy. In this operation both pectoral muscles are preserved and the highest axillary nodes are not removed. Such operations are more properly listed as mastectomy and axillary gland dissection. It is not possible to determine from available data whether the

Patey modified radical mastectomy is actually a superior operation in terms of recurrence rates and survival.

The advantages of modified radical mastectomy are cosmetic and functional in that preservation of the pectoralis major muscle avoids a hollow beneath the clavicle and appears to be associated with a somewhat lower incidence of shoulder dysfunction and edema of the arm. There is now considerable evidence that morbidity, mortality, local recurrence, and survival rates for standard and modified radical mastectomy are not much different for stage I and II breast cancer. There are, however, strong advocates for the superiority of standard radical mastectomy in relation to local recurrence and survival (Anglem TJ, Leber RE: Ann Surg 176:625, 1972; Haagensen CD: JAMA 224:1181, 1973). Prospective controlled clinical studies will be needed to settle the issue in a definitive manner, but there is already a notable shift in major centers to the use of modified radical mastectomy and other more conservative procedures in patients who, a few years ago, would have been treated by standard radical mastectomy.

D. Simple Mastectomy: If the malignancy is confined to the breast without spread to the adjacent muscles or to the regional nodes or beyond (true clinical stage I disease), simple mastectomy (or even wide local excision) should be effective in eradicating the cancer. Clinical experience bears this out. The problem is the inability to determine with certainty, prior to their resection and pathologic examination, that the axillary nodes are uninvolved. Reference has already been made to the fact that physical examination is highly unreliable in detecting axillary metastases. Nevertheless, Crile (JAMA 199:736, 1967) has advanced the controversial argument that simple mastectomy may be safely performed for stage I breast cancer, with axillary dissection undertaken only if axillary nodes are suspect when palpated through the wound or become clinically involved at a later date. The rationale for leaving the axillary nodes until they become clinically positive is that, theoretically, the regional lymph nodes are repositories of systemic immunity, which prevents the spread of early cancer.

Miller (Ann Surg 170:879, 1969) has reported that the 10-year survival rate and the local recurrence rate in patients treated by simple mastectomy alone are distinctly inferior to the results obtained by radical mastectomy. There is no question that simple mastectomy is inadequate definitive treatment for breast cancer except for use in certain carefully selected cases of noninvasive (type I) carcinoma.

E. Local Excision: Limited procedures such as local excision ("lumpectomy"), quadrant excision, partial mastectomy, and subcutaneous mastectomy have been suggested as definitive treatment for early breast cancer such as small stage I lesions in the periphery of the breast laterally, particularly if the tumor is of histologic type I. Crile (Crile G Jr, Hoerr SO: Surg Gynecol Obstet 132:780, 1971; Crile G Jr: Lancet 1:549, 1972) has been the most prominent recent advocate of limited resection. Although patients with strictly localized disease adequately excised will be cured by local excision, the hazards of local recurrence and of leaving unsuspected metastases in axillary nodes are serious (Anglem TJ, Leber RE: Ann Surg 176:625, 1972; Anglem TJ, Leber RE: CA 23:330, 1973). Limited surgical procedures which remove less than the entire breast have not been shown to be as effective as mastectomy and are not recommended for operable breast cancer.

F. Radiotherapy: In recent years, the proved efficacy of irradiation in sterilizing the primary lesion and the axillary and internal mammary nodes (Guttman RJ: Am J Roentgenol Radium Ther Nucl Med 96:560, 1966; Cancer 20:1046, 1967) has made radiation therapy with or without simple mastectomy (or wedge resection) a reasonable option for primary treatment of certain breast cancers, particularly those that are locally advanced or when the patient refuses mastectomy. The capability of radical irradiation to destroy or confine metastases in unresected regional nodes has largely eliminated the difference in survival between standard or modified radical mastectomy and simple mastectomy plus irradiation. McWhirtir's policy (since 1941) of treating almost all stages of mammary cancer with simple mastectomy and radical irradiation has been much debated and contested, but the method appears to produce crude survivals at 10 and 15 years which approximate those of radical mastectomy for comparable stages of disease (McWhirtir R: Am J Roentgenol Radium Ther Nucl Med 92:3, 1964).

More recently, an increasing number of stage I and II patients have been successfully treated entirely by irradiation after biopsy or local excision of the primary tumor. A dose of 4500–5000 rads is delivered over a period of 4–5 weeks. This is followed 2–3 weeks later by an additional dose of 1500–2000 rads by iridium 192 implantation in those patients with gross residual disease after biopsy (Weichselbaum RR, Hellman S: Page 69 in: *Controversy in Surgery.* Varco RL, Delaney JP [editors]. Saunders, 1976.)

Orthovoltage irradiation has been used in the past but has in recent years been entirely supplanted by supervoltage irradiation for the primary or adjunctive treatment of breast cancer.

Choice of Primary Treatment for Breast Cancer

There is evidence that mammary cancer confined to the breast and axillary nodes can be controlled by a number of different approaches including standard radical mastectomy, modified radical mastectomy, and radical irradiation with or without simple mastectomy. The variability in tumor-host relationship from patient to patient and the unpredictability of occult metastases make it impossible to determine with precision the relative merits of current competing forms of treatment without additional controlled prospective clinical trials.

Relying on evidence now at hand, modified radical mastectomy is recommended as the primary treatment of choice in stage I and II lesions. Results are apparently comparable to those obtained with standard radical mastectomy. Chest wall deformity and problems with shoulder mobility are less with modified radical mastectomy because the pectoralis major muscle is not removed. The best cosmetic result is achieved when a transverse incision can be used.

Stage III lesions are a borderline group and may or may not be suitable for surgical treatment by either a standard or modified radical mastectomy. Radical surgical treatment is usually contraindicated in stage III lesions with the following characteristics:

(1) Extensive edema involving more than one-third of the skin of the breast.
(2) Satellite nodules on the skin.
(3) Carcinoma of the inflammatory type.
(4) Parasternal tumor nodules.
(5) Edema of the ipsilateral arm.
(6) Palpable ipsilateral infraclavicular lymph nodes (metastases suspected or proved by biopsy).
(7) Two or more of the following grave signs of locally advanced carcinoma:
　(a) Ulceration of the skin.
　(b) Limited edema involving less than one-third of the skin of the breast.
　(c) Fixation of axillary lymph nodes to the skin or the deep structures of the axilla.
　(d) Axillary lymph nodes measuring 2.5 cm or more in transverse diameter.
　(e) Pectoral muscle or chest wall attachment.

The features listed above are signs of advanced disease and are almost invariably associated with spread to the internal mammary or supraclavicular nodes or other distant sites outside the scope of either standard or modified radical mastectomy. Under these circumstances, operation is not curative and may actually disseminate the disease locally or systemically. Radiotherapy with or without simple mastectomy (or wedge resection) is a more effective approach in these advanced stage III cases.

There remain those stage III lesions which do not exhibit the advanced signs listed above. A modified radical mastectomy may be performed if the primary tumor and the enlarged axillary nodes can clearly be excised with an adequate margin by this procedure. Attachment to the pectoral muscles, high axillary nodes, large primary tumor or nodes, or other technically unfavorable conditions would make standard radical mastectomy the preferred operation.

A. Follow-Up After Radical Mastectomy: Patients with breast cancer should be followed for life after radical mastectomy or other curative treatment for at least 2 reasons: to detect recurrences and to observe the opposite breast for a second carcinoma. Local and distant metastases often occur during the first 3 years after radical mastectomy or other curative procedure. During this period the patient is examined every 3–4 months. Examination is then done every 6 months until 5 years postoperatively and every 6–12 months thereafter. Special attention is given to the remaining breast because of the increased risk of developing a second primary. The patient should examine her own breast monthly, and a mammogram should be obtained annually. In some cases, metastases are dormant for long periods and may appear up to 10–15 years or longer after removal of the primary tumor.

B. Breast Reconstruction: Breast removal is emotionally disturbing, and women may ask about the possibility of reconstruction. Breast reconstruction, usually involving multiple operations and the implantation of a prosthesis, may be technically feasible after standard or modified radical mastectomy provided there has been no skin graft or radiotherapy to the chest wall (Lewis JR: Surg Clin North Am 51:429, 1971). However, it should only be considered when there is a negligible likelihood of recurrence. Patients who are initially interested in reconstruction often decide after a period of adjustment and the use of an external prosthesis that they are no longer interested in the procedure.

C. Pregnancy: There are insufficient data to determine with certainty whether abortion improves the prognosis of a patient who develops breast cancer during pregnancy or whether subsequent pregnancy in a patient who has had breast cancer has an adverse effect. It is theoretically possible that the high level of estrogen produced by the placenta would be detrimental to the patient with an estrogen-dependent breast cancer. It is therefore reasonable to advise abortion when the patient develops breast cancer during the first trimester, with progressively less rationale for the procedure as the later stages of pregnancy are reached. Obviously, the decision must be individualized.

Advice regarding pregnancy must sometimes be given to women who have undergone radical mastectomy or other treatment for cancer of the breast. The weight of the somewhat contradictory evidence is that pregnancy is hazardous and should be avoided or interrupted until the patient has been free of the disease for 10 years. The more favorable the clinical stage and pathologic type of disease, the less the theoretic risk of the presumed stimulating effect of pregnancy on occult metastases.

Radiotherapy as Adjunct to Radical Mastectomy

The purposes of preoperative or postoperative radiotherapy in association with modified or standard radical mastectomy are (1) to reduce the incidence of local recurrence from residual cancer in the operative field and (2) to destroy metastatic cancer in the internal mammary and supraclavicular lymph nodes. Patients are, therefore, selected for radiotherapy on the basis of the likelihood of local recurrence or of the existence of disease in unresected regional nodes. According to these criteria, completely resectable lesions confined to the breast (stage I) do not call for radiotherapy. On the other hand, stage II and stage III patients may be considered for radiotherapy before or after modified or standard radical mastectomy. Only supervoltage (not orthovoltage) irradiation should be advised as adjunctive therapy.

A. Preoperative Radiotherapy: The beneficial results of preoperative radiotherapy are more definite than those of postoperative radiotherapy. Preoperative irradiation reduces the incidence of local recurrence and may improve the 10-year survival rate. One investigator (Fletcher GH: JAMA 200:140, 1967; Cancer 29:545, 1972) demonstrated a 5% local recurrence rate after preoperative radiotherapy—compared to a 16% local recurrence rate following postoperative radiotherapy. Preoperative radiotherapy is possibly also of value in making inoperable patients curable by radical mastectomy, although in such patients the results may not be superior to those obtainable by radiotherapy alone.

Indications for preoperative irradiation include the following: (1) a primary tumor larger than 5 cm, (2) limited skin edema or direct skin involvement over the tumor, (3) multiple low or midaxillary nodes, and (4) a prior operation which may have disseminated the tumor locally. A 4500–5000 rad tumor dose is delivered to the axillary, supraclavicular, and internal mammary nodes, and the chest wall and breast are treated tangentially. Radical mastectomy is performed 5–6 weeks after completion of radiotherapy.

B. Postoperative Radiotherapy: The efficacy of postoperative irradiation in improving survival or recurrence rates has not been conclusively demonstrated. However, in view of the proved ability of supervoltage radiotherapy to destroy cancer cells in the breast and regional nodes, postoperative radiotherapy is recommended in some centers under the following conditions: (1) The tumor is cut through or there is a high likelihood that residual tumor has been left in the operative field. (2) The tumor is larger than 5 cm or is located in the central or medial portion of the breast. (3) There are metastases to the axillary nodes. Radiotherapy is begun as soon after operation as the patient's general condition and state of the wound permit. A tumor dose in the range of 4500–5000 rads is delivered in 4–5 weeks, primarily to the internal mammary, supra-, and infraclavicular nodal areas and to the chest wall. The axilla may or may not be irradiated.

When irradiation is properly managed, delayed wound healing and pulmonary damage are infrequent problems. If the axilla is not irradiated, any tendency to lymphedema of the arm will not be accentuated.

Chemotherapy as Adjunct to Radical Mastectomy

Chemotherapy is currently under investigation as an adjunct to the surgical treatment of patients found at radical mastectomy to have positive axillary nodes. The poor prognosis of this group of patients has already been noted. In 1958, a clinical trial was begun by the National Surgical Adjuvant Breast Project to determine whether thiotepa, when administered on the day of and for 2 successive days following radical mastectomy, would reduce treatment failure and increase patient survival. Follow-up studies at 5 years and 10 years showed a significant decrease in recurrence rate for premenopausal women with 4 or more positive nodes who received thiotepa. There was a 20% improvement in survival in this group (Fisher B, Wolmark

N: Cancer [Suppl] 36:627, 1975; Carbone PP: Cancer [Suppl] 36:633, 1975). Another more recent multi-institutional, randomized, prospective cooperative clinical trial was undertaken to evaluate the efficacy of prolonged oral administration of melphalan (Alkeran) as an adjuvant to radical mastectomy (conventional or modified) in lengthening the disease-free interval of women with potentially curable breast cancer having one or more axillary nodes involved with cancer (Fisher B & others: N Engl J Med 292:117, 1975). In premenopausal women, the difference with respect to disease-free interval between treated and control groups was highly significant. A treatment failure occurred in 30% of premenopausal patients receiving placebo and in only 3% of those treated with melphalan. A similar trend was observed in postmenopausal patients. This demonstration of the effectiveness of melphalan as an adjuvant to radical mastectomy, and reports of comparable results with the use of combination chemotherapy (Bonadonna G & others: N Engl J Med 294:405, 1976), indicate that adjuvant chemotherapy should be given serious consideration in the management of patients who are found on radical mastectomy to have positive axillary nodes. Studies are continuing in order to develop improved treatment programs and to determine the possible long-range adverse effects of the chemotherapeutic agents themselves.

Pre- & Postoperative Management of Radical Mastectomy

A. Preoperative Preparation: A prime objective prior to mastectomy is to establish the histologic diagnosis of the primary tumor. Treatment should never be undertaken until this is done. It is appropriate to accomplish this by open biopsy performed under local or general anesthesia in the operating room without admitting the patient to the hospital. Needle biopsy may be adequate in some cases. If the tumor is malignant, the patient is scheduled for early hospital admission and definitive surgery. As an alternative, the patient is admitted to the hospital and the diagnosis is established by open biopsy with frozen section, usually under general anesthesia. If the frozen section is positive, the surgeon proceeds immediately with mastectomy.

Another major objective prior to mastectomy is to determine that the tumor is clinically localized to breast and axillary nodes and warrants an attempt to cure by resection. Specifically, the cancer should be "staged," which requires that distant metastases be ruled out by the various observations—x-ray, scanning, and others—described on pp 276–277.

In addition to the above, the patient's general health and operative risk are evaluated in the usual manner. The immediate preoperative orders consist essentially of skin preparation and preanesthetic medication. Transfusion is rarely required during mastectomy, but if the need for blood is anticipated, typing and cross-matching should be requested.

Preoperatively, full discussion with the patient regarding the rationale for mastectomy and the manner of coping with the cosmetic and psychologic effects of the operation is essential. Patients often have questions about possible alternatives to standard or modified radical mastectomy such as local excision, simple mastectomy, and radiotherapy and may wish detailed explanation of the risks and benefits of the various procedures. Time spent preoperatively in assuring the understanding of the patient and her husband is well spent.

It is important to obtain an estrogen receptor assay on the breast cancer tissue removed at operation, if possible, unless this was done at the time of biopsy (see p 284). Special handling of the specimen for the assay, such as immediate freezing in liquid nitrogen, is necessary for reliable results. Therefore, advance planning may be required in cooperation with the laboratory performing the examination.

B. Postoperative Care: Wound complications following modified or standard radical mastectomy such as marginal slough, fluid collection under the flaps, and infection are minimized by attention during operation to viability of skin flaps and to closure without tension. Suction drainage of the wound by means of catheters placed beneath the skin flaps usually prevents the collection of blood and serum. Bulky compression dressings are unnecessary. When fluid collects beneath the skin flaps in spite of suction drainage, it is removed by repeated needle aspiration.

Active motion of the arm and shoulder on the operated side should be encouraged after the first few days, so that by 10–14 days postoperatively there is a full range of motion. Failure of the patient to cooperate or to make progress may necessitate physical therapy. The Service Committee of the American Cancer Society sponsors a rehabilitation program for postmastectomy patients called Reach for Recovery and will provide useful literature upon request. The patient's morale is improved by early provision of a breast prosthesis held in place by a comfortably fitted brassiere.

Complications of Radical Mastectomy

Mortality and morbidity rates following radical mastectomy are low, and the procedure is generally well tolerated even by elderly patients. The operative mortality rate is in the range of 0.5–1%, with cause of death in most cases being cardiovascular or pulmonary complications. Occasional wound complications such as hematoma or serum collection under the skin flaps and necrosis of skin margins are usually easily managed. They are minimized by suction drainage of the wound and avoidance of undue tension on the skin flaps at closure—by the use of a skin graft if necessary. The most serious complications or sequelae are local recurrence and edema of the arm.

A. Local Recurrence: Recurrence of cancer within the operative field following radical mastectomy is due to incomplete removal of tumor or involved nodes, to cutting across infiltrated lymphatics, or to spillage of tumor cells into the wound. The rate of local recurrence correlates with tumor size, the presence and number of involved axillary nodes, the histologic type of tumor, and the presence of skin edema or skin and fascia fixation with the primary. In one series of 704 patients treated with radical mastectomy without ancillary therapy and uniformly followed for at least 5 years, 17% developed local recurrence. When the axillary nodes were not involved at the time of mastectomy, the local recurrence rate was 7%, but the rate was 26% when they were involved. A similar difference in local recurrence rate was noted between small and large tumors. In general, local recurrence rate is a function of the stage of the patient's disease. (Spratt JS Jr, Donegan WL: *Cancer of the Breast.* Saunders, 1967.)

Chest wall recurrences usually appear within the first 2 years, with a peak incidence in the second year, but may occur as late as 15 or more years after radical mastectomy. Suspect nodules should be biopsied. If the biopsy is positive, disseminated disease must be suspected and a search for metastases made by chest x-ray and bone and liver scans. Local excision or localized radiotherapy may be feasible if an isolated nodule is present. If lesions are multiple or accompanied by evidence of regional involvement in the internal mammary or supraclavicular nodes, the disease is best managed by comprehensive radiation treatment of the whole chest wall including the parasternal, supraclavicular, and axillary areas. Local recurrence usually signals the presence of widespread disease, but when there is no evidence of metastases beyond the chest wall and regional nodes, radical irradiation for cure should be attempted.

B. Edema of the Arm: Except for local recurrence, the only important late complication of standard radical mastectomy is edema of the arm. Significant edema occurs in 10–30% of cases. When it appears in the early postoperative period, it is usually caused by lymphatic obstruction due to infection in the axilla. Postoperative radiotherapy to the axilla increases the incidence of arm edema. Late or secondary edema of the arm may develop years after radical mastectomy as a result of axillary recurrence or of infection in the hand or arm with obliteration of lymphatic channels. After radical mastectomy, the lymphatic drainage of the arm is always compromised and the extremity becomes more than normally susceptible to infection following minor injuries. The patient should be warned of this and treatment by antibiotic, heat, rest, and elevation instituted promptly if infection occurs. Specific instruction should be given to the patient who has had radical mastectomy to avoid breaks in the skin of the hand and arm on the operated side and to refrain from tasks likely to cause superficial wounds and infections. Injections for inoculation and immunization should not be given in that arm. Chronic edema is managed by elevation and by a snugly fitted elastic sleeve which is slipped over the arm from hand to shoulder.

Palliative Treatment

A. Radiotherapy: Palliative radiotherapy may be advised for locally advanced cancers with distant metastases in order to control ulceration, pain, and other manifestations in the breast and regional nodes. Radical irradiation of the breast and chest wall and the axillary, internal mammary, and supraclavicular nodes should be undertaken in an attempt to cure locally advanced and inoperable lesions when there is no evidence of distant metastases. A certain number of patients in this group are cured in spite of extensive breast and regional node involvement.

Palliative irradiation is also of value in the treatment of localized bone or soft tissue metastases to control pain or avoid fracture, particularly when hormonal, endocrine ablation, and chemical therapy are inappropriate or ineffective. Radiotherapy is especially useful in treatment of the isolated bony metastasis.

B. Hormone Therapy: When distant metastases have occurred in breast cancer, the patient is incurable, but disseminated disease may be kept under control or made to regress for prolonged periods by various forms of endocrine therapy including administration of hormones or ablation of the ovaries, adrenals, or pituitary. About one-third of breast cancer patients will respond to one or more of these endocrine measures. The incidence of hormonal responsiveness is approximately the same in premenopausal women as in older postmenopausal women, although the methods of treatment used may be quite different. The frequency of favorable response to hormone manipulation can be increased to about 60% if treatment is confined to patients known to have estrogen receptor in their tumors (see p 284).

Endocrine therapy is employed when surgery and irradiation have failed or when widespread metastases have rendered them useless. Many patients are candidates for a trial of hormone treatment because about half of all patients with breast cancer and 60–80% of those having positive axillary nodes at the time of mastectomy will develop metastatic lesions. The major forms of hormone treatment are (1) estrogen, (2) androgen, (3) corticosteroid therapy, and (4) endocrine ablation.

1. Estrogen therapy—Estrogens should be reserved for postmenopausal women. The best results of estrogen administration are obtained in women more than 5 years past the menopause. Estrogen is capable of causing exacerbation of tumor growth in 50% of premenopausal women and should not be given to them or to recently postmenopausal women until the vaginal smear ceases to show evidence of estrogenic activity. Tumor remission rates from estrogen (and androgen as well) tend to increase with increasing number of years past the menopause.

Estrogen administered as primary therapy will induce tumor regression in over 30% of postmenopausal patients with advanced breast cancer. Objective evidence of tumor regression is seen most commonly in soft tissue metastases in older patients, and over 40% of this group show remission of tumor growth. Both local soft tissue and visceral lesions show a higher remission rate from estrogen than from androgen therapy. The reverse is true for bone metastases. When estrogen receptor assay of the cancer is positive, the response rate to estrogen therapy is about 65%. When the assay is negative for estrogen receptors, the response rate is only about 9% (McGuire WL: Cancer [Suppl] 36:638, 1975).

Treatment usually consists of giving diethylstilbestrol, 5 mg 3 times daily orally (or equivalent), and should be continued as long as it is beneficial.

Initial evidence of regression of metastatic cancer is usually not seen until about 4 weeks after beginning estrogen therapy, but the trial of estrogen should not be abandoned in less than 2 months except in case of obvious exacerbation or serious side-effects. The average duration of remission is about 16 months, but remissions of soft tissue lesions of over 5 years are occasionally seen. The survival time of those who respond to estrogen therapy is about twice that of nonresponders.

The commonest side-effects are anorexia, nausea, and vomiting. These usually disappear within a few weeks, but when symptoms of toxicity are severe the dosage should be reduced temporarily until tolerance is acquired. Pigmentation of nipples, areolas, and axillary skin, enlargement of the breasts, and sodium and water retention are other side-effects of estrogen therapy. Uterine bleeding occurs in the majority of postmenopausal patients when estrogen therapy is stopped, and patients should be told of this possibility to avoid anxiety. Severe bleeding can usually be controlled by administration of testosterone propionate, 100 mg IM daily for 3 or 4 doses.

There is evidence that various synthetic progestins with antiestrogenic action such as megestrol acetate (Megace) are also moderately effective in the treatment of disseminated breast cancer (Ansfield FJ & others: Cancer 33:607, 1974).

2. Androgen therapy—Androgen administration causes temporary amenorrhea in premenopausal women. Tumor regression is noted in 20% of such patients with advanced breast cancer. However, because of the more frequent and prolonged remission from castration, this procedure is preferred as initial treatment in the premenopausal group. Androgen therapy may be usefully added to castration in patients under 35 years of age, or in the presence of bone metastases, because of the poor results from castration alone in such patients. Failure of response to castration may be considered an indication for a trial of androgen therapy because of the low likelihood of a favorable response by these patients to adrenalectomy or hypophysectomy.

Estrogen therapy is not advisable in recently postmenopausal women until the vaginal smear ceases to show evidence of estrogenic activity because of the danger of exacerbating the disease. A trial of androgen therapy is warranted in this group, but a favorable response can be expected in only about 15% of patients.

Since bone metastases are commonly more responsive to androgen than to estrogen therapy, a trial of androgen may be advantageous when osseous lesions are present, particularly before adrenalectomy or hypophysectomy. About 25% of patients more than 5 years past the menopause with bone metastases will respond to androgen therapy. Patients failing to respond can still be subjected to operation if indicated, and surgery will usually have been delayed only about 6 weeks.

Postmenopausal patients who have shown a favorable response to castration or estrogen therapy and have then relapsed may be given a trial of androgen therapy with a 20–30% chance of favorable response. In patients more than 5 years past the menopause, bone metastases which have failed to respond to estrogens are more likely to regress on secondary androgen therapy than are soft tissue metastases. Occasionally, androgen administration will cause tumor regression in the completely hypophysectomized patient.

When estrogen receptor assay of the cancer is positive, the response rate to androgen therapy is about 45%. When the assay is negative, the response rate is only about 8% (McGuire WL: Cancer [Suppl] 36:638, 1975).

Androgen may be given continuously as long as tumor regression persists. It is probably preferable, however, to administer androgen until the tumor has regressed maximally and then discontinue administration until reactivation occurs, at which time resumption of androgen therapy will often lead to another regression. Intermittent therapy of this kind has the advantage of reducing the tendency to virilization while varying the hormonal environment of the tumor, thereby possibly postponing the development of autonomy in the tumor.

The androgen preparation frequently employed is testosterone propionate, 100 mg IM 3 times a week. However, it is simpler and equally effective to give fluoxymesterone (Halotestin), 20–40 mg daily orally. An orally administered nonvirilizing androgen, testolactone (Teslac), in a dosage of 1–2 g daily, is reported to be slightly less effective than testosterone propionate in causing tumor regression. The major interest in this compound is that, since it appears to be relatively inert hormonally, it may have a direct effect on the breast cancer.

About 3 months of androgen therapy are usually required for maximal response. Pain relief may be achieved in up to 80% of patients with osseous metastases. In addition, androgen therapy usually results in a sense of well-being and an increase in energy and weight, particularly in postmenopausal patients. The principal adverse side-effects are increased libido and masculinization, eg, hirsutism, hoarseness, loss of scalp hair, acne, and ruddy complexion. Virilization occurs in practically all women taking testosterone propionate for longer than 6 months but in only about one-third of patients taking fluoxymesterone. Fluid retention, anorexia, vomiting, and hepatotoxicity are among the side-effects of androgen therapy.

Estrogen and androgen therapy are generally of limited value in patients with metastases to the liver or lung.

3. Corticosteroids—Corticosteroids are especially valuable in the management of the serious acute symptoms which may result from such conditions as hypercalcemia, brain and lung metastases, and hepatic metastases with jaundice. Corticosteroid therapy is also indicated for patients who are too ill for major endocrine ablation therapy and for those whose tumors do not respond to other endocrine therapy.

The patient's age and previous response to sex hormone therapy are not correlated with response to corticosteroid therapy, which probably acts through a local effect upon the tumor or the tumor bed. Previous response to corticosteroids does not predict a similar response to adrenalectomy. Objective evidence of tumor regression following corticosteroid administration is less than that following adrenalectomy. Remission on corticosteroid therapy averages about 6 months; following adrenalectomy, over 12 months.

The subjective response of the seriously ill patient to corticosteroids is often striking. Appetite, sense of well-being, and pain from bone or visceral metastases may be markedly improved. However, objective regression of soft tissue lesions occurs in only about 15% of patients. The relief of coma from brain metastases and dyspnea from lung metastases is often encouraging but transient. Hypercalcemia is probably improved by specific action on calcium metabolism.

Average daily oral doses are cortisone, 150 mg, or prednisone or prednisolone, 30 mg. Twice or 3 times these dosages may be required temporarily for control of severe, acute symptoms. Other corticosteroids have been employed in equivalent dosage with similar results. The dosage of corticosteroids must be reduced slowly if they have been used for prolonged periods because of the adrenocortical atrophy that is induced.

Adrenocortical hormones may cause numerous complications such as uncontrollable infection, bleeding peptic ulcer, muscle weakness, hypertension, diabetes, edema, and features of Cushing's syndrome.

The best overall tumor remission rate from hormonal therapy in postmenopausal patients can be obtained when treatment is individualized. In general, patients with soft tissue and intrathoracic metastases will respond best to estrogen therapy. Androgen therapy is usually more effective in patients with bone metastases. Corticosteroid therapy should be considered in particular for brain and liver metastases.

4. Therapeutic endocrine ablation—

a. Castration—Oophorectomy in premenopausal women with advanced, metastatic, or recurrent breast cancer results in temporary regression in about 35% of cases, with objective improvement lasting an average of about 10 months. Life is definitely prolonged in those who respond favorably. Patients not responding to castration usually fail to respond favorably to adrenalectomy, hypophysectomy, or specific hormones. Authorities differ on whether castration should be given a trial in all premenopausal women before advising bilateral adrenalectomy or hypophysectomy. Of those patients responding favorably to castration, 40–50% will respond to bilateral adrenalectomy or hypophysectomy. Of those not responding to oophorectomy, only 10–15% show tumor regression after one of those major procedures. According to some authorities, simultaneous oophorectomy and adrenalectomy is the palliative treatment of choice in premenopausal women with disseminated breast cancer.

Prophylactic castration of premenopausal women with breast cancer is not of value and is not recommended.

Castration can be performed by bilateral oophorectomy or irradiation. Surgical removal of the ovaries is preferable because it rules out the possibility of residual ovarian function. Therapeutic castration is essentially confined to premenopausal women and is of no value in truly postmenopausal women. Ovarian function may persist for a few years after cessation of menses, and this can be determined by means of the vaginal smear; if evidence of persistent estrogenic activity is found, castration may be beneficial.

b. Adrenalectomy or hypophysectomy—Regression of advanced breast cancer occurs in about 30% of patients after either of these procedures. Patients who respond to castration or to hormone administration are most likely to benefit from removal of the adrenals or pituitary. This information is helpful in the selection of patients for one of these major ablation procedures.

Adrenalectomy is usually preferred over hypophysectomy because of its wider availability and greater ease of postoperative endocrine management. The mortality rate of both procedures is in the range of 5%. In some centers, transnasal transsphenoidal microsurgical hypophysectomy is the initial treatment of choice for postmenopausal patients with metastatic breast carcinoma (Pearson OH: CA 26:165, 1976). In experienced hands, this procedure is well tolerated and associated with low morbidity and mortality rates and a low incidence of side-effects. The response rate after adrenalectomy and hypophysectomy would appear to be about the same. A slight advantage for hypophysectomy has been claimed, but this has not been firmly established.

Corticosteroid replacement therapy is required after bilateral adrenalectomy. The following regimen is suggested:

Day before operation, 6 pm: Hydrocortisone sodium succinate, 100 mg IM
Day of operation:
    Preoperatively: 100 mg IM
    During operation: 100 mg IM
    Postoperatively: 50 mg IM every 4 hours
Postoperative day:
    First day: 100 mg IM every 8 hours
    Second day: 50 mg IM every 6 hours
    Third day: 50 mg IM every 12 hours
    Fourth day: 25 mg IM every 8 hours, or cortisone acetate, 25 mg orally every 8 hours
    Fifth day and thereafter as maintenance dose: Cortisone acetate, 25 mg orally twice daily

The maintenance dose of cortisone must be supplemented in some patients by fludrocortisone, 0.1–0.25 mg orally daily or every other day, for its sodium-retaining effect. Diet following adrenalectomy should include at least 3 g of salt daily, which may be achieved by liberal salting of food. Adrenal insufficiency will occur if the cortisone maintenance regimen is inadequate or is neglected. Resulting symptoms may include extreme weakness, nausea and vomiting, rapid weight loss, or hypotension. Increased stress calls for increased cortisone dosage. Acute crises of adrenal insufficiency require immediate hospitalization and intensive treatment.

Following hypophysectomy, the above regimen is followed to prevent adrenal insufficiency. In addition, thyroid hormone replacement is required. A maintenance dose of thyroid, 60–120 mg daily, or levothyroxine, 0.1–0.2 mg daily, is used. Transient (in some cases permanent) diabetes insipidus may follow hypophysectomy. Under these circumstances, polyuria may be controlled, depending upon its severity and persistence, by vasopressin tannate (Pitressin Tannate), 0.5–1 ml in oil IM (effective 24–72 hours) or a nasal spray of synthetic vasopressin (lypressin or arginine vasopressin).

In premenopausal women, when oophorectomy alone is followed by remission and adrenalectomy is withheld until progression of the tumor resumes, the overall palliation and length of survival are better than when adrenals and ovaries are removed at the same operation. Menopausal and postmenopausal women should be treated by simultaneous oophorectomy and adrenalectomy.

The response of metastatic breast carcinoma to administration of hormones or to ablation of endocrine glands is most likely to be favorable under the following circumstances: (1) slowly growing tumor (eg, free interval between diagnosis and development of metastases exceeds 24 months); (2) hormone therapy is begun promptly when metastases appear; (3) metastases localized to soft tissues, bones, and pleuropulmonary region (as opposed to visceral areas such as liver and brain); (4) advanced age; and (5) previous response to hormone therapy or castration. However, favorable responses may occur occasionally when none of these conditions exist.

Adrenalectomy or hypophysectomy will be of no benefit to two-thirds of randomly selected patients on whom the operation is performed. Obviously, it is of great importance to develop methods of selection which will identify the patients who will respond and thus avoid unnecessary major surgery in the remainder. Recent studies (McGuire WL: Cancer [Suppl] 36:638, 1975) emphasize the significance of estrogen receptors in breast cancer tissue as an indicator of responsiveness to endocrine therapy by either hormone administration or endocrine ablation. In 94 patients with negative tumor estrogen receptor values, only 8 responded to endocrine ablation (adrenalectomy, hypophysectomy, or castration), whereas, in 107 patients with positive tumor estrogen receptor values, 59 responded to endo-

crine ablation. About 30% of patients with borderline tumor estrogen receptor values also responded. The prognostic significance of endocrine receptor assay does not appear to depend upon the type of tissue examined. Estrogen receptor values from primary tumors or metastatic lesions predict equally well. The percentage of primary tumors reported to contain estrogen receptors has risen in recent years from 50% to 70–85%, probably because of increased sensitivity of assay methods. In view of these findings, it is advisable to obtain an estrogen receptor assay on the tumor of every patient with primary or metastatic breast cancer as a guide to future treatment, particularly when adrenalectomy or hypophysectomy is under consideration.

In an effort to improve further the selection of patients for hormone manipulation, the significance of progesterone receptors in breast cancer tissue is currently being studied (Horwitz KB & others: Science 189:726, 1975). Progesterone receptors were found in 56% of a small series of breast cancers all of which contained estrogen receptors, but progesterone receptors were absent from cancers that did not contain estrogen receptors. Preliminary clinical trials showed that only those cancers with progesterone receptors regressed after endocrine therapy. If these results are confirmed, the presence of progesterone receptors in breast cancer may prove to be a sensitive predictor of responsiveness to endocrine therapy.

C. Chemotherapy: Anticancer chemotherapy should be considered for palliation of advanced breast cancer when visceral metastases are present or when hormone treatment is unsuccessful or the patient becomes unresponsive to it. Chemotherapy is most likely to be effective in patients who previously responded to hormonal therapy. The most useful single chemotherapeutic agent to date is doxorubicin (Adriamycin), an anthracycline antibiotic administered intravenously, with a response rate of 40–50%. The remissions tend to be brief, and, in general, experience with single agent chemotherapy in patients with disseminated disease has not been too encouraging.

Combination chemotherapy using multiple agents has proved to be more effective, with objectively observed favorable responses achieved in 60–80% of patients with stage IV disease. Various combinations of drugs have been used, and clinical trials are continuing in an effort to improve results and to reduce undesirable side-effects of treatment. Doxorubicin and cyclophosphamide produced an objective response in 87% of 46 patients who had an adequate trial of therapy (Jones SE & others: Cancer 36:90, 1975). Other chemotherapeutic regimens have consisted of various combinations of drugs including cyclophosphamide, vincristine, methotrexate, and fluorouracil with response rates ranging up to 60–70% (Otis PT, Armentrout SA: Cancer 36:311, 1975). The value of chemotherapy has been underestimated in the past because it has typically been reserved for use after hormone administration and endocrine ablation have failed.

D. Malignant Pleural Effusion: This condition

develops at some time in almost half of patients with breast cancer. When severe and persistent, the effusion is best controlled by closed tube drainage of the chest and intrapleural chemotherapy. An intercostal tube is inserted and placed on suction and water-seal drainage until as much fluid as possible has been removed. Then mechlorethamine (0.4 mg/kg, up to 20 mg) or thiotepa (30–45 mg, or 0.8 mg/kg) in 40 ml of saline is injected through the tube, which is clamped for 6 hours. Suction drainage is then reinstituted for 4–6 days–or until no further fluid is obtained–before removing the catheter. The procedure may be repeated in 3–4 weeks if necessary. Toxicity due to intrapleural mechlorethamine or thiotepa is usually mild and consists of occasional nausea or vomiting and infrequent bone marrow depression.

E. Hypercalcemia in Advanced Breast Cancer: Hypercalcemia occurs transiently or terminally in about 10% of women with advanced disease. The hypercalcemia of breast cancer is usually but not always associated with osteolytic metastases. Increased blood calcium may be related in some cases to the occurrence in the patient's blood of phytosteryl esters which have calcium-mobilizing properties similar to that of vitamin D. Immobilization exaggerates the tendency of direct bony invasion or humoral processes to produce hypercalcemia. Breast cancers do not produce parathyroid hormone, and the hypercalcemia is therefore not associated with low serum phosphate or low tubular reabsorption of phosphate (TRP) (unless artifactually produced by glucose or corticosteroid administration). Thus, the presence of hypercalcemia, hypophosphatemia, and low TRP in a patient with breast cancer indicates an additional diagnosis such as parathyroid adenoma. Although estrogens and androgens were once erroneously thought to cause hypercalcemia in breast cancer, it now appears that they are actually beneficial in the condition. It is possible, however, that acute hypercalcemia may be precipitated by the nausea, vomiting, and dehydration which may occur with hormone therapy–particularly estrogens–and radiotherapy.

The symptoms of hypercalcemia are protean, and its course is treacherous. Initial symptoms usually include diffuse central nervous system changes, alterations of renal function, vomiting, and dehydration. Rapid deterioration, anuria, coma, and death may occur.

Prevention is important and consists of (1) adequate hydration (at least 2 liters of fluid per day), (2) maintenance of as much physical activity as possible, and (3) a low-calcium diet (avoidance of milk, cheese, ice cream, and vitamin D).

Treatment for mild hypercalcemia in patients with only moderate elevation of serum calcium (eg, 11–12 mg/100 ml) consists of hydration to induce diuresis, preferably with sodium-containing fluids to facilitate tubular rejection of calcium. In severe hypercalcemia with calcium levels above 12 mg/100 ml, corticosteroid is administered orally or intravenously in the form of prednisone, 30–100 mg/day (or equivalent), in order to decrease calcium mobilization from bone. Corticosteroid treatment is usually required only until restoration of a normal serum calcium level, which is subsequently maintained by 3 liters daily of oral fluids, avoidance of milk and cheese, and maintenance of an adequate activity status.

When the above measures prove inadequate to control high levels of serum calcium, the administration of isotonic solution of sodium sulfate intravenously is valuable. Sodium sulfate forms a calcium complex which is readily excreted by the kidney. There is current interest in mithramycin as an antitumor agent which regularly lowers both normal and elevated serum calcium levels at dosages which are relatively nontoxic. Major endocrine ablation may be advisable after hypercalcemia is controlled or may rarely be necessary as a control measure.

After subsidence of an episode of hypercalcemia, many patients survive for months or years with essentially the same relationship to their disease.

Prognosis

The clinical stage and pathologic type of breast cancer are the most reliable indicators of prognosis. Initial therapy also influences prognosis critically in potentially curable patients. There is evidence that several different treatment programs achieve approximately the same results when the disease is limited to the breast and regional nodes. Physicians have tended to adopt and actively espouse one or another therapeutic approach depending upon their personal experience or their interpretation of the conflicting reports in the literature regarding the procedure which offers the most favorable outlook for long-term survival. As a result, there is considerable controversy and confusion as to optimal primary treatment of breast cancer. It is well to keep this point in mind when advising the patient on prognosis in relation to treatment.

As a guide to prognosis in individual patients, it is useful to refer to crude 10-year survival statistics for various types of treatment by stage of disease as shown in Table 20–14.

Regrettably, such retrospective surveys as those summarized in Table 20–14 do not permit valid conclusions regarding the relative merits of competing modes of therapy such as radiotherapy and radical mastectomy. A few prospective, randomized, controlled clinical studies have been successfully completed in which 2 methods of treatment are compared in patients with potentially curable or "operable" breast cancer. These have not demonstrated the superiority of radical mastectomy or extended radical mastectomy over radiotherapy combined with a limited surgical procedure such as simple mastectomy.

For example, Brinkley D, Haybittle JL (Lancet 2:1086, 1971) in Cambridge, England, compared the results of simple mastectomy plus radiotherapy with radical mastectomy plus radiotherapy. Patients were UICC stage II and were randomly assigned for treatment to a simple or a radical mastectomy group between 1958 and 1965. Accessible axillary lymph nodes

Table 20—14. Results of treatment of breast cancer—10-year survival.

Authors	Procedure	Stage of Columbia Clinical Classification	Number of Patients	Local Recurrence (%)	Crude 10-Year Survival (%)
Miller E (Ann Surg 170:879, 1969)	Simple mastectomy*	A	115		40
		B	34		26
		C	18		22
		D	45		9
			Total 212		
Handley RS (Breast 2:16, 1976)	Modified (Patey) radical mastectomy	A	280	12	60
		B	133	24	42
		C	11	64	18
		D	1		0
			Total 425		
Haagensen CD & Cooley E (Ann Surg 170:884, 1969)	Standard (Halsted) radical mastectomy†	A	344	7	70
		B	138	18	40
		C	63	29	27
		D	11	64	18
			Total 556		
Dahl-Iversen E & Tobiassen T (Ann Surg 170:889, 1969)	Extended radical mastectomy‡ (internal mammary and supra-clavicular dissection)	A	352	20	57
		B	75	32	24
		C	34	. . .	35
		D	15	. . .	7
			Total 476		
Kaae V & Johansen H (Ann Surg 170:895, 1969)	Simple mastectomy plus irradiation orthovoltage 4200—4500 rads	A	159	19	50
		B	28	29	32
		C	9	33	0
		D	3	33	0
			Total 199		

*Most patients received 1000 R or less of 250 kV irradiation.
†8.8% of patients received prophylactic postoperative irradiation.
‡8.6% of patients received prophylactic postoperative irradiation.

were removed with the breast in some of the simple mastectomy patients, but there was no formal block dissection of the axilla in these cases. Simple mastectomy was done on 91 patients and radical mastectomy on 113. Crude 5-year survival rates for simple and radical mastectomy groups were 63% and 58%, respectively. This study showed that the only significant difference between the 2 groups was an increased incidence of edema on the side of operation in patients who had radical mastectomy.

Another relevant prospective randomized clinical trial was conducted in Copenhagen between 1951 and 1957 by Kaae S, Johansen H (p 93 in: *Prognostic Factors in Breast Cancer.* Forrest APM, Kunkler PB [editors]. Williams & Wilkins, 1968). They compared the results of simple mastectomy plus radiotherapy with extended radical mastectomy (standard radical mastectomy plus removal of internal mammary and supraclavicular nodes). The extended radical mastectomy patients received no irradiation. Staging was done in part according to the UICC clinical staging system and in part according to the Columbia criteria. All patients may be considered to fall within UICC stages I and II. Treatment was simple mastectomy plus radiotherapy in 149 patients and extended radical mastectomy in 153 patients. Crude 10-year survival rates for simple and extended radical mastectomy groups

were 46% and 49%, respectively; and the crude 10-year recurrence-free survival rate was 42% in each group. As in the study by Brinkley and Haybittle, radiotherapy plus simple removal of the breast proved as effective as radical surgery in controlling regional recurrence of disease.

Orthovoltage irradiation was used in the above 2 clinical trials. Supervoltage radiotherapy as now available is more effective and is associated with fewer complications. Thus there is little doubt that radiotherapy is as efficient in the control of metastases to regional nodes as is surgical excision. This being the case, the progress of current clinical trials involving minimal surgery such as simple removal of the breast lump or partial mastectomy plus supervoltage radiotherapy will be followed with interest.

Coincidental with increased diversity in approach to treatment of operable breast cancer in recent years has been wider recognition of the fact that breast cancer is in most cases already a systemically disseminated disease when the diagnosis is made. Therefore, failure of cure is not necessarily related to the type of primary treatment but rather to the fact that procedures on breast and regional nodes do not eradicate occult metastases which already exist in bone, lung, liver, or elsewhere. This is illustrated by survival data obtained from a 10-year follow-up of patients in the National

Surgical Adjuvant Breast Project clinical trial begun in 1958. This study showed that following radical mastectomy, 75% of all patients with positive axillary nodes (65% with 1−3 and 86% of those with 4 or more positive) were treatment failures by 10 years. The survival of those with 1−3 positive nodes was 37.5%; it was only 13.4% when more than 3 nodes contained tumor. Especially disturbing was the observation that 25% of patients with negative nodes were treatment failures by 10 years as the result of distant metastases (Fisher B, Wolmark N: Cancer [Suppl] 36:627, 1975). These findings underscore the significance of recent clinical trials which showed that adjuvant chemotherapy after mastectomy increases the tumor-free period in patients with positive axillary nodes (see p 287).

The fact remains that no alternative form of treatment is superior to surgical removal of breast and axillary nodes for properly selected patients. Therefore, there is continued widespread reliance on radical mastectomy, or a modification of it, in spite of the inevitable cosmetic and occasional functional disadvantages compared to lesser procedures with or without radiotherapy.

As treatment options and complexity of management have increased, so has the importance of close cooperation of surgeon, radiotherapist, and oncologist in order to assure the best possible therapeutic regimen and outlook for patients with breast cancer. At the same time it is clear that earlier diagnosis, through public and professional education and programs of screening, is necessary if the overall mortality rate from breast cancer is to be reduced by existing methods of therapy.

CARCINOMA OF THE MALE BREAST

Essentials of Diagnosis

- A painless lump beneath the areola in a man, usually over 50 years of age.
- Nipple discharge, retraction, or ulceration may occur.

General Considerations

Breast cancer in men is a rare disease; the incidence is only about 1% of that in the female. The average age at occurrence is about 60—somewhat older than the commonest presenting age in the female. The prognosis, even in stage I cases, is worse in the male than in the female. Blood-borne metastases are commonly present when the male patient appears for initial treatment. These metastases may be latent and may not become manifest for many years.

As in the female, hormonal influences are probably related to the development of male breast cancer. A high estrogen level (as in liver disease), a shift in the androgen-estrogen ratio, or an abnormal susceptibility of breast tissue to normal estrogen concentrations may be of etiologic significance.

Clinical Findings

A painless lump, occasionally associated with nipple discharge, retraction, erosion, or ulceration, is the chief complaint. Examination usually shows a hard, ill-defined, nontender mass beneath the nipple or areola. Gynecomastia not uncommonly precedes or accompanies male breast cancer.

There is a high incidence of both breast cancer and gynecomastia in Bantu males, theoretically due to failure of estrogen inactivation by a damaged liver associated with vitamin B deficiency. Breast cancer is staged in the male as in the female patient. Gynecomastia and metastatic cancer from another site (eg, prostate) must be considered in the differential diagnosis of a breast lesion in the male patient. Biopsy settles the issue.

Treatment

Treatment consists of radical mastectomy in operable patients, who should be chosen by the same criteria as for female breast carcinoma. Radiation therapy is also advised as in female patients according to similar indications. Irradiation is the first step in the treatment of localized metastases in the skin, lymph nodes, or skeleton which are causing symptoms.

Since male breast cancer is so frequently a disseminated disease, endocrine therapy is of considerable importance in its management. Castration in advanced breast cancer is the most successful palliative measure and more beneficial than the same procedure in the female. Objective evidence of regression may be seen in 60−70% of male patients who are castrated—approximately twice the proportion seen in females. The average duration of tumor growth remission is about 30 months, and life is undoubtedly prolonged. Bone is the most frequent site of metastases from breast cancer in the male (as it is in the female also), and castration relieves bone pain in the vast majority of patients so treated. The longer the interval between mastectomy and recurrence, the longer the tumor growth remission following castration. As in the female, there is no correlation between the histologic type of the tumor and the likelihood of remission following castration. In view of the marked benefits of castration in advanced disease, prophylactic castration has been suggested in stage II male breast cancer, but there is no certainty that this approach is warranted.

Bilateral adrenalectomy (or hypophysectomy) has been proposed as the procedure of choice when tumor has reactivated after castration. Corticosteroid therapy is considered by some to be more efficacious than major endocrine ablation. Male breast cancer is too rare to enable this issue to be decided in a definitive manner at this time. Either approach may be temporarily beneficial. It is probably preferable to reserve corticosteroid therapy for those patients unfit for major endocrine ablation. The recommended dosage of prednisolone or prednisone is 30 mg daily orally, increased to 100 mg daily for urgent symptoms. The dosage is reduced to 20 mg daily when control is established, but it may be necessary to increase the dosage to maintain control over a long period. The side-effects of corticosteroid therapy must be kept in mind.

Estrogen therapy—5 mg of diethylstilbestrol 3 times daily orally—may rarely be effective. Androgen therapy may exacerbate bone pain. Castration, bilateral adrenalectomy, and corticosteroids are the main lines of therapy for advanced male breast cancer at the present time. Nonhormonal combination chemotherapy will probably be used with increasing frequency in the future as an alternative mode of treatment.

Examination of the breast cancer for estrogen receptor protein may in future prove to be of value in predicting response to endocrine ablation (Rosen PP & others: Cancer 37:1866, 1976). Adjuvant chemotherapy for the same indications as in female breast cancer (see p 287) may be useful, but experience with this form of treatment is lacking at present.

Prognosis

The prognosis of male breast cancer is poorer than that of female breast cancer owing to occurrence at older ages and with more unfavorable features. The crude 5- and 10-year survival rates for UICC stage I male breast cancer are about 58% and 38%, respectively. For clinical stage II disease the 5- and 10-year survival rates are approximately 38% and 10%. The overall survival rates at 5 and 10 years are 36% and 17% (Scheike O: Br J Cancer 30:261, 1974).

MAMMARY DYSPLASIA

Essentials of Diagnosis

- Painful, often multiple, frequently bilateral masses in the breast.
- Rapid fluctuation in the size of the masses is common.
- Frequently, pain occurs or increases and size increases during premenstrual phase of cycle.
- Most common age is 30—50. Rare in postmenopausal women.

General Considerations

This disorder, also known as chronic cystic mastitis of the breast, is the most frequent lesion of the breast. It is common in women 30—50 years of age but rare in postmenopausal women, which suggests that it is related to ovarian activity. Estrogen hormone is considered an etiologic factor. The typical pathologic change in the breast is the formation of gross and microscopic cysts from the terminal ducts and acini. Large cysts are clinically palpable and may be several centimeters or more in diameter.

Clinical Findings

Mammary dysplasia may produce an asymptomatic lump in the breast which is discovered by accident, but pain or tenderness often calls attention to the mass. There may be discharge from the nipple. In many cases discomfort occurs or is increased during the premenstrual phase of the cycle, at which time the cysts tend to enlarge. Fluctuation in size and rapid appearance or disappearance of a breast tumor are common in cystic disease. Multiple or bilateral masses are not unusual, and many patients will give a past history of transient lump in the breast or cyclic breast pain. Pain, fluctuation in size, and multiplicity of lesions are the features most helpful in differentiation from carcinoma. However, if skin retraction is present, the diagnosis of cancer should be assumed until disproved by biopsy.

Differential Diagnosis

Pain, fluctuation in size, and multiplicity of lesions help to differentiate these lesions from carcinoma and adenofibroma. Final diagnosis often depends on biopsy. Mammography may be helpful.

Treatment

Because mammary dysplasia is frequently indistinguishable from carcinoma on the basis of clinical findings, it is advisable to biopsy suspicious lesions in the operating room. General anesthesia is usually required, but small lesions may be suitable for excision under local anesthesia. Provision is often made for immediate diagnosis by frozen section. If cancer is present, definitive surgery such as mastectomy may be deferred for a few days without risk pending further discussion with the patient and additional studies as needed. When it is planned to proceed at once with mastectomy if the biopsy is positive, the patient must be prepared preoperatively. Discrete cysts or small localized areas of cystic disease should be excised when cancer has been ruled out by microscopic examination. Surgery in mammary dysplasia should be conservative, since the primary objective of surgery is to exclude cancer. Simple mastectomy or extensive removal of breast tissue is rarely, if ever, indicated.

When the diagnosis of mammary dysplasia has been established by previous biopsy or is practically certain because the history is classical, aspiration of a discrete mass suggestive of a cyst is indicated. The skin and overlying tissues are anesthetized by infiltration with 1% procaine, and a No. 21 gauge needle is introduced (see Fig 20—8). If a cyst is present, typical watery fluid (straw-colored, gray, greenish, brown, or black) is easily evacuated and the mass disappears. Cytologic examination of the fluid should be considered. The patient is reexamined at intervals of 2—4 weeks for 3 months and every 6—12 months thereafter throughout life. If no fluid is obtained, if a mass persists after aspiration, if cytology is suspicious, or if at any time during follow-up an atypical persistent lump is noted, biopsy should be performed without delay.

Breast pain associated with generalized mammary dysplasia is best treated by avoidance of trauma and by wearing (night and day) a brassiere which gives good support and protection. Hormone therapy is not advisable because it does not cure the condition and has undesirable side-effects.

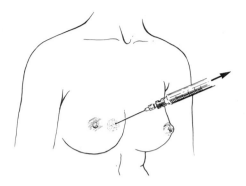

Figure 20—8. Needle aspiration of cyst.

Prognosis

Exacerbations of pain, tenderness, and cyst formation may occur at any time until the menopause, when symptoms subside. The patient should be advised to examine her own breasts each month just after menstruation and to inform her physician if a mass appears (see p 278). David HB & others (Cancer 17:957, 1964) concluded from a thorough review of the world literature that the risk of breast cancer in women with mammary dysplasia is about twice that of women in general. Follow-up examinations at regular intervals should therefore be arranged.

FIBROADENOMA OF THE BREAST

This common benign neoplasm occurs most frequently in young women, usually within 20 years after puberty. It is somewhat more frequent and tends to occur at an earlier age in black than in white women. Multiple tumors in one or both breasts are found in 10—15% of patients.

The typical fibroadenoma is a round, firm, discrete, relatively movable, nontender mass 1—5 cm in diameter. The tumor is usually discovered accidentally. Clinical diagnosis in young patients is generally not difficult. In women over 30, cystic disease of the breast and carcinoma of the breast must be considered. Fibroadenoma does not normally occur after the menopause, but postmenopausal women may occasionally develop fibroadenoma after administration of estrogenic hormone.

Treatment in all cases is excision and pathologic examination to determine if the lesion is cancerous.

Cystosarcoma phyllodes is a type of fibroadenoma with cellular stroma which tends to grow rapidly. This tumor may reach a large size, and if inadequately excised will recur locally. The lesion is rarely malignant. Treatment is usually by local excision of the mass with a margin of surrounding breast tissue.

DIFFERENTIAL DIAGNOSIS OF NIPPLE DISCHARGE

In order of frequency, the following lesions cause nipple discharge: intraductal papilloma, carcinoma, mammary dysplasia, and ectasia of the ducts. The discharge is usually serous or bloody. It should be checked for occult blood with the benzidine or guaiac test. When papilloma or cancer is the cause, a tumor can frequently (but not always) be palpated beneath or close to the areola.

The site of the duct orifice from which the fluid exudes is a guide to the location of the involved duct. Gentle pressure on the breast is made with the fingertip at successive points around the circumference of the areola (Fig 20—9). A point will often be found at which pressure produces discharge. The dilated duct or a small tumor may be palpable here. The involved area should be excised by a meticulous technic which ensures removal of the affected duct and breast tissues immediately adjacent to it. If a tumor is present it should be biopsied and a frozen section done to determine whether cancer is present.

When localization is not possible and no mass is palpable, the patient should be reexamined every week for 1 month. When unilateral discharge persists, even without definite localization or tumor, exploration must be considered. The alternative is careful follow-up at intervals of 1—3 months. Mammography should be done. Cytologic examination of nipple discharge for exfoliated cancer cells occasionally may be helpful in differential diagnosis.

Although none of the benign lesions causing nipple discharge are precancerous, they may coexist with cancer and it is not possible to distinguish them definitely from cancer on clinical grounds. Patients with carcinoma almost always have a palpable mass, but in rare instances a nipple discharge may be the only sign. For these reasons chronic nipple discharge, especially if bloody, is usually an indication for resection of the involved ducts.

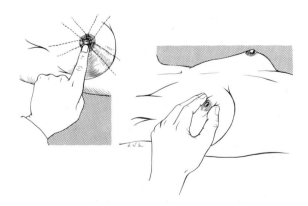

Figure 20—9. In patients with nipple discharge, the involved duct can usually be localized by fingertip pressure at successive points around the areola.

FAT NECROSIS

Fat necrosis is a rare lesion of the breast but is of clinical importance because it produces a mass, often accompanied by skin or nipple retraction, which is indistinguishable from carcinoma. Trauma is presumed to be the cause, although only about half of patients give a history of injury to the breast. Ecchymosis is occasionally seen near the tumor. Tenderness may or may not be present. If untreated, the mass associated with fat necrosis gradually disappears. As a rule the safest course is to obtain a biopsy. When carcinoma has been ruled out, the mass should be excised.

BREAST ABSCESS

During nursing, an area of redness, tenderness, and induration not infrequently develops in the breast. In the early stages the infection can often be reversed by continuing nursing with that breast and administering an antibiotic. If the lesion progresses to form a localized mass with local and systemic signs of infection, an abscess is present and should be drained.

A subareolar abscess may develop in young or middle-aged women who are not lactating. These infections tend to recur after incision and drainage unless the area is explored in a quiescent interval with excision of the involved collecting ducts at the base of the nipple.

Except for the subareolar type of abscess, infection in the breast is very rare unless the patient is lactating. Therefore, findings suggestive of abscess in the nonlactating breast require incision and biopsy of any indurated tissue.

•   •   •

General References

Carcinoma of the Breast

Anderson CB, Philpott GW, Ferguson TB: The treatment of malignant pleural effusion. Cancer 33:916, 1974.

Cady B: Total mastectomy and partial axillary dissection. Surg Clin North Am 53:313, 1973.

Egan RL: *Mammography,* 2nd ed. Thomas, 1972.

Farrow JH: Current concepts in the detection and treatment of the earliest of the early breast cancers. Cancer 25:468, 1970.

Fisher ER & others: The pathology of invasive breast cancer. Cancer 36:1, 1975.

Goldenberg IS & others: Androgenic therapy for advanced breast cancer in women: A report of the Cooperative Breast Cancer Group. JAMA 223:1267, 1973.

Haagensen CD: *Diseases of the Breast,* 2nd ed. Saunders, 1971.

Kennedy BJ: Hormone therapy in inoperable breast cancer. Cancer 24:1345, 1969.

Lee JM & others: An evaluation of five drug combination chemotherapy in the management of recurrent carcinoma of the breast. Surg Gynecol Obstet 138:77, 1974.

Marty R, Hoffman HC: Bone scan helps detect breast cancer metastases. JAMA 221:1215, 1972.

McGuire WL: *Estrogen Receptors in Human Breast Cancer.* Raven Press, 1975.

Oberfield RA & others: A multidisciplined approach for the management of breast cancer. Med Clin North Am 56:651, 1972.

O'Brien PH: Preoperative irradiation in cancer therapy [breast]. Surg Clin North Am 51:66, 1971.

Papaioannou AN: Etiologic factors in cancer of the breast in humans. Surg Gynecol Obstet 138:257, 1974.

Pearson OH: Endocrine treatment of breast cancer. CA 26:165, 1976.

Robbins GF & others: Metastatic bone disease developing in patients with potentially curable breast cancer. Cancer 29:1702, 1972.

Torres JE, Mickal A: Carcinoma of the breast in pregnancy. Clin Obstet Gynecol 18:219, 1975.

Welbourne RB, Burn JI: Treatment of advanced mammary cancer. N Engl J Med 287:398, 1972.

Wolfe JN: *Xeroradiography of the Breast.* Thomas, 1972.

Carcinoma of the Male Breast

Cortese AF, Cornell GN: Carcinoma of the male breast. Ann Surg 173:275, 1971.

Crichlow RW: Breast cancer in males. Breast 2:12, 1976.

Mammary Dysplasia

Fechner RE: Fibrocystic disease in women receiving oral contraceptive hormones. Cancer 25:1332, 1970.

Sartwell PE, Arthes FG, Tonascia JA: Epidemiology of benign breast lesions: Lack of association with oral contraceptive use. N Engl J Med 288:551, 1973.

Differential Diagnosis of Nipple Discharge

Funderburk WW, Syphax B: Evaluation of nipple discharge in benign and malignant breast disease. Cancer 24:1290, 1969.

Leis HP Jr, Dursi J, Mersheimer WL: Nipple discharge: Significance and treatment. NY State J Med 67:3105, 1967.

Breast Abscess

Benson EA, Goodman MA: Incision with primary suture in the treatment of acute puerperal breast abscess. Br J Surg 57:55, 1970.

Habif DV & others: Subareolar abscess associated with squamous metaplasia of lactiferous ducts. Am J Surg 119:523, 1970.

21...
Thoracic Wall, Pleura, Lung, & Mediastinum

Arthur N. Thomas, MD

ANATOMY OF THE CHEST WALL & PLEURA

The chest wall is an air-tight, expandable, cone-shaped cage. Lung ventilation is accomplished by the generation of negative pressure within it by simultaneous expansion of the rib cage and downward diaphragmatic excursion.

The ventral wall of the bony thorax is the shortest dimension. It extends from the suprasternal notch to the xiphoid—a distance of approximately 18 cm. It is formed by the vertically aligned manubrium, sternum, and xiphoid and the costal cartilages of the first 10 ribs. The sides of the chest wall consist of the upper 10 ribs, which slope downward and forward from their posterior attachments. The posterior chest wall is formed by the 12 thoracic vertebrae, their transverse processes, and the 12 ribs (Fig 21–1). The upper ventral portion of the thoracic cage is covered by the clavicle and subclavian vessels. Laterally, it is covered by the shoulder and axillary nerves and vessels; dorsally, it is covered by the scapula.

The superior aperture of the thorax (also called either the thoracic inlet or the thoracic outlet), is a 5 × 10 cm kidney-shaped opening bounded by the first costal cartilages and ribs laterally, the manubrium anteriorly, and the body of the first thoracic vertebra posteriorly. The inferior aperture of the thorax is bounded by the twelfth vertebra and ribs posteriorly and the cartilages of the seventh to twelfth ribs and the xiphisternal joint anteriorly. It is much wider than the superior aperture and is occupied by the diaphragm.

The blood supply and innervation of the chest wall are via the intercostal vessels and nerves (Figs 21–2 and 21–3), but the upper thorax also receives vessels and nerves from the cervical and axillary regions.

The parietal pleura is the innermost lining of the chest wall and is divided into 4 parts: the cervical pleura (cupula), costal pleura, mediastinal pleura, and diaphragmatic pleura. The visceral pleura is the serous layer investing the lungs and joins the parietal pleura at the hilus of the lung. The pleural space is compressed to a capillary gap and normally contains only a few drops of serous fluid. This space may be enlarged when

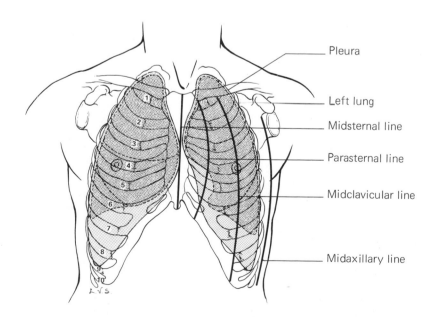

Figure 21—1. The thorax, showing rib cage, pleura, and lung fields.

Pleura

Left lung

Midsternal line

Parasternal line

Midclavicular line

Midaxillary line

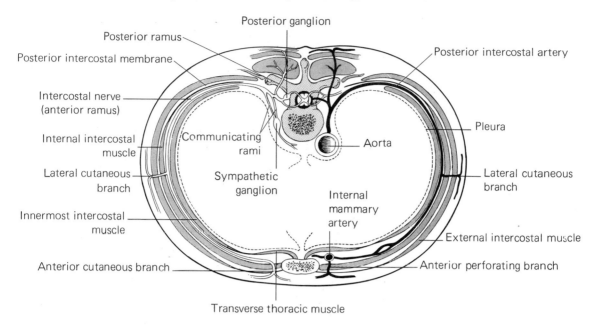

Figure 21–2. Transverse section of thorax.

fluid (hydrothorax), blood (hemothorax), pus (pyothorax or empyema), or air (pneumothorax) is present.

PHYSIOLOGY OF THE CHEST WALL & PLEURA

Mechanics of Respiration*

Breathing entails expansion of thoracic volume by elevation of the rib cage and descent of the diaphragm. The former predominates in men and the latter in women. In infants, because the ribs have not yet assumed their oblique contour, diaphragmatic breathing is required to provide sufficient ventilation.

Expiration is mainly passive and depends upon elastic recoil of the lungs. With deep breathing, the abdominal musculature contracts and pulls the rib cage downward and simultaneously elevates the diaphragm by compressing the abdominal viscera against it.

Wade OL: Movements of the thoracic cage and diaphragm in respiration. J Physiol 124:193, 1954.

Physiology of the Pleural Space

A. Pressure: The pleural cavity pressure is normally negative due to the elastic recoil of the lung and chest wall. During quiet respiration, it varies from −15 cm water with inspiration to 0–2 cm water during expiration. Deep breathing may cause large pressure changes (eg, −60 cm water during forced inspiration to

+30 cm water during vigorous expiration). Because of gravity, pleural pressure at the apex is more negative when the body is erect and changes about 0.2 cm water per centimeter of vertical height.

B. Fluid Formation and Reabsorption: Transudation and absorption of fluid within the pleural space normally follow the Starling equation, which depends on hydrostatic, colloid, and tissue pressures. In health,

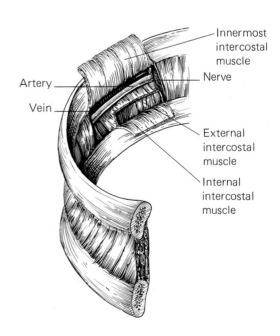

Figure 21–3. Intercostal muscles, vessels, and nerves.

*Pulmonary physiology and ventilation are described in Chapter 3.

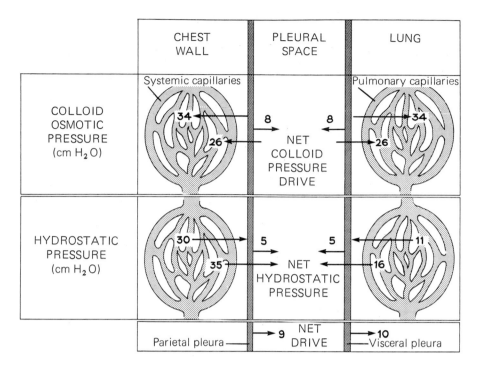

Figure 21—4. Movement of fluid across the pleural space, showing production and absorption of pleural fluid.

fluid is formed by the parietal pleura and absorbed by the visceral pleura (Fig 21—4). Systemic capillary hydrostatic pressure is 30 cm water and intrapleural negative pressure averages −5 cm water. Together these give a net hydrostatic pressure of 35 cm water that causes fluid transudation from the parietal pleura. The colloid osmotic pressure of the systemic capillaries is 34 cm water; this is opposed by 8 cm water pleural space osmotic pressure. Thus, a net 26 cm water osmotic pressure draws fluid back into systemic capillaries. Systemic hydrostatic pressure (35 cm water) exceeds osmotic pressure (26 cm water) by 9 cm water; thus, there is a 9 cm water net drive of fluid into the pleural space by systemic capillaries in the chest wall. Similar calculations for the visceral pleura involving the low pressure pulmonary circulation will show that there is a resulting net drive of 10 cm water that attracts pleural fluid into pulmonary capillaries.

In health, pleural fluid is low in protein (100 mg/100 ml). When it increases in disease to about 1 g/100 ml, the net colloid osmotic pressure of the visceral pleural capillaries is equalled and pleural fluid reabsorption becomes dependent on lymphatic drainage. Thus, abnormal amounts of pleural fluid may accumulate (1) when hydrostatic pressure is increased, such as in heart failure; (2) when capillary permeability is increased, as in inflammatory or neoplastic disease; or (3) when colloid osmotic pressure is decreased.

Robin ED, Cross CE, Zelis R: Pulmonary edema. (2 parts.) N Engl J Med 288:239, 292, 1973.

Rutishauser WJ & others: Pleural pressures at dorsal and ventral sites in supine and prone body position. J Appl Physiol 21:1500, 1966.

Stewart PB: The rate of formation and lymphatic removal of fluid in pleural effusions. J Clin Invest 42:258, 1963.

DISEASES OF THE CHEST WALL

Defects of development are described in Chapter 48. Neuromuscular syndromes of the inlet or shoulder are described in Chapter 38. Injuries to the chest wall are described in Chapter 16.

LUNG HERNIA (PNEUMATOCELE)

Pneumatocele or herniation of the lung can occur through defects in the chest wall caused by abnormal development, trauma, or surgery. Most lung hernias are thoracic in location, but cervical (defect of Sibson's fascia) or diaphragmatic herniation may occasionally occur. They are usually asymptomatic, but some patients experience local tenderness, pain, or mild dyspnea. Diagnosis is based on physical examination.

Although treatment has included various truss-like devices, operative repair is best if symptoms are present.

Shocket E, Hudseon TR: Lung hernia. Indust Med 26:556, 1957.

CHEST WALL INFECTIONS

Infections that appear to involve only the skin may actually represent outward extensions of deeper infection of the ribs, cartilage, sternum, or even the pleural space (empyema necessitatis). Inadequate drainage of superficial infection can lead to inward extension into the pleural space, causing empyema.

Subpectoral abscess is caused by suppurative adenitis of the axillary lymph nodes, rib or pleural infection, or posterior extension of a breast abscess, or may occur as a complication of chest wall surgery (eg, mastectomy, pacemaker placement). Hemolytic streptococci and *Staphylococcus aureus* are the usual organisms. The patient appears septic and the pectoral region is red and swollen, obliterating the normal infraclavicular depression. Shoulder movement is painful. Treatment consists of antibiotics and drainage by an incision along the lateral border of the pectoralis major muscle.

Subscapular abscess may arise from osteomyelitis of the scapula but most commonly follows thoracic operations such as thoracotomy or thoracoplasty. Winging of the scapula or paravertebral bulging of the trapezius muscle is usually present. The pus collection can be made more apparent by the bulge produced in adjacent soft tissues when the scapula is pressed against the chest wall. A pleural communication is suggested if a cough impulse is present or if the size of the mass varies with position or direct pressure. The diagnosis is established by needle aspiration. Treatment consists of open drainage for pyogenic infections not involving the pleura. Tuberculosis should be treated by chemotherapy and drainage, which can sometimes be accomplished by needle aspiration.

Sternal Osteomyelitis

Infection of the sternum now most commonly follows sternotomy incisions and presents as a postoperative wound infection or mediastinitis. Various gram-positive cocci and gram-negative bacilli have been isolated in individual cases. Treatment consists of antibiotics and either open drainage or closed drainage plus irrigation with antibiotic solution. In some cases, resection of involved sternum and a margin of adjacent normal bone is necessary.

Wray TW, Bryant RE, Killen DA: Sternal osteomyelitis and costochondritis after median sternotomy. J Thorac Cardiovasc Surg 65:227, 1973.

Osteomyelitis of the Ribs

In the past, osteomyelitis of the ribs was often caused by typhoid fever and tuberculosis. Except for a few cases in children, hematogenous osteomyelitis of the ribs is uncommon today. Most rib infections now occur as complications of thoracotomy incisions or occur in ribs adjacent to a draining empyema.

Infection of the Costal Cartilages & Xiphoid

Costal cartilage infections are relatively unresponsive to antibiotic therapy because once perichondral vascularity is interrupted the cartilage dies and remains as a foreign body to perpetuate the infection and sinus tract formation. The infection may be established during the course of septicemia, but the most common cause is direct extension of other surgical infections (eg, wound infection, subphrenic abscess). Surgical division of costal cartilages, as in a thoracoabdominal incision, may predispose to cartilage infection postoperatively if local sepsis develops. A wide variety of organisms have been implicated.

Pain, swelling, and erythema of overlying skin and subcutaneous tissue may be marked. This may be followed by fluctuance, spontaneous drainage, and sinuses which chronically discharge pus. The course may be fulminant or may be indolent over months or years with periodic exacerbations. There may be an associated osteomyelitis of the sternum, ribs, or clavicle.

The differential diagnosis includes local bone or cartilage tumors, Tietze's syndrome, chest wall metastasis, eroding aortic aneurysm, and bronchocutaneous fistula.

As a rule, the upper 5 costal cartilages (Fig 21–1) articulate separately with the sternum, but the sixth through the tenth cartilages are contiguous. Therefore, when one of the upper 5 costal cartilages is involved, local excision will usually suffice; but when cartilages 6 through 10 are involved, removal of the entire costal arch is usually required. If adjacent osteomyelitis is present, only grossly diseased bone need be excised.

Cure can be expected if operation removes all the infected cartilage, but in many instances recurrence is prompt due to underestimation of the extent of the disease and inadequate resection.

Payne WS, Cardoza F, Weed LA: Chronic draining sinuses of the chest wall. Surg Clin North Am 53:927, 1973.

Williams CD & others: Chronic infection of the costal cartilages after thoracic surgical procedures. J Thorac Cardiovasc Surg 66:592, 1973.

TIETZE'S SYNDROME

Tietze's syndrome is a painful nonsuppurative inflammation of costochondral cartilages of unknown cause. It affects adults of either sex. Local tenderness is the only symptom. The swelling and tenderness eventually disappear without therapy. The syndrome may recur.

Treatment is symptomatic and may include analgesics and local or systemic corticosteroids. When symptoms persist longer than 3 weeks and tumefaction suggests neoplasm, excision of the involved cartilage may be indicated and is usually curative.

Wehrmacher WH: Significance of Tietze's syndrome in differential diagnosis of chest pain. JAMA 157:505, 1955.

MONDOR'S DISEASE
(Thrombophlebitis of the Thoracoepigastric Vein)

Mondor's disease consists of localized thrombophlebitis of the anterolateral chest wall. It is more common in women than in men and occasionally follows radical mastectomy. There are few symptoms other than the presence of a tender cord-like structure in the subcutaneous tissues of the abdomen, thorax, or axilla. The disease is self-limited and devoid of complications such as thromboembolism.

Abramson DJ: Mondor's disease and string phlebitis. JAMA 196:1087, 1966.

CHEST WALL TUMORS

Except for those of the breast, primary tumors of the chest wall are all sarcomas; carcinoma in this area not of breast origin is always metastatic. Only about 5–8% of skeletal and soft tissue tumors that occur in humans involve the chest wall.

Most soft tissue tumors of the chest wall are benign, whereas half of skeletal tumors are malignant; most of the latter represent metastases from remote primaries. Benign tumors often occur in young adults; primary malignant tumors during middle age; and metastatic tumors in elderly people. Tumors in this area occur more often in males than females.

Clinical Findings
A. Symptoms and Signs: Many tumors are asymptomatic and are first noted on a routine chest x-ray. When symptomatic, they present with local swelling or pain. In general, pain is more often associated with malignancy.

B. Laboratory Findings: There are no diagnostic findings on blood count, urinalysis, serum calcium, acid or alkaline phosphatase, or bone marrow biopsy. Radioactive ^{85}Sr or other bone scans may be useful to localize tumors not visible by ordinary roentgenographic studies.

C. X-Ray Findings: X-rays may be valuable for detection, diagnosis, or evaluation of tumors, but the diagnosis usually depends on complete histologic study.

D. Biopsy: Incisional biopsy or needle biopsy may not recover tissue representative of the most malignant portion of the tumor, and seeding of the adjacent soft tissue with malignant tumor cells sometimes occurs. Therefore, whenever possible, wide excisional biopsy is preferred.

Differential Diagnosis
Chest wall tumors may be simulated by enlarged costal cartilages, chest wall infections, fractures, rickets, scurvy, hyperparathyroidism, and other conditions.

Specific Neoplasms
A. Benign Soft Tissue Tumors:
1. Lipomas–Lipomas are the most common benign tumors of the chest wall. Occasionally they are very large, lobulated, and may have dumbbell-shaped extensions that indent the endothoracic fascia beneath the sternum through a vertebral foramen. They may on occasion communicate with a large mediastinal or supraclavicular component.

2. Neurogenic tumors–These may arise from intercostal or superficial nerves. Solitary neurofibromas are most common, followed by neurolemmomas.

3. Cavernous hemangiomas–Hemangiomas of the thoracic wall are usually painful and occur in children. They may be isolated tumors or may involve other tissues (eg, lung), suggesting Rendu-Osler-Weber syndrome.

4. Lymphangiomas–This rare lesion is seen most often in children. It may have poorly defined borders that make complete excision difficult.

B. Malignant Soft Tissue Tumors:
1. Fibrosarcomas–Fibrosarcoma is the most common primary soft tissue malignancy of the chest wall. It is most common in young adults.

2. Liposarcomas–These tumors account for approximately one-third of all primary malignancies of the chest wall. They occur more often in men.

3. Neurofibrosarcomas–Neurofibrosarcomas involve the thoracic wall almost twice as often as other parts of the body. They often occur in patients with Recklinghausen's disease and usually originate from intercostal nerves.

C. Benign Skeletal Tumors:
1. Chondromas, osteochondromas, and myxochondromas–The combined frequency of these 3 cartilaginous tumors is nearly the same as that of fibrous dysplasia (ie, they comprise about 30–45% of all benign skeletal tumors). Cartilaginous tumors are usually single and occur with equal frequency in males and females between childhood and the fourth decade. The tumors are usually painless and tend to occur anteriorly along the costal margin or in the parasternal area. Wide local excision is curative.

2. Fibrous dysplasia–Fibrous dysplasia (bone cyst, osteofibroma, fibrous osteoma, fibrosis ossificans) accounts for a third or more of benign skeletal tumors of the chest wall. This cystic bone tumor can occur in any portion of the skeletal system, but approximately half involve the ribs. They must be clinically differentiated from cystic bone lesions associated with hyperparathyroidism. The tumor is usually single and may be related to trauma. Some patients complain of swelling, tenderness, or vague pain or discomfort, but the lesion is usually silent and is detected on routine chest x-ray. Treatment consists of local excision.

3. Eosinophilic granuloma—Eosinophilic granuloma may occur in the clavicle, scapula, or (rarely) in the sternum. There may be coexisting infiltrative lung involvement. It often represents a more benign form of Letterer-Siwe disease or Hand-Schüller-Christian syndrome. The patient may have fever, malaise, leukocytosis, eosinophilia, or bone pain. Rib involvement presents as a swelling with cortical bone destruction and periosteal new growth. The clinical picture can resemble osteomyelitis or Ewing's sarcoma. When the disease is localized, excision will result in cure.

4. Hemangioma—Cavernous hemangioma of the ribs presents as a painful mass in infancy or childhood. The tumor appears on x-ray as either multiple radiolucent areas or a single trabeculated cyst.

5. Miscellaneous—Fibromas, lipomas, osteomas, and aneurysmal bone cysts are all relatively rare lesions of the skeletal chest wall. The diagnosis is established after excisional biopsy.

D. Malignant Skeletal Tumors:

1. Chondrosarcomas—Chondrosarcomas are the most common primary malignant tumors of the chest wall. About 15–20% of all skeletal chondrosarcomas occur in the ribs or sternum. Most appear in patients 20–40 years of age. They tend to occur anteriorly at the costochondral junction of the rib cage but may occur anywhere along the rib. Local involvement of pleura, adjacent ribs, muscle, diaphragm, or other soft tissue may develop. There may be pain, but most patients complain only of the mass. Chest x-ray shows destroyed cortical bone, usually with diffuse mottled calcification, and the border of the tumor is indistinct. Treatment consists of wide radical excision. Only occasionally are regional lymph nodes involved. The 5-year survival rate is 10–30%, depending largely upon the adequacy of the initial excision.

2. Osteosarcoma (osteogenic sarcoma)—Osteosarcoma occurs in the second and third decades, and 60% occur in males. It is more malignant than chondrosarcoma. X-ray findings consist of bone destruction and recalcification at right angles to the bony cortex which gives the characteristic "sunburst" appearance. Hematogenous metastasis with pulmonary involvement is common. Treatment consists of radical local excision, but the prognosis is poor and 5-year survivals are rare.

3. Myeloma (solitary plasmacytomas)—These tumors are often found as a manifestation of systemic multiple myeloma, and patients with myeloma of the chest wall usually develop manifestations of systemic disease. The roentgenographic findings are punched-out, osteolytic lesions without evidence of new bone formation. The disease affects adults in the fifth to seventh decades and is seen nearly twice as often in males as in females. Solitary myeloma is quite rare, and systemic involvement eventually occurs in all cases. Treatment with antimetabolites relieves bone pain,

although life is not prolonged. The 5-year survival rate is only about 5%.

4. Ewing's sarcoma (hemangioendothelioma, endothelioma)—Ewing's tumors are associated with systemic symptoms such as fever and malaise and, locally, a painful, warm chest wall mass. Roentgenographic findings often show a characteristic "onion skin" calcification. These tumors are highly malignant, and evidence of other skeletal lesions is present in 30–75% when first seen. The diagnosis should be established by needle biopsy since surgical excision does not improve survival. X-ray irradiation is the only treatment available. Survival for as long as 5 years is rare.

5. Lymphoma—The diagnosis and treatment of chest wall lymphomas are essentially the same as for those lesions found elsewhere in the body.

E. Metastatic Chest Wall Tumors: Metastases to bones of the thorax are often multiple and are usually from tumors of the kidney, thyroid, lung, breast, prostate, stomach, uterus, or colon (Fig 21–5). Involvement by direct extension occurs in carcinoma of the breast and lung. Some cases of lung carcinoma involving the chest wall by direct extension have been cured by radical resection.

Groff DB III, Adkins PC: Chest wall tumors: A collective review. Ann Thorac Surg 4:260, 1967.

Martini N & others: Primary malignant tumors of the sternum. Surg Gynecol Obstet 138:391, 1974.

Omell GH & others: Chest wall tumors. Radiol Clin North Am 11:197, 1973.

Teitelbaum SL: Twenty years' experience with intrinsic tumors of the bony thorax at a large institution. J Thorac Cardiovasc Surg 63:776, 1972.

Teitelbaum SL: Twenty years' experience with soft tissue sarcomas of the chest wall in a large institution. J Thorac Cardiovasc Surg 63:585, 1972.

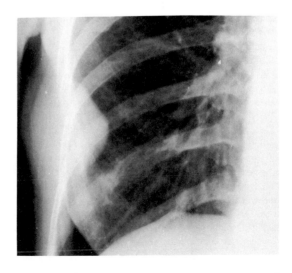

Figure 21–5. Rib metastasis and extrapleural mass from leiomyosarcoma of the uterus.

DISEASES OF THE PLEURA

The most common symptom of pleural disease is **pleuritic pain**—chest pain associated with respiratory excursion which sometimes reflexly inhibits respiration. Pleural pain is mediated through nerves to the parietal pleura or diaphragm since the visceral pleura does not contain pain fibers. When pulmonary processes become painful, it indicates involvement of both the visceral and parietal pleura. Pleuritic pain is felt in the shoulder over the distribution of the third through fifth cervical segments. Diseases involving the pleural surfaces can also produce an audible friction rub on auscultation. Both pleuritic pain and friction rubs may diminish if a pleural effusion forms.

Respiratory movement may lag on the affected side. Fullness or even bulging may appear with effusion. Long-standing pleural disease can even cause contraction and immobility of the involved hemithorax. The intercostal spaces are narrowed, and the ribs have a shingled relationship. Acute inflammation of the pleura may be associated with tenderness of the intercostal spaces or, in advanced cases, with swelling, redness, and local warmth. Tactile fremitus to the spoken voice is diminished with effusion, and there is dullness to percussion. Breath sounds may be exaggerated, bronchial, or amphoric in quality over a lung compressed by pleural effusion.

PLEURAL EFFUSIONS

The term pleural effusion denotes endogenous fluid in the pleural space. A more exact terminology is used when the character of the fluid is known. **Hydrothorax** denotes serous effusions, either transudates or exudates. **Pyothorax (empyema), hemothorax,** and **chylothorax** are other categories. These are discussed separately below.

Pleural effusions may occur with disease of the lungs, mediastinum, or chest wall. Identification of the specific type of effusion often depends on examination of fluid obtained by thoracentesis (Table 21–1). If this procedure is unsuccessful, either needle or open pleural biopsy must be considered.

Transudates have a specific gravity less than 1.016 and a protein content of less than 3 g/100 ml. Transudates contain only a few cells and are most often clear and yellow but occasionally are blood-tinged. Transudates occur in congestive heart failure, nephritis, and cirrhosis of the liver. Exudates, which have a higher specific gravity and protein content than transudates, may look clear, cloudy, or bloody. Examination of sediment after centrifugation may show tumor cells, bacteria, fungi, tubercle bacilli, or parasites such as amebas.

Committee on Therapy, American Thoracic Society: Therapy of pleural effusion. Am Rev Respir Dis 97:479, 1968.

PLEURAL EFFUSION FROM NONPULMONARY DISEASES

Immunologic Diseases

Systemic lupus erythematosus is associated with pleural effusion in about half of cases. Only 10% represent isolated pleural involvement, and these are usually small (though they may be massive). In about 30–50% of cases, the heart is enlarged on x-ray.

Pleural effusion in patients with rheumatoid arthritis occurs almost exclusively in middle-aged men. The effusions are usually unilateral and involve the right side somewhat more often than the left. There appears to be no relationship between the pulmonary manifestations of rheumatoid disease and pleural effusion.

Cardiovascular Diseases

Pleural effusion is seen in constrictive pericarditis and congestive heart failure (Fig 21–6). The right hemithorax alone is most often affected, though the effusion may be bilateral. Fluid occasionally localizes in interlobar fissures, giving "phantom tumors" or "disappearing tumors." Interlobar effusions involve the right horizontal fissure in most cases but may be bilateral.

Pancreatitis

Pleural effusion secondary to pancreatitis usually affects only the left side but sometimes is on the right. The diagnosis rests on finding an amylase concentration in the fluid substantially above that in the serum.

Meigs' Syndrome

Meigs' syndrome (ascites and hydrothorax) was first described in patients with fibroma of the ovary. Since then, a wide variety of pelvic tumors such as fibromas, thecomas, granulosa cell tumors, Brenner tumors, cystadenomas, adenocarcinomas, and fibromyomas of the uterus have also been implicated.

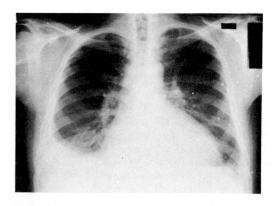

Figure 21–6. Pleural effusion secondary to heart failure (myocarditis).

Table 21—1. Differential diagnosis of pleural effusions.*

	Tuberculosis	Malignancy	Congestive Failure	Pneumonia and Other Non-tuberculous Infections	Rheumatoid Arthritis and Collagen Disease	Pulmonary Embolism
Clinical context	Younger patient with history of exposure to tuberculosis.	Older patient in poor general health.	Presence of congestive failure.	Presence of respiratory infection.	History of joint involvement; subcutaneous nodules.	Postoperative, immobilized, or venous disease.
Gross appearance	Usually serous; often sanguineous.	Often sanguineous.	Serous.	Serous.	Turbid or yellow-green.	Often sanguineous.
Microscopic examination	May be positive for acid-fast bacilli; cholesterol crystals.	Cytology positive in 50%.	. . .	May be positive for bacilli.	. . .	. . .
Cell count	Few have > 10,000 erythrocytes; most have > 1000 leukocytes, mostly lymphocytes.	Two-thirds bloody; 40% > 1000 leukocytes, mostly lymphocytes.	Few have > 10,000 erythrocytes or > 1000 leukocytes.	Polymorphonuclears predominate.	Lymphocytes predominate.	Erythrocytes predominate.
Culture	Many have positive pleural effusion; few have positive sputum or gastric washings.	. . .	. . .	May be positive.	. . .	. . .
Specific gravity	Most > 1.016.	Most > 1.016.	Most < 1.016.	> 1.016.	> 1.016.	> 1.016.
Protein	90% 3 g/100 ml or more.	90% 3 g/100 ml or more.	75% < 3 g/100 ml.	3 g/100 ml or more.	3 g/100 ml or more.	3 g/100 ml or more.
Sugar	60% < 60 mg/100 ml.	Rarely < 60 mg/100 ml.	. . .	Occasionally 60 mg/100 ml.	5—17 mg/100 ml (rheumatoid arthritis).	. . .
Other	No mesothelial cells on cytology. Tuberculin test usually positive. Pleural biopsy positive.	If hemorrhagic fluid, 65% will be due to tumor; tends to recur after removal.	Right-sided in 55—70%.	Associated with infiltrate on x-ray.	Rapid clotting time; LE cell or rheumatoid factor may be present.	Source of emboli may be noted.

Other exudates: (Sp gr > 1.016.)

    Fungal infection: Exposure in endemic area. Serous fluid. Microscopy and culture may be positive for fungi. Protein 3 g/100 ml or more. Skin and serologic tests may be helpful.

    Trauma: Serosanguineous fluid. Protein 3 g/100 ml or more.

    Chylothorax: History of injury or cancer. Chylous fluid with no protein but with fat droplets.

*Modified from: Therapy of pleural effusion: A statement by the Committee on Therapy of the American Thoracic Society. Am Rev Respir Dis 97:479, 1968.

Removal of the pelvic tumor is invariably followed by clearing of both effusions.

Cirrhosis of the Liver

Right-sided hydrothorax occurs in about 5% of patients with cirrhosis and ascites.

Renal Disease

Hydronephrosis, nephrotic syndrome, and acute glomerulonephritis are sometimes associated with hydrothorax.

Thromboembolic Disease

Pleural effusion following pulmonary embolism is usually serosanguineous and may be grossly bloody. These effusions are occasionally massive but usually are small and associated with characteristic x-ray findings in the lung. Treatment of the pleural effusion is usually not necessary, and the fluid is reabsorbed in a few days.

Dunn JM, Sloan H: Pleural effusion and fibrosis secondary to Sansert administration. Ann Thorac Surg 15:295, 1973.

Levine BW, Castleman B: Recurrent pleural effusion. N Engl J Med 290:152, 1974.

Prabhaker KN & others: Pseudocyst of the pancreas associated with hydrothorax: Report of a case and review of the literature. J Thorac Cardiovasc Surg 61:885, 1971.

MALIGNANT PLEURAL EFFUSION

About half of all patients with carcinoma of the breast or lung develop pleural effusion during the course of their disease, and 25% of all effusions are the result of malignancy. Cytologic examination of pleural fluid is positive in 70% and pleural biopsy in 80% of malignant effusions. A definitive diagnosis is nearly always achieved by using both procedures if needed.

About 10% of malignant effusions are due to pleural mesotheliomas and the rest to metastatic tumors. About half of bilateral effusions associated with normal heart size are due to malignancy, and these are almost invariably associated with hepatic metastases.

The clinical findings are pleuritic pain, cough, fever, chest pain, dyspnea, and weakness. Occasionally, patients have large effusion without any symptoms.

Treatment

Multiple technics are used to treat malignant pleural effusions (Fig 21–7). The usual objective is to obtain full lung expansion and pleural symphysis so that the effusion does not recur. The most commonly used regimens are closed tube drainage for 4–7 days, with or without instillation of a sclerosing solution (eg, mechlorethamine) into the pleural space. Thoracentesis or tube drainage may be complicated by pneumothorax, fever, fluid loculation, and infection. Only rarely are thoracotomy, pleurectomy, and other aggressive surgical approaches indicated.

Prognosis

Recurrence of the effusion is inevitable after needle aspiration alone but drops to 15% in patients treated by tube drainage. However, the overall prognosis is very poor. The average duration of life in patients with malignant effusions due to solid tumors is about 6 months; with lymphomas, the average duration is 16 months.

Adler RH, Sayek I: Treatment of malignant pleural effusion: A method using tube thoracostomy and talc. Ann Thorac Surg 22:8, 1976.

Dollinger MR: Management of recurrent malignant effusions. CA 22:138, 1972.

Lambert CJ & others: The treatment of malignant pleural effusion by closed trochar tube drainage. Ann Thorac Surg 3:1, 1967.

Mark JBD & others: Intrapleural mechlorethamine hydrochloride therapy for malignant pleural effusion. JAMA 187:858, 1964.

EMPYEMA

Essentials of Diagnosis

- Chest pain, hemoptysis, shortness of breath, weakness.
- Fever.
- Patient may be toxic.
- Findings of pleural effusion.

General Considerations

The initial pleural response to infection may be an exudate, depending somewhat on the organism involved. Pleural exudates can form with nearby infec-

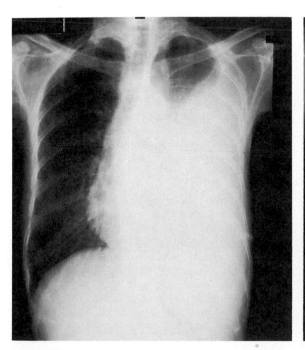
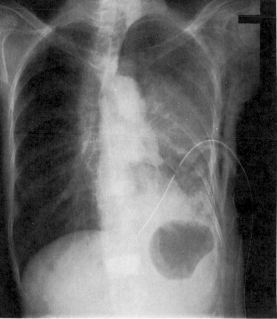

Figure 21–7. Malignant pleural effusion (carcinoma of lung). *Left:* Posteroanterior projection before treatment. *Right:* After chest tube drainage. Note left hilar mass and osteoblastic metastasis to the first lumbar vertebra.

tion even before organisms have entered the pleural spaces; however, this is either transitory or bacterial invasion follows. **Empyema thoracis** is an acute or chronic suppurative pleural exudate which may be caused by many organisms, eg, pneumococci, streptococci, staphylococci, bacteroides, *Escherichia coli, Proteus vulgaris,* tubercle bacilli, fungi, and amebas.

Infections may involve the pleural spaces by (1) direct extension of pneumonia; (2) lymphatic spread from neighboring infections of the lungs, mediastinum, chest wall, or diaphragm; (3) hematogenous spread from a remote infection; (4) direct inoculation by penetrating trauma or surgical incision of a pulmonary abscess (Fig 21–8); (5) ruptured thoracic viscera (eg, esophagus) or displaced abdominal viscera (eg, strangulated traumatic diaphragmatic hernia); or (6) extension of subdiaphragmatic processes such as subdiaphragmatic abscesses, hepatic abscesses, or perinephric abscesses.

When empyema follows pneumonia, it is known as **metapneumonic empyema.** In children, cystic fibrosis of the pancreas, congenital biliary atresia, agammaglobulinemia, Hodgkin's disease, and leukemia are predisposing factors. In adults, empyema usually develops in association with another debilitating disease.

Clinical Findings

A. Symptoms and Signs: Chest pain, shortness of breath, fever, weakness, and hemoptysis are usually

Table 21–2. Incidence of various complications of staphylococcal pneumonia in adults and children (in %).

	Adults	Children
Abscess	25	50
Empyema	15	15
Pneumatocele	1	35
Effusion	30	55
Bronchopleural fistula	2	5

present. Some patients are severely toxic or even comatose when first seen. They may be cyanotic, hypotensive, dehydrated, and oliguric. Temperature may reach 40.6 C (105 F) but is usually less. Respirations may be grunting. The physical findings of a pleural effusion are present (see above). In the absence of fever, empyema must be differentiated from pulmonary edema or pulmonary embolus with effusion.

B. Laboratory Findings: The hematocrit may be in the low 30s, particularly after rehydration. The white blood count is in the range of 14,000–18,000/μl, with a shift to the left.

The bacteriologic diagnosis is the most important part of the evaluation:

1. *Staphylococcus aureus*–*S aureus* is the most common organism involved in empyema in all age groups and accounts for over 90% of cases in infants and children. Staphylococcal pneumonia has a tendency to lead to empyema, abscesses, and pneumatoceles (Table 21–2). **Pneumatoceles** are thin-walled cystic spaces that form as a result of a check valve type of obstruction of small bronchi. They can produce localized overexpansion and rupture. The term pneumatocele is also used to refer to hernia of the chest wall, an unrelated condition.

2. *Streptococcus pyogenes*–Empyema is an especially frequent complication of streptococcal pneumonia. It is characterized by thick green pus which tends to become loculated within 2 or 3 days. Streptococcal organisms can often be diagnosed by sputum culture (60%), but throat culture is negative in about 80% of cases and blood cultures are rarely positive. The diagnosis is best made by culture of the pleural effusion. The antistreptolysin titer is greater than 250 Todd units in 97% of cases. The pneumonic component of streptococcal empyema may be minimal, and empyema may be the initial manifestation (Fig 21–9).

3. Bacteroides–Bacteroides empyema seems especially to affect young females with pelvic infections and elderly men with underlying respiratory disease, alcoholism, or malignancy. Identification of this organism is sometimes difficult because of its strict anaerobic requirement and slow growth. Its antibiotic sensitivities are discussed in Chapter 11. Empyema with these bacteria develops more rapidly than with *Escherichia coli* or *Pseudomonas aeruginosa,* and loculation may be present almost from the beginning. The accumulation of pus is massive, thick, and foul-smelling, and it tends to return rapidly after evacuation. Mixed

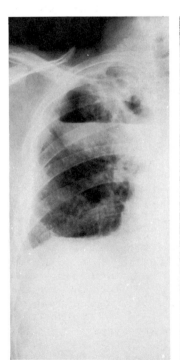
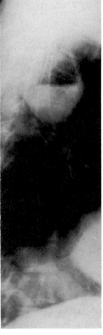

Figure 21–8. Postoperative loculated empyema with bronchopleural fistula. *Left:* Posteroanterior projection. *Right:* Lateral projection.

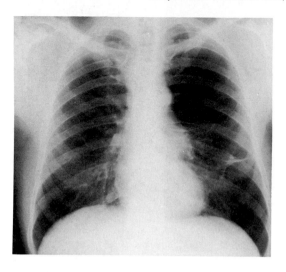 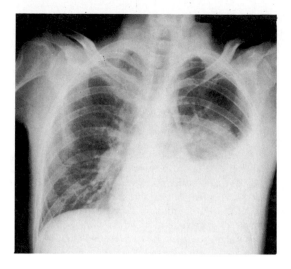

Figure 21–9. Streptococcal empyema. *Left:* Normal x-ray when admitted with high fever. *Right:* Chest x-ray 3 days after admission.

infection with anaerobic streptococci is common.

4. Klebsiella pneumoniae—Pneumonia and empyema from this organism principally affect debilitated, elderly, chronically ill, or alcoholic patients. One should suspect *K pneumoniae* when an effusion is associated with massive parenchymal consolidation. Abscess and cavitation occur in half of patients, and one-third of these develop empyema. Treatment must be aggressive but is often unsuccessful because of extensive parenchymal necrosis and the frequent development of a bronchopleural fistula.

5. Other bacteria—*Streptococcus pneumoniae* is now less often a cause of empyema than it was in the preantibiotic era. Pleural involvement following pneumococcal pneumonia usually occurred 7–10 days after onset, and most patients now have received effective antibiotic therapy by this time.

Escherichia coli, pseudomonas, and proteus may cause empyema in patients with underlying systemic disease.

C. X-Ray Findings: The roentgenographic appearance is characterized by opacification of a portion of the pleural space, sometimes with a fluid level. A pneumonic infiltrate is usually present but may be obscured by the effusion.

Complications

The complications of empyema are **empyema necessitatis** (invasion of the chest wall), bronchopleural fistula, pericardial extension, mediastinal abscess, osteomyelitis of ribs or cartilage, septicemia, and chronicity. Formation of a bronchial fistula into an empyema requires emergency treatment to avoid flooding of the opposite lung with pus and subsequent fatal pneumonia.

Metastatic abscesses, particularly to the brain, are unusual when antibiotic coverage is adequate but can occur in neglected cases. Prolonged suppuration such as may occur in postpneumonectomy empyema can

result in amyloid deposition, particularly in the liver and kidneys.

Treatment

A. Antibiotic Treatment: Prompt diagnosis and treatment are essential. Cultures of throat, sputum, pleural fluid, and blood should be obtained. Initial antibiotic treatment should be chosen on the basis of the clinical findings and the results of smears. When not contraindicated by allergy, high doses of penicillin should be used since the organisms that most commonly cause empyema are sensitive to penicillin. When staphylococcal infection is suspected, penicillinase resistance must be considered and a drug such as methicillin included in the regimen. Drainage should be done promptly in all cases to prevent empyema necessitatis and to obviate general toxicity and other septic sequelae.

B. Drainage of Pleural Space: Evacuation of the pus by needle aspiration may be elected in cases where the pleural effusion is minimal and watery and a prompt response to antibiotic therapy can be expected. However, even in favorable cases such as streptococcal empyema in young men, hospitalization time is almost 2 weeks longer when needle aspiration is used rather than closed tube drainage. In general, inadequate early drainage is the most frequent cause of subsequent therapeutic intractability from loculations, etc.

Prompt closed tube drainage of the pleural space to underwater seal is preferred in most cases (see Thoracentesis in Chapter 51). In cases failing to respond to simple drainage or where roentgenographic demonstration of multiple air-fluid levels indicates that loculation has already occurred, insertion of the tube may be combined with local rib resection (2.5–5 cm) and limited thoracic exploration to remove necrotic material and break down loculations. The chest tube can be brought through the chest wall by a separate incision or through the same incision, made airtight with layered absorbable sutures. Closed tube drainage with negative pressure minimizes the size of the residual pleural space.

When empyema is associated with parenchymal necrosis or lung trapping, the pleural space may not be obliterated by the above measures and the residual space may require prolonged drainage to prevent sealing off and reactivation of the infection. By 5–7 days, the space communicating with the chest tube is usually isolated from the remaining pleural space and the underwater seal is no longer necessary to prevent lung collapse. At this point, the chest tube can be cut, leaving a portion protruding from the chest wall to maintain a chronic draining tract. Later, if the space does not seem to be shrinking or if debridement is required, it can be managed by a larger chest wall and rib resection, known as an **Eloesser flap.** This procedure consists of suturing a flap of skin to the pleura, creating a epithelium-lined sinus into the empyema cavity for simpler long-term care.

C. Other Surgical Measures: More aggressive surgical approaches are reserved for unusual cases. Thoracoplasty, which involves collapsing the chest wall to obliterate pleural space, is rarely indicated. This procedure is discussed further in the section on tuberculosis. Empyemectomy involves resection of the empyema cavity en bloc and is usually reserved for empyemas localized to a lower lobe. This procedure may be especially appropriate when the associated lower lobe is destroyed and also requires resection. Decortication, or removal of the residual pleural peel, is indicated in the occasional case when ventilation of normal lung is prevented by a thick inelastic pleural scar or diaphragmatic fixation.

In occasional cases, bronchopleural fistula will not respond to therapy or may be so massive that pulmonary resection or reclosure of the postoperative bronchial stump is required. Bronchial stump closure may be buttressed by pedicle grafts of muscle or pleura, or other special procedures may be used. Postpneumonectomy empyema can occur with or without bronchopleural fistula. Initial treatment is by closed tube drainage, but once mediastinal stability is achieved an Eloesser flap can be performed to facilitate drainage. When pleural sepsis is controlled, the chest wall opening (Eloesser flap) may be closed without risk of recurrent empyema. This must be done by instillation of an appropriate antibiotic solution into the pleural space at the time of closure. This procedure is possible provided there is no bronchopleural fistula. In postpneumonectomy empyema without bronchopleural fistula, sterilization of the space is sometimes possible by antibiotic irrigation using chest tubes, thus eliminating the need for open drainage.

Chronic persistence of an empyema space is sometimes due to remediable causes of incomplete lung expansion. In cases with atelectasis due to aspiration of blood or mucus or when clearing of endobronchial secretions is inadequate, bronchoscopy should be performed early and repeated if necessary.

Prognosis

The average duration of hospitalization is 30–70 days. The mortality rate is higher in patients over age 40 and in those with predisposing conditions as outlined above. Those who arrive comatose, hypotensive, in pulmonary edema, or without leukocytosis have a poorer prognosis. Patients who succumb usually do so during the early part of the illness. The mortality rate is higher in infections with gram-negative organisms than with gram-positive ones.

The mortality rate in currently reported series ranges from 10–20% of patients developing empyema in association with pneumonia and from 25–55% in postoperative patients.

Rare Causes of Empyema

Almost any organism that infects the lungs can cause pleural effusion or empyema. *Mycobacterium tuberculosis* will be discussed with pulmonary tuberculosis. *Pasteurella tularensis* (causing tularemia) is associated with pleural involvement in 50% of cases of the typhoidal form. Organisms of the salmonella and clostridial groups have occasionally caused empyema.

Actinomyces israelii and Nocardia species may also cause pleural effusion and empyema. Pneumonitis is invariably present and usually is nonsegmentally distributed (homogeneous). The course of the disease may consist of lung abscesses followed by empyema and chest wall involvement with rib destruction (empyema necessitatis).

Entamoeba histolytica may cause secondary pleuropulmonary involvement by extension from a liver abscess. Lung cavitation and occasionally bronchobiliary fistula may occur. Sputum and pleural fluid may appear as "chocolate sauce." Amebic abscess often becomes secondarily infected with pyogenic organisms, in which case purulent empyema tends to mask the underlying amebiasis. *Paragonimus westermani* and *Echinococcus granulosus* (see Chapter 11) are rare causes of pleural effusions or empyema.

Basiliere JL, Bistrong HW, Spence WF: Streptococcal pneumonia: Recent outbreaks in military recruit populations. Am J Med 44:580, 1968.

Cattaneo SM, Kilman JW: Surgical therapy of empyema. Arch Surg 106:564, 1973.

Coon JL, Shuck JM: Failure of tube thoracostomy for post-traumatic empyema: An indication for early decortication. J Trauma 15:588, 1975.

Dines DE: Diagnostic significance of pneumotocele of the lung. JAMA 204:1169, 1968.

Geha AS: Pleural empyema: Changing etiologic, bacteriologic, and therapeutic aspects. J Thorac Cardiovasc Surg 61:626, 1971.

Kevy SU, Lowe BA: Streptococcal pneumonia and empyema in childhood. N Engl J Med 264:738, 1961.

Morin JE, Munro DD, MacLean LD: Early thoracotomy for empyema. J Thorac Cardiovasc Surg 64:530, 1972.

Stafford EG, Clagett OT: Postpneumonectomy empyema. J Thorac Cardiovasc Surg 63:771, 1972.

Sullivan KM & others: Anaerobic empyema thoracis. Arch Intern Med 131:521, 1973.

Symbas PN & others: Nontuberculous pleural empyema in adults: The role of a modified Eloesser procedure in its management. Ann Thorac Surg 12:69, 1971.

Tillotson JR, Lerner AM: Bacteroides pneumonias: Characteristics of cases with empyema. Ann Intern Med 68:308, 1968.

Tillotson JR, Lerner AM: Characteristics of pneumonias caused by *Escherichia coli.* N Engl J Med 277:115, 1967.

Vianna NJ: Nontuberculous bacterial empyema in patients with and without underlying diseases. JAMA 215:69, 1971.

Young D, Simon J, Pomerantz M: Current indications for and status of decortication for "trapped lung." Ann Thorac Surg 14:631, 1972.

CHYLOTHORAX

Accumulation of chyle in the pleural space may be (1) congenital, (2) traumatic postoperative, (3) traumatic nonsurgical, or (4) nontraumatic.

Congenital chylothorax is relatively rare. It is due primarily to congenital abnormalities of the lymphatic system such as absence of the thoracic duct or a fistula between the thoracic duct and the pleural space. Traumatic postoperative chylothorax follows operations or diagnostic procedures that injure the thoracic duct, most commonly cardiovascular and esophageal operations. Traumatic nonsurgical chylothorax follows either penetrating, blunt, or blast injuries. Fractures are not necessary for thoracic duct injury to occur. The usual mechanism is thought to be a shearing of the duct by the right crus of the diaphragm. This may occur with violent coughing or hyperextension of the spine. Nontraumatic chylothorax is generally regarded as ominous, since malignancy is the most frequent cause. However, there are many other causes such as hepatic cirrhosis, thoracic aortic aneurysm, and filariasis.

The treatment of nonmalignant chylothorax usually consists of removing sufficient fluid by needle or closed tube drainage to obtain full lung expansion. In many cases, the irritating nature of chyle will promote pleural symphysis and plug the leakage of chyle. During this time, the patient should be given a low-fat diet. In some cases, the patient may be fasted for several weeks and nutrition maintained by intravenous hyperalimentation. Surgical division and ligation of the duct should be considered early if drainage does not lead to prompt improvement. See Chapter 16 for further discussion.

Crosby IK, Crouch J, Reed WA: Chylopericardium and chylothorax. J Thorac Cardiovasc Surg 65:935, 1973.

Joyce LD, Lindsay WG, Nicoloff DM: Chylothorax after median sternotomy for intrapericardial cardiac surgery. J Thorac Cardiovasc Surg 71:476, 1976.

HEMOTHORAX

Accumulation of blood in the pleural space is most commonly due to trauma, pulmonary infarction, neoplasms, or tuberculosis. It may also occur as a complication of surgery or diagnostic procedures.

Treatment consists of closed tube drainage to evacuate the blood before clotting occurs. If no other specific treatment is required, relatively large amounts of blood or clot may be absorbed from the pleural space without significant sequelae if secondary infection does not occur. Occasionally, a persistent blood clot may result in fibrosis that impairs pulmonary function, in which case decortication should be considered. See Chapter 16 for further discussion.

PRIMARY PLEURAL TUMORS

There are 2 kinds of primary pleural tumors: localized mesothelioma and diffuse malignant mesothelioma. **Localized mesothelioma** most often arises from visceral pleura, is either pedunculated or sessile, and may either protrude into the pleural cavity or be embedded within the lung. It may achieve a gigantic size. Microscopically, this tumor is composed mainly of spindle cells and appears quite malignant, but usually the tumor is well encapsulated. Most do not recur after local excision, but about 30% of solitary mesotheliomas are malignant. Pleural effusion is present in only 10–15% of cases. The presence of blood in the effusion does not indicate incurability. The roentgenographic findings consist of a peripheral, well-demarcated mass, often forming an obtuse angle with the chest wall. Bone and joint pain, swelling, and arthritis have been described in as many as two-thirds of localized mesotheliomas.

Diffuse mesothelioma may arise anywhere within the pleura. It rapidly proliferates along the pleural surface to encase the lung. Pleural effusion is almost always present and is usually bloody. In cases without effusion, this lesion may present as diffuse pleural thickening. It is more common in areas where asbestos is mined.

All diffuse lesions are malignant. There is little evidence that they arise from originally benign localized mesothelioma. Diffuse mesotheliomas occur in all age groups but are often seen in relatively young patients, especially males, between 40–50 years. The patients complain of pleural pain, malaise, weight loss, weakness, anemia, fever, irritative cough, or dyspnea. The physical findings are those of pleural thickening or effusion.

Treatment of diffuse mesothelioma is rarely surgical but consists principally of relief of symptoms by controlling the pleural effusion, which may rapidly reaccumulate. Radiotherapy and intrapleural radioactive isotopes occasionally provide long-term remissions.

McDonald AD, Magner D, Eyssen G: Primary mesothelial tumors in Canada, 1960-1968: A pathologic review by the

Mesothelioma Panel of the Canadian Reference Center. CA 31:869, 1973.

Shearin JC Jr, Jackson D: Malignant pleural mesothelioma: Report of 19 cases. J Thorac Cardiovasc Surg 71:621, 1976.

Taryle DA & others: Pleural mesotheliomas: An analysis of 18 cases and review of the literature. Medicine 55:153, 1976.

PNEUMOTHORAX

Essentials of Diagnosis

- Chest pain referred to the shoulder or arm on the involved side.
- Dyspnea.
- Hyperresonance, decreased chest motion, decreased breath and voice sounds on involved side.
- Mediastinal shift away from involved side.
- Chest x-ray revealing retraction of the lung from the parietal pleura is diagnostic.

General Considerations

Air or gas in the pleural space (pneumothorax) may originate from rupture of the respiratory system (eg, lung, bronchus, trachea), esophagus, or the chest wall or it may be generated by microorganisms in a pleural infection. Pneumothorax may be classified as spontaneous, traumatic, or iatrogenic, depending on the cause. It is referred to as "closed" when the chest wall is intact or "open" when a breach in the chest wall exists. The magnitude of pneumothorax is expressed as an estimate of the percentage of collapse of the lung. For example, a small rim of air around the lung would represent about a 5–10% pneumothorax. When the visceral and parietal pleuras are not adherent, pressure in the pleural space may be sufficient to displace the mediastinum to the opposite side (**tension pneumothorax**). Both open ("sucking") chest wounds and tension pneumothorax are surgical emergencies since they seriously compromise total ventilation.

In trauma patients, pneumothorax is often associated with blood in the pleural space (hemopneumothorax). (Traumatic pneumothorax is discussed in Chapter 16.) With esophageal rupture, the combination of pleural suppuration and air is known as pyopneumothorax. (Esophageal rupture is discussed in Chapter 23.)

Iatrogenic pneumothorax may occur as a result of inadvertent introduction of air into the pleural space, inadvertent puncture or rupture of the lung, or intentional introduction of air into the pleural space or mediastinum. Thoracentesis, placement of a subclavian vein catheter for central venous pressure monitoring, operations on the chest wall, neck, back, or upper abdomen, lung or pleural biopsy, thoracentesis, brachial block, arteriography, and intercostal nerve block are procedures that are often complicated by pneumothorax. Inadvertent rupture of the lung may occur with assisted ventilation for anesthesia or respiratory support. Pneumothorax may intentionally be induced

for diagnosis or treatment.

Spontaneous pneumothorax may occur in any age group but is most common in males 15–35 years of age (Fig 21–10). In newborn infants, it may be asymptomatic and discovered as an incidental finding on a chest x-ray, or it may cause acute respiratory distress. In young adults, spontaneous pneumothorax develops without known cause in association with localized emphysematous blebs near the apex of the upper lobe. In elderly patients, generalized emphysema, bullous emphysema, or some other predisposing cause is usually present. The left and right sides are involved with approximately equal frequency. Bilateral involvement and tension pneumothorax are both uncommon. Males predominate over females 10:1. An associated effusion which may contain blood is present in 10%.

About 30% of patients with spontaneous pneumothorax have chronic pulmonary disease, consisting largely of chronic bronchitis or emphysema. A history of smoking, pneumonia, recent upper respiratory infection, or asthma is often obtained. Secondary spontaneous pneumothorax (pneumothorax related to active disease) may occur in staphylococcal pneumonia, lung abscess, or a multitude of other less common pulmonary conditions ranging from sarcoidosis to thoracic endometriosis.

Clinical Findings

A. Symptoms and Signs: In one-third of cases, the pneumothorax occurs during mild to moderate exercise. Symptoms are chest pain, shortness of breath, cough, and shoulder pain, but in 5% of cases there are no symptoms at all. Severe cases may be associated with syncope, nausea, vomiting, or shock. Physical findings include evidence of diminished ventilation of the affected lung and hyperresonance, but the diagno-

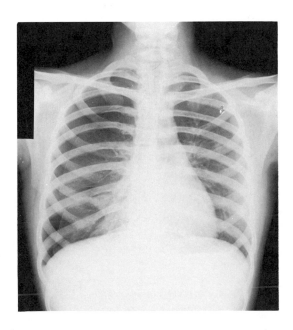

Figure 21–10. Spontaneous pneumothorax on right side.

sis may elude the examiner unless a chest x-ray is obtained. Tension pneumothorax may produce mediastinal shift and tracheal displacement away from the affected side with neck vein distention, cyanosis, and shock.

B. X-Ray Findings: X-ray shows the extent of pneumothorax (Fig 21–10).

C. Differential Diagnosis: In tension pneumothorax, the main disorders that must be differentiated are cardiac tamponade and acute congestive heart failure. The physical findings of tension pneumothorax are occasionally obscure, and the condition in such cases is first suspected only after a chest x-ray has been obtained. The x-ray appearance of giant lung cyst and of a distended stomach within the thorax after traumatic rupture of the diaphragm is similar.

Complications

Pneumothorax may be complicated by tension pneumothorax, simultaneous bilateral pneumothorax, recurrent or persistent pneumothorax, pleural effusion or hemothorax, empyema, or pneumonitis.

Treatment

The objective of treatment is to promptly reexpand the lung by means of thoracentesis, closed tube drainage, or thoracotomy. General measures include bed rest, treatment of underlying diseases, relief of pain, and management of shock and hypoxia. Thoracentesis is used for diagnosis and as a definitive measure for reexpansion in mild cases when continuous observation is possible to detect recurrence. However, closed tube drainage is the most reliable treatment. The tube is usually inserted anteriorly via the second anterior intercostal space into the apex of the pleural cavity. Air leaks that persist for 5–7 days and recurrent pneumothorax are usually treated by thoracotomy to excise apical blebs and to achieve pleural symphysis through pleural scarification, pleurectomy, or the use of pleural irritants.

Prognosis

The prognosis in properly managed patients with primary spontaneous pneumothorax is excellent. In patients with spontaneous pneumothorax secondary to another condition, the prognosis is determined by the underlying disease but the overall mortality rate is 10–15%.

Recurrence is the most common indication for operative treatment, and the probability of another recurrence increases with each attack. The average interval between attacks is 2–3 years, but pneumothorax can recur almost immediately or as long as 20 years afterward. Asynchronous bilateral involvement occurs in about 10%.

Brooks JW: Open thoracotomy in the management of spontaneous pneumothorax. Ann Surg 177:798, 1973.

Clark TA & others: Spontaneous pneumothorax. Am J Surg 124:728, 1972.

Mercier C & others: Outpatient management of intercostal tube drainage in spontaneous pneumothorax. Ann Thorac Surg 22:163, 1976.

Stier M & others: Iatrogenic causes of pneumothorax: Increasing incidence with advances in medical care. NY State J Med 73:1296, 1973.

PLEURAL CALCIFICATION OR PLAQUES

Pleural calcification occasionally occurs after long-term pleural infections, in organized collections of pleural blood, following empyema, in tuberculosis, and in asbestosis or silicosis. The costal and diaphragmatic pleura are involved more often than the visceral pleura.

Hyaline plaques may be seen at thoracotomy and may be confused with pleural metastatic implants. The cause of pleural plaques is not known, but the condition may follow tuberculosis or inhalation of asbestos fibers.

Pairolero PC, Bernatz PH, Harrison EG: Surgical implications of parietal pleural plaques. Surg Clin North Am 53:867, 1973.

THE LUNGS

SURGICAL ANATOMY
(See Fig 21–11.)

Clinical recognition of segmental anatomy has permitted thoracic surgeons to devise operative procedures that minimize unnecessary removal of normal lung parenchyma. Bronchopulmonary segments make up large lung units called the lobes. The right lung has 3 lobes: upper, middle, and lower. The left lung consists of 2 lobes: upper and lower. On the left, the lingular portion of the upper lobe is the homologue of the right middle lobe. Two fissures separate the lobes on the right side. The major or oblique fissure divides the upper and middle lobes from the lower lobe. The minor or horizontal fissure separates the middle from the upper lobe. On the left side, the single oblique fissure separates the upper and lower lobes.

The bronchopulmonary segmental anatomy is designated by numbers (Boyden) or by name (Jackson and Huber). The bronchial tree undergoes sequential division until the smallest unit of ventilation, the alveolus, is reached. The trachea and the main stem bronchi and their branches are prevented from collapse by horseshoe-shaped cartilages in their walls. Cartilaginous reinforcement of the airway gradually becomes less complete as the branches get smaller and ceases altogether with bronchi of 1–2 mm.

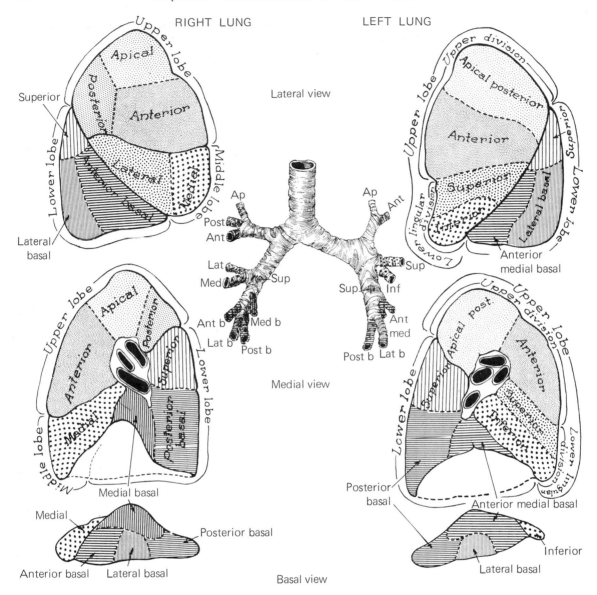

Figure 21–11. Segmental anatomy of the lungs. (Modified and reproduced, with permission, from Krupp MA & others: *Physician's Handbook,* 18th ed. Lange, 1976.)

THE PULMONARY VASCULAR SYSTEM

The lungs have a dual blood supply: the pulmonary and the bronchial arterial systems. The pulmonary arteries transmit venous blood from the right ventricle for oxygenation. They closely accompany the bronchi. The bronchial arteries usually arise directly from the aorta or nearby intercostal arteries and are variable in number. They transmit oxygenated blood at systemic arterial pressure to the bronchial wall to the level of the terminal bronchioles.

The pulmonary veins travel in the interlobar septa and do not correspond to the distribution of the bronchi or the pulmonary arteries. The large bronchi may have bronchial veins that drain into the azygous system or—as occurs more distally in the bronchial tree—drain directly into the pulmonary venous system. Multiple rudimentary anastomoses exist between the pulmonary arteries and veins, the bronchial and pulmonary arteries, and the bronchial and pulmonary veins that may expand to transmit significant flow in disease.

THE LYMPHATICS

From the parenchyma, the lymphatics travel in intersegmental septa; those which reach the parenchymal surface from subpleural networks. Drainage continues toward the hilus in channels which follow the bronchi and pulmonary arteries. They eventually enter lymph nodes in the major fissures of the lungs, the hilus, and the paratracheal regions.

The direction of lymphatic drainage—irrespective of the primary site—is cephalad and usually ipsilateral, but contralateral flow may occur from any lobe. It appears from the spread of left lower lobe neoplasms that the lymphatics from this lobe may be almost equally distributed to the left and right. Otherwise, the usual sequence of lymphatic spread of pulmonary cancer is first to regional parabronchial nodes and then to the ipsilateral paratracheal, scalene, or inferior deep cervical nodes.

Nohl-Oser HC: Anatomy of the lymphatic drainage of the lungs. Ann R Coll Surg Engl 51:165, 1972.

PHYSIOLOGY OF THE LUNG

The 7 major functions of the lung are as follows:

(1) Respiration and acid-base regulation, ie, to exchange oxygen and CO_2 between blood and the atmosphere. (See Chapter 12 for further discussion.)

(2) Blood reservoir.

(3) Excretion, eg, water vapor, ethanol, hydrocarbons.

(4) Temperature regulation.

(5) Detoxification and metabolic degradation.

(6) Secretion, eg, histamine, thromboplastin, prostaglandins.

(7) Cleansing and filtering, eg, carbon, silica in air; blood clots, particulate matter in blood.

SYMPTOMS & SIGNS
OF RESPIRATORY DISEASE

Occasionally, patients with advanced pulmonary disease have no symptoms.

Cough

Cough is a defensive mechanism mediated by the trigeminal, glossopharyngeal, superior laryngeal, and vagus nerves. It may be the first symptom of bronchial irritation by pulmonary disease. Cough is either dry or productive. Dry cough may be caused by any respiratory disease and often precedes a productive cough. Productive cough indicates bronchial irritation. Sputum should be described as to color, consistency, amount, time of occurrence, and special characteristics such as the presence of food particles or blood. Cough is sometimes described as hacking, loose, brassy, bovine, violent, spasmodic, irritative, persistent, or severe, but these features are rarely of diagnostic value.

Wynder EL, Lemon FR, Mantel N: Epidemiology of persistent cough. Am Rev Respir Dis 91:679, 1965.

Hoarseness or Voice Change

Voice change occurs when there is irritation or inflammation of the vocal cords or obstruction of nasal passages, or after interference with laryngeal innervation. Vocal cord paralysis may occur, especially on the left side, with carcinoma of the lung or esophagus, but also can be idiopathic or due to benign disease. Persistent voice change warrants examination of the vocal cords to rule out intrinsic lesions and abductor nerve paresis.

Maisel RH, Ogura JH: Evaluation and treatment of vocal cord paralysis. Laryngoscope 84:302, 1974.

Shortness of Breath (Dyspnea)

Dyspnea must be distinguished from sighing, malaise, or anxiety. The character of the dyspnea, its duration, and its relationship to position, exertion, or other symptoms should be determined. Shortness of breath may be caused by chest pain (eg, angina pectoris, pleurisy, or peritonitis).

Chest Pain

Pleuritic pain is discussed on p 305.

The lung is relatively insensitive to pain, but in inflammatory diseases the tracheobronchial tree may be sensitive to contact or change in temperature.

Mediastinal pain is often felt retrosternally and may radiate to the back, neck, or arms. It may resemble myocardial ischemia and be described as squeezing, boring, pressing, or choking—much as in pulmonary embolism, pulmonary hypertension, pericarditis, or dissecting aneurysm. Esophageal pain is usually burning but may be spasmodic.

Chest wall pain, not pleuritic in origin, may be distinguished from pleuritic pain because it is not aggravated by cough and deep breathing and is usually poorly localized, constant, and dull or aching.

Hemoptysis

Hemoptysis must always be investigated (by bronchoscopy) since it is often the first sign of serious disease such as carcinoma, tuberculosis, or pulmonary infarction. It must be differentiated from nasal, upper airway, and gastrointestinal tract bleeding. Hemoptysis does not always indicate severe lung disease since it may be due to bronchitis or mitral stenosis or may be an idiopathic nonrecurrent event in a person without demonstrable disease. In general, about 90% of patients with hemoptysis have an identifiable underlying disease. Sometimes the amount of blood lost may be massive (ie, > 600 ml), as in tuberculosis, mitral stenosis, or bronchiectasis; or even exsanguinating, as when a thoracic aortic aneurysm ruptures into a bronchus.

Gourin A, Garzon AA: Operative treatment of massive hemoptysis. Ann Thorac Surg 18:52, 1974.

Mattox KL, Guinn GA: Emergency resection for massive hemoptysis. Ann Thorac Surg 17:377, 1974.

Wheezing

Diffuse wheezing occurs in patients with asthma, allergies, bronchitis, emphysema, or heart failure. A localized wheeze denotes isolated bronchial obstruction due to secretions, foreign bodies, strictures, or tumors.

Signs of Respiratory Disease

The physical findings in respiratory disease include local changes of the chest wall or diaphragm, evidence of mediastinal shift or widening, supraclavicular adenopathy, or percussive and auscultatory findings in the lungs themselves. Extrathoracic manifestations of pulmonary disease such as clubbing or hypertrophic pulmonary osteoarthropathy may be present. Cyanosis indicates at least 5 g/100 ml of reduced hemoglobin in the blood, often due to ventilatory insufficiency; right-to-left shunting, as in cardiac disease; excessive hemoglobin, as in polycythemia; abnormal hemoglobin, as in methemoglobinemia; or circulatory stasis due to cardiac disease or hypothermia.

Cohen MH: Signs and symptoms of bronchogenic carcinoma. Semin Oncol 1:183, 1974.

SPECIAL DIAGNOSTIC STUDIES

Skin Tests

Skin tests are used in the diagnosis of tuberculosis, histoplasmosis, and coccidioidomycosis. Tuberculin testing is usually done with purified protein derivative (PPD) injected intradermally. Intermediate strength PPD should be used in patients who seem likely to have active disease. Induration of 10 mm or more at the injection site after 48–72 hours is called positive and indicates either active or arrested disease. Mumps antigen is usually placed on the opposite forearm to test for anergy. Because false-negative reactions are rare, a negative test fairly reliably rules out tuberculosis. Skin tests for histoplasmosis and coccidioidomycosis are carried out in a similar way, but tests for fungal infections are unreliable, and serologic tests should be done.

Freedman SO: Tuberculin testing and screening: A critical evaluation. Hosp Practice May 1972, p 63.
Howard WL & others: The loss of tuberculin sensitivity in certain patients with active pulmonary tuberculosis. Dis Chest 57:530, 1970.

Endoscopy

A. Laryngoscopy: Indirect laryngoscopy is used to assess vocal cord mobility in patients suspected of having lung carcinoma, especially when there has been a voice change. It should also be performed to search for an otherwise occult source for malignant cells in sputum or metastases in cervical lymph nodes.

B. Bronchoscopy: Roentgenographic evidence of bronchial obstruction, unresolved pneumonia, foreign body, suspected carcinoma, undiagnosed hemoptysis, aspiration pneumonia, and lung abscess are only a few of the indications for bronchoscopy. The procedure can be done using either the standard hollow metal or the flexible fiberoptic bronchoscope and local or general anesthesia. Washings are usually obtained for bacterial or fungal culture and cytologic examination. Visible lesions are biopsied directly, and occasionally biopsies are taken of the carina even though it appears normal. Brush biopsies are obtained from specific bronchopulmonary segments. Occasionally, transcarinal needle biopsy of a subcarinal node is obtained. Thirty to 50% of lung tumors are visible bronchoscopically. Brushing, random biopsies, and sputum cytology may still yield a positive diagnosis of cancer or tuberculosis in the absence of a visible lesion.

C. Mediastinoscopy: Mediastinoscopy permits direct biopsy of paratracheal and carinal lymph nodes without thoracotomy. Tumor is found by this technic in about 40% of cases of lung cancer, and such a finding may indicate surgical incurability. Persons with a negative biopsy have a relatively favorable prognosis with surgical treatment.

Mediastinoscopy is almost invariably accurate in the diagnosis of sarcoidosis. It is also useful to diagnose tuberculosis, histoplasmosis, silicosis, metastatic carcinoma, lymphoma, and carcinoma of the esophagus. It should not be used in primary mediastinal tumors, which should be approached by an incision permitting definitive excision.

Mediastinoscopy is done through a suprasternal, parasternal, or subxiphoid incision. The mortality rate is 0.09% and the morbidity rate 1.5%. The main complications are hemorrhage, pneumothorax, injury to the recurrent laryngeal nerve, and infection.

D. Pleuroscopy: Pleuroscopy, either direct or combined with mediastinoscopy, may increase the accuracy of diagnosis of thoracic disease or improve assessment of the extent of malignancy.

Deslauriers J & others: Mediastinopleuroscopy: A new approach to the diagnosis of intrathoracic diseases. Ann Thorac Surg 22:265, 1976.
Fishman NH, Bronstein MH: Is mediastinoscopy necessary in the evaluation of lung cancer? Ann Thorac Surg 20:678, 1975.
Fosburg RG & others: Positive mediastinoscopy: An ominous finding. Ann Thorac Surg 18:346, 1974.
Goldberg EM, Shapiro CM, Glicksman AS: Mediastinoscopy for assessing mediastinal spread in clinical staging of lung carcinoma. Semin Oncol 1:205, 1974.
Lewis RJ & others: Direct diagnostic thoracoscopy. Ann Thorac Surg 21:536, 1976.
Naruke T, Suemasu K, Ishikawa S: Surgical treatment for lung cancer with metastasis to mediastinal lymph nodes. J Thorac Cardiovasc Surg 71:279, 1976.
Solomon DA & others: Cytology in fiberoptic bronchoscopy. Chest 65:616, 1974.
Stoloff IL: The prognostic value of bronchoscopy in primary lung cancer. JAMA 227:299, 1974.
Yrigoyen E, Fujikawa YF: Flexible fiberoptic bronchoscopy: Anesthesia, technique and results. West J Med 122:117, 1975.

Scalene Lymph Node Biopsy

Scalene lymph node biopsy has been largely replaced by mediastinoscopy in the evaluation of pulmonary disease since it offers the same information but is less reliable. In the evaluation of lung cancer, about 15% of scalene node biopsies are positive when the cervical nodes are not palpable compared with 85% when the nodes are palpable. The risk of major complications is about 5%. Deaths are rare.

Boyd AD: Mediastinoscopy: Comparison with scalene fat pad biopsy. NY State J Med 71:445, 1971.

Pleural Biopsy

A. Needle Biopsy: This procedure is indicated when the cause of a pleural effusion cannot be determined by analysis of the fluid or when tuberculosis is suspected. Any one of 3 needles can be used: the Vim-Silverman, Cope, or Abrams (Harefield) needle. A positive diagnosis can be obtained in 60–85% of cases of tuberculosis or malignancy. The principal complication is pneumothorax. Five to 10% of biopsy specimens are inadequate for diagnosis.

B. Open Biopsy: Open pleural biopsy is especially useful in those without pleural effusion, or when needle biopsy has failed. The quality of the specimen and the likelihood of its representing the pathology are better than with needle biopsy, but open biopsy is a more extensive procedure.

Hill HE, Hensler NM, Breckler IA: Pleural biopsy in diagnosis of effusion: Results in 50 cases of pleural disease observed consecutively. Am Rev Respir Dis 78.8, 1958.

Scerbo J, Keltz J, Stone DJ: A prospective study of closed pleural biopsies. JAMA 218:377, 1971.

Lung Biopsy

A. Needle Biopsy: The indications for percutaneous needle biopsy are not well established. It may be indicated in diffuse parenchymal disease and in some patients with localized lesions. The diagnosis of interstitial pneumonia, carcinoma, sarcoidosis, hypersensitivity lung disease, lymphoma, pulmonary alveolar proteinosis, and miliary tuberculosis has been established by this method.

In localized disease—particularly when carcinoma is suspected—there is controversy concerning the risks of spreading the tumor by needle biopsy. Until this is settled, needle biopsy of possible carcinoma should be reserved for patients with surgically incurable disease. Needle biopsies are done by any of 3 technics: aspiration with a cutting needle, by trephine, or by air drill. Needle biopsy of the lung is also possible by a transbronchial technic using a modified Vim-Silverman needle.

Complications following percutaneous needle biopsy include pneumothorax (20–40%), hemothorax, hemoptysis, and air embolism. Pulmonary hypertension or cysts and bullae are contraindications. Several deaths have been reported. There is about a 60% chance of success of obtaining useful information.

B. Open Lung Biopsy: A limited intercostal or anterior parasternal incision is used to remove a 3–4 cm wedge of lung tissue in diffuse parenchymal lung disease. The site of incision is selected for accessibility and the promise of giving information of diagnostic value. General or local anesthesia may be used. Open lung biopsy has a lower mortality rate, fewer complications, and greater diagnostic yield than needle biopsy. When a focal lesion is biopsied, a larger incision is used; peripheral lesions are totally excised by wedge or segmental resection; deeply placed lesions may be removed by lobectomy in suitable candidates.

Becker RM, Munro DD: Transaxillary minithoracotomy: The optimal approach for certain pulmonary and mediastinal lesions. Ann Thorac Surg 22:254, 1976.

Berger RL, Dargan EL, Huang BL: Dissemination of cancer cells by needle biopsy of the lung. J Thorac Cardiovasc Surg 63:430, 1972.

Ellis JH Jr: Transbronchial lung biopsy via the fiberoptic bronchoscope: Experience with 107 consecutive cases and comparison with bronchial brushing. Chest 68:524, 1975.

Gaensler EA, Moister VB, Hamm J: Open lung biopsy in diffuse pulmonary disease. N Engl J Med 270:1319, 1964.

Nelems JM & others: Emergency open lung biopsy. Ann Thorac Surg 22:260, 1976.

Steel SJ, Winstanley DP: Trephine biopsy of the lung and pleura. Thorax 24:576, 1969.

Sputum Analysis

Exfoliative sputum cytology is most valuable for detection of lung cancer. Specimens are obtained by deep coughing, bronchial washings by either bronchoscopic or percutaneous transtracheal washing technics, or by abrasion with a brush. Specimens should be collected fresh in the morning and delivered to the laboratory promptly. Centrifugation or filtration can be used to concentrate the cellular elements.

In primary lung cancer, sputum cytology is positive in 30–60% of cases. Repeated sputum examination improves the diagnostic return. Examination of the first bronchoscopic washing material yields a diagnosis in 60% of cases. Postbronchoscopy sputum analysis may yield positive findings when previous tests were negative.

Clark RE, Kyriakos M, Hendrix Y: The effect of anesthetic method upon the results of bronchial washing cytology. J Thorac Cardiovasc Surg 63:930, 1972.

Erozan YS, Frost JK: Cytopathologic diagnosis of cancer in pulmonary material: A critical histopathologic correlation. Acta Cytol 14:560, 1970.

Ozgelen FN, Brodsky SL, DeGroat A: An examination of the merits and intrinsic limitations of exfoliative cytology in 465 cases of lung cancer. J Thorac Cardiovasc Surg 49:221, 1965.

Struve-Christensen E, Michaelsen M, Mossing N: The diagnostic value of bronchial washing in lung cancer. J Thorac Cardiovasc Surg 68:313, 1974.

Immunologic Assessment

It is now recognized that immunologic factors play an important role in thoracic disease. The status of the immunologic system influences the results of skin tests, the host's resistance to infection or malignant disease, and virulence of metabolic diseases such as myasthenia gravis.

Holmes CE: Immunology and lung cancer. Ann Thorac Surg 21:250, 1976.

McKneally MF & others: Regional immunotherapy with intrapleural BCG for lung cancer: Surgical considerations. J Thorac Cardiovasc Surg 72:333, 1976.

Olkowski ZL: Immunocompetence of patients with bronchogenic carcinoma. Ann Thorac Surg 21:546, 1976.

Skinner DB, DeMeester TR: Immunology and thoracic surgery. Ann Thorac Surg 21:462, 1976.

Wanebo HJ & others: Immune reactivity in primary carcinoma of the lung and its relation to prognosis. J Thorac Cardiovasc Surg 72:339, 1976.

Other Methods

Specialized procedures may become useful to evaluate patients with pulmonary disease. At present, however, the value of azygography, selective bronchial arteriography, lung scan, and cinebronchography is not established.

DeMeester TR & others: Gallium-67 scanning for carcinoma of the lung. J Thorac Cardiovasc Surg 72:699, 1976.

Gutierrez AC & others: Radioisotope scans in the evaluation of metastatic bronchogenic carcinoma. J Thorac Cardiovasc Surg 69:934, 1975.

Jereb M, Sinner W: The use of some special radiologic procedures in chest disease. Radiol Clin North Am 11:109, 1973.

Macumber HH, Calvin JW: Perfusion lung scan patterns in 100 patients with bronchogenic carcinoma. J Thorac Cardiovasc Surg 72:299, 1976.

Muggia FM, Chervu LR: Lung cancer: Diagnosis in metastatic sites. Semin Oncol 1:217, 1974.

DISEASES OF THE LUNGS

CYSTIC LESIONS OF THE LUNG

Broad usage of the term pulmonary cyst would include the following:

(1) Bronchogenic cysts: Congenital epithelium-lined developmental abnormalities.

(2) Pneumatoceles: Nonepithelized cavities in the parenchyma, often associated with staphylococcal pneumonia.

(3) Emphysematous bullae: Nonepithelized lung cavities resulting from degenerative changes in emphysema (Fig 21–12).

(4) Cystic bronchiectasis: Cyst-like bronchial dilatation which may be acquired or congenital.

(5) Lung cavities: Acquired lung spaces following destructive lung disease such as abscess, tuberculosis, fungal infection, malignancy.

(6) Parasitic cysts.

(7) Diffuse cystic disease: Seen in mucoviscidosis and Letterer-Siwe disease.

Fitzgerald MX & others: Long-term results of surgery for bullous emphysema. J Thorac Cardiovasc Surg 68:566, 1974.

CONGENITAL CYSTIC LESIONS

Congenital cystic lesions of the lung are uncommon and usually not associated with cysts of other organs. The terminology of these lesions is confusing. Cysts that involve the lung can be derived from 3 sources: the air passages, pulmonary lymphatics, or

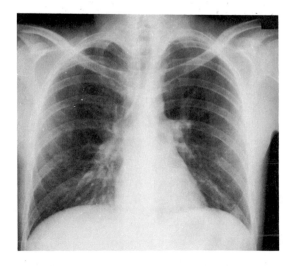 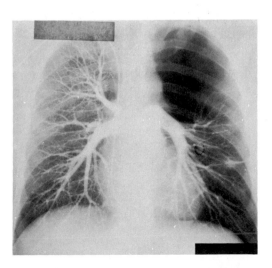

Figure 21–12. Emphysematous bullae of left lung. *Left:* Posteroanterior projection. *Right:* Pulmonary angiogram.

pleural surfaces. Four distinct types of congenital cysts arising from the air passages are recognized: (1) bronchogenic cysts, (2) sequestration of the lung, (3) congenital cystic adenomatoid malformation, and (4) infantile lobar emphysema. Except for the latter, all can present at any age but are more common in children and young adults. These lesions must sometimes be distinguished from pneumatoceles, blebs, bullae, or tumors.

The lungs and the trachea develop from the ventral bud of the primitive foregut. Abnormalities of ventral budding cause various types of bronchogenic cysts and pulmonary sequestrations. The ultimate location of the cyst or sequestration depends upon the extent of differentiation of the foregut. Early anomalies of budding lead to peripheral lung cysts or intralobar sequestration; later anomalies may cause cysts to remain extrapleural (bronchogenic) or sequestrations to be separate from the rest of the lung and to possess their own pleural coverings (extralobar sequestration). Abnormalities of development of the terminal bronchioles and alveolar ducts result in cystic adenomatoid formation. Alveoli develop by the 28th week of gestation, and abnormal alveolar development accounts for most cases of infantile lobar emphysema.

1. BRONCHOGENIC CYSTS

The term bronchogenic cyst includes both bronchial and lung cysts. They may be located in the mediastinum or hilus, but 50–70% are located in the lung. The more proximal cysts (bronchial) seldom have a bronchial communication and therefore are less likely to become secondarily infected. These cysts, usually considered mediastinal, are often in the right paratracheal, carinal, hilar, or paraesophageal locations. More peripheral bronchogenic cysts (congenital lung cysts) are thin-walled, often multiloculated or multiple, and usually have bronchial communications. They tend to become infected and to result in recurrent pneumonia, fever, sepsis, or other types of respiratory distress.

Clinical Findings

Congenital pulmonary cysts are manifested in infancy with respiratory embarrassment, pneumothorax, or compression atelectasis. If air trapping is the main feature, there will be dyspnea, cyanosis, and subcostal retraction. Less severe cases present as recurrent infection, hemoptysis, or an undiagnosed finding on chest roentgenogram.

Congenital lung cysts may occur anywhere in the lungs but involve the lower lobes twice as often as other sites. In adults, the lesion may be asymptomatic when detected by a chest roentgenogram. The mass may appear as a homogeneous density, a cavity with an air-fluid level, or an air cyst. It may be difficult to distinguish lung cysts from benign or malignant tumors, cavitary lesions due to fungi or tuberculosis, or pulmonary abscess.

Treatment

Treatment consists of local removal by enucleation, segmental resection, or in some cases lobectomy.

2. SEQUESTRATION OF THE LUNG

Masses of lung tissue that have no communication with the tracheobronchial tree are termed sequestrations. Two types are recognized. In intralobar sequestration, the abnormal lung is surrounded by normal lung and is supplied by anomalous systemic arteries; the venous drainage is into the pulmonary veins. Bronchial communication may be acquired through infection (about 15% of cases), but it is difficult to demonstrate radiologically. Repeated infections frequently occur because of poor drainage. Eighty-five percent of sequestrations are of the intralobar type. Extralobar sequestration consists of a separate or accessory mass of lung tissue invested by its own pleura. Anatomic and physiologic separation from adjacent lung tissue is complete, but vascular supply is the same as with intralobar sequestration.

The diagnosis is verified by arteriographic demonstration of a systemic arterial supply to the sequestered segment. Some cases are asymptomatic and are first discovered on chest x-rays.

After infection is controlled, resection of the sequestration is indicated to prevent recurrent suppuration. Intralobar sequestration usually requires lobectomy; extralobar sequestrations can usually be locally excised. The main technical hazard is the aberrant blood supply.

3. CONGENITAL CYSTIC ADENOMATOID MALFORMATION

Congenital cystic adenomatoid malformation presents with manifestations of air trapping, progressive distention of the abnormal lung, and multiple cysts. It may be found in stillborns with anasarca, neonates with respiratory distress, or in older children and young adults as an asymptomatic chest x-ray finding, recurrent infection, or following pneumothorax.

4. INFANTILE LOBAR EMPHYSEMA

Infantile lobar emphysema with acute overinflation of the upper lobes or middle lobe is a cause of acute respiratory distress in infants. It is discussed in Chapter 48.

Khalil KG, Kilman JW: Pulmonary sequestration. J Thorac Cardiovasc Surg 70:928, 1975.

Sade RM, Clouse M, Ellis FH Jr: Collective review: The spectrum of pulmonary sequestration. Ann Thorac Surg 18:644, 1974.

White JJ & others: Cardiovascular and respiratory manifestations of pulmonary sequestration in childhood. Ann Thorac Surg 18:286, 1974.

Zumbro GL & others: Pulmonary sequestration: A broad spectrum of bronchopulmonary foregut abnormalities. Ann Thorac Surg 20:161, 1975.

VASCULAR LESIONS OF THE LUNG

Pulmonary arteriovenous fistulas of the lung are either congenital or acquired. Angiography is useful to determine if the arterial supply is from the pulmonary artery or from a systemic artery.

Arom KV, Lyons GW: Traumatic pulmonary arteriovenous fistula. J Thorac Cardiovasc Surg 70:918, 1975.

Dines DE & others: Pulmonary arteriovenous fistulas. Mayo Clin Proc 49:460, 1974.

INFECTIONS OF THE LUNGS

BACTERIAL INFECTIONS

For many years, treatment of pleuropulmonary infections required a considerable portion of a thoracic surgeon's time, but drainage of pus from lung abscess, resection of bronchiectasis, and surgical treatment of tuberculosis have become relatively rare since the advent of effective antimicrobial therapy. Pulmonary infections are still common, but modern treatment is usually capable of preventing them from progressing to complications that require surgical treatment.

Among the infections, pneumonia is still the most lethal. At least half of all cases are bacterial, and 90% of these (40% of all cases) are due to pneumococci. Pneumococcal pneumonias are effectively treated with penicillin, but the other bacterial pneumonias are usually more resistant to therapy. *Staphylococcus aureus* (1–5%), *Klebsiella pneumoniae* (1–5%), *Haemophilus influenzae* (1%), *Neisseria meningitidis* (< 1%), *Streptococcus pyogenes* (< 1%), and the enterobacteriaceae (< 1%) are the pyogenic organisms most likely to lead to surgical complications. A major consideration in lung abscess and suppurative pneumonitis today is exclusion of bronchial carcinoma as an underlying cause.

Cattaneo SM & others: Selective sputum cultures. J Thorac Cardiovasc Surg 69:152, 1975.

LUNG ABSCESS

Essentials of Diagnosis

- Development of pulmonary symptoms about 2 weeks after possible aspiration, bronchial obstruction, or previous pneumonia.
- Septic fever and sweats.
- Periodic sudden expectoration of large amounts of purulent, foul-smelling or "musty" sputum.
- Hemoptysis may occur.
- X-ray density with central radiolucency and fluid level.

General Considerations

Lung abscess may result from aspiration (50%), bronchial obstruction (eg, from carcinoma), necrotizing pneumonia (20%), infection of cysts or bullae, or extension of infection from the subdiaphragmatic spaces or liver; or it may occur as a postembolic phenomenon or after trauma. In England, tuberculosis and carcinoma are the most common causes of lung abscess; the latter predominates in men over age 50.

To a large extent, the cause of lung abscess determines its location. In abscess secondary to aspiration, the patient's position at the time of aspiration is important. When the patient is supine, there is a tendency for aspirated material to enter the posterior segment of the right upper lobe or the superior segment of the right lower lobe. Carcinomatous abscess more frequently involves the anterior segments of the upper lobes. Embolic abscesses are often small and multiple and tend to involve the lower lobes. Basilar abscesses may suggest prior pneumonia. Abscesses often occur in alcoholics and other debilitated persons. Some follow aspiration during anesthesia and surgery. In other cases, aspiration may be a complication of esophageal diseases such as hiatal hernia, carcinoma, achalasia, or tracheoesophageal fistula. Pneumonia occurs in debilitated persons being given broad-spectrum antibiotics, those requiring tracheal tubes and ventilation therapy, those with systemic diseases, or those requiring treatment that affects host resistance. Diabetes, preexisting lung disease, dental caries, and epilepsy are also predisposing causes.

Although staphylococci, streptococci, and neisseriae are frequently found, the original causative organisms are often unknown because so many patients are treated with antibiotics without cultures and eventually a variety of gram-negative organisms emerge during antibiotic therapy. Pulmonary infarcts may become infected in patients with septic bacterial endocarditis or drug addicts who use intravenous administration. Bland pulmonary infarcts also may become infected from adjacent bronchial disease. Lung abscesses following emboli are often near pleural surfaces; bronchopleural fistulas and emphysema can result.

Clinical Findings

A. Symptoms and Signs: The predisposing cause

of lung abscess often contributes prominently to the clinical picture. During the development of an abscess, the clinical findings are indistinguishable from those of severe acute bronchopneumonia. The patient usually has fever, chills, pleuritic chest pain, and prostration. Sputum production may initially be minimal but can become putrid or fetid, which strongly suggests the diagnosis. Hemoptysis occasionally precedes the onset of productive cough. Physical findings may be indistinguishable from those of pneumonia.

B. Laboratory Findings: Leukocytosis is present.

C. X-Ray Findings: Chest x-ray initially shows only collapse or consolidation. If a solid or dense infiltrate is present, the diagnosis of carcinoma or tuberculosis may be suggested. Air-fluid levels develop once bronchial communication is established (Fig 21–13).

Differential Diagnosis

An abscess differs from bronchiectasis in that in abscess the infection is extrabronchial. The most common conditions causing abscess of the lung are tuberculosis, fungal infections, and carcinoma. Since carcinoma underlies 10–20% of lung abscesses, this should always be excluded. Bronchoscopy, sputum cytologic examination, and close follow-up are essential. The x-ray appearance may resemble lung cysts or blebs.

Complications

The complications of lung abscess are local spread, causing loss of additional parenchyma or even loss of an entire lobe; hemorrhage into the abscess, which can be massive; bronchopleural fistula; and emphysema, tension pneumothorax, pyopneumothorax, and pericarditis. Metastatic abscesses may occur, especially to the brain. Failure to heal, the most common complication, requires resection. Late complications are residual bronchiectasis, chronic abscess, chronic bronchopleural fistula, and recurrent pneumonitis.

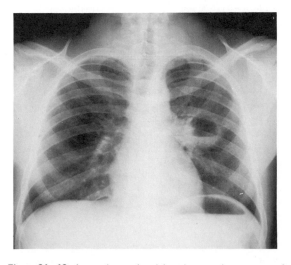

Figure 21–13. Lung abscess involving the superior segment of the left lower lobe.

Treatment

A. General Measures: Severely ill patients in shock, dehydration, or toxemia should receive immediate resuscitative measures. Sputum should be sent immediately for culture for aerobic and anaerobic organisms. Examination of stained smears of sputum or tracheal aspirates can suggest appropriate antibiotic therapy. Bronchoscopy may be repeated at regular intervals to maintain drainage.

Postural drainage, assisted ventilation, and bronchodilators may be indicated. It is rare for a patient not to respond to such a regimen. The cavity will usually diminish in size within 2–3 weeks. If fever persists for 4 weeks, antibiotic therapy is often required for 6–8 weeks. However, failure to observe improvement on this regimen within 2–3 weeks should strongly suggest the presence of another disease, especially carcinoma.

B. Surgical Treatment: Occasionally, external closed drainage may be considered in severely ill patients with acute disease who are poor operative risks and have persistent sepsis because of inadequate bronchial drainage. Closed tube drainage is indicated only when it can be established that the drainage tract will traverse an area of symphysis of the parietal and visceral pleura so that empyema will not result.

Fewer than 5% of patients require surgical therapy unless an underlying carcinoma exists. Surgery is reserved for patients who show inadequate resolution radiologically or clinically or who cannot be withdrawn from antibiotic therapy. As long as improvement occurs on medical therapy, surgery is unnecessary. Large size of the abscess (> 6 cm), total lobe destruction, persistent bronchopleural fistula, persistent sepsis, or persistence of the abscess over several weeks is a surgical indication. Lobectomy is the usual procedure. Rarely, massive hemoptysis will make emergency lobectomy mandatory.

Prognosis

Medical therapy is successful in about 95% of cases; the remaining few require surgical treatment. There is a 10–15% mortality rate in those who need operation because of an inadequate response to antibiotics.

Chidi CC, Mendelsohn HJ: Lung abscess: A study of the results of treatment based on 90 consecutive cases. J Thorac Cardiovasc Surg 68:168, 1974.

Medical Staff Conference: Lung abscess. West J Med 124:476, 1976.

BRONCHIECTASIS

The dilatation of the bronchial tree in bronchiectasis used to be considered irreversible, but this is now known to be false. Bronchiectasis often coexists with chronic bronchitis. Involvement is bilateral in

50% of cases, usually in the lower lobes, and in only 10% of cases is the lingular or middle lobe involved without ipsilateral lower lobe involvement. Cases requiring surgical treatment are rare because antimicrobial therapy of pulmonary infections has largely prevented this disease.

Bronchiectasis is mainly a pediatric disease, with 50% of cases having onset of symptoms before 3 years of age. Most cases begin with pneumonia complicating one of the childhood contagious diseases such as pertussis. Rarely, congenital defects such as mucoviscidosis and Kartagener's triad (situs inversus, sinusitis, and bronchiectasis) are involved in the pathogenesis. Patients with immunologic deficits and preexisting pulmonary disease such as lung abscess or bronchial obstruction by tuberculosis, tumors, or foreign body sometimes develop bronchiectasis. The common feature in many of these is long-standing destructive bronchial infection.

The diagnosis of bronchiectasis depends on radiologic demonstration by bronchography of the typical irregular cylindric or saccular bronchial dilatations.

Patients with bronchiectasis have cough, sputum production, and sometimes dyspnea; the symptoms are aggravated by frequent upper respiratory infections. Hemoptysis occurs in 50% of older patients. A few patients have little sputum ("dry bronchiectasis"). There may be associated pulmonary fibrosis or emphysema in advanced cases. Clubbing of the fingers is seen in about a third of cases.

Attacks of pneumonitis are often due to pneumococci or *Haemophilus influenzae.* Involvement of other segments of the bronchial tree, pulmonary fibrosis, and pulmonary insufficiency occur in advanced cases or when medical treatment has been inadequate.

Medical treatment consists of postural drainage, cessation of smoking, antibiotic therapy, and treatment of underlying conditions such as sinusitis. Humidification, bronchodilators, and expectorants may facilitate clearing of secretions. Upper respiratory infections may be treated with broad-spectrum antibiotics such as tetracyclines or ampicillin.

Surgical therapy is reserved for patients with localized disease (ie, involving one lobe) who have failed to respond to a strict medical regimen. The presence of diffuse pulmonary emphysema may limit the feasibility of surgery. In well-selected cases resection for bronchiectasis shows improvement in 95% with lobar disease. Bilateral involvement—particularly if the middle lobe or lingula is involved—has a poor prognosis following surgery.

Ferguson TB, Burford TH: The changing pattern of pulmonary suppuration. Dis Chest 53:396, 1968.
Sealy WC & others: The treatment of multisegmental and localized bronchiectasis. Surg Gynecol Obstet 123:80, 1966.
Tager I, Speizer FE: Role of infection in chronic bronchitis. N Engl J Med 292:563, 1975.

MIDDLE LOBE SYNDROME

The middle lobe syndrome consists of repeated infections in this lobe which usually respond to antibiotics. It can be a manifestation of partial bronchial obstruction, to which the middle lobe is particularly susceptible. However, recurrent segmental infections can occur in other areas of the lung by a similar process. Secondary bronchiectasis is a frequent complication.

Broncholithiasis (see below) and middle lobe syndrome have been considered to be caused by compression or erosion of the bronchus by adjacent diseased lymph nodes. The middle lobe syndrome is seen less frequently now than formerly, and in some recently reported cases it was not associated with obstruction of the middle lobe bronchus. Other factors, such as poor natural drainage and lack of collateral ventilation, probably explain the frequency of middle lobe involvement and in some cases are sufficient to cause symptoms even though the bronchus is entirely patent. Bronchial obstruction may be demonstrable in as few as one-fourth of cases. It appears that in the middle lobe the presence of complete fissures limits collateral ventilation and favors the persistence of collapse, retained secretions, and infection.

Most patients who require surgical treatment are women over age 20 with symptoms of recurrent infectious bronchiectasis which include cough, hemoptysis, chest pain, and fever. Wheezing is occasionally reported. Chest roentgenography shows a midlung field density, middle lobe atelectasis, a small contracted middle lobe, or consolidated middle lobe. Bronchoscopy and bronchography show bronchiectasis in 40% of cases, incomplete filling in 20%, and occasionally a narrowed middle lobe orifice. Granulomatous disease, including tuberculosis and occasionally histoplasmosis, may be found.

Endobronchial tumors and foreign bodies must be ruled out by bronchoscopy or bronchography.

Most patients respond to intensive medical therapy (similar to that for bronchiectasis), and only a few require surgery. When surgery is required, lobectomy is performed. Indications for surgery include bronchiectasis, fibrosis (bronchostenosis), abscess, unresolved or intractable recurrent pneumonia, and suspicion of neoplasm.

Bradham RR, Sealy WC, Young WG Jr: Chronic middle lobe infection: Factors responsible for its development. Ann Thorac Surg 2:611, 1966.
Johnson RM, Lindskog GE: Further studies on factors influencing collateral ventilation. J Thorac Cardiovasc Surg 62:321, 1971.

BRONCHOLITHIASIS

Broncholithiasis is an unusual condition in which a calcified parabronchial lymph node erodes into the bronchus and is either coughed up or lodges there. Rarely, inspissated and impacted mucoid material may undergo calcification and form a broncholith or "lung stone." In Europe, 10% of operated patients had documented tuberculosis. Histoplasmosis may be an equally important or even more important cause in the USA.

The criteria for diagnosis of broncholithiasis are (1) bronchoscopic evidence of peribronchial disease, (2) significant hilar calcifications, and (3) absence of associated pulmonary disease to explain the patient's symptoms.

Sudden unexpected hemoptysis in an otherwise healthy patient is the cardinal manifestation. The bleeding stops without specific measures and only rarely is massive.

Other frequent symptoms are cough, fever and chills, and purulent sputum. There may be localized pleuritic pain or localized wheezing. A history of expectoration of stones is present in one-third of cases. The chest roentgenogram invariably shows hilar calcification. One-third of cases have obstructive pneumonitis. Bronchoscopy demonstrates broncholiths in over 25%, and other endobronchial abnormalities in about 10% of cases.

The complications of broncholithiasis are suppurative lung disease, life-threatening hemoptysis, and bronchoesophageal fistula.

Medical treatment combined with bronchoscopic removal of the broncholith is usually indicated. In most patients symptoms are limited to a single attack of hemoptysis, since the invading lymph node becomes encased in scar tissue. Surgery is indicated to treat complications of broncholithiasis or when malignancy cannot be excluded. Of the 25% of patients that require surgery, most have lobectomy. Patients with bronchoesophageal fistula may require only fistula repair.

With adequate medical and surgical treatment, the prognosis has been greatly improved in recent years.

Arrigoni MG, Bernatz PE, Donoghue FE: Broncholithiasis. J Thorac Cardiovasc Surg 62:231, 1971.
Faber LP & others: The surgical implication of broncholithiasis. J Thorac Cardiovasc Surg 70:779, 1975.

MUCOVISCIDOSIS & MUCOID IMPACTION OF THE BRONCHI

Mucoviscidosis is a serious pulmonary disorder of children which may lead to bronchitis, bronchiectasis, pulmonary fibrosis, emphysema, or lung abscess.

Mucoid impaction occurs in adults and is associated with asthma and bronchitis. The mucoid plugs are rubbery, semisolid, gray to greenish-yellow in color, and round, oval, or elongated in shape. There is often a history of recurrent upper respiratory infection, fever, and chest pain. Expectoration of hard mucus plugs or hemoptysis may occur.

Most patients present with a history of respiratory infections, but nearly one-half have findings suggestive of bronchogenic carcinoma. The chest x-ray shows U-shaped lesions involving the second order bronchi. Bronchography helps to delineate the mass. Bronchoscopy is done to assess for malignancy and obtain cultures and for therapeutic purposes.

Bronchogenic carcinoma, fungal disease, tuberculosis, bronchiectasis, abscess, bacterial pneumonia, lipoid pneumonia, pulmonary eosinophilic granuloma, Löffler's syndrome, and cystic fibrosis must be ruled out.

Treatment is usually medical and includes expectorants, detergents, bronchodilators, antibiotics, and aerosol inhalation therapy. Acetylcysteine (Mucomyst) has largely converted this condition to a purely medical disease. Surgery is indicated when malignancy cannot be ruled out, for destroyed lung, or in the treatment of abscess.

Laforet EG: Mucoid impaction of a stem bronchus. J Thorac Cardiovasc Surg 68:309, 1974.
Urschel HC Jr, Paulson DL, Shaw RR: Mucoid impaction of bronchi. Ann Thorac Surg 2:1, 1966.

TUBERCULOSIS

Essentials of Diagnosis

- Minimal symptoms: malaise, lassitude, easy fatigability, anorexia, mild weight loss, afternoon fever, cough, apical rales, and hemoptysis.
- Positive tuberculin skin test; especially recent change from negative to positive.
- Apical lung infiltrates, often with cavities on chest films.
- *Mycobacterium tuberculosis* in sputum or in gastric or tracheal washings.

General Considerations

Several species of the genus Mycobacterium may cause lung disease, but 95% are due to *M tuberculosis*. *M bovis* and *M avium* are seldom found in humans. Several less common species of Mycobacterium that are chiefly soil-dwellers have become clinically more important in recent years and have been less responsive to preventive and therapeutic measures.

Although tuberculosis is declining as a cause of death, an estimated 35 million persons are tuberculin-positive in the USA and form a reservoir from which about 5000–8000 clinical cases are expected. In addition, about 30,000 new cases occur annually. About one-third of cases are first reported at death. Although in the USA less than 20% of the population is tuberculin-positive, tuberculosis remains the most common infectious cause of death worldwide.

The initial infection involves pulmonary parenchyma in the midzone of the lung. When hypersensitivity develops after several weeks, the typical caseation appears. Regional hilar lymph nodes become enlarged. Most cases arrest spontaneously at this stage. If the infection progresses, caseation necrosis develops and giant cells produce a typical tubercle. Although this has been called reinfection tuberculosis, postprimary tuberculosis, and secondary tuberculosis, it usually consists of continued activity or reactivation of a focus of latent disease. True reinfection or "superinfection" from repeated exposure seldom occurs. Destruction of additional tissue produces the varied clinical pattern. At this stage, the apical and posterior segments of the upper lobes and the superior segments of the lower lobes are the usual sites of infection.

Clinical Findings

A. Symptoms and Signs: In the vast majority of primary infections, there is no clinical evidence of disease. When present, symptoms may include fever, cough, anorexia, weight loss, night sweats, excessive perspiration, chest pain, lethargy, or dyspnea. More severe symptoms may occur in extrapulmonary disease such as with involvement of the pericardium, bones, joints, urinary tract, meninges, lymph nodes, or pleural space. Erythema nodosum is seen occasionally in patients with active disease.

B. Laboratory Findings: The skin test with intermediate strength PPD is positive in more than 90% of patients with active tuberculosis. False-negatives are usually due to anergy or to improper testing or outdated tuberculin. Anergy is sometimes associated with disseminated tuberculosis, measles, sarcoidosis, lymphomas, or recent vaccination with live viruses (eg, poliomyelitis, measles, German measles, mumps, influenza, or yellow fever). Immunosuppressive drugs (eg, corticosteroids or azathioprine) may also cause false-negative responses.

Culture of sputum, gastric aspirate, and pleural fluid and pleural or lung biopsies are important to establish the diagnosis.

C. X-Ray Findings: Pulmonary tuberculosis often predominantly involves the apical and posterior segments of the upper lobes (85%) or the superior segments of the lower lobes (10%). Seldom is the anterior segment of the upper lobe solely involved, as in other granulomatous diseases such as histoplasmosis. Involvement of the basal segments of the lower lobes is uncommon except in women, blacks, and diabetics, but endobronchial disease usually involves the lower lobes, producing atelectasis or consolidation. Differing roentgenographic patterns are found which correspond to the pathologic variations of the disease: the local exudative lesion, the local productive lesion, cavitation, acute tuberculous pneumonia, miliary tuberculosis, bronchiectasis, bronchostenosis, and tuberculoma.

D. Bronchoscopy: Bronchoscopy may be required to rule out other diseases, improve the quality of specimens for culture, or assess endobronchial disease.

Differential Diagnosis

Localized tuberculosis is sometimes indistinguishable from bronchogenic carcinoma, particularly when it presents as a tuberculoma without calcification. When there is cavitation, carcinoma, coccidioidomycosis, and other granulomatous diseases must be considered as well as pyogenic abscess or cavitation of a pulmonary infarct. The manifestations of tuberculosis are so variable that in patients with a positive tuberculin test this disease is often difficult to totally exclude. One should suspect tuberculosis more strongly when there has been recent heavy exposure or when the tuberculin reaction has only recently converted or is very strong.

Prevention

Ideally, prevention of tuberculosis would consist of elimination of contact with tubercle bacilli so that implantation is prevented. In the USA this is approaching reality, as shown by the fact that only 3.5% of young adults have positive reactions to intermediate strength PPD.

BCG vaccination is warranted to induce relative immunity in tuberculin-negative individuals subject to exposure. It is about 80% effective in preventing infection and almost 100% effective in preventing lethal infections.

Chemoprophylaxis is advocated in the following cases: (1) Patients whose skin test recently converted from negative to positive. (2) Persons with known recent exposure, especially children and young adults. Chemoprophylaxis should be given for 6–12 weeks until retesting demonstrates a negative skin test. (3) Persons with positive skin tests and x-ray evidence for dormant tuberculosis. (4) Persons who are tuberculin-positive and especially predisposed to active tuberculosis, ie, patients with severe diabetes mellitus or nodular silicosis, those undergoing treatment with corticosteroids, postgastrectomy patients, patients with malignancies (especially lymphoma), strong tuberculin reactors, patients subject to continued heavy exposure, undernourished people, and alcoholics.

The regimen used for prophylaxis is isoniazid, 300 mg/day, given as a single dose.

Treatment

A. Medical Treatment: Chemotherapy is usually started while the patient is hospitalized to establish the diagnosis, determine baseline laboratory values (white blood counts, hematocrit, BUN, and SGOT levels), and detect drug toxicity. Smears and cultures are best done and sensitivities of the organism determined where close medical supervision is possible. Prolonged bed rest, hospitalization, and isolation are no longer recommended in the average case. The impact of this changed approach can be appreciated by noting that in 1945 the average hospital stay was over 2 years; by 1970, it was reduced to 3 months or less.

Therapy (Table 21–3) usually consists of 2 or 3 drugs in combination to prevent the emergence of resistant strains and minimize toxicity. The duration of antituberculosis drug treatment is at least 18 months or until radiologic signs of activity are gone, whichever is longer.

The principal causes of failure of chemotherapy are as follows: (1) failure of the patient to take the medications; (2) single drug therapy interruptions, often caused by drug toxicity or hypersensitivity; (3) inadequate initial drug treatment; and (4) primary resistance (including atypical mycobacteria).

B. Surgical Treatment: The role of surgery in treatment of tuberculosis has diminished dramatically since chemotherapy became available. It is now confined to the following indications: (1) failure of chemotherapy, (2) diagnosis, (3) destroyed lung, (4) postsurgical complications, (5) persistent bronchopleural fistula, and (6) tuberculous bronchiectasis.

The surgical procedures available consist of (1) diagnostic procedures such as bronchoscopy, mediastinoscopy, scalene node biopsy, lung biopsy, lymph node biopsy, and pleural biopsy; (2) pleural drainage operations such as closed tube drainage or open drain-

Table 21–3. Antituberculosis drugs and their side-effects.*

Drug	Dosage (Adult Daily)	Side-Effects (Usual)	Monitoring†	Remarks
Isoniazid (INH)	5–10 mg/kg; 300–600 mg	Peripheral neuritis, hepatitis, hypersensitivity, convulsions.	SGOT/SGPT (not as routine).	For neuritis, pyridoxine, 25–50 mg as prophylaxis; 50–100 mg as treatment.
Ethambutol (EMB)	25 mg/kg for 60 days, then 15 mg/kg‡	Optic neuritis (reversible with discontinuation of drug; very rare at 15 mg/kg); skin rash.	Visual acuity, red-green color discrimination (Snellen chart).	Ocular history and funduscopic examination before use; contraindicated with optic neuritis; use with caution if serious ocular problems.
Streptomycin (SM)	0.75–1 g (frequently given for initial 60 days with advanced disease)	Otic and vestibular toxicity, decreased hearing, vertigo, tinnitus (nephrotoxicity—rare).	Gross hearing (ticking of watch); if abnormal audiograms, BUN and creatinine.	More common in older patients (> 60); decrease dose or avoid drug if renal function is not adequate.
Aminosalicylic acid (PAS)	12–15 g	Gastrointestinal, hypersensitivity (rash), hepatotoxicity, sodium load.	SGOT/SGPT.	For gastrointestinal irritation, temporarily reduce dose or use calcium, potassium, ascorbic acid, or resin combinations; avoid sodium salt in elderly patients or renal disease.
Rifampin	600 mg once daily (children, 10–20 mg/kg to a maximum of 600)	Minimal; liver dysfunction rarely.	SGOT/SGPT.	Extremely effective.
Ethionamide§	750–1000 mg	Gastrointestinal, hepatotoxicity, hypersensitivity (rash).	SGOT/SGPT.	Temporarily stop or reduce dose with gastrointestinal irritation and hepatotoxicity.
Pyrazinamide§ (PZA)	20–35 mg/kg; not over 3 g	Hyperuricemia, hepatotoxicity, arthralgia.	Uric acid, SGOT/SGPT.	Probenecid or allopurinol to reduce serum uric acid.
Cycloserine§	750 mg	Psychosis, personality changes, convulsions, rash.	Drug blood levels if poor renal function.	Pyridoxine, 50–300 mg/day, may help; mental problems more common with predisposition.
Capreomycin§	1 g daily for 60–120 days, followed by 1 g 2–3 times weekly	Nephrotoxicity, ototoxicity, hepatotoxicity, hypersensitivity.	Same as streptomycin with SGOT/SGPT in addition.	Effective, newly released drug; not for pediatric use.
Viomycin§	1 g every 12 hours twice a week	Similar to streptomycin but nephrotoxicity more common.	As for streptomycin, plus urinalysis.	As for streptomycin.
Kanamycin§	0.5–1 g			Rarely used.

*Reproduced, with permission, from Weg JG: Treatment and control of tuberculosis. National Tuberculosis and Respiratory Disease Association, 1972.

†The most important monitoring device is an informed patient having ready access to medical care supplemented by a careful history and appropriate physical examination.

‡FDA recommends 15 mg/kg for entire treatment period except for re-treatment cases, when 25 mg/kg is recommended for the initial 60 days.

§These are the so-called second-line drugs which have more frequent and more severe side-effects; knowledge and experience in their use are desirable prerequisites.

age (eg, Eloesser flap); (3) collapse therapy, including phrenic nerve crush, pneumoperitoneum, pneumothorax, thoracoplasty, or plombage; (4) decortication; and (5) pulmonary resection, which may be pleuropneumonectomy, pneumonectomy, lobectomy, segmentectomy, or wedge resection. Resection is the preferred method of surgical treatment whenever feasible since the infection is actually removed.

Surgical resection for diagnosis may be necessary to rule out other diseases such as malignancy or to obtain material for cultures. Patients with destroyed lobes (Fig 21–14) or cavitary tuberculosis of the right upper lobe (Fig 21–15) containing large infected foci may sometimes be candidates for resection. Thin-walled cavities ("open negative") have a relapse rate of less than 2%, whereas infection relapses in about 10% of cases with thick-walled cavities, and selected patients in the latter category may occasionally be surgical candidates.

The disease becomes reactivated in some patients who have had thoracoplasty, plombage, or resection, and a few will require operation. The most common indications for surgery after plombage therapy are pleural infection (pyogenic or tuberculous) and migration of the plombage material, causing pain or compression of other organs. Following pulmonary resection, tuberculous empyema may develop in the postpneumonectomy space, sometimes associated with a bronchopleural fistula or bony sequestration. Persistent bronchopleural fistula after chemotherapy and closed tube drainage may require direct operative closure. Tuberculosis-related bronchiectasis, particularly if localized to a lower lobe, may sometimes require surgery, particularly if there has been significant bronchial scarring or stricture.

Tuberculous empyema poses unique problems of management. Treatment depends upon whether the empyema is (1) with or without parenchymal disease, (2) mixed tuberculous and pyogenic or purely tuberculous, and (3) with or without bronchopleural fistula. In all cases, the ultimate objective is complete expansion of the lung and obliteration of the empyema space. Pulmonary decortication or resection may be used for tuberculosis, but open or closed drainage is necessary when the process is complicated by pyogenic infection or bronchopleural fistula. Extrapleural thoracoplasty may be used in rare cases to obliterate a cavity but should be avoided if possible.

Prognosis

The prognosis is excellent in most cases treated medically; the mortality rate decreased from 25% in 1945 to 10% in 1970. The operative mortality rate in pulmonary resections for tuberculosis is about 10% for pneumonectomy, 3% for lobectomy, and 1% for segmentectomy and subsegmental resections.

The relapse rate following modern chemotherapy is about 4%; following combined resectional therapy and chemotherapy, relapse occurs in about 2%.

Cryer PE, Kissane J (editors): Miliary tuberculosis. Am J Med 58:847, 1975.

Delarue NC, Gale G: Surgical salvage in pulmonary tuberculosis. Ann Thorac Surg 18:38, 1974.

Dineen P, Homan WP, Grafe WR: Tuberculous peritonitis: 43 years' experience in diagnosis and treatment. Ann Surg 184:717, 1976.

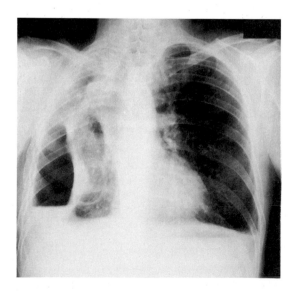

Figure 21–14. Tuberculosis of the right lung with empyema and bronchopleural fistula.

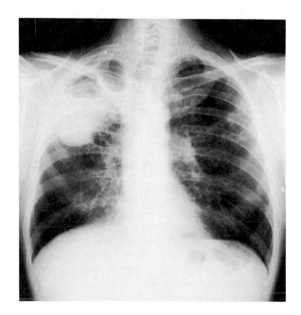

Figure 21–15. Cavitary tuberculosis of the right upper lobe.

Elkadi A & others: Surgical treatment of atypical pulmonary tuberculosis. J Thorac Cardiovasc Surg 72:435, 1976.

Hobby GL, Johnson PM, Boytar-Papirnyik V: Primary drug resistance: A continuing study of drug resistance in tuberculosis in a veteran population within the U.S. Am Rev Respir Dis 110:95, 1974.

Hyde L: Clinical significance of the tuberculin skin test. Am Rev Respir Dis 105:453, 1972.

Lefrak SS & others: Chemoprophylaxis of tuberculosis. Arch Intern Med 135:606, 1975.

McConville JH, Rapoport MI: Tuberculosis management in the mid-1970s. JAMA 235:172, 1976.

McLaughlin JS, Hankins JR: Current aspects of surgery for pulmonary tuberculosis. Ann Thorac Surg 17:513, 1974.

Oseasohn R: Current use of BCG. Am Rev Respir Dis 109:500, 1974.

MYCOTIC INFECTION OF THE LUNGS

The increasing frequency of fungal disease is related to the widespread use of broad-spectrum antibiotics, corticosteroids, and immunosuppressive drugs. In the USA, each of the 3 most commonly encountered mycoses of surgical importance—histoplasmosis, coccidioidomycosis, blastomycosis—has a rather restricted endemic area. The surgeon becomes involved with fungal disease of the lung in 3 situations: (1) during diagnostic procedures, eg, bronchoscopy or biopsy; (2) in treatment of a lesion (eg, excisional biopsy) where the diagnosis is uncertain but neoplasm cannot be ruled out; and (3) in treatment of known fungal disease unresponsive to medical therapy. Special stains, special culture media, and special technics are essential for isolation and identification.

HISTOPLASMOSIS

Histoplasma capsulatum is found in soil contaminated by pigeon, chicken, or bat droppings. It is most prevalent in states bordering the Mississippi, Missouri, and Ohio River valleys. In the USA, 30 million persons are estimated to have been infected as shown by histoplasmin skin tests. Histoplasmosis has also been reported in South and Central America, India, Malaysia, and Cyprus. It is rare in Europe and Australia and almost nonexistent in England and Japan.

The symptoms and roentgenographic findings of histoplasmosis resemble those of tuberculosis, although the disease appears to progress more slowly. There may be cough, malaise, hemoptysis, low-grade fever, and weight loss. As many as 30% of cases coexist with tuberculosis. Pulmonary fibrosis, bulla formation, and

pulmonary insufficiency occur in advanced cases. Mediastinal involvement is quite frequent and may take the form of granuloma formation, fibrosis with superior vena caval syndrome, or dysphagia. Erosion of inflammatory lymph nodes into bronchi may cause expectoration of broncholiths, hemoptysis, wheezing, or bronchiectasis. Traction diverticula of the esophagus may lead to development of tracheoesophageal fistula. Pericardial involvement may lead to constrictive pericarditis.

Histoplasmosis is a major diagnostic possibility in lesions that present as solitary pulmonary nodules, constituting about 15–20% of the total.

Radiologically, early infections appear as diffuse mottled parenchymal infiltrations surrounding the hili and enlargement of hilar lymph nodes. Cavitation indicates advanced infection and is the complication for which the surgeon is most often consulted. The diagnosis rests upon finding a positive skin test or complement fixation test and culturing the fungus from sputum or a bronchial aspirate.

Medical therapy with amphotericin B may be indicated.

Many cases appearing as solitary pulmonary nodules will require excisional biopsy to rule out neoplasm. Surgical therapy for unresolved cavitary disease or specific complications of mediastinal involvement must be planned to meet the criteria of feasibility of surgical correction.

Forrest JV: Common fungal diseases of the lung. 2. Histoplasmosis. Radiol Clin North Am 11:163, 1973.

Saab SB, Ungaro R, Almond C: The role and results of surgery in the management of chronic pulmonary histoplasmosis J Thorac Cardiovasc Surg 68:159, 1974.

COCCIDIOIDOMYCOSIS

Coccidioides immitis is endemic to the southwestern part of the USA, especially the San Joaquin Valley of California. A few cases have been reported in Mexico and Central and South America. This soil-dweller produces arthrospores that are carried in the air and inhaled. Half of persons living in the endemic area have positive skin tests, and 25% of newly arrived individuals have a positive coccidioidin skin test after 1 year. Most conversions are asymptomatic, but about one-third develop flu-like symptoms. One percent of these go on to a prolonged illness lasting weeks or months. About 10 million people in the USA are estimated to have been infected.

Symptoms may be "flu-like," consisting of malaise, headache, and fever. There may be pleuritic pain and cough productive of mucoid bloody sputum. Physical signs are not helpful. The diagnosis is based on culture of sputum, fluids, or tissues obtained by biopsy. Roentgenographic findings are often indistinguishable from those of other granulomatous infec-

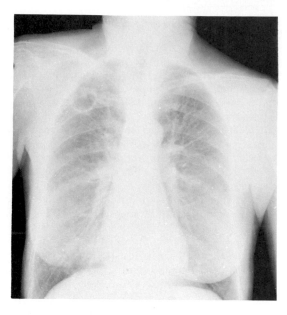

Figure 21—16. Thin-walled cavity of coccidioidomycosis.

tions. Nodules may excavate to form thin- or thick-walled cavities (Fig 21—16), particularly in the upper lobes. Unlike tuberculosis, the anterior segments of the upper lobes are frequently involved. Cavitary disease is associated with pneumothorax and empyema in 2% of cases.

The only effective treatment is amphotericin B. Because of the drug's toxicity, it is given only on specific indications, ie, severe disease, disseminated disease, threat of dissemination, progressive pulmonary lesions, for surgical coverage, in patients with known disease who require corticosteroids, during pregnancy, or in diabetics.

Surgical treatment is reserved for patients with cavities that rupture into the pleural space, produce recurrent hemoptysis, or which are large or enlarging. Some bleeding occurs in 65% of coccidioidal cavities. Surgery may also be performed for undiagnosed solid lesions suspicious of carcinoma. Wide surgical excision of cavities or nodules—preferably lobectomy—is advised because of the frequent presence of satellite lesions which predispose to postoperative complications. Ten to 15% of cases develop bronchopleural fistulas, coccidioidal empyema, or reactivation when wedge or localized excision is used.

Franz JL & others: Pulmonary coccidioidomycosis presenting by direct extension through the chest wall. J Thorac Cardiovasc Surg 67:474, 1974.
Nelson AR: The surgical treatment of pulmonary coccidioidomycosis. Curr Probl Surg, Oct 1974.

NORTH AMERICAN BLASTOMYCOSIS

Blastomyces dermatitidis has a mycelial phase in soil and a yeast phase in humans and animals. Endemic areas are in the Western Hemisphere, particularly the central and southeastern USA and in Canada. It is considerably less common than histoplasmosis, but the exact incidence is not known. The disease has a cutaneous and a pulmonary form.

Pulmonary blastomycosis presents with symptoms of cough, chest pain, hemoptysis, and fever. Chest roentgenographic findings are nonspecific and may show cavitation, unresolved infiltrates, or consolidation. Calcification of parenchymal lesions is very rare. Skin lesions usually have a specific appearance, consisting of chronic indolent enlarging papulopustules with thick adherent crusts and elevated violaceous edges. The diagnosis is made by culture of the organism from sputum, skin lesions, abscesses, or biopsy material. The organism may also be demonstrated in urine, CSF, or blood. Pleural effusion occurs in 2% of cases, bony lesions in 25% of cases, and genitourinary tract lesions in 10% of males. When untreated, the clinical course is one of frequent remissions and exacerbations and a mortality rate of 30%. A positive blastomycin skin test should be considered significant only when stronger than that to histoplasmin and coccidioidin. Serologic tests may also be helpful.

Hydroxystilbamidine and amphotericin B should be considered for treatment.

Surgery is rarely indicated. It is more often employed for diagnosis to rule out bronchogenic carcinoma. Postoperative dissemination is minimized if drug therapy is used concomitantly with surgery; when not accompanied by adequate drug therapy, operative spread is common.

Sarosi GA & others: Clinical features of acute pulmonary blastomycosis. N Engl J Med 290:540, 1974.
Witorsch P, Utz JP: North American blastomycosis: A study of 40 patients. Medicine 47:169, 1968.

CRYPTOCOCCOSIS
(Torulosis)

Cryptococcus neoformans is a soil-dweller—particularly soil contaminated by pigeon droppings—that has a worldwide distribution. The organism enters the blood via the lungs and has a predilection for the CNS. It is a primary pathogen but also an opportunistic invader in debilitated patients, particularly those with lymphoma or collagen disease or those receiving antimetabolites, corticosteroids, or antibiotics.

Pulmonary symptoms are nonspecific or so insidious that they may not receive clinical recognition. When it affects patients ill from another disease, symptoms of the latter often overshadow those due to cryptococcosis. The disease is often discovered inadvertently on chest x-ray or by a pathologist examining tissue removed at thoracotomy. Cultures of sputum, bronchial washings, and spinal fluid may establish the diagnosis, but false-negatives are fairly common. Chest x-rays usually show a fairly well circumscribed mass, 2–8 cm in diameter, often single, in a lower lobe. Cavitation occurs in about 15% of cases. Pleural involvement is unusual and calcification is rare.

When extrapulmonary (especially CNS) disease is present, amphotericin B coverage is indicated. In the absence of CNS disease, amphotericin B may be withheld when cryptococcosis is found in a specimen of lung resected for diagnosis of a solitary nodule.

Hatcher CR Jr & others: Primary pulmonary cryptococcosis. J Thorac Cardiovasc Surg 61:39, 1971.
Sutliff WD: Histoplasmosis cooperative study. 5. Amphotericin B dosage for chronic pulmonary histoplasmosis. Am Rev Respir Dis 105:60, 1972.

ACTINOMYCOSIS

Actinomyces israelii is a normal inhabitant of the oral cavity of man. The diagnosis is made from cultures of yellow-brown granules called "sulfur granules" from suppurative material or draining sinuses.

In man, cervicofacial, thoracic, and abdominal forms are recognized. The infections with this organism produce a marked fibroplastic response. Thoracic involvement, characteristically manifested by empyema or draining chest wall sinuses, is often associated with nonspecific pulmonary infiltrates, consolidation, or hilar manifestations.

Treatment

Penicillin is the drug of choice. Surgical treatment (with antibiotic coverage) may be required, ie, open drainage or wide excision. The diagnosis is sometimes made after thoracotomy for a lesion suspected to be bronchogenic carcinoma.

Eastridge CE & others: Actinomycosis: A 24-year experience. South Med J 65:839, 1972.

NOCARDIOSIS

Nocardia asteroides and, less commonly, *N brasiliensis* or *N madurae* cause human infections. The organisms are found worldwide in soil, grasses, and in several species of animals. The lesions may resemble actinomycosis with sulfur granules and there is an acid-fast bacillus-like form resembling tuberculosis. They are often opportunistic.

Symptoms are often flu-like. Empyema develops in 25% of cases, often forming subcutaneous abscesses or fistulous tracts and sinuses. Nocardia has been isolated from broncholiths almost as often as histoplasma.

Sulfadiazine is the drug of choice. Pulmonary resection is rarely indicated. As a rule, surgical treatment is restricted to drainage of empyema or abscesses.

Freese JW & others: Pulmonary infection with *Nocardia asteroides:* Findings in eleven clinical cases. J Thorac Cardiovasc Surg 46:537, 1963.

ASPERGILLOSIS

Aspergillus fumigatus is the most commonly found species, but *A flavus, A niger,* and *A nidulans* also cause clinical disease. Three clinical forms occur: (1) bronchitis secondary to aspergillus sensitivity; (2) aspergillomas or fungus balls, which present as saprophytes in long-standing cavitary lung disease (Fig 21–17); and (3) opportunistic invasive infections causing a necrotizing pneumonia, infarction, and hematogenous dissemination.

Medical treatment has been unsatisfactory but iodides, nystatin, hydroxystilbamidine, and amphotericin B have all been reported to produce cures. Surgical therapy is indicated in suitably selected patients with aspergilloma, particularly if recurrent hemoptysis has occurred.

Henderson RD & others: Surgery in pulmonary aspergillosis. J Thorac Cardiovasc Surg 70:1088, 1975.
Karas A & others: Pulmonary aspergillosis: An analysis of 41 patients. Ann Thorac Surg 22:1, 1976.

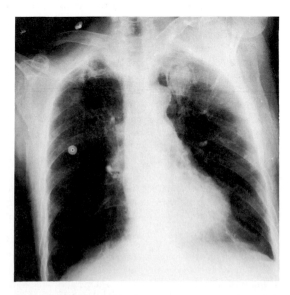

Figure 21–17. Aspergilloma (fungus ball) in tuberculous cavity of the left upper lobe.

Saab SB, Almond C: Surgical aspects of pulmonary aspergillosis. J Thorac Cardiovasc Surg 68:455, 1974.

OTHER MYCOTIC INFECTIONS

Candida albicans and other species of Candida usually cause opportunistic infections involving the lungs of patients treated by endotracheal tube, assisted ventilation, and broad-spectrum antibiotics. Localized bronchopulmonary candidiasis is extremely rare. Other relatively rare mycotic infections of thoracic surgical interest are sporotrichosis, which produces a localized cavity; phycomycosis, monosporosis, or mucormycosis; South American blastomycosis; and geotrichosis.

Bennett JE: Chemotherapy of systemic mycoses. (2 parts.) N Engl J Med 290:30, 320, 1974.

Jung JY & others: The role of surgery in the management of pulmonary monosporosis: A collective review. J Thorac Cardiovasc Surg 73:139, 1977.

Razzuk MA, Urschel HC Jr, Paulson DL: Systemic mycosis: Primary pathogenic fungi. Ann Thorac Surg 15:644, 1973.

PARASITIC DISEASES*

Pneumocystis Carinii Infection

Pneumocystis carinii is an opportunistic protozoon organism afflicting patients with impaired immunity. Pulmonary involvement leads to progressive pneumonia and respiratory insufficiency. In the past, patients with impaired immune mechanisms or lymphatic and leukemic malignancy were most frequently affected. Now, most recipients of organ transplants undergo immunosuppressive therapy to prevent organ rejection and many have become infected with pneumocystis. The most reliable means of diagnosis is lung biopsy. Without treatment, the clinical course is one of relentless progression. Therapy with pentamidine isethionate is usually effective.

Pulmonary & Pleural Amebiasis

Entamoeba histolytica is a protozoan infection that may have pleuropulmonary involvement in 10–20% of cases. About 75% of cases of thoracic involvement are secondary to transdiaphragmatic rupture of hepatic abscesses and only about 15% of cases of thoracic involvement occur without hepatic abscesses.

Clinical and roentgenographic manifestations are those of pleurisy, pleural effusion, empyema (25% have secondary pyogenic infection), bronchopleural fistula, or pulmonary abscess. There may be right

---

*Echinococcosis and amebiasis are discussed in Chapter 11.

upper quadrant pain, pleuritic pain, dry cough, or a cough productive of material resembling "chocolate sauce" or "anchovy sauce."

Medical treatment consists of metronidazole, dehydroemetine, chloroquine, and antibiotics for secondary bacterial infections (see Chapter 11).

Thoracentesis is used if no secondary infection is present. Surgical treatment in secondarily infected cases usually consists of closed tube drainage (occasionally followed by open drainage), decortication, or pulmonary resection.

The survival rate with pulmonary involvement is 90%. About 25% need only medical treatment, 35% chemotherapy and thoracentesis, 15% closed drainage, and 12% require more extensive procedures. Deaths are most common in patients with secondary bacterial infection.

Drew WL & others: Diagnosis of *Pneumocystis carinii* pneumonia by bronchopulmonary lavage. JAMA 230:713, 1974.

Geelhoed GW & others: The diagnosis and management of *Pneumocystis carinii* pneumonia. Ann Thorac Surg 14:335, 1972.

Herrera-Lierandi R: Thoracic repercussions of amebiasis. J Thorac Cardiovasc Surg 52:361, 1966.

Tyras DH & others: The role of early lung biopsy in the diagnosis and treatment of *Pneumocystis carinii* pneumonia. Ann Thorac Surg 18:571, 1974.

Walzer PD & others: *Pneumocystis carinii* pneumonia in the United States: Epidemiologic, diagnostic, and clinical features. Ann Intern Med 80:83, 1974.

SARCOIDOSIS
(Boeck's Sarcoid, Benign Lymphogranulomatosis)

Sarcoidosis is a noncaseating granulomatous disease of unknown cause involving the lungs, liver, spleen, lymph nodes, skin, and bones. The distribution is worldwide, but the largest series are reported from Scandinavia, England, and the USA. Sarcoidosis is more prevalent in rural areas, particularly in the southeastern USA. The incidence in blacks (especially females) is 10–17 times that in whites. Half of patients are between the ages of 20 and 40.

Clinical Findings

A. Symptoms and Signs: Sarcoidosis may present with symptoms of pulmonary infection, but usually these are insidious and nonspecific. Erythema nodosum may herald the onset, and weight loss, fatigue, weakness, and malaise may appear later. Fever occurs in 15% of cases. Pulmonary symptoms occur in 20–30% and include dry cough and dyspnea. Hemoptysis is rare. One-fifth of cases have myocardial involvement, and heart block or failure may occur. Peripheral lymph nodes are enlarged in 75%; scalene lymph nodes are microscopically involved in 80%; mediastinal nodes in 90%; and cutaneous involvement is present in 30%. Hepatic and splenic involvement can be shown by biopsy in 70% of cases. There may be migratory or persistent polyarthritis, and CNS involvement occurs in a few patients.

B. Laboratory Findings: Laboratory findings are hypercalciuria (30%), hypercalcemia (15%), abnormal serum proteins, elevated alkaline phosphatase, leukopenia, and eosinophilia. The Kveim test is positive in 75% of cases.

C. X-Ray Findings: Chest roentgenographic findings are bilateral, symmetric hilar and paratracheal lymph node involvement (75–90%), diffuse pulmonary disease without enlargement of hilar nodes (25%), combined diffuse pulmonary disease and hilar lymph node involvement, or pulmonary fibrosis (20%). Pleural effusion is rare unless due to heart failure.

D. Biopsy: If peripheral adenopathy or skin lesions are present, histologic diagnosis should be sought by biopsy of these lesions. Otherwise, biopsy via mediastinoscopy or of scalene lymph nodes will provide the answer in over 90% of cases.

Differential Diagnosis

Tuberculosis, coccidioidomycosis, histoplasmosis, cryptococcosis, and brucellosis may present a picture identical to that of sarcoidosis. Metastatic cancer, foreign body granulomas (especially in heroin addicts), or hamartomatosis may be difficult to exclude.

Treatment

Medical treatment consists of observation, general supportive measures, and, in severe cases, corticosteroids. Preventive antituberculosis therapy should be used when corticosteroids are given or when a positive tuberculin reaction is present. Surgical management, in addition to procedures to establish the diagnosis and rule out other diseases (eg, biopsies of lymph nodes, lung, or liver), involves treatment of heart block by pacemaker implantation or, rarely, treatment of the complications of bullous emphysema in advanced cases.

Prognosis

The prognosis is poorer in blacks and when relapses have occurred. The mortality rate is about 5–10% in patients followed for 20 years. Cardiac failure is the leading cause of death. Superimposed tuberculosis is common and should be anticipated. About 65% of patients recover fully; 20–25% have some degree of permanent disability.

Israel HL & others: A controlled trial of prednisone treatment of sarcoidosis. Am Rev Respir Dis 107:609, 1973.

Mitchell DN, Scadding JG: Sarcoidosis. Am Rev Respir Dis 110:774, 1974.

Siltzbach LE & others: Course and prognosis of sarcoidosis around the world. Am J Med 57:847, 1974.

PULMONARY THROMBOEMBOLIC DISEASE

Essentials of Diagnosis

- Large pulmonary embolus: Sudden onset of dyspnea and anxiety, with or without substernal pain. Signs of acute right heart failure and circulatory collapse may follow shortly after.
- Pulmonary infarction: Less severe dyspnea, pleuritic pain, cough, hemoptysis, and an x-ray density in the lung are characteristic of pulmonary infarction.
- Recurrent minor emboli: gradually developing, unexplained, with or without pulmonary x-ray densities.
- History or clinical findings of thrombophlebitis are common in patients with pulmonary embolism.

General Considerations

Pulmonary embolism is a frequent autopsy finding. Half of cases are not suspected clinically, and in 20% no physical findings preceded the embolism. Pulmonary thromboembolism does not necessarily result in pulmonary infarction, which occurs in only 10–15% of cases. The site of origin of the clot is usually the lower extremity or pelvic veins; rarely, the upper extremities or cervical veins. The right atrium is the source in some cases. Clot may even originate within the lungs by intravascular coagulation in chronic low output states or in diseases involving the arterial wall.

Clotted blood is by far the most common embolus to the pulmonary vasculature, but fat, air, bits of tumor, amniotic fluid, bone marrow, parasites, and, in addicts, foreign materials such as starch, cotton, glass, rubber, etc may be found. Bacterial vegetations may embolize in bacterial endocarditis.

Clinical Findings

A. Symptoms and Signs: Pulmonary thromboembolism is manifested in 4 ways: (1) acute massive embolism, (2) segmental emboli with or without infarction, (3) multiple small emboli that present as pulmonary insufficiency, and (4) silent or asymptomatic emboli. The clinical findings of pulmonary embolism or infarction are usually either cardiac or respiratory; hypoxia may lead to restlessness or anxiety. When 65–70% of the pulmonary vasculature is occluded, acute pulmonary hypertension occurs, cardiac output decreases, and hypotension, cardiac arrhythmias, shock, and death may ensue. This may occur within a few minutes or a few days. When embolism results in infarction, dyspnea, tachycardia, fever, pleuritic chest pain, cough, and sometimes hemoptysis develop. Dyspnea and chest pain are the most common symptoms, and dyspnea is always present in severe cases. When emboli are recurrent and small, the onset of dyspnea may be insidious. Chest pain is of 2 types. Retrosternal pain may be identical to that of myocardial infarction and is due to acute pulmonary hypertension or coronary insufficiency caused by diminished cardiac output. The second type of pain is pleuritic. Hemoptysis occurs in 20–35% of cases, and cough is present primarily as a result of hemoptysis.

Physical signs include decreased breath sounds, rales, rhonchi, rubs, or signs of pleural effusion. Evidence of right heart failure and pulmonary hypertension may be present, eg, a loud second pulmonic sound, venous distention, and acute liver enlargement. Cyanosis is often present.

B. Laboratory Findings: Laboratory tests are usually not diagnostic. Arterial blood gases may reveal a low oxygen tension, and there may be a gradient in P_{CO_2} between arterial blood and the end tidal gas. Electrocardiographic changes are helpful only in one-third of cases, but classically show an S wave in lead I, an inverted Q wave or T wave (or both) in lead III, and T wave inversion over the right side of the heart.

Roentgenographic findings may show either nothing abnormal, evidence of diminished vascularity, or, later, typical wedge-shaped peripheral infiltrates with or without effusion. The lower lobes are most often involved, especially the right. Ten to 15% of cases involve primarily the upper lobes. Evidence of acute enlargement of the pulmonary artery or a sudden termination of the pulmonary artery may be present. There may be signs of cor pulmonale in severe cases.

Pulmonary angiography is the only means of definitive diagnosis and should precede surgery in all patients being considered for thoracotomy (Fig 21–18). It may be necessary to institute cardiopulmonary bypass to accomplish this procedure. The angiogram shows the clot or an occlusion in the pulmonary arteries.

Radioisotope scanning using macroaggregated albumin tagged with ^{131}I is useful in less severe or doubtful cases. A normal scan rules out a massive embolism, but the presence of a defect does not prove the diagnosis. Diminished perfusion may occur for many reasons, including bullae, atelectasis, pneumonia, diminished cardiac output, etc. Serial scans may be more valuable.

Differential Diagnosis

The most common mistaken diagnosis in massive embolism is myocardial infarction. Thoracotomy in these patients carries a high mortality rate and must be avoided. In less severe cases, congestive heart failure, pneumonia, and asthma must be considered.

Treatment

The patient is immediately given heparin as anticoagulant (see p 739) to prevent further thrombosis and for the pharmacologic effect of heparin that reduces pulmonary vascular resistance. Acid-base abnormalities are corrected. The patient is constantly monitored. Treatment should include cardiopulmonary resuscitative measures to support circulation and improve oxygenation. Hypotension is treated by pressor agents and hypoxia by intubation, assisted ventilation, or oxygen mask.

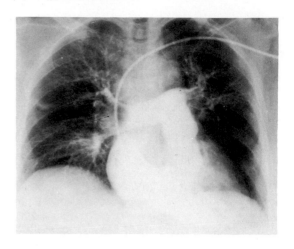

Figure 21–18. Pulmonary angiogram in a patient with massive thromboembolism.

Surgical treatment is used to prevent recurrent episodes of embolism in patients who have emboli while adequately anticoagulated. The procedures available include caval ligation or caval filters (see p 740).

Embolectomy requiring thoracotomy and cardiopulmonary bypass is reserved for patients receiving adequate medical therapy whose deterioration is indicated by hypotension, severe hypoxemia, or cardiac arrest and arteriographic evidence of occlusion of 50% or more of the pulmonary vasculature. Prolonged extracorporeal bypass with membrane oxygenation may prove valuable since the acutely induced myocardial and pulmonary effects are reversible.

Prognosis

The overall prognosis is poor. About 47,000 people die every year of pulmonary embolism in the USA, and most of these are not clinically detected or treated. It is estimated that 75% of patients die within 1 hour. In recognized cases of massive embolism, the extent of embolism is most critical. In patients who withstand the initial episode, resolution and recanalization of the pulmonary vasculature can occur promptly, and most patients do not have lasting disability.

Accumulated statistics since 1967 for embolectomy with cardiopulmonary bypass show that survival was 70% using cardiopulmonary bypass and 60% with medical therapy.

Alpert JS & others: Mortality in patients treated for pulmonary embolism. JAMA 236:1477, 1976.

Eberlein TJ, Carey LC: Comparison of surgical managements for pulmonary emboli. Ann Surg 179:836, 1973.

Greenfield LJ: Pulmonary embolism: Diagnosis and management. Curr Probl Surg 13 (4), April 1976.

Hill JD & others: Prognostic factors in the treatment of acute respiratory insufficiency with long-term extracorporeal oxygenation. J Thorac Cardiovasc Surg 68:905, 1974.

Houk VN & others: Chronic thrombotic obstruction of major pulmonary arteries. Am J Med 35:269, 1963.

Paraskos JA & others: Late prognosis of acute pulmonary embolism. N Engl J Med 289:55, 1973.

Turnier E & others: Massive pulmonary embolism. Am J Surg 125:611, 1973.

THE SOLITARY PULMONARY NODULE
("Coin Lesions")

Solitary pulmonary nodules or "coin lesions" are peripheral circumscribed pulmonary lesions that are due either to granulomatous diseases or neoplasms. The latter include benign or malignant primary or secondary tumors. Many characteristics denote probable benignity or malignancy, but often the diagnosis is not certain. Since 5-year survival following resection of a solitary nodule that turns out to be bronchogenic carcinoma may be as high as 90%, prompt surgical therapy is warranted when malignancy cannot be excluded. In the average patient, the risk of thoracotomy is less than 1%, and if the chance of malignancy is 5% the probability of cure will outweigh the risk of thoracotomy.

The overall incidence of malignancy in solitary nodular lesions seen on x-ray is about 5–10%. However, in patients ultimately selected for resection of the nodules, the probability of malignancy is considerably higher. The breakdown is as follows: 35% primary carcinomas, 35% nonspecific granulomas, 20% tuberculous granulomas, about 5% mixed tumors (hamartomas), and 5% metastatic carcinomas. A small miscellaneous category includes adenomas, cysts, and other lesions. The overall incidence of solitary nodules is 3–9 times higher in males than females. Malignancy is almost twice as frequent in males as in females.

Clinical Findings

A. Symptoms: Symptoms are usually absent, but cough, weight loss, chest pain, or hemoptysis favors a diagnosis of malignancy.

B. Past History: There may be a history of living in an endemic granuloma area. Previous tuberculosis favors granuloma, whereas smoking favors malignancy. Ninety percent of patients with solitary metastatic lesions have a history of extrapulmonary malignancy.

C. Signs: Clubbing is uncommon in benign lesions and is seen occasionally in malignant ones. Hypertrophic osteoarthropathy signifies an 80% or greater probability of malignancy.

D. Laboratory Findings: Positive skin tests do not rule out malignancy, but granulomatous disease is less likely when skin tests are negative. In granuloma of known cause, the skin test is positive in 90% of cases of tuberculosis, 80% of cases of histoplasmosis, and 70% of cases of coccidioidomycosis.

Sputum cultures are usually negative. Cytologic examination of sputum yields a diagnosis in only 5–20% of cases.

E. X-Ray Findings: Coin lesions can rarely be diagnosed with certainty—whether benign or malignant—by radiologic findings (Fig 21–19). Some useful x-ray features are as follows.*

1. Size—Lesions 1 cm or less in diameter are probably granulomas; those greater than 1 cm have a significant probability of cancer, and a lesion 4 cm or more in diameter is very likely malignant (Fig 21–20A and B).

2. Cavitation and radiolucent areas—These are seen in both benign and malignant lesions (Figs 21–19 and 21–20).

3. Calcification—The presence of calcification tends to favor granuloma but does not exclude carcinoma unless it appears as concentric laminations. Calcification may be misinterpreted on plain films, and tomograms should be obtained when considered important. Calcifications of the "target" or "popcorn" variety are very unlikely to be malignant (Fig 21–19B and C). Lesions that are completely or heavily calcified are most likely benign. Malignant lesions with calcifications are most often squamous cell carcinomas. Adenocarcinomas are next most common. Calcification in malignancies generally consists of small flecks located eccentrically or at the periphery of the nodule.

4. Density—Dense lesions less than 3 cm in diameter favor a diagnosis of malignancy (Fig 21–19D and E).

5. Margins—Irregular shape is often seen in inflammatory lesions and benign lung tumors (Fig 21–19F). A rounded lesion with umbilication suggests malignancy (Fig 21–19G). Indistinct margins favor malignancy (Fig 21–20H), whereas discrete margins favor benignity (Fig 21–19B), although circumscribed margins are seen in about 30% of malignant lesions.

6. Growth—Documented absence of growth for more than 1 year means that malignancy is highly unlikely, but slow growth has been seen in malignant lesions followed for 6 years or more.

7. Satellites—The presence of satellite densities favors a diagnosis of granuloma.

F. Other Studies: Probably the most useful study is a previous chest film for comparison. Bronchoscopy is of value in about 10% of solitary cases, and mediastinoscopy may be diagnostic of malignancy in 6–15% of cases. In the absence of a pertinent history, a search should not be made for a primary lesion by roentgenographic studies of the upper gastrointestinal tract, urinary tract, or skeletal system. Percutaneous needle biopsy should not be done in potentially curable surgical candidates because of possible intrathoracic dissemination of the tumor.

---

*The most persuasive radiologic evidences of benignity are (1) calcification, especially if concentric or laminated; and (2) documented absence of growth for 1 year.

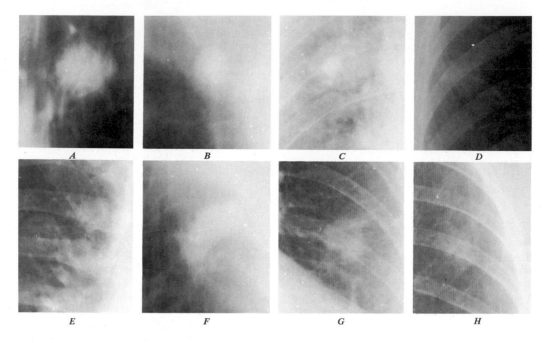

Figure 21–19. Coin lesions. *A:* Large cell undifferentiated carcinoma in RUL (tomogram). *B:* Histoplasmosis (tomogram). *C:* Harmartoma. *D:* Solitary metastasis from epidermoid carcinoma of the cervix. *E:* Tuberculoma (tomogram). *F:* Foreign body granuloma in heroin addict (tomogram). *G:* Adenocarcinoma of LUL (present 6 years). *H:* Alveolar cell carcinoma of LUL (present 3 years). (RUL = right upper lobe; LUL = left upper lobe.)

Treatment

A decision must often be made about whether or not to give therapy for tuberculosis. The risks of the patient's being lost to follow-up, indecisive results even after 3–6 months, and the possibility of spread of tumor are factors favoring early resolution of the diagnostic dilemma by excisional biopsy. The overall risk of thoracotomy is less than 1%. Patients with a higher operative risk are in the age group of 50 years or older, but these patients also have a 50–60% chance of having carcinoma.

Surgical diagnosis may be made by excisional wedge biopsy in peripheral lesions and may constitute definitive therapy for benign lesions, for solitary metastasis, and for primary malignancy in poor-risk patients. Centrally placed lesions or those suspected of being coccidioidomycosis should be treated by lobectomy. Primary malignancies are treated by lobectomy in good-risk patients with regional node dissection. Pneumonectomy should not be done until a tissue diagnosis of malignancy has been established.

Prognosis

The prognosis for malignant coin lesions is 3–6 times more favorable than that for lung cancer in general. The 5-year survival rate in those less than 2 cm in diameter is about 70%.

Bateson EM: An analysis of 155 solitary lung lesions illustrating the differential diagnosis of mixed tumours of the lung. Clin Radiol 16:51, 1965.

Burdette WJ, Evans C: Management of coin lesions and carcinoma of the lung. Ann Surg 161:649, 1965.

Jackman RJ & others: Survival rates in peripheral bronchogenic carcinomas up to four centimeters in diameter presenting as solitary pulmonary nodules. J Thorac Cardiovasc Surg 57:1, 1969.

Lillington GA: The solitary pulmonary nodule–1974. Am Rev Respir Dis 110:699, 1974.

Nathan MH: Management of the solitary pulmonary nodule. JAMA 227:1141, 1974.

O'Connor TM & others: The malignant solitary nodule: Follow-up study. Arch Surg 86:985, 1963.

Steele JD: The solitary pulmonary nodule. J Thorac Cardiovasc Surg 46:21, 1963.

LUNG NEOPLASMS

BENIGN NEOPLASMS

Benign tumors of the lung are very uncommon and account for only 1–2% of all pulmonary neoplasms. Over half of the cases that are included in this category are bronchial adenomas, which are in fact low-grade malignant tumors since about 15% metastasize. Considering only coin lesions of the lungs, 5–10% are benign neoplasms.

Most truly benign lesions of the lung are hamartomas (mixed tumors). Other types are fibrous mesotheliomas, xanthomatous and inflammatory pseudotumors, and miscellaneous rare lesions such as lipomas and benign granular cell myoblastomas.

Benign lung tumors may occur at almost any age. Hamartomas occur in males twice as often as females. Symptoms are absent in 60% and nonspecific in many other cases. Bronchial obstruction by the lesion, pneumonitis, and hemoptysis may occur. Clubbing or hypertrophic osteoarthropathy does not occur in benign tumors except in fibrous mesotheliomas. X-ray may show calcification.

The differential diagnosis is discussed in the context of solitary pulmonary nodules in the preceding section.

Surgical excision should be conservative, and enucleation or wedge excision done when possible. The prognosis is excellent.

Arrigoni MG & others: Benign tumors of the lung: A ten-year surgical experience. J Thorac Cardiovasc Surg 60:589, 1970.

Bateson EM: An analysis of 155 solitary lung lesions illustrating the differential diagnosis of mixed tumours of the lung. Clin Radiol 16:51, 1965.

Steele JD: The solitary nodule. J Thorac Cardiovasc Surg 46:21, 1963.

MALIGNANT LUNG NEOPLASMS

Essentials of Diagnosis

- Insidious onset with cough, localized wheeze, or hemoptysis; often asymptomatic.
- May present as an unresolved pneumonia, atelectasis, or pleurisy with bloody effusion, or as a pulmonary nodule seen on x-ray.
- Metastases to other organs may produce initial symptoms.
- Endocrine, biochemical, and neuromuscular disorders (see below) may be the presenting features of bronchogenic carcinoma.

General Considerations

The incidence of lung cancer is increasing, and lung cancer has become the most common fatal malignancy in males. In England during 1966, 39% of all male cancer deaths and 8% of all deaths were caused by lung cancer. The United Kingdom mortality rates are the highest of all, and Finland, Austria, several western European countries, and the Union of South Africa all have higher mortality rates from lung cancer than the USA.

It is believed that the rate of increase has reached a peak and that the twentieth century increase was due to cigarette smoking, air pollution, and specific industrial hazards. By far the most important etiologic factor in lung cancer is cigarette smoking. Cigarette smoking is related causally to bronchogenic carcinoma of the squamous cell and oat cell types but not to adenocarcinoma or alveolar cell carcinomas. Various materials in mining and industrial exposure that have been associated with bronchogenic carcinoma include asbestos, radioactive materials, arsenic, chromates, and nickel.

Classification

The classification of malignant lung tumors proposed in 1958 by the World Health Organization is shown in Table 21–4. This classification is still the one most widely used today.

Pathologic Features

A. Squamous Cell Carcinomas: These tumors may be well differentiated or not depending upon the presence of keratin and epithelial pearls; intracellular bridges; cell size and uniformity; or mitosis. About 45% of all lung tumors are squamous cell. Two-thirds are located centrally near the hilus and one-third peripherally. Growth rate and rate of metastases tend to be slower than those of other lung tumors.

B. Oat Cell Carcinomas: These are highly malignant tumors composed of small round or oval cells that often resemble lymphocytes. The origin of these cells is unknown, but they resemble carcinoid tumors and also have a similar distribution and propensity to cause endocrine disturbances. Anaplastic tumors of this type represent approximately 35% of all bronchial carcinomas. About 80% are centrally located and 20% peripheral.

C. Adenocarcinomas: Adenocarcinomas containing glandular elements comprise about 15% of malignant lung tumors. Histologically, they are acinar, papillary, or large giant cell in type. Tumors arising in the

Table 21–4. WHO classification (1958) of malignant tumors of the lung.

Epidermoid carcinoma (squamous cell).
    Keratinizing squamous carcinoma.
Oat cell carcinoma.
Adenocarcinoma.
Bronchiolar or bronchoalveolar carcinoma.
Undifferentiated large cell carcinoma.
Bronchial carcinoid.
Tumors of tracheobronchial mucous glands.
    Adenoid cystic carcinoma (cylindroma).
    Mucoepidermoid carcinoma.
    Bronchial mucous gland adenocarcinoma.
Papilloma and papillary carcinoma.
Sarcoma.
    Malignant lymphoma.
    Leiomyosarcoma.
    Others.
Teratomas, embryonal tumors, and mixed tumors.
Pleural mesothelioma.
    Epithelial or diffuse.
    Fibrosarcomas.
    Other pleural sarcomas.

periphery and in scars are often adenocarcinomas. Adenocarcinomas are peripheral in 75% of cases and central in 25%. They are intermediate in malignant potential between squamous cell and oat cell types. They often spread along vascular channels. Bronchiolar or alveolar cell carcinomas are well-differentiated papillary adenocarcinomas and represent perhaps 2.5% of all malignant tumors. Giant cell tumors are highly malignant. They have pleomorphic or multinucleated cells and represent about 1% of all lung carcinomas.

D. Large Cell Undifferentiated Tumors: This is a poorly defined group of tumors. Some resemble anaplastic or squamous cell tumors with cells characterized by abundant cytoplasm—unlike the oat cell undifferentiated tumors. These tumors are seen more often peripherally; comprise 3—5% of all lung tumors; and are less malignant than small cell undifferentiated tumors.

E. Bronchial Adenomas: These comprise about 1% of lung tumors. They are slow-growing and have a low propensity to metastasize. They are sometimes erroneously classified as benign tumors. Bronchial carcinoid is the most common (85%); adenoid cystic carcinomas (cylindromas) are next in frequency (10—15%); and mucoepidermoid tumors are rare. Carcinoid tumors are usually centrally located in the main stem or lobar bronchi, but 5—10% may be located peripherally. The clinical course is often indolent, extending over years. Adenoid cystic tumors or cylindromas resemble analogous neoplasms in the salivary gland and are either pseudoacinar or medullary in type. These tumors are more malignant than carcinoid tumors but also tend to grow slowly. They have a distribution similar to that of the carcinoids. Mucoepidermoid tumors are most often centrally located and are usually of low-grade malignancy, resembling their salivary gland counterpart. Three cell types may be identified: squamous cells with keratin, mucin-producing cells, and intermediate cells arranged in nests or cords. Bronchial adenomas—especially carcinoid tumors—are twice as common in women as in men.

F. Isolated Bronchial Papilloma and Papillary Carcinomas: These rare tumors are usually part of generalized papillomatosis of the larynx or trachea.

G. Sarcomas: Sarcomas of the lung constitute less than 1% of all lung cancers. Involvement of the lung is not uncommon (7—40%) in disseminated lymphoma but rarely is seen confined to the lung. Most are lymphosarcomas or reticulum cell sarcomas. Other sarcomas arising from soft tissues or primitive mesenchymal cells may be (1) spindle cell sarcomas of the fibro-, lipo-, or myxosarcomatous type; (2) myosarcomas of either smooth or skeletal muscle type; (3) neurosarcomas; (4) chondrosarcomas or osteosarcomas; (5) vascular tumors of hemangiosarcomatous or lymphangiosarcomatous types; or (6) malignant histiocytomas.

Clinical Findings

A. Symptoms and Signs: In 10—20% of patients, no symptoms are present when lung cancer is first diagnosed. The malignancy is usually detected by chest roentgenogram or, very occasionally, by positive cytology. The first symptom may be cough (29%), chest pain (13%), dyspnea (12%), or hemoptysis (6%). A few cases present with pneumonia and malaise, symptoms of brain metastases, bronchitis, epigastric pain or anorexia, weight loss, pain from bone metastases, swelling of the upper body, shoulder pain, flu, hoarseness, or pleurisy.

When symptoms become established, the principal complaints are cough (usually productive) and hemoptysis.

The symptoms can be divided into thoracic and extrathoracic categories. Thoracic symptoms include cough, hemoptysis, wheezing, and pneumonia. Bronchial occlusion may cause dyspnea or tightness of the chest. Extension to the pleura may cause pleuritic pain and symptoms of pleural effusion. Pleural effusion is seen in bronchial obstruction or lymphatic obstruction and is more likely to be serous than bloody. Bloody effusion is usually caused by direct pleural involvement. Oat cell carcinoma most frequently invades the lymphatics and has the highest incidence of pleural effusion. Mediastinal involvement may give symptoms of retrosternal pain, hoarseness from recurrent laryngeal involvement (usually the left), or vena caval obstruction (often oat cell).

Tumors involving the thoracic or superior pulmonary sulcus at the root of the neck may cause **Pancoast's syndrome,** which consists of an apical lung tumor that involves the brachial plexus, the sympathetic ganglia at the base of the neck, and sometimes destruction of ribs and vertebrae. Symptoms are pain, loss of strength in the arm, and **Horner's syndrome** (ptosis, miosis, enophthalmos, and ipsilateral decreased sweating on the involved side). There may be swelling of the involved arm.

Extrathoracic manifestations of lung cancer may be due either to metastatic or to nonmetastatic causes. Extrathoracic metastases occur from either hematogenous or lymphatic dissemination. Lung cancer commonly metastasizes to the cervical and abdominal lymph nodes, liver, adrenals, kidneys, brain, or bone. The exact sequence of metastases differs somewhat with different pathologic types, but the patterns are the same. Lymph node involvement at autopsy is 75% hilar, 60% mediastinal, 15% mesenteric, 5% pancreatic, 3% axillary, and 1% inguinal. Blood-borne metastases at autopsy are to the brain (85%), adrenals (45%), liver (45%), and bone (35%). The bones most frequently involved are the vertebrae (20%), ribs (10%), pelvis (5%), and skull (less than 1%). Metastases are commonly widespread; the pancreas, heart, pericardium, thyroid, spleen, and bowel are often involved.

Nonmetastatic extrathoracic manifestations related to lung cancer include the following: (1) Connective tissue syndromes: dermatomyositis, scleroderma, hypertrophic pulmonary osteoarthropathy. (2) Neuromyopathies: cerebellar degeneration, encephalomyelopathy, polyneuropathy, and myopathy. (3) Endocrine effects and associated metabolic disorders:

hyperadrenocorticism (oat cell), inappropriate anti-diuretic hormone secretion (oat cell), hypercalcemia (with or without skeletal metastases), gynecomastia, hypoglycemia, excessive gonadotropin secretion, and carcinoid syndrome (weight loss, anorexia, explosive diarrhea, cutaneous flushing, and tachycardia) second-ary to excessive secretion of 5-hydroxytryptamine. (4) Vascular and hematologic manifestations: migra-tory thrombophlebitis, thrombocytopenia, anemias, and chronic consumptive coagulopathies. The prog-nostic importance of these must be individually deter-

mined since some, eg, clubbing or hypertrophic osteo-arthropathy, have no adverse prognostic implications whereas others—particularly hormone-secreting tu-mors—are often associated with oat cell carcinoma and for that reason have a poor prognosis.

B. X-Ray Findings: The roentgenographic mani-festations of lung cancer are quite variable (Fig 21–20). They have been classified as hilar, parenchy-mal, and intrathoracic and extrapulmonary. A hilar abnormality with or without a mass is present in about 40% of cases; a parenchymal mass greater than 4 cm in

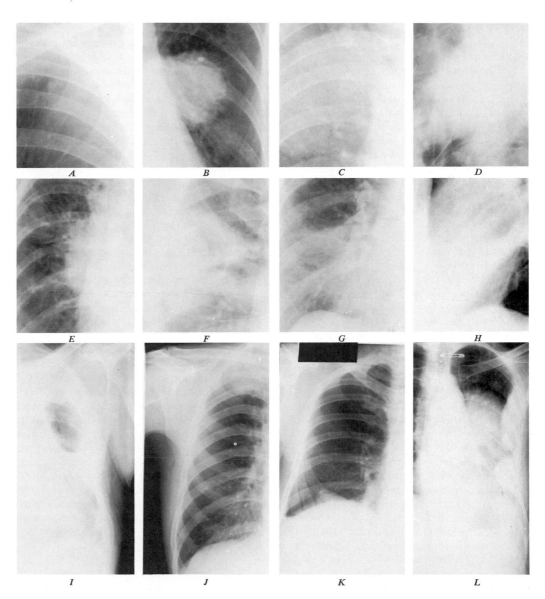

Figure 21—20. X-ray manifestations of lung cancer. *A:* Small epidermoid carcinoma in LUL (posteroanterior projection). *B:* Large coin lesion; adenocarcinoma in superior segment of LLL (lateral projection). *C* and *D:* Epidermoid carcinoma in RUL. *E:* Right hilar mass; oat cell carcinoma. *F:* Large cavitary epidermoid carcinoma in RUL. *G* (posteroanterior projection) and *H* (lateral projection): Middle lobe atelectasis from bronchial carcinoid (not visible). *I:* Opacification of left hemithorax; large cavitary epidermoid carci-noma. *J:* Pancoast's tumor; poorly differentiated epidermoid carcinoma with erosion of third rib and pathologic fracture of fourth rib. *K:* Right phrenic nerve paralysis caused by epidermoid carcinoma. *L:* Pleural metastasis caused by adenocarcinoma of LLL. (LUL = left upper lobe; LLL = left lower lobe; etc.)

diameter in 20% and smaller than 4 cm in 20%; and an apical mass in 2.5%. Extrapulmonary intrathoracic manifestations are present in 10%.

Treatment

Evaluation for treatment must be individualized. The objectives are to establish the diagnosis of lung cancer and to assess the curability of the tumor and the general health and suitability of the patient as a surgical candidate. This assessment must be done without undue delay since the only chance for cure is with surgery. It is very important to determine if the extent of tumor will permit possible cure so that unnecessary thoracotomy is avoided.

Unfortunately, two-thirds of patients with lung cancer are incurable when first seen. Evidence of incurability is as follows: (1) Regional lymph node involvement (enlarged supraclavicular, axillary, or abdominal lymph nodes). (2) Malignant pleural effusion diagnosed by cytologic examination. (3) Recurrent laryngeal nerve paralysis. (4) Phrenic nerve paralysis. (5) High paratracheal, contralateral hilar extension, or lymph node involvement. (6) Any distant metastasis synchronous with the appearance of the primary (most commonly the brain, adrenals, liver, and skeleton). (7) Superior vena cava syndrome. (8) Involvement of the main pulmonary artery.

The prognosis is less favorable if the lesion is bronchoscopically visible; if the chest wall is involved by direct extension; if Pancoast's tumor (superior sulcus tumor) is present; if cytologic examination of the sputum has established the presence of oat cell tumor; or if a biopsy diagnosis has been made. Some consider oat cell carcinoma to be incurable, and it is true that 90% of patients will be incurable by the above criteria when properly evaluated. However, in those patients who undergo resection for cure, the overall 5-year survival rate is 10%. Patients with peritracheal node involvement, carinal involvement in adenocarcinoma, or undifferentiated tumor are very unlikely to be curable.

The medical condition of the patient may contraindicate surgery, but the assessment must be based on general health status, not on chronologic age.

Despite careful preoperative assessment, 5–10% of patients who undergo thoracotomy are found to be incurable. It is essential that low-risk diagnostic procedures such as bronchoscopy, laryngoscopy, scalene or mediastinal lymph node biopsy, and examination of pleural fluid for malignant cells be used liberally to minimize unnecessary thoracotomy since the operative mortality rate in such patients is 2–3 times higher than in patients who undergo curative resection.

At operation the surgeon may be unable to proceed safely with a chance for cure because of parietal pleural seeding, vena caval involvement, vertebral body extension, contralateral or high peritracheal lymph node involvement, aortic arch involvement, or hepatic metastases palpable through the diaphragm, and in some cases the need is clearly for pneumonectomy in a patient who will tolerate only a lobectomy.

A. General Measures: There is no curative medical therapy for lung cancer. Medical treatment should be limited to preoperative preparation of the patient for surgery and must include assessment and measures to improve pulmonary function, heart failure, nutrition, and metabolic or acid-base disturbances.

B. Radiotherapy: Radiotherapy in lung cancer is used for palliation, as adjuvant therapy in combination with surgery, or occasionally for cure. Palliation of symptoms is the most frequent use of radiotherapy; it may be used for pain, for symptoms due to metastases to bone or brain, or for relief of obstruction of the airway or of the superior vena cava. Radiotherapy when used as an adjuvant to surgery may be given either pre- or postoperatively. Preoperative radiotherapy has not been proved to be of value except possibly preceding resection of Pancoast tumors. Preoperative therapy (exceeding 3000 rads) has been implicated in bronchial stump complications when the operative area is treated directly. Postoperative radiotherapy may be of benefit for patients who have mediastinal involvement or Pancoast tumors. Radiotherapy is curative of lung cancer in only 1–2% of cases, and these occur most often in undifferentiated tumors. Oat cell carcinoma has a grim outlook with any form of therapy, but surgery is preferable if patients are selected for operation by the criteria outlined above.

C. Surgical Treatment: If there is no evidence of incurability, the surgical treatment of lung cancer consists of thoracotomy and resection of the involved lung with regional lymph nodes or contiguous structures. Lobectomy is the procedure of choice in good-risk patients with localized disease. Pneumonectomy or bilobectomy (eg, right upper and middle lobes or right lower and middle lobes) is used when the tumor is situated at a fissure or in such a way as to require wide excision. Wedge resection or segmentectomy is used for localized disease in poor-risk patients, for low-grade malignancy, and when conservative surgery is indicated because the tumor is probably metastatic.

Bronchoplastic procedures such as sleeve resection are used to conserve lung tissue, eg, in the resection of a tumor involving the take-off of the upper lobe bronchus when pulmonary function is limited or the tumor is of low-grade malignancy (eg, carcinoid).

Extended resections are sometimes indicated in special situations. In-continuity resection of a lobe or lung with the chest wall, intrapericardial resection, extrapleural dissection, and, rarely, other procedures are sometimes warranted if the tumor is well differentiated.

Prognosis

Improvements in patient evaluation, anesthesia, and postoperative care in the past decade have made most reported operative morbidity and mortality statistics obsolete. Intensive care facilities with trained personnel, monitoring equipment, ventilatory support, blood gas analysis, and around-the-clock laboratory and radiologic facilities have greatly improved results. These advances, together with better selection of curable patients, permit many centers to report 5% or less operative mortality rates following major pulmonary resections in patients 40–60 years of age. In young good-risk patients or when thoracotomy is done for diagnostic purposes or for benign disease, the mortality rate should approach zero.

Five-year survival is about 35% following lobectomy and 20% after pneumonectomy. These rates are determined largely by the histologic type of tumor and operative or pathologic evidence of extension or invasiveness. The age of the patient, the anatomic location of the tumor, tumor doubling time, and the presence or absence of symptoms also have a bearing on the outcome. The prognosis is poor in children, young adults, and women, but adenocarcinoma and undifferentiated tumors predominate in these patients. Histologic evidence of lymph node involvement and blood vessel invasion adversely affect the prognosis.

It must be emphasized that overall curability of lung cancer is less than postoperative 5-year survival since two-thirds of all patients with lung cancer are not candidates for surgical treatment. Overall survival is only about one-fourth to one-third of the cure rate of surgically treated patients.

The natural history of lung cancer varies with the histologic type, the age of the patient, the location of the tumor, and other factors. Without surgery, 95% of patients with primary lung cancer are dead in 2 years. The average reported delay between the first visit to a physician and the operation is 4–6 months.

Arrigoni MG & others: Benign tumors of the lung: A ten-year experience. J Thorac Cardiovasc Surg 60:589, 1970.

Dowell AR: Primary pulmonary leiomyosarcoma: Report of 2 cases and review of the literature. Ann Thorac Surg 17:384, 1974.

Hersh EM, Mavligit GM, Gutterman JU: Immunotherapy as related to lung cancer: A review. Semin Oncol 1:273, 1974.

Hilaris BS & others: Interstitial irradiation for unresectable carcinoma of the lung. Ann Thorac Surg 20:491, 1975.

Hodgkin JE: Evaluation before thoracotomy. West J Med 122:104, 1975.

James EC & others: Preferred surgical treatment for alveolar cell carcinoma. Ann Thorac Surg 22:157, 1976.

Jensik RJ & others: Bronchoplastic and conservative resectional procedures for bronchial adenoma. J Thorac Cardiovasc Surg 68:556, 1974.

Katsuki H & others: Long-term intermittent adjuvant chemotherapy for primary, resected lung cancer. J Thorac Cardiovasc Surg 70:590, 1975.

Kennedy JH: Extrapulmonary effects of cancer of the lung and pleura: Endocrine, muscular, cutaneous, hematologic and cardiovascular manifestations not due to metastases. J Thorac Cardiovasc Surg 61:514, 1971.

Kirsh MM & others: Carcinoma of the lung: Results of treatment over ten years. Ann Thorac Surg 21:371, 1976.

Kirsh MM & others: Complications of pulmonary resection. Ann Thorac Surg 20:215, 1975.

Kirsh MM & others: Major pulmonary resection for bronchogenic carcinoma in the elderly. Ann Thorac Surg 22:369, 1976.

Martini N, Melamed MR: Multiple primary lung cancers. J Thorac Cardiovasc Surg 70:606, 1975.

Meyer JA: The concept and significance of growth rates in human pulmonary tumors. Ann Thorac Surg 14:309, 1972.

Miller RE, Hopeman AR: Bronchial adenoma. Ann Thorac Surg 19:378, 1975.

Mountain CF: Surgical therapy in lung cancer: Biologic, physiologic, and technical determinants. Semin Oncol 3:253, 1974.

Okike N, Bernatz PE, Woolner LB: Carcinoid tumors of the lung. Ann Thorac Surg 22:270, 1976.

Overholt RH, Neptune WB, Ashraf MM: Primary cancer of the lung. Ann Thorac Surg 20:511, 1975.

Paulson DL: Carcinomas in the superior pulmonary sulcus. J Thorac Cardiovasc Surg 70:1095, 1975.

Primack A: The production of markers by bronchogenic carcinoma: A review. Semin Oncol 1:236, 1974.

Rassam JW, Anderson G: Incidence of paramalignant disorders in bronchogenic carcinoma. Thorax 30:86, 1975.

Shields TW & others: Relationship of cell type and lymph node metastasis to survival after resection of bronchial carcinoma. Ann Thorac Surg 20:501, 1975.

Stanford W & others: Results of treatment of primary carcinoma of the lung: Analysis of 3,000 cases. J Thorac Cardiovasc Surg 72:441, 1976.

Vincent RG & others: Surgical therapy of lung cancer. J Thorac Cardiovasc Surg 71:581, 1976.

Weiss W: Operative mortality and five-year survival rates in men with bronchogenic carcinoma. Chest 66:483, 1974.

Woolner LB & others: In situ and early invasive bronchogenic carcinoma. J Thorac Cardiovasc Surg 60:275, 1970.

Yashar J, Yashar JJ: Factors affecting long-term survival of patients with bronchogenic carcinoma. Am J Surg 129:386, 1975.

SECONDARY MALIGNANT NEOPLASMS OF THE LUNG

Lung metastases occur in about 30% of all patients with malignancy. Depending upon the primary lesion, the number of metastases may be limited, and a few of these patients may be surgically curable. The most frequent sources of solitary metastatic lesions are the colon, kidneys, uterus and ovaries, testes, malignant melanoma, pharynx, and bone. In coin lesions, solitary metastasis is the ultimate diagnosis in about 5%. Ten percent of malignant coin lesions are solitary metastases, and in 90% of these cases a history of the primary is available.

Certain criteria for selection of patients suitable for resection have been developed: (1) The initial primary must be controlled, and no other metastases can be present. (2) When the initial primary was a squamous cell tumor, the lung lesion should be evaluated as a new primary. (3) When the initial lesion was an adenocarcinoma, other common sites of metastasis must be sought. (4) A waiting period of 3–6 months is advisable before thoracotomy if the primary lesion was treated within 2 years. (5) Total lung tomograms or stereoscopic views of the lung must be obtained to rule out additional metastases. (6) Synchronous appearance of a pulmonary metastasis and the primary lesion must be evaluated individually, but in general the prognosis improves as the interval between control of the primary and the appearance of the lung metastasis increases. (7) Multiple lesions, particularly when bilateral or involving different lobes, usually mean that the prognosis is poor. Recently, however, multiple resections for metastases from osteogenic sarcoma have been shown to be worthwhile.

About 80% of solitary metastases meeting the above criteria are found to be resectable. Eighty percent are carcinomas and 20% sarcomas. The 5-year survival rate following removal of the carcinomas is 35%; for the sarcomas, 25%. Only a few 5-year survivals following removal of lung cancers metastatic from malignant melanoma or the breasts have been reported.

Cahan WG, Castro EB: Significance of a solitary lung shadow in patients with breast cancer. Ann Surg 181:137, 1975.

Magilligan DJ Jr & others: Pulmonary neoplasm with solitary cerebral metastasis: Results of combined excision. J Thorac Cardiovasc Surg 72:690, 1976.

Martini N & others: Multiple pulmonary resections in the treatment of osteogenic sarcoma. Ann Thorac Surg 12:271, 1971.

Morton DL & others: Surgical resection and adjunctive immunotherapy for selected patients with multiple pulmonary metastases. Ann Surg 178:360, 1973.

Turney SZ, Haight C: Pulmonary resection for metastatic neoplasms. J Thorac Cardiovasc Surg 61:784, 1971.

THE MEDIASTINUM

The mediastinum is a complex part of the thorax that may become involved in a wide variety of primary and secondary pathologic processes. Anatomically, the mediastinum is the central compartment between the pleural cavities. It extends anteriorly from the suprasternal notch to the xiphoid process and posteriorly from the first to the eleventh thoracic vertebrae. Superiorly, fascial planes in the neck are in direct communication; inferiorly, the mediastinum is limited by the diaphragm, although extensions through diaphragmatic apertures communicate with retroperitoneal fascial planes.

Many mediastinal clinical lesions are asymptomatic and are discovered by chest x-ray. It becomes of clinical interest to topographically catalogue cysts, tumors, and other radiologic findings.

In Burkell's classification (Fig 21–21), the **anterior mediastinum** contains the thymus gland, lymph nodes, ascending and transverse aorta, the great vessels, and areolar tissue. The **middle mediastinum** contains the heart, pericardium, trachea, hili of lungs, phrenic nerves, lymph nodes, and areolar tissue. The **posterior mediastinum** contains sympathetic chains, vagus nerves, esophagus, thoracic duct, lymph nodes, and descending aorta.

Congenital abnormalities within the mediastinum are numerous. A defect in the anterior mediastinal pleura with communication of the right and left hemi-

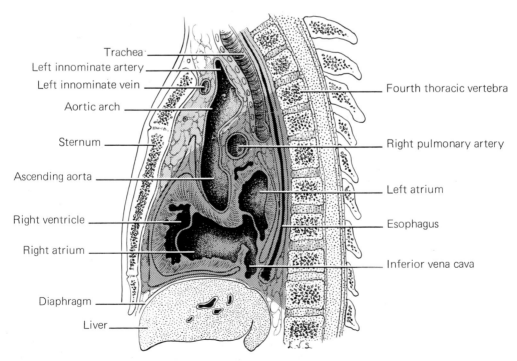

Figure 21–21. Divisions of the mediastinum (Burkell's classification). Upper mediastinum; light screening: anterior mediastinum; lower dark screening: middle mediastinum; dotted area at right: posterior mediastinum.

thorax is rare in humans. This retrosternal part of the anterior mediastinum is normally thin, and overexpansion of one pleural space may cause "mediastinal herniation" or a bulge of mediastinal pleura toward the opposite side.

Displacements of the mediastinum occur from masses, accumulations of air, fluid, blood, chyle, etc and can interfere with vital functions. Tracheal compression, vena caval obstruction, and esophageal obstruction cause clinical symptoms. The mediastinum can also be displaced laterally when pathologic processes of one hemithorax cause mediastinal shift. Fibrosis and previous pneumonectomy can shift the mediastinum toward the affected side. Open pneumothorax and massive hemothorax shift the mediastinum away from the affected side. Open pneumothorax produces alternating paradoxical mediastinal shifts with respiration and will adversely affect ventilation. Acute mediastinal displacement may produce hypoxia or reduce venous return and cause low cardiac output, tachycardia, arrhythmias, or hypotension.

MEDIASTINITIS

Mediastinal infections may be acute or chronic. There are 4 sources of mediastinal infection: direct contamination; hematogenous or lymphatic; extension of infection from the neck or retroperitoneum; and extension from the lung or pleura. The most common direct contamination is esophageal perforation. Acute mediastinitis may follow esophageal, cardiac, and other mediastinal operations. Rarely, the mediastinum is directly infected by suppurative conditions involving the ribs or vertebrae. Most direct mediastinal infections are caused by pyogenic organisms. Most mediastinal infections that invade via the hematogenous and lymphatic routes are granulomas. Contiguous involvement of the mediastinum along fascial planes from cervical infection is relatively frequent; this occurs less commonly from the retroperitoneum. Empyema often loculates to form a paramediastinal abscess, but extension to form a true mediastinal abscess is uncommon. Extension of mediastinal infections to involve the pleura is common.

1. ACUTE MEDIASTINITIS

Esophageal perforation, the source of 90% of acute mediastinal infections, can be caused by vomiting (Boerhaave's syndrome), iatrogenic trauma (endoscopy, dilatation, operation), external trauma (penetrating or blunt), cuffed tracheal tubes, ingestion of corrosives, carcinoma, or other esophageal disease. Mediastinal infection secondary to cervical disease may follow oral surgery, cellulitis, external trauma involving the pharynx, esophagus, or trachea, and cervical operative procedures such as tracheostomy.

Clinical Findings

Acute mediastinitis usually occurs after a known predisposing cause. Emetogenic esophageal perforation is usually associated with a history of vomiting but in some cases is insidious in onset. Severe, boring pain located in the substernal, left or right chest, or epigastric regions is the chief complaint in over 90% of cases. One-third have radiation to the back, and in some cases pain in the back may predominate. Low thoracic mediastinitis can sometimes be confused with acute abdominal diseases. Acute mediastinitis may be ushered in by chills, fever, or shock. If pleurisy develops, breathing may aggravate the pain or give shoulder radiation. Swallowing increases the pain, and dysphagia may be present. The patient is febrile and sweaty and the pulse may be thready. About 60% have subcutaneous emphysema or pneumomediastinum. A pericardial crunching sound with systole (Hamman's sign) is often a late sign. Fifty percent of patients with esophageal perforation have pleural effusion or hydropneumothorax. Neck tenderness and crepitation are more often found in cervical perforations.

The diagnosis may be confirmed by contrast x-ray examination of the esophagus, preferably using water-soluble media, or by endoscopic visualization of the perforation. Myocardial infarction is sometimes mistakenly diagnosed in patients with esophageal perforation when a predisposing cause or pneumomediastinum is not apparent.

Complications

Complications include pericarditis and shock. Following operative closure of esophageal perforation leaks, empyema, abscess, and fistula may occur.

Prevention

Esophageal perforation occurs significantly less often with fiberoptic endoscopy than when a rigid endoscope is used. When possible, anastomosis of the esophagus in the cervical region is safer than anastomosis within the thorax.

Treatment

Patients in shock are resuscitated, broad-spectrum antibiotics are given, and a nasogastric tube passed. In emetogenic esophageal perforations, there is a vertical tear located posteriorly just proximal to the esophagogastric junction. These patients require thoracotomy because gastric or esophageal contents are extravasated into the mediastinum. Instrumental perforation of the cervical or thoracic esophagus requires wide drainage and closure of the perforation if the esophagus is not too friable. The mediastinum is drained via the pleural cavity using large-bore catheters. Postoperatively, nutritional needs must be provided by either intravenous alimentation or feeding via nasogastric, gastrostomy, or jejunostomy tube. Gastrostomy may help to minimize reflux into the esophagus.

Prognosis

Following operative treatment for perforations of the esophagus, complications occur in about 40% of cases. The frequency of leaks may be reduced by buttressing the esophageal suture line. The mortality rate is about 10% in instrumental, 20% in emetogenic, 35% in postoperative, and 75–80% in corrosive perforation. Prompt drainage and repair are the most important factors in determining outcome. The mortality rate after cervical perforations is less than after endothoracic perforation.

Hardy JD & others: Esophageal perforations and fistulas: Review of 36 cases with operative closure of four chronic fistulas. Ann Surg 177:788, 1973.

Mansour KA, Teaford H: Atraumatic rupture of the esophagus into the pericardium simulating acute myocardial infarction. J Thorac Cardiovasc Surg 65:458, 1973.

Rea WJ & others: Traumatic esophageal perforation. Ann Thorac Surg 14:671, 1972.

Rosoff L, White EJ: Perforation of the esophagus. Am J Surg 128:207, 1974.

Tesler MA, Eisenberg MM: Spontaneous esophageal rupture: Collective review. Internat Abstr Surg 117:1, 1973.

2. CHRONIC MEDIASTINITIS

Chronic mediastinitis usually involves specific granulomatous processes, with mediastinal fibrosis and cold abscesses of the mediastinum. Histoplasmosis, tuberculosis, actinomyces, nocardia, blastomyces, and syphilis have been incriminated. Amebic abscesses and parasitic disease such as echinococcal cysts are rare causes. Usually, the infectious process is due to histoplasmosis or tuberculosis and involves the mediastinal lymph nodes. Adjacent mediastinal structures becomes secondarily involved. It is thought that granulomatous mediastinitis and fibrosing mediastinitis are different manifestations of the same disease. Mediastinal fibrosis is a term used synonymously with idiopathic, fibrous, collagenous, or sclerosing mediastinitis. Eighty or more cases of mediastinal fibrosis have been reported, but the cause has been determined in only 16%, and of these over 90% were due to histoplasmosis. In only 25% of 103 cases of granulomatous mediastinitis has the cause been identified. Histoplasmosis was the most common known cause (60%) and tuberculosis the second most common (25%).

About 85% of patients with mediastinal fibrosis have symptoms from entrapment of mediastinal structures as follows: superior vena caval obstruction in 82%; tracheobronchial obstruction, 9%; pulmonary vein obstruction, 6%; pulmonary artery occlusion, 6%; and esophageal obstruction, 3%. Rarely, inferior vena caval obstruction or involvement of the thoracic duct, atrium, recurrent laryngeal nerve, or stellate ganglion is found. Multiple structures may be simultaneously involved.

Seventy-five percent of patients with granulomatous mediastinitis have no symptoms and are discovered by chest x-ray, which shows a mediastinal mass. The mass is in the right paratracheal region in 75% of cases. In the 25% of patients with symptoms, about half have superior vena cava obstruction and a third have esophageal obstruction. Occasional patients have bronchial obstruction, bronchoesophageal fistula, or pulmonary venous obstruction.

A mediastinal tubercular or fungal (especially actinomyces) abscess occasionally dissects long distances to present on the chest wall paravertebrally or parasternally. Secondary rib or costal cartilage infections with multiple draining sinus tracts occur.

Clinical Findings

A. Symptoms and Signs: Granulomatous and fibrosing mediastinitis involves both sexes equally, and the average age is 35–40 years. A discussion of the clinical manifestations of mediastinal masses and superior vena cava obstruction will follow later in this chapter. Patients with esophageal involvement have dysphagia or hematemesis. Tracheobronchial involvement may cause severe cough, hemoptysis, dyspnea, wheezing, and episodes of obstructive pneumonitis. Pulmonary vein obstruction, the most serious manifestation, produces congestive heart failure resembling advanced mitral stenosis. It is usually fatal. Although not diagnostic, in cases due to histoplasmosis or tuberculosis the respective skin tests are strongly positive.

B. X-Ray Findings: In granulomatous mediastinitis, there is often a right paratracheal or anterior mediastinal mass. There may be spotty or subcapsular calcification. Calcification also can occur in thymoma or teratoma located in this region.

Treatment

Specific medical treatment may be indicated. In general, depending on the cause, mediastinal masses should be resected. Superior vena caval obstruction will be discussed in the section that follows. Treatment of obstructive pneumonitis is specific antibiotics. Definitive surgical treatment may occasionally be indicated when bronchiectasis, bronchostenosis, abscess, or intractable pneumonia occurs.

Prognosis

The prognosis following surgical excision of granulomatous mediastinal masses is good. Operative procedures do not appear to activate fibrosing mediastinitis, but success in treatment has been unpredictable. Most patients with fibrosing mediastinitis, whether treated or not, survive but have persistent symptoms.

Ferguson TB, Burford TH: Mediastinal granuloma: A 15-year experience. Ann Thorac Surg 1:125, 1965.

Garcia JM & others: Technique for reconstruction of superior vena cava in fibrosing mediastinitis. J Thorac Cardiovasc Surg 65:547, 1973.

Goodwin RA, Nickell JA, DesPrez RM: Mediastinal fibrosis complicating healed primary histoplasmosis and tuberculosis. Medicine 51:227, 1972.

Gopalrao T & others: Surgical treatment of obstruction of the superior vena cava and right pulmonary artery. J Thorac Cardiovasc Surg 63:394, 1972.

Miller RE, Sullivan FJ: Superior vena caval obstruction secondary to fibrosing mediastinitis. Ann Thorac Surg 15:483, 1973.

Payne WS, Cardoza F, Weed LA: Chronic draining sinuses of the chest wall. Surg Clin North Am 53:927, 1973.

Schowengerdt CG, Suyemoto R, Main FB: Granulomatous and fibrous mediastinitis: A review and analysis of 180 cases. J Thorac Cardiovasc Surg 57:365, 1969.

SUPERIOR VENA CAVAL SYNDROME

Superior vena caval obstruction produces a distinctive clinical syndrome. Malignant tumors are the cause in 80–90% of cases; lung cancer accounts for about 90%, and most of these are lesions of the right upper lobe. The incidence of superior vena caval syndrome in lung cancer patients is 3–5%. The male/female ratio is about 5:1. Other primary mediastinal tumors that may cause superior vena caval obstruction include thymoma, Hodgkin's disease, and lymphosarcoma. Metastatic tumors from the breast, thyroid, or melanoma may also occasionally cause superior venal caval obstruction. Benign tumors are unusual, but substernal goiter, any large benign mediastinal masses, and atrial myxoma have been implicated. Thrombotic conditions, either idiopathic or associated with polycythemia, mediastinal infection, or indwelling catheters, are unusual causes. The association of superior vena caval obstruction with chronic mediastinitis is discussed in the preceding section. Trauma may produce acute venous obstruction (eg, traumatic asphyxia, mediastinal hematoma).

The clinical manifestations depend on the abruptness of onset, location of obstruction, completeness of occlusion, and availability of collateral pathways. Venous pressure measured in the arms or head varies from 200–500 mm water, and severity of symptoms is correlated with the pressure. Fatal cerebral edema can occur within minutes of an acute complete obstruction, whereas a slowly evolving one permits development of collaterals and may be only mildly symptomatic. Symptoms are milder when the azygous vein is patent. Azygous blood flow, normally about 11% of the total venous return, can increase to 35% of the venous return from the head, neck, and upper extremities. Thus, the most severe cases occur when occlusion is complete and the azygous vein is involved. The thrombus may propagate proximally to occlude the innominate and axillary veins.

Clinical Findings

Symptoms include puffiness of the face, arms, and shoulders and a blue or purple discoloration of the skin. CNS symptoms include headache, nausea, dizziness, vomiting, distortion of vision, drowsiness, stupor, and convulsions. Respiratory symptoms include cough,

hoarseness, and dyspnea, often due to edema of the vocal cords or trachea. These symptoms are made worse by lying flat or bending over. In long-standing cases, esophageal varices may develop and produce gastrointestinal bleeding. The veins of the neck and upper extremities are visibly distended, and in long-standing cases there are marked collateral venous channels over the anterior chest and abdomen. Onset of symptoms in fibrosing mediastinitis may be insidious, consisting initially of early morning edema of the face and hands. Occasionally, symptoms and findings are localized to one side when the level of obstruction is above the cava and only one innominate vein is blocked. In this situation, symptoms are mild because communicating veins in the neck usually decompress the affected side.

The diagnosis is confirmed by measuring upper extremity venous pressure; in patients with severe symptoms, a pressure of 350 mm water or more is usual. The location and extent of the obstruction is best determined by venography. When patients with malignant vena caval obstruction are studied by venography, 35% have thrombosis involving the innominate or axillary veins, 15% complete caval obstruction without thrombosis, and 50% partial superior vena caval obstruction. In cases where patency of the azygous vein is in question, interosseus azygography may be useful. Chest x-ray may show a right upper lobe lung lesion or right paratracheal mass. Aortography may occasionally be required to exclude aortic aneurysm. The methods for diagnosis of bronchogenic carcinoma are discussed elsewhere. The differential diagnosis may include angioneurotic edema, congestive heart failure, and constrictive pericarditis. Effort thrombosis of the axillary vein and innominate vein obstruction from elongation and buckling of the innominate artery can be considered in unilateral cases.

Complications

In patients with partial superior vena caval obstruction, thrombosis may suddenly change mild symptoms to marked venous distention, cyanotic swelling, vocal cord edema, and impaired cerebration. Bleeding from esophageal varices is rare except in severe long-standing cases.

Treatment

Superior vena caval obstruction caused by malignancy should be treated with diuretics, fluid restriction, and prompt radiation therapy. Because of the possibility of thrombosis in malignant cases, anticoagulants or fibrinolytic agents have been suggested. Chemotherapy is sometimes used alone or with radiotherapy. Most cases of malignant superior vena caval obstruction are not remediable by operation.

In benign incomplete superior vena caval obstruction, surgical excision of the compressing mass can provide an excellent result. In total obstruction, such as occurs in fibrosing mediastinitis, most patients will gradually improve without treatment. There are numerous surgical procedures designed to bypass caval obstruction, replace the superior vena cava, or recanalize the vena caval lumen. The results following these procedures have been dramatically effective in some cases, but only recently have these procedures been of sufficient success to warrant consideration.

Prognosis

Radiotherapy is most effective when superior vena caval obstruction is incomplete. Mean survival of patients with malignant caval obstruction from lung cancer is 6–8 months. The mortality rate from causes related to vena caval obstruction itself is only 1–2%.

Barrett NR: Idiopathic mediastinal fibrosis. Br J Surg 46:207, 1958.

Boruchow IB, Johnson J: Obstruction of the vena cava: Collective review. Surg Gynecol Obstet 134:115, 1971.

Gomes MN, Hufnagel CA: Superior vena cava obstruction: A review of the literature and report of 2 cases due to benign intrathoracic tumors. Ann Thorac Surg 20:344, 1975.

Miller DB: Palliative surgery for benign superior vena caval syndrome. Am J Surg 129:361, 1975.

Salsali M, Clifton EE: Superior vena caval obstruction with lung cancer. Ann Thorac Surg 6:437, 1968.

Scherck JP, Kerstein MD, Stansel HC Jr: The current status of vena caval replacement. Surgery 76:209, 1974.

Taylor GA & others: Bypassing the obstructed superior vena cava with a subcutaneous long saphenous vein graft. J Thorac Cardiovasc Surg 68:237, 1974.

TRAUMATIC ASPHYXIA

Traumatic asphyxia or "ecchymotic mask" is a condition of sudden superior vena caval obstruction produced by sustained thoracic compression such as when the victim is pinned beneath an automobile, machinery, or lumber. This injury is produced by acute venous hypertension from mechanical obstruction of the superior vena cava. A deep violaceous discoloration of the face and neck occurs which is sharply demarcated on the upper chest. There may be striking conjunctival congestion, punctate cutaneous ecchymotic areas, or evidence of CNS involvement. Restlessness, confusion, irritability, or convulsions may occur. In severe cases, there may be unconsciousness or paraplegia. Associated injuries are fractures of ribs or vertebrae, pulmonary contusion, and hemopneumothorax. Treatment is supportive, with the focus primarily on the associated injuries. Most cases improve if they survive the original injury, although the mortality rate at the time of injury is high.

Moore JD, Meyer JH, Gaxo O: Traumatic asphyxia. Chest 62:634, 1972.

MEDIASTINAL MASS LESIONS

Mediastinal masses may be of congenital, traumatic, infectious, degenerative, or neoplastic origin. Thyroid goiters occasionally can be at least partially substernal; skeletal tumors may grow into the mediastinum; or diaphragmatic lesions may involve the mediastinum.

An extensive work-up of a mediastinal lesion is usually not required for diagnosis. Surgery is usually required to establish the diagnosis and provide effective treatment. Numerous preoperative studies may delay effective treatment and may not be especially valuable since an operation is virtually inevitable. A standard posteroanterior and lateral chest film will often provide all the information required. However, special technics are useful in some cases.

Oblique or overpenetrated x-rays are sometimes helpful. Fluoroscopy may show pulsation or variation of shape or location with change of position and respiration. Tomography may reveal calcification or airfluid levels. Barium swallow is used to evaluate intrinsic esophageal lesions or esophageal displacement by extrinsic masses. Contrast studies of the intestinal tract may reveal the stomach, colon, or small bowel in a hernia. Myelography can be of crucial importance in neurogenic tumors to explain symptoms or plan operative management. Bronchography may be useful to differentiate lung tumors mimicking a mediastinal mass.

Venography is used to evaluate distortion, obstruction, or collateral channels. Angiocardiography and aortography help identify aneurysms or displacement. Pulmonary arteriography may be useful to distinguish mediastinal and pulmonary tumors. Interosseus azygography may be useful in evaluation of vena caval obstruction.

Bronchoscopy and esophagoscopy are occasionally useful to identify primary lung lesions or lesions of the esophagus. Mediastinoscopy and mediastinal biopsy must be used cautiously in mediastinal tumors that are potentially curable. Excisional biopsy is preferable in lesions such as thymoma that are histologically difficult to evaluate since a curable malignancy might be seeded. Mediastinoscopy is useful in sarcoidosis or disseminated lymphoma.

Scintiscan is an important method of evaluating possible substernal goiter in anterior mediastinal lesions, since goiters can almost always be removed by a cervical approach. Skin tests and serologic studies may be used in suspected granuloma. Bone marrow, hormone assays, etc are occasionally indicated.

When substernal goiter is excluded, neurogenic tumors constitute 26%, cysts 21%, teratodermoids 16%, thymomas 12%, lymphoma 12%, and all other lesions 12% of mediastinal masses. About 25% are malignant. In children, the incidence of malignancy is about the same, but teratodermoids and vascular tumors are more common.

The distribution of mediastinal tumors is as shown in Table 21–5.

Table 21—5. Distribution of tumors and other mass lesions in the mediastinum.

All parts of mediastinum
Lymph node lesions
Bronchogenic cysts

Middle mediastinum	
Teratoma	
Thymoma	
Parathyroid adenoma	
Aneurysms	**Posterior mediastinum**
Lipoma	Neurogenic tumors
Myxoma	Pheochromocytoma
Goiter	Aneurysms
	Enterogenous cysts
	Spinal lesions
Anterior mediastinum	Hiatus hernia
Teratoma	
Lymphangiomas	
Angiomas	
Pericardial cysts	
Esophageal lesions	

Clinical Findings

Symptoms are much more frequent in malignant than benign lesions. About one-third of patients have no symptoms. Fifty percent of patients have respiratory symptoms such as cough, wheezing, dyspnea, and recurrent pneumonias. Hemoptysis and, rarely, expectoration of cyst contents may occur. Chest pain, weight loss, and dysphagia are found with equal frequency, each in about 10% of patients. Myasthenia, fever, and superior vena caval obstruction are each found in about 5% of patients.

Some symptoms suggest malignancy and thus have a poorer prognosis: hoarseness, Horner's syndrome, severe pain, and superior vena caval obstruction. Malignant tumors may produce chylothorax. Fever may be intermittant in Hodgkin's disease. Thymoma produces myasthenia, hypogammaglobulinemia, Whipple's disease, red blood cell aplasia, and Cushing's disease. Hypoglycemia is a rare complication of mesotheliomas, teratomas, and fibromas. Hypertension and diarrhea occur with pheochromocytoma and ganglioneuroma. Neurogenic tumors may produce specific neurologic findings from cord pressure or may be associated with hypertrophic osteoarthropathy and peptic ulcer disease.

A. Neurogenic Tumors: Neurogenic tumors almost always occur in the posterior mediastinum, often the upper part arising from intercostal or sympathetic nerves. Rarely, the vagus or phrenic nerve can be involved. The most common variety arises from the nerve sheath (schwannoma) and is usually benign. Ten percent of neurogenic tumors are malignant, and malignancy is more frequent in children. Most malignant tumors arise from the nerve cells. Neurogenic tumors may be multiple or dumbbell in type, with widening of the intervertebral foramen. In these cases, myelography is necessary to determine if a portion of the growth is within the spinal canal. If a dumbbell tumor is found, it is best to remove the intraspinal portion first to avoid possible spinal cord injury.

B. Mediastinal Cystic Lesions: Cysts of the mediastinum may arise from the pericardium, bronchi, esophagus, or thymus. Pericardial cysts are also called springwater or mesothelial cysts. Seventy-five percent are located near the cardiophrenic angles; of these, 75% are on the right side. Ten percent are actually diverticula of the pericardial sac which communicate with the pericardial space. Bronchogenic cysts arise close to the main stem bronchus or trachea. A favorite site is just below the carina. Histologically, they contain elements found in bronchi such as cartilage and are lined by respiratory epithelium. Enterogenous cysts are known by several names, including esophageal cyst, enteric cyst, or duplication of the alimentary tract. They arise along the surface of the esophagus and may be embedded within its wall. They may be lined by squamous epithelium similar to the esophagus or gastric mucosa. Enterogenous cysts are occasionally associated with congenital abnormalities of the vertebrae. About 10% of cysts in the mediastinum are nonspecific, without a recognizable lining.

C. Teratodermoid Tumors: Teratodermoid tumors are the most common mass lesion of the anterior mediastinum. They are both solid and cystic and may contain hair or teeth. Microscopically, ectodermal, endodermal, and mesodermal elements are present. Occasionally they rupture into the pleural space, lung, pericardium, or vascular structures.

D. Thymomas: Thymomas are uncommon in childhood, but in adults they are the most common anterior mediastinal mass. Their association with myasthenia gravis is well known, but most patients with myasthenia do not have thymoma. It is now usual procedure to remove the thymus in patients with severe myasthenia whether or not a tumor is present. The benefit from thymectomy seems best in female patients without thymoma whose disease is of short duration. One of the most difficult aspects of thymic tumors is establishing a histologic diagnosis of malignancy. The behavior of the tumor is more reliable than its histology, ie, whether or not invasion of adjacent structures such as pericardium or lung occurs.

E. Lymphomas: Lymphomas are usually associated with disseminated disease metastatic to the mediastinum. Occasionally, lymphosarcoma, Hodgkin's disease, or reticulum cell sarcoma arises as a primary mediastinal lesion. Surgical excision is indicated, although radiation therapy and chemotherapy are also used in treatment.

Treatment

Operation is usually indicated for an undiagnosed mediastinal mass to determine the histologic diagnosis and provide a chance for surgical cure. In malignant lesions, surgery is combined with radiotherapy or chemotherapy as indicated.

Prognosis

The postoperative mortality rate is 1—4% in several reports. Most fatalities are from postoperative respiratory complications in patients with myasthenia gravis. About one-third of patients with malignant mediastinal tumors survive 5 years.

Benjamin SP & others: Primary lymphatic tumors of the mediastinum. Cancer 30:708, 1972.

Gale AW & others: Neurogenic tumors of the mediastinum. Ann Thorac Surg 17:434, 1974.

Grob D: Myasthenia gravis. Ann NY Acad Sci 274:1, 1976.

Medical Staff Conference: Myasthenia gravis and the thymus gland. West J Med 123:123, 1975.

Mulder DG, Herman C, Buckberg GD: Effect of thymectomy in patients with myasthenia gravis. Am J Surg 128:202, 1974.

Rubush JL & others: Mediastinal tumors: Review of 186 cases. J Thorac Cardiovasc Surg 65:216, 1973.

Whittaker LD Jr, Lynn HB: Mediastinal tumors and cysts in the pediatric patient. Surg Clin North Am 53:893, 1973.

Wychulis AR & others: Surgical treatment of mediastinal tumors: A 40-year experience. J Thorac Cardiovasc Surg 62:379, 1971.

●   ●   ●

General References

Baum GL (editor): *Textbook of Pulmonary Diseases,* 2nd ed. Little, Brown, 1974.

Blades B: *Surgical Diseases of the Chest,* 3rd ed. Mosby, 1974.

Borrie J: *Management of Emergencies in Thoracic Surgery,* 2nd ed. Appleton-Century-Crofts, 1972.

D'Abreu AL, Collis JL, Clarke DB: *A Practice of Thoracic Surgery,* 3rd ed. Arnold, 1971.

Felson B: *Chest Roentgenology.* Saunders, 1973.

Fraser RG, Paré JAP: *Diagnosis of Diseases of the Chest.* Saunders, 1970.

Fraser RG, Paré JAP: *Structure and Function of the Lung.* Saunders, 1971.

Glenn WWL, Liebow AE, Lindskog GE: *Thoracic and Cardio-*

vascular Surgery With Related Pathology, 3rd ed. Appleton-Century-Crofts, 1975.

Johnson J & others: *Surgery of the Chest,* 4th ed. Year Book, 1970.

Kubik S: *Surgical Anatomy of the Thorax.* Saunders, 1970.

Leigh TF, Weens HS: *The Mediastinum.* Thomas, 1959.

Sabiston DC Jr, Spencer FC: *Gibbon's Surgery of the Chest,* 3rd ed. Saunders, 1976.

Shields TW: *General Thoracic Surgery.* Lea & Febiger, 1972.

Spencer H: *Pathology of the Lung,* 2nd ed. Pergamon Press, 1968.

Watson WL: *Lung Cancer.* Mosby, 1968.

22...
The Heart:
I. Acquired Diseases

Benson B. Roe, MD, & Daniel J. Ullyot, MD

GENERAL CONSIDERATIONS

During the past decade, the surgeon's role in the management of acquired heart disease has progressed from crude attempts at palliation by removing mechanical obstructions to his present ability to offer definitive therapy of all but the rarest forms of cardiac disease. We can now reasonably expect that even the patient with diffuse coronary artery disease or advanced myocardiopathy will be treated satisfactorily by replacement pumps or improved methods of managing cardiac transplantation. Not only must the cardiac surgeon be able to recognize the subtle nuances of cardiac symptoms and physical signs; he must also be able to detect ECG and radiographic abnormalities which characterize the primary disease and its postoperative complications.

Information obtained under operative conditions is not reliably diagnostic, and surgical success is predicated upon accurate anatomic and physiologic identification of disease before operation. The essential information provided by cardiac catheterization and cineradiography is as crucial to the cardiac surgeon as are the guidance and navigational instruments to the aircraft pilot. The rash surgeon who makes action decisions "by the seat of his pants" is destined to failure.

The selection of patients, choice of operative procedure, reduction of surgical risk, and prognosis for functional improvement are significantly aided by quantitative assessment of obstructive processes, regurgitant flow, ventricular ejection, pulmonary hypertension, and coronary artery patency in addition to the usual pressure and shunt measurements.

These methods of evaluation and long-term postoperative assessment have made it possible to identify operable heart disease before it causes irreversible secondary complications and is beyond surgical treatment. Surgical benefits have been greatly extended while becoming more sharply defined, and the lower operative mortality has lessened the tendency to defer operation.

EXTRACORPOREAL CIRCULATION

There are obvious temporal and technical limitations to operating within the heart while it remains beating or during brief periods of inflow occlusion. Satisfactory substitution technics to support circulation and oxygenation were long sought but slowly achieved. The functions provided by the enormous surface area of the human lung were not easy to reproduce mechanically, and unpredictable pathologic damage often followed the early use of extracorporeal oxygenation.

Several types of pumping mechanisms have been used, but all have now given way to the simple roller pump which damages blood only slightly.

Extracorporeal oxygenation by cross-circulation between parent (donor) and child (patient) was used clinically by Lillehei in a small series of operations in 1953. Experimental attempts were made to utilize an animal lung as an oxygenator, but these technics were abandoned when mechanical oxygenators became available. An important step in this achievement was the recognition by DeWall that tubing and containers made of plastic material were far less damaging to blood elements than were those made of glass.

Three basic methods of oxygenation have been employed clinically, and each has important advantages and disadvantages. Blood-gas exchange can occur (1) on the surface of a **film** of blood, (2) on the surface of gas **bubbles** in a column of blood, or (3) across a thin plastic **membrane** separating alternating thin layers of blood and oxygen. The filming technic is further subdivided into (a) gravity flow down a stainless steel **screen** with a cascade effect which supposedly keeps the surface layer mixed and changed, and (b) repeated reexposure on a series of rotating **disks** which dip into a trough of moving blood. Because the diffusion rate of oxygen through blood is less than 10 μm/second and the thinnest film is about 100 μm thick, the method is inefficient and requires multiple reexposures of the poorly mixed blood. Priming volumes are large and oxygenation is slow, but many consider this method less destructive to blood elements than the bubble technic.

Bubble oxygenation has the advantage of a large cumulative surface area and more efficient gas exchange; thus, priming volumes are smaller and recirculation is not required. However, embolization of residual microbubbles or of the antifoaming agent is a potential hazard. Furthermore, some surgeons contend that blood is damaged by this method, which renders it dangerous for perfusions of more than 1 hour. (Our own satisfactory experience with patients who have

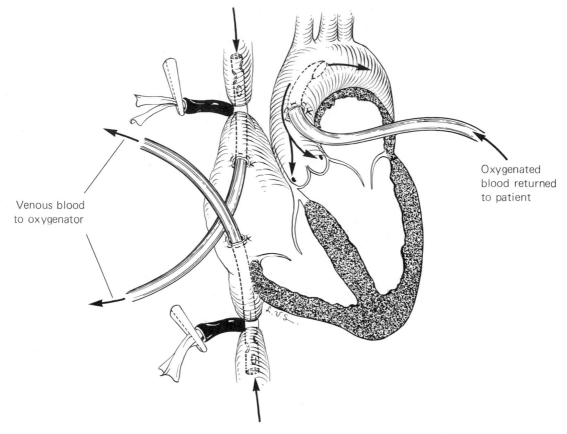

Venous blood
to oxygenator

Oxygenated
blood returned
to patient

Figure 22—1. Cannulation sites commonly used in connecting the extracorporeal circuit. Venous blood is drained through tubes introduced into both vena cavas. Oxygenated blood is returned to the arterial system through a tube in the aorta.

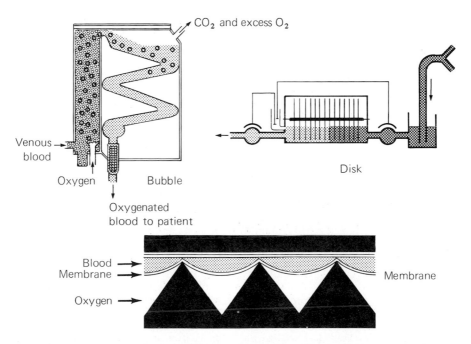

CO_2 and excess O_2

Venous
blood

Oxygen   Bubble

Oxygenated
blood to patient

Disk

Blood →
Membrane →   Membrane

Oxygen →

Figure 22—2. Three clinically employed types of oxygenation: bubble, disk, and membrane.

sustained few or no complications after 4 or 5 hours of bubble oxygenation does not support this belief.) The availability of relatively inexpensive disposable bubble oxygenators has added to the popularity of this method. Generous heparinization (3500 units/kg plus a constant heparin infusion at a rate of half the initial dose per hour of bypass), high flow rates (2–2.5 liters/sq m), and hemodilution (priming the oxygenator with acellular physiologic solutions) have contributed to the reduction of complications. While technical variations in extracorporeal circulation still cover a wide spectrum, the fundamentals are now well established and complications are rare.

Membrane oxygenators have the theoretical advantage of minimizing damage to blood elements and are expected to be the eventual method of choice. Until recently they have been cumbersome, expensive, and resistant to flow and have required a large priming volume. Thus, their use has been principally for long-term perfusion in treating pulmonary insufficiency.

No method of extracorporeal circulation is without its complications. Hemorrhagic consolidation of the lung and other tissues is the ultimate result of prolonged (12 hours or more) perfusion by bubble and film technics. However, recognition and avoidance of the many pitfalls in technical application have reduced what was once a formidable undertaking to a safe routine method which has few detrimental effects even after 6 hours or more of total body perfusion. Air embolization, intravascular coagulation, inadequate perfusion, ventricular distention, hypokalemia, and myocardial damage are usually caused by faulty application of the method rather than by the method itself. In the last few years, very few cardiac surgical deaths have been attributed to problems related to the extracorporeal system per se.

Postoperative Complications & Management Following Extracorporeal Circulation

During the early use of extracorporeal circulation, serious and fatal pulmonary, renal, and neurologic complications were common. Improved technics and better knowledge have materially reduced both the incidence and severity of these problems, many of which were related to unrecognized microembolism, inadequate heparinization, poor flow rates, and neglected intracardiac decompression.

Some degree of pulmonary shunting and congestion is invariably present after open heart procedures but is effectively managed with a brief period of positive pressure respiration in the postoperative period and now only rarely causes severe respiratory insufficiency. The histopathology of this phenomenon consists of alveolar wall thickening with deposition of leukocytes and cellular debris with red cells in the alveolar spaces.

Neurologic sequelae are now seen only rarely and usually can be correlated with systemic air embolization. Meticulous and extensive procedures are routinely employed to evacuate air from its multiple areas of potential entrapment within the heart and pulmo-

nary veins before restoring cardiac output. Despite these efforts, however, we have identified the passage of air bubbles through the ascending aorta (with a Doppler flow probe) for 10 or 15 minutes after discontinuing bypass. This finding, in conjunction with a low incidence of neurologic complications, suggests that the body tolerates micro air embolism quite well.

Low cardiac output syndrome (cardiogenic shock) is the most common cause of postoperative death, particularly after manipulation or replacement of the mitral valve. The complication is recognized by delayed responsiveness, oliguria, peripheral constriction, and hypotension. For this reason, it is customary to monitor central arterial pressure, venous pressure, and urinary output with close observation of the patient's general appearance and peripheral color changes.

The many explanations advanced for this development have had little to substantiate them. Undoubtedly, coronary air emboli, iatrogenic damage to the coronary arteries, prolonged cardiac ischemia, and underlying myocardial disease all play a role. Hypovolemia certainly accounts for most cases with this difficulty. The postperfusion state is associated with "third space" sequestration of blood, and large volumes of additional fluid are necessary to maintain adequate circulating blood. The left atrial pressure should be monitored and fluid replacement continued until this value is elevated above 20 mm Hg to push the output "up the Starling curve."

Excessive postoperative bleeding is a common complication which in many cases requires reopening the incision for evacuation of clot and further hemostatic control. Although it is not uncommon to discover a surgical source, such as bleeding from a suture line, a transected coronary vessel, or a cannulation site, in most cases only diffuse oozing is found, and the probability of inadequate neutralization of heparin must be considered. Before reoperation, the clotting time and prothrombin time should be determined to reveal any correctable deficiency in protamine or vitamin K. It is interesting, however, that persistent and unremitting bleeding usually subsides after reexposure of the operative field and evacuation of clot, even when no significant bleeding point is identified.

Varying degrees of cardiac arrhythmia are exceedingly common and require constant monitoring for recognition. Their occurrence is related to the operative procedure, the underlying disease, and the medications in use. Repairs in the region of the conduction system (aortic valve replacement) may produce transient or permanent third degree heart block. Mitral valve disease is likely to be associated with atrial fibrillation, which, if not present preoperatively, may develop postoperatively; postperfusion hypokalemia can lead to digitalis toxicity and ventricular fibrillation; and tachycardia can result from inadequate digitalization.

Disseminated intravascular coagulation with secondary pulmonary consolidation and diffuse bleeding into the gastrointestinal tract is a devastating complication which is sometimes difficult to recognize. Its cause is not well established but may be related to a homologous blood reaction, infection, low output with sludging, inadequate heparinization during perfusion, or hypoxia.

Cohen LS: Current status of circulatory assist devices. Am J Cardiol 33:316, 1974.

Roe BB: Whole body perfusion with heart-lung machines: Present status and future trends. Chap 1 in: *Cardiovascular Surgery, Current Practice.* Vol 1. Burford TH, Ferguson TB (editors). Mosby, 1969.

VALVULAR HEART DISEASE

Valvular heart disease manifesting itself for the first time in adult life has usually been attributed to rheumatic fever in childhood. It is evident, however, that in a significant proportion of cases the disorder is congenital or degenerative. Some congenital anatomic variations produce no hemodynamic abnormalities or even murmurs in early life when the leaflet structure is relatively flexible. Later, deposition of fibrin and calcium, presumably a consequence of turbulent flow around the tethered leaflets, results in loss of flexibility and narrowing of the orifice. However, no information is available to explain how or why fibrocalcific deposits develop in and around valves. The resulting clinical lesions are described as valvular stenosis or insufficiency depending on the mechanics of the pathologic process. Pure stenosis can occur in a totally competent valve, and a regurgitant valve may be unrestrictive, but the latter is seldom rheumatic in origin. In many instances, the anatomic abnormality consists of a fixed orifice which may both restrict forward flow and fail to prevent backward flow. The size, shape,

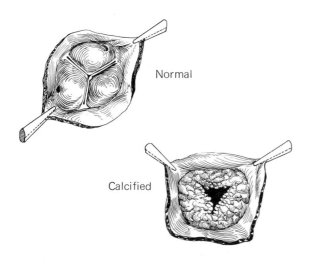

Figure 22–3. Aortic valve (normal and calcified).

flexibility, and position of the opening determine the relative degrees of stenosis and regurgitation.

From a prognostic standpoint, aortic valvular stenosis is less well tolerated than incompetence because the impairment to flow raises intraventricular pressure. More cardiac work is required to overcome increased pressure than is required to handle the increased volume load resulting from regurgitation.

AORTIC STENOSIS

Essentials of Diagnosis

- Loud, harsh basal systolic murmur, often radiating to the neck.
- Evidence of left ventricular strain or overactivity by ECG or physical examination.
- Diminished or dampened peripheral pulse wave.

General Considerations

Aortic stenosis may appear at any stage of adulthood, and there is no clear distinction between the congenital and acquired forms of the disease. It is more common in men than in women. Symptoms are characteristically absent or minimal until myocardial failure heralds the terminal stages of the disease. Transient bouts of syncope or angina during exertion may occur when limited cardiac output cannot meet the requirements of muscular activity or other demands along with the basic perfusion needs of the brain or heart. Sudden unheralded cardiac arrest (presumably due to ventricular fibrillation) is a common complication of aortic stenosis and adds to the urgency for elective correction.

Clinical Findings

A. Symptoms and Signs: A systolic ejection type of murmur is heard in the right second interspace and frequently is transmitted to the neck vessels. Peripheral pulses may be dampened, with a delayed upstroke, and left ventricular hypertrophy is manifested by cardiac enlargement with a left ventricular lift. The shock-like symptoms and moist palms in patients with peripheral vasoconstriction occur when obstruction has critically reduced cardiac output. The effects of gradually impaired cardiac output are not as clinically dramatic or distressing as those of congestive failure and may lead to dangerous complacency about the severity of the disease.

B. X-Ray Findings: The chest film shows left ventricular enlargement after long-standing stenosis, but (remarkably) there may be little or no visible hypertrophy in far-advanced disease of recent onset. Calcific deposits are frequently seen in the aortic valve area on fluoroscopy or in overpenetrated films, but neither hypertrophy nor calcium is essential to making the diagnosis.

C. Cardiac Catheterization: Left ventricular systolic pressure is significantly higher than in the aorta. It is sometimes difficult or impossible to pass a catheter retrograde through a stenotic valve, so that this determination may have to be made by a transseptal or percutaneous approach. In advanced disease, the early evidence of left ventricular failure will be reflected by an elevated left ventricular end-diastolic pressure to levels as high as 30 mm Hg or more. Pulmonary wedge pressures without ventricular tracings might, therefore, misleadingly suggest mitral disease. When severe myocardial failure is thus manifested, the prognosis is grave and the operative risk is high. Interpretation of the systolic gradient across the aortic valve must be based on a knowledge of cardiac output. In advanced disease, a low output (below 2 liters/sq m/minute) may reduce this gradient. Aortic pressure curves have a slow upstroke and a characteristic anacrotic notch (Fig 22–4).

Treatment

Surgical replacement of the diseased valve is recommended when the disease first becomes symptomatic. Evidence of decompensation should be interpreted as end stage disease, and prompt response to supportive treatment does not obviate the need for surgery. When a characteristic systolic murmur is associated with left ventricular hypertrophy or signs of failure, cardiac catheterization should be performed to identify a stenosis which can be treated before it reaches the dangerous symptomatic stage. A resting systolic gradient above 50 mm Hg warrants surgical consideration, but this criterion should not be used alone because its magnitude is influenced by the flow rate; such a gradient at basal resting cardiac output

may double or treble during exercise. In advanced disease, the murmur may be deceptively diminished since the output and gradient are depressed by the impaired performance of the failing ventricle.

Attempts to reconstruct the diseased valve by opening commissures and excising calcific deposits have been virtually abandoned because of unsatisfactory long-term results and rapid recurrence. The pathologic process usually obliterates any semblance of valve structure, and it is futile to expect that function can be restored.

Prognosis

Early experience with this high-risk group of patients was associated with a significant operative mortality, but recently the risk has been reduced to less than 5% and patients over 70 have tolerated the procedure remarkably well. Associated coronary artery disease or secondary cor bovinum militates against a good long-term functional result, but (surprisingly) these disorders have not been a major surgical hazard.

Long-term results are difficult to assess in a disease process in the older age groups with a wide spectrum of severity. Replacement devices (or homografts) are undergoing constant change, and the risk factors of thromboembolism versus anticoagulation are not yet established. Embolization or thrombus formation on the prosthesis, hemorrhagic complications of anticoagulation, disruption or mechanical failure of the prosthesis, and arrhythmias account for late deaths at a rate of 1–3% per year. There seems little doubt, however, that life expectancy has been extended by surgical replacement of the calcified, stenotic aortic valve. The value of several mechanical prostheses and the glutaraldehyde preserved xenograft is now well documented. Homografts and some prostheses have been abandoned and there is still disagreement about which is the most durable and functionally effective replacement device.

Eddleman EE Jr & others: Critical analysis of clinical factors in estimating severity of aortic valve disease. Am J Cardiol 31:687, 1973.

Glancy DL, Epstein SE: Differential diagnosis of type and severity of obstruction to left ventricular outflow. Prog Cardiovasc Dis 14:153, 1971.

Perloff JK: Clinical recognition of aortic stenosis: The physical signs and differential diagnosis of the various forms of obstruction to left ventricular outflow. Prog Cardiovasc Dis 10:323, 1968.

Roberts WC: The congenitally bicuspid aortic valve: A study of 85 autopsy cases. Am J Cardiol 26:72, 1970.

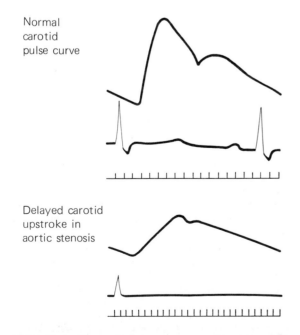

Normal carotid pulse curve

Delayed carotid upstroke in aortic stenosis

Figure 22–4. Abnormal aortic pressure curve in aortic stenosis with delayed upstroke.

AORTIC INSUFFICIENCY

Essentials of Diagnosis

- Visible overactivity of the left ventricle.
- Left ventricular heave with an apical impulse displaced to the axilla.

- Peripheral pulses collapse in diastole, and a diminuendo blowing diastolic murmur is heard along the left sternal border.

General Considerations

When aortic incompetence develops gradually, even severe hemodynamic derangement may be tolerated for long periods without disability. The muscle development and energy requirements for increased volume work are significantly less than those needed for the greater pressure load imposed by aortic stenosis.

Acute aortic insufficiency, on the other hand, is very poorly tolerated, and a much less severe degree of valve leakage may be fatal unless it is corrected promptly. Impaired coronary perfusion secondary to the lowered diastolic (coronary-filling) pressure and the normally small ventricular chamber whose volume is inadequate to accommodate increased output requirements are major factors complicating the acute illness. One must not apply the traditional criterion of compensatory cardiac enlargement as an index of severity in the acute state. Congestive failure and aortic diastolic murmur are alone sufficient to justify valve replacement if salvage is to be expected. In the presence of bacterial endocarditis, the hazards of embolization from bacterial vegetation or sudden further loss of valve integrity by erosion may offset the theoretical desirability of deferring operation until the infection is controlled.

Clinical Findings

In the chronic state of aortic insufficiency, the chest film shows gross cardiac enlargement with a prominent left ventricular shadow. In advanced disease, evidence of pulmonary congestion may be present, and wedge pressure (ventricular end-diastolic pressure) is elevated (as high as 45 mm Hg) on cardiac catheterization. Arterial pressure curves are sharply peaked, and the dicrotic notch is delayed or absent. It is a deceptive paradox that the arterial diastolic pressure, which may have been nearly zero, rises as the patient becomes symptomatically worse. This rise is a manifestation of failure with elevated ventricular end-diastolic pressure below which the arterial pressure cannot fall, even with wide-open incompetence. Whenever a patient with aortic insufficiency begins to have symptoms or shows radiographic progression of his heart size, he should be studied by cardiac catheterization. If the left ventricular end-diastolic pressure is elevated significantly above 15 mm Hg, valve replacement should be recommended.

Treatment

Surgery is recommended when the first evidence of decompensation is recognized and certainly should not be delayed after the first episode of frank failure. Although most patients will respond promptly to digitalization, this does not justify postponing valve replacement because left ventricular function will deteriorate progressively and the functional benefit of valve

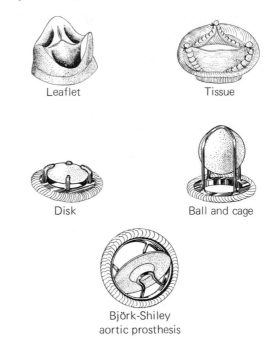

Figure 22—5. Examples of artificial heart valves.

replacement will be significantly impaired. The hospital mortality rate for valve replacement in aortic insufficiency is well below the 5% estimate for aortic stenosis, but long-term survival has been disappointing when the process has been allowed to progress to the "cor bovinum" stage; a successful operative result merely delays the inexorable progress of myocardial fibrosis and intractable muscular failure. For this reason, replacement is now recommended as soon as progressive and significant ventricular enlargement is recognized.

Procedures directed at preserving and reconstituting the patient's own valve have now been abandoned because of poor long-term results. Plications, suspensions, and other reconstruction devices have all broken down and have required later replacement. Except in small children, diseased aortic valves are best removed. Replacement may employ prostheses, homografts, or heterografts.

Prognosis

The immediate surgical risk is low. Long-term rehabilitation after correcting valve dysfunction is impaired by the degree of preoperative myocardial degeneration and thus tends to respond inversely to the degree of preoperative chronic cardiomegaly.

Late complications and death can occur from malfunction of the replacement valve, paravalvular leakage, thrombotic occlusion, congestive failure, arrhythmia, embolism, or hemorrhage secondary to prophylactic anticoagulation. Surgical experience, improved valve construction, earlier operation, better management practices, and the use of tissue valve replacements are helping to reduce these hazards.

These authors have not experienced significant para-valvular leakage in their patients in the absence of pre-existing infection, and no valve dysfunctions have occurred with the Smeloff-Cutter ball valve during 8 years of experience. Some other prosthetic valves, however, have malfunctioned.

Griffin FM Jr, Jones G, Cobbs CG: Aortic insufficiency in bacterial endocarditis. Ann Intern Med 76:23, 1972.

Lee SJK & others: Circulatory changes in severe aortic regurgitation before and after surgical correction. Am J Cardiol 28:442, 1971.

Najafi H: Aortic insufficiency: Clinical manifestations and surgical treatment. Am Heart J 82:120, 1971.

Spagnuolo M & others: Natural history of rheumatic aortic regurgitation: Criteria predictive of death, congestive heart failure, and angina in young patients. Circulation 44:368, 1971.

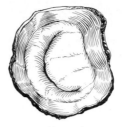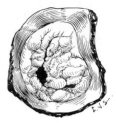

Normal   Calcified

Figure 22—6. Mitral valve (normal and calcified) as viewed from the left atrium.

MITRAL STENOSIS

Essentials of Diagnosis

- Dyspnea, orthopnea, and paroxysmal nocturnal dyspnea.
- Radiographic evidence of prominent superior pulmonary vessels.
- Enlarged left atrium.
- Prominent mitral first sound, opening snap (usually), and apical crescendo diastolic rumble.

General Considerations

The most common lesion caused by rheumatic fever is stenotic scarring of the mitral valve which is involved in the inflammatory process of rheumatic disease. It is usually years or decades after the bout of active carditis before progressive scarring and contracture produce a significant functional abnormality. Why the frequency and severity of late rheumatic pathologic change is greatest in the mitral valve, less in the aortic valve, uncommon in the tricuspid valve, and virtually absent in the pulmonic valve is not known. Because the incidence parallels the relative stress sustained by the 4 valves, this factor has been invoked as a possible basis but without valid explanation. Symptoms are often well controlled by unconscious or deliberate restriction of activity; thus, advanced stenosis can develop insidiously without apparent disability until late in the disease.

Clinical Findings

A. Symptoms and Signs: The characteristic murmur of mitral stenosis is sometimes difficult to localize at the cardiac apex, but the diagnosis should be suspected in the presence of an accentuated mitral first sound, a loud opening snap at the beginning of diastole, and an increased intensity of the pulmonic second sound. The diastolic murmur is a low-pitched rumble with presystolic accentuation. Development of atrial

fibrillation with consequent loss of atrial systole to overcome the obstruction characteristically precipitates symptoms. Dyspnea, wheezing, orthopnea, and paroxysmal nocturnal dyspnea are characteristic complaints; hemoptysis, chest pain (not anginal), and peripheral edema are manifestations of chronic congestion.

B. X-Ray Findings: The cardiac silhouette is enlarged in the region of the left atrial appendage and pulmonary artery. Left atrial and right ventricular enlargement are sometimes seen in the lateral view. Penetrated films may show calcific deposits in the region of the mitral valve. In advanced stages, pulmonary congestion is evident and the pulmonary venous shadows become prominent in the upper lobes. Kerley "B" lines may be present in the lung periphery, manifesting lymphatic engorgement.

C. Cardiac Catheterization: Cardiac catheterization shows elevation of pulmonary artery and pulmonary capillary wedge pressures from normal values of 25/10 mm Hg and 7—10 mm Hg (respectively) to resting values of more than double those figures, which characteristically rise with mild exercise to values as high as systemic pressure in the pulmonary artery and 45 mm Hg in the capillary wedge.

Differential Diagnosis

Because auscultatory findings are often subtle, the symptoms of congestive heart failure are often attributed to myocardial or pericardial disease. The characteristic murmurs of mitral stenosis are similar to those heard with atrial tumors or tricuspid stenosis.

Complications

Chronic mitral stenosis commonly causes atrial fibrillation, and the latter may contribute to the development of atrial thrombi which can produce arterial embolization. Pulmonary hypertension with vascular changes and impaired ventilation ("cardiac asthma") can occur in the late stages of the disease.

Treatment

Symptoms precipitated by arrhythmia can be temporarily controlled with digitalis or quinidine. Diuretics and salt restriction will reduce pulmonary congestion. However, since the disease is one of mechanical obstruction, definitive therapy is necessarily surgical.

Mitral commissurotomy (reopening of the fused valve leaflet) has been accomplished with significant success by closed technics consisting of blind fracture of the valve structures with a finger or instrument in the heart. Because symptoms develop at a critical degree of valve stenosis, significant functional improvement can be derived from a slight increase in the effective valve area from slightly more than 1 sq cm to perhaps 2 sq cm, even though considerable obstruction remains. Before the days of safe, effective extracorporeal circulation, closed commissurotomy was usually preferable. However, the complex and extensive nature of the valvular pathologic process, the embolic hazard from unsuspected atrial thrombi, and the danger of producing mitral insufficiency are all reasons to recommend the open approach to every diseased valve. This method provides for meticulous mobilization of the valve leaflets, removal of thrombi before they become dislodged, and repair of any secondary commissural leakage. Direct visualization has focused attention on the intricate and extensive nature of subvalvular fusion. Short chordae tendineae to both leaflets from a single papillary muscle may tether valve mobility and require meticulous sharp separation. Thickened chordal and papillary structures frequently show no evidence of cleavage and must be divided deeply into the ventricle before an effective orifice can be developed.

Many surgeons will undertake commissurotomy for primary isolated mitral stenosis even with the expectation that eventual valve replacement will be necessary. However, growing satisfaction with replacement devices and the predictability of their performance have led to valve replacement in a higher proportion of patients with mitral stenosis. It is now considered desirable to replace almost all recurrently stenotic valves, almost all stenotic valves in patients over 55 or 60 years of age, and most heavily calcified valves or stenotic valves associated with significant aortic valve disease requiring replacement.

Prognosis

Mitral stenosis characteristically recurs after valvotomy in 3–10 years, presumably because of the behavior of scar tissue which is an integral part of the lesions. The incidence of systemic embolization is reduced but not obliterated by valvotomy. Some degree of mitral insufficiency is a frequent consequence of valvotomy, and its severity may be incorrectly assessed; subsequent replacement may be necessitated by this complication.

Atrial fibrillation is reversible in less than one-third of patients who had this condition before operation, and medical management is necessary indefinitely.

Ellis LB & others: Fifteen to twenty-year study of one thousand patients undergoing closed mitral valvuloplasty. Circulation 48:357, 1973.

Mullin EM Jr & others: Current results of operation for mitral stenosis: Clinical and hemodynamic assessments in 124 consecutive patients treated by closed commissurotomy, open commissurotomy or valve replacement. Circulation 46:298, 1972.

Rowe JC & others: The course of mitral stenosis without surgery: Ten- and twenty-year perspectives. Ann Intern Med 52:741, 1960.

Selzer A, Cohn KE: Natural history of mitral stenosis: A review. Circulation 45:878, 1972.

MITRAL INSUFFICIENCY

Essentials of Diagnosis

- Loud systolic murmur at the apex, radiating into the axilla.
- Pulmonary congestion from elevated left atrial pressure.
- Cardiac enlargement consisting of left ventricular distention with hypertrophy and giant left atrium.

General Considerations

In mitral insufficiency, the valve fails to close because of (1) rheumatic inflammation, secondary scarring, and leaflet retraction (usually associated with mitral stenosis); (2) myxomatous degeneration with prolapse of leaflets; (3) attenuation and elongation of subvalvular structures with prolapse; (4) rupture of chordae tendineae or papillary muscles; (5) myocardiopathy with annular distention and secondary leaflet insufficiency; and (6) bacterial endocarditis.

Clinical Findings

A. Symptoms and Signs: Symptoms characteristically occur late in the disease and consist of dyspnea, orthopnea, wheezing, and paroxysmal nocturnal dyspnea. Insidious fatigability may precede any of these. Cardiac enlargement, left ventricular heave, and apical systolic murmurs are easily identified. Atrial fibrillation is common.

B. X-Ray Findings: The enlarged left atrium and left ventricular hypertrophy are identifiable on the chest film. Vascular congestion in the lungs is accompanied by prominent superior pulmonary veins and Kerley "B" lines in advanced disease.

C. Cardiac Catheterization and Cineangiocardiography: Cardiac catheterization shows an elevated mean left atrial pressure of 20–30 mm Hg with a high V wave up to 60 mm Hg, but the magnitude and distensibility of the enlarged atrial chamber have a significant damping effect on this regurgitant jet. Thus, the volume of regurgitation does not correlate well with the height of the V wave, particularly in the acute lesions of sudden onset where an undistended atrium may reflect a high pressure wave with a relatively small backflow.

Cineangiocardiography will demonstrate a regurgitant jet of contrast medium through the mitral valve when it is injected into the left ventricle. It is sometimes possible to identify the location of the jet.

Differential Diagnosis

Characteristic findings are not often mistaken for other diseases, but the systolic murmur can easily be confused with that of aortic or pulmonic stenosis. In the postinfarction state, it is often difficult to distinguish the systolic murmur of a ruptured ventricular septum from that of a ruptured papillary muscle (see p 360) and mitral regurgitation. When the anterior leaflet of the mitral valve is incompetent, the regurgitant jet is directed anteriorly and may easily be mistaken for the murmur of aortic stenosis. Since definitive identification of the lesion by angiographic and cardiac catheterization technics has become a standard procedure, the surgeon is seldom concerned with problems in differential diagnosis.

Treatment

Medical supportive measures such as digitalization, diuretics, and salt restriction can control symptoms satisfactorily for many years. If disability progresses or if cardiomegaly increases, surgical correction is indicated.

A wide variety of reconstructive surgical procedures have been attempted and advocated for the regurgitant mitral valve, but nearly all have been abandoned in favor of replacement. The thick muscular cone that constitutes the left ventricle does not lend itself to the distortion of true "annuloplasty." There are, however, tethered leaflets that can be mobilized by dividing subvalvular structures and by inserting a gusset of autogenous tissue to correct incompetence. However, the only circumstance in which success can be expected with nonreplacement technics is a ruptured chorda tendinea on the mural leaflet; the long concave curve of this valve edge lends itself admirably to wedge resection, shortening the curve and providing apposition to the septal leaflet in systole without impairing diastolic flow. Most operations for mitral insufficiency now result in replacement because of its more predictable outcome and generally acceptable long-term results. It remains to be determined which mechanical device or tissue valve will have the best long-term performance. Several alternatives can provide a 5-year life expectancy in at least 70% of patients, and the choice of method remains a matter of surgical judgment.

Prognosis

The secondary effects of elevated left atrial pressure and left atrial distention are progressive, and the patient will eventually die in congestive heart failure if the defect is not corrected. Operative mortality from valve replacement in this disease is less than that in stenosis (5–10%), but long-term complications are similar and the functional result, although almost invariably one of improvement, is variable; the size and performance of the replacement device and the degree of underlying myocardial disease are undoubtedly fac-

tors. For reasons not clearly understood, the left ventricular performance after mitral valve replacement is characteristically impaired for some weeks or months, in sharp contrast to the performance after replacement of the aortic valve. It has been thought by some that the cage of the ball valve extending into the ventricle interferes with ventricular function; this stimulated the development of so-called "low-profile" disk valves, but recent studies have indicated that there is no functional difference between the 2 mechanisms. However, the inability of the valve annulus to contract against a rigid ring could cause functional impairment.

Braunwald E: Mitral regurgitation: Physiologic, clinical, and surgical considerations. N Engl J Med 281:425, 1969.

Kirklin JW: Replacement of the mitral valve for mitral incompetence. Surgery 72:827, 1972.

Littler WA, Epstein EJ, Coulshed N: Acute mitral regurgitation resulting from ruptured or elongated chordae tendineae. Q J Med 42:87, 1973.

Roberts WC, Perloff JK: Mitral valvular disease: A clinicopathologic survey of the conditions causing the mitral valve to function abnormally. Ann Intern Med 77:939, 1972.

TRICUSPID STENOSIS & INSUFFICIENCY

Malfunction of the tricuspid valve is much less common than aortic and mitral valve malfunction, but the principles of recognition and management are similar to those in mitral disease, with less emphasis on replacement.

Clinical Findings

Right-sided heart failure is manifested by elevated venous pressure, hepatic enlargement, edema, and ascites. Murmurs of tricuspid valve disease are heard on the right side of the sternum and are similar to those of the mitral valve. Tricuspid insufficiency results in a venous pulse wave which produces a pulsating liver. X-rays show an enlarged right atrium. Cardiac catheterization demonstrates elevation of right atrial pressure with a high V wave of 10–20 mm Hg in the presence of valve incompetence (with variable factors similar to those of mitral insufficiency according to chamber size).

The functional significance of tricuspid insufficiency is influenced by the degree of concomitant pulmonary vascular resistance (either primary or secondary to mitral valve disease). In the presence of normal pulmonary arterial pressure, pulmonary perfusion can be maintained by modest elevation of systemic venous pressure without requiring effective pumping action of the right ventricle; thus, the need for definitive treatment is limited to patients with additional hemodynamic abnormalities.

Treatment

Tricuspid valve disease is seldom seen without

associated mitral or aortic disease (or both). The exceptions are bacterial endocarditis (frequently associated with narcotic addiction) and associated tumor. Symptoms may respond to medical management as readily as in mitral disease. Surgical correction is sometimes indicated in conjunction with operations on the mitral valve.

Tricuspid stenosis usually appears as a conical structure with a central fibrous ring which presents no evident commissural lines for simple incisional relief, and some cardiac surgeons tend to replace the diseased tricuspid valve with the same alacrity as in mitral disease. It is evident, however, that the systemic effects of tricuspid insufficiency (or even total tricuspid excision) are well tolerated in the absence of high pulmonary vascular resistance and that the right ventricle is less suitable for the usual prosthetic devices. For these reasons, most surgeons are conservative about tricuspid replacement except in the presence of advanced organic disease.

Functional tricuspid insufficiency with flexible, intact leaflets lends itself well to improvement with true annuloplasty because of the crescentic shape of the valve annulus which (unlike the mitral annulus) provides for effective plication.

Prognosis

Tricuspid valve disease alone may be well tolerated. Congestive symptoms which do not involve the lung are less likely to be fatal, and the necessity for replacement is less pressing. Because of disputed indications for replacement, greater adaptability to annuloplasty, lower incidence of disease, and the almost invariable association with mitral valve disease, it is difficult to assess the surgical experience. Tricuspid valve replacement in combination with mitral or aortic valve replacement (or both) has an immediate surgical mortality rate of 10–15%, which reflects the risk of multivalve disease. Even so, it is apparent that the right ventricular cavity is less suited to a round (and particularly a caged) replacement device than is the left ventricle, and that late thrombosis in this area is more common. It is also notable that all fascia lata valves in the tricuspid position deteriorate. Successful total excision of the tricuspid valve for acute bacterial endocarditis has been reported.

Braunwald NS, Ross J Jr, Morrow AG: Conservative management of tricuspid regurgitation in patients undergoing mitral valve replacement. Circulation 35:63, 1967.

Carpentier A & others: Surgical management of acquired tricuspid valve disease. J Thorac Cardiovasc Surg 67:53, 1974.

Kay JH, Maselli-Campagna G, Tsuji HK: Surgical treatment of tricuspid insufficiency. Ann Surg 162:53, 1965.

Pluth JR, Ellis FH Jr: Tricuspid insufficiency in patients undergoing mitral valve replacement. J Thorac Cardiovasc Surg 58:484, 1969.

Starr A, Herr R, Wood J: Tricuspid replacement for acquired valve disease. Surg Gynecol Obstet 122:1295, 1966.

•   •   •

THORACIC AORTIC ANEURYSM

Essentials of Diagnosis

- Enlarged mediastinal silhouette.
- Chest pain radiating to the back (not invariable).
- Angiographic demonstration of abnormal aorta.

General Considerations

Pathologic distention of the aorta tends to be progressive because, at a given pressure, tension on the diseased aortic wall increases in direct proportion to its diameter.

Thoracic aortic aneurysm may be due to (1) syphilis, (2) arteriosclerosis, (3) a degenerative process (cystic medial necrosis, Marfan's syndrome), or (4) trauma.

Aneurysms may be saccular outpouchings of an otherwise normally contoured aorta (usually syphilitic) but more commonly are a fusiform enlargement of the entire lumen. The latter are sometimes localized, but diffuse enlargement and tortuosity of the aorta also occur.

Clinical Findings

A. Symptoms and Signs: The manifestations of thoracic aortic aneurysm are related to its size and location. Bony erosion of the sternum or vertebral bodies can cause pain. Stretching of the recurrent laryngeal nerve may result in hoarseness. Coughing may occur because of compression of bronchi, and erosion into a lung may cause hemoptysis.

B. X-Ray Findings: Aortography is the only definitive study which can verify and delineate the aneurysm. Multiple views may be necessary to identify the nature and relationship of the arch vessels as well as the nature of the aorta at the limits of the aneurysm.

Differential Diagnosis

A space-occupying lesion in the mediastinum can be any of several mediastinal tumors or cysts as well as

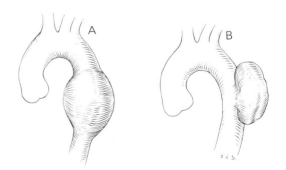

Figure 22–7. Types of thoracic aortic aneurysms. *A:* Fusiform. *B:* Saccular.

an aortic aneurysm. The signs, symptoms, and appearance on plain roentgenograms are often indistinguishable, so that aortography is always mandatory when the slightest doubt exists.

Treatment

Supportive measures to treat the secondary effects of an expanding mass are obviously of no avail since response is based on removal of the offending process. Systemic hypertension must be controlled because it compounds the hazard and accelerates the expansion of an aneurysm; however, surgical relief provides the only opportunity for definitive management. Replacement with a polyester tube graft is necessary for fusiform aneurysm. Saccular aneurysms can frequently be obliterated by closure of the neck at its connection to the aorta without total excision. Because of the related structures, the surgical hazards and results vary according to the location and pathologic nature of the disease process. Localized aneurysms of the ascending and descending aorta are more easily and safely treated than those of the arch, which require establishment of new connections to the head vessels. Aneurysms involving the sinuses of Valsalva are frequently associated with malfunction of the aortic valve and invariably result in displacement of the coronary ostia. It is, therefore, frequently necessary to replace the aortic valve and to transpose the coronary ostia into the cloth graft.

Operations for thoracic aortic aneurysm pose many technical and logistical challenges. A large aneurysmal mass may displace the heart and mediastinal structures so as to preclude the usual cannulation routes or to prevent access for clamping the aorta beyond the aneurysm. Under these circumstances, it is essential to initiate perfusion through the groin in order to induce profound total body hypothermia, which permits extended circulatory arrest; thus, the hazardous dissection can be carried out under "cadaveric" conditions.

Aneurysms of the distal aortic arch and descending aorta which must be approached from the left side require either left heart bypass (left atrium to femoral artery) or lower body cardiopulmonary perfusion (femoral vein to femoral artery through an oxygenator). Both of these technics require far greater skill than total body perfusion because of the distributional problem between the 2 pumping systems (the normal heart and lungs for the upper extremities and the extracorporeal perfusion system for the lower body).

Prognosis

Without surgical correction, progressive distention and eventual rupture are inevitable, but the course is unpredictable. Evidence of progressive enlargement should make operation compelling.

Cooley DA & others: Surgical management of aneurysms of the ascending aorta, including those associated with aortic valvular incompetence. Surg Clin North Am 46:1033, 1966.

Crisler C, Bahnson HT: Aneurysms of the aorta. Curr Probl Surg, Dec 1972.

Mannick JA: Surgical treatment of aneurysms of the abdominal and thoracic aorta. Prog Cardiovasc Dis 16:69, 1973.

AORTIC DISSECTION
("Dissecting Aneurysm")

Essentials of Diagnosis

- Sudden severe chest pain with radiation to the back, abdomen, and extremities.
- Shock may be present, though often not until the later stages.
- CNS changes may occur.
- A history of hypertension is common.
- Dissection occurs most frequently in males.

General Considerations

Intramural splitting or dissection of the aorta usually arises from an intimal tear either just distal to the aortic valve or adjacent to the take-off of the left subclavian artery. Over 60% of dissections arise in the ascending aorta, roughly 20% in the transverse or distal arch, and the remainder in the descending thoracic or abdominal aorta. The process is commonly called dissecting aneurysm, but the term is inappropriate because aortic dissection does not always result in significant dilatation. The disease process consists of a degenerative weakness of the muscularis layer of the aorta (cystic medial necrosis). Hypertension is usually the triggering mechanism, but the patient may present in a state of shock with deceptively "normal" blood pressure.

Clinical Findings

A. Symptoms and Signs: Silent "dissections" have been encountered, but characteristically the onset is accompanied by chest pain (sometimes described as "tearing") which may extend into the back and abdomen. Discrepancies in character, timing, and magnitude of pulse waves may be present among the extremities, depending upon the location and consequences of the dissection. When the dissecting process selectively obliterates the central lumen, obstructing pulsatile flow to major vessels of the extremities, the brain, or abdominal organs, there will be varying degrees of impaired perfusion to these areas depending upon the circulatory mechanics. If the dissection process provides effective flow into the peripheral false lumen and if the false lumen communicates with the involved pathways, there may be little or no evidence of impaired organ function. If, however, the dissection effectively obliterates the flow to the involved organ system, evidence of ischemia or infarction will be seen, prompting immediate operation.

B. X-Ray Findings: Chest films do not always show mediastinal widening. Aortography may opacify the true lumen, false lumen (external pathway), or both. Multiple injections at different sites may be necessary to locate the intimal tear and to establish patency of essential vascular pathways. Several views may also be required to identify these landmarks.

Differential Diagnosis

The presenting signs and symptoms of acute myocardial infarction are similar to those of aortic dissection, so that the latter diagnosis may be missed. A normal ECG and abnormal pulse pattern suggest dissection.

Treatment

In simple dissection, both immediate salvage and long-term survival are greater after nonsurgical treatment and vigorous antihypertensive management than after surgical replacement. Because of its diffuse nature and the poor aortic tissue which characterizes the disease, the technical problems of surgical reconstruction are significant and the operative risk is high (15–20%). However, surgery is necessary if the patient develops secondary aortic insufficiency, obstruction of a major vascular pathway, or evidence of impending rupture suggested by intrapleural bleeding—or if, in spite of therapy, further extension is suggested by continued pain or expanding mediastinal shadow. It is desirable—though not always feasible—to resect the origin of the dissection and to obliterate the false lumen which may extend in both directions from this point. Occasionally the 2 ends can be reconnected, but the space usually must be filled with a synthetic graft. If the dissection is chronic or of long standing, it is important to map and identify the outflow to each of the major aortic branches because of the possibility that the false lumen has become the only pathway to one or more of these vessels. Obliteration of the false lumen in the procedure will then result in necrosis of the involved organ.

Prognosis

After prompt and vigorous antihypertensive therapy in uncomplicated cases, the immediate survival rate is 85% and the long-term survival rate 58%. Operative intervention, where indicated, results in a salvage rate of approximately 80%, depending on the origin and extent of dissection. The prognosis is necessarily guarded because of the diffuse and degenerative nature of the underlying disease process. Uncontrolled hypertension in the presence of a diseased arterial tree has a predictable outcome, and yet clinically unrecognized dissections are not infrequently discovered at autopsy, either with reentry pathways and patency of both lumens or with thrombosis and scarring of the false lumen.

Anaguostopoulos CE, Manakavalan JS, Kittle CF: Aortic dissections and dissecting aneurysms. Am J Cardiol 30:263, 1972.

Gore I, Hirst AE Jr: Dissecting aneurysm of the aorta. Prog Cardiovasc Dis 16:103, 1973.

Symbas PN & others: Rupture of the aorta: A diagnostic triad. Ann Thorac Surg 15:405, 1973.

Wheat MW Jr: Treatment of dissecting aneurysms of the aorta: Current status. Prog Cardiovasc Dis 16:87, 1973.

ISCHEMIC HEART DISEASE

Coronary atherosclerosis may impair myocardial blood flow, causing left ventricular ischemia and infarction. The effects of myocardial ischemia include decreased ventricular compliance, depressed contractility, exertional chest pain (angina pectoris), rest pain (angina decubitus), prolonged chest pain at rest without ECG or enzyme evidence of infarction (preinfarction angina, unstable angina, coronary insufficiency, intermediate coronary syndrome), and irreversible myocardial damage (myocardial infarction). Early deaths from myocardial infarction are secondary to arrhythmia or low cardiac output. The present hospital mortality rate of myocardial infarction is approximately 20%, usually related to left ventricular failure. Patients dying in cardiogenic shock following acute myocardial infarction commonly show destruction of more than 40% of left ventricular muscle. Mechanical sequelae of myocardial infarction such as impairment of mitral valvular competence, ventricular septal perforation, left ventricular aneurysm, and left ventricular rupture are associated with a high mortality rate.

Surgical management includes coronary artery bypass for angina pectoris, mitral valve replacement for postinfarction mitral imcompetence, repair of postinfarction rupture of the ventricular septum or free wall, and left ventricular aneurysmectomy.

ANGINA PECTORIS

Essentials of Diagnosis

- Precordial chest pain.
- ECG evidence of ischemia during pain or on exercise testing.
- Angiographic demonstration of significant obstruction of major coronary vessels.

Clinical Findings

A. Symptoms and Signs: Patients typically present with substernal chest pain of short duration (less than 15 minutes) radiating to the arm, neck, or jaw and occurring with exertion, emotion, or exposure to cold. Symptoms promptly disappear with rest and the administration of nitroglycerin. The history may disclose previous myocardial infarction and the presence of risk factors associated with coronary artery disease (hypertension, hypercholesterolemia, and a family history of ischemic heart disease). Physical examination usually shows nothing abnormal. The finding of ear lobe creases has been associated with the presence of coronary artery disease. Evidence of coronary artery risk factors such as hypertension or hyperlipoproteinemia (eg, xanthelasma) may be found. A third heart sound or findings of congestive heart failure suggest left ventricular ischemic damage.

B. Laboratory and Special Studies: The results of routine laboratory studies are usually normal. Serum cholesterol values are likely to be elevated. The resting ECG will show nonspecific abnormalities or evidence of previous myocardial infarction in 30–40% of cases. The multiple lead, graded exercise ECG will be positive for ischemia (ST segment depression during or immediately following exercise) in 85% of patients presenting with anginal chest pain and with subsequently proved coronary artery obstruction. Other studies helpful in establishing the presence of myocardial ischemia include myocardial scintigraphy (eg, perfusion imaging using rapidly diffusible radionuclides such as thallium 201) and metabolic studies (determination of abnormal myocardial lactate metabolism during atrial pacing). Because of the wide prevalence of asymptomatic coronary artery disease, it is important to document ischemia by one or more of the above technics (exercise ECG, perfusion imaging, metabolic studies), especially in patients with atypical anginal pain syndromes.

Patients with more severe coronary insufficiency (prolonged chest pain occurring at rest) often manifest ST segment depression on the resting ECG during episodes of pain. These patients are not subjected to exercise or atrial pacing because of the risk of precipitating arrhythmia or myocardial infarction.

A small percentage of patients will present with "variant" (Prinzmetal) angina. Such patients characteristically have chest pain at rest and not with exercise and show reversible ST segment elevation on the resting ECG during pain. This syndrome is associated with a high incidence of subsequent myocardial infarction and death comparable to that in patients with unstable angina. These patients are frequently found to have evidence of coronary artery spasm with or without fixed coronary artery obstruction.

Approximately 80% of patients with a clinical diagnosis of angina pectoris will have demonstrable abnormalities on coronary angiography. The remainder are presumed to have symptoms unrelated to myocardial ischemia. However, myocardial ischemia is possible even in the presence of angiographically normal coronary arteries. Atrial pacing studies in some patients have shown abnormal myocardial lactate metabolism suggesting ischemia despite apparently normal coronary arteries. The prognosis in such patients is excellent with medical therapy.

Left ventricular cineangiography is done at the time of coronary angiography and will show normal or slightly impaired wall motion in most cases. Patients with poor left ventricular function (systolic ejection fraction less than 0.3 or left ventricular end diastolic pressure elevation above 20 mm Hg) are considered high operative risks. The presence of left ventricular aneurysm or valve defects such as mitral regurgitation are important findings, especially when operation is being considered.

Differential Diagnosis

Other causes of chest pain must be considered, such as esophageal spasm, peptic ulcer disease, pericarditis, costochondritis, visceral artery ischemia, biliary colic, cervical spine disease, thoracic outlet syndrome, and aortic valvular disease.

Treatment

A. Medical Treatment: Most patients respond to short-acting nitrates (nitroglycerin), long-acting nitrates (isosorbide dinitrate), or β-adrenergic blocking agents (propranolol) for relief of pain. General medical measures include proscription of smoking, treatment of hypertension or hyperlipidemia if present, and dietary measures to attain ideal weight.

B. Surgical Treatment: The most common clinical indication for coronary artery bypass is disabling angina pectoris refractory to medical management. Patients fitting the definition of unstable or preinfarction angina pectoris are considered strong candidates for surgical management because of the poor prognosis with medical therapy. Other clinical indications for surgery include postmyocardial infarction angina (patients having ischemic chest pain at rest refractory to medical therapy within days or weeks of acute myocardial infarction), myocardial ischemia not accompanied by angina pectoris, precocious ischemic heart disease (eg, one or more myocardial infarctions occurring in patients age 45 or less), and patients with or without angina pectoris undergoing other cardiac surgery such as valve replacement.

Patients with clinical indications for surgery undergo selective coronary angiography and left ventriculography. If greater than 70% stenosis of one or more major coronary arteries (left main, left anterior descending, left circumflex, right) is demonstrated, along with satisfactory distal vessels and acceptable left ventricular function, surgery is recommended.

Operation consists of placing bypass grafts from the ascending aorta to the coronary arteries beyond the obstruction using autogenous saphenous vein and employing cardiopulmonary bypass. Direct internal mammary artery to coronary artery anastomosis may be used, especially to the LAD and its branches. Coronary artery endarterectomy in combination with bypass graft is occasionally used when diffuse distal coronary atherosclerosis is present.

Relative contraindications to surgery are extensive distal coronary atherosclerosis and poor left ventricular function.

Prognosis Following Surgical Treatment

The operative mortality rate (any death within 30 days of operation constitutes an operative death) is 4% or less in elective coronary artery bypass. The single best determinant of the operative mortality rate is left ventricular function. The operative mortality rate is currently 10–15% in patients with poor left ventricular function (defined above). It increases in temporal proximity to acute myocardial infarction. Elective coronary artery bypass is not advised within 6 weeks of acute myocardial infarction. Patients manifesting prolonged chest pain and ECG evidence of acute myocardial infarction during cardiac catheterization or in hospital awaiting elective coronary artery bypass are considered candidates for emergency coronary artery bypass. If such patients are operated upon within 6—8 hours of the onset of chest pain, the operative mortality rate is low, and some fail to manifest the electrocardiographic findings of infarction. The application of emergency coronary artery bypass to patients presenting to the hospital with acute myocardial infarction and to patients in cardiogenic shock (without evidence of mechanical complications) following acute myocardial infarction is considered investigational at this time.

Eighty to 90% of patients operated upon for relief of angina pectoris experience good to excellent palliation, 60—70% having complete relief of symptoms. Objective improvement in exercise tolerance can be shown in approximately 80% of surviving patients. The saphenous graft patency rate is 70—85% at 1 year. Approximately 95% of patients studied will have one or more grafts open. There is a slight (5%) fall in patency rate in grafts open at 1 year when studied at 3 years. Late (> 3 year) graft patency rates have not been established. Individual case reports document vein graft patency 7 years after implantation.

Data on the effects of operation on left ventricular function are conflicting. On the one hand, 6—15% of patients will manifest ECG evidence of transmural myocardial infarction (new Q wave) perioperatively, and most of these will show localized deterioration of wall motion on subsequent left ventriculogram. Requisites for showing improvement in left ventricular function, on the other hand, are the presence of ischemic depression of myocardial contractility occurring at the time of preoperative study, a patent graft to the ischemic segment, and absence of perioperative myocardial infarction. When these conditions are met, improved wall motion can usually be demonstrated postoperatively.

The effects of coronary artery bypass on the rate of progression of the atherosclerotic process are not known. Not unexpectedly, high-grade proximal lesions will often close following coronary artery grafting, since blood will preferentially flow through the graft rather than across the stenotic segment.

The impact of coronary artery bypass on the rate of occurrence of myocardial infarction has not been established. There are few data on the myocardial infarction rate in medically managed patients with angiographic confirmation of extent of disease for comparison. The late myocardial infarction rate in surgically managed patients appears low, however (around 1—3% per year).

The mortality rate in ischemic heart disease is best correlated with the extent of coronary artery disease shown angiographically. The yearly mortality rate for 1-, 2-, and 3-vessel disease is about 2%, 7%, and 11%, respectively. The mortality rate for patients with left main stem obstruction is similar to that of patients with three vessel involvement.

Prospective randomized studies have shown improved survival with surgical management in patients with left main stem lesions. Studies of surgically treated patients with triple vessel disease strongly suggest improved survival when compared to studies of patients with a similar extent of coronary artery disease treated medically.

It appears that in certain subsets of patients, ie, those with extensive anatomic coronary artery disease, surgical management offers the best opportunity for improved survival as well as relief of chest pain.

Bruschke AVG & others: Progress study of 590 consecutive nonsurgical cases of coronary disease followed 5—9 years. Circulation 47:1147, 1973.

Campeau L & others: Postoperative changes in aortocoronary saphenous vein grafts revisited. Circulation 52:369, 1975.

Cannom DS & others: The long-term follow-up of patients undergoing saphenous vein surgery. Circulation 49:77, 1974.

Gazes PC & others: Preinfarctional (unstable) angina: A prospective study—ten year follow-up. Circulation 48:331, 1973.

Humphries JO & others: Natural history of ischemic heart disease in relation to arteriographic findings. A twelve year study of 224 patients. Circulation 49:489, 1974.

Kannel WB & others: Natural history of angina pectoris in the Framingham study. Am J Cardiol 29:154, 1972.

Ross RS: Ischemic heart disease: An overview. Am J Cardiol 36:496, 1975.

Sternberg L & others: Significance of new Q waves after aortocoronary bypass surgery: Correlation with changes in ventricular wall motion. Circulation 52:1037, 1975.

Talano JV & others: Influence of surgery on survival in 145 patients with left main coronary artery disease. Circulation 52 (Suppl 1):105, 1975.

Ullyot DJ & others: The impact of coronary artery bypass on late myocardial infarction. J Thorac Cardiovasc Surg 73:165, 1977.

Ullyot DJ & others: Improved survival after coronary artery surgery in patients with extensive coronary artery disease. J Thorac Cardiovasc Surg 70:405, 1975.

MECHANICAL COMPLICATIONS OF MYOCARDIAL INFARCTION

1. VENTRICULAR SEPTAL RUPTURE

The incidence of ventricular septal rupture—characterized by a pansystolic murmur in the week following acute myocardial infarction—is around 1%. Perforation occurs in the muscular portion of the septum and is localized to the anterior septum in two-thirds of cases. The resultant left-to-right shunt commonly exceeds a flow ratio of 2:1. The clinical course is that of sudden deterioration followed either by cardiogenic shock and death or by gradual stabilization and chronic congestive heart failure. The prognosis is poor: there is a 50% mortality at one week and an 80% mortality at 2 months in unoperated patients.

The important differentiation is between ventricular septal rupture and mitral insufficiency. The distinction can be made at the bedside using a Swan-Ganz catheter to demonstrate a left-to-right shunt. Additional studies for preoperative evaluation include left ventriculography to assess left ventricular function and selective coronary angiography.

Initial therapy consists of medical measures to treat shock and congestive heart failure. Recent reports suggest that circulatory support with intra-aortic balloon assistance may stabilize the patient's condition, reduce myocardial ischemia, and lower the risk of diagnostic studies. The operative risk is greatly reduced when surgery can be delayed for 3—6 weeks to allow fibrous healing to occur. Surgical management consists of closing the defect, resection of associated ventricular aneurysm if present, and coronary artery bypass when appropriate. The 1-year survival in patients operated on within 6 weeks of infarction is around 10%, whereas after 6 weeks it is 35—50%.

Buckley MJ & others: Surgical management of ventricular septal defects and mitral regurgitation complicating acute myocardial infarction. Ann Thorac Surg 16:598, 1973.

Giuliani ER & others: Postinfarction ventricular septal rupture: Surgical considerations and results. Circulation 49:455, 1974.

Kitamura S, Mendez A, Kay JH: Ventricular septal defect following myocardial infarction: Experience with surgical repair through a left ventriculotomy and review of literature. J Thorac Cardiovasc Surg 61:186, 1971.

Selzer A, Gerbode F, Kerth WJ: Clinical, hemodynamic, and surgical considerations of rupture of the ventricular septum after myocardial infarction. Am Heart J 78:598, 1969.

2. MITRAL INSUFFICIENCY

Approximately 1% of early deaths from acute myocardial infarction are associated with severe mitral insufficiency. The manifestations are a systolic murmur, prominent V waves seen on pulmonary artery wedge tracing, and mitral incompetence documented by left ventriculography. This complication is less common but more likely to be fatal than ventricular septal rupture. Valvular incompetence may be due to discrete papillary muscle rupture or, more commonly, to extensive myocardial damage involving the inferior left ventricular wall (papillary muscle dysfunction). The mortality rate associated with mitral insufficiency complicating acute myocardial infarction is approximately 70% within 24 hours of the onset of the murmur and 90% within 2 weeks.

Initial management consists of medical measures to improve left ventricular failure monitoring systemic arterial, pulmonary arterial, and pulmonary artery wedge pressure and urine output. The distinction between mitral insufficiency and ventricular septal perforation can be made at the bedside by right heart catheterization using a Swan-Ganz catheter. Patients in cardiogenic shock are perhaps best managed by intra-aortic balloon pumping allowing temporary (24-hour) hemodynamic improvement while diagnostic studies are undertaken. Studies include left ventriculography to confirm mitral insufficiency and to evaluate left ventricular function and selective coronary angiography.

The clinical indication for surgery is cardiogenic shock or intractable left ventricular failure.

Surgical treatment consists of mitral valve replacement and coronary artery bypass when appropriate. Rarely, mitral valvuloplasty is done rather than valve replacement.

The operative mortality rate is related to the extent of myocardial damage. Patients with extensive left ventricular injury requiring surgery in the acute phase for cardiogenic shock have a very high operative mortality rate, but survivals have been reported. Patients operated on after 2 months have an operative mortality rate of about 25%.

Late deaths are related to the extent of coronary artery disease and are usually due to recurrent myocardial infarction.

The quality of palliation is good in surviving patients. Most patients in functional class III—IV preoperatively will be in class I—II postoperatively.

Buckley MJ & others: Surgical management of ventricular septal defects and mitral regurgitation complicating acute myocardial infarction. Ann Thorac Surg 16:598, 1973.

Merin G & others: Surgery for mitral valve incompetence after myocardial infarction. Am J Cardiol 32:322, 1973.

Mundth ED & others: Surgery for complications of acute myocardial infarction. Circulation 45:239, 1972.

3. LEFT VENTRICULAR ANEURYSM

Left ventricular aneurysm is defined as a localized protrusion of the left ventricular wall beyond the normal outer and cavitary contours. It occurs in approximately 4% of cases of acute myocardial infarction. The manifestations are abnormal precordial pulsation sustained throughout ventricular systole, ECG evidence of myocardial infarction with persistent ST segment elevation, localized left ventricular bulge seen on chest film or fluoroscopy, and demonstration of localized protrusion on left ventriculogram. By cineangiographic criteria, the incidence is about 20%. The majority of aneurysms involve the anteroseptal portion of the left ventricle. Over 50% contain mural thrombus.

The primary clinical manifestation is left ventricular failure, which is related to the extent of myocardial damage and to the degree of impairment of the efficiency of left ventricular contraction.

The prognosis is poor. Less than 20% of unoperated patients live 5 years. Survival is related to the degree of impairment of left ventricular function and to the severity of the associated coronary artery disease. Death is secondary to left ventricular failure or recurrent myocardial infarction. Rupture is rare. Other clinical sequelae include angina pectoris, ventricular tachyarrhythmias, and systemic emboli from mural thrombi.

Indications for surgery are intractable congestive heart failure, disabling angina pectoris, recurrent ventricular tachyarrhythmia, and, rarely, systemic thromboembolism.

Left ventriculography is necessary to localize the aneurysm and to evaluate residual myocardial function. The principal contraindication to surgery is generalized myocardial dysfunction. Selective coronary angiography is done to assess the coronary circulation for possible concomitant bypass grafting.

Surgical treatment consists of excision of the aneurysm combined with coronary artery bypass when appropriate.

Reports of operative mortality rates vary from 7–20%. Improvement in symptoms of congestive heart failure is seen in about 80% of surviving patients. Objective improvement in left ventricular function can be shown in two-thirds of patients studied postoperatively. Ninety percent of patients with angina pectoris experience good to excellent palliation. Improvement in survival is striking. In the largest surgical series reported, 76% of patients were alive 4 years postoperatively (see Loop reference, below). Ventricular aneurysmectomy combined with coronary artery bypass has been shown to result in better late mortality statistics than aneurysmectomy alone even though the operative mortality rate is not affected.

Chesler E, Beck W, Schrire V: Left ventricular aneurysm: A cardiologist's view. Ann Thorac Surg 13:407, 1972.
Cooley DA, Hallman GL: Surgical treatment of left ventricular aneurysm: Experience with excision of postinfarction lesions in 80 patients. Prog Cardiovasc Dis 2:222, 1968.
Loop FD & others: Aneurysms of the left ventricle: Survival and results of a ten-year surgical experience. Ann Surg 178:399, 1973.
Merin G & others: Surgery for postinfarction ventricular aneurysm. Ann Thorac Surg 15:588, 1973.
Stoney WS & others: Repair of anteroseptal ventricular aneurysm. Ann Thorac Surg 15:394, 1973.

.   .   .

PERICARDITIS

Pericarditis is an inflammatory process involving the parietal and visceral layers of pericardium and the outer myocardium. It may occur as an isolated process or as a local manifestation of systemic disease. The most common variety is idiopathic—probably viral— occurring in young adults and having a generally favorable prognosis. Other common causes are acute myocardial infarction, tuberculosis, direct bacterial contamination, rheumatic fever, postpericardiotomy syndrome, and uremia. Complications of pericarditis such as cardiac tamponade and fibrous constriction may require operative management.

Clinical Findings

A. Symptoms and Signs: Patients with acute pericarditis typically present with precordial pain or discomfort, a pericardial friction rub, evidence of cardiac tamponade, right heart failure, and fever.

B. Laboratory Findings: Leukocytosis is often present. The ECG characteristically shows ST segment elevation without reciprocal depression. The chest x-ray is usually normal.

C. Special Examinations: The presence and nature of pericardial fluid can be demonstrated by radioisotope scanning, echocardiography, pericardiocentesis, and, less commonly, angiocardiography using CO_2 or iodinated contrast material. The specific etiologic diagnosis may require open pericardial biopsy.

Differential Diagnosis

Other conditions which must be considered in the differential diagnosis of acute pericarditis are angina pectoris (particularly the Prinzmetal type), acute myocardial infarction, pleuritis, spontaneous pneumothorax, pulmonary embolism, aortic dissection, and mediastinal emphysema. Acute pericarditis may simulate peritonitis, especially in children.

Complications

A. Cardiac Tamponade: Rapid development of pericardial effusion may interfere with diastolic filling and result in diminished cardiac output and circulatory failure. Recent experimental evidence shows that increased pericardial pressure may interfere directly with coronary blood flow.

The intensity of the heart tones is diminished; the neck veins are distended, and distend even more on inspiration (Kussmaul's sign); and the paradoxical pulse (defined as a lowering of systolic pressure of greater than 10 mm Hg on normal inspiration) is accentuated. Peripheral signs of circulatory failure may be present and demand prompt treatment.

Noninvasive studies such as echocardiography and radioisotope scanning are preferred to angiocardiography in documenting effusion.

Early pericardiocentesis is indicated, especially when evidence of diminished cardiac output is present.

B. Constrictive Pericarditis: Patients with chronic constrictive pericarditis typically present with congestive heart failure, hepatomegaly, ascites, and peripheral edema. The neck veins are distended. Kussmaul's sign is commonly present; an accentuated paradoxical pulse is present in about 30% of cases. The heart sounds are quiet and the apex impulse is usually absent. A pericardial knock may be heard corresponding to fast ventricular filling in early diastole.

Low QRS voltage may be seen on the ECG. Pericardial calcification is present in 40–50% of patients but is not diagnostic of constriction. Cardiac catheterization may show characteristic early, rapid elevation of diastolic pressure and high end-diastolic pressure in both ventricles.

In some instances, open pericardial biopsy is required to distinguish between chronic constrictive pericarditis and cardiomyopathy.

Treatment

A. Medical Measures: Medical treatment of acute pericarditis consists of bed rest, salicylate analgesics for pain, and therapy directed against specific etiologic factors. Occasionally, corticosteroids are employed in idiopathic acute pericarditis, but relapse on withdrawal of therapy is common.

The results of therapy depend on the cause. Relapsing acute pericarditis may develop in as many as 10% of patients treated for acute idiopathic pericarditis.

B. Surgical Treatment: Surgical management includes pericardiocentesis (see p 217) for cardiac tamponade, open pericardial drainage for acute suppurative pericarditis, and pericardiectomy for chronic constrictive pericarditis, recurrent cardiac tamponade, and some patients with relapsing acute pericarditis.

Approximately 75% of surviving patients experience long-term benefit from pericardiectomy for chronic constrictive pericarditis. The procedure has an operative mortality rate of about 10%. Results seem to be related to the extent of associated myocardial fibrosis and atrophy and to the completeness of pericardiectomy. An adequate epicardiectomy as well as pericardiectomy over both ventricles must be accomplished to relieve chronic constriction. Hemodynamic improvement is not seen immediately after decortication, but normal intracardiac pressures are usually found on studies performed later. When the development of chronic constrictive pericarditis can be anticipated—as, for example, in tuberculous pericarditis with delayed medical treatment—early pericardiectomy is encouraged before dense fibrosis and myocardial atrophy occur.

Baue AE, Blakemore WS: The pericardium. Ann Thorac Surg 14:81, 1972.

Ellis K, King DL: Pericarditis and pericardial effusion. Radiol Clin North Am 11:393, 1973.

Engle MA & others: The postpericardotomy syndrome and anti-heart antibodies. Circulation 49:401, 1974.

Feigenbaum H, Chang S: Pericardial effusion. In: *Echocardiography.* Feigenbaum H. Lea & Febiger, 1972.

Fowler NO, Manitsas GT: Infectious pericarditis. Prog Cardiovasc Dis 16:323, 1973.

Schmid R, Goldman MJ: Pericarditis. Medical Staff Conference. West J Med 123:467, 1975.

Spodick DH: Differential diagnosis of acute pericarditis. Prog Cardiovasc Dis 14:192, 1971.

Staab EV, Patton DD: Nuclear medicine studies in patients with pericardial effusion. Semin Nucl Med 3:191, 1973.

Viola AR: The influence of pericardiectomy on the hemodynamics of chronic constrictive pericarditis. Circulation 48:1038, 1971.

Wychulis AR, Connolly DC, McGoon DC: Surgical treatment of pericarditis. J Thorac Cardiovasc Surg 62:608, 1971.

CARDIAC TUMORS

As with tumors elsewhere in the body, tumors of the heart are manifested primarily by their space-occupying effects and may remain asymptomatic until they become large. If pedunculated, a tumor can produce transient symptoms of obstruction to blood flow; if friable, it can deliver emboli into the blood stream; and if rapidly invasive on the epicardial surface, it can produce hemopericardium and pericardial tamponade.

Tumors can occur at any age. They have been reported in children as young as 6 and in adults over 70.

Benign **myxoma** is by far the most common lesion and accounts for nearly 75% of primary benign cardiac tumors (Table 22–1). Its physical characteristics range from a smooth, firm, spherical, encapsulated mass to a loose conglomeration of gelatinous material with the cohesiveness of jellied consommé. Eighty percent are pedunculated. Over 75% are attached to the septum in the left atrium, but they do also occur in the right atrium and rarely in the ventricles.

Malignant tumors are predominantly sarcomas, most commonly rhabdomyosarcoma and angiosarcoma. Malignant teratomas of the heart occur rarely.

A full spectrum of metastatic tumors to the heart has been reported. Hepatomas will extend directly into the heart through the hepatic veins.

Clinical Findings

Systemic symptoms reported with some myxomas include fever, weight loss, and anemia. Laboratory studies may show an increased sedimentation rate,

Table 22–1. Types of heart tumors.

I. Primary
A. Benign—75%
1. Myxoma
2. Rhabdomyoma (Purkinje hamartoma)
3. Papillary tumor of heart valve (Lambl excrescence)
4. Fibroma
5. Lipoma
6. Teratoma
B. Malignant—25%
1. Sarcoma: angiosarcoma, rhabdomyosarcoma, fibrosarcoma, liposarcoma, neurosarcoma, leiomyosarcoma
2. Teratoma
II. Metastatic
A. Carcinoma—67%
B. Sarcoma—20%
C. Melanoma—12%

increased gamma globulin, and variable elevations of SGOT and LDH.

The onset and clinical findings of cardiac tumors are variable, and the latter are frequently bizarre. Classically, a pedunculated left atrial myxoma has a ball valve action in the mitral orifice which obstructs flow and mimics mitral stenosis or distorts a leaflet to produce mitral insufficiency. Subtle differences in the murmurs produced may identify a tumor, particularly when the position of the patient alters the murmur.

Sudden onset of vascular obstruction, particularly in a young person with no history of cardiovascular disease, should raise a suspicion of fragmenting left atrial myxoma. If the diagnosis is verified histologically from the embolus, immediate intervention is indicated without further study.

Bizarre cardiac symptoms, distortions of the cardiac silhouette, or unexplained tamponade or signs of obstruction should lead to angiographic study, which usually makes the diagnosis.

Differential Diagnosis

A cardiac tumor may be mistaken for a variety of valvular lesions, and even angiocardiography cannot distinguish it from an atrial thrombus.

Treatment

Surgical removal of the tumor is indicated because of its obvious hemodynamic hazards. The malignant potential of a myxoma is uncertain, but recurrences have been reported. For this reason, excision of the pedicle with its base should be done whenever possible. The urgency of the necessity for removal depends upon how the tumor manifests itself. Embolization represents an imminent hazard of being repeated and should be considered an emergency. Severe hemodynamic symptoms, even if intermittent, should also be considered pressing; but mild intermittent symptoms can be dealt with electively. An asymptomatic calcified mass discovered incidentally can probably be observed without risk.

In contrast to intraluminal myxomas, sarcomas are seldom favorably localized by the time they are identified, and complete resection is almost never possible. Surgery is indicated to provide palliative relief of tumor compression and to obtain a tissue diagnosis. Radiation therapy may provide effective palliation in some instances.

Casteneda AR, Varco RL: Tumors of the heart: Surgical considerations. Am J Cardiol 21:357, 1968.

Fine G: Primary tumors of the pericardium and heart. Cardiovasc Clin 5:207, 1973.

Kabbani S, Cooley DA: Atrial myxoma: Surgical considerations. J Thorac Cardiovasc Surg 65:731, 1973.

Selzer A, Sakai FJ, Popper RW: Protean clinical manifestations of primary tumors of the heart. Am J Med 52:9, 1972.

CARDIOPULMONARY RESUSCITATION

Cardiac arrest is either a precipitous event which may lead to immediate death or the terminal result of a gradual dying process. Experience derived largely from the management of patients undergoing chest surgery has demonstrated that circulatory arrest is both preventable and reversible in a substantial number of patients, particularly when it is not the consequence of progressive and irreversible disease. It is now feasible to deal effectively with this disaster when it occurs elsewhere in the hospital. Every physician must, therefore, be familiar with the measures which may salvage the patient who "dies" unexpectedly. This responsibility includes being able to use a laryngoscope and pass an endotracheal tube, to administer effective external cardiac compression, and to apply electrical defibrillation, as well as familiarity with the drugs and fluids that should be given.

"Cardiac arrest" is manifested by asystole, ventricular fibrillation, or profound cardiovascular collapse with continued but ineffective cardiac function. Many of these terminal events may be precipitated by or associated with severe pulmonary dysfunction, and it is obviously essential to consider the heart and lungs as a single unit in providing the body's oxygen needs. Thus, attention must be directed to both organs in considering the cause and administering resuscitation.

Etiology of Cardiac Arrest

Although unrecognized or unpreventable hypoxia probably accounts for the substantial majority (perhaps 75%) of cardiac arrests, much remains to be learned about the neurohumoral and electrical mechanisms which precipitate the event. It is almost impossible to reconstruct a complete picture of the patient's cardiac status immediately prior to cardiopulmonary arrest. Nevertheless, a number of causative factors have been recognized and are worthy of attention. Conduction abnormalities are produced by hyperkalemia and hypermagnesemia. Myocardial irritability and digitalis toxicity are augmented by hypokalemia, and vasodilatation and impaired perfusion can result from sedatives, narcotics, and anesthetic agents. Respiratory acidosis and hypoxia result from the ventilatory depression produced by narcotics.

Diagnosis of Cardiac Arrest

Any patient who fails to respond to commands or painful stimulus, who becomes pale without palpable pulse or blood pressure, whose respiratory activity ceases, or whose ECG shows ventricular fibrillation or absent electrical activity should be considered to be in cardiac arrest, and resuscitation should be started. Prompt treatment produces the best results. Confirmation of the arrest is made by palpating for the carotid or femoral pulses.

Treatment of Cardiac Arrest

Suspected cardiopulmonary arrest requires that a

series of effective measures be instituted immediately without moving the patient but while simultaneously calling for assistance. Results will be closely related to prompt recognition of the problem and to the performance of a well-trained resuscitation team which should be on 24-hour call in every hospital. Persistence of resuscitative efforts should be encouraged. Patients have been saved after more than 80 depolarizing shocks or after efforts lasting over 1 hour.

Resuscitation consists of the following steps:

A. Airway: (See Fig 16–4.) The essential first step in the treatment of cardiac arrest is to establish an open airway. This can often be done by simply tilting the head backward and pulling the lower jaw forward. If the airway is still blocked, it may be necessary to manually extract vomitus or a foreign body (eg, false teeth) from the pharynx with a finger, at the same time displacing the tongue to secure an open airway. Insertion of an endotracheal tube is preferable since it gives better control of ventilation.

B. Breathing: Oxygen should be administered through the endotracheal tube or with a tight-fitting mask. If oxygen is not immediately available, ventilation can be maintained by mouth-to-mouth breathing either directly or via a Resuscitube.

C. Cardiac Resuscitation: (Fig 22–8.) Closed chest massage should be started at once. This is accomplished by placing the patient on a hard surface, being certain that adequate ventilation has been established. A sharp blow with the fist to the sternum may stimu-

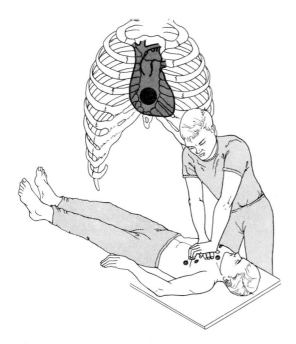

Figure 22–8. Technic of closed chest cardiac massage. Heavy circle in heart drawing shows area of application of force. Circles on supine figure show points of application of electrodes for defibrillation. (Reproduced, with permission, from Krupp MA, Chatton MJ (editors): *Current Medical Diagnosis & Treatment 1977.* Lange, 1977.)

late the heart to beat. If this is not effective, place the base of the hand on the lower end of the sternum (not the xiphoid process) and press directly downward 4–5 cm toward the spine about once per second. The pressure exerted should be enough to depress the sternum but not enough to fracture a rib. Positive action requires more than arm motion, especially in robust adult patients; it is recommended that the physician kneel on the bed astride the patient so the weight of the shoulders can be exerted against the patient's chest.

An attempt should be made to coordinate the massage with respiratory assistance so that one respiratory cycle is interposed between every 5 cardiac compressions. The carotid or femoral pulse should be palpated between each compression to determine the pressure necessary to produce a palpable pulse. Observe the pupils; persistent dilatation is a sign that adequate ventilation and perfusion have not been achieved.

Excessively vigorous compression can fracture ribs or costal cartilage and may even rupture the liver or spleen. Damage to other organs such as the lung and stomach has also been reported.

If flail chest, bilateral pneumothorax, or lacerations of the heart make external massage impossible, immediate thoracotomy and direct cardiac massage may be required.

D. Drug Therapy: Medications and electrolytes must all be administered intravenously, since absorption from the tissues in this state is limited and delayed. Persistent ventricular irritability should be treated with injections of 50–100 mg of lidocaine followed, if necessary, by an intravenous drip of this drug. If there is reason to suspect hypokalemia, potassium chloride can be administered in doses of 10–20 mEq. Impaired perfusion will result in metabolic acidosis, which should be treated by injection of 1 ampule of sodium bicarbonate intravenously. (Ampules usually contain 44 mEq.) Except in severe degrees (pH < 7.2), acidosis itself is not particularly harmful, and it is recommended that more attention be directed toward treating its cause (poor perfusion).

Inotropic drugs may be essential to stimulate adequate cardiac contraction or may be necessary to initiate systolic activity. Isoproterenol is the drug of choice because of its ancillary vasodilatory action, but epinephrine is an excellent substitute. The dosage of isoproterenol is 2 mg IV in 500 ml of 0.5 N saline or 5% dextrose and water at a rate of 10–20 drops per minute. It may be necessary to double or quadruple this dose—or, conversely, the drug may induce ventricular fibrillation and have to be discontinued.

E. Defibrillation: If the patient is in ventricular fibrillation, restoration of normal cardiac rhythm is essential but should not be attempted until effective circulation has been provided to the heart and brain (manifested by the patient's responsiveness). An ischemic heart will neither defibrillate nor respond to inotropic drugs. During the initial resuscitation efforts, while circulation and ventilation are being supported, ECG leads can be connected, effective intravenous pathways established, and arterial pressure monitoring provided.

Defibrillation should be attempted only after it is determined that the heart is fibrillating and after sufficient circulatory support has been provided to perfuse the heart and reverse hypoxia. Defibrillator electrodes must be applied with conductive jelly or over wet saline sponges. The electrodes should be placed in the midaxillary line of the left lower rib cage and over the upper sternum. The defibrillator (usually a condenser discharge system) should be set between 200 and 400 watt-seconds. Respiratory support is temporarily suspended during the shock but instantly resumed thereafter while the result is being assessed. Only one or 2 attempts at defibrillation should be made without an interval to attempt further improvement of circulation, volume loss, acidosis, or electrolyte imbalance.

Skin burns from the electrodes can be minimized by making certain that their entire surfaces are covered with conductive paste and are completely in contact with the body surface, leaving no gap for a spark to cross. On the other hand, the paste must not be smeared so as to form a conductive bridge between the 2 electrodes and thus cause a short circuit.

F. Pacemaker: Electrical pacing may be necessary when an asystole total heart block or sinus bradycardia persists. Conventional electrodes may be introduced intravenously, and percutaneous electrodes can be introduced through the apex.

Goldberg AH: Cardiopulmonary arrest. N Engl J Med 290:381, 1974.

Jude JR, Nagel EL: Cardiopulmonary resuscitation, 1970. Mod Concepts Cardiovasc Dis 39:133, 1970.

Lemire JG, Johnson AL: Is cardiac resuscitation worthwhile? A decade of experience. N Engl J Med 286:970, 1972.

Standards for cardiopulmonary resuscitation (CPR) and emergency cardiac care (ECC). 3. Advanced life support. JAMA 227 (Suppl):852, 1974.

CARDIAC PACEMAKER THERAPY

Cardiac conduction disturbances include defective impulse formation (sino-atrial node dysfunction, "sick sinus syndrome") and delay or interruption of impulse propagation (block). Symptoms are due to low cardiac output secondary to bradycardia, asystole, or escape tachyarrhythmias. The most common cause is idiopathic degeneration of the specialized conductive tissue of the heart. Other causes are myocardial infarction or ischemia secondary to coronary atherosclerosis, cardiomyopathy, drug effects, operative injury, and congenital defects.

Indications for Pacemaker Therapy

Electrical control of heart rate (pacing) may improve cardiac output, prevent asystole, and suppress ventricular irritability or ectopic rhythms.

A. Permanent: Permanent electrical pacing is indicated in symptomatic patients with bradyarrhythmia or block. Symptoms include Adams-Stokes attacks, exertional dizziness, confusion, fatigue, congestive heart failure, and angina pectoris. ECG findings include sinus bradycardia, tachycardia-bradycardia syndrome, atrial fibrillation or flutter with slow ventricular response, junctional bradycardia, second or third degree AV block, and bifascicular or trifascicular block.

B. Temporary: Temporary pacing is employed (1) in emergencies in which bradycardia is accompanied by syncope, myocardial ischemia, or hypotension; (2) for potentially reversible heart block, as in drug toxicity (digitalis, quinidine, propranolol), acute myocardial infarction, or cardiac surgical procedures; (3) for suppression of ventricular irritability and treatment of refractory tachyarrhythmias, especially in acute myocardial infarction; (4) for asymptomatic patients with heart block undergoing surgery; and (5) for patients with or without heart block having cardiac catheterization. It is common for asystole to occur in patients undergoing coronary angiography even without baseline electrocardiographic abnormalities.

Treatment

The pacemaker generator, consisting of a power source and a timing device, transmits an electrical impulse along a wire electrode which has been placed in contact with either the endocardium or the myocardium. The permanent pacemakers in use today depend on batteries using mercury-zinc, lithium, nickel-cadmium (rechargeable), or plutonium cells. Mercury-zinc cells provide power for up to 5 years, lithium to 7 years, and plutonium or rechargeable, potentially to 20 years. The timing device may be fixed rate (asynchronous), atrial synchronous, demand, or AV sequential. More than 80% of implanted pacemakers today are the ventricular-inhibited demand type which sense the patient's QRS complex and emit pulses only if the heart rate falls below a predetermined level. Demand pacing avoids pacemaker-induced ventricular fibrillation, a complication sometimes seen with fixed rate devices. Electrode wires are designed for either temporary or permanent use.

A. Temporary: Temporary pacemaker electrodes are of 2 types: (1) wires placed directly in the myocardium at the time of cardiac surgery; and (2) catheters inserted into a peripheral vein and advanced to contact the endocardium, usually of the right ventricle. The latter are of 2 types: a soft catheter which is floated into the heart using electrocardiographic monitoring, and a stiffer catheter requiring fluoroscopic control for insertion. The electrodes are connected to an external pacemaker generator which is usually maintained in the demand mode. Temporary pacing may be used for as long as 4 weeks, which, in most instances, is sufficient to determine if permanent pacemaker implantation will be needed.

B. Permanent: Permanent pacemaker electrodes

are of 2 types: myocardial wires placed usually on the left ventricle and transvenous electrodes wedged in the right ventricular endocardium under fluoroscopic control. Transvenous insertion is generally preferred because it does not require exposure of the heart and can be performed under local anesthesia. Epicardial placement is favored in children and is employed in adults when attempts at transvenous insertion fail. The electrodes are connected to an implantable pacemaker which is buried in the subcutaneous tissues of the chest wall or abdominal wall.

Results of Therapy

Permanent pacemaker implantation can be done with very low operative risk even in elderly patients and results in good palliation of symptoms. Electronic failure is rare, although present pacemaker generators must be replaced every 3–5 years. Many patients are currently followed by physician-supervised services which maintain direct or telephone contact with patients. Patients are observed for evidence of pacemaker failure and are reminded to undergo generator change prior to the expected time of battery failure. The incidence of transvenous electrode displacement is around 5%, occurring usually within 48 hours of initial insertion. Complications such as wire fracture, pacemaker extrusion, infection, ventricular perforation accompanied by cardiac tamponade, or external interference with pacemaker function are rare.

Conklin EF & others: Use of the permanent transvenous pacemaker in 168 consecutive patients. Am Heart J 82:4, 1971.

Kaltman AJ: Indications for temporary pacemaker insertion in acute myocardial infarction. Am Heart J 81:837, 1971.

Parsonnet V & others: Implantable cardiac pacemakers. Status report and resource guidelines. Report of the Inter-Society Commission for Heart Disease Resources. Circulation 50:A21, 1974.

Williams GD & others: Electric control of the heart. (2 parts.) Curr Probl Surg, Feb, March, 1974.

Wright KE Jr, McIntosh HD: Artificial pacemakers, indications and management. Circulation 47:1108, 1973.

● ● ●

General References

Behrendt DM, Austen WG: Current status of prosthetics for heart valve replacement. Prog Cardiovasc Dis 15:369, 1973.

Behrendt DM, Austen WG: *Patient Care in Cardiac Surgery,* 2nd ed. Little, Brown, 1976

Braunwald E & others: Effects of mitral valve replacement on the pulmonary vascular dynamics of patients with pulmonary hypertension. N Engl J Med 273:509, 1965.

Kirklin JW, Pacifico AD: Surgery for acquired valvular heart disease. (2 parts.) N Engl J Med 288:133, 194, 1973.

Levine FH, Copeland JG, Morrow AG: Prosthetic replacement of the mitral valve: Continuing assessments of the 100 patients operated upon during 1961–1965. Circulation 47:518, 1973.

Pluth JR, McGoon DC: Current status of heart valve replacement. Mod Concepts Cardiovasc Dis 43.63, 1974.

Reichek N, Shelburne JC, Perloff JK: Clinical aspects of rheumatic valvular disease. Prog Cardiovasc Dis 15:491, 1973.

Symbas PN: *Traumatic Injuries of the Heart and Great Vessels.* Thomas, 1972.

22...
The Heart:
II. Congenital Diseases

L. Henry Edmunds, Jr., MD

GENERAL CONSIDERATIONS

Developmental defects of the heart and great vessels encompass a wide spectrum of anatomic malformations that produce varying degrees of circulatory dysfunction. The different malformations are classified by anatomic characteristics, but the severity of individual lesions within each classification varies widely. Most importantly, the severity of the anatomic malformation often does not correlate with the degree of circulatory dysfunction. The same type of anatomic malformation may cause disabling symptoms in one patient and no symptoms in another. For proper management of patients with congenital heart disease, both the anatomic diagnosis and the pathologic physiology of the abnormal circulatory system must be understood.

The cardiac surgeon must clearly understand the pathologic anatomy of a given lesion in order to correct the structural deformity. However, the pathologic physiology of the abnormal circulation is far more important for understanding the symptoms, signs, laboratory findings, and complications of a particular anatomic lesion and the basis of medical or surgical management. To facilitate this understanding, congenital heart defects have been classified as (1) obstructive lesions, (2) lesions which increase pulmonary blood flow, (3) lesions which reduce pulmonary blood flow, and (4) complex malformations. A few rare anomalies that are not easily included in the above classification are grouped as miscellaneous lesions.

Incidence

Approximately 8–10 newborns out of every 1000 have some type of congenital heart disease. In the USA, about 12–15 thousand babies are born with congenital heart disease each year. Without treatment, about 40% of these infants will die before they are 3 months old. Some lesions are more common in one sex than the other; however, no racial predilection is recognized. High mortality rates in the first weeks and months after birth and occasional spontaneous cures reduce the incidence of congenital heart disease in school-age children to approximately 4.5 per 1000. The most reliable figures for the frequency of lesions at birth and at school age are presented in Table 22–2.

Etiology

Most congenital heart lesions occur sporadically and are not associated with other disease. With few exceptions, the cause is not known. Maternal rubella causes 1–2% of all congenital heart lesions. Characteristically, these babies have patent ductus arteriosus and peripheral pulmonary stenosis (with or without ventricular septal defect), deafness, and cataracts. Other lesions occur in association with chromosomal anomalies; the most common is the association of persistent atrioventricular canal with 21 trisomy (Down's syndrome). Some diseases such as Marfan's syndrome, gargoylism, and certain cases of supravalvular aortic stenosis are inherited diseases.

In families without known genetic defects, 14% of persons with congenital heart lesions have a relative with a congenital heart defect. This incidence is much higher than that of the general population but much lower than can be explained by genetic laws.

Clinical Diagnosis

A congenital heart lesion may produce different degrees of circulatory dysfunction and different clinical features at different ages. The clinical manifes-

Table 22–2. Frequency of various lesions in children with congenital heart disease.*

	Percentage at Birth	Percentage at School Age
Ventricular septal defect	30.8	12.5–28.1
Patent ductus arteriosus	8.0	11.2–14.1
Atrial septal defect†	10.9	15.1–20.0
Pulmonary stenosis and atresia	8.9	17.5–20.0
Aortic stenosis and atresia	6.5	11.7–17.5
Coarctation of aorta	6.0	2.5–7.5
Tetralogy of Fallot	6.1	3.8
Transposition of great arteries	4.6	
Truncus arteriosus	0.9	
Tricuspid atresia	1.2	
Miscellaneous	7.0	7.2–7.5
Undiagnosed	9.1	

*From Hoffman JIE: Natural history of congenital heart disease: Problems of its assessment with special reference to ventricular septal defects. Circulation 37:97, 1968.

†Includes ostium secundum, ostium primum, and total anomalous pulmonary venous connection.

tations of different types of anatomic malformations vary widely, and few lesions produce pathognomonic symptoms or signs. Although anatomic changes in some lesions occur during infancy and early childhood, most of the variation in symptoms and signs is due to changes in circulatory dynamics. The circulatory physiology of a newborn differs from that of an older infant or child. At birth, pulmonary vascular resistance is nearly equal to systemic resistance and both the foramen ovale and the ductus arteriosus are patent. As the ductus closes and pulmonary vascular resistance decreases, profound changes in circulatory dynamics may occur in patients with congenital heart defects. Similarly, activity affects circulatory physiology and the clinical manifestations of most congenital heart lesions.

Some newborns have obvious heart disease; others—even those with complex lesions—may appear normal at birth and show no evidence of abnormal circulation for days or weeks. In some cases, the possibility of congenital heart disease is not suspected until a murmur or abnormal finding is discovered at well baby, routine, or school examinations weeks or years after birth. Respiratory and feeding problems, cyanosis, absent or weak femoral pulses, murmurs, enlargement of the liver or heart, and failure to gain weight suggest the presence of heart disease in newborns. Frequent respiratory infections, irritability, fatigue, and poor growth and weight gain are common manifestations of congenital heart disease in older infants.

The diagnostic process should start with a thorough history and physical examination, ECG, posteroanterior and lateral chest x-rays, and hematocrit. Arterial blood P_{O_2}, P_{CO_2}, and pH determinations are often helpful. Clinical information frequently leads to an accurate diagnosis in children, but in newborns and infants these data usually only narrow the differential diagnosis. "Classical" findings of specific anatomic lesions often are absent or masked in newborns and young infants, and the differential diagnosis must include complex and potentially lethal malformations which are seldom observed in older children.

Recently, echocardiography has proved helpful in the diagnosis of congenital heart lesions. Current M-mode instruments can provide information about chamber dimensions and wall thickness, valve and vessel locations, the thickness of the ventricular septum, and the relationship of various intracardiac structures to each other. The technic is noninvasive, and echocardiographic descriptions of most congenital heart lesions are now available.

Cardiac catheterization and cineangiocardiography add the necessary information to define the anatomic and physiologic derangements. Definition of both the structural and functional abnormalities is essential for proper management of congenital heart lesions in patients of all ages.

Cardiac Catheterization & Cineangiocardiography

These special studies can be performed at any time after birth in all infants, including small prematures. Local anesthesia with or without sedation is used routinely. There are virtually no contraindications to the procedure in patients with suspected heart disease regardless of the severity of circulatory dysfunction. Catheters are introduced percutaneously through the saphenous, femoral, or brachial vein for study of the right heart chambers. The aorta and left heart are usually catheterized from the femoral or umbilical artery (occasionally the axillary or brachial artery). In this approach, the catheter is passed retrograde across the aortic valve into the left ventricle and occasionally into the left atrium. The left atrium can also be entered by passing a catheter from the right atrium across a patent foramen ovale or by perforating the interatrial septum with a special needle (older children only). Catheters are maneuvered into specific chambers and vessels under fluoroscopic vision to obtain phasic and mean pressures and blood samples and to inject contrast material for biplane (usually anteroposterior and lateral) cineangiocardiograms. During the catheterization procedure, accumulated data may prompt additional measurements, cineangiocardiograms, or special studies to make certain that the anatomic and functional abnormalities of the lesion are clearly defined.

Mean and phasic pressures in various cardiac chambers provide quantitative information that is diagnostic of many lesions. In normal individuals, mean and phasic pressures in the different cardiac chambers differ with age (Table 22–3).

Cardiac output is generally measured by either the Fick or Stewart-Hamilton method. Both measurements are subject to considerable error (15–100%). Cardiac output is corrected for differences in body size by dividing the measured cardiac output (liters/min) by body surface area (sq m) to produce the cardiac index (liters/min/sq m). Normal cardiac indices range from 3–5 liters/min/sq m.

Pulmonary vascular resistance (PVR) in Wood units is calculated by dividing the difference between mean pulmonary arterial (PA) and left atrial (LA) pressures (mm Hg) by the cardiac index. Normal pulmonary vascular resistances are 1–3 Wood units. Systemic vascular resistance is calculated by dividing the difference between mean aortic and right atrial pressures by the cardiac index. Normal systemic vascular resistances are 12–20 Wood units. The arbitrary Wood unit can be converted into dyne-sec/cm^{-5} by multiplying by 80.

Table 22–3. Normal phasic and mean pressures.*

Location	Newborn (mm Hg)	One Month After Birth (mm Hg)	Children (mm Hg)
Right atrium	(2)	(2)	(1–5)
Right ventricle	50/3	30/3	15–28/0–5
Pulmonary artery	50/30 (38)	30/12 (18)	15–28/5–15
Left atrium	(4)	(4)	(5–8)
Left ventricle	70/5	80/5	80–120/0–8
Aorta	70/45 (55)	80/50 (60)	80–120/60–75

*Numbers in parentheses are mean pressures. Other numbers are systolic/diastolic pressures.

Abnormal communications or shunts between the left and right heart chambers and great vessels can be detected by indicator dyes. More commonly, shunts are calculated by measurements of blood oxygen saturations (the percentage of hemoglobin that is saturated with oxygen). Normally, blood oxygen saturations are 70–75% in the right heart chambers and above 96% in the left heart chambers and systemic arteries. An increase in the blood oxygen saturation in the right heart chambers indicates a left-to-right shunt; similarly, a decrease in oxygen saturation in the left heart chambers indicates a right-to-left shunt. The increase in blood oxygen saturation required to diagnose a left-to-right shunt varies between 5–15% depending upon the chamber sampled and the number of measurements.

Using the Fick principle, both pulmonary blood flow (Qp) and systemic blood flow (Qs) can be calculated from measurements of blood oxygen saturation. Blood oxygen content is calculated by multiplying the saturation percentage by 1.34 and by the hemoglobin concentration (g/liter).

$$\frac{Qp}{(\text{liters/min})} = \frac{\text{Oxygen consumption (ml/min)}}{\text{Pulmonary venous } O_2 \text{ content (ml/liter)} - \text{Pulmonary arterial } O_2 \text{ content (ml/liter)}}$$

$$\frac{Qs}{(\text{liters/min})} = \frac{\text{Oxygen consumption (ml/min)}}{\text{Systemic arterial } O_2 \text{ content (ml/liter)} - \text{Mixed venous } O_2 \text{ content (ml/liter)}}$$

Effective pulmonary blood flow is defined as the amount of mixed systemic venous blood (upstream to any shunt) that passes through the lungs. Effective pulmonary blood flow (Qep) is calculated as follows:

$$\frac{Qep}{(\text{liters/min})} = \frac{\text{Oxygen consumption (ml/min)}}{\text{Pulmonary venous } O_2 \text{ content (ml/liter)} - \text{Mixed venous } O_2 \text{ content (ml/liter)}}$$

The magnitude of a left-to-right shunt equals Qp minus Qep, and the amount of a right-to-left shunt equals Qs minus Qep.

Since oxygen uptake by the lungs always equals oxygen consumption by the tissues, the relative magnitudes or ratio of pulmonary and systemic blood flows can be calculated without measuring oxygen consumption. The flow ratio is inversely proportionate to the arteriovenous differences in oxygen saturation:

$$\frac{Qp}{Qs} = \frac{\text{Systemic arterial } O_2 \text{ saturation} - \text{Systemic venous } O_2 \text{ saturation}}{\text{Pulmonary venous } O_2 \text{ saturation} - \text{Pulmonary arterial } O_2 \text{ saturation}}$$

Flow ratios can be calculated directly from oxygen saturations because the constants (1.34 and the hemoglobin concentration) used to convert blood oxygen saturation to blood oxygen content cancel out.

Cardiac catheterization is associated with an overall mortality rate of 0.06–0.44%. Infrequent complications include cardiac arrhythmias and arrest, perfora-tion of the heart, adverse reactions to contrast material, injection of contrast material into the myocardial wall, embolism, thrombosis or injury of a peripheral vessel, local hematoma formation, false aneurysm, arteriovenous fistula formation, and sepsis.

Medical Management

Drugs, diet, and activity are regulated to achieve optimal performance of the abnormal circulation and maximal growth and development of the child. Special care is required for emergencies such as congestive heart failure, arrhythmias, hypoxic spells, syncopal episodes, and infections. Careful observation may prevent development of irreversible complications such as pulmonary vascular disease, cerebral thrombosis, and bacterial endocarditis. The timing of special diagnostic and surgical procedures, recommendations to parents and school authorities, and care during unrelated illnesses are important factors in good medical management.

Operative Management

Some operations completely correct all anatomic malformations and result in the restoration of a normal circulation (eg, division of patent ductus, closure of ventricular septal defect). Other procedures improve anatomic deformities and circulatory function but fail to restore normal circulatory physiologic mechanisms and thus do not result in complete cure (eg, valvulotomy or correction of tetralogy of Fallot). Other operations require replacement of missing or deformed parts with man-made valves or conduits to achieve improvement in circulatory function. Lastly, some operations, generally called palliative procedures, actually create additional anatomic defects in order to improve circulatory function. These latter procedures are generally reserved for patients with severe lesions that cannot be anatomically improved or substituted or for patients in whom the risk of a more extensive operation is high. In general, palliative operations are designed to either reduce or increase pulmonary blood flow.

Cardiac operations may or may not require the use of the heart-lung machine. Lesions of the great vessels (eg, coarctation, vascular ring anomalies) and certain extracardiac lesions (eg, anomalous left coronary artery) can be anatomically corrected without the use of the heart-lung machine. These operations are commonly called "closed heart procedures." "Open heart procedures" require the use of the heart-lung machine in order to correct or improve intracardiac malformations. During open heart operations, venous blood is shunted from both vena cavas or the right atrium into a mechanical oxygenator and then is pumped to the patient via a cannula in the aorta or femoral artery. Cardiopulmonary bypass provides satisfactory conditions for intracardiac surgery and may be combined with moderate (28–32 C) or deep (18–22 C) hypothermia to provide periods of low perfusion flow or complete circulatory arrest.

The small size of newborns and young infants, the

complexity of many anatomic lesions that require repair, poor tolerance of prolonged periods of cardiopulmonary bypass, and better tolerance of cerebral ischemia have prompted the use of technics to temporarily arrest the circulation during corrective operations in newborns and infants. Although the circulation cannot be interrupted safely at 37 C (98.6 F) for more than 3 or 4 minutes, very short procedures such as incision of a stenotic pulmonary valve or creation of an atrial septal defect can be performed during temporary occlusion of both vena cavas. In infants, careful anesthesia and hypercapnia permit surface cooling to 18–22 C without the onset of cardiac arrhythmias that usually occur in older children and adults at around 28–32 C. In surface-cooled infants, the circulation can be arrested safely for up to 50 minutes. Although these patients can be rewarmed by surface means, surface cooling is more commonly combined with short periods of perfusion cooling using cardiopulmonary bypass. This technic speeds cooling and rewarming and ensures adequate perfusion of the entire body during rewarming. Circulatory arrest is not used unless the speed and accuracy of the intracardiac repair are greatly enhanced. Permanent neurologic sequelae are infrequent (less than 4%) after up to 50 minutes of circulatory arrest at 18–20 C.

The choice of operation requires consideration of many factors. Obviously, curative procedures are preferable to all others if the risk of operation is low. When cure cannot be achieved, such factors as residual circulatory dysfunction, early and late complications of the procedure, effects of growth, and the psychologic and sociologic burdens of the patient and parents must be considered in addition to risk. In many instances, selection and timing of operation for a given patient require the knowledge and experience of several experts and detailed anatomic and physiologic information about the lesion.

A. Intraoperative Care: At present, halothane or intravenous morphine is most commonly used for anesthesia during cardiac operations in newborns, older infants, and children. ECG, arterial blood pressure, pulse, and rectal and nasopharyngeal temperatures are monitored continuously. An arterial catheter can be inserted into the radial, brachial, femoral, dorsalis pedis, or temporal arteries by percutaneous (usually) or cutdown technics. The umbilical artery can be used in newborns. A venous catheter and one additional intravenous line are inserted for administration of blood, fluids, and drugs. During open heart surgery, central venous pressure is monitored constantly and arterial pH, P_{O_2}, and P_{CO_2} are measured intermittently. Serum potassium and ionized calcium and hematocrit are measured during and after cardiopulmonary bypass. A defibrillator, blood, sodium bicarbonate, isoproterenol, epinephrine, calcium, lidocaine, heparin, and protamine sulfate should be available in the operating room. Activated clotting times are helpful in regulating heparin dosage and protamine reversal of heparin. Fresh frozen plasma and platelet concentrates may help restore important coagulation factors

after bypass. Blood replacement and administration of fluids must be carefully controlled, particularly in very small patients. A sterile needle (No. 20, thin-walled) connected to a pressure transducer and recorder is useful for measuring particular vessel or chamber pressures during operation. Before closing the wound, the surgeon may elect to leave insulated wires attached to the atrium and small polyvinyl catheters or multiple lumen catheters (Swan-Ganz catheters) in the atria or pulmonary artery (or both).

B. Postoperative Care: Operation for congenital heart disease requires careful postoperative nursing care and observation. This is best carried out in an intensive care unit where specially trained nurses and doctors and monitoring and resuscitative equipment are constantly available. In the early postoperative period, cardiac output, ventilation, and fluid and electrolyte balances require particular attention. The management program is designed to detect abnormalities early, before irreversible damage occurs, and to support organs and organ systems that have reduced or marginal function.

Upon arrival of the patient in the intensive care unit, several monitors are connected to the patient and blood is sent for laboratory examination. The ECG and the arterial blood pressure are continuously displayed on an oscilloscope. Often central venous pressure, left atrial or pulmonary capillary wedge pressure, and pulmonary arterial pressure are continuously monitored also. Measured pressures, rectal temperature, pulse rate, and respiratory rate are charted frequently. A portable chest x-ray and a 12-lead ECG are taken. Arterial blood is analyzed for pH, P_{O_2}, and P_{CO_2}. The hematocrit and serum electrolytes (including calcium and magnesium) are measured.

1. Blood and fluid balance—Blood losses are carefully measured and replaced with filtered, fresh heparinized blood or citrated blood less than 5 days old. If blood loss has been excessive (over 3–5 ml/kg/hour), an activated clotting time (Hemochron Co.) with or without added protamine is done and blood is sent to the laboratory for platelet count, partial thromboplastin time, prothrombin time, fibrinogen concentration, and detection of fibrin split products. Deficiencies in platelet count or function and reduction of plasma clotting factors are improved by platelet transfusions and fresh frozen plasma.

Bladder catheters are not used in infants and children unless urine flow must be monitored to assess the adequacy of the circulation postoperatively. When used, bladder catheters are removed as soon as possible to avoid urethral irritation, urinary retention, or infection. When catheters are not used, urine is collected in adhesive plastic bags and diapers are weighed. Intravenous fluids and flush solutions are carefully measured and recorded.

In infants, intravenous and intra-arterial fluids are best administered by a precision pump. Drug dosages are calculated and measured carefully and are usually given intravenously early after operation. The stomach is aspirated periodically of air and fluid. Oral feedings are started as soon as peristalsis returns.

2. Cardiac output—Special attention is required to evaluate and maintain an adequate cardiac output early after operation. Cardiac output is a function of heart rate and ventricular stroke volume. Arrhythmias reduce ventricular filling, and bradycardia (less than 60) or rapid tachycardia (over 180) reduces cardiac output. Arrhythmias require prompt treatment with appropriate drugs, electrical pacing wires, and, occasionally, electrical defibrillation. The amount of blood ejected with each beat is affected by the volume of blood within the heart during diastole (end-diastolic volume), the force of the myocardial contraction, and ventricular wall tension during systole (afterload). Within limits, expansion of the blood volume and elevation of atrial pressures increase ventricular end-diastolic volume. A variety of drugs (including digoxin, catecholamines, and calcium) and pathologic states (hypoxia, acidosis, hypercapnia) alter the contractility of myocardial sarcomeres. Afterload is reduced by systemic and pulmonary vasodilators. Reduction of afterload combined with additional blood or colloids can increase cardiac output 10–25%. The ECG, atrial pressures, arterial pressure, peripheral pulses, urine output, arterial pH, and P_{CO_2} provide indirect information about the adequacy of the cardiac output. More objective information can be obtained from measurements (in duplicate) of cardiac output by dye or thermal dilution. Cardiac outputs less than 1.8 liters/sq m/min or mixed venous (pulmonary arterial) oxygen saturation less than 25% is inadequate and is associated with a high mortality rate.

3. Respiratory care—The objectives of postoperative respiratory care are to maintain pulmonary gas transfer and to prevent pulmonary complications. After operation, the soft polyvinyl endotracheal tube is not removed or is replaced by a nasoendotracheal tube if more than 12–24 hours of respiratory support is anticipated. If cardiac output is adequate and if the patient is satisfactorily awake, the patient may be extubated. In most cases, respiratory support is provided for a few hours to several days. Three levels of respiratory support are commonly used in infants and children after heart surgery. Controlled ventilation provides total respiratory support and is used in sedated and pharmacologically paralyzed patients. Intermittent mandatory ventilation is a new technic that provides 4–20 breaths per minute in sedated patients who otherwise breathe spontaneously. The third level of support is a system to provide continuous positive airway pressure (CPAP) throughout the respiratory cycle in spontaneously breathing patients. Positive end-expiratory pressures are generally used with all respiratory support systems to increase functional residual capacity and often arterial P_{O_2} and to prevent atelectasis. Arterial P_{O_2}, P_{CO_2}, and pH are measured frequently, and these values and clinical signs of excessive respiratory work are used to determine the level of respiratory support. Clinical signs of excessive respiratory work or obstruction of the endotracheal tube or major airway include flaring nares, subcostal retraction, rest-

lessness, asymmetric chest expansion, bradycardia, cyanosis, or inability to pass the tip of the aspirating catheter beyond the tip of the endotracheal tube. As soon as possible, inspired oxygen concentration is reduced below 60% to avoid oxygen toxicity. Later, mechanical ventilation and end-expiratory airway pressure are withdrawn in steps using serial blood gas measurements to guide changes.

Outward transport of mucus is extremely important in the prevention of airway obstruction and pulmonary infection. Inspired gases are warmed and humidified, and the patient's position is changed each hour. Chest physical therapy, hyperinflation of the lungs, and instillation of small amounts of 0.9% saline solution into the endotracheal tube aid mucus transport. Aspiration of the endotracheal tube is performed frequently with sterile catheters and gloves. Suspicious mucus is examined by stained smear and culture, and appropriate antibiotics are given if organisms are found.

Extubation is not performed until the patient's cardiac output is adequate and circulatory dynamics are stable. Arterial blood gases must be in the normal range when the inspired oxygen concentration is 0.4 or less. After extubation, the patient is carefully observed for evidence of respiratory insufficiency or hypoventilation. Arterial blood gases are measured every 2–4 hours, and the patient is reintubated if P_{O_2} falls below 50 mm Hg or if severe respiratory acidosis develops. Chest physical therapy, encouragement of cough, and gentle oropharyngeal aspiration are continued until respiratory function is clearly adequate.

4. Prevention of complications—Careful observation and monitoring are necessary to prevent postsurgical complications. The most frequently observed respiratory complications are hypoventilation, hypoxia due to airway obstruction, pulmonary edema, pneumothorax (in infants), aspiration of stomach contents, and pneumonia.

Arrhythmias, hypovolemia, hypervolemia, and low cardiac output, pericardial tamponade, and continuing blood losses are the most common postoperative circulatory problems.

Relatively infrequent complications include oliguria, anuria, severe electrolyte imbalance, jaundice, wound infection, seizures, coma, and CNS deficits. Septicemia from contamination of multiple catheter sites is a serious, occasionally lethal complication which must be recognized early and treated aggressively.

Campbell M: The causes of malformations of the heart. Chap 6, pp 84–88, in: *Paediatric Cardiology*. Watson H (editor). Mosby, 1968.

Edmunds LH Jr, Downes JJ: Respiratory therapy in infants. In: *Gibbon's Surgery of the Chest*, 3rd ed. Sabiston DC Jr, Spencer FC (editors). Saunders, 1976.

Hoffman JIE: Natural history of congenital heart disease: Problems of its assessment with special reference to ventricular septal defects. Circulation 37:97, 1968.

Kidd BSL, Keith JD (editors): *The Natural History and Progress in Treatment of Congenital Heart Defects*. Thomas, 1971.

Parr GVS, Blackstone EH, Kirklin JW: Cardiac performance and mortality early after intracardiac surgery in infants and young children. Circulation 51:867, 1975.

I. OBSTRUCTIVE CONGENITAL HEART LESIONS

Obstructive lesions impede the forward flow of blood, increase ventricular afterloads, and cause turbulence within the vascular system. The impedance of the obstructive lesion is inversely proportionate to the cross-sectional area or squared diameter of the lumen. A 60% reduction in cross-sectional area causes a small pressure difference across the lesion during peak systole. Further obstruction causes progressively higher pressure differences which vary in proportion to changes in blood flow velocity during the cardiac cycle. Turbulence and cavitation develop when the degree of obstruction and velocity of flow exceed critical values.

In the absence of a ventricular septal defect, an obstructive lesion at the aortic or pulmonary valve initially causes the proximal ventricle to hypertrophy. Progressive hypertrophy compensates for the increased systolic pressure and ventricular work required to maintain forward flow but eventually may cause the heart to become "muscle-bound." Severe ventricular hypertrophy reduces diastolic filling volume, ventricular wall compliance, and the contractile force of myocardial sarcomeres. Under certain physiologic conditions, subendocardial areas of the hypertrophied muscle may become ischemic. Eventually, the ventricle fails when the systolic pressure required to maintain adequate forward flow exceeds that which the ventricle can produce. Ventricular end-diastolic volume and pressure increase, ventricular stroke volume decreases, and blood accumulates in the atrium and veins upstream to the decompensated ventricle.

The most common congenital obstructive lesions of the heart and great vessels are aortic and pulmonary valvular stenosis and coarctation of the aorta. Tricuspid atresia and pulmonary atresia are discussed below in the section on lesions that decrease pulmonary blood flow. Congenital mitral stenosis and cor triatriatum—rare lesions which produce pulmonary venous hypertension—are included in this section.

PULMONARY STENOSIS

Essentials of Diagnosis

- No symptoms in patients with mild or moderately severe lesions.
- Cyanosis and right-sided heart failure in patients (usually infants) with severe lesions.
- High-pitched systolic ejection murmur that is maximal in the second left interspace. S_2 delayed and soft. Ejection click often present. Increased right ventricular impulse.
- No ejection click and inaudible S_2 in severe cases.

General Considerations

Pulmonary stenosis with intact ventricular septum is a relatively common congenital heart lesion (Table 22–2) that affects boys and girls with equal frequency. There are 2 main types: valvular and infundibular (Fig 22–9).

Valvular pulmonary stenosis occurs in approximately 95% of patients. In most patients, the commis-

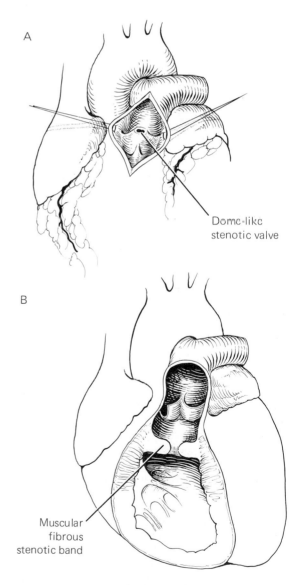

Figure 22–9. Pulmonary stenosis. *A:* Valvular pulmonary stenosis. *B:* Infundibular pulmonary stenosis.

Dome-like stenotic valve

Muscular fibrous stenotic band

sures of a flexible tricuspid semilunar valve fuse to produce a dome-like structure with a central opening of varying size (Fig 22–9A). Rarely, the valve is bicuspid, severely malformed, or associated with a hypoplastic pulmonary annulus. Infundibular stenosis associated with a normal pulmonary valve occurs infrequently and is most often caused by a distinct fibrous or muscular band in the outflow tract of the right ventricle below the pulmonary valve (Fig 22–9B). More often, hypertrophy of the right ventricular musculature narrows the infundibulum upstream to valvular pulmonary stenosis.

Most patients with pulmonary stenosis have a patent foramen ovale; a few have a true atrial septal defect. Turbulence produced by blood passing through the narrowed valvular orifice at high velocity causes poststenotic dilatation of the main pulmonary artery. As the child grows, the stenotic orifice sometimes fails to enlarge proportionately, and right ventricular pressure increases disproportionately to the increase in resting cardiac output.

In infants, severe valvular pulmonary stenosis may be associated with underdevelopment of the right ventricle.

Clinical Findings

A. Symptoms and Signs: Most children with pulmonary stenosis and an intact ventricular septum have no symptoms and grow and develop normally. A few complain of fatigue and dyspnea on exertion. Patients with very severe pulmonary stenosis may have anterior chest pain (angina), dizziness, and episodic dyspnea. These patients occasionally die suddenly. Patients with less severe obstruction who develop right ventricular failure often develop slight cyanosis. Infants with severe pulmonary stenosis feed poorly, are often lethargic, and occasionally have hypoxic spells.

Pulmonary stenosis causes a high-pitched systolic ejection murmur which is maximal in the second left anterior interspace and widely transmitted. An ejection click is frequently present but may not be audible in patients with severe stenosis. The pulmonary second sound is delayed and is usually soft. The right ventricular impulse is usually increased.

In early infancy, severe pulmonary stenosis may cause right ventricular failure and cyanosis from right-to-left shunting of blood through a patent foramen ovale. These infants have a systolic ejection murmur (which may be less intense than that found in older children), hepatomegaly, cardiomegaly, cyanosis, and poor peripheral perfusion.

B. X-Ray Findings: Most children have abnormal chest roentgenograms. Dilatation of the main pulmonary artery and enlargement of the right ventricle, atrium, or entire heart are the most common findings. The degree of cardiac enlargement is not always proportionate to the severity of the right ventricular hypertension. The aortic arch is on the left. In infants with right-to-left shunting, pulmonary vascular markings may be reduced.

C. Electrocardiography: ECGs indicate right atrial and ventricular hypertrophy, and with few exceptions the changes are proportionate to the severity of the obstructive lesion and the pressure in the right ventricle. In neonates, the ECG may show left ventricular or biventricular hypertrophy.

D. Cardiac Catheterization and Cineangiocardiography: Cardiac catheterization reveals the magnitude of the right ventricular pressure, which may exceed left ventricular pressure, and the site of the obstruction. Cineangiocardiograms demonstrate severe malformations, hypoplastic annuli, secondary infundibular muscular hypertrophy, and other lesions.

Differential Diagnosis

In children, pulmonary stenosis must be differentiated from aortic stenosis, small ventricular septal defect, and tetralogy of Fallot. In neonates, severe pulmonary stenosis must be distinguished from aortic stenosis, pulmonary atresia, tricuspid atresia, tetralogy of Fallot, and hypoplastic right ventricle.

Natural History

Approximately half of deaths due to pulmonary stenosis occur in infants under 1 year of age. The remainder occur in asymptomatic children or adults who develop severe right ventricular hypertension and reduced cardiac output. The frequency with which moderate pulmonary stenosis progresses to severe pulmonary stenosis is not known. Available evidence suggests that progressive stenosis, severe right ventricular hypertension, and failure rarely develop in patients with right ventricular-pulmonary arterial pressure differences below 50–60 mm Hg.

Treatment

Infants who have severe right ventricular failure or hypoxic spells require urgent operation. Cardiac catheterization and angiographic studies are necessary to exclude other lesions such as pulmonary atresia or hypoplastic right ventricle. Open pulmonary valvulotomy and closure of the foramen ovale are carried out using cardiopulmonary bypass and hypothermia. A patent ductus, if present, should be ligated. Less satisfactorily, valvulotomy may be performed under direct vision while the venous return (both vena cavas) to the heart is interrupted for 2 or 3 minutes at 37 C (inflow occlusion). Less frequently, a valvulotome (a spear-like instrument) is introduced through the right ventricle of the beating heart and guided through the stenotic pulmonary valve (Brock procedure). After blind incision of the fused leaflets, a dilator is used to open the orifice further. Infants with associated underdevelopment of the right ventricle require a systemic-pulmonary arterial anastomosis in addition to the pulmonary valvotomy.

Operation is generally recommended for children or adults who have a pressure difference of 60 mm Hg or more across the pulmonary valve. Temporary cardiopulmonary bypass is used. The stenotic valve is exposed through a pulmonary arteriotomy. Every effort is made to completely relieve the obstruction without causing pulmonary regurgitation, but a small amount of regurgitation is preferable to incomplete relief of the stenosis. The infundibulum is palpated through the opened pulmonary valve to detect the presence of a localized muscular or fibrotic obstruction. Severe infundibular obstructions can be excised through a right ventriculotomy or, preferably, through a right atriotomy with careful retraction of the tricuspid leaflets. Most often, hypertrophied infundibular muscle without fibrosis need not be excised since it regresses after the valvular obstruction is adequately removed. Occasional patients who have a hypoplastic pulmonary annulus require a pericardial patch across the annulus. At operation, the atrial septum should be explored to close possible atrial septal defects or a patent foramen ovale.

Prognosis After Surgery

The hospital mortality rate following operations for relief of pulmonary stenosis in children and adults is 2–3%. Patients with severe stenosis who do not have resection of secondarily hypertrophied infundibular muscle often have right ventricular hypertension at the operating table and for weeks or months postoperatively; this regresses, but it may cause some degree of right ventricular failure postoperatively. Serious operative complications include neurologic injuries, hemorrhage, wound infection, postpericardiotomy syndrome, transient arrhythmias, and respiratory problems.

In over 90% of patients, operation relieves symptoms and results in regression of ECG and x-ray abnormalities. Most patients have postoperative systolic murmurs and often diastolic murmurs which were not present preoperatively. Only 10% of patients have significant residual abnormalities.

Gilbert JW, Morrow AG, Talbert JL: The surgical significance of hypertrophic infundibular obstruction accompanying valvular pulmonic stenosis. J Thorac Cardiovasc Surg 46:457, 1963.

Mustard WT, Jain SC, Trusler GA: Pulmonic stenosis in the first year of life. Br Heart J 30:255, 1968.

Nadas AS: Pulmonic stenosis: Indications for surgery in children and adults. N Engl J Med 287:1196, 1972.

Tandon R, Nadas AS, Gross RE: Results of open-heart surgery in patients with pulmonic stenosis and intact ventricular septum. Circulation 31:190, 1965.

AORTIC STENOSIS

Four types of congenital aortic stenosis are generally recognized (Fig 22–10). Valvular aortic stenosis is the most common; subaortic and supravalvular aortic stenosis and asymmetric septal hypertrophy occur infrequently.

1. VALVULAR AORTIC STENOSIS

Essentials of Diagnosis

- Usually asymptomatic in children; angina and syncope indicate severe stenosis.
- May cause severe heart failure in infants.
- Prominent left ventricular impulse, narrow pulse pressure.
- Harsh systolic murmur and thrill along left sternal border; systolic ejection click.

General Considerations

Valvular aortic stenosis occurs predominantly in males. In about 20% of patients, the lesion is associated with other congenital heart defects (endocardial fibroelastosis, patent ductus arteriosus, coarctation of the aorta, ventricular septal defect, and pulmonary stenosis). The aortic leaflets are thickened, fibrotic, and malformed. All 3 commissures may be fused, but more often one commissure is absent or poorly formed, so that the aortic valve is bicuspid. Stenosis results if the remaining commissures are fused or if the leaflet tissue becomes stiff and calcified in adult life. Calcification of the valve does not occur in childhood, but poststenotic dilatation of the ascending aorta may occur. Occasionally, hypoplasia of the aortic annulus, absence of 2 commissures, or aortic regurgitation may be associated with valvular aortic stenosis.

Newborns with symptomatic valvular aortic stenosis often have poor left ventricular function due to subendocardial ischemia or endocardial fibroelastosis. In many cases the aortic annulus is small, and a patent foramen ovale is usually present.

Clinical Findings

A. Symptoms and Signs: Many individuals have bicuspid aortic valves which are not stenotic during childhood and early adult life. Most children with congenital valvular aortic stenosis are asymptomatic and have normal growth. A few patients with relatively severe stenosis develop dyspnea, angina, or syncope with effort. Neonates with severe aortic stenosis develop severe heart failure and cyanosis with associated feeding difficulties and respiratory distress.

A harsh, basal systolic murmur with a palpable thrill, a prominent left ventricular impulse, and a narrow pulse pressure are characteristic physical findings. The heart may not be enlarged. The murmur is usually transmitted into the neck, but in infants the murmur may not be audible because of heart failure and low cardiac output. Infants have tachypnea, hepatomegaly, cardiomegaly, cyanosis, poor peripheral perfusion, and often an increased right ventricular impulse.

B. X-Ray Findings: In children, chest x-rays are normal or show some degree of left ventricular hypertrophy. In some patients, the elevated left ventricular end-diastolic and atrial pressures cause pulmonary venous congestion. The ascending aorta may be dilated (poststenotic dilatation). Infants with severe aortic stenosis usually have dilated cardiac silhouettes and

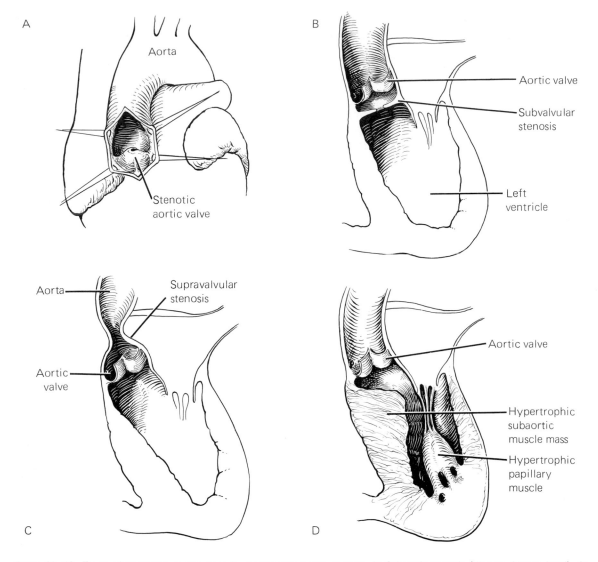

Figure 22–10. Types of congenital aortic stenosis. *A:* Valvular aortic stenosis. *B:* Subaortic stenosis (discrete fibrous band). *C:* Supravalvular aortic stenosis. *D:* Idiopathic hypertrophic subaortic stenosis.

pulmonary venous congestion.

C. Electrocardiography: The vectorcardiogram correlates better with peak left ventricular pressure than does the ECG. The ECG usually shows left ventricular hypertrophy in children who have a pressure difference across the aortic valve of more than 50 mm Hg, but occasionally the ECG is normal in these patients. In infants, the ECG does not show left ventricular hypertrophy with aortic stenosis and may show right ventricular hypertrophy. The presence of symptoms or ECG evidence of left ventricular strain indicates severe aortic stenosis.

D. Cardiac Catheterization and Cineangiocardiography: With patience, a catheter can usually be passed retrograde through the stenotic aortic valve into the left ventricle. These studies are necessary to confirm the diagnosis, to differentiate valvular stenosis from

other types, to measure pressure differences, and to identify associated lesions. Neonates may shunt left to right across a stretched patent foramen ovale.

Differential Diagnosis

Valvular aortic stenosis must be differentiated by cardiac catheterization and cineangiocardiography from subvalvular and supravalvular aortic stenosis and pulmonary stenosis. In newborns, the absence of a murmur and the difficulty in detecting cyanosis may cause confusion between aortic stenosis and other lesions such as total anomalous pulmonary venous connection or double outlet right ventricle.

Natural History

About 10% of infants born with congenital aortic stenosis develop heart failure within the first year of life, and most of these will die without operation. Neonates who develop severe failure within 1 month of birth have a particularly poor prognosis because of the severity of the lesion and poor left ventricular function. A few patients who survive the neonatal period develop heart failure, but the majority do not develop symptoms until later childhood or adulthood.

Serial measurements show that the severity of aortic stenosis often increases with growth. Sudden death occurs in 1–7% of children who have congenital aortic stenosis. Most of these children develop symptoms before death. About 20% of patients with congenital aortic stenosis develop some degree of aortic valvular regurgitation. Patients with bicuspid aortic valves and minimal aortic stenosis may develop symptomatic aortic stenosis after their fifth decade from fibrosis and calcification of the abnormal valve. All patients are susceptible to bacterial endocarditis of the deformed valve.

Treatment

Infants who develop severe heart failure which cannot be controlled with digoxin and diuretics require urgent operation. Successful operations have been performed utilizing either inflow occlusion at 34–37 C or a short period of cardiopulmonary bypass. Cardiopulmonary bypass provides better operative conditions and therefore permits the surgeon to produce the best possible aortic valve with the tissue at hand. Commissures of the stenotic valve are incised to relieve the obstruction caused by the thickened abnormal valve. Undeveloped commissures cannot be cut because unsupported leaflets will prolapse to produce aortic regurgitation, which is poorly tolerated. Successful relief of the obstruction is directly related to the structural pathologic characteristics of the valve.

Asymptomatic children with congenital aortic stenosis should refrain from severe exercise. Most of these children do not require operation until after 8–10 years of age. The appearance of symptoms (particularly syncope or angina) or signs of left ventricular strain on the ECG indicates the need for cardiac catheterization and cineangiocardiography. Patients with a systolic pressure difference of over 50 mm Hg at rest are candidates for aortic valvotomy. Operation is always performed with temporary cardiopulmonary bypass. With few exceptions, incision of fused commissures results in partial or complete relief of the aortic stenosis without producing severe aortic regurgitation. Rarely, a prosthesis must be inserted for a badly deformed or torn valve or for associated hypoplasia of the aortic annulus.

Prognosis After Surgery

Valvotomy during the first 2–3 weeks after birth salvages some infants, but many die of inoperable lesions or severe malfunction of the left ventricle. Results are usually related to the preoperative condition of the patient, left ventricular function, and whether or not the surgeon can relieve the obstruction without producing aortic regurgitation. After the first

month, the prognosis improves, and over 80% of infants less than 1 year of age survive valvotomy. During childhood, the mortality rate of elective valvotomy is less than 5%. Late deaths occur in approximately 10% of infant survivors. About 40% of older children who have aortic valvotomy have postoperative aortic regurgitation. Within 10 years, about 25% of patients with aortic valvotomy require reoperation or develop significant restenosis. Since the valve leaflets are deformed, most if not all patients will eventually require reoperation and probably prosthetic replacement of the aortic valve in adult life.

Braunwald E & others: Congenital aortic stenosis: Clinical and hemodynamic findings in 100 patients. Circulation 27:426, 1963.

Friedman WF: Serial hemodynamic observations in asymptomatic children with valvar aortic stenosis. Circulation 43:91, 1971.

Keane JF & others: Aortic stenosis surgery in infancy. Circulation 52:1138, 1975.

Lakier JB & others: Isolated aortic stenosis in the neonate: Natural history and hemodynamic considerations. Circulation 50:801, 1974.

2. SUBAORTIC STENOSIS

A discrete muscular or fibrous membrane or a diffusely narrowed segment of the left ventricular outflow tract (Fig 22–10B) causes a pressure difference between the body of the left ventricle and the aortic valve. The lesion seldom causes symptoms in infants, but in children the symptoms and findings are similar to those in patients with valvular aortic stenosis. The majority of patients with subvalvular aortic stenosis have both systolic and diastolic basal murmurs and frequently have additional cardiac defects. Turbulence in the left ventricular outflow tract often causes thickening of the normal aortic leaflets and poststenotic dilatation of the ascending aorta. Occasionally, valvular and subvalvular aortic stenosis may occur simultaneously. The diffuse or tunnel type of subvalvular aortic stenosis is sometimes associated with anomalous insertion of the anterior leaflet of the mitral valve. At cardiac catheterization, a pressure difference is found as the catheter is withdrawn from the body of the left ventricle to the ascending aorta. Cineangiocardiograms and the absence of pressure changes after administration of isoproterenol differentiate subaortic stenosis from valvular aortic stenosis and asymmetric septal hypertrophy.

Approximately two-thirds of patients have a discrete subvalvular fibrous or muscular membrane which is attached to the lateral edges of the anterior leaflet of the mitral valve and ventricular septum. This membrane is excised during temporary cardiopulmonary bypass after the aorta has been opened and the normal aortic leaflets have been retracted. Excision of the tunnel type of subvalvular aortic stenosis is more difficult. Occasionally, the left ventricle must be opened to excise obstructive tissue deep within the ventricular cavity, and sometimes the mitral valve must be excised and replaced. Recently, older children with severe tunnel type subaortic stenosis have been successfully treated using a valved prosthetic conduit from the apex of the left ventricle to the subdiaphragmatic aorta. In patients with discrete subvalvular aortic stenosis, the operative mortality rate is less than 5%; the pressure difference is relieved; and the lesion does not recur. The operative mortality rate is considerably higher in patients with the tunnel type of subaortic stenosis, and some of the survivors do not get satisfactory relief of the obstruction.

Cooley DA & others: Surgical treatment of left ventricular outflow tract obstruction with apico-aortic valved conduit. Surgery 80:674, 1976.

Reis RL & others: Congenital fixed subvalvular aortic stenosis. Circulation 43 (Suppl 1):11, 1971.

3. SUPRAVALVULAR AORTIC STENOSIS

In most patients, supravalvular aortic stenosis is an isolated lesion and is not associated with mental retardation or genetic factors. The sexes are affected with equal frequency. Occasional patients have familial supravalvular aortic stenosis which occurs as an isolated lesion or in association with peripheral pulmonary arterial stenoses. Mental retardation, "elfin facies," strabismus, dental anomalies, inguinal hernia, and narrowing of peripheral systemic and pulmonary arteries occur in approximately 20% of patients with supravalvular aortic stenosis. Hypercalcemia in early infancy has been found in many of these patients.

The aorta usually has an hourglass deformity just above the aortic valve (Fig 22–10C); less commonly, the lesion is caused by a localized fibrotic membrane or hypoplasia of the ascending aorta. Symptoms and physical findings are similar to those of valvular aortic stenosis with the exception that the aortic second sound may be accentuated. The diagnosis is confirmed by cardiac catheterization and cineangiocardiography.

Localized fibrotic membranes and discrete hourglass deformities can be alleviated by insertion of a prosthetic patch in the ascending aorta. Hypoplasia of the ascending aorta cannot be corrected by operation. Asymptomatic patients who have pressure gradients less than 70 mm Hg at rest are not candidates for operation.

Rastelli GC & others: Surgical treatment of supravalvular aortic stenosis. J Thorac Cardiovasc Surg 51:873, 1966.

4. ASYMMETRIC SEPTAL HYPERTROPHY (ASH)

This genetically transmitted disease of cardiac muscle features disproportionate thickening of the ventricular septum as compared to the ventricular free wall. Myocardial sarcomeres are hypertrophied and arranged in a bizarre pattern. The asymmetric muscle mass may or may not cause obstruction of the left ventricular outflow tract (Fig 22–10D). Symptomatic patients nearly always have some degree of obstruction during systole. Abnormal forward motion of the anterior leaflet of the mitral valve during systole brings this leaflet against the asymmetric hypertrophied septal mass. The severity of the obstruction increases during systole and is proportionate to the volume of the left ventricular cavity, the force of ventricular contraction, and the cross-sectional area of the left ventricular outflow tract during systole. Exercise, digitalis, isoproterenol, epinephrine, and nitroglycerin alter these dynamic relationships and generally increase the pressure difference across the obstructive area. During the normal systole which follows the premature ventricular beat, arterial pulse pressure decreases in patients with ASH and increases in patients with valvular aortic stenosis. The hypertrophied muscle occasionally obstructs the right ventricular outflow tract as well as the left and may interfere with the function of the mitral valve. The cause of the progressive muscular hypertrophy is not known. A basal systolic murmur which was not previously present may be the first clinical sign of ASH. Many new cases and asymptomatic patients without obstructive ASH are discovered by echocardiography of relatives of known patients with the disease. The most common symptoms are fatigue, syncope, angina, and dyspnea on exertion. Variable physical findings include prominent left ventricular impulse, a basal systolic murmur with thrill, and a bifid carotid arterial pulse.

Heart size is often normal but may be enlarged on chest roentgenograms. The ECG is nearly always abnormal. Left ventricular hypertrophy, prolongation of the Q–T interval, ST and T abnormalities, and abnormal Q waves are the most common findings. The diagnosis is made by echocardiography. During cardiac catheterization, the diagnosis is confirmed by finding characteristic pressure changes in response to premature ventricular contraction and infusion of isoproterenol. Lateral cineangiocardiograms demonstrate systolic narrowing of the left ventricular outflow tract opposite the mitral valve.

The natural history of the disease is variable but tends to be progressive. Sudden death occurs, and most patients do not reach their fifth decade. In symptomatic children, the risk of death is approximately 4% per year. Propranolol may alleviate symptoms in many patients with left ventricular outflow obstruction but does not reverse the progressive hypertrophy. Symptomatic patients must not be given digitalis, isoproterenol, or nitroglycerin.

Operation requires temporary cardiopulmonary bypass. Several operations have been devised, but most commonly the abnormal hypertrophied muscle beneath the right coronary cusp of the aortic valve is incised with parallel incisions. The intervening muscle tissue is removed. The operation is preferably performed through an aortotomy, but occasionally a left ventriculotomy is necessary. Some surgeons have recommended excision and replacement of the mitral valve to completely relieve left ventricular outflow obstruction, but this is rarely necessary.

The operative mortality rate is less than 10%. Complications include residual stenosis and iatrogenic heart block, ventricular septal defect, or mitral regurgitation. Left bundle branch block is nearly always produced. Although operation usually alleviates or abolishes the obstruction, occasional patients may still suffer sudden death.

Epstein SE & others: The role of operative treatment in patients with idiopathic hypertrophic subaortic stenosis. Circulation 48:677, 1973.

Muron BJ & others: Asymmetric septal hypertrophy in children. Circulation 53:9, 1976.

COARCTATION OF THE AORTA

Essentials of Diagnosis

- Infants may have severe heart failure; children are usually asymptomatic.
- Absent or weak femoral pulses.
- Systolic pressure higher in upper extremities than in lower extremities; diastolic pressures are similar.
- Harsh systolic murmur heard in the back.

General Considerations

Coarctation or stenosis of the aorta is a relatively common congenital heart lesion (Table 22–2) that occurs twice as frequently in males as in females. Ninety-eight percent of all aortic coarctations are located at or near the aortic isthmus (the segment of aorta adjacent to the ligamentum arteriosum or ductus arteriosus). Rarely, coarctation may occur in other aortic locations or in multiple sites. In over 50% of patients, the aortic valve is bicuspid.

Patients with coarctation of the aorta are divided into 2 relatively distinct groups by the clinical course of the disease during the first year after birth. Some infants develop severe life-threatening heart failure. Over 60% of those infants have major associated cardiac lesions including patent ductus arteriosus, which is common. Tubular hypoplasia of the aortic arch, anomalous origin of the right subclavian artery, ventricular and atrial septal defects, left ventricular outflow obstructions, fibroelastosis, transposition of the great arteries, and double outlet right ventricle (Taussig-Bing type) are the most frequently encoun-

tered associated lesions.

The majority of patients with coarctation of the aorta do not develop life-threatening symptoms during infancy. With the exception of bicuspid aortic valves and patent ductus arteriosus, associated lesions are not common, but approximately 2% of patients have congenital mitral regurgitation. The aortic constriction is usually well localized and produced by both external narrowing and an intraluminal diaphragm. In nearly half of patients with coarctation, the internal diameter of the constricted segment is between 0.5 and 5 mm. About one-fourth are larger, and another fourth are atretic. In older children, the aortic wall upstream to the fibrous diaphragm develops intimal thickening and atheroma formation. Downstream, the aorta usually dilates and may have a plaque of intimal thickening where the jet of blood passing through the coarctation hits the aortic wall. In older children and adults, the aorta downstream to the coarctation becomes thin, friable, and eventually calcified. In these patients, intercostal arteries frequently become aneurysmal.

Coarctation causes systolic and diastolic hypertension in the proximal aorta and upper extremities and stimulates the enlargement of collateral vessels that connect branches of the subclavian arteries to arteries that originate from the aorta downstream to the coarctation. In most patients, blood flow to the lower body is not reduced, but pulse pressure downstream to the aortic coarctation is decreased and peak systolic pressure is delayed after peak pressure in the upstream aorta. Left ventricular work is increased.

The pathophysiology of the proximal hypertension is not understood. In some infants who have poorly developed collateral vessels, blood flow to the lower body is reduced, but even in these patients the presence of the coarcted segment does not explain the magnitude of the proximal hypertension. Most patients with aortic coarctation have normal plasma angiotensin concentrations and normal renal blood flow and function. The possibility that the sensitivity of aortic and carotid baroreceptors changes in coarctation has not been confirmed in animal experiments.

Clinical Findings

A. Symptoms and Signs: Most patients with aortic coarctation are asymptomatic and well developed. Occasionally, children complain of headaches, fatigue, pains in the calves when running, or frequent nosebleeds. The disease is usually detected during routine physical examination by detecting weak or absent femoral pulses, measuring elevated arm blood pressures, or auscultating a harsh systolic murmur along the left sternal border and in the back. The femoral pulse, if palpable, is delayed as compared to the radial pulse. In the upper extremities, systolic blood pressure is 20 mm Hg or more higher than that in the lower extremities, but diastolic pressures are similar. A systolic murmur with thrill in the suprasternal notch is usually present; occasionally, the murmur is continuous. If collateral vessels are well developed, flow murmurs may be heard in the axillas, medial to the scapulas, and over the lateral ribs. A few patients have apical systolic murmurs from mitral regurgitation or precordial systolic murmurs from aortic stenosis.

Most symptomatic infants with coarctation develop severe heart failure within the first 6 weeks after birth. Signs include tachypnea, dyspnea, respiratory distress, pulmonary rales, hepatomegaly, poor feeding, poor weight gain, and poor peripheral perfusion. The heart is enlarged and usually has a gallop rhythm. Murmurs are generally not diagnostic because of associated lesions. Femoral pulses are generally weak or absent, but the amplitude may vary at different observations. Infrequently, right-to-left shunting through a patent ductus arteriosus that is downstream to the coarctation causes cyanosis of the lower body.

B. X-Ray Findings: Chest x-rays usually show left ventricular enlargement with or without notching of ribs between T3 and T8 in children with coarctation. Occasionally, the aorta bulges proximal and distal to the coarcted segment to produce a 3 sign in the plain chest film. The reverse, or E sign, is seen in the barium-filled esophagus.

The heart is greatly enlarged in symptomatic infants, and the peripheral lung fields appear congested. Rib notching is not present, and the contour of the descending thoracic aorta is usually obscured by the thymus gland.

C. Electrocardiography: The ECG shows left ventricular hypertrophy which is proportionate to the severity of the coarctation and proximal hypertension in children. In infants, particularly those less than 6 months of age, the ECG shows an abnormal increase in right ventricular hypertrophy with or without left ventricular hypertrophy. Isolated left ventricular hypertrophy is rare in infants with aortic coarctation.

D. Cardiac Catheterization and Cineangiocardiography: These studies document the pressure difference across the coarctation, illustrate the local anatomy and the adequacy of collateral vessels, and often are diagnostic of an associated bicuspid aortic valve. In symptomatic infants, cardiac catheterization and cineangiocardiography are necessary to demonstrate the length of the coarcted segment and to define associated intracardiac and extracardiac lesions. Left ventricular end-diastolic pressures are always greatly elevated in these patients. Pulmonary venous blood is often partially unsaturated because of associated respiratory problems.

Differential Diagnosis

Clinical signs, particularly proximal hypertension and reduced, delayed femoral pulses, establish the diagnosis of coarctation in children. In symptomatic infants, the differential diagnosis must include other diseases which cause severe heart failure, particularly aortic stenosis, interrupted aortic arch, hypoplastic left heart, and fibroelastosis.

Natural History

Children who survive infancy rarely die before their second decade; however, the mean age at death in these patients is about 40 years. Patients die of congestive heart failure, cerebral hemorrhage or thrombosis, ruptured intercostal arterial aneurysms, or dissecting aneurysms of the ascending aorta. Pregnant women with coarctation are more susceptible to complications. Since the advent of antibiotics, bacterial infections of the coarcted segment or bicuspid aortic valve are rare causes of death.

In symptomatic infants, heart failure is the most common cause of death. Cerebral hemorrhage and hypertensive encephalopathy are rare causes.

Treatment

Resection of the stenotic segment of the aorta is recommended for nearly every patient with coarctation of the aorta. The optimal age for elective operation is between 4 and 8 years. In children, the elastic aorta can be brought together for a primary anastomosis in nearly all cases. Infrequently, the coarcted segment may be enlarged or a prosthetic graft may be used to bridge the distance between the 2 ends of the aorta. If collateral vessels are poorly developed or if operation is required for restenosis of the aorta, hypothermia to 31 C, partial cardiopulmonary bypass, or a temporary shunt is recommended to protect the spinal cord from ischemic injury during cross-clamping of the aorta. For most children, well-developed collateral vessels supply the distal aorta during temporary aortic cross-clamping.

An intensive trial of medical measures (digoxin, diuretics, morphine, and oxygen) is recommended for all infants with severe heart failure associated with coarctation of the aorta. The infant often improves dramatically within a few hours, and operation can be postponed until childhood. Infants who do not respond to medical therapy within 12–24 hours require immediate operation, since otherwise the mortality rate approaches 100%. Operation consists of resection of the aortic coarctation and division of a patent ductus arteriosus if this lesion is also present. Additional palliative procedures (eg, pulmonary arterial banding) are added depending upon specific associated intracardiac lesions.

Prognosis After Surgery

In children, operative mortality for elective resection of aortic coarctation is 1–2%. The operative mortality rate increases in adult patients who have friable, atheromatous aortas. All patients obtain some relief of the proximal hypertension, and over 80% of children eventually have normal systolic blood pressures. However, blood pressures may remain elevated immediately after operation and gradually decrease over a 6-month period.

Hemorrhage is the most frequent postoperative complication. Paraplegia or paraparesis is a rare (0.4%) but catastrophic complication and is related to the adequacy of the collateral circulation and the duration of aortic cross-clamping during construction of the anastomosis. Necrotizing arteritis of mesenteric vessels develops rarely, although up to one-fourth of patients develop abdominal pain 2–7 days postoperatively. Some patients have paradoxical hypertension after operation which is often associated with abdominal pain. The hypertension and pain are thought to be due to increased sympathetic activity and possibly increased plasma renin. These patients nearly always respond to sympatholytic drugs which reduce blood pressure and reduce the likelihood of severe necrotizing arteritis with gangrenous bowel. Injury to the left recurrent laryngeal nerve and chylothorax are infrequent complications.

The operative mortality rate is 15–25% in symptomatic infants who require resection of aortic coarctation for heart failure that is unresponsive to medical therapy. The mortality rate is lowest in the occasional infant who develops severe heart failure and does not have associated intracardiac lesions. The mortality rate increases in proportion to the severity of the associated lesions, and occasional patients with hypoplastic left hearts or severe fibroelastosis are inoperable.

Restenosis develops at the suture line in a few patients–particularly infants who require emergency operation. In children, restenosis is usually due to technical factors, the use of continuous sutures, or progressive fibrosis and scarring. Rarely, infants may develop rapid restenosis and recurrence of the symptoms of heart failure within a few weeks or months after operation. More commonly, progressive stenosis occurs, and most infants who survive resection of aortic coarctation have small systolic pressure differences across the anastomosis at follow-up cardiac catheterization during childhood. The pathogenesis of rapid or progressive restenosis is not known.

Brewer LA III & others: Spinal cord complications following surgery for coarctation of the aorta. J Thorac Cardiovasc Surg 64:368, 1972.

Fishman NH & others: Surgical management of severe aortic coarctation and interrupted aortic arch in neonates. J Thorac Cardiovasc Surg 71:35, 1976.

Freed MD & others: Coarctation of the aorta with congenital mitral regurgitation. Circulation 49:1175, 1974.

Hartmann AF Jr & others: Recurrent coarctation of the aorta after successful repair in infancy. Am J Cardiol 25:405, 1970.

Rocchini AP & others: Pathogenesis of paradoxical hypertension after coarctation resection. Circulation 54:382, 1976.

Schuster SR, Gross RE: Surgery for coarctation of the aorta: A review of 500 cases. J Thorac Cardiovasc Surg 43:54, 1962.

Sinha SN & others: Coarctation of the aorta in infancy. Circulation 40:385, 1969.

INTERRUPTED AORTIC ARCH

Absence of the aortic arch distal to the left subclavian artery (type A) or between the left carotid and left subclavian arteries (type B) causes approximately 4% of deaths due to congenital heart disease in infants. Almost any intracardiac anomaly may coexist with interrupted aortic arch, and all patients have an associated intracardiac lesion. Ventricular septal defect is most common. The distal aorta receives blood from a patent ductus arteriosus which often constricts shortly after birth. Severe heart failure with acidosis develops, and most infants die within the first month after birth.

Reconstruction of the aortic arch by direct anastomosis or bridging vessels with or without simultaneous palliation of the intracardiac lesion has produced survival in up to 60% of patients. Occasional patients have survived simultaneous correction of the intracardiac anomaly and reconstruction of the arch.

Fishman NH & others: Surgical management of severe aortic coarctation and interrupted aortic arch in neonates. J Thorac Cardiovasc Surg 71:35, 1976.

Van Praagh R & others: Interrupted aortic arch: Surgical treatment. Am J Cardiol 27:200, 1971.

AORTIC ATRESIA

Atresia of the aortic valve is associated with hypoplasia of the ascending aorta, hypoplasia or atresia of the left ventricle, and atresia or severe stenosis of the mitral valve. Coronary arteries arise from the base of the hypoplastic ascending aorta. A large patent ductus and an atrial septal defect are required for life, and most patients die within a few days. Systemic and pulmonary venous blood are mixed in the atria and then pumped by the right ventricle to the pulmonary arteries and systemic arteries via a patent ductus arteriosus. Aortic atresia and other variants of hypoplastic left heart are the most common causes of death from congenital heart disease in the first week of life. Infants may appear normal at birth but soon develop congestive heart failure with poor peripheral pulses and variable cyanosis. Physical, radiographic, and electrocardiographic findings are not diagnostic; cardiac catheterization and cineangiocardiography are required to establish the diagnosis and to rule out other lesions for which effective therapy exists. At present, medical management is ineffective, and operations are not usually recommended.

Cayler GG, Smeloff EA, Miller GE Jr: Surgical palliation of hypoplastic left side of the heart. N Engl J Med 282:780, 1970.

MITRAL ATRESIA & STENOSIS

In approximately 50% of patients with congenital mitral stenosis, the lesion is associated with hypoplasia of the left heart and aortic atresia. Patients who have mitral atresia with a normal aortic valve often have a hypoplastic left ventricle that communicates with the large right ventricle through a ventricular septal defect. Other anomalies—particularly of the systemic and pulmonary veins—are often present. Patients with mitral atresia with normal aortic valves seldom survive early infancy.

In congenital mitral stenosis not associated with aortic atresia, the funnel-shaped valve is thickened, with short, fused chordae tendineae and poorly defined commissures. Patients frequently have associated lesions (patent ductus arteriosus, aortic stenosis, coarctation of the aorta). The principal symptoms are dyspnea and frequent respiratory infections due to pulmonary hypertension and pulmonary congestion. An apical diastolic rumble with associated thrill is invariably present; an opening snap, loud first sound, and mitral systolic murmurs are also usually present. Chest x-rays show a dilated left atrium and increased pulmonary venous markings. In time, pulmonary vascular disease can occur if the stenosis is not relieved.

Over half of these infants die in their first year, and few survive childhood. A few mitral valves can be improved by valvuloplasty; more often, the deformed valve must be excised and replaced with a prosthesis. A few infants and young children have survived mitral valve replacement.

Tsuji HK & others: Congenital mitral stenosis. J Thorac Cardiovasc Surg 53:850, 1967.

COR TRIATRIATUM

In this rare anomaly, pulmonary veins enter a small accessory left atrial chamber which communicates with the normal-sized true left atrium through a small opening. Pulmonary venous hypertension causes pulmonary congestion and, eventually, increased pulmonary arterial and right ventricular pressures. Patients have severe dyspnea and frequent respiratory infections but do not have an apical diastolic rumble. An elevated pulmonary arterial or pulmonary capillary (wedge) pressure and a normal left atrial pressure at cardiac catheterization strongly suggest the diagnosis, which is proved by cineangiocardiography. Operation requires cardiopulmonary bypass and consists of excision of the obstructing membrane between the accessory chamber and the normal left atrium. Without operation, over half of patients die in infancy.

Brickman RD & others: Cor triatriatum. J Thorac Cardiovasc Surg 60:523, 1970.

II. CONGENITAL HEART LESIONS WHICH INCREASE PULMONARY ARTERIAL BLOOD FLOW

Approximately 50% of all congenital heart lesions shunt blood from the systemic arterial circulation into the pulmonary circulation (left-to-right shunt). The most common lesions in this group are patent ductus arteriosus and defects of the atrial septum, atrioventricular canal, and ventricular septum. Rare lesions include ruptured sinus of Valsalva, aortic-pulmonary window, truncus arteriosus, and some types of transposition of the great vessels, double outlet right ventricle, and other complex lesions.

Because compliance of the thick-walled left ventricle is less than that of the right ventricle and because systemic vascular resistance is normally about 10 times higher than pulmonary vascular resistance, pressures in the left heart chambers and systemic arteries are higher than corresponding pressures in the right heart and pulmonary arteries. These higher pressures cause some of the oxygenated blood in the left heart and systemic arteries to shunt through abnormal anatomic communications and to recirculate through the lungs without passing through systemic capillaries. The excessive pulmonary circulation causes pulmonary vascular congestion, resulting in frequent respiratory infections, and places an additional burden on the involved ventricle (the right ventricle in atrial septal defects; the left ventricle in patent ductus arteriosus; and both ventricles in atrioventricular canal and ventricular septal defects). The increased "volume load" or "preload" increases the diastolic volume of the involved ventricle. As the ventricle dilates, end-diastolic pressure increases; eventually, the ventricle may fail (ie, at the point at which an increase in ventricular volume at end-diastole no longer causes an increase in ventricular stroke volume).

In the circulation, resistance, flow, and pressure are related by the formula $R = P/F$, where R is resistance of a specified segment of the circulatory system (impedance when flow is pulsatile), P is the pressure difference across the resistance (in mm Hg), and F is the flow in liters/min/sq m. Conventionally, resistance is calculated in "Wood units" (mm Hg/liter/min/sq m). Resistances vary in different segments of the circulatory system. When no abnormal communications or shunts are present, blood passes through these resistances serially. When an abnormal communication is present, the relative downstream resistances of the normal and abnormal pathways largely determine relative blood flows in each pathway. This simplistic but useful concept is clearly illustrated in patients who have large ventricular septal defects in which the pressures in the right and left ventricles are nearly equal throughout the cardiac cycle. If we assume equal atrial pressures, the mean pressure difference across the pulmonary vascular bed is the same as that across the systemic vascular bed. Under these conditions, the ratio of pulmonary to systemic blood flow (10:1) is inversely proportionate to the ratio of the pulmonary to systemic resistance (1:10). In actual practice, the pulmonary-systemic flow ratio is less because of blood streaming within the ventricles, unequal atrial pressures, compliance of the pulmonary vasculature and ventricles, and other dynamic factors.

Because blood flow is pulsatile, pressures, flow, velocity, and impedance within the circulatory system change throughout the cardiac cycle. As indicated above, if dynamic factors are ignored by using mean pressures, flows, and resistances, the ratio of downstream resistances largely determines the ratio of net flows through normal and abnormal (shunt) pathways. Because the mean left atrial pressure is 2–3 mm Hg higher than the mean right atrial pressure, the net flow across an atrial septal defect is from left to right. However, during the cardiac cycle, phasic tracings of right and left atrial pressures show moments when right atrial pressure exceeds the simultaneous left atrial pressure. At these times, blood flows from right to left across the defect. Thus, although the net shunt is from left to right, atrial septal defects and many other shunts within the vascular system are actually bidirectional because of dynamic factors.

Increased pulmonary blood flow increases pulmonary arterial blood pressure. Although pulmonary vessels are very distensible (and therefore compliant), pulmonary arterial pressure in the normal lung approximately doubles when pulmonary blood flow triples. Elevation of left atrial pressure from excessive flow or increased left ventricular end-diastolic pressure increases pulmonary arterial pressure, interstitial lung water, and probably pulmonary vascular resistance. If pulmonary arterioles also constrict in response to the increased blood flow, pulmonary vascular resistance increases (hyperkinetic pulmonary hypertension) and pulmonary arterial pressure may increase further unless flow decreases. Pulmonary vasoconstriction can be reversed by inhalation of oxygen or intravenous tolazoline, and this test is used to differentiate hyperkinetic pulmonary hypertension from pulmonary vascular disease. The elevation in pulmonary arterial pressure increases the afterload of the right ventricle, which already may have an increased "volume" or "preload" if the septal defect is in the atrium or ventricle.

In some patients, increased pulmonary blood flow and increased pulmonary arterial pressure eventually cause muscular hypertrophy of the media of pulmonary arterioles (stage 1), proliferation of intima (stage 2), and, eventually, hyalinization and fibrosis of the media and adventitia (stage 3). These morphologic changes, termed "pulmonary vascular disease," are acquired, but they are more likely to occur in congenital lesions which produce both high pulmonary arterial pressure and large flows (ventricular septal defect, complete atrioventricular canal, truncus arteriosus) than in those that produce increased pulmonary blood flow only (atrial septal defect, total anomalous pulmonary venous connection). Pulmonary venous hypertension and chronic hypoxemia from residence at high altitudes also favor the development of pulmonary vascular disease. As the cross-sectional area of the pulmonary vascular bed decreases as a result of the morphologic changes, pulmonary vascular resistance increases and the ratio of pulmonary vascular resistance to systemic vascular resistance increases. The amount of blood shunted from left to right decreases. When pulmonary vascular resistance equals or exceeds systemic vascular resistance, left-to-right blood flow across the lesion ceases or reverses. The term Eisenmenger's syndrome describes the condition in which obstruction of the pulmonary vasculature reduces pulmonary blood flow and causes blood to shunt from right to left. Patients who have advanced pulmonary vascular disease (stage 3) and balanced or reversed shunts (Eisenmenger's syndrome) cannot be helped by operation and frequently do not survive the attempt. Often these patients live many years as they develop progressive cyanosis and polycythemia from their lesion which now shunts blood from right to left.

Pulmonary arterial banding is a palliative operation which is designed to reduce pulmonary arterial blood flow by increasing the total resistance to blood flow across the lungs (Fig 22–11). The band constricts the main pulmonary artery downstream to the valve and adds a resistance in series to the vascular resistance of the lung. Ideally, total resistance of the band and the lungs should equal systemic vascular resistance. If vascular resistance in the lungs is already high, only a small resistance can be added by the band. Because of dynamic changes in cardiac output pressures and resistances within the circulation, addition of a fixed resistance (the band) cannot produce balanced pulmonary and systemic flows under all physiologic conditions. However, a good band can reduce pulmonary arterial blood flow sufficiently to alleviate ventricular failure and prevent rapid progression of pulmonary vascular disease. Unfortunately, preexisting pulmonary vascular disease may not regress after banding.

Congenital heart lesions which thoroughly mix

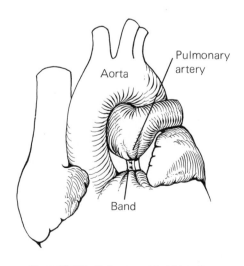

Figure 22–11. Pulmonary arterial banding.

systemic and pulmonary venous blood (eg, total anomalous pulmonary venous connection, single ventricle, truncus arteriosus) cause cyanosis. In these lesions, the oxygen saturation of aortic and pulmonary arterial blood may be similar, and the severity of the cyanosis is directly proportionate to the relative amounts of fully saturated pulmonary venous blood and unsaturated systemic venous blood that are mixed. If the amount of blood which flows through the lungs is 3 or more times the amount of systemic blood flow, the resulting oxygen saturation of the mixed blood will be high and cyanosis will be minimal. (For example, 3 parts oxygenated blood [20 ml O_2/100 ml] added to 1 part systemic venous blood [14 ml O_2/100 ml] saturates 92% of the hemoglobin in the mixed blood [18.5 ml O_2/100 ml].) Conversely, if an associated obstructive lesion or pulmonary vascular disease reduces the amount of pulmonary arterial blood flow in relation to systemic arterial blood flow, the mixed systemic and pulmonary venous blood will be much less saturated and cyanosis will be severe. (For example, 1 part oxygenated blood [20 ml O_2/100 ml] added to 3 parts systemic venous blood [14 ml O_2/100 ml] saturates only 77% of the hemoglobin in the mixed blood [15.5 ml O_2/100 ml].)

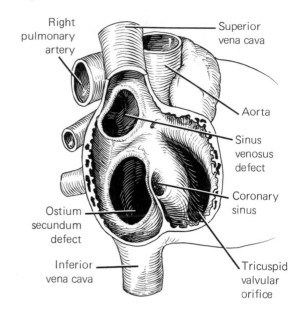

Figure 22–12. Sinus venosus and ostium secundum defects in the atrial septum as viewed from the opened right atrium.

ATRIAL SEPTAL DEFECT, OSTIUM SECUNDUM TYPE

Essentials of Diagnosis

- Acyanotic, asymptomatic.
- Right ventricular lift.
- S_2 widely split and fixed.
- Grade 1–3/6 ejection pulmonary systolic murmur.
- Diastolic flow murmur at the lower left sternal border.

General Considerations

These defects occur in the region of the fossa ovalis. They may be single or multiple and vary in size from a few millimeters to 5 cm in diameter. Secundum defects are distinguished from (1) sinus venosus defects, which occur cephalad at the inlet of the superior vena cava into the right atrium; (2) patent foramen ovale, which is present in approximately 20% of the population; (3) right hemianomalous pulmonary veins with an intact atrial septum; and (4) ostium primum defects, which are discussed below (Fig 22–12). In approximately 10% of patients, atrial septal defects are associated with either right hemianomalous pulmonary veins or persistent left superior vena cava.

Clinical Findings

A. Symptoms and Signs: Uncomplicated atrial septal defects seldom cause symptoms. Rarely, infants will develop heart failure, and children will become fatigued and dyspneic upon exertion more easily than normal children. Characteristic physical signs include a midsystolic ejection murmur over the upper left heart border with a loud and widely split second heart sound which does not change with respiration. The systolic murmur is due to turbulence at the pulmonary valve caused by the high-velocity ejection from the right ventricle. Fixed splitting of the second sound is an important diagnostic sign and is due to the fact that inspiration delays the sound of aortic valve closure (A_2) in patients with atrial septal defect. Thus, inspiration delays both A_2 and P_2; consequently, the interval between the 2 sounds does not change during the respiratory cycle. In patients with large left-to-right shunts (> 2:1), a soft diastolic murmur caused by blood passing through the tricuspid valve is also heard.

B. X-Ray Findings: Plain chest films reveal increased pulmonary vascularity and often an enlarged right atrium and ventricle.

C. Electrocardiography: The ECG is either normal or shows right axis deviation and right ventricular hypertrophy without conduction abnormalities.

D. Cardiac Catheterization and Cineangiocardiography: At cardiac catheterization, the catheter usually passes easily into both atria across the atrial septum. Blood samples from the right atrium and ventricle show an increase in oxygen saturation of at least 10% as compared to samples from the superior vena cava. Cineangiocardiograms after left atrial injection show simultaneous opacification of both atria.

Differential Diagnosis

Ostium secundum defects must be distinguished from common atrioventricular canal, total anomalous pulmonary venous connection, small ventricular septal defects, left ventricular to right atrial shunts, and hemianomalous pulmonary veins with an intact septum. Ostium primum defects, sinus venosus defects, and hemianomalous pulmonary veins are easily recognized and corrected at operation; preoperative recognition is not essential. In total anomalous pulmonary venous connection, blood oxygen saturation is the same in the right atrium, both ventricles, the pulmonary artery, and the aorta. Cineangiocardiograms after left ventricular injections are particularly useful for detecting small ventricular septal defects or left ventricular-right atrial shunts.

Natural History

Heart failure from uncomplicated ostium secundum defects is rare in childhood but occurs in approximately 40% of adults over 30 years of age. Pulmonary vascular disease does not occur in children but does occur in 5–10% of adults with untreated lesions. Patients who have small left-to-right shunts (< 2:1) do not require operation. Bacterial endocarditis is rare, but atrial arrhythmias may occur in adults and can precipitate severe heart failure in the aged.

Treatment

Ostium secundum defects are closed during temporary cardiopulmonary bypass. The heart is approached through a midline sternotomy or a right thoracotomy. The margins of the defect usually can be approximated by direct suture; occasionally, a patch of pericardium is necessary. Hemianomalous veins are redirected into the left atrium by shifting the atrial septum to the right of the orifices of the pulmonary veins. Sinus venosus defects are usually patched, and occasionally the entrance of the superior vena cava must be enlarged as well.

Prognosis After Operation

The mortality rate following open repair of ostium secundum defects should be less than 1%. Complications include air embolism with subsequent CNS damage, postoperative atrial arrhythmias, wound infection, and hemorrhage.

Sellers RD & others: Secundum type atrial septal defects: Results with 275 patients. Surgery 59:155, 1966.

Zaver AG, Nadas AS: Atrial septal defect—secundum type. Circulation 31 (Suppl 3):24, 1965.

ATRIAL SEPTAL DEFECT, OSTIUM PRIMUM TYPE

Essentials of Diagnosis

- Acyanotic; asymptomatic, or dyspnea on exertion.
- Fixed, widely split second sound.
- Apical systolic murmur (often).
- ECG shows left axis deviation; QRS frontal vector is counterclockwise.

General Considerations

Ostium primum defects are part of a group of lesions which occur during development of the atrioventricular canal. Ostium primum defects (occasionally called incomplete atrioventricular canal) are less severe than complete atrioventricular canal defects, which involve the interventricular septum as well as the atrial septum. Ostium primum defects are located low in the atrial septum, caudad to the fossa ovalis and adjacent to the coronary sinus and the orifice of the tricuspid valve. The aortic leaflet of the mitral valve is usually cleft; occasionally, the septal leaflet of the tricuspid valve is cleft also. The septal defect is usually 2–4 cm in diameter. The incidence of ostium primum defects is approximately one-third that of ostium secundum defects.

Clinical Findings

A. Symptoms and Signs: Most children are asymptomatic or complain of dyspnea on exertion and easy fatigability. Occasional infants develop severe congestive heart failure from mitral regurgitation and a large left-to-right shunt across the ostium primum defect. Physical signs include a systolic ejection murmur which is maximal in the second left intercostal space, fixed wide splitting of the second sound, and often a systolic murmur at the apex of the heart which is transmitted to the left axilla.

B. X-Ray Findings: Plain chest films usually show cardiomegaly with increased pulmonary vasculature. Both atria and both ventricles may be enlarged.

C. Electrocardiography: The ECG is characteristically abnormal: the mean QRS axis is shifted to the left (usually 0 to −60 degrees); the P–R interval is often prolonged; and P waves are often tall. The frontal QRS loop of the vectorcardiogram is oriented superiorly and is inscribed in a counterclockwise direction. These findings are suggestive (but not pathognomonic) of an ostium primum defect or persistent atrioventricular canal.

D. Cardiac Catheterization and Cineangiocardiography: During cardiac catheterization, an increase in oxygen saturation nearly always occurs in the right atrium. Left atrial pressures may be elevated, and the *v* wave may be prominent. Cineangiocardiograms taken after left ventricular injection often demonstrate mitral incompetence and opacification of the atria before the right ventricle is seen. In the posteroanterior projection, the abnormally low attachment of the anterior leaflet of the mitral valve produces a characteristic "gooseneck" deformity of the left ventricular outflow tract.

Differential Diagnosis

Ostium primum defects must be distinguished from more severe defects of the atrioventricular canal, ventricular septal defects, ostium secundum defects, and congenital mitral valvular regurgitation. The ECG, vectorcardiogram, and cineangiocardiographic findings are particularly important in the differential diagnosis.

Natural History

Ostium primum defects with associated severe mitral regurgitation or tricuspid regurgitation may cause heart failure in infancy and childhood. Bacterial endocarditis is rare, and pulmonary vascular disease generally does not develop until adult life.

Treatment

Ostium primum defects in children are repaired through a median sternotomy using cardiopulmonary bypass. When mitral regurgitation is present, the cleft in the mitral valve is approximated with interrupted sutures in such a way as to correct regurgitation without narrowing the mitral valvular annulus. If the valve is not incompetent, no sutures are placed in the cleft. The primum defect is closed with a pericardial patch.

Prognosis After Operation

The mortality rate of repair of ostium primum defects in children is approximately 3%. Aside from air embolism, the most important operative complication is complete heart block due to ligature of the conduction bundle during repair of the primum defect.

Many patients have a residual apical systolic murmur after operation, but mitral regurgitation is usually trivial.

Braunwald NS, Morrow AG: Incomplete persistent atrioventricular canal. J Thorac Cardiovasc Surg 51:71, 1966.

Gerbode F & others: Endocardial cushion defects. Ann Surg 166:486, 1967.

COMPLETE ATRIOVENTRICULAR CANAL

Essentials of Diagnosis

- Heart failure common in infancy.
- Cardiomegaly, blowing pansystolic murmur, other variable murmurs.
- Loud S_2 with fixed splitting.
- ECG shows left axis deviation and counterclockwise frontal QRS vector loop.

General Considerations

Abnormal development of the atrioventricular endocardial cushions in utero causes a central deficiency of both the atrial and ventricular septa and deficiencies of the mitral and tricuspid valves. Partial and complete atrioventricular canal defects differ in whether or not the septal leaflets of the mitral and tricuspid valves attach firmly to the crest of the interventricular septum. In partial atrioventricular canal, the tricuspid valve is firmly attached to the ventricular septum so that there is no direct communication between the left and right ventricles. The anatomy is essentially that of an ostium primum defect with varying degrees of atrioventricular valvular deficiencies. In complete atrioventricular canal (CAVC), mitral and tricuspid leaflets are either not attached to the ventric-

ular septum or are attached by chordae (Fig 22−13). Thus, a direct communication between the 2 ventricles exists. Furthermore, the mitral and tricuspid valves are not separately formed but exist as part of a common atrioventricular valve. Complete atrioventricular canal defects have been classified under 3 surgically important types by Rastelli and his colleagues. About one-third of patients with CAVC have additional cardiovascular anomalies.

The common atrioventricular valve is incompetent, and blood is shunted from left to right at both the atrial and ventricular levels. Right ventricular pressure equals left ventricular pressure, and pulmonary arterial pressure is elevated, often to systemic levels.

Clinical Findings

A. Symptoms and Signs: Most infants with complete atrioventricular canal develop heart failure during the first few weeks or months of life. Symptoms include poor feeding, failure to grow, and frequent respiratory problems. These babies have tachypnea, hepatomegaly, an active, enlarged heart, and a blowing pansystolic murmur which is often associated with a thrill at the left sternal border. Slight cyanosis may be apparent during crying or feeding. If pulmonary arterial flow is greatly increased, the second sound is loud and split through all phases of respiration. An apical systolic murmur, a fourth left interspace soft systolic murmur, and a diastolic murmur are present.

B. X-Ray Findings: Plain chest films show moderate to severe cardiomegaly, increased pulmonary vasculature, and pulmonary congestion. Heart size may be normal at birth.

C. Electrocardiography: The ECG nearly always shows left axis deviation with superior orientation and counterclockwise inscription of the frontal QRS vector. Biventricular hypertrophy and prolongation of the P−R interval are usually present.

D. Echocardiography: Echocardiograms show abnormal motion of the anterior mitral leaflet, may indicate separation of the leaflet by the cleft, and may show lack of continuity between the atrioventricular valves and ventricular septum.

E. Cardiac Catheterization and Cineangiocardiography: Cardiac catheterization reveals arterialized blood in the right atrium. The venous catheter can be easily pushed into all cardiac chambers. Ventricular pressures are often identical; atrial pressure and pulmonary arterial pressures are elevated. Pulmonary vascular resistance is often increased. Severe increased pulmonary vascular resistance decreases the magnitude of the left-to-right shunt and may reduce arterial oxygen saturation. Cineangiocardiograms after left ventricular injection reveal a characteristic "gooseneck" deformity of the mitral valve and left ventricular outflow tract in the anteroposterior projection. Contrast material frequently regurgitates from both ventricles into both atria. Cineangiography in left and right anterior oblique projections may be helpful in determining the presence or absence of a direct interventricular communication.

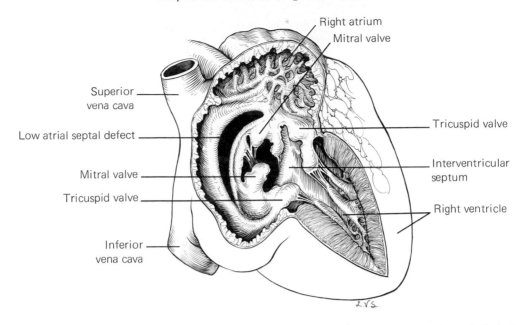

Figure 22-13. Complete atrioventricular canal. The most common type has a divided anterior common atrioventricular leaflet. Both the mitral and tricuspid portions are attached to the interventricular septum with long, nonfused chordae tendineae. The mitral and tricuspid portions of the common posterior atrioventricular leaflet are not separated. (Modified from Rastelli & others, 1968.)

Differential Diagnosis

The ECG, vectorcardiogram, echocardiogram, and clinical findings of heart failure, pansystolic murmur with loud, split S_2, and increased pulmonary arterial blood flow are sufficiently distinctive to make the diagnosis in most instances. Cardiac catheterization and cineangiocardiography confirm the diagnosis and help to define the amount of pulmonary overcirculation, the degree of pulmonary hypertension, and the severity of the anatomic lesion.

Natural History

Many infants with complete atrioventricular canal die, and those that do survive have repeated episodes of heart failure and respiratory infection. Pulmonary hypertension and vascular disease generally develop during childhood in patients who survive infancy and are not treated. Patients with less severe atrioventricular canal malformations may remain well. These patients generally have diminished growth, easy fatigability, and dyspnea on exertion and frequently must take digitalis and diuretics.

Treatment

Occasional infants with increased pulmonary arterial blood flow, pulmonary hypertension, and heart failure may benefit from pulmonary arterial banding. Unfortunately, heart failure usually persists after pulmonary arterial banding for CAVC, and growth and development are limited. Patients who have direct left ventricular-right atrial shunts or severe atrioventricular valvular regurgitation are not helped by banding.

Complete repair of CAVC defects can be carried out at any age using cardiopulmonary bypass, deep hypothermia, and circulatory arrest. Results are directly proportionate to the severity of the valvular malformations and whether or not adequate valvular tissue is available for reconstruction of a reasonably competent mitral valve. Some infants have severely malformed, primitive deformities which cannot be formed into a competent functioning mitral valve.

For successful correction, pulmonary vascular resistance should be 70% or less than systemic vascular resistance. The repair is generally carried out through a right atriotomy. Three anatomic types of persistent atrioventricular canal defects are recognized, and the 2 most common types can be repaired using a patch (pericardium or Dacron) sutured to the cephalad margin of the ventricular septum, the atrioventricular valves, and the atrial margin of the defect. Septal portions of the mitral and tricuspid leaflets are sutured to the patch. In the third type, some of the chordae tendineae of each atrioventricular valve arise from the opposite ventricular cavity; thus, the ventricular septal defect cannot be closed without interfering with the function of the atrioventricular valves. In these patients, either a small hole in the ventricular patch must be left for the chordae, or the mitral valve must be excised and replaced. Since severe mitral regurgitation is the most common cause of death after operation, mitral valve replacement is required if the mitral valve cannot be reconstructed. The tricuspid valve often cannot be completely repaired, but a small amount of regurgitation is generally well tolerated.

Prognosis After Operation

The hospital mortality rate of pulmonary arterial banding during infancy for common atrioventricular canal is approximately 20%. The mortality rate for complete repair of common atrioventricular canal defects (excluding ostium primum) is 5–15% in children. Occasional infants have survived complete repair of this defect, but the mortality rate of the operation is very high. Some patients have residual mitral or tricuspid valvular stenosis or regurgitation, and nearly all have a residual apical systolic murmur. Complete heart block occurs in 5–10% of patients. Most surviving patients are improved, with increased exercise tolerance, reduced heart size, and reduced pulmonary vascularity. Occasional patients (5–10%) die months or years later of unexplained causes.

Casteneda AR & others: Surgical correction of complete atrioventricular canal utilizing ball valve replacement of the mitral valve. J Thorac Cardiovasc Surg 62:926, 1971.

Hunt CE & others: Banding of the pulmonary artery: Results in 111 children. Circulation 43:395, 1971.

McGoon DC & others: Correction of complete atrioventricular canal in infants. Mayo Clin Proc 48:169, 1973.

Rastelli GC & others: Surgical repair of the complete form of persistent common atrioventricular canal. J Thorac Cardiovasc Surg 55:299, 1968.

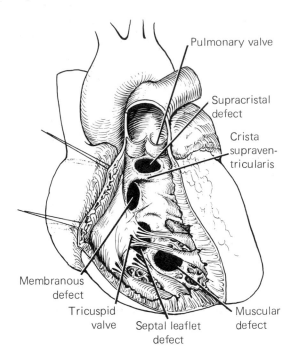

Figure 22–14. Anatomic locations of various ventricular septal defects. The wall of the right ventricle has been excised to expose the ventricular septum.

VENTRICULAR SEPTAL DEFECT

Essentials of Diagnosis

- Asymptomatic if defect is small.
- Heart failure with dyspnea, frequent respiratory infections, and poor growth if the defect is large.
- Grade 2–6/6 pansystolic murmur maximal at the left sternal border.
- S_2 loud with apical diastolic flow murmur and biventricular enlargement if the defect is large.

General Considerations

Approximately 85% of ventricular septal defects occur in the membranous septum, which is located just beneath portions of the right coronary and noncoronary aortic cusp adjacent to the anterior and septal leaflets of the tricuspid valve and caudad to a muscular ridge in the outflow tract of the right ventricle called the crista supraventricularis (Fig 22–14). A small number of ventricular defects occur anterior to the crista supraventricularis just beneath the pulmonary valve (supracristal defects), beneath the septal leaflet of the tricuspid valve, or in the muscular ventricular septum. Muscular septal defects (about 10% of patients) are frequently multiple and may occur in association with other types of ventricular septal defects.

Membranous or high ventricular septal defects vary in size from a few millimeters to more than 3 cm in diameter. The conduction bundle is located at the posterior and caudal margins of these defects, usually near the endocardium of the left ventricle. Anomalies commonly associated with ventricular septal defects include patent ductus arteriosus, coarctation of the aorta, and atrial septal defect. Ventricular septal defects which are associated with pulmonary stenosis are discussed under tetralogy of Fallot. Occasionally, supracristal or membranous ventricular septal defects are associated with significant aortic regurgitation, which is usually due to elongation and prolapse of the noncoronary aortic cusp. Rarely, ventricular septal defect may be associated with absence of the pulmonary valve.

Clinical Findings

A. Symptoms and Signs: The clinical features of ventricular septal defects are directly related to the size of the defect and the amount of pulmonary blood flow. The patient with a small ventricular septal defect is asymptomatic and has a normal ECG and chest film. A systolic murmur with thrill can be heard over the third and fourth left interspace, but no diastolic murmur is present at the apex. Left ventricular pressure is higher than right ventricular pressure, and pulmonary arterial blood flow is seldom more than twice systemic blood flow.

Children with moderate or large ventricular septal defects may be asymptomatic or may complain of dyspnea on exertion and easy fatigability. On physical examination, a loud pansystolic murmur with thrill is present along the lower left sternal border, and the heart is hyperactive. A soft diastolic flow murmur is present at the apex. P_2 is sometimes normal or decreased, but if pulmonary hypertension is present P_2 may be increased and delayed and the apical diastolic murmur is absent. The heart is usually enlarged; the pericardium may bulge; and growth is often slightly retarded. A few patients with associated aortic insufficiency also have a diastolic murmur in the third and fourth left sternal interspaces.

Infants with moderate or large ventricular septal defects often have severe heart failure. Failure is particularly likely if a patent ductus arteriosus is also present. Dyspnea, tachycardia, feeding problems, liver enlargement, and respiratory distress may occur 2–3 months after birth as the normally increased pulmonary vascular resistance of the newborn begins to decrease. The heart is enlarged and hyperactive and may have a gallop rhythm. A pansystolic murmur and apical diastolic murmur are present, and P_2 is loud and delayed.

B. X-Ray Findings: Chest films in patients with moderate or large ventricular septal defects show increased pulmonary vasculature with large pulmonary arteries and enlargement of both ventricles. If pulmonary vascular disease is present, the main pulmonary vessels appear very large, vessels of moderate size appear clubbed, and fine markings are reduced in peripheral lung fields. The right ventricle is greatly enlarged.

C. Electrocardiography: The ECG usually shows left ventricular hypertrophy and may show biventricular hypertrophy if pulmonary vascular resistance is moderately increased or if pulmonary blood flow is exceptionally large. If the ratio of pulmonary to systemic vascular resistance is high (> 0.75), large, notched R waves are present in the right precordial leads.

D. Cardiac Catheterization and Cineangiocardiography: The diagnosis is made or confirmed at cardiac catheterization by finding an increase in right ventricular blood oxygen saturation of more than 10%. The catheter often passes through the defect into the opposite ventricle. Ventricular pressures are equal or nearly equal in patients who have large ventricular septal defects and large pulmonary arterial blood flows. Right ventricular and pulmonary arterial pressures are elevated but are below systemic pressures in patients with moderate-sized ventricular septal defects. Cineangiocardiograms (particularly the left anterior oblique view) demonstrate the location of ventricular septal defects and the existence of multiple or atypical defects.

Differential Diagnosis

Ventricular septal defects must be distinguished from other lesions which produce left-to-right shunts. In infancy, ventricular septal defects must also be distinguished from aortic or pulmonary stenosis, which produces similar murmurs. Definitive diagnosis is made by cardiac catheterization and cineangiocardiography; however, it is not always possible (nor necessary) to rule out the possibility of a small ventricular septal defect.

Natural History

About two-thirds of all patients with isolated ventricular septal defects who are seen in the first year after birth have small defects which are generally asymptomatic and do not threaten life. Approximately one-fourth of these defects close spontaneously within 7 or 8 years. These patients, generally with less than 1.5:1 left-to-right shunts, have no risk of pulmonary vascular disease and approximately one chance in 6 of developing bacterial endocarditis during their lifetime.

In the approximate one-third of patients with large or multiple ventricular septal defects, about 5% will die in infancy of heart failure or respiratory infection. Most of these symptomatic infants will have repeated episodes of heart failure and pulmonary infections during the first year of life; however, after the first birthday, heart failure due to isolated ventricular septal defect is unusual. One of 3 developments causes the reduced incidence of heart failure after early infancy. In 25–40% of patients, the ventricular septal defect becomes smaller, and many (but not all) of these defects close spontaneously during infancy and early childhood. Few are known to close after adolescence. About 10% of infants with large ventricular septal defects develop infundibular muscular hypertrophy which reduces pulmonary blood flow.

Pulmonary vascular disease develops in 50% or more of patients with large ventricular septal defects. This dire complication may occur during the second year of life or at any time thereafter. As the arteriolar changes of pulmonary vascular disease develop, pulmonary vascular resistance increases and eventually equals or exceeds systemic resistance. In time, the flow of blood across the ventricular septal defect balances or becomes right-to-left (Eisenmenger's syndrome). These patients seldom live past age 30–40 years but may survive 15–20 years before dying of progressive hypoxia and polycythemia.

Treatment

Patients with small ventricular septal defects and pulmonary blood flow that is less than twice systemic flow have a slight risk of bacterial endocarditis, no risk of pulmonary vascular disease and probably no decrease in longevity. Operative closure of the defect is optional and can be performed at a very low (but not zero) risk.

Infants who have congestive heart failure due to ventricular septal defect and patent ductus arteriosus should have operative division of the patent ductus arteriosus. Infants who do not have patent ductus arteriosus and who have severe heart failure that cannot be controlled by medical measures should have operation. Single defects in the membranous septum, beneath the tricuspid septal leaflet and above the crista supraventricularis, are preferably closed in infancy. Infants with multiple muscular ventricular septal defects or defects associated with other symptomatic lesions (eg, coarctation) are preferably treated by pulmonary arterial banding. Muscular defects are often difficult to locate in infants.

Total correction of ventricular septal defects is most easily performed during cardiopulmonary bypass with or without deep hypothermia and circulatory arrest. High defects in the membranous septum are repaired through the right atrium and tricuspid valvular orifice. The atrial approach avoids incision and subsequent necrosis of right ventricular muscle. Over 80% of septal defects require patching with prosthetic material (Dacron or Teflon); the remainder can be closed by direct suture.

A right ventriculotomy is recommended for most other types of defects and for a technically easier repair of high septal defects. Supracristal defects can be repaired by working through a pulmonary arteriotomy and retracting the pulmonary valvular cusps. If the supracristal defect is associated with aortic regurgitation, closure of the septal defect may be performed by working through the aortic root or via right ventriculotomy. One or more cusps of the incompetent aortic valve generally are elongated. Competence can usually be restored by plication of the elongated aortic cusps; rarely, the aortic valve must be replaced. Muscular ventricular septal defects are often multiple and may be difficult to locate from the right ventricular side of the septum. Some surgeons prefer to close these holes via a left ventriculotomy. Others close muscular defects with patches and buttressed mattress sutures from the right ventricular approach. Muscular defects near the apex of the heart may be closed through a left ventriculotomy or by suturing the posterior margins of the defects to the anterior ventricular wall with mattress sutures that are tied outside the right ventricle.

All patients with unoperated ventricular septal defects must be followed closely during infancy and childhood. Although heart failure is infrequent after 1 year of age, pulmonary vascular disease may develop in any patient with a moderate or large ventricular septal defect. Change in the quality of the pulmonary second sound, increasing right ventricular hypertrophy, and decrease in heart size on a chest roentgenogram suggests the onset of pulmonary vascular disease. These patients require cardiac catheterization and operation to prevent progression of pulmonary vascular disease.

Prognosis After Surgery

The mortality rate of pulmonary arterial banding for ventricular septal defects is 1–3%. Patients who have correction of ventricular septal defects and removal of a previous pulmonary arterial band have a slightly higher mortality rate (approximately 5%). The mortality rate in patients with multiple muscular ventricular septal defects is higher than that associated with other types. Furthermore, the rate of recurrence or failure to close all of the defects is higher. Up to 14% of patients with closed membranous or ventricular septal defects have a residual left-to-right shunt after operation, but only a small percentage require reoperation. Less than 1% of patients develop permanent complete heart block, but approximately 50% develop right bundle branch block due to disturbance of some of the peripheral pathways of the conduction system.

Nearly all patients who do not have significant pulmonary vascular disease improve postoperatively: heart size decreases and growth rate is accelerated. Successful repair of a ventricular septal defect is thought to reduce the incidence of subsequent bacterial endocarditis.

The mortality rate of total corrective operations in patients with pulmonary vascular disease is increased. The hospital mortality rate is 15–30% when the ratio of pulmonary vascular to systemic vascular resistance is greater than 0.75. Another 25% of patients die later; in 25%, pulmonary vascular disease does not change; and only 25% are improved. Pulmonary vascular resistance decreases postoperatively in 70% of patients who have a preoperative ratio of pulmonary vascular resistance to systemic vascular resistance between 0.45 and 0.75.

Barratt-Boyes BG & others: Repair of ventricular septal defect in the first two years of life using profound hypothermia-circulatory arrest techniques. Ann Surg 184:376, 1976.

Cartmill TB & others: Results of repair of ventricular septal defects. J Thorac Cardiovasc Surg 52:46, 1966.

Girod DA & others: Recent results of two-stage surgical treatment of large ventricular septal defect. Circulation 50 (Suppl 2):9, 1974.

Griepp E & others: Is pulmonary artery banding for ventricular septal defects obsolete? Circulation 50 (Suppl 2):14, 1974.

Keith JD & others: Ventricular septal defect: Incidence, morbidity and mortality in various age groups. Br Heart J 33 (Suppl):81, 1971.

Lillehei CW & others: Pre and postoperative cardiac catheterization in 200 patients undergoing closure of ventricular septal defects. Surgery 63:69, 1968.

Subramanian S: Primary definitive intracardiac operations in infants: Ventricular septal defect. Page 141 in: *Advances in Cardiovascular Surgery*. Kirklin JW (editor). Grune & Stratton, 1973.

Trusler GA & others: Repair of ventricular septal defect with aortic insufficiency. J Thorac Cardiovasc Surg 66:394, 1973.

Wood P: The Eisenmenger syndrome. (2 parts.) Br Med J 2:701, 755, 1958.

PATENT DUCTUS ARTERIOSUS

Essentials of Diagnosis

- Patients with small or moderately large patent ducts are asymptomatic and have a continuous murmur over the pulmonary area, loud S_2, and bounding peripheral pulses.
- Poor feeding, respiratory distress, and frequent respiratory infections in infants with heart failure.
- Murmur usually systolic, sometimes continuous.
- Widened pulse pressure.

General Considerations

Normally, smooth muscle in the wall of the ductus arteriosus and increased blood oxygen tension cause the ductus arteriosus to constrict in the first days of life and to close completely with progressive fibrosis by 3 months of age. For unknown reasons, some ducts remain patent. The inside diameter of the ductus arteriosus varies from a few millimeters up to 10 mm and increases as the patient grows. With rare exceptions, the ductus arteriosus is to the left of the esophagus and trachea even when the aorta descends on the right. About 15% of patients with patent ductus arteriosus have associated anomalies, particularly ventricular septal defect or coarctation of the aorta.

Clinical Findings

A. Symptoms and Signs: Clinical findings are related to the size of the left-to-right shunt, which in turn is related to the diameter of the patent ductus arteriosus. Over 15% of premature infants and a few full-term infants with large shunts develop feeding problems, heart failure, enterocolitis, and respiratory distress in the first weeks of life, when the elevated pulmonary vascular resistance of the newborn begins to decrease. Cyanosis may occur if hyaline membrane disease, congestive atelectasis, or pneumonia occurs simultaneously. A murmur may not be present initially; later (at 1–4 weeks of age), a systolic murmur may appear. The liver and heart are generally enlarged. Peripheral pulses are bounding when the left-to-right shunt is large. Some of these patients are severely ill; others develop recurrent episodes of heart failure and respiratory distress during the first year of life. After the first year, heart failure is unusual.

Most infants and nearly all children with isolated patent ductus arteriosus are asymptomatic and have normal growth. A continuous murmur which is maximal in the second left intercostal space and widely transmitted is characteristic. An associated thrill may be present; the left ventricular impulse is increased; S_2 is loud; pulse pressure is widened; and peripheral pulses are increased.

B. X-Ray Findings: Chest films show increased pulmonary vascularity, prominent pulmonary arteries, and sometimes enlargement of the left ventricle in patients with moderate or large patent ducts. Young infants who are in heart failure may have a ground glass appearance of the peripheral lung fields, areas of atelectasis, and pulmonary infiltrates.

C. Electrocardiography: The ECG is often normal but may show left ventricular hypertrophy in older infants and children with large shunts.

D. Cardiac Catheterization and Cineangiocardiography: The catheter may pass through the ductus at catheterization. Pulmonary arterial pressures are normal or only slightly elevated in over 90% of asymptomatic patients. Pulmonary arterial pressures may approach or equal systemic pressures in symptomatic neonates. Blood oxygen saturation in the pulmonary arteries is greater than that in the right ventricle. Cineangiocardiograms demonstrate the ductus best after contrast material is injected into the aorta near the aortic isthmus. In premature infants, the clinical diagnosis can be confirmed by echocardiography.

Differential Diagnosis

In symptomatic premature infants, clinical signs and echocardiography may be sufficient to establish the diagnosis. Occasionally, cardiac catheterization is performed to rule out other associated lesions. In older patients, the classic clinical signs are sufficient to make the diagnosis.

In older infants and children, patent ductus arteriosus must be differentiated from venous hums and from the following rare lesions which produce a continuous murmur and an extracardiac left-to-right shunt: aortic-pulmonary window, ruptured sinus of Valsalva, and coronary arteriovenous fistula. Atypical location of the murmur and unusual findings on the chest film and ECG are indications for catheterization and cineangiocardiography in these patients.

Natural History

In most symptomatic premature infants, patent ductus arteriosus occurs in association with respiratory distress syndrome. In these patients, the ductus increases the severity of the respiratory disease and contributes to the development of bronchopulmonary dysplasia. A few premature infants develop heart failure with mild or no respiratory disease. Survival is greatly influenced by respiratory complications and complications of prematurity. If the infant survives the neonatal period, the ductus usually closes spontaneously.

Approximately 5% of full-term infants with untreated patent ductus arteriosus will die from heart failure and pulmonary complications in the first year of life. Another 5–10% of patients have large shunts and elevated pulmonary arterial pressures and may develop pulmonary vascular disease in late childhood or early adult life. The remainder are generally asymptomatic but have an increased incidence of subacute bacterial endocarditis at the ductus arteriosus. Adults 30–40 years of age who do not have pulmonary vascular disease often develop heart failure from the large left-to-right shunt through the ductus arteriosus.

Treatment

Surgical ligation of the ductus arteriosus in premature infants controls heart failure and, if performed early, generally reduces the severity of any associated respiratory disease. The operation can be performed extrathoracically and has been proved to have a very low operative mortality rate. Successful operations have been performed in 700–800 g infants for heart failure, enterocolitis, and respiratory distress. Indomethacin, a prostaglandin E_1 inhibitor, has recently been shown to produce closure of the patent ductus arteriosus in premature infants. Early reports indicate some degree of renal toxicity which may be related to dosage.

Division of the patent ductus arteriosus is recommended at any age for symptomatic infants and young children who have poorly controlled heart failure or repeated respiratory infections. The operation is contraindicated in patients with balanced or right-to-left shunts through the ductus arteriosus. Patients who have subacute bacterial endocarditis are preferably operated on after a course of antibiotics. Patients who have infected, recurrent, or aneurysmal ducts are best approached with cardiopulmonary bypass to permit temporary occlusion of the descending thoracic aorta when the ductus is divided.

Prognosis After Surgery

In uncomplicated cases, the mortality rate in full-term infants and older children from division of patent ductus arteriosus is less than 1% and approaches 0.2%. Causes of death are related to associated cardiac lesions and operative or postoperative hemorrhage. Operation reduces the susceptibility to subacute bacterial endocarditis.

In premature infants the mortality rate is high, but it is directly related to complications or prematurity and associated respiratory distress or enterocolitis. Early operation before severe morbidity occurs reduces the overall mortality rate since death from an operative complication is unusual even in premature infants. If early good results with indomethacin are confirmed and serious side-effects absent, operative closure in premature infants will be reserved for those few babies in whom the drug fails.

Edmunds LH Jr & others: Surgical closure of the ductus arteriosus in premature infants. Circulation 48:856, 1973.

Heymann MA & others: Closure of the ductus arteriosus in premature infants by inhibition of prostaglandin synthesis. N Engl J Med 295:530, 1976.

Jones JC: Twenty-five years' experience with the surgery of patent ductus arteriosus. J Thorac Cardiovasc Surg 50:149, 1965.

Rudolph AM & others: Hemodynamic basis for clinical manifestations of patent ductus arteriosus. Am Heart J 68:447, 1964.

AORTIC-PULMONARY WINDOW

A hole 5–30 mm in diameter between the ascending aorta and the main pulmonary artery produces a left-to-right shunt and physical findings identical with those of patent ductus arteriosus. Location of a continuous or systolic murmur in the third interspace near the left sternal border may suggest the correct diagnosis, which should be confirmed by cardiac catheterization and cineangiocardiography. Patients with large shunts have severe heart failure and are prone to develop pulmonary vascular disease at an early age. Division and closure of the aorta and main pulmonary artery during cardiopulmonary bypass produce good results in patients of all ages who do not have advanced pulmonary vascular disease.

Deverall PB & others: Aortopulmonary window. J Thorac Cardiovasc Surg 57:479, 1969.

RUPTURED SINUS OF VALSALVA

Rupture of the thin membranous tissue between an aortic sinus of Valsalva and an intracardiac chamber causes an immediate left-to-right shunt, a well-localized parasternal continuous murmur with associated thrill, wide pulse pressure, and increased heart size. In normal individuals, rupture is rare and generally occurs during the third or fourth decade. The cause is not known, but ruptured sinus of Valsalva occurs more frequently in patients with Marfan's syndrome or other abiotrophic diseases of connective tissue. Seventy-five percent of cases involve the right coronary sinus, which ruptures into the right ventricle (70%), right atrium (20%), or, rarely, the left ventricle or pulmonary artery. The remaining cases involve the noncoronary sinus, which ruptures into the right atrium or, less frequently, the right or left ventricle. About 20% of patients have an associated small ventricular septal defect. There are usually no symptoms, but when rupture occurs these patients suddenly develop chest pain and signs of congestive heart failure with a left-to-right shunt.

The lesion is repaired by closing the fistulous opening from the right atrium, right ventricle, or aorta during temporary cardiopulmonary bypass. The operative mortality rate is less than 5%.

Paton BC & others: Ruptured sinus of Valsalva. Arch Surg 90:209, 1965.

LEFT VENTRICULAR-RIGHT ATRIAL SHUNT

A defect in the membranous septum near the annulus of the septal leaflet of the tricuspid valve and a perforation or cleft of the septal leaflet produces a left ventricular to right atrial shunt. The lesion is uncommon, and the size of the shunt is variable. Symptoms of heart failure may be present in infancy or may not develop until late childhood. The systolic murmur is not diagnostic. At cardiac catheterization, blood oxygen saturation is increased in the right atrium, and on cineangiocardiograms the right atrium opacifies after injection of contrast material into the left ventricle.

In symptomatic patients, the defect is closed by direct sutures from the right atrium during cardiopulmonary bypass. The operative mortality rate is less than 5%.

Barclay RS & others: Communication between the left ventricle and right atrium. Thorax 22:473, 1967.

CORONARY ARTERIAL FISTULA

A fistulous communication between the right (60%) or left (40%) coronary arteries and the right ventricle (90%), right atrium, or coronary sinus produces a left-to-right shunt and increased pulmonary blood flow. The involved coronary vessels are dilated, and the fistulous openings may be multiple. Many patients are asymptomatic; some develop evidence of myocardial ischemia, and others have some degree of heart failure. A continuous murmur is usually present over the heart. Angiograms are required to determine the number and location of the fistulas.

The fistulous connections are ligated at operation without interrupting the coronary artery. Cardiopulmonary bypass is sometimes required. The operative mortality rate is below 5%.

Oldham HN Jr & others: Surgical management of congenital coronary artery fistula. Ann Thorac Surg 12:503, 1971.

TOTAL ANOMALOUS PULMONARY VENOUS CONNECTION (TAPVC)

Essentials of Diagnosis

- Pulmonary congestion, tachypnea, cardiac failure, and variable cyanosis.
- Severe heart failure, cyanosis, poor pulses, acidosis in infants.
- Pulmonary midsystolic murmur present with loud, fixed splitting of S_2 in some patients.
- Enlargement of right atrium and ventricle with severe pulmonary vascular congestion.
- Blood oxygen saturation similar in aorta and pulmonary artery.
- Pulmonary arterial and wedge pressures often elevated.

General Considerations

The term total anomalous pulmonary venous connection (TAPVC) indicates that pulmonary veins do not make a direct connection with the left atrium. Blood reaches the left atrium only through an atrial septal defect or patent foramen ovale. Pulmonary and systemic venous blood are mixed in the right atrium; thus, except for streaming, blood oxygen saturations in the aorta and pulmonary artery are similar. The degree of cyanosis varies and is inversely proportionate to pulmonary blood flow and directly proportionate to pulmonary venous desaturation from lung disease, pulmonary hypertension, and low systemic cardiac output in patients who occasionally are obstructed at the interatrial communication.

Three fairly distinct physiologic groups of patients have been identified. Over half of the patients with TAPVC have partial obstruction of the anomalous connections that carry pulmonary venous blood to the right atrium. Pulmonary arterial pressures equal or exceed 50% of systemic arterial pressures, and pulmonary capillary wedge pressure is usually higher than 15 mm Hg. In these patients, pulmonary blood flow may be slightly greater than, equal to, or less than systemic blood flow. About 20% of patients with TAPVC have pulmonary hypertension but do not have obstruction of the pulmonary veins. Pulmonary blood flow is more than twice systemic, and pulmonary capillary wedge pressure is below 15 mm Hg. Approximately 25% of patients with TAPVC do not have pulmonary hypertension or pulmonary venous obstruction. These patients have mild cyanosis.

Most cases of total anomalous pulmonary venous connection can be grouped into one of 3 different anatomic types (Fig 22–15). In type 1 (55% of patients), the pulmonary veins enter a common vein in the transverse sinus behind the heart and drain into the right atrium via a supracardiac pathway consisting of a persistent left vertical vein, the innominate vein, and the right superior vena cava. In type 2 (30% of patients), pulmonary venous blood enters the right atrium directly or via the coronary sinus. In type 3 (12% of patients), the common pulmonary vein behind the heart passes through the esophageal hiatus to enter the inferior vena cava, portal vein, or ductus venosus. Many mixed and complex varieties of total anomalous pulmonary venous connection have been described. About one-third of patients with TAPVC have other major cardiac anomalies excluding atrial septal defect and patent ductus arteriosus. Up to 50% of patients with TAPVC have patent ductus arteriosus.

Clinical Findings

A. Symptoms and Signs: Clinical findings vary according to the amount of pulmonary arterial blood flow and the degree of pulmonary venous hypertension. In the 25% of patients who have mild or no pulmonary venous hypertension, pulmonary arterial blood flow is greater than systemic and symptoms and signs are similar to those found in patients with large atrial septal defects. Cyanosis is minimal.

Approximately 60% of patients have significant obstruction of the anomalous pulmonary venous pathway. This group includes essentially all infants with infradiaphragmatic connections and many patients with supracardiac or mixed connections. These infants develop heart failure with severe cyanosis, poor peripheral perfusion, respiratory distress, poor feeding, and lethargy within the first few months after birth. Growth and development are poor. The right ventricular impulse is often prominent, and the liver is usually enlarged. The second heart sound is loud and single or closely split. Murmurs are not diagnostic. Pulmonary rales may be heard.

A third clinical group, comprising approximately 15% of patients with TAPVC, develop hyperkinetic pulmonary hypertension without pulmonary venous obstruction. These infants usually develop symptoms of heart failure during the first year after birth. Cyanosis is moderate. Tachypnea, feeding difficulties,

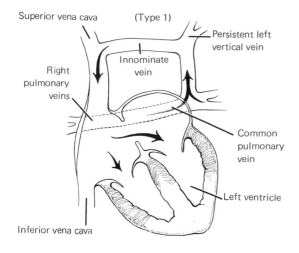

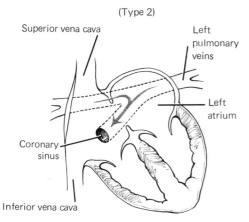

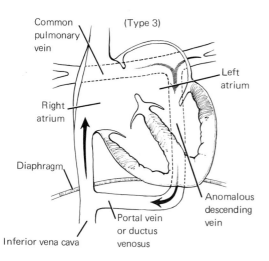

Figure 22–15. Common types of total anomalous pulmonary venous connection. *Type 1:* The pulmonary veins connect to a persistent left vertical vein, the innominate vein, and the right superior vena cava. *Type 2:* The pulmonary veins connect to the coronary sinus and the right atrium. *Type 3:* The pulmonary veins connect to an anomalous descending vein, a portal vein or persistent ductus venosus, and eventually the inferior vena cava.

respiratory infections, prominent right ventricular impulse, hepatomegaly, and cardiac enlargement are present. The second heart sound is widely split and fixed with a loud pulmonary component. Pulmonary flow murmurs and gallop rhythm are common.

B. X-Ray Findings: Plain chest films are diagnostic when 2 superior vena cavas cause the "snowman" or "figure-of-eight" appearance in the anterior posterior projection (type 1). Infants with pulmonary venous obstruction have severe pulmonary vascular congestion and ground glass appearance in the peripheral lung fields, but the heart is not enlarged or only slightly enlarged. Infants with pulmonary hypertension without pulmonary venous obstruction have enlarged hearts due to enlargement of the right atrium and ventricle and prominent pulmonary vasculature.

C. Electrocardiography: The ECG is not diagnostic and shows right axis deviation, right ventricular hypertrophy, and, after 1 month of age, right atrial hypertrophy.

D. Cardiac Catheterization and Cineangiocardiography: At cardiac catheterization, a catheter often can be passed from the right atrium into the anomalous veins in the lungs. Increase in blood oxygen saturation is found at the entrance of the pulmonary veins into the anomalous connection. Few patients have more than a 3 mm Hg pressure difference between the left and right atria. Pulmonary arterial and pulmonary capillary wedge pressures are helpful in determining the presence of significant pulmonary venous obstruction or pulmonary arterial hypertension.

Significant pulmonary venous obstruction is present when pulmonary capillary wedge pressures exceed 15 mm Hg. Pulmonary hypertension is diagnosed if pulmonary arterial pressure exceeds half of systemic pressure. Blood oxygen saturations are similar in the aorta and pulmonary artery but often vary slightly because of streaming. Complete catheterization studies are technically difficult to obtain in these patients, and estimates of pulmonary systemic flows are guesses because of difficulties in obtaining well-mixed venous samples. The anatomy of the anomalous veins is best determined by selective cineangiocardiography after injection of contrast material into the pulmonary veins and the common anomalous vein behind the heart.

Differential Diagnosis

Cyanotic infants with total anomalous pulmonary venous connection must be differentiated from patients with tetralogy of Fallot, transposition of the great vessels, and ventricular septal defect with associated respiratory disease. Patients with minimal cyanosis have findings which are similar to those in patients with large atrial septal defects. The anatomy and type of anomalous venous drainage must be determined by cardiac catheterization and cineangiocardiography.

Natural History

Without treatment, over 80% of infants born with TAPVC die within 1 year of birth. Fewer than 10% of infants with pulmonary venous obstruction survive their first 3 months. Approximately 50% of infants with pulmonary hypertension without pulmonary venous obstruction die in their first year. Survivors may develop pulmonary vascular disease, which reduces the symptoms of heart failure but has an ominous long-term prognosis. Over 80% of infants without pulmonary hypertension or pulmonary venous obstruction survive their first year, but many require treatment for heart failure. Anatomically, patients with types 1 and 2 have the best prognosis, but the physiologic classification is a more important prognosticator than the anatomic type.

Treatment

Seriously ill infants with all types of TAPVC and pulmonary venous hypertension require emergency operation with cardiopulmonary bypass and deep hypothermia. Occasional infants with insufficient atrial septal defects may benefit from balloon septostomy performed during cardiac catheterization. Early operation without allowing progressive deterioration to occur during a trial of medical management has produced the best results.

In patients with type 2 lesions, the orifice of the coronary sinus is enlarged and the atrial septal defect is patched so that all of the coronary sinus blood (and pulmonary venous return) is directed into the left atrium. When pulmonary veins enter the right atrium directly, the atrial septum is repositioned. In patients with types 1 and 3, an anastomosis is made between the common pulmonary vein behind the heart and the left atrium. This operation can be performed through a left or right thoracotomy or a median sternotomy during a brief period of circulatory arrest or low perfusion rate.

Prognosis After Surgery

The mortality rate of corrective operations is approximately 30–50% in infants under 3 months of age. The mortality rate is highest in patients with infradiaphragmatic anomalous veins (type 3) and mixed types and in those with pulmonary venous obstruction and severe pulmonary hypertension. In older infants, the operative mortality rate is considerably less, and in children it is less than 5%. Postoperative respiratory problems are particularly troublesome in patients with venous hypertension and congestive atelectasis. A few patients develop low cardiac output after operation.

Barratt-Boyes BG: Primary definitive operations in infants: Total anomalous pulmonary venous connection. Page 127 in: *Advances in Cardiovascular Surgery*. Kirklin JW (editor). Grune & Stratton, 1973.

Darling RC & others: Total pulmonary venous drainage into the right side of the heart. Lab Invest 6:44, 1957.

Gathman GE & Nadas AS: Total anomalous pulmonary venous connection: Clinical and physiologic observations of 75 pediatric patients. Circulation 42:143, 1970.

Gomes MMR & others: Total anomalous pulmonary venous connection. J Thorac Cardiovasc Surg 60:116, 1970.

TRUNCUS ARTERIOSUS

In truncus arteriosus, a single large vessel with 4–6 semilunar valves overrides the ventricular septum and distributes all of the blood which is ejected from the heart. A large ventricular septal defect is present beneath the truncal valve, which may be incompetent. The main pulmonary artery (Fig 22–16A), separate right and left pulmonary arteries, or multiple pulmonary arteries originate from the ascending or descending truncal aorta and provide blood flow to the lungs.

In most infants pulmonary blood flow is increased and signs and symptoms of severe heart failure are present. A minority of patients, particularly those in whom pulmonary arteries arise from the descending thoracic aorta, have reduced pulmonary blood flow and are clinically cyanotic. Most patients do not survive infancy. A few patients who have nearly balanced systemic and pulmonary blood flows may do well during infancy and childhood.

Palliative operations include pulmonary arterial banding and systemic to pulmonary arterial shunts in patients with reduced pulmonary blood flow. Pulmonary arterial bands often must be placed on the right and left pulmonary vessels separately because of the absence or very short length of the main pulmonary artery. Palliative operations have high early and late mortality rates and salvage few patients for corrective operations in late childhood.

Corrective operation consists of separation of the aorta and pulmonary arteries, closure of the ventricular septal defect, and placement of a valved conduit between the right ventricle and distal pulmonary arteries (Fig 22–16). Most commonly, a Dacron conduit containing a glutaraldehyde-preserved porcine heterograft valve is used to substitute for the missing cardiac anatomy. In patients over 2 years of age, the conduit operation has generally excellent results (mortality rate less than 10%) in patients with pulmonary-systemic resistance ratios less than 0.6. In infants, results of the conduit operation are variable, with mortality rates in relatively small series ranging from 15–80%.

Appelbaum A & others: Surgical treatment of truncus arteriosus with emphasis on infants and small children. J Thorac Cardiovasc Surg 71:436, 1976.

Ebert PA & others: Pulmonary artery conduits in infants younger than six months of age. J Thorac Cardiovasc Surg 72:351, 1976.

McGoon DC, Wallace RB, Danielson GK: The Rastelli operation: Its indications and results. J Thorac Cardiovasc Surg 65:65, 1973.

Poirier RA, Berman MA, Stansel HC Jr: Current status of the surgical treatment of truncus arteriosus. J Thorac Cardiovasc Surg 69:169, 1975.

Van Praagh R, Van Praagh S: The anatomy of common aortico-pulmonary trunk (truncus arteriosus communis) and its embryologic implications. Am J Cardiol 16:406, 1965.

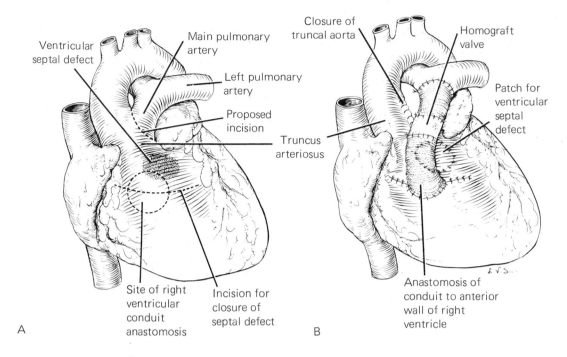

Figure 22–16. Type 1 truncus arteriosus. *A:* The main pulmonary artery arises from the truncus arteriosus downstream to the truncal semilunar valve. A ventricular septal defect is always present. *B:* The main pulmonary artery is incised from the truncus. The ventricular septal defect is closed with a patch. A conduit of Dacron which contains a homograft aortic valve is sutured to the anterior wall of the right ventricle and the distal pulmonary artery. A conduit between the right ventricle and pulmonary artery was successfully introduced by J.W. Kirklin in 1964 during correction of severe tetralogy of Fallot.

III. CONGENITAL HEART LESIONS WHICH DECREASE PULMONARY ARTERIAL BLOOD FLOW

The combination of an obstructive lesion of the right heart and a septal defect reduces pulmonary arterial blood flow and causes some systemic venous blood to enter the systemic arterial circulation directly (right-to-left shunt). The degree of cyanosis is directly proportionate to the amount of the right-to-left shunt and inversely proportionate to the amount of pulmonary arterial blood flow. Tetralogy of Fallot is the most common lesion in this group, which also includes pulmonary atresia, tricuspid atresia, Ebstein's anomaly, certain complex malformations, and patients with total anomalous pulmonary venous connection and truncus arteriosus who have reduced pulmonary arterial blood flow. Pulmonary vascular disease due to acquired hyperplasia of the intimal and medial layers of pulmonary arterioles develops in some patients who have lesions which initially produce excessive pulmonary blood flow. As pulmonary arterioles become obstructed, pulmonary blood flow decreases and causes blood to shunt from right to left (Eisenmenger's syndrome).

Severe cyanosis stimulates red cell production, which increases blood hematocrit and hemoglobin concentration. This improves oxygen transport because blood which reaches the lungs will bind more oxygen per 100 ml. The elevated hematocrit, which may reach 80% or more, increases the viscosity of blood and may reduce certain clotting factors, particularly platelets and fibrinogen. Dehydration in patients with a very high hematocrit may cause systemic and pulmonary venous thrombosis in spite of the reduced concentration of clotting factors.

Changes in the degree of cyanosis, hypoxic spells, squatting, and clubbing are frequently associated with lesions that reduce pulmonary blood flow. Several factors may alter the degree of cyanosis by altering the ratio of pulmonary and systemic resistances. Exercise decreases systemic vascular resistance, increases systemic blood flow, and, in tetralogy of Fallot, decreases pulmonary blood flow and arterial oxygen saturation. Increased catecholamines or acidosis can also reduce pulmonary blood flow in patients with tetralogy of Fallot.

Hypoxic spells indicate severe cerebral hypoxia and are due to acute reduction of pulmonary blood flow. Spasm of the infundibular muscle is the most likely cause of hypoxic spells, which can occur without warning. Infants and young children become unconscious for varying periods of time and occasionally die. The most effective treatment is to administer oxygen and small doses of morphine, place the patient in the knee-chest position with his head down, and correct the associated metabolic acidosis.

Children who have reduced pulmonary arterial blood flow and cyanotic heart disease squat frequently. In the squatting position (sitting on the heels), systemic vascular resistance increases. The increased systemic vascular resistance decreases right-to-left shunting and temporarily increases pulmonary arterial blood flow.

Clubbing of fingers and toes develops in late infancy and early childhood and is due to proliferation of capillaries and small arteriovenous fistulas in the distal phalanges. The mechanism and teleologic advantage (if any) of clubbing are not known.

Reduced pulmonary arterial blood flow stimulates enlargement of the bronchial and mediastinal arteries. These vessels connect with pulmonary arteries and, in some children, may provide most of the pulmonary blood flow. At birth, the ductus arteriosus is patent and provides substantial blood flow to the pul-

monary arteries of patients with obstructive lesions of the right heart. Unfortunately, this useful vessel nearly always closes during the first few hours and days after birth.

Several palliative operations that shunt blood from the systemic to the pulmonary arterial circulation have been devised for infants and young children who have insufficient pulmonary arterial blood flow. The Blalock-Taussig operation connects the subclavian artery to the ipsilateral pulmonary artery with an end-to-side anastomosis (Fig 22–17A). The Waterston aortic to right pulmonary arterial anastomosis connects the posterior portion of the ascending aorta to the anterior wall of the right pulmonary artery (Fig 22–17B). The Potts operation joins the left pulmonary artery and the descending thoracic aorta by a side-to-side anastomosis (Fig 22–17C). In neonates, injection of the wall of the ductus arteriosus with 10% formalin has delayed closure of this valuable vessel for weeks or

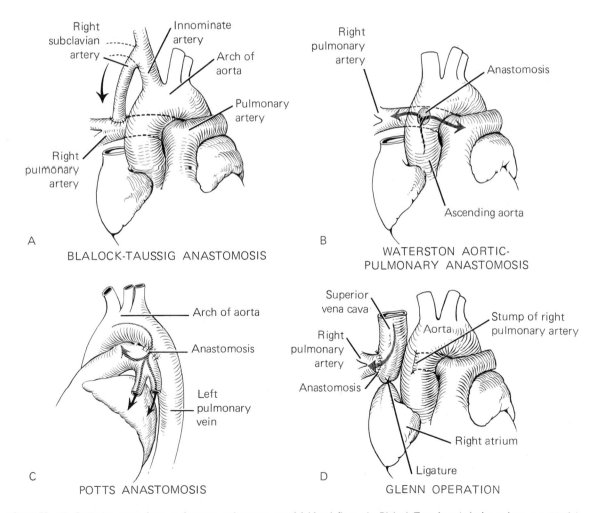

Figure 22–17. Palliative operations to increase pulmonary arterial blood flow. *A:* Blalock-Taussig subclavian-pulmonary arterial anastomosis. *B:* Waterston aortic to right pulmonary arterial anastomosis. *C:* Potts anastomosis between the left pulmonary artery and the descending thoracic aorta. *D:* The Glenn operation. The end of the right pulmonary artery is connected to the side of the superior vena cava, which is ligated caudad to the anastomosis.

months. All of these connections increase pulmonary blood flow because of the pressure difference between the systemic arterial and pulmonary circulations. The Glenn operation (Fig 22–17D) connects the superior vena cava to the right pulmonary artery in such a way that superior vena caval blood must enter the right pulmonary artery without passing through the heart.

TETRALOGY OF FALLOT

Essentials of Diagnosis

- History of hypoxic spells and squatting.
- Cyanosis and clubbing.
- Prominent right ventricular impulse, single S_2.
- Grade 1–3/6 ejection murmur in third left intercostal space.
- Systolic murmur softens or disappears during cyanotic spell.

General Considerations

Tetralogy of Fallot is a cardiac malformation with 4 anatomic abnormalities (Fig 22–18). The lesion is due to underdevelopment of the right ventricular infundibulum (that portion of the right ventricle that is just upstream to the pulmonary valve). Parietal and septal muscular bands that attach to the crista supraventricularis (a muscular ridge between the infundibulum and the body of the right ventricle) obstruct the underdeveloped infundibulum. The ventricular septal defect is large (equal pressures in both ventricles) and is located upstream to the crista supraventricularis in the membranous septum just caudad to the aortic valve. The aorta arises partially but not wholly from the right ventricle. Right ventricular hypertrophy is the fourth anomaly of the tetrad and is a secondary development.

The infundibular stenosis is located upstream to the pulmonary valve and downstream to the ventricular septal defect. An infundibular "chamber" may be present between the hypertrophied muscle tissue and the pulmonary valve. In approximately two-thirds of patients, the pulmonary valve is also stenotic and rarely is atretic. Occasionally, the pulmonary valvular annulus and the main pulmonary artery are hypoplastic. Occasional patients have stenotic lesions within the pulmonary arteries, usually at the junction of the right and left main pulmonary vessels. Rarely, the left pulmonary artery is absent or the pulmonary valvular cusps are rudimentary or absent.

Atrial septal defect and right aortic arch occur frequently with tetralogy of Fallot. In patients with severe obstruction, the bronchial arteries enlarge and dilate in response to the diminished pulmonary arterial blood flow. Occasionally, the anterior descending coronary artery originates from the right coronary artery and crosses the right ventricular outflow tract.

Although the functional pathology and operative treatment of ventricular septal defect with acquired infundibular obstruction are similar to those of tetralogy of Fallot, the 2 lesions differ in developmental and pathologic anatomy.

Clinical Findings

A. Symptoms and Signs: Clinical findings are directly related to the severity of the right ventricular obstructive lesion and the amount of pulmonary blood flow. Severe right ventricular obstruction or pulmonary atresia causes cyanosis in early infancy. A large

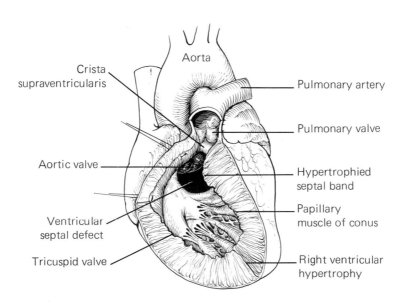

Figure 22–18. Tetralogy of Fallot. The aorta overrides the ventricular septum. A large ventricular septal defect is present, and the hypoplastic infundibulum with hypertrophied parietal and septal muscle bands obstructs blood flow to the pulmonary arteries.

patent ductus arteriosus may mask the lesion for the first few days after birth, but as the ductus constricts cyanosis increases. Infants feed poorly, tire easily, hyperventilate, and have episodic hypoxic spells. Murmurs are not diagnostic, but a systolic murmur is usually present along the left sternal border. The heart and liver are usually not enlarged in infants with severe tetralogy of Fallot, and heart failure is absent. During a hypoxic spell, the infant becomes deeply cyanotic, tachypneic, lethargic, or unconscious, and a systolic murmur over the right ventricular outflow tract softens or disappears.

Less severe right ventricular outflow obstruction and greater pulmonary arterial blood flow produce different clinical findings. Newborns do not become hypoxic and acidotic, and cyanosis may not be striking. These infants generally feed and grow well and do not have heart failure, but they do develop increasing cyanosis. Some babies develop hypoxic spells at 3–4 months of age; others do not have such spells until later, and some never have hypoxic spells. During the first year, clubbing and polycythemia develop. Later, exercise tolerance is reduced, growth rate is below normal, and squatting may occur. A systolic murmur and thrill are usually present along the left sternal border, and the pulmonary second sound is generally decreased. A continuous murmur discovered in late infancy or childhood suggests either greatly increased bronchial arterial flow or associated patent ductus arteriosus.

B. X-Ray Findings: Chest films show reduced pulmonary vascularity, hypertrophy of the right ventricle, and little or no cardiac enlargement. Right ventricular hypertrophy elevates the apex of the heart. Central pulmonary vessels may be normal or small. In approximately 20% of patients, the aortic arch is on the right side.

C. Electrocardiography: The electrocardiogram shows right ventricular hypertrophy, which is a normal finding in newborns. In older infants, the electrocardiogram shows moderate to severe right ventricular hypertrophy.

D. Cardiac Catheterization and Cineangiocardiography: In tetralogy of Fallot, ventricular pressures are equal and the major shunt is from right to left at the ventricular level. Occasionally, a small left-to-right ventricular shunt may also be present, and a right-to-left shunt may be present in the atria. Pressure differences are present between the body of the right ventricle and the infundibulum and may be present across the pulmonary valve and, occasionally, across a segment of the pulmonary arteries. The percentage of oxyhemoglobin in left ventricular and aortic blood is directly related to the ratio of pulmonary to systemic blood flow. Cineangiocardiograms after right ventricular injection of contrast material demonstrate the size of the right ventricle, the severity and location of the infundibular and pulmonary valvular stenoses, the size of the pulmonary valvular annulus and main pulmonary artery, and the presence of peripheral pulmonary stenosis.

Differential Diagnosis

In early infancy, severe forms of tetralogy of Fallot may be difficult to distinguish from other complex cyanotic malformations such as transposition of the great vessels with pulmonary stenosis and ventricular septal defect, severe pulmonary stenosis with patent foramen ovale, double outlet right ventricle, and tricuspid atresia. The ECG is helpful in identifying tricuspid atresia, and the absence of heart failure suggests tetralogy of Fallot or pulmonary atresia with ventricular septal defect. Cardiac catheterization and cineangiocardiography are required for accurate diagnosis. The diagnosis of tetralogy of Fallot is more easily made in older infants and children on the basis of clinical findings; however, cardiac catheterization and cineangiocardiography provide important anatomic and physiologic information which relates to the management of the patient.

Natural History

A few patients who have relatively large pulmonary arterial blood flows during childhood reach age 30–40 before increasing cyanosis, polycythemia, and clinical signs of heart failure develop. Most patients with tetralogy of Fallot do not survive past age 20; the average age at death is 12 years in patients who survive infancy. Infants with severe right ventricular outflow obstruction or pulmonary atresia usually succumb in the first few months of life during a hypoxic spell. Progressive hypertrophy of infundibular muscle and thrombosis of pulmonary vessels during infancy and childhood increase the severity of cyanosis and polycythemia and the likelihood of a fatal hypoxic spell. Hypoxia is the cause of death in most patients who die of tetralogy of Fallot.

Infection is the second most common cause of death. Rare causes include cerebrovenous thrombosis secondary to polycythemia, cerebral abscess resulting from bacteria in venous blood passing through the shunt directly into the arterial circulation, and subacute bacterial endocarditis.

A few infants with tetralogy of Fallot develop pulmonary atresia but survive because of concurrent development of large bronchial vessels which provide sufficient pulmonary blood flow to sustain life. These patients have well-developed right ventricles, but the true pulmonary arteries are often hypoplastic or even vestigial.

Treatment

The selection of operation for symptomatic infants with tetralogy of Fallot is controversial in those who have anatomic features which are favorable for total correction. If the main pulmonary artery and pulmonary annulus are not severely hypoplastic, and if the patient has not been taking propranolol, total correction can be carried out.

Total correction for Fallot's tetralogy is performed during total cardiopulmonary bypass. In infants, deep hypothermia and circulatory arrest are helpful but not essential. A patent ductus arteriosus or a previously constructed systemic artery to pulmonary artery shunt is closed just before cardiopulmonary bypass begins. The right ventricle may be opened through a vertical or transverse ventriculotomy. The fibrous and muscular obstruction of the outflow tract is excised widely to create an unobstructed channel to the pulmonary valve. The pulmonary valve is inspected, and incised if stenotic. A patch of pericardium is used to enlarge the right ventricular outflow tract in most infants. In older infants and children, outflow patches are used in 25–60% of cases. Resection of the infundibular stenosis can be performed without ventriculotomy by working through the tricuspid valve in over half of children who have tetralogy of Fallot. If the pulmonary annulus and main pulmonary artery are severely hypoplastic or atretic, a conduit (Fig 22–16B) is used. The infundibular resection and pulmonary angioplasty must be sufficient to reduce the ratio between right and left ventricular systolic pressures to 0.9 or less. The ventricular septal defect is closed with a prosthetic patch. Associated atrial septal defects are also closed during the operation.

A palliative shunt may be preferred by some surgeons who feel that the mortality rate and complications of total correction, particularly in infants less than 3 months of age, are higher than the combination of a palliative shunt and later corrective operation. The Blalock-Taussig subclavian-pulmonary arterial anastomosis (Fig 22–17A) on the side opposite the aortic arch is strongly preferred to other shunts. It is now possible to construct tiny (2 mm) anastomoses in newborns with a high rate of patency. The Blalock-Taussig anastomosis rarely causes pulmonary congestion from excessive pulmonary blood flow and is generally easy to ligate at the time of total correction. The Waterston aortic-right pulmonary arterial anastomosis (Fig 22–17B) is easier to construct, but the amount of flow through the anastomosis is difficult to control. Furthermore, as the child grows, stenosis or occlusion of the right pulmonary artery occurs frequently and complicates removal of the shunt at the time of the corrective operation. The Potts anastomosis (Fig 22–17C) consists of anastomosing the descending aorta to the left pulmonary artery. This procedure is little used today because it too is difficult to close at a subsequent corrective operation.

Patients with acquired pulmonary atresia, ventricular septal defect, and abundant bronchial arterial blood flow can be successfully operated on if the pulmonary arteries are sufficiently well developed to receive the entire cardiac output. A valved Dacron conduit is used to connect the right ventricle and the distal pulmonary arteries, and the ventricular septal defect is closed. The bronchial arteries, which are multiple and arise from the descending thoracic aorta and aortic arch, must be interrupted and any previously constructed systemic-pulmonary arterial shunts must be taken down. Occasionally, small pulmonary arteries may be stimulated to enlarge by construction of a systemic-pulmonary arterial shunt as a first stage operation.

Prognosis After Surgery

The mortality rate of Blalock-Taussig or Waterston shunts is less than 5% for patients of any age who have tetralogy of Fallot. A successful shunt causes a continuous murmur, increases heart size, improves pulmonary vascularity, and reduces both cyanosis and the hematocrit. All systemic artery-pulmonary artery shunts cause the majority of flow to enter the lung on the same side as the shunt. Over a period of 10 years, nearly a third of patients with Blalock-Taussig anastomoses will undergo stenosis or occlusion of the shunt. Arm complications and uncontrolled heart failure after Blalock-Taussig anastomoses are extremely rare; early occlusion requiring reoperation occurs in about 5% of older infants and children and up to 10% of newborns.

The overall mortality rate for elective correction of tetralogy of Fallot in children is now about 5%. The mortality rate in infants less than 1 year of age is only slightly higher. Right ventricular failure, heart block, arrhythmias, and infection are the most common causes of death. A previous Potts anastomosis, single pulmonary artery, or massive bronchial blood flow increases the operative mortality rate approximately 2-fold.

Approximately 35% of surviving patients have no exercise limitations; 55% have no limitations of ordinary activity; and only 10% have residual disability. Cardiac outputs obtained during maximum exercise are less than those obtained in normal subjects and most patients continue to have right ventricular-pulmonary arterial pressure differences during exercise. Many patients have some degree of pulmonary valvular regurgitation and paradoxic movement of the right ventricular outflow tract. Patients with residual disability often are found to have residual ventricular septal shunts or elevated right ventricular pressures; some of these patients have had a successful second operation. Considering the complexity of the lesion and the magnitude of the repair, the overall clinical results of operation are excellent.

Castaneda AR & others: Open heart surgery during the first three months of life. J Thorac Cardiovasc Surg 68:719, 1974.

Edmunds LH Hr & others: Transatrial repair of tetralogy of Fallot. Surgery 80:681, 1976.

Epstein SE & others: Hemodynamic abnormalities in response to mild and intense upright exercise following operative correction of an atrial septal defect or tetralogy of Fallot. Circulation 47:1065, 1973.

Gay WA Jr, Ebert PA: Aorta-to-right pulmonary artery anastomosis causing obstruction of the right pulmonary artery. Ann Thorac Surg 16:402, 1973.

Kirklin JW, Karp RB: *The Tetralogy of Fallot from a Surgical Viewpoint.* Saunders, 1970.

Laks H, Marco JD, Willman VL: The Blalock-Taussig shunt in the first six months of life. J Thorac Cardiovasc Surg 70:687, 1975.

McGoon DC, Baird DK, Davis GD: Surgical management of large bronchial collateral arteries with pulmonary stenosis or atresia. Circulation 52:109, 1975.

Starr A, Bonchek LI, Sunderland CO: Total correction of tetralogy of Fallot in infancy. J Thorac Cardiovasc Surg 65:45, 1973.

Taussig HB & others: Ten to thirteen year follow-up on patients after a Blalock-Taussig operation. Circulation 25:630, 1962.

PULMONARY ATRESIA WITH INTACT VENTRICULAR SEPTUM

Atresia or hypoplasia of the pulmonary artery associated with ventricular septal defect represents a severe malformation of tetralogy of Fallot. This lesion (also called pseudotruncus) has been discussed with tetralogy of Fallot.

Pulmonary atresia with an intact ventricular septum is usually associated with a hypoplastic or rudimentary right ventricle (type 1), but it may occur with a normal or dilated right ventricle in association with an incompetent and sometimes malformed tricuspid valve (type 2). The pulmonary valve is small and imperforate; distal pulmonary arteries are patent, and blood is shunted from right to left across the inter-atrial septum. A patent ductus is mandatory for survival, but the ductus is often small and constricts during the first few days or weeks after birth. The degree of cyanosis is inversely proportionate to the amount of pulmonary blood flow through the ductus arteriosus.

Cyanosis may be present at birth or may appear within a few days along with heart failure, hypoxic spells, and acidosis. The ECG generally shows left ventricular dominance in patients with a hypoplastic (type 1) right ventricle. Serial x-rays usually indicate a progressive increase in heart size and diminished pulmonary vasculature. The condition must be differentiated from tricuspid atresia, severe tetralogy of Fallot, severe pulmonary stenosis, and transposition of the great arteries with associated pulmonary stenosis. Cineangiocardiograms show a blind right ventricle with contrast material escaping through dilated myocardial sinusoids or through the tricuspid valve.

If the right ventricle is grossly underdeveloped, a Waterston or Blalock-Taussig anastomosis (Fig 22–17A and B) is required. At the same time or later, a pulmonary valvulotomy performed blindly (Brock procedure) is recommended to establish a connection between the right ventricle and pulmonary artery in hope of inducing growth of the hypoplastic ventricle. In a few instances, growth of the right ventricle has permitted a second operation to establish continuity between the right ventricle and pulmonary artery with a valved conduit. If the right ventricle and infundibulum are reasonably well developed, a valved conduit can be used during infancy as the primary procedure.

Late deaths from arrhythmia, heart failure, closure of the shunt, and pulmonary infection occur frequently in infants with hypoplastic right ventricles who survive shunt operations in the neonatal period. However, without treatment nearly all infants die within their first year.

Dhanavaravibul S, Nora JJ, McNamara DG: Pulmonary valvular atresia with intact ventricular septum: Problems in diagnosis and results of treatment. J Pediatr 77:1010, 1970.

Dobell ARC, Grignon A: Early and late results in pulmonary atresia. Ann Thorac Surg 24, 1977. (In press.)

Ebert PA & others: Pulmonary artery conduits in infants younger than six months of age. J Thorac Cardiovasc Surg 72:351, 1976.

Edmunds LH Jr & others: Anastomoses between aorta and right pulmonary artery (Waterston) in neonates. N Engl J Med 284:464, 1971.

TRICUSPID ATRESIA

The tricuspid valve is completely absent in 1–2% of newborns with congenital heart disease. In the majority of patients, the great vessels are not transposed, the right ventricle is hypoplastic, a small muscular ventricular septal defect is present, and the pulmonary valve is stenotic or hypoplastic. Blood passes across the foramen ovale (or atrial septal defect if it is present), is mixed with pulmonary venous blood in the left atrium, and is pumped by the left ventricle into the great vessels. Occasionally, the ventricular septum is intact. Sometimes a large ventricular septal defect is present without associated pulmonary valvular obstruction. About 25% of patients have transposition of the great arteries.

Infants with tricuspid atresia and reduced pulmonary blood flow (80% of the total) develop cyanosis within the first week after birth. Tachypnea, dyspnea, hypoxic spells, acidosis, and feeding difficulties are additional findings. Most patients have a systolic precordial murmur. Polycythemia and clubbing develop later; liver enlargement and systemic venous hypertension may develop in older infants and children who have partial obstruction to flow at the atrial septum.

Heart size is sometimes normal, but the left heart border has a boxlike contour as a result of left atrial enlargement on chest x-rays taken during infancy. Pulmonary vascular markings are decreased. The ECG and vectorcardiogram show left ventricular hypertrophy and left axis deviation. This finding, which is present from birth in virtually all patients with tricuspid atresia and diminished pulmonary blood flow, strongly suggests the diagnosis in cyanotic infants. At cardiac catheterization, right atrial pressure usually exceeds left atrial pressure and blood oxygen saturation increases in the left atrium. After injection into the right atrium or systemic veins, contrast material opacifies the left atrium and ventricle and both great arteries in sequence. The right ventricle may appear only as a filling defect between the right atrium and the left ventricle. Tricuspid atresia is differentiated from tetralogy of Fallot by the ECG. Other lesions which must be included in the differential diagnosis are hypoplastic right heart, pulmonary atresia, and a variety of lesions (single ventricle, persistent atrioventricular canal, transposition of the great arteries) associated with pulmonary stenosis.

Most patients with tricuspid atresia and reduced pulmonary arterial blood flow die during a hypoxic spell within 3 months after birth when the ductus arteriosus constricts or closes. In rare types in which pulmonary arterial blood flow is adequate or increased, the prognosis is better. Infants who have reduced pulmonary blood flow may benefit from a systemic to pulmonary arterial anastomosis. A Blalock-Taussig anastomosis is preferred, but sometimes a Waterston or Potts anastomosis is necessary. A balloon atrial septostomy or operative excision of the atrial septum may be required in occasional patients who have partial obstruction at the atrial septum.

The Glenn operation (Fig 22–17D) is an alternative procedure to a systemic artery-pulmonary artery anastomosis. This operation reduces the amount of blood which must be ejected by the left ventricle and increases pulmonary blood flow. The operation is not recommended for newborns because pulmonary vascular resistance may still be elevated as a result of the fetal anatomic configuration of the pulmonary arterioles. Although the operation reduces left ventricular work and improves most patients, late complications from the development of collaterals around the ligated superior vena cava occur. The operation is difficult to take down if a later corrective operation is carried out.

A new operation, developed by Fontan, creates a connection between the right atrium and pulmonary arteries using a valved Dacron conduit. The atrial septal defect is closed so that all systemic venous blood that reaches the right atrium must pass through the conduit into the pulmonary arteries. The main pulmonary artery is ligated. The conduit connects the right atrium to the left pulmonary artery if a previous superior vena cava-right pulmonary arterial anastomosis (Glenn) is present. Pulmonary vascular resistance must be normal, and previously constructed systemic-pulmonary arterial shunts must be taken down. The operative mortality rate of the Fontan operation is approximately 33%, and nearly all patients have ascites, pleural effusions, and hepatomegaly in the immediate postoperative period.

Deverall PB & others: Surgical management of tricuspid atresia. Thorax 24:239, 1969.

Edwards WS, Bargeron LM Jr: The superiority of the Glenn operation for tricuspid atresia in infancy and childhood. J Thorac Cardiovasc Surg 55:60, 1968.

Fontan F, Baudet E: Surgical repair of tricuspid atresia. Thorax 26:240, 1971.

Fontan F & others: Repair of tricuspid atresia: Surgical considerations and results. Circulation 50 (Suppl 3):72, 1974.

Kyger ER III & others: Surgical palliation of tricuspid atresia. Circulation 52:685, 1975.

Tatooles CJ: Operative repair for tricuspid atresia. Ann Thorac Surg 21:499, 1976.

EBSTEIN'S ANOMALY

In this malformation, the septal and posterior leaflets of the tricuspid valve are small and deformed and arise from the wall of the right ventricle below the normal tricuspid annulus. The anterior leaflet is often large and is attached to the tricuspid annulus. The malformation causes the upper portion of the right ventricle to be a part of the right atrium. This portion of the right ventricle is generally thin and contracts poorly. The downstream portion of the right ventricle is usually small, and the tricuspid valve is usually incompetent. Most patients have an associated atrial septal defect (50%) or patent foramen ovale. A minority of patients have associated pulmonary stenosis, ventricular septal defect, tetralogy of Fallot, or transposition of the great arteries.

About half of patients develop right heart failure, systemic venous hypertension, hepatomegaly, arrhythmias, and cyanosis in infancy. A systolic murmur associated with a poor right ventricular impulse is often present. Associated lesions reduce life expectancy, and few of these patients survive infancy. Other patients are asymptomatic or have mild symptoms during infancy and childhood but develop progressive cardiomegaly, arrhythmias, cyanosis, and severe right heart failure in the third and fourth decades of life. Massive enlargement of the entire heart—but particularly the right atrium—may develop. The ECG characteristically shows large P waves, prolonged P–R conduction, and low voltage in the right ventricular leads. Right atrial pressure is usually increased during cardiac catheterization, and the atrial *v* wave is large. Most patients have a right-to-left shunt between the atria. The abnormal position of the tricuspid valve is best demonstrated by a right ventricular angiogram.

A superior vena cava to right pulmonary arterial anastomosis (Glenn operation) has provided effective palliation for some patients, but this operation is not often successful in infants. In older patients, the atrial septal defect or patent foramen ovale is closed, and an annuloplasty is performed if the anatomy of the tricuspid valve is favorable. In other patients, the tricuspid valve is not disturbed. Rarely, the tricuspid valve is replaced. Occasional patients are strikingly improved, but the overall results are generally unsatisfactory because of the inherent inability of the diseased right ventricle to contract effectively.

Kumar AE & others: Ebstein's anomaly: Clinical profile and natural history. Am J Cardiol 28:84, 1971.

McFaul RC & others: Ebstein's malformation: Surgical experience at the Mayo Clinic. J Thorac Cardiovasc Surg 72:910, 1976.

HYPOPLASTIC RIGHT VENTRICLE

Underdevelopment of the right ventricle commonly occurs with pulmonary and tricuspid atresia and may occur with valvular pulmonary stenosis. Rarely, hypoplasia of the right ventricle may occur as an isolated lesion. The right ventricle may have a small cavity, hypertrophied ventricular walls, and a patent, deformed tricuspid valve—or may have a large cavity, thin, fibrotic ventricular walls, and an incompetent tricuspid valve. The pulmonary artery and valve are small but well formed. These lesions are part of a spectrum of right ventricular and pulmonary arterial malformations which range from tricuspid atresia and Ebstein's anomaly to pulmonary stenosis, tetralogy of Fallot, and pulmonary atresia. Older patients with thin, dilated right ventricles may benefit from superior vena cava to right pulmonary arterial (Glenn) anastomosis. A systemic to pulmonary arterial anastomosis is recommended in infants.

Hollman A: Underdevelopment of the right ventricle. Chap 32, pp 501–509, in: *Paediatric Cardiology*. Watson H (editor). Mosby, 1968.

IV. COMPLEX CONGENITAL HEART MALFORMATIONS

This imprecise term denotes a group of lesions which have complicated anatomic features that involve abnormal relationships between different parts of the heart and great vessels. The abnormal relationships of different subunits to each other distinguish the complex lesions from more localized defects in septation or development of specific structures. Pulmonary blood flow may be increased or decreased in complex lesions, and obstructive lesions may be present.

Most patients with complex congenital heart lesions die in infancy or early childhood, but a few live to adult life.

The principal structures of the heart and great vessels are formed and aligned between the third and seventh weeks of gestation. Normally, the straight cardiac tube develops 5 segments which are labeled (from caudad to cephalad) sinus venosus, atrial canal, ventricular canal, bulbus cordis, and truncus arteriosus. Toward the end of the third week, the segmented cardiac tube normally loops to the right (*d*-loop) and folds on itself to begin the process of septation. By the fifth week, the apex of the heart swings leftward to bring the right ventricle to an anterior position. The sinus venosus becomes part of the right atrium, and the atrial canal forms the right and left atria. At the other end, truncal ridges divide the truncus arteriosus into the aorta and main pulmonary artery.

Endocardial cushions—which form the atrioventricular valves—and conal ridges of the bulbus cordis participate in the development of the ventricular septum and division of the primitive ventricular canal. In addition, the bulbus cordis forms the semilunar valves and parts of the inflow and outflow portions of the right ventricle. A part of the bulbus cordis called the conus arteriosus normally forms the parietal band and part of the free wall of the right ventricular infundibulum (outflow portion of the right ventricle immediately upstream to the pulmonary valve). After birth, the structures formed by the conus arteriosus appear to be integral parts of the right ventricle and ventricular septum, but in early fetal life the conus arteriosus may develop or fail to develop independently of other portions of the bulbus cordis. When a conus is present, it forms an integral unit with the adjacent aortic or pulmonary valve; changes in the relationship between the conus and adjacent semilunar valve do not occur. Abnormalities in the independent development of the conus arteriosus and in the looping of the cardiac tube explain the development of many complex congenital heart lesions.

Certain normal relationships deserve emphasis before individual complex lesions are considered. Normally, *d*-looping causes the aortic valve to be located to the right of the pulmonary valve. *D*-looping and subsequent shift of the apex of the heart cause the right ventricle to be located anterior to and to the right of the left ventricle. Development of the conus arteriosus beneath the pulmonary valve causes the pulmonary valve to be more cephalad in relation to the aortic valve. Normally, muscular conal tissue separates the annuli of the pulmonary and tricuspid valves. Involution of the conus arteriosus beneath the aortic valve causes the aortic annulus adjacent to the noncoronary cusp of the aortic valve to be contiguous with the annulus of the anterior leaflet of the mitral valve.

Certain rules have proved useful in the diagnostic analysis of patients with complex congenital heart lesions. With 2 rare exceptions (asplenia and polysplenia), the position of the viscera determines the location of the atria. When the stomach bubble is left and the liver is right (situs solitus), the right atrium and inferior vena cava are right-sided. In situs inversus totalis, the positions of both the viscera and the atria are reversed. The right atrium is defined as the structure receiving systemic venous blood; the left atrium is the chamber receiving pulmonary venous blood. The ventricles are designated by their structure; thus, angiocardiograms are necessary to locate the anatomic ventricles and to determine their relationship to the atria. The right ventricle is coarsely trabeculated and usually has a rounded, globular shape, whereas the left ventricle has few trabeculae and has a more conical shape, particularly in systole. The atrioventricular valves are parts of the morphologic ventricles rather than the atria.

The atria and ventricles develop independently. When the right atrium connects with the right ventricle and the left atrium connects with the morphologic left ventricle, the atria and ventricles have a *concordant* relationship. A *discordant* atrioventricular relationship exists when the right atrium connects with the left ventricle.

The direction of the looping of the cardiac tube determines the location of the ventricles (*d*-loop, right ventricle anterior to and to the right of the left ventricle). Usually, the direction of ventricular looping is concordant with the direction of conotruncal twisting, either both rightward or both leftward. Conotruncal twisting, persistence or involution of subsemilunar valve coni (see below), and ventricular looping determine the relationships of the semilunar valves to each other. When ventricular looping and conotruncal twisting are concordant, the location of the aortic valve (in relation to the pulmonary valve—right or left) indicates the direction of ventricular looping. Thus, if the aortic valve is to the right of the pulmonary valve, a *d*-loop is present and the right ventricle is anterior and to the right of the left ventricle. However, since the conus arteriosus and ventricular canal develop independently, the direction of ventricular looping and conotruncal twisting can be discordant, and the location of the semilunar valves to each other will not indicate the direction of ventricular looping. The term "malposition of the great arteries" describes discordance between ventricular looping and the location of the semilunar valves.

Persistence or involution of conal tissue beneath each semilunar valve explains many of the common cardiac anomalies as well as some very rare specimens. Normally, the subpulmonary conus remains and the subaortic conus involutes to produce fibrous continuity of the aortic and mitral valves. Tetralogy of Fallot and truncus arteriosus are explained by normal involution of the subaortic conus and subnormal development of the subpulmonary conus. In complex malformations, either the subaortic or subpulmonary conus may persist or involute, or both may persist, or both may involute. Angiocardiograms are necessary to determine conal development beneath the semilunar valves and the presence or absence of continuity between semilunar and atrioventricular valves.

The classification and terminology of complex lesions remain unsettled because many variations can exist in the positional relationships of the atria, ventricles, great arteries, cardiac axes, and heart positions. For the sake of simplicity, complex lesions can be divided into 3 large groups: conotruncal malformations, single ventricle, and cardiac malposition.

CONOTRUNCAL MALFORMATIONS

Conotruncal malformations result from different combinations of cardiac tube looping (location of the ventricles), conotruncal twisting, and persistence or involution of the subaortic and subpulmonary coni. This broad category of lesions includes transposition of

the great arteries, malpositions of the great arteries, and double outlet ventricles as well as tetralogy of Fallot, pulmonary atresia, and truncus arteriosus. To reduce confusion and to concentrate on the more common and important conotruncal malformations, typical transposition of the great arteries, corrected transposition, malposition of the great arteries, and double outlet ventricles will be presented here.

VanPraagh R: Conotruncal malformations. Page 139 in: *Heart Disease in Infancy*. Barratt-Boyes BG & others (editors). Livingstone, 1973.

TYPICAL TRANSPOSITION OF THE GREAT ARTERIES
(*D*-Transposition)

Essentials of Diagnosis

- Situs solitus, levocardia.
- Cyanosis from birth; hypoxic spells sometimes present.
- Heart failure often present.
- Murmurs variable: often absent and not diagnostic.
- Cardiac enlargement and diminished pulmonary artery segment on x-ray.

General Considerations

Transposition of the great arteries is defined strictly and requires the presence of an interventricular septum, the origin of the aorta from the morphologic right ventricle, and the origin of the pulmonary arteries from the left ventricle. The plane of the ventricular septum is used to determine the ventricular origin of each great artery.

Approximately 60% of all patients with transposition of the great arteries have typical transposition with situs solitus and levocardia. The lesion is more common in males. During development of the heart, the segmented cardiac tube loops to the right (*d*-loop), the conotruncus twists rightward, but the conus arteriosus beneath the pulmonary valve disappears and the conal tissue beneath the aortic valve usually (but not always) develops well. The *d*-loop and development of the subaortic conus arteriosus cause the aortic valve to be anterior to and slightly to the right of the pulmonary valve. The aorta arises from the normally placed anterior morphologic right ventricle (Fig 22–19). Involution of the subpulmonary conus arteriosus places the annuli of the pulmonary and mitral valves in continuity. The pulmonary artery arises from the posterior left ventricle. The atria and ventricles are concordant: the right atrium empties into the right ventricle and the left atrium into the left ventricle. The coronary arteries arise from the aorta, but usually the right coronary orifice is anterior and slightly to the left.

Transposition of the great arteries causes the systemic and pulmonary circulations to be independent. Anatomic communication (ventricular septal defect, patent ductus arteriosus, atrial septal defect) between the separate circulations is required to mix oxygenated and unoxygenated blood. The degree of cyanosis is proportional to the relative amount of oxygenated pulmonary venous blood that reaches the right ventricle and aorta. Nearly half of patients with typical transposition have an associated ventricular septal defect. The ductus arteriosus, which may mix pulmonary and systemic blood at birth, closes during early infancy in most patients. Atrial septal defects provide the third common anatomic communication between the independent circulations, but relatively few babies have large atrial septal defects. Approximately 30% of infants with transposition and ventricular septal defects also have obstruction of the left ventricular outflow tract. About 5% of patients have left ventricular outflow obstruction with an intact ventricular septum. Single ventricle, persistent atrioventricular canal, total anomalous pulmonary venous connection, tricuspid atresia, and coarctation are less common anomalies associated with typical transposition of the great arteries.

Clinical Findings

A. Symptoms and Signs: Clinical findings in infancy are related to the presence or absence of a ventricular septal defect and subpulmonary stenosis. Infants with transposition and an intact ventricular septum are cyanotic at birth and develop severe cyanosis (arterial P_{O_2} 15–30 mm Hg), acidosis, and hypoxic spells when the ductus arteriosus begins to close. Signs of heart failure—tachypnea, hepatomegaly, and cardiomegaly—are also present. Cardiac murmurs are usually not heard and, if present, are generally soft and nondiagnostic.

When a ventricular septal defect is present, cyanosis is less severe and hypoxic spells are generally absent. Heart failure may be severe, with hyperactive ventricles and severe respiratory distress. A faint systolic murmur or no murmur may be present. When transposition of the great arteries is combined with ventricular septal defect and subpulmonary stenosis, the heart is usually quiet and small and cyanosis is present without signs of heart failure. A faint or harsh systolic murmur is sometimes present over the precordium.

Older infants and children develop polycythemia and clubbing and grow slowly. The heart and liver are usually enlarged. The full clinical picture varies with specific associated lesions and previous palliative operations.

B. X-Ray Findings: In newborns, the heart may not appear enlarged and the thymic shadow may obscure the narrow mediastinal vascular pedicle. The aorta arises on the patient's right, and the pulmonary arterial segment is absent or diminished in the posteroanterior projection. After 1 or 2 weeks, cardiomegaly develops, and if pulmonary arterial blood flow is increased the lungs appear congested.

C. Electrocardiography: The ECG findings vary with the patient's age and associated lesions. In newborns, the ECG may be normal; older infants usually have some abnormal right ventricular hypertrophy. If subpulmonary stenosis is present, left ventricular hypertrophy may also be present.

D. Cardiac Catheterization and Cineangiocardiography: These studies are required to define the pathologic anatomy and physiology in patients with transposition of the great arteries. Systemic pressures are found in the right ventricle, and the catheter passes directly into the aorta. The pulmonary artery cannot be entered easily except when a large ventricular septal defect is present or when a special balloon catheter is

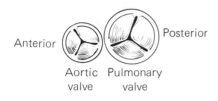

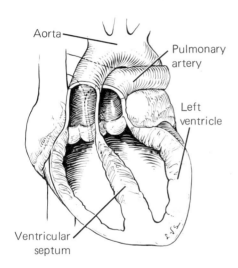

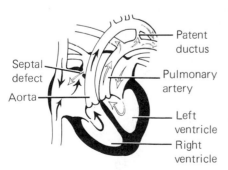

Figure 22–19. Typical transposition of the great arteries. The aorta arises from the morphologic right ventricle and is anterior to and slightly to the right of the pulmonary artery, which originates from the morphologic left ventricle. Inset at bottom illustrates the independent systemic and pulmonary circulations, which may be connected by a patent ductus arteriosus or atrial septal defect. Inset at top illustrates a common relationship of the 2 great arteries in typical transposition.

used. In the absence of lung disease, arterial oxygen saturation in the pulmonary veins is normal. Pulmonary venous and left atrial pressures are usually elevated when pulmonary arterial blood flow exceeds systemic blood flow. Oxygen saturation of blood in the left ventricle is higher than that found in the aorta and right ventricle. Ventricular pressures are identical when a large ventricular septal defect is present. The route of the catheter and changes in blood oxygen saturation define the sites of mixing of the 2 circulations. Since the pulmonary and systemic circulations are independent, reliable calculations of shunt flows are not possible.

Cineangiocardiograms show that the aorta is located anterior to and slightly to the right of the pulmonary artery and that it fills from the right ventricle. The aortic valve is more superior than normal and is near the level of the fourth or fifth thoracic vertebra. The trabeculated, globular right ventricle is anterior to and to the right of the posterior left ventricle. Selective injections of contrast material and lateral and oblique views are necessary to demonstrate the conal anatomy and the presence of atrial and ventricular septal defects, pulmonary stenosis, patent ductus arteriosus, and other more complex cardiac anomalies.

Differential Diagnosis

In newborns, cyanosis may be caused by respiratory disease, tetralogy of Fallot, pulmonary or tricuspid atresia, total anomalous pulmonary venous connection with pulmonary venous obstruction, truncus arteriosus, Ebstein's anomaly, and atresia of the left heart. Newborns with tetralogy of Fallot usually do not develop heart failure early, and the aortic arch may be on the right. The combination of definite cyanosis and heart failure in a newborn suggests transposition of the great arteries and is sufficient indication for cardiac catheterization and cineangiocardiography.

Natural History

Without treatment, 50% of newborns with transposition of the great arteries die by 1 month of age and 90% die within 1 year after birth. Patients with intact ventricular septa have the worst prognosis, and survival beyond 1 year occurs only if a large atrial septal defect is also present. Patients with large ventricular septal defects and excessive pulmonary blood flow usually succumb during their first year from severe heart failure. Patients who have ventricular septal defect and mild or moderate subpulmonary stenosis have the best prognosis. The prognosis is particularly poor when more severe associated lesions are also present.

The combination of heart failure and severe hypoxia is the most common cause of death in infancy. Respiratory infections, systemic emboli, systemic infection, progressive pulmonary vascular disease, cerebral abscess, and occasionally cerebral venous thrombosis may cause death at any time in older infants and young children.

Patients who survive palliative procedures or operations may close their ventricular septal defects or may

develop subpulmonary stenosis or pulmonary vascular disease. Approximately 15–20% of patients will close their ventricular septal defect or develop subpulmonary stenosis within the first 2 years after birth. Patients with transposition of the great arteries and increased pulmonary arterial blood flow develop pulmonary vascular disease more quickly than other patients who have increased pulmonary arterial blood flow from less complicated defects. Irreversible pulmonary vascular disease may develop in the first year.

Treatment

Infants who are deeply cyanotic ($Pa_{O_2} < 35$ mm Hg) or who develop heart failure should be given oxygen and digoxin and should have cardiac catheterization. Enlargement or creation of an atrial septal defect by balloon catheter (Rashkind procedure) is recommended for virtually every patient who has transposition and who requires catheterization. The atrial septum is torn by rapidly pulling an inflated balloon from the left atrium into the right atrium. A large atrial septal defect improves blood mixing and obliterates the pressure difference between the left and right atria. A balloon septostomy is difficult to perform after 2 or 3 months of age because of increased thickness and strength of the atrial septum. These patients require operation.

Palliative operations for transposition of the great arteries are used infrequently and only for patients with severe associated lesions such as pulmonary atresia or single ventricle. Palliative procedures are used to increase or reduce pulmonary blood flow. The Blalock-Hanlon operation to create an atrial septal defect is no longer recommended for typical transposition.

At any age, systemic venous blood can be redirected through the mitral valve, left ventricle, and pulmonary artery by insertion of a pericardial or Dacron partition in the atrium (Mustard operation; Fig 22–20). This baffle, which is sewn in place after the atrial septum is excised, redirects pulmonary venous blood into the right ventricle and aorta. This "corrective" operation converts the independent pulmonary and systemic circulations into a single circulatory system in series, but the morphologic right ventricle must support systemic blood pressure. Associated ventricular septal defects may be closed transatrially, or closure may be deferred. Obstructive lesions of the left ventricular outflow tract are usually, but not always, resected via a pulmonary arterotomy.

In transposition, ventricular septal defects may be located anywhere within the ventricular septum. Defects are preferably closed transatrially, but this is not always possible. Low defects of the muscular septum can be closed via a left ventriculotomy, but others must be closed through an incision in the right ventricle. In patients with pulmonary vascular disease (greater than 10 units), "palliative Mustard" operations are recommended. The interatrial baffle is sewn in place, but no attempt is made to close the ventricular septal defect.

In selected older patients with transposition of

the great arteries, ventricular septal defect, and obstruction of the left ventricular outflow tract, blood flow from the left ventricle is redirected through the ventricular septal defect into the aorta by insertion of a patch within the right ventricle. A Dacron tube (conduit) that contains a heterograft or homograft aortic valve is used to connect the right ventricle to the main pulmonary artery downstream to the obstruction and pulmonary valve (conduit operation; Fig 22–16B). The proximal pulmonary artery is closed. This procedure has the advantage that the morphologic left ventricle supports the systemic blood pressure and obviates the often impossible task of relieving the left ventricular outflow tract obstruction. A similar operation can be performed for transposition of the great arteries, ventricular septal defect, and pulmonary atresia if the pulmonary arteries are sufficiently large to accept the total cardiac output.

Anatomic correction of typical transposition of the great arteries with ventricular septal defect has been attempted and in a few instances has been successful. The procedure requires transfer of the ostia of the coronary arteries to the root of the great vessel arising from the left ventricle and anastomosis of this vessel to the distal ascending aorta. The aortic root arising from the right ventricle is connected to the distal main pulmonary artery.

Prognosis After Surgery

After balloon atrial septostomy (Rashkind procedure), arterial oxygen saturation generally increases from about 40% to approximately 65%. Operative fatalities are rare, and over 90% of patients survive the initial hospitalization. After balloon septostomy, only 50% of patients reach 30 months of age unless the Mustard operation is performed.

The mortality rate of the Mustard operation is 5–10% in infants over 3 months of age who have transposition of the great arteries without ventricular septal defect, left ventricular outflow tract obstruction, or other lesions. Interestingly, the mortality rate of the operation may be lower in infants 3–12 months of age than in older infants and children.

An associated ventricular septal defect or obstruction of the left ventricular outflow tract increases the mortality rate of the Mustard operation to 20–30%. The mortality rate for palliative Mustard operations is 10–15% in selected patients. Approximately 50% of patients have supraventricular arrhythmias following Mustard's operation. The high incidence of arrhythmias is due to interference with the sinus node and coronary sinus, both of which can be avoided, and incisions and suture lines across multiple conduction pathways in the atrium. Late postoperative complications include obstruction of the superior vena cava and pulmonary venous hypertension. Patch enlargement of the anatomic right atrium reduces the likelihood of pulmonary venous hypertension.

Ebert PA, Gay WA Jr, Engle MA: Correction of transposition of the great arteries. Ann Surg 74:433, 1974.

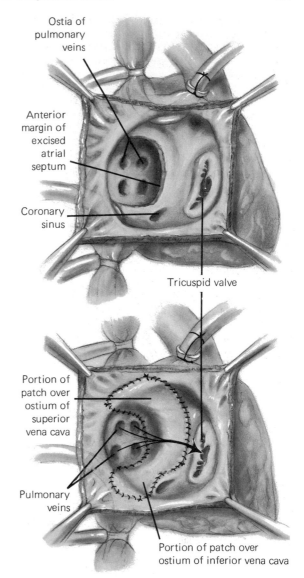

Figure 22–20. The Mustard operation. *A:* The atrial septum has been excised except for the anterior portion that contains the anterior intra-atrial conduction pathway. Pulmonary venous openings are visible at the posterior left atrial wall. *B:* A partition of pericardium or Dacron cloth is sutured around the left and right pulmonary venous openings, around the openings of the superior and inferior vena cavas, and to the anterior margin of the interatrial septum. Systemic venous blood then passes posterior to the partition toward the mitral valve. Pulmonary venous blood and blood from the coronary sinus pass anterior to the partition toward the tricuspid valve. A patch of Dacron or pericardium is often used to enlarge the right (now functional left) atrium when the atriotomy (not shown) is closed.

Jatene AD & others: Anatomic correction of transposition of the great vessels. J Thorac Cardiovasc Surg 72:364, 1976.

Lindesmith GG & others: The Mustard operation as a palliative procedure. J Thorac Cardiovasc Surg 63:75, 1972.

Mustard WT & others: The surgical management of transposition of the great vessels. J Thorac Cardiovasc Surg 48:953, 1964.

Parr GVS & others: Cardiac performance early after interatrial transposition of venous return in infants and small children. Circulation 50 (Suppl 2):2, 1974.

Paul MH, Van Praagh S, Van Praagh R: Transposition of the great vessels. Chap 40, pp 576–610, in: *Paediatric Cardiology*. Watson H (editor). Mosby, 1968.

Rashkind WJ, Miller WW: Transposition of the great arteries: Results of palliation by balloon atrial septostomy in 31 infants. Circulation 38:453, 1968.

Rastelli GC, McGoon DC, Wallace RB: Anatomic correction of transposition of the great arteries with ventricular septal defect and subpulmonary stenosis. J Thorac Cardiovasc Surg 58:545, 1969.

Trusler GA, Mustard WT: Palliative and reparative procedures for transposition of the great arteries: Current review. Ann Thorac Surg 17:410, 1974.

CORRECTED TRANSPOSITION OF THE GREAT ARTERIES

Corrected transposition is a physiologic term which indicates that systemic venous blood reaches the lungs and pulmonary venous blood reaches the systemic arteries in the presence of transposition or malposition of the great arteries. Most commonly in patients with situs solitus and levocardia, this rare anomaly develops from *l*-looping of the cardiac tube, rightward twisting of the conotruncus, and overdevelopment of the subaortic conus arteriosus. The aorta is anterior to and to the left of the posterior pulmonary artery (*l*-transposition). *l*-Looping causes the morphologic left ventricle to be located anterior to and to the right of the posterior morphologic right ventricle. Corrected transposition also occurs very rarely with other combinations of conotruncal malformations and in patients with cardiac and visceral malpositions. Involution of the subpulmonary conus and development of the subaortic conus cause fibrous continuity of the pulmonary and anatomic mitral valve (functional right atrioventricular valve). The coronary arteries are inverted with the ventricles, so that the left coronary artery is anterior. When no associated lesions are present, systemic venous blood passes through the right atrium, mitral valve, and left ventricle and into the pulmonary artery. Pulmonary venous blood passes through the left atrium, tricuspid valve, and right ventricle and into the left-sided aorta. Thus, the atria and ventricles are discordant, and the ventricles and great arteries are also discordant. The normal physiologic circulation gives the lesion its name ("corrected transposition"). Unfortunately, malformations of the morphologic tricuspid valve (functional left atrioventricular valve), ventricular septal defect, arrhythmias, or subpulmonary or pulmonary valvular stenosis occur in over 90% of patients.

The clinical manifestations of corrected transpositions vary in relation to the associated lesions. Asymptomatic patients have small hearts, atrioventricular conduction delays, and occasionally mild incompetence of the anatomic tricuspid valve, and they very rarely live a long life. Patients with large ventricular septal defects or tricuspid valvular incompetence (or both) develop severe heart failure and massive cardiomegaly in infancy and early childhood. Pulmonary stenosis with ventricular septal defect causes cyanosis with or without heart failure. Partial or complete atrioventricular block occurs in a high percentage of cases. More than half of patients with complicated lesions die in early childhood of heart failure or heart block.

In symptomatic patients, the posteroanterior chest film may suggest the diagnosis. The aortic knob is absent from the right mediastinal border, and the ascending aorta is displaced to the patient's left where it forms a straight left superior mediastinal border that tapers to a narrow waist. The heart may be massively enlarged, and pulmonary venous congestion may be increased. The ECG frequently shows atrioventricular conduction block. Inversion of the ventricles causes the normal q waves in the left ECG leads to be absent.

Cardiac catheterization and cineangiocardiography establish the diagnosis and the presence of associated lesions. Atrioventricular conduction disturbances occur frequently during catheterization. The passage of the catheter or angiocardiograms show the aorta anterior to and to the left of the pulmonary artery. Subaortic conal tissue pushes the aortic valve superiorly and separates the aorta and morphologic tricuspid annuli. The inverted positions of the ventricle can be determined from their anatomic characteristics. The lesion must be distinguished from typical *d*-transposition, tetralogy of Fallot, congenital mitral incompetence, and congenital heart block.

Operative management of symptomatic patients with corrected transposition is directed toward the associated lesions, but in general the results have not been satisfactory. Complete heart block with a slow ventricular rate and uncontrolled heart failure requires an implanted pacemaker with (preferably) epicardial leads. Ventricular septal defects can be closed, but technical difficulties due to the position of the coronary arteries, large size of the defects, and poorly functioning atrioventricular valves greatly increase the operative risk. Severe tricuspid (functional left atrioventricular valve) insufficiency requires prosthetic valve replacement. Subpulmonary stenosis is usually complicated, and a palliative systemic to pulmonary arterial anastomosis is recommended in preference to excision of the stenotic lesion. Intraoperative mapping of the conduction system reduces the risk of operative heart block.

Friedberg DZ, Nadas AS: Clinical profile of patients with congenital corrected transposition of the great arteries. N Engl J Med 282:1053, 1970.

MALPOSITION OF THE GREAT ARTERIES

Discordance between the directions of cono-truncal twisting and ventricular looping causes malposition of the great arteries. Semilunar valves of the great vessels have abnormal relationships with each other. Physiologically, the circulation may function normally, as in corrected transposition, or abnormally, as in typical transposition. Examples of malposition of the great arteries are rare and frequently occur in association with situs inversus, dextrocardia, pulmonary atresia, single ventricle, and other severe cardiac lesions. Because of the variations and the degree of conal development, the direction of ventricular looping, conotruncal twisting, and associated anomalies, the pathologic anatomy of these lesions varies greatly.

Most patients with malposition of the great arteries do not survive infancy; however, a few patients reach childhood. The great variation in pathologic anatomy causes similar variations in circulatory dysfunction; thus, each individual must be carefully studied. The anatomic relationships of the cardiac subunits must be defined according to the diagnostic "rules" described previously. Although many lesions are inoperable, some carefully selected patients can be helped by operation.

DOUBLE OUTLET RIGHT VENTRICLE

In double outlet right ventricle, both great arteries arise from the right ventricle. A ventricular septal defect is invariably present, although in rare instances it may be small. Most often, the aorta is in the *d*-position and the atria and ventricles are concordant. However, *l*-position of the aorta may occur and the atria and ventricles may be discordant with either aortic position. Valvular or subvalvular pulmonary stenosis and coarctation of the aorta are the most common associated anomalies. The ventricular septal defect may be located beneath the aortic or pulmonary valves, or both, or neither.

Most commonly, the atria and ventricles are concordant and the aorta is in the *d*-position. If the ventricular septal defect is beneath the aortic valve and pulmonary stenosis is not present, blood from the left ventricle streams through the septal defect into the aorta. These patients are acyanotic, often develop heart failure in infancy, have equal pressures in left and right ventricles, and are likely to develop pulmonary vascular disease. A systolic murmur is present along the left sternal border. The ECG shows right ventricular hypertrophy. Chest x-rays are not diagnostic, but the diagnosis can be made by echocardiography with or without cineangiocardiography. Cineangiocardiograms show that the aorta is displaced anteriorly and that the aortic and pulmonary valves are at the same level. Clinically, the lesion is similar to a large ventricular septal

defect. This lesion can be repaired by placing a prosthetic intraventricular conduit between the ventricular septal defect and the aortic annulus so that the left ventricular blood passes directly into the aorta. Pulmonary arterial banding may be necessary for small infants to control heart failure; however, primary repair is possible even in infants. The operative mortality rate in older infants and children is proportionate to the severity of coexisting pulmonary vascular disease.

If the ventricular septal defect is beneath the pulmonary valve and anterior (and cephalad) to the crista supraventricularis, left ventricular blood streams preferentially into the pulmonary artery. These patients are cyanotic from birth and may develop severe heart failure, and they must be differentiated from patients with transposition of the great arteries with ventricular septal defect. If pulmonary stenosis is not present, pulmonary vascular disease may develop rapidly. The anatomic diagnosis is made by angiograms. Repair can be achieved by placing a prosthetic patch over the ventricular septal defect and pulmonary annulus so that the left ventricular blood enters the pulmonary artery. A Mustard operation to reverse systemic and pulmonary venous return at the atrium completes the repair.

Pulmonary stenosis and coarctation are the most common associated lesions. Coarctation may be severe enough to require operation in early infancy. Pulmonary stenosis protects against the development of pulmonary vascular disease but increases cyanosis and hypoxia. A systemic-pulmonary arterial anastomosis (preferably a Blalock-Taussig anastomosis) may be required in infants. Corrective operations usually require an external valved conduit to bypass the pulmonary stenosis, combined with an intraventricular conduit as described above for subaortic or subpulmonary ventricular septal defects.

Kirklin JW, Harp RA, McGoon DC: Surgical treatment of origin of both vessels from right ventricle, including cases of pulmonary stenosis. J Thorac Cardiovasc Surg 48:1026, 1964.

Pacifico AD, Kirklin JW, Bargeron LM Jr: Complex congenital malformations: Surgical treatment of double outlet right ventricle and double outlet left ventricle. Page 57 in: *Advances in Cardiovascular Surgery.* Kirklin JW (editor). Grune & Stratton, 1973.

DOUBLE OUTLET LEFT VENTRICLE

Origin of both great arteries from a morphologic left ventricle is a rare anomaly. Like double outlet right ventricle, double outlet left ventricle may exist with the aorta to the right, anterior to, or to the left of the pulmonary artery, with or without a muscular conus beneath either or both great arteries. A ventricular septal defect must be present for survival. Pulmonary stenosis is usually present. Total correction by closing the ventricular septal defect and pulmonary valve and constructing a valved conduit from the right ventricle to the pulmonary artery has been performed in children. Occasionally, an intraventricular repair can be performed by closing the ventricular septal defect so that the pulmonary artery is connected to the right ventricle.

Pacifico AD & others: Surgical treatment of double outlet left ventricle. Circulation 48 (Suppl 3):19, 1973.

SINGLE VENTRICLE

Single ventricle describes a heart with one ventricular chamber which receives blood from both the tricuspid and mitral valves or a common atrioventricular valve. The lesion is present in up to 3% of congenital heart defects. Atypical or typical transposition of the great arteries occurs in approximately 85% of patients. Twenty-five to 35% of patients have a common atrioventricular valve, and another 25% have stenosis or regurgitation of one of the atrioventricular valves. One-third to one-half of patients have pulmonary stenosis or atresia, and another third have aortic stenosis. The lesion occurs in association with situs inversus, dextrocardia, and asplenia in approximately 20% of patients. Defects of the atrial septum, total anomalous pulmonary venous connection, and truncus arteriosus are occasionally seen with single ventricle.

Single ventricle has been subdivided into 4 anatomic groups by the morphology of the ventricle. In approximately 75% of patients, single ventricle develops from the left ventricular portion of the ventricular canal and from the conus arteriosus and infundibulum of the right ventricle. The right ventricular contribution forms a small outflow chamber from which the great vessels originate. The diagnosis of single ventricle and specific associated lesions must be made by cardiac catheterization and cineangiocardiography. Absence of the ventricular septum and information about the atrioventricular valves can be obtained by echocardiography.

Clinical findings and prognosis are related to the relative amounts of pulmonary and systemic arterial blood flow. Some patients have survived into their second decade, but most die in infancy. Infants may be palliated by pulmonary arterial banding or shunt operations. In older children with 2 atrioventricular valves, the ventricle can be partitioned using a thick prosthetic patch. A valved external conduit is often necessary to provide pulmonary blood flow. Operative mapping of the ventricular conduction system is necessary to prevent heart block. The most suitable anatomic types for operation are patients with an anatomic left ventricle and outflow chamber and those with a common ventricle formed from both ventricular sinuses. Currently the operation has a high hospital mortality rate.

Edie RN & others: Surgical repair of single ventricle. J Thorac Cardiovasc Surg 66:350, 1973.

Lev M & others: Single (primitive) ventricle. Circulation 39:577, 1969.
McGoon DC & others: The problem of correcting single and common ventricle. Circulation 54 (suppl 2):101, 1976.
Van Praagh R, Omgley PA, Swan HJC: Anatomic types of single or common ventricle in man. Am J Cardiol 13:367, 1964.

CARDIAC MALPOSITION

Situs inversus totalis is a rare anomaly in which the stomach and other abdominal organs occupy positions which are the mirror images of normal (situs solitus). Except in asplenia and polysplenia (see below), the position of the viscera determines the location of the atrium; thus, in situs inversus, the atria are reversed and the heart is right-sided (dextrocardia). The morphologic left atrium is on the right. When the ventricles and atria are concordant, the right atrium (on the patient's left) empties into the anatomic right ventricle. If transposition is not present, the circulation is normal and the cardiac chambers and vessels are the mirror image of normal structures. If transposition is present, the aorta is anterior to the pulmonary artery in the right-sided heart.

Rather severe associated anomalies usually occur with situs inversus, dextrocardia, and malposition of the great arteries. If the atria and ventricles are discordant, transposition or malposition of the great arteries is always present and the lesion may be physiologically "corrected." In most cases, the aorta arises to the left of the pulmonary artery and severe associated anomalies are present.

Isolated levocardia is the remaining condition that occurs with situs inversus totalis. The heart is located in the left chest, and most patients have severe associated cardiac anomalies and agenesis of the left lung.

Isolated dextrocardia is the term used to designate mirror image position of the heart when the viscera are in normal position (situs solitus). Agenesis of the right lung is present in many of these patients.

Cardiac catheterization and cineangiocardiography are essential to understand the pathologic anatomy and physiology of these lesions. The diagnostic rules for locating the visceral situs, morphologic ventricles, and positions of the great vessels must be used to label each structure and chamber opacified by the contrast material.

Life expectancy is dependent upon the severity of the circulatory handicap. Some patients live to advanced age, and others can be helped by specific palliative operations to improve circulatory function. A few patients are candidates for totally corrective operations of less severe associated lesions.

Kirklin JW: Surgery for transposition, corrected transposition, and related complex anomalies. Pages 26–31 in: *Lecture Outlines, Postgraduate Course on Cardiovascular Surgery.* American College of Surgeons, 1970.

ASPLENIA & POLYSPLENIA

Absence of the spleen, midline position of the stomach and liver (indeterminate situs), distinct middle lobes of both right and left lungs, and Howell-Jolly bodies within red cells are associated with severe cardiac anomalies. About a third of such patients have dextrocardia. Single atrium, single ventricle, atrioventricular canal, transposition, pulmonary atresia, and anomalies of systemic and pulmonary venous return may occur. These patients are abnormally susceptible to bacterial infections, particularly pneumococcal infections.

Many small spleens, interruption of the hepatic portion of the inferior vena cava, absence of middle pulmonary lobes in both lungs, and absence of the gallbladder are associated with the same severe cardiac anomalies listed above with the exception of transposition.

Moller JH & others: Congenital cardiac disease associated with polysplenia. Circulation 36:789, 1967.

V. MISCELLANEOUS CONGENITAL HEART LESIONS

CONGENITAL HEART BLOCK

Complete atrioventricular dissociation occurs as an isolated lesion or in association with other congenital cardiac anomalies, particularly corrected transposition of the great vessels, atrial septal defect, and endocardial fibroelastosis. The cardiac rate is generally higher (40–80 beats per minute) than that which occurs in adults or in children who have complete heart block as a result of intracardiac surgery. The diagnosis is made by ECG. A few patients will develop Adams-Stokes syncopal attacks; others—particularly those with associated lesions—develop heart failure. Sudden death may occur in patients who have Adams-Stokes attacks. Digoxin is not recommended in these patients, but diuretics may help to control heart failure. Medical therapy also includes sublingual isoproterenol, but symptomatic patients are best treated with an implanted electrical pacemaker with epicardial electrodes.

Nakamura FF, Nadas AS: Complete heart block in infants and children. N Engl J Med 270:1261, 1964.

CONGENITAL MITRAL INSUFFICIENCY

Isolated congenital mitral insufficiency is a rare lesion and is due to deformed mitral leaflets, short, thick chordae tendineae, dilatation of the mitral annulus, or cleft leaflets. More commonly, congenital mitral insufficiency occurs in association with other lesions such as persistent atrioventricular canal, coarctation of the aorta, or corrected transposition of the great arteries.

The severity of the insufficiency is variable. In severe cases, left heart failure with pulmonary venous congestion causes fatigue, poor weight gain, dyspnea, and palpitations. A pansystolic murmur is maximal at the apex and is transmitted to the left axilla. The ECG shows left ventricular hypertrophy, and chest films show cardiomegaly with left atrial enlargement and pulmonary venous congestion. The diagnosis and severity of the mitral incompetence can be assessed at cardiac catheterization; however, cineangiocardiograms do not provide sufficient detail to indicate whether or not mitral valvuloplasty is possible.

Children with poorly controlled heart failure require operation. Operation is not recommended for those with mild or moderate symptoms. If additional left-sided lesions are present such as coarctation or aortic stenosis, these defects are usually corrected first. Valvuloplasty and annuloplasty are preferable to valve replacement. Unfortunately, almost half of patients require valve replacement.

A variety of mitral prostheses have been successfully inserted into infants and children. The operative mortality rate approximates 10%, and, unless a glutaraldehyde-preserved heterograft valve is used, anticoagulants are required to control thromboembolism. Infants with prosthetic mitral valves require replacement with a larger prosthesis in early adolescence. Late complications include sudden death, stroke, and bleeding problems.

Bernhard WF, Litwin SB: The surgical treatment of unusual congenital mitral anomalies. Circulation 46 (Suppl 2):35, 1972.

Berry BE & others: Cardiac valve replacement in children. J Thorac Cardiovasc Surg 68:705, 1974.

ANOMALOUS LEFT CORONARY ARTERY

Origin of the left coronary artery from the pulmonary artery causes myocardial ischemia and heart failure in infancy. The right coronary artery is normal and supplies blood to the entire myocardium via intracoronary collaterals. Blood flow in the anomalous left coronary artery is usually retrograde into the pulmonary artery; however, the amount of left-to-right shunting is small. The left ventricle is dilated and fibrotic, has paradoxic motion, and contracts poorly. During feeding or other activity, infants develop episodic pain, pallor, sweating, and tachypnea, which suggest angina pectoris. The heart progressively enlarges, and an apical systolic murmur of mitral insufficiency occasionally develops if the papillary muscle is infarcted. The ECG often shows evidence of myocardial infarction in the left limb and precordial leads. Chest films confirm the gross cardiomegaly and pulmonary venous congestion. The diagnosis is made by cineangiocardiography. Contrast material opacifies only the right coronary artery after injection into the aortic root. The left coronary artery can often be faintly seen in late frames. An increase in oxygen saturation in the main pulmonary artery is not always found and is seldom diagnostic.

A few infants with mild symptoms can be managed medically, but most have severe heart failure and arrhythmias which do not respond to medical management. A few infants have had successful anastomosis of the left subclavian artery to the detached anomalous left coronary artery. Older children have had aorto-left coronary saphenous vein grafts. Previously, ligation of the anomalous left coronary artery at its origin was recommended to improve myocardial blood flow from the right coronary artery.

Patients with left-to-right shunts generally survive ligation of the anomalous left coronary artery, and those with little or no left-to-right shunting do not. Follow-up information after antegrade left coronary arterial flow is restored is sparse, but most patients continue to have abnormal function of the left ventricle.

Askenazi J, Nadas AS: Anomalous left coronary artery originating from the pulmonary artery. Circulation 51:976, 1975.
Meyer BW & others: A method of definitive surgical treatment of anomalous origin of left coronary artery. J Thorac Cardiovasc Surg 56:104, 1968.

PULMONARY ARTERIOVENOUS FISTULA

In 50% of patients, this rare vascular anomaly is associated with multiple telangiectases (Rendu-Osler-Weber syndrome). One or more large arteriovenous fistulas that do not communicate with alveolar capillaries may occur anywhere in the lungs but are most commonly present in the lower lobes. Pulmonary arterial blood shunts through the fistula into the pulmonary veins to cause mild to moderate cyanosis. Pulmonary arterial and venous pressures are low. Occasional infants develop dyspnea, cyanosis, and right heart failure. Cyanosis, clubbing, and polycythemia are usually most pronounced in late childhood. A soft systolic or continuous murmur is occasionally present over the fistula. Chest x-rays show irregular opacified lesions in the peripheral lung fields at the site of the fistulas. The lesion is confirmed by cineangiocardiography after right ventricular or pulmonary arterial injection. Excision of the fistula is indicated in symptomatic patients and in patients with solitary lesions but is not generally recommended for patients with multiple lesions. Localized resections or lobectomy is most commonly performed.

Shumacker HB Jr, Waldhausen JA: Pulmonary arteriovenous fistulas in children. Ann Surg 158:713, 1963.

PULMONARY ARTERIAL STENOSIS

Single or multiple stenoses of the pulmonary arteries occur commonly at the bifurcation of the main pulmonary artery but may occur anywhere between the pulmonary valve and the tertiary pulmonary arteries. About two-thirds of patients have pulmonary valvular stenosis, tetralogy of Fallot, ventricular septal defects, or patent ductus arteriosus. The stenotic lesions produce harsh systolic murmurs which are not well localized. The location of the stenotic areas is determined by observation of a pressure difference during catheterization of the main pulmonary arteries and by cineangiocardiograms after injection of contrast material into the right ventricle.

Patients without associated congenital heart lesions usually do not require operation. Supravalvular stenosis or hypoplasia of the main pulmonary artery or proximal portions of the right or left pulmonary arteries is usually treated by enlargement with pericardial or Dacron patches during correction of associated intracardiac lesions.

Watson H: Stenosis of the pulmonary arteries. Page 534 in: *Paediatric Cardiology*. Watson H (editor). Mosby, 1968.

PERSISTENT LEFT SUPERIOR VENA CAVA

Persistence of a left superior vena cava which connects the left jugular and subclavian veins to the coronary sinus causes no symptoms but is not uncommon. The anomaly is important to the surgeon since a separate catheter must be inserted through the coronary sinus into the left superior vena cava to collect systemic venous blood during cardiopulmonary bypass. Rarely, the right superior vena cava is absent; in most cases, an innominate vein and both left and right cavas are present and each cava is adequate to carry all of the systemic venous return from the upper body.

ENDOCARDIAL FIBROELASTOSIS

This lesion is not operable, but it may occur in association with operable lesions such as coarctation of the aorta, aortic stenosis, anomalous left coronary artery, and mitral valvular disease. Hyperplasia of subendocardial elastic and collagenous tissue and proliferation of capillaries cause marked thickening of the ventricular wall and a smooth, glistening lining of the left ventricle. Trabeculae are obliterated, and papillary muscles and chordae tendineae are contracted. The disease affects principally the left ventricle and left atrium; involvement of the right heart chambers is rare. There is some evidence that the disease results from subendocardial ischemia in utero.

Fibroelastosis affects 1–2% of patients with congenital heart disease and may occur primarily without other cardiac lesions. Nearly all infants die of left heart failure within the first year. No specific therapy is available.

Moller JH & others: Endocardial fibroelastosis: A clinical and anatomic study of 47 patients with emphasis on its relationship to mitral insufficiency. Circulation 30:759, 1964.

CARDIAC TUMORS

Cardiac tumors are rare in infancy and childhood. Metastatic malignant sarcomas are the most common cardiac tumors. Most are inoperable, and none can be cured.

Benign tumors of the heart may cause cardiomegaly, heart failure, murmurs, arrhythmias, and conduction disturbances. The heart silhouette may be irregular. Functional pathologic changes are directly related to the location and size of the intracardiac tumor mass.

Rhabdomyomas are most common in infants and are often associated with tuberous sclerosis. These tumors involve the ventricular wall, are often multiple, and to date have not been cured.

Fibromas and hamartomas usually present as intracavitary masses attached to the wall of a cardiac chamber. The left ventricle is most frequently involved. Intracavitary fibromas can be successfully excised; intramural tumors cannot.

Myxomas are unknown in infants and rare in children. Intracavitary myxomas are attached to either the atrial or ventricular septum, obstruct flow, and may shed peripheral emboli. Myxomas are usually easily excised but may recur if excision is incomplete.

Teratomas are often extracardiac and attached to the aortic root. Symptoms are produced by cardiac compression. Extracardiac teratomas are easily excised; intracardiac lesions may involve indispensable portions of the heart.

Nadas AS, Ellison RC: Cardiac tumors in infancy. Am J Cardiol 21:363, 1968.
Van Der Hauwaert LG: Cardiac tumors in infancy and childhood. Br Heart J 33:125, 1971.

●   ●   ●

General References

Kirklin JW (editor): *Advances in Cardiovascular Surgery.* Grune & Stratton, 1973.
Nadas AS, Fyler DC: *Pediatric Cardiology.* Saunders, 1972.

Rudolph AM: *Congenital Heart Disease.* Year Book, 1974.
Watson H (editor): *Paediatric Cardiology.* Mosby, 1968.

23...
Esophagus & Diaphragm

Orville F. Grimes, MD

THE ESOPHAGUS

Surgery of the esophagus has made significant progress in the past 25 years as improvements in anesthesia and other refinements have allowed esophageal operations to be performed with acceptable morbidity and mortality rates. Before the early 1930s, surgical procedures involving the esophagus were limited largely to the cervical and intra-abdominal segments.

ANATOMY
(Fig 23–1)

The esophagus is a muscular tube which serves as a conduit for the passage of food from the pharynx to the stomach. It originates at the level of the sixth cervical vertebra posterior to the cricoid cartilage. In the thorax, the esophagus passes behind the aortic arch and the left main stem bronchus, enters the abdomen through the esophageal hiatus of the diaphragm, and

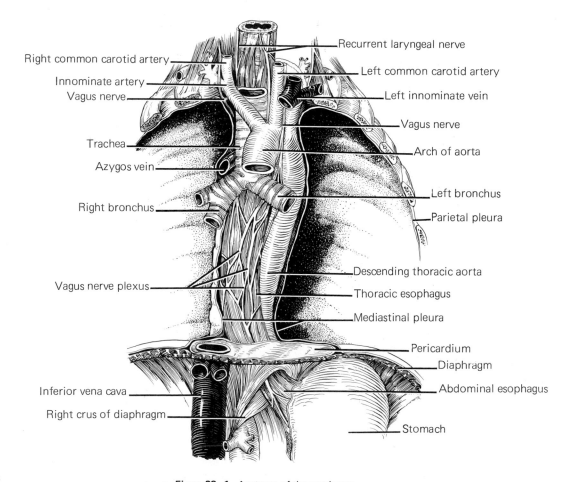

Right common carotid artery

Innominate artery

Vagus nerve

Trachea

Azygos vein

Right bronchus

Vagus nerve plexus

Inferior vena cava

Right crus of diaphragm

Recurrent laryngeal nerve

Left common carotid artery

Left innominate vein

Vagus nerve

Arch of aorta

Left bronchus

Parietal pleura

Descending thoracic aorta

Thoracic esophagus

Mediastinal pleura

Pericardium

Diaphragm

Abdominal esophagus

Stomach

Figure 23–1. Anatomy of the esophagus.

414

terminates in the fundus of the stomach. Its muscle fibers originate from the cricoid cartilage and pharynx above and interdigitate with those of the stomach below. About 2–4 cm of esophagus normally lie below the diaphragm. The junction between the esophagus and stomach is maintained in its normal intra-abdominal position by reflections of the peritoneum onto the stomach and the phrenoesophageal ligament onto the esophagus. The latter is a fibroelastic membrane which lies beneath the peritoneum, on the inferior surface of the diaphragm. When it reaches the esophageal hiatus, the ligament is reflected orad onto the lower esophagus, where it inserts into the circular muscle layer above the gastroesophageal sphincter, 2–4 cm above the diaphragm.

Three anatomic areas of narrowing occur in the esophagus: (1) at the level of the cricoid cartilage (pharyngoesophageal sphincter); (2) in the midthorax, from compression by the aortic arch and the left main stem bronchus; and (3) at the level of the esophageal hiatus of the diaphragm (gastroesophageal sphincter).

In the adult, the length of the esophagus as measured from the upper incisor teeth to the cricopharyngeus muscle is 15–20 cm; to the aortic arch, 20–25 cm; to the inferior pulmonary vein, 30–35 cm; and to the cardioesophageal junction, approximately 40–45 cm.

The musculature of the pharynx and upper third of the esophagus is skeletal in type; the remainder is smooth muscle. Physiologically, the entire organ behaves as a single functioning unit so that no distinction can be made between the upper and lower esophagus from the standpoint of propulsive activity. As in the intestinal tract, the muscle fibers are arranged into inner circular and outer longitudinal layers.

The arterial supply to the esophagus is quite consistent. The upper end is supplied by branches from the inferior thyroid arteries. The thoracic portion receives elements from the bronchial arteries and from esophageal branches originating directly from the aorta. The intercostal arteries may also contribute. The diaphragmatic and abdominal segments are nourished by the left inferior phrenic artery and by the esophageal branches of the left gastric artery.

The venous drainage is more complex and variable. The most important veins are those that drain the lower esophagus. Blood from this region passes into the esophageal branches of the coronary vein, a tributary of the portal vein. This connection constitutes a direct communication between the portal circulation and the venous drainage of the lower esophagus and upper stomach. When the portal system is obstructed, as in cirrhosis of the liver, blood is shunted upward through the coronary vein and the esophageal venous plexus, to eventually pass by way of the azygos vein into the superior vena cava. As they become distended from the increased blood flow and pressure, the esophageal veins may eventually form varices.

The mucosal lining of the esophagus consists of stratified squamous epithelium which contains scat-tered mucous glands throughout. The esophagus has no serosal layer, and for this reason does not heal as readily after injury or surgical anastomosis as other portions of the gastrointestinal tract.

PHYSIOLOGY

Advances have been made in recent years in understanding the physiology and pathophysiology of the esophagus using cineradiography and measurements of intraluminal pressures. Manometric technics have found valuable application in the study of a variety of diseases of the esophagus, and facilities for esophageal manometry are now available in many hospitals. The examination consists of passing into the esophagus a bundle of 2 or 3 fine polyethylene catheters each of which contains a small distal opening. Continuous perfusion of these tubes with small volumes of saline solution ensures patency of their orifices and offers a slight resistance to squeeze. The openings are situated 5 cm apart so that simultaneous recording of pressure can be made at intervals over a segment of known length. Pressures are measured in the resting state by slowly withdrawing the catheters from the stomach toward the pharynx. Pressures are recorded within the stomach, the gastroesophageal sphincter, the body of the esophagus, and the pharyngoesophageal sphincter. Additional data are obtained during swallowing and other movements which may shed light on the suspected disorder.

Correlation of the findings of esophageal motility studies and cineradiology provides a great deal of data on which to base opinions about the causes of dysphagia and odynophagia. Measurement of intraesophageal pH and electrical potential differences may be of clinical value in some instances, but the extent of their usefulness remains to be determined.

The function of the esophagus is to transport food and fluids from the mouth to the stomach and occasionally in the reverse direction. The esophagus contains a sphincter at the junction of the pharynx and esophagus (pharyngoesophageal sphincter) and another between the esophagus and stomach (gastroesophageal sphincter). Pressures in the resting state as measured by manometry are higher in the region of these sphincters than on either side. Pressures in the mouth and pharynx are atmospheric; those within the body of the resting esophagus are slightly subatmospheric, a reflection of normal intrathoracic pressure. Pressure within the stomach is slightly greater than atmospheric.

The structures at the gastroesophageal junction normally function efficiently to prevent reflux of gastric acid and food from the stomach into the esophagus. The mechanism of gastroesophageal competence is complex and, despite intensive study, is incompletely understood at present.

The gastroesophageal sphincter comprises the lower 4 cm of esophagus, where resting pressure within the lumen normally exceeds intragastric pressure by 15–25 cm water owing to tonic contraction of the esophageal musculature. Sphincteric competence is greatly aided by the <u>normal intra-abdominal location</u> of the terminal esophagus. <u>Dislocation of the sphincter by a sliding hiatal hernia is the major cause of sphincteric incompetence and reflux esophagitis.</u> The failure of excision of periesophageal structures to change the pressure indicates that it originates from the sphincter itself rather than the diaphragmatic crura or phrenoesophageal ligament. Careful dissection of the terminal esophagus has not demonstrated a separate anatomic counterpart of the special function of this area, and it is often referred to as a physiologic sphincter. However, if the esophageal muscle is injured at this point, gastroesophageal reflux may result.

Experimentally, the gastroesophageal sphincter is strengthened by gastrin and weakened by cholecystokinin, secretin, and glucagon. After a protein meal, contraction of the sphincter increases and after a fat meal it becomes weaker; whether these effects reflect the actions of gastrin, cholecystokinin, or other hormones is unclear. However, gastrin is no longer thought to be a major determinant of sphincter strength.

Cholinergic and α-adrenergic stimuli enhance and β-adrenergic stimuli inhibit contraction of the sphincter. Recent experiments suggest that a system of nonadrenergic inhibitory nerves involving ATP (or a related compound) as a neurotransmitter and cyclic AMP as an intracellular second messenger may be responsible for sphincter relaxation under physiologic circumstances.

Many kinds of normal daily activity transiently increase intra-abdominal pressure. It was thought for years that the lack of reflux of gastric contents under these circumstances was normally due to the presence of an intra-abdominal segment of esophagus which transmitted the pressure increment to the sphincter, thus counterbalancing rises within the stomach. Later studies have now shown that pressure in the sphincter increases in response to induced rises in gastric pressure regardless of the position of the gastroesophageal junction relative to the diaphragm. For example, asymptomatic subjects with large hiatal hernias have an elevation of sphincteric pressure following abdominal compression which is quantitatively identical with that in patients whose sphincter resides below the diaphragm. The mechanism of this response has not yet been elucidated, but its rapid onset suggests a neural reflex.

When swallowing is begun, the tongue propels the bolus of food into the pharynx. Coordinated voluntary movement of the pharyngeal structures results in closure of the glottis and the nasopharynx. The glottis and pharynx rise during this maneuver, and the normal resting high-pressure zone at the pharyngoesophageal sphincter decreases, permitting entry of the food into the upper esophagus. After the food has traversed the pharynx and the pharyngoesophageal sphincter, the pharyngeal musculature relaxes and the high-pressure zone returns at the pharyngoesophageal sphincter. As

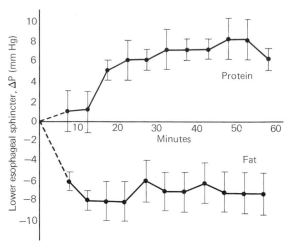

Figure 23–2. Changes in lower esophageal sphincter pressure after eating a meal consisting predominantly of protein or fat. (Data of Nebel OT, Castell DO: Gastroenterology 63:778, 1972.)

the bolus of food enters the esophagus, a peristaltic wave begins which travels toward the stomach at a speed of 4–6 cm/sec, propelling the food before it. The act of swallowing is a reflex response integrated in the medulla oblongata. When the subject is in the upright position, liquids and semisolid foods usually fall to the distal esophagus by gravity ahead of the slower peristaltic wave. The gastroesophageal sphincter relaxes in anticipation of the advancing food and peristalsis, thereby allowing the bolus to be transported into the stomach. After the food passes through, the sphincter regains its tone until another peristaltic wave arrives from above.

The term primary peristalsis denotes the wave of contraction initiated by swallowing which begins in the upper esophagus and travels the entire length of the organ (Fig 23–3). Local stimulation by distention at any point in the body of the esophagus will elicit a peristaltic wave from the point of the stimulus. This is

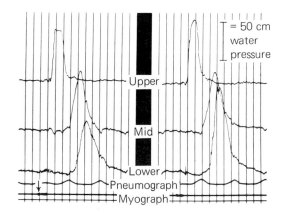

Figure 23–3. Deglutition. Normal esophageal peristaltic waves and pressures during consecutive swallows. Note the orderly downward progression of the waves.

called secondary peristalsis and aids esophageal emptying when the primary wave has failed to clear the lumen of ingested food or when gastric contents reflux from the stomach. Tertiary waves are stationary nonpropulsive contractions that may occur in any portion of the esophagus. Tertiary waves are considered abnormal, but they are frequently present in elderly subjects who have no symptoms of esophageal disease.

Incompetence of the gastroesophageal sphincter takes place normally during vomiting. During this event, the gastroesophageal junction rises above the level of the diaphragmatic hiatus. Ascent is probably the result of contraction of the longitudinal musculature of the esophagus; an additional result is effacement of the mucosal rosette which ordinarily fills the lumen of the gastroesophageal junction. Expulsion of gastric contents by the violent contractions of the gastric antrum and abdominal wall then becomes possible. After vomiting has subsided, the structures resume their ordinary relationships with the gastroesophageal junction below the level of the diaphragm.

The buccopharyngeal and esophageal structures engaged in swallowing and transmission of food to the stomach are innervated by motor fibers from the fifth, seventh, ninth, tenth, 11th, and 12th cranial nerves. Afferent sensory impulses are important in maintaining coordination of the motor activity.

Biancani P & others: Pressure, tension, and force of closure of the human lower esophageal sphincter and esophagus. J Clin Invest 56:476, 1975.

Castell DO: The lower esophageal sphincter. Ann Intern Med 83:390, 1975.

Davenport HW: Chewing and swallowing. Chap 1, pp 13—27, in: *Physiology of the Digestive Tract.* Year Book, 1971.

Diamant NE, El-Sharkawy TY: Neural control of esophageal peristalsis. Gastroenterology 72:546, 1977.

Dodds WJ & others: Effect of increased intraabdominal pressure on lower esophageal sphincter pressure. Am J Dig Dis 20:298, 1975.

Goyal RK, Rattan S: Genesis of basal sphincter pressure: Effect of tetrodotoxin on lower esophageal sphincter pressure in opossum in vivo. Gastroenterology 71:62, 1976.

Mukhopadhyay AK, Weisbrodt NW: Neural organization of esophageal peristalsis: Role of vagus nerve. Gastroenterology 68:444, 1975.

Nebel OT, Castell DO: Lower esophageal sphincter pressure changes after food ingestion. Gastroenterology 63:778, 1972.

Rattan S, Goyal RK: Neural control of the lower esophageal sphincter. J Clin Invest 54:899, 1974.

Tuch A, Cohen S: Lower esophageal sphincter relaxation: Studies on the neurogenic inhibitory mechanism. J Clin Invest 52:14, 1973.

Walker CO & others: Effect of continuous infusion of pentagastrin on lower esophageal sphincter pressure and gastric acid secretion in normal subjects. J Clin Invest 56:218, 1975.

Weinstein WM & others: The normal human esophageal mucosa: A histological reappraisal. Gastroenterology 68:40, 1975.

Weisbrodt NW: Neuromuscular organization of esophageal and pharyngeal motility. Arch Intern Med 136:524, 1976.

Winans CS: The pharyngoesophageal closure mechanism: A manometric study. Gastroenterology 63:768, 1972.

ESOPHAGEAL MOTILITY DISORDERS

Disturbances of the neuromuscular function of the esophagus can result either in hypermotility or hypomotility disorders.

CRICOPHARYNGEAL ACHALASIA

Essentials of Diagnosis

- Cervical dysphagia.
- Cricopharyngeal bar on barium swallow.
- Zenker's diverticulum in some patients.

General Considerations

Cricopharyngeal achalasia, the most common motility disorder of the proximal esophagus, is an acquired condition of unknown cause that occurs principally in patients over 60 years of age. It may occur as an isolated abnormality or in association with Zenker's diverticulum. Some experts believe that cricopharyngeal achalasia is an important factor in the pathogenesis of Zenker's diverticulum, a concept which has led to recommendations for concomitant cricopharyngeal myotomy at the time of diverticulectomy for the latter condition. This theory has not been universally accepted.

Clinical Findings

A. Symptoms and Signs: Cervical dysphagia, more pronounced for solids than for liquids, is the main symptom. A chronic cough develops in some patients from minor aspirations of saliva and ingested food.

B. X-Ray Findings: Barium swallow nearly always shows a prominent cricopharyngeal bar, which is sometimes so striking as to suggest mechanical obstruction.

C. Endoscopy: The findings on endoscopy are of an extrinsic constriction which allows passage of the endoscope as it is advanced.

D. Manometry: Manometry of the cricopharyngeal sphincter, hypopharynx, and upper esophagus reveals either incomplete relaxation of the sphincter with swallowing, imperfect coordination of relaxation following pharyngeal contraction, or both.

Differential Diagnosis

Esophageal neoplasms must be ruled out by endoscopy. Cervical dysphagia is occasionally the predominant complaint in reflux due to lower esophageal sphincter incompetence. In such cases, surgical correction of the reflux relieves the cervical dysphagia.

Treatment

Treatment consists of myotomy of the cricopharyngeus and upper 3—4 cm of the esophageal musculature. Although general anesthesia is used for most cases, the procedure may even be performed under local anesthesia. The esophagus is approached through an incision parallel to the anterior border of the sternomastoid muscle. The myotomy is made in the midline posteriorly, dividing all fibers of the muscle layers until the submucosa is reached.

Prognosis

Complications are uncommon, and relief of symptoms is usually complete and permanent postoperatively. The procedure should probably not be performed in patients with gastroesophageal reflux because of an increased risk of aspiration.

Helsper JT & others: Cricopharyngeal achalasia. Am J Surg 128:521, 1974.

Hiebert CA: Surgery for cricopharyngeal dysfunction under local anesthesia. Am J Surg 131:423, 1976.

Hurwitz AL & others: Oropharyngeal dysphagia. Am J Dig Dis 20:313, 1975.

Palmer ED: Disorders of the cricopharyngeus muscle: A review. Gastroenterology 71:510, 1976.

MISCELLANEOUS NEUROMUSCULAR SWALLOWING DISTURBANCES

Disturbances in the swallowing mechanism may occur in patients with neuromuscular disorders, especially those of the myotonic type. In myasthenia gravis, the peristaltic waves have a decrease in amplitude, and, on repetitive swallowing, peristalsis disappears in the lower esophagus. In myotonia dystrophica, in which both smooth and striated muscles are involved, motor failure of the esophagus is common.

Nonspecific abnormalities in peristalsis of the esophageal musculature may occur in many central or peripheral neurologic disorders. Simultaneous waves, spasms, and weak contractions can be observed in patients with such conditions as parkinsonism, hemiplegic states, multiple sclerosis, and amyotrophic lateral sclerosis.

Fisher RA & others: Esophageal motility in neuromuscular disorders. Ann Intern Med 63:229, 1965.

Kelley ML: Dysphagia and motor failure of the esophagus in myotonia dystrophica. Neurology 14:955, 1964.

Mukhopadhyay AK: Esophageal motor dysfunction in systemic diseases. Arch Intern Med 136:583, 1976.

Olsen AM, Schlegel JF: Neuromuscular problems of the esophagus in the elderly. Geriatrics 28:48, 1973.

Stewart IM & others: Oesophageal motor changes in diabetes mellitus. Thorax 31:278, 1976.

DIFFUSE ESOPHAGEAL SPASM

Essentials of Diagnosis

- Dysphagia, substernal pain.
- Nervousness, intermittent symptoms.
- Fluoroscopic, cineradiographic, and manometric evidence of hyperperistalsis.

General Considerations

Diffuse spasm of the esophagus is accompanied by irregular uncoordinated peristaltic movements and intermittent spasm of the cardioesophageal junction. Hypermotility is probably caused by an abnormal interplay of the sympathetic and parasympathetic nerve impulses to the lower esophagus, although the exact mechanism remains obscure. It has no known relationship to the development of esophageal cancer.

Clinical Findings

A. Symptoms and Signs: Weight loss is uncommon despite the presence of dysphagia. Intermittency of symptoms is characteristic. Substernal distress varying from slight discomfort to severe, colicky pain occurs frequently. The pain often simulates that of coronary artery disease and may result in a highly nervous temperament, so that a diagnosis of psychoneurosis often is made.

B. X-Ray Findings: The esophagogram is abnormal in 60% of these patients. Fluoroscopic studies show segmental spasms, areas of narrowing, and irregular uncoordinated peristalsis described as "curling" or "corkscrew esophagus." A small hiatal hernia is frequently demonstrated; less commonly, an epiphrenic diverticulum is present.

C. Manometry: Manometric studies show wide variations in pressure measurements with abolition of normal peristaltic waves. Occasionally, the lower esophagus alone may have irregular, uncoordinated muscular contractions while the proximal portions show normal peristaltic waves. More often, however, the entire esophagus is involved. Many of the patients with symptomatic diffuse spasm have a demonstrable hypersensitivity to methacholine.

Differential Diagnosis

The symptoms produced by diffuse spasm must be distinguished from those produced by heart disease, mediastinal masses, benign and malignant esophageal tumors, and scleroderma. Although radiologic and pressure studies are diagnostically accurate, esophagoscopy should be performed to confirm the absence of intraluminal lesions such as esophagitis which often produce esophageal spasm.

Complications

Sliding hiatal hernia and epiphrenic diverticula may be secondary complications of the uncoordinated and severe contractions of the esophagus. Regurgitation and aspiration may occur, possibly leading to repeated pneumonic infections. In general, however, the condition is usually mild and does not lead to serious complications. The syndrome of gastroesophageal hypercontracting sphincter is not a separate entity from diffuse spasm, although in the latter the sphincter is usually normal.

Treatment

Long acting nitrates (eg, Isordil, Cardilate) may give symptomatic relief. A soft diet taken in 5–6 small feedings daily may be required, especially when dysphagia is the most prominent symptom. Recently, a lengthy extramucous cardiomyotomy extending along the entire body of the esophagus has been used, with benefit to 50–60% of patients. The esophageal musculature is divided in a linear fashion to the level of the submucosa throughout the thoracic esophagus to include the cardioesophageal sphincter. In this way, the abnormal muscular motility affects only a portion of the circumference of the esophagus, thereby diminishing the severity of the muscular spasm.

Bennett JR, Hendrix TR: Diffuse esophageal spasm: A disorder with more than one cause. Gastroenterology 59:273, 1970.

Castell DO: Achalasia and diffuse esophageal spasm. Arch Intern Med 136:571, 1976.

DiMarino AJ Jr, Cohen S: Characteristics of lower esophageal sphincter function in symptomatic diffuse spasm. Gastroenterology 66:1, 1974.

Garrett JM, Godwin DH: Gastroesophageal hypercontracting sphincter. JAMA 208:992, 1969.

Henderson RD, Pearson FG: Reflux control following extended myotomy in primary disordered motor activity (diffuse spasm) of the esophagus. Ann Thorac Surg 22:278, 1976.

Kramer P & others: Oesophageal sensitivity to Mecholyl in symptomatic diffuse spasm. Gut 8:120, 1967.

Paris F & others: Pre- and postoperative manometric studies in diffuse esophageal spasm. J Thorac Cardiovasc Surg 70:126, 1975.

Swamy N. Esophageal spasm: Clinical and manometric response to nitroglycerine and long acting nitrites. Gastroenterology 72:23, 1977.

GASTROESOPHAGEAL ACHALASIA

Essentials of Diagnosis

- Dysphagia.
- Retention of ingested food in the esophagus.
- Radiologic evidence of absent primary peristalsis, dilated body of the esophagus, and a conically narrow cardioesophageal junction.
- Absent primary peristalsis by manometry and cineradiography.

General Considerations

Achalasia of the esophagus is a neuromuscular disorder in which esophageal dilatation and hypertrophy occur without organic stenosis. Primary peristalsis is absent and the cardioesophageal sphincter fails to relax in response to swallowing. The circular muscle layer hypertrophies, while the longitudinal coat retains its normal thickness. Although the cause is not clearly understood, it is now generally accepted that achalasia develops on a neurogenic basis. The absence, atrophy, or disintegration of the ganglion cells of Auerbach's myenteric plexuses in many patients with achalasia

lends support to this concept. The causes of the changes in the ganglia are obscure. Selective destruction of the dorsal motor nuclei of the vagus nerves in the medulla in experimental animals has produced similar changes. Achalasia affects males more often than females and may develop at any age. The peak years are 30–60. Carcinoma in association with achalasia is uncommon but occurs with greater frequency than in the general population.

Clinical Findings

A. Symptoms and Signs: Dysphagia is the dominant symptom, but weight loss is not usually marked despite the functional obstruction. The dilated esophagus is able to contain large quantities of food which only gradually pass into the stomach, largely by gravity. Pain is infrequent even though shallow ulcerations may be produced in the mucosa by the retention and disintegration of ingested food. Regurgitation of retained esophageal contents is common, especially during the night while the patient sleeps in a recumbent position. Aspiration may lead to repeated bouts of pneumonia.

A variant called **vigorous achalasia** is characterized by chest pain and esophageal spasms that generate nonpropulsive high pressure waves in the body of the esophagus. Sphincteric dysfunction is the same as in ordinary achalasia.

During esophagoscopy, the instrument can be advanced through the narrow sphincter without increased force, a feature that distinguishes achalasia from carcinoma or benign peptic stricture.

B. X-Ray Findings: Radiologic studies demonstrate the classic features even in early achalasia. The narrowing at the cardia has a characteristic contour. The dilated body of the esophagus blends into a smooth cone-shaped area of narrowing 3–6 cm long (Fig 23–4). On fluoroscopy the peristaltic waves are weak, simultaneous, irregular, uncoordinated, or absent. As the disease progresses, the esophagus dilates further, becomes tortuous, and, in far-advanced cases, sigmoid in shape. The lowermost segment retains the classic long linear narrowing even in the late stages of the disease. The column of barium is held up at the narrowed area because the sphincteric mechanism fails to relax normally.

C. Manometry: Manometric studies are of value in confirming the diagnosis and are more sensitive than cineradiography, although in practice both are often obtained. The motility pattern is as follows: The pharyngoesophageal sphincter has a normal action; the body of the esophagus is devoid of primary peristaltic waves, but simultaneous disorganized muscular activity may be present. Occasionally, no peristalsis of any sort can be observed. The pressure in the gastroesophageal sphincter is greater than normal, and relaxation after swallowing is incomplete. The subcutaneous administration of bethanecol results in a forceful sustained contraction of the lower two-thirds of the esophagus which is often briefly painful. This response is a manifestation of autonomic denervation of the organ and

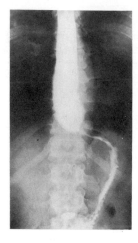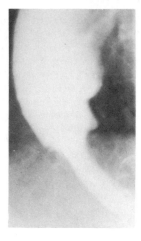

Figure 23–4. Achalasia of the esophagus. *Left:* Moderately advanced achalasia. Note dilated body of esophagus and smoothly tapered lower portion. *Right:* Widely patent cardioesophageal region following extramucous cardiomyotomy.

does not occur in normal subjects. A positive response is not entirely specific for achalasia but is also noted in symptomatic diffuse spasm, which suggests that the 2 conditions share some pathophysiologic characteristics. In fact, progression of typical diffuse spasm to typical achalasia has been documented, although it must be fairly uncommon.

Differential Diagnosis

Clinically and radiographically, scleroderma is the esophageal lesion which most closely mimics achalasia. In both instances, dilatation and lack of peristalsis are noted. However, in early scleroderma the long, conical, smoothly tapered region in the lower esophagus is not seen. Furthermore, the cardioesophageal sphincter in scleroderma is widely patent instead of narrowed, so that free reflux of gastric contents can frequently be observed fluoroscopically in scleroderma but is almost totally absent in achalasia. The incompetent sphincter in scleroderma results in peptic esophagitis, which often leads to distal narrowing by stricture. When this stage is reached, the radiologic appearances of achalasia and scleroderma may be identical, consisting of a widely dilated body and a narrow distal segment. Cineradiography, manometry, and esophagoscopy may be required to differentiate the two. In scleroderma, peristalsis is usually preserved in the skeletal muscle portion of the esophagus, whereas the entire organ is affected in achalasia. The esophagus in scleroderma does not contract in response to methacholine.

Benign strictures of the lower esophagus and carcinoma at or near the cardioesophageal junction are important conditions to be distinguished from achalasia. In both, however, the huge dilatation of the proximal esophagus seen frequently in both achalasia and in scleroderma does not occur. Motility studies are helpful since in organic stenosis vigorous peristalsis occurs in response to the obstruction. Esophagoscopy

should always be performed to aid in establishing the diagnosis and also to rule out other intraluminal conditions. Esophageal cytologic studies should also be performed to rule out carcinoma.

Complications

Small mucosal ulcerations may develop from the irritation caused by retained food, but true peptic ulceration or massive hemorrhage is rare in achalasia. Aspiration of regurgitated esophageal contents may lead to repeated episodes of pneumonitis, tracheobronchitis, and, rarely, asphyxiation. Malnutrition is rarely severe in spite of the functional obstruction at the cardia. Although carcinoma may occasionally be seen in association with achalasia, it is not yet known if earlier treatment of the esophageal stasis would prevent malignant degeneration.

Treatment

Antispasmodic drugs exert no appreciable benefit. The aim of therapy is to relieve the functional obstruction at the cardia. This can be accomplished by either forceful dilatation or direct surgical division of the muscle fibers of the lower esophageal sphincter.

Forceful dilatation involves rapid pneumatic expansion of an inflatable bag placed at the esophagogastric junction. The procedure is accompanied by pain and is thought to disrupt some of the sphincteric musculature.

Although most patients are treated initially by forceful bougienage, those with far-advanced achalasia in which the esophagus has become hugely dilated and tortuous are best treated surgically. Forceful dilatation as the first therapeutic maneuver is successful in approximately 50% of patients. An additional 35% achieve an adequate swallowing mechanism by a second forceful bougienage.

Approximately 15% of patients with achalasia will require an operative procedure either because of failure of forceful dilatation or because the esophagus is so deformed and distorted that bougienage would be extremely hazardous. Forceful dilatation is not without danger since esophageal perforation occurs in 3–5% of cases.

Occasionally in elderly or poor-risk patients, the cardia can be kept reasonably patent with the use of mercury-weighted (Hurst) dilators which the patient may swallow as necessary. The column of mercury inside the smooth-tipped rubber dilator slowly allows the instrument to pass safely into the stomach by gravity.

The extramucous cardiomyotomy of Heller provides good overall results and is now the surgical procedure used almost exclusively throughout the world. The longitudinal myotomy extends from the level of the inferior pulmonary ligament downward onto the upper stomach. The incision is about 10–12 cm long and extends no more than 1 cm in its gastric portion. Care is taken to divide all of the muscular fibers since, if a few tiny circular fibers remain undivided, dysphagia may continue. Reflux is uncommon following cardiomyotomy if the gastric extension of the incision is strictly limited; results are good to excellent in 90% of patients. In the remaining few patients, some degree of swallowing difficulty may remain—due either to an inadequate myotomy or to the extensive paralysis of the body of the esophagus.

Prognosis

Relief of obstructive symptoms can be obtained by forceful dilatation or by surgery in at least 85% of patients. A properly performed modified Heller procedure overcomes the functional obstruction and only rarely leads to esophageal reflux. The addition of vagotomy and gastric drainage operations to the myotomy procedure is unnecessary.

Arvanitakis C: Achalasia of the esophagus: A reappraisal of esophagomyotomy vs forceful pneumatic dilatation. Am J Dig Dis 20:841, 1975.

Carter R, Brewer L: Achalasia and esophageal carcinoma: Studies in early diagnosis for improved surgical management. Am J Surg 130:114, 1975.

Cohen S & others: The site of denervation in achalasia. Gut 13:556, 1972.

Ellis FG: The natural history of achalasia. Proc R Soc Med 53:663, 1960.

Ellis FH Jr: Esophagomyotomy for esophageal achalasia. Surg Clin North Am 53:319, 1973.

Ellis FH Jr, Gibb SP: Reoperation after esophagomyotomy for achalasia of the esophagus. Am J Surg 129:407, 1975.

Grimes OF, Stephens HB, Margulis AR: Achalasia of the esophagus. Am J Surg 120:198, 1970.

Kramer P & others: Transition from symptomatic diffuse spasm to cardiospasm. Gut 8:115, 1967.

Sanderson DR & others: Syndrome of vigorous achalasia: Clinical and physiologic observations. Dis Chest 52:508, 1967.

Vantrappen G & others: Treatment of achalasia with pneumatic dilatations. Gut 12:268, 1971.

ESOPHAGEAL MANIFESTATIONS IN SCLERODERMA & DERMATOMYOSITIS

Scleroderma and several other systemic diseases occasionally involve the esophagus. When the esophageal symptoms overshadow other manifestations of the disease, the diagnosis may sometimes be difficult.

Esophageal dysfunction occurs commonly in patients with scleroderma. The initial symptoms are usually those of reflux: regurgitation, heartburn, and, occasionally, bleeding. Dysphagia is a less common complaint until esophagitis progresses to stricture formation. The esophageal symptoms usually appear in patients with the characteristic skin changes and Raynaud's syndrome. However, a number of cases have been reported where the motility defects were noted long before other findings of the disease.

The principal abnormality is atrophy and fibrosis of the esophageal smooth muscle, resulting in progressively weakening function. The changes affect the smooth muscle portion of the esophagus and are most marked at the gastroesophageal sphincter. The motility disorder can be recognized by manometry and cineradiography as relatively specific for this disease. The most noticeable abnormality is a patulous gastroesophageal sphincter which permits free reflux of gastric contents. Primary peristaltic waves become progressively weaker as they approach the sphincter. As time passes, peristalsis becomes more and more feeble and the severe esophagitis may produce a stricture. Esophageal shortening may draw the sphincter above the diaphragmatic hiatus, producing a hiatal hernia.

Antacids and elevation of the head of the patient's bed are useful in preventing reflux esophagitis. Nothing has been found which will delay the deterioration of esophageal function. Strictures can often be managed with repeated dilatations. The Collis-Belsey operation to prevent reflux is successful in the majority of patients even in the face of stricture formation.

Dysphagia occurs in about 60% of patients with dermatomyositis. Motility studies show a generalized muscular defect in which weakness of the cricopharyngeal sphincteric mechanism predominates. Although the dysfunction in the body of the esophagus resembles that of scleroderma, the cardioesophageal sphincter in dermatomyositis is usually unaffected. Corticosteroids may be beneficial in controlling symptoms.

Donoghue FE, Winkleman RK, Moersch HJ: Esophageal defects in dermatomyositis. Ann Otol Rhinol Laryngol 69:1139, 1960.

Henderson RD, Pearson FG: Surgical management of esophageal scleroderma. J Thorac Cardiovasc Surg 66:686, 1973.

McLaughlin JS & others: Surgical treatment of strictures of the esophagus in patients with scleroderma. J Thorac Cardiovasc Surg 61:641, 1971.

Orringer MB & others: Gastroesophageal reflux in esophageal scleroderma: Diagnosis and implications. Ann Thorac Surg 22:120, 1976.

Ramirez-Mata M & others: Esophageal motility in systemic lupus erythematosus. Am J Dig Dis 19:132, 1974.

Rodman GP, Fennell RH Jr: Progressive systemic sclerosis *sine* scleroderma. JAMA 180:665, 1962.

Turner R & others: Esophageal dysfunction in collagen disease. Am J Med Sci 265:191, 1973.

DIVERTICULA

Diverticula of the esophagus are commonly associated with motor dysfunction. They are acquired lesions which result from the protrusion of mucosa and submucosa through a weakness or defect in the musculature (pulsion type) or from the pulling outward of the esophageal wall from inflamed and scarred peribronchial mediastinal lymph nodes (traction type).

PHARYNGOESOPHAGEAL (ZENKER'S) DIVERTICULUM

Essentials of Diagnosis

- Dysphagia, pressure symptoms, and gurgling sounds in the neck.
- Regurgitation of undigested food, halitosis.
- Manual emptying of the diverticulum by the patient.

General Considerations

Pharyngoesophageal pulsion diverticulum is the most common of the esophageal diverticula and is 3 times more frequent in men than in women. It arises posteriorly in the midline of the neck—above the cricopharyngeus muscle and below the inferior constrictor of the pharynx. Between these 2 muscle groups is a weakened area through which the mucosa and submucosa gradually evaginate as a result of the high pressures generated during swallowing. Zenker's diverticulum is rarely seen in patients below age 30; most patients are over 60. Although its mouth is in the midline, the sac projects laterally, usually into the left paravertebral region. The body of the esophagus often shows abnormal motility patterns in patients with Zenker's diverticulum.

Clinical Findings

A. Symptoms and Signs: Dysphagia is the most common symptom and is related to the size of the diverticulum. Undigested food is regurgitated into the mouth, especially in the recumbent position, and the patient may manually massage the neck after eating to empty the sac. Swelling of the neck, gurgling noises after eating, halitosis, and a sour metallic taste in the mouth are common symptoms.

B. X-Ray Findings: Fluoroscopic examination demonstrates a smoothly rounded outpouching arising posteriorly in the midline of the neck (Fig 23–5).

Differential Diagnosis

The dysphagia produced by pharyngoesophageal diverticula must be distinguished from that produced by malignant lesions, although carcinoma at this level is uncommon. Achalasia of the cricopharyngeus muscle may produce symptoms similar to those of Zenker's diverticulum. Cervical esophageal webs must also be considered. However, the radiologic discovery of a smoothly rounded blind pouch is diagnostic and is rarely confused with other lesions at this level. Esophagoscopy is usually unnecessary and may be hazardous because the instrument may enter the ostium of the diverticulum instead of the true esophageal lumen. Since the diverticulum is composed only of mucosa and submucosa, it is easily perforated.

Regurgitation and aspiration may produce tracheobronchial irritation and pneumonitis. This usually occurs while in the recumbent position, as during sleep. Food may become trapped in the diverticulum and rarely may lead to perforation, mediastinitis, or a paraesophageal abscess. Retained food may ulcerate the mucosa and cause bleeding. Rarely, a fistula may form between the diverticulum and the trachea as a result of infection. Pulmonary infection is the most frequent serious complication, and many patients are first seen after experiencing repeated episodes of pneumonitis.

Treatment

Surgical removal of the diverticulum is curative. A one-stage procedure is employed. It has recently been suggested that in addition to the diverticulectomy, the cricopharyngeus muscle should be transected; the

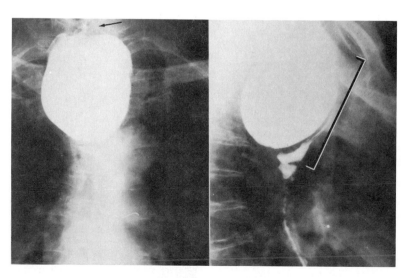

Figure 23–5. Large pharyngoesophageal diverticulum. Note origin in midline *(arrow, left)* and compression of esophagus *(bracket, right)*.

rationale of this procedure is that spasticity of the musculature may contribute to the continuation of symptoms after excision of the diverticulum.

Prognosis

A temporary fistula occasionally develops postoperatively, but this usually heals spontaneously. The mortality rate after surgical excision is low, and the results are good.

Ellis FH Jr & others: Cricopharyngeal myotomy for pharyngo-esophageal diverticulum. Ann Surg 170:340, 1969.

Hansen JB & others: Pharyngo-oesophageal diverticula: A clinical and cineradiographic follow-up study of 23 cases treated by diverticulectomy. Scand J Thorac Cardiovasc Surg 7:81, 1973.

Palmer ED: Disorders of the cricopharyngeus muscle: A review. Gastroenterology 71:510, 1976.

Perrott JW: Anatomical aspects of hypopharyngeal diverticula. Aust NZ J Surg 31:307, 1962.

Welsh GF, Payne WS: The present status of one-stage pharyngo-esophageal diverticulectomy. Surg Clin North Am 53:953, 1973.

EPIPHRENIC DIVERTICULUM

Essentials of Diagnosis

- Dysphagia and a sensation of pressure in the lower esophagus after eating.
- Intermittent vomiting, substernal pain.
- Typical radiologic contour.
- Disturbed motility of the lower esophagus.
- Associated hiatal hernia on occasion.

General Considerations

Epiphrenic pulsion diverticula are usually located just above the diaphragm but may occur as high as the midthorax. They are usually associated with motility disturbances and are frequently larger than diverticula which arise elsewhere in the esophagus. Esophagitis may develop at the ostium. Peridiverticular localized mediastinitis may be seen, especially if ulceration of the mucosa of the sac occurs.

Differential Diagnosis

The appearance on x-ray films and on fluoroscopy is so distinctive that a definitive diagnosis can usually be made. Associated conditions such as benign or malignant stenoses, webs, hiatal hernia, achalasia, and other motility disorders must be ruled out. The most common conditions associated with epiphrenic diverticula are achalasia and esophageal spasm below the diverticulum, and symptoms are more apt to be due to the abnormal motility than to the diverticulum itself.

Complications

Esophagitis, periesophagitis, and occasional bleeding from ulceration are the most frequent complications. Tracheobronchial aspiration of regurgitated esophageal contents is uncommon. Perforation occurs rarely.

Treatment

Most patients have minor symptoms that do not require surgery. Surgery is indicated when symptoms become progressively more severe. The operation consists of a thoracotomy, excision of the diverticulum, and procedures for underlying motility abnormalities. A linear division of the esophageal musculature below the diverticulum should be performed in most cases because of the frequent association of epiphrenic diverticulum with diffuse spasm or achalasia. If a hiatal hernia is present, it should be repaired.

Prognosis

Surgery is successful in 80–90% of cases.

Allen TH, Clagett OT: Changing concepts in the surgical treatment of pulsion diverticula of the lower esophagus. J Thorac Cardiovasc Surg 50:455, 1965.

Bruggeman LL, Seaman WB: Epiphrenic diverticula: An analysis of 80 cases. Am J Roentgenol Radium Ther Nucl Med 119:266, 1973.

TRACTION DIVERTICULUM

Essentials of Diagnosis

- Usually an incidental radiologic finding.
- Dysphagia.
- Episodes of coughing due to fixation to the trachea or bronchus or peribronchial lymph nodes.
- Typical x-ray.

General Considerations

Traction diverticula occur in the midthoracic esophagus. Inflamed lymph nodes near the tracheal bifurcation become adherent to the esophagus, and, as fibrosis and contraction occur with healing, the esophageal wall is pulled anteriorly to form a sac. The diverticulum is at first cone-shaped, with its apex fixed to the fibrotic lymph node; later, a pulsion effect from the intraluminal pressure may be added, so that the contour becomes rounded.

Traction diverticula are usually discovered after age 40 and occur with equal frequency in both sexes. They are rarely multiple, frequently asymptomatic, and are often found during a routine gastrointestinal x-ray study.

Clinical Findings

Most diverticula of this type are asymptomatic, but occasionally the diverticulum may become inflamed and may then produce dysphagia and a sense of pulling on the tracheobronchial tree during swallowing.

Differential Diagnosis

The radiologic discovery (usually during an upper gastrointestinal fluoroscopic study) of an outpouching in the midthoracic esophagus is not likely to be misinterpreted. If associated inflammation causes narrowing of the esophageal lumen, carcinoma or benign stricture must be ruled out by esophagoscopy.

Complications

In rare instances the diverticulum may perforate into neighboring structures, causing fistula or abscess formation. Bleeding is uncommon.

Treatment

Since most traction diverticula are asymptomatic, no specific treatment is necessary. An occasional patient may develop symptoms, in which case surgical excision is warranted.

Boyd DP, Adams HD: Esophageal diverticulum. N Engl J Med 264:641, 1961.

INSTRUMENTAL PERFORATION OF THE ESOPHAGUS

Essentials of Diagnosis

- History of recent instrumentation, sudden elevation of temperature, and pain in the neck or chest.
- Leukocytosis, change of voice into bass-like tone.
- Crepitus in the neck due to extravasation of air.
- Subcutaneous emphysema (mainly in the cervical region).
- Localization of injury by fluoroscopic studies with water-soluble opaque media.
- Pneumothorax if perforation involves the thoracic esophagus.

General Considerations

Instrumental perforation during diagnostic esophagoscopy accounts for most esophageal injuries. Similar injuries may occur during gastroscopy, gastroesophageal balloon tamponade, and esophageal dilation with various instruments. Even simple intubation of the esophagus for diagnostic or therapeutic purposes may result in perforation. Perforations are most likely to occur in the cervical esophagus. The esophagoscope may press the posterior wall of the esophagus against osteoarthritic spurs of the cervical vertebrae, causing contusion or laceration. The cricopharyngeal area is the most common point of perforation. The resistance of the muscular sphincter must be overcome in order to insert the esophagoscope into the esophageal lumen. The pressure necessary to obliterate the sphincteric tone may result in a rapid descent of the instrument to produce a tear of the esophagus.

Perforations of the intrathoracic esophagus may occur at any level but are most common at the natural sites of narrowing, ie, at the level of the left main stem bronchus and at the diaphragmatic hiatus.

Clinical Findings

A. Symptoms and Signs: Pain, fever, dysphagia, and hypotension bordering on shock are the most common early findings after perforation of the esophagus. The severity of each of these manifestations is dependent largely on the site and extent of the perforation and the rapidity of the inflammatory reaction that develops. Hyperpnea is almost always noted, but dyspnea most often indicates that the perforation has occurred in the thoracic esophagus, with laceration of the pleura to produce pneumothorax, chest pain, and a rapidly developing pleural effusion.

Cervical tenderness is a common early sign, and pain upon attempted swallowing may be severe. Crepitation in the soft tissues of the neck can almost always be demonstrated, although it may be minimal. If the thoracic esophagus is perforated, the symptoms and signs are usually limited to the chest; occasionally, crepitus is palpable in the neck but tenderness in the cervical region is not often present. Because of the escape of air into the mediastinum, a "mediastinal crunch" may be heard as the heart beats against the air-filled tissues (Hamman's sign). Shock develops earlier in thoracic perforations than in injuries to the cervical esophagus because of the rapid flooding of the mediastinum and pleural space with highly infective salivary secretions.

B. X-Ray Findings: X-ray studies are important not only in demonstrating that perforation has occurred but also in locating the exact site of the injury. In perforations of the cervical esophagus, x-ray films show air in the soft tissues, especially along the cervical spine. The trachea may be displaced anteriorly by air and fluid in the space behind the esophagus (retrovisceral space). Later, widening of the superior mediastinum may be seen. Mediastinal widening and emphysema and pleural effusion with or without pneumothorax are often present in perforations of the body of the esophagus in the thorax. Fluoroscopic examination using water-soluble opaque media should always be obtained to localize the site of the injury (Fig 23–6). Esophagoscopy is unnecessary except when the perforation has been caused by the ingestion of a foreign body.

Complications

Wounds of the esophagus may be fatal because regional tissues quickly become contaminated with highly virulent oropharyngeal bacteria. Fulminant mediastinitis, bronchopneumonia, pericarditis, and septicemia may occur in rapid succession. Abscess is uncommon in intrathoracic perforations because the mediastinal pleura is almost always lacerated so that the esophageal contents drain directly into the pleural space. Empyema, mediastinitis, and severe sepsis may develop if an intrathoracic perforation is not recog-

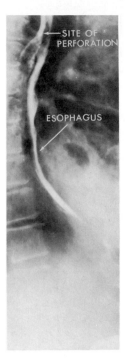

Figure 23—6. Extravasation of contrast material through instrumental perforation of upper thoracic esophagus. Note locules of air and fluid anterior to esophagus, indicating that mediastinitis had already developed.

nized and treated immediately. Since the prevertebral fascia and spaces of the neck are continuous into the mediastinum, mediastinitis may occur as a result of perforations in the cervical esophagus.

Differential Diagnosis

Wounds resulting from instrumentation are unlikely to be misinterpreted since the typical symptoms and signs occur so rapidly. When mediastinal or cervical abscesses develop slowly as a result of small tears or perforations, they must be differentiated from other masses or growths largely by fluoroscopic studies using water-soluble contrast media.

Prevention

The flexible fiberoptic esophagoscope is much safer than the rigid instruments and should be used whenever feasible. Even in skilled hands, perforation is a recognized risk with metal esophagoscopes; however, they allow strictures to be dilated with bougies passed through the lumen which is not possible with the fiberoptic instruments. Careful, gentle technic and the use of a lumen finder are mandatory. General anesthesia to provide complete relaxation is preferred, although the procedure can be accomplished under topical anesthesia. Food or fluids by mouth should not be allowed for 12—24 hours or until it can be determined with absolute certainty that no injury has occurred.

Treatment

Immediate operation is advisable. Closure of the perforation and external drainage should be accomplished. Occasionally, in perforations of the cervical esophagus, simple drainage may suffice since the tears are often small and difficult to identify in the presence of inflammatory edema. Although antibiotics alone have occasionally been successful, this method of treatment is more risky than direct surgical repair and should be employed only in patients in whom a general anesthetic is strongly contraindicated.

Nonoperative management of intrathoracic perforations is extremely hazardous and rarely tried. If the perforation is contained entirely within the mediastinum and toxicity is minimal—indicating that a minor laceration has been produced—conservative therapy with nasogastric decompression and massive doses of antibiotics may be permissible.

Prognosis

With prompt operative repair, external drainage, and adjuvant antibiotics, most patients who sustain instrumental perforations of the esophagus will recover. Although intrathoracic perforations have a less favorable outlook because of the rapid development of mediastinitis and empyema, immediate operation to repair the injury is usually lifesaving.

Berry BE, Ochsner JL: Perforation of the esophagus: A 30 year review. J Thorac Cardiovasc Surg 65:1, 1973.

Boyd DP, Wittman CJ Jr: Some principles in treating perforation of esophagus. Surg Clin North Am 51:567, 1971.

Hardy JD & others: Esophageal perforations and fistulas. Ann Surg 177:788, 1973.

Rosoff L, White EJ: Perforation of the esophagus. Am J Surg 128:207, 1974.

SPONTANEOUS (POSTEMETIC) PERFORATION OF THE ESOPHAGUS (Boerhaave's Syndrome)

Essentials of Diagnosis

- Usually in males.
- History of alcoholic debauch, excessive food intake, or both.
- Violent vomiting or retching followed by agonizing pain in the epigastrium and lower anterior thorax.
- Rigid abdomen.
- Pneumothorax, mediastinal widening, and emphysema.
- Crepitus in the neck.
- Radiographic evidence of mediastinal, pleural, or intra-abdominal air.
- Demonstration of rupture of the lower esophagus by esophagogram.

General Considerations

Spontaneous perforations often occur in patients

who have had no previous esophageal disease. The rupture involves all layers of the esophageal wall and most frequently occurs in the left posterolateral aspect of the lower esophagus. The second most common site is in the midthoracic esophagus on the right side at the level of the azygos vein. The tear results from excessive pressure exerted directly upon the esophagus by violent retching and vomiting.

Clinical Findings

A. Symptoms and Signs: Shock develops rapidly. The diagnosis is suggested by a history of bouts of vomiting or retching, especially in an alcoholic male of middle age or older, followed by sudden and severe abdominal and lower chest pain. Hematemesis may occur (see Mallory-Weiss syndrome, p 486).

B. X-Ray Findings: Pneumothorax, usually on the left side, can be demonstrated on plain chest films. The rent can be localized by x-rays taken during a swallow of water-soluble contrast medium.

Differential Diagnosis

Especially if an accurate history cannot be obtained, the shock which almost always develops must be distinguished from shock due to other causes such as myocardial infarction, pulmonary embolus, ruptured intra-abdominal viscus, and sepsis. When an immediate diagnosis is not forthcoming, the patient may be thought to have either a perforated peptic ulcer or acute pancreatitis.

Treatment

Antibiotic therapy should always be employed. Immediate thoracotomy to repair the rupture is mandatory if the patient's condition permits. Ordinarily, however, primary repair is not feasible if 12 hours or more have elapsed. In these instances, drainage of the pleural space is accomplished by multiple thoracostomy tubes. In addition, bypassing of the perforated area by cervical esophagostomy and gastrostomy or jejunostomy may be lifesaving. Definitive repair can be accomplished at a later time. The ruptured area can also be sutured around a T tube whose long arm is brought out through the lower thorax. The esophagocutaneous fistula can be repaired later.

Prognosis

If an early diagnosis can be made, the outlook is excellent since repair of the perforation can be accomplished with minimal contamination. However, one series showed that in only 2 of 34 patients who had spontaneous perforations was a premortem diagnosis made. In most of these, the patients were admitted in shock or severe sepsis and their problem was thought to be due to other catastrophes such as myocardial infarction, severe pancreatitis, pneumonia, or peritonitis due to a ruptured viscus.

Abbott AA & others: Atraumatic so-called "spontaneous" rupture of the esophagus. J Thorac Cardiovasc Surg 59:67, 1970.

Hamilton SGI: Spontaneous rupture of the esophagus. Br J Surg 54:304, 1967.

Thompson NW & others: The spectrum of emetogenic injury to the esophagus and stomach. Am J Surg 113:13, 1967.

Watts DH: Lesions brought on by vomiting: The effect of hiatus hernia on the site of injury. Gastroenterology 71:683, 1976.

FOREIGN BODIES OF THE ESOPHAGUS

Essentials of Diagnosis

- History of recent ingestion of food or foreign material.
- Vague discomfort in the midline of the chest or neck, progressing to pain if infection develops.
- Dysphagia.
- Occasionally, respiratory distress.
- Radiographic discovery of foreign matter or of esophageal obstruction.

General Considerations

Most cases occur in children. Mentally disturbed patients often ingest foreign bodies. The esophagus may become obstructed by impactions of meat, especially in the edentulous patient. Many of these objects become engaged in the esophagus as it enters the superior thoracic strait. Others arrest at the level of the aortic arch, at the left main stem bronchus, or just above the cardioesophageal junction—ie, at the natural anatomic areas of narrowing.

Clinical Findings

A. Symptoms and Signs: Pain in the midline of the thorax or neck is prominent when large objects are ingested, especially when infection surrounds the foreign body. Dysphagia, varying from mild distress to complete obstruction, may occur. Pressure on the tracheobronchial tree often produces respiratory distress. In most cases, the diagnosis can be made on the basis of the history.

B. X-Ray Findings: Roentgenography, either by plain films or by the use of radiopaque liquids, provides specific information regarding the type of foreign body and its location. Esophagoscopy is not only diagnostic but also therapeutic since the direct observation of the foreign body allows its safe removal.

Differential Diagnosis

Obstructive foreign bodies in the esophagus that cannot be identified must be differentiated from other causes of obstruction such as stenosis, caustic strictures, and tumors.

Complications

Esophageal inflammation and infection often occur around the foreign object. Perforation into the surrounding mediastinal structures may occur, leading to mediastinitis, hemorrhage from adjacent major blood vessels, or abscess formation. Neglected foreign bodies may erode through the esophageal wall to form a tracheoesophageal fistula. Late strictures may develop from the contraction of fibrous tissue incident to the inflammatory process.

Treatment

Many foreign objects will dislodge themselves and pass through the intestinal tract without difficulty. This is especially true in children, who often ingest smooth objects such as coins and marbles. Most foreign bodies in the esophagus, however, should be removed by endoscopy following proper roentgenographic studies. Esophagotomy to remove an impacted foreign body is rarely necessary.

The use of proteolytic enzymes to dissolve a bolus of impacted meat is usually successful, but occasionally the esophageal wall may be injured, and esophageal perforation has been reported.

Spitz L: Management of ingested foreign bodies in childhood. Br Med J 4:469, 1971.

CORROSIVE ESOPHAGITIS

Essentials of Diagnosis

- History of ingestion of caustic liquids or solids.
- Burns of the lips, mouth, and tongue.
- Pain and dysphagia.

General Considerations

Ingestion of strong solutions of acid or alkali or of solid substances of similar nature produces extensive chemical burns, often leading to corrosive esophagitis. Depending upon the concentration and the length of time the irritant remains in contact with the mucosa, various pathologic changes occur. Sloughing of the mucous membrane, edema and inflammation of the submucosa, thrombosis of esophageal vessels, infection, perforation, and mediastinitis may develop if the injury is severe.

Clinical Findings

Systemic symptoms roughly parallel the severity of the caustic burns. If the damage is severe, the patient appears toxic, with high fever, prostration, and shock. Inflammatory edema of the lips, mouth, tongue, and oropharynx may cause respiratory distress. Pain on attempted swallowing may be intense. Tracheobronchitis accompanied by coughing and increased bronchial secretions is frequently noted. Complete esophageal obstruction due to edema, inflammation, and mucosal sloughing may develop within the first few days.

The corrosive injury may be so severe that large areas of mucosa are destroyed, including that of the stomach. The burns are most often linear, but they may be patchy and irregular in outline. Many are circular and involve considerable lengths of the esophagus. Circular burns are prone to lead to early stricture. Caustic injuries tend to be more severe at the areas of anatomic narrowing of the esophagus.

Complications

Complications include perforation, bleeding, mediastinitis, tracheoesophageal fistulas, and stricture formation.

Treatment

A. Emergency Treatment: Emergency treatment consists of washing the esophagus with large volumes of water. Dilute acid or alkaline solutions may be used to neutralize the ingested liquid.

B. Medical Treatment: Broad-spectrum antibiotics are given immediately to prevent bacterial invasion of the esophageal wall. Corticosteroids are used in the acute phase to reduce fibrous tissue proliferation and thereby to decrease the possibility of stricture formation.

C. Esophagoscopy and Dilatation: Early esophagoscopy is recommended to determine the initial extent of the injury and may be repeated as necessary to assess the progress of healing. Although the procedures must be performed with extreme caution, dilatation by esophagoscopy or bougienage should be performed in patients in whom esophageal narrowing or actual stenosis appears to be developing.

D. Surgical Treatment: In spite of the prompt and efficient use of corticosteroids, antibiotics, and dilatations, the process may progress to stricture formation—especially when extensive destruction and fibrosis of the esophagus have occurred. In these instances, the esophagus must be replaced by segments of stomach, jejunum, or colon.

Prognosis

Early and proper management of caustic burns provides satisfactory results in most cases. The ingestion of strong acid or alkaline solutions with extensive immediate destruction of the mucosa produces such profound pathologic changes that the development of fibrous strictures is almost inevitable.

Campbell GS & others: Treatment of corrosive burns of the esophagus. Arch Surg 112:495, 1977.
Haller JA & others: Pathophysiology and management of acute corrosive burns of the esophagus. J Pediatr Surg 6:578, 1971.
Ragheb MI & others: Management of corrosive esophagitis. Surgery 79:494, 1976.

BENIGN TUMORS OF THE ESOPHAGUS

Essentials of Diagnosis

- Dysphagia often present but frequently mild.

- Sense of pressure in thorax or neck.
- Radiographic demonstration of intra- or extraluminal mass, smooth in outline.

General Considerations

Benign growths may arise in any layer of the esophagus. Inflammatory polyps or granulomas are occasionally associated with esophagitis and may be mistakenly interpreted as neoplastic lesions. Papillomas arising from the mucosa are either sessile or pedunculated; although they are usually small lesions, occasionally they become large enough to produce obstruction. They may slough off spontaneously into the esophageal lumen.

Leiomyoma is the most frequent benign lesion of the esophagus. Leiomyomas are intramural lesions which narrow the esophageal lumen extrinsically. The mucosa overlying the tumor is generally intact, but occasionally it may become ulcerated as a result of pressure by an enlarging lesion. Other tumors such as fibromas, lipomas, fibromyomas, and myxomas are rare.

Congenital cysts or reduplications of the esophagus (the second most common benign lesion after leiomyoma) may occur at any level, although they are most commonly in the lower esophageal segment.

Clinical Findings

Many benign lesions are asymptomatic and are discovered incidentally during upper gastrointestinal fluoroscopic examination. Cysts and leiomyomas may be of sufficient size to appear as a density, usually round or ovoid, in the mediastinum on routine chest x-rays. Benign tumors or cysts grow slowly and become symptomatic only after sufficient encroachment of the esophageal lumen has occurred. Radiographic study of the intramural leiomyoma shows a smoothly rounded, often spherical mass which causes extrinsic narrowing of the esophageal lumen (Fig 23–7). The overlying mucosa is almost always intact. Peristalsis is not affected by leiomyomas but is often abnormal in the presence of cysts or reduplications. Spasm of the musculature adjacent to the cyst or duplication is the most common abnormality of peristalsis. Dilatation of the esophagus proximal to any of the benign lesions is rarely seen. Intraluminal growths can be recognized at esophagoscopy, and a specific tissue diagnosis should always be obtained. Attempts to biopsy intramural lesions through an intact overlying mucous membrane are hazardous because of the possibility of inducing hemorrhage into the lesion with resulting increase of its size; pressure upon the adjacent mediastinal structures may produce cardiorespiratory embarrassment.

Differential Diagnosis

Leiomyomas, cysts, and reduplications can be distinguished from cancerous growths by their classic radiographic appearance. Intraluminal papillomas, polyps, or granulomas may be indistinguishable radiographically from early carcinoma, and their exact nature must be confirmed histologically.

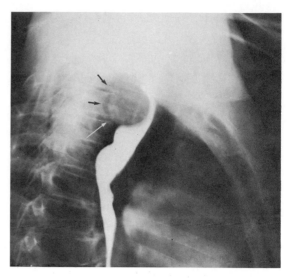

Figure 23–7. Leiomyoma of esophagus. Note smooth, rounded density causing extrinsic compression of esophageal lumen.

Complications

Cysts and duplications derive their arterial supply directly from the aorta. Hemorrhage into these lesions may occur, especially following infection, although this complication is uncommon. Adhesions which form between the cystic lesions and the adjacent esophagus often produce progressive dysphagia. Pedunculated intraluminal tumors may cause sudden obstruction by torsion of their pedicles, which is followed by edema, infection, and bleeding. In the upper esophagus, pedunculated polypoid growths may be regurgitated upward into the hypopharynx and occasionally may fall into the glottic chink and produce laryngeal obstruction.

Bleeding may occur from ulcerations of the mucosa overlying a leiomyoma. Symptoms related to benign lesions of the esophagus are usually due to the presence of the lesion itself; the severity of the dysphagia is accentuated by the development of swelling, infection, hemorrhage, or obstruction.

Treatment

Small polypoid intraluminal lesions may be removed completely with biopsy forceps during esophagoscopy. The intramural lesions, reduplications, and cysts should be excised either by thoracotomy or through a cervical approach when located in the neck.

Schmidt A, Lockwood K: Benign neoplasms of the esophagus. Acta Chir Scand 133:640, 1967.

Schmidt HW, Clagett OT, Harrison EG Jr: Benign tumors and cysts of the esophagus. J Thorac Cardiovasc Surg 41:717, 1961.

Seremetis MG & others: Leiomyoma of the esophagus. Ann Thorac Surg 16:308, 1973.

MALIGNANT TUMORS OF THE ESOPHAGUS

Essentials of Diagnosis

- Progressive dysphagia, initially during ingestion of solid foods and later from liquids.
- Progressive weight loss and inanition.
- Classic radiographic outlines: irregular mucosal pattern with narrowing, with shelf-like upper border or concentrically narrowed esophageal lumen.
- Definitive diagnosis established by biopsy or cytology.

General Considerations

Most malignant tumors of the esophagus are carcinomas; sarcomas and carcinosarcomas are rare. Esophageal carcinoma occurs more frequently in males. The peak incidence is between 50–60 years. Malignant tumors located at the esophagogastric junction are usually adenocarcinomas and are probably largely of gastric origin. Those arising proximal to the cardia, ie, the true esophageal tumors, are almost all squamous cell carcinomas.

Carcinoma of the esophagus constitutes about 4% of all malignant lesions arising along the gastrointestinal tract. Twenty percent occur in the upper third, approximately 35% in the middle third, and 45% in the lower esophagus, including those developing at the cardia.

The carcinoma usually appears as a fungating growth extending irregularly into the esophageal lumen. Ulceration of its central portion is common. Annular lesions with extensive infiltration of the esophageal wall produce obstruction earlier than those which involve only a portion of the circumference of the esophagus. Regardless of their cell type, malignancies disseminate by direct invasion into surrounding mediastinal structures, through the blood stream by local vascular involvement, and by lymphatic dissemination. Lymph nodes at some distance from the primary lesion often contain metastatic deposits, and intramural extension, both upward and downward, frequently involves considerable lengths of the esophagus. Lower esophageal lesions metastasize primarily to the celiac and suprapancreatic lymph nodes. Lung, bone, liver, and brain are frequent sites of metastases.

Clinical Findings

A. Symptoms and Signs: Dysphagia is the most prominent symptom, and as a result the loss of weight is often striking. Solid foods initially cause difficulty; later, even liquids may be difficult to swallow. Weight loss, weakness, anemia, and inanition are almost always present. Pain is not common unless invasion of somatic structures occurs.

B. X-Ray Findings: Fluoroscopic studies provide a high degree of diagnostic accuracy. The malignancy appears as an irregular mass of variable size and length whose upper border is roughly horizontal and resembles a "shelf." Annular lesions appear as constricting bands with a narrowed lumen which contains an irregular mucosal outline (Fig 23–8). Dilatation of the esophagus may occur proximal to the growth, although it is not as great as that which occurs in chronic benign obstructive disease.

C. Esophagoscopy: Esophagoscopy with biopsy provides an accurate tissue diagnosis in most cases. However, the mucosa immediately proximal to the lesion may be so redundant, edematous, and inflamed that the tumor may not be directly visualized at esophagoscopy. In this case, esophageal washings to obtain cellular material are rewarding. Lesions as far distally as the midthoracic esophagus may involve the tracheobronchial tree by direct invasion. For this reason, bronchoscopy in addition to esophagoscopy is always indicated in the assessment of growths at these levels.

Differential Diagnosis

The fungating type of esophageal cancer presents a typical radiographic picture consisting of an irregular mucosal contour and the uppermost "shelf." Annular carcinomas may be mistaken for benign strictures, especially if most of the growth is largely intramural. Benign papillomas, polyps, or granulomatous masses can be distinguished from early carcinomas only on histologic examination.

Complications

Cancer of the esophagus rarely bleeds massively, although occult anemia is frequently observed. The most common complications result from invasion of important mediastinal structures such as the superior vena cava, aorta, trachea, major bronchi, and pericardium. Fatal hemorrhage, tracheal obstruction, and cardiac arrhythmias may result. A fistula may develop between the esophagus and the tracheobronchial tree and lead to aspiration pneumonitis, purulent bronchitis, and pulmonary abscesses.

Prevention

The cause of esophageal cancer is not known. Agents that have been suggested are hot liquids, alcohol, spicy foods, and tobacco. Available data do not support a cause and effect relationship with either cigarettes or pipe smoking. The incidence of esophageal cancer varies considerably throughout the world in countries with highly variable diets and customs. No basic cause has been identified in China, Japan, Russia, and Scandinavia, where the incidence is especially high.

Treatment

Esophageal carcinoma is treated by surgery, irradiation, or both. In recent years, preoperative radiation has been utilized in an effort to sterilize the soft tissues and lymphatics around the primary growth. Radiation therapy will often permit excision of an otherwise nonresectable growth and will increase the percentage of curative resections. Malignant lesions in the middle and upper thirds of the esophagus are quite likely to be nonresectable because of their propensity

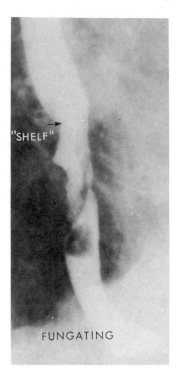

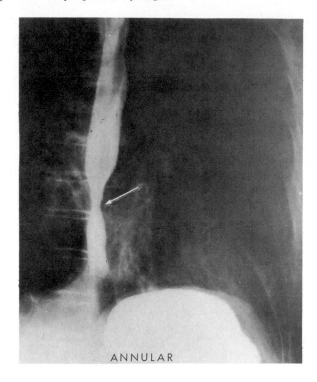

Figure 23–8. Two common types of esophageal carcinoma.

to invade vital nearby structures such as the aorta, pericardium, superior vena cava, and the tracheobronchial tree. Carcinomas of the lower third of the esophagus are often resected primarily; even in this area, however, preoperative radiation therapy is being given. General opinion is that radiation therapy followed by resection has improved the outlook, although the available statistics do not constitute proof.

A complete cancericidal course of radiation (5000–6000 R) is administered to the entire mediastinum, and surgery is undertaken 6–8 weeks later. Variable amounts of viable carcinoma usually remain after irradiation. Esophagogastrostomy in one stage through a 2-cavity abdominal and right thoracic approach is the most commonly employed procedure. Through an abdominal incision, an assessment is made for metastatic deposits, which occur mainly in the celiac and suprapancreatic lymph nodes and in the liver. If no metastases are found, the entire stomach is mobilized with its blood supply maintained by the right gastric and right gastroepiploic vessels. The short gastric arteries and the left gastric arteries are ligated to further free up the stomach as a pouch to be used as a replacement for the resected esophagus. A pyloroplasty completes the abdominal portion of the procedure. After the abdominal incision is closed, the patient is turned so that a right thoracotomy can be accomplished. The right-sided approach is preferable since the arch of the aorta does not obscure the operative field and also because the better exposure

facilitates safe removal of the growth from adjacent structures. The esophagus and the growth are resected high in the thorax and an anastomosis is created between the transected end of the esophagus and the fundus of the stomach. The high resection prevents esophagitis and allows for the resection of as much esophagus as possible to make certain that submucosal metastatic spread of the cancer has been removed. As an alternative to the stomach, colon or small bowel may be used to restore intestinal continuity.

In patients with far-advanced malignancies, distant metastases, or recurrence after radiotherapy, palliation to allow the patient to swallow can be obtained by bougienage or occasionally by intraluminal plastic tubes.

Prognosis

Esophageal cancer is a dread disease, and the operative mortality is about 20%. The 3-year survival rate is approximately 5%. Carcinoma of the lower esophagus has a somewhat better prognosis than do lesions in the middle and upper thirds. The overall resectability rate is approximately 30%.

Ellis FH Jr: Surgery for malignant lesions of the esophagogastric junction. Surg Clin North Am 56:571, 1976.

Gunnlaughsson G & others: Analysis of the records of 1657 patients with carcinoma of the esophagus and cardia of the stomach. Surg Gynecol Obstet 130:997, 1970.

Orringer MB, Sloan H: Substernal gastric bypass of the excluded thoracic esophagus for palliation of esophageal carcinoma.

J Thorac Cardiovasc Surg 70:836, 1975.

Parker EF, Gregorie HB: Carcinoma of the esophagus: Long term results. JAMA 235:1018, 1976.

Rubin P: Cancer of the gastrointestinal tract. 1. Esophagus: Detection and diagnosis. 2. Esophagus: Treatment— localized and advanced. JAMA 226:1544, 1973; 227:175, 1974.

Skinner DB: Esophageal malignancies: Experience with 110 cases. Surg Clin North Am 56:137, 1976.

Thomas AN: Treatment of malignant esophageal obstruction by endoesophageal intubation. Am J Surg 128:306, 1974.

ESOPHAGEAL BANDS, WEBS, OR RINGS

Congenital bands or webs may develop at any level but are more frequent in the subcricoid region. Others form in the lower esophageal segment. These bands cause dysphagia and may be treated by endoscopic dilatation in which the thin, web-like band is usually fractured, followed by complete relief of symptoms. Resection and primary anastomosis are occasionally necessary for the more fibrous unyielding concentric bands. The latter are more likely to be in the lower esophagus.

Band-like narrowing, usually associated with hiatal hernia, was described by Schatzki. Most patients are relatively free from symptoms unless the ring is less than 12 mm in diameter. Occasionally, dysphagia is severe. Endoscopy often fails to reveal the smooth concentric narrowing since the overlying mucosa is intact. Esophagitis is often present together with hiatal hernia and the Schatzki ring. Repair of the associated hiatal hernia is insufficient to control the dysphagia; the ring

must be dilated or excised. In some cases the ring can be ruptured by rapidly inflating a balloon in its lumen, as is done for achalasia. Afterward, the patient should be treated for esophagitis.

Goyal RK & others: Lower esophageal ring. (2 parts.) N Engl J Med 282:1298, 1355, 1970.

Kelley ML Jr, Frazer JP: Symptomatic mid-esophageal webs. JAMA 197:143, 1966.

Lam CR & others: The nature and surgical treatment of lower esophageal ring (Schatzki's ring). J Thorac Cardiovasc Surg 63:34, 1972.

The Patterson-Kelly lesion. Br Med J 2:530, 1969.

Postlethwait RW, Sealy WC: Experiences with the treatment of 59 patients with lower esophageal web. Ann Surg 165:786, 1967.

THE DIAPHRAGM
(Fig 23—9)

The diaphragm is a musculotendinous dome-shaped structure attached posteriorly to the first, second, and third lumbar vertebrae, anteriorly to the lower sternum, and laterally to the costal arches. It separates the abdominal and the thoracic cavities. The diaphragm allows the passage of various normal structures through anatomic foramens. The aortic hiatus lies posteriorly at the level of the 12th thoracic vertebra, and through it pass the aorta, the thoracic duct, and the azygos venous system. The esophageal hiatus lies immediately anteriorly and slightly to the left at the level of the tenth thoracic vertebra and is

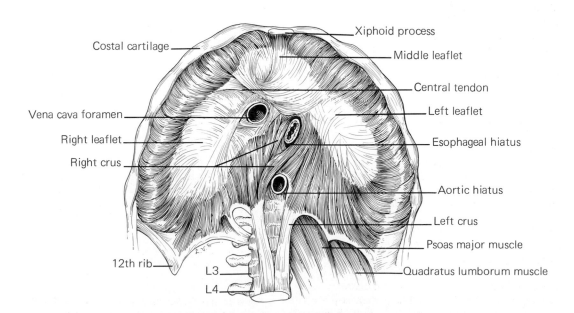

Figure 23—9. Inferior surface of diaphragm.

separated from the aortic hiatus by the decussation of the right crus of the diaphragm. Through this hiatus pass the esophagus and the vagus nerves. At the level of the ninth thoracic vertebra and slightly to the right of the esophageal hiatus is the vena cava foramen, which allows passage of the inferior cava and small branches of the phrenic nerve. The phrenic arteries arising directly from the aorta supply the diaphragm along with the lower intercostal arteries and the terminal branches of the internal mammary arteries.

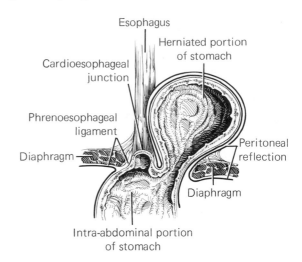

Figure 23—10. Paraesophageal hernia.

ESOPHAGEAL HIATAL HERNIA

There are 2 types of esophageal hiatal hernia: paraesophageal and sliding. Symptoms usually develop in adult life. Obesity, aging, and general weakening of the musculofascial structures set the stage for enlargement of the esophageal hiatus.

1. PARAESOPHAGEAL HIATAL HERNIA
(Figs 23—10 and 23—11)

Essentials of Diagnosis
- Often asymptomatic.
- Symptoms from mechanical obstruction: dysphagia, strangulation, stasis gastric ulcer.

General Considerations
In the paraesophageal type of diaphragmatic hernia, all or part of the stomach herniates into the thorax immediately adjacent and to the left of an undisplaced gastroesophageal junction (Fig 23—11). Since the gastroesophageal sphincteric mechanism functions normally, reflux of gastric contents does not occur. In those uncommon instances in which the paraesophageal hernia occurs in association with the sliding type, gastroesophageal reflux may occur along with other symptoms of an otherwise pure paraesophageal type. Paraesophageal hernia accounts for less than 10% of hernias of the esophageal hiatus.

Clinical Findings
The most common symptoms of uncomplicated paraesophageal hernia usually develop in adult life and consist of gaseous eructations, a sense of pressure in the lower chest after eating, and, occasionally, palpitations due to cardiac arrhythmias. All of these are pressure phenomena caused by enlargement of the herniated gastric pouch by food displacing the fundic air bubble. As noted, heartburn due to gastroesophageal reflux is uncommon.

Complications
The most frequent complications of paraesophageal hernia are hemorrhage, incarceration, obstruction, and strangulation. The herniated portion of the stom-

ach often becomes congested, and bleeding occurs from erosions of the mucosa. Obstruction may occur, most often at the esophagogastric junction as a result of torsion and angulation at this point—especially if a large portion (or all) of the stomach herniates into the chest. In paraesophageal hiatal hernia—in contrast to the sliding type—other viscera such as the small and large intestine and spleen may also enter the mediastinum along with the stomach.

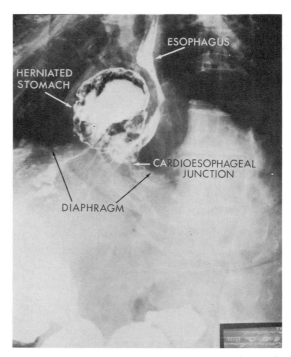

Figure 23—11. Paraesophageal hernia. Note that the cardioesophageal junction remains in its normal anatomic position below the diaphragm.

Treatment

Since complications are frequent even in the absence of symptoms, operative repair is indicated in most cases. The usual method is to return the herniated stomach to the abdomen and fix it there by sutures to the posterior rectus sheath (anterior gastropexy). The enlarged hiatus is closed snugly around the gastroesophageal junction with interrupted sutures.

Prognosis

The results of surgical management are generally good unless the diaphragmatic musculature has become weakened and tenuous.

Culver GJ & others: Mechanism of obstruction in paraesophageal diaphragmatic hernias. JAMA 181:933, 1962.

Hill LD: Incarcerated paraesophageal hernia. Am J Surg 126:286, 1973.

Hill LD, Tobias JA: Paraesophageal hernia. Arch Surg 96:735, 1968.

Larson NE & others: Mechanism of obstruction and strangulation in hernias of the esophageal hiatus. Surg Gynecol Obstet 119:835, 1964.

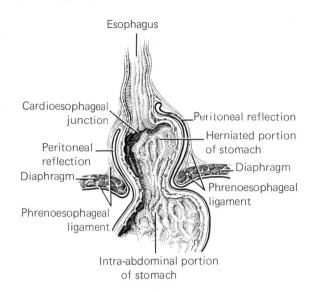

Figure 23—12. Sliding esophageal hernia.

2. SLIDING HIATAL HERNIA & REFLUX ESOPHAGITIS
(Figs 23—12 and 23—13)

Essentials of Diagnosis

- Heartburn, often worse on recumbency.
- Regurgitation ("water brash").
- Sliding hiatal hernia on upper gastrointestinal series.
- Decreased resting pressure in lower esophageal sphincter.

General Considerations

The sliding type of hiatal hernia comprises more than 90% of hernias at the esophageal hiatus. The upper stomach, along with the cardioesophageal junction, is displaced upward into the posterior mediastimun. The hernia is partially surrounded by a peritoneal sac similar to that of a sliding hernia in the inguinal region. Often the displacement is stationary, but in some cases the stomach may actually slide in and out of the thorax with changes in body position, alterations of pressure in the abdominal and thoracic cavities, and after a large meal.

Concomitant with displacement, the normal competence of the gastroesophageal sphincter is often compromised, and reflux of gastric contents into the esophagus is a frequent result. Regurgitation is accentuated in the supine position or by anything that increases intra-abdominal pressure such as lifting, stooping forward, straining, overeating, and the late stages of pregnancy.

Esophageal motility studies in patients with symptomatic hiatal hernia reveal low pressures in the gastroesophageal sphincter and failure of sphincter pressure to increase sufficiently to prevent reflux following elevations in intra-abdominal pressure. It is not yet clear why a weakened sphincter develops so often in association with a hiatal hernia. Sphincter strength is thought to be at least partly regulated by circulating levels of gastrin, and several reports indicate that both basal and postprandial gastrin concentrations are lower in patients with reflux than in normal subjects. Although reflux may occur in the absence of a hiatal

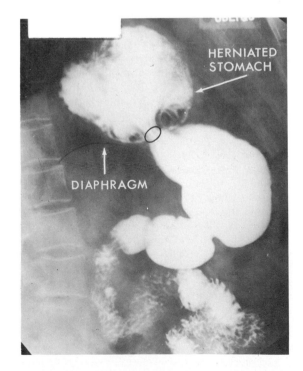

Figure 23—13. Large sliding hiatal hernia. Diaphragmatic hiatus is circled.

hernia, a substantial majority of patients with reflux esophagitis have hernias, but why they should also have diminished gastrin release is obscure. Surgical procedures which correct the hernia have been shown to eliminate reflux and increase basal sphincteric pressure and the rise in pressure following elevation of abdominal pressure.

Clinical Findings

A. Symptoms and Signs: In spite of the deranged anatomy at the cardioesophageal junction, at least 50% of sliding esophageal hernias are asymptomatic. Reflux of gastric contents into the esophagus accounts for most of the symptoms and complications that do occur. Retrosternal and epigastric burning pain—often referred to as heartburn—frequently occurs after eating and while sleeping or lying in a recumbent position. This distress is relieved partially or completely by drinking water or other liquids, by antacids, or, in many instances, by standing or sitting. Patients with severe regurgitation often report that bitter or sour-tasting fluid may regurgitate as far as the throat and mouth, especially at night when they are supine.

Dysphagia may be a prominent complaint and results from the inflammatory edema incident to the lower esophagus, but its presence indicates a more advanced stage of the disease and a greater likelihood that complications will eventually develop.

B. X-Ray Findings: The diagnosis of sliding esophageal hiatal hernia is made by the radiographic demonstration of a portion of the stomach protruding upward through the esophageal hiatus (Fig 23–13). Repeated fluoroscopic studies may be required. The presence of hiatal hernia may be suggested on routine chest films by the discovery of a gas-filled portion of stomach above the level of the diaphragm; this is often best observed in the lateral projection, since in the anteroposterior view the cardiac shadow may obliterate the hernia outline.

C. Special Examinations: In symptomatic patients—especially those with dysphagia—esophagoscopy and esophageal biopsy should be performed to assess the severity of the esophagitis and to rule out associated conditions such as strictures, polyps, ulcers, and malignancies. Esophageal motility studies, by showing abnormally low sphincter pressures and proximal displacement of the gastroesophageal junction, may aid in the diagnosis, and pH determinations may be necessary to determine whether or not true reflux exists.

The **standard acid reflux** test is the most accurate way to diagnose abnormal gastroesophageal reflux. 300 ml of 0.1 N hydrochloric acid are instilled into the stomach through a manometry catheter, and a pH probe is positioned 5 cm proximal to the lower esophageal sphincter. Esophageal pH is monitored while the patient performs the following: rests in the supine position, breathes deeply, executes the Valsalva maneuver, the Müller maneuver (inspiration against a closed glottis), and coughs. Each of these is repeated in the right and left lateral decubitus positions and with the head down. A positive result, signifying abnormal reflux, consists of a drop in pH below 4.0 in 3 or more of the 16 possible test situations. The number of reflux episodes correlates positively with the clinical severity of the esophagitis.

The **Bernstein test** provides a reasonably reliable means of determining whether the patient's symptoms are actually due to esophagitis: Through a tube placed in the body of the esophagus, either 0.15 M NaCl or 0.1 N HCl solution is slowly infused and the symptomatic response of the patient is noted. If esophagitis is present, the HCl solution produces discomfort and heartburn similar to the patient's clinical complaints but the NaCl solution does not; dilute HCl does not cause burning in persons without esophagitis. Gastritis or peptic ulcer disease of the stomach or duodenum can give false-positive tests.

Differential Diagnosis

Sliding esophageal hiatal hernia has been called the great masquerader of the upper abdomen. Other conditions may present symptoms which mimic those of hiatal hernia, and vice versa. The symptoms caused by a variety of abdominal and intrathoracic diseases are often difficult to differentiate from each other and from those of an uncomplicated sliding hernia. Cholelithiasis, diverticulitis, peptic ulcer, achalasia, and coronary artery disease are common examples. Not infrequently, 3 conditions exist together: hiatal hernia, gallbladder disease, and colonic diverticular disease (Saint's triad).

Since esophageal pain may be referred upward into the neck, shoulders, or arms, angina pectoris must be considered. The Bernstein test is often valuable in the differentiation.

Complications

As indicated above, esophagitis due to reflux is the most common complication. Small, shallow ulcerations may develop, and true callous ulcers may at times be observed in neglected cases, but, in general, ulceration is uncommon. The principal problem in advanced disease is stricture formation. Carcinoma is occasionally associated with sliding hiatal hernia.

Treatment

A. Medical Treatment: At least half of sliding esophageal hiatal hernias are asymptomatic and require no treatment. The great majority of patients with esophagitis can be managed by a conservative program of high-protein, low-fat diet, frequent small feedings, and antacids. The antacid regimen should follow the principles outlined in Chapter 26. Anticholinergic drugs are contraindicated in this condition because they weaken the lower esophageal sphincter.

Every effort must be made to enlist the aid of gravity in preventing reflux. The patient should not lie down after meals and should not eat a late meal before bedtime. The head of the patient's bed should be elevated on 4- to 6-inch blocks; attempting to sleep propped up on pillows is a compromise that almost never succeeds.

Clinical trials are presently being conducted with metoclopramide and bethanechol, both of which increase the strength of the lower esophageal sphincter. Preliminary reports on the use of bethanechol, 25 mg orally 4 times daily, are optimistic.

B. Surgical Treatment: Repair can be accomplished either transthoracically or through an abdominal approach. In patients in whom intra-abdominal disease is suspected, the transabdominal approach is mandatory. In obese patients or in patients with a shortened esophagus that requires more mobilization than can be achieved through the abdomen, a transthoracic approach is preferable. In either approach, the operative technic is similar.

Repair of sliding hernias is more complicated than for the paraesophageal type. The objective is to restore the cardioesophageal junction to its correct anatomic position in the abdomen and to secure it firmly in place. The enlarged hiatus is closed so that it approximates the crural columns of the diaphragm posteriorly with heavy nonabsorbable sutures. The lower esophagus is extensively mobilized so that about 5 cm of esophagus will reside in the abdomen at the conclusion of the repair. After the crura have been approximated, the upper part of the lesser curvature of the stomach and the cardioesophageal junction are firmly sutured to the closed crura posteriorly (Hill procedure).

Another effective technic—fundoplication—can be used alone or sometimes in combination with the above method. Transabdominal fundoplication (Nissen procedure) consists of wrapping part of the fundus completely around the lower 4–6 cm of esophagus and fixing it in place so that the esophagus passes through a short tunnel of stomach before it ends. The Belsey (Mark IV) fundoplication is somewhat similar except that the fundus is wrapped only 270 degrees around the esophageal circumference and the operation is performed through a left thoracotomy.

The Hill, Nissen, and Belsey procedures are all effective in preventing reflux. The fundoplication operations, particularly the Nissen procedure, have gained most in popularity in the past few years.

A procedure to reduce gastric acidity should not routinely be added to the hiatal hernia repair but should be reserved for patients with known peptic ulcer disease. A parietal cell vagotomy combined with a Nissen fundoplication is probably best in such cases.

Mild strictures can be managed by dilatations with orally passed bougies (eg, Hurst or Maloney dilators) and an intensive medical regimen for the esophagitis. Sometimes—usually in tight strictures—one or more dilatations must be performed under direct vision using a rigid metal esophagoscope. If this approach fails to result in improvement, surgery should be considered. Hiatal hernia repair plus occasional dilatations will provide relief in all but the most advanced cases. In the latter, excision of the strictured lower esophagus is required with restoration of continuity either by an esophagogastrostomy or, preferably, by interposing a 15 cm isoperistaltic segment of jejunum between the esophagus and the stomach.

Prognosis

About 90% of patients experience a good result following surgery; the remaining 10% have persistent or recurrent reflux. Relief of symptoms is accompanied by an increase in resting pressure in the lower esophageal sphincter of about 10 mm Hg. Recurrence of symptoms is more frequent than an anatomic recurrence. The latter may be due to an inadequate technical repair initially; to excessive tension on the point of fixation of the cardioesophageal junction due to shortening of the esophagus; or to weakening of the musculofascial structures by aging, atrophy, or obesity.

Bahadorzadeh K, Jordan PH Jr: Evaluation of the Nissen fundoplication for treatment of hiatal hernia: Use of parietal cell vagotomy as an adjunctive procedure. Ann Surg 181:402, 1975.

Behar J: Reflux esophagitis: Pathogenesis, diagnosis, and management. Arch Intern Med 136:560, 1976.

Cohen S, Booth GH Jr: Gastric acid secretion and lower-esophageal-sphincter pressure in response to coffee and caffeine. N Engl J Med 293:897, 1975.

DeMeester TR, Johnson LF: The evaluation of objective measurements of gastroesophageal reflux and their contribution to patient management. Surg Clin North Am 56:39, 1976.

DeMeester TR & others: Evaluation of current operations for the prevention of gastroesophageal reflux. Ann Surg 180:511, 1974.

DeMeester TR & others: Patterns of gastroesophageal reflux in health and disease. Ann Surg 184:459, 1976.

Ellis FH Jr & others: The effect of fundoplication on the lower esophageal sphincter. Surg Gynecol Obstet 143:1, 1976.

Fisher RS & others: The lower esophageal sphincter as a barrier to gastroesophageal reflux. Gastroenterology 72:19, 1977.

Herrington JL Jr, Mody B: Total duodenal diversion for treatment of reflux esophagitis uncontrolled by repeated antireflux procedures. Ann Surg 183:636, 1976.

Herrington JL Jr & others: Conservative surgical treatment for reflux esophagitis and esophageal stricture. Ann Surg 181:552, 1975.

Hollenbeck JI, Woodward ER: Treatment of peptic esophageal stricture with combined fundic patch-fundoplication. Ann Surg 182:472, 1975.

Larrain A & others: Surgical correction of reflux: An effective therapy for esophageal strictures. Gastroenterology 69:578, 1975.

Lipshutz WH & others: Normal lower-esophageal-sphincter function after surgical treatment of gastroesophageal reflux. N Engl J Med 291:1107, 1974.

Lipshutz WH & others: Pathogenesis of lower-esophageal-sphincter incompetence. N Engl J Med 289:182, 1973.

McCallum RW & others: Comparative effects of metoclopramide and bethanechol on lower esophageal sphincter pressure in reflux patients. Gastroenterology 68:1114, 1975.

Orringer MB, Sloan H: Collis-Belsey reconstruction of the esophagogastric junction. J Thorac Cardiovasc Surg 71:295, 1976.

Ottinger LW: Clinical management of hiatus hernias and gastroesophageal reflux. Surg Clin North Am 54:475, 1974.

Pearson FG, Henderson RD: Long-term follow-up of peptic strictures managed by dilatation, modified Collis gastroplasty, and Belsey hiatus hernia repair. Surgery 80:396, 1976.

Rees JR & others: Management of transmural peptic strictures of the esophagus. Ann Surg 179:382, 1974.

Rex JC & others: Esophageal hiatal hernia: A 10-year study of medically treated cases. JAMA 178:271, 1961.

Skinner DB, DeMeester TR: Gastroesophageal reflux. Curr Probl Surg 13 (1), Jan 1976.

Strug BS & others: Surgical management of benign esophageal strictures. Surg Gynecol Obstet 138:74, 1974.

COLUMNAR-LINED ESOPHAGUS WITH OR WITHOUT HIATAL HERNIA
(Barrett's Esophagus)

In 1950, Barrett of England described a pathologic condition in which the lower esophagus is lined with columnar epithelium similar to that of the cardiac portion of the stomach except that acid- and pepsin-producing cells are not usually present. It appears to be a form of epithelial metaplasia which results from reflux esophagitis. The abnormal epithelium should be considered premalignant since adenocarcinoma develops in about 10% of patients. Most patients have an associated hiatal hernia.

Although columnar-lined esophagus occasionally occurs in children and young adults, it is more commonly encountered in older people.

The most frequent complication is stricture formation at the squamocolumnar junction. Large ulcers occasionally develop, usually at the squamocolumnar junction, causing massive bleeding. Management depends upon the pathologic changes that occur. Rarely, resection may be necessary to control bleeding or to remove large, painful, penetrating ulcers.

Berquist TH & others: Radioisotope scintigraphy in diagnosis of Barrett's esophagus. Am J Roentgenol Radium Ther Nucl Med 123:401, 1975.

Borrie J, Goldwater L: Columnar cell-lined esophagus: Assessment of etiology and treatment. J Thorac Cardiovasc Surg 71:825, 1976.

Hill LD & others: Simplified management of reflux esophagitis with stricture. Ann Surg 172:638, 1970.

Mangla JC & others: Pepsin secretion, pepsinogen, and gastrin in "Barrett's esophagus." Gastroenterology 70:669, 1976.

Naef AP & others: Columnar-lined esophagus: An acquired lesion with malignant potential. J Thorac Cardiovasc Surg 70:826, 1975.

Paull A & others: The histologic spectrum of Barrett's esophagus. N Engl J Med 295:476, 1976.

PARASTERNAL OR RETROSTERNAL (FORAMEN OF MORGAGNI) HERNIA
(Fig 23–14)

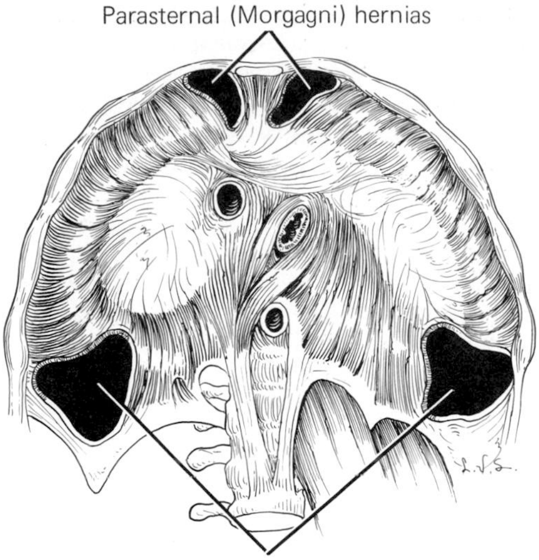

Failure of fusion of the sternal and costal portions of the diaphragm anteriorly in the midline creates a defect (foramen of Morgagni) through which hernias can occur. Normally, the diaphragm becomes fused,

Figure 23–14. Sites of congenital diaphragmatic herniation.

allowing only the internal mammary arteries and their superior epigastric branches, along with lymphatics, to pass through this area.

Although this condition is congenital, symptoms usually do not develop until middle life or later. Most patients are women. The symptomatology is variable, but substernal fullness or pain predominates. In infants, if the hernia is large and contains considerable abdominal viscera, the cardiorespiratory distress may simulate that of the more common Bochdalek's hernia and immediate repair becomes mandatory. In adults, complications are rare and many cases are asymptomatic. Routine chest films may show a retrosternal mass or an air-filled viscus.

Elective surgical repair is indicated in most instances to prevent complications. An emergency operation may become necessary in the newborn infant who develops progressive cardiorespiratory insufficiency. Repair of the defect by a transabdominal approach is preferable, and the results are excellent.

Thomas TV: Subcostosternal diaphragmatic hernia. J Thorac Cardiovasc Surg 63:279, 1972.

TRAUMATIC DIAPHRAGMATIC HERNIA

Traumatic rupture of the diaphragm may occur as a result of penetrating wounds or severe blunt external trauma. Lacerations usually occur in the tendinous portion of the diaphragm, most often on the left side. The liver provides protection to diaphragmatic injury on the right side except from penetrating wounds. Abdominal viscera may immediately herniate through the defect in the diaphragm into the pleural cavity or may gradually insinuate themselves into the thorax over a period of months or years.

Clinical Findings

The symptoms are related to the amount of viscera which herniate into the thorax. Some degree of intestinal obstruction may be present. Plain films of the chest will show either a solid mass shadow if the omentum is the primary herniated structure, or a number of fluid levels if hollow viscera herniate. Passage of a nasogastric tube into the herniated stomach above the diaphragm is diagnostic. Fluoroscopic studies often will show the stomach protruding through the diaphragmatic rent. Barium study of the colon may show irregular patches of barium in the colon above the diaphragm or a smooth colonic outline if the colon does not contain feces.

Differential Diagnosis

Traumatic rupture of the diaphragm must be differentiated from atelectasis, space-consuming tumors of the lower pleural space, pleural effusion, and intestinal obstruction due to other causes.

Complications

Hemorrhage and obstruction may occur. If herniation is massive, progressive cardiorespiratory insufficiency may threaten life. The most severe complication is strangulating obstruction of the herniated viscera.

Treatment

Transthoracic repair of the ruptured diaphragm is recommended. In the asymptomatic patient in whom a definite diagnosis of a previous traumatic rupture of the diaphragm can be established—and if other conditions simulating traumatic diaphragmatic hernia can be ruled out—operative repair can be delayed until definite symptoms develop. In acute rupture of the diaphragm, associated injuries often take precedence over the diaphragmatic injury; in these instances, however, the acute traumatic tear in the diaphragm should be repaired when feasible.

Prognosis

Surgical repair of the rent in the diaphragm is curative, and the prognosis is excellent. The diaphragm supports sutures well, so that recurrence is practically unknown.

Ebert PA & others: Traumatic diaphragmatic hernia. Surg Gynecol Obstet 125:59, 1967.

Gourin A, Garzon AA: Diagnostic problems in traumatic diaphragmatic hernia. J Trauma 14:20, 1974.

Grimes OF: Traumatic injuries of the diaphragm: Diaphragmatic hernia. Am J Surg 128:174, 1974.

Hood RM: Traumatic diaphragmatic hernia. Ann Thorac Surg 12:311, 1971.

DUPLICATION OF THE DIAPHRAGM

Duplication—usually of the left hemidiaphragm—is rare. It is frequently associated with an anomaly of the vasculature of the lower lobe of the left lung.

TUMORS OF THE DIAPHRAGM

Primary tumors of the diaphragm are not common. The majority are benign lipomas. Pericardial cysts develop in the interval between the heart and the diaphragm and are usually unilocular and on the right side. Fibrosarcoma, the most common primary malignant diaphragmatic tumor, is extremely rare.

Benign tumors are usually asymptomatic. Since their benign nature cannot be established except by histologic study, all lesions of this type should be excised through an appropriate thoracotomy.

DIAPHRAGMATIC FLUTTER

Diaphragmatic flutter is the most common functional disorder of the diaphragm. The cause is not known. It is characterized by diaphragmatic contraction, either continuously or paroxysmally, at a rate of 50—300 per minute or more. Hyperventilation and respiratory alkalosis may result.

Treatment is difficult and often unsatisfactory. Injection of anesthetic solutions into the phrenic nerve may provide temporary relief. Excision of 2—4 cm of the phrenic nerve is frequently curative.

● ● ●

General References

Morson BC, Dawson IMP: *Gastrointestinal Pathology.* Blackwell, 1972.

Payne WS, Olsen AM: *The Esophagus.* Lea & Febiger, 1974.

Skinner DB, DeMeester TR: Gastroesophageal reflux. Curr Probl Surg 13 (1), Jan 1976.

Sleisenger M, Fordtran J: *Gastrointestinal Disease.* Saunders, 1973.

Smith RA, Smith RE (editors): *Surgery of the Esophagus.* Appleton-Century-Crofts, 1972.

24...

Acute Abdomen

J. Englebert Dunphy, MD

Acute abdominal diseases are usually manifested by pain, anorexia, nausea, vomiting, and fever. On physical examination, tenderness, muscle spasm, and changes in peristalsis are important signs. A correct diagnosis depends upon the precision and care with which the history is taken and the physical examination performed.

HISTORY

The history determines the direction of the investigation, and physical examination often furnishes the definitive data. Laboratory and x-ray studies provide important confirmatory evidence.

Mode of Onset of Abdominal Pain

If the patient is well one moment and seized with agonizing (explosive) pain the next, the most probable diagnosis is either free rupture of a hollow viscus or vascular accident. Renal and biliary colic may be very sudden in onset but are not likely to cause such severe and prostrating pain.

If the pain is rapid in onset—moderately severe at first and rapidly becoming worse—consider acute pancreatitis, mesenteric thrombosis, or strangulation of the small bowel.

Gradual onset of slowly progressive pain is characteristic of peritoneal infection or inflammation. Appendicitis and diverticulitis often start in this way.

Character of the Pain (Fig 24—1)

One must determine the exact character of the abdominal pain.

Excruciating pain not relieved by narcotics indicates a vascular lesion such as massive infarction of the intestine or rupture of an abdominal aneurysm.

Very severe pain, readily controlled by medication, is more typical of acute pancreatitis or the peritonitis associated with a ruptured viscus. Obstructive appendicitis and incarcerated small bowel without extensive infarction occasionally produce the same type of pain. The pain of biliary or renal colic is usually promptly alleviated by medication.

If the pain is **dull, vague, and poorly localized,** it is also likely to have been gradual in onset. These findings strongly suggest an inflammatory process or a low-grade infection. Appendicitis commonly presents in this fashion.

An occasional patient will say that he has no abdominal pain but only a sense of fullness, and feels that he would feel better if he could only have a bowel movement. Sometimes he has taken an enema but has had no relief despite the fact that his bowels moved. This symptom complex—the "gas stoppage sign"—is characteristic of retrocecal appendicitis but may be present when any inflammatory lesion is walled off from the free peritoneal cavity.

Intermittent pain with cramps and rushes is commonly seen in gastroenteritis. However, if the pain comes in regular cycles, rising in crescendo fashion and then subsiding to a pain-free interval, the most likely diagnosis is mechanical small bowel obstruction. This type of pain occurs occasionally in early subacute pancreatitis. If auscultation reveals intermittent peristaltic rushes, rising in crescendo fashion and synchronous with the pain, small bowel obstruction is very likely. In the colic of gastroenteritis, on the other hand, peristaltic rushes have little or no relation to abdominal cramps.

Radiation or a shift in localization of the pain has particular significance. Pain in the shoulder follows diaphragmatic irritation due to air, peritoneal fluid, or blood. Biliary pain is often referred to the right scapula and rarely to the left epigastrium and left shoulder, simulating angina pectoris. Classically, the pain of appendicitis begins in the epigastrium and settles in the right lower quadrant. A shift or spread of abdominal pain often indicates spreading peritonitis.

Anorexia; Nausea & Vomiting

Anorexia, nausea, and vomiting are common symptoms of acute abdominal disease, and careful analysis of the character of these symptoms may be of great value in arriving at the correct diagnosis. However, there may be advanced abdominal disease without anorexia, nausea, or vomiting. If the peritoneum is well protected from infection or inflammation, as in retrocecal appendicitis or when the appendix is completely isolated by omentum, the patient may not only have no anorexia but insist that he is hungry. The time of onset of these symptoms is important because,

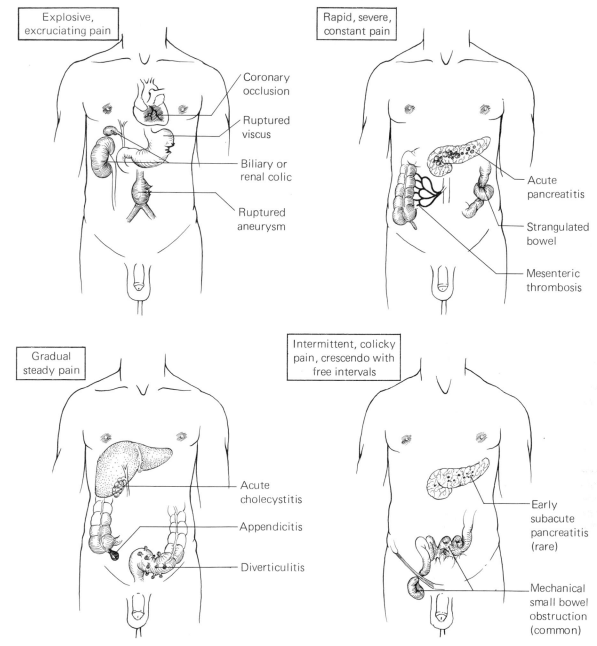

Figure 24—1. Precise identification of the nature of pain is of critical importance in differential diagnosis.

if they precede the onset of pain, gastroenteritis or some systemic illness is much more likely than an acute abdominal emergency requiring operation.

When nausea and vomiting are very prominent symptoms, the most likely possibilities are gastroenteritis, acute gastritis, acute pancreatitis, common duct stone, and high intestinal obstruction. In most other acute surgical emergencies, nausea and vomiting are not dominant symptoms though they may be present.

Severe vomiting with retching—particularly following a dietary indiscretion or an alcoholic bout—

should immediately suggest laceration of the gastroesophageal junction (Mallory-Weiss syndrome) or an esophageal perforation (Boerhaave's syndrome; see Chapter 23). Massive hematemesis or severe pain radiating into the chest and left shoulder in association with severe vomiting and retching make these critical emergencies very likely.

Diarrhea, Constipation, & Obstipation

Some alteration of bowel function is common in most cases of acute abdominal emergencies, but the variations are extraordinary. There are several important clues. If it can be ascertained for certain that a patient has passed no gas and had no bowel movements for 24–48 hours, he has intestinal obstruction. Under these circumstances, however, there will also be either obvious distention or persistent vomiting. If the patient insists that he has not passed gas for 24–48 hours but there is no vomiting and no distention, it is likely that he has been unaware of the passage of gas. Diarrhea is the classic manifestation of gastroenteritis, but it also may be a dominant symptom of pelvic appendicitis. Bloody and repetitive diarrhea indicates ulceration of the colon. Ulcerative colitis, Crohn's disease, and bacillary and amebic dysenteries must be considered first. Bloody diarrhea is a common sign of colonic ischemia, but it is often absent in superior mesenteric thrombosis with extensive gangrene of small and large bowel.

Chills & Fever

Some degree of fever is common to most acute surgical emergencies. In appendicitis, fever is not usually very high, and high fever should suggest either pylephlebitis or some other diagnosis. A very high fever with peritoneal signs in a female patient with no apparent general systemic illness is characteristic of acute pelvic inflammatory disease.

Repeated chills and fever characterize pylephlebitis and bacteremia. Their presence in suspected appendicitis strongly suggests perforation. Repeated chills and fever are most common in infections of the biliary or renal tracts. Acute cholangitis and acute pyelitis usually present with intermittent chills and fever. Chills, fever, jaundice, and hypotension indicate suppurative cholangitis—a surgical emergency.

PHYSICAL EXAMINATION

Having taken note of diagnostic possibilities in the history, the physician proceeds to the physical examination. This must be complete, with particular emphasis on the abdominal examination. The care with which the examination is performed often establishes the diagnosis. The appropriate approach is outlined in Table 24–1.

Initial Abdominal Examination

The abdomen should first be inspected, looking for such striking features as the scaphoid, contracted abdomen of an early perforated viscus, the visible peristalsis of mechanical obstruction, or the soft, doughy distention of early ileus.

The next step is to examine the inguinal and femoral canals in both sexes and the genitalia in the male. This must be done very gently, asking the patient to cough but causing as little discomfort as possible. In most acute inflammatory conditions, coughing will elicit pain not in the groin but in the abdomen. If the patient is then asked to point one finger to where he

Table 24–1. Routine for physical examination of the acute abdomen.

(1) Inspection.	(6) Deep palpation.
(2) Cough tenderness. Examine hernial rings and male genitalia.	(7) Rebound tenderness.
(3) Feel for spasm.	(8) Auscultation.
(4) One-finger palpation.	(9) Special signs.
(5) Costovertebral tenderness.	(10) Rectal and pelvic examination.

feels the pain, an objective localization of the lesion is obtained. With this information in hand, the examiner can proceed to examine the abdomen, deliberately avoiding the area which he now knows to be most tender.

Spasm

The next step is to establish the presence or absence of true spasm. This is done by placing the hand gently over the rectus abdominis muscle and depressing it slightly and gently, without causing pain (Fig 24–2). Properly performed, this maneuver is a comforting one to the patient. Now ask the patient to take a long breath. If the spasm is voluntary, the muscle will immediately relax underneath the gentle pressure of the palpating hand. If there is true spasm, however, the muscle will remain taut and rigid throughout the respiratory cycle. This maneuver alone is sufficient to establish the presence of peritonitis. Except for rare neurologic disorders—and, for reasons that no one understands, renal colic—only peritoneal inflammation produces abdominal muscle rigidity. In renal colic, the spasm is confined to the entire rectus muscle on one side. The distinction is important because marked rigidity of the entire length of one rectus muscle with relaxation of the opposite cannot occur in peritonitis since there is no compartmentalization of the peritoneal cavity. It is possible, however, to have segmental spasm of a rectus muscle involving only the upper or lower portion on one side, or to have

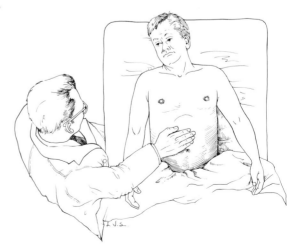

Figure 24–2. Testing for spasm.

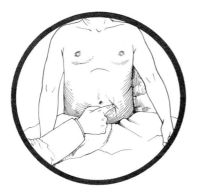

Figure 24—3. Gentle systematic palpation with one finger is the best way to localize an area of tenderness.

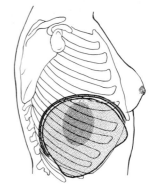

Figure 24—4. Darker shaded area shows area of decreased liver dullness due to free air in the peritoneal cavity.

segmental spasm of both rectus muscles in upper or lower abdominal peritonitis. In generalized peritonitis, both muscles are usually involved to the same degree.

Test for Abdominal Tenderness

The test for abdominal tenderness must be done with one finger and not with the entire hand (Fig 24—3). It is impossible to accurately localize peritoneal inflammation if palpation for tenderness is done with the entire hand. Careful one-finger palpation, beginning as far away as possible from the area of localized cough-elicited pain and gradually working toward it, will usually enable the examiner to determine precisely the limitations of abdominal tenderness. In early acute appendicitis, this is often no larger than a silver dollar and sometimes smaller. Whenever there is diffuse abdominal tenderness without associated involuntary rigidity of the muscles, one should suspect gastroenteritis or some other inflammatory process of the intestines without peritonitis. Gastroenteritis is characteristically accompanied by diffuse abdominal tenderness with no muscular rigidity.

Percussion

In free perforation of a hollow viscus with air under the diaphragm, there may be diminished or absent liver dullness (Fig 24—4). Tympany laterally in the midaxillary line 5 cm or more above the costal margin is due to free air; tympany anteriorly over the liver may be due to air in distended loops of bowel.

Masses

Having established the presence or absence of muscular rigidity and localized the area of tenderness, the examiner now palpates more deeply for the presence of abdominal masses. Among the more common lesions identifiable by careful palpation in patients with acute abdominal pain are cholecystitis, appendicitis with early abscess formation, sigmoid diverticulitis, and leaking abdominal aneurysm.

Peristaltic Sounds

Auscultation is an essential part of the abdominal examination. The absence of audible peristalsis—ie, a completely silent abdomen—means diffuse peritonitis. It may be necessary to listen for as long as 2 or 3 minutes to establish the absence of peristalsis. Other manifestations of diffuse peritonitis such as rigidity and distention are usually present also in such cases. It should be remembered that there may be persistent peristalsis in the presence of established peritonitis (see Chapter 25).

Intermittent crescendo peristaltic rushes with regular free intervals are diagnostic of acute mid small bowel obstruction. For reasons that are not entirely clear, the only other lesion that produces peristalsis of this type is early acute pancreatitis, in which the dilated sentinel loop seen on x-ray appears to undergo cyclic peristaltic contractions simulating those of acute mechanical obstruction.

In gastroenteritis, fulminating ulcerative colitis, and the dysenteries, there is abnormal high-pitched peristalsis with rushes, but these are not synchronous with the episodes of pain.

Special Signs

There are several maneuvers in physical examination which may elicit confirmatory evidence of an acute abdominal lesion:

A. Iliopsoas Sign: The patient flexes his thigh against the resistance of the examiner's hand (Fig

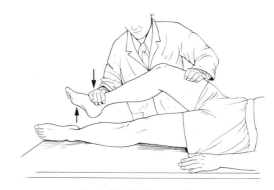

Figure 24—5. Iliopsoas sign.

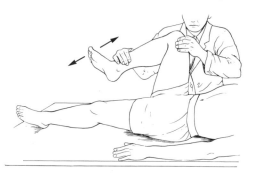

Figure 24—6. Obturator sign.

24—5). A painful response indicates an inflammatory process involving the psoas muscle.

B. Obturator Sign: The patient's thigh is flexed to a right angle and is gently rotated internally and externally (Fig 24—6). If pain is elicited, there is an inflammatory lesion involving the obturator internus muscle (pelvic appendicitis, diverticulitis).

C. Fist Percussion Sign: Gentle percussion with the fist over the anterior chest wall elicits sharp pain if there is an acute inflammation involving the space between the diaphragm and liver on the right and the stomach or spleen on the left (Fig 24—7).

D. Inspiratory Arrest (Murphy's Sign): The patient is asked to take a deep breath as the examiner gently palpates the right upper quadrant. With descent of the diaphragm, an acutely inflamed gallbladder comes in contact with the examining fingers, causing the patient pain and arresting the breath.

Other Examinations

The examination is completed by pelvic and rectal examination. The importance of pelvic and rectal examinations, particularly in acute pelvic appendicitis, will be discussed in Chapter 32.

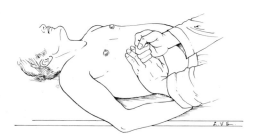

Figure 24—7. Fist percussion of lower anterior chest wall. A gentle blow will elicit pain in the presence of any inflammatory lesion involving the diaphragm or liver on the right or the diaphragm, spleen, or stomach on the left. This sign is often positive in acute hepatitis. A negative response is rare in acute cholecystitis.

LABORATORY EXAMINATION

Hematocrit, complete blood count, and urine examination should be obtained in all cases.

Blood

The hematocrit is of critical importance, reflecting in a significant way changes in plasma volume—particularly dehydration due to excessive vomiting or loss of fluids into the peritoneum or intestinal lumen. A low hematocrit may indicate preexisting anemia or bleeding.

The white blood count may be helpful if significantly elevated. However, normal or even low counts can be obtained in the presence of established peritonitis. A low blood count, particularly with lymphocytosis, may suggest viral infection or gastroenteritis. Marked leukopenia may suggest a blood dyscrasia or severe sepsis. A progressively rising white count is of considerable value and usually indicates progression of an inflammatory or septic process. A shift to the left on a blood smear may be a clue to an inflammatory reaction in the presence of a normal or only moderately elevated count.

Serum Electrolytes

Serum electrolytes are often required to document the nature and extent of fluid losses.

Serum Amylase

Serum amylase requires careful evaluation. If elevated, it may be a clue to acute pancreatitis, but it may be low or normal in hemorrhagic pancreatitis. It is often high in cases of mesenteric thrombosis, intestinal obstruction, or perforated duodenal ulcer. A persistently high amylase level is often seen in the presence of acute pseudocysts.

Acute pancreatitis may occur in association with hyperlipemia—especially type I or V hyperlipoproteinemia—but there may be suppression or inhibition of serum amylase activity so that a low or normal value is measured (see Chapter 29).

Urine

Examination of the urine is of critical importance to exclude urinary tract sepsis and diabetes. A low urine specific gravity in the presence of severe vomiting may be the earliest clue to associated renal disease and requires prompt evaluation of the BUN and creatinine.

Peritoneal Fluid

In obscure cases, examination of the peritoneal fluid for blood and pus may be required. This is particularly true in elderly obtunded patients in whom the physical signs are very difficult to interpret and the presence of peritonitis cannot be excluded. It may be best to tap a single quadrant of the abdomen. In other cases, particularly if intraperitoneal bleeding is suspected, insertion of a catheter is more reliable (see Chapter 51).

RADIOLOGIC EXAMINATION

Radiologic examination often provides extremely important evidence in the diagnosis of acute abdominal disease. The closest cooperation and communication between the surgeon and the radiologist is essential. Each must have maximum information available to him, and joint review of films is frequently of critical importance.

In most cases of acute abdominal disease—and in all cases in which the diagnosis is obscure—the following x-ray films should be obtained: plain films, supine and upright, of the abdomen; kidneys, ureters, and bladder (KUB); and a film of the chest. In reviewing these films, the following questions should be asked: (1) Are the outlines of the liver, spleen, kidneys, and psoas muscle clearly defined? (2) Are the peritoneal fat lines identifiable? (3) Is the gas pattern in the stomach, small bowel, and colon within normal limits? (4) Is there evidence of air outside of the bowel or beneath the diaphragm? (5) Is there air in the biliary radicals? (6) Are there abnormal opaque shadows such as gallstones, fecaliths, or calcification in lymph nodes, pancreas, aorta, or other soft tissue masses.

In addition to these studies, special contrast studies, barium swallow, judicious introduction of barium into the rectum, intravenous urograms, or intravenous cholangiograms are sometimes indicated. A liver scan may be indicated because of suspicion of acute hepatic abscess. An unsuspected mass or the nature of a palpable mass may be demonstrated by ultrasound or CT scan.

On the basis of these examinations, the following important bits of evidence may be obtained: Obliteration of the psoas shadow may indicate a retroperitoneal hematoma or an abscess (Fig 24–8). An enlarged or displaced kidney shadow may indicate a urologic lesion simulating an acute abdominal process. Enlargement of the splenic shadow with displacement of stomach or colon may suggest blood clot due to delayed rupture of the spleen.

Gas patterns are of particular importance. They are more readily characterized if a nasogastric tube has been passed and the stomach emptied. Residual gas and fluid within the stomach suggest pyloric obstruction. Dilated loops of small bowel with air-fluid levels and no gas in the colon are indicative of small bowel obstruction (Fig 24–9). An enlarged gallbladder, fluid-filled pseudocyst, or a solid retroperitoneal tumor may be detected by ultrasound or CT scan.

The position of the cecum may be a clue to appendicitis in an unusual location. Marked dilatation and rotation of the cecum or sigmoid are typical of volvulus. (See Chapter 34.)

Marked dilatation of the entire colon suggests colonic obstruction. Massive dilatation of the colon in acute colitis indicates toxic megacolon.

Distention of both small and large bowel is characteristic of ileus, peritonitis, and pseudo-obstruction of the bowel (Fig 24–10).

Free air under the diaphragm indicates a perforated viscus, most commonly seen in perforated gastric or duodenal ulcer (Fig 24–11). Massive amounts of air beneath both diaphragms suggest colonic perforation. An encapsulated air shadow outside the contours of

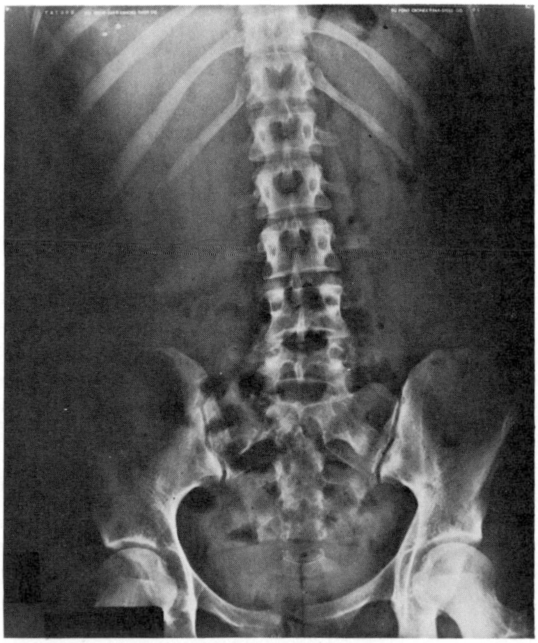

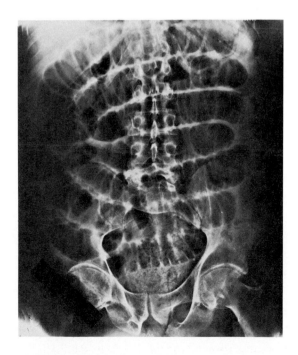

Figure 24–8. Obliteration of the psoas shadow by a right subhepatic abscess.

Figure 24–9. Small bowel obstruction. Note dilated loops of small bowel with air-fluid levels and no gas in the colon.

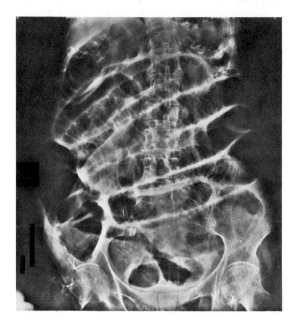

Figure 24—10. Distention of both small and large bowel as seen in ileus and peritonitis.

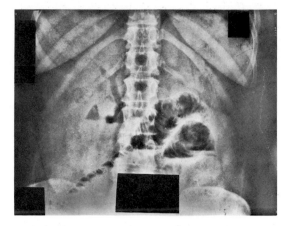

Figure 24—12. Air in the biliary tract indicating free communication between the gastrointestinal tract and the biliary tree. The common duct is well outlined.

small or large bowel may indicate localized perforation of the intestine. Air in the biliary tract is diagnostic of a free communication between some portion of the gastrointestinal tract and the biliary tree (Fig 24–12). If there is evidence of intestinal obstruction, it is characteristic of gallstone ileus. Air in the portal venous system indicates pylephlebitis with a gas-forming organism.

The differentiation between distended small and large bowel may at times be difficult. In advanced cases, the clinical signs may be more reliable in the differentiation between intestinal obstruction and peritonitis.

Plain films of the abdomen may establish the diagnosis of gallstones, pancreatic calcification, retroperitoneal calcification, and vascular calcification. Such findings must be carefully correlated with the history and physical examination to establish their significance.

Rarely, a swallow of meglumine diatrizoate (Gastrografin) may be necessary to confirm or exclude a diagnosis of high intestinal obstruction or perforation of the stomach or duodenum.

Barium enema should be avoided if possible in the presence of acute abdominal disease and peritonitis. In rare cases it is required—most frequently for establishing a diagnosis of diverticulitis, sigmoid volvulus, or low partial colonic obstruction due to carcinoma.

Angiograms are being used more frequently and may be of value in cases of rupture of a solid viscus such as the spleen or kidney. An angiogram may be the only way to recognize a subcapsular or central rupture of the liver. Mesenteric angiography is the best way to identify the site of bleeding in massive lower gastrointestinal hemorrhage.

Finally, large soft tissue masses, retroperitoneal tumors, metastatic carcinoma of the testicle, and other malignant lesions undergoing necrosis may simulate an acute abdomen. Abnormal contours detected by x-ray, ultrasound, or CT scan may help in diagnosis.

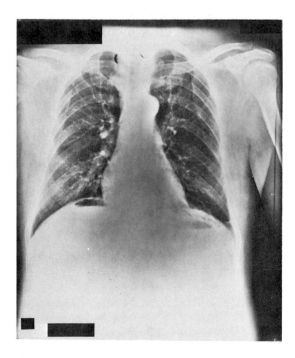

Figure 24—11. Free air under the diaphragm resulting from perforated viscus—in this case, duodenal ulcer.

DIFFERENTIAL DIAGNOSIS
OF ACUTE ABDOMEN

Although the factors in differential diagnosis of the major acute surgical conditions are discussed in relation to each particular disease elsewhere in this book, the following clues should be borne in mind:

(1) Appendicitis is the commonest cause of bizarre peritoneal findings with ileus or apparent intestinal obstruction. In the presence of a suspected septic or inflammatory lesion, it should never be lower than number 2 on the list of causes.

(2) Pelvic appendicitis frequently presents with vomiting, diarrhea, and mild abdominal pain. It is easily confused with gastroenteritis. Initially, abdominal signs may be minimal and the rectal or pelvic examination may be negative. A high white count makes gastroenteritis unlikely. Repeated rectal or pelvic examinations are essential to early diagnosis.

(3) When the patient says he has no pain but only "abdominal pressure" and he is sure that passage of flatus or a good bowel movement would relieve him, remember the "gas stoppage sign" in appendicitis.

(4) Unremitting, severe deep-seated abdominal pain with minimal physical findings should always raise the question of a vascular lesion, particularly mesenteric vascular occlusion.

(5) Nausea, vomiting, and retching as the **dominant** symptoms suggest acute gastritis or pancreatitis.

(6) Intermittent colicky abdominal pain, increasing to a peak and then subsiding to a pain-free interval, is characteristic of mild small bowel obstruction. Hyperactive peristalsis occurring simultaneously is essentially diagnostic.

(7) Intestinal obstruction in an old woman who has had no previous operations strongly suggests a strangulated femoral hernia. There may be no pain referred to the hernia, and the palpable sac may not be tender. Examine and reexamine the femoral rings. If there is no hernia in this type of patient, suspect gallstone ileus.

(8) Upper abdominal pain (which may be so mild that the patient does not seek medical advice) followed many hours or several days later by signs of intestinal obstruction is typical of gallstone ileus. Look for an opaque gallstone and air in the biliary tract on x-ray.

(9) An acute illness characterized by jaundice, high fever with chills, and hypotension means suppurative cholangitis—a critical surgical emergency.

(10) Severe vomiting of food or gastric contents followed later by retching and hematemesis is almost diagnostic of gastroesophageal laceration (Mallory-Weiss syndrome).

(11) Abdominal pain in patients with cloudy lactescent serum suggests acute pancreatitis, but serum amylase is often normal.

Disorders which must be commonly considered in the differential diagnosis of a patient who presents with acute abdominal pain are discussed in the following paragraphs.

Myocardial Infarction

Acute myocardial infarction may simulate perforated ulcer or acute cholecystitis, particularly if the pain is epigastric. Careful examination will indicate that abdominal rigidity is absent and peristalsis is not altered. Other manifestations of coronary occlusion, including ECG changes, should make the diagnosis.

The problem is more difficult when the patient with known coronary artery disease develops acute cholecystitis or a perforated ulcer.

Acute Hepatitis

Acute hepatitis in its initial phases is sometimes associated with severe right upper quadrant pain and tenderness. In all instances of suspected acute cholecystitis, diffuse tenderness over the liver should immediately raise the question of acute hepatitis. Appropriate laboratory studies will make the diagnosis.

Rheumatic Fever

Rheumatic fever is not infrequently accompanied by vague, ill-defined abdominal pain simulating appendicitis. A careful history and physical examination, as described above, will indicate that no acute abdominal lesion is present.

Polyarteritis Nodosa

Many types of vasculitis may cause abdominal pain simulating acute surgical abdominal disease. At times vasculitis may involve the appendix or small bowel, so that surgery is mandatory. The diagnosis can sometimes be established by examination of the surgical specimen. In most instances, however, careful examination will indicate that there is no evidence for a progressive intraperitoneal lesion. The diagnosis is established by muscle or skin biopsy.

Acute Porphyria

Severe abdominal pain may accompany various forms of porphyria and porphyrinuria. A critical appraisal of the abdominal findings will usually cast doubt on the diagnosis of abdominal disease, and examination of the urine (Watson-Schwartz test) will reveal the presence of porphobilinogen.

Acute Epidemic Pleurodynia

Particularly in young people, acute epidemic pleurodynia may strongly suggest acute appendicitis. The condition appears from time to time in children's camps, and all too often the first few patients are subjected to appendectomy before the true nature of the condition is recognized. Careful examination of the abdomen is the surest way of avoiding this error. Tenderness is high and is often present over the lower thoracic wall rather than over the peritoneum.

Acute Spontaneous Pneumothorax

Acute spontaneous pneumothorax has been mistaken for acute cholecystitis. Careful physical examination again provides the answer. Chest x-ray is diagnostic.

Pneumonia, Pleurisy, & Empyema

Pneumonia, pleurisy, and empyema—or, indeed, any thoracic lesion resulting in diaphragmatic irritation—will produce right upper quadrant pain simulating an abdominal condition. Careful history and physical examination, together with appropriate x-ray studies, readily clarify the diagnosis provided the examiner bears the possibility of thoracic disease in mind.

Lesions of the Spine

Osteoarthritis with compression of the thoracic spine and spinal nerves may produce severe, ill-defined abdominal pain simulating a variety of intraperitoneal lesions, particularly biliary colic. Some degree of involuntary rigidity of the rectus abdominis muscle may be present as an additional confusing factor. Careful analysis of the nature of the pain, its radiating character, and the presence of hyperesthesias will lead to appropriate further studies necessary to establish the diagnosis—particularly x-ray examination of the involved vertebrae.

A spinal cord tumor may also produce radiating pain simulating biliary or renal colic.

Diseases of the Hip Joint

A variety of diseases of the hip may produce pain radiating into the right or left lower quadrant. Acute bursitis, in particular, may simulate pelvic appendicitis. Absence of true abdominal tenderness and rigidity, together with examination of the hip joint, readily clarifies the diagnosis.

TREATMENT OF ACUTE ABDOMEN

When the diagnosis is in doubt but the patient is not critically ill, a period of "dynamic" or "active" observation is in order. Frequent checks for progression of symptoms combined with careful, gentle reexaminations of the abdomen will avoid many unnecessary operations without risking dangerous delays.

Analgesics for the relief of severe pain should be given without hesitation. Indeed, the evaluation of acute abdominal disease can be performed more accurately after severe pain is relieved and the cooperation of the patient obtained. What at first appeared to be very diffuse tenderness may now be better localized. Abdominal masses which could not be felt before often become obvious after moderate sedation and relief of pain.

Antibiotics should be withheld until the diagnosis is established. In obscure cases, heavy antibiotic therapy may mask progression of the disease and lead to the development of serious complications with marked morbidity.

Laboratory and physical examination should be repeated at frequent intervals.

If the diagnosis is in doubt but the patient clearly has signs of peritonitis, operation must be undertaken as soon as fluid and electrolyte imbalance has been corrected. Nasogastric suction should be initiated as soon as it is recognized that the patient has evidence of peritonitis, ileus, or intestinal obstruction. This is preferably done before any diagnostic measures are undertaken.

Particularly in the good-risk patient, a right or left rectus or midline incision may be preferable to a horizontal or oblique incision since the former permit more extensive exploration of the peritoneal cavity and can be adjusted more readily if the most likely diagnosis is proved to be incorrect after the peritoneal cavity is opened.

On the other hand, in the elderly, obese, poor-risk patient, it often is preferable to make a small, well-localized incision over the most likely site of the cause of the peritonitis. This can be closed and another incision made with less total risk to the patient than if a long midline or rectus incision is used. In the elderly poor-risk patient, an extensive incision is prone to infection, suppuration, and dehiscence—complications which may prove fatal. Multiple small incisions under these circumstances are less likely to break down, and even if infection occurs dehiscence and evisceration are less likely.

●   ●   ●

General References

Botsford TW, Wilson RE: *The Acute Abdomen,* 2nd ed. Saunders, 1977.

Cope Z: *The Early Diagnosis of the Acute Abdomen,* 14th ed. Oxford Univ Press, 1972.

Dunphy JE, Botsford TW: *Physical Examination of the Surgical Patient,* 4th ed. Saunders, 1975.

Gelin L, Nyhus LM, Condon RE: *Abdominal Pain: A Guide to Rapid Diagnosis.* Lippincott, 1969.

Jones PF: *Emergency Abdominal Surgery in Infancy, Childhood and Adult Life.* Blackwell, 1974.

Leaper DJ & others: Computer-assisted diagnosis of abdominal pain using "estimates" provided by clinicians. Br Med J 4:350, 1972.

Staniland JR & others: Clinical presentation of acute abdomen: Study of 600 patients. Br Med J 3:393, 1972.

Steinheber FV: Medical conditions mimicking the acute surgical abdomen. Med Clin North Am 57:1559, 1973.

Way LW: Abdominal pain. Chap 24 in: *Gastrointestinal Disease.* Sleisenger MH, Fordtran JS (editors). Saunders, 1973.

Yajko RD, Steele G: Exploratory celiotomy for acute abdominal pain. Am J Surg 128:773, 1974.

25 . . .
Peritoneal Cavity

J. Englebert Dunphy, MD

The abdomen is lined by a thin layer of endo-thelium which covers the interior of the abdominal wall (parietal peritoneum) and all of the organs within the abdominal cavity (the visceral peritoneum). As the peritoneum envelops the viscera in the course of embryologic development, numerous compartments are formed. The lesser peritoneal cavity lies behind the stomach and the lesser omentum or gastrohepatic ligament, communicating with the main peritoneal cavity through the foramen epiploicum (foramen of Winslow). (See Fig 25–1.) The endothelial surface of the peritoneum is smooth and glistening and is normally lubricated by a small amount of fluid. In its deeper layers, there is a rich network of capillaries and lymphatics.

The peritoneum is normally quite resistant to infection. Bacteria injected into the peritoneal cavity are rapidly phagocytosed and eliminated. The same quantity of bacteria injected subcutaneously or retro-peritoneally would produce abscess formation or a spreading cellulitis. Bacterial peritonitis, therefore, can occur only as a result of continuous or persistent con-

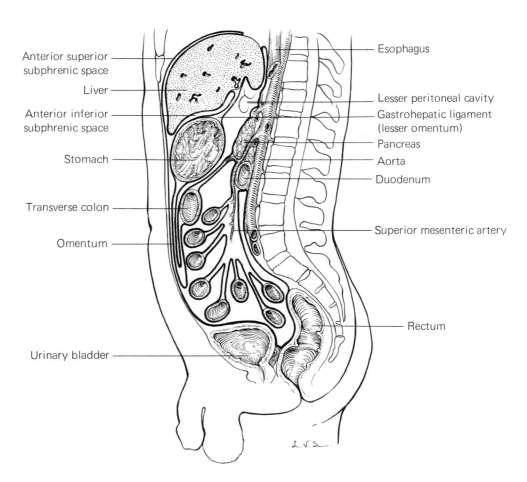

Figure 25–1. The peritoneal reflections and location of the lesser peritoneal cavity.

tamination or as a result of contamination with an unusually virulent bacterial strain or species. Foreign bodies or free fluids as in ascites also reduce the resistance of the peritoneum to infection.

The omentum is a double fold of peritoneum, usually loaded with fat, which hangs from the stomach and the transverse colon as an apron over the small intestine. It is a very mobile, highly specialized tissue and plays an active role in the control of suppurative inflammation and infection within the peritoneal cavity.

ACUTE PERITONITIS

Primary or "spontaneous" bacterial peritonitis is caused by direct hematogenous invasion of the peritoneal cavity. Before the introduction of antibiotics, primary peritonitis with streptococci or pneumococci occurred not infrequently in otherwise healthy adults as well as children. Today this condition is seen principally in patients with cirrhosis and ascites or nephrosis. Recently, primary peritonitis has been recognized in patients with systemic lupus erythematosus.

Secondary peritonitis is caused by acute infections such as appendicitis or diverticulitis or by perforation of a viscus from duodenal or gastric ulcer or abdominal wounds.

Acute generalized peritonitis due to a ruptured viscus is characterized by severe abdominal pain, vomiting, and variable degrees of fever. On physical examination, the abdomen is rigid and silent. Laboratory studies show leukocytosis and hemoconcentration. Progressive abdominal distention, ileus, hypotension, and shock follow.

Peritonitis secondary to infection, as in appendicitis or diverticulitis, is more gradual in onset. Initial manifestations are those of the underlying disease, with gradual development of spreading peritonitis manifested by increasing tenderness, abdominal rigidity, and distention. In the very old and very young, peritonitis may develop insidiously, so that marked ileus and abdominal distention are present when the patient is first seen.

BACTERIAL & CHEMICAL PERITONITIS

The first result of perforation of the stomach due to peptic ulcer is chemical peritonitis, but infection soon follows. Bile, pancreatic juice, and gastric juice combined produce a severe irritation of the peritoneum, leading to profound shock which can cause death before bacterial invasion develops. The massive loss of fluid within the peritoneal cavity is comparable to that seen in an extensive burn.

Peritonitis due to bile alone has unique characteristics. If the bile is infected, as in rupture of an inflamed gallbladder, there may be profound shock and collapse. Normal, uninfected bile without pancreatic or intestinal fluid is remarkably innocuous. Bile peritonitis due to traumatic rupture of the common duct may produce a picture similar to slowly progressive ascites with very little abdominal pain.

Blood and sterile urine evoke a mild peritoneal reaction. The shock of intraperitoneal hemorrhage is due principally to loss of blood rather than peritoneal irritation. Similarly, sterile urine may produce only a mild peritoneal reaction, whereas infected urine can lead to a rapidly progressive bacterial peritonitis.

In nearly every case of peritonitis, bacterial invasion ultimately occurs. Perforation of the colon, however, produces a massive bacterial invasion of the peritoneal cavity which may lead to septicemia and overwhelming sepsis with a mixed infection, often with gas-forming organisms. Rupture of the cecum due to unrelieved large bowel obstruction, for example, produces a particularly fulminating form of peritonitis.

Depending upon the cause, peritonitis may be localized, diffuse, or generalized. Localization is dependent upon the nature of the primary lesion and the natural defenses of the host. Classically, it is seen most often in appendicitis. The omentum plays a major role in localization, but the virulence of the organisms may also determine localization or diffuse spread. The liver is an important organ in the systemic reaction to peritonitis, as bacteria picked up by the lymphatics and portal system are destroyed in the liver. In the presence of hepatic insufficiency, as in cirrhosis, this function is limited and generalized septicemia rapidly ensues. If the invading organisms are highly virulent, as are clostridia, generalized septicemia may dominate the picture of peritonitis.

Clinical Findings

A. Symptoms and Signs: Regardless of the cause, abdominal pain, nausea, vomiting, and fever are present. The severity of the manifestations is directly related to the extent of the contamination. In acute generalized peritonitis, some degree of shock is always present, and shock may be profound.

There is diffuse, exquisite abdominal tenderness and board-like rigidity of the abdomen. In acute generalized peritonitis due to a ruptured viscus, the abdomen is silent from the onset. When peritonitis develops gradually, peristalsis may persist and be hyperactive in areas isolated from the localized area of peritoneal inflammation and infection. Without treatment, the condition rapidly progresses to marked ileus, abdominal distention, hypotension, and toxemia with ultimate respiratory, renal, and cardiac failure.

B. Laboratory Findings: There is marked leukocytosis and hemoconcentration. The serum electrolyte concentrations vary, but marked metabolic acidosis with respiratory alkalosis is a characteristic feature of bacterial or chemical peritonitis.

C. X-Ray Findings: Plain films of the abdomen show distention of both large and small bowel with fluid levels. There is a thickened appearance to loops of bowel due to the presence of fluid between loops. Air may be seen beneath the diaphragm if free perforation of a hollow viscus has occurred.

D. Special Examinations: Abdominal paracentesis may be helpful in obscure cases. It is particularly valuable following nonpenetrating abdominal injury and in the aged, when symptoms and signs may be equivocal. Aspiration of the 4 quadrants of the abdomen may be carried out, but a single tap and insertion of a catheter for peritoneal lavage is more reliable, especially in cases of suspected peritonitis due to nonpenetrating trauma.

Common Surgical Causes of Peritonitis

The problem of differential diagnosis relates to the primary cause. Is it perforated ulcer? Acute pancreatitis? Mesenteric thrombosis? In more slowly progressive peritonitis, is it due to appendicitis, acute cholecystitis, or diverticulitis? The diagnosis and differential diagnosis of each of these entities are discussed in more detail elsewhere in this book.

Intestinal obstruction may produce abdominal distention and tenderness without peritonitis, but the history and physical findings usually make the diagnosis clear. The differentiation is important because, although both intestinal obstruction and peritonitis require prompt operation, a different timing and operative approach may be required.

Common Causes of Acute Peritonitis

Although each clinical entity is discussed in more detail under separate headings, a brief overview is given here. (See Fig 25–2.)

A. Acute Perforated Ulcer: Acute free perforation of the stomach or duodenum produces the classical findings of generalized peritonitis. Severe generalized abdominal pain and some degree of shock are characteristic. The abdomen is board-like, often scaphoid, and rigid throughout. Tenderness (including rectal tenderness) is diffuse. Pain often radiates to the right or left shoulder. Within a few minutes of the onset of perforation, peristalsis ceases. Air is found beneath the diaphragm in 80% of cases. The area of liver dullness is decreased anteriorly and laterally. In perforated duodenal ulcer, most of the air will be found on the right side. Whenever a film shows a massive amount of air on the left side of the diaphragm, a high gastric or colonic perforation should be suspected.

B. Acute Pancreatitis: Acute pancreatitis is more gradual in onset; vomiting is often a dominant feature; pain is steady, gradually increasing in severity; and hypotension and shock develop gradually. The physical findings are also less striking in acute pancreatitis because the disease begins in a retroperitoneal organ. In the early stages, although there may be upper abdominal tenderness, spasm and rigidity are usually not present. Peritonitis due to acute pancreatitis is easily overlooked until the disease process is well established.

C. Acute Appendicitis: Acute appendicitis is the most common cause of peritonitis, but fortunately today this is usually localized rather than diffuse and generalized. Generalized peritonitis secondary to appendicitis usually develops gradually. At times, however, there is an acute exacerbation of pain, which, having arisen in the epigastrium and settled in the right lower quadrant, suddenly becomes generalized, indicating perforation. More commonly, however, when perforation occurs it is already partially walled off, and a diffusing peritonitis develops gradually over a period of hours. It is said that in no case of peritonitis should appendicitis be listed lower than second among the

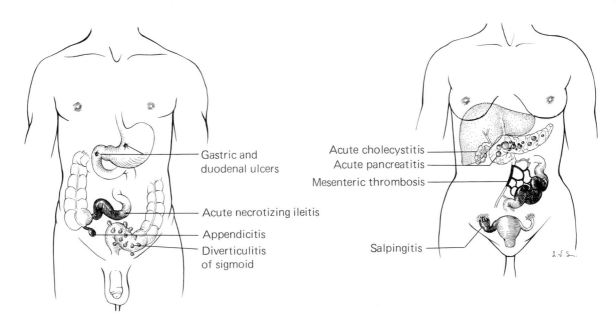

Figure 25–2. Common primary causes of peritonitis.

possible causes since it is capable—because of the varied position of the appendix—of simulating any other acute abdominal inflammatory lesion. More details are given in Chapter 32.

D. Acute Salpingitis: Acute salpingitis may produce diffuse abdominal pain and marked tenderness and spasm throughout the lower abdomen, indicative of a rapidly advancing peritoneal inflammation. The temperature is often high, but the pulse is slow and the patient exhibits a state of well-being quite out of place with the physical findings.

E. Acute Mesenteric Vascular Occlusion: Vascular lesions are characterized by severe abdominal pain with limited findings of peritonitis in the early stages. It may be exceedingly difficult to distinguish between pancreatitis and mesenteric thrombosis. Early and marked elevation of serum amylase suggests pancreatitis, but there may be an elevation of amylase in mesenteric thrombosis.

F. Acute Cholecystitis: Acute cholecystitis produces a localized peritonitis as the condition advances. In contrast to perforated ulcer and acute appendicitis, peristalsis in acute cholecystitis tends to be active and sometimes hyperactive. The finding of very active peristalsis with right upper quadrant signs is a good clue to acute cholecystitis as opposed to perforated ulcer.

G. Gallbladder Perforation: Perforation of the gallbladder may produce a diffuse, rapidly progressive form of peritonitis which simulates perforation of a duodenal or gastric ulcer. The condition is rare because gangrene of the gallbladder develops so slowly that the inflammatory process is usually walled off.

H. Trauma to Abdomen: The differential diagnosis of peritonitis is often clearly established by the history, as in penetrating or nonpenetrating abdominal wounds.

I. Acute Diverticulitis: Acute diverticulitis is a fairly common cause of peritonitis. There may be free perforation of the diverticulum, producing a rapid diffusing peritonitis with generalized abdominal pain, tenderness, and spasm. Leakage of air from the colon may result in rapidly progressive abdominal distention with large amounts of air under the diaphragm. A massive amount of air under the left diaphragm should suggest perforated diverticulum.

More commonly, diverticulitis progresses gradually and produces signs and symptoms suggestive of left-sided appendicitis. The sigmoid loop may extend to the right side of the abdomen and closely simulate appendicitis, just as a long appendix may produce inflammatory signs on the left suggestive of diverticulitis. The details of the differential diagnosis are discussed elsewhere.

Differential Diagnosis
(Nonsurgical Conditions Simulating Peritonitis)

Many systemic diseases result in marked intestinal ileus closely resembling intestinal obstruction or peritonitis. Pneumonia, particularly in the aged, is often accompanied by marked abdominal distention and

ileus simulating slowly progressive peritonitis. Diaphragmatic pleurisy may also be associated with abdominal pain suggestive of acute cholecystitis or perforated ulcer.

Uremia commonly is associated with abdominal distention and ileus. Since patients with chronic renal failure may develop primary intraperitoneal diseases, such as appendicitis or perforated ulcer, the differential diagnosis may be very difficult, particularly if the history is unobtainable or unreliable. Abdominal tap may be required but is conclusive only if positive.

As discussed in the differential diagnosis of appendicitis (Chapter 32), a variety of other medical conditions may produce abdominal pain simulating early acute peritonitis.

"Periodic peritonitis" (familial Mediterranean fever, familial paroxysmal polyserositis) is a rare, obscure entity which produces all the manifestations of acute peritonitis but without any identifiable cause. The disease is characterized by recurring episodes of abdominal pain with exquisite direct and rebound tenderness. Fever (38—38.5 C [100.4—101.3 F]) and leukocytosis accompany the attack. Colchicine is highly effective in preventing acute attacks. In fact, a favorable response to chronic administration of colchicine is the most definitive diagnostic test. There appears to be a familial incidence among Mediterranean populations, notably Armenians, Jews, and Arabs. Laparotomy is often performed for the first episode. At operation, the peritoneal surfaces may be inflamed and there is free fluid, but smears and cultures are negative. Even though it is normal, the appendix should be removed to rule out the possibility of acute appendicitis in the differential diagnosis of recurrent episodes.

Complications

The principal acute complications of peritonitis are shock, high-output respiratory failure, acute renal tubular necrosis, and hepatic failure associated with liver abscesses and pylephlebitis.

If the acute complications are prevented or corrected—and if death does not result early—the principal late complication is intraperitoneal abscess formation. Abscesses commonly form in the pelvis and in the subdiaphragmatic and subhepatic areas but may develop anywhere within the peritoneal cavity. The end result is intraperitoneal adhesion formation, particularly after operations for peritonitis. These adhesions are common causes of intestinal obstruction.

Abscesses and adhesions as complications of peritonitis are discussed separately below.

Prevention

Prevention depends upon early recognition and treatment. Prompt use of massive wide-spectrum antibiotic therapy also contributes to the prevention of generalized peritonitis regardless of cause.

Treatment

In primary peritonitis, if the diagnosis can be established by the clinical findings and abdominal paracentesis, antibiotic therapy is the treatment of choice. If appendicitis and other surgical lesions cannot be excluded, operation may be necessary. In early secondary peritonitis, treatment consists of removing the cause by operation. Appendectomy, cholecystectomy, closure of perforated ulcer, and resection of gangrenous intestine are the most common surgical procedures in the control of early peritonitis. Combined with antibiotic therapy, early operation has a negligible mortality rate referable to peritonitis.

Advanced and established peritonitis also requires surgery for control in most cases. Sometimes, however, patients are seen in whom the peritonitis is localizing, and a course of cautious observation and nonsurgical treatment may be indicated.

Very rarely, especially in the aged or debilitated, the patient's condition has deteriorated to the point where anesthesia and any type of surgery would be lethal. The only hope is that antibiotics and major supportive measures will permit localization and formation of abscesses which can be drained later.

A. Preoperative Management: All patients with advanced peritonitis require a period of preoperative preparation. More complete details regarding the treatment of septic surgical shock are presented in Chapter 15. As soon as the circulation is stable and reasonable respiratory exchange has been established, operation should be performed.

1. Fluids—Nasogastric suction and fluid therapy should be started immediately after the patient arrives in the emergency room.

Fluid therapy should be initiated with balanced salt solution or lactated Ringer's injection. Potassium should be restricted initially since there is likely to be poor renal function due to shock and hypovolemia.

When an adequate urinary output has been established, potassium may be given as required. Final adjustment of electrolyte administration can be made on the basis of the laboratory findings and measurement of fluid losses.

2. Laboratory tests—At the time fluid therapy is initiated in the emergency ward, blood should be drawn for complete blood count and serum sodium, potassium, chloride, bicarbonate, creatinine, and amylase. In critically ill patients, P_{O_2}, P_{CO_2}, and arterial pH determinations should also be obtained.

3. Urinary flow—In early or moderately advanced peritonitis, urinary catheterization should be avoided because it establishes one more portal of entry for bacteremia. In advanced peritonitis with shock and renal failure, an indwelling catheter is advisable in order to determine the hourly urinary output and to estimate fluid requirements.

4. Central venous pressure—Central venous pressure should be monitored in critically ill patients with threatened renal or circulatory failure. However, CVP alone is not a reliable index of blood volume or cardiac function. (See Chapter 14.)

5. Analgesics—Narcotics and sedatives should be administered as needed to control pain. Initial sedation with morphine, 10–15 mg IM, is usually adequate, and

repeated administration should be avoided in the preoperative period. If the patient is in severe pain and also in shock, morphine should be administered intravenously in small doses (1–3 mg) repeated as needed.

6. Antibiotics—Antibiotic therapy is a mainstay of treatment and should be initiated as soon as the diagnosis is made. Combining an agent effective against coliforms with one active against anaerobes is the accepted approach. Many experienced surgeons still prefer massive doses of penicillin combined with tetracycline initially. After type specificity has been determined, kanamycin or clindamycin may prove more effective.

7. Oxygen—Peritonitis imposes marked increases in metabolic demands which are accompanied by proportionately increased demands for ventilation and oxygenation ("high output respiratory failure"). Because of the marked abdominal distention, elevation of the diaphragms, and possibly associated pulmonary insufficiency from emphysema, the patient is unable to meet these expanded oxygen requirements. Determination of blood gases is essential and may indicate more advanced respiratory insufficiency than the clinical findings suggest. Oxygen therapy, assisted respiration, and, in some cases, tracheostomy may be required. Nasogastric suction may not relieve the distention sufficiently to improve the vital capacity. Consequently, operation with release of distention and decompression of the intestine may be an essential part of improving respiratory exchange. Unrecognized severe respiratory insufficiency has in the past been mistaken for the "toxemia" of peritonitis. Marked improvement of respiratory function can be expected as soon as the abdomen is opened, peritoneal fluid aspirated, and (if necessary) distended loops of bowel decompressed.

B. Operative Technic: Although the operative procedure in peritonitis is determined by the nature of the primary cause, there are several additional points in the management of generalized peritonitis which require emphasis.

1. Peritoneal toilet—At the completion of the operation, an effort should be made to remove all necrotic material and contaminated fluid from the peritoneal cavity.

2. Intestinal decompression—If there is massive intestinal distention—and particularly if the loops of small bowel contain large amounts of fluid—intestinal decompression should be employed. This may be done either by the use of a tube (the Baker tube is the most effective and can be left down postoperatively) or by aspiration of the small bowel through one or more needle points introduced through small purse-string sutures of silk, which can be tied afterward.

3. Irrigation of the peritoneal cavity—If there has been gross contamination, particularly with bowel contents, the peritoneal cavity should be thoroughly irrigated with lactated Ringer's or normal saline solution to remove as much foreign material, detritus, and clumps of fibrin as possible. Most authorities no longer recommend the one-shot instillation of an antibiotic into the peritoneal cavity since appropriate high-dosage systemic therapy started before operation assures a high concentration in the peritoneal fluid.

4. Drainage—Drainage of the general peritoneal cavity is in most cases unnecessary, ineffective, and undesirable. Drainage should be employed only where there are localized masses of necrotic material or debris which cannot be removed, or actual abscess formation. Prophylactic drainage will not prevent the formation of intraperitoneal abscesses and may even encourage abscess formation. The principal indication for drainage is an actual or potential source of continued contamination. Wounds and inflammatory disorders of the pancreas or biliary tract are examples. When an opening into a viscus cannot be securely closed, sump drains with continuous suction are required.

Every effort should be made to isolate the wound from the contaminated peritoneal fluid, preferably by impermeable plastic drapes. If significant contamination of the wound cannot be avoided, the skin and subcutaneous tissues should be left open. Wound closure in patients with peritonitis calls for the use of retention sutures since ileus and distention are likely complications and the risk of dehiscence is decreased.

A method of closure with retention sutures which permits the skin and subcutaneous tissues to be left open is described in Chapter 10.

5. Binders—Scultetus binders of all types should be avoided because they restrict the chest wall and compound existing respiratory insufficiency. Adhesive tapes (Fig 25–3) will provide excellent support to the wound, enable the patient to cough with less discomfort, and do not restrict the thoracic cage.

C. Postoperative Management: After operation, all of the measures instituted preoperatively should be continued. The patient should be given nothing by mouth; nasogastric suction must be continuous; and fluid and electrolyte balance must be carefully monitored. Narcotics should be used as required to control pain. Meperidine (pethidine) is not as effective as morphine for pain.

As soon as cultures and sensitivity tests have been obtained, type-specific antibiotic therapy should be instituted.

Although the patient is usually hemoconcentrated due to fluid losses in the early phase of peritonitis, significant degrees of anemia soon develop following correction of the hypovolemia. Transfusions of whole blood or packed red cells may have been required during the operation, and additional blood may be needed postoperatively.

Prognosis

The prognosis in all forms of peritonitis depends upon the cause. In acute peritonitis, the age of the patient and the duration of the illness before operation are critical factors. In the very young and the very old, generalized peritonitis has a grave prognosis. In early acute peritonitis, regardless of cause, the prognosis is favorable.

Prognosis is discussed in more detail under specific disease headings.

Altemeier WA & others: Intra-abdominal sepsis. Adv Surg 5:281, 1971.

Clowes GHA & others: Circulating factors in the etiology of pulmonary insufficiency and right heart failure accompanying severe sepsis (peritonitis). Ann Surg 171:663, 1970.

Fullen WD & others: Prophylactic antibiotics in penetrating wounds of the abdomen. J Trauma 12:282, 1972.

Golden GT, Shaw A: Primary peritonitis. Surg Gynecol Obstet 135:513, 1972.

Gorbach SL, Bartlett JG: Anaerobic infections. (3 parts.) N Engl J Med 290:1177, 1237, 1289, 1974.

Hunt TK & others: Antibiotics in surgery. Arch Surg 110:148, 1975.

Skillman J & others: Peritonitis and respiratory failure after abdominal operations. Ann Surg 170:122, 1969.

Sohar E & others: Familial Mediterranean fever. Am J Med 43:227, 1967.

Zemer D & others: A controlled trial of colchicine in preventing attacks of familial Mediterranean fever. N Engl J Med 291:932, 1974.

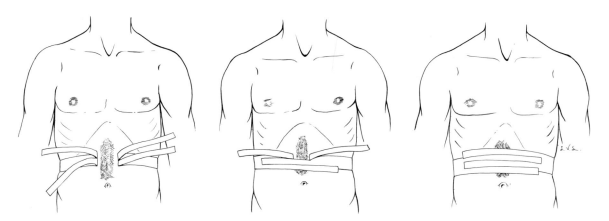

Figure 25–3. Adhesive binders after abdominal surgery, applied "Scultetus fashion" without restriction of the thoracic cage.

GONOCOCCAL PERITONITIS

Gonococcal peritonitis (discussed in greater detail in Chapter 44) has unique characteristics. It often produces severe abdominal pain, fever, and peritoneal signs without tachycardia, hypotension, or shock. Characteristically, the patient does not look ill. A unique feature is the extent of the inflammation throughout the peritoneal cavity with the formation of adhesions between the liver and diaphragm. In the early stages, acute right upper quadrant abdominal pain may occur, simulating acute cholecystitis.

TUBERCULOUS PERITONITIS

Tuberculous peritonitis is a chronic granulomatous lesion of the peritoneal cavity. It often appears as a primary abdominal infection without pulmonary, intestinal, or fallopian tube involvement in the early stages. The available evidence supports the concept of reactivation of a latent peritoneal focus as the most attractive explanation for most cases, although others appear as a manifestation of systemic spread of extraabdominal infection.

The patient commonly presents with a 2- to 4-month history of weakness, night sweats, anorexia, weight loss, and abdominal distention. On physical examination, the only finding may be that of free fluid in the peritoneal cavity. At times there is a "doughy" feeling to the abdomen, and vague masses may be noted. If there are associated tuberculous lesions of the bowel, a distinct mass may be palpated, particularly in the right colon.

Paracentesis will reveal fluid which is pale or greenish-yellow. The protein content of the fluid nearly always exceeds 3 g/100 ml, and microscopy shows predominantly lymphocytes. Acid-fast bacilli are rarely identified on smear, but cultures of the ascitic fluid are positive in over 80% of cases. Percutaneous biopsy of the peritoneum is the most expeditious means of establishing the diagnosis, but diagnostic laparotomy may be necessary if that fails.

The course of the disease tends to be chronic, but the response to antituberculosis therapy is usually excellent. There is evidence that the addition of corticosteroids to the treatment regimen may lower the incidence of late intestinal obstruction from adhesive bands.

Borhanmanesh F & others: Tuberculous peritonitis. Ann Intern Med 76:567, 1972.

Dineen P & others: Tuberculous peritonitis. Ann Surg 184:717, 1976.

CHYLOUS PERITONITIS

Another form of chronic peritonitis is due to the presence of chyle in the peritoneal cavity. This may be of congenital origin, appearing in childhood as a chronic swelling of the abdomen.

In adults, chylous peritonitis (ascites) is usually due to obstruction of the flow of chyle by malignant tumors of the upper abdomen or thorax, although in almost half of cases no cause is uncovered. Lymphoma is a common cause, but the condition is also seen in cancer of the pancreas or stomach and in retroperitoneal sarcomas. Any abdominal neoplasm that spreads retroperitoneally may ultimately produce chylous ascites.

If chylous peritonitis is discovered at laparotomy, a retroperitoneal dissection to locate a ruptured lymph vessel is not required; the chyle leak generally seals without specific therapy.

Treatment is unsatisfactory if the primary cause is an inoperable malignant tumor. X-ray treatment, however, may result in dramatic improvement in cases of lymphoma.

Congenital chylous ascites is due to a developmental abnormality of intestinal lymphatics which may be markedly enlarged and communicate freely with the peritoneal cavity. There may be channels involving the extremities so that chyle appears in the skin ("cutaneous chylous reflux"). If ascites is minimal or absent, chylous cutaneous reflux can be corrected by an operation which divides the large incompetent lymphatic channels between the mesentery of the intestine and the lymphatics of the thigh.

Kinmonth JB: *The Lymphatics.* Williams & Wilkins 1972.

Kinmonth JB, Cox SJ: Protein-losing enteropathy in primary lymphoedema: Mesenteric lymphography and gut resection. Br J Surg 61:589, 1974.

Krizek TJ, Davis JH: Acute chylous peritonitis. Arch Surg 91:253, 1965.

GRANULOMATOUS PERITONITIS

A peculiar type of acute or chronic granulomatous peritonitis has been identified as occurring secondary to a variety of substances used in the preparation of surgical gloves. Talc produces a chronic granulomatous lesion and has not been used for some years in the preparation of surgical gloves.

More recently, substitutes for talc, particularly starch powders from corn or rice, have been used. A peculiar syndrome characterized by severe abdominal pain, fever, and marked peritoneal irritation but with a normal white blood count appears within 2–3 weeks of what has appeared to be an otherwise uncomplicated abdominal operation. The pain may be so severe and the clinical findings so disturbing that immediate laparotomy is undertaken. Experience has shown that reexploration merely aggravates the syndrome by disseminating the inciting agent with reactivation of the process.

The exact cause of the reaction is not known, and it appears to be limited to a relatively small number of patients who react in a hypersensitive manner to the presence of the foreign material. Upon recognition of the syndrome, reoperation should be avoided. Good immediate results have followed corticosteroid therapy.

The condition can be prevented by carefully washing all foreign material from surgical gloves prior to operation.

Aarons J, Fitzgerald W: The persisting hazards of surgical glove powder. Surg Gynecol Obstet 138:385, 1974.
Sugarbaker PH & others: Glove starch granulomatous disease: An unsolved problem. Am J Surg 128:3, 1974.

PERITONEAL ABSCESSES

Intraperitoneal abscesses are common complications of peritonitis and may also follow major abdominal operations without established peritonitis. Inadequately drained leakage following biliary or pancreatic surgery, small subclinical leaks from intestinal anastomoses, collections of blood, and contaminated peritoneal fluid all tend to settle in dependent parts of the abdomen, and abscess formation may be a sequel. Detritus, foreign material, and necrotic tissue are more important factors in abscess formation than bacteria alone.

The common sites are under the diaphragm, along the undersurface of the right lobe of the liver, along the lateral gutters, and in the pelvis (Fig 25–4).

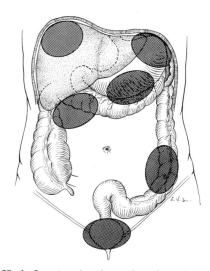

Figure 25—4. Common locations of peritoneal abscess formation.

Persistent fever is the classic sign of a developing intraperitoneal abscess. As the fever following a major peritoneal insult subsides, instead of returning to normal it persists and gradually rises in a stepwise fashion. A progressively rising temperature that does not return to normal over a period of several days is typical of abscess formation. With threatened perforation or extension into adjacent structures, chills, fever, and hypotension may develop.

Special methods of scanning as with gallium, ultrasound, and CT scans have opened up an important approach to the recognition and localization of peritoneal abscesses (see Chapter 9).

Midabdominal Abscesses

These abscesses may occur anywhere within the abdominal cavity from just below the transverse colon to the pelvis. The right and left gutters are the most common sites, but an abscess may form wherever a collection of foreign material or blood has occurred.

Midabdominal abscesses are particularly difficult to identify. Knowing the cause of the original peritoneal disease is of considerable help in identifying the presence of an abscess—diverticulitis being more likely to involve the left gutter and appendicitis the right gutter. Perforations from regional enteritis or ulcerative colitis may result in centrally placed abscesses.

Abscesses develop at the root of the mesentery between loops of bowel and are protected from the anterior abdominal wall by the mesentery of the small intestine.

Repeated careful and gentle examination of the abdomen, feeling for a developing mass, is the most reliable method of identifying a midabdominal abscess. Plain x-ray films of the abdomen may be helpful: A mass shadow may be identified, collections of gas or air may be seen, or persistently dilated irregular loops of bowel may indicate the presence of the abscess. Ultrasound is becoming increasingly more reliable in the detection of intraperitoneal abscesses.

Midabdominal abscesses may subside spontaneously. Prolonged postoperative ileus is a common major complication, and continuous gastric suction, sometimes with the use of a long tube, may be required.

A progressively enlarging abdominal mass is an indication for drainage. Frequently this will be delayed for 2–3 days until the mass appears to be well localized and in close contact with the abdominal wall. On other occasions, with deep-seated midabdominal abscesses, the patient may become so ill, with high fever, chills, and hypotension, that laparotomy to find and drain the abscess becomes essential.

Open transabdominal drainage of an intraperitoneal abscess, while not ideal, can be safely done under cover of antibiotics and peritoneal irrigation. It is absolutely essential to explore the peritoneal cavity for residual abscesses if the patient is clearly deteriorating. Huge abscesses containing more than a liter of pus may occur without significant physical findings.

between the liver and the diaphragm (anterior superior) or anteriorly below the liver (anterior inferior) or posteriorly above the kidney (posterior inferior). On the left, an abscess may develop anteriorly between the left lobe of the liver, spleen, or stomach and the diaphragm (superior). Inferiorly on the left, pus may develop below the stomach anterior to the transverse colon or posteriorly in the lesser peritoneal cavity (posterior superior). The posterior space on the right is called superior by some authorities and inferior by others. The important anatomic feature is that this space is best approached through the 12th rib from behind (see below).

The recognition of subphrenic abscess and its precise localization require a combination of repeated physical and x-ray examinations and scanning. Unexplained fever after peritoneal infection of any type without evident wound infection or peritoneal abscesses should immediately arouse suspicion of a subphrenic abscess.

The primary cause is often a clue to localization. Appendicitis commonly produces a right posterior inferior abscess. Infections of the gallbladder, stomach, and duodenum are more apt to produce anterior superior or subhepatic (right inferior) abscesses. Pancreatitis commonly produces a left inferior posterior abscess. Diverticulitis, particularly of the descending colon, may result in a left anterior inferior abscess. Perforation of a high greater curvature ulcer and injuries or abscesses of the spleen are more apt to produce superior left-sided subphrenic abscesses lying close to the dome of the diaphragm. The old adage "Pus somewhere, pus nowhere, pus under the diaphragm" is often appropriate.

All too often, subphrenic abscesses develop insidiously, but on occasion there may be pain and tenderness anteriorly or posteriorly on the affected side. Motion of the diaphragm on the affected side is restricted, and in superior space involvement there usually is a pleural effusion. In advanced cases, there may be widening of the intercostal spaces with fullness and palpable edema.

Management with antibiotics usually suppresses the physical signs, so that a persistent spiking fever, tachycardia, and malaise are the only manifestations.

X-ray examination is of the greatest importance. Demonstration of an air-fluid level below the diaphragm with a pleural effusion above it is diagnostic. Unfortunately, this represents an advanced abscess and more commonly the only findings are fixation and elevation of the diaphragm and a pleural effusion on the involved side. Lateral films may be of great help in localizing the abscess to an anterior or posterior position.

Inferior abscesses are more difficult to recognize than superior ones and are less apt to be associated with diaphragmatic immobility and pleural effusion.

Diagnostic aspiration of suspected abscesses is very hazardous, as pus may be transferred from the abscess to the free peritoneal or pleural spaces, compounding the sepsis. If there is a large pleural effusion, it can be tapped very high, taking only a few milliliters of fluid to identify its character. In subphrenic abscess, the

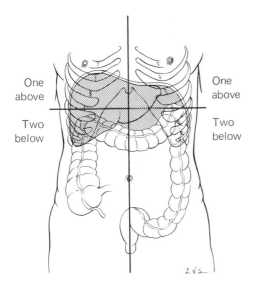

Figure 25–5. Simple scheme for remembering the subphrenic spaces. There is one space above the line on the right: the anterior superior. On the left, there is one space above the line (between the liver and the diaphragm) and 2 below: one anterior to the lesser sac and the lesser sac itself. On the right, the inferior subphrenic space extends from the bare area posteriorly to the subhepatic area anteriorly. Its posterior portion was formerly designated the posterior superior space.

Subphrenic Abscess

Subphrenic abscesses pose special problems in diagnosis and treatment. Although there is much argument about the anatomic nature of the subphrenic spaces, from a practical point of view abscesses may occur in any one of 6 areas (Fig 25–5).

On the right side (Fig 25–6), pus may be found

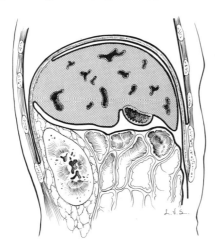

Figure 25–6. Right subphrenic spaces. The anterior superior space extends from the anterior edge of the liver to the bare area. The right inferior space extends from the bare area posteriorly to the anterior subhepatic area. Although anatomically in continuity, abscesses tend to localize either anteriorly or posteriorly.

pleural fluid is straw-colored and sterile.

Unless recognized and treated, subphrenic abscesses may rupture into a bronchus or the peritoneum or the pleura. The mortality in neglected cases is very high.

Treatment. The treatment of subphrenic abscess is surgical. As noted earlier, however, limited infection in the subphrenic spaces with elevation and fixation of the diaphragm may resolve following antibiotic therapy.

The absolute indication for drainage is obvious progressive sepsis, often with deterioration of the general condition of the patient. Ideally, subphrenic abscesses should be identified and drained before the patient becomes gravely ill. It may be necessary to explore the subphrenic spaces surgically in order to establish the diagnosis.

The ideal treatment of subphrenic abscess is extraperitoneal extrapleural drainage. Posterior abscesses may be drained through the bed of the 12th rib on the affected side (Fig 25–7). The incision must be transverse and not parallel to the bed of the rib to avoid entering the pleura. Recently, a lateral extraperitoneal approach has been shown to be simpler and more direct than the posterior route.

Anteriorly, a subcostal incision is made and carried through the transversalis fascia. The abscess cavity is located by blunt dissection and drained without entering the peritoneal cavity (Fig 25–7).

It is not essential to avoid a transperitoneal approach; in all cases in which the abscess cannot be identified or adequately drained by an extraperitoneal approach, transperitoneal or transpleural drainage must be used. In transpleural drainage, it is essential that the pleura be fused or that the operation be staged. Transperitoneal operations can be performed in one stage.

The prognosis after adequate drainage of subphrenic abscesses is excellent. However, adequate drainage is often difficult to obtain, particularly in some right ante-

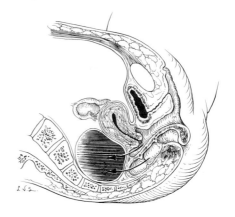

Figure 25–8. A pelvic abscess may be drained through the rectum or vagina.

rior superior and left posterior inferior abscesses. Transpleural drainage in one or 2 stages may be required in very large right superior abscesses. Repeated reoperation may be required in left posterior inferior abscess, especially when pancreatitis is the cause.

Pelvic Abscess

A pelvic abscess is usually readily recognized. In addition to fever, there may be lower abdominal discomfort and diarrhea. Rectal examination will disclose tenderness and a fullness in the pouch of Douglas. With a very high pelvic abscess, rectal examination may initially be negative, so that repeated daily examinations become necessary. This is essential if the patient appears seriously ill, with high fever and pulse rate.

Pelvic abscesses may subside spontaneously or progress to a large, tense, slightly fluctuant mass protruding into the anterior rectal wall or vagina. Diarrhea is an indication that the abscess is mature.

Pelvic abscesses may be drained through the rectum or vagina (Fig 25–8). Needle aspiration before introducing scissors or a clamp is a wise precaution in most cases. Drains should be left in the cavity but may be removed in several days if the clinical response is good. In general, drainage of pelvic abscess provides a very gratifying result with rapid recovery.

Altemeier WA & others: Intra-abdominal abscesses. Am J Surg 125:70, 1973.

Boyd DP: The subphrenic spaces and the emperor's new robes. N Engl J Med 275:911, 1966.

DeCosse JJ & others: Subphrenic abscess. Surg Gynecol Obstet 138:841, 1974.

Halasz NA: Subphrenic abscesses: Myths and facts. JAMA 214:724, 1970.

Roberts EAB, Nealon TF Jr: Subphrenic abscess: Comparison between operative and antibiotic management. Ann Surg 180:209, 1974.

Stone HH, Hester TR Jr: Incisional and peritoneal infection after emergency celiotomy. Ann Surg 177:669, 1973.

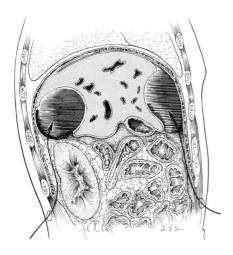

Figure 25–7. Extraperitoneal approaches to the right subphrenic spaces. An abscess in the anterior portion of the inferior space must be drained transperitoneally. Posterior abscesses may be drained laterally.

PERITONEAL ADHESIONS

Intraperitoneal adhesions are a late result of peritoneal trauma or peritonitis. They may occur following abdominal operations in which there was no clinical evidence of peritonitis. Adhesions may occur following peritonitis without operation—the classic example being gonococcal peritonitis (see above), which frequently results in extensive adhesions between the liver and diaphragm. Other low-grade peritoneal infections not requiring surgery (eg, tuberculosis) may produce extensive intraperitoneal adhesions.

Intraperitoneal adhesions are commonest after operations in which there is localized or generalized peritonitis. They are not the result of simple defects in peritoneal coverage. In the absence of trauma, hemorrhage, or bacterial contamination, large defects in the peritoneum heal very rapidly by metamorphosis of in situ mesodermal cells. A new peritoneal surface arises from the raw area.

The major factors contributing to intraperitoneal adhesions appear to be a combination of mechanical injury, ischemia, bacterial contamination, venous stasis, and the presence of blood. Foreign material of any kind is likely to stimulate the formation of adhesions. Talc and various starches used in the preparation of surgeons' gloves (see above) have been identified as a cause of severe postoperative peritoneal reaction with extensive adhesion formation. Cellulose fibers from disposable surgical drapes have also been implicated.

Short, fat females are particularly likely to develop postoperative adhesions.

Peritoneal adhesions may produce no symptoms. Very rarely, extensive adhesions may form between the abdominal wall and a loop of bowel, the stomach, or the anterior surface of the liver, producing abdominal pain. Most intraperitoneal adhesions, however, are asymptomatic until intestinal obstruction occurs.

Scrupulous surgical technic is the only way of avoiding postoperative adhesions with or without associated peritonitis. Traumatized areas of peritoneum should be protected by interposing omentum between the area and loops of small bowel. All foreign material and blood should be carefully aspirated from the peritoneal cavity at the completion of the operation.

Management of recurrent intestinal obstruction associated with adhesions is discussed in Chapter 33.

Ellis H: The cause and prevention of postoperative intraperitoneal adhesions. Surg Gynecol Obstet 133:497, 1971.

Milligan DW, Raftery AT: Observations on the pathogenesis of peritoneal adhesions. Br J Surg 61:274, 1974.

Tinker MA & others: Granulomatous peritonitis due to cellulose fibers from disposable surgical fabrics. Ann Surg 180:831, 1974.

Weibel MA, Majno G: Peritoneal adhesions and their relation to abdominal surgery. Am J Surg 126:346, 1973.

TUMORS OF THE PERITONEUM & RETROPERITONEUM

A variety of tumors may involve the peritoneum. In most instances, these are secondary cancerous implants from various abdominal organs—characteristically, the stomach and ovary. At times the primary lesion is small and the peritoneal seeding is disseminated widely as tiny implants. Ascites may be associated with intraperitoneal metastases, and the clinical picture may simulate chronic peritonitis due to other causes.

Diffuse abdominal carcinomatosis has a desperate prognosis except in the case of cancer of the ovary (see Chapter 44).

Peritoneal Mesothelioma

Mesothelioma, the only primary malignancy of the peritoneum, has attracted increased attention recently because of a rising incidence and demonstration that exposure to asbestos is responsible for more than half of cases. A long latent period (30–40 years) from contact with asbestos to appearance of the tumor raises fears that many more persons may develop mesothelioma in the future despite adoption of more stringent precautions by industrial users of the material. About 65% of mesotheliomas arise from the pleura and 25% from the peritoneum; about 10% affect both. In the abdomen, the tumor presents either as a bulky mass, usually in the epigastrium, with discrete implants elsewhere in the peritoneum, or as diffuse involvement of the peritoneal surfaces with numerous adhesions. Abdominal pain, ascites, distention, and marked weight loss are the usual presenting findings. A palpable mass is present in only 15% of cases. Differential diagnosis involves tuberculous peritonitis and carcinomatosis from a visceral primary. The diagnosis can be established by cytologic examination of the ascitic fluid. Some patients have thrombocytosis and fibrin split products in their serum. Metastases to liver or lungs occur late. No form of treatment has been shown to be beneficial, and the patients generally succumb within 12 months after diagnosis.

Moertel CG: Peritoneal mesothelioma. Gastroenterology 63: 346, 1972.

Pseudomyxoma Peritonei

This is a rather obscure disease which may begin by intraperitoneal dissemination of mucus and implantation of cells from a mucocele of the appendix or mucous cystadenoma of the ovary. In either case, the abdomen is filled with masses of gelatinous, partially encysted mucin. The patient may present with ascites or signs of low-grade intestinal obstruction.

At operation, huge masses of jelly-like material are easily evacuated from the abdominal cavity. The disease tends to run a chronic course, and patients are often palliated by periodic operations to remove mucin or relieve intestinal obstruction. Instillation of alkylating agents (mechlorethamine, 20 mg, or thiotepa, 60 mg) into the peritoneal cavity after removal of mucoid masses appears to have been beneficial.

With the passage of time, the disease assumes the course of a low-grade diffuse peritoneal malignancy. Distant metastases do not occur, but death ensues from malnutrition and recurrent intestinal obstruction. X-ray therapy and systemic chemotherapy have not been of benefit.

Limber GK & others: Pseudomyxoma peritonei. Ann Surg 178:587, 1973.
Little JM & others: Pseudomyxoma peritonei. Lancet 2:659, 1969.
Long RTL & others: Pseudomyxoma peritonei. Am J Surg 117:162, 1969.

Cysts of the Mesentery

Mesenteric cysts are rare lesions of developmental origin. They are variable in size, usually filled with straw-colored fluid, and have scant blood supply. Most mesenteric cysts are benign and can be shelled out without injury to the mesenteric blood vessels or intestine. Since the patient often presents with a fixed abdominal mass, the condition, though rare, must be carefully distinguished from retroperitoneal sarcoma. Laparotomy and excision or biopsy is essential.

Hardin W, Hardy J: Mesenteric cysts. Am J Surg 119:640, 1970.

Retroperitoneal Tumors

There are a variety of retroperitoneal tumors, usually of connective tissue origin. Fibrosarcoma, leiomyosarcoma, liposarcoma, and lymphoma may present primarily as retroperitoneal lesions. The course is usually characterized by low-grade pain or discomfort, fever, and eventually the appearance of a palpable mass on physical examination. In the early stages, x-ray studies are usually not helpful; later, as the mass enlarges, displacement of bowel or ureters may be seen.

Rarely, the lesion proves to be benign or of such low-grade malignancy that good results follow surgical excision. In malignant lesions—except for lymphosarcoma—treatment is usually unsatisfactory. Palliation may be achieved by aggressive but incomplete removal of some liposarcomas and leiomyosarcomas. Abdominal exploration and biopsy are essential in all cases because the response to irradiation may be gratifying if a lymphoma is discovered.

Braasch JW, Mon AB: Primary retroperitoneal tumors. Surg Clin North Am 47:663, 1967.
Lowman RM & others: Lumbar angiography in the diagnosis of primary retroperitoneal tumors. Surg Gynecol Obstet 132:597, 1971.
Riches E: The Gordon-Taylor tradition in the surgery of cancer with an account of paramesenteric tumors. Ann R Coll Surg Engl 42:71, 1968.

Mesenteric Panniculitis
(Mesenteric Lipodystrophy)

A bizarre form of chronic fat necrosis may in-volve the retroperitoneum and root of the mesentery. Histologically, the lesion is similar to that found in Weber-Christian disease and other forms of subcutaneous fat necrosis.

The course is characterized by low-grade fever, malaise, and vague recurrent abdominal pain. As in the case of other retroperitoneal tumors, plain films of the abdomen are often negative. Mesenteric arteriograms and CT scans may help to localize the lesions, and a mass may be evident on barium or x-ray studies of the gut. Sooner or later, an abdominal mass is palpable. Operation is usually required to establish the diagnosis, and it may be difficult to distinguish the lesion from a retroperitoneal neoplasm or a retroperitoneal dissection of a pancreatic pseudocyst. Biopsy will show the characteristic appearance of chronic fat necrosis. Attempts at resection are not indicated.

In most cases, the disease regresses spontaneously. No specific form of therapy is known, but systemic corticosteroids seem to have helped in some patients. In a rare variant of this syndrome called **retractile mesenteritis**, fibrosis produces mesenteric retraction, obstruction of mesenteric lymphatics and veins, and a fatal outcome.

Durst AL & others: Mesenteric panniculitis. Surgery 81:203, 1977.
Kipfer RE & others: Mesenteric lipodystrophy. Ann Intern Med 80:582, 1974.

RETROPERITONEAL FIBROSIS

Retroperitoneal fibrosis usually affects the urinary tract (see Chapter 43), but on occasion it has been identified with sclerotic lesions involving the small and large bowel. It is thought to be a hypersensitivity reaction to drugs (notably methysergide) or an autoimmune process. The mesentery may be involved, and the condition may be confused with mesenteric panniculitis.

The clinical manifestations are usually those of low-grade small bowel or colonic obstruction. If retroperitoneal fibrosis is not kept in mind as a possibility, it may be mistaken for malignancy. The diagnosis can usually be established by biopsy.

Favorable results have been reported following lysis of the constricting bands and the use of corticosteroids.

Koep L, Zuidema GD: The clinical significance of retroperitoneal fibrosis. Surgery 81:250, 1977.
Mitchell RJ: Alimentary complications of non-malignant retroperitoneal fibrosis. Br J Surg 58:254, 1971.

THE OMENTUM

The omentum may be the site of infection or tumor formations. It is also subject to torsion and frequently is involved in adhesions, producing intestinal obstruction.

Infection

The omentum is involved in all instances of peritonitis and provides an important protective mechanism against spreading peritonitis. In certain chronic diseases such as tuberculosis, the omentum may itself become infected and appear as a rolled-up tumorous mass instead of having its usual apron-like appearance.

Nonspecific inflammation of the omentum (epiploitis) may cause vague abdominal pain. At operation, the only finding is a rolled-up portion of thickened, edematous omentum. Microscopic study will show only mild inflammation. This lesion may be the result of a previous torsion.

Infarction & Torsion of the Omentum

Torsion of the omentum usually occurs when one portion of it is fixed by an adhesion or is caught in the opening of a hernia. The omentum rotates on itself, so that the blood supply becomes compressed.

Acute torsion produces severe abdominal pain, nausea, vomiting, and tenderness localized to the involved area. There may be a palpable mass. The condition is rare and is usually mistaken for some more common acute abdominal disorder such as intestinal obstruction or acute appendicitis.

At operation, the omentum will be found as a twisted mass with impaired blood supply and varying degrees of infarction. Excision is required. The prognosis is good.

Infarction of the omentum may be secondary to trauma or vascular lesions such as polyarteritis nodosa. Treatment is the same as for infarction caused by torsion.

Adams JT: Primary torsion of the omentum. Am J Surg 126:102, 1973.

DeLaurentis DA & others: Idiopathic segmental infarction of the greater omentum. Arch Surg 102:474, 1971.

Tumors & Cysts of the Omentum

The omentum is frequently involved by secondary deposits of cancer, and at times this may appear as a primary lesion because of the small size of the original growth. More often, it is clear that the involvement is secondary to an obvious gastrointestinal carcinoma. Rarely, primary cysts or vascular anomalies of the omentum may be found incidental to operation for other disorders.

●   ●   ●

26 ...
Stomach & Duodenum

Lawrence W. Way, MD

I. STOMACH

The stomach receives food from the esophagus and serves 4 functions: (1) It acts as a reservoir which permits eating reasonably large quantities of food at intervals of several hours. (2) Food contained in the stomach is mixed, triturated, and delivered into the duodenum in amounts regulated by its chemical nature and texture. (3) The first stages of protein and carbohydrate digestion are carried out in the stomach. (4) A few substances are absorbed across the gastric mucosa.

ANATOMY
(Figs 26–1, 26–2, 26–3)

The **cardia** is located at the gastroesophageal junction. The **fundus** is the portion of the stomach that lies cephalad to the gastroesophageal junction. The **corpus** or body of the stomach is the capacious central part; division of the corpus from the pyloric antrum is marked by the angular incisure, a crease on the lesser curvature just proximal to the "crow's-foot" terminations of the nerves of Latarjet. The **pylorus** is the boundary between the stomach and the duodenum.

The **cardiac gland area** is the small segment located at the gastroesophageal junction. Histologically, it contains principally mucus-secreting cells, although a few parietal cells are sometimes present. The **oxyntic gland area** is the portion containing parietal (oxyntic) cells and chief cells (Fig 26–2). The boundary between this region and the adjacent pyloric gland area is reasonably sharp since the zone of transition spans a segment of only 1–1.5 cm. The **pyloric gland area** comprises about the distal 30% of the stomach and contains G cells which manufacture the hormone gastrin. Mucous cells are common in the oxyntic and pyloric gland areas.

As in the rest of the gastrointestinal tract, the muscular wall of the stomach is composed of an outer longitudinal and an inner circular layer. An additional incomplete inner layer of obliquely situated fibers is most prominent near the lesser curvature but is of less substance than the other 2 layers.

Blood Supply

The blood supply of the stomach and duodenum is illustrated in Fig 26–3. The left gastric artery supplies the lesser curvature and connects with the right gastric artery, a branch of the hepatic artery. The greater curvature is supplied by the right gastroepiploic artery (a branch of the gastroduodenal artery) and the

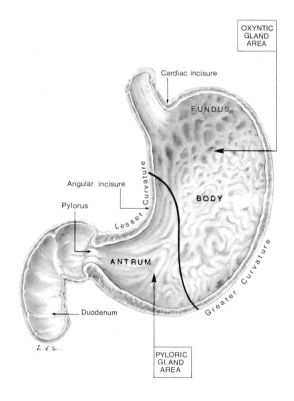

Figure 26–1. Names of the parts of the stomach. The line drawn from the lesser to the greater curvature depicts the approximate boundary between the oxyntic gland area and the pyloric gland area. No prominent landmark exists to distinguish between antrum and body (corpus). The fundus is the portion craniad to the esophagogastric junction.

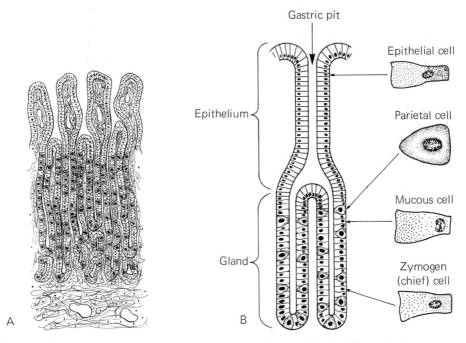

Figure 26—2. Histologic features of the mucosa in the oxyntic gland area. Each gastric pit drains 3—7 tubular gastric glands. The neck of the gland contains many mucous cells. Oxyntic (parietal) cells are most numerous in the midportion of the glands; peptic (chief) cells predominate in the basal portion. *A:* Drawing from photomicrograph of the gastric mucosa.

left gastroepiploic artery (a branch of the splenic artery). The midportion of the greater curvature corresponds to a point at which the gastric branches of this vascular arcade change direction. The fundus of the stomach along the greater curvature is supplied by the vasa brevia, branches of the splenic and left gastro-epiploic arteries.

The blood supply to the duodenum is from the superior and inferior pancreaticoduodenal arteries, which are branches of the gastroduodenal artery and the superior mesenteric artery, respectively. The stomach contains a rich submucosal vascular plexus. Venous blood from the stomach drains into the coronary, gastroepiploic, and splenic veins before entering the portal vein. The lymphatic drainage of the stomach, which largely parallels the arteries, partially determines the direction of spread of gastric neoplasms.

Nerve Supply

The parasympathetic nerves to the stomach are shown in Fig 26—3. As a rule, 2 major vagal trunks pass through the esophageal hiatus in close approximation to the esophageal muscle. These nerves are originally located to the right and left of the esophagus and stomach during embryonic development. When the foregut rotates, the lesser curvature turns to the right and the greater curvature to the left, and corresponding shifts in location of the vagal trunks follow. Hence, the right vagus supplies the posterior and the left the anterior gastric surface. About 90% of the vagal fibers are sensory afferent; the remaining 10% are efferent.

In the region of the gastroesophageal junction, each trunk bifurcates. The anterior trunk sends a division to the liver which travels in the lesser omentum. The bifurcation of the posterior trunk gives rise to fibers which enter the celiac plexus and supply the parasympathetic innervation to the remainder of the gastrointestinal tract as far as the mid transverse colon. Both trunks, after giving rise to their extragastric divisions, send some fibers directly onto the surface of the stomach and others along the lesser curvature (anterior and posterior nerves of Latarjet) which supply the distal part of the organ. As shown in Fig 26—3, a variable number of vagal fibers ascend with the left gastric artery after having passed through the celiac plexus.

The preganglionic motor fibers of the vagal trunks synapse with ganglion cells in Auerbach's plexus (plexus myentericus) between the longitudinal and circular muscle layers. Postganglionic cholinergic fibers are distributed to the cells of the smooth muscle layers and the mucosa.

The adrenergic innervation to the stomach consists of postganglionic fibers which pass along the arterial vessels from the celiac plexus.

PHYSIOLOGY

Motility

Storage, mixing, trituration, and regulated empty-

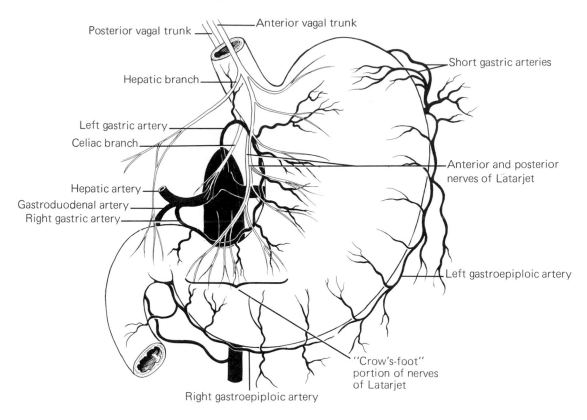

Figure 26–3. Blood supply and parasympathetic innervation of the stomach and duodenum.

ing are accomplished by the muscular apparatus of the stomach. Peristaltic waves originate in the fundus and pass toward the pylorus. The thickness of the smooth muscle increases in the antrum and corresponds to the stronger contractions that can be measured in the distal stomach. The pylorus behaves as a sphincter, although it normally allows a little to-and-fro movement of chyme across the junction.

An electrical pacemaker is situated in the fundal musculature near the greater curvature. Regular (3/minute) electrical impulses (pacesetter potential or basic electrical rhythm) arise from this area and pass toward the pylorus in the outer longitudinal layer. Every impulse is not always followed by a peristaltic muscular contraction, but the impulses determine the maximal peristaltic rate. The frequency of peristalsis is governed by a variety of stimuli mentioned below. Each contraction follows sequential depolarization of the underlying circular muscle resulting from arrival of the pacesetter potential.

Peristaltic contractions are more forceful in the antrum than the body and travel faster as they progress distally. Gastric chyme is forced into the funnel-shaped antral chamber by peristalsis; the volume of contents delivered into the duodenum by each peristaltic wave depends on the strength of the advancing wave and the extent to which the pylorus closes. Most of the gastric contents which are pushed into the antral funnel are propelled backward as the pylorus closes and pressure

within the antral lumen rises. Five to 15 ml enter the duodenum with each gastric peristaltic wave.

The volume of the empty gastric lumen is only 50 ml. By a process called receptive relaxation, the stomach can accommodate about 1000 ml before intraluminal pressure begins to rise. Receptive relaxation is an active process mediated by vagal reflexes and abolished by vagotomy. Peristalsis is initiated by the stimulus of distention after eating. Various other factors have positive or negative influences on the rate and strength of contractions and the rate of gastric emptying. Vagal reflexes from the stomach have a facilitating influence on peristalsis. The texture of the meal participates in the regulation of emptying; small particles are emptied more rapidly than large ones which the organ attempts to reduce in size (trituration). The osmolality of gastric chyme and its chemical makeup are monitored by duodenal receptors. If osmolality is greater than 200 mOsm/liter, a long vagal reflex (the enterogastric reflex) is activated, delaying emptying. Of the known hormonal effects, gastrin enhances gastric emptying whereas cholecystokinin, secretin, and other enterogastrones delay it.

Gastric Juice

The output of gastric juice in a fasting subject varies between 500 and 1500 ml/day. After each meal, about 1000 ml are secreted by the stomach.

The components of gastric juice are as follows:

A. Mucus: Mucus is a heterogeneous mixture of glycoproteins manufactured in the mucous cells of the oxyntic and the pyloric gland areas. Mucus does not provide a barrier to the diffusion of H^+ and cannot be thought of as protective of the mucosa on that basis. It probably acts as a lubricant and may impede diffusion of pepsin.

B. Pepsinogen: Pepsinogens are synthesized in the chief cells of the oxyntic gland area (and to a lesser extent in the pyloric area) and are stored as visible granules. Cholinergic stimuli, either vagal or intramural, are the most potent pepsigogues, although gastrin and secretin are also effective. The precursor zymogen is activated when pH falls below 5.0, a process that entails severance of a polypeptide fragment from the larger molecule. Pepsin cleaves peptide bonds, especially those containing phenylalanine, tyrosine, or leucine. Its optimal pH is about 2.0. Pepsin activity is abolished at $pH > 5.0$, and the molecule is irreversibly denatured at $pH > 8.0$.

C. Intrinsic Factor: Intrinsic factor, a mucoprotein secreted by the parietal cells, binds with vitamin B_{12} of dietary origin and greatly enhances absorption of the vitamin. Absorption occurs by an active process in the terminal ileum.

Intrinsic factor secretion is enhanced by stimuli that produce H^+ output from parietal cells. Pernicious anemia is characterized by atrophy of the parietal cell mucosa, deficiency in intrinsic factor, and anemia. Subclinical deficiencies in vitamin B_{12} have been described after operations that reduce gastric acid secretion, and abnormal Schilling tests in these patients can be corrected by the administration of intrinsic factor. Total gastrectomy creates a dependence on parenteral administration of vitamin B_{12}.

D. Blood Group Substances: Seventy-five percent of people secrete blood group antigens into gastric juice. The trait is genetically determined and is associated with a lower incidence of duodenal ulcer than in nonsecretors.

E. Electrolytes: The unique characteristic of gastric secretion is its high concentration of hydrochloric acid, a product of the parietal cells. As the concentration of H^+ rises during secretion, that of Na^+ drops in a reciprocal fashion. K^+ remains relatively constant at 5–10 mEq/liter. Chloride concentration remains near 150 mEq/liter and gastric juice maintains its isotonicity at varying secretory rates.

**Mechanism of Gastric Acid Secretion
& the Mucosal Barrier**

Parietal cells secrete hydrochloric acid (150 mEq/liter), which can reduce gastric pH to 1.0 or less. Not much is known about the intracellular biochemical events that precede acid secretion. Stimulation and inhibition of secretion may be regulated intracellularly by cyclic GMP (guanosine monophosphate) and cyclic AMP (adenosine monophosphate), respectively, the ultimate effect depending on the relative amounts of the two. Both H^+ and Cl^- are actively transported into the gastric lumen by separate pumps which are coupled

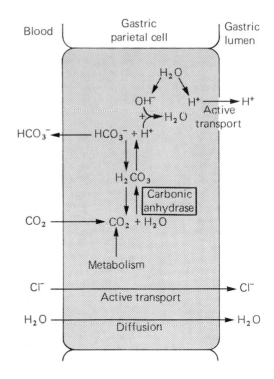

Figure 26–4. Intracellular processes in the formation of gastric hydrochloric acid.

(Fig 26–4). A negative electrical potential (30 mV) on the mucosal surface is generated by the chloride transport mechanism. The H^+ may be thought of as a product of the dissociation of H_2O. Carbonic acid is formed from the hydration of CO_2, a reaction which is facilitated by the large amount of carbonic anhydrase in these cells. The carbonic acid dissociates, and the resulting bicarbonate is excreted into the blood stream. Water enters the gastric lumen passively following the actively transported ions, and the secretion is isotonic or nearly so.

The concentration of acid secreted by parietal cells is 150 mEq/liter—a million times greater than the hydrogen ion concentration in blood. The ability of the stomach to secrete and hold this highly concentrated solution within its lumen is intrinsic to the mucosa itself and not the consequence of any special anatomic structure. Thus, it is not surprising that barrier efficiency should vary in relation to mucosal disease or injury. Disruption of the barrier occurs experimentally after hemorrhage, shock, topical aspirin, alcohol, bile salts, and several types of detergents. Aspirin and alcohol are synergistic in their damaging effects. As hydrogen ions enter the submucosa, they release histamine from mast cells and activate intramural cholinergic fibers (Fig 26–5). The histamine leads to edema formation and probably further increases acid production. Pepsinogen secretion and muscular contraction are stimulated by the cholinergic activity. The result of these events is a weakened mucosa susceptible to ulceration (Figs 26–10 and

Table 26–1. Gastrointestinal polypeptide hormones.

	Number of Amino Acid Residues	MW	Homologous Hormone	Cellular Location	Stimulus for Release	Actions
A. Established hormones						
Gastrin circulates in 3 or more forms; referred to as little gastrin (G17), big gastrin (BG, G34), and big big gastrin (BBG)	17 34 ?	2100, 3900, 20,000	CCK-PZ	G cells of antrum and duodenum	Gastric distention and protein in the stomach	Stimulates acid and pepsin secretion; stimulates gastric mucosal growth.
Cholecystokinin-pancreozymin (CCK-PZ)	33	3883	Gastrin	Mucosa of entire small intestine	Fat, protein, and their digestion products in the intestine	Stimulates gallbladder contraction; stimulates pancreatic enzyme secretion; stimulates pancreatic growth; inhibits gastric emptying.
Secretin	27	3056	Glucagon	Mucosa of duodenum and jejunum	Low pH in the duodenum; threshold pH 4.5	Stimulates pancreatic and biliary HCO_3^- secretion; augments action of CCK-PZ on pancreatic enzyme secretion.
B. Candidate hormones*						
Gastric inhibitory polypeptide (GIP)	43	5105	Secretin	Mucosa of duodenum and jejunum	Glucose or fat in the duodenum	Stimulates release of insulin from pancreas; inhibits gastric H^+ secretion and gastric motility.
Vasoactive intestinal polypeptide (VIP)	28	3100	Secretin	Mucosa of entire small intestine and colon	Stimulus-induced release has not been demonstrated	Inhibits gastric H^+ and pepsin secretion; stimulates pancreatic HCO_3^- secretion and secretion from intestinal mucosa; inhibits gastric and gallbladder motility.
Motilin	22	2700	?	Mucosa of duodenum and jejunum	Alkaline pH (8.2) in the duodenum	Stimulates gastric motility.
Enterogastrone	?	?	?	Mucosa of small intestine	Fat in the intestine	Inhibits gastric H^+ secretion.
Entero-oxyntin (mediator of the "intestinal phase" of H^+ secretion)	?	?	?	Mucosa of small intestine	Protein in the intestine	Stimulates gastric H^+ secretion.
Enteroglucagon	?	3500–7000	Glucagon	Mucosa of small intestine	Glucose or fat in the intestine	Glycogenolysis.
Chymodenin	43	4900	?	Mucosa of small intestine	Fat in the intestine	Specific stimulation of chymotrypsin secretion by the pancreas.
Bulbogastrone	?	?	?	Duodenal bulb	Acid in the duodenal bulb	Inhibits gastric H^+ secretion.

*The candidate hormones are either (1) peptides extracted from the gut which have not yet been proved to have a physiologic role or (2) physiologic actions postulated as being due to as yet unidentified hormones.

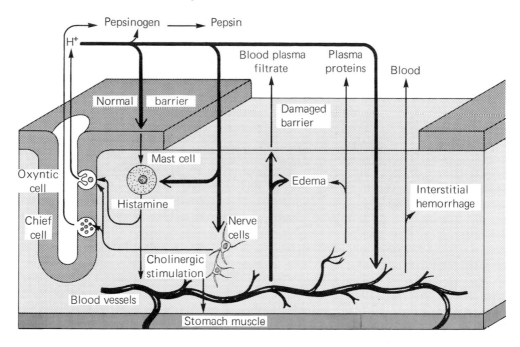

Figure 26–5. Effects of intraluminal acid on a normal or broken gastric mucosal barrier. If the barrier is intact, back diffusion of H^+ is minimal and causes no harm. When the barrier is disrupted, H^+ diffuses rapidly into the submucosa, histamine is released locally, and cholinergic fibers are stimulated. The consequences are increased H^+ and pepsinogen secretion, stimulation of gastric motility, and production of submucosal edema and hemorrhage.

26–11). The extent to which back diffusion is actually involved in the pathogenesis of gastric mucosal disease (eg, stress ulcer, gastric ulcer) is unknown.

Gastrointestinal Hormones

The hormones gastrin, cholecystokinin-pancreozymin (CCK-PZ), and secretin have been studied in great detail and are known to have important roles in regulation of gastrointestinal function. Some of the characteristics of these hormones are described in Table 26–1 along with those of the candidate hormones, so called because they have not yet earned full recognition as physiologic substances. Reliable radioimmunoassays have been developed for gastrin, glucagon, GIP, and VIP, and knowledge of the physiology of these hormones has grown rapidly. Difficulties in developing assays for secretin and CCK-PZ have made it necessary to continue to rely on indirect experimental evidence concerning their endogenous release.

Regulation of Acid Secretion

The regulation of acid secretion can best be described by considering separately those factors that enhance gastric acid production and those that depress it. The interaction of these forces is what determines the levels of secretion observed while fasting and after meals.

A. Stimulation of Acid Secretion: Acid production is usually presented as the result of 3 phases which are excited simultaneously after a meal. The separation

into phases is of value principally for descriptive purposes.

1. Cephalic phase—Stimuli that act upon the brain lead to increased vagal efferent activity and acid secretion. The sight, smell, taste, or even the thought of appetizing food may elicit this response. The effect is entirely vagally mediated and is abolished by vagotomy. The vagal stimuli have a direct effect on the parietal cells to increase acid output.

2. Gastric phase—The arrival of food in the stomach, through both mechanical and chemical stimulation, releases gastrin. Distention of the antrum is the major mechanical stimulus. By contact with the antral mucosa, products of protein digestion also liberate gastrin.

The presence of food in the stomach excites long vagal reflexes, impulses that pass to the CNS via vagal afferents and return to stimulate the parietal cells.

A third aspect of the gastric phase involves the sensitizing effect of distention of the parietal cell area to gastrin which is probably mediated through local intramural cholinergic reflexes.

3. Intestinal phase—The role of the intestinal phase in the stimulation of gastric secretion has been incompletely investigated. Various experiments have shown that the presence of food in the small bowel releases a humoral factor, recently named enterooxyntin, which evokes acid secretion from the stomach.

B. Inhibition of Acid Secretion: Without strategically located systems which limit secretion, unchecked acid production could become a serious clinical problem. Examples can be found (eg, Billroth II gastrectomy with retained antrum) where acid production rose after surgical procedures that interfered with these inhibitory mechanisms.

1. Antral inhibition—pH below 2.5 in the antrum inhibits the release of gastrin regardless of the stimulus. When the pH reaches 1.2, gastrin release is almost completely blocked. If the normal relationship of parietal cell mucosa to antral mucosa is changed so that acid does not flow past the site of gastrin production, serum gastrin may increase to high levels with marked acid stimulation.

2. Intestinal inhibition—The intestine participates in controlling acid secretion by liberating hormones that inhibit both the release of gastrin and its effects on the parietal cells. Secretin and CCK-PZ block acid secretion under experimental conditions, but current thinking is that neither has this as a physiologic action. Fat in the intestine is the most potent method of inhibition, affecting gastrin release and stimulation. Neither CCK-PZ nor GIP, both released by fat, seems capable of explaining all of the features of fat inhibition, and the term enterogastrone is used to refer to the still unidentified hormone which is presumably responsible. Bulbogastrone is a hypothetical hormone postulated to explain the unique potency of acidification of the duodenal bulb to reduce acid secretion.

Integration of Gastric Physiologic Function

Ingested food is mixed with salivary amylase before it reaches the stomach. The mechanisms stimulating gastric secretion are activated. Serum gastrin levels increase from a mean fasting concentration of about 50 pg/ml to 200 pg/ml, the peak occurring about 30 minutes after the meal (Fig 26–6). Food in the lumen of the stomach is exposed to high concentrations of acid and pepsin at the mucosal surface. Food settles in layers determined by sequence of arrival, but fat tends to float to the top. The greatest mixing occurs in the antrum. Antral contents therefore become more uniformly acidic than those in the body of the organ, where the central portion of the meal tends to remain alkaline for a considerable time, allowing continued activity of the amylase.

Peptic digestion of protein in the stomach is only about 5–10% complete. Carbohydrate digestion is more complete and may reach 30–40%. Gastric juice contains a lipolytic enzyme, but gastric digestion of triglycerides appears to be small.

The gastric contents are delivered to the duodenum at a rate that is determined by the texture of the meal, its osmolality and acidity, and its content of fat. A meal of lean meat, potatoes, and vegetables leaves the stomach within 3 hours. A meal with a very high fat content may remain in the stomach for 6–12 hours.

Cooke AR: Control of gastric emptying and motility. Gastroenterology 68:804, 1975.

Davenport HW: *A Digest of Digestion.* Year Book, 1975.

Grossman MI: Candidate hormones of the gut. Gastroenterology 67:730, 1974.

Malagelada JR & others: Measurement of gastric functions during digestion of ordinary solid meals in man. Gastroenterology 70:203, 1976.

Pearse AGE & others: The newer gut hormones. Gastroenterology 72:746, 1977.

Richardson CT & others: Studies on the mechanisms of food-stimulated gastric acid secretion in normal human subjects. J Clin Invest 58:623, 1976.

Samloff IM: Pepsinogens, pepsins, and pepsin inhibitors. Gastroenterology 60:586, 1971.

Walsh JH, Grossman MI: Gastrin. (2 parts.) N Engl J Med 292:1324, 1377, 1975.

PEPTIC ULCER

Peptic ulcers result from the corrosive action of acid gastric juice on a vulnerable epithelium. Depending on circumstances, they may occur in the esophagus, duodenum, the stomach itself, in the jejunum after surgical construction of a gastrojejunostomy, or in the ileum in relation to ectopic gastric mucosa in Meckel's diverticulum. When the term peptic ulcer was first used, it was thought that the most important factor was the peptic activity in gastric juice. Since then, evidence has accumulated that implicates acid as the chief causative agent; in fact, it is axiomatic that if gastric juice contains no acid a (benign) peptic ulcer cannot be present. Appreciation of the central role of acid has led to the emphasis on antacid therapy as the mainstay of medical therapy of ulcers and to operations logically designed to reduce acid secretion as the major surgical approach.

It has been estimated that about 5% of the adult population in the USA suffer from active peptic ulcer disease. Men are affected 3 times as often as women. Duodenal ulcers are 10 times more common than gastric ulcers in young patients, but in the older age groups the frequency is about equal. The incidence in men has been declining steadily and is now less than half what it was 20 years ago. The reasons for this are completely unknown. In the USA, peptic ulcer disease annually causes about 15,000 deaths and about 15 million days lost from work. The loss to the nation's economy—considering deaths, costs of hospitalization, and days of work lost—is over $1 billion a year.

In general terms, the ulcerative process can lead to 4 types of disability: (1) **Pain** is the most common. (2) **Bleeding** may occur due to erosion of submucosal or extraintestinal vessels as the ulcer becomes deeper. (3) Penetration of the ulcer through all layers of the affected gut results in **perforation** if other viscera do not seal the ulcer. (4) **Obstruction** may result from inflammatory swelling and scarring and is most likely to occur with ulcers located at the pylorus or gastroesophageal junction because the lumen is narrowest at those sites.

The causes, clinical features, and prognosis of duodenal ulcer and gastric ulcer are sufficiently different to suggest that they are fundamentally different diseases whose major common feature is acid-pepsin-dependent ulceration.

1. DUODENAL ULCER

Essentials of Diagnosis

- Epigastric pain relieved by food or antacids.
- Epigastric tenderness.
- Normal or increased gastric acid secretion.
- Signs of ulcer disease on upper gastro-intestinal x-rays.

General Considerations

Duodenal ulcers may occur in any age group but are most common in the young and middle-aged (20–45 years). They appear in men more often than women, but the incidence in men is decreasing while that in women is on the rise. Most clinicians note that fewer chronic painful duodenal ulcers are being seen but that bleeding ulcers are becoming a greater clinical problem.

About 95% of duodenal ulcers are situated within 2 cm of the pylorus, in the duodenal bulb.

Several clues are available regarding the causes of duodenal ulcer, but a satisfactory comprehensive theory remains elusive. The disease has apparently emerged as a major clinical entity in Western society only since the latter part of the 19th century. The incidence reached a peak about 25 years ago, then declined at a rate of 8% per year until the past few years, when it seems to have plateaued. The rising prevalence in women in recent years parallels their acceptance of increased responsibilities outside the home. Duodenal ulcer is rare in most tribal African cultures, whereas in the USA the incidence in blacks equals or is greater than that in the white population.

Increased gastric acid secretion is present in many patients with duodenal ulcer. Both basal and maximal outputs are high, indicating a sustained increased drive to the parietal cells and an enlarged parietal cell mass. The latter presumably reflects a response to increased stimulation over a prolonged period. Gastrin levels in fasting patients with duodenal ulcer are about the same as those in people without ulcers, but the postprandial rise is greater than normal (Fig 26–6). Since acid hypersecretion could normally be expected to inhibit gastrin release, the elevation may be etiologically significant. The traditional explanation for the hypersecretion seen in this disease is increased vagal activity, said to be a reflection of underlying psychic stresses. Data to support this speculation are unavailable.

Another possible explanation for the increased acid secretion in peptic ulcer might be deficiencies in the production of enterogastrones. Several studies comparing duodenal ulcer patients with normal subjects show no differences in the response to

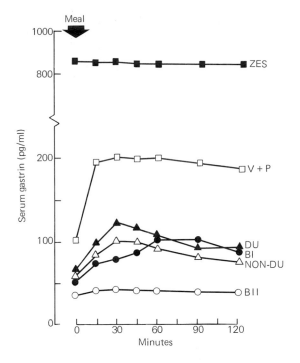

Figure 26–6. Postprandial gastrin values in patients with Zollinger-Ellison syndrome (ZES), vagotomy and pyloroplasty (V + P), unoperated duodenal ulcer (DU), Billroth I gastrectomy (BI), normals (NON-DU), and Billroth II gastrectomy (BII). (Data courtesy of Dr John Walsh.)

intestinal stimulation, but this hypothesis has not yet been fully explored.

Another theoretical cause of peptic ulcer is decreased resistance of the duodenal mucosa to the action of gastric acid and pepsin. A major weakness of this theory is that it fails to account for the known acid hypersecretion. Several other clinical factors are known to be associated with enhanced susceptibility to duodenal ulcer. The disease is more common in individuals with blood group O and in those who fail to secrete blood group antigens H, A, or B in their gastric juice. An antipeptic activity of these substances may account for this relationship.

Chronic liver disease, chronic lung disease, and chronic pancreatitis have all been implicated as increasing the possibility of duodenal ulceration. Except for patients with pancreatic exocrine insufficiency who have decreased bicarbonate secretion into the duodenum, the mechanism is unclear.

Clinical Findings

A. Symptoms and Signs: Pain is the presenting symptom in most patients with uncomplicated duodenal ulcer. It is usually located in the epigastrium and is variably described as aching, burning, or gnawing, but radiologic survey studies indicate that as many as a third of patients with active duodenal ulcer may be entirely free of gastrointestinal complaints.

The daily cycle of the pain is characteristic. The patient usually has no pain in the morning until an hour or more after breakfast. It is relieved by the noon meal, only to recur in the later afternoon. Pain may appear again in the evening, and in about half of cases it arouses the patient during the night. Food, milk, or antacid preparations temporarily relieve the discomfort.

When the ulcer **penetrates** posteriorly into the head of the pancreas, back pain is noted; concomitantly, the cyclic pattern of pain may change to a more steady discomfort, with less relief from food and antacids.

Varying degrees of nausea and vomiting accompany the pain. Vomiting may be a major feature even in the absence of obstruction. For unknown reasons, such patients are sometimes less responsive to medical or surgical therapy.

The abdominal examination may reveal localized epigastric tenderness to the right of the midline, but in many instances no tenderness can be elicited.

The activity of duodenal ulcer and its accompanying symptoms typically remit and recur at intervals of several years. Relapses last for 2–4 months, but the variation is great. The natural tendency toward remission must be kept in mind when attributing improvement in symptoms to any particular therapeutic regimen.

B. Laboratory Findings:

1. Test for occult blood–The stool should be examined for occult blood even in the absence of clinical or laboratory evidence of gastrointestinal bleeding.

2. Gastric analysis–A gastric analysis need not be performed in every ulcer patient but should be ordered (1) in patients who do not respond promptly to an antacid regimen; (2) in patients under consideration for elective surgery; (3) in patients suspected on the basis of other findings (eg, x-rays) of having Zollinger-Ellison syndrome; and (4) in patients with recurrent ulcer after previous ulcer operation.

a. Standard gastric analysis– The standard gastric analysis consists of the following: (1) Measurement of acid production by the unstimulated stomach under basal fasting conditions; the result is expressed as H^+ secretion in mEq/hour and is termed the **basal acid output (BAO)**. (2) Measurement of acid production during stimulation by histamine, betazole (Histalog), or pentagastrin given in a dose that is maximal for this effect. The result is expressed as H^+ secretion in mEq/hour and is termed the **maximal acid output (MAO)**.

The test is performed as follows: The patient fasts for 12 hours before the study, except that he may have water. Antacids, anticholinergic drugs, or other agents known to affect gastric section must be withheld. The reliability of the procedure is enhanced by having the examination performed by a specially trained technician. A nasogastric tube is passed into the stomach. Fluoroscopic verification of positioning improves results but is impractical in most instances. The stomach is emptied of its contents, which are discarded; subsequent secretions are preserved. The

Table 26–2. Mean values for acid output during gastric analysis for normals and patients with duodenal ulcer. The upper limits of normal are: Basal (BAO), 5 mEq/hour; maximal (MAO), 30 mEq/hour.

	Sex	Mean Acid Output (mEq/Hour)	
		Normal	Duodenal Ulcer
Basal	Male	2.5	5.5
	Female	1.5	3.0
Maximal	Male	30	40
(betazole)	Female	20	30

patient should be supine, positioned somewhat on his left side, and instructed to expectorate all saliva. Aspiration of gastric juice must be made continuously. The specimens are divided into 15-minute aliquots.

At the end of the basal hour of collection, betazole (Histalog), 1.5 mg/kg, or pentagastrin, 6 μg/kg, is given by subcutaneous injection. Gastric juice is subsequently collected for an additional 1½ hours. Acid concentration in each 15-minute specimen is then titrated to pH 7.0. Output (in mEq) is obtained as the product of concentration and volume of the specimen. BAO is determined as the sum of the 4 periods before betazole injection. MAO is calculated by adding the 4 highest consecutive periods after stimulation.

Interpretation of the results of gastric analysis is outlined in Table 26–2. Over half of patients with duodenal ulcer have maximal secretory values that overlap those of people without ulcers.

The term **achlorhydria** denotes no acid (pH > 6.0) after maximal stimulation. Achlorhydria is incompatible with a diagnosis of benign peptic ulcer. In patients in whom x-ray studies have demonstrated gastric ulcer, this finding would indicate the presence of underlying gastric cancer. Malignancy in duodenal ulcers is extremely rare.

In Zollinger-Ellison syndrome, basal acid secretion is often greater than 15 mEq/hour, and the ratio of BAO to MAO is characteristically 0.6 or greater. Confirmation of the diagnosis requires direct measurement of elevated serum gastrin levels by immunoassay.

In the past, gastric acid output was collected during a 12-hour overnight period for clinical analysis. This method is less accurate than the basal 1-hour collection and has been abandoned. The terms "free" acid, "combined" acid, and "degrees" of acidity have generally been discarded since they were confusing and without pathophysiologic significance. Free acid was the amount of acid in milliequivalents on titration to pH 3.5; combined acid, the amount from pH 3.5–7.0. The degrees of acidity of a specimen were the number of milliliters of 0.1 N NaOH solution required to titrate 100 ml of gastric juice to neutrality; by chance, it equaled the concentration of H^+ in mEq/liter.

b. Hollander insulin gastric analysis–The Hollander test involves the intravenous administration of regular insulin and measurement of gastric acid secretion. The procedure is based on the assumption that acid after insulin hypoglycemia is entirely the result of vagal impulses arising from CNS stimulation. The Hollander test has principally been used as a means of determining the completeness of vagotomy postoperatively. Recent evidence indicates a poor relationship between the results of the Hollander test and recurrence of ulcer after vagotomy, so it appears to be of little clinical usefulness. The trend is to perform a standard gastric analysis to study acid secretion in patients with recurrent ulcer.

The patient is studied first under basal conditions as described above. Collections of gastric juice are made for 1 hour, and regular insulin, 0.2 unit/kg, is then given by rapid IV injection. A blood sample is taken for glucose determination before the insulin is given and again 30 and 60 minutes afterward. Gastric juice is aspirated for 2 hours after insulin, and each 15-minute sample is titrated to pH 7.0.

The interpretation of the Hollander test uses the concentrations of acid in the secreted juice rather than the quantity in milliequivalents. The standard criteria for a positive test, meaning that significant vagal innervation persists, are as follows: If the basal secretion contained no acid, a level of 10 mEq/liter after insulin is positive; if the basal secretion contained acid, an elevation of its concentration by 20 mEq/liter over basal, after insulin, is positive.

3. Serum gastrin—Serum gastrin determinations are now readily available. Depending on the laboratory doing the test, normal basal levels average 50–100 pg/ml, and levels over 200 pg/ml can almost always be considered elevated.

Gastrin concentrations may rise in hyposecretory and hypersecretory states. In the former conditions (eg, atrophic gastritis, pernicious anemia), the cause is higher antral pH with loss of antral inhibition for gastrin release. Much more important clinically are elevated gastrins with concomitant hypersecretion, where the high gastrin is responsible for the increased acid and resulting peptic ulceration. The best-defined clinical conditions in this category are Zollinger-Ellison syndrome (gastrinoma) and retained antrum after Billroth II gastrectomy. Whether some cases of duodenal ulcer are due to antral hypersensitivity with abnormally high gastrins is presently being studied.

A fasting serum gastrin determination should be obtained in patients with peptic ulcer disease and any of the following: (1) basal acid secretion > 10 mEq/hour (intact stomach) or > 5 mEq/hour (after gastrectomy); (2) patients with a ratio of basal to maximal acid output (BAO/MAO) over 0.4; (3) all patients with recurrent ulcer after previous ulcer operation; (4) any patient with concomitant hyperparathyroidism or other endocrine tumor.

Gastrin concentrations under 200 pg/ml are considered normal. Patients with Zollinger-Ellison syndrome or retained antrum usually have basal concentrations above 500 pg/ml. In the range 200–500 pg/ml, the patient should be studied by intravenous infusion of calcium (4–5 mg/kg/hour for 3 hours) or bolus injection of secretin (2 units/kg). In Zollinger-Ellison syndrome, the gastrin response to calcium and secretin is greater than 300 pg/ml and 100 pg/ml, respectively. Maximal response after calcium occurs during the third hour of infusion; after secretin, the peak is reached in 5–15 minutes.

C. X-Ray Findings: Radiologic examination of the gastroduodenal region is done after the patient swallows a barium sulfate suspension. The changes induced by duodenal ulcer consist of duodenal deformities and an ulcer niche. Distortion of the normal duodenal configuration results from inflammatory swelling and scarring and leads to findings such as distortion of the duodenal bulb, eccentricity of the pyloric channel, or pseudodiverticulum formation. The ulcer itself may be seen either in profile or, more commonly, en face.

The reliability of x-ray diagnosis appears to be high, but accurate figures are not available to support this clinical impression. In the routine case, response to therapy should be judged mainly on symptomatic changes rather than evidence of healing demonstrated on serial x-ray examinations.

D. Special Examinations: Gastroscopy is useful to evaluate patients with an uncertain diagnosis, bleeding from the upper intestine, or those who have obstruction of the gastroduodenal segment.

Differential Diagnosis

The differential diagnosis of peptic ulcer includes any other abdominal disorder that causes epigastric pain and indigestion. The most common diseases simulating peptic ulcer are (1) chronic cholecystitis, in which cholecystograms show either nonfunction of the gallbladder or stones in a functioning gallbladder; (2) pancreatitis, in which the serum amylase is elevated (not elevated in peptic ulcer disease unless the ulcer penetrates through into the pancreas); (3) functional indigestion, in which x-rays are normal; and (4) hiatal hernia, which can be seen on x-rays.

X-ray is the most important diagnostic adjunct in verifying the presence and character of the underlying peptic ulcer disease.

Complications

Other than the morbidity caused by pain, the common complications of duodenal ulcer are hemorrhage, perforation, and duodenal obstruction. Each of these is discussed in a separate section. Less common complications consist of pancreatitis and biliary obstruction.

Prevention

Prevention of ulcer disease entails avoidance of ulcerogenic drugs and other substances in susceptible individuals: nicotine, alcohol, reserpine, caffeine, and other xanthines found in cola drinks. No other special dietary precautions are thought to be significant. Elimination of unusually stressful environmental factors may be helpful.

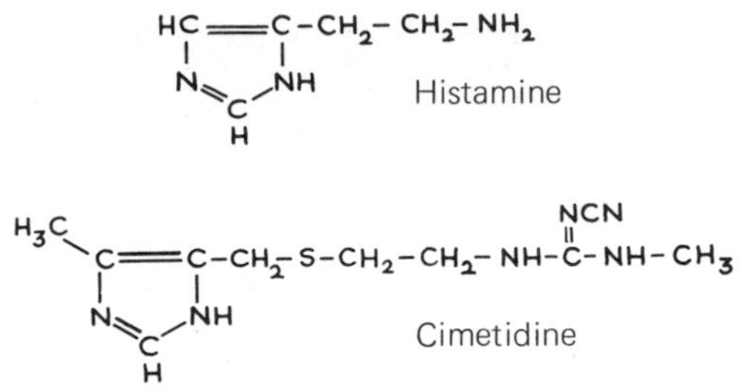

Treatment

Duodenal ulcer can be controlled by medical treatment in a substantial majority of patients. Surgical treatment is reserved for those whose ulcer disease persists in the face of an adequate medical regimen (called an **intractable** ulcer) or in whom bleeding, perforation, or obstruction develops.

A. Medical Treatment: The goals of medical treatment are to remove ulcerogenic factors and to neutralize gastroduodenal pH so that healing may occur.

1. Diet—Ulcerogenic agents must be proscribed. Nicotine, corticosteroids, reserpine, alcohol, salicylates, and caffeine and other xanthines (coffee, tea, and cola beverages) have all been shown to have theoretical or actual adverse effects in duodenal ulcer.

Food buffers gastric acid principally via the carboxyl groups in protein and the patient should be taught the importance of frequent meals of a palatable and nutritious character. A snack between each of the 3 main meals and again in the late evening is a convenient schedule during treatment of an acute ulcer.

A bland diet based on use of soft foods, including custards, creams, milk, etc, has not been shown to benefit the ulcer patient. The physician must make every attempt to enlist the patient's informed cooperation in the therapeutic program since in most instances it is the patient who makes many of the therapeutic decisions over the protracted course of the disease. In discussing dietary restrictions—which most patients assume to be the cornerstone of therapy—it is useful to recommend only that the patient avoid items that seem to aggravate his symptoms.

2. Antacids—The criteria for adequate antacid therapy consist of selecting an effective preparation, prescribing the proper dose and dosage interval, and obtaining patient compliance with the regimen.

An adequate antacid regimen heals about 75% of duodenal ulcers after 1 month of treatment. Treatment regimens that rely on self-regulated doses in response to pain or taking antacids on a 3-times-a-day schedule are inadequate.

After it has been verified that the patient is eating 3 meals a day, the antacid should be prescribed for 1 and 3 hours after each meal. Treatment should continue for at least 6 weeks. Magnesium oxide, which is often combined with aluminum hydroxide (eg, Maalox, Mylanta), is probably the antacid of choice. If diarrhea becomes a problem with one of these compounds they can be alternated with aluminum hydroxide gel. Calcium carbonate, once a popular antacid, has fallen into disuse because it is associated with rebound acid hypersecretion as its neutralizing capacity dissipates, and it may produce hypercalcemia.

The liquid forms of all antacids are more effective than tablets and should always be used for intensive treatment of an acute ulcer. On the other hand, for occasional dyspepsia while at work, shopping, and in other social situations, patients will find that the convenience of tablets compensates for their inferiority to liquid antacids. In such cases, the tablets should be chewed or dissolved in the mouth for maximum effect.

Figure 26–7. Structures of histamine and cimetidine, an H_2 blocker.

3. H_2 receptor antagonists—(Fig 26–7.) The H_2 blocking agent cimetidine reduces acid secretion and is effective in the treatment of duodenal and gastric ulcers. For duodenal ulcers, the efficacy of this agent is about the same as that of vigorous antacid therapy. However, cimetidine can also control acid hypersecretion in Zollinger-Ellison syndrome, providing for the first time a nonsurgical treatment for that condition. The usual dose is 300 mg after meals and at bedtime.

Metiamide, the first of the H_2 blockers tried in man, was associated with several cases of agranulocytosis and was withdrawn from use. When taken for several months, cimetidine has caused no side-effects. Whether more prolonged ingestion of cimetidine will be as safe is as yet unknown. Of concern is the fact that T cells possess H_2 receptors, suggesting the possibility that H_2 blockers might interfere with cell-mediated immunity. Studies to date have not shown changes in immune function in humans taking these drugs.

4. Anticholinergic drugs— These compounds have logical attractiveness for the treatment of peptic ulcer, but in practice they have not been shown to have therapeutic benefit. Anticholinergic drugs have theoretic value because they decrease acid secretion and delay gastric emptying. Earlier studies suggested a decreased incidence of recurrence in patients placed on anticholinergic agents after an initial remission was achieved, but attempts to repeat this observation have not been successful. They are often prescribed before bedtime to delay emptying of an evening snack.

Several anticholinergics seem to have greater gastric effect than peripheral action. Propantheline (Pro-Banthine), glycopyrrolate (Robinul), and oxyphencyclimine (Daricon) are superior to belladonna or atropine in this respect. Dosage should be sufficient to produce dryness of the mouth.

5. Rest and sedation—Severe anxiety calls for treatment with sedatives such as phenobarbital or diazepam, but the routine use of sedatives is not known to hasten healing of ulcers. It is occasionally necessary to recommend to the patient that he temporarily or even permanently withdraw from an anxiety-producing environment or occupation if control of ulcer cannot be achieved otherwise.

Admission to the hospital speeds healing of gastric ulcers and may have similar value for duodenal ulcer. This action removes the patient from his environment, provides an opportunity for physical and emotional rest, and ensures greater accuracy in administration of an intensive antacid regimen. The major expense incurred by this measure demands that it be used only for those patients who do not respond to outpatient treatment or who are in imminent danger of developing complications.

6. Gastric irradiation—Irradiation of the parietal cell mucosa diminishes acid secretion and can be used to treat peptic ulcers in selected patients. A total dose of 1600–2000 rads is delivered to the tissues over a 10-day period. The mean secretory depression of about 50% usually appears within 3–6 weeks after completion of therapy and leads to healing of the ulcer in the majority of cases. The histologic appearance and function of the mucosa recover in a large portion of patients over several years thereafter; recurrent ulceration develops in 30% by 5 years. Hypertension due to radiation nephritis has been detected in some patients treated more than 5 years earlier by this regimen. For these reasons, this technic should be restricted to the elective treatment of elderly patients who are unacceptably poor risks for surgery.

7. Experimental drugs—Under investigation is the possible clinical use of prostaglandin analogues for depressing acid secretion. There is also renewed interest in bismuth compounds following reports that tripotassium dicitrato bismuthate (DeNol) accelerates healing of gastric and duodenal ulcers. Bismuth compounds cannot function as antacids, and their mechanism of action is completely unknown.

B. Surgical Treatment: If medical management fails to control the patient's symptoms, one must first consider whether the therapeutic regimen has taken full advantage of the potential of antacids and avoidance of aggravating situations and drugs. If medical treatment has been optimal, the ulcer may be judged **intractable** and surgical treatment is indicated. There are unanswered questions regarding precise definition of the clinical state of intractability because it is difficult to conclude, for example, how many episodes of recurrence represent morbidity equivalent to that which may be expected in a large series of patients electively treated by surgery. Individual interpretation of the situation by the patient and his physician should entail a consideration of the patient's suffering, the extent to which it compromises his personal way of life, and accurate appreciation of the benefits and risks of elective surgery.

The management of hemorrhage, perforation, and obstruction due to peptic ulcer is discussed separately in later sections of this chapter. These complications frequently are manifestations of intractability in the broader sense of the word.

All of the successful surgical procedures for curing peptic ulcer are aimed at reduction of gastric acid secretion. Excision of the ulcer itself is not sufficient either with duodenal or gastric ulcer; recurrence is nearly inevitable with such procedures.

The 5 fundamentally different surgical methods of treating ulcer are as follows: subtotal gastrectomy, vagotomy, antrectomy, gastrojejunostomy, and total gastrectomy. Except in special circumstances, the choice of operation today for the average patient with duodenal ulcer is among (1) vagotomy (truncal or selective) with a drainage procedure, (2) parietal cell vagotomy without a drainage procedure, (3) vagotomy and antrectomy, and (4) subtotal gastrectomy (Fig 26–8). However, an understanding of the physiology of gastric secretion and motility makes it possible for the surgeon to modify his technics to handle unusual findings and still control the the ulcer diathesis.

1. Subtotal gastrectomy—This operation consists of resection of two-thirds to three-fourths of the distal stomach. The proximal remnant may be reanastomosed to the duodenum (**Billroth I** resection) or to the side of the proximal jejunum (**Billroth II** resection). For duodenal ulcer, the Billroth II technic is preferable because recurrent ulceration is less frequent. One reason may be that, owing to release of duodenal gastrin, postprandial gastrin levels are higher after Billroth I than Billroth II gastrectomy (Fig 26–6).

When creating a Billroth II (gastrojejunostomy) reconstruction, the jejunal loop may be brought up to the gastric remnant either anterior to the transverse colon or posteriorly through a hole in the transverse mesocolon. Since either method is satisfactory, an antecolic anastomosis is elected in most cases because it is simpler. One must verify carefully that the segment of small intestine being used actually is proximal jejunum, because inadvertent gastroileal anastomosis will lead to serious malabsorption. In fact, the length of the jejunal segment between the ligament of Treitz and the site of gastrojejunostomy should be as short as possible (about 15 cm) to avoid postoperative nutritional problems.

It appears not to matter whether the gastrojejunostomy is performed with the afferent jejunal limb at the greater curvature edge of the gastric remnant ("isoperistaltic") or at the lesser curvature ("antiperistaltic").

In most instances, the surgeon will be able to remove the ulcerated portion of duodenum in the course of the resection. However, it is not imperative that this be done, and in some cases it would be hazardous or ill-advised. The duodenal stump is closed after a Billroth II gastrectomy, and if an ulcer must be left in place it usually heals promptly.

The principal technical challenge in gastrectomy for duodenal ulcer is presented by the location of the ulcerated, inflamed duodenum at the site where the bowel must be transected. The dissection must avoid injury to the pancreas and the extrahepatic biliary ducts. After the specimen has been removed, gastroduodenal anastomosis requires a healthy cuff of duodenum about 1 cm long distal to the previous location of the ulcer. If this criterion cannot be met, a gastrojejunal anastomosis reestablishes gastrointestinal continuity by anastomosing healthy portions of bowel, thus avoiding the risks of anastomotic disruption. When

Antrectomy and vagotomy   Subtotal gastrectomy   Total gastrectomy

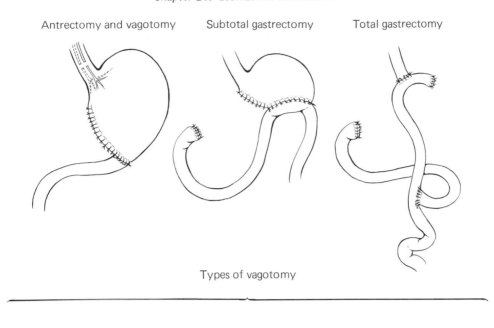

Types of vagotomy

Truncal   Selective   Parietal cell

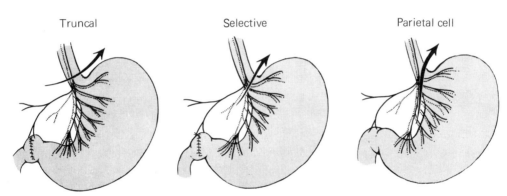

Figure 26—8. Various types of operations currently popular for treating duodenal ulcer disease. Total gastrectomy is reserved for Zollinger-Ellison syndrome. The choice among the other procedures should be individualized according to principles discussed in the text.

performing a Billroth II resection, the surgeon must be certain that the duodenal closure is secure. Occasionally, if a secure closure is impossible, a tube should be sewn snugly into the duodenal stump and brought out through the abdominal wall as a temporary controlled decompressing fistula.

Physiologically, subtotal gastrectomy accomplishes complete removal of the major source of gastrin (the antrum) and of about half of the parietal cell area of the stomach.

The Billroth II subtotal gastrectomy has the advantages of low incidence of recurrent ulceration (about 2%) and generally good long-term outcome when all factors are taken into account. Its disadvantages are that it is a longer, more extensive surgical procedure, and it may aggravate poor nutrition in already underweight persons.

2. Vagotomy and drainage—Truncal vagotomy consists of resection of a 1 or 2 cm segment of each vagal trunk as it enters the abdomen on the distal esophagus. The resulting vagal denervation of the gastric musculature produces delayed emptying of the stomach in many patients unless a drainage procedure is performed. The method of drainage most often selected in the USA is (Heineke-Mikulicz) **pyloroplasty** (Fig 26—9); in Great Britain, **gastrojejunostomy** is more popular. Neither gives a superior functional result, and pyloroplasty is less time-consuming. Various types of pyloroplasties are technically feasible, but their description is beyond the scope of this text.

Selective vagotomy possesses theoretical advantages over truncal vagotomy because vagal innervation of the viscera other than the stomach is preserved. The procedure entails transection of each abdominal vagus at a point just beyond its bifurcation into gastric and extragastric divisions. Thus, the hepatic branch of the anterior vagus and the celiac branch of the posterior vagus are maintained.

Vagal denervation of just the parietal cell area of the stomach is a procedure only recently given widespread trial. In addition to **parietal cell vagotomy,** the operation has been called proximal gastric vagotomy, highly selective vagotomy, and superselective vagotomy. The technic spares the main nerves of Latarjet (Fig 26—8) but divides all vagal branches that terminate on the proximal two-thirds of the stomach. Since antral innervation is preserved, gastric emptying is relatively unimpaired and a drainage procedure is unnecessary.

Selective vagotomy causes less postvagotomy diarrhea than truncal vagotomy, but the incidence of dumping syndrome is probably higher. Both procedures are about equally effective in controlling ulcer disease. Parietal cell vagotomy appears to have about the same effectiveness as truncal or selective vagotomy for curing the ulcer disease, but dumping and diarrhea are much less frequent. After truncal vagotomy, the risk of recurrence is substantially greater in patients whose preoperative maximal acid output exceeds 40—45 mEq/hour, and for them gastrectomy might be preferable.

Physiologically, all types of vagotomy eliminate direct vagal stimulation of the parietal cells and decrease parietal cell sensitivity to gastrin. Interestingly, basal and postprandial serum gastrin levels are increased because the effects of antral denervation are more than offset by the drop in gastric pH (Fig 26—6). Basal and stimulated acid secretion are both reduced to about one-third of preoperative levels.

The vagotomy procedures have the advantages of technical simplicity and preservation of the entire gastric reservoir capacity. The principal disadvantage is recurrent ulceration in about 10% of patients.

3. Antrectomy and vagotomy—This operation entails a 50% distal gastrectomy, with the line of gastric transection carried high on the lesser curvature to conform with the boundary of the gastrin-producing mucosa. Vagotomy is performed as described in the preceding section; antrectomy by itself is insufficient to prevent a high recurrence rate.

After vagotomy and antrectomy, either a Billroth I or II reconstruction may be accomplished. The Billroth I type has been used by most surgeons, but there is no evidence that its results are really superior.

Vagotomy and antrectomy is associated with a low incidence of marginal ulceration (2%) and a generally good overall outcome. The major disadvantage compared with vagotomy and a drainage procedure is the increased time and effort required to perform the gastric resection.

4. Gastrojejunostomy—Gastrojejunostomy was the first operation that was extensively used for the treatment of duodenal ulcer. It has been generally discarded as definitive therapy because about 20% of patients developed recurrent ulcers on the jejunal side of the stoma.

The physiologic explanation for the good results with gastrojejunostomy is that it decreases the gastric phase of gastric secretion and lowers acid output.

Despite its long-term unsatisfactory results, gastrojejunostomy may still be advisable when one is forced to do as little as possible because of technical difficulties or because of the precarious condition of the patient.

5. Total gastrectomy—Complete removal of the stomach is not required to cure the usual forms of peptic ulcer disease. From the technical standpoint, the operation is of significantly greater magnitude than any form of partial gastrectomy, and short-term postoperative morbidity is greater. Nutritional difficulties are experienced by some of the patients afterward.

Total gastrectomy is the procedure of choice for patients with Zollinger-Ellison syndrome (gastrin-producing tumors). Occasionally it must be done to save a patient who is bleeding from erosive gastritis.

Complications of Surgery for Peptic Ulcer

A. Early Complications: The complications in the immediate postoperative period consist of duodenal stump leakage, gastric retention, and hemorrhage.

1. Duodenal stump leakage—Blowout of the duodenal stump is the most common cause of death after Billroth II gastrectomy. This complication can be prevented by resorting to catheter drainage of the duodenum if the degree of inflammation jeopardizes the duodenal closure. Equally important is selection of vagotomy and a drainage procedure in preference to gastric resection in any patient with a badly damaged or inflamed duodenum. Obstruction of the afferent limb of the gastrojejunostomy may contribute to this complication by increasing intraluminal pressure in the duodenum.

The clinical picture is characterized by sudden severe upper abdominal pain during the third to sixth days after surgery. The pain often radiates to the shoulder and the patient develops abdominal rigidity, high fever, and leukocytosis.

Immediate reoperation is mandatory. Drains—or, preferably, a sump suction device—should be placed in the region of the leaking duodenal closure. Attempts to resuture the duodenum at this time are unsuccessful. If the afferent loop is obstructed, this must be corrected, but not necessarily at the same time that the drains are inserted.

Large fluid and electrolyte losses through the fistula may be a clinical problem. Once drainage has been established, the patient should be managed as any case of high-output intestinal fistula. Spontaneous closure usually occurs if the patient survives the acute phase; if it does not, the fistula should be surgically closed after the patient has been stable for 4—6 weeks.

2. Gastric retention—An occasional patient is unable to tolerate oral feedings when they are started 5 or 6 days after surgery. He may become nauseated and complain of fullness and abdominal and shoulder pain, and will vomit if nasogastric suction is not reestablished. If this is due to edema of the stoma aggravated by gastric atony resulting from the vagotomy, resolution will gradually occur if the stomach is decompressed for several more days.

In some cases, organic obstruction underlies these symptoms. It may be due to a small anastomotic leak, excessive inversion of tissue at the anastomosis, perianastomotic hematoma, or anastomotic entrapment by omentum. Even in these cases, the gastric obstruction may improve with time, although as much as 3–4 weeks may be necessary.

The best way to handle this situation is to temporize. Gastrointestinal x-rays may suggest whether the cause is functional or organic. If a prolonged delay is anticipated before the patient will be able to resume adequate oral nourishment, intravenous hyperalimentation is a useful adjunct. In most cases, loss of gastric tone is the principal cause. After decompression of the overdistended stomach by 48 hours of continuous aspiration, the tube should be removed and feeding begun with small amounts of palatable solid food. Intermittent aspiration at intervals of 4–8 hours is required to make certain that the stomach is not becoming overdistended. Occasionally, when no improvement has occurred after 3–4 weeks and it is clear that obstruction is present, reoperation is required. Chronic delayed emptying from functional causes may respond to metoclopramide.

3. Hemorrhage—Hemorrhage within 24 hours after surgery results from failure to adequately ligate the vessels in the seromuscular coats of the stomach or jejunum. Hemorrhage may also occur on the fourth to seventh postoperative days as a result of slough of tissue at the suture line and erosion into the seromuscular blood vessels. Less commonly, postoperative bleeding results from unsuspected blood dyscrasias.

Initial attempts to stop the hemorrhage consist of ice water lavage of the stomach. Blood loss should be replaced. If 1500–2000 ml of blood have been lost and the bleeding persists, reoperation is indicated.

B. Late Complications:

1. Anastomotic ulcer (marginal ulcer, stomal ulcer, recurrent ulcer)—Recurrent ulcers form in about 10% of duodenal ulcer patients treated by vagotomy and pyloroplasty; in 2–3% after vagotomy and antrectomy or subtotal gastrectomy; and in 15–20% after gastroenterostomy alone. Recurrence is quite unusual after gastrectomy for gastric ulcer. Recurrent ulcers nearly always develop immediately adjacent to the anastomosis on the intestinal side.

The usual complaint is upper abdominal pain, which is often aggravated by eating and improved by antacids. In some patients, the pain is felt more to the left in the epigastrium, and left axillary or shoulder pain is occasionally reported. About a third of patients with stomal ulcer will experience a major episode of gastrointestinal hemorrhage. Free perforation is much less common (5%).

a. Causes—It is often possible to explain in pathophysiologic terms why the ulcer has returned. The following causes should be considered depending on which surgical procedure was used as primary treatment.

(1) Insufficient operation—Most recurrent ulcers probably develop because the original operation was insufficient to control the ulcer diathesis. In the case of vagotomy, recurrences occur most often in patients whose preoperative maximal acid output is greater than 40–45 mEq/hour, where the reduction in secretion following this procedure (60%) may be insufficient. Acid output is decreased even more by subtotal gastrectomy or antrectomy and vagotomy (80%), and recurrences after these procedures are correspondingly less common.

(2) Inadequate gastric resection—The size of the gastric remnant as shown on x-rays will demonstrate with reasonable accuracy whether a full two-thirds resection has been done in the case of subtotal gastrectomy or if a complete antrectomy was done in the case of antrectomy and vagotomy.

(3) Incomplete vagotomy—When truncal vagotomy is performed for duodenal ulcer, acid secretion is reduced by 60%. If secretion greater than 40% of the preoperative value persists, a major vagal trunk may have been overlooked. Such a patient should exhibit a rise in his output after insulin (Hollander test) of at least several mEq/hour. The classical Hollander criteria for "incomplete vagotomy" have not withstood critical analysis, ie, a positive Hollander test does not establish the presence of intact vagal fibers in the sense that another vagotomy can be expected to cure the patient.

(4) Inadequate drainage procedure—Chronic partial gastric outlet obstruction is responsible for some cases of recurrent ulcer after vagotomy and a drainage procedure. In these patients, the ulcer appears in the stomach instead of the small bowel.

(5) Retained antrum—During gastric resection, the distal line of transection should be through the duodenum so that the entire antrum is removed. If the operation has been done so that a portion of antrum remains attached to the duodenum after a Billroth II gastrectomy, the pH in the antral remnant is not affected by acid produced in the residual parietal cell mucosa. Gastrin production increases unchecked, and persistent acid stimulation leads to marginal ulceration.

(6) Loss of alkaline secretions near the anastomosis—The alkaline pancreatic and biliary secretions normally flow near the point where gastric acid enters the small bowel. If the afferent loop is especially long after a Billroth II gastrectomy, considerable absorption may occur before these juices reach the anastomosis, and an ulcer may be the result. Another ulcer of similar cause follows side-to-side anastomosis of the afferent and efferent limbs of the gastrojejunostomy.

(7) Zollinger-Ellison syndrome—This condition, which is dealt with in detail in a later section, must always be considered in the differential diagnosis of stomal ulceration. Characteristic findings on gastrointestinal x-rays, gastric analysis, or high concentrations of serum gastrin should suggest the diagnosis.

b. Diagnosis—The patient generally presents with recurrent dyspepsia, pain, or gastrointestinal bleeding. Barium x-ray studies should be ordered, but it must be remembered that only 50% of marginal ulcers can be demonstrated on x-rays. Thus, a negative gastrointestinal series is of little value in excluding the diagnosis. Gastroscopy should usually be performed since many marginal ulcers that were not demonstrated by x-ray can be seen through the gastroscope.

Serum gastrin measurements should probably be performed on every patient with recurrent ulcer. On gastric analysis, elevated basal secretion of acid might suggest the Zollinger-Ellison syndrome or retained antrum. Since each of these is due to excessive gastrin, the findings on gastric analysis are similar: high basal secretion (greater than 5 mEq/hour after previous surgery) and a high ratio of basal to stimulated secretion (BAO/MAO > 0.6). Retained antrum can sometimes be shown on the x-rays, but inspection of the duodenal stump during laparotomy may be necessary if the afferent loop cannot be filled with barium.

c. Treatment—Medical treatment has a low record of success for marginal ulcer. Unless some major ulcerogenic factor can be eliminated, nearly all patients require additional surgery.

Vagotomy alone is effective treatment for marginal ulcers which appear after subtotal gastrectomy. If the patient's original operation entailed a vagotomy, persistent hypersecretion may indicate incomplete vagotomy. In these cases, intact vagal fibers should be sought at laparotomy and divided. If a good-sized vagal trunk is not found, a gastric resection should be performed.

Preoperative suspicion of retained antrum should lead to examination of the duodenal stump and re-resection, depending on what is found. Retained antrum is an infrequent cause of marginal ulcer in modern practice, and elevated gastrin levels usually signify Zollinger-Ellison syndrome.

2. Gastrojejunocolic and gastrocolic fistula—A deeply eroding ulcer may occasionally produce a fistula between the stomach and colon. Most examples have resulted from recurrent peptic ulcer after an operation that included a gastrojejunal anastomosis. Rarely, spontaneous fistulas have developed between the stomach and colon from malignant gastric tumors, ulcerative colitis, or granulomatous colitis.

Severe diarrhea and weight loss are the presenting symptoms in over 90% of cases. Abdominal pain typical of recurrent peptic ulcer often precedes the onset of the diarrhea. Sometimes the pain suddenly improves at the moment the fistula is produced and diarrhea begins. Intestinal bleeding complicates the marginal ulceration in a few patients. Bowel movements number 8–12 or more per day; they are watery and often contain particles of undigested food. The patient's breath or eructations may be unusually foul-smelling, and emesis may be feculent.

Malnutrition is often severe and may produce emaciation and dependent edema due to hypoproteinemia. Intestinal motility is hyperactive, and intestinal obstruction may be suggested by the combination of visible peristalsis and occasional feculent vomiting.

Laboratory studies reveal low serum proteins and manifestations of fluid and electrolyte depletion. Appropriate tests may reflect deficiencies in both water-soluble and fat-soluble vitamins.

An upper gastrointestinal series reveals the marginal ulcer in only 50% of patients who have one. In only 15% is the fistula shown on x-rays after oral ingestion of barium. The diagnosis ultimately depends on barium enema which demonstrates the fistulous tract unfailingly.

The ill effects of gastrocolic fistula are due to the enormous load of bacteria which enters the proximal intestine from the colon. Short circuit of food past the intestine via the fistula is almost never an important factor. The mechanisms by which the bacteria so severely hinder absorption include deconjugation of bile salts, production of diarrheogenic hydroxy fatty acids, mucosal damage, and others as yet unknown.

Initial treatment should replenish fluid and electrolyte deficits. Severely malnourished patients may benefit from a period of intravenous hyperalimentation, but surgery must be performed as soon as the patient's condition permits. Definitive surgical correction can usually be accomplished as a single procedure. In the past, procedures that diverted the fecal stream from the fistula were used to allow the patient to repair his nutritional defects before more difficult corrective operations were performed. Proximal colostomy, division of the ileum and ileosigmoidostomy, and exclusion of the fistula with colocolostomy were all effective. A single-stage correction avoids one or more additional operations. The involved colon and ulcerated gastrojejunal segment are excised and colonic continuity reestablished. Vagotomy, partial gastrectomy, or both are required to treat the ulcer diathesis and prevent another recurrent ulcer. Results are excellent in benign disease. In general, the outlook for patients with malignant fistulas is poor.

3. Dumping syndrome—Symptoms of the dumping syndrome are noted to some extent by most patients who have an operation that impairs the ability of the stomach to regulate its rate of emptying. Weeks or months after surgery, dumping is a clinical problem in only 1 or 2% of patients. Symptoms fall into 2 categories: cardiovascular and gastrointestinal. Shortly after eating, the patient may experience palpitations, sweating, weakness, dyspnea, flushing, nausea, abdominal cramps, belching, vomiting, diarrhea, and, rarely, syncope. The degree of severity varies widely among patients, and not all symptoms are reported by all patients. In severe cases, the patient must lie down for 30–40 minutes until his discomfort passes.

Dumping can be elicited in normal subjects by instilling hypertonic solutions into the proximal small intestine or by mechanical distention of the jejunum. Appearance of the syndrome after gastric surgery can be explained on the basis of rapid entry of hypertonic food into the small bowel. Decreased blood volume, increased splanchnic blood flow, decreased blood pressure, and increased hematocrit can be measured by appropriate technics but are probably not directly responsible for the symptoms. The incidence of dumping correlates loosely with the amount of stomach removed, the size of the gastrointestinal anastomosis, and preoperative psychologic instability.

Diet therapy to reduce jejunal osmolality is successful in all but a few cases. The diet should be low in carbohydrates and high in fat and protein content. Sugars and carbohydrates are least well tolerated; some patients are especially sensitive to milk. Meals should be taken dry, with fluids restricted to between meals. This dietary regimen ordinarily suffices, but anticholinergic drugs may be of additional help in some patients, and others have reported improvement with serotonin antagonists.

If dumping symptoms are refractory to dietary treatment, further surgery should be considered. Good results are most often achieved by inserting an antiperistaltic 10 cm segment of jejunum between the gastric remnant and the duodenum. The procedure delays gastric emptying and diverts food into the less sensitive duodenum rather than the jejunum. A marginal ulcer may appear after this operation unless vagotomy is included.

Unfortunately, the term "dumping" has also been applied to an unrelated phenomenon sometimes seen in postgastrectomy patients, ie, late postprandial **reactive hypoglycemia**. This condition partially mimics early dumping syndrome, but the onset of symptoms coincides with hypoglycemia 3–4 hours after eating and the patient is relieved by eating sugar.

4. Weight loss and malabsorption—Some patients gain weight when gastrectomy relieves postprandial ulcer discomfort, but, on the average, a 5–10% loss in weight can be expected after gastric resection. Both decreased intake and decreased efficiency of digestion and absorption are responsible. Patients are usually comfortable at their lower weight and do not consider it a problem. In an occasional case, serious malnutrition complicates gastrectomy and the clinician is faced with a complicated set of variables that must be recognized and evaluated. The major factors that may contribute to malnutrition after gastrectomy are as follows:

a. Small gastric reservoir—Patients note that hunger is satisfied after smaller meals because the size of the stomach is reduced. Attempts to eat amounts equivalent to their preoperative capacity lead to uncomfortable fullness and nausea. More frequent meals may be recommended to attain increased intake.

b. Perianastomotic obstruction—Partial obstruction may occur at several points on a Billroth II anastomosis. Narrowing may follow scarring or may herald an anastomotic ulcer. Kinks and stenoses have been described at the junction of either the afferent or efferent loop with the stomach. Rarely, one of the jejunal limbs may intussuscept into the gastric remnant. The common result of these various mechanical obstructions is postprandial vomiting and pain. Patients who find that they vomit after eating voluntarily limit their intake.

The **afferent loop syndrome** in patients with a Billroth II gastrectomy consists of abdominal pain appearing 15–30 minutes after eating which is relieved suddenly by vomiting bilious fluid free of food. This is thought to be caused by partial obstruction of the afferent loop at the anastomosis and presumably is due to unimpeded passage of food from the stomach into the efferent loop, release of secretin and cholecystokinin, and stimulation of pancreatic secretion and gallbladder contraction. Bile accumulates in the afferent loop until the obstruction is suddenly overcome and the empty stomach is flooded with bile, causing vomiting. However, this classic picture is seldom present.

Standard radiologic studies with barium may be supplemented by cineradiography using a "motor meal" in attempts to delineate partial obstructions about the anastomosis.

c. Alkaline gastritis—Reflux of duodenal juices into the stomach is an invariable and usually innocuous situation after operations that interfere with pyloric function but in some patients may cause marked gastritis. The principal symptom is postprandial pain, and the diagnosis rests on endoscopic and biopsy demonstration of an edematous inflamed perianastomotic gastric mucosa. Since a minor degree of gastritis is found in most patients after Billroth II gastrectomy, the endoscopic findings must be striking to justify this diagnosis. Stools may be positive when tested for occult blood, but melena or hematemesis is rare. Although this entity is sometimes called bile gastritis, it is not certain that bile salts are solely responsible for the pathologic features, and cholestyramine rarely gives symptomatic improvement. Persistent severe pain is an indication for surgical reconstruction. Any procedure that diverts duodenal juices from the stomach will give relief: the ones most commonly used are Roux-en-Y gastrojejunostomy or insertion of a 15 cm isoperistaltic segment of jejunum between stomach and duodenum. If the preoperative diagnosis is correct, postoperative relief is usually rewarding.

d. Malabsorption—A decrease in the efficiency of fat absorption can be detected in most patients with a Billroth II gastrectomy. Normally, no more than 5% of ingested fat is excreted in the stool, but nearly all patients who have had a Billroth II excrete 10–15%. Steatorrhea of this degree is not usually accompanied by weight loss or diarrhea and remains subclinical in most patients. The principal cause is uncoordinated mixing of food and pancreatic enzymes in the bowel.

Some patients have afferent loop stasis which fosters bacterial proliferation and creates a variant of the **blind loop syndrome.** The bacteria deconjugate bile salts, which then precipitate or are absorbed, making them unavailable for micellar solubilization of lipolytic products. A block in the absorption mechanism for fat is thus superimposed on the defective lipolysis. Weight loss and diarrhea may be marked and accompanied by deficiencies of fat-soluble vitamins (A, D, E, and K). Symptomatic and biochemical improvement in fat absorption often results from administration of antibiotics to lower the bacterial concentration in the afferent loop. Tetracycline and lincomycin have given the best results because they attack bacteroides, the organism that accounts for the bile salt deconjugation. Oral replacement of pancreatic enzymes may give further benefit.

Although short-term control of steatorrhea can be achieved by these means, they are too expensive and unreliable for prolonged therapy. Bacterial resistance develops to one antibiotic after another. Therefore, in the absence of major contraindications to surgery, the Billroth II should be converted to a Billroth I anastomosis. This procedure eliminates the afferent loop responsible for the blind loop syndrome, improves mixing of food with enzymes, and will substantially improve most patients with well-documented postgastrectomy malabsorption.

5. Anemia—Iron deficiency anemia develops in about 30% of patients within 5 years after partial gastrectomy. It is caused by failure to absorb food iron bound in an organic molecule. Before this diagnosis is accepted, the patient should be checked for blood loss from the gastrointestinal tract. Slow bleeding from a marginal ulcer or an unsuspected tumor must be sought by appropriate endoscopic and radiologic tests. Inorganic iron—ferrous sulfate or ferrous gluconate—is indicated for treatment and is absorbed normally after gastrectomy.

Vitamin B_{12} deficiency and megaloblastic anemia appear in a few cases after gastrectomy. One cause is inadequate production of intrinsic factor, since addition of intrinsic factor corrects the abnormal Schilling test found in some patients. Inefficient mixing of food with gastric secretion may produce incomplete binding of intrinsic factor and the vitamin. In other cases, vitamin B_{12} deficiency is a manifestation of afferent loop stasis and the blind loop syndrome. In this situation, the bacteria in the intestine compete with the host for the vitamin B_{12} contained in food. Parenteral vitamin B_{12} should be given if vitamin B_{12} deficiency is present. Surgical correction of the blind loop syndrome will ordinarily be indicated to improve absorption.

6. Postvagotomy diarrhea—The daily frequency of bowel movements is increased in about two-thirds of patients who have had a truncal vagotomy. In the great majority, this is either accepted as an improvement by the patient or is considered of no significance. About 5–10% of patients who have had truncal vagotomy will require treatment with antidiarrheal agents at some time or another, and perhaps 1% are seriously troubled by this complication. The diarrhea may be episodic, in which case the onset is unpredictable after symptom-free intervals of weeks to months. An attack may consist of only one or 2 watery movements or, in severe cases, may last for a few days. Other patients may continuously produce 3–5 loose stools per day.

Postvagotomy diarrhea is probably due to increased gastric emptying (following the drainage procedure) and the effects of vagal denervation on intestinal motility, but the pathophysiology has not been fully explained. Selective gastric vagotomy was introduced in the hope that preservation of the extragastric vagal fibers would lower the frequency of this complication. The operation has been partly successful in this regard, but even more encouraging is the observation that diarrhea seems to be almost entirely avoided by parietal cell vagotomy.

Most mild cases of postvagotomy diarrhea can be treated satisfactorily with kaolin-pectin compounds (eg, Kaopectate). Codeine or diphenoxylate with atropine (Lomotil) may be needed for more severe cases. If these measures are inadequate and the patient's morbidity is substantial, a reversed 10 cm segment of jejunum may be inserted at the gastric outlet or in the jejunum 100 cm distal to the ligament of Treitz.

Summary Statement on Duodenal Ulcer

Duodenal ulcer disease is characterized by exacerbations and remissions. In the average case, activity of the symptoms reaches a peak 5–10 years after the initial diagnosis and subsides slightly thereafter. Patients with severe symptoms, those who require hospitalization, and those with high acid secretion tend to do less well with medical treatment. The onset of back pain is a bad prognostic sign. Some degree of bleeding will be seen in 15%, perforation in 5%, and obstruction in less than 5%. About 15% of all patients who develop duodenal ulcer will eventually need surgery, and as many as 50% who have been hospitalized will come to operation.

The results of elective surgery for duodenal ulcer are satisfactory to excellent in about 90% of cases. The mortality rate following elective surgery should be approximately 1–2% regardless of which operation the surgeon favors. We consider vagotomy the best operation for the average patient whose stimulated acid secretion is under 40 mEq/hour. A discussion of the relative merits of the different types of vagotomy was presented earlier. For a healthy, well-nourished, hypersecreting man undergoing elective operation, vagotomy and antrectomy combines the virtues of a low rate of recurrent ulcer with minimal early and late complications. However, if the patient's general condition is suboptimal or technical difficulties can be anticipated during gastric resection, vagotomy and pyloroplasty will minimize the immediate morbidity and mortality. This procedure offers slightly poorer long-term results than vagotomy and antrectomy or subtotal gastrectomy, principally because of the higher incidence of recurrent ulcer after vagotomy and drainage.

The most common causes of late morbidity after surgery for peptic ulcer are marginal ulcer, dumping syndrome, anemia, malnutrition, and diarrhea. Each has been discussed above.

In summary, the overall results of elective surgery for duodenal ulcer are good in 85–90% of patients. In poor-risk patients, pyloroplasty and vagotomy or parietal cell vagotomy offers the lowest mortality rate. In good-risk patients, all 3 of the popular operations should have equally low mortality rates; vagotomy is recommended except for those with especially high acid secretion; in the latter case, vagotomy and antrectomy or subtotal gastrectomy may give better long-term results.

Duodenal Ulcer

Edwards FC, Coghill NF: Clinical manifestations in patients with chronic atrophic gastritis, gastric ulcer, and duodenal ulcer. Q J Med 37:337, 1968.

Ganguli PC & others: Antral-gastrin-cell hyperplasia in peptic-ulcer disease. Lancet 1:583, 1974.

Gray GR & others: Oral cimetidine in severe duodenal ulceration. Lancet 1:4, 1977.

Grossman MI (moderator): A new look at peptic ulcer. Ann Intern Med 84:57, 1976.

Grossman MI: Some minor heresies about vagotomy. Gastroenterology 67:1016, 1974.

Hallenbeck GA: The natural history of duodenal ulcer disease. Surg Clin North Am 56:1235, 1976.

Herrington JL Jr: Truncal vagotomy with antrectomy. Surg Clin North Am 56:1335, 1976.

Ippoliti A, Walsh J: Newer concepts in the pathogenesis of peptic ulcer disease. Surg Clin North Am 56:1479, 1976.

Isenberg JI: Therapy of peptic ulcer. JAMA 233:540, 1975.

Johnston D, Goligher JC: Selective, highly selective, or truncal vagotomy? Surg Clin North Am 56:1313, 1976.

Jordan PH Jr: Current status of parietal cell vagotomy. Ann Surg 184:659, 1976.

Jordan PH Jr: A follow-up report of a prospective evaluation of vagotomy-pyloroplasty and vagotomy-antrectomy for treatment of duodenal ulcer. Ann Surg 180:259, 1974.

Kronborg O: Assessment of completeness of vagotomy. Surg Clin North Am 56:1421, 1976.

Kronborg O: Gastric acid secretion and risk of recurrence of duodenal ulcer within six to eight years after truncal vagotomy and drainage. Gut 15:714, 1974.

Tanner NC: Personal observations and experiences in the diagnosis and management of ulcer disease and disabilities that follow peptic ulcer operations. Surg Clin North Am 56:1349, 1976.

Wise L, Ballinger WF: The elective surgical treatment of chronic duodenal ulcer: A critical review. Surgery 76:811, 1974.

Wormsley KG: The pathophysiology of duodenal ulceration. Gut 15:59, 1974.

Marginal Ulcer

Amdrup E: Selective vagotomy of the gastric remnant for extragastric ulcer recurrence following resection. Scand J Gastroenterol 6:489, 1971.

Cleator IGM, Holubitsky IB, Harrison RC: Anastomotic ulceration. Ann Surg 179:339, 1974.

Cody JH & others: Gastrocolic and gastrojejunocolic fistulae. Ann Surg 181:376, 1975.

Holst-Christensen J & others: Recurrent ulcer after proximal gastric vagotomy for duodenal and pre-pyloric ulcer. Br J Surg 64:42, 1977.

Keighley MRB & others: A symptomatic discriminant to identify recurrent ulcer in patients with dyspepsia after gastric surgery. Lancet 2:278, 1976.

Kronborg O: A follow-up of patients operated upon for recurrence after vagotomy and drainage for duodenal ulcer. Scand J Gastroenterol 8:123, 1973.

Kronborg O: Influence of the number of parietal cells on risk of recurrence after truncal vagotomy and drainage for duodenal ulcer. Scand J Gastroenterol 2:423, 1972.

Passaro E Jr & others: Marginal ulcer: A guide to management. Surg Clin North Am 56:1435, 1976.

Van Heerden JA, Bernatz PE, Rovelstad RA: The retained gastric antrum: Clinical considerations. Mayo Clin Proc 46:25, 1971.

Postgastrectomy Syndromes

Allan JG, Russell RI: Cholestyramine in treatment of postvagotomy diarrhea. Br Med J 1:674, 1977.

Browning GG, Buchan KA, Mackay C: Clinical and laboratory study of postvagotomy diarrhoea. Gut 15:644, 1974.

Buchwald H: The dumping syndrome and its treatment. Am J Surg 116:81, 1968.

Buskin FL, Woodward ER: *Postgastrectomy Syndromes.* Saunders, 1976.

Cohen AM, Ottinger LW: Delayed gastric emptying following gastrectomy. Ann Surg 184:689, 1976.

Cooperman AM: Postoperative alkaline reflux gastritis. Surg Clin North Am 56:1445, 1976.

Donovan I, Alexander-Williams J: Postoperative gastric retention and delayed gastric emptying. Surg Clin North Am 56:1413, 1976.

Harvey HD: Complications in hospital following partial gastrectomy for peptic ulcer: 1936 to 1959. Surg Gynecol Obstet 117:211, 1963.

Hines JD, Hoffbrand AV, Mollin DL: The hematologic complications following partial gastrectomy. Am J Med 43:555, 1967.

MacGregor IL & others: Gastric emptying of solid food in normal man and after subtotal gastrectomy and truncal vagotomy with pyloroplasty. Gastroenterology 72:206, 1977.

Metzger WH & others: Effect of metoclopramide in chronic gastric retention after gastric surgery. Gastroenterology 71:30, 1976.

Reber HA, Way LW: Surgical treatment of late postgastrectomy syndromes. Am J Surg 129:71, 1975.

Shultz KT & others: Mechanism of postgastrectomy hypoglycemia. Arch Int Med 128:240, 1971.

Van Heerden JA & others: Postoperative reflux gastritis. Am J Surg 129:82, 1975.

Wirts CW & others: The correction of postgastrectomy malabsorption following a jejunal interposition operation. Gastroenterology 49:141, 1965.

ZOLLINGER-ELLISON SYNDROME
(Gastrinoma)

Essentials of Diagnosis

- Peptic ulcer disease (often severe).
- Gastric hypersecretion.
- Elevated serum gastrin.
- Nonbeta islet cell tumor of the pancreas.

General Considerations

Zollinger-Ellison (ZE) syndrome consists of peptic ulcer disease caused by a gastrin-producing tumor (gastrinoma). The gastrin-producing lesions in the pancreas are nonbeta islet cell carcinomas (60%), solitary adenomas (25%), and hyperplasia or microadenomatosis (10%); the remaining cases (5%) are due to solitary submucosal gastrinomas in the first or second portion of the duodenum.

About a third of patients have other endocrine tumors—most commonly of the parathyroid and pituitary glands. When associated with tumors in other endocrine organs, the condition is known as multiple endocrine adenomatosis I (MEA-I) syndrome.

Clinical Findings

A. Symptoms and Signs: Abdominal pain is an almost invariable manifestation of peptic ulceration. Diarrhea occurs in 30% of cases and is caused by hypersecretion of acid: flooding of the duodenum with acid may destroy pancreatic lipase and produce steatorrhea, damage the small bowel mucosa, and overload the intestine with gastric and pancreatic secretions. About 5% of patients present with only diarrhea.

Symptoms are often refractory to large doses of antacids. The patient may drink 3 or 4 quarts of milk daily in search of relief from pain. Hemorrhage, perforation, and obstruction are common complications. Marginal ulcers appear after surgical procedures that would cure the ordinary ulcer diathesis.

B. Laboratory Findings: Serum gastrin levels should be obtained in any patient suspected of harboring a gastrinoma. In most laboratories, normal values by radioimmunoassay are under 200 pg/ml, whereas patients with this condition have levels that usually exceed 500 pg/ml and may reach 10,000 pg/ml or more. Patients with borderline gastrin values (eg, 200–500 pg/ml) whose acid secretion is in the duodenal ulcer range should have gastrin measurement after intravenous calcium or secretin. After intravenous administration of calcium (15 mg/kg/3 hours), a rise in gastrin of 300 pg/ml is diagnostic of gastrinoma; after giving secretin (2 units/kg IV as a bolus), a rise of 100 pg/ml is diagnostic.

Serum calcium determinations may reveal hypercalcemia and lead to the discovery of one or more parathyroid adenomas.

Gastric analysis shows hypersecretion of > 15 mEq H^+ per hour basally in most ZE patients who have an intact stomach. In patients with a previous gastrectomy, basal acid output of 9 mEq/hour would be highly suggestive. Since the parietal cells are already near to maximal stimulation by endogenous gastrin, during gastric analysis there is little increase in acid production after betazole (Histalog) or pentagastrin, and the ratio of basal to maximal acid output (BAO/MAO) characteristically exceeds 0.6.

C. X-Ray Findings: Upper gastrointestinal series usually shows ulceration in the duodenal bulb, although ulcers sometimes appear in the distal duodenum or proximal jejunum. The finding of ulcers in these distal locations is nearly pathognomonic for gastrinoma. The x-ray appearance is highly suggestive. The stomach contains prominent rugal folds, and secretions are present in the lumen despite the overnight fast. The duodenum may be dilated and exhibit hyperactive peristalsis. Edema may be detected in the small bowel mucosa. The barium flocculates in the intestine, and transit time is accelerated. Selective angiography can sometimes demonstrate the pancreatic tumor.

Treatment

H_2 blocking agents (eg, cimetidine) will usually suppress acid secretion and control the clinical manifestations of the disease, at least for a while. Whether there is any place for long-term therapy with H_2 blockers for patients with Zollinger-Ellison syndrome is problematic. Nevertheless, these drugs should prevent complications while the patients are being prepared for surgery.

At present, total gastrectomy with a Roux-en-Y esophagojejunostomy is the best treatment for most patients. Removal of the tumor may seem a more attractive choice at first but runs a high risk of being incomplete since 75% of patients have multiple tumor foci. Surgical dissection frequently fails to reveal all the tumor deposits, and incomplete removal in the presence of an intact stomach may result in stormy exacerbations of the ulcer disease postoperatively, with perforation or hemorrhage.

Localized pancreatic tumors should be resected if this can be accomplished by distal pancreatectomy. The growth of many of these tumors is so indolent that few surgeons believe a radical pancreatectomy is justified for a gastrinoma in the head of the pancreas.

Prognosis

Most patients lead a relatively normal life after total gastrectomy. Weight loss and dumping are rarely severe. Children who have total gastrectomy for this disease maintain normal growth rates. Although two-thirds of gastrinomas are malignant, after total gastrectomy they generally tend to be dormant and, in the absence of residual stomach, are of no clinical significance. A few malignant gastrinomas grow, metastasize, and ultimately kill the patient.

Lifelong oral iron and parenteral vitamin B_{12} replacement are required after total gastrectomy.

Fox PS & others: The influence of total gastrectomy on survival in malignant Zollinger-Ellison tumors. Ann Surg 180:558, 1974.

Fox PS & others: Surgical management of the Zollinger-Ellison syndrome. Surg Clin North Am 54:395, 1974.

Isenberg JI & others: Zollinger-Ellison syndrome. Gastroenterology 65:140, 1973.

Richardson CT, Walsh JH: The value of a histamine H_2-receptor antagonist in the management of patients with the Zollinger-Ellison syndrome. N Engl J Med 294:133, 1976.

Way LW, Goldman L, Dunphy JE: Zollinger-Ellison syndrome. Am J Surg 116:293, 1968.

Zollinger RM & others: Observations on the postoperative tumor growth behavior of certain islet cell tumors. Ann Surg 184:525, 1976.

GASTRIC ULCER

Essentials of Diagnosis

- Epigastric pain relieved by food or antacids.
- Ulcer demonstrated by x-ray.
- Acid present on gastric analysis.

General Considerations

The peak incidence of gastric ulcer is in patients age 40–60 years, or about 10 years older than the average for those with duodenal ulcer. Ninety-five percent of gastric ulcers are located on the lesser curvature, and 60% of these are within 6 cm of the pylorus. The symptoms and complications of gastric ulcer closely resemble those of duodenal ulcer.

Gastric ulcers may be separated into 2 groups with different causes and different treatments. One type occurs in patients who have had duodenal ulcer in the past and whose x-rays show duodenal deformity in addition to gastric ulcer. Acid secretion measured by gastric analysis is in the range for duodenal ulcer. The gastric ulcer is located close to the pylorus. Surgical treatment for these patients should follow the guidelines for duodenal ulcer.

Most gastric ulcers appear de novo without an earlier history of duodenal ulcer or radiologic evidence of duodenal scarring. They are usually located within 2 cm of the boundary between parietal cell and pyloric mucosa, but always in the latter. As noted above, 95% are on the lesser curvature.

Antral gastritis is universally present in gastric ulcer, being most severe near the pylorus and gradually diminishing in sections taken progressively farther from the pylorus. Regurgitation of duodenal contents into the stomach commonly occurs in patients with gastric ulcer and is associated with pyloric sphincter dysfunction characterized by failure to contract following hormonal stimulation with secretin or cholecystokinin. Experimentally, when bile and pancreatic juice in combination bathe the gastric mucosa, atrophic gastritis ensues. These findings suggest that duodenal juice weakens the mucosal resistance of the antrum and that ulceration follows the action of acid and pepsin at the site on the pyloric mucosa where they are most concentrated.

Increasingly of late, ingestion of salicylates has been implicated as a cause of acute gastric bleeding and chronic gastric ulcers. Salicylates in an acid pH are known to damage the gastric mucosal barrier which normally prevents diffusion of acid out of the lumen of the stomach. The deleterious effects of salicylates have been demonstrated experimentally, and epidemiologic evidence reinforces the belief that these agents are a significant cause of gastric ulcer.

Dragstedt proposed that gastric ulcers were caused by stasis and an increased gastric phase of secretion. This arose from his observation that gastric ulcers sometimes developed in patients with gastric retention after vagotomy (without a drainage procedure). Stasis is a plausible explanation for gastric ulcers in patients with duodenal deformity after many years of duodenal ulcer disease but seems less likely to account for those not associated with duodenal disease. In fact, gastric emptying is unimpaired in patients with gastric ulcer. Gastrin levels are slightly higher than normal, a reflection of the low rates of acid secretion with less inhibition of the antrum.

A critical diagnostic consideration in dealing with gastric ulcer is the possibility that the niche seen on x-ray represents an ulcerated malignancy rather than a simple benign ulcer. Efforts must be expended during the *initial* stages of the work-up to establish this distinction. Despite the generally discouraging results of surgery for gastric adenocarcinoma, those whose tumors are difficult to separate from benign ulcer by x-ray have a 50–75% chance of cure after gastrectomy.

Clinical Findings

A. Symptoms and Signs: The principal symptoms are epigastric pain relieved by food or antacids, as in duodenal ulcer. Epigastric tenderness is a variable finding. Compared with duodenal ulcer, the pain in gastric ulcer tends to appear earlier after eating, often within 30 minutes. The attacks generally last longer (over 4 weeks) than those of duodenal ulcer, and the severity of symptoms is more liable to lead to loss of time from work. Vomiting, anorexia, and aggravation of pain by eating also occur with greater frequency with gastric ulcer. However, the overlap of symptoms between the 2 diseases is so great that historical information does not permit an accurate diagnosis without x-rays.

B. Laboratory Findings:

1. Gastric analysis—If gastric ulcer is accompanied by signs of active or old duodenal ulcer, the gastric analysis may show hypersecretion. If the gastric ulcer is unrelated to duodenal disease, basal and maximal acid secretion will be low or normal. Refer to pp 462–463 for details of interpreting the gastric analysis.

Achlorhydria is defined as no acid (pH > 6.0) after betazole (Histalog) stimulation. Achlorhydria is incompatible with the diagnosis of benign peptic ulcer and would imply malignancy in a gastric ulcer. About 5% of malignant gastric ulcers will be associated with this finding.

2. Biopsy and cytology—Examination of cells in gastric washings should be done in all patients with gastric ulcer shortly after diagnosis. In expert hands, cytologic examination can detect 90–95% of gastric malignancies. The errors of cytology tend to be false negatives; a positive report for malignancy is highly reliable. Biopsy and cytology specimens obtained directly from the lesion during endoscopy are even more valuable in differentiating benign from malignant ulcers.

C. X-Ray Findings: Upper gastrointestinal x-rays will show an ulcer usually on the lesser curvature in the pyloric area. In the absence of a tumor mass, the following suggest that the ulcer is malignant: (1) the deepest penetration of the ulcer is not beyond the expected border of the gastric wall; (2) presence of the meniscus sign, a prominent rim of radiolucency surrounding the ulcer, caused by heaped-up edges of tumor; and (3) malignancy is more common (10%) in ulcers greater than 2 cm in diameter. Coexistence of duodenal deformity or ulcer favors a diagnosis of benign ulcer in the stomach.

D. Gastroscopy: Gastroscopy should be performed as part of the initial work-up of patients with gastric ulcer to attempt to find malignant lesions. The rolled-up margins of the ulcer that produce the meniscus sign on x-ray can be distinguished from the flat edges characteristic of a benign ulcer. Multiple (3–6) biopsy specimens and brush biopsy should be routinely obtained from the edge of the lesion.

Differential Diagnosis

The characteristic symptoms of gastric ulcer are often clouded by numerous nonspecific complaints. In fact, it is impossible to rely on historical information alone for diagnosis in the average patient who presents with dyspepsia as a chief complaint. Uncomplicated hiatal hernia, atrophic gastritis, chronic cholecystitis, irritable colon syndrome, and undifferentiated functional problems are distinguishable from peptic ulcer only after appropriate radiologic studies and sometimes not even then.

X-rays, gastroscopy, gastric cytology, and gastric analysis should all be performed to attempt to rule out malignant gastric ulcer. Even after the results of these tests have been considered and the ulcer is judged to be benign, about 4% will prove to be malignant.

At this point, treatment is instituted. Healing of the ulcer is desirable not only to rid the patient of his symptoms but also to demonstrate that the ulcer was in fact benign. Failure of the ulcer to heal after 6–12 weeks suggests that it may be malignant.

Complications

Bleeding, obstruction, and perforation are the principal complications of gastric ulcer. They are discussed separately under those headings elsewhere in this chapter.

Treatment

A. Medical Treatment: Medical management of gastric ulcer is the same as for duodenal ulcer. The patient should be questioned regarding the use of ulcerogenic agents, and they should be eliminated as far as possible. Detailed inquiry should be made for excessive use of salicylates. The physician may have to list each of the popular remedies which contain this compound, because patients often fail to appreciate the thrust of the questioning and deny taking aspirin when large amounts of Anacin or Alka-Seltzer are a daily habit.

The diet and antacid regimen outlined in the section on treatment of duodenal ulcer should be started if the severity of symptoms does not require hospitalization. If symptomatic relief does not result within 1–2 weeks, hospitalization is advisable. Repeat x-rays should be obtained to document the rate of healing. After 6 weeks, healing usually has reached a plateau. At this point, treatment must be individualized according to circumstances. The medical regimen might be continued for the elderly poor-risk patient. Gastrectomy is recommended for the patient who has no contraindications to surgery. Whenever one elects to prolong medical treatment at this stage, he must understand that the failure to heal indicates a significant possibility that the ulcer is malignant. Therefore,

gastroscopy and cytologic studies should be repeated.

The ulcerative process in small carcinomas may well be due to acid-peptic digestion since partial healing on a regimen of antacids is common for lesions subsequently shown to be tumors. Therefore, healing should be followed to completion in all cases before the ulcer can be accepted as truly benign. Even then, a follow-up x-ray is advisable 6–12 months later as a further check on the absence of malignancy.

Carbenoxolone sodium and deglycyrrhizinated licorice have both been shown by randomized clinical trials to hasten healing of gastric ulcers. These drugs are in widespread use in many countries but are not yet available in the USA.

In general, gastric ulcers are difficult to cure medically, recur frequently, and cause more severe symptoms than duodenal ulcers. In ulcers which fail to heal, malignancy cannot be excluded. For these reasons–plus the fact that gastrectomy cures gastric ulcer so efficiently–surgical treatment is advised in many of these patients.

B. Surgical Treatment: Patients with gastric ulcers located near the pylorus associated with increased acid secretion and x-ray changes similar to those of duodenal ulcer should be treated as outlined in the section on duodenal ulcer.

For patients with simple gastric ulcer not related to duodenal ulcer, a 40–50% gastrectomy and Billroth I reconstruction should be performed. The absence of duodenal disease facilitates the surgeon's task and reduces the risk of immediate postoperative complications. The recurrence rate is negligible (about 1%), and the long-term results are excellent. All late postgastrectomy problems except anemia are less common than after gastrectomy for duodenal ulcer.

Ordinarily, the ulcer is easily encompassed by the usual resection. When the ulcer is higher on the lesser curvature than the resection would otherwise extend, it is not necessary to remove 75% or more of the stomach; in these cases, a distal gastrectomy can be performed and the ulcer either locally excised or biopsied and oversewn (Kelling-Madlener procedure).

In recent years, vagotomy and pyloroplasty has been tried for gastric ulcer. The operation is highly successful, but the overall results are not quite as good as with gastrectomy. Unless an additional step is taken to excise the ulcer, an occasional patient will be left with a malignancy intact. Failure of the ulcer to heal or recurrent ulceration has been more frequent, and postvagotomy diarrhea complicates the course in a small percentage of cases. The place of vagotomy and pyloroplasty would seem to be in those patients who are poor risks for the additional surgical manipulation and operating time entailed in gastrectomy. Most of these are patients with acute complications from their ulcers such as hemorrhage or perforation.

Davis Z & others: The surgically treated chronic gastric ulcer: An extended follow-up. Ann Surg 185:205, 1977.
Duthie HL, Kwong NK: Vagotomy or gastrectomy for gastric ulcer. Br Med J 4:79, 1973.

Fisher RS, Boden G: Reversibility of pyloric sphincter dysfunction in gastric ulcer. Gastroenterology 69:591, 1975.

Grossman MI: The Veterans Administration cooperative study on gastric ulcer. Chapter 10: Resumé and comment. Gastroenterology 61:635, 1971.

Ivey KJ, Clifton JA: Back diffusion of hydrogen ions across gastric mucosa of patients with gastric ulcer and rheumatoid arthritis. Br Med J 1:16, 1974.

Jensen H-E & others: Bleeding gastric ulcer. Scand J Gastroenterol 7:535, 1972.

Kraus M & others: Prognosis of gastric ulcer: Twenty-five year follow-up. Ann Surg 184:471, 1976.

Langman MJS, Knapp DR, Wakley EJ: Treatment of chronic gastric ulcer with carbenoxolone and gefarnate: A comparative trial. Br Med J 3:84, 1973.

Montgomery RD, Richardson BP: Gastric ulcer and cancer. Q J Med 44:591, 1975.

Rhodes J: Etiology of gastric ulcer. Gastroenterology 63:171, 1972.

Sapala JA, Ponka JL: Operative treatment of benign gastric ulcers. Am J Surg 125:19, 1973.

Wilson WJ & others: The computer analysis and diagnosis of gastric ulcers. Radiology 85:1064, 1965.

UPPER GASTROINTESTINAL HEMORRHAGE

Upper gastrointestinal hemorrhage may be mild or severe but should always be considered an ominous manifestation that deserves thorough evaluation. Bleeding is the most common serious complication of peptic ulcer, portal hypertension, and gastritis, and these conditions taken together account for most episodes of upper gastrointestinal bleeding in the average hospital population.

The major factors that determine the diagnostic and therapeutic approach are the amount and rate of bleeding. Estimates of both should be made promptly and monitored and revised continuously until the episode has been resolved.

Hematemesis or melena is present except when the rate of blood loss is minimal. **Hematemesis** of either bright-red or dark blood indicates that the source is proximal to the ligament of Treitz. It is more common from bleeding that originates in the stomach or esophagus. In general, hematemesis denotes a more rapidly bleeding lesion, and a high percentage of patients who vomit blood require surgery. Coffee-ground vomitus is due to vomiting of blood which has been in the stomach long enough for gastric acid to convert hemoglobin to methemoglobin.

Most patients with **melena** (passage of black or tarry stools) are bleeding from the upper gastrointestinal tract, but melena can be produced by blood entering the bowel at any point from mouth to cecum. The conversion of red blood to dark depends more on the time it resides in the intestine than the site of origin. The black color of melenic stools is probably caused by hematin, the product of oxidation of heme by intestinal and bacterial enzymes. Melena can be produced by as little as 50–100 ml of blood in the stomach. When 1 liter of blood was instilled into the upper intestine of experimental subjects, melena persisted for 3–5 days, which points out that the rate of change in character of the stool is a poor guide to the time bleeding stopped after an episode of hemorrhage.

Hematochezia is defined as the passage of bright-red blood from the rectum. Bright-red rectal blood can be produced by bleeding from the colon, rectum, or anus. However, if intestinal transit is rapid during brisk bleeding in the upper intestine, bright-red blood may be passed unchanged in the stool.

Tests for Occult Blood

Normal subjects lose about 2.5 ml of blood per day in their stools, presumably from minor mechanical abrasions of the intestinal epithelium. Between 50 and 100 ml of blood per day will produce melena. Tests for occult blood in the stool should be able to detect amounts between 10 and 50 ml/day. False-positive results may be due to dietary hemoglobin, myoglobin, or peroxidases of plant origin. Iron ingestion does not give positive reactions. The various tests using guaiac, benzidine, phenolphthalein, or orthotolidine have similar specificities. The sensitivity of the guaiac slide test (Hemoccult) is in the desired range and is the best one available at present.

Initial Management

In an apparently healthy patient, melena of a week or more suggests that the bleeding is slow. In this type of patient, admission to the hospital should be followed by a deliberate but nonemergent work-up. However, patients who present with hematemesis or sudden melena should be handled as if exsanguination were imminent until this possibility has been investigated thoroughly. The clinical approach entails a simultaneous series of diagnostic and therapeutic steps with the following initial goals: (1) Rapidly assess the status of the circulatory system and replace blood loss as necessary. (2) Determine the amount and rate of bleeding. (3) Slow or stop the bleeding by ice water lavage. (4) Discover the lesion responsible for the episode. The last step may lead to more specific treatment appropriate to the underlying condition.

The patient should be admitted to the hospital promptly regardless of the initial apparent severity of bleeding. Historical information should be gathered about the acute problem and other major health data. Peptic ulcer, acute gastritis, esophageal varices, esophagitis, and Mallory-Weiss tear account for over 90% of cases, and questions concerning the major symptoms and predisposing factors of each may be asked in a few moments' time. The patient should be asked about salicylate intake and any history of a bleeding tendency. This information should be obtained while resuscitation is in progress if the patient requires immediate treatment.

Of the diseases commonly responsible for acute upper gastrointestinal bleeding, only portal hypertension is associated with diagnostic findings on physical examination. However, the clinician must be careful not to automatically attribute gastrointestinal bleeding in a patient with jaundice, ascites, splenomegaly, spider angiomas, or hepatomegaly to esophageal varices; over half of cirrhotic patients who present with acute hemorrhage are bleeding from gastritis or peptic ulcer. Therefore, additional diagnostic information must be obtained in these patients before specific therapy can be planned.

Blood should be drawn for cross-matching, packed cell volume, hemoglobin, creatinine, and tests of liver function. An intravenous infusion of 0.15 N NaCl solution should be started and, in the massive bleeder, a large-bore (32–36F) Ewald nasogastric tube inserted. In cases of melena, the gastric aspirate should be examined to verify the gastroduodenal source of the hemorrhage, but about 25% of patients with bleeding duodenal ulcers have gastric aspirates that test negatively for the presence of blood. The tube must be larger than the standard nasogastric tube (16F) so the stomach can be lavaged free of liquid blood and clots. After the gastric contents have been removed, the stomach should be irrigated with a large syringe and copious amounts of ice water or saline solution until blood no longer returns. Then the tube should be attached to continuous suction so that further blood loss can be measured. When the bleeding has stopped, the large tube may be replaced with a smaller one.

If the patient was bleeding at the time the nasogastric tube was inserted, iced saline irrigation usually stops it. If bleeding continues or if tachycardia or lowered blood pressure is present, the patient should be monitored and treated as for hemorrhagic shock. A central venous pressure line should be inserted to serve as a guide to blood replacement and an indwelling urinary catheter placed for hourly determination of urine output—an indication of tissue perfusion.

The most critical signs indicating the need for rapid transfusion are syncope, shock, tachycardia, and hypotension. Any of these combined with a history of acute blood loss demands prompt transfusion.

In acute rapid hemorrhage, the hematocrit may be normal or only slightly lowered. A very low hematocrit without obvious signs of shock indicates more prolonged blood loss. Shock requires whole blood transfusion, but packed cells are preferable to raise a chronically low hematocrit to normal.

All of these steps can be made within 1 or 2 hours after the acutely bleeding patient has entered the hospital. In most instances, this aggressive approach will result in a patient whose bleeding is at least temporarily under control, whose blood volume has been restored to normal, and who is being adequately monitored so that recurrent bleeding can be detected immediately and its rate determined. When this stage is reached, additional diagnostic tests should be performed.

Diagnosis of Cause of Bleeding

In most cases, when the patient becomes stable enough for further evaluation, the first diagnostic measure is endoscopic examination of the upper gastrointestinal region. The examination can be performed at the patient's bedside, but a more satisfactory study can usually be obtained if the patient can be moved to a special endoscopy suite. The patient should be studied as soon as practical after his condition has become stable so that the source can be identified while bleeding is still active. Thus, if it is successful, endoscopy provides a direct estimate of cause of hemorrhage rather than the indirect evidence available from barium upper gastrointestinal x-rays. Fiberoptic endoscopy has been shown to be more accurate than x-rays in demonstrating bleeding from peptic ulcers, acute gastritis, Mallory-Weiss tears, and esophagitis. The 2 methods are about equally useful in demonstrating esophageal varices, but endoscopy is more likely than x-ray to settle the question whether the varices were actually responsible for the bleeding episode. In most patients, an upper gastrointestinal x-ray examination should be obtained sometime within 24 hours of endoscopy.

Several new technics to control gastroduodenal bleeding without operation are presently being developed and evaluated. One of these, selective angiography, has both diagnostic and therapeutic usefulness. For diagnosis, it is most helpful when other studies fail to demonstrate the cause of bleeding, a situation most commonly encountered when the site is distal to the ligament of Treitz. Infusion through the angiographic catheter of vasoconstrictors (eg, vasopressin) and embolization of the bleeding vessel with autologous clot or Gelfoam have been tried as ways to halt the bleeding. The former, which has received a wider trial, seems to be effective if the source of the bleeding is a small vessel (eg, gastritis, stress ulcer, Mallory-Weiss tear), but it is ineffective for chronic peptic ulcers that bleed. From the practical standpoint, angiography is logistically complicated and the examination usually requires several hours even when performed by experienced personnel. Considerable judgment is required to decide when it is more likely to be a benefit rather than a hindrance in patient management. Other methods being investigated include use of topical vasoconstrictors (eg, levarterenol) in the gastric lumen, electrocoagulation and laser beam coagulation via the endoscope, and topical application of tissue adhesives.

Later Management

Although a precise diagnosis of the cause of the bleeding may be valuable in later management, the patient must not be allowed to slip out of clinical control during the search for definitive diagnostic information. The indication for emergency surgery depends more on the response to immediate gastric lavage and the rate of blood loss than the specific cause of bleeding. The major exception to this rule is bleeding from esophageal varices. For varices, both nonsurgical and surgical approaches vary significantly from those pertaining to the other common causes of massive hemorrhage. Endoscopy should be performed as early as feasible in patients who seem to have varices, keeping in mind that no segment of the population is entirely free of alcoholism or other causes of portal hypertension.

The need for transfusion should be determined on a continuing basis, and blood volume must be maintained. Blood pressure, pulse, central venous pressure, hematocrit, hourly urinary volume, and amount of blood obtained from the gastric tube or from the rectum all enter into this assessment. Older notions that bleeding might subside more often if the blood volume were incompletely replenished have been rejected. However, many clinical studies have documented the tendency to underestimate blood loss and inadequately transfuse massively bleeding patients who truly need aggressive therapy. Continued slow bleeding is best followed by serial determinations of the hematocrit.

Several factors are associated with a worse prognosis with continued medical management of the bleeding episode. Most of these are not absolute indications for laparotomy, but they should alert the clinician that emergency surgery may be required.

High rates of bleeding or amounts of blood loss predict high failure rates with medical treatment. Hematemesis is usually associated with more rapid bleeding and a greater blood volume deficit than melena. The presence of hypotension on admission to the hospital or the need for more than 4 units of blood to obtain circulatory stability implies a worse prognosis; if bleeding continues and subsequent transfusion requirements exceed 1 unit every 8 hours, continued medical management is usually unwise.

Total transfusion requirements also correlate with mortality. Death is uncommon when less than 7 units of blood have been used, and the mortality rate rises progressively thereafter. This observation has sometimes been misinterpreted to mean that operation should be considered only after the patient has required 7 units, a policy that would regularly result in a 9–12 unit hemorrhage before surgical control could be achieved in rapid bleeders.

In general, bleeding from a gastric ulcer is more dangerous than bleeding from gastritis or duodenal ulcer, and patients with gastric ulcer should be always considered for early surgery. Regardless of the cause, if bleeding recurs after it had initially stopped, the chances of success without operation are low. Recurrent bleeding in the hospital is accepted by most clinicians as a clear indication for immediate laparotomy.

Lastly, patients over age 60 tolerate continued blood loss less well than younger patients and should not be permitted to bleed until secondary cardiovascular, pulmonary, or renal complications arise.

HEMORRHAGE FROM PEPTIC ULCER

Approximately 20% of patients with peptic ulcer will experience a bleeding episode, and this complication is responsible for about 40% of the deaths from

Table 26—3. Causes of massive upper gastrointestinal hemorrhage. Note that malignancies are rarely the cause of massive bleeding.

	Relative Incidence*	
Common causes		
Peptic ulcer		55%
Duodenal ulcer	40%	
Gastric ulcer	15%	
Esophageal varices		10%
Gastritis		20%
Mallory-Weiss syndrome		10%
Uncommon causes		5%
Gastric carcinoma		
Esophagitis		
Pancreatitis		
Hematobilia		
Duodenal diverticulum		

*Considerable variation can be expected in the relative incidence between different patient populations. The incidence of gastritis as a cause of bleeding reflects the frequency of early endoscopy as a diagnostic measure.

peptic ulcer. Peptic ulcer is the most common cause of massive upper gastrointestinal hemorrhage, accounting for over half of all cases. Other causes are listed in Table 26—3. Chronic gastric and duodenal ulcers have about the same tendency to bleed, but the former produce more severe episodes. Bleeding ulcers are more common in persons with blood group O, although the reason for this association is not known.

Bleeding ulcers in the duodenum are usually located on the posterior surface of the duodenal bulb. As the ulcer penetrates, the gastroduodenal artery is exposed and may become eroded. Since no major blood vessels lie on the anterior surface of the duodenal bulb, ulcerations at this point are not as prone to bleed. Patients with concomitant bleeding and perforation usually have 2 ulcers, a bleeding posterior ulcer and a perforated anterior one. Postbulbar ulcers (those in the second portion of the duodenum) bleed frequently, although ulcers in this area are much less common than those near the pylorus.

In some patients, the bleeding is sudden and massive, manifested by hematemesis and shock. In others, chronic anemia and weakness due to slow blood loss may be the only findings. The diagnosis is often suggested by a history of typical ulcer pain. In fact, the presence of a chronic ulcer has in some cases been well documented before the patient presents with acute bleeding. However, previous ulcer symptoms may not be present. Although there may be epigastric tenderness on abdominal examination, the finding is not of much diagnostic value.

In the preceding section, the management of acute upper gastrointestinal hemorrhage, the selection of diagnostic tests, and the factors suggesting the need for operation were discussed. Most patients (75%) with bleeding peptic ulcer can be successfully managed by medical means alone. Initial therapeutic efforts usually halt the bleeding. At this point, antacids should be given hourly, although some prefer to drip them continuously into the stomach through the nasogastric tube. After 12–24 hours have passed and the bleeding has clearly stopped, the patient should be fed at frequent intervals if he feels hungry. Twice daily hematocrit readings should be ordered as a check on slow continued blood loss. Anticholinergic drugs are of uncertain value and are avoided by some because their effect on the heart rate may interfere with the assessment of persistent or recurrent bleeding. Stools should be tested daily for the presence of blood, remembering that they will usually remain guaiac-positive for several days after the bleeding stops.

Rebleeding in the hospital has been attended by a mortality rate of about 25%, and a policy of early surgery for those who rebled would improve this figure. Patients who present with hematemesis and those whose hemoglobin falls below 8 g/100 ml have a higher risk of rebleeding. About 3 times as many patients with gastric ulcer (30%) rebled compared with those with duodenal ulcer. Most instances of rebleeding occur within 2 days from the time the first episode stopped. In one study, only 3% of patients who stopped bleeding for this long bled again.

Emergency Surgery

About 25% of patients bleeding from a peptic ulcer will require emergency surgery. Selection of those most likely to survive with surgical compared with medical treatment rests on the rate of blood loss and the other factors associated with a poor prognosis.

The patient should be brought into as good hemodynamic balance as possible. Sometimes it is not possible to entirely replace the blood deficit because bleeding is too rapid, but this is rare. Elderly patients are particularly difficult to manage because cardiac disability may make the line between too little and too much blood transfusion a fine one. Emergency treatment with digitalis may be useful at times.

The type of operation most appropriate for the emergency control of bleeding ulcer has been a subject of considerable controversy in the past 15 years. The question was whether vagotomy and pyloroplasty with suture of the bleeding site is preferable to gastrectomy. Vagotomy and pyloroplasty has the advantage of technical simplicity and therefore, perhaps, a lower operative mortality but was also thought to be less effective in preventing rebleeding. Convincing evidence has gradually accumulated to show that the overall mortality is significantly less after vagotomy and pyloroplasty and that rebleeding appears with about equal frequency after either procedure.

When laparotomy is performed, the first step should be to make a pyloroplasty incision. If a duodenal ulcer is present, the bleeding vessel should be ligated with sutures of nonabsorbable material and the duodenum and antrum inspected for additional ulcers. The pyloroplasty incision should then be closed and a truncal vagotomy performed. If the posterior wall of the duodenal bulb has been destroyed by a giant duodenal ulcer, a gastrectomy and Billroth II gastrojejunostomy would be preferable since these somewhat uncommon ulcers are especially prone to bleed again if left in continuity with the stomach. Gastric ulcers can be handled either by gastrectomy or vagotomy and pyloroplasty. A thorough search should always be made for second ulcers or other causes of bleeding.

On occasion, the bleeding point is not immediately found after the first inspection through the pyloroplasty incision. In these patients, the surgeon must consider uncommon causes of bleeding such as postbulbar ulcers, hematobilia, and bleeding esophagitis. Mallory-Weiss tears of the gastroesophageal mucosa are especially difficult to locate because they are small, unaccompanied by surrounding inflammation, and hidden within the rugae of the proximal stomach. A separate long gastrotomy and painstaking exploration are required to find these lesions.

Elective Surgery for Bleeding Ulcer

Since most patients stop bleeding under medical therapy, a plan must be made for their subsequent management. About a third of patients who bleed once do so for a second time within the next 5 years. Patients who have bled twice in the past have double the risk of rebleeding. Elective surgery can reduce the chances of additional hemorrhage to about 5–8%. The inability to achieve even better results probably reflects the more virulent nature of the ulcer diathesis in these patients. Early surgical treatment should generally be recommended for those who have had substantial chronic disability preceding their acute hemorrhage or for those with a giant duodenal ulcer. Young patients whose hemorrhage was the first manifestation of disease, those in whom an ulcerogenic agent is detected such as excessive salicylate ingestion, and those whose bleeding was minor might be expected to do better with good medical therapy. The large group of patients between these extremes must be individualized, since there is no proved best course. In general, they should be given vigorous medical treatment but referred for elective surgery if remissions cannot be achieved or maintained. If a second bleeding attack occurs on medical therapy, early surgery would be advisable.

Prognosis

The mortality rate for an acute massive hemorrhage is about 15% in most reported series. Careful study of the causes of death suggests that this figure could be improved by (1) more precise blood replacement—since undertransfusion is the cause of some of the morbidity and mortality; and (2) earlier surgery in selected patients who fall into serious-risk categories—since the tendency has been to perform surgery on too few patients and to do it too late in the illness.

Conn JH & others: Massive hemorrhage from peptic ulcer: Evaluation of methods of surgical control. Ann Surg 169:784, 1969.

Douglass HO Jr: Levarterenol irrigation: Control of massive gastrointestinal bleeding in poor-risk patients. JAMA 230:1653, 1974.

Eisenberg H, Steer ML: The nonoperative treatment of massive pyloroduodenal hemorrhage by retracted clot embolization. Surgery 79:414, 1976.

Foster JH, Hickok DF, Dunphy JE: Factors influencing mortality following emergency operation for massive upper gastrointestinal hemorrhage. Surg Gynecol Obstet 117:257, 1963.

Hallenbeck GA: Elective surgery for treatment of hemorrhage from duodenal ulcer. Gastroenterology 59:784, 1970.

Halmagyi AF: A critical review of 425 patients with upper gastrointestinal hemorrhage. Surg Gynecol Obstet 130:419, 1970.

Harvey RF, Langman MJS: The late results of medical and surgical treatment for bleeding duodenal ulcer. Q J Med 39:539, 1970.

Himal HS & others: The management of upper gastrointestinal hemorrhage: A multiparametric computer analysis. Ann Surg 179:489, 1974.

Irving JD, Northfield TC: Emergency arteriography in acute gastrointestinal bleeding. Br Med J 1:929, 1976.

Johnson WC, Widrich WC: Efficacy of selective splanchnic arteriography and vasopressin perfusion in diagnosis and treatment of gastrointestinal hemorrhage. Am J Surg 131:481, 1976.

Levy M: Aspirin use in patients with major upper gastrointestinal bleeding and peptic-ulcer disease: A report from the Boston Collaborative Drug Surveillance Program. N Engl J Med 290:1158, 1974.

Lightdale CJ & others: Cancer and upper gastrointestinal tract hemorrhage. JAMA 226:139, 1973.

Malt RA: Control of massive upper gastrointestinal hemorrhage. N Engl J Med 286:1043, 1972.

McGregor DB & others: Massive gastrointestinal hemorrhage: A twenty-five year experience with vagotomy and drainage. Surgery 80:530, 1976.

Morris DW & others: Prospective randomized study of diagnosis and outcome in acute upper-gastrointestinal bleeding: Endoscopy versus conventional radiography. Am J Dig Dis 20:1103, 1975.

Northfield TC: Factors predisposing to recurrent hemorrhage after acute gastrointestinal bleeding. Br Med J 1:26, 1971.

Palmer ED: Upper gastrointestinal hemorrhage. JAMA 231:853, 1975.

Read RC, Huebl HC, Thal AP: Randomized study of massive bleeding from peptic ulceration. Ann Surg 162:561, 1965.

Schiller KFR, Truelove SC, Williams DG: Haematemesis and melaena, with special reference to factors influencing the outcome. Br Med J 2:7, 1970.

Stafford ES & others: Benign gastric ulcer with life-threatening hemorrhage. Ann Surg 165:967, 1967.

MALLORY-WEISS SYNDROME

Mallory-Weiss syndrome is responsible for about 10% of cases of acute hemorrhage from the upper gastrointestinal region. This lesion consists of a 1–4 cm longitudinal tear in the gastric mucosa near the esophagogastric junction which usually follows a bout of forceful retching. The disruption extends through the mucosa and submucosa but not usually into the muscularis mucosae. About 75% are confined to the stomach; 20% straddle the esophagogastric junction; and 5% are entirely within the distal esophagus. Two-thirds of patients have a hiatal hernia.

The majority of patients are alcoholics, but the lesion may appear after severe retching for any reason. Several cases have been reported following closed chest cardiac massage.

Clinical Findings

If a good history can be obtained, it is of more diagnostic importance in this condition than in the other major causes of acute gastric bleeding. Typically, the patient first vomits food and gastric contents. This is followed by forceful retching, and then bloody vomitus. Rapid increases in gastric pressure, sometimes aggravated by hiatal hernia, undoubtedly cause the mucosal rift. Actual rupture of the distal esophagus can also be produced by vomiting (Boerhaave's syndrome), but the difference seems to depend on vomiting of food in rupture and nonproductive retching in gastric mucosal tear. During retching, the esophagogastric sphincter does not relax, and the sudden rise in pressure from abdominal and antral contraction is focused at the point where Mallory-Weiss tears appear.

The diagnosis may be strongly suspected if a typical history is obtained. Esophagogastroscopy is the most practical means of making the diagnosis before operation. Barium x-ray examination cannot demonstrate the lesion, but there have been reports on the successful use of selective angiography to show the site of bleeding.

Treatment & Prognosis

Initially the patient is handled according to the general measures prescribed for upper gastrointestinal hemorrhage. In about 90% of patients, the bleeding stops spontaneously after ice water lavage of the stomach. An intravenous infusion of vasopressin (0.4–0.6 units/minute) may be useful in a few patients. If bleeding persists, surgical repair of the tear will be required. The gastric balloon of the Sengstaken-Blakemore tube fails to tamponade the hemorrhage, and in several instances where it was used it was thought to further extend the tear.

If the diagnosis has been made before laparotomy, the surgeon should make a long (10–12 cm), high gastrotomy after the abdomen is opened. The tear may be difficult to adequately expose. The search must be meticulous, since in about 25% of patients there are 2 tears. A running suture of nonabsorbable material should be used to oversew the lesion. Postoperative recurrence is rare.

Foster DN & others: Diagnosis of Mallory-Weiss lesions. Lancet 2:483, 1976.

Holmes KD: Mallory-Weiss syndrome: Review of 20 cases and literature review. Ann Surg 164:810, 1966.

Knauer CM: Mallory-Weiss syndrome. Gastroenterology 71:5, 1976.

St. John DJB & others: The Mallory-Weiss syndrome. Br Med J 1:140, 1974.

Weaver DH, Maxwell JG, Castleton KB: Mallory-Weiss syndrome. Am J Surg 118:887, 1969.

PYLORIC OBSTRUCTION DUE TO PEPTIC ULCER

The cycles of inflammation and repair in peptic ulcer disease may cause obstruction of the gastroduodenal junction as a result of edema, muscular spasm, and scarring. To the extent that the first 2 factors are involved, the obstruction may be reversible with medical treatment. Obstruction is usually due to duodenal ulcer and is less common than either bleeding or perforation. The few gastric ulcers that obstruct are close to the pylorus. Obstruction due to peptic ulcer must be differentiated from that caused by an antral malignancy.

Clinical Findings

A. Symptoms and Signs: The great majority of patients with obstruction have a long history of symptomatic peptic ulcer, and as many as 30% have been treated for perforation or obstruction in the past. The patient often notes gradually increasing ulcer pains over weeks or months with the eventual development of anorexia, vomiting, and failure to gain relief from antacids. The vomitus often contains food ingested several hours previously, and absence of bile staining reflects the site of blockage. Weight loss may be marked if the patient has delayed seeking medical care.

Dehydration and malnutrition may be obvious on physical examination but are not always present. A succussion splash can usually be elicited from the retained gastric contents. Peristalsis of the distended stomach may be visible on gross inspection of the abdomen, but this sign is relatively rare. Most patients have upper abdominal tenderness. Tetany may appear with advanced alkalosis.

B. Laboratory Findings: A significant degree of anemia is found in about 25% of patients. Prolonged vomiting leads to a unique form of metabolic alkalosis with dehydration. Measurement of serum electrolytes shows hypochloremia, hypokalemia, hyponatremia, and increased bicarbonate. Vomiting depletes the patient of Na^+, K^+, and Cl^-; the latter is lost in excess of Na^+ and K^+ as HCl. Gastric HCl loss causes extracellular HCO_3^- to rise, and renal excretion of HCO_3^- increases in an attempt to maintain pH. Large amounts of Na^+ are excreted in the urine with the HCO_3^-. Increasing Na^+ deficit evokes aldosterone secretion, which in turn brings about renal Na^+ conservation at the expense of more renal loss of K^+ and H^+. GFR may drop and produce a prerenal azotemia. The eventual result of the process is a marked deficit of Na^+, Cl^-, K^+, and H_2O. Treatment involves replacement of water and NaCl until a satisfactory urine flow has been established. KCl replacement should then be started. Details of management are found in Chapter 12.

C. Saline Load Test: This is a simple means to assess the degree of pyloric obstruction and is useful in following the patient's progress during the first few days of nasogastric suction.

Through the nasogastric tube, 700 ml of normal saline (at room temperature) are infused over 3–5 minutes and the tube is clamped. Thirty minutes later, the stomach is aspirated and the residual volume of saline recorded. Recovery of more than 350 ml indicates obstruction.

D. X-Ray Findings: Plain abdominal x-rays may show a large gastric fluid level. An upper gastrointestinal series should not be performed until the stomach has been emptied because dilution of the barium in the retained secretions makes a worthwhile study impossible.

E. Special Examinations: Gastroscopy is usually indicated to rule out the presence of an obstructing neoplasm.

Treatment

A. Medical Treatment: A large (32F) Ewald tube should be passed and the stomach emptied of its contents and lavaged until clean. A large tube is necessary because particles of food cannot be withdrawn through the regular nasogastric tube. After completely decompressing the stomach, a smaller tube should be inserted and placed on suction for several days to allow pyloric edema and spasm to subside and to permit the gastric musculature to regain its tone. A saline load test may be performed at this point as a baseline for later comparison. Anticholinergic drugs should be withheld.

The gastric aspirate should be examined for acid content and malignant cells. Absence of acid (pH > 6.0) would suggest that the block is caused by a malignancy.

After decompressing the stomach for 48–72 hours, the tube should be withdrawn and the saline load test repeated. If this indicates sufficient improvement, a liquid diet may be started. Gradual resumption of a solid diet is permitted as tolerated.

An upper gastrointestinal series should be performed at the end of the period of recovery. If a malignancy is still suspected—and especially if gastric emptying does not improve—the obstruction should be examined by gastroscopy.

B. Surgical Treatment: If 3–4 days of gastric aspiration do not result in some relief of the obstruction, the patient should be treated surgically. Persistence of nonoperative effort beyond this period in the absence of progress rarely achieves the hoped-for result and often allows the patient to deteriorate as an operative candidate.

Surgical treatment may consist either of a vagotomy and drainage procedure (Fig 26–9) or gastrectomy. Earlier fears that vagotomy in this type of patient would be complicated by delayed gastric emptying have not been realized. Either procedure is satisfactory provided gastric tonus has been restored by adequate decompression.

Prognosis

About two-thirds of patients with acute obstruction fail to improve sufficiently on medical therapy and require operation to relieve the blockage. The need for surgery in those whose acute obstruction resolves

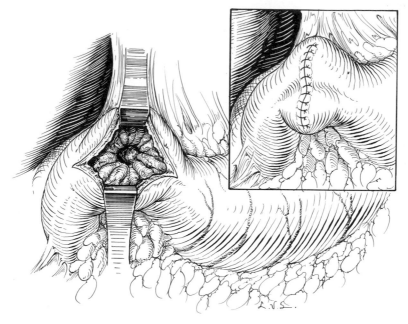

Figure 26—9. Heineke-Mikulicz pyloroplasty. A longitudinal incision has been made across the pylorus, revealing an active ulcer in the duodenal bulb. The insert shows the transverse closure of the incision which widens the gastric outlet. The accompanying vagotomy is not shown.

with suction may be based on the severity of persistent symptoms.

Boyle JD, Goldstein H: Management of pyloric obstruction. Med Clin North Am 52:1329, 1968.

DeMatteis RA, Hermann RE: Vagotomy and drainage for obstructing duodenal ulcers. Am J Surg 127:237, 1974.

Hermann RE: Obstructing duodenal ulcer. Surg Clin North Am 56:1403, 1976.

Howe CT, LeQuesne LP: Pyloric stenosis: The metabolic effects. Br J Surg 51:923, 1964.

Kozoll DD, Meyer KA: Obstructing gastroduodenal ulcers: Symptoms and signs. Arch Surg 89:491, 1964.

PERFORATED PEPTIC ULCER

Perforation complicates peptic ulcer about half as often as hemorrhage. Most perforated ulcers are located anteriorly, although occasionally gastric ulcers perforate into the lesser sac. The 15% mortality rate correlates with increased age, female sex, and gastric perforations. The diagnosis is overlooked in about 5%, most of whom do not survive.

Anterior ulcers tend to perforate instead of bleed because of the absence of protective viscera and major blood vessels on this surface. In less than 10%, acute bleeding from a posterior "kissing" ulcer complicates the anterior perforation, an association which carries a high mortality rate. Immediately after the perforation occurs, the peritoneal cavity is flooded with gastroduodenal secretions which elicit a chemical peritonitis.

Early cultures show either no growth or a light growth of streptococci or enteric bacilli. Gradually, over 12 hours or more, the process evolves into a full-blown bacterial peritonitis. The morbidity and mortality are directly related to the interval between the acute event and surgical closure of the perforation.

In an unknown percentage of cases, the perforation becomes sealed by adherence to the undersurface of the liver. In such patients, the process may be self-limited, but a subphrenic abscess will develop in many.

Clinical Findings

A. Symptoms and Signs: The perforation usually elicits a sudden, severe upper abdominal pain whose onset can be recalled precisely. The patient may or may not have had preceding chronic symptoms of peptic ulcer disease. Perforation rarely is heralded by nausea or vomiting, and it typically occurs several hours after the last meal. Shoulder pain, if present, reflects diaphragmatic irritation. Back pain is uncommon.

The initial reaction consists of a chemical peritonitis caused by gastric acid or bile and pancreatic enzymes. The peritoneal reaction dilutes these irritants with a thin exudate, and as a result the patient's symptoms may temporarily improve before progressing to bacterial peritonitis. If the physician sees the patient for the first time during this symptomatic lull, he must not be misled into interpreting it as representing bona fide improvement.

The patient appears severely distressed, lying quietly with his knees drawn up and breathing shallowly to minimize abdominal motion. Fever is absent at the start. The abdominal muscles are rigid owing to severe involuntary spasm. Epigastric tenderness may not be as marked as expected because the board-like rigidity protects the abdominal viscera from the palpating hand. Air escaped from the stomach may enter the space between the liver and abdominal wall, and upon percussion the normal dullness over the liver will be tympanitic. Peristaltic sounds are reduced or absent. If delay in treatment allows continued escape of air into the peritoneal cavity, this may lead to abdominal distention and diffuse tympany.

The above description applies to the typical case of perforation with classical findings. In as many as one-third of patients the presentation is not as dramatic, diagnosis is less obvious, and serious delays in treatment may result from failure to consider this condition and obtain the appropriate abdominal x-rays. Many of these atypical perforations occur in patients already hospitalized for some unrelated illness, and the significance of the new symptom of abdominal pain is not appreciated. The only way to improve this record is to routinely obtain abdominal films on patients with abdominal pain of recent onset.

Lesser degrees of shock with minimal abdominal findings occur if the leak is small or rapidly sealed. A small duodenal perforation may leak fluid slowly which runs down the lateral peritoneal gutter, producing pain and muscular rigidity in the right lower quadrant and thus raising a problem of confusion with acute appendicitis.

Perforations may be sealed by omentum or by the liver, with the later development of a subhepatic or subdiaphragmatic abscess.

B. Laboratory Findings: A mild leukocytosis in the range of 12,000/μl is common in the early stages. After 12–24 hours, this may rise to 20,000/μl or more if treatment has been inadequate. The mild rise in the serum amylase value that occurs in many patients is probably caused by absorption of the enzyme from duodenal secretions within the peritoneum. Direct measurement of fluid obtained by paracentesis may show very high levels of amylase.

C. X-Ray Findings: Plain x-rays of the abdomen reveal free air in 85% of patients. Films should be taken with the patient supine and upright. A film in the left lateral decubitus position may be a more practical way to demonstrate free air in the uncomfortable patient who cannot tolerate the upright position for long. Most patients can lie in this position for 10–15 minutes before an x-ray is taken. This allows scattered small amounts of air to accumulate between the liver and the lateral chest wall where they are more readily demonstrated. Free air in the abdomen in a patient with sudden upper abdominal pain should clinch the diagnosis.

If no free air is demonstrated and the clinical picture suggests perforated ulcer, an emergency upper gastrointestinal series should be made with a water-soluble contrast agent. If the perforation has not sealed, the diagnosis is established by noting escape of the contrast material from the lumen.

Differential Diagnosis

The differential diagnosis must include acute pancreatitis and acute cholecystitis. The former does not have as explosive an onset as perforated ulcer and is usually accompanied by a high serum amylase level. Acute cholecystitis with perforated gallbladder could mimic perforated ulcer closely but free air would not be present with ruptured gallbladder. Intestinal obstruction has a more gradual onset and is characterized by less severe pain which is crampy and accompanied by vomiting.

The simultaneous onset of pain and free air in the abdomen in the absence of trauma usually means perforated peptic ulcer. Free perforation of colonic diverticulitis or acute appendicitis is another rare cause.

Treatment

The proper diagnosis is often suspected before the patient is sent for confirmatory x-rays. Whenever a perforated ulcer is considered possible, the first step should be to pass a nasogastric tube and empty the stomach to reduce further contamination of the peritoneal cavity. Blood should be drawn for laboratory studies and an intravenous infusion of crystalloid solution started. The patient should be given high doses of antibiotics effective against a wide spectrum of enteric organisms. If the patient's overall condition is precarious owing to delay in treatment, fluid resuscitation should precede diagnostic measures. X-rays should then be obtained as soon as his status will permit. The clinician must always keep in mind the penalty for delay in treating this disease.

The simplest treatment, laparotomy and suture closure of the perforation, solves the immediate problem but has no definitive effect on the ulcer disease. For many years this was the standard treatment for all patients, although it has been increasingly challenged in the past decade. The suture closure should be reinforced by incorporating a healthy tab of omentum, and all fluid should be aspirated from the peritoneal cavity. Drainage is not indicated. Reperforation is rare in the immediate postoperative period.

About three-fourths of patients whose perforation is the culmination of a history of chronic symptoms continue to have clinically severe ulcer disease after simple closure. Recognition of this fact has gradually led to a more aggressive treatment policy, involving a definitive ulcer operation, for many patients with acute perforation. The indications for a definitive procedure are good general condition of the patient and presence of symptoms of ulcer disease (including previous complications) for more than 1 month. Under these circumstances, most surgeons would perform a truncal vagotomy and incorporate the site of perforation in a Heineke-Mikulicz pyloroplasty; others prefer vagotomy and partial gastrectomy. Parietal cell vagotomy and closure of the perforation has not had sufficient trial on which to base any statement about whether it gives better results than the other procedures. A definitive surgical procedure should not be attempted when the patient's general condition is precarious or when purulent peritonitis has developed.

Concomitant hemorrhage and perforation are most often due to 2 ulcers, an anterior perforated one and a posterior one that is bleeding. At operation, a definitive procedure for the ulcer disease is mandatory in addition to control of the bleeding point with sutures. Perforated ulcers that also obstruct obviously cannot be treated by suture closure of the perforation alone. Vagotomy plus gastroenterostomy or pyloroplasty should be performed. Perforated anastomotic ulcers require a vagotomy or gastrectomy since in the long run closure alone is nearly always inadequate.

Nonoperative treatment consists of continuous gastric suction and the administration of antibiotics in high doses. Although this has been shown to be effective therapy with a low mortality rate, it is accompanied by a significant incidence of peritoneal and subphrenic abscess with greater morbidity than operative closure. For this reason, it is employed only for certain selected poor-risk patients or those seen very late with extensive peritonitis and toxemia. Even in advanced cases, operation is the best treatment if the condition of the patient permits.

Prognosis

About 15–18% of patients with perforated ulcer die, and about a third of these are undiagnosed before surgery. The mortality rate of perforated ulcer seen early is negligible. Delay in treatment, advanced age, and associated systemic diseases account for most deaths.

Cleator IGM, Holubitsky IB, Harrison RC: Perforated anastomotic ulcers. Ann Surg 177:436, 1973.

Coutsoftides T, Himal HS: Perforated gastroduodenal ulcers. Am J Surg 132:575, 1976.

Felix WR Jr, Stahlgren LH: Death by undiagnosed perforated peptic ulcer: Analysis of 31 cases. Ann Surg 177:344, 1973.

Griffen GE, Organ CH Jr: The natural history of the perforated duodenal ulcer treated by suture plication. Ann Surg 183:382, 1976.

Jordon GL Jr, DeBakey ME, Duncan JM Jr: Surgical management of perforated peptic ulcer. Ann Surg 179:628, 1974.

Jordon PH Jr & others: Vagotomy of the fundic gland area of the stomach without drainage: A definitive treatment for perforated duodenal ulcer. Am J Surg 131:523, 1976.

Kirkpatrick JR: The role of definitive surgery in the management of perforated duodenal ulcer disease. Arch Surg 110:1016, 1975.

Sawyers JL & others: Acute perforated duodenal ulcer. Arch Surg 110:527, 1975.

Steiger E, Cooperman AM: Considerations in the management of perforated peptic ulcers. Surg Clin North Am 56:1395, 1976.

Taylor H: The non-surgical treatment of perforated peptic ulcer. Gastroenterology 33:353, 1957.

STRESS GASTRODUODENITIS & STRESS ULCER
(Stress Ulceration)

The term stress ulcer has been used to refer to a heterogeneous group of acute gastric or duodenal ulcers which develop following physiologically stressful illnesses. There are 4 major etiologic factors associated with such lesions: (1) shock, (2) sepsis, (3) burns, and (4) CNS tumors or trauma.

Etiology

A. Stress Ulcer: Acute ulcers following shock, sepsis, and burns have enough common features to suggest they evolve by a similar pathogenetic mechanism, and present practice confines use of the term stress ulcer to this group.

Hemorrhage is the major clinical problem, although perforation occurs in about 10%. Despite their predilection to develop in the parietal cell mucosa, in about 30% of patients the duodenum is affected and sometimes both stomach and duodenum are involved. Morphologically, the ulcers are shallow discrete lesions with congestion and edema but little inflammatory reaction at their margins. Gastroduodenal endoscopy performed early in traumatized or burned patients has shown acute gastric erosions in the majority of patients within 72 hours of the injury. Such studies illustrate how frequently the disease process remains subclinical; clinically apparent ulcers develop in about 20% of susceptible patients. Clinically evident bleeding is usually not seen until 3–5 days after the injury, and when massive bleeding occurs it generally does not appear until 4–5 days later.

Mucosal ischemia, which decreases mucosal metabolic activity and energy stores, is thought to be the primary etiologic factor. The mucosa is then rendered more vulnerable to acid-pepsin ulceration by the effects of bile reflux, sepsis, malnutrition, ileus, gastric dilatation, and renal and respiratory insufficiency. Acid hypersecretion may be involved to some extent since burned patients who manifest serious bleeding have higher gastric acid output than patients with a more benign course. Disruption of the gastric mucosal barrier to back diffusion of acid has been found in less than half of the patients and is now thought to be a manifestation of the disease rather than a cause.

B. Cushing's Ulcers: Acute ulcers associated with CNS tumors or injuries differ from stress ulcers because they are associated with elevated levels of serum gastrin and increased gastric acid secretion. Morphologically, they are similar to ordinary gastroduodenal peptic ulcers. Cushing's ulcers are more prone to perforate than other kinds of stress ulcers.

C. Hemorrhagic Alcoholic Gastritis: This disorder may share some etiologic factors with the above conditions, but the natural history is different and the response to treatment is considerably better. Most of these patients can be controlled medically. By contrast with stress ulcer, when surgery is required for alcoholic

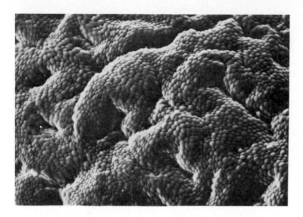

Figure 26—10. Scanning electron photomicrograph of the surface epithelium of a normal subject showing individual cells and numerous gastric pits. (Reduced from × 350.) (Courtesy of Jeanne M. Riddle.)

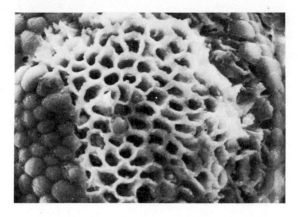

Figure 26—11. Scanning electron photomicrograph of the surface epithelium of a patient with acute gastric mucosal erosions showing a patch of cellular defoliation. Lesions such as this may account for back diffusion of H$^+$. (Reduced from × 1145.) (Courtesy of Jeanne M. Riddle.)

gastritis, a high proportion are cured by pyloroplasty and vagotomy.

D. Aspirin: Aspirin ingestion can aggravate most types of acute and chronic peptic ulceration. In severely ill, hospitalized patients, this drug is contraindicated because of its potentially deleterious effects on the gastric mucosal barrier and on platelet adhesiveness. However, lesions produced principally by salicylates should not be termed stress ulcers.

Clinical Findings

Hemorrhage is nearly always the first manifestation. Pain rarely occurs. Physical examination is not contributory except to reveal gross or occult fecal blood or signs of shock.

Prevention

Intensive antacid therapy in high-risk patients appears to prevent bleeding from stress ulcers. The antacids should be given at hourly intervals or by continuous drip to maintain gastric neutrality, and the pH of gastric contents should be checked every 30—60 minutes by aspirating an aliquot and testing it with litmus paper. Dosage of the antacid should be adjusted to keep the gastric pH above 4.0 or 5.0. Milk will not elevate gastric pH to the desired level and should not be used as a substitute.

Treatment

Initial management should consist of gastric lavage with chilled solutions and measures to combat sepsis if present.

Some success has been reported with the selective infusion of vasoconstricting agents (eg, vasopressin) into the left gastric artery through a percutaneously placed catheter. In the sickest patients, if facilities and trained personnel are available, this technic should probably be attempted before operation is considered.

Laparotomy must be performed if the nonopera-

tive regimen fails to halt the bleeding. Surgical treatment should consist of vagotomy and pyloroplasty with suture of the bleeding points or vagotomy and subtotal gastrectomy. Most experts recommend a high subtotal gastrectomy, excising as much of the ulcerated parietal cell mucosa as possible, if the patient's condition will permit. When it occurs, rebleeding is nearly always from an ulcer left behind at the initial procedure. Rarely, total gastrectomy has had to be used because of the extent of the ulceration and the severity of the bleeding.

Athanasoulis CA & others: Control of acute gastric mucosal hemorrhage: Intra-arterial infusion of posterior pituitary extract. N Engl J Med 290:597, 1974.

Czaja AJ & others: Acute gastroduodenal disease after thermal injury: An endoscopic evaluation of incidence and natural history. N Engl J Med 291:925, 1974.

Fischer RP & others: The maintenance of gastric mucosal barrier during the early erosive gastritis component of stress ulceration. Surgery 80:40, 1976.

Goodman AA & others: Symposium on the current status of the treatment of stress ulcers. Am J Surg 125:461, 1973.

Kirtley JA & others: The surgical management of stress ulcers. Ann Surg 169:801, 1969.

Lucas CE & others: Natural history and surgical dilemma of "stress" gastric bleeding. Arch Surg 102:266, 1971.

MacDonald AS, Steele BJ, Bottomley MG: Treatment of stress-induced upper gastrointestinal haemorrhage with metiamide. Lancet 1:68, 1976.

McAlhany JC Jr & others: Antacid control of complications from acute gastroduodenal disease after burns. J Trauma 16:645, 1976.

Menguy R (Moderator): Symposium on stress ulceration. Hosp Physician 8:50, 1976.

Menguy R, Master YF: Gastric mucosal energy metabolism and "stress ulceration." Ann Surg 180:538, 1974.

Menguy R, Gadacz T, Zatchuk R: The surgical management of acute gastric mucosal bleeding. Arch Surg 99:198, 1969.

Moody FG, Cheung LY: Stress ulcers: Their pathogenesis, diagnosis, and treatment. Surg Clin North Am 56:1469, 1976.

Rosenthal A & others: Gastrin levels and gastric acidity in the pathogenesis of acute gastroduodenal disease after burns. Surg Gynecol Obstet 144:232, 1977.

Silen W: New concepts of the gastric mucosal barrier. Am J Surg 133:8, 1977.

Silen W: Potpourri dissected. N Engl J Med 291:974, 1974.

Simonian SJ, Curtis LE: Treatment of hemorrhagic gastritis by antacid. Ann Surg 184:429, 1976.

GASTRIC CARCINOMA

Carcinoma of the stomach causes 15,000 deaths in the USA annually. The incidence has dropped dramatically to one-third what it was 30 years ago. The reason for this is not known, nor is it completely understood why the incidence varies so greatly between countries. The present incidence in American males is 10 new cases per 100,000 population per year. The highest rate of 70 per 100,000 males is seen in Japan; in eastern and central European countries, it is about 40 per 100,000 per year. Epidemiologic studies suggest that the incidence of gastric carcinoma is related to low dietary intake of vegetables and fruits and high intake of starches. Carcinoma of the stomach is rare under the age of 40, from which point the risk gradually climbs. The mean age at discovery is 63. It is about twice as common in men as in women.

Gastric epithelial malignancies are nearly always adenocarcinomas. Squamous cell tumors of the proximal stomach involve the stomach secondarily from the esophagus. Five morphologic subdivisions correlate loosely with the natural history and outcome.

(1) **Ulcerating carcinoma (25%).** This consists of a deep, penetrating ulcer-tumor which extends through all layers of the stomach. It may involve adjacent organs in the process. The edges are shallow by contrast with overhanging edges noted in benign ulcers.

(2) **Polypoid carcinomas (25%)** are large, bulky intraluminal growths that tend to metastasize late.

(3) **Superficial spreading carcinoma (15%).** Superficial spreading tumor is confined to the mucosa and submucosa (carcinoma in situ). Metastases are uncommon.

(4) **Linitis plastica (10%).** This variety of spreading tumor involves all layers with a marked desmoplastic reaction in which it may be difficult to identify the malignant cells. The stomach loses its pliability. Cure of this lesion is rare because of early spread.

(5) **Advanced carcinoma (35%).** This largest category contains the big tumors which are found partly within and partly without the stomach. They may originally have qualified for inclusion in the preceding groups but have outgrown that early stage.

Gastric adenocarcinomas can also be classified by the degree of differentiation of their cells. In general, rate and extent of spread correlate with lack of differentiation. Some tumors are found histologically to excite an inflammatory cell reaction at their borders, and this feature indicates a relatively good prognosis.

Extension occurs by intramural spread, direct extraluminal growth, and lymphatic metastases. Three-fourths of patients have metastases when first seen. Within the stomach, proximal spread exceeds distal. The pylorus acts as a partial barrier, but tumor is found in 25% of cases in the first few centimeters of the bulb.

Sixty percent of tumors are in the pyloric region, predominantly on the lesser curvature; 30% arise in the body, 5% at the cardia, and 5% involve the entire organ. Benign ulcers develop at the greater curvature and cardia less commonly than malignant ones. Ulcers at these points are particularly suspect for neoplasm.

Clinical Findings

A. Symptoms and Signs: The earliest symptom is usually vague postprandial abdominal heaviness which the patient does not identify as a pain. Sometimes the discomfort is no different from other vague dyspeptic symptoms which had been intermittently present for years. However, the frequency and persistence are new.

Anorexia develops early and may be most pronounced for meat. Weight loss is the most common symptom; when the patient is first seen by a physician, it averages about 5–7 kg (11–15 lb). True postprandial pain suggesting a benign gastric ulcer is relatively uncommon, but one may be misled if subsequent x-rays show an ulcer. Vomiting may be present and becomes a major feature if pyloric obstruction occurs. It may be coffee-ground in appearance due to bleeding by the tumor. Dysphagia may be the presenting symptom of lesions at the cardia. An epigastric mass can be felt on examination in about one-fourth of cases. Hepatomegaly is present in 10%. The stool will be positive for occult blood in half of patients, and melena is seen in a few. Otherwise, abnormal physical findings are confined to signs of distant spread of the tumor. Metastases to the neck along the thoracic duct may produce a Virchow node. Rectal examination may reveal a Blumer shelf, a solid peritoneal deposit anterior to the rectum. Enlarged ovaries (Krukenberg tumors) may be caused by intraperitoneal metastases. Further dissemination may involve the liver, lungs, brain, or bone.

B. Laboratory Findings:

1. Anemia is present in 40% of patients. CEA levels are elevated in 65%, usually indicating extensive spread of the tumor.

2. Gastric analysis—About 20% of patients with adenocarcinoma of the stomach are achlorhydric after maximal stimulation. This finding would eliminate the possibility of benign ulceration.

3. Gastric cytology—A good cytology laboratory can make the proper diagnosis in over 90% of malignant gastric tumors. False-positive reports are rare. Adenocarcinoma can be differentiated from lymphoma and squamous cell carcinoma. Only leiomyosarcomas cannot be diagnosed regularly. Direct biopsy and brush biopsy specimens obtained during gastroscopy are even more reliable than gastric washings as methods of making a histologic diagnosis.

C. X-Ray Findings: Upper gastrointestinal series may be diagnostic for some tumors. Major diagnostic problems are posed by ulcerating tumors, a few of which may not be distinguishable radiologically from benign peptic ulcers. The differential features are listed in the section on gastric ulcer, but x-rays alone are insufficiently reliable to establish a diagnosis of benign ulcer. It is strongly recommended that all patients with a newly discovered gastric ulcer undergo gastroscopy, gastric analysis, and gastric cytology.

D. Gastroscopy: Gastric carcinoma can usually be identified as such by its gross appearance during gastroscopy. All gastric lesions thought possibly to be neoplastic should be biopsied (6–10) times and brushed to obtain a specimen for cytologic examination.

Treatment

Surgical resection is the only curative treatment. Patients who have lost more than 10% of their body weight in the few months before diagnosis should probably be nutritionally resuscitated by a 2-week course of high-caloric (eg, 3000–4000 Cal/day) parenteral nutrition before being subjected to a major surgical resection.

The surgical objectives should be to remove the tumor, an adjacent uninvolved margin of stomach and duodenum, the regional lymph nodes, and, if necessary, portions of involved adjacent organs. For example, if the tumor is located in the pylorus, a curative resection would entail distal gastrectomy with en bloc removal of the omentum and, in some instances, excision of the left gastric artery and nearby lymph nodes. Reconstruction after gastrectomy may be by either a Billroth I or II procedure, but the latter is often preferable because postoperative growth of residual tumor near the pylorus would obstruct a gastroduodenal anastomosis early.

Esophagogastrectomy may be performed for tumors at the cardia. Total gastrectomy cannot be recommended except where the resection is curative, ie, will leave no gross tumor behind.

The propensity for proximal submucosal spread must be appreciated at surgery. It is often advisable to perform a frozen section at the proximal margin before constructing the anastomosis. If tumor is found, the gastrectomy should be extended.

Palliation is sometimes possible even though cure is not. Palliative resections may be performed for distal tumors which are obstructing or those which may soon become so. A Billroth II resection is preferable to a diverting gastrojejunostomy.

For advanced disease, the most effective chemotherapeutic regimen, which elicits an objective response in 40% of patients, consists of a combination of methyl-CCNU (semustine) and fluorouracil (5-FU, Efudex).

Prognosis

In the USA, the overall 5-year survival rate is about 12%. For localized tumors, the figure is 40%. In the absence of lymph node involvement, surgical cure can be predicted in two-thirds.

Death from tumor may follow dissemination to other organs or may be the result of progressive gastric obstruction and malnutrition.

Bjelke E: Epidemiologic studies of cancer of the stomach, colon, and rectum. Scand J Gastroenterol 9 (Suppl 31):1, 1974.

Black MM & others: Prognostic significance of microscopic structure of gastric carcinomas and their regional lymph nodes. Cancer 27:703, 1971.

Cady B & others: Gastric cancer. Am J Surg 133:423, 1977.

Cassell P, Robinson JO: Cancer of the stomach: A review of 854 patients. Br J Surg 63:603, 1976.

Hawley PR, Westerholm P, Morson BC: Pathology and prognosis of carcinoma of the stomach. Br J Surg 57:877, 1970.

Hoerr SO: Prognosis for carcinoma of the stomach. Surg Gynecol Obstet 137:205, 1973.

Inberg MV & others: Surgical treatment of gastric carcinoma. Arch Surg 110:703, 1975.

Kennedy BJ: TNM classification for stomach cancer. Cancer 26:971, 1970.

Lilienfeld A: Epidemiology of gastric cancer. N Engl J Med 286:316, 1972.

Moertel CG & others: Sequential and combination chemotherapy of advanced gastric cancer. Cancer 38:678, 1976.

Myren J & others: Gastroscopy with directed biopsy and routine x-ray examination in the diagnosis of the malignancies of the stomach. Scand J Gastroenterol 10:193, 1975.

Rubin P & others: Gastric cancer diagnosis. JAMA 228:883, 1974.

Rubin P & others: Gastric cancer: Treatment principles. JAMA 228:1283, 1974.

Stern JL & others: Evaluation of palliative resection in advanced carcinoma of the stomach. Surgery 77:291, 1975.

Zacho A & others: Surgical treatment of gastric malignancies. Ann Surg 179:94, 1974.

GASTRIC POLYPS

Adenomatous polyps of the stomach are single or multiple benign tumors which occur predominantly in the elderly. Those located in the distal stomach are more apt to cause symptoms. Whenever gastric polyps are discovered, gastric malignancy must be ruled out. Many adenomatous polyps are found in stomachs which contain a separate distinct carcinoma, but it is generally agreed that benign polyps do not themselves turn malignant. Lesions with a stalk and those less than 2 cm in diameter have little risk of malignancy. The incidence of malignancy rises with increasing size.

Anemia may develop from chronic blood loss or deficient iron absorption. Over 90% of patients are achlorhydric after maximal stimulation. Deficient vitamin B_{12} absorption exists in 25%, although megaloblastic anemia is present in only a few of these. Exfoliative cytologic examination of specimens obtained by endoscopy and brush biopsy should be performed in all patients.

Excision with a snare through the endoscope may

be performed safely for some pedunculated polyps. Otherwise, laparotomy is indicated for polyps greater than 1 cm in diameter or when the radiologist or cytologist suspects malignancy. Single polyps may be excised through a gastrotomy and a frozen section performed. If the polyp is found to be carcinoma, an appropriate type of gastrectomy is indicated. Partial gastrectomy should be performed for multiple polyps in the distal stomach. If 10–20 polyps are distributed throughout the stomach, the antrum should be removed and the fundic polyps excised. Total gastrectomy may be required for diffuse multiple polyposis, a rare condition in which the entire gastric mucosa is involved.

The patient should be followed by occasional x-rays. Recurrence is uncommon after surgery.

Bone GE, McClelland RN: Management of gastric polyps. Surg Gynecol Obstet 142:933, 1976.

GASTRIC LYMPHOMAS

Lymphoma is the second most common primary malignancy of the stomach but comprises only 2% of the total, 95% being adenocarcinomas. Lymphomas are classified as lymphosarcomas or reticulum cell sarcomas according to cellular characteristics.

The principal symptoms are epigastric pain and weight loss, similar to those of carcinoma. Characteristically, the tumor has attained bulky proportions by the time it is discovered; by comparison with adenocarcinoma of the stomach, the symptoms from a gastric lymphoma are usually mild in relation to the size of the lesion. A palpable epigastric mass is present in 50% of patients. Barium x-ray studies will demonstrate the lesion, although it usually is mistaken for adenocarcinoma or, in 10% of cases, for benign gastric ulcer. Gastroscopy with biopsy and gastric cytologic examination should provide the correct diagnosis. Gastric lymphomas can trap the clinician into thinking he is dealing with inoperable carcinoma, judged so because the tumor is so large. It is important to avoid this mistake since resection and postoperative radiotherapy result in 5-year survival in over 50% of cases.

Hertzer NR, Hoerr SO: An interpretive review of lymphoma of the stomach. Surg Gynecol Obstet 143:113, 1976.

Naqvi MS, Burrows L, Kark AE: Lymphoma of the gastrointestinal tract. Ann Surg 170:221, 1969.

GASTRIC LEIOMYOMAS & LEIOMYOSARCOMAS

Leiomyomas are common submucosal growths which are usually asymptomatic but may cause intestinal bleeding. Leiomyosarcomas may grow to a large size and most often present with bleeding. Radiologically, the tumor contains a central ulceration caused by necrosis from outgrowth of its blood supply. In most cases the tumor arises from the proximal stomach. It may grow into the gastric lumen, remain entirely on the serosal surface, or even become pedunculated within the abdominal cavity. Spread is by direct invasion or blood-borne metastases. Leiomyomas should be removed by enucleation or wedge resection. After the more radical resections required for leiomyosarcomas, the 5-year survival rate is 50%. The tumor is resistant to radiotherapy.

Morrissey K & others: Muscular tumors of the stomach. Ann Surg 178:148, 1973.

Welch JP: Smooth muscle tumors of the stomach. Am J Surg 130:279, 1975.

GASTRITIS

Acute Gastritis

This condition has been recognized with greater frequency since the use of gastroscopy in acute upper gastrointestinal bleeding has become widespread. Ingestion of large amounts of alcohol or other injurious agents such as salicylates is an important causative factor. It is not entirely clear what important differences exist (if any) between acute hemorrhagic gastritis and acute gastric stress ulcers, although gastritis runs a milder course. The patient may experience epigastric pain, or the gastritis may be asymptomatic.

The lamina propria contains a variable number of inflammatory cells consisting principally of polymorphonuclear leukocytes. Punctate superficial mucosal ulceration may develop and occasionally leads to massive hemorrhage. When healing begins, the abnormal mucosal appearance may improve rapidly.

Diagnosis can be made by gastroscopy, sometimes supplemented by gastric mucosal biopsy.

Initial management should follow the guidelines presented for upper gastrointestinal hemorrhage. Fortunately, gastric lavage with cold solutions is usually effective in halting the blood loss. As in other conditions with acute gastric hemorrhage, the decision for operation depends on the rate of continuing hemorrhage after treatment.

Vagotomy, in addition to reducing acid secretion, has been shown to divert blood away from the gastric mucosa by opening submucosal shunts. Vagotomy with a drainage procedure would be the first effort of many surgeons. If this fails, subtotal or, in rare cases, total gastrectomy might be necessary to save the patient.

The prognosis after bleeding stops is good if intake of harmful substances can be prevented.

Chronic Gastritis

Chronic gastritis embraces a wide variety of

lesions, in some cases related only by virtue of their gastric location. Chronic atrophic gastritis of the parietal cell mucosa is found in patients with pernicious anemia who also have achlorhydria and antibodies against intrinsic factor and parietal cells. Atrophic gastritis with achlorhydria also occurs without pernicious anemia. Within 5 years, adenocarcinoma of the stomach develops in 12% of patients with atrophic gastritis and achlorhydria. Patients with atrophic gastritis should undergo gastroscopy and gastric cytologic studies yearly to detect neoplasms early.

Chronic gastritis is invariably found in patients with benign gastric ulcer. It has been suggested that this is caused by regurgitation of duodenal secretions.

Chatterjee D: Idiopathic chronic gastritis. Surg Gynecol Obstet 143:986, 1976.
Cheli R & others: A clinical and statistical follow-up study of atrophic gastritis. Am J Dig Dis 18:1061, 1973.
Strickland RG, Mackay IR: A reappraisal of the nature and significance of chronic atrophic gastritis. Am J Dig Dis 18:426, 1973.

MENETRIER'S DISEASE

Menetrier's disease, a form of hypertrophic gastritis, consists of giant hypertrophy of the gastric rugae, normal or low acid secretion, and excessive loss of protein into the gut with resulting hypoproteinemia. Chronic blood loss may also be a problem. The patient complains of indigestion which responds to antacids, but this treatment does not improve the gastric pathology or secondary hypoproteinemia. The hypertrophic rugae present as enormous filling defects on upper gastrointestinal series and are frequently misinterpreted as carcinoma. In a few cases the protein leak from the gastric mucosa has responded to atropine or hexamethonium bromide. Partial or, sometimes, total gastrectomy is indicated for hypoproteinemia, anemia, or inability to exclude malignancy. When these problems are not severe enough to justify surgery, the disease gradually evolves into atrophic gastritis.

Berenson MM & others: Menetrier's disease. Gastroenterology 70:257, 1976.
Davis JM & others: Menetrier's disease. Ann Surg 185:456, 1977.

ACUTE GASTRIC DILATATION

Acute gastric dilatation usually follows surgery on the upper abdomen, particularly in patients who have received oxygen by nasal catheter or those who have been placed on a respirator using a face mask. Swallowed air produces gastric distention and increased intragastric pressure. As pressure exceeds that in the mucosal veins, acute bleeding may occur.

Anorexia, hiccuping, vomiting of brownish, dark-stained or bloody gastric contents, epigastric tympany, and tachycardia are important early diagnostic signs. Shock due to acute gastric dilatation can be rapidly fatal. Death may result from dehydration, bleeding, acute pulmonary edema, or aspiration of gastric contents into the tracheobronchial tree.

Treatment consists of the insertion of a nasogastric tube with decompression of the stomach and restoration of fluids and electrolytes.

PROLAPSE OF THE GASTRIC MUCOSA

This uncommon lesion occasionally accompanies small prepyloric gastric ulcers. Episodes of vomiting and abdominal pain simulate peptic ulcer disease. X-ray shows prolapse of antral folds into the duodenum. One must be alert to the presence of gastric or duodenal ulcer as the underlying cause.

Antrectomy with a Billroth I anastomosis is occasionally required. Generally, conservative treatment suffices.

GASTRIC VOLVULUS

The stomach may rotate about its longitudinal axis (organo-axial volvulus) or a line drawn from the mid lesser to the mid greater curvature (mesenterio-axial volvulus). The former is the most common and is often associated with a paraesophageal hiatal hernia. In other patients, eventration of the left diaphragm allows the colon to rise upward and twist the stomach by pulling on the gastrocolic ligament.

Acute gastric volvulus produces severe abdominal pain accompanied by a diagnostic triad (Brochardt's triad): (1) vomiting followed by retching and then inability to vomit, (2) epigastric distention, and (3) inability to pass a nasogastric tube. The situation calls for immediate laparotomy to prevent death from acute gastric necrosis and shock. An emergency upper gastrointestinal series will show a block at the point of the volvulus. The mortality rate is high.

Chronic volvulus is more common than acute. It may be asymptomatic or may cause crampy intermittent pain. Cases associated with paraesophageal hiatal hernia should be treated by repair of the hernia and anterior gastropexy. When cases are due to eventration of the diaphragm, the gastrocolic ligament should be divided the entire length of the greater curvature. The colon rises to fill the space caused by the eventration, and the stomach will resume its normal position, to be fastened by a gastropexy.

Tanner NC: Chronic and recurrent volvulus of the stomach. Am J Surg 115:505, 1968.
Wastell C, Ellis H: Volvulus of the stomach. Br J Surg 58:557, 1971.

GASTRIC DIVERTICULA

Gastric diverticula are uncommon and usually asymptomatic. Most are pulsion diverticula consisting of mucosa and submucosa only, located on the lesser curvature within a few centimeters of the esophagogastric junction. Those in the prepyloric region generally possess all layers and are more likely to be symptomatic. A few patients have symptoms from hemorrhage or inflammation within a gastric diverticulum, but for the most part these lesions are incidental findings on upper gastrointestinal series. Radiologically, they can be confused with a gastric ulcer.

Hughes W, Pierce WS: Surgical implications of gastric diverticula. Surg Gynecol Obstet 131:99, 1970.

BEZOAR

Bezoars are concretions formed in the stomach. Trichobezoars are composed of hair and are usually found in young girls who pick at their hair and swallow it. Phytobezoars consist of agglomerated vegetable fibers. Pressure by the mass can create a gastric ulcer which is prone to bleed or perforate.

The postgastrectomy state predisposes to bezoar formation because pepsin and acid secretion are reduced and the triturating function of the antrum is gone. Orange segments or other fruits which contain a large amount of cellulose have been implicated in most cases. Improper mastication of food is a contributing factor which can sometimes be obviated by providing the patient with well-fitting dentures. The fruit may remain in the stomach or pass into the small intestine and cause obstruction. Some surgeons routinely warn postgastrectomy patients to avoid citrus fruits.

Large semisolid bezoars of *Candida albicans* have also been found in postgastrectomy patients. Some can be fragmented with the gastroscope. The patient should also be treated with oral nystatin.

Patients with symptomatic gastric bezoars may complain of abdominal pain. Ulceration and bleeding are associated with a mortality rate of 20%.

Oral administration of papain and cellulase usually will digest the mass. This treatment must not be allowed to delay surgery indicated to prevent imminent complications. Symptomatic patients should be treated by operative removal of the bezoar and excision of secondary gastric ulcers.

Davis RC, Faruqui AMA: Endoscopic enzymatic dissolution: Nonsurgical therapy for gastric phytobezoars. JAMA 229:1332, 1974.

Jaffe BM, Sasser WF: Management of gastric persimmon bezoars. Am J Surg 114:962, 1967.

Pollard HB, Block GE: Rapid dissolution of phytobezoar by cellulase enzyme. Am J Surg 116:933, 1968.

II. DUODENUM*

Duodenal Diverticula

Diverticula of the duodenum are found in 20% of autopsies and 5–10% of upper gastrointestinal series. Symptoms are uncommon, and only 1% of those found by x-ray warrant surgery.

Duodenal pulsion diverticula are acquired outpouchings of the mucosa and submucosa, 90% of which are on the medial aspect of the duodenum. Most are solitary and within 2.5 cm of the ampulla of Vater. They are not seen in the first portion of the duodenum, where diverticular configurations are due to scarring by peptic ulceration or cholecystitis.

A few patients have chronic postprandial abdominal pain or dyspepsia caused by a duodenal diverticulum. Treatment is with antacids and anticholinergics.

Serious complications are hemorrhage or perforation from inflammation, pancreatitis, and biliary obstruction. Bile acid-bilirubinate enteroliths are occasionally formed by bile stasis in a diverticulum. Enteroliths can precipitate diverticular inflammation or biliary obstruction and rarely have caused bowel obstruction after entering the intestinal lumen.

Surgical treatment is required for complications and, rarely, for persistent symptoms. Excision and a 2-layer closure are usually possible after mobilization of the duodenum and dissection of the diverticulum from the pancreas. Removal of the diverticulum and closure of the defect are superior to simple drainage in the case of perforation. If biliary obstruction appears in a patient whose bile duct empties into a diverticulum, excision might be more hazardous than a side-to-side choledochoduodenostomy.

The rare wind sock type of intraluminal diverticulum usually presents with vague epigastric pain and postprandial fullness, although intestinal bleeding or pancreatitis is occasionally seen. The diagnosis can be made by barium x-ray studies. The diverticulum can be excised through a nearby duodenotomy.

Economides NG & others: Intraluminal duodenal diverticulum in the adult. Ann Surg 185:147, 1977.

Luler GL & others: Perforating duodenal diverticulitis. Arch Surg 99:572, 1969.

Neill SA, Thompson NW: The complications of duodenal diverticula and their management. Surg Gynecol Obstet 120:1251, 1965.

Duodenal Tumors

Tumors of the duodenum are rare. Carcinoma of the ampulla of Vater is discussed in Chapter 30.

A. Malignant Tumors: Most malignant duodenal tumors are adenocarcinomas, leiomyosarcomas, and lymphomas. They appear in the descending duodenum more often than elsewhere. Pain, obstruction, bleeding,

---

*Duodenal ulcer is discussed under Peptic Ulcer earlier in this chapter.

obstructive jaundice, and an abdominal mass are the modes of presentation. Duodenal carcinomas, particularly those in the third and fourth portions of the duodenum, are often missed on barium x-ray studies. Endoscopy and biopsy will usually be diagnostic if the examiner is suspicious enough and can reach the lesion.

If possible, adenocarcinomas and leiomyosarcomas should be resected. Pancreaticoduodenectomy is usually necessary if the tumor is localized. Unresectable lesions should be treated by radiotherapy. Biopsy and radiotherapy are recommended for lymphoma.

After curative resections, the 5-year survival rate is 30%. The overall 5-year survival rate is 18%.

B. Benign Tumors: These are encountered even less often than duodenal malignancies. Brunner's gland adenomas are those most likely to be symptomatic. They are small submucosal nodules which have a predilection for the posterior duodenal wall at the junction of the first and second portions. Sessile and pedunculated variants are seen. Symptoms are due to bleeding or obstruction. Leiomyomas and carcinoids may also be found in the duodenum and ordinarily are symptomatic.

Ectopic islet cell adenomas (gastrinomas) in the duodenal submucosa are responsible for a small number of cases of Zollinger-Ellison syndrome.

Kibbey WE & others: Primary duodenal tumors. Arch Surg 111:377, 1976.

Lawrence W Jr & others: Benign duodenal tumors. Ann Surg 172:1015, 1970.

Moss WM & others. Primary adenocarcinoma of the duodenum. Arch Surg 108:805, 1974.

Sakker S, Ware CC: Carcinoma of the duodenum: Comparisons of surgery, radiotherapy, and chemotherapy. Br J Surg 60:867, 1973.

Superior Mesenteric Artery Obstruction of the Duodenum

Rarely, obstruction of the third portion of the duodenum is produced by compression between the superior mesenteric vessels and the aorta. It most commonly appears after rapid weight loss following injury. Patients in body casts are particularly susceptible.

The superior mesenteric artery normally leaves the aorta at an angle of 50–60 degrees, and the distance between the 2 vessels where the duodenum passes between them is 10–20 mm. These measurements in patients with the superior mesenteric artery syndrome average 18 degrees and 2.5 mm. Acute loss of mesenteric fat is thought to permit the artery to drop posteriorly, trapping the bowel like a scissors.

Skepticism exists regarding the frequency of this condition in adults who have not experienced acute loss of weight. Most often the patient in question is a thin, nervous woman whose complaints of dyspepsia and occasional emesis are more properly explained on a functional basis. When a clear-cut example is encountered, it may actually represent a form of intestinal malrotation with duodenal bands.

The patient complains of epigastric bloating and crampy pain which is relieved by vomiting. The symptoms may remit in the prone position. Anorexia and postprandial pain lead to additional malnutrition and weight loss.

Upper gastrointestinal x-rays demonstrate a widened duodenum proximal to a sharp obstruction at the point where the artery crosses the third portion of the duodenum. When the patient moves to the knee-chest position, the passage of barium is suddenly unimpeded. Further verification can be provided if angiography shows an angle of 25 degrees or less between the superior mesenteric artery and the aorta. However, this procedure is not recommended for routine evaluation of obvious cases.

Many patients whose superior mesenteric artery makes a prominent impression on the duodenum are asymptomatic, and in ambulatory patients one should hesitate to attribute vague chronic complaints to this finding.

Involvement of the duodenum by scleroderma leads to duodenal dilatation and hypomotility and an x-ray and clinical picture highly suggestive of the superior mesenteric artery syndrome. In the latter, increased duodenal peristalsis should be demonstrable proximal to the arterial blockage, whereas diminished peristalsis characterizes scleroderma. Patients with duodenal scleroderma usually have dysphagia from concomitant esophageal involvement.

Malrotation with duodenal obstruction by congenital bands can mimic this syndrome.

Postural therapy may suffice. The patient should be placed prone when symptomatic or in anticipation of postprandial difficulties. Ambulatory patients should be instructed to assume the knee-chest position, which allows the viscera and the artery to rotate forward off the duodenum.

Chronic obstruction may require section of the suspensory ligament and mobilization of the duodenum, or a duodenojejunostomy to bypass the obstruction. Patients with various forms of malrotation should be treated by mobilizing the duodenojejunal flexure, which releases the duodenum from entrapment by congenital bands.

Akin JT Jr & others: Vascular compression of the duodenum. Surgery 79:515, 1976.

Louw JH: Intestinal malrotation and duodenal ileus. J R Coll Surg Edinb 5:101, 1960.

Regional Enteritis of the Stomach & Duodenum

The proximal intestine and stomach are rarely involved in regional enteritis, although this disease has now been reported in every part of the gastrointestinal tract from the lips to the anus. Most patients with Crohn's disease in the stomach or duodenum have ileal involvement as well.

Pain can in many instances be relieved by antacids. Intermittent vomiting from duodenal stenosis or pyloric obstruction is frequent. The x-ray finding of a cobblestone mucosa or stenosis would be suggestive when associated with typical changes in the ileum. The endoscopic appearance is fairly characteristic, and biopsy with the peroral suction device usually gives an adequate specimen for histologic confirmation of the diagnosis.

Medical treatment is nonspecific and consists principally of corticosteroids during exacerbations. Surgery may be indicated for disabling pain or obstruction. If localized to the stomach, a partial gastrectomy can be performed. However, when the stomach is affected, the duodenum is usually involved as well. Bypass gastrojejunostomy has provided symptomatic relief for this type of patient.

Danzi JT & others: Endoscopic features of gastroduodenal Crohn's disease. Gastroenterology 70:9, 1976.

Fielding JF & others: Crohn's disease of the stomach and duodenum. Gut 11:1001, 1970.

Thompson WM & others: Regional enteritis of the duodenum. Radiology 123:252, 1975.

Wise L & others: Crohn's disease of the duodenum. Am J Surg 121:184, 1971.

● ● ●

General References

Buskin FL, Woodward ER: *Postgastrectomy Syndromes.* Saunders, 1976.

Cooperman AM (editor): Symposium on peptic ulcer disease. Surg Clin North Am 56:1231, Dec 1976. [Entire issue.]

Davenport HW: *Digest of Digestion.* Year Book, 1975.

McNeer G, Pack GT: *Neoplasms of the Stomach.* Lippincott, 1967.

Menguy R: *Surgery of Peptic Ulcer.* Saunders, 1976.

Nyhus LM, Harkins HN: *Surgery of the Stomach and Duodenum,* 3rd ed. Little, Brown, 1977.

Sleisenger M, Fortran JS: *Gastrointestinal Disease.* Saunders, 1973.

Wormsley KG: *Duodenal Ulcer.* Eden Press, 1977.

27...
Liver

Lawrence W. Way, MD, & Robert C. Lim, Jr., MD

Liver transplantation is still an experimental operation and is discussed in Chapter 50. The physiology of bilirubin metabolism and the diagnostic approach to the jaundiced patient are covered in Chapter 29.

SURGICAL ANATOMY

Segments

The liver develops as an embryologic outpouching from the duodenum by a process which is described in Chapter 29. The liver is one of the largest organs in the body, representing 2% of the total body weight. In classic descriptions, the liver was characterized as having 4 lobes: right, left, caudate, and quadrate. However, these traditional lobes do not describe the true segmental anatomy of the liver, which is depicted in Fig 27–1. The main lobar fissure can be thought of as represented by an oblique plane passing posteriorly from the gallbladder bed to the vena cava, dividing the anatomic right and left lobes. This primary division is to the right of the falciform ligament. The right lobe is subdivided into anterior and posterior segments by the right segmental fissure. The left lobe is subdivided into medial and lateral segments by the left segmental fissure, marked by the position of the falciform ligament.

The relationship of the liver to the other abdominal organs is shown in Fig 27–2.

Venous Blood Supply (Fig 27–3)

Both the portal and hepatic venous systems lack valves. The portal vein terminates in the porta hepatis by dividing into right and left lobar branches. The right lobar branch immediately follows the course of the segmental ducts and arteries. The left lobar branch has 2 portions: the transverse part and the umbilical part. The former is a short segment coursing through the porta hepatis. The latter descends into the umbilical fossa and supplies the medial and lateral segments of the left lobe.

The hepatic veins represent the final common pathway for the central veins of the lobules of the liver. There are 3 major hepatic veins: left, right, and middle. The middle hepatic vein lies in the major lobar fissure and drains blood from the medial segment of the left lobe and the inferior portion of the anterior

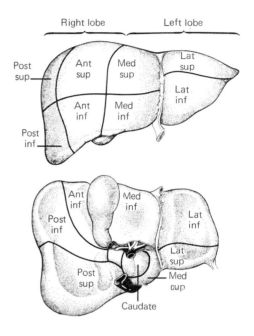

Figure 27–1. Segmental anatomy of the liver. The major lobar fissure, separating the right and left lobes, passes from the inferior vena cava through the gallbladder bed.

segment of the right lobe. The left hepatic vein drains the lateral segment of the left lobe and the right hepatic vein the posterior segment and much of the anterior segment of the right lobe. Several small accessory veins enter the inferior vena cava directly from the posterior segment of the right lobe and must be carefully ligated during a right hemihepatectomy. The middle hepatic vein usually joins the left hepatic vein before they meet the inferior vena cava.

Arterial Blood Supply

The common hepatic artery arises from the celiac axis, ascends in the hepatoduodenal ligament, and gives rise to the right gastric and gastroduodenal arteries before dividing into right and left branches in the hilus. The hepatic artery supplies approximately 25% of the 1500 ml of blood which enter the liver each minute; the remaining 75% is supplied by the portal vein. In 10% of individuals, the common hepatic artery

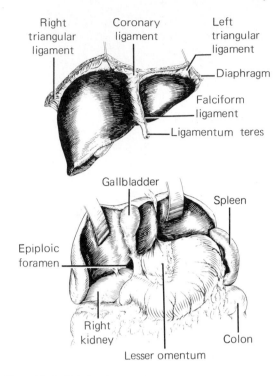

Right triangular ligament Coronary ligament Left triangular ligament

Diaphragm

Falciform ligament

Ligamentum teres

Gallbladder

Spleen

Epiploic foramen

Right kidney

Colon

Lesser omentum

Figure 27—2. Relationships of the liver to adjacent abdominal organs.

Elias H, Sherrick JC: *Morphology of the Liver.* Academic Press, 1969.

Goldsmith NA, Woodburne RT: The surgical anatomy pertaining to liver resection. Surg Gynecol Obstet 105:310, 1957.

Michels NA: Newer anatomy of the liver and its variant blood supply and collateral circulation. Am J Surg 112:337, 1966.

DIAGNOSTIC PROCEDURES

Liver Biopsy

A specimen of liver adequate for histologic diagnosis can be obtained by the percutaneous insertion of a variety of biopsy needles. The Menghini needle is preferred unless the liver substance is unusually hard (eg, advanced cirrhosis, hepatic fibrosis), in which case the Vim-Silverman needle may be more likely to obtain a satisfactory specimen.

Liver biopsy is of greatest value in the diagnosis of parenchymal disease such as viral hepatitis. Tumors can often be sampled, and increased accuracy can be obtained by consulting the hepatic scan before performing the biopsy. It is usually impossible to reliably differentiate among the various causes of cholestasis by histologic appearances.

The procedure is hazardous in the presence of defective coagulation, ascites, hepatic adenoma, or hydatid disease of the liver. If the prothrombin time is below 50%, vitamin K should be given and the biopsy postponed until a response is observed. Patients with suspected extrahepatic biliary obstruction should be premedicated with antibiotics to prevent an exacerbation of cholangitis.

The reported mortality rate is about 0.1%.

Menghini G: One-second biopsy of the liver. N Engl J Med 283:582, 1970.

has an anomalous origin. In the most common variants, the common hepatic or the right hepatic artery arises from the superior mesenteric artery. The left hepatic originates from the left gastric artery in 15% of subjects. The common hepatic artery divides to follow the segmental ducts. Once they enter the liver and divide, the various segmental branches are termed end-arteries since they do not communicate with each other via collaterals.

Biliary Drainage

Segmental bile ducts drain each segment. The right anterior and right posterior segmental ducts unite to form the right hepatic duct, and the left lateral and left medial segmental ducts form the left hepatic duct. These lobar ducts join outside the parenchyma to form the common hepatic duct. Anatomic variations are common. In over 25% of specimens, the duct from the right posterior segment joins the left hepatic duct independently. Variations are far less common on the left side.

Lymphatics

Superficial lymphatics arise from superficial portions of the lobules and pass beneath the capsule to enter the posterior mediastinum via the diaphragm and the suspensory ligaments of the liver. Some enter the porta hepatis and others enter the coronary chain. Other lymphatics arise deep in the liver lobules and pass either with the hepatic veins along the vena cava or with the portal veins into the porta hepatis.

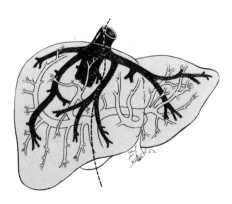

Figure 27—3. Anatomy of the veins of the liver. The major lobar fissure is represented by the dashed line. Branches of the hepatic artery and biliary ducts follow those of the portal vein. The darker vessels represent the hepatic veins and vena cava; the lighter system represents the portal vein and its branches.

Liver Scans

Scintillation scans of the liver may be performed using numerous radionuclides. At present, technetium-99m and gold-198 colloids give the best quality pictures. Lateral as well as anterior views should be routinely obtained. Space-occupying lesions in the liver such as tumors, abscesses, or cysts may be demonstrated as filling defects. Lesions with a diameter less than 2.5 cm cannot usually be detected. The accuracy of the technic is around 60%; 20% are false-positive and 20% false-negative. Substantial observer variation has been demonstrated in interpretation of individual scans, and they should be judged of indeterminate value unless the abnormal findings are well defined and compatible with other clinical and laboratory data. In general, hepatic scans are greatly overused, particularly to screen for metastases in patients with known or suspected malignant disease, where they rarely contribute to patient management.

Hepatic scans are occasionally of value to demonstrate the extent of hepatomegaly or the position of the liver in relation to a subphrenic abscess.

Drum DE: Scintigraphy of the liver and spleen. Postgrad Med 54:118, July 1973.

Ludbrook J & others: Observer error in reporting on liver scans for space-occupying lesions. Gastroenterology 62:1013, 1972.

Rosenthal S: Are hepatic scans overused? Dig Diseases 21:659, 1976.

Arteriography

The hepatic artery may be opacified with contrast media selectively injected through a catheter inserted percutaneously through the femoral or axillary artery. Sequential x-rays demonstrate a hepatic arterial phase, a parenchymal phase, and a portal venous phase. The procedure is useful to outline space-occupying lesions in the liver as well as abnormal vascular patterns. Since lesions smaller than the resolution of the hepatic scan can sometimes be shown, arteriography can be used as an adjunct to scanning when the results of the latter are equivocal. Advanced cirrhosis may be recognized by a characteristic corkscrew configuration of the intrahepatic vessels. Primary hepatomas and hemangiomas have distinctive vascular appearances. Metastatic tumors and adenomas vary in vascularity, but in general they have a less pronounced arterial blush than hepatomas and frequently appear as filling defects that displace the arterial vessels. Cholangiocarcinoma, cysts, and abscesses present as avascular filling defects without specific identifying features. Angiography has been of major value in the diagnosis of hematobilia. Its use in the management of selected cases of liver trauma appears promising.

Baum S: Hepatic angiography. Chap 27, pp 444–465, in: *Progress in Liver Diseases*. Vol 3. Popper H, Schaffner F (editors). Grune & Stratton, 1970.

Pollard JJ: Abdominal angiography. N Engl J Med 279:1093, 1968.

HEPATIC RESECTION

Increased understanding of the anatomy and physiology of the liver has made resection of more than 50% of the organ possible with an acceptably low mortality rate. The indications for resections of major segments of the liver are relatively uncommon and include primary and secondary malignant tumors, benign tumors, traumatic rupture, cysts, and abscesses.

Removal of as much as 80–85% of the normal liver is consistent with survival. Liver function is reduced for several weeks after extensive resections, but the extraordinary regenerative capacity of the liver rapidly provides new functioning hepatocytes. Although hepatic regeneration—or, more aptly, "restorative hyperplasia"—has been the subject of intense study, the process is only vaguely understood. Normally mitoses among hepatocytes are exceedingly rare, and it has been estimated that individual cells may survive for the lifetime of the organism. However, within 24 hours after partial hepatectomy, cell replication becomes active and continues until the original weight of the organ is restored. Studies in man indicate that considerable regeneration occurs within 10 days and that the process is essentially complete by 4–5 weeks. Excised lobes are not re-formed as such. Rather, the growth consists of formation of new lobules and expansion of residual lobules. The stimulus for restorative hyperplasia is known to be humoral, but it has not been further characterized.

Preoperative Evaluation

Since liver function is compromised after major hepatic resections, the decision to perform such operations must take into account the preoperative functional status. Cirrhosis is a relative contraindication for hepatectomy because the limited reserve of the residual cirrhotic liver is usually insufficient to meet essential metabolic demands and it has little capacity for regeneration. These factors prohibit resection of some primary hepatic tumors which develop in cirrhotics.

The level of serum albumin before operation should be greater than 3 g/100 ml if complications are to be avoided. If the value is lower, the patient should be prepared by parenteral albumin infusions.

Active hepatocellular disease at the time of hepatectomy would seriously diminish the chances of postoperative recovery. Therefore, a markedly elevated SGOT (above 400 IU/liter) or demonstration of substantial necrosis or inflammation on liver biopsy would usually rule out hepatic resection until the active process subsided.

Technic of Hepatic Resections

Based upon the lobar anatomy, hepatic resections are classified as segmental or nonsegmental. Wedge resections and resectional debridement of devitalized tissue are examples of the latter. Major lobar resections must be planned in accordance with the segmental vascular anatomy (Fig 27–3). The terminology and extent of the common types of resections are depicted in Fig 27–4. The operation entails removal of a lobe or segment with its afferent and efferent vessels while avoiding injury to vessels and bile ducts supplying the residual tissue. An extended right hepatectomy–the most extensive–removes all but 15–20% of the hepatic mass.

Left lobectomy or left lateral hepatectomy can usually be performed through an abdominal incision, but procedures involving extirpation of the right lobe require a thoracoabdominal approach. The key to technical success is hemostasis. The appropriate hilar vessels are divided before beginning the dissection, and the liver tissue is then transected bluntly with the finger fracture technic or the handle of a scalpel. Copious bleeding can be temporarily controlled by compressing the portal triad, and individual vessels can then be suture ligated.

The space created by removing a part of the liver must be drained with a large sump tube and numerous soft rubber drains. To be adequate, the drain must be aided by gravity by being dependent. This is best accomplished through the bed of the 12th rib. Despite precautions, about 20% of patients develop abscesses in or near this space and require additional operations for drainage some time in the postoperative period.

Postoperative Course

If 50% or more of the liver has been removed, the patient will require close monitoring and metabolic support for the first 1 or 2 weeks after operation.

A. Blood Glucose: The blood glucose level may fall immediately after surgery if it is not maintained by parenteral infusions. The glucose concentration should be measured twice daily for the first 2 days and 5% or 10% glucose administered intravenously in quantities sufficient to avoid hypoglycemia.

B. Plasma Protein: The serum albumin concentration drops in most patients. Hypoalbuminemia should be corrected by the intravenous route to avoid pulmonary edema or ascites. The albumin deficit presumably results from loss of functioning liver tissue plus depressed synthetic capacity of the residual liver. The usual requirement is 50–100 g of salt-poor albumin daily for about 1 week.

C. Clotting Factors: The concentrations of several clotting factors invariably drop after partial hepatectomy. To prevent complications, surgical hemostasis must be meticulous. The prothrombin level falls to about 50% of normal, and vitamin K must be given. Low concentrations of fibrinogen and factor IX usually improve spontaneously and require no treatment. If there is oozing of blood postoperatively, fresh frozen plasma should be given to replenish depleted clotting factors. Serious complications sometimes follow disseminated intravascular coagulation. This condition usually develops after severe trauma to many organs.

D. Liver Function Studies: The serum bilirubin rises to an average peak of 5–6 mg/100 ml several days after resection but usually returns to normal within 1–2 weeks. The absolute height of bilirubin is affected by the amount of blood transfused, the presence or absence of disease in the residual liver, sepsis, and trauma to other areas. The alkaline phosphatase usually remains normal after partial hepatectomy unless functioning bile ducts have been traumatized or obstructed. SGOT and serum LDH rise for several days and then return to normal levels.

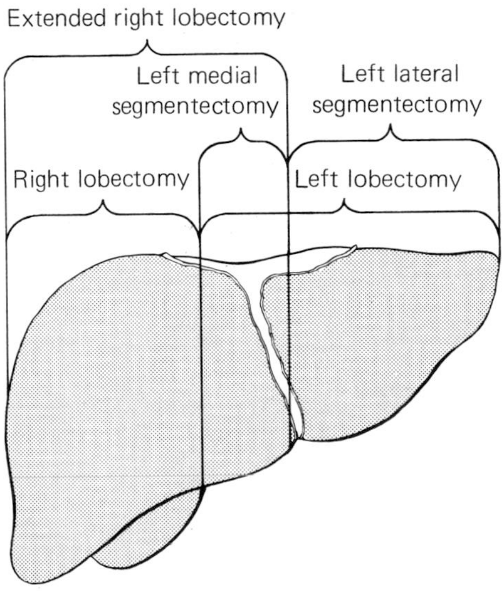

Complications

Atelectasis and pneumonitis of the right lung are frequent after partial hepatectomy, especially when a thoracoabdominal approach has been used.

Fever of 39 C (102.2 F) or greater occurs in over half of patients. Fever may be due to pulmonary complications or perihepatic abscess, but in many cases no cause can be identified and convalescence in the latter patients may be otherwise unmarred. Abscess formation is a major problem in the space created by the resection and requires reexploration and drainage.

Partial hepatectomy is attended by a relatively high incidence of postoperative stress ulcers. Prophylactic antacids should be given routinely through the nasogastric tube after operation.

Liver failure may result if the residual tissue is diseased or has been compromised by prolonged ischemia during the operation. Ascites, varices, and coma are the manifestations.

Prognosis

The mortality rate is about 25% but is largely related to the underlying disease. The various prognostic factors will be discussed under the separate disease headings.

Figure 27–4. Terminology of various segmental resections of the liver. Lobectomy is sometimes referred to as hemihepatectomy.

Aronsen KF & others: Metabolic changes following major hepatic resection. Ann Surg 169:102, 1969.

Blumgart LH & others: Observations on liver regeneration after right hepatic lobectomy. Gut 12:922, 1971.

Gans H & others: Evaluation of the effects of the finger fracture technique used in hepatic resection. Surg Gynecol Obstet 138:885, 1974.

Lin TY: Results in 107 hepatic lobectomies with a preliminary report on the use of a clamp to reduce blood loss. Ann Surg 177:413, 1973.

Longmire WP Jr: Hepatic resection. Adv Surg 8:29, 1974.

Pinkerton JA & others: A study of the postoperative course after hepatic lobectomy. Ann Surg 173:800, 1971.

Stone HH & others: Physiologic considerations in major hepatic resections. Am J Surg 117:78, 1969.

DISEASES & DISORDERS OF THE LIVER

HEPATIC TRAUMA

Based on the mechanism of injury, liver trauma is classified as penetrating or blunt. Penetrating wounds, comprising more than half of cases, are due to bullets, knives, etc which lacerate the liver or its afferent or efferent vessels. In civilian practice, most of these tend to be clean wounds—dangerous because of abdominal bleeding but not producing much devitalization of liver substance. In contrast, high-velocity missiles, in addition to piercing the liver, shatter the parenchyma for a variable distance from the track of the missile.

Blunt trauma can be inflicted by a direct blow to the upper abdomen or lower right rib cage or can follow sudden deceleration, as occurs with a fall from a great height. Most often a consequence of automobile accidents, direct blunt trauma tends to produce explosive bursting wounds or linear lacerations of the hepatic surface, often with considerable parenchymal destruction. The stellate bursting type of injury tends to affect the posterior superior segment of the right lobe because of its relatively vulnerable location, convex surface, fixed position, and concentration of hepatic mass. Damage to the left lobe is much less common than damage to the right. Injuries that involve shearing forces can tear the hepatic veins where they enter the liver substance, producing an exsanguinating retrohepatic injury in an area that is difficult to surgically expose and repair. The principal surgical goals are to stop bleeding and debride devitalized liver. Studies of large numbers of liver injuries indicate that all but a few are surgically manageable. Because some degree of liver failure is common postoperatively, efforts should be made during each stage of management to maintain adequate oxygenation of blood and perfusion of the liver by avoiding hypoxia and hypovolemia.

Clinical Findings

With penetrating wounds of the abdomen, diagnosis of liver injury is rarely a problem because laparotomy should be routine. If it is not certain whether a wound actually enters the abdomen, it may be explored initially under local anesthesia.

A. Symptoms and Signs: The clinical manifestations of liver injury are those of hypovolemic shock, ie, hypotension, decreased urinary output, low CVP, and, in some cases, abdominal distention. Early documentation of intra-abdominal bleeding following blunt injury is sometimes possible by peritoneal tap. Because false-negative results can occur with this test, peritoneal lavage should be performed if blood is not obtained with the tap (see Chapter 51).

B. Laboratory Findings: The rate of blood loss is usually so rapid that anemia does not develop. Leukocytosis greater than $15,000/\mu l$ is common following rupture of either the liver or spleen from blunt trauma.

C. X-Ray Findings: In most cases, x-ray evaluation is of minor importance. Hepatomegaly may be evident on plain abdominal films, or the right diaphragm may be elevated. Fractured ribs over the liver should suggest liver injury.

Angiography is not routine because it is so time-consuming. However, it may be useful to delineate the extent of central rupture and is diagnostic in hematobilia.

D. Special Examinations: Hepatic scan may show filling defects in cases of central rupture or subcapsular hematoma without active bleeding.

Treatment

In severely traumatized patients, abdominal exploration should be accepted as a legitimate part of the diagnostic work-up, indicated whenever strong suspicion exists that liver or other visceral injury has occurred. The morbidity caused by delay while waiting for diagnostic certainty is far greater than that due to a negative diagnostic laparotomy. When the abdomen is entered, thorough exploration requires palpation and inspection of all of the liver surfaces; if signs of injury are noted, the ligamentous attachments should be divided to permit full evaluation.

Depending on the depth and location of the wound, bleeding may be either simple or difficult to control. Subcapsular hematomas so often overlie an active bleeding site or parenchyma in need of debridement that they should be explored even though it appears superficially that the injury is effectively tamponaded and of limited severity.

Most lacerations have stopped bleeding by the time operation is performed. In the absence of active hemorrhage, these wounds should not be sutured because a closed space would be created which is susceptible to abscess formation or hematobilia. Several soft rubber drains placed in the vicinity of the injury should be brought out through a separate incision, usually at the tip of the 12th rib.

Active bleeding from liver lacerations should be managed by direct suture of identifiable vessels and electrocautery of bleeding parenchyma. The full extent of the wound must be inspected, and this means that a short, deep laceration may require extension of its length on the surface. Deep mattress sutures to tamponade liver bleeding should be used only when attempts at direct suture ligation and hepatic artery ligation have failed. After bleeding is stopped, no attempt should be made to restore continuity of the surface by closing the wound. Only drainage is needed.

If rapid bleeding obscures its source, temporary occlusion of the hepatic artery and portal vein with a soft tourniquet or vascular clamp (Pringle maneuver) for periods of 15–20 minutes may permit more accurate ligation of the vessels in the wound. In some cases, persistent arterial hemorrhage can only be controlled by ligation of the hepatic artery or one of the accessible lobar branches in the hilus. Collaterals from the remaining arterialized segments and through ligamentous attachments develop over several weeks to resupply the dearterialized area. After arterial ligation, the hepatic ligaments should not be divided if that can be avoided, but the gallbladder should be removed.

The most difficult problems with bleeding involve lacerations of the major hepatic veins. Temporary clamping of the inflow vessels may or may not slow blood loss enough to allow inspection and suture of the bleeding point. Occasionally, packs placed behind the liver for 20–30 minutes will stop the bleeding. For persistent bleeding from retrohepatic tears, the abdominal incision can be extended into a median sternotomy and a shunt placed via the atrial appendage into the inferior vena cava past the origin of the hepatic veins. This will permit total isolation of the liver circulation without interrupting the return of venous blood from the lower extremities to the heart. Lobectomy, usually of the right lobe, may be required to manage this type of injury.

Blunt injuries associated with substantial amounts of parenchymal destruction are the most difficult to manage. Debridement of devitalized tissue must be adequate but generally involves piecemeal removal of tissue rather than segmental or lobar resections. Rarely (eg, 1% of cases), a particularly severe pulverizing injury will require formal lobectomy.

Adequate postoperative drainage is of critical importance and is best obtained through the bed of the resected 12th rib. Theoretically, a T tube in the common duct should prevent bile leaks by reducing biliary pressure, but experience has shown that this is associated with many complications and it cannot be recommended except in special circumstances.

Penetrating injuries that involve the hepatic flexure of the colon as well as the liver are especially prone to severe subhepatic sepsis if managed by primary colonic anastomosis. After the liver is repaired and the injured colon resected, a temporary ileostomy and mucous fistula may avoid this complication.

Postoperative Complications

With present technics, hemorrhage at laparotomy is rarely uncontrollable except with retrohepatic venous injuries. Patients who rebleed from the liver wound after initial suture ligation should be treated by reexploration and lobectomy. Angiography and scintiscanning may provide useful diagnostic information preoperatively in such patients.

Subhepatic sepsis develops in about 20% of patients and is more frequent if lobectomy has been performed. Many cases of local postoperative infection can be attributed to faulty drainage.

Hematobilia may be responsible for gastrointestinal bleeding in the postoperative period and can be diagnosed by selective angiography of the hepatic artery. Treatment consists of ligation of the artery supplying the bleeding vessel, or, if that fails, segmental resection.

Bleeding from stress ulcers is common after hepatic trauma and seems especially prone to occur in patients with ancillary T tube drainage of the common duct. All patients with liver injuries should be given antacids after operation.

Prognosis

The mortality rate of 10–15% following hepatic trauma depends largely on the type of injury and the extent of associated injury to other organs. About one-third of patients admitted in shock cannot be saved. Only 1% of penetrating civilian wounds are lethal, whereas a 20% mortality rate attends blunt trauma. The mortality rate in blunt hepatic injury is 10% when only the liver is injured. If 3 major organs are damaged, the death rate is close to 70%.

Aaron S & others: Selective ligation of the hepatic artery for trauma of the liver. Surg Gynecol Obstet 141:187, 1975.

Ayella RJ & others: Contrast roentgenography in the management of major liver injury. Surg Gynecol Obstet 139:545, 1974.

Bismuth H: Hemobilia. N Engl J Med 288:617, 1973.

DeFore WW Jr & others: Management of 1,590 consecutive cases of liver trauma. Arch Surg 111:493, 1976.

Hardy KJ: Patterns of liver injury after fatal blunt trauma. Surg Gynecol Obstet 134:39, 1972.

Lim RC Jr & others: Postoperative treatment of patients after liver resection for trauma. Arch Surg 112:429, 1977.

Lim RC Jr & others: Prevention of complications after liver trauma. Am J Surg 132:156, 1976.

Longmire WP Jr, Cleveland RJ: Surgical anatomy and blunt trauma of the liver. Surg Clin North Am 52:687, 1972.

Lucas CE, Ledgerwood AM: Controlled biliary drainage for large injuries of the liver. Surg Gynecol Obstet 137:585, 1973.

Lucas CE, Ledgerwood AM: Prospective evaluation of hemostatic techniques for liver injuries. J Trauma 16:442, 1976.

Madding GF, Kennedy PA: *Trauma to the Liver,* 2nd ed. Saunders, 1971.

Mays ET: The hazards of suturing certain wounds of the liver. Surg Gynecol Obstet 143:201, 1976.

Mays ET: Hepatic trauma. Curr Probl Surg, Nov 1976.

Mays ET: Lobectomy, sublobar resection, and resectional debridement for severe liver injuries. J Trauma 12:309, 1972.

Trunkey DD & others: Management of liver trauma in 811 consecutive patients. Ann Surg 179:722, 1974.

SPONTANEOUS HEPATIC RUPTURE

Spontaneous rupture of the liver is not common. Most cases are due to preeclampsia-eclampsia, but spontaneous rupture has also been reported in association with hepatic hemangioma, gallstone obstruction, primary and metastatic liver carcinoma, hepatic adenoma, typhoid fever, malaria, tuberculosis, syphilis, polyarteritis nodosa, and diabetes mellitus. Rupture of the liver in the newborn is related to birth trauma in larger infants after difficult deliveries. The common course is intrahepatic hemorrhage expanding to capsular rupture.

Treatment consists of emergency surgery as for traumatic rupture (see above).

Baumwol M, Park W: An acute abdomen: Spontaneous rupture of the liver during pregnancy. Br J Surg 63:718, 1976.

PRIMARY MALIGNANT TUMORS OF THE LIVER

Primary hepatic malignancy is uncommon in the USA. However, the incidence is high in parts of the Orient and Africa, and in some regions hepatoma is the single most frequent abdominal tumor. The etiologic factors in these high-risk areas are environmental or cultural, since persons of similar racial background in the USA are at only slightly greater risk than Caucasians. About 7100 cases—distributed equally between men and women—occurred in the USA in 1972. Most arise in persons over 50 years of age, but a small number are found in children, mainly under 2 years of age.

Three cellular types are recognized: hepatocellular carcinoma (hepatoma), cholangiocellular carcinoma (cholangiocarcinoma), and a mixed form (hepatocholangioma). In children, the hepatocellular tumor is sometimes termed a hepatoblastoma because of its cellular similarity to fetal liver and the occasional presence of hematopoiesis.

Hepatomas comprise about 80% of primary hepatic malignancies. Their gross morphology allows separation into 3 classes: a **massive** form, characterized by a single predominant mass which may have small satellite nodules; a **nodular** form, composed of multiple nodules, often distributed throughout the liver; and a **diffuse** variety, characterized by infiltration of tumor throughout the remaining parenchyma.

In 70% of patients, tumor has spread outside the liver when hepatoma is first diagnosed. Metastases are almost invariably present with the nodular or diffuse forms, but 40% of the massive type are confined to the liver. The hilar and celiac lymph nodes are most commonly involved. Metastases to lung and the peritoneal surface also occur frequently. The portal or hepatic veins may be invaded by tumor, and venous occlusion may occur in either case.

Microscopically, there is little stroma between the malignant cells, and the tumor has a soft consistency. The tumor may be highly vascularized, a feature which sometimes produces massive intraperitoneal hemorrhage following spontaneous rupture. Hepatocellular function occurs in some, as indicated by the presence of bile pigment between or in the tumor cells.

Cholangiocarcinomas make up about 15% of hepatic carcinomas. They are usually well-differentiated tumors which spread invasively in the liver substance. Extrahepatic metastases are the rule by the time the tumor is detected.

The mixed tumors resemble hepatomas in their pathologic and clinical behavior.

Postnecrotic or posthepatic cirrhosis is a predisposing factor in about two-thirds of reported cases, although cirrhosis was found in only 15% in a recent large series from the USA. Hepatoma is a late complication of alcoholic (nutritional) cirrhosis and correlates more closely with alcohol ingestion than with overt alcoholic liver disease. Patients who are chronically seropositive for $HB_S Ag$ constitute a high-risk group for development of hepatoma, which in some cases may be detected at an early stage by periodic measurement of alpha-fetoprotein levels. Widespread infestation with liver flukes *(Clonorchis sinensis)* is at least partly responsible for the increased incidence of these tumors in the Orient, although other factors may also be important. Certain fungus products called aflatoxins have been shown to be capable of producing liver tumors experimentally. These substances have been detected in ground nuts and grain in some parts of the world where hepatomas are common.

Angiosarcoma of the liver, a rare fatal tumor, has developed in a number of workers intensively exposed to vinyl chloride for prolonged periods in polymerization plants.

Clinical Findings

A. Symptoms and Signs: The clinical diagnosis is usually quite difficult, and until recently the majority of primary hepatic carcinomas were not diagnosed until after death. Abdominal pain and distention are the most common symptoms. The pain can be felt in the epigastrium or right upper quadrant and sometimes is associated with referred pain in the right shoulder. Weight loss is usually present, and jaundice is evident in about one-third of cases.

Hepatomegaly can be detected in 80% of cases, and a mass is palpable in most of the rest. An arterial bruit can be heard over the liver in about 25% of cases and is a useful clue to the diagnosis if acute alcoholic hepatitis can be excluded. The systolic accentuation should enable it to be easily distinguished from the venous collateral hum found in portal hypertension. In a few patients, a friction rub is present over the liver. Ascites or gastrointestinal bleeding from varices is found in about 30%. Blood in ascites is highly suggestive of hepatoma. Intermittent fever is sometimes a prominent presenting feature.

The patterns of clinical presentation are as follows: (1) rapid progression of hepatic neoplasm with pain and hepatomegaly; (2) sudden deterioration of the condition of a cirrhotic due to the appearance of hepatic failure, bleeding varices, or ascites; (3) sudden, massive intraperitoneal hemorrhage; (4) acute illness with fever and abdominal pain; (5) distant metastases; and (6) no specific clinical findings.

B. Laboratory Findings: The serum bilirubin is elevated in one-third of patients. In another 25%, serum alkaline phosphatase is increased but the serum bilirubin is normal. Since many of these patients have cirrhosis, the significance of these alterations is often difficult to assess.

C. Liver Scan: Hepatic scintiscans are abnormal in about 90% of patients.

D. Arteriography: Hepatomas are usually supplied by the hepatic artery, and in 80% of cases selective angiography demonstrates increased tumor vascularity compared with adjacent parenchyma. In about 20%, the picture is diagnostic and consists of multiple tortuous tumor vessels and an intense blush on the hepatogram phase. In some cases, the center of the tumor has become necrotic and only the peripheral areas display the dense tumor blush. Cholangiocarcinomas rarely have a substantial arterial supply and appear less vascular compared with adjacent tissue. Although 10% of metastatic adenocarcinomas show greatly increased vascularity, they do not develop the typical vessel pattern of hepatomas. Some metastatic carcinoids and hepatic hamartomas are extremely vascular, and hemangiomas display a characteristic picture of patchy vascular pooling.

Portal venograms can be obtained by observing the venous phase after splanchnic arterial injections. These may show displacement of intrahepatic portal venous branches or, in some cases, invasion or occlusion of the vein by tumor. If esophageal varices are present, they may also be seen.

E. Special Tests: Alpha-fetoprotein (AFP) is an a_1 globulin normally present only in the fetal circulation. AFP measured by immunoassay is present in high concentrations in the serum of about 80% of patients with primary hepatomas and a few others with testicular tumors. It is also elevated to a lesser degree in chronic active hepatitis and acute viral and alcoholic hepatitis, where it seems to reflect the extent of liver regeneration. The theory that AFP functions normally during pregnancy as an immunosuppressant to protect the fetus from its maternal host suggests that AFP could serve an analogous function favoring growth of hepatomas in adults.

Changes in AFP levels in patients with hepatoma correlate well with growth activity of the tumor and can be used postoperatively as an index of the success of curative hepatic resection. The possible use of specific AFP antibodies as carriers for therapeutic radionuclides is being evaluated.

F. Liver Biopsy: The diagnosis can be established by percutaneous liver biopsy in most patients if the biopsy site is selected according to the scan. Percutaneous biopsy is safe if clotting factors are normal, and

early fears about implantation or dissemination of tumor during the procedure appear to have been unwarranted. The accuracy of biopsy can apparently be increased using the peritoneoscope.

Differential Diagnosis

The clinical picture is usually nonspecific. Because of weight loss and weakness, liver cancer is most often confused with other abdominal carcinomas. Once hepatomegaly and a filling defect in the liver are found, it must be determined whether the liver harbors a primary neoplasm or metastases. Arteriography, biopsy, and serum alpha-fetoprotein determination supply data to establish the exact diagnosis in most cases. However, it may be difficult to distinguish hepatic malignancy from benign tumors or cysts or, if the patient is febrile, from liver abscess.

When complications develop suddenly in a cirrhotic patient, the possibility of hepatoma must always be considered. Numerous examples have been reported where portacaval shunts were performed for recent variceal hemorrhage in a cirrhotic patient without suspecting that a hepatoma was responsible for the portal hypertension.

In rare instances, primary hepatocellular malignancy is associated with metabolic or endocrine abnormalities such as hypoglycemic attacks, Cushing's syndrome, or virilization.

Complications

Sudden intra-abdominal hemorrhage may occur from spontaneous bleeding. Obstruction of the portal vein may produce portal hypertension, and obstruction of the hepatic veins may produce the Budd-Chiari syndrome. Liver failure is a common cause of death.

Treatment

Surgical resection is the only treatment that offers a possibility of cure. Partial hepatectomy should be considered if the tumor is localized and would be encompassed by the proposed resection. Extension of tumor into the opposite lobe or involvement of the vena cava or hepatic veins of the opposite lobe eliminates the possibility of curative resection. Cirrhosis should be considered a relative contraindication because the limited functional reserve of the diseased parenchyma greatly increases the risk of postoperative liver failure. About 75% of patients with hepatic tumors are unsuitable for resection for these reasons.

Palliation can be obtained in certain cases by selective hepatic arterial infusion of chemotherapeutic agents. Fluorouracil and methotrexate have given the best results.

Ligation of the hepatic artery has been used as treatment for hepatomas since the artery serves as the principal source of blood supply. The goal of this approach is to bring about selective ischemic necrosis of tumor. Palliation has occasionally resulted from this treatment, but residual tumor continues to multiply until the patient succumbs.

Arterial ligation and local chemotherapy have

been used in combination. The hepatic artery is divided and a perfusion catheter inserted into the distal end for administration of antineoplastic drugs.

Prognosis

Despite the development in the past decade of newer technics that have permitted earlier diagnosis, there has been no appreciable improvement in survival. The average life expectancy after diagnosis is about 6 months. The patients generally die from the effects of the expanding hepatic neoplasm rather than from metastases. Fewer than 100 five-year survivors have been reported following partial hepatectomy. Several patients have survived for 2–3 years following selective perfusion of antitumor agents through the hepatic artery.

Liver transplantation could become a successful method of treatment if the problems discussed in Chapter 50 can be solved.

Adson MA, Sheedy PF: Resection of primary hepatic malignant lesions. Arch Surg 108:599, 1974.

Almersjö O & others: Selective celiac angiography and surgical exploration for suspected liver cancer. Am J Surg 131:676, 1976.

Balasegaram M: Management of primary liver cell carcinoma. Am J Surg 130:33, 1975.

Berk PD & others: Vinyl chloride-associated liver disease. Ann Intern Med 84:717, 1976.

Clatworthy HW Jr & others: Primary liver tumors in infancy and childhood. Arch Surg 109:143, 1974.

Fortner JG & others: Surgery in liver tumors. Curr Probl Surg, June 1972.

Ihde DC & others: Clinical manifestations of hepatoma. Am J Med 56:83, 1974.

Kew MC & others: Diagnosis of primary cancer of the liver. Br Med J 4:408, 1971.

Kohn J, Weaver PC: Serum-alpha$_1$-fetoprotein in hepatocellular carcinoma. Lancet 2:334, 1974.

Malt RA & others: Manifestations and prognosis of carcinoma of the liver. Surg Gynecol Obstet 135:361, 1972.

Nagasue N & others: Angiographic evaluation of hepatoma for surgical treatment. Surg Gynecol Obstet 143:184, 1976.

Okezie O, DeAngelis G: Spontaneous rupture of hepatoma: A misdiagnosed surgical emergency. Ann Surg 179:133, 1974.

Ong GB, Chan PKW. Primary carcinoma of the liver. Surg Gynecol Obstet 143:31, 1976.

Parks LC & others: Alpha fetoproteins: An index of progression or regression of hepatoma, and a target for immunotherapy. Ann Surg 180:599, 1974.

Ramming KP & others: Hepatic artery ligation and 5-fluorouracil infusion for metastatic colon carcinoma and primary hepatoma. Am J Surg 132:236, 1976.

Ruoslahti E & others: Serum a-fetoprotein: Diagnostic significance in liver disease. Br Med J 2:527, 1974.

METASTATIC NEOPLASMS OF THE LIVER

Metastatic malignancy is 20 times more common than primary tumors in the liver. Cancers of the breast, lung, pancreas, stomach, large intestine, kidney, ovary, and uterus account for about 75% of cases. Spread to the liver may be via the systemic circulation, portal vein, or, less often, the lymphatics. Interestingly, the cirrhotic liver, which often gives rise to primary hepatic tumors, is less susceptible than normal liver to implantation of metastases.

Over 90% of patients with hepatic metastases have tumor implants in other organs. The lung is most commonly involved and contains tumor in 30% of cases. It may be useful for the surgeon to appreciate that 10% of patients with hepatic metastases have gross tumor deposits demonstrable on hepatic section which cannot be seen or felt from the surface of the liver during laparotomy.

Weight loss, fatigue, and anorexia are the presenting general complaints. Right upper abdominal pain, ascites, and jaundice are the usual symptoms referable to the liver. The pain may radiate around the costal margin or straight through to the back. Fever without demonstrable infection is present in 15–20% of cases and bears only a loose relationship to leukocytosis.

In about two-thirds of cases, physical examination reveals hepatomegaly or a palpable metastatic tumor in the upper abdomen. Either may be tender to palpation. If portal hypertension is present, it may be manifested by abdominal venous collaterals or splenomegaly. A friction rub is sometimes heard and is always highly suggestive of hepatic tumor.

Laboratory investigation reveals a hematocrit between 30–36%. The serum bilirubin is elevated in almost half of patients, and half of these have values over 4 mg/100 ml. Sulfobromophthalein (BSP) retention is abnormal in most patients, and the alkaline phosphatase is also usually increased.

The diagnosis can be established by percutaneous liver biopsy or fine needle aspiration for malignant cells in most cases, especially if the hepatic scan is used to direct the site of the biopsy. Selective hepatic angiography may be diagnostic in puzzling cases. Metastatic lesions are principally supplied by the hepatic artery but on angiograms are usually shown to be less vascular than hepatomas.

Little effective treatment is available for the average patient. Partial hepatic resection may be justified for solitary or localized multiple metastases if there are no signs of tumor elsewhere. Patients who are candidates for this approach usually have a colorectal primary tumor. Partial hepatectomy is also sometimes worthwhile to extirpate a tumor invading directly from a contiguous organ.

Systemic chemotherapy does not improve survival. Recent attempts at palliation have concentrated on delivery of high levels of chemotherapeutic agents by infusion directly into the hepatic artery or portal vein. Hepatic artery ligation has also benefited some by causing necrosis of the bulk of the tumor mass.

Without treatment, the median survival time after detection of hepatic metastases is 75 days. Only 5% are alive after 2 years. Survival is slightly longer in patients with metastases from colonic cancer than in patients with metastases from pancreatic or gastric tumors.

Fenster LF, Klatskin G: Manifestations of metastatic tumors of the liver. Am J Med 31:238, 1961.

Jaffe BM & others: Factors influencing survival in patients with untreated hepatic metastases. Surg Gynecol Obstet 127:1, 1968.

Larmi TKI & others: Treatment of patients with hepatic tumors and jaundice by ligation of the hepatic artery. Arch Surg 108:178, 1974.

Massey WH & others: Hepatic artery infusion for metastatic malignancy using percutaneously placed catheters. Am J Surg 121:160, 1971.

Rapoport AH, Burleson RL: Survival of patients treated with systemic fluorouracil for hepatic metastases. Surg Gynecol Obstet 130:773, 1970.

Sparks FC & others: Hepatic artery ligation and postoperative chemotherapy for hepatic metastases. Cancer 35:1074, 1975.

Stehlin JS Jr & others: Experience with infusion and resection in cancer of the liver. Surg Gynecol Obstet 138:855, 1974.

Wilson SM, Adson MA: Surgical treatment of hepatic metastases for colorectal cancers. Arch Surg 111:330, 1976.

BENIGN TUMORS & CYSTS OF THE LIVER*

Hemangiomas

Hemangioma is the most common of the benign hepatic tumors, and—except for the skin and mucous membranes—the liver is the most common location for hemangiomas. Women are affected more often than men in a ratio of 6:1. Histologically, hepatic hemangiomas are of the cavernous type. Most are small solitary subcapsular growths which are found incidentally during laparotomy or at autopsy. Those greater than 4 cm in diameter may cause abdominal pain or a palpable mass. Some patients have presented with hemorrhagic shock resulting from spontaneous rupture. Large congenital hemangiomas of the liver may be associated with others in the skin. Occasionally, a hemangioma may behave as an arteriovenous fistula and produce cardiac hypertrophy and congestive heart failure. Selective hepatic arteriography reveals a vascular tumor containing spaces that trap the contrast media longer than surrounding parenchyma.

Symptomatic hemangiomas should be excised. If discovered as an incidental finding during laparotomy, a hemangioma should not be biopsied or removed because difficulties with hemostasis can be extreme. Radiotherapy has been effective in limiting enlargement of unresectable tumors. Patients with congestive failure due to arteriovenous fistula have been helped by ligation of the hepatic artery.

Hepatic Adenoma

These benign tumors occur almost exclusively in women and appear to be increasing in frequency be-

*Echinococcal cysts are discussed in Chapter 11.

cause of the widespread use of oral contraceptives. Mestranol-containing compounds have been singled out as etiologically important by one report, but the evidence implicating this specific hormone is still inconclusive.

The tumors are soft, yellow-tan, well-circumscribed masses that measure about 2–15 cm in diameter. Most of those that cause symptoms are in the 8–15 cm range. Two-thirds of hepatic adenomas are solitary; the remainder are multiple. A few are pedunculated. It is currently believed that hepatic adenomas rarely if ever become malignant. Histologically, hepatic adenomas consist of an encapsulated homogeneous mass of normal-appearing hepatocytes without bile ducts or central veins. The fibrous septa characteristic of focal nodular hyperplasia are absent. Hemorrhage may be present.

About half of patients discovered to have hepatic adenomas are asymptomatic. Most of those with symptoms present acutely with sudden right upper quadrant pain or intra-abdominal hemorrhage and shock. These complications are due to spontaneous hemorrhage into the substance of the tumor, which may rupture into the peritoneal cavity. There is a strong association of acute bleeding episodes with menstruation. The presentation of one-third of patients is less acute, with pain over the liver associated with nausea and vomiting. Patients with symptoms usually have a palpable mass in the liver.

Liver function tests and alpha-fetoprotein levels are usually normal. Hepatic scans may show a focal defect but often are deceptively normal. Hepatic angiography demonstrates a hypervascular lesion with numerous feeding vessels entering from the periphery. Dense opacification persists into the venous phase. This picture cannot usually be distinguished from that of a malignant hepatoma. Liver biopsy is contraindicated because of the danger of bleeding.

Symptomatic hepatic adenomas must be resected, which in acutely bleeding patients may be lifesaving. They cannot be enucleated but require a partial hepatectomy. The high potential for serious complications justifies prophylactic excision of asymptomatic hepatic adenomas. At laparotomy, it may be difficult to distinguish hepatic adenoma from hepatoma by gross inspection or even frozen section examination.

Most patients recover without sequelae after surgical removal; recurrence is rare. Radiotherapy and chemotherapy are of no therapeutic value.

Focal Nodular Hyperplasia

Focal nodular hyperplasia is a benign lesion with no malignant potential. It is found in women twice as often as men but, unlike hepatic adenomas, is not thought to be related to the use of birth control pills.

Grossly, the lesion is a well-circumscribed, firm, tan, usually subcapsular mass measuring 2–3 cm in diameter. In patients with symptoms, the lesions average 4–7 cm in diameter and occasionally are multiple. Eighty percent are solitary. The appearance on cut section is pathognomonic, consisting of a central stellate scar with radiating fibrous septa that compartmentalize the lesion into lobules. Histologically, there are nodular aggregations of normal-appearing hepatocytes without central veins or portal triads. Bile duct proliferation is present in the nodules.

Seventy-five percent of patients with focal nodular hyperplasia are asymptomatic. Those with symptoms present with a right upper quadrant mass, discomfort, or both. Unlike hepatic adenomas, these lesions rarely bleed because of their abundant connective tissue stroma. A few patients with diffuse focal nodular hyperplasia develop portal hypertension.

Hepatic function tests are usually normal. Hepatic scans may or may not show a filling defect. The arteriographic pattern is of a vascular tumor similar in appearance to a hepatic adenoma.

Symptomatic lesions should be removed; asymptomatic ones may be left undisturbed since their growth is indolent and complications are rare. Focal nodular hyperplasia can be reliably identified on examination of frozen sections.

Cysts

Hepatic cysts are usually solitary unilocular anomalies which produce no symptoms. The occasional large cyst may present as an upper abdominal mass or discomfort. Polycystic liver disease is associated in about half of cases with polycystic renal disease. It is probably a variant of the disease called congenital hepatic fibrosis.

Large symptomatic cysts should be subtotally excised or drained by a Roux-en-Y limb of jejunum if they are situated deep within the liver. The possibility of echinococcosis (see Chapter 11) should always be ruled out by performing serologic studies before operation. Multiple cysts do not usually require treatment, but several cases have been managed by surgically creating windows between the large cysts and allowing them to drain into the abdominal cavity.

Adam YG & others: Giant hemangiomas of the liver. Ann Surg 172:239, 1970.

Ameriks JA & others: Hepatic cell adenomas, spontaneous liver rupture, and oral contraceptives. Arch Surg 110:548, 1975.

Coutsoftides T, Hermann RE: Nonparasitic cysts of the liver. Surg Gynecol Obstet 138:906, 1974.

Edmondson HA & others: Liver-cell adenomas associated with use of oral contraceptives. N Engl J Med 294:470, 1976.

Foster JH: Primary benign solid tumors of the liver. Am J Surg 133:536, 1977.

Ishak KG, Rabin L: Benign tumors of the liver. Med Clin North Am 59:995, 1975.

Knowles DM II, Wolff M: Focal nodular hyperplasia of the liver. Hum Pathol 7:533, 1976.

Park WC, Phillips R: The role of radiation therapy in the management of hemangiomas of the liver. JAMA 212:1496, 1970.

Rake MO & others: Ligation of the hepatic artery in the treatment of heart failure due to hepatic haemangiomatosis. Gut 11:512, 1970.

Sanfelippo PM, Beahrs OH, Weiland LH: Cystic disease of the liver. Ann Surg 179:922, 1974.

Sewell JH, Weiss K: Spontaneous rupture of hemangioma of the liver. Arch Surg 83:105, 1961.

Sherlock S: Hepatic adenomas and oral contraceptives. Gut 16:753, 1975.

HEPATIC ABSCESS

Hepatic abscesses may be bacterial, parasitic, or fungal in origin. In the USA, pyogenic abscesses are the most common, and amebic abscesses (see Chapter 11) are next most common. Unless otherwise specified, the following remarks refer to bacterial abscesses.

Cases are about evenly divided between those with a single abscess and those with many abscesses. Solitary abscesses affect the right lobe 5 times more commonly than the left and are particularly prone to develop in patients with diabetes mellitus. Multiple abscesses are usually distributed throughout both lobes. Therapy is usually successful for a solitary abscess that is diagnosed early and treated, whereas multiple abscesses are often incurable. Many of the latter are terminal manifestations of untreatable hepatobiliary malignancy.

In most cases, the development of a hepatic abscess follows a suppurative process elsewhere in the body. Many abscesses are due to direct spread from biliary infections such as empyema of the gallbladder or protracted cholangitis. Abdominal infections such as appendicitis or diverticulitis may spread through the portal vein to involve the liver with abscess formation. Other cases develop after generalized sepsis from bacterial endocarditis, renal infection, or pneumonitis. In 10–15% of cases, no antecedent infection can be documented ("cryptogenic" abscesses). Other rare causes include secondary bacterial infection of an amebic abscess, hydatid cyst, or congenital hepatic cyst.

In some patients, the hepatic abscess supervenes as a complication of another active infection; in others, months or even years may elapse between resolution of the original sepsis and the infection in the liver. Detection of the liver abscess is usually not difficult in the former, but when the primary disease and the abscess are temporally separated there is often considerable delay in diagnosis.

Clinical Findings

A. Symptoms and Signs: When liver abscess develops in the course of another intra-abdominal infection such as diverticulitis, it is accompanied by increasing toxicity, higher fever, jaundice, and a generally deteriorating clinical picture. Right upper quadrant pain may appear.

In other cases, the diagnosis is much less obvious since the illness develops insidiously in a previously healthy person. In these, the first symptoms are usually malaise and fatigue, followed after several weeks by fever. Epigastric or right upper quadrant pain is present in about half of cases. The pain may be aggravated by motion or may be referred to the right shoulder.

The course of fever is often erratic, and spikes to 40–41 C (104–105.8 F) are common. Chills are present in about 25% of cases. The liver is usually enlarged and may be tender to palpation. If tenderness is severe, the condition may be confused with cholecystitis.

Jaundice is unusual in solitary abscesses unless the patient's condition is seriously worsening. It is often present in patients with multiple abscesses and in general is a bad prognostic sign.

B. Laboratory Findings: Leukocytosis is present in most cases and is usually over $15,000/\mu l$. A small group of patients—containing some of the most seriously ill—fail to develop leukocytosis. Anemia is present in most patients. The average hematocrit is 33%.

The serum bilirubin is usually normal except in patients with multiple abscesses or when hepatic failure has supervened. The alkaline phosphatase is often elevated even in the presence of a normal bilirubin—a pattern characteristic of segmental obstruction of the bile ducts.

C. X-Ray Findings: X-ray changes are present in the right lung in about one-third of cases and consist of basilar atelectasis or pleural effusion. The right diaphragm may be elevated and less mobile than the left.

Plain films of the abdomen are usually normal or show only hepatomegaly. In a few patients, an air-fluid level in the region of the liver reveals the presence and location of the abscess. Distortion of the contour of the stomach on upper gastrointestinal series may be seen with large abscesses involving the left lobe.

Intravenous cholangiograms and oral cholecystograms fail to outline the bile ducts and are of no diagnostic value.

Selective hepatic arteriography may add valuable supplemental information to that obtained from the scan. Abscesses smaller than the 2.5 cm limit of resolution of the scan may sometimes be shown. Avascularity of the defect suggests abscess rather than tumor except in the rare case where there has been extensive necrosis within the tumor.

D. Liver Scan: The radioisotope liver scan is of great diagnostic value. If several views are obtained, the site and size of a solitary abscess can be clearly established. Multiple small abscesses are usually impossible to diagnose on scan.

Ultrasonic scans are of help to differentiate abscess from tumor.

Differential Diagnosis

In many cases, the early findings may be so vague that hepatic abscess is not even considered. The multiple other causes of malaise, weight loss, and anemia would enter into the differential diagnosis. When spiking fevers appear, the physician must consider all the causes of fever of unknown origin. Failure to entertain the possibility of hepatic abscess and to obtain the necessary hepatic scans and arteriograms leads to most errors in diagnosis. Many patients are not diagnosed until exploratory laparotomy is performed for fever

and abdominal pain. Abdominal lymphoma is a common preoperative diagnosis in these cases.

After the hepatic scan has revealed an abscess, the infectious agent—amebic or bacterial—must be determined. If blood cultures are positive, a pyogenic cause can be inferred, but it is often impossible to differentiate between amebic and bacterial abscesses until after treatment has been instituted for both possibilities. Positive serologic tests would verify amebiasis, but the results may not be available for several weeks. Whenever there is doubt, the patient should receive both metronidazole for amebiasis and antibiotics for bacterial infection.

Complications

Complications result either from further dissemination of infection or from progressive impairment of liver function. Intrahepatic spread of infection may create multiple additional abscesses and is responsible for some failures after surgical treatment of an apparently solitary abscess. As the untreated abscess expands, rupture may occur into the pleural or peritoneal cavity, usually with catastrophic results. Septicemia and septic shock are common terminal complications of diffuse hepatic infection. Hepatic failure may develop in addition to uncontrolled sepsis or it may predominate over signs of infection.

Hematobilia may follow bleeding from the vascular wall into the abscess cavity. In this case, drainage of the abscess may be inadequate treatment, and lobectomy may be required to control bleeding.

Treatment

After blood cultures have been obtained, parenteral antibiotics should be administered in high doses. If the bacteria and its sensitivities have been identified, the choice of drug should be made on that basis. In the absence of such information, antibiotics should be selected according to the presumptive source of the infection. In most cases, the organism is of enteric origin. *Escherichia coli,* bacteroides, and anaerobic streptococci are most frequently recovered. Gram-positive cocci, staphylococci, or hemolytic streptococci are usually recovered if the primary infection was bacterial endocarditis or pneumonitis.

If the possibility of amebic abscess cannot be excluded, the patient should be treated with metronidazole until more definitive information becomes available. (See Chapter 11 for details of the treatment regimen for amebiasis.)

Pyogenic abscesses must be surgically drained since nonoperative management is almost uniformly fatal. Abscesses in the dependent posterior superior segment of the right lobe can be drained extraperitoneally through the bed of the 12th rib. In most cases, however, drainage can be more satisfactorily achieved at laparotomy. This allows inspection of the liver for possible additional undisclosed abscesses and permits preliminary exploration of other areas of the abdomen before drainage. The results of treatment in recent years suggest that it is not of major importance to establish drainage extraperitoneally as was once thought.

At operation the contents of the abscess should be initially evacuated using a large needle or trocar attached to a suction device. Care should be taken to avoid spilling pus into the abdomen. Samples should be sent for culture and sensitivity tests and investigation for amebas. Surprisingly, some apparently pyogenic abscesses give no growth when the contents are cultured. After the cavity is emptied, an incision is made into the abscess and a large sump drain inserted which is brought out through the abdominal wall. Additional soft rubber drains should be placed in the subhepatic region. Postoperatively, the sump is left in place until the cavity begins to shrink around the tube, after which it is gradually withdrawn.

Several groups have reported that pyogenic abscesses may be definitively treated by percutaneous needle aspiration combined with specific antibiotics, but this approach has received insufficient evaluation to permit a judgment about whether it would be as successful as open drainage in the average case.

In most cases, multiple abscesses cannot be drained satisfactorily. Rarely, multiple abscesses are confined to a single lobe and can be cured by lobectomy. It has been suggested that administration of high concentrations of antibiotics through the umbilical vein may be more effective for multiple abscesses than antibiotic infusion into a peripheral vein. In any event, biliary obstruction or other causes of the sepsis must also be corrected if there is to be any hope for cure.

Prognosis

The overall mortality rate is about 40% and is related to 2 problems: delay in diagnosis of solitary abscesses and multiple abscesses for which there is no effective treatment. The appearance of jaundice and a falling serum albumin are both bad prognostic signs. Prompt diagnosis and treatment of a solitary abscess is associated with a mortality rate of about 10%.

Altemeier WA & others: Abscesses of the liver: Surgical considerations. Arch Surg 101:258, 1970.

De la Maza LM & others: The changing etiology of liver abscess. JAMA 227:161, 1974.

Holt JM, Spry CJF: Solitary pyogenic liver abscess in patients with diabetes mellitus. Lancet 2:198, 1966.

Pai ST, Bakk YW: Radioisotope scanning in the diagnosis of liver abscess. Am J Surg 119:330, 1970.

Pitt HA, Zuidema GD: Factors influencing mortality in the treatment of pyogenic hepatic abscess. Surg Gynecol Obstet 140:228, 1975.

Ranson JH & others: New diagnostic and therapeutic techniques in the management of pyogenic liver abscesses. Ann Surg 181:508, 1975.

Rubin RH & others: Hepatic abscess: Changes in clinical, bacteriologic and therapeutic aspects. Am J Med 57:601, 1974.

● ● ●

General References

Cameron HM, Linsell DA, Warwick GP: *Liver Cell Cancer.* Elsevier, 1976.

Foster JH, Berman MM: *Solid Liver Tumors.* Saunders, 1977.

Madding GF, Kennedy PA: Symposium on hepatic surgery. Surg Clin North Am 57 (2), 1977. [Entire issue.]

Sandblom P: *Hemobilia.* Thomas, 1972.

Schiff L (editor): *Diseases of the Liver,* 4th ed. Lippincott, 1975.

Schwartz SI: *Surgical Diseases of the Liver.* McGraw-Hill, 1964.

Sherlock S: *Diseases of the Liver and Biliary System,* 5th ed. Blackwell, 1975.

28 . . .
Portal Hypertension

Lawrence W. Way, MD

Portal hypertension is most commonly caused by cirrhosis of the liver, but various other diseases are occasionally implicated. The rise in portal pressure is usually a result of increased resistance to flow (eg, cirrhosis); rarely, massively increased portal flow is an important contributing factor. The high portal pressure stimulates expansion of rudimentary venous collaterals between the portal and systemic venous systems. The most significant is the venous plexus at the gastroesophageal junction, which drains into the azygos veins. Under the stimulus to transport greater volumes, these may develop into large fragile submucosal varices susceptible to spontaneous rupture and massive hemorrhage. This is the major complication of portal hypertension and the usual reason the surgeon becomes involved in the care of these patients. The other common clinical sequelae include ascites, hepatic encephalopathy, and secondary hypersplenism. If the surgeon can construct a large-diameter anastomosis (shunt) between the portal and systemic venous circulations, the elevated portal pressure drops and the risk of variceal hemorrhage is eliminated. However, decisions about the care of these patients are rarely simple since portacaval shunts tend to impair hepatic function and lower the threshold for encephalopathy. Potential candidates for operation must be carefully evaluated to ensure optimal surgical results.

ANATOMY OF THE PORTAL CIRCULATION

The portal vein is formed by the confluence of the splenic and superior mesenteric veins at the level of the second lumbar vertebra behind the head of the pancreas (Fig 28–1). It runs for 8–9 cm to the hilus of the liver, where it divides into lobar branches. The coronary (left gastric) vein usually enters the portal vein on its anteromedial aspect just cephalad to the margin of the pancreas, in which case it usually must be ligated during the surgical construction of a portacaval shunt; in 25% of cases, the coronary vein joins the splenic vein. Other small venous tributaries from the pancreas and duodenum are less constant but must be anticipated during surgical mobilization of the portal vein.

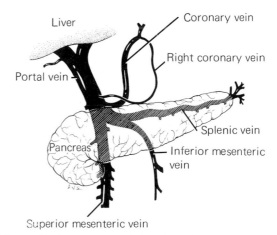

Figure 28–1. Anatomic relationships of portal vein and branches.

The inferior mesenteric vein generally drains into the splenic vein several centimeters to the left of the junction with the superior mesenteric vein; not uncommonly, it empties directly into the superior mesenteric vein.

In the hepatoduodenal ligament, the portal vein lies dorsal and slightly medial to the common bile duct. A large lymph node is often encountered lateral to the vein and must be dissected off before a shunt can be performed.

PHYSIOLOGY

Total hepatic blood flow is about 1500 ml/minute and comprises 25% of the cardiac output. Two-thirds of the flow enters through the portal vein and one-third through the hepatic artery. Pressure in the portal vein is normally 10–15 cm water (7–11 mm Hg). The liver derives half of its oxygen from hepatic arterial blood and half from portal venous inflow.

Portal venous and hepatic arterial blood become pooled after entering the periphery of the hepatic sinusoid (Fig 28–2). There is evidence that sphincters regulate flow from the hepatic arterioles into the low-

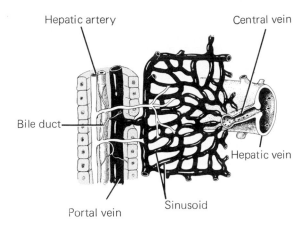

Hepatic artery

Central vein

Bile duct

Hepatic vein

Portal vein

Sinusoid

Figure 28–2. Vascular anatomy of the liver lobule.

Table 28–1. Causes of portal hypertension.

I. Increased resistance to flow
  A. Prehepatic (portal vein obstruction)
    1. Congenital atresia or stenosis
    2. Thrombosis of portal vein
    3. Thrombosis of splenic vein
    4. Extrinsic compression (eg, tumors)
  B. Hepatic
    1. Cirrhosis
      a. Portal cirrhosis (nutritional, alcoholic, Laennec's)
      b. Postnecrotic cirrhosis
      c. Biliary cirrhosis
      d. Others (Wilson's disease, hemochromatosis, late schistosomiasis)
    2. Acute alcoholic liver disease
    3. Congenital hepatic fibrosis
    4. Idiopathic portal hypertension (hepatoportal sclerosis)
    5. Schistosomiasis
  C. Posthepatic
    1. Budd-Chiari syndrome
    2. Constrictive pericarditis
II. Increased portal blood flow
  A. Arterial-portal venous fistula
  B. Increased splenic flow
    1. Banti's syndrome
    2. Splenomegaly (eg, tropical splenomegaly, myeloid metaplasia)

pressure sinusoids, although they have not been convincingly demonstrated by histologic technics. Flow within the sinusoids is erratic since at any given moment the blood may be stationary in as many as 40% of them. The regulatory mechanisms governing sinusoidal blood flow are not well understood, but the normal sinusoidal bed can accommodate large variations in portal flow without significant changes in portal pressure.

Sudden occlusion of the portal vein results in an immediate 60% rise in hepatic arterial flow. In a matter of weeks, total flow gradually returns toward normal. On the other hand, sudden reductions in hepatic arterial supply are not immediately met by significant increases in portal vein flow. In both normal subjects and cirrhotics, total hepatic flow and portal pressure drop following hepatic arterial occlusion. Arterial collaterals develop over the ensuing months, and arterial perfusion is ultimately restored.

Bloch EH: The termination of hepatic arterioles and the functional unit of the liver as determined by microscopy of the living organ. Ann New York Acad Sci 170:78, 1970.
Greenway CV, Stark RD: Hepatic vascular bed. Physiol Rev 51:23, 1971.
Marks C: Developmental basis of the portal venous system. Am J Surg 117:671, 1969.

ETIOLOGY

The causes of portal hypertension are listed in Table 28–1. In all but a few instances, the basic lesion is increased resistance to portal flow. Those associated with increased resistance can be subclassified according to the site of the block as prehepatic, hepatic, and posthepatic. Cirrhosis accounts for about 85% of cases of portal hypertension in the USA, and the most common form is that due to alcoholism. Postnecrotic cirrhosis is next in frequency, followed by biliary cirrho-

sis. The other intrahepatic causes of portal hypertension are relatively rare in this country, although in some parts of the world hepatic schistosomiasis comprises the largest single group. Idiopathic portal hypertension appears with greater frequency in southern Asia.

Next to cirrhosis, extrahepatic portal venous occlusion is the most common cause of portal hypertension. These patients are generally younger than the cirrhotics, and many are children. Posthepatic obstruction due to Budd-Chiari syndrome or constrictive pericarditis is rare.

PATHOPHYSIOLOGY

Portal hypertension is defined as portal pressure of 20 cm water (15 mm Hg) or more.

The greater resistance to portal flow presented by the cirrhotic liver is a result of parenchymal fibrosis and changes in vascular anatomy. Portal inflow is partially obstructed by scar formation. As much as one-third of portal flow may bypass sinusoids through shunts traversing areas bridged by fibrosis between portal areas and central veins. A great deal more remains to be learned about hemodynamics through the cirrhotic liver, but it is noteworthy that the regenerative nodule is associated with a postsinusoidal* type of resistance as measured by wedged hepatic vein pressure. Regenerative nodules are supplied with blood mainly from the hepatic artery, and blood escapes from the sinusoids of these nodules through abnormal hepatic venous channels at the periphery of the nodule. An interesting phenomenon is presented by hepatic schistosomiasis which evolves through 2 pathophysiologic phases. Early in the disease, granulomas from parasitic involvement are seen in the triads, and the portal hypertension is presinusoidal. Eventually, fibrosis and regenerative nodules appear, and the block shifts to a postsinusoidal position.

Even in the absence of cirrhosis, acute alcoholism can raise portal pressure by producing centrolobular swelling and fibrosis. Sinusoidal resistance to flow is also increased by engorgement of adjacent hepatocytes with fat and resultant distortion and narrowing of the vascular pathway. Examples have been documented where the elevated portal pressure dropped with resolution of the pathologic changes.

Fluctuations in the level of portal hypertension also occur in conjunction with changes in blood volume, and patients with ascites are especially sensitive. Administration of colloid solutions to a patient with a normal or expanded blood volume could theoretically aggravate the clinical manifestations of portal hypertension.

Budd-Chiari syndrome (see p 522) is produced by restriction to flow through the hepatic veins or the inferior vena cava above the liver. The resulting sinusoidal hypertension produces prominent ascites and hepatomegaly.

Total splenic blood flow is usually increased in splenomegaly regardless of the cause. Although increased portal inflow may contribute to portal hypertension in cirrhosis, it is not a decisive factor since splenectomy has no permanent effect on portal pressure. **Banti's syndrome** was originally defined as liver injury secondary to primary splenic disease, but most of the original cases actually consisted of cirrhosis as the primary disease with congestive splenomegaly. The greatly increased splenic blood flow in some cases of myeloid metaplasia and tropical splenomegaly with portal hypertension resembles the effects of an arterial-portal venous fistula, and splenectomy alone may cure the portal hypertension in some cases. Except in these terms, Banti's syndrome must be quite rare.

The average portal flow in cirrhotic patients with complications of portal hypertension is about 30% of

normal, ranging from 0–700 ml/minute. On the average, hepatic arterial flow is reduced by a similar proportion. The range of portal flow rates in different patients may vary greatly; in a few, blood in the portal vein moves only sluggishly, and in rare instances the direction of flow may even be reversed so that the portal vein functions as an outflow tract from the liver. These states of low flow predispose to spontaneous thrombosis of the portal vein, an occasional complication of cirrhosis which usually renders the portal vein unsuitable for a shunt.

The obstacle to flow through the liver stimulates expansion of collateral channels between the portal and systemic venous systems. As the pathologic process develops, portal pressure increases until a level of about 40 cm water (30 mm Hg) is reached. At this point, increasing hepatic resistance, even to the point of occlusion of the portal vein, diverts a greater fraction of portal flow through the collaterals without significant increments in portal pressure.

The type of collaterals which develop depends partly on the cause of the portal hypertension. In extrahepatic portal vein thrombosis (without liver disease), collaterals (hepatopetal) in the diaphragm, in the hepatocolic and hepatogastric ligaments, etc transport blood into the liver around the occluded vein. In both cirrhosis and portal thrombosis, collaterals (hepatofugal) appear which carry blood around the liver into the systemic circulation, and it is these that produce esophageal and gastric varices. Other common spontaneous collaterals are through a recanalized umbilical vein to the abdominal wall, from the superior hemorrhoidal vein into the middle and inferior hemorrhoidal veins, and through numerous small veins (of Retzius) connecting the retroperitoneal viscera with the posterior abdominal wall. Although spontaneous hemorrhage may occur from duodenal, cecal, or hemorrhoidal varices, only rarely does such an event present clinically as massive bleeding.

Blendis LM & others: Spleen blood flow and splanchnic haemodynamics in blood dyscrasia and other splenomegalies. Clin Sci 38:73, 1970.

Greenway CV, Stark RD: Hepatic vascular bed. Physiol Rev 51:23, 1971.

Lebrec D & others: Splanchnic hemodynamics in cirrhotic patients with esophageal varices and gastrointestinal bleeding. Gastroenterology 70:1108, 1976.

Leevy CM, Kiernan T: The hepatic circulation and portal hypertension. Clin Gastroenterol 4:381, 1975.

Moreno AH & others: Portal blood flow in cirrhosis of the liver. J Clin Invest 46:436, 1967.

Moreno AH & others: Spontaneous reversal of portal blood flow: The case for and against its occurrence in patients with cirrhosis of the liver. Ann Surg 181:346, 1975.

Zimmon DS, Kessler RE: The portal pressure-blood volume relationship in cirrhosis. Gut 15:99, 1974.

---

*A catheter wedged in a tributary of the hepatic vein estimates the pressure in the afferent veins to the sinusoid. The gradient between the wedged pressure and that in the hepatic vein reflects resistance at any point between the wedged position and the periphery of the sinusoid. Therefore, in the absence of definite pathologic evidence for the precise location of the block, it is impossible by this technic to distinguish between a sinusoidal and postsinusoidal lesion. The literature, however, often refers with unjustified precision to cirrhosis as producing a postsinusoidal block, whereas a combination of postsinusoidal and sinusoidal resistance is actually involved.

CIRRHOSIS OF THE LIVER

The death rate from cirrhosis of the liver exceeds 23,000 per year in the USA. The incidence of the disease is increasing, and at present it is the third most common cause of death in men in the fifth decade of life.

The alcoholic satisfies caloric needs from dietary alcohol to the exclusion of other important nutrients such as protein, vitamins, and minerals. Alcohol exerts direct toxic effects on the liver which are magnified in the presence of protein deficiency, but it is not known why only 15% of alcoholics develop cirrhosis. Hepatic steatosis and alcoholic hepatitis are stages of alcoholic liver injury that precede cirrhosis. Alcoholic hyalin, a glycoprotein, accumulates in centrolobular hepatocytes of patients with alcoholic hepatitis. There is some evidence that immunologic responses to alcoholic hyalin may be important in the pathogenesis of cirrhosis.

Collagen deposition in cirrhosis results from primary increased fibroblastic activity as well as from repair following hepatocellular necrosis. The ultimate result is a liver containing regenerative nodules and connective tissue septa linking portal fields with central canals.

The natural history of cirrhosis is imperfectly understood because major discrepancies exist in survival statistics. Nevertheless, once the diagnosis has been established, 30% or more of patients are dead within a year. A group of cirrhotics with varices followed by the Boston Interhospital Liver Group experienced a 1-year mortality rate of 66%. Cirrhotics without varices may benefit substantially by returning to a nutritious diet and abstaining from alcohol. However, once bleeding has occurred, survival is only slightly improved by nonoperative therapy. Bleeding occurs in about 40% of all patients with cirrhosis, and the initial episode of variceal hemorrhage is fatal to 50–80%. At least two-thirds of those who survive their initial hemorrhage will bleed again, and the risk of dying from the second is about the same as from the first episode. It is principally for such patients that portacaval shunts are recommended.

Garceau AJ, Chalmers TC: The natural history of cirrhosis. 1. Survival with esophageal varices. N Engl J Med 268:469, 1963.

Leevy CM & others: Liver disease of the alcoholic. Med Clin North Am 59:909, 1975.

Lieber CS: Alcohol and malnutrition in the pathogenesis of liver disease. JAMA 233:1077, 1975.

Popper H (editor): Symposium on cirrhosis. Clin Gastroenterol 4:225, May 1975. [Entire issue.]

Powell WJ Jr, Klatskin G: Duration of survival in patients with Laennec's cirrhosis. Am J Med 44:406, 1968.

ACUTE MASSIVELY BLEEDING VARICES

About two-thirds of patients with massive bleeding from varices die as a result of the acute event. The high mortality rate reflects not only the amount and rate of hemorrhage but also the frequent presence of severely compromised liver function and other systemic disease which may or may not be related to alcoholism. Malnutrition, pulmonary aspiration and infection, and coronary artery disease are frequently coexistent factors presaging a fatal outcome. The alcoholic patient often does not cooperate during therapy, and if delirium tremens ensues even his physical control may present a major clinical management problem.

Clinical Findings

A. Symptoms and Signs: The initial management of the patient with massive gastrointestinal hemorrhage is discussed in Chapter 26. It must be emphasized that bleeding from varices cannot be accurately diagnosed on clinical grounds alone even though the history or the appearance of the patient may strongly suggest the presence of cirrhosis or portal hypertension. Most patients with bleeding varices have alcoholic cirrhosis, and the diagnosis may seem obvious in a patient with hepatomegaly, jaundice, and vascular spiders who admits to a recent alcoholic binge. Splenomegaly, the most constant physical finding, is present in 80–90% of patients with portal hypertension regardless of the cause. Ascites is frequently present. Massive ascites and hepatosplenomegaly in a nonalcoholic would suggest the rare Budd-Chiari syndrome. If cirrhosis or varices have been documented on previous examinations, hematemesis later may point toward bleeding varices.

B. Laboratory Findings: Most alcoholics with acute upper gastrointestinal bleeding have compromised liver function. The bilirubin is usually elevated; it may be normal, but BSP retention will be found if there is cirrhosis. Serum albumin is often below 3 g/100 ml. The leukocyte count may be elevated. Anemia may be a reflection of chronic alcoholic liver disease or hypersplenism as well as acute hemorrhage. The development of a hepatoma by a cirrhotic sometimes is first manifested by bleeding varices, and this possibility should be checked by testing for serum α-fetoglobulin. The prothrombin time and partial thromboplastin time may be abnormal.

C. Special Examinations:

1. Esophagogastroscopy—Emergency esophagogastroscopy is the most useful procedure for diagnosing bleeding varices and should be scheduled as soon as the patient's general condition is stabilized by blood transfusion and other supportive measures. Varices appear as 3–4 large, tortuous submucosal bluish vessels running longitudinally in the distal esophagus. The bleeding site may be identified, but sometimes the lumen fills with blood so rapidly that the lesion is obscured. Acute hemorrhagic gastritis and Mallory-Weiss tears are 2 lesions in the differential diagnosis that can be seen on endoscopy but cannot be detected on upper gastrointestinal series.

2. Upper gastrointestinal series—A barium swallow will outline the varices in about 90% of affected patients, and if the patient's condition remains satisfactory x-rays should be performed after endoscopy. If both varices and a peptic ulcer are found on x-ray, the source of the bleeding is indeterminate unless endoscopy has settled the question.

Treatment of Acute Bleeding

After varices have been definitely incriminated as the cause of the bleeding, specific therapy can be instituted. The therapeutic options include administration of vasopressin, insertion of a Sengstaken-Blakemore (SB) tube, and emergency surgery (either variceal ligation or emergency portacaval shunt).

A. Vasopressin: Vasopressin (Pitressin) lowers mesenteric blood flow by constricting mesenteric arterioles. The action is relatively specific, since the hepatic artery is affected only slightly. Vasopressin is given as a peripheral intravenous infusion of 0.4–0.6 units/min for 1 hour. This regimen has been shown to be safer and more effective than more rapid bolus injections. The reduction in flow lowers portal venous pressure by 25%, which helps to stop variceal bleeding. The dose can be repeated every 3–4 hours if necessary.

The technic of selective infusion of vasopressin into the superior mesenteric artery is much more complicated and is no more effective than a peripheral venous infusion.

The cardiovascular complications of vasopressin (ie, reduced cardiac output and coronary blood flow, bradycardia) may be offset without affecting its portal actions by simultaneously administering isoproterenol (0.1 mg/hour IV).

B. Balloon Tamponade: (Fig 28–3.) These tubes have 2 balloons attached which can be inflated in the lumen of the gut to tamponade bleeding varices. There are 3–4 lumens in the tube: 2 are for filling the balloons and the third permits aspiration of gastric contents. A fourth lumen in the new Minnesota tube is used to aspirate the esophagus orad to the esophageal balloon. Since the task of placement and subsequent care is complicated and time-consuming, tube tamponade should generally be used only after the diagnosis of bleeding varices has been definitely established by endoscopy. However, in some cases of massive hemorrhage, there may not be time for endoscopy and the tube may be used on the basis of clinical suspicion alone. However, if inflating the balloons controls the bleeding, this does not prove that it originated from varices. As a treatment device, balloon tamponade has not been regularly effective for Mallory-Weiss tears and would not be expected to affect other causes of gastroduodenal hemorrhage.

A new Davol 20F Sengstaken-Blakemore tube or the Minnesota 4-lumen tube should be used, and both balloons must be checked under water for leaks. Before the SB tube is inserted, a standard nasogastric tube should be tied alongside with its tip located just orad to the esophageal balloon. The patient's stomach should be emptied as completely as possible to avoid aspiration before inserting the tube. The entire assembly is then passed through the patient's mouth into his stomach. To verify that the tube has entered the stomach, inject 25–50 ml of air rapidly into the gastric balloon while listening over the epigastrium with a stethoscope. The gastric balloon is then inflated with air (250–275 ml for the SB tube; 450–500 ml for the 4-lumen tube), and traction is applied until a snug fit is obtained between the balloon and the gastroesophageal junction. If the patient develops substernal pain while the gastric balloon is being inflated, stop immediately and determine that it is not in the esophagus. The position is fixed to maintain tension by taping a mouth guard to the tube (Fig 28–3), and a film obtained with a portable x-ray unit provides a final check on the location of the balloon. The esophageal balloon should be inflated only if bleeding continues after compression by the gastric balloon. The esophageal balloon should be distended with a manometer to 33–60 cm water (25–45 mm Hg), maintaining the lowest pressure that produces hemostasis.

The patient must be under continuous observation, preferably in the intensive care unit or by special nurses on the ward. A heavy pair of scissors should be kept at the bedside, and those responsible for the patient's care should be instructed to cut across the tube (which rapidly deflates the balloons) and remove it quickly if respiratory obstruction develops.

The most common serious problem is aspiration of pharyngeal secretions and pneumonitis. This has been largely obviated by tying on the additional tube which maintains the hypopharynx clear of secretions.

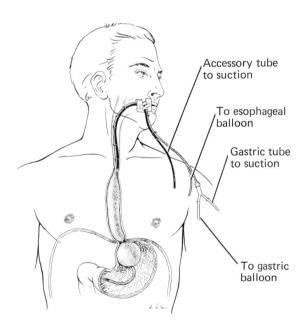

Figure 28–3. Sengstaken-Blakemore (SB) tube with both gastric and esophageal balloons inflated.

Accessory tube to suction

To esophageal balloon

Gastric tube to suction

To gastric balloon

Allowing the patient to move around in bed and to breathe comfortably also helps to preserve pulmonary function.

Another serious hazard is the occasional instance of esophageal rupture caused by inflation of the esophageal balloon. To avoid this risk, the latter should not be inflated beyond the pressures listed above. With these precautions and expert nursing care, the incidence of complications is negligible.

About 85–90% of actively bleeding patients can be controlled by balloon tamponade. When bleeding has stopped, the ballons are left inflated for another 24 hours. They are then decompressed, leaving the tube in place. If bleeding does not recur in the subsequent 24 hours, the tube should be withdrawn. If a tamponade tube has been used but bleeding either continues or recurs with the balloons inflated, emergency surgical treatment must be considered. The return of bleeding after successful balloon tamponade should be treated by reinsertion of another tube.

Several groups that have relied heavily on the SB tube report a hospital mortality rate below 40% for acute variceal bleeding. Patients who survive may then be considered as candidates for elective portacaval shunt.

C. Emergency Operation: The 2 operations to control active bleeding are variceal ligation and portacaval shunt.

1. Variceal ligation—In the past this was usually performed through a left thoracotomy, but most surgeons prefer an abdominal approach because concomitant gastric varices or other causes of bleeding are easier to manage. The lumen of the lower esophagus is entered, and the varices are oversewn with a running suture of chromic catgut. When a thoracotomy is used, gastric varices can be exposed by a diaphragmatic incision and proximal gastrotomy.

Variceal ligation usually stops acute bleeding, but since it does nothing to lower portal pressure recurrent bleeding is common before the patient can be prepared for definitive portacaval shunt. For this reason, the operation is seldom used.

2. Emergency portacaval shunt—Since the bleeding is a direct consequence of elevated portal pressure, reduction of pressure by a shunt is usually successful treatment. The disadvantages of this approach are that the diagnostic work-up may have to be abbreviated in emergency circumstances; liver function is often acutely compromised; and the patient's general condition (eg, cardiac, pulmonary, and renal status) is frequently suboptimal. Despite these drawbacks, operation is sometimes necessary if bleeding continues despite tamponade or vasopressin infusion. It has been argued by some that, since the patient's overall condition so frequently deteriorates during the initial 24–48 hours of medical management, earlier surgery might be preferable for nearly all patients after initial resuscitation. This proposition needs more empirical support before being accepted.

Portacaval shunt, either end-to-side, side-to-side, or H-mesocaval, is the procedure of choice since these are easier to perform than splenorenal shunts. Angiograms are not usually available, so at laparotomy a thrombosed portal vein is occasionally discovered which is unsuitable for anastomosis. In this situation, the best operation would probably be an H-mesocaval shunt using a segment of arterial Dacron graft.

The overall mortality for emergency shunts is about 50%. The result in the individual patient is largely determined by the quality of liver function, the extent of blood loss before and during operation, the duration of operation, and the technical result (ie, whether the shunt remains patent). In general, patients with good liver function, minimal or no encephalopathy, and mild or no ascites do well, but this describes only a minority of acute bleeders. Alcoholics seem to fare better than nonalcoholic cirrhotics since liver function in the former can be expected to improve postoperatively with restoration of good nutrition. However, patients with acute alcoholic hepatitis experience a high mortality from emergency operations and may go unrecognized preoperatively among a nonselected group of patients with bleeding varices.

Summary: There is considerable disagreement about the best way to manage the acutely bleeding patient. Each of the following 3 options has its proponents: (1) Nonoperative management with vasopressin or Sengstaken-Blakemore tube for all patients initially, and emergency operation if this fails to control bleeding. (2) Emergency portacaval shunt for those who appear to be "good risks" and nonoperative management of "poor-risk" patients. (3) Emergency portacaval shunt for all patients. At present, most clinicians probably adhere to the notion that emergency surgery should be performed only after an attempt at nonoperative treatment. However, adherents to the other 2 policies report what they interpret to be improved results so that the final judgment awaits controlled clinical trials. Transesophageal ligation of varices has fallen into relative disuse because the patient is exposed to the morbidity of a major operation which often is only transiently successful in controlling the hemorrhage.

NONBLEEDING VARICES
(Elective Portosystemic Shunts)

The goal of a portacaval shunt is to prevent bleeding from varices, and in these terms the operation is successful in 95% of cases. Those who rebleed usually are found to have developed thrombosis at the anastomosis. Theoretically, an elective shunt should be considered for any patient with a substantial future risk of bleeding from varices. Although about 30% of all patients with varices will bleed within 5 years, imperfect knowledge of the determining factors makes it impossible to predict the likelihood of this event in any individual patient. The principal side-effects limiting more general use of shunts are decreased liver function, increased susceptibility to encephalopathy, and an operative mortality rate of 5–10%. When making a judgment about the advisability of performing a shunt for a given patient, the physician must attempt to balance the risk of these untoward effects with that of future hemorrhage.

A. Prophylactic Shunt: Since about one-third of cirrhotics with varices who have not bled eventually die of this complication, prophylactic construction of a shunt was proposed to avoid the high mortality rate of the acute episode. Several controlled clinical trials were performed to investigate the results of such a policy, and each showed that prophylactic portacaval shunts in unselected patients with varices did not improve longevity. The shunted group was protected from hemorrhage but experienced a completely offsetting rise in mortality from liver failure. Encephalopathy was greater among the treated group than in the controls. Unfortunately, a detailed analysis of the control groups did not turn up clues to indicate which of the patients would go on to bleed without surgery. Presumably, if a high-risk group could be identified, another trial of the prophylactic shunt would be warranted.

B. Therapeutic Shunt: The results of the studies on prophylactic shunts revealed more adverse effects from the operation than had been anticipated and raised questions regarding the value of shunts in patients who had bled previously, the so-called therapeutic shunt. Although it had long been believed that survival of these patients was prolonged by operation, controlled trials comparing end-to-side and side-to-side portacaval shunts to nonoperative management were instituted to scientifically examine the question. The results demonstrate slightly increased longevity of those who were shunted compared with nonshunted controls. A reciprocal relationship was found between reduction of liver function following operation and the protection from bleeding. Those with good liver function seemed to fare better with a shunt. Unexpectedly, the incidence of encephalopathy was about the same in the medical and surgical groups, chiefly owing to the tendency for nonshunted patients to develop this complication in conjunction with additional episodes of variceal bleeding.

These findings added further emphasis to the need for a means of reducing portal pressure without compromising liver function.

Other means being explored to improve the care of patients with varices involve development of tests that more accurately predict the hepatic effects of a shunt (eg, preoperative quantification of hepatic blood flow); trials with shunts that are technically simpler (H-mesocaval shunt); and operations that destroy the varices directly without disturbing portahepatic blood flow (eg, sclerotherapy, gastroesophageal venous devascularization).

In summary: An end-to-side or distal splenorenal shunt should generally be recommended for patients under age 60 with good liver function who have bled previously. The distal splenorenal (Warren) shunt is presently being studied in controlled clinical trials and increasingly appears to have advantages over other

shunting procedures. Although the evidence is still inconclusive, many consider the Warren shunt in properly selected patients to be the best available operation for portal hypertension.

Preoperative Management

After an acute hemorrhage has stopped—especially in alcoholics—the patient's condition can usually be improved by giving a high-calorie, high-protein diet for several weeks. If acute liver damage is present as a result of alcoholism, it should be allowed to subside.

Table 28–2 shows the general relationship between operative mortality and quality of liver function. The detrimental effect of a shunt on liver function is thought to be due to nutritional deprivation from loss of portal venous blood flow. Diversion of portal blood is virtually complete after portacaval shunts but is substantially less after a central splenorenal shunt or the distal splenorenal (Warren) shunt.

Tolerance of a portacaval shunt also appears related to the degree that hepatic resistance and flow through collaterals have preoperatively reduced hepatopetal portal flow. Thus, when residual portal flow into the liver is slight, performance of a shunt would have less of an effect on hepatic nutrition and patient survival may be greater. The incidence of postoperative encephalopathy also correlates with the quantitative effect of the shunt on portal flow, and this complication is less after a central splenorenal than portacaval anastomosis. The segmental diversion of blood in the distal splenorenal shunt appears to totally avoid encephalopathy.

Unfortunately, at present the easiest shunts to perform are associated with the highest incidence of late side-effects.

Preoperative evaluation must verify the diagnosis of varices, measure portal pressure, and radiographically demonstrate the portal venous anatomy. Whether the blood loss in an earlier acute hemorrhage was actually from varices must be questioned since acute gastritis, peptic ulcer, and the Mallory-Weiss lesion account for more than half of the episodes of acute upper gastrointestinal bleeding in cirrhotics. Esophagoscopic recognition of bleeding varices is the most convincing

Table 28–2. Relation of hepatic function and nutrition to operative mortality after portacaval shunt.

Group	A	B	C
Operative Mortality	2%	10%	50%
Serum bilirubin (mg/100 ml)	< 2.0	2.0–3.0	> 3.0
Serum albumin (g/100 ml)	> 3.5	3.0–3.5	< 3.0
Ascites	None	Easily controlled	Poorly controlled
Encephalopathy	None	Minimal	Advanced
Nutrition	Excellent	Good	Poor

evidence. If esophagoscopy and upper gastrointestinal x-rays were performed acutely and failed to reveal any abnormalities other than varices although a definitive bleeding point was not seen, this can nevertheless be taken as fairly reliable proof. Of dubious reliability is evidence that use of an SB tube was responsible for controlling the bleeding. When nothing more is available than a history of melena or hematemesis and x-rays showing varices, other causes of the bleeding cannot be excluded with certainty. Thus, the diagnosis is often based on indirect evidence and judgment.

Optimal preoperative preparation should aim for a serum albumin above 3 g/100 ml, serum bilirubin less than 2 mg/100 ml, and a normal prothrombin time. Ascites should be absent or minimal. However, after diet therapy has been tried, nothing further is achieved by using diuretics for stable ascites. There should be no signs of encephalopathy. If these criteria cannot be met, the increased operative and late morbidity will correlate with the degree of residual hepatic dysfunction (Table 28–2).

A. Measurement of Portal Pressure: Measurement of portal pressure should be obtained to establish the presence and height of portal hypertension. Bleeding from varices is nearly always associated with a wedged hepatic vein-free hepatic vein pressure gradient of 15 cm water or greater. If the hepatic vein wedged pressure does not verify portal hypertension, either the diagnosis is incorrect or the block is presinusoidal. In the latter case, a direct percutaneous measurement of splenic pulp pressure should be obtained.

Three methods are available for measuring portal pressure preoperatively: wedged hepatic vein pressure (WHVP), direct percutaneous splenic pulp manometry, and cannulation of the umbilical vein remnant. They all reliably reflect portal pressure with the exception that WHVP remains normal in the presence of a presinusoidal block. Since most patients have sinusoidal (or postsinusoidal) lesions and because the procedure has almost no morbidity, WHVP is usually the method of choice.

1. Wedged hepatic vein pressure (WHVP)—A catheter is passed percutaneously via the brachial or axillary vein into the vena cava and then, under fluoroscopic control, one of the hepatic veins is entered. The pressure is measured in the free hepatic vein (FHVP), and the catheter is advanced until it becomes wedged in a peripheral tributary. The reading in the wedged position measures the pressure across any resistance up to the first system of collaterals that allows flow around the stagnated column of blood. For a catheter wedged in the hepatic vein, this point is at the periphery of the sinusoid. Subtraction of FHVP from WHVP gives the portal-hepatic pressure gradient. The normal value is about 4 cm water (3 mm Hg); a gradient above 8 cm water (6 mm Hg) is considered to represent portal hypertension; in bleeding varices, the gradient is usually greater than 20 cm water (15 mm Hg).

Although a satisfactory anatomic explanation is unavailable, it has been shown that the WHVP accurately reflects portal vein pressure (PVP) in all types of cirrhosis. If the lesion is located on the splanchnic side of the sinusoid (presinusoidal), whether it is prehepatic or intrahepatic, portal pressure is not measured by this technic. After the pressure readings are obtained, diatrizoate (Hypaque) is injected through the catheter for x-ray verification of the wedged position and to check the flow behavior of contrast refluxed into the portal vein. If portal flow is retrograde or sluggish, this suggests that portal diversion would not further impair liver function.

2. Splenic pulp manometry—Except for special cases, this method has largely been supplanted by hepatic vein wedged pressure. The patient should be positioned supine on an x-ray cassette changer, mildly sedated, and instructed to breathe shallowly and regularly to avoid sudden wide diaphragmatic excursions. A needle or cannula is inserted percutaneously into the estimated center of the splenic surface, which usually corresponds to a site on the skin in the eighth, ninth, or tenth intercostal space in the midaxillary line. It is best to use a plastic catheter with a metal trocar because—after insertion into the spleen—removal of the trocar allows flexibility in response to respiratory motion. Pressure readings are obtained with a water manometer using the midaxillary line as the zero reference. Fifty ml of diatrizoate are then injected over 5 seconds to opacify the portal venous system, and x-rays are taken with an automatic cassette changer every 2 seconds for 8 exposures. The quality of films is excellent, but the varices themselves are not always well opacified. This technic will usually demonstrate whether or not the portal vein is patent. When considered only from the standpoint of diagnosis, this method is less accurate than esophagoscopy or barium swallow for demonstrating varices.

Direct splenic puncture entails greater morbidity than the other methods of measuring pressure or outlining the venous anatomy. Abdominal bleeding from the splenic surface requires blood transfusion in about 5% of cases, and splenectomy is sometimes necessary. Nevertheless, this is still the best means of determining portal pressure in patients with presinusoidal block.

3. Umbilical vein cannulation—The remnant of umbilical vein passes in the falciform ligament from the umbilicus to the left branch of the portal vein. Its lumen usually remains obliterated, although in some patients spontaneous recanalization allows it to serve as a portal systemic collateral. The lumen of the obliterated vessel can be reopened with a probe and used to enter the portal circulation. This has recently been exploited as a means of measuring portal pressure and obtaining venous angiograms. The procedure can usually be done with local anesthesia and sedation. The obliterated umbilical vein is surgically located in the falciform ligament, and a dilator is forced down the lumen until the left branch of the portal vein is broken into. A catheter is inserted into the portal vein for measuring pressure and for injecting x-ray contrast medium.

Umbilical vein catheterization can be successfully performed in most patients with portal hypertension not associated with extrahepatic portal vein thrombosis. Its place in the evaluation of the average patient is not yet clear, but the procedure does provide direct access to the portal circulation, and the morbidity rate is low.

B. Angiography: Selective splenic and superior mesenteric angiography is usually the best way to visualize the vascular anatomy unless a decision has already been made to measure portal pressure by splenic puncture. If the latter is necessary, a splenoportogram should be obtained simultaneously. In nearly all cases, the portal vein should be outlined angiographically before proceeding with plans for a portacaval shunt since in about 10% of cirrhotics the vein is thrombosed and cannot be used for this shunt. The behavior of contrast media in the portal vein may provide a semiquantitative impression of the rate of hepatopetal flow. The varices are often demonstrated, but angiograms are less reliable than barium swallow or esophagoscopy for the diagnosis of varices.

Selective angiography is performed by inserting a catheter percutaneously into the femoral or axillary artery and advancing it into the celiac artery and, if possible, the splenic artery. Contrast medium is injected, and films are exposed during the arterial and venous phases. Complications are rare, and the quality of the x-rays is good.

C. Liver Biopsy: In the majority of patients, the preoperative evaluation should include a percutaneous liver biopsy. Biopsy should verify the clinical diagnosis of cirrhosis but is especially important to uncover acute liver disease such as alcoholic hepatitis. Biopsy is also helpful to diagnose the less common causes of portal hypertension such as schistosomiasis, hepatic fibrosis, hepatoma, etc.

Types of Shunts

Fig 28–4 depicts the various shunts in use at this time. Although they differ technically in many ways, physiologically there are only 3 different types: end-to-side, side-to-side, and distal splenorenal (Warren).

A. End-to-Side Anastomosis: The end-to-side shunt completely disconnects the liver from the portal system. The portal vein is transected near its bifurcation in the liver hilus and anastomosed to the side of the inferior vena cava. The hepatic stump of the vein is oversewn. Postoperatively, the hepatic vein wedged pressure (sinusoidal pressure) drops slightly after this procedure, reflecting the inability of the hepatic artery to fully compensate for the loss of portal inflow.

B. Side-to-Side Anastomosis: The side-to-side portacaval, mesocaval, mesorenal, and central splenorenal shunts are all physiologically similar since the shunt preserves continuity between the hepatic limb of the portal vein, the portal system, and the anastomosis. It was thought that the side-to-side portacaval shunt might permit continued hepatic perfusion with portal blood, but, in fact, flow through the hepatic limb of the standard side-to-side shunt is nearly always away from the liver and toward the anastomosis. The extent to which hepatofugal flow is produced by other types of "side-to-side" shunts listed above is not known. The physiologic consequences of this reversed flow in the average case are uncertain, but it probably accounts for the somewhat poorer results of this procedure compared with the end-to-side anastomosis.

Although ascites itself is rarely an indication for portacaval shunt, a side-to-side shunt more effectively eliminates this problem than an end-to-side shunt. The necessity for decompressing intrahepatic portal pressure makes the side-to-side shunt imperative for **Budd-Chiari syndrome**.

C. Distal Splenorenal (Warren) Shunt: The Warren shunt diverts only a section of the portal bed from the liver and preserves hepatic perfusion by blood arriving from the superior mesenteric vein. The usual method consists of transecting the mobilized splenic vein and anastomosing the splenic end to the side of the renal vein. The operation is technically difficult, and several modifications have been proposed. One involves a side-to-side anastomosis between splenic and renal veins followed by ligation of the portal (hepatic) limb of the splenic. Lastly, in some cases where mobilization of the splenic vein appeared to be hazardous, the renal

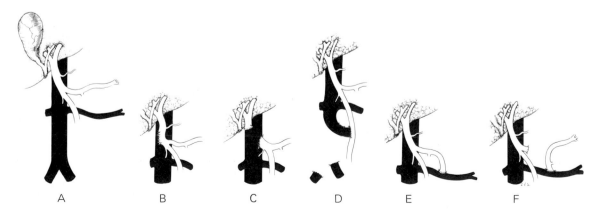

Figure 28–4. Types of portacaval anastomoses: *A:* Normal. *B:* Side-to-side. *C:* End-to-side. *D:* Mesocaval. *E:* Central splenorenal. *F:* Distal splenorenal (Warren).

vein has been transected and the end of the caval segment sutured to the side of the undisturbed splenic vein. The segment of splenic vein between the anastomosis and the portal vein is then ligated. Surprisingly, this seems to have little permanent effect on function or the kidney as long as the adrenal and other tributaries are preserved on the oversewn renal vein stump.

Choice of Shunt

In the past, side-to-side or end-to-side portacaval and central splenorenal shunts have been considered the "standard" operations, the others being reserved for special application. Recent clinical trials support this conclusion and suggest that the differences between these 3 procedures on late follow-up are minor.

The relatively new distal splenorenal (Warren) shunt has especially attractive physiologic advantages since it does not further impair liver function and avoids encephalopathy altogether. The operation is more difficult technically and for this reason cannot always be successfully accomplished; it should not be used in the presence of ascites. Except in these instances, however, the continued good results reported by Warren warrant increasing optimism regarding this procedure. The results after 3 years of a controlled trial comparing the distal splenorenal with the H-mesocaval shunt showed substantially less encephalopathy with the former technic. Eventually, it may be generally accepted as the best choice for the average candidate undergoing elective portosystemic decompression.

The mesocaval and mesorenal shunts are useful when neither portacaval nor splenorenal anastomosis is feasible. This is most commonly seen after failure of other operations, in young children with portal vein occlusion when the splenic vein is too small, and in patients with unsuitable portal and splenic veins.

The H-mesocaval shunt has recently been advocated as worthy of more widespread trial. The operation consists of suturing a segment of prosthetic vascular graft or autogenous vein between the superior mesenteric vein and inferior vena cava, a procedure that can be accomplished quickly because the veins need little mobilization. Several reports suggest that these grafts remain patent for prolonged periods. The claim that postoperatively the patients have less encephalopathy than after end-to-side or side-to-side portacaval shunts is hard to understand and awaits substantiation. At present, the principal usefulness of this procedure is for emergency shunts where technical simplicity is especially desirable.

Complications

Encephalopathy and diminished liver function are the major complications of portacaval shunts. The incidence of peptic ulcer may be increased by the operation, but the evidence is contradictory. An increased incidence would presumably be due to the diversion of portal blood containing a gastric secretagogue of intestinal origin, normally destroyed by the liver. Hemosiderosis develops in the livers of some shunted patients over many years.

General

Boyer JL & others: Idiopathic portal hypertension. Ann Intern Med 66:41, 1967.

Burchell AR & others: Hemodynamic variables and prognosis following portacaval shunts. Surg Gynecol Obstet 138:359, 1974.

Gall EA, Kierle AM: Portal systemic venous shunt: Pathological factors contributing to postoperative survival. Gastroenterology 49:656, 1965.

Lopez-Torres A, Waye JD: The safety of intubation in patients with esophageal varices. Am J Dig Dis 18:1032, 1973.

McCray RS & others: Erroneous diagnosis of hemorrhage from esophageal varices. Am J Dig Dis 14:755, 1969.

Pitcher JL: Safety and effectiveness of the modified Sengstaken-Blakemore tube: A prospective study. Gastroenterology 61:291, 1971.

Schramek A & others: New observations in the clinical spectrum of the Budd-Chiari syndrome. Ann Surg 180:368, 1974.

Siegel JH, Goldwyn RM: Hyperdynamic states and the physiologic determinants of survival in patients with cirrhosis and portal hypertension. Arch Surg 108:282, 1974.

Emergency Portacaval Shunts

Edmondson HT & others: Clinical investigation of the portacaval shunt. 4. A report of early survival from the emergency operation. Ann Surg 173:372, 1971.

Orloff MJ & others: Portacaval shunt as emergency procedure in unselected patients with alcoholic cirrhosis. Surg Gynecol Obstet 141:59, 1975.

Elective Portosystemic Shunts

Britton RC: The clinical effectiveness of selective portal shunts. Am J Surg 133:506, 1977.

Burchell AR & others: Hepatic artery flow improvement after portacaval shunt: A single hemodynamic clinical correlate. Ann Surg 184:289, 1976.

Drapanas T & others: Hemodynamics of the interposition mesocaval shunt. Ann Surg 181:523, 1975.

Galambos JT & others: Selective and total shunts in the treatment of bleeding varices. A randomized controlled trial. N Engl J Med 295:1089, 1976.

Hutson DG & others: The fate of esophageal varices following selective distal splenorenal shunt. Ann Surg 183:496, 1976.

Jackson FC & others: A clinical investigation of the portacaval shunt. 5. Survival analysis of the therapeutic operation. Ann Surg 174:672, 1971.

Malt RA: Portasystemic venous shunts. (2 parts.) N Engl J Med 295:24, 80, 1976.

Malt RA & others: Risk in therapeutic portacaval and splenorenal shunts. Ann Surg 184:279, 1976.

Mikkelsen WP: Therapeutic portacaval shunt: Preliminary data on controlled trial and morbid effects of acute hyaline necrosis. Arch Surg 108:302, 1974.

Nay HR, Fitzpatrick HF: Mesocaval "H" graft using autogenous vein graft. Ann Surg 183:114, 1976.

Reynolds TB: The role of hemodynamic measurements in portasystemic shunt surgery. Arch Surg 108:276, 1974.

Smith GW: Use of hemodynamic selection criteria in the management of cirrhotic patients with portal hypertension. Ann Surg 179:782, 1974.

EXTRAHEPATIC PORTAL VENOUS OCCLUSION

Idiopathic portal vein thrombosis (in the absence of liver disease) accounts for most cases of portal hypertension in childhood and for a few cases in adults. Neonatal septicemia, omphalitis, umbilical vein catheterization for exchange transfusion, and dehydration have all been incriminated as possible causes, but collectively they can be implicated in less than half of cases.

The patient presents with variceal hemorrhage, splenomegaly, or hypersplenism. Ascites is uncommon except transiently after bleeding. Liver function is either normal or only slightly impaired, which probably accounts for the low incidence of overt encephalopathy. There is an increased frequency of neuropsychiatric problems, which may be a subtle form of encephalopathy.

Because the patient's general condition and liver function are good, the mortality rate for sudden massive bleeding is about 20%, much below the rate in other types of portal hypertension. The diagnosis can be confirmed radiologically by percutaneous mesenteric angiography. Hepatic vein wedged pressure is normal.

Emergency treatment consists of the administration of vasopressin to reduce portal pressure, blood transfusion to restore circulating blood volume, and tamponade with the Sengstaken-Blakemore tube. If these measures fail and bleeding continues, transesophageal ligation of varices should be considered as a lifesaving measure. In general, however, the bleeding episodes are self-limited and uncommonly fatal, so emergency operations are rarely necessary.

The thrombosed portal vein is unsuitable for a shunt. A mesocaval shunt is best for young children whose vessels are small. In older individuals a central splenorenal shunt is most commonly used. Splenectomy alone has no permanent effect and sacrifices the splenic vein, which might be needed later for a shunt. Because shunts in patients under 9–10 years of age have a high rate of spontaneous thrombosis, variceal bleeding is preferably managed without a shunt until the child has grown to a suitable size. If previous operations have used all the major veins in unsuccessful shunts, an esophagogastrectomy with colon interposition may be performed to eliminate the varices.

Owing to technical problems, an adequate shunt is more difficult to accomplish in patients with portal vein block than in cirrhotics. Since they tolerate sudden blood loss much better than those with liver disease, their survival without a shunt is considerably better too.

Isolated **thrombosis of the splenic vein** can be caused by pancreatitis or trauma. The resulting venous hypertension of the splenic veins spills over into the gastroesophageal venous plexus via the short gastric vessels; the portal and mesenteric venous pressures are normal. In this condition, splenectomy alone is curative.

Fonkalsrud EW & others: Management of extrahepatic portal hypertension in children. Ann Surg 180:487, 1974.

Pinkerton JA & others: Portal hypertension in childhood. Ann Surg 175:870, 1972.

Rothwell-Jackson RL, Hunt AH: Proximal gastric resection in the treatment of bleeding gastroesophageal varices in patients with portal hypertension due to extrahepatic obstruction. Br J Surg 57:487, 1970.

Salam A & others: Splenic vein thrombosis: A diagnosable and curable form of portal hypertension. Surgery 74:961, 1973.

Voorhees AB Jr, Price JB Jr: Extrahepatic portal hypertension. Arch Surg 108:338, 1974.

BUDD-CHIARI SYNDROME

This rare syndrome resulting from obstruction of hepatic venous outflow has been seen with greater frequency in recent years, presumably because of widespread use of birth control pills. Most cases are caused by spontaneous thrombosis of the hepatic veins (some of these patients have polycythemia vera) or venous obstruction from neoplasms. In the Orient, membranous stenosis of the suprahepatic inferior vena cava of obscure cause has been responsible for some cases.

The posthepatic (postsinusoidal) obstruction raises sinusoidal pressure, which is transmitted upstream to cause portal hypertension. Because the parenchyma is relatively free of fibrosis, filtration across the sinusoids and hepatic lymph formation increase greatly, producing marked ascites.

Clinical symptoms usually begin with a mild prodrome consisting of vague right upper quadrant abdominal pain, postprandial bloating, and anorexia. After weeks or months, a more florid picture develops consisting of gross ascites, hepatomegaly, and hepatic failure. At this stage the SGOT is usually markedly increased, the serum bilirubin is slightly elevated, and the alkaline phosphatase is inconsistently abnormal.

Liver scan usually demonstrates absent function through most of the liver except for a small central area representing the caudate lobe, whose venous outflow is spared because it is separate from that of the rest of the liver. Liver biopsy reveals grossly dilated central veins and sinusoids, pericentral necrosis, and replacement of hepatocytes by red blood cells. Centrolobular fibrosis develops late. The diagnosis must be confirmed by venography which demonstrates the occluded hepatic veins.

If the correct diagnosis can be made before serious complications of hepatic failure or portal hypertension supervene, a side-to-side portacaval shunt should be performed. The postoperative results are excellent in patients without malignant neoplasms.

Langer B & others: Clinical spectrum of the Budd-Chiari syndrome and its surgical management. Am J Surg 129:137, 1975.

ASCITES

Ascites in hepatic disease results from (1) increased formation of hepatic lymph (from sinusoidal hypertension), (2) increased formation of splanchnic lymph, (3) hypoalbuminemia, and (4) salt and water retention by the kidneys. Ascites generally can be controlled by salt and water restriction and careful use of diuretics (especially spironolactone).

Surgical Treatment

A. Portacaval Shunt: When planning surgery for a patient with varices, shunt selection can ignore ascites unless it has been a major problem. However, when ascites has been severe, the side-to-side shunts (portacaval, H-mesocaval, central splenorenal) are more effective because they reduce sinusoidal as well as splanchnic venous pressure.

B. Peritoneal-Jugular Shunt (LeVeen Shunt): In specially selected patients, severe ascites may be treated by permanent implantation of a Silastic tube to shunt fluid continuously from the peritoneal cavity to the jugular vein. A small Silastic valve buried in the abdominal wall is inserted in the line to ensure a unidirectional flow of ascitic fluid from the abdomen to the blood stream. Only 3–5 cm of water pressure is required to open the valve and permit flow. Increased venous pressure closes the valve, a feature that limits excessive flow if cardiac function is impaired.

The procedure is contraindicated if there has been recent variceal bleeding because it seems to predispose to recurrent hemorrhage. To be sure that it is sterile, the ascites should be checked within 48 hours before implanting the valve. Antibiotics are given pre- and postoperatively, and the procedure is performed under local anesthesia.

Postoperatively, the patient is outfitted with an abdominal binder and instructed to perform respiratory exercises against mild pressure to increase abdominal pressure and flow through the shunt. Dietary salt should not be restricted. Diuretics (furosemide) are usually given for 10 days.

An average of 10 lb of weight is lost in the first 10 days after the operation. Particularly gratifying has been the improved renal function noted in many patients with the hepatorenal syndrome. The major complication (in about 5% of cases) has been thrombosis of the valve. Lethal septicemia may occur if the ascites is infected. It is too early to judge the long-term effectiveness of this procedure, but in some patients good results have persisted for over 2 years.

LeVeen HH & others: Further experience with peritoneo-venous shunt for ascites. Ann Surg 184:574, 1976.

Orloff MJ: Effect of side to side portacaval shunt on intractable ascites, sodium excretion, and aldosterone metabolism in man. Am J Surg 112:287, 1966.

Wapnick S & others: LeVeen continuous peritoneal-jugular shunt. Improvement of renal function in ascitic patients. JAMA 237:131, 1977.

Witte MH & others: Physiological factors involved in the causation of cirrhotic ascites. Gastroenterology 61:742, 1971.

HEPATIC ENCEPHALOPATHY

CNS symptoms, either episodic or continuous, are seen in patients with chronic liver disease and are especially prone to develop after portacaval shunt. Portal-systemic encephalopathy, ammonia intoxication, hepatic coma, and meat intoxication are terms which have been used synonymously to refer to this condition.

The possible symptoms span a wide range from lethargy to coma—from minor personality changes to psychosis—from asterixis to paraplegia. A toxic action of ammonia on the CNS has been considered the most likely cause since in affected patients ammonia levels, especially in arterial blood or CSF, are elevated and experimental administration of ammonia has produced similar symptoms. Ammonia is formed in the gut—principally the colon—by the action of bacteria on urea. It is absorbed and transported in portal venous blood to the liver, where normally about 80% is extracted and converted to glutamine, a nontoxic storage compound. Absorbed ammonia may reach the systemic circulation in increased amounts through spontaneous portal systemic collaterals or surgically created shunts, or as a result of decreased hepatic extraction due to parenchymal liver disease.

Another mechanism may be excessive exposure of the CNS to β-hydroxylated phenylethyl amines or their precursor amino acids, which displace the normal neurotransmitters norepinephrine and dopamine. These false neurotransmitters are inactive at synapses and result in CNS dysfunction. These compounds are also produced in the gut by bacterial action, and thus a positive correlation of symptoms with ammonia levels would be expected.

Serum levels of branched chain amino acids (leucine, isoleucine, valine) are decreased and levels of aromatic amino acids (tryptophan, phenylalanine, tyrosine) are elevated in patients with encephalopathy. One hypothesis attributes this to a decreased insulin/glucagon ratio accompanying the catabolic state so characteristic of these patients. Branched chain amino acids are catabolized by fat and muscle for fuel and aromatic amino acids accumulate as a consequence of decreased hepatic degradation. Because these 2 classes of amino acids compete for transport across the blood-brain barrier, the result is increased access to the CNS of the aromatic amino acids, which serve as precursors for false neurotransmitters. As a corollary, it has been shown that total parenteral nutrition of patients with encephalopathy using a special formula rich in branched chain amino acids can induce anabolism and improve cerebral function.

Encephalopathy is a major unwanted side-effect of portacaval shunt. Since it can be socially incapacitating or even lethal, the risks in the individual patient must be carefully considered before operation. The most important factors in predicting the postoperative chance of developing this complication are the quality of liver function, the extent of reduction in hepatic parenchymal blood flow through the portal vein (ie, the extent to which the disease has already shunted portal blood), the type of liver disease, and the age of the patient. The factors contributing to the development of encephalopathy are listed in Table 28–3. Those just mentioned are patient- and disease-determined, whereas the others are at least partially under the control of the physician.

Elderly patients are considerably more susceptible—so much so that the standard shunts are rarely performed in persons over age 60. Alcoholics fare better than those with postnecrotic or cryptogenic cirrhosis, apparently owing to the invariable progression of liver dysfunction in the latter.

Good liver function partially protects the patient from encephalopathy if other variables are held constant. If the liver has adapted to complete or nearly complete diversion of portal blood before operation, a surgical shunt is less apt to depress liver function further. For example, patients with thrombosis of the portal vein (complete diversion and normal liver function) do not experience encephalopathy after portal-systemic shunt.

Increased intestinal protein, whether of dietary origin or from intestinal bleeding, aggravates encephalopathy by providing more substrate for intestinal bacteria. Constipation allows greater time for bacterial action on colonic contents. Azotemia results in higher concentrations of blood urea which diffuses into the intestine, is converted to ammonia, and then reabsorbed. Hypokalemia and metabolic alkalosis aggravate encephalopathy by shifting ammonia from extracellular to intracellular sites where the toxic action occurs.

Electroencephalography is more sensitive than clinical evaluation in detecting minor involvement. The changes are nonspecific and consist of slower mean frequencies. Studies performed at different times can be compared to assess the effects of therapy.

Acute encephalopathy is often precipitated by episodes of intestinal hemorrhage. Treatment consists of removing the blood by suction and purgation, halting the bleeding if possible, and administering intestinal antibiotics (eg, neomycin). Blood volume must be maintained to avoid prerenal azotemia.

Table 28–3. Factors contributing to encephalopathy.

A. Increased Systemic Ammonia Levels
1. Extent of portal-systemic venous shunt
2. Depressed liver function
3. Intestinal protein load
4. Intestinal flora
5. Azotemia
6. Constipation

B. Increased Sensitivity of CNS
1. Age of patient
2. Hypokalemia
3. Alkalosis
4. Diuretics
5. Sedatives, narcotics, tranquilizers
6. Infection
7. Hypoxia, hypoglycemia, myxedema

Chronic encephalopathy is treated by restriction of dietary protein to 40–60 g/day, avoidance of constipation, and sometimes by continuous administration of intestinal antibiotics to reduce bacterial action. Lactalose, a disaccharide unaffected by intestinal enzymes, is the drug of choice for long-term control. When given orally (20–30 g 3–4 times daily) it lowers pH in the colonic lumen to 4.5–5.5; this favors conversion of ammonia to nonabsorbable ammonium ion and has an analogous action on other toxic amines. An osmotic cathartic action by the unabsorbed sugar induces mild diarrhea and excretion of the ammonia. If these measures are insufficient, ileostomy or colonic exclusion by ileosigmoid anastomosis may be justified.

Fischer JE: Hepatic coma in cirrhosis, portal hypertension, and following portacaval shunt: Its etiologies and the current status of its treatment. Arch Surg 108:325, 1974.

Fischer JE, Baldessarini RJ: Pathogenesis and therapy of hepatic coma. Prog Liver Dis 5:363, 1976.

Fischer JE & others: The effect of normalization of plasma amino acids on hepatic encephalopathy in man. Surgery 80:77, 1976.

Resnick RH & others: A controlled trial of colon bypass in chronic hepatic encephalopathy. Gastroenterology 54:1057, 1968.

Schenker S & others: Hepatic encephalopathy: Current status. Gastroenterology 66:121, 1974.

Soeters PB, Fischer JE: Insulin, glucagon, amino acid imbalance, and hepatic encephalopathy. Lancet 2:880, 1976.

•   •   •

General References

Child CG III: *Portal Hypertension.* Saunders, 1974.

Leevy CM, Britton RC (editors): The hepatic circulation and portal hypertension. Ann New York Acad Sci 170:1, 1970.

McDermott WV Jr: *Surgery of the Liver and Portal Circulation.* Lea & Febiger, 1974.

Schiff L (editor): *Diseases of the Liver,* 4th ed. Lippincott, 1975.

Sedgwick CE, Poulantzas JK: *Portal Hypertension.* Little, Brown, 1967.

Sherlock S: *Diseases of the Liver and Biliary System,* 5th ed. Blackwell, 1975.

29 . . .
Biliary Tract

Lawrence W. Way, MD, & J. Englebert Dunphy, MD

EMBRYOLOGY & ANATOMY

The anlage of the biliary ducts and liver consists of a diverticulum which appears on the ventral aspect of the foregut in 3 mm embryos. The cranial portion becomes the liver; a caudal bud forms the ventral pancreas; and an intermediate bud develops into the gallbladder. Originally hollow, the hepatic diverticulum becomes a solid mass of cells which later recanalizes to form the ducts. The smallest ducts—the bile canaliculi—are first seen as a basal network between the primitive hepatocytes, which eventually expands throughout the liver (Fig 29–1). Numerous microvilli increase the canalicular surface area. Bile secreted here passes through the interlobular ductules (canals of Hering) and the lobar ducts and then into the hepatic duct in the hilus. In most cases, the common hepatic duct is formed by the union of a single right and left duct, but in 25% of individuals the anterior and posterior divisions of the right duct join the left duct separately. The origin of the common hepatic duct is close to the liver but always outside its substance. It runs about 4 cm before joining the cystic duct to form the common bile duct. The common duct begins in the hepatoduo-

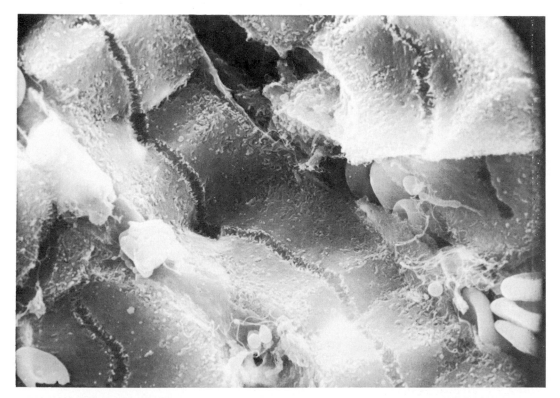

Figure 29–1. Scanning electron photomicrograph of a hepatic plate with adjacent sinusoids and sinusoidal microvilli and a bile canaliculus running in the center of the liver cells. Although their boundaries are indistinct, about 4 hepatocytes comprise the section of the plate in the middle of the photograph. Occasional red cells are present within the sinusoids. (Reduced from X 2000.) (Courtesy of Dr James Boyer.)

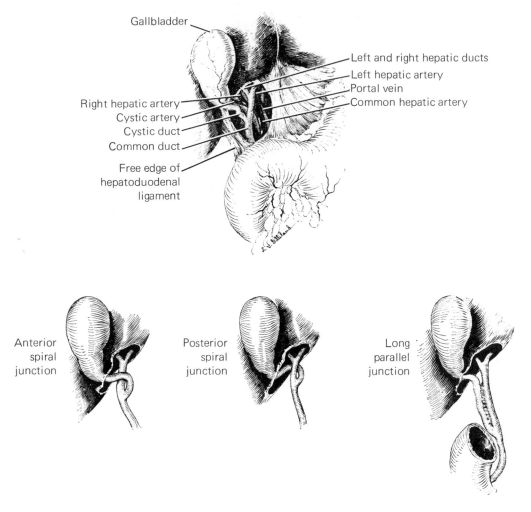

Gallbladder

Left and right hepatic ducts
Left hepatic artery
Portal vein
Common hepatic artery

Right hepatic artery
Cystic artery
Cystic duct
Common duct

Free edge of
hepatoduodenal
ligament

Anterior
spiral
junction

Posterior
spiral
junction

Long
parallel
junction

Figure 29–2. Anatomy of gallbladder and variations in anatomy of the cystic duct.

denal ligament, passes behind the first portion of the duodenum, and runs in a groove on the posterior surface of the pancreas before entering the duodenum. Its terminal 1 cm is intimately adherent to the duodenal wall. The total length of the common duct is about 9 cm (3½ inches).

In 80–90% of individuals, the main pancreatic duct joins the common duct to form a common channel about 1 cm long. The intraduodenal segment of the duct is called the hepatopancreatic ampulla or ampulla of Vater—somewhat of a misnomer since the lumen is not wider here.

The gallbladder is a pear-shaped organ adherent to the undersurface of the liver in a groove separating the right and left lobes. The fundus projects 1–2 cm below the hepatic edge and can often be palpated when the cystic or common duct is obstructed. It rarely has a complete peritoneal covering, but when this variation does occur it predisposes to infarction by torsion. The gallbladder holds about 50 ml of bile when fully distended. The neck of the gallbladder tapers into the narrow cystic duct which connects with the common

duct. The lumen of the cystic duct contains a thin mucosal septum, the spiral valve of Heister, which offers mild resistance to bile flow. In 75% of persons, the cystic duct enters the common duct at an angle. In the remainder, it runs parallel to the hepatic duct or winds around it before joining (Fig 29–2).

In the hepatoduodenal ligament, the hepatic artery is to the left of the common duct and the portal vein is posterior and medial. The right hepatic artery usually passes behind the hepatic duct and then gives off the cystic artery before entering the right lobe of the liver, but variations are common.

The mucosal epithelium of the bile ducts varies from cuboidal in the ductules to columnar in the main ducts. The gallbladder mucosa is thrown into prominent ridges when the organ is collapsed, and these flatten during distention. The tall columnar cells of the gallbladder mucosa are covered by microvilli on their luminal surface. Wide channels, which play an important role in water and electrolyte absorption, separate the individual cells.

The walls of the bile ducts contain only small

amounts of smooth muscle, but the termination of the common duct is enveloped by a complex sphincteric muscle. The gallbladder musculature is composed of interdigitated bundles of longitudinal and spirally arranged fibers.

The biliary tree receives parasympathetic and sympathetic innervation. The former contains motor fibers to the gallbladder and secretory fibers to the ductal epithelium. The afferent fibers in the sympathetic nerves mediate the pain of biliary colic.

Kune GA: The influence of structure and function in the surgery of the biliary tract. Ann R Coll Surg Engl 47:78, 1970.

Lindner HH, Green RB: Embryology and surgical anatomy of the extrahepatic biliary tract. Surg Clin North Am 44:1273, 1964.

PHYSIOLOGY

Bile Flow

Bile is produced at a rate of 500–1500 ml/day by secretory mechanisms in the hepatocytes and the cells of the ducts. Active secretion of bile salts into the biliary canaliculus is responsible for most of the volume of bile and its fluctuations. Na^+ and water follow passively to establish isosmolality and electrical neutrality. Lecithin and cholesterol (Fig 29–8) enter the canaliculus at rates that correlate with variations in bile salt output. Bilirubin and a number of other organic anions—estrogens, sulfobromophthalein, etc—are actively secreted by the hepatocyte by a different transport system from that which handles bile salts.

The columnar cells of the ducts add a fluid rich in

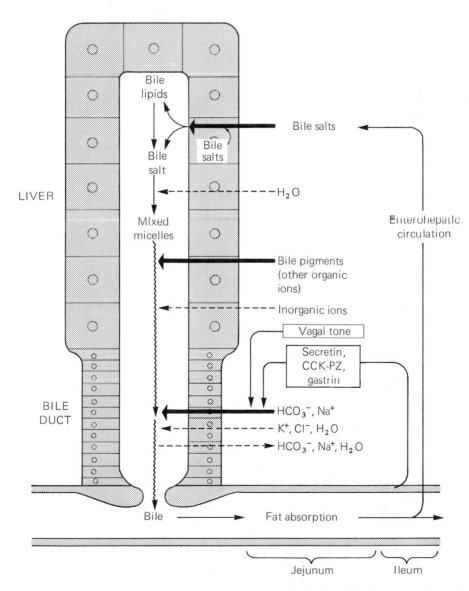

Figure 29–3. Bile formation. Solid lines into the ductular lumen indicate active transport; dotted lines represent passive diffusion.

HCO_3^- to that produced in the canaliculus. This involves active secretion of Na^+ and HCO_3^- by a cellular pump which is stimulated by secretin, gastrin, and cholecystokinin. K^+ and water are distributed passively across the ducts (Fig 29–3).

Between meals, bile is stored in the gallbladder, where it may be concentrated at rates up to 20% per hour. Na^+ and either HCO_3^- or Cl^- are actively transported from its lumen during absorption. The changes in composition brought about by concentration are shown in Fig 29–4.

Three factors regulate bile flow: hepatic secretion, gallbladder contraction, and choledochal sphincteric resistance. In the fasting state, pressure in the common bile duct is 5–10 cm water and bile produced in the liver is diverted into the gallbladder. After a meal, the gallbladder contracts, the sphincter relaxes, and bile is forced into the duodenum in squirts as ductal pressure intermittently exceeds sphincteric resistance. During contraction, pressure within the gallbladder reaches 25 cm water and that in the common bile duct 15–20 cm water.

Cholecystokinin-pancreozymin (CCK-PZ) is the major physiologic stimulus for gallbladder contraction and relaxation of the sphincter, but vagal impulses facilitate its action. The hormone is released into the blood stream from the mucosa of the small bowel by fat or lipolytic products in the lumen. Amino acids and small polypeptides are weaker stimuli, and carbohydrates are ineffective. Bile flow during a meal is augmented by increased turnover of bile salts in the enterohepatic circulation and stimulation of ductal secretion by secretin, gastrin, and CCK-PZ.

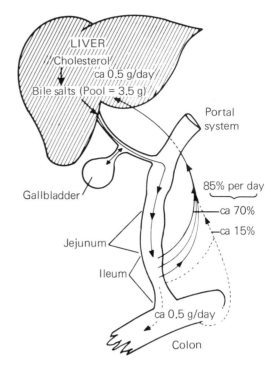

Figure 29–5. Enterohepatic circulation of bile salts. (Courtesy of M. Tyor.)

Bile Salts & the Enterohepatic Circulation (Fig 29–5)

Bile salts are steroid molecules formed by hepatocytes from cholesterol. The rate of synthesis is under feedback control and can be increased a maximum of about 10-fold. Two **primary** bile salts—cholate and chenodeoxycholate—are produced by the liver cells. Before excretion into bile, they are conjugated with either glycine or taurine to enhance water solubility. Intestinal bacteria may alter these compounds to produce the **secondary** bile salts, deoxycholate and lithocholate. The former is reabsorbed and enters bile, but lithocholate is insoluble and is excreted in the stool. Bile is composed of 40% cholate, 40% chenodeoxycholate, and 20% deoxycholate, conjugated with glycine or taurine in a ratio of 3:1.

The principal function of bile salts in the intestine is to solubilize lipids and lipolytic products and facilitate their absorption. Bile salts are detergents: molecules with water-soluble and fat-soluble groups at opposite poles. In an aqueous solution they spontaneously aggregate in groups called micelles, composed of 8–10 molecules. The molecules in the micelle are arranged with the hydrophobic poles in the center and the hydrophilic groups on the surface facing the water. Micelles can solubilize lipids within their hydrophobic centers and still remain in aqueous solution.

Lecithin and cholesterol, the other major solids, are transported in bile within the micelles. Lecithin is a polar phospholipid which is incapable itself of forming micelles and is only slightly soluble in water. However, when incorporated into bile salt micelles, it expands

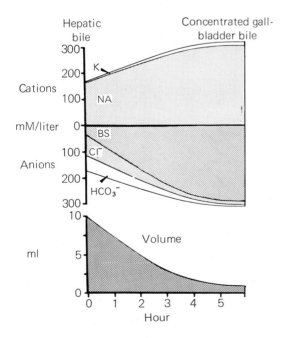

Figure 29–4. Changes in gallbladder bile composition with time. (Courtesy of J. Dietschy.)

the hydrocarbon center of the micelles and enhances their capacity to solubilize nonpolar lipids such as cholesterol.

Bile salts, lecithin, and cholesterol comprise about 90% of the solids in bile, the remainder consisting of bilirubin, fatty acids, and inorganic salts. Gallbladder bile contains about 10% solids and has a bile salt concentration between 200–300 mM/liter (Fig 29–4).

Bile salts remain in the intestinal lumen throughout the jejunum, where they participate in fat absorption. Upon reaching the distal small bowel, they are reabsorbed by an active transport system located in the terminal 200 cm of ileum. Over 95% of bile salts arriving from the jejunum are transferred by this process into portal vein blood; the remainder enter the colon, where they are converted to secondary bile salts. The entire bile salt pool of 2.5–4 g circulates twice through the enterohepatic circulation during each meal, and 6–8 cycles are made each day. The normal daily loss of bile salts in the stool amounts to 10–20% of the pool and is restored by hepatic synthesis.

Carey MC, Small DM: Micelle formation by bile salts. Arch Intern Med 130:506, 1972.

Dowling RH: The enterohepatic circulation. Gastroenterology 62:122, 1972.

Hallenbeck GA: Biliary and pancreatic intraductal pressures. Chap 57, pp 1007–1025, in: *Handbook of Physiology.* Vol 2: *Secretion.* American Physiological Society, 1967.

Javitt NB: Hepatic bile formation. (2 parts.) N Engl J Med 295:1464, 1511, 1976.

Wheeler HO: Concentrating function of the gallbladder. Am J Med 51:588, 1971.

Bilirubin

About 250–300 mg of bilirubin are excreted each day in the bile, most of it from breakdown of red cells in the reticuloendothelial system. First, heme is liberated from hemoglobin, and the iron and globin are removed for reuse by the organism. Biliverdin, the first pigment formed from heme, is reduced to unconjugated bilirubin, the indirect-reacting bilirubin of the van den Bergh test. Unconjugated bilirubin is insoluble in water and is transported in plasma bound to albumin.

Bilirubin is extracted from blood by the liver cells and after entering the cytoplasm is bound to one of 2 molecules, the Y and Z proteins, for which it and several other organic anions have high affinity. Unconjugated bilirubin is then conjugated with glucuronic acid to form bilirubin diglucuronide, the water-soluble, direct bilirubin. Conjugation is catalyzed by glucuronyl transferase, an enzyme on the endoplasmic reticulum. Bilirubin diglucuronide is actively transported into the biliary canaliculus by a mechanism shared by several organic anions but separate from that responsible for excretion of bile salts.

After entering the intestine, bilirubin is reduced by intestinal bacteria to several compounds known as urobilinogens which are subsequently oxidized and converted to pigmented urobilins. The term urobilino-

gen is often used to refer to both urobilins and urobilinogens.

About 300 mg of bilirubin enter the gut each day, but daily fecal urobilinogen amounts to only 200 mg. The discrepancy between bilirubin input and urobilinogen excretion has not yet been accounted for. About 1% of the intestinal pigment load is reabsorbed as urobilinogen and enters the enterohepatic circulation. The small amount of urobilinogen in the portal blood which escapes extraction and reexcretion in the bile is disposed of in the urine.

Fleischner G, Arias IM: Recent advances in bilirubin formation, transport, metabolism and excretion. Am J Med 49:576, 1970.

Schmid R: Bilirubin metabolism in man. N Engl J Med 287:703, 1972.

JAUNDICE

Jaundice can be categorized as prehepatic, hepatic, or posthepatic based upon the site of the underlying disease. Hemolysis is the most common form of prehepatic jaundice and is due to increased production of bilirubin. Less common prehepatic examples are Gilbert's disease and the Crigler-Najjar syndrome.

Hepatic parenchymal jaundice is subdivided into hepatocellular and cholestatic varieties. The former includes acute viral hepatitis and chronic alcoholic cirrhosis. Some cases of intrahepatic cholestasis may be indistinguishable clinically and biochemically from cholestasis due to common duct obstruction. Primary biliary cirrhosis, toxic drug jaundice, cholestatic jaundice of pregnancy, and postoperative cholestatic jaundice are the most commonly seen forms.

Extrahepatic jaundice most often results from biliary obstruction by a malignant tumor, choledocholithiasis, or biliary stricture. Pancreatic pseudocyst, sclerosing cholangitis, metastatic malignancy, and duodenal diverticulitis are less common causes.

History

The age, sex, and parity of the patient and possible deleterious habits should be noted. Most cases of infectious hepatitis occur in patients under 30 years. A history of drug addiction may suggest serum hepatitis transmitted by shared hypodermic equipment. Chronic alcoholism can usually be documented in patients with cirrhosis, and acute jaundice in alcoholics usually follows a recent binge. Obstructing gallstones or tumors are more common in older people.

Patients with jaundice due to choledocholithiasis may have associated biliary colic, fever, and chills and may report previous similar attacks. The pain in malignant obstruction is deep-seated and dull and may be affected by changes in position. Pain in the region of the liver is frequently experienced in the early stages of viral hepatitis and acute alcoholic liver injury. The patient with extrahepatic obstruction may report that his stools have become lighter in color and his urine dark.

Cholestatic diseases are often accompanied by **pruritus**—a symptom that may overshadow all others in the discomfort it causes. Pruritus may precede jaundice, but usually they appear at about the same time. The itching is most severe on the extremities and is aggravated by warm, humid weather. It is caused by an excess of bile salts in the system and correlates fairly well with amounts that can be recovered from the surface of the skin. Cholestyramine (Cuemid, Questran), an anion exchange resin, may provide dramatic symptomatic relief by binding bile salts in the intestinal lumen and preventing their reabsorption.

Physical Examination

Hepatomegaly is common in both hepatic and posthepatic jaundice. In some cases, palpation of the liver may suggest cirrhosis or metastatic malignancy, but impressions of this sort tend to be unreliable. Secondary stigmas of cirrhosis usually accompany acute alcoholic jaundice: liver palms, spider angiomas, ascites, collateral veins on the abdominal walls, and splenomegaly suggest cirrhosis. A nontender, palpable gallbladder in a jaundiced patient strongly suggests malignant obstruction of the common duct (Courvoisier's law), but absence of a palpable gallbladder is of little significance in ruling out malignancy.

Laboratory Tests

In hemolytic disease, the increased bilirubin is principally in the unconjugated indirect fraction. Since unconjugated bilirubin is insoluble in water, the jaundice in hemolysis is acholuric. The total bilirubin in hemolysis rarely exceeds 4–5 mg/100 ml because the rate of excretion increases as the total bilirubin rises and a plateau is quickly reached. Greater values suggest concomitant hepatic parenchymal disease.

Jaundice due to hepatic parenchymal disease is characterized by elevations of both conjugated and unconjugated serum bilirubin. An increase in the conjugated fraction always signifies disease within the hepatobiliary system. The direct bilirubin predominates in about half of cases of hepatic parenchymal disease.

Both intrahepatic cholestasis and extrahepatic obstruction raise the direct bilirubin, although the indirect fraction also increases somewhat. Since direct bilirubin is water-soluble, bilirubinuria develops. With complete extrahepatic obstruction, the total bilirubin rises to a plateau of 25–30 mg/100 ml, at which point loss in the urine equals the additional daily production. Higher values suggest concomitant hemolysis or decreased renal function. Obstruction of a single hepatic duct does not usually cause jaundice.

In malignant extrahepatic obstruction, the serum bilirubin is about 20 mg/100 ml, and these patients display the highest average concentrations. Obstructive jaundice due to common duct stones often produces transient bilirubin increases in the range of 2–4 mg/100 ml, and the level rarely goes over 15 mg/100

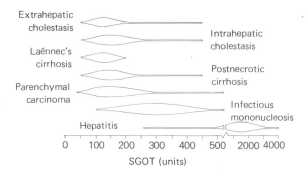

Figure 29—6. Range of SGOT values in various hepatobiliary disorders.

ml. Serum bilirubin values in patients with alcoholic cirrhosis and acute viral hepatitis vary widely in relation to the severity of the parenchymal damage. Hemolysis generally increases fecal urobilinogen, and complete extrahepatic biliary obstruction reduces both fecal and urinary urobilinogen. In the presence of hepatocellular jaundice, urobilinogen reabsorbed from the intestine is poorly excreted by the diseased liver, and urinary output rises.

Fig 29—6 depicts the range of serum SGOT determinations in a variety of conditions associated with jaundice. In extrahepatic obstruction, modest rises are common, but SGOT levels as high as 1000 units have been seen (though rarely) in patients with common duct stones. In the latter patients, the high value lasted for only a few days and was associated with 10-fold increases in LDH concentrations.

Serum alkaline phosphatase comes from 3 sites: liver, bone, and intestine. In normal subjects, liver and bone contribute about equally, and the intestinal contribution is small. Hepatic alkaline phosphatase is a product of the epithelial cells of the cholangioles, and increased alkaline phosphatase associated with liver disease is the result of increased enzyme production. Alkaline phosphatase levels go up with intrahepatic cholestasis, cholangitis, or extrahepatic obstruction. Since the elevation is from overproduction, it may occur with focal hepatic lesions in the absence of jaundice. For example, a solitary hepatic metastasis or pyogenic abscess in one lobe may fail to obstruct enough to cause jaundice but usually is associated with an increased alkaline phosphatase. In cholangitis with incomplete extrahepatic obstruction, serum bilirubin may be normal or mildly elevated but serum alkaline phosphatase may be very high.

Bone disease may complicate the interpretation of abnormal alkaline phosphatase levels (Fig 29—7). If one suspects that the increased serum enzyme may be from bone, serum calcium and phosphorus and a 5′-nucleotidase or leucine aminopeptidase level should be determined. These enzymes are also produced by cholangioles and are elevated in cholestasis, but their serum concentrations remain unchanged with bone disease.

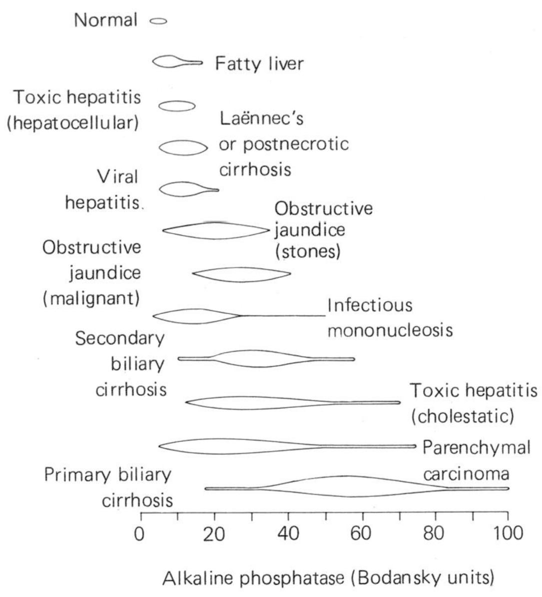
Normal
Fatty liver
Toxic hepatitis
(hepatocellular)
Laënnec's
or postnecrotic
cirrhosis
Viral
hepatitis
Obstructive
jaundice
(stones)
Obstructive
jaundice
(malignant)
Infectious
mononucleosis
Secondary
biliary
cirrhosis
Toxic hepatitis
(cholestatic)
Parenchymal
carcinoma
Primary biliary
cirrhosis
0 20 40 60 80 100
Alkaline phosphatase (Bodansky units)

Figure 29–7. Range of alkaline phosphatase values in various hepatobiliary disorders.

Changes in serum protein levels may reflect hepatic parenchymal dysfunction. In cirrhosis, the serum albumin falls and the globulins increase. Serum globulins reach high values in some patients with primary biliary cirrhosis. Biliary obstruction generally produces no changes unless secondary biliary cirrhosis has developed. The various serum flocculation tests measure relative alterations in serum protein fractions and are markedly abnormal only in hepatocellular disease.

Javitt NB: Cholestatic jaundice. Med Clin North Am 59:817, 1975.

Kaplan MM: Alkaline phosphatase. N Engl J Med 286:200, 1972.

Lorenzo GA, Beal JM: Recent advances in obstructive jaundice. Surg Clin North Am 51:211, 1971.

Ostrow JD: Jaundice in older children and adults. JAMA 234:522, 1975.

Schenker S & others: Differential diagnosis of jaundice. Am J Dig Dis 7:449, 1962.

Zimmerman HJ: The differential diagnosis of jaundice. Med Clin North Am 52:1417, 1968.

PATHOGENESIS OF GALLSTONES

More than 15 million people in the USA have gallstones in their gallbladders; about 300,000 operations are performed annually for this disease, and at least 6000 deaths result from its complications or treatment. The incidence rises with age, so that between 50 and 65 years of age about 20% of women and 5% of men are affected.

The gallstones in 75% of patients are composed predominantly (70–95%) of cholesterol and are referred to as cholesterol stones. The remaining 25% are pigment stones. Regardless of composition, all gallstones give rise to similar clinical sequelae.

Cholesterol Gallstones

Cholesterol gallstones result from secretion by the liver of bile supersaturated with cholesterol. If conditions are favorable, the cholesterol precipitates from solution and the newly formed crystals grow to macroscopic stones. Except when the common bile duct is dilated or partially obstructed, the stones in this disease form almost exclusively within the gallbladder. Those found in the ducts usually reach that location after passing through the cystic duct.

The incidence of cholesterol gallstone disease is highest in American Indians, lower in Caucasians, and lowest in Negroes, with a 2-fold gradient from one group to the next. More than 75% of American Indian women over age 40 are affected. Before puberty, the disease is rare but of equal frequency in both sexes. Thereafter, women are more commonly affected than men until after menopause, when the discrepancy lessens. Hormonal effects are also reflected in the increased incidence of gallstones with multiparity and the increased cholesterol saturation of bile and greater incidence of gallstones following ingestion of oral contraceptives.

As noted previously, cholesterol is insoluble and in bile must be transported within the bile salt micelles. Lecithin incorporated into the bile salt micelle enhances its cholesterol-carrying capacity. Using ordinates on which the relative amount of each of these bile components is expressed as a molar percentage, their relationship can be depicted on a triangular graph where any possible mixture is represented as a point (Fig 29–8). In a solution comprising 10% solids, similar to gallbladder bile, the curved line in Fig 29–8 demarcates the area (clear space) where cholesterol is entirely in micellar solution from that (shaded space) where it must exist as a precipitate or supersaturated solution.

When the relative composition of specimens of gallbladder or hepatic bile from patients with cholesterol gallstones is plotted on this graph, the location falls outside the zone of solubility, whereas bile from normal subjects usually falls inside the zone. However, the rate of bile salt secretion from the liver increases with meals and drops during fasting. Lecithin and bile salt output rise and fall together, but, because cholesterol secretion is largely independent, the saturation of bile with cholesterol rises during fasting and in many otherwise healthy persons transiently exceeds the limit of cholesterol solubility. These individuals are presumably at risk of developing gallstones if their gallbladder provides the nidus for crystallization and other favorable conditions.

A reduction in cholesterol solubility obviously could result either from lowered cholesterol-holding capacity (the micelles) or increased cholesterol secretion. The bile salt pool in patients with cholesterol

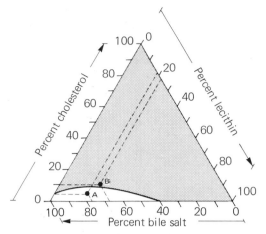

Figure 29–8. Triangular coordinates for depicting combination of bile salts, lecithin, and cholesterol. Point A represents the mean values for gallbladder bile from normal subjects: 77% bile salts, 18% lecithin, and 5% cholesterol. Point B represents the mean values for gallbladder bile from patients with cholesterol gallstones: 68% bile salts, 22% lecithin, and 10% cholesterol.

gallstone disease (1.5 g) is about half the size of normal subjects. This results in lower bile salt secretion from the liver and seems to be the principal mechanism by which cholesterol supersaturation occurs. Other patients, especially obese women, appear to excrete increased quantities of cholesterol in their bile.

Pigment Stones

Pigment stones account for 25% of gallstones in the USA and 60% of those in Japan. Pigment stones are black to dark brown, 2–5 mm in diameter, and amorphous. They are composed of a mixture of calcium bilirubinate, bile acids, and other unidentified substances. About 50% of pigment stones are radiopaque, and in the USA they comprise two-thirds of all radiopaque gallstones. The incidence is similar in men and women and in blacks and whites. Pigment stones are rare in American Indians.

Predisposing factors are cirrhosis, bile stasis (eg, a strictured or markedly dilated common duct), and chronic hemolysis. Some patients with pigment stones have increased concentrations of unconjugated bilirubin in their bile. In the Orient this may be the result of the action of β-glucuronidase produced by *E coli*, which secondarily invades the ductal system when it becomes infested with *Clonorchis sinensis* or *Ascaris lumbricoides*. Except as a secondary invader, *E coli* is absent from the bile ducts of persons in Western cultures and the pathogenesis is largely unknown. Stone formation may involve increased production by the gallbladder mucosa of sulfated glycoproteins upon which calcium precipitates, eventually giving rise to macroscopic stones.

Bennion LJ, Grundy SM: Effects of obesity and caloric intake on biliary lipid metabolism in man. J Clin Invest 56:996, 1975.

Bennion LJ & others: Effects of oral contraceptives on the gallbladder bile of normal women. N Engl J Med 294:189, 1976.

Small DM: The etiology and pathogenesis of gallstones. Adv Surg 10:63, 1976.

Soloway RD & others: Pigment gallstones. Gastroenterology 72:167, 1977.

Sutor DJ, Wooley SE: The organic matrix of gallstones. Gut 14:487, 1974.

Sutor DJ, Wooley SE: The sequential deposition of crystalline material in gallstones: Evidence for changing gallbladder bile composition during the growth of some stones. Gut 15:130, 1974.

Trotman BW, Ostrow JD, Soloway RD: Pigment vs cholesterol cholelithiasis: Comparison of stone and bile composition. Am J Dig Dis 19:585, 1974.

Trotman BW, Soloway RD: Pigment vs cholesterol cholelithiasis: Clinical and epidemiological aspects. Am J Dig Dis 20:735, 1975.

DIAGNOSTIC EXAMINATION OF THE BILIARY TREE

Plain Abdominal Film

The posteroanterior supine view of the abdomen will show gallstones in the 10–15% of cases where they are radiopaque. The bile itself sometimes contains sufficient calcium (milk of calcium bile) to be seen. An enlarged gallbladder can occasionally be identified as a soft tissue mass in the right upper quadrant indenting an air-filled hepatic flexure.

In several types of biliary disease, the diagnosis may be suggested by air seen in the bile ducts on a plain film. This would usually signify the presence of a biliary-intestinal fistula (from disease or surgery) but also occurs rarely in severe cholangitis, emphysematous cholecystitis, and biliary ascariasis.

Oral Cholecystogram

Tyropanoate (Bilopaque) or iopanoic acid (Telepaque) is taken orally the night before the examination, preferably along with a light meal containing fat. The drug is absorbed, bound to albumin in portal blood, extracted by hepatocytes, and secreted in bile. Opacification occurs only with concentration in the gallbladder and on the average is optimal 17 hours after taking the iopanoate. Posteroanterior and oblique supine views and an upright or lateral decubitus film are obtained, a meal containing fat is given, and the x-rays are repeated. The fat releases cholecystokinin, which empties the gallbladder and may outline the bile ducts. Gallstones appear as radiolucent filling defects in the gallbladder lumen.

Oral cholecystograms are unsatisfactory if the contrast agent is inefficiently absorbed from the intestine or poorly excreted by the liver. Absorption is often impaired in acute abdominal illnesses with ileus, vomiting, or diarrhea. If the bilirubin level is over 3 mg/100 ml, hepatic excretion will probably be inadequate. False-negative results are obtained in 5% of tests. A normal gallbladder may not opacify for several weeks after severe trauma or a major illness.

Nonopacification occurs in 20% of patients after the usual single-dose regimen. When a second dose is given and x-rays repeated the following day, opacification is obtained in 65% of these patients. Persistent nonopacification is a highly reliable (> 95% true positive) indication of gallbladder disease. Instead of performing a double-dose oral cholecystogram as the next step when a single dose fails to opacify, it may be simpler to first obtain an ultrasound scan, which will demonstrate gallstones in 85% of patients who have them. Then a second dose of iopanoate and additional x-rays may be reserved for those whose ultrasound scans are negative or equivocal.

Intravenous Cholangiography (IVC)

Intravenous iodipamide (Cholografin) is excreted by the hepatocyte in sufficient concentration to opacify the bile ducts, and, if the cystic duct is not obstructed, the gallbladder will also be demonstrated. The degree of opacification never approaches that of oral cholecystography, and IVC cannot be considered an alternative method for investigating the gallbladder.

The success of intravenous cholangiography is critically dependent on efficient hepatic excretion of the contrast agent; if the serum bilirubin concentration is greater than 4 mg/100 ml, the chances of a satisfactory examination are negligible. Between 2 and 4 mg/100 ml, the incidence of opacification is no more than 20%. In this bilirubin range, the likelihood of obtaining a useful study is greater if the bilirubin is dropping rapidly than if it is stationary or increasing.

Tomography is an essential part of the study, but even with tomography and good liver function there is a 15–20% incidence of false-negative results. Obvious strictures and stones can be missed, and a negative study does not have the same reliability as one in which a defect is demonstrated.

Intravenous cholangiography is of greatest value in (1) patients suspected of having biliary colic who have had a previous cholecystectomy and (2) patients with acute abdominal pain in whom acute cholecystitis is suspected.

Percutaneous Transhepatic Cholangiography

Percutaneous transhepatic cholangiography may opacify the biliary tree in patients too jaundiced for oral or intravenous studies. The examination is performed by passing a fine needle through the right lower rib cage, the hepatic parenchyma, and into the lumen of a bile duct. Water-soluble contrast material is injected, and x-ray films are taken.

The technical success is related to the degree of dilatation of the intrahepatic bile ducts. Transhepatic cholangiography is especially valuable in demonstrating obstruction from tumors, stones, and strictures. Failure to enter a duct does not prove that obstruction is absent, but there is rarely a problem in obtaining a good study with malignant obstruction. Transhepatic

cholangiography should not be done in patients with cholangitis until the infection has been controlled with antibiotics. Septic shock has been produced by sudden inoculation of organisms from bile into the systemic circulation. Otherwise, the contraindications are the same as for percutaneous liver biopsy.

Retrograde Endoscopic Cholangiography

This technic involves cannulating the sphincter of Oddi under direct vision through a side-viewing duodenoscope. It is a difficult procedure and requires special training involving more than familiarity with the use of fiberoptic endoscopes. It is often possible to obtain opacification of the pancreatic as well as the bile ducts. This method of cholangiography is especially applicable to patients with an abnormal clotting mechanism who would not be candidates for transhepatic puncture of the ducts. Its major drawback involves the potential of contaminating the sterile bile and producing cholangitis in patients with high-grade obstruction.

Transjugular Cholangiography

This method involves passing a catheter under radiographic control from the jugular vein into the liver via the hepatic veins. Free and wedged venous pressure measurements, hepatic venography, and even liver biopsy (using a suction needle) can all be performed through the same catheter. When the tip of the catheter reaches the center of the liver, it is forced into the parenchyma until a bile duct is entered. Because a direct communication is made between the obstructed duct and the systemic circulation, the danger of septicemia is high if the bile is heavily contaminated with bacteria. Active cholangitis is a strong contraindication to this procedure. Of the 3 technics of direct nonoperative cholangiography, this one may have special value for studying patients with neoplastic obstruction whose coagulation tests are abnormal.

Ultrasound

Ultrasonography is useful to detect gallbladder stones and dilated bile ducts. The examination is relatively inexpensive and singularly free of morbidity and has rapidly assumed a prominent place in clinical practice. When studying the gallbladder, false-positives for stones are rare but false-negatives, due to small stones or a contracted gallbladder, occur in about 15% of patients. Thus, only positive studies are completely reliable. Ultrasound can be especially useful to verify the presence of gallstones in patients with a nonopacifying gallbladder on oral cholecystography or in acute cholecystitis.

The ability to demonstrate dilated bile ducts may help select patients for transhepatic cholangiography. Depending on the clinical picture, the finding of dilated bile ducts by ultrasound may occasionally be enough evidence to lead directly to operation.

Addison NV & others: Evaluation of biliary tract disease by ultrasonic B-mode scanning. Br J Surg 63:784, 1976.

Bartrum RJ Jr & others: Ultrasonic and radiographic cholecystography. N Engl J Med 296:538, 1977.

Berk RN: Radiology of the gallbladder and bile ducts. Surg Clin
North Am 53:973, 1973.

Elias E & others: A randomized trial of percutaneous transhepatic cholangiography with the Chiba needle versus endoscopic retrograde cholangiography for bile duct visualization in jaundice. Gastroenterology 71:439, 1976.

Ferrucci JT Jr, Eaton SB Jr: Radiologic evaluation of obstructive jaundice. Surg Clin North Am 54:537, 1974.

Ferrucci JT Jr & others: Fine needle transhepatic cholangiography: A new approach to obstructive jaundice. Am J
Roentgenol Radium Ther Nucl Med 127:403, 1976.

Loeb PM & others: Endoscopic pancreatocholangiography in
the diagnosis of biliary tract disease. Surg Clin North Am
53:1007, 1973.

Mujahed Z, Evans JA, Whalen JP: The nonopacified gallbladder
on oral cholecystography. Radiology 112:1, 1974.

Rosch J & others: Transjugular approach to the liver, biliary
system, and portal circulation. Am J Roentgenol Radium
Ther Nucl Med 125:602, 1975.

Scholz FJ & others: Intravenous cholangiography. Radiology
114:513, 1975.

DISEASES OF THE
GALLBLADDER & BILE DUCTS

ASYMPTOMATIC GALLSTONES

Data on the prevalence of gallstones in the USA indicate that only about 30% of people with chole-lithiasis come to surgery. To date there are no satisfactory studies on the natural history of asymptomatic gallstones, but it must be a relatively benign condition. Moreover, the available information demonstrates that few people pass rapidly from an asymptomatic state to one of life-threatening complications; an initial period of episodic biliary colic occurs in the majority. For these reasons, the present practice of operating only on symptomatic patients, leaving the millions without symptoms alone, seems justified. A burning question to many clinicians is what to advise the asymptomatic patient found to have gallstones during the course of unrelated studies. The presence of any of the following portends a more serious course and should probably serve as reasons for prophylactic cholecystectomy: (1) diabetes mellitus, because of the frequency of serious complications and a high mortality rate (10−15%) in acute cholecystitis; (2) a nonvisualizing gallbladder, because this signifies more advanced disease; (3) large stones (greater than 2 cm in diameter), because they more often produce acute cholecystitis than small stones; and (4) a calcified gallbladder, because it so often is associated with carcinoma. However, most asymptomatic patients have none of these special features. Certainly, if coexistent cardiopulmonary or other problems raise the risk of surgery, operation

should not be considered. For the average asymptomatic patient it is not reasonable to make a strong recommendation for cholecystectomy. The tendency is to operate on younger patients and temporize in the elderly.

Carey JB Jr: Natural history of gallstone disease. Mod Treat
5:493, 1968.

Wenckert A, Robertson B: The natural course of gallstone disease: Eleven-year review of 781 nonoperated cases. Gastroenterology 50:376, 1966.

Wilbur RS, Bolt RJ: Incidence of gallbladder disease in "normal" men. Gastroenterology 36:251, 1959.

GALLSTONES &
CHRONIC CHOLECYSTITIS
(Biliary Colic)

Essentials of Diagnosis

- Episodic abdominal pain.
- Dyspepsia.
- Gallstones on cholecystography.

General Considerations

Chronic cholecystitis is the most common form of symptomatic gallbladder disease and is associated with gallstones in nearly every case. In general, the term cholecystitis is applied whenever gallstones are present regardless of the histologic appearance of the gallbladder. Repeated minor episodes of obstruction of the cystic duct cause intermittent biliary colic and contribute to inflammation and subsequent scar formation. Gallbladders from patients with gallstones who have never had an attack of acute cholecystitis are of 2 types: (1) In some, the mucosa may be slightly flattened, but the wall is thin and unscarred and, except for the stones, appears normal. (2) Others exhibit obvious signs of chronic inflammation with thickening, cellular infiltration, loss of elasticity, and fibrosis. The clinical history in these 2 groups cannot always be distinguished, and inflammatory changes may also be found in patients with asymptomatic gallstones.

Clinical Findings

A. Symptoms and Signs: Biliary colic, the most characteristic symptom, is caused by transient gallstone obstruction of the cystic duct. The pain usually begins abruptly and subsides gradually, lasting for a few minutes to several hours. The pain of biliary colic is usually steady—not intermittent, like intestinal colic. In some patients, attacks occur postprandially; in others, there is no relationship to meals. The frequency of attacks is quite variable, ranging from nearly continuous trouble to episodes many years apart. Nausea may accompany the pain, but vomiting is not as common as in choledocholithiasis.

Biliary colic is usually felt in the right upper quadrant, but epigastric and left abdominal pain are

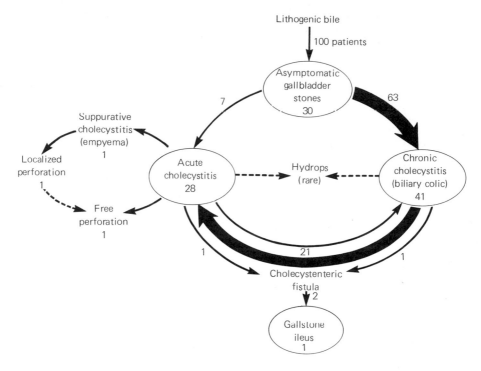

Figure 29—9. The natural history of gallbladder stones. The numbers approximate the percentage of patients in each category. Note that most patients with acute cholecystitis have previously had biliary colic.

common and in some cases precordial pain occurs. The pain may radiate around the costal margin into the back or may be referred to the region of the scapula. Pain on top of the shoulder is unusual and suggests direct diaphragmatic irritation. In a severe attack, the patient usually curls up in bed, changing position frequently in search of a more comfortable position.

During an attack, there may be tenderness in the right upper quadrant and, rarely, the gallbladder is palpable.

Fatty food intolerance, dyspepsia, indigestion, heartburn, flatulence, nausea, and eructations are other symptoms associated with gallstone disease. Because they are also frequent in the general population, their presence in any given patient may only be incidental to the gallstones.

B. Laboratory Findings: An oral cholecystogram will usually show stones in the gallbladder. If hepatic function and intestinal absorption are normal, failure to visualize the gallbladder after 2 separate oral cholecystograms indicates nonfunction from gallbladder disease. An intravenous cholangiogram may be ordered if the clinical picture is atypical or if malabsorption of the dye cannot be ruled out.

Differential Diagnosis

Gallbladder colic may be strongly suggested by the history, but the clinical impression should always be verified by x-rays. Biliary colic may simulate the pain of duodenal ulcer, hiatal hernia, pancreatitis, and myocardial infarction.

ECG and a chest x-ray should be obtained to investigate cardiopulmonary disease. It has been suggested that biliary colic may sometimes aggravate cardiac disease, but recent reviews of the relationship conclude that angina pectoris or an abnormal ECG should rarely be indications for cholecystectomy.

Right-sided radicular pain in the T6—T10 dermatomes may be confused with biliary colic. Osteoarthritic spurs, vertebral lesions, or tumors may be shown on x-rays of the spine or may be suggested by hyperesthesia of the abdominal skin.

An upper gastrointestinal series should be performed in a search for esophageal spasm, hiatal hernia, peptic ulcer, or gastric tumors. In some patients the irritable colon syndrome may be mistaken for gallbladder discomfort. Carcinoma of the cecum or ascending colon may be overlooked on the assumption that the postprandial pain in these conditions is due to gallstones.

Complications

Chronic cholecystitis predisposes to acute cholecystitis, common duct stones, and adenocarcinoma of the gallbladder. The incidence of all of these complications increases the longer the stones have been present.

Treatment

A. Medical Treatment: At present, no effective nonsurgical treatment is available for chronic cholecystitis and cholelithiasis. In some cases, symptoms occur after ingestion of certain foods. Avoidance of these foods may be symptomatically helpful, but change in diet will not reduce the risk of complications.

Chenodeoxycholic acid, one of the primary bile salts, when given orally to gallstone patients (15 mg/kg/day), expands the bile salt pool to normal, desaturates the bile with respect to cholesterol, and slowly dissolves cholesterol gallstones. Cholic acid does not produce the same changes. In a pilot study at the Mayo Clinic, after 18 months of continuous treatment, total dissolution occurred in one-third of patients with radiolucent stones. It is noteworthy that after treatment was stopped the bile promptly resumed its supersaturated quality, and in several patients gallstones recurred which responded once again to resumption of the drug. Chenodeoxycholate is ineffective for radiopaque stones and for those in a gallbladder that fails to opacify on oral cholecystography. With present knowledge it is considered unsafe for women capable of bearing children because of fears of hepatotoxicity to the fetus. A nationwide trial is being conducted in the USA to determine the safety and efficacy of this drug before it is released for general use.

B. Surgical Treatment: Cholecystectomy should be performed in most patients with symptoms. The procedure can be scheduled at the patient's convenience, within weeks or months after diagnosis. Active concurrent disease which increases the risk of surgery should be treated before operation. In some chronically ill patients, surgery should be deferred indefinitely.

After the abdomen is opened, the common duct is examined for the presence of stones before cholecystectomy is begun. (The indications for common duct exploration are discussed below.) An operative cholangiogram should be used as a routine check on the presence of stones in the duct.

Prognosis

Serious morbidity and deaths related to the operation itself are rare and are almost confined to the elderly. Relief of symptoms postoperatively is related to the extent to which they were typical of gallstone disease and the degree of chronic inflammation found in the gallbladder. In general, the operation can be considered to be successful in 95% of cases.

Boquist L & others: Mortality after gallbladder surgery: A study of 3257 cholecystectomies. Surgery 71:616, 1972.

Bremner DN & others: A study of cholecystectomy. Surg Gynecol Obstet 138:752, 1974.

Edlund Y, Zettergren L: Histopathology of the gallbladder in gallstone disease related to clinical data. Acta Chir Scand 116:450, 1959.

French EB, Robb WAT: Biliary and renal colic. Br Med J 3:121, 1963.

Gunn A, Keddie N: Some clinical observations on patients with gallstones. Lancet 2:239, 1972.

Higgins JA: Nonfunctioning gallbladder. Mod Treat 5:500, 1968.

Lahana DA, Schoenfield LJ: Progress in medical therapy of gallstones. Surg Clin North Am 53:1053, 1973.

Price WH: Gall-bladder dyspepsia. Br Med J 3:138, 1963.

ACUTE CHOLECYSTITIS

Essentials of Diagnosis

- Acute right upper quadrant pain and tenderness.
- Mild fever and leukocytosis.
- Palpable gallbladder in one-third of cases.
- Nonvisualized gallbladder on intravenous cholangiogram.

General Considerations

In 98% of cases, acute cholecystitis results from obstruction of the cystic duct by a gallstone impacted in Hartmann's pouch. The gallbladder becomes inflamed and distended, creating abdominal pain and tenderness. The natural history of acute cholecystitis varies considerably depending on whether the obstruction becomes relieved, the extent of secondary bacterial invasion, the age of the patient, and the presence of other aggravating factors such as diabetes mellitus. Most attacks resolve spontaneously without surgery or other specific therapy, but some progress to abscess formation or free perforation with generalized peritonitis.

The pathologic changes in the gallbladder evolve in a typical pattern. Subserosal edema and hemorrhage and patchy mucosal necrosis are the first changes. Later, polymorphonuclear leukocytes appear. The final stage involves development of fibrosis. Gangrene and perforation may occur as early as 3 days after onset, but most perforations occur during the second week. In those cases that resolve spontaneously, acute inflammation has largely cleared by 4 weeks, but some residual evidence of inflammation may last for several months. About 90% of gallbladders removed during an acute attack show chronic scarring, although many of these patients deny having had any previous symptoms.

The cause of acute cholecystitis is still partially conjectural. Obstruction of the cystic duct is present in most cases, but experimentally produced obstruction does not cause inflammation unless gallstones are present—nor does cholecystitis always develop after obstruction even if stones are present. Pancreatic juice, concentrated bile salts, or bacterial cultures, when injected into the gallbladders of animals with an occluded cystic duct, may produce cholecystitis. The extent to which these experiments are relevant to the pathogenesis of the disease in humans remains hazy. Bacteria can be cultured from the bile of 50% of patients with acute cholecystitis, but the frequent absence of bacteria and the lack of suppuration in general have led to an emphasis on nonbacterial theories of etiology.

About 2% of cases of acute cholecystitis occur in the absence of cholelithiasis. Some of these are due to cystic duct obstruction by another process such as a malignant tumor. Rarely, acute acalculous cholecystitis results from cystic artery occlusion or primary bacterial infection by *E coli,* clostridia, or occasionally

Salmonella typhosa. Acute acalculous cholecystitis has also been reported as a complication of prolonged fasting after an unrelated operation. It has been postulated that the inflammation is caused by high concentrations of bile salts which develop in the gallbladder under these circumstances.

Clinical Findings

A. Symptoms and Signs: The first symptom is sudden abdominal pain in the right upper quadrant, sometimes associated with referred pain in the region of the right scapula. In 75% of cases, the patient will have had previous attacks of biliary colic, at first indistinguishable from the present illness. However, in acute cholecystitis the pain persists and becomes associated with abdominal tenderness. Nausea and vomiting are present in about half of patients, but the vomiting is rarely severe. Mild icterus occurs in 10%. The temperature usually ranges from 38—38.5 C (100.4—101.3 F). High fever and chills are uncommon and should suggest the possibility of complications or an incorrect diagnosis.

Right upper quadrant tenderness is present, and in about a third of patients the gallbladder is palpable in a position usually somewhat lateral to its normal one. Voluntary guarding during examination may prevent detection of an enlarged gallbladder. In others, the gallbladder is not enlarged because scarring of the wall restricts distention. If the patient is instructed to breathe deeply during palpation in the right subcostal region, he experiences accentuated tenderness and sudden inspiratory arrest (Murphy's sign).

B. Laboratory Findings: The leukocyte count is usually elevated to 12—15 thousand/μl. Normal counts are common, but if the count goes much above 15,000 one should suspect complications. A mild elevation of the serum bilirubin (in the range of 2—4 mg/100 ml) is common, presumably due to secondary inflammation of the common duct by the contiguous gallbladder. Bilirubin values above this range would most likely indicate the associated presence of common duct stones. A mild increase in alkaline phosphatase, 5'-nucleotidase, and leucine aminopeptidase may accompany the attack. Occasionally, the serum amylase concentration transiently reaches 1000 units/100 ml or more.

C. X-Ray Findings: A plain x-ray of the abdomen may occasionally show an enlarged gallbladder shadow. In 15% of patients, the gallstones contain enough calcium to be seen on the plain film.

An oral cholecystogram cannot be relied on during acute cholecystitis or other acute abdominal disorders characterized by vomiting and should be postponed until 4—6 weeks after the acute attack.

Intravenous cholangiography may be diagnostic: except for mild transient cases, opacification of the gallbladder excludes the diagnosis; demonstration of contrast in the bile ducts but none in the gallbladder confirms the diagnosis of acute cholecystitis. An ultrasound scan may verify the presence of gallbladder stones.

Differential Diagnosis

The differential diagnosis includes other common causes of acute upper abdominal pain and tenderness. An acute peptic ulcer with or without perforation might be suggested by a history of epigastric pain relieved by food or antacids. Most cases of perforated ulcer demonstrate free air under the diaphragm on x-ray. Intravenous cholangiography or emergency upper gastrointestinal series with water-soluble contrast may help in puzzling situations.

Acute pancreatitis can easily be confused with acute cholecystitis, especially if cholecystitis is accompanied by an elevated amylase. Intravenous cholangiograms would outline the gallbladder in most cases of acute pancreatitis. Sometimes the 2 diseases coexist, but pancreatitis should not be accepted as a second diagnosis without specific findings.

Acute appendicitis in patients with a high cecum may closely simulate acute cholecystitis.

Severe right upper quadrant pain with high fever and local tenderness may develop in acute gonococcal perihepatitis (Fitz-Hugh and Curtis syndrome). Clues to the proper diagnosis may be found in tenderness in the adnexa, vaginal discharge which contains gonococci on a gram-stained smear, and a disparity between the patient's high fever and her general lack of toxicity.

Acute viral hepatitis has a more gradual onset and is accompanied by sustained elevations of SGOT and SGPT. Although hepatic enzymes may rise in acute cholecystitis, they become normal within 24—48 hours and in all but a few cases the absolute levels do not approach those seen in hepatitis. Alcoholic hepatitis may be clinically indistinguishable from acute cholecystitis because it produces marked right upper quadrant tenderness and leukocytosis and the SGOT is usually normal or only mildly elevated. Liver biopsy may be diagnostic if it shows acute parenchymal necrosis and inflammation.

Severe pneumonitis in the right lung or an acute myocardial infarction occasionally masquerades as an acute abdominal disorder.

Complications

The major complications of acute cholecystitis are empyema, gangrene, and perforation. In **empyema** (suppurative cholecystitis), the gallbladder contains frank pus and the patient becomes more toxic with high spiking fever (39—40 C [102.2—104 F]), chills, and leukocytosis greater than 15,000/μl. Parenteral antibiotics should be given, and surgery, either cholecystostomy or cholecystectomy, performed promptly.

Perforation may take any of 3 forms: (1) localized perforation with pericholecystic abscess; (2) free perforation with generalized peritonitis; and (3) perforation into an adjacent hollow viscus with the formation of a fistula. Perforation may occur as early as 3 days after the onset of acute cholecystitis, or late in the second week. The total incidence of perforation is about 10%.

Pericholecystic abscess, the most common form of perforation, should be suspected when the signs and symptoms progress, especially when accompanied by the appearance of a palpable mass. The patient often becomes toxic, with fever to 39 C (102.2 F) and a leukocyte count above 15,000/μl, but sometimes there is no correlation between the clinical signs and the development of local abscess. Cholecystectomy and drainage of the abscess can be performed safely in many of these patients, but if the patient's condition is unstable, cholecystostomy is preferable.

Free perforation occurs in only 1−2% of patients, more often early in the disease when gangrene develops before adhesions wall off the gallbladder. The diagnosis is made preoperatively in less than half of cases. In some patients with localized pain, sudden spread of pain and tenderness to other parts of the abdomen suggests the diagnosis. Whenever it is suspected, free perforation must be treated by emergency laparotomy. Abdominal paracentesis may be misleading and has proved to be of little diagnostic usefulness. Cholecystectomy should be performed if the patient's condition will permit; otherwise, cholecystostomy is done. The mortality rate depends partly on whether the cystic duct remained obstructed or the stone was dislodged after perforation. The former leads to a purulent peritonitis which is lethal in 20% of cases. In the latter, a true bile peritonitis ensues and over 50% of patients die. The earlier operation is performed, the better the prognosis.

Cholecystenteric fistula. If the acutely inflamed gallbladder becomes adherent to adjacent stomach, duodenum, or colon and necrosis develops at the site of one of these adhesions, perforation may occur into the lumen of the gut. The resulting decompression often allows the acute disease to resolve. If the gallbladder stones discharge through the fistula and if they are large enough, they may obstruct the small intestine (gallstone ileus; see below). Rarely, patients vomit gallstones which entered the stomach through a cholecystogastric fistula. In most patients, the acute attack improves and the cholecystenteric fistula is clinically unsuspected.

Cholecystenteric fistulas do not usually cause symptoms unless the gallbladder is still partially obstructed by stones or scarring. Neither oral nor intravenous cholangiograms will opacify the gallbladder or the fistula, but the latter may be shown on upper gastrointestinal series, where it must be differentiated from a fistula due to perforated peptic ulcer. Malabsorption and steatorrhea have been reported in isolated cases of cholecystocolonic fistulas. Steatorrhea in this situation could be due either to absence of bile in the proximal bowel following diversion into the colon or deconjugation of bile salts in the duodenum by excess colonic bacteria.

Symptomatic cholecystenteric fistulas should be treated by cholecystectomy and closure of the fistula. The majority are discovered incidentally during cholecystectomy for symptomatic gallbladder disease.

Treatment

Acute cholecystitis will resolve in most cases whether the patient is managed expectantly (medical treatment) or by cholecystectomy. The nonsurgical regimen eventually requires interval operation, whereas the surgical approach is definitive. The choice should be individualized for each patient. Intravenous fluids should be given to correct dehydration and electrolyte imbalance, and a nasogastric tube should be inserted. For pain relief, morphine and meperidine have the theoretical disadvantage of elevating biliary pressure by contracting the sphincter of Oddi. Pentazocine does not share this action, but if relief is unsatisfactory with this drug one of the others may be prescribed.

Antibiotics are not usually required and should be reserved for patients in jeopardy of developing complications. Ampicillin, tetracycline, chloramphenicol, and cephaloridine have been recommended for the treatment of biliary infections because they are normally excreted in the bile. However, in biliary disease they may be blocked from reaching the infection by this route. For the expectant treatment of acute cholecystitis of average severity, parenteral ampicillin (4 g daily) or cephaloridine (2−4 g daily) should be given. Parenteral penicillin (20 million units daily) and kanamycin (15 mg/kg daily) or penicillin and gentamicin (2−4 mg/kg daily) should be given for severe disease.

The following are the major factors that affect the decision for early surgery (Fig 29−10): (1) whether the diagnosis is established; (2) the general health of the patient as modified by coexistent disease or the present illness; and (3) signs of local complications of acute cholecystitis. The diagnosis should be clear-cut and the patient optimally prepared; if perforation is suspected, emergency surgery is indicated.

About 30% of cases satisfy the criteria for early definitive operation with little delay after admission to the hospital. An example might be a healthy young patient who is admitted within 24 hours of the onset of symptoms. If the history and physical findings are typical and if the distended, tender gallbladder is palpable, the diagnosis can be accepted. This patient might be scheduled for operation in the next open position on the surgery list. This does not mean that an emergency is present, as in the case of acute appendicitis or perforated peptic ulcer, because acute cholecystitis does not usually threaten complications within short, rigid time intervals. Left untreated, most cases would resolve without sequelae. Therefore, the operation need not be done in the middle of the night but under the better circumstances during the regular operating schedule with a prepared team.

In another 30% of patients, however, the correct diagnosis is not obvious. The diagnosis of acute cholecystitis based upon clinical criteria alone is in error in 5−10% of cases. In most instances these are patients whose clinical findings consist of upper abdominal pain without a palpable gallbladder. Many of the conditions listed in the section on differential diagnosis may have to be ruled out. If early surgery is being considered and the bilirubin is normal, emergency intravenous cholangiograms can be diagnostic. Gallstones may be demonstrable by an ultrasound scan.

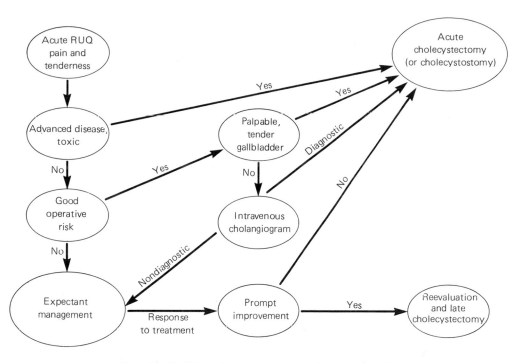

Figure 29—10. Scheme for the management of acute cholecystitis.

In another 30%, the diagnosis of acute cholecystitis may be definitely established but the general condition of the patient is unsatisfactory. This situation most often involves elderly patients who have been admitted to the hospital after being sick for several days. Dehydration may be severe, and the patient's cardiovascular system may be in suboptimal balance. In some cases congestive heart failure has developed, and a period of time will be required for digitalization. As a general rule, anything that may materially increase the risk of general anesthesia and laparotomy should be corrected, if possible, before cholecystectomy. The decision for expectant management cannot be rigidly adhered to, however, if the patient fails to improve as anticipated. Impending complications must be suspected and surgical intervention reconsidered under these circumstances.

About 10% of patients with acute cholecystitis require emergency operation. These are generally clinical situations where the disease appears to have become complicated or is about to. High fever (39 C [102.2 F]), marked leukocytosis (> 15,000/μl), or chills should alert one to the possibility of suppurative progression. The sudden appearance of generalized abdominal pain may indicate free perforation. A mass that develops in the gallbladder area where it was not felt previously may be a sign of local perforation and abscess formation. Changes of this sort are indications for emergency laparotomy.

Since acute cholecystitis in a patient with diabetes mellitus is often a fulminating disease with a high incidence of serious complications and a mortality rate of about 15%, cholecystectomy should be considered

an urgent matter in the diabetic.

Cholecystectomy is the preferable operation in acute cholecystitis and can be safely performed in about 90% of patients. Operative cholangiography should be performed in most cases and the common bile duct explored if appropriate indications are present (see section on choledocholithiasis). Cholecystostomy is reserved for those whose general condition is precarious or when local complications are present; most of those who require cholecystostomy are over 60 years of age. The decision to perform cholecystostomy should usually be made before the abdomen is opened since it depends on factors apparent during preoperative evaluation. It should rarely be the result of having initially embarked upon cholecystectomy and then changing to a lesser operation; in such cases, cholecystostomy should have been the original choice.

Cholecystostomy consists of emptying the contents of the gallbladder through an incision in the fundus and then suturing a large-bore tube within the lumen for continued postoperative drainage. If possible, all gallstones should be removed, for this allows subsequent removal of the tube with a good chance that the patient will not require cholecystectomy. After the patient has recovered, x-rays should be obtained after injecting diatrizoate (Hypaque) into the cholecystostomy tube. If the gallbladder or common duct contains stones, elective cholecystectomy should be scheduled when the patient can be optimally prepared. If the biliary tree is free of stones, the tube can be removed and the patient followed for development of new symptoms. Gallstones recur in about 50% of cases within 5 years. Many would plan routinely for cholecystectomy, but elderly patients with concomitant disease are probably managed best nonoperatively until symptoms develop. If this rule is followed, about half of such patients will need an operation.

Prognosis

The overall mortality rate of acute cholecystitis is about 5%. Nearly all of the deaths are in patients over age 60 or those with diabetes mellitus. In the older age group, secondary cardiovascular or pulmonary complications contribute substantially to mortality. Uncontrolled sepsis with peritonitis or intrahepatic abscesses are the most important local conditions responsible for deaths.

Common duct stones are present in about 15% of patients with acute cholecystitis, and some of the more seriously ill patients have simultaneous cholangitis from biliary obstruction. Acute pancreatitis may also complicate acute cholecystitis, and the combination carries a greater risk.

Patients who develop the suppurative forms of gallbladder disease such as empyema or perforation are less likely to recover. Earlier admission to the hospital and early cholecystectomy reduce the chances of these complications.

Acute Cholecystitis: General

Bulow S & others: Reappraisal of surgery for suppurative cholecystitis. Arch Surg 112:282, 1977.

Cafferata HT & others: Acute cholecystitis in a municipal hospital. Arch Surg 98:435, 1969.

Dumont AE: Significance of hyperbilirubinemia in acute cholecystitis. Surg Gynecol Obstet 142:855, 1976.

Du Plessis DJ, Jersky J: The management of acute cholecystitis. Surg Clin North Am 53:1071, 1973.

Gagic N & others: Acute cholecystitis. Surg Gynecol Obstet 140:868, 1975.

Glenn F: Cholecystostomy in the high risk patient with biliary tract disease. Ann Surg 185:185, 1977.

Hoerr SO, Hazard JB: Acute cholecystitis without gallbladder stones. Am J Surg 111:47, 1966.

McArthur P & others: Controlled clinical trial comparing early with interval cholecystectomy for acute cholecystitis. Br J Surg 62:850, 1975.

Ottinger LW: Acute cholecystitis as a postoperative complication. Ann Surg 184:162, 1976.

Raine PAM, Gunn AA: Acute cholecystitis. Br J Surg 62:697, 1975.

Thorpe CD: Emergency intravenous cholangiography in patients with acute abdominal pain. Am J Surg 125:46, 1973.

Van der Linden W, Sunzel H: Early versus delayed operation for acute cholecystitis: A controlled clinical trial. Am J Surg 120:7, 1970.

Welch JP, Malt RA: Outcome of cholecystostomy. Surg Gynecol Obstet 135:717, 1972.

Acute Cholecystitis: Complications

Essenhigh DM: Perforation of the gallbladder. Br J Surg 55:175, 1968.

Haff RC & others: Biliary-enteric fistulas. Surg Gynecol Obstet 133:84, 1971.

McCarthy JD, Picazo JG: Bile peritonitis. Am J Surg 116:664, 1968.

MacDonald JA: Perforation of the gallbladder associated with acute cholecystitis. Ann Surg 164:849, 1966.

Piedad OH, Wels PB: Spontaneous internal biliary fistula, obstructive and nonobstructive types: 20-year review of 55 cases. Ann Surg 175:75, 1972.

Rosato EF & others: Bile ascites. Surg Gynecol Obstet 130:494, 1970.

Stull JR, Thomford NR: Biliary intestinal fistula. Am J Surg 120:27, 1970.

EMPHYSEMATOUS CHOLECYSTITIS

Emphysematous cholecystitis is a rare condition in which bubbles of gas from anaerobic infection appear in the lumen of the gallbladder, its wall, the pericholecystic space, and on occasion the bile ducts. Clostridia species are the most commonly implicated organisms, but other gas-forming anaerobes such as *E coli* or anaerobic streptococci may be found. Men outnumber women by 3:1, and 20% of all patients have diabetes mellitus. In contrast to the usual form of acute cholecystitis, the disease probably is a bacterial infection from the earliest moment. In many reported cases, the gallbladder contained no stones. These characteristics suggest the possibility that cystic artery occlusion and ischemia may initiate emphysematous cholecystitis.

The disease begins with sudden and rapidly progressive right upper quadrant pain. Fever and leukocytosis reach high levels quickly, and the patient is considerably more toxic than is usually the case in acute cholecystitis. On examination, a mass can usually be found in the right upper quadrant.

Plain films of the abdomen show tissue emphysema outlining the gallbladder and, in some cases, an air-fluid level in the lumen. The clinical and x-ray pictures are characteristic enough so that the diagnosis is usually obvious.

The patient should be treated with high doses of antibiotics effective against clostridia and the other species mentioned above. Emergency surgical treatment should follow the initial resuscitative measures. Cholecystectomy can be safely performed in most cases, but the most critically ill might fare better with cholecystostomy. The types of complications are the same as in other forms of acute cholecystitis, but the morbidity and mortality rates are higher.

May RE, Strong R: Acute emphysematous cholecystitis. Br J Surg 58:453, 1971.

Rosoff L, Meyers H: Acute emphysematous cholecystitis. Am J Surg 111:410, 1966.

GALLSTONE ILEUS

Gallstone ileus is mechanical intestinal obstruction caused by a large gallstone lodged in the lumen. It is seen most often in women, and the average age is about 70 years. However, gallstone ileus may occur in any age group where cholesterol stones are found.

Clinical Findings

A. Symptoms: The patient usually presents with obvious small bowel obstruction, either partial or complete. The obstructing gallstone enters the intestine through a cholecystenteric fistula located in the duodenum, colon, or, rarely, the stomach or jejunum. Usually it is between the gallbladder and the duodenum. Oddly, a history compatible with a recent episode of acute cholecystitis can be obtained in only a third of cases. This suggests that in the others the stone may erode into the neighboring viscus by pressure necrosis rather than by producing acute cholecystitis. The gallbladder may contain one or several stones, but stones that cause gallstone ileus are almost always 2.5 cm or more in diameter. The lumen in the proximal bowel will allow most of these large calculi to pass caudally until the ileum is reached. Rarely, the stone obstructs the duodenum at the site of the fistula. Obstruction of the large intestine may follow passage of a gallstone through a fistula at the hepatic flexure or may occur even after the stone has traversed the entire small bowel. Gallstone ileus of the colon is rare because the normal colonic lumen is large; many reported cases have had colonic narrowing by diverticular disease as a predisposing factor.

As the gallstone moves down the small intestine, it may temporarily block the lumen and create obstructive symptoms only to dislodge and pass farther along. This creates an intermittent or tumbling obstruction that is characteristic of gallstone ileus and is reflected clinically by intermittency of signs and symptoms. When a segment of intestine is reached where further passage is impossible, complete obstruction develops. The episodic symptoms may occur for days and lead the physician to optimistically predict a spontaneous resolution of the problem. In fact, before operation is performed, symptoms have been present for longer than 1 week in the average case.

The diagnosis of gallstone ileus should always be considered whenever small bowel obstruction is encountered in an elderly patient. If the patient has never previously had a laparotomy that might have produced adhesions and if incarceration of an external hernia can be excluded by physical examination, gallstone ileus should be high on the list. A history of recent right upper quadrant pain which preceded the bowel obstruction may provide a helpful clue, as would the tumbling type of obstruction if it can be recognized clinically.

B. Signs: In most patients the findings on physical examination are typical of distal small bowel obstruction since the stone usually becomes wedged in the ileum. Obstruction of the duodenum or jejunum may give a perplexing clinical picture because of the lack of distention. Right upper quadrant tenderness and a mass may be present in some cases, but the distended abdomen may be difficult to examine accurately. The stone can occasionally be palpated within the ileum on abdominal, pelvic, or rectal examination, but it is seldom recognized for what it is.

C. X-Ray Findings: In addition to dilated small intestine, plain films of the abdomen may show a radiopaque gallstone, and unless one is alert to the possibility of gallstone ileus the ectopic stone can be a puzzling finding. In about 40% of cases, careful examination of the film will reveal gas in the biliary tree, a manifestation of the cholecystenteric fistula. When the clinical picture is unclear, an upper gastrointestinal series should be obtained which will demonstrate the cholecystoduodenal fistula and verify intestinal obstruction.

Treatment

The proper treatment is emergency laparotomy and removal of the obstructing stone through a small enterotomy. The proximal intestine must be carefully inspected for the presence of a second calculus which might cause a postoperative recurrence. The gallbladder should be left undisturbed at the original operation. Although some have claimed that cholecystectomy can be performed safely at this point, it is not recommended for the following reasons: (1) The emergency operation would be converted from a simple procedure into one that may last 4–5 hours, and (2) the patient rarely obtains tangible immediate benefit from having the gallbladder out anyway. Prevention of recurrent gallstone ileus has been offered as an argument for cholecystectomy during the emergency procedure, but recurrence has been reported in only 4% of patients, and this figure could probably be reduced by careful palpation and extraction of additional calculi from the intestine proximal to the obstruction.

Once the patient has recovered from the operation, an elective cholecystectomy should be scheduled if the patient complains of chronic gallbladder symptoms. On this basis, interval cholecystectomy will be required in about 30% of patients. The fistula itself is rarely the source of trouble and closes spontaneously in many patients.

Prognosis

The mortality rate of gallstone ileus remains about 20% largely because of the poor general condition of the elderly patients at the time of laparotomy. In many cases the patient has developed cardiac or pulmonary complications during a preoperative delay when the diagnosis was unclear. The mortality rate can be reduced by being alert for the diagnosis in appropriate circumstances because—once considered—the clinical and radiologic data can usually be pieced together.

Andersson A, Zederfeldt B: Gallstone ileus. Acta Chir Scand 135:713, 1969.

Räf L, Spangen L: Gallstone ileus. Acta Chir Scand 137:665, 1971.

Raiford TS: Intestinal obstruction caused by gallstones. Am J Surg 104:383, 1962.

CHOLEDOCHOLITHIASIS

Essentials of Diagnosis
- Biliary pain.
- Jaundice
- Episodic cholangitis.
- Gallstones in gallbladder or previous chole-
  cystectomy.

General Considerations

Gallstones may traverse the cystic duct and enter the common bile duct but are often prevented from reaching the duodenum by the narrowing in the hepatopancreatic (Vater's) ampulla. In the duct they cause symptoms by obstructing the flow of bile. Approximately 15% of patients with stones in the gallbladder are found to harbor calculi within the bile ducts. Common duct stones are usually accompanied by others in the gallbladder, but in rare cases the gallbladder is empty. The number of duct stones may vary from 1 to more than 100. Gallstones occasionally form within the ductal system de novo after prolonged ductal infection or stasis. They sometimes pass spontaneously into the duodenum.

Little is known about the natural history of common duct stones. The principal clinical syndromes are biliary colic, cholangitis, jaundice, pancreatitis, or combinations of these (Fig 29–11). It seems likely, however, that as many as 50% of patients with choledocholithiasis remain asymptomatic.

Cholangitis is caused by bacterial infection of an obstructed biliary tree. The block to flow may be partial or, less commonly, complete. The most common predisposing causes are choledocholithiasis and biliary stricture. Involvement of the duct by neoplasm, pancreatic cysts, duodenal diverticula, or invasion by parasites is less common. The symptoms (referred to in older texts as **Charcot's triad**) are biliary colic, jaundice, and chills and fever.

Cholangitis virtually always signifies biliary obstruction since, in the absence of obstruction, even heavy bacterial contamination of ducts does not produce symptoms or pathologic changes. With obstruction, ductal pressure rises and bacteria proliferate and escape into the systemic circulation via the hepatic sinusoids. Experimentally, the incidence of positive blood cultures with ductal infection varies directly with the absolute height of biliary pressure—an observation that underscores the importance of decompression of the duct in the treatment of cholangitis.

The common duct may dilate to 2–3 cm proximal to an obstructing lesion, and truly huge ducts develop in patients with biliary tumors. In biliary stricture or choledocholithiasis, the inflammatory reaction restricts dilatation so that the ducts tend to be somewhat smaller. Dilatation of the ductal system also can be limited by cirrhosis.

Biliary colic results from rapid rises in biliary pressure whether the block is in the common duct or neck of the gallbladder. Gradual occlusion of the

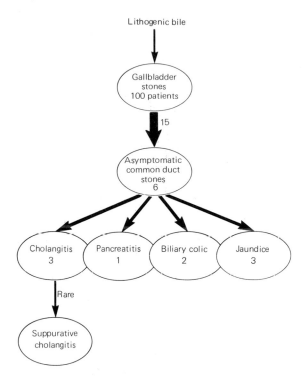

Figure 29–11. The natural history of common duct stones. Note that the individual syndromes overlap, indicating they may appear together in various combinations.

duct—as in malignancy—rarely produces the same kind of pain as gallstone disease.

Clinical Findings

A. Symptoms: Choledocholithiasis may be asymptomatic or may produce sudden overwhelming toxicity with a rapid demise. The seriousness of the disease parallels the degree of obstruction, the length of time it has been present, and the extent of secondary bacterial infection. Biliary colic, jaundice, or pancreatitis may be isolated findings or may occur in any combination along with signs of infection.

Acute (nonsuppurative) cholangitis, one of the major syndromes produced by choledocholithiasis, is characterized by biliary colic, fever, chills, leukocytosis, and jaundice. There is a continuous spectrum of increasing severity of cholangitis ending in acute suppurative cholangitis, which has shock and mental confusion as additional manifestations. Suppurative cholangitis, which accounts for less than 10% of all cases of cholangitis, is discussed below in the section on complications.

Biliary colic from common duct obstruction cannot be distinguished from that caused by stones in the gallbladder. The pain is felt in the right subcostal region, epigastrium, or even the substernal area. Referred pain to the region of the right scapula is common.

Choledocholithiasis should be strongly suspected if intermittent chills, fever, or jaundice accompany biliary colic. Some patients notice transient darkening of their urine during an attack even though jaundice is not evident. Light stools may be reported.

Pruritus is usually the result of persistent long-standing obstruction. The itching is more intense in warm weather when the patient perspires and is usually worse on the extremities than on the trunk.

B. Signs: The patient may be icteric and toxic, with high fever and chills, or he may appear to be perfectly healthy. A palpable gallbladder is unusual in patients with obstructive jaundice from common duct stone because scarring of the gallbladder renders it inelastic and nondistensible. Thus, a palpable non-tender gallbladder in a jaundiced patient usually indicates malignant obstruction of the duct. Tenderness may be present in the right upper quadrant but is not often as marked as in acute cholecystitis, perforated peptic ulcer, or acute pancreatitis. Tender hepatic enlargement may occur, especially if obstruction has been present for more than several days.

C. Laboratory Findings: In cholangitis, leukocytosis of 15,000/µl is usually present, and values above 20,000/µl are common. A rise in serum bilirubin often appears within 24 hours of the onset of symptoms. The absolute level usually remains under 10 mg/100 ml, and most are in the range of 2–4 mg/100 ml. The direct fraction exceeds the indirect, but the latter becomes elevated in most cases. Bilirubin levels do not ordinarily reach the high values seen in malignant tumors because the obstruction is usually incomplete and transient. In fact, fluctuating jaundice is so characteristic of choledocholithiasis that it fairly reliably differentiates between benign and malignant obstruction.

The 24-hour urinary urobilinogen will usually exceed 4 mg. Fecal urobilinogen may be low.

The serum alkaline phosphatase, leucine aminopeptidase, and 5'-nucleotidase levels usually rise and may be the only chemical abnormalities in patients without jaundice. When the obstruction is relieved, the alkaline phosphatase returns rapidly toward normal after brief obstruction but may remain elevated for weeks or even permanently after prolonged obstruction.

Mild increases in SGOT and SGPT are often seen with extrahepatic obstruction of the ducts; rarely, SGOT levels transiently reach 1000.

D. X-Ray Findings: Radiopaque gallstones may be seen on plain abdominal films. Intravenous cholangiography may be successful if the patient is not jaundiced but is rarely satisfactory during an attack of cholangitis. It is better to delay the cholangiogram until the acute symptoms have subsided and the serum bilirubin has returned to normal.

Differential Diagnosis

The work-up should consider the same possibilities in differential diagnosis as for cholecystitis.

Serum amylase levels above 500 units/100 ml can be from acute pancreatitis, acute cholecystitis, or choledocholithiasis. Other manifestations of pancreatic disease should be documented before an unqualified diagnosis of pancreatitis is subscribed to.

In viral hepatitis, the SGOT and SGPT reach high levels and the indirect bilirubin fraction may predominate. A history of exposure to hepatitis and a young patient are additional clues.

Alcoholic cirrhosis or acute alcoholic hepatitis may present with jaundice, right upper quadrant tenderness, and leukocytosis. The differentiation from cholangitis may be impossible from clinical data. A history of a recent binge suggests acute liver disease. A percutaneous liver biopsy may be specific.

Intrahepatic cholestasis from drugs, pregnancy, chronic active hepatitis, or primary biliary cirrhosis may be quite difficult to distinguish from extrahepatic obstruction. Transhepatic or retrograde cholangiography is required in many. If jaundice has persisted for 4–6 weeks, a mechanical cause is probable. Since most patients improve during this interval, persistent jaundice should never be assumed to be the result of intrahepatic disease unless a normal cholangiogram rules out obstruction of the major ducts.

Intermittent jaundice and cholangitis after cholecystectomy are compatible with biliary stricture, and the distinction may be impossible without a good cholangiogram or direct surgical exploration. The history may help, since symptoms due to stricture usually appear within several months after the cholecystectomy and cholangitis due to stones is frequently not seen for several years.

Biliary tumors usually produce jaundice without biliary colic or fever, and, once it begins, the jaundice rarely remits. The stools may be positive for occult blood when the obstruction is due to tumor.

Complications

Long-standing ductal infection can produce multiple intrahepatic abscesses. Hepatic failure or secondary biliary cirrhosis may develop in unrelieved obstruction of long duration. Since the obstruction is usually incomplete and intermittent, cirrhosis develops only after several years in untreated disease. Acute pancreatitis, a fairly common complication of calculous biliary disease, is discussed in detail in Chapter 30. Rarely, a stone in the common duct may erode through the ampulla, resulting in gallstone ileus. Hemorrhage is also a rare complication.

Acute suppurative cholangitis (acute obstructive suppurative cholangitis) results from a combination of obstruction and virulent infection. The common bile duct contains pus instead of bile. Choledocholithiasis is the cause of the biliary obstruction in most cases, but in a few it is neoplasm, ampullary stenosis, or congenital cystic disease. It is a critical surgical emergency manifested by septicemia and shock. The diagnostic pentad consists of abdominal pain, jaundice, fever and chills, mental confusion or lethargy, and shock. Jaundice may be mild, and the serum bilirubin is often only slightly abnormal (2–5 mg/100 ml). Based on clinical findings, the diagnosis is appropriate when signs of sepsis, including hypotension, are more prominent than those of biliary obstruction (eg, jaundice, abdominal pain, and tenderness). The diagnosis is often missed and treatment delayed because the significance of the manifestations of biliary disease are not appreciated. The white blood count is usually above 15,000/μl. Blood cultures are nearly always positive.

The treatment of suppurative cholangitis should consist of circulatory resuscitation, preoperative preparation, and emergency laparotomy. Parenteral antibiotics must be started as soon as possible. The principal surgical objective is to relieve the pressure within the common duct proximal to the obstruction. The most direct method is to perform a choledochotomy, a more successful technic for decompression than cholecystostomy. When the choledochotomy incision is made, pressure in the duct may cause the pus to spurt out. If the patient has been moribund or rapidly deteriorating before operation, simple cleansing of the duct and insertion of a T tube will suffice. On the other hand, if the patient's condition has been stable, thorough exploration, removal of the common duct stones, and cholecystectomy may be done.

Treatment

Patients with acute cholangitis should be treated with systemic antibiotics according to the guidelines given for acute cholecystitis (see above); this usually controls the attack within 24–48 hours. If the patient's condition worsens or if marked improvement is not observed within 2–4 days, laparotomy and exploration of the common bile duct should be performed. Lack of response may indicate that suppurative cholangitis is imminent.

Once cholangitis resolves, additional attempts should be made to confirm the diagnosis. In the meantime, antibiotic treatment should be continued. An intravenous cholangiogram may reveal the cause of the symptoms. Transhepatic cholangiography should be delayed until infection has subsided.

The patient with cholangitis and common duct stones should be scheduled for operation shortly after the attack has resolved and any other medical problems have been investigated. If the prothrombin time is abnormal, it should be corrected by parenteral vitamin K before laparotomy.

The classic indications for common duct exploration during cholecystectomy are the following: (1) preoperative jaundice, (2) demonstration of stones on intravenous or transhepatic cholangiography, (3) pancreatitis in association with the biliary disease, (4) dilated common duct (> 1 cm in diameter), (5) presence of small stones in the gallbladder, (6) a palpable stone in the duct, and (7) ductal stone demonstrated by operative cholangiography. It is useful to divide these indications into absolute ones and relative ones based on their proved reliability as indications of common duct stone (Fig 29–12). Thus, the *absolute* indications are preoperative demonstration of stones by x-ray, preoperative history of cholangitis with jaundice, jaundice alone (if the bilirubin exceeds 7 mg/100 ml), palpable stone in the duct, and a positive operative cholangiogram. The *relative* indications are mild jaundice without fever and chills, small stones, and a dilated duct. With relative indications, stones are present in only 20% of cases, and the decision to explore the duct can be based upon the results of an operative cholangiogram.

After exploration of the duct is completed and all stones have been removed, a T tube is inserted. A postexploratory operative cholangiogram through the T tube should be obtained in all cases. It will often reveal overlooked stones which can be removed by reopening the duct. Cholecystectomy should be performed after the duct has been explored.

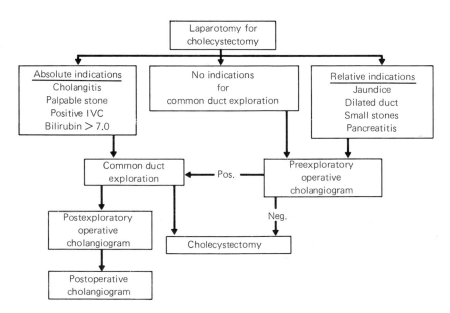

Figure 29–12. Diagnostic and therapeutic management of choledocholithiasis.

About a week after the operation, a postoperative cholangiogram should be performed through the T tube. About 3–5% of patients who have had stones removed from the duct will be found to have a residual stone on the postoperative x-ray. However, if the duct is clear, the tube should be clamped overnight to make certain that the ductal system is functional; if no symptoms appear, the tube can be pulled out the next morning.

Two methods have recently been developed for treating retained stones found on postoperative T tube cholangiograms. One technic is based on the ability of bile salt solutions to resolubilize cholesterol and is not useful for treating pigment stones. Sodium cholate solution (150 mM/liter, pH 7.5) is infused at a rate of 30 ml/hour directly into the T tube. The solution bathes the stone and passes into the duodenum. Cholestyramine resin (Cuemid, Questran), 4 g every 2 hours, is given orally to bind the bile salts in the intestine and prevent diarrhea. If the retained stones are obstructing the duct, the solution can be administered into the vicinity of the stone through a small catheter passed through the lumen of the T tube and positioned under radiologic control. The cholate solution runs out the residual lumen of the T tube. This regimen has eliminated retained stones in about two-thirds of cases.

An even simpler method is to attempt to extract the stones with a ureteral stone basket. About 1 month should be allowed to elapse after surgery for the tract of the T tube to fully mature. The T tube is then removed in the x-ray department, and, using image intensification fluoroscopy, a ureteral stone basket is passed down the tract into the duct and the wire cage expanded to trap the stone. The apparatus is drawn backward, and the stone will usually lodge within its grasp so that it can be extracted. Improvements in the success rate of this method can be expected with refinements in instrumentation. We currently try mechanical extraction first and use cholic acid infusion if that fails.

Bartlett MK, Warshaw AL, Ottinger LW: The removal of biliary duct stones. Surg Clin North Am 54:599, 1974.

Doran FSA: The sites to which pain is referred from the common bile-duct and its implication for the theory of referred pain. Br J Surg 54:599, 1967.

Herman AH & others: Problems engendered by a "standard approach" to all patients with jaundice or biliary pain. Am J Surg 127:404, 1974.

Hinshaw DB: Acute obstructive suppurative cholangitis. Surg Clin North Am 53:1089, 1973.

Mazzariello RM: Residual biliary tract stones: Nonoperative treatment of 570 patients. Surg Annu 8:113, 1976.

Saharia PC, Cameron JL: Clinical management of acute cholangitis. Surg Gynecol Obstet 142:369, 1976.

Way LW: Retained common duct stones. Surg Clin North Am 53:1139, 1973.

Way LW & others: Management of choledocholithiasis. Ann Surg 176:347, 1972.

Welch JP, Donaldson GA: The urgency of diagnosis and surgical treatment of acute suppurative cholangitis. Am J Surg 131:527, 1976.

POSTCHOLECYSTECTOMY SYNDROME

This term has been used to designate the heterogeneous group of patients who continue to complain of symptoms after cholecystectomy. It is not really a syndrome, and the term is confusing.

The usual reason why relief is incomplete after cholecystectomy is that the preoperative diagnosis of chronic cholecystitis was incorrect. The only symptom entirely characteristic of chronic cholecystitis is biliary colic. When a calculous gallbladder is removed in the hope that the patient will gain relief from dyspepsia, fatty food intolerance, belching, etc, the operation may leave the symptoms unchanged. The amount of scarring in the gallbladder wall correlates fairly well with the extent of symptomatic improvement after cholecystectomy; patients with vague postoperative complaints are more likely to have had a thin-walled, unscarred organ or a gallbladder without stones.

In other cases, an organic diagnosis has been overlooked during the preoperative evaluation. Pancreatitis, peptic ulcer, gastritis, or esophagitis may have actually been the origin of symptoms attributed to the gallstones. These possibilities should be reinvestigated when symptoms persist.

Choledocholithiasis or biliary stricture is sometimes responsible for abdominal pain after cholecystectomy. Liver function studies and an intravenous cholangiogram should be obtained. One normal intravenous cholangiogram does not eliminate the possibility of a common duct stone; in suspicious cases the above studies should be repeated, and in some cases a transhepatic or retrograde cholangiogram is indicated.

Stenosis of the hepatobiliary ampulla, a long cystic duct remnant, and neuromas are other conditions that have been blamed for continued symptoms, but well-verified cases are uncommon.

Berge T, Haeger K: Clinical significance of the amputation neuroma and length of the cystic duct remnant. Acta Chir Scand 133:55, 1967.

Bodvall B: The postcholecystectomy syndromes. Clin Gastroenterol 2:103, 1973.

Bodvall B, Overgaard B: Computer analysis of postcholecystectomy biliary tract symptoms. Surg Gynecol Obstet 124:723, 1967.

Christiansen J, Schmidt A: The postcholecystectomy syndrome. Acta Chir Scand 137:789, 1971.

Glenn F: Postcholecystectomy choledocholithiasis. Surg Gynecol Obstet 134:249, 1972.

CARCINOMA OF THE GALLBLADDER

Carcinoma of the gallbladder is an uncommon neoplasm that appears in elderly patients, 80% of whom have cholelithiasis. Cholelithiasis may be an etiologic factor, for the risk of malignant degeneration correlates with the length of time gallstones have been present. The tumor is 3 times more common in women than in men, as one would expect from the association with gallstones.

Most primary tumors of the gallbladder are adenocarcinomas which appear histologically to be scirrhous (60%), papillary (25%), or mucoid (15%). Dissemination of the tumor occurs early by direct invasion of the liver and hilar structures and by metastases to the liver and lungs. Spread is virtually certain by the time symptoms appear.

Clinical Findings

The presenting complaint is of right upper quadrant pain similar to previous episodes of biliary colic but more persistent. Obstruction of the cystic duct by tumor sometimes initiates an attack of acute cholecystitis. Other cases are first seen after obstructive jaundice has resulted from secondary involvement of the common duct, and cholangitis may be present in these.

Examination usually reveals a mass in the region of the gallbladder. It may not be recognized as a neoplasm if the patient has acute cholecystitis. If cholangitis is the principal symptom, a palpable gallbladder would be an unusual finding with choledocholithiasis alone and should suggest gallbladder carcinoma.

Complications

Obstruction of the common duct may produce multiple intrahepatic abscesses. Abscesses in or next to the tumor-laden gallbladder are frequent.

Prevention

Prevention of adenocarcinoma of the gallbladder has been offered in the past as an argument for performing cholecystectomy in patients with asymptomatic cholelithiasis. The reasoning appears to be sound if used in relation to young patients with the disease.

Treatment

Detailed pathologic studies indicate that in 25% of patients all detectable tumor would be removed by a resection of the gallbladder and adjacent liver bed and the lymph nodes along the common bile duct. Although this is the operation recommended in the absence of distant spread of tumor, pessimism regarding the curability of gallbladder cancer has impeded the adoption of any procedure more extensive than cholecystectomy. The addition of a right hepatic lobectomy offers little hope of improving survival rates because liver metastases occur only in the presence of spread to areas outside the limits of surgical resection.

For patients with more advanced disease, surgical decompression of an obstructed common duct can sometimes provide palliation.

The 5% of patients who presently survive more than 5 years are mainly those whose carcinoma was an incidental finding after cholecystectomy for chronic symptomatic gallstone disease.

Prognosis

Radiotherapy and chemotherapy are not effective palliative agents. About 90% of patients are dead within a year after diagnosis.

Adson MA: Carcinoma of the gallbladder. Surg Clin North Am 53:1203, 1973.

Hardy MA, Volk H: Primary carcinoma of the gallbladder. Am J Surg 120:800, 1970.

Hart J & others: Cholelithiasis in the aetiology of gallbladder neoplasms. Lancet 1:1151, 1971.

MALIGNANT TUMORS OF THE BILE DUCT

Essentials of Diagnosis

- Cholestatic jaundice.
- Biliary colic or cholangitis (rare).
- Transhepatic cholangiogram usually diagnostic.

General Considerations

Primary malignant tumors of the bile duct are even less common than adenocarcinoma of the gallbladder. Unlike the latter, bile duct tumors are not more common in patients with cholelithiasis, and men and women are affected with equal frequency. Several hepatobiliary diseases, including malignant bile duct tumors, are found with greater frequency in ulcerative colitis, but it is not certain whether colectomy would prevent them. Chronic parasitic infestation of the bile ducts in the Orient may be responsible for the greater incidence of bile duct tumors in that area.

Most malignant biliary tumors are adenocarcinomas located in the hepatic or common bile duct. The histologic pattern varies from typical adenocarcinoma to tumors composed principally of fibrous stroma and few cells. The acellular tumors may be mistaken for benign strictures or sclerosing cholangitis if adequate biopsies are not obtained.

Clinical Findings

A. Symptoms and Signs: The illness presents with gradual onset of jaundice or pruritus. Chills, fever, and biliary colic are usually absent, and except for a deep discomfort in the right upper quadrant the patient feels well. Bilirubinuria is present from the start, and light-colored stools are usual. Anorexia and weight loss develop insidiously with time.

Icterus is the most obvious physical finding. If the tumor is confined to the common duct, the gallbladder distends and becomes palpable in the right upper quadrant. Patients with tumors of the hepatic or cystic ducts do not develop palpable gallbladders. If obstruction is unrelieved, the liver may become cirrhotic and splenomegaly, ascites, or bleeding varices become secondary manifestations.

B. Laboratory Findings: Since the duct is often completely obstructed, the serum bilirubin is usually over 15 mg/100 ml. Serum alkaline phosphatase, leucine aminopeptidase, and 5'-nucleotidase are also increased. Fever and leukocytosis are not common since the bile is sterile in most cases. Urobilinogen excretion is reduced in both urine and feces. The stool may contain occult blood, but this is more common with tumors of the pancreas or hepatopancreatic ampulla than those of the bile ducts.

C. X-Ray Findings: The upper gastrointestinal series occasionally shows extrinsic impingement by the tumor upon the duodenum. Oral or intravenous cholangiography is usually of no value because of the high-grade obstruction. Ultrasound scans usually detect the dilated bile ducts. Transhepatic cholangiograms clearly depict the lesion and are indicated in most cases.

Differential Diagnosis

The differential diagnosis must consider other causes of extrahepatic and intrahepatic cholestatic jaundice. Choledocholithiasis is characterized by intermittent partial obstruction and cholangitis which contrasts sharply with the generally unremitting but painless jaundice of malignant obstruction. Dilatation of the gallbladder characterizes tumors, whereas the gallbladder is usually too scarred to dilate with calculous obstruction.

The combination of an enlarged gallbladder with obstructive jaundice is usually recognized as due to tumor. If the gallbladder cannot be felt, primary biliary cirrhosis, drug-induced jaundice, chronic active hepatitis, metastatic hepatic malignancy, and common duct stone must be ruled out. As a general rule, whenever one is faced with cholestatic jaundice, no fever, and a normal upper gastrointestinal series, a transhepatic cholangiogram, ultrasound examination, and liver biopsy should be seriously considered. If an extrahepatic tumor is present, ultrasound will usually demonstrate dilated bile ducts and a transhepatic cholangiogram will show the point of obstruction. If the patient is still undiagnosed after an evaluation which included an unsuccessful transhepatic cholangiogram, exploratory laparotomy is usually indicated if jaundice has been present for more than 3–4 weeks and is not improving. The chances of finding a mechanical occlusion are good.

Treatment

Jaundice appears early but even so the tumor usually involves contiguous structures or has metastasized so that surgical cure is rarely possible. Nevertheless, laparotomy is indicated and substantial palliation may follow procedures to relieve the obstruction. At operation, the extent of the tumor in the bile duct should be investigated by choledochoscopy, which in some cases has demonstrated otherwise occult multicentricity.

Tumors of the distal common duct should be treated by radical pancreaticoduodenectomy (Whipple procedure) if it appears that all of the tumor would be removed. Secondary involvement of the portal vein is the usual reason for unresectability for tumors in this location. If the tumor cannot be excised, bile flow should be reestablished into the intestine by means of cholecystojejunostomy, side-to-side choledochoduodenostomy, or Roux-en-Y choledochojejunostomy. The first 2 are used more often than the latter because they are technically easier.

Mid common duct or hepatic duct tumors should also be removed if possible. Otherwise, palliative procedures for unobstructing the flow of bile should be performed.

Tumors at the junction of the hepatic ducts may not be obvious to gross inspection when the abdomen is first explored. The gallbladder and common duct are normal in caliber, and the initial impression may be that the block is intrahepatic. It is important to identify these bifurcation tumors because permanent insertion of a U tube stent, which allows bile to flow past the tumor into the duodenum, has resulted in survival for several years. Decompression may also be possible in some cases by splitting the hepatic parenchyma to expose one of the dilated intrahepatic ducts to which a Roux-en-Y limb of jejunum is then anastomosed.

Prognosis

The average patient with adenocarcinoma of the bile duct may survive a year or so. Biliary cirrhosis, intrahepatic infection, and general debility with terminal pneumonitis are the usual causes of death. Palliative measures play an important role in improving the length and quality of survival even though surgical cure is rare.

Altemeier WA, Culbertson WR: Sclerosing carcinoma of the hepatic bile ducts. Surg Clin North Am 53:1229, 1973.

Anderson A & others: Malignant tumors of the extrahepatic bile ducts. Surgery 81:198, 1977.

Bismuth H, Corlette MB: Intrahepatic cholangioenteric anastomosis in carcinoma of the hilus of the liver. Surg Gynecol Obstet 140:170, 1975.

Ritchie J & others: Biliary tract carcinoma associated with ulcerative colitis. Q J Med 43:263, 1974.

Terblanche J, Louw JH: U tube drainage in the palliative therapy of carcinoma of the main hepatic duct junction. Surg Clin North Am 53:1245, 1973.

Tompkins RK & others: Operative endoscopy in the management of biliary tract neoplasms. Am J Surg 132:174, 1976.

BENIGN TUMORS & PSEUDOTUMORS OF THE GALLBLADDER

Various unrelated lesions appear on the cholecystogram as projections from the gallbladder wall. The differentiation from gallstones is based upon observing whether a shift in position of the projections follows changes in posture of the patient since stones are not fixed.

Polyps

Most of these are not true neoplasms but cholesterol polyps, a local form of cholesterosis. Histologically, they consist of a cluster of lipid-filled macrophages in the submucosa. They become easily detached from the wall when the gallbladder is handled at surgery. It is not known whether cholesterol polyps are important in the genesis of gallstones. Some patients experience gallbladder pain, but whether this is related to the presence of the polyps per se or is a manifestation of functional gallbladder disease has not been established.

Inflammatory polyps have also been reported, but they are quite rare.

Adenomyomatosis

On cholecystography, this entity presents as a slight intraluminal convexity that is often marked by a central umbilication. It is usually found in the fundus but may occur elsewhere. It is unclear whether adenomyomatosis is an acquired degenerative lesion or a developmental abnormality (ie, hamartoma). The following synonyms for this lesion appear in the literature: adenomatous hyperplasia, cholecystitis glandularis proliferans, and diverticulosis of the gallbladder. Although the condition is probably asymptomatic in many cases, adenomyomatosis can cause abdominal pain. Cholecystectomy should be performed in such patients.

Adenomas

These appear as pedunculated adenomatous polyps, true neoplasms which may be papillary or nonpapillary histologically. In a few cases they have been found in association with carcinoma in situ of the gallbladder.

Christensen AH, Ishak KG: Benign tumors and pseudotumors of the gallbladder. Arch Pathol 90:423, 1970.
Ram MD, Midha D: Adenomyomatosis of the gallbladder. Surgery 78:224, 1975.

BENIGN TUMORS OF THE BILE DUCTS

Benign papillomas and adenomas may arise from the ductal epithelium. Only 90 cases have been reported to date. The neoplastic propensity of the ductal epithelium is widespread, so the tumors are often multiple and recurrence is common after excision. The affected duct must be radically excised for permanent cure to result.

Bruhans R, Myers RT: Benign neoplasms of the extrahepatic biliary ducts. Am Surg 37:161, 1971.

BILIARY STRICTURE

Essentials of Diagnosis

- Episodic cholangitis.
- Previous biliary surgery.
- Transhepatic cholangiogram often diagnostic.

General Considerations

Benign biliary strictures are caused by surgical trauma in about 95% of cases. The remainder result from external abdominal trauma or, rarely, from erosion of the duct by a gallstone. Prevention of injury to the duct depends on a combination of technical skill, experience, and a thorough knowledge of the normal anatomy and its variations in the hilus of the liver. Biliary stricture was more frequent in the past when many cholecystectomies were performed by incompletely trained surgeons.

The varieties of injury consist of transection, incision, excision of a segment, or occlusion of the duct by a ligature. The accident can sometimes be attributed to technical difficulties presented by advanced disease. The surgeon may or may not recognize immediately that he has damaged the duct. If he finds that it has been transected, an end-to-end anastomosis should be performed with insertion of a T tube through a nearby choledochotomy. However, the injury often goes unnoticed.

Clinical Findings

A. Symptoms: Manifestations of injury to the duct may or may not be evident in the postoperative period. If complete occlusion has been produced, jaundice will develop rapidly, but more often a rent has been made in the side of the duct and the earliest sign is excessive or prolonged drainage of bile from the abdominal drains.

Depending on the severity of the trauma and the amount of aggravating infection, cholangitis develops within 2 weeks or as late as a year or more after the operation. However, it is rare that more than 2 years separate the trauma and its initial symptoms.

In the typical case, the patient has episodic pain, fever, chills, and mild jaundice within a few weeks to months after cholecystectomy. Antibiotics are usually successful in controlling symptoms, but additional attacks occur at irregular intervals. The pattern of symptoms varies between patients from mild transient attacks to severe toxicity with suppurative cholangitis.

Documentation of an operative injury is sometimes available, and there may even have been previous operative procedures for stricture. When cholangitis develops in either of these kinds of patients, a diagnosis of recurrence of stricture is virtually certain.

B. Signs: Findings are not distinctive. The right upper quadrant may be tender but usually is not. Jaundice is usually present during an attack of cholangitis.

C. Laboratory Findings: The alkaline phosphatase, leucine aminopeptidase, and 5′-nucleotidase are elevated in most cases. The bilirubin fluctuates in relation to symptoms but usually remains below 10 mg/100 ml.

Blood cultures may be positive during acute cholangitis.

D. X-Ray Findings: An intravenous cholangiogram may outline the stricture if the study can be done at a time when the bilirubin is normal. In other cases, transhepatic or retrograde endoscopic cholangiograms are necessary. Failure to enter the intrahepatic bile ducts when attempting a transhepatic cholangiogram would not rule out stricture as the cause of symptoms.

Differential Diagnosis

Choledocholithiasis is the condition which most often must be differentiated from biliary stricture because the clinical and laboratory findings can be identical. A history of trauma to the duct would point toward stricture as the more likely diagnosis. The final distinction must await radiologic or surgical findings in many instances. An intravenous cholangiogram or, if that fails, a transhepatic or retrograde cholangiogram may answer the question. If not, laparotomy is probably indicated once episodic cholangitis has been verified.

Other causes of cholestatic jaundice may have to be ruled out in some cases.

Complications

Complications develop if the stricture is not corrected. Persistent cholangitis may progress to multiple intrahepatic abscesses and a septic death.

Other patients gradually develop biliary cirrhosis, portal hypertension, and esophageal varices over many years. When portal hypertension has developed, operations in the hilus of the liver are bloody and technical problems are often insurmountable. A prophylactic splenorenal shunt should be performed and the stricture repair scheduled for several months later.

Treatment

Strictures of the bile duct should be surgically repaired in all but the few patients whose poor general condition dictates a nonoperative approach. Symptomatic treatment with antibiotics should be used to control acute cholangitis, but long-term antibiotic treatment is not recommended as a definitive regimen. Although the attacks may regularly respond to antibiotics, this therapy does not protect the liver from the damaging effect of the partial biliary obstruction, and, if uncorrected, secondary biliary cirrhosis or hepatic failure will gradually develop.

The surgical procedure should be selected on the basis of technical considerations presented by the individual patient. The general goals of the repair should be to reestablish biliary flow by anastomosing normal duct from the hepatic side of the stricture to either the intestine or the residual normal duct below the stricture. Excision of the strictured segment and end-to-end repair may seem the simplest solution but frequently entails more technical problems than connecting the proximal duct directly to the intestine. The duct can be reimplanted into the duodenum or a Roux-en-Y loop of jejunum. Roux-en-Y hepaticojejunostomy will more often provide a suitable anastomosis without tension. A side-to-side choledochoduodenostomy is adequate for the uncommon case with

stricture of the retroduodenal portion of the duct. Rarely, when a definitive repair is technically impossible, the stricture may be chronically stented (eg, with a U tube).

Prognosis

The death rate from biliary stricture is about 10−15%, and the morbidity is high. If the stricture is not repaired, episodic cholangitis and secondary liver disease are inevitable.

Surgical correction of the stricture is successful in about 75% of cases. Experience at centers with a special interest in this problem indicates that good results can be obtained even if several previous attempts did not relieve the obstruction. Therefore, if a stricture is present, the patient should be considered for correction despite a history of surgical failure.

Cameron JL & others: Long term transhepatic intubation for hilar hepatic duct strictures. Ann Surg 183:488, 1976.

Longmire WP Jr: Early management of injury to the extrahepatic biliary tract. JAMA 195:111, 1966.

Sedgwick CE & others: Management of portal hypertension secondary to bile duct strictures. Ann Surg 163:949, 1966.

Warren KW, Jefferson MF: Prevention and repair of strictures of the extrahepatic bile ducts. Surg Clin North Am 53:1169, 1973.

Way LW, Dunphy JE: Biliary stricture. Am J Surg 124:287, 1972.

UNCOMMON CAUSES OF BILE DUCT OBSTRUCTION

Congenital Choledochal Cysts

About 30% of congenital choledochal cysts produce their first symptoms in adults, usually presenting with jaundice, cholangitis, and a right upper quadrant mass. Diagnosis can be made by transhepatic or retrograde cholangiography. The optimal procedure is excision of the cyst and construction of a Roux-en-Y hepaticojejunostomy. If this is not technically possible or the patient's condition will not permit a prolonged procedure, the cyst should be emptied of precipitated biliary sludge and a cystenteric anastomosis constructed.

Fonkalsrud EW: Choledochal cysts. Surg Clin North Am 53: 1275, 1973.

Ishida M & others: Primary excision of choledochal cysts. Surgery 68:884, 1970.

Caroli's Disease

Caroli's disease, another form of congenital cystic disease, consists of saccular intrahepatic dilatation of the ducts. In some cases the biliary abnormality is an isolated finding, but more often it is associated with congenital hepatic fibrosis and medullary sponge kidney. The latter patients often present in childhood or as young adults with complications of portal hypertension. Others have cholangitis and obstructive jaundice as initial manifestations. There is no definitive surgical solution to the problem except in rare cases with isolated involvement of one hepatic lobe where lobectomy is curative. Intermittent antibiotic therapy for cholangitis is the usual regimen.

Caroli J: Diseases of the intrahepatic biliary tree. Clin Gastroenterol 2:147, 1973.
Watts DR & others: Congenital dilitation of the intrahepatic biliary ducts. Arch Surg 108:592, 1974.

Hematobilia

Hematobilia presents with the triad of biliary colic, obstructive jaundice, and occult or gross intestinal bleeding. Most cases in Western cultures follow several weeks after hepatic trauma with bleeding from an intrahepatic branch of the hepatic artery into a duct. It is seen with less frequency now because the general principles of the management of hepatic trauma are better understood. In the Orient, hematobilia usually follows ductal parasitism *(Ascaris lumbricoides)* or Oriental cholangiohepatitis. Other causes are hepatic neoplasms, rupture of a hepatic artery aneurysm, hepatic abscess, and choledocholithiasis. Diagnosis can be established by selective hepatic arteriograms. Depending on the cause, either direct ligation of the bleeding point in the liver or proximal ligation of an upstream branch of the hepatic artery in the hilus is required.

Sandblom P: Hemobilia. Surg Clin North Am 53:1191, 1973.

Pancreatitis

Pancreatitis can cause obstruction of the intrapancreatic portion of the bile duct by inflammatory swelling, encasement with scar, or compression by a pseudocyst. The patient may present with painless jaundice or cholangitis. The diagnosis may be difficult in an alcoholic where chronic painless jaundice, especially in the absence of pancreatic calcification, is almost automatically attributed to hepatic cirrhosis. Occasionally a distended gallbladder can be felt on abdominal examination. Differentiation from choledocholithiasis and secondary acute pancreatitis depends on biliary x-rays or surgical exploration if the jaundice persists. Jaundice due to inflammation alone rarely lasts more than 2 weeks; persistent jaundice following an attack of acute pancreatitis suggests the development of a pseudocyst, underlying chronic pancreatitis with obstruction by fibrosis, or even an obstructing neoplasm. Obstruction of the common bile duct by a pseudocyst usually responds to drainage of the cyst. Obstruction by chronic pancreatitis can be managed by side-to-side choledochoduodenostomy or Roux-en-Y choledocho- or cholecystojejunostomy.

McCollum WB, Jordan PH Jr: Obstructive jaundice in patients with pancreatitis without associated biliary tract disease. Ann Surg 182:116, 1975.
Warshaw AL & others: Persistent obstructive jaundice, cholangitis, and biliary cirrhosis due to common bile duct stenosis in chronic pancreatitis. Gastroenterology 70:562, 1976.

Duodenal Diverticula

Duodenal diverticula usually arise on the medial aspect of the duodenum within 2 cm of the orifice of the bile duct, and in some individuals the duct empties directly into a diverticulum. Even in the latter circumstance, duodenal diverticula are usually innocuous. Occasionally, distortion of the duct entrance or obstruction by enterolith formation in the diverticulum produces symptoms. Either choledochoduodenostomy or Roux-en-Y choledochojejunostomy is usually a safer method of reestablishing biliary drainage than attempts to excise the diverticulum and reimplant the duct.

McSherry CK, Glenn F: Biliary tract obstruction and duodenal diverticula. Surg Gynecol Obstet 130:829, 1970.

Ascariasis

When the worms invade the duct from the duodenum, ascariasis can produce symptoms of ductal obstruction. Air may sometimes be seen within the ducts on plain films. Antibiotics should be used until cholangitis is controlled, and then a regimen of piperazine should be given. The acute symptoms usually subside with antibiotics, but, if they do not, emergency exploration and removal of the worms is indicated. Intravenous cholangiograms after treatment with piperazine will demonstrate whether the duct has been emptied of intact worms and fragments. Residual foreign bodies in the ducts should be surgically removed.

Louw JH: Abdominal complications of *Ascaris lumbricoides* infestation in children. Br J Surg 53:510, 1966.
Wright RM, Dorrough RL, Ditmore HB: Ascariasis of the biliary system. Arch Surg 86:72, 1963.

Oriental Cholangiohepatitis

Oriental cholangiohepatitis is a type of chronic recurrent cholangitis prevalent in coastal areas from Japan to Southeast Asia. In Hong Kong it is the third most common indication for emergency laparotomy and the most frequent type of biliary disease. The disease is endemic in areas in Asia where parasitic infestation of the biliary tract is common. The parasites create an inflammatory process that becomes secondarily infected with enteric bacilli. Calcium bilirubinate stones are formed by mechanisms described earlier in the chapter.

In contrast with cholesterol cholelithiasis, which starts in the gallbladder, Oriental cholangiohepatitis is primarily a disease of the bile ducts. Only 15% of patients with Oriental cholangiohepatitis have cholecystolithiasis. The gallbladder is usually distended during an acute attack because it is not chronically scarred.

Chronic recurrent infection often leads to biliary strictures and hepatic abscess formation. The strictures are usually located in the intrahepatic bile ducts, and for some unknown reason the left lobe of the liver is more severely involved. Intrahepatic gallstones are common, and their surgical removal may be difficult or impossible. Acute abdominal pain, chills, and high fever are usually present, and jaundice develops in about half of cases. Right upper quadrant tenderness is usually marked, and in about 80% of cases the gallbladder is palpable.

Systemic antibiotics should be given for acute cholangitis. Surgical treatment consists of cholecystectomy, common duct exploration, and removal of stones. A side-to-side choledochoduodenostomy is required in most patients because the huge duct drains so poorly.

Although some patients can be cured, prolonged morbidity from repeated infection is almost unavoidable once strictures have appeared or the intrahepatic ducts have become packed with stones.

Fung J: Liver fluke infestation and cholangiohepatitis. Br J Surg 48:404, 1961.

Maki T, Sato T, Matsushiro T: A reappraisal of surgical treatment for intrahepatic gallstones. Ann Surg 175:155, 1972.

Sclerosing Cholangitis

Sclerosing cholangitis is a rare chronic disease of unknown cause which is characterized by nonbacterial inflammatory narrowing of the bile ducts. About 25% of cases are in patients with ulcerative colitis. Other less commonly associated conditions are thyroiditis, retroperitoneal fibrosis, and mediastinal fibrosis. In most cases the entire biliary tree is affected by the inflammatory process, which causes irregular partial obliteration of the lumen of the ducts. The woody-hard duct walls contain increased collagen and lymphoid elements and are thickened at the expense of the lumen.

The clinical onset usually consists of the gradual appearance of mild jaundice and pruritus. Laboratory findings are typical of cholestasis. The total serum bilirubin averages about 4 mg/100 ml and rarely exceeds 10 mg/100 ml. Oral or intravenous cholangiography will not opacify the biliary anatomy, transhepatic cholangiograms are usually unsuccessful because the ducts are too small to be entered with the percutaneous needle, but retrograde endoscopic cholangiograms may be diagnostic. Liver biopsy may show pericholangitis and bile stasis, but the changes are nonspecific.

At operation the lumen is usually so small that it is difficult to locate in the center of the thickened duct. By careful dissection, a pinpoint opening can be found which contains bile. An operative cholangiogram should be obtained to verify the diagnosis and to determine the extent of the disease. Although most patients have generalized disease, in one-third it affects only one portion of the biliary tree and the other areas appear normal. Both isolated extrahepatic and intrahepatic involvement have been described.

Sclerosing cholangitis is a diffuse process that can be closely mimicked by certain desmoplastic primary biliary malignancies. Thus, focal strictures of the bile duct in the absence of previous surgery will usually be discovered to be due to a malignant tumor. Malignant neoplasms sometimes cause more diffuse narrowing which may be mistaken for sclerosing cholangitis. Because of this potential diagnostic pitfall, it is always advisable to biopsy the wall of the duct whenever either of these entities is suspected.

A T tube should be placed into the common duct after the lumen has been dilated and should be left in place for an extended period after surgery (eg, 12 months). Dramatic relief of pruritus and jaundice sometimes follows this procedure, and a few patients remain free of symptoms for years.

Systemic corticosteroids have been advocated, but it is not yet certain that they have a positive effect. Nevertheless, the present practice is to begin a regimen of prednisone, 30–40 mg/day postoperatively. This dosage is maintained for several months, gradually tapered downward over a year, and the drug is then withdrawn.

The natural history of sclerosing cholangitis is one of chronicity and unpredictable severity. Some patients seem to obtain nearly complete remission after treatment, but this is not common. Bacterial cholangitis may develop after operation if adequate drainage has not been established. In these cases, antibiotics will be required at intervals. Most patients experience the gradual evolution of secondary biliary cirrhosis after many years of mild to moderate jaundice and pruritus. Hepatic failure, ascites, or esophageal varices are late complications and may be lethal.

Schwartz SI: Primary sclerosing cholangitis: A disease revisited. Surg Clin North Am 53:1161, 1973.

•   •   •

General References

Bouchier IAD (editor): Diseases of the biliary tract. Clin Gastro-enterol 2:1, 1973. [Entire issue.]

Glenn F, McSherry CK: Calculous biliary tract disease. Curr Probl Surg, June 1975.

Kune GA: *Current Practice of Biliary Surgery.* Little, Brown, 1972.

Longmire WP Jr (editor): Symposium on gallstones. Adv Surg 10:61, 1976.

Orloff MJ (editor): Symposium on surgery of the biliary tree.

Surg Clin North Am 53:961, 1973. [Entire issue.]

Paumgartner G (editor): Bile acids. Clin Gastroenterol 6:1, Jan 1977. [Entire issue.]

Schein CJ: *Acute Cholecystitis.* Harper, 1972.

Sherlock S: *Diseases of the Liver and Biliary System,* 5th ed. Blackwell, 1975.

Thorbjarnarson B: *Surgery of the Biliary Tract.* Saunders, 1976.

White TT, Sarles H, Benhamou J-P: *Liver, Bile Ducts, and Pancreas.* Grune & Stratton, 1977.

30 . . .

Pancreas

Howard A. Reber, MD, & Lawrence W. Way, MD

EMBRYOLOGY

The pancreas arises in the fourth week of fetal life from the caudal part of the foregut as dorsal and ventral pancreatic buds. Both anlagen rotate to the right and fuse near the point of origin of the ventral pancreas. Later, as the duodenum rotates, the pancreas shifts to the left. In the adult, only the caudal portion of the head and the uncinate process are derived from the ventral pancreas. The cranial part of the head and all of the body and tail are derived from the dorsal pancreas. Most of the dorsal pancreatic duct joins with the duct of the ventral pancreas to form the main pancreatic duct (**duct of Wirsung**); a small part persists as the accessory duct (**duct of Santorini**).

ANATOMY

The pancreas is a thin elliptical organ which lies within the retroperitoneum in the upper abdomen (Figs 30–1 and 30–2). In the adult, it is 12–15 cm long and weighs 70–110 g. The gland can be divided into 3 portions—head, body, and tail. The head of the pancreas is intimately adherent to the medial portion of the duodenum and lies in front of the inferior vena cava and superior mesenteric vessels. A small tongue of tissue called the uncinate process lies behind the superior mesenteric vessels as they emerge from the retroperitoneum. Anteriorly, the stomach and first portion of the duodenum lie partly in front of the pancreas. The common bile duct passes through a posterior groove in the head of the pancreas adjacent to the duodenum. The body of the pancreas is in contact posteriorly with the aorta, the left crus of the diaphragm, the left adrenal gland, and the left kidney. The tail of the pancreas lies in the hilus of the spleen. The main pancreatic duct (the duct of Wirsung) courses along the gland from the tail to the head and joins the common bile duct just before entering the duodenum at the ampulla of Vater. The accessory pancreatic duct (the duct of Santorini) enters the duodenum 2–2.5 cm proximal to the ampulla of Vater (Fig 30–1).

The blood supply of the pancreas is derived from branches of the celiac and superior mesenteric arteries (Fig 30–2). The superior pancreaticoduodenal artery arises from the gastroduodenal artery, runs parallel to the duodenum, and eventually meets the inferior pancreaticoduodenal artery to form an arcade. The splenic artery provides tributaries which supply the body and tail of the pancreas. The main branches are termed the dorsal pancreatic, pancreatica magna, and caudal pancreatic arteries. The venous supply of the gland parallels the arterial supply. Lymphatic drainage is into the peripancreatic nodes located along the veins.

The visceral efferent supply to the pancreas is derived from the vagal and splanchnic nerves. The efferent fibers pass through the celiac plexus from the celiac branch of the right vagal nerve to terminate in ganglia located in the interlobular septa of the pancreas. Postganglionic fibers from these synapses innervate the acini, the islets, and the ducts. The visceral efferent fibers from the pancreas also travel in the vagal and splanchnic nerves, but those which mediate pain are confined to the latter. Sympathetic fibers to the pancreas pass from the splanchnic nerves through the celiac plexus and innervate the pancreatic vasculature.

Silen W: Surgical anatomy of the pancreas. Surg Clin North Am 44:1253, 1964.

PHYSIOLOGY

Exocrine Function

The external secretion of the pancreas consists of a clear, alkaline (pH 7.0–8.3) solution of 1–2 liters per day which contains digestive enzymes.

The water and electrolyte secretion is formed by the centroacinar and intercalated duct cells principally in response to secretin stimulation. The secretion is modified by exchange processes and active secretion in the ductal collecting system. The cations sodium and potassium are present in the same concentrations as in plasma. The anions bicarbonate and chloride vary in concentration according to the rate of secretion: with increasing rate of secretion, the bicarbonate concentra-

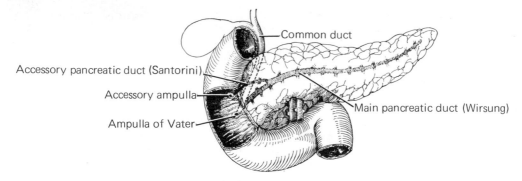

Figure 30—1. Anatomic configuration of pancreatic ductal system. (Courtesy of W Silen.)

tion increases and chloride concentration falls so that the sum of the 2 is the same throughout the secretory range. Pancreatic juice helps neutralize gastric acid in the duodenum and adjusts luminal pH to the level which gives optimal activity of pancreatic enzymes.

Pancreatic enzymes are synthesized, stored (as zymogen granules), and released by the acinar cells of the gland. Pancreatic enzymes are proteolytic, lipolytic, and amylolytic. Lipase and amylase are stored and secreted in active forms. The proteolytic enzymes are secreted as inactive precursors and are activated by the duodenal enzyme enterokinase. Other enzymes secreted by the pancreas include ribonucleases and phospholipase A. Phospholipase A is secreted as an inactive proenzyme which is activated in the duodenum by trypsin. It catalyzes the conversion of biliary lecithin to lysolecithin.

Turnover of protein in the pancreas exceeds that of any other organ in the body. Intravenously injected amino acids are incorporated into enzyme protein and may appear in the pancreatic juice within 1 hour. Three mechanisms prevent autodigestion of the pan-

creas by its proteolytic enzymes: (1) They are stored in acinar cells as zymogen granules, where they are separated from other cell proteins. (2) They are secreted in an inactive form. (3) Inhibitors of proteolytic enzymes are present in pancreatic juice and tissue.

The hormones that affect exocrine secretion (secretin, cholecystokinin-pancreozymin, gastrin, and glucagon) are discussed in Chapter 26 (Table 26—1).

Endocrine Function

The function of the endocrine pancreas is to facilitate storage of foodstuffs by release of insulin after a meal and to provide a mechanism for their mobilization by release of glucagon during periods of fasting. Both hormones are produced by the islets of Langerhans.

Insulin, a polypeptide (MW 5734) consisting of 51 amino acid residues, is formed in the beta cells of the pancreas via the precursor proinsulin. Insulin secretion is stimulated by rising or high serum concentrations of metabolic substrates such as glucose, amino acids, and perhaps short chain fatty acids. The major

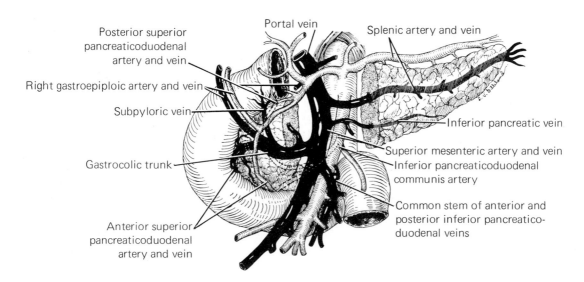

Figure 30—2. Arterial supply and venous drainage of the pancreas. (Courtesy of W Silen.)

normal stimulus for insulin release appears to be glucose, which in the gut liberates the hormone GIP (gastric inhibitory polypeptide). GIP in turn releases insulin from the beta cells. The release and synthesis of insulin are stimulated by the activation of specific glucoreceptors located on the surface membrane of the beta cell. Insulin release is also stimulated by glucagon, secretin, CCK-PZ, VIP (vasoactive intestinal polypeptide), and gastrin, all of which sensitize the receptors on the beta cell to glucose. Epinephrine, tolbutamide, and chlorpropamide release insulin by acting on the adenylate cyclase system.

The short-term regulation of gluconeogenesis depends on the balance between insulin (inhibits) and glucagon (stimulates) or catecholamines. Insulin increases lipolysis in adipose tissue, which increases the supply of fatty acids to the liver, where they are oxidized to ketone bodies. Insulin deficiency results in decreased protein synthesis. Studies on the mechanism of insulin action suggest that the hormone exerts its effect via receptors on the cell membrane.

Beck IT: The role of pancreatic enzymes in digestion. Am J Clin Nutr 26:311, 1973.

Brooks FP: The neurohumoral control of pancreatic exocrine secretion. Am J Clin Nutr 26:291, 1973.

Janowitz HD: Pancreatic secretion of fluid and electrolytes. Page 925 in: *Handbook of Physiology.* Section 6, Vol 2. American Physiological Society, 1967.

Krahl ME: Endocrine function of the pancreas. Annu Rev Physiol 36:331, 1974.

CONGENITAL ANOMALIES OF THE PANCREAS

Annular Pancreas

In this rare condition, a ring of pancreatic tissue from the head of the pancreas surrounds the descending duodenum. The abnormality usually presents in infancy as duodenal obstruction with postprandial vomiting. There is bile in the vomitus if the constriction is distal to the entrance of the common bile duct. X-rays show a dilated stomach and proximal duodenum (double bubble sign) and little or no air in the rest of the small bowel. After correction of fluid and electrolyte imbalance, the obstructed segment should be bypassed by a duodenojejunostomy or other similar procedure. No attempt should be made to resect the obstructing pancreas because a pancreatic fistula or acute pancreatitis often develops postoperatively. Occasionally, annular pancreas will present in adult life with similar symptoms.

PANCREATITIS

Pancreatitis is a common nonbacterial inflammatory disease which results from activation, interstitial liberation, and autodigestion of the pancreas by its own enzymes. The process may or may not be accompanied by permanent morphologic and functional changes in the gland. Much is known about the causes of pancreatitis, but despite the accumulation of a considerable amount of experimental data, our understanding of the pathogenesis of this disorder is still incomplete.

Acute pancreatitis is characterized by sudden upper abdominal pain, nausea, vomiting, and elevated serum amylase. **Chronic pancreatitis** is characterized by chronic pain, pancreatic calcification on x-ray, or exocrine (steatorrhea) or endocrine (diabetes mellitus) insufficiency. Attacks of acute pancreatitis can and often do occur in patients with chronic pancreatitis. **Acute relapsing pancreatitis** is defined as multiple attacks of pancreatitis without permanent pancreatic scarring, a picture most often associated with biliary pancreatitis. The unsatisfactory term **chronic relapsing pancreatitis**, denoting recurrent acute attacks, superimposed on chronic pancreatitis, will not be used in this chapter. Alcoholic pancreatitis often behaves in this way. **Subacute pancreatitis** has also been used by some to describe the minor acute attacks which typically appear late in alcoholic pancreatitis.

Etiology

Most cases of pancreatitis are caused by gallstone disease or alcoholism; a few result from hyperparathyroidism, trauma, hyperlipidemia, and genetic predisposition; and the remainder are idiopathic. Important differences exist in the manifestations and natural history of the disease as produced by these various factors.

A. Biliary Pancreatitis: About 40% of cases of acute pancreatitis are associated with gallstone disease, which, if untreated, usually gives rise to additional acute attacks. For unknown reasons, even repeated attacks of acute biliary pancreatitis fail to produce chronic pancreatitis. Eradication of the biliary disease nearly always prevents recurrent pancreatitis. The etiologic mechanism most likely consists of transient obstruction of the ampulla of Vater and pancreatic duct by a gallstone. Choledocholithiasis is found in only 25% of cases, but because over 90% of patients excrete a gallstone in feces passed within 10 days of an acute attack, it is assumed that most attacks are caused by a gallstone traversing the common duct and ampulla of Vater. Other possible steps in pathogenesis initiated by passage of the gallstone are discussed below.

B. Alcoholic Pancreatitis: In the USA, alcoholism accounts for about 40% of cases of pancreatitis. Characteristically, the patients have been heavy users of hard liquor or wine; the condition is relatively infrequent in countries where beer is the most popular alcoholic beverage. Most commonly, 6 years or more of alcoholic excess precede the initial attack of pancreatitis, and, even with the first clinical manifestations, signs of chronic pancreatitis can be detected if the gland is examined microscopically. Thus, alcoholic pancreatitis is often considered to be synonymous with chronic pancreatitis no matter what the clinical findings are.

Both direct and indirect effects of alcohol have been etiologically implicated. In experimental studies, alcohol reduces incorporation of ^{32}P into parenchymal phospholipids, decreases zymogen synthesis, and produces ultrastructural changes in acinar cells. Acute administration of alcohol stimulates pancreatic secretion and induces spasm in the sphincter of Oddi. This has been compared with experiments that produce acute pancreatitis by combining partial ductal obstruction and secretory stimulation. If the patient can be persuaded to stop drinking, acute attacks may be prevented, but parenchymal damage continues to occur as a consequence of persistent ductal obstruction and fibrosis.

C. Hyperparathyroidism: Hyperparathyroidism and other clinical disorders accompanied by hypercalcemia are occasionally complicated by acute pancreatitis. With time, chronic pancreatitis and ductal calculi appear. It is thought that the increased calcium concentrations in pancreatic juice which result from hypercalcemia may prematurely activate proteases. They also may facilitate calculous precipitation in the ducts.

D. Hyperlipidemia: In some patients—especially alcoholics—hyperlipidemia appears transiently during an acute attack of pancreatitis; in others with primary hyperlipidemia (especially types I and V), pancreatitis seems to be a direct consequence of the metabolic abnormality. Hyperlipidemia during an acute attack of pancreatitis is usually associated with a normal serum amylase due to interference by the lipid with the chemical determination for amylase; urinary output of amylase may still be high. It is important to inspect the serum of a patient with acute pain because if it is lactescent, pancreatitis will almost always be the correct diagnosis. If a primary lipid abnormality is present, dietary control reduces the chances of additional attacks of pancreatitis as well as the other complications of hyperlipidemia.

E. Familial Pancreatitis: In this condition, attacks of abdominal pain usually begin in childhood. The genetic defect appears to be transmitted as a non-X-linked dominant with variable penetrance. Some affected families also have aminoaciduria, but this is not a universal finding. Chronic calcific pancreatitis develops eventually, and many patients become candidates for operation for chronic pain. Pancreatic carcinoma is reported to be more frequent in patients with familial pancreatitis.

F. Protein Deficiency: In certain populations where dietary protein intake is markedly deficient, the incidence of chronic pancreatitis is high. The reason for this association is obscure, especially in view of the observation that alcoholic pancreatitis afflicts alcoholics with higher dietary protein and fat intake than those who escape pancreatic disease.

G. Postoperative Pancreatitis: The rare case of pancreatitis that occurs after Billroth II gastrectomy is due to acute obstruction of the afferent loop and reflux of duodenal secretions under high pressure into the pancreatic ducts. The condition has been recreated experimentally in dogs (Pfeffer loop preparation).

Other cases of postoperative pancreatitis may follow biliary or gastric surgery or even operations remote from the pancreas. In most cases, however, the procedure includes direct manipulation of the pancreas or biliary ducts. At one time it was common practice to leave a long-armed T tube in the common bile duct after choledochotomy until it was recognized that the presence of the tube in the ampulla of Vater often caused acute pancreatitis postoperatively.

H. Idiopathic Pancreatitis and Miscellaneous Causes: In about 15% of patients, representing the third largest group after biliary and alcoholic pancreatitis, there is no identifiable cause of the condition. If followed for a few years, about one-third of these patients will develop gallstone disease.

Miscellaneous uncommon causes include the administration of corticosteroids, thiazide diuretics, other drugs, and scorpion stings.

Pathogenesis

The concept that pancreatitis is due to enzymatic digestion of the gland is supported by the finding of proteolytic enzymes in ascitic fluid and increased amounts of phospholipase A and lysolecithins in pancreatic tissue from patients with acute pancreatitis. Experimentally, pancreatitis can be created readily if activated enzymes are injected into the pancreatic ducts under pressure. Trypsin has not been found in excessive amounts in pancreatic tissue from affected humans, possibly because of inactivation by trypsin inhibitors. Nevertheless, although the available evidence is inconclusive, the autodigestion theory is almost universally accepted. Other proposed factors are vascular insufficiency, lymphatic congestion, and activation of the kallikrein-kinin system.

For many years, trypsin and other proteases were held to be the principal injurious agents, but recent evidence has emphasized phospholipase A, lipase, and elastase as possibly of greater importance. Trypsin, it was noted, ordinarily does not attack living cells, and even when trypsin is forced into the interstitial spaces the resulting pancreatitis does not include coagulation necrosis, which is so prominent in human pancreatitis.

Phospholipase A, in the presence of small amounts of bile salts, attacks free phospholipids (eg, lecithin) and those bound in cellular membranes to produce extremely potent lyso- compounds. Lysolecithin, which would result from the action of phospholipase A on biliary lecithin or phospholipase A itself, plus bile salts, comprises a mixture capable of producing severe necrotizing pancreatitis, as experiments in several species have shown. Trypsin is important in this scheme because small amounts are needed to activate phospholipase A from its inactive precursor.

Elastase, which is both elastolytic and proteolytic, is secreted in an active form. Because it can digest the walls of blood vessels, elastase has been thought to be important in the pathogenesis of hemorrhagic pancreatitis.

If autodigestion is the final common pathway in pancreatitis, earlier steps must account for the presence of active enzymes and their reaction products in the ducts and their escape into the interstitium. The following are the most popular theories which attempt to link the known etiologic factors with autodigestion:

A. Obstruction-Secretion: In animals, ligation of the pancreatic duct generally produces a mild edema of the pancreas which resolves within a week. Thereafter, atrophy of the secretory apparatus occurs. On the other hand, partial or intermittent ductal obstruction, which more closely mimics what seems to happen in humans, can produce frank pancreatitis if the gland is simultaneously stimulated to secrete. The major shortcoming of these experiments has been the difficulty encountered in attempting to cause severe pancreatitis in this way. However, since the human pancreas manufactures 10 times as much phospholipase A as dogs or rats, the consequences of obstruction in humans conceivably could be more serious.

B. Common Channel Theory: Opie, having observed pancreatitis in a patient with a gallstone impacted in the ampulla of Vater, speculated that reflux of bile into the pancreatic ducts might have initiated the process. Flow between the biliary and pancreatic ducts requires a common channel connecting these 2 systems with the duodenum. Although these ducts converge in 90% of humans, only 10% have a common channel long enough to permit biliary-pancreatic reflux if the ampulla contained a gallstone. By itself, fresh normal bile is innocuous in the pancreatic duct. If mixed with bacteria or incubated with pancreatic juice—or if the bile salts are deconjugated—bile is rendered more harmful. These observations have led to the suggestion that pancreatic juice initially might enter the bile ducts and gallbladder and incubate and the mixture then be discharged back into the pancreas. Another suggestion is that infected bile containing deconjugated bile salts is refluxed to produce pancreatitis.

C. Duodenal Reflux: The above theories fail to supply an explanation for activation of pancreatic enzymes, a process which normally takes place through the action of enterokinase in the duodenum. In experimental animals, if the segment of duodenum into which the pancreatic duct empties is surgically converted to a closed loop, reflux of duodenal juice initiates severe pancreatitis (Pfeffer loop). Pancreatitis associated with acute afferent loop obstruction after Billroth II gastrectomy is probably the result of similar factors. Other than in this specific example, duodenal reflux seems unlikely to be etiologically important since it would be difficult to produce and there are no direct observations to support the notion.

It must be admitted that a satisfactory explanation of pathogenesis of pancreatitis is not presently available. In biliary pancreatitis, transient obstruction of the ampulla of Vater by a gallstone is most likely the first event. Whether bile reflux follows is problematic. Alcoholic pancreatitis probably has several causes, including partial ductal obstruction, secretory stimulation, and chronic toxic actions of alcohol on parenchymal cells.

Acosta JM, Ledesma CL: Gallstone migration as a cause of acute pancreatitis. N Engl J Med 290:484, 1974.

Anderson MC & others: Further inquiry into the pathogenesis of acute pancreatitis: Role of pancreatic enzymes. Arch Surg 99:185, 1969.

Creutzfeldt W, Schmidt H: Aetiology and pathogenesis of pancreatitis (current concepts). Scand J Gastroenterol 6:47, 1970.

Elmslie R & others: The significance of reflux of trypsin and bile in the pathogenesis of human pancreatitis. Br J Surg 53:809, 1966.

Geokas MC: Acute pancreatitis. Calif Med 117:25, Aug 1972.

Kattwinkel J & others: Hereditary pancreatitis: Three new kindreds and a critical review of the literature. Pediatrics 51:55, 1973.

Pirola RC, Davis AE: The sphincter of Oddi and pancreatitis. Am J Dig Dis 15:583, 1970.

Sarles H & others: Observations on 205 confirmed cases of acute pancreatitis, recurring pancreatitis, and chronic pancreatitis. Gut 6:545, 1965.

ACUTE PANCREATITIS

Essentials of Diagnosis

- Abrupt onset of epigastric pain, frequently with back pain.
- Nausea and vomiting.
- Elevated serum or urinary amylase.
- Cholelithiasis or alcoholism (many patients).

General Considerations

While edematous and hemorrhagic pancreatitis are manifestations of the same pathologic processes and the general principles of treatment are the same, hemorrhagic pancreatitis has more complications and a higher mortality rate. In edematous pancreatitis, the glandular tissue and surrounding retroperitoneal structures are engorged with interstitial fluid and the pancreas is infiltrated with inflammatory cells which surround small foci of parenchymal necrosis. Hemorrhagic pancreatitis is characterized by bleeding into the parenchyma and surrounding retroperitoneal structures and extensive pancreatic necrosis. In both forms, the peritoneal surfaces may be studded with small calcifications representing areas of fat necrosis.

Clinical Findings

A. Symptoms and Signs: The acute attack frequently begins following a large meal and consists of severe epigastric pain that radiates through to the back. The pain is unrelenting and usually associated with vomiting and retching. In severe cases, the patient may collapse from shock.

Depending on the severity of the disease, there may be profound dehydration, tachycardia, and postural hypotension. Examination of the abdomen reveals decreased or absent bowel sounds and tenderness which may be generalized but more often is localized to the epigastrium. Temperature is usually normal or slightly elevated in uncomplicated pancreatitis. Clinical evidence of pleural effusion may be present, especially on the left. If an abdominal mass is found, it probably represents swollen pancreas (phlegmon), a pseudocyst, or abscess. There may be bluish discoloration in the flank (Grey Turner's sign) or periumbilical area (Cullen's sign), indicating hemorrhagic pancreatitis with dissection of blood retroperitoneally into these areas.

B. Laboratory Findings: The hematocrit may be elevated as a consequence of dehydration or low as a result of abdominal blood loss in hemorrhagic pancreatitis. There is usually a moderate leukocytosis, but total white blood cell counts over 12,000/μl are unusual in the absence of suppurative complications. Liver function studies are usually normal, but there may be a mild elevation of the serum bilirubin concentration (usually below 2 mg/100 ml). Elevated serum lipase is detectable early and for several days after the acute attack, but the test is done infrequently because it requires up to 24 hours to perform and is difficult to standardize.

The serum amylase level rises above 200 IU/100 ml within 6 hours of the onset of an acute episode and generally remains elevated for about 2 days. Although it is the most valuable and most frequently performed diagnostic study, it is not completely reliable for the following reasons: (1) Elevated amylase levels also occur in other acute abdominal conditions such as gangrenous cholecystitis, small bowel obstruction, mesenteric infarction, and perforated ulcer. (2) Episodes of acute pancreatitis may occur unaccompanied by rises in serum amylase; this is the rule if hyperlipidemia is present. (3) The high level may have returned to normal before the blood was drawn.

Urine amylase excretion is a similar but somewhat more accurate test for pancreatitis; values above 5000 IU/24 hours are abnormal. Urinary clearance of amylase increases during pancreatitis, and its expression as a percentage of creatinine clearance is said to distinguish hyperamylasemia in pancreatitis from that due to other conditions in which amylase clearance is unchanged. The ratio of amylase clearance to creatinine clearance is below 5% in normal persons and those with nonpancreatic causes of hyperamylasemia and is usually 5–10% in persons with pancreatitis. The clearance ratio is calculated as follows:

$$\frac{(\text{Urine amylase})}{(\text{Serum amylase})} \times \frac{(\text{Serum creatinine})}{(\text{Urine creatinine})} \times 100\%$$

In severe pancreatitis, the serum calcium concentration may fall as a result of combination of calcium with fatty acids (liberated from retroperitoneal fat by lipase) and impaired reabsorption from bone due to the action of calcitonin (liberated by high levels of glucagon). Relative hypoparathyroidism and hypoalbuminemia have also been implicated.

C. X-Ray Findings: In about two-thirds of cases of acute pancreatitis, a plain abdominal film will reveal some abnormality. The most frequent finding is isolated dilatation of a segment of gut **(sentinel loop)** consisting of jejunum, transverse colon, or duodenum adjacent to the pancreas. Gas distending the right colon which abruptly stops in the mid or left transverse colon **(colon cutoff sign)** is due to colonic spasm adjacent to the pancreatic inflammation. An upper gastrointestinal series may show a widened duodenal loop, swollen ampulla of Vater, and occasionally evidence of gastric irritability. Chest films may reveal a pleural effusion on the left side.

Occasionally, a radiopaque gallstone will be apparent on plain x-rays. In all cases, after the attack is over, one must search for gallstone disease by oral or intravenous cholecystography.

Differential Diagnosis

Acute pancreatitis is actually a diagnosis of exclusion in which other acute upper abdominal conditions such as acute cholecystitis, penetrating or perforated duodenal ulcer, high small bowel obstruction, and mesenteric infarction must be seriously considered. In most cases, the distinction is possible on the basis of the clinical picture and laboratory findings. The critical point is that the diseases with which acute pancreatitis are most likely to be confused are often lethal if not treated surgically. Therefore, diagnostic laparotomy is indicated if they cannot be ruled out on clinical grounds.

In **macroamylasemia**, serum amylase levels are elevated, but the pancreas is normal. Neither the amylase-creatinine clearance ratio nor urinary amylase excretion is increased. The elevated serum levels are due to impaired renal amylase excretion of a large complex amylase molecule. Macroamylasemia should be suspected when serum amylase levels are high, renal excretion is low, and the patient does not appear to have pancreatitis. The diagnosis can be confirmed by serum protein electrophoresis. No treatment is required, and the significance of macroamylasemia is unknown.

Complications

The principal complications of acute pancreatitis are abscess formation and pseudocyst. These are discussed in separate sections. Gastrointestinal bleeding may occur from adjacent inflamed stomach or duodenum, ruptured pseudocyst, or peptic ulcer. Intraperitoneal bleeding may occur spontaneously from the celiac or splenic artery or from the spleen following acute splenic vein thrombosis.

Even with mild disease, arterial hypoxia develops in two-thirds of patients, but in those with severe pancreatitis respiratory insufficiency may be progressive and is associated with a high mortality rate. Early endotracheal intubation with assisted ventilation, careful attention to fluid and acid-base balance, and perhaps peritoneal lavage may improve the prognosis. The cause is unclear but may be related to alteration of pulmonary surfactant by elevated serum levels of pancreatic lecithinase or to alterations in coagulation leading to diffuse pulmonary microembolism. Other factors such as hypocalcemia with tetany, abdominal distention, pain and guarding, and diaphragmatic elevation may also play a role.

Treatment

A. Medical Treatment: The goals of medical therapy are reduction of pancreatic secretory stimuli and correction of fluid and electrolyte derangements.

1. Gastric suction—Oral intake is withheld, and a nasogastric tube is inserted to aspirate gastric secretions. Although there is no solid empirical support for the theory, this is thought to eliminate release of secretin and CCK-PZ and—by avoiding pancreatic stimulation, to hasten resolution of the disease. Nasogastric aspiration also eliminates vomiting.

2. Fluid replacement—Patients with acute pancreatitis sequester fluid in the retroperitoneum, and the volume in some cases may be so great that large amounts of saline or colloid solutions are necessary to maintain circulating blood volume and renal function. In severe hemorrhagic pancreatitis, blood transfusion may also be required. The adequacy of fluid replacement may be judged most accurately by monitoring the volume and specific gravity of urine.

3. Analgesics—Morphine or meperidine may occasionally be required, but, because these drugs cause spasm of the sphincter of Oddi, pentazocine is preferable if it provides relief of pain.

4. Anticholinergics—The known stimulatory effect of the vagus nerve on pancreatic secretion provides a theoretical basis for the use of anticholinergic agents in this disease. There is, however, no proof that the clinical course of patients given these drugs is improved.

5. Antibiotics—Antibiotics are not thought to be useful in the average case and should be reserved for the treatment of specific suppurative complications.

6. Calcium—In severe attacks, hypocalcemia may require parenteral calcium replacement in amounts determined by serial calcium measurements. In some instances, when hypocalcemia is refractory to treatment, parathyroid extract, 200 units IV every 4 hours for 6 doses, has successfully reversed it. Recognition is important not only because hypocalcemia may produce cardiac arrhythmias but because the degree of hypocalcemia is closely correlated with the death rate: patients with serum calcium levels under 7.5 mg/100 ml rarely survive.

7. Oxygen—In severely ill patients (eg, those with hypocalcemia and large fluid requirements), arterial hypoxemia is almost always present and supplemental oxygen should be given by mask. In the most severe cases, endotracheal intubation and mechanical ventilation with positive end-expiratory pressure may be necessary. Diuretics may be useful in decreasing lung water and improving arterial oxygen saturation.

8. Miscellaneous methods of treatment—

a. Peritoneal lavage has been employed in severe refractory cases of acute pancreatitis to remove toxins in the peritoneal fluid which would otherwise have been absorbed into the systemic circulation. The value of lavage has not been firmly established, but it appears to most observers to have a significant positive effect in many severely ill patients. The technic involves infusing and withdrawing 1 liter of lactated Ringer's solution through a peritoneal dialysis catheter every hour. If a response occurs, it will be seen within 8 hours. If the patient improves following lavage, laparotomy can be avoided; if improvement does not occur, laparotomy may be required.

b. Glucagon—Intravenous glucagon, 1–1.5 mg every 4 hours during the acute attack, has been reported to relieve abdominal pain and speed resolution of the inflammation and return of elevated serum enzyme levels toward normal. More recent evidence fails to support these claims.

c. Trasylol—A decade ago, Trasylol, a proteolytic enzyme inhibitor, was tested extensively for treating acute pancreatitis, but the results were conflicting. In general, the better studies failed to show a useful effect; recently, however, a well-designed randomized trial suggested that Trasylol reduced the mortality rate, particularly in elderly patients.

d. Nutrition—Total parenteral nutrition avoids pancreatic secretory stimulation and should be used for nutritional support in patients with protracted illness. Elemental diets ingested orally or given by tube into the small intestine do not avoid secretory stimulation. Neither form of nutrition directly affects recovery from an episode of pancreatic inflammation.

B. Surgical Treatment: Surgery is generally contraindicated in uncomplicated acute pancreatitis. However, when the diagnosis is uncertain, diagnostic laparotomy is not thought to aggravate pancreatitis. In biliary pancreatitis, elective cholecystectomy and search for common duct stones should be performed several weeks after the acute attack has resolved. Occasionally, a patient with acute pancreatitis and choledocholithiasis fails to improve and may require removal of common duct stones during the acute attack.

When laparotomy is required for differential diagnosis and acute pancreatitis is found, choledochotomy and insertion of a T tube should be performed if there is any suggestion of biliary obstruction, and large drains should be laid down to the pancreas. Additional procedures are probably not beneficial.

In patients with acute hemorrhagic pancreatitis not responding to medical therapy, laparotomy is indicated. Necrotic pancreas and other nonviable tissue should be debrided, a choledochotomy performed and a T tube inserted if there is common duct obstruction, and large drains should be placed near the pancreas. The literature on this subject is misleading since it suggests that an anatomic total pancreatectomy may be indicated in some patients. In fact, total pancreatectomy is not technically feasible in acute pancreatitis, and the operation consists of aggressive debridement of devitalized pancreatic parenchyma. The mortality rate is very high with any form of therapy.

Surgery for complications of acute pancreatitis such as abscess, pseudocyst, and pancreatic ascites is discussed below.

Prognosis

The mortality rate in acute pancreatitis is about 10%. Respiratory insufficiency and hypocalcemia indicate a poor prognosis. The mortality rate of acute hemorrhagic pancreatitis exceeds 50%.

Blackburn GL & others: New approaches to the management of severe acute pancreatitis. Am J Surg 131:114, 1976.

Burk JE & others: Macroamylasemia: A newly recognized cause for elevated serum amylase activity. N Engl J Med 277:941, 1967.

Cameron JL & others: Acute pancreatitis with hyperlipemia: Evidence for a persistent defect in lipid metabolism. Am J Med 56:482, 1974.

Cameron JL & others: Acute pancreatitis with hyperlipidemia: The incidence of lipid abnormalities in acute pancreatitis. Ann Surg 177:483, 1972.

Glazer G: Hemorrhagic and necrotizing pancreatitis. Br J Surg 62:169, 1975.

Hermann RE, Hertzer NR: Time of biliary surgery after acute pancreatitis due to biliary disease: Report of six illustrative cases. Arch Surg 100:71, 1970.

Howard JM, Ehrlich EW: Gallstone pancreatitis: A clinical entity. Surgery 51:177, 1962.

Johnson SG & others: Mechanism of increased renal clearance of amylase/creatinine in acute pancreatitis. N Engl J Med 295:1214, 1976.

Jordan GL Jr, Spjut HJ: Hemorrhagic pancreatitis. Arch Surg 104:489, 1972.

Kelly TR & others: Methemalbumin in acute pancreatitis: An experimental and clinical appraisal. Ann Surg 175:15, 1972.

Norton L, Eiseman B: Near total pancreatectomy for hemorrhagic pancreatitis. Am J Surg 127:191, 1974.

Peterson LM & others: Acute pancreatitis occurring after operation. Surg Gynecol Obstet 127:1, 1968.

Ranson JHC & others: Prognostic signs and nonoperative peritoneal lavage in acute pancreatitis. Surg Gynecol Obstet 143:209, 1976.

Ranson JHC & others: Prognostic signs and the role of operative management in acute pancreatitis. Surg Gynecol Obstet 139:69, 1974.

Ranson JHC & others: Respiratory complications in acute pancreatitis. Ann Surg 179:557, 1974.

Robertson GM Jr & others: Inadequate parathyroid response in acute pancreatitis. N Engl J Med 294:512, 1976.

Rosato EF & others: Peritoneal lavage therapy in hemorrhagic pancreatitis. Surgery 74:106, 1973.

Salt WB II, Schenker S: Amylase—its clinical significance: A review of the literature. Medicine 55:269, 1976.

Storck G & others: A study of autopsies upon 116 patients with acute pancreatitis. Surg Gynecol Obstet 143:241, 1976.

Trapnell J: The natural history and management of acute pancreatitis. Clin Gastroenterol 1:147, 1972.

Warshaw AL, Fuller AF Jr: Specificity of increased renal clearance of amylase in diagnosis of acute pancreatitis. N Engl J Med 292:325, 1975.

Warshaw AL & others: The pathogenesis of pulmonary edema in acute pancreatitis. Ann Surg 182:505, 1975.

PANCREATIC PSEUDOCYST

Essentials of Diagnosis

- Epigastric mass and pain.
- Mild fever and leukocytosis.
- Pancreatic cyst by ultrasound or CT scan.

General Considerations

Pancreatic pseudocysts are encapsulated collections of fluid with high enzyme concentrations which arise from the pancreas. They are usually located either within or adjacent to the pancreas in the lesser sac, but pancreatic pseudocysts have also been found in the neck, mediastinum, and pelvis. The walls of a pseudocyst are formed by inflammatory fibrosis of the peritoneal, mesenteric, and serosal membranes, which limits spread of the pancreatic juice as the lesion develops. The term pseudocyst denotes absence of an epithelial lining, whereas true cysts are lined by epithelium.

Two somewhat different processes are involved in the pathogenesis of pancreatic pseudocysts. Many occur as complications of severe acute pancreatitis, where extravasation of pancreatic juice and glandular necrosis form a sterile pocket of fluid which is not reabsorbed as inflammation subsides. Superinfection of such collections leads to pancreatic abscess instead of pseudocyst. In other patients, usually alcoholics or trauma victims, pseudocysts appear without preceding acute pancreatitis. The mechanism in these cases consists of ductal obstruction and formation of a retention cyst which loses its epithelial lining as it grows beyond the confines of the gland. In posttraumatic pseudocyst, symptoms usually do not appear until several weeks after the injury. Some are iatrogenic, occurring during splenectomy; others follow an external blow to the abdomen.

Pseudocysts develop in about 2% of cases of acute pancreatitis. The cysts are single in 85% of cases and multiple in the remainder.

Clinical Findings

A. Symptoms and Signs: A pseudocyst should be suspected when a patient with acute pancreatitis fails to recover after a week of treatment or when, after improving for a time, his symptoms return. In acute pancreatitis, the initial manifestation is often a palpable tender mass in the epigastrium consisting of swollen pancreas and contiguous structures (phlegmon). On repeated examinations, the phlegmon may disappear. If a mass persists, it most likely represents a pseudocyst.

In other cases, the pseudocyst develops insidiously without an obvious attack of acute pancreatitis.

Regardless of the type of prodromal phase, pain is the most common finding. Fever, weight loss, tenderness, and a palpable mass are present in about half of patients. A few have jaundice, a manifestation of obstruction of the intrapancreatic segment of the bile duct.

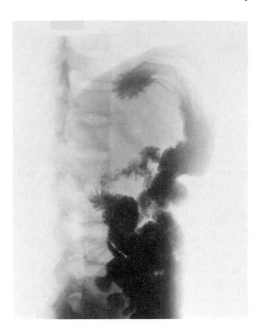

Figure 30—3. A pancreatic pseudocyst has displaced the stomach anteriorly, producing a smooth crescentic impression on the lesser curvature.

B. Laboratory Findings: An elevated serum amylase and leukocytosis are present in about half of patients. When present, elevated bilirubin levels reflect biliary obstruction. Of those patients with acute pancreatitis whose serum amylase remains elevated for as long as 3 weeks, about half will have a pseudocyst.

C. X-Ray Findings: In the majority of instances, an upper gastrointestinal series will reveal a mass in the lesser sac which distorts the stomach or duodenum (Fig 30—3). Pseudocyst, pancreatic swelling (phlegmon), and pancreatic abscess cannot be distinguished on the basis of the x-rays.

D. Special Examinations: Ultrasound scanning can distinguish between a fluid-filled and solid mass. The course of a phlegmon may be followed with repeated studies to determine if a pseudocyst is developing. Masses in the upper abdomen revealed by abdominal examination or x-rays should be investigated to learn if they are cystic. If so, they will often be pancreatic pseudocysts or, rarely, cystic neoplasms. CT scans appear to be useful for the diagnosis of pancreatic pseudocysts. Endoscopic retrograde cannulation of the pancreatic duct with injection of dye and x-ray opacification (ERCP) may demonstrate pseudocysts but carries a risk of serious infection of the cyst. The presence of a pancreatic pseudocyst is considered a relative contraindication for ERCP. With wider use of ultrasound and ERCP in the diagnosis of pancreatic disease, small asymptomatic pseudocysts are being demonstrated. Although the natural history of these subclinical lesions is presently unknown, it is presumed to be relatively benign and there is no indication for active surgical treatment.

Differential Diagnosis

Pancreatic pseudocysts must be distinguished from pancreatic abscess and acute pancreatic phlegmon. Patients with an abscess are clinically toxic, with high fever (39—40 C) and marked leukocytosis (greater than 15,000/μl).

In rare cases, patients with pseudocyst present with weight loss, jaundice, and a nontender palpable gallbladder and are first thought to have pancreatic carcinoma. Ultrasound scanning, by indicating that the lesion is fluid-filled, suggests the correct diagnosis.

Neoplastic cysts—either cystadenoma or cystadenocarcinoma—account for about 10% of all cases of cystic pancreatic masses and may be indistinguishable preoperatively from pseudocyst. The correct diagnosis can be made from histologic study of a biopsy of the cyst wall obtained at operation.

Complications

A. Infection: Infection is a rare complication resulting in high fever, chills, and leukocytosis. Surgical drainage is required as soon as the diagnosis is suspected. Infected pseudocysts intimately adherent to the stomach can be drained by cystogastrostomy; otherwise, drainage should be external because the suture line of a Roux-en-Y cystojejunostomy may not heal.

B. Rupture: Sudden perforation into the free peritoneal cavity produces severe chemical peritonitis with boardlike abdominal rigidity and severe pain. Rapid enlargement of the pseudocyst is sometimes noted before it ruptures. The treatment is emergency surgery with irrigation of the peritoneal cavity and a drainage procedure for the pseudocyst. This complication occurs in less than 5% of cases, but even with prompt treatment it is often fatal.

C. Hemorrhage: Bleeding may occur into the cyst cavity or an adjacent viscus into which the cyst has eroded. Intracystic bleeding may present as an enlarging abdominal mass with anemia resulting from blood loss. If the cyst has eroded into the stomach, there may be hematemesis, melena, and blood in the nasogastric aspirate. The rapidity of the blood loss often produces hemorrhagic shock and usually precludes arteriography. Emergency laparotomy is required as a lifesaving measure. The source of the hemorrhage may be the splenic or gastroduodenal artery as it passes through the cyst wall and is eroded by enzymes in the pseudocyst fluid.

Treatment

Operation is required for pancreatic pseudocysts to prevent complications and eliminate symptoms. Ultrasound scans suggest that some very young pseudocysts which form during acute pancreatitis may resolve spontaneously. However, after the first few weeks of the disease, resolution occurs only in very rare cases where adequate drainage follows rupture of the cyst into a viscus.

An acute pseudocyst arising from pancreatitis should be allowed to mature for 4—6 weeks while the cyst wall becomes firm enough to hold sutures. Excision, external drainage, and internal drainage are the 3 types of surgical procedures used in treatment.

A. Excision: Excision is the most definitive method of treatment but is usually feasible only for pseudocysts in the tail of the gland. This approach is recommended especially for cysts which follow trauma, where the head and body of the gland are normal. Most cysts should be drained either externally or internally into the gut.

B. External Drainage: External drainage is best for critically ill patients or when the cyst wall has not matured sufficiently for anastomosis to other organs. A large tube is sewn into the cyst lumen and its end is brought out through the abdominal wall. Occasionally, the edges of the open cyst can be sutured to the peritoneum, and the cyst is said to be "marsupialized." This technic has largely been discarded. External drainage is complicated in a third of patients by a pancreatic fistula which sometimes drains for several years but on the average closes in about 5 months.

C. Internal Drainage: The preferred method of treatment is internal drainage, in which the cyst is anastomosed to a Roux-en-Y limb of jejunum (cystojejunostomy), to the posterior wall of the stomach (cystogastrostomy), or to the duodenum (cystoduodenostomy). During the procedure, the interior of the cyst should be inspected for evidence of tumor and a piece of the cyst wall should be obtained for microscopic study. X-rays obtained after filling the cyst with contrast medium give useful anatomic information and outline the pancreatic ducts in about 10% of cases. Cystogastrostomy is preferable for cysts behind and densely adherent to the stomach. To accomplish free, dependent drainage, Roux-en-Y cystojejunostomy has the advantage of adaptability to cysts in various other locations. Following an internal drainage procedure, the cyst cavity becomes obliterated within a few weeks. Even after cystogastrostomy, the patient can be allowed to eat an unrestricted diet within a week of surgery, and x-rays taken at this time usually show only a small residual cyst cavity.

Prognosis

The recurrence rate for pancreatic pseudocyst is about 10%, and recurrence is more frequent after treatment by external drainage. Serious postoperative hemorrhage from the cyst occurs rarely—most often after cystogastrostomy. In most cases, however, surgical treatment of pseudocysts is uncomplicated and definitively solves the immediate problem. Many patients later experience chronic pain as a manifestation of underlying chronic pancreatitis.

Anderson MC: Management of pancreatic pseudocyst. Am J Surg 123:209, 1972.

Folk FA, Freeark RJ: Reoperations for pancreatic pseudocyst. Arch Surg 100:430, 1970.

Hanna WA: Rupture of pancreatic cysts: Report of a case and review of the literature. Br J Surg 47:495, 1960.

Rosenberg IK & others: Surgical experience with pancreatic pseudocysts. Am J Surg 177:11, 1969.

Sankaran S, Walt AJ: The natural and unnatural history of pancreatic pseudocysts. Br J Surg 62:37, 1975.

Schumer W & others: Transgastric cystogastrostomy. Surg Gynecol Obstet 137:48, 1973.

Stanley JC & others: Major arterial hemorrhage, a complication of pancreatic pseudocysts and chronic pancreatitis. Arch Surg 111:435, 1976.

Tucker PC, Webster PD: Traumatic pseudocysts of the pancreas. Arch Intern Med 129:583, 1972.

Warren KW & others: Surgical treatment of pancreatic cysts: Review of 183 cases. Ann Surg 163:886, 1966.

Weinstein BR & others: Obstructive jaundice as a complication of pancreatitis. Ann Intern Med 58:245, 1963.

PANCREATIC ABSCESS

Pancreatic abscess, which complicates about 5% of cases of acute pancreatitis, is invariably fatal if untreated. It tends to develop in severe cases accompanied by hypovolemic shock and pancreatic necrosis and is an especially frequent complication of postoperative pancreatitis. Abscess formation follows secondary bacterial contamination of necrotic pancreatic debris and hemorrhagic exudate, but where the organisms come from is not known. There is no evidence that prophylactic antibiotics given early in the course of acute pancreatitis decrease the incidence of abscess.

Clinical Findings

An abscess should be suspected when a patient with severe acute pancreatitis fails to improve and develops rising fever (39–40 C) and leukocytosis (15–20 thousand/μl) or when symptoms return after a period of recovery. In most cases, there is improvement for a while before sepsis appears 2–4 weeks after the attack began. Epigastric pain and tenderness and a palpable tender mass are the principal clues to diagnosis. Vomiting or jaundice may be present, but in some cases fever and leukocytosis are the only findings. The serum amylase may be elevated but usually is normal. Characteristically the serum albumin is below 2.5 g/100 ml and the alkaline phosphatase is elevated. Pleural fluid and diaphragmatic paralysis may be evident on chest x-rays. An upper gastrointestinal series usually shows deformity of the stomach or duodenum by a mass. Diagnostic ultrasound scanning will usually indicate the presence of a cyst in the area of the pancreas. The distinction between noninfected pseudocyst and pancreatic abscess depends on clinical evidence of suppuration. In about 10% of cases, a plain film of the abdomen will reveal gas bubbles ("soap bubble sign") in the area of the pancreas, a diagnostic finding.

In general, the diagnosis is difficult, treatment is often instituted late, and morbidity and mortality rates are high.

Treatment

Surgical drainage of the pus is mandatory; laparotomy should be undertaken whenever abscess is strongly suspected. Preoperatively, the patient should be given broad-spectrum antibiotics since the organisms are usually a mixed flora, most often *Escherichia coli,* bacteroides, staphylococcus, klebsiella, proteus, etc. A transabdominal approach is best, and wide exploration of the peripancreatic and retroperitoneal area is necessary since the necrotizing process may have spread broadly through tissue planes. Necrotic debris should be removed and external drainage instituted. Internal drainage into the gut is neither wise nor practical.

Postoperatively, recurrent or additional abscesses may require reoperation. Postoperative hemorrhage (immediate or delayed) from the abscess cavity occurs occasionally.

Prognosis

The mortality rate is about 30%, a consequence of the severity of the condition and the inability in some cases to make the proper diagnosis.

Bolooki H & others: Pancreatic abscesses and lesser omental sac collections. Surg Gynecol Obstet 126:1301, 1968.

Holden JL & others: Pancreatic abscess following acute pancreatitis. Arch Surg 111:858, 1976.

Miller TA & others: Pancreatic abscess. Arch Surg 108:545, 1974.

PANCREATIC ASCITES

Pancreatic ascites consists of accumulated pancreatic fluid in the abdomen without peritonitis or severe pain. Since many of these patients are alcoholic, they are often thought at first to have cirrhotic ascites. The syndrome is most often due to chronic leakage of a pseudocyst, but a few cases are due to disruption of one of the pancreatic ducts. The principal etiologic factors are alcoholic pancreatitis in adults and traumatic pancreatitis in children. Marked recent weight loss is a major clinical manifestation, and unresponsiveness of the ascites to diuretics is an additional diagnostic clue. The ascitic fluid, which ranges in appearance from straw-colored to blood-tinged, contains elevated protein ($>$ 2.9 g/100 ml) and amylase levels. Once this condition is suspected, definitive diagnosis is based on chemical analysis of the ascites and endoscopic retrograde pancreatography (ERCP). ERCP frequently demonstrates the point of fluid leak and allows a rational surgical approach if operation is required.

Particularly when malnutrition is severe, initial therapy should consist of a period of intravenous hyperalimentation which in some cases results in spontaneous cure. If substantial improvement has not occurred after 2 weeks of nutritional resuscitation, surgery should be performed. The site of origin of the fluid may be grossly evident at operation, but in some patients it can only be demonstrated by operative pan-

creatography. Internal drainage into the gut by means of a Roux-en-Y segment of jejunum is the best procedure in most cases, but for technical reasons external drainage is all that can be done in some. The jejunum is anastomosed to the site of ductal leak or, more often, the leaking pseudocyst. Eighty percent of patients experience relief of symptoms. The mortality rate is low if the patient is treated before debilitation becomes severe.

Chronic pleural effusions of pancreatic origin resulting from communication between the pleural space and the pancreatic ductal system have also been described. Diagnosis and treatment are based upon the same principles as pancreatic ascites.

Sankaran S, Walt AJ: Pancreatic ascites: Recognition and management. Arch Surg 111:430, 1976.

Smith RB III & others: Pancreatic ascites: Diagnosis and management, with particular reference to surgical technics. Ann Surg 177:538, 1973.

CHRONIC PANCREATITIS

Essentials of Diagnosis

- Persistent or recurrent abdominal pain.
- Pancreatic calcification on x-ray in 50%.
- Pancreatic insufficiency in 30%: malabsorption and diabetes mellitus.
- Most often due to alcoholism.

General Considerations

Chronic alcoholism causes most cases of chronic pancreatitis, but a few are due to hyperparathyroidism, hyperlipidemia, or inherited predisposition (familial pancreatitis). Direct trauma to the gland, either from an external blow or from surgical injury, can produce chronic pancreatitis, often localized to one section of the gland. Although gallstone disease may cause repeated attacks of acute pancreatitis, these patients rarely develop the permanent glandular scarring and pancreatic insufficiency typical of alcoholism.

Alcoholic pancreatitis is thought to be due to the toxic effects of alcohol on the acinar cells. There is an increase in the concentration of enzyme protein in pancreatic secretion. The protein precipitates in the ducts, thus forming obstructing plugs which subsequently calcify. Pathologic changes within the gland include destruction of glandular parenchyma with acinar fibrosis, reduplication of the smaller ducts, ductal calcification, and stenoses with proximal ductal dilatation.

Clinical Findings

A. Symptoms and Signs: The typical patient with advanced chronic pancreatitis has persistent deep-seated upper abdominal pain that waxes and wanes from day to day. Sometimes, however, there may be no symptoms at all even though the pancreas is markedly fibrotic. In other patients, episodes of abdominal pain may be separated by painless intervals lasting weeks to months. Patients with chronic pancreatitis may also experience acute attacks of pancreatitis superimposed on one of these other clinical patterns. If the pancreatic destruction has progressed far enough, there may be diabetes mellitus, weight loss, and malnutrition resulting from malabsorption. Because of chronic debilitating pain, narcotic addiction occurs often.

B. Laboratory Findings:

1. Amylase—Serum and urinary amylase levels may be elevated, but in many cases pancreatic fibrosis is advanced and enzyme-forming capacity so impaired that episodes of pain occur without elevation of enzymes.

2. Pancreatic function tests—Clinically evident pancreatic insufficiency does not occur until 90% of the functional pancreatic parenchyma has been destroyed; this occurs in about 30% of cases. However, with chronic pancreatitis, 80–90% of individuals have abnormal pancreatic exocrine function. Because tests of pancreatic function are abnormal in other pancreatic diseases, their diagnostic value is somewhat limited.

In the standard test meal which is given by mouth **(Lundh test)**, pancreatic secretion is collected by duodenal intubation and the tryptic activity of the juice is determined. In chronic pancreatitis, mean tryptic activity is decreased from 17 IU/liter to less than 6 IU/liter.

In the direct pancreatic stimulatory test, secretin (1 U/kg IV) is given, duodenal contents are collected, and total volume and bicarbonate output of pancreatic juice are determined. With chronic pancreatitis, bicarbonate concentration is less than 90 mEq/liter (normal, 90–130 mEq/liter) and volume flow is less than 2 ml/kg/80 minutes (normal, 2–4 ml/kg/80 minutes).

A new test which is easier to perform involves the oral administration of a synthetic peptide which is specifically cleaved by chymotrypsin. The urinary excretion of *p*-aminobenzoic acid (PABA) released by this cleavage is determined. In patients with chronic pancreatitis, urine recovery of PABA is lower (40%) than in patients with no pancreatic disease (75%).

3. Diabetes—The patient may have an abnormal glucose tolerance curve or overt diabetes mellitus indistinguishable from the usual form of diabetes of adult onset not associated with chronic pancreatitis. Serum insulin values in patients with diabetes and chronic pancreatitis are abnormally low.

4. Malabsorption—Steatorrhea may be documented by placing the patient on a diet containing 100 g of fat per day and then measuring fecal fat excretion over 72 hours (normal excretion < 5 g/day). Daily fecal nitrogen is normally less than 1.5 g/day on a daily intake of 70 g of protein. Severe pancreatic insufficiency may produce excessive fecal nitrogen loss, but, because of the action of proteolytic enzymes contained in the intestinal mucosa, creatorrhea is not as prominent as steatorrhea.

5. Jaundice—Rarely, obstructive jaundice with a serum bilirubin level as high as 10–20 mg/100 ml can be caused by compression of the distal common bile duct from pancreatic fibrosis, but persistently high bilirubin levels are usually caused by a pseudocyst or pancreatic neoplasm.

6. Miscellaneous—Vitamin B_{12} malabsorption has been demonstrated in some patients with pancreatic insufficiency but is rare in chronic pancreatitis. It can be corrected by oral administration of trypsin.

C. X-Ray Findings: X-rays of the abdomen reveal pancreatic calcification in 50% of patients with chronic pancreatitis. Pancreatic pseudocyst, a common complication of chronic pancreatitis, can be demonstrated on upper gastrointestinal series by displacement of the stomach or widening of the duodenal sweep. An oral cholecystogram should be performed to search for gallstone disease. Occasionally, intravenous cholangiography may be required to outline more accurately a distal common duct distorted by pancreatic scarring. ERCP may demonstrate characteristic duct abnormalities (eg, stricture, dilatation).

Complications

The principal complications of chronic pancreatitis are pancreatic pseudocyst, malnutrition, and diabetes mellitus. Adenocarcinoma of the pancreas occurs with greater frequency in patients with familial chronic pancreatitis than the general population. Occasionally, development of a neoplasm is heralded by disappearance of pancreatic calcification previously seen on plain x-ray films.

Treatment

A. Medical Treatment: Attacks of acute pancreatitis are managed as described in the preceding section.

Alcoholic patients with chronic pancreatitis should be strongly advised against the continued use of alcohol. If this can be successfully accomplished, it will relieve chronic or episodic pain in more than half of cases even though irreversible damage to the pancreas has occurred. Psychiatric treatment may be beneficial.

Diarrhea resulting from malabsorption can be managed by increasing the proportion of carbohydrate and protein in the diet and limiting fat intake. In general, fat intake should be allowed as tolerated. Supplementary pancreatic enzymes (Viokase or Cotazym, 4–12 g daily) should be given in divided doses 1 hour before and again with each meal throughout the day. Diabetes in these patients usually requires insulin.

B. Surgical Treatment: (Fig 30–4) Surgical therapy is principally of value for relief of chronic pain intractable to other measures. As a preliminary in alcoholics, it is essential that every effort be made to eliminate alcohol abuse. The best surgical candidates are those whose pain persists after alcohol has been abandoned.

1. Drainage procedures—A dilated ductal system implies obstruction, and with this finding procedures that facilitate ductal drainage are usually successful. Calcific alcoholic pancreatitis is the most common con-

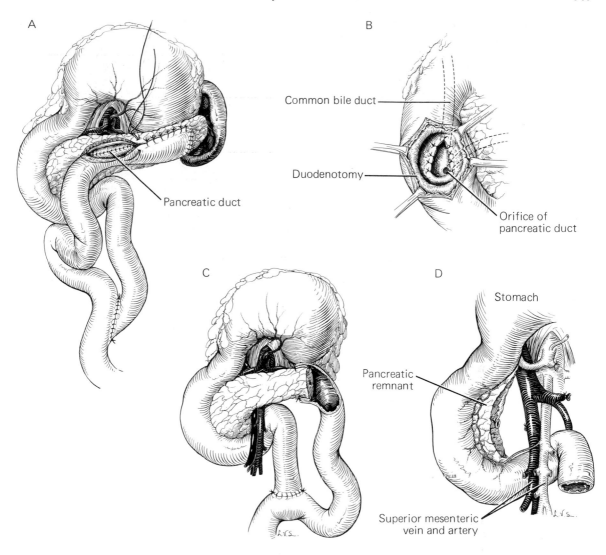

Figure 30—4. Operations for chronic pancreatitis. Indications for the various procedures are discussed in the text. *A:* Longitudinal pancreaticojejunostomy (Puestow). *B:* Sphincteroplasty. *C:* Caudal pancreaticojejunostomy (DuVal). *D:* 95% pancreatectomy.

dition that falls in this category. Ductal dilatation can be demonstrated preoperatively by retrograde endoscopic cannulation, by direct operative pancreatography, or by operative inspection where it may be grossly obvious as a prominent ridge on the surface of the gland. Even without pancreatography, multiple calcifications in the region of the pancreas on plain x-ray films reliably suggest the presence of a dilated duct. Thus, the patients most in need of preoperative pancreatography are those without obvious pancreatic calculi.

In the usual situation, ductal calculi and adjacent stenoses obstruct the main duct at multiple points (chain of lakes appearance). For these patients, longitudinal pancreaticojejunostomy **(Puestow procedure)** is the simplest effective procedure to improve drainage (Fig 30—4A). The duct is opened anteriorly from the tail into the head of the gland and anastomosed side-to-side to a Roux-en-Y segment of proximal jejunum. Postoperatively, about 80% of patients are permanently relieved of pain, and pancreatic insufficiency even improves on occasion.

A variety of less common types of ductal obstruction can be dealt with according to the site of the lesion. For example, a uniformly dilated duct without stenoses or calculi is occasionally due to fibrosis of the sphincter of Oddi, and **sphincteroplasty** is the appropriate procedure (Fig 30—4B). A single point of obstruction in mid-duct might suggest a distal pancreaticojejunostomy **(DuVal procedure)**, an operation which is performed like the Puestow procedure except that the jejunal limb is anastomosed to the stump of the gland and its dilated duct after part of the tail has been removed (Fig 30—4C).

2. Pancreatectomy—Another approach to pain relief is extirpation of the diseased tissue. If chronic pancreatitis is localized to the tail, as is often the case after trauma, resection is simple, definitive, and the procedure of choice. Functional insufficiency is not a problem after such limited resections.

Subtotal pancreatectomy, removing 80–95% of the pancreas except for a rim adjacent to the duodenum, is a more aggressive procedure which is useful in carefully selected patients (Fig 30–4D). It is preferable to total pancreatectomy or pancreaticoduodenectomy (Whipple procedure) if a major resection is indicated. Most surgeons believe that subtotal pancreatectomy should be reserved for patients without a dilated duct since the technically simpler Puestow procedure is usually successful in patients with ductal dilatation. If the Puestow procedure fails, subtotal pancreatectomy should be considered. Diabetes mellitus and exocrine insufficiency are inevitable consequences which should be considered when contemplating a major pancreatic resection in irresponsible alcoholic patients.

Prognosis

Except in advanced cases with continuous pain, alcoholics who can be persuaded to stop drinking often experience relief from pain and recurrent attacks of pancreatitis. In familial pancreatitis, the progress of the disease is inexorable and many of these patients require surgery. Narcotic addiction, diabetes, and malnutrition are serious problems in many patients.

Arvanitakis C, Greenberger NJ: Diagnosis of pancreatic disease by a synthetic peptide: A new test of exocrine pancreatic function. Lancet 1:663, 1976.

Bilbao MK & others: Complications of endoscopic retrograde cholangiopancreatography (ERCP): A study of 10,000 cases. Gastroenterology 70:314, 1976.

Frey CF, Child CG III, Fry W: Pancreatectomy for chronic pancreatitis. Ann Surg 184:403, 1976.

Howard JM, Nedwich A: Correlation of the histologic observations and operative findings in patients with chronic pancreatitis. Surg Gynecol Obstet 132:387, 1971.

Ogoshi K & others: Endoscopic pancreatocholangiography in the evaluation of pancreatic and biliary disease. Gastroenterology 64:210, 1973.

Sarles H: Chronic calcifying pancreatitis: Chronic alcoholic pancreatitis. Gastroenterology 66:604, 1974.

Sarles H & others: Observations on 205 confirmed cases of acute pancreatitis, recurring pancreatitis, and chronic pancreatitis. Gut 6:545, 1965.

Stobbe KC & others: Pancreatic lithiasis. Surg Gynecol Obstet 131:6, 1970.

Way LW, Gadacz T, Goldman L: Surgical treatment of chronic pancreatitis. Am J Surg 127:202, 1974.

White TT, Keith RG: Long term follow-up study of fifty patients with pancreaticojejunostomy. Surg Gynecol Obstet 136:353, 1973.

CARCINOMA OF THE PANCREAS

For unknown reasons, the incidence of carcinoma of the pancreas is increasing in the USA at an annual rate of 15%. In 1977, an estimated 22,000 new cases of pancreatic cancer will occur. After tumors of the lung and colon, pancreatic carcinoma is the third leading cause of cancer death in men between 35 and 54 years of age. It occurs with increased frequency in cigarette smokers and diabetics. The peak incidence is in the fifth and sixth decades. In two-thirds of cases, the tumor is located in the head of the gland; the remainder occur in the body or tail. Ductal adenocarcinoma, mainly of a poorly differentiated cell pattern, accounts for 80% of the malignancies, and the remainder are islet cell tumors and cystadenocarcinomas. Pancreatic adenocarcinoma is characterized by early local extension to contiguous structures and metastases to regional lymph nodes and the liver. Pulmonary, peritoneal, and distant nodal metastases occur later.

Clinical Findings

A. Symptoms and Signs:

1. Carcinoma of the head of the pancreas–About 75% of patients with carcinoma of the head of the pancreas present with weight loss and obstructive jaundice. To emphasize the difference from choledocholithiasis which causes biliary colic, the clinical findings used to be characterized as "painless jaundice." In fact, most patients have deep-seated, vague, nauseating abdominal pain. Back pain occurs in 25% of patients and is associated with a worse prognosis. In general, smaller tumors confined to the pancreas are associated with less pain. Hepatomegaly is present in half of patients but does not necessarily indicate spread to the liver. A palpable mass, which is found in 20%, nearly always signifies surgical incurability. Jaundice is unrelenting in most patients but fluctuates in about 10%. In contrast to common duct obstruction by gallstones, where fever and chills are common, sepsis occurs in only 10–15% of patients with malignant obstruction. A palpable nontender gallbladder in a jaundiced patient suggests neoplastic obstruction of the common duct (Courvoisier's law), most often from pancreatic malignancy; this finding is present in about half of cases. Jaundice is often accompanied by pruritus, especially of the hands and feet.

2. Carcinoma of the body and tail of the pancreas–Since carcinomas of the body and tail of the pancreas are remote from the bile duct, less than 10% of patients are jaundiced. The presenting complaints are weight loss and pain, which sometimes occurs in excruciating paroxysms. In the few patients with hepatomegaly, metastatic involvement has usually occurred. Migratory thrombophlebitis develops in 10% of cases. Once considered relatively specific as a clue to pancreatic cancer, this complication is now known to affect patients with other types of malignant disease.

The diagnosis of pancreatic carcinoma may be extremely difficult. The typical patient who presents with abdominal pain, weight loss, and obstructive jaundice rarely presents a problem, but those with just weight loss, vague abdominal pain, and nondiagnostic x-rays are occasionally labeled psychoneurotics until the existence of malignancy becomes obvious. If back pain predominates, orthopedic or neurosurgical causes may be sought at first. One characteristic feature is the tendency for the patient to seek relief of pain by assuming a sitting position with the spine flexed. Recumbency, on the other hand, aggravates the discomfort and sometimes makes sleeping in bed impossible.

B. Laboratory Findings: Elevated alkaline phosphatase and bilirubin levels reflect either common duct obstruction or hepatic metastases. The bilirubin values with neoplastic obstruction average 18 mg/100 ml, much higher than generally seen with benign disease of the bile ducts. Only rarely are serum transaminase levels markedly elevated. Repeated examination of stool specimens for occult blood gives a positive reaction in most cases. Cytologic studies of pancreatic secretions collected from the duodenum after secretin stimulation may show malignant cells. Unfortunately, this test is rarely positive in small, surgically curable tumors. An oncofetal antigen specific for pancreatic carcinoma has recently been detected in the serum of affected patients, but further studies are necessary before the value of this test in clinical diagnosis is clear.

C. X-Ray Findings: Upper gastrointestinal series with hypotonic duodenography may show a filling defect in the duodenum or early mucosal abnormalities suggestive of invasion by tumor. Angiography of the pancreas uncommonly shows accentuated vascular opacification within the tumor (tumor "blush") or, more often, encasement or distortion of vessels by the tumor mass. Radionuclide scanning of the pancreas is not yet a reliable test. Retrograde cannulation of the pancreaticobiliary system or transhepatic cholangiography may demonstrate common duct obstruction. So far, CT scanning has not been better than other technics in diagnosing small pancreatic neoplasms.

Differential Diagnosis

The other periampullary neoplasms—carcinoma of the ampulla of Vater, distal common bile duct, or duodenum—may also present with pain, weight loss, obstructive jaundice, and a palpable gallbladder. Preoperative cholangiography and gastrointestinal x-rays may suggest the correct diagnosis, but laparotomy is sometimes required. If obstructive jaundice is the major finding, intrahepatic cholestasis must be ruled out, usually by direct (transhepatic or retrograde) cholangiography.

Complications

Obstruction of the splenic vein by tumor may cause splenomegaly and segmental portal hypertension with bleeding esophageal varices. Hepatic vein obstruction is one cause of Budd-Chiari syndrome.

Treatment

Pancreatic resection for pancreatic cancer is justifiable only for cure, and inability to remove all gross tumor precludes this approach. The lesion is considered resectable if the following areas are free of tumor:

(1) the hepatic artery near the origin of the gastroduodenal artery; (2) the portal and superior mesenteric veins as they pass through the uncinate process and behind the body of the pancreas; (3) the superior mesenteric artery where it courses under the body of the pancreas; and (4) the liver and regional lymph nodes. Since the pancreas is so close to the portal vein and the superior mesenteric vessels, involvement of these structures occurs early and prohibits cure because they cannot be surgically sacrificed. Cancers of the head of the pancreas can be resected in about 15% of cases, but, because of local and distant spread, this is possible for only about 5% of cases of lesions of the body and tail.

In most cases, histologic confirmation of the diagnosis is possible at operation by direct biopsy of the primary lesion or metastases. With small lesions within the head of the gland, it may be difficult to obtain a specimen for histologic diagnosis because as much as two-thirds of the palpable mass may consist of a shell of inflamed pancreatic tissue which surrounds the tumor. One approach is needle biopsy through the duodenal wall. The complication of pancreatic fistula would then have little consequence since it would drain into the duodenum, but hemorrhage or pancreatitis could still occur. A newer and safer method is insertion of a fine needle into the pancreatic mass and aspiration of its contents into a syringe. The aspirate is examined for malignant cells. Occasionally, histologic diagnosis is impossible and clinical decisions must rest on inferences derived from indirect proof of the existence of cancer.

For the rare lesion of the body or tail which is resectable, a distal pancreatectomy to the left of the superior mesenteric vessels may be sufficient.

For curable lesions of the head, pancreaticoduodenectomy (**Whipple operation**) is required (Fig 30—5). This involves resection of the distal stomach, common bile duct, gallbladder, duodenum, and the pancreas to mid-body. Truncal vagotomy should be performed to obviate peptic ulceration of the jejunum postoperatively. The operative mortality rate of 15% is attributable to complications such as pancreatic and biliary fistulas, hemorrhage, and infection.

Low cure rates after pancreaticoduodenectomy have encouraged a trial of total pancreatectomy for pancreatic cancer based on the following observations: (1) pancreatic carcinoma is multicentric in approximately 40% of cases; (2) the frequency of intraductal and perineural dissemination within the gland means that tumor is often left behind after partial pancreatectomy; and (3) total pancreatectomy eliminates pancreaticojejunostomy, a major source of morbidity from anastomotic disruption. However, total pancreatectomy produces a brittle type of diabetes mellitus, and unless increased cure rates result from this more aggressive approach it will be difficult to justify.

For incurable lesions producing obstructive jaundice, cholecystojejunostomy or choledochojejunostomy provides relief of the cosmetic problem and the annoying pruritus. Before performing cholecystojeju-

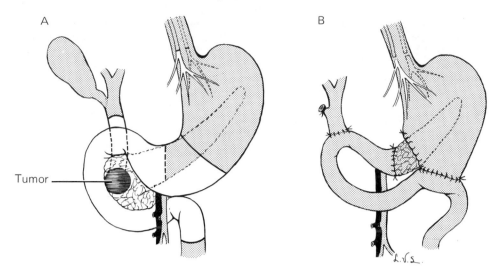

Figure 30—5. Pancreaticoduodenectomy (Whipple procedure). *A:* Preoperative anatomic relationships showing a tumor in the head of the pancreas. *B:* Postoperative reconstruction showing pancreatic, biliary, and gastric anastomoses. A cholecystectomy and bilateral truncal vagotomy are also part of the procedure.

nostomy, a cholangiogram should be obtained to verify patency between the cystic and common bile ducts unless it is grossly obvious. If malignant duodenal obstruction is present, gastrojejunostomy should be performed to bypass the malignancy. We do not feel that, in the absence of obstruction, gastrojejunostomy should be performed prophylactically because very few such patients actually develop obstruction before they succumb to other effects of the tumor.

Neither radiotherapy nor chemotherapy prolongs survival, but they are sometimes effective for pain relief. Recent reports suggest that combinations of chemotherapeutic agents may be more effective than single agents, but this remains to be verified.

Prognosis

Most patients with pancreatic adenocarcinoma are dead within a year after the diagnosis is made. Overall 5-year survival for carcinoma of the head of the pancreas is about 10%, but only a few of these patients are actually free of tumor. Cures of tumors of the body and tail are exceedingly rare.

Banwo O & others: New oncofetal antigen for human pancreas. Lancet 1:643, 1974.

Baylor SM, Berg JW: Cross-classification and survival characteristics of 3,000 cases of cancer of the pancreas. J Surg Oncol 5:335, 1973.

Becker WF & others: Cystadenoma and cystadenocarcinoma of the pancreas. Ann Surg 161:845, 1965.

Brooks JR, Calevras JM: Cancer of the pancreas: Palliative operation, Whipple procedure, or total pancreatectomy? Am J Surg 131:516, 1976.

Crile G Jr: The advantages of bypass operations over radical pancreatoduodenectomy in the treatment of pancreatic carcinoma. Surg Gynecol Obstet 130:1049, 1970.

Douglass HO Jr, Holyoke ED: Pancreatic cancer: Initial treatment as the determinant of survival. JAMA 229:793, 1974.

Fortner JG: Recent advances in pancreatic cancer. Surg Clin North Am 54:859, 1974.

Haslam JB & others: Radiation therapy in the treatment of irresectable adenocarcinoma of the pancreas. Cancer 32:1341, 1973.

Howard JM: Pancreatico-duodenectomy: Forty-one consecutive Whipple resections without an operative mortality. Ann Surg 168:629, 1968.

Levin DL, Connelly RR: Cancer of the pancreas: Available epidemiologic information and its implications. Cancer 31:1231, 1973.

Lightwood R & others: The risk and accuracy of pancreatic biopsy. Am J Surg 132:189, 1976.

Macdonald JS & others: Current diagnosis and management of pancreatic carcinoma. J Natl Cancer Inst 56:1093, 1976.

Spratt JS Jr: Improving trends with pancreaticoduodenectomy. Am J Surg 131:239, 1976.

Warren KW & others: Results of radical resection for periampullary cancer. Ann Surg 181:534, 1975.

Wise L & others: Periampullary cancer. Am J Surg 131:141, 1976.

CARCINOMA OF THE AMPULLA OF VATER

Ampullary adenocarcinoma accounts for about 10% of neoplasms which obstruct the distal bile duct. This tumor spreads locally and metastasizes more slowly than pancreatic carcinoma. The symptoms are similar to those associated with carcinoma of the head of the pancreas, but weight loss and pain are less prominent. Jaundice occurs early in most patients, which is one reason why ampullary carcinomas are often diagnosed while still curable. The stools often contain occult blood from the ulcerating neoplasm. Hypotonic duodenography may reveal a fungating or polypoid intraluminal mass, and the lesion may be visible by fiberoptic duodenoscopy. Treatment consists of pancreaticoduodenectomy as for pancreatic carcinoma. The 5-year survival rate is about 35%. The lesion may be locally excised through a duodenotomy if the patient is too poor a risk for pancreaticoduodenectomy.

Crane JM & others: Surgical experience with malignant tumors of the ampulla of Vater and duodenum. Surg Gynecol Obstet 137:937, 1973.

Makipour H & others: Carcinoma of the ampulla of Vater. Ann Surg 183:341, 1976.

PANCREATIC ISLET CELL TUMORS

Insulinoma, the most common islet cell neoplasm, arises from beta cells and produces insulin and symptoms of hypoglycemia. Tumors of the delta or alpha$_1$ cells produce gastrin and the Zollinger-Ellison syndrome. Alpha$_2$ cell neoplasms may produce excess glucagon and hyperglycemia. Nonbeta islet cell tumors may secrete serotonin, ACTH, MSH, and kinins (and evoke the carcinoid syndrome). Some produce pancreatic cholera, a severe diarrheal illness.

1. INSULINOMA

Insulinomas have been reported in all age groups. About 80% are solitary and benign. About 10% are malignant, and metastases are usually evident at the time of diagnosis. The remainder are either multiple benign adenomas or islet cell hyperplasia.

The symptoms (related to cerebral glucose deprivation) are bizarre behavior, memory lapse, or unconsciousness. Patients may be mistakenly treated for psychiatric illness. There may be profuse sympathetic discharge with palpitations, sweating, and tremulousness. Hypoglycemic episodes are usually precipitated by fasting and are relieved by food. The classical diagnostic criteria (**Whipple's triad**) are present in most cases: (1) hypoglycemic symptoms produced by fasting; (2) blood glucose below 50 mg/100 ml during symptomatic episodes; and (3) relief of symptoms by intravenous glucose. Because other hypoglycemic states can produce this triad, definitive diagnosis depends upon demonstration of an abnormally high serum level of insulin in the presence of hypoglycemia. This requires that the patient fast for 72 hours or until hypoglycemic symptoms appear and that blood glucose and serum immunoreactive insulin (IRI) levels then be determined. A glucose:insulin ratio of less than 1 indicates insulinoma.

Drugs that release insulin (glucagon, leucine, arginine, tolbutamide) have been used for provocative tests but are diagnostic in only about half of cases.

A useful suppression test involves the administration of fish insulin to produce hypoglycemia. Normal subjects respond by suppressing endogenous insulin secretion, but in patients with insulinoma suppression does not occur. Measurement of serum IRI detects circulating endogenous insulin but not fish insulin.

After the diagnosis is certain, arteriography should be performed. Accurate localization is extremely valuable to the surgeon if the tumor is small.

Some mesenchymal tumors, principally fibrosarcomas, can also produce hypoglycemia, probably due to secretion of an insulin-like substance.

Treatment

Surgery should be done promptly because with repeated hypoglycemic attacks permanent cerebral damage occurs, the patient becomes progressively more obese, and the tumor may be malignant. Medical treatment is reserved for surgically incurable lesions.

A. Medical Treatment: Medical therapy consists principally of administration of diazoxide, which suppresses release of tumor insulin. For incurable islet cell carcinomas, promising results have been obtained with streptozocin, an antibiotic which inhibits DNA synthesis. Approximately 60% of patients with metastatic islet cell carcinomas improve with streptozocin, and those who do live twice as long as nonresponders (average 3.5 years vs 1.4 years). Since toxicity is considerable, streptozocin is not recommended as a routine adjunct to surgical therapy.

B. Surgical Treatment: At surgery, the entire pancreas must be meticulously palpated because the tumors are frequently small and difficult to find. If the tumor can be identified, it may either be enucleated or a partial pancreatectomy performed. If the tumor cannot be identified grossly, a distal pancreatectomy should be performed and the specimen inspected after serial sectioning. If no tumor is found, additional pancreas should be removed until an 80% pancreatectomy is performed. Since insulinomas occur with equal frequency throughout the gland, this cures about 80% of cases which require a blind resection. Distal pancreatectomy avoids the higher morbidity and mortality rates associated with pancreaticoduodenectomy, an operation which some have advocated. Unfortunately, intraoperative monitoring of blood glucose is an unreliable means of determining if the tumor has been excised. For islet cell hyperplasia or multiple benign adenomas, subtotal pancreatectomy will usually remove enough diseased tissue so that symptoms will disappear or regress and the patient can be more easily managed medically. In 90% of cases of islet cell carcinoma, metastasis to liver or extrapancreatic extension has already occurred at the time of surgery. Resection of as much metastatic and primary tumor as can be accomplished safely is useful for palliation even when surgical cure is impossible.

Diagnosis of insulinoma. (Editorial.) Lancet 2:385, 1974.

Edis AJ & others: Insulinoma: Current diagnosis and surgical management. Curr Probl Surg 12(10), Oct 1976.

Fajans SS, Floyd JC Jr: Fasting hypoglycemia in adults. N Engl J Med 294:766, 1976.

Fulton RE & others: Preoperative angiographic localization of insulin-producing tumors of the pancreas. Am J Roentgenol Radium Ther Nucl Med 123:367, 1975.

Harrison TS & others: Current surgical management of functioning islet cell tumors of the pancreas. Ann Surg 178:485, 1973.

Stefanini P & others: Beta-islet cell tumors of the pancreas: Results of a study on 1,067 cases. Surgery 75:597, 1974.

2. PANCREATIC CHOLERA
(WDHA Syndrome: Watery Diarrhea, Hypokalemia, & Achlorhydria)

Pancreatic cholera is characterized by profuse watery diarrhea, massive fecal loss of potassium, low serum potassium, and extreme weakness. Gastric acid secretion is usually low or absent even after stimulation with betazole or pentagastrin. Stool volume losses average about 5 liters/day during acute episodes and contain over 300 mEq of potassium (20 times normal). Severe metabolic acidosis is frequently caused by loss of bicarbonate in the stool. Many of these patients are hypercalcemic, possibly from secretion by the tumor of a parathyroid hormone-like substance. Other patients have abnormal glucose tolerance as a result of hypokalemia and altered sensitivity to insulin. Patients who complain of severe diarrhea must be carefully studied for other causes before the diagnosis of WDHA syndrome is seriously entertained. Chronic laxative abuse is a frequent explanation for such symptoms.

Pancreatic cholera is caused by one or more hormones elaborated by a nonbeta islet cell tumor of the pancreas. Although the mediator has not been identified with certainty, many cases seem to be caused by VIP (vasoactive intestinal polypeptide), a compound structurally related to secretin which causes diarrhea in experimental animals. PGE (prostaglandin E) has also been implicated in a few cases. Systemic administration of PGE increases intestinal motility and causes diarrhea.

Preoperative angiography should be used in an attempt to localize the tumor. Approximately 80% of the tumors are solitary and located in the body or tail and can be easily removed. About half of the lesions are benign. Of the malignant cases, three-fourths have metastasized by the time of exploration. Even if all of the tumor cannot be removed, resection of the bulk of it alleviates symptoms in about 40% of patients even though the average survival is only 1 year. If the neoplasm cannot be identified grossly at operation, distal pancreatectomy should be performed. If severe diarrhea continues, corticosteroid therapy may be of benefit. Streptozotocin has also produced remissions in several cases, but nephrotoxicity may limit its effectiveness. Selective arterial administration is preferred when renal function is impaired.

Jaffe BM, Condon S: Prostaglandins E and F in endocrine diarrheagenic syndromes. Ann Surg 184:516, 1976.

Kahn CR & others: Pancreatic cholera: Beneficial effects of treatment with streptozotocin. N Engl J Med 292:941, 1975.

Krejs GJ & others: Intractable diarrhea. Am J Dig Dis 22:280, 1977.

Said SI, Faloona GR: Elevated plasma and tissue levels of vasoactive intestinal polypeptide in the watery-diarrhea syndrome due to pancreatic, bronchogenic, and other tumors. N Engl J Med 293:154, 1975.

Verner JV, Morrison AB: Endocrine pancreatic islet disease with diarrhea. Arch Intern Med 133:492, 1974.

3. GLUCAGONOMA

Glucagonoma produces a characteristic clinical syndrome which includes necrolytic dermatitis (usually involving the legs and perineum), stomatitis, weight loss, and in most cases diabetes. A normochromic normocytic anemia is frequent. The patients are usually middle-aged women who seek medical treatment for the skin lesions. The diagnosis is made by recognition of the symptom complex, demonstration of elevated serum glucagon levels, and pancreatic arteriography, which may demonstrate the tumor. The tumors arise from a_2 cells in the pancreatic islets. Most of them are benign, and surgical resection is curative. Streptozotocin may be effective when the tumor is unresectable.

Danforth DN & others: Elevated plasma proglucagon-like component with a glucagon-secreting tumor: Effect of streptozotocin. N Engl J Med 295:242, 1976.

Mallinson CN & others: A glucagonoma syndrome. Lancet 2:1, 1974.

•   •   •

General References

Carey LC (editor): The Pancreas. Mosby, 1973.

Gambill EE: Pancreatitis. Mosby, 1973.

Howat HT (editor): The exocrine pancreas. Clin Gastroenterol, Jan 1972.

Mercadier MP, Clot JP, Russell TR: Chronic recurrent pancreatitis and pancreatic pseudocysts. Curr Probl Surg, July 1973.

31 . . .
Spleen

Jerry Goldstone, MD, & Lawrence W. Way, MD

The spleen is a dark purplish, highly vascular, coffeebean- to comma-shaped organ situated in the left upper quadrant of the abdomen at the level of the 8th to 11th ribs between the fundus of the stomach, the diaphragm, the splenic flexure of the colon, and the left kidney (Fig 31–1). The adult spleen weighs 100–150 g, measures about 12 × 7 × 4 cm, and usually cannot be felt on palpation of the abdomen. It is attached to and supported by adjacent viscera and the abdominal wall by numerous peritoneal folds, remnants of the embryologic dorsal mesogastrium. The folds or ligaments are normally avascular, but they may carry large collateral veins in patients with portal hypertension.

The splenic capsule consists of peritoneum overlying a 1–2 mm fibroelastic layer which contains a few smooth muscle cells. The fibroelastic layer sends into the pulp numerous fibrous bands (trabeculae) which form the framework of the spleen. In dogs and cats, but not humans, the spleen stores blood that is autotransfused when the organ contracts in response to circulating catecholamines.

The splenic artery enters the hilus of the spleen and sends branches along the trabeculae (trabecular arteries) which terminate in branches that enter the white and red pulp. The white pulp consists of lymphatic tissue and lymphoid follicles containing predominantly lymphocytes, plasma cells, and macrophages distributed throughout a reticular network. The red pulp is made up of cords of reticular cells and sinuses forming a honeycombed vascular space. The vascular spaces of the marginal zone between the red and white pulp contain mostly plasma and are a preferential location for sequestration of foreign material and abnormal cells.

PHYSIOLOGY

Although its physiology is incompletely understood, the human spleen has reticuloendothelial, immunologic, and storage functions. Nevertheless, normal life is possible without a spleen.

Senescent, faulty, or damaged red cells unable to pass through 3–4 μm pores are trapped and removed by splenic reticulum cells. Although it contains only 25 ml of red cells (1% of total red cell mass), 250–350 liters of blood flow through the spleen daily; each red cell averages 1000 passes through the spleen each day. Blood traverses the spleen via several routes, with normal cells passing rapidly and abnormal and aged cells being retarded and entrapped. As they travel through the hypoxic, acidotic, glucose-deprived splenic channels, red cells are "conditioned," becoming more susceptible to subsequent trapping and destruction. In the presence of splenomegaly and other disease states, the flow patterns of the spleen become more circuitous, so that even normal cells may be pooled.

The adult spleen produces monocytes, lymphocytes, and plasma cells. Hematopoiesis of other blood elements occurs in the fetal spleen and, in adult life, in certain diseases (eg, myeloid metaplasia) in which the spleen serves as a site of extramedullary hematopoiesis.

Lymphocytes, the predominant cells of the spleen, produce antibodies (immunoglobulins). The spleen is particularly well suited to facilitate antibody formation, since plasma is skimmed by the trabecular arteries and delivered to the lymphoid follicles, bringing soluble antigens into direct contact with immunologically competent cells. Cells and particulate matter,

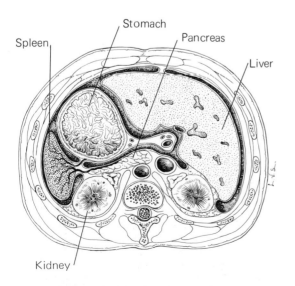

Figure 31–1. Normal anatomic relations of the spleen.

including particulate antigens (eg, bacteria), travel through the sluggish sinuses and cords and make direct contact with the macrophages which line these vascular channels. Although phagocytosis and synthesis of immunoglobulins also occur in other organs, the spleen appears to have a central role in the development of new antibodies after initial exposure to foreign antigens. This is especially important in infancy and explains the increased incidence of infections that follows splenectomy in children under 2 years of age. Even in adults, splenectomy leads to a slight but temporary reduction in antibody formation.

Normally, about 30% of the total platelet pool is sequestered in the spleen, but as much as 80% can be sequestered in patients with splenomegaly. Sequestration and increased splenic destruction of platelets account for the thrombocytopenia so often produced by splenomegaly.

Doan CA: The spleen: Its structure and functions. Postgrad Med 43:126, May 1968.

Harker LA & others: Thrombokinetics in man. J Clin Invest 48:963, 1969.

Weiss L: A scanning electron microscopic study of the spleen. Blood 43:665, 1974.

Weiss L: The structure of the normal spleen. Semin Hematol 2:205, 1965.

Wennberg E & others: The structure of the spleen and hemolysis. Annu Rev Med 20:29, 1969.

HYPERSPLENISM

Essentials of Diagnosis

- Large spleen.
- Pancytopenia.
- Active marrow.
- Cured by splenectomy.

General Considerations

Hypersplenism is characterized by one or more of the following hematologic findings: anemia, leukopenia, and thrombocytopenia. It is accompanied by excessive splenic sequestration or destruction of blood cells, hyperplasia of the respective precursors in the marrow, and splenomegaly and is always ameliorated by splenectomy. If the life span of the blood cells does not increase following splenectomy, the diagnosis of hypersplenism was incorrect.

The defects in hypersplenism are exaggerations of normal splenic functions, such as removal and destruction of aged or defective cells, sequestration of normal cells, and production of immunoglobulins. There is no convincing evidence to support the theory that the spleen in this condition produces a hormone that inhibits the bone marrow. The principal cause of cytopenias in hypersplenism is increased sequestration and destruction of blood cells in the spleen. Etiologic factors include (1) splenic enlargement, (2) intrinsic defects in blood cells, or (3) autoimmune destruction

of blood cells. Splenic sequestration of blood cells produces work hypertrophy of the spleen, an increase in its reticuloendothelial mass, further sequestration, and further work hypertrophy. The hyperplastic spleen is not selective in its hyperfunction. For example, even though the splenomegaly may have been induced by sequestration of abnormal red cells (eg, hemolytic anemia), platelets and leukocytes may also be destroyed more rapidly than normal.

Splenic enlargement is the most common cause of hypersplenism and is the only type in which primary changes in the spleen or splenic circulation are solely responsible for excessive destruction of blood cells. Hypersplenism from this cause is classified as primary or secondary.

Primary hypersplenism, formerly called primary splenic neutropenia or pancytopenia, is a diagnosis of exclusion reached after a careful search (including a study of the splenic pathology) for conditions that can produce secondary hypersplenism. True primary hypersplenism is probably rare; most cases diagnosed as primary hypersplenism involve intrinsic defects in the blood cells or the presence of unrecognized blood cell antibodies. What appears to be primary hypersplenism may be an early manifestation of lymphoma or leukemia, since these malignancies develop in some patients late after splenectomy.

Secondary hypersplenism is most often due to congestive splenomegaly from portal hypertension (cirrhosis or portal or splenic vein obstruction) or from neoplastic diseases involving the spleen (eg, Hodgkins disease, lymphomas, myeloid metaplasia, leukemia) (Table 31–1).

About 60% of patients with cirrhosis develop splenomegaly and 15% develop hypersplenism. Splenomegaly is in part due to elevated portal pressures and "passive congestion," but other factors must be involved since splenic size does not correlate well with

Table 31–1. Causes of hypersplenism.

Splenic enlargement
Congestion (cirrhosis; portal or splenic vein obstruction)
Neoplasm (Hodgkin's disease, lymphoma, leukemia, myeloid metaplasia)
Inflammation (mononucleosis, subacute bacterial endocarditis, tuberculosis, malaria, sarcoid, systemic lupus erythematosus, Felty's syndrome)
Infiltration (histiocytosis, Gaucher's disease, Letterer-Siwe disease, amyloidosis)
Intrinsic defects of blood cells
Congenital hemolytic anemia (spherocytosis, thalassemia, pyruvate kinase deficiency, G6PD deficiency, elliptocytosis)
Immune destruction of blood cells
Acquired autoimmune hemolytic anemia (eg, methyldopa, lymphoproliferative disorders, systemic lupus erythematosus, bacterial infection)
Immunologic thrombocytopenic purpura (toxic or drug reaction, viral infection, systemic lupus erythematosus)
Thrombotic thrombocytopenic purpura

the level of portal pressure. Nevertheless, the size of the splenic artery and the magnitude of splenic arterial flow are proportionate to the splenic enlargement. The hypersplenism of cirrhosis is seldom of clinical significance; the anemia and thrombocytopenia are usually mild and rarely are indications for splenectomy.

If portal decompression is indicated for bleeding esophageal varices, selection of the type of shunt should be made without considering the presence of hypersplenism; any procedure that lowers the portal pressure tends to improve the thrombocytopenia and anemia and reduce the size of the spleen. It is rare for hypersplenism to develop after a successful portal-systemic shunt. In the rare case of portal hypertension caused by massive splenomegaly and huge splenic blood flow, splenectomy alone will cure the hypersplenism and portal hypertension.

Some cases of secondary hypersplenism are due to inflammatory diseases involving the spleen such as tuberculosis, malaria, brucellosis, and kala-azar (all uncommon in the USA) or mononucleosis, hepatitis, and subacute bacterial endocarditis. Boeck's sarcoid is complicated by splenomegaly in 25% of patients and secondary hypersplenism in about 5%. Patients with chronic rheumatoid arthritis may develop splenomegaly and neutropenia, an association known as **Felty's syndrome.** Systemic lupus erythematosus and the reticuloendothelioses (Gaucher's disease, Letterer-Siwe disease, etc) are other causes of reticuloendothelial hyperplasia, splenomegaly, and secondary hypersplenism.

Clinical Findings

A. Symptoms and Signs: The clinical findings depend largely on the underlying disorder. Manifestations of hypersplenism usually develop gradually, and the diagnosis often follows a routine physical or laboratory examination. Some patients experience left upper quadrant fullness or discomfort, which can be severe. Others have hematemesis due to gastroesophageal varices.

Purpura, bruising, and diffuse mucous membrane bleeding are unusual symptoms despite the presence of thrombocytopenia. Recurrent infections and chronic leg ulcers are sometimes seen in patients with Felty's syndrome and severe leukopenia.

B. Laboratory Findings: The normocytic normochromic anemia is usually only moderately severe. Hemoglobin values below 10 g/100 ml suggest one of the following complications: (1) chronic blood loss, usually from esophageal varices secondary to portal hypertension; (2) simultaneous hemolysis in the liver; (3) autoimmune hemolytic anemia; or (4) relative marrow failure (as in cirrhosis). Rarely, secondary folic acid deficiency and megaloblastic anemia may develop. If the patient has a primary condition such as myelofibrosis or thalassemia, the red cells have the characteristic morphologic abnormalities of these disorders. Despite the anemia, the total red cell mass may be normal or even increased, because so much blood is pooled in the big spleen. In some cases, expansion of

plasma volume is a factor aggravating the anemia. The reticulocyte count is usually slightly elevated. The white blood count is usually 2000–4000/μl but may be lower; the leukopenia is confined to the granulocytes, especially the polymorphonuclear cells, and some leftward shift is common. Platelet counts are usually about 100,000/μl but may fall to as low as 50,000/μl. The bone marrow shows varying degrees of generalized hyperplasia.

C. Evaluation of Splenic Size: Before it becomes palpable, an enlarged spleen may cause dullness to percussion above the left ninth intercostal space. Splenomegaly is manifested on supine x-rays of the abdomen by medial displacement of the stomach and downward displacement of the transverse colon and splenic flexure. Radioisotopic splenic scans using ^{51}Cr-tagged, heated red cells or ^{99m}Tc sulfur colloid are more accurate methods of demonstrating splenic size and of differentiating the spleen from other abdominal masses. Splenic arteriography, which will delineate the intrasplenic vasculature, is especially useful to identify mass lesions.

D. Evaluation of Splenic Function: Reduced red cell or platelet survival can be measured by labeling the patient's cells with ^{51}Cr and measuring the rate of disappearance of radioactivity from the blood. The spleen's role in producing the anemia or thrombocytopenia can be determined by measuring the ratio of radioactivity that accumulates in the liver and spleen during destruction of the tagged cells; a spleen/liver ratio greater than 2:1 indicates significant splenic pooling and suggests that splenectomy would be beneficial.

Differential Diagnosis

Leukemia and lymphoma are diagnosed by marrow aspiration, lymph node biopsy, and examination of the peripheral blood (white count and differential). In hereditary spherocytosis there are spherocytes, osmotic fragility is increased, and platelets and white cells are normal. The hemoglobinopathies with splenomegaly are differentiated on the basis of hemoglobin electrophoresis or the demonstration of an unstable hemoglobin. Thalassemia major becomes apparent in early childhood, and the blood smear morphology is characteristic. In myelofibrosis the bone marrow shows proliferation of fibroblasts and replacement of normal elements. In idiopathic thrombocytopenic purpura the spleen is normal or only slightly enlarged. In aplastic anemia the spleen is not enlarged and the marrow is fatty.

Treatment & Prognosis

The course, response to treatment, and prognosis of the hypersplenic syndromes differ widely depending on the underlying disease, whose treatment may cure the hypersplenism. For example, hypersplenism in malaria responds to antimalarial therapy. In some diseases, especially those involving immune reactions, corticosteroids are effective. In practice, most patients with hypersplenism are given a therapeutic trial of corticosteroids.

Table 31—2. Indications for splenectomy in hypersplenism.

(1) Primary hypersplenism (usually)
(2) Secondary hypersplenism
    (a) Depending upon the primary disease, the patient's medical status, and the prognosis.
    (b) Most cases of secondary hypersplenism with the following manifestations are an indication for splenectomy:
        (i) Major hemolysis with symptomatic anemia and need for transfusions.
        (ii) Marked neutropenia (< 1000 PMNs) with recurrent infections.
        (iii) Thrombocytopenia causing purpura or hemorrhage.
        (iv) Massive splenomegaly causing severe symptoms.

Table 31—3. Indications for splenectomy.

Splenectomy always indicated
  Splenic injury (common)
  Primary splenic tumor (rare)
  Splenic abscess (rare)
  Hereditary spherocytosis (congenital hemolytic anemia)
Splenectomy usually indicated
  Primary hypersplenism
  Chronic idiopathic thrombocytopenic purpura
Splenectomy sometimes indicated
  Autoimmune hemolytic disease
  Ovalocytosis with hemolysis
  Nonspherocytic congenital hemolytic anemias (eg, pyruvate kinase deficiency)
  Hemoglobin H disease
  Hodgkin's disease (for staging)
Splenectomy rarely indicated
  Chronic lymphatic leukemia
  Lymphosarcoma
  Hodgkin's disease (except for staging)
  Macroglobulinemia
  Myelofibrosis
  Thalassemia major
  Splenic artery aneurysm
  Sickle cell anemia
Splenectomy not indicated
  Asymptomatic hypersplenism
  Splenomegaly with infection
  Splenomegaly associated with elevated IgM
  Hereditary hemolytic anemia of moderate degree
  Acute leukemia
  Agranulocytosis

The indications for splenectomy in hypersplenism are listed in Table 31—2. Splenectomy should be performed for primary hypersplenism. In secondary hypersplenism, the severity and prognosis of the primary disease and the risk of surgery must be considered. Because the longer the hypersplenism is present the worse it gets (work hypertrophy), many hematologists believe that splenectomy should be performed early in the course of the illness rather than waiting for the clinical manifestations to become severe. Splenectomy will decrease transfusion requirements, decrease the incidence and number of infections, prevent hemorrhage, and reduce pain.

Splenectomy may not be necessary when the hypersplenism is mild (Table 31—3). Operation is also contraindicated in the following diseases where it has been shown to have no therapeutic benefit: acute leukemia, agranulocytosis, paroxysmal nocturnal hemoglobinuria, and Wiscott-Aldrich syndrome. In sickle cell anemia, splenectomy is rarely necessary because in most patients autosplenectomy has occurred by age 10.

Some of the best results have followed splenectomy for Felty's syndrome, myeloid metaplasia, chronic malaria, and tuberculosis of the spleen. Less satisfactory results have been achieved in thalassemia major, sickle cell anemia, and the secondary hypersplenism of lymphoma and the leukemias.

The course of congestive splenomegaly due to portal hypertension depends upon the degree of venous obstruction and liver damage. Without hematemesis, the course may be relatively benign and splenectomy may not be necessary.

Amorosi EL: Hypersplenism. Semin Hematol 2:249, 1965.

Aster RH: Pooling of platelets in the spleen: Role in the pathogenesis of thrombocytopenia. J Clin Invest 45:645, 1966.

Breitfeld V & others: Pathology of the spleen in hematologic disease. Surg Clin North Am 55:233, 1975.

Christensen BE: Pathophysiology of "hypersplenism syndrome." Scand J Haematol 11:5, 1973.

Crosby WH: Splenectomy in hematologic disorders. N Engl J Med 286:1252, 1972.

Dameshek HL & others: Hematologic indications for splenectomy. Surg Clin North Am 55:253, 1975.

Ellis LD & others: The dilemma of hypersplenism. Surg Clin North Am 55:277, 1975.

Felix WR & others: The effect of portacaval shunt on hypersplenism. Surg Gynecol Obstet 139:899, 1974.

Gomes MMR & others: Indications for splenectomy in hematologic disease. Surg Gynecol Obstet 125:106, 1967.

Gritlin N & others: Splenic blood flow and resistance in patients before and after portacaval anastomosis. Gastroenterology 59:208, 1970.

Herrmann RE & others: Splenectomy for the diagnosis of splenomegaly. Ann Surg 168:896, 1968.

Hypersplenism: Medical Staff Conference, University of California School of Medicine San Francisco. Calif Med 118:24, Jan 1973.

Jacob HS: Hypersplenism: Mechanisms and management. Br J Haematol 27:1, 1974.

Jandl JH & others: Increased splenic pooling and the pathogenesis of hypersplenism. Am J Med Sci 253:383, 1967.

McGarity WC & others: Brucellosis: Indications for splenectomy. Am J Surg 115:355, 1968.

Riley SM & others: Role of splenectomy in Felty's syndrome. Am J Surg 130:51, 1975.

Witte CL & others: Splenic circulatory dynamics in congestive splenomegaly. Gastroenterology 67:498, 1974.

HYPERSPLENIC DISORDERS POTENTIALLY AMENABLE TO SPLENECTOMY

1. HEREDITARY SPHEROCYTOSIS

Essentials of Diagnosis

- Malaise, abdominal discomfort.
- Jaundice, anemia, splenomegaly.
- Spherocytosis, increased osmotic fragility of red cells, negative Coombs test.

General Considerations

Hereditary spherocytosis (congenital hemolytic jaundice, familial hemolytic anemia), the commonest congenital hemolytic anemia, is transmitted as an autosomal dominant trait. The basic defect is increased permeability of the red cell membrane to Na^+. This produces small, dense, round red cells with increased osmotic fragility and a rigid nondeformable shape. The lack of deformability delays the cells as they pass through the normal gaps and channels in the splenic pulp, resulting in glucose and ATP deprivation, damage to the red cell membranes, and, finally, membrane fragmentation and cell disruption. Significant cell destruction occurs only in the presence of the spleen.

The condition is seen in all races but is more frequent in whites than in blacks. When discovered early in infancy, it may resemble hemolytic disease of the newborn due to ABO incompatibility. Occasionally the diagnosis is not made until later in adult life, but the highest incidence is in the first 3 decades.

Clinical Findings

A. Symptoms and Signs: The principal manifestations are splenomegaly and mild to moderate anemia and jaundice. The patient may complain of easy fatigability. The spleen is almost always enlarged and may cause fullness and discomfort in the left upper quadrant. However, most patients are diagnosed during a family survey at a time when they are asymptomatic.

Periodic exacerbations of hemolysis can occur. The rare hypoplastic crises, which often follow acute viral illnesses, may be associated with profound anemia, headache, nausea, abdominal pain, pancytopenia, and hypoactive marrow.

B. Laboratory Findings: The red cell count (3–4 million/μl) and hemoglobin (9–12 g/100 ml) are moderately reduced. Some of the asymptomatic patients detected by family surveys have normal red cell counts when first seen. The red cells are small (MCV = 70–80 fl) and hyperchromic (MCHC = 36–40%). Spherocytes in varying numbers, sizes, and shapes are seen on a Wright-stained smear. The reticulocyte count is increased to 5–20%.

The indirect serum bilirubin and stool urobilinogen are usually elevated, and serum haptoglobin is usually decreased to absent. The Coombs test is negative. Osmotic fragility is increased; hemolysis of 5–10% of cells may be observed at saline concentrations of 0.6%. Occasionally, the osmotic fragility is normal but the incubated fragility test (defibrinated blood incubated at 37 C for 24 hours) will show increased hemolysis. Autohemolysis of defibrinated blood incubated under sterile conditions for 48 hours is usually greatly increased (10–20%, compared to a normal value of less than 5%). The addition of 10% glucose before incubation will decrease the abnormal osmotic fragility and autohemolysis. Infusion of the patient's own blood labeled with ^{51}Cr shows a greatly shortened red cell life span and sequestration in the spleen. Normal red cells labeled with ^{51}Cr have a normal life span when transfused into a spherocytotic patient, indicating that splenic function is normal.

Differential Diagnosis

At present there is no pathognomonic test for hereditary spherocytosis. Spherocytes in large numbers may occur in autoimmune hemolytic anemias, in which osmotic fragility and autohemolysis may be increased but are usually not improved by incubation with glucose. The positive Coombs test, negative family history, and sharply reduced survival of normal donor red cells are diagnostic of autoimmune hemolysis. Spherocytes are also seen in hemoglobin C disease, in some alcoholics, and in some cases of severe burns.

Complications

Pigment gallstones occur in about 85% of adults with spherocytosis but are uncommon under age 10. On the other hand, gallstones in a child should suggest congenital spherocytosis.

Chronic, usually bilateral leg ulcers unrelated to varicosities are a rare complication but, when present, will heal only after the spleen is removed.

Treatment

Splenectomy is the sole treatment for hereditary spherocytosis and is indicated even when the anemia is fully compensated and the patient is asymptomatic. The longer the hemolytic process persists, the greater the potential risk of complications such as hypoplastic crises and cholelithiasis. When there is associated cholelithiasis, splenectomy should precede cholecystectomy unless both procedures are performed during the same laparotomy (the most common approach). Unless the clinical manifestations are severe, splenectomy should be delayed in children until the fourth or fifth year of life to avoid the risk of increased infection due to loss of reticuloendothelial function. At operation, the gallbladder should be inspected for stones and accessory spleens should be sought.

Prognosis

Splenectomy cures the anemia and jaundice in all patients. The membrane abnormality, spherocytosis, and increased osmotic fragility persist, but red cell life span becomes almost normal. An overlooked accessory spleen is an occasional cause of failure of splenectomy. The presence of Howell-Jolly bodies in red cells makes the presence of accessory spleens unlikely.

Chapman RG: Red cell life span after splenectomy in hereditary spherocytosis. J Clin Invest 47:2263, 1968.

Jacob HS: Hereditary spherocytosis: A disease of the red cell membrane. Semin Hematol 2:139, 1965.

Lawrie GM & others: The surgical treatment of hereditary spherocytosis. Surg Gynecol Obstet 139:208, 1974.

Macpherson AS & others: The role of the spleen in congenital spherocytosis. Am J Med 50:35, 1971.

Mayman D & others: Hereditary spherocytosis: The metabolism of erythrocytes in the peripheral blood and in the splenic pulp. Br J Haematol 27:201, 1974.

2. HEREDITARY NONSPHEROCYTIC HEMOLYTIC ANEMIA

This is a heterogeneous group of rare hemolytic anemias caused by inherited intrinsic red cell defects. Included in the group are pyruvate kinase (PK) deficiency and glucose-6-phosphate dehydrogenase (G6PD) deficiency. They are usually manifested in early childhood with anemia, jaundice, reticulocytosis, erythroid hyperplasia of the marrow, and normal osmotic fragility. As with other hemolytic anemias, there may be associated cholelithiasis.

Multiple blood transfusions are often required. Splenectomy, while not curative, may ameliorate some of these conditions, especially pyruvate kinase deficiency.

DeGruchy GC & others: The non-spherocytic congenital hemolytic anemias. Br J Haematol 23 [Suppl]:19, 1972.

Nathan DG & others: Life-span and organ sequestration of the red cells in pyruvate-kinase deficiency. N Engl J Med 278:73, 1968.

Valentine WN: Hereditary hemolytic anemias associated with specific erythrocyte enzymopathies. West J Med 108:280, 1968.

THALASSEMIA MAJOR
(Mediterranean Anemia; Cooley's Anemia)

In this autosomal dominant disorder a structural defect in one of the globin chains of the hemoglobin molecule produces abnormal red cells (eg, target cells). Heterozygotes usually have mild anemia (thalassemia minor); however, starting early in infancy, homozygotes have severe chronic anemia accompanied by jaundice, hepatosplenomegaly (often massive), retarded body growth, and enlargement of the head. The peripheral blood smear reveals target cells, nucleated red cells, and a hypochromic microcytic anemia. Gallstones are present in about 25% of patients. A characteristic feature is the persistence of fetal hemoglobin (Hb F).

Splenectomy is helpful in some patients by reducing hemolysis and transfusion requirements and by removing an enlarged, uncomfortable spleen.

Nathan D: Thalassemia. N Engl J Med 286:586, 1972.

Orkin SH & others: The thalassemias. N Engl J Med 295:710, 1976.

4. HEREDITARY ELLIPTOCYTOSIS

This familial disorder, also known as ovalocytosis, is usually of little clinical significance. Normally, up to 15% oval or elliptical red blood cells can be seen on peripheral blood smear. In elliptocytosis, at least 25% and up to 90% of circulating erythrocytes are elliptical. As with hereditary spherocytosis, an abnormally permeable red cell membrane is responsible for the abnormal shape and the increased splenic destruction.

Most affected individuals are asymptomatic; about 10% have clinical manifestations consisting of moderate anemia, slight jaundice, and a palpable spleen.

Symptomatic patients should have splenectomy, and cholecystectomy if gallstones are present. The red cell defect persists after splenectomy, but the hemolysis and anemia are cured.

Cutting HO & others: Autosomal dominant hemolytic anemia characterized by ovalocytosis. Am J Med 39:21, 1965.

Lipton EL: Elliptocytosis with hemolytic anemia: The effects of splenectomy. Pediatrics 15:67, 1955.

ACQUIRED HEMOLYTIC ANEMIA

Essentials of Diagnosis

- Fatigue, pallor, jaundice.
- Splenomegaly.
- Persistent anemia and reticulocytosis.
- Positive Coombs test.

General Considerations

Nonhereditary hemolytic anemias can be acquired during life by exposure to a variety of chemicals, drugs, bacteria, and physical agents. Administration of high doses of penicillin, quinidine, and methyldopa has been implicated in many cases. In fact, about 20% of patients treated with methyldopa develop a positive Coombs test, though only 2% of these develop hemolytic anemia. The mechanism responsible for the hemolysis is not clear since most of the antibodies are hemagglutinins rather than hemolysins, but it is thought that the immunologically altered red cells are trapped in the reticuloendothelial system, including the spleen. Treatment includes removal of the offending agent, administration of corticosteroids, and blood transfusions.

When patients develop antibodies to their own red cells, the condition is called **autoimmune hemolytic anemia**. The antibodies are thought to be produced in the spleen. Both warm and cold antibodies have been described. Only the hemolytic anemia associated with warm antibodies (IgG) requires splenectomy; patients with cold (nongamma or complement) antibody usually do not respond to splenectomy. Autoimmune hemolytic anemia may be associated with other diseases, especially lymphoproliferative disorders and collagen vascular diseases (eg, systemic lupus erythematosus).

Hemolysis without demonstrable antibody (Coombs test negative) can develop in uremia, cirrhosis, cancer, and certain bacterial infections.

Clinical Findings

A. Symptoms and Signs: Autoimmune hemolytic anemia may be encountered at any age but is most common after age 50; it occurs twice as often in women. The onset is usually acute, consisting of anemia, mild jaundice, and sometimes fever. The spleen is palpably enlarged in over 50% of patients, and pigment gallstones are present in about 25%. Rarely, a sudden severe onset produces hemoglobinuria, renal tubular necrosis, and a 40–50% mortality rate.

B. Laboratory Findings: Hemolytic anemia is diagnosed by demonstrating a normocytic normochromic anemia, reticulocytosis (over 10%), erythroid hyperplasia of the marrow, and elevation of serum indirect bilirubin. Stool urobilinogen may be greatly increased, but there is no bile in the urine. Serum haptoglobin is usually low or absent. The direct Coombs test is positive because the patient's red cells are coated with immunoglobulins or complement (or both).

Treatment

Associated diseases must be carefully sought and appropriately treated. Corticosteroids produce a remission in about 75% of patients, but only 25% of remissions are permanent. Transfusion should be avoided as far as possible since cross-matching may be extremely difficult, requiring washed red cells and saline-active antisera.

Splenectomy is indicated for patients who fail to respond to 4–6 weeks of high-dose corticosteroid therapy, for patients who relapse after an initial response when steroids are withdrawn, and for patients in whom steroid therapy is contraindicated (eg, those with active pulmonary tuberculosis). Patients who require chronic high-dose steroid therapy should also be considered for splenectomy since the risks of long-term steroid administration are substantial.

Splenectomy is effective because it removes a site of hemolytic antibody production as well as the principal site of red cell destruction. Occasionally, splenectomy discloses the presence of an underlying disorder such as lymphoma. [51]Cr red cell survival and splenic sequestration studies should be performed preoperatively. A spleen/liver sequestration ratio of more than 2:1 usually implies a favorable response. Complete clinical remission is achieved following splenectomy in about 50% of unselected cases and in 80% of cases with significant splenic sequestration.

Prognosis

Relapses may occur after splenectomy but are less frequent if the initial response was good. The ultimate prognosis in the secondary cases depends upon the underlying disorder.

Allgood JW & others: Idiopathic acquired autoimmune hemolytic anemia. Am J Med 43:254, 1967.

Dacie JV: Autoimmune hemolytic anemias. Br Med J 2:381, 1970.

Garratty G, Petz LD: Drug-induced hemolytic anemia. Am J Med 58:398, 1975.

Goldberg A & others: Radiochromium in the selection of patients with hemolytic anemia for splenectomy. Lancet 1:109, 1966.

IMMUNOLOGIC THROMBOCYTOPENIC PURPURA
(Idiopathic Thrombocytopenic Purpura, ITP)

Essentials of Diagnosis

- Petechiae, ecchymoses, epistaxis, easy bruising.
- No splenomegaly.
- Decreased platelet count, prolonged bleeding time, poor clot retraction, normal coagulation time.

General Considerations

ITP is a hemorrhagic syndrome with diverse causes characterized by marked reduction in the number of circulating platelets, abundant megakaryocytes in the bone marrow, and a shortened platelet life span. It may be idiopathic or secondary to a lymphoproliferative disorder, drugs or toxins, bacterial or viral infection (especially in children), systemic lupus erythematosus, or other conditions. Thrombocytopenia with no apparent cause is termed idiopathic.

Whether the disorder is primary or secondary, the pathogenesis involves a circulatory antiplatelet factor (ie, antibody) which leads to increased platelet destruction in the reticuloendothelial system, predominantly the spleen. Normal platelets are rapidly destroyed when transfused to patients with ITP. The rate of platelet destruction determines the magnitude of thrombocytopenia and increased megakaryocyte production. Most patients, especially those with chronic ITP, also have platelet-agglutinating and complement-fixing antibodies. Splenomegaly, present in only 2% of cases, generally is a manifestation of an underlying disorder such as lymphoma or systemic lupus erythematosus. Radioactivity rapidly increases over the spleen and liver following infusion of ^{51}Cr-tagged platelets to patients with ITP.

Clinical Findings

A. Symptoms and Signs: The onset may be acute, with ecchymoses or showers of petechiae, accompanied by one or more of the following (in order of frequency): bleeding gums (with blood blisters), vaginal bleeding, gastrointestinal bleeding, and hematuria. CNS bleeding occurs in 3% of patients. The acute form is most common in children, usually occurring before 8 years of age, and often begins 1–3 weeks after a viral upper respiratory illness.

The chronic form, which may start at any age, is 3 times more common in women. It characteristically has an insidious onset, often with a long history of easy bruisability and menorrhagia. Showers of petechiae may occur, especially over pressure areas. Cyclic remissions and exacerbations may continue for several years, but the platelet count is always one-third to one-half normal.

B. Laboratory Findings: The platelet count is moderately to severely decreased (always below 100,000/μl), and platelets may be absent from the peripheral blood smear. Although white and red cell counts are usually normal, iron deficiency anemia may be present as a result of bleeding. The bone marrow shows increased numbers of abnormal megakaryocytes not surrounded by platelets.

The bleeding time is prolonged, capillary fragility (Rumpel-Leede test) greatly increased, and clot retraction poor. PTT, PT, and coagulation time are normal. Normal ^{51}Cr-labeled platelets transfused into patients with ITP manifest a shortened survival (normal = 10 days; ITP = 1–3 days) and splenic sequestration.

Differential Diagnosis

Other causes of nonimmunologic thrombocytopenia must be ruled out, such as leukemia, aplastic anemia, and macroglobulinemia. Thrombocytopenia and purpura may be caused by ineffective thrombocytopoiesis (eg, pernicious anemia, preleukemic states) or by nonimmune platelet destruction (eg, septicemia, disseminated intravascular coagulation, or other causes of hypersplenism). Bone marrow and platelet survival studies will usually not identify the cause of a destructive thrombocytopenia. The diagnosis of the immune variety of ITP is usually made by exclusion since tests for specific antibodies are not generally available except for some drug-induced immune purpuras (eg, quinidine, penicillin).

Treatment

The treatment of ITP depends on the age of the patient, the severity of the disease, the duration of the thrombocytopenia, and the clinical variant. Secondary immune thrombocytopenias are best managed by treating the underlying primary disorder (eg, if it is drug-induced, the drug should be stopped).

Patients with mild or no symptoms need no specific therapy but should avoid contact sports, elective surgery, and all unessential medications. Corticosteroids are indicated in patients with moderate to severe purpura of short duration. Steroids increase the platelet count in 75% of cases, which will avert the danger of severe hemorrhage. Usually, 40 mg/day of prednisone (or equivalent) are required. This dosage is continued until the platelet count returns to normal

and then is gradually tapered after 4–6 weeks. Corticosteroids produce sustained remissions in about 20% of adults.

Splenectomy is indicated for patients who do not respond to corticosteroids, for those who relapse after an initial remission on steroids, and for those whose disease has lasted for more than 1 year. Corticosteroid therapy is not necessary in the immediate preoperative period unless bleeding is severe or the patient was receiving steroids before the operation. Intracranial bleeding is an indication for emergency splenectomy.

Splenectomy produces a sustained remission in about 70% of patients. As with corticosteroids, success rates are better with acute than chronic ITP. The platelet count rises promptly following splenectomy (eg, it may double in 24 hours) and reaches a peak after 1–2 weeks. If the platelet count remains elevated after 2 months, the patient can be considered cured. Occasionally, the platelet count reaches 1–2 million/μl. Although this is generally considered to be harmless and not an indication for anticoagulation, some recommend the administration of anti-platelet aggregating agents (eg, aspirin). When corticosteroids and splenectomy have failed, immunosuppressive drugs (azathioprine, vincristine) will achieve a remission in 25% of cases.

Prognosis

Acute ITP in children under 16 years of age has an excellent prognosis; approximately 80% of patients have a complete and permanent spontaneous remission. This occurs in only 25% of adults. Splenectomy is successful in about 85% of patients, but more often in idiopathic cases than those secondary to another disorder.

Baldini M: Idiopathic thrombocytopenic purpura. N Engl J Med 274:1245, 1966.

Baldini M: Idiopathic thrombocytopenic purpura and the ITP syndrome. Med Clin North Am 56:47, 1972.

Bergin JJ & others: Compelling splenectomy in medically comprised patients. Ann Surg 178:761, 1973.

Block GE & others: Splenectomy for idiopathic thrombocytopenic purpura. Arch Surg 92:484, 1966.

Harker LA: Thrombokinetics in idiopathic thrombocytopenic purpura. Br J Haematol 19:95, 1970.

Harker LA & others: Thrombokinetics in man. J Clin Invest 48:963, 1969.

Karpatkin S: Autoimmune thrombocytopenic purpura. Am J Med Sci 261:127, 1971.

MacPherson AI & others: Planned splenectomy in the treatment of idiopathic thrombocytopenic purpura. Br Med J 1:64, 1975.

Ries CA & others: Cr[51] platelet kinetics in thrombocytopenia: Correlation between splenic sequestration of platelets and response to splenectomy. Ann Intern Med 80:702, 1974.

THROMBOTIC THROMBOCYTOPENIC PURPURA (TTP)

Thrombotic thrombocytopenic purpura is an acute, usually fatal disease of short duration with a pentad of clinical features: (1) fever, (2) thrombocytopenic purpura, (3) hemolytic anemia, (4) neurologic manifestations, and (5) renal failure. The cause is unknown, but autoimmunity has been implicated. It is most common between ages 10 and 40.

The thrombocytopenia is probably due to shortened platelet life span. The microangiopathic hemolytic anemia is produced by passage of red cells over damaged small blood vessels containing fibrin strands. Rigid red cells are trapped and fragmented in the spleen, whereas those that escape the spleen may be more vulnerable to damage and destruction in the abnormal microvasculature. Frequently the anemia is severe and may be aggravated by hemorrhage secondary to thrombocytopenia.

Neurologic manifestations, due to involvement of small cerebral vessels, are frequent and tend to fluctuate rapidly. Cerebral infarction is rare, but intracerebral hemorrhage is a common cause of death. Renal dysfunction is manifested by proteinuria, gross or microscopic hematuria, and elevated BUN and serum creatinine. Acute renal failure is common. Microinfarctions in the pancreas and gastrointestinal tract commonly cause abdominal pain. Hepatomegaly and splenomegaly occur in 35% of cases.

The clinical diagnosis can only be confirmed by biopsy, which shows a characteristic histologic vascular lesion located at arteriolocapillary junctions consisting of subintimal deposition of PAS-positive material, hyaline thrombi, and vessel wall weakening, leading to aneurysmal dilatations. The lesions are widespread and may be seen in muscle, skin, bone marrow, kidney, and lymph nodes. The diagnosis is most easily made by bedside biopsy of the gingiva.

Prognosis & Treatment

About two-thirds of patients are dead within 3 months of onset, usually from renal failure or intracerebral hemorrhage.

There have been reports of remissions and recoveries following heparin, dextran, corticosteroids, fibrinolytic agents, dipyridamole, aspirin, antimetabolites, or splenectomy, but term survival rate is less than 10% with any form of treatment. The best results follow combination therapy with corticosteroids in high doses (1200 mg/day hydrocortisone sodium succinate [Solu-Cortef] or equivalent), dextran 70, and prompt splenectomy.

Amorosi EL & others: Thrombotic thrombocytopenic purpura: Report of 16 cases and review of the literature. Medicine 45:139, 1966.

Bernard RP & others: Splenectomy for thrombotic thrombocytopenic purpura. Ann Surg 169:616, 1969.

Cuttner J: Splenectomy, steroids, and dextran 70 in thrombotic thrombocytopenic purpura. JAMA 227:397, 1974.

Goldenfarb PB & others: Thrombotic thrombocytopenic purpura: A ten-year survey. JAMA 226:644, 1973.

Hill JB & others: Thrombotic thrombocytopenic purpura: Treatment with corticosteroids and splenectomy. Arch Intern Med 122:353, 1968.

AGNOGENIC MYELOID METAPLASIA

Agnogenic myeloid metaplasia is a myeloproliferative disorder of unknown cause ("agnogenic") that is closely related to myelofibrosis, polycythemia vera, and myelogenous leukemia. It is characterized by moderate to massive splenomegaly, leukoerythroblastic blood reaction, and hypocellularity and fibrosis of the bone marrow.

Pathologically, the bone marrow is almost completely replaced by fibrous tissue, although in some cases the marrow is hyperplastic and fibrosis is minimal. Extramedullary hematopoiesis develops mainly in the spleen, liver, and long bones. Symptoms are attributable to anemia—weakness, fatigue, dyspnea; and to splenomegaly—abdominal fullness and pain, which may be severe. Spontaneous bleeding, secondary infection, bone pain, and a hypermetabolic state are frequent. Portal hypertension develops in some cases, due to fibrosis of the liver, greatly increased splenic blood flow, or both.

Hepatomegaly is present in 75% and splenomegaly in 100% of cases. Striking changes are seen in the peripheral blood. Red cells vary greatly in size and shape and many are distorted and fragmented. The white count is usually high (20–50 thousand/μl). The platelet count may be elevated, but values less than 100,000/μl are seen in 30% of cases. Secondary hypersplenism is common and may lead to thrombocytopenia and hemolytic anemia. It was once incorrectly thought that the spleen performed a crucial function of extramedullary hematopoiesis in this disease and that splenectomy could be lethal. In fact, many patients with myeloid metaplasia feel better if the massive spleen is removed, and their hypersplenism is often corrected.

About 30% of patients are asymptomatic at the time of initial diagnosis and require no therapy. When anemia and splenomegaly produce symptoms, transfusions, androgenic steroids, antimetabolites, and radiation therapy are indicated. Splenectomy is indicated for the following: (1) major hemolysis unresponsive to medical management, (2) severe symptoms from massive splenomegaly, (3) life-threatening thrombocytopenia, and (4) portal hypertension with variceal hemorrhage. This is one of the rare occasions when portal hypertension can be cured by splenectomy.

Splenectomy in myeloid metaplasia is associated with a 13% mortality rate and frequent complications, but operation gives better long-term survival than medical management. For unknown reasons, women have fewer complications and live longer following splenectomy than men. A prospective clinical trial comparing splenectomy early in the disease to medical therapy is now being conducted. The high operative mortality rate of splenectomy in the past was at least partly related to overlong delay in performing the operation.

Gomes MR & others: Splenectomy for myeloid metaplasia. Surg Gynecol Obstet 125:106, 1967.

Silverstein MN: *Agnogenic Myeloid Metaplasia.* Publishing Sciences Group, 1975.

Silverstein MN & others: Sex, splenectomy, and myeloid metaplasia. JAMA 227:424, 1974.

ANEURYSM OF THE SPLENIC ARTERY

Splenic artery aneurysm is uncommon even though this is the second most frequent abdominal artery to undergo aneurysmal change. It occurs twice as often in women as in men. The patients can be divided into 2 groups: (1) elderly people whose aneurysms are manifestations of atherosclerosis and (2) young women with apparently congenital aneurysms which have a predilection for rupture during pregnancy, perhaps related to hormonal and hemodynamic changes of pregnancy. Portal hypertension and splenomegaly may be associated with some cases, and inflammatory processes involving the vessel wall (eg, pancreatitis) occasionally lead to aneurysm. These lesions are usually asymptomatic and noted on abdominal x-rays as an eggshell rim of calcification in the left upper quadrant. Sometimes they are responsible for pain, nausea, and vomiting. Symptoms suggest impending rupture, and splenectomy with ligation of the splenic artery is indicated.

When a calcified atherosclerotic aneurysm is discovered in a patient over age 60, surgical excision is not indicated in the absence of symptoms or splenic enlargement. In younger patients, aneurysmectomy and splenectomy are advisable to prevent rupture. Sudden intra-abdominal hemorrhage during pregnancy suggests rupture of the splenic artery and calls for prompt laparotomy. The aneurysm is usually found within several centimeters of the hilus of the spleen. Control of bleeding followed by excision of the aneurysm and splenectomy is the treatment of choice.

Moore SW & others: Splenic artery aneurysms. Ann Surg 153:1033, 1961.

Stanley JC & others: Splanchnic artery aneurysms. Arch Surg 101:689, 1970.

Westcott JL & others: Aneurysms of the splenic artery. Surg Gynecol Obstet 136:541, 1973.

CYSTS & TUMORS OF THE SPLEEN

Parasitic cysts are almost always echinococcal (see Chapter 11). They may be asymptomatic, but usually the patient notices splenomegaly. Calcification of the cyst wall may be seen on x-ray. Eosinophilia may be found and serologic tests may confirm the diagnosis. The treatment of choice is splenectomy.

Other cysts are dermoid, epidermoid, endothelial, and pseudocysts. The latter are thought to be the result of infarction or delayed splenic rupture from previous trauma. Splenectomy is indicated to exclude the presence of a primary tumor or other rare causes of splenomegaly.

The rare primary tumors of the spleen include lymphoma, sarcoma, hemangioma, and hamartoma. These lesions are usually asymptomatic until splenomegaly causes abdominal discomfort or a palpable mass. The benign vascular tumors of the spleen (angiomas) can produce hypersplenism because the spleen functions as an arteriovenous shunt. Spontaneous rupture with massive hemorrhage can occur. Splenectomy is indicated if the tumor appears to be limited to the spleen.

The spleen is a common site for metastases in advanced malignancies, especially of the lung and breast. Splenic metastases are common autopsy findings but are rarely clinically significant.

Ahmann DL & others: Malignant lymphoma of the spleen. Cancer 19:461, 1966.

Asbury GF: Calcified pseudocysts of the spleen. Arch Surg 76:148, 1958.

O'Brien PH & others: Splenectomy for hypersplenism in malignant lymphoma. Arch Surg 101:348, 1970.

Skarin AT & others: Lymphosarcoma of the spleen. Arch Intern Med 127:259, 1971.

ABSCESS OF THE SPLEEN

Splenic abscesses are uncommon but are important because the mortality rate is so high. They may be caused by hematogenous seeding of the spleen with bacteria from remote sepsis, by direct spread of infection from adjacent structures, or by splenic trauma resulting in a secondarily infected splenic hematoma. In 80% of cases one or more abscesses exist in organs other than the spleen, and the splenic abscess develops as a terminal manifestation of uncontrolled sepsis of other organs. In some patients, unexplained sepsis, progressive splenic enlargement, and abdominal pain are the presenting manifestations. The spleen may not be palpable because of left upper quadrant tenderness and guarding. Many of these abscesses are solitary and potentially curable. Splenic scans or arteriograms should be performed on all suspected cases. The finding of gas in the spleen on plain abdominal x-ray is pathognomonic of splenic abscess.

Most splenic abscesses remain localized, periodically seeding the blood stream with bacteria, but spontaneous rupture and peritonitis may occur. Splenectomy is essential for cure if sepsis is localized to the spleen. Splenotomy and drainage are indicated rarely for large complicated abscesses when splenectomy would be technically hazardous.

Chulay JD, Lankerani MR: Splenic abscess. Am J Med 61:513, 1976.
Gadacz T & others: Changing clinical spectrum of splenic abscess. Am J Surg 128:182, 1974.

ACCESSORY & ECTOPIC SPLEEN

Ectopic spleen (wandering spleen) is an unusual condition in which a long splenic pedicle allows the spleen to move about the abdomen. The mass can be identified as spleen by radionuclide scan. It often resides in the lower abdomen or pelvis, where even a normal-sized spleen can be felt as a mass. The condition is 13 times more common in women than men. Acute torsion of the pedicle occurs occasionally, necessitating emergency splenectomy.

Removal of pelvic spleens is recommended in all cases, especially in women of childbearing age to prevent splenic rupture by the enlarging uterus during pregnancy and to eliminate any chance of volvulus of the long splenic pedicle.

Accessory spleens are found in about 10% of routine postmortem autopsies. Ordinarily of no significance, they may play a role in the recurrence of certain hematologic disorders for which splenectomy was performed.

The majority of accessory spleens are located near the hilus of the spleen and the tail of the pancreas. They may display the same pathologic features as the main spleen, but this is not always the case. During splenectomy for hematologic diseases, accessory spleens should be sought and removed.

Appel MF & others: The surgical and hematologic significance of accessory spleens. Surg Gynecol Obstet 143:191, 1976.
Hatfield PM & others: Ectopic pelvic spleen. Arch Surg 111:603, 1976.

SPLENECTOMY FOR STAGING HODGKIN'S DISEASE

To plan curative radiation therapy of Hodgkin's disease, precise knowledge of the extent of the disease is essential, since the outcome depends to a significant degree upon the recognition and treatment of all sites of disease. At present, clinical assessment short of laparotomy cannot accurately estimate the extent of ab-dominal involvement. Lymphangiography to visualize the abdominal nodes has not proved to be reliable. At laparotomy, about 25% of patients who are clinically stage I or II are found to have unsuspected disease in the abdomen. The presence of splenic involvement changes the clinical stage from I or II to at least III. Laparotomy for staging is only indicated when the results may influence therapy; Hodgkin's disease involving bone marrow or viscera other than the spleen (stage IV) signifies diffuse disease that cannot be cured by x-ray and is an indication for chemotherapy.

Staging laparotomy involves splenectomy, liver biopsy, and thorough abdominal exploration with generous biopsy of periaortic lymph nodes and any others that appear abnormal on lymphangiogram or by gross inspection. Metallic clips placed next to involved nodes at the time of surgery will aid the radiation therapist. In addition to the diagnostic information obtained, removal of the spleen improves tolerance to chemotherapy. Radiation injury to the left kidney and lung is avoided because the spleen need not be irradiated. Inadvertent radiation castration in females can be avoided if oophoropexy is performed at the time of staging laparotomy.

Enright LP & others: The surgical diagnosis of abdominal Hodgkin's disease. Surg Gynecol Obstet 130:853, 1970.
Glatstein E & others: Surgical staging of abdominal involvement in unselected patients with Hodgkin's disease. Radiology 97:425, 1970.
Meeker SR & others: Critical evaluation of laparotomy and splenectomy in Hodgkin's disease. Arch Surg 104:222, 1972.
O'Connel & others: Staging laparotomy in Hodgkin's disease. Am J Med 57:36, 1974.
Paglia MA & others: Surgical aspects and results of laparotomy and splenectomy in Hodgkin's disease. Am J Roentgenol 117:44, 1972.

RUPTURE OF THE SPLEEN

Essentials of Diagnosis

- Trauma to the abdomen or flank; often a fractured rib on the left.
- Abdominal pain and tenderness.
- Pain in the left shoulder or left side of the neck.
- Tachycardia.
- Anemia or hypotension.

General Considerations

Disruption of the parenchyma, capsule, or blood supply of the spleen is termed rupture. It is the most common indication for splenectomy and the most common major injury from blunt abdominal trauma.

The spleen may be ruptured by penetrating, nonpenetrating, or operative thoracic or abdominal trauma, or it may rupture spontaneously. Even trivial trauma has been reported to cause splenic rupture. The spleen is highly vascular but friable and bleeds profusely when injured.

Most penetrating abdominal injuries are obvious, and surgical exploration is routine; if a splenic rupture is present it will be readily discovered. Penetrating thoracic injuries must penetrate the lung, pleura, and diaphragm before reaching the spleen.

Automobile accidents are the most common cause of blunt trauma to the spleen. With blunt injury the spleen may be fractured through the parenchyma and capsule, avulsed from its pedicle, or disrupted beneath an intact capsule to produce a subcapsular or contained hematoma. Approximately 5% of blunt injuries to the spleen result in **delayed rupture,** which begins as a subcapsular hematoma that grows and becomes manifest days to weeks later. Delayed splenic rupture is believed to evolve as follows: There is a minor rupture of the splenic pulp, but the lesion is either intraparenchymal, subcapsular, or contained within peritoneal folds. As the red cells disintegrate, the hematoma liquifies and increased osmolality of its contents attracts additional fluid. This leads to expansion of the cavity, secondary hemorrhage, and eventually rupture. It frequently produces sudden shock from profuse bleeding. Approximately 75% of delayed ruptures occur within 2 weeks of the initial injury, but in rare instances months or years may pass before secondary bleeding occurs. Some patients present with anemia and a left upper quadrant mass suggesting a retroperitoneal tumor.

Operative trauma to the spleen, which accounts for about 20% of splenectomies, is most common during upper abdominal operations on adjacent viscera (stomach, esophageal hiatus, vagus nerves, splenic flexure of the colon, etc). The usual mechanisms of injury are avulsion of the splenic capsule by traction on the peritoneal attachments and direct injury by a misplaced retractor.

The spleen may also rupture spontaneously (no antecedent trauma). Spontaneous rupture of a normal spleen is rare; it most frequently occurs in malaria, mononucleosis, lymphoma, leukemia, typhoid fever, and other conditions accompanied by an enlarged, diseased spleen. Spontaneous rupture is a rare complication of pregnancy and of oral anticoagulant therapy.

Deaths from splenic rupture may be attributed to delay in diagnosis and concomitant injuries. The diagnosis may be difficult even when suspected. Associated injuries are often present and may mask the physical signs. Abdominal pain and tenderness are usually present, but the peritoneal reaction to bleeding varies greatly and some patients will have minimal findings even when intraperitoneal bleeding is massive.

Clinical Findings

A. Symptoms and Signs: The clinical spectrum varies from severe hypovolemic shock to minimal or no symptoms. Most patients fall between these extremes. There is usually a history of a blow to the upper abdomen, particularly to the left flank, but the trauma may have seemed so trivial as to be overlooked by the patient. This is especially true in children. Most patients complain of generalized abdominal pain which is most severe in the left upper quadrant. About one-third of patients have pain confined to the left upper quadrant. Referred pain is often felt in the left shoulder or cervical region (Kehr's sign). This is a reliable indication of diaphragmatic irritation and can often be elicited by placing the patient in the Trendelenburg position or by palpation in the left upper quadrant. Mild nausea and vomiting may occur.

The abdominal findings are those of low-grade peritoneal irritation (ie, tenderness, mild spasm, and distention). The area of splenic dullness may be increased to percussion, or a mass may be palpable in the left upper quadrant. With marked bleeding, the abdomen may distend rapidly and the characteristic signs of acute blood loss (ie, tachycardia, hypotension, and shock) will appear. An important early diagnostic clue is tenderness over the ninth and tenth ribs on the left. A fractured rib in that area should arouse a strong suspicion of the possibility of a ruptured spleen. It occurs in about 20% of cases.

In doubtful cases, paracentesis is indicated to look for free intra-abdominal blood. The method and interpretation of this test are described in Chapter 51.

B. Laboratory Findings: With acute rupture, the initial hematocrit is usually normal, but serial determinations will show a fall. The leukocyte count is often increased to $15,000-20,000/\mu l$ with a shift to the left.

C. X-Ray Findings: Plain films of the abdomen may show fractured ribs or an enlarged spleen. The gastric air bubble may be displaced medially and the transverse colon inferiorly. A serrated appearance of the greater curvature of the stomach due to dissection of blood into the gastrosplenic ligament is a useful radiographic sign but is uncommon.

Technetium-sulfur colloid nuclide scans may demonstrate splenic enlargement and intraparenchymal hematomas and have the advantage of being noninvasive. Selective splenic arteriograms are helpful in doubtful cases and are particularly useful in evaluating for delayed rupture. Good quality films with multiple views should identify even small splenic injuries.

Treatment & Prognosis

Splenectomy is always indicated as soon as the diagnosis is made. Diagnostic laparotomy should be performed whenever splenic injury is strongly suspected. Small iatrogenic capsular tears can sometimes be successfully treated by application of a hemostatic agent such as microcrystalline collagen. The mortality rate of isolated splenic rupture is 10%; if there are other serious concomitant injuries, the mortality rate approaches 25%.

Awe WC & others: Selective angiography in splenic trauma. Am J Surg 126:171, 1973.

Benjamin CI & others: Delayed rupture or delayed diagnosis of rupture of the spleen. Surg Gynecol Obstet 142:171, 1976.

Burrington JD: Surgical repair of a ruptured spleen in children.

Arch Surg 112:417, 1977.

Lieberman RC & others: A study of 248 instances of traumatic rupture of the spleen. Surg Gynecol Obstet 127:961, 1968.

Lowenfels AB & others: Kehr's sign: A neglected aid in rupture of the spleen. N Engl J Med 274:1019, 1966.

Olsen WR, Polley TZ Jr: A second look at delayed splenic rupture. Arch Surg 112:422, 1977.

Olsen WR & others: Surgical injury to the spleen. Surg Gynecol Obstet 131:57, 1970.

Steele M & others: Advances in management of splenic injuries. Am J Surg 130:159, 1975.

SPLENOSIS

In splenosis, multiple small implants of splenic tissue grow in scattered areas on the peritoneal surfaces throughout the abdomen. They arise from dissemination and autotransplantation of splenic fragments following traumatic rupture of the spleen. Splenosis is usually an incidental finding discovered much later during laparotomy for an unrelated problem. However, the implants stimulate formation of adhesions and may be a cause of intestinal obstruction. They must be distinguished from peritoneal nodules of metastatic carcinoma and from accessory spleens. Histologically, they differ from accessory spleens by the absence of elastic or smooth muscle fibers in the delicate capsule.

Whether splenosis performs the functions of normal splenic tissue has not been settled, but aggressive attempts at surgical excision are probably not warranted.

Brewster DC: Splenosis: Report of two cases and review of the literature. Am J Surg 126:14, 1973.

Widmann WD & others: Splenosis: A disease or a beneficial condition? Arch Surg 102:152, 1971.

SPLENECTOMY

Preoperative preparation of patients undergoing elective splenectomy should correct coagulation abnormalities and deficits in red cell mass, treat infections, and control immune reactions. Because platelets are removed so rapidly from the circulation, they usually are not given for thrombocytopenia until after the splenic artery has been ligated. Antibodies in the patient's serum may complicate cross-matching of blood. Many patients require corticosteroid coverage in the perioperative period. For emergency splenectomy, hypovolemia should be corrected by whole blood transfusions.

Details of surgical technic are not within the scope of this text, but it should be noted that there are 2 methods of splenectomy (Fig 31–2). In one, primarily of value in traumatic rupture of the spleen, the organ is immediately mobilized and the splenic artery is secured from behind as it enters the hilus. In the other, of vital importance in the removal of massively enlarged spleens, the organ is left in situ. The gastrocolic ligament is opened and the splenic artery ligated as it courses along the upper edge of the pancreas. This permits blood to leave the spleen through the splenic vein while all other attachments (ie, the short gastric vessels and colic attachments) are divided before the spleen is delivered. This method permits the removal of massively enlarged vascular spleens with practically no loss of blood.

In elderly or cardiac patients, care must be taken that the large amount of blood trapped in the spleen does not overload the circulation when the splenic artery is ligated and the venous return is left intact.

Ballinger WF II & others: Splenectomy: Indications, technique, complications. Curr Probl Surg, Feb 1965.

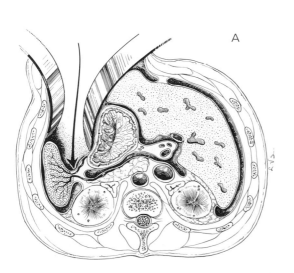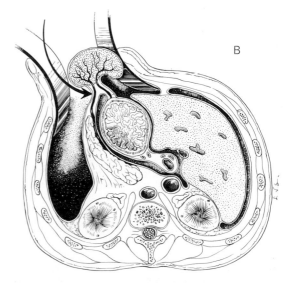

Figure 31–2. *A:* Anterior approach to splenic artery. *B:* Mobilization of spleen with posterior exposure of splenic artery.

Brooks DH: Surgery of the spleen. Surg Clin North Am 55:287, 1975.

Dunphy JE: Splenectomy for trauma. Am J Surg 71:450, 1946.

Kiesewetter WB: Pediatric splenectomy: Indications, technique, complications, and mortality. Surg Clin North Am 55:449, 1975.

Diamond LK: Splenectomy in childhood and the hazard of overwhelming infection. Pediatrics 43:886, 1969.

Dickerman JD: Bacterial infection and the asplenic host: A review. J Trauma 16:662, 1976.

McBride JA & others: The effect of splenectomy on the leukocyte count. Br J Haematol 14:225, 1968.

Pedersen B & others: On the late effects of removal of the normal spleen. Acta Chir Scand 131:89, 1966.

Swartz SL & others: Splenectomy for hematologic disorders. Curr Probl Surg, May 1971.

HEMATOLOGIC EFFECTS OF SPLENECTOMY

Because the spleen has no unique functions, its removal in a normal adult has few clinical consequences. Red cell count and indices do not change, but a few cells with cytoplasmic inclusions may appear, eg, Heinz bodies, Howell-Jolly bodies, and siderocytes. Postoperatively there is a temporary leukocytosis, predominantly involving an increase in lymphocytes. Platelets are usually increased, occasionally markedly so, and may stay at levels of $400-500,000/\mu l$ for over a year. A platelet count of over a million is not an indication for anticoagulants, but antiplatelet agents such as aspirin may help prevent thrombosis in this situation. Even more striking thrombocytosis (eg, $2-3$ million/μl) may develop after splenectomy for hemolytic anemia. These patients require no treatment.

Splenectomy can lead to temporary reduction in antibody production in adults but in young children under age 2 it has been associated with an increased frequency of severe infections, especially pneumococcal and meningococcal. The increased risk may correlate better with the type of disease than with the age of the patient, but, in general, splenectomy should be deferred until age 4 unless the hematologic problem is especially severe.

Crosby WH: Splenectomy in hematologic disorders. N Engl J Med 286:1252, 1972.

OTHER POSTSPLENECTOMY PROBLEMS

Complications related to splenectomy per se are relatively few, with atelectasis, pancreatitis, and postoperative hemorrhage being the most common. If splenectomy is done for thrombocytopenia, secondary bleeding may occur even though the platelet count usually rises promptly. Platelet transfusions should be given if primary hemostasis is abnormal (ie, oozing occurs) and the platelet count remains low. Thromboembolic complications may be more common following splenectomy, but this complication does not correlate positively with the degree of thrombocytosis.

Claret I & others: Immunological studies in the post-splenectomy syndrome. J Pediatr Surg 10:59, 1975.

Dickerman JD: Bacterial infection and the asplenic host: A review. J Trauma 16:662, 1976.

Hodam RP: The risk of splenectomy. A review of 310 cases. Am J Surg 119:709, 1970.

Naylor R & others: Morbidity and mortality from injuries to the spleen. J Trauma 14:773, 1974.

Schimpff SC & others: Infections in 92 splenectomized patients with Hodgkin's disease. A clinical review. Am J Med 59:695, 1975.

Steele M & others: Advances in management of splenic injuries. Am J Surg 130:159, 1975.

●   ●   ●

General References

Ballinger WF II, Erslev AJ: Splenectomy. Curr Probl Surg, Feb 1965.

Eraklis AJ, Filler RM: Splenectomy in childhood. J Pediatr Surg 7:382, 1972.

Fabri PJ & others: A quarter century with splenectomy. Arch Surg 108:569, 1974.

Harris JW, Kellermeyer RW: The Red Cell. Production, Metabolism, Destruction: Normal and Abnormal, revised ed. Harvard Univ Press, 1970.

Lennert K: The Spleen. Springer-Verlag, 1970.

Schwartz SI & others: Splenectomy for hematologic disorders. Curr Probl Surg, May 1971.

32 . . .
Appendix

J. Englebert Dunphy, MD

ANATOMY & PHYSIOLOGY

In infants, the appendix is a conical diverticulum at the apex of the cecum, but with differential growth and distention of the cecum the appendix ultimately arises on the left and dorsally approximately 2.5 cm (1 inch) below the ileocecal valve. The teniae of the colon converge at the base of the appendix, an arrangement which helps to locate this structure at operation.

The position of the appendix has important clinical implications (Fig 32–1). The appendix is fixed retrocecally in 16% of adults and is freely mobile in the remainder, so that precise location varies with distention and emptying of the cecum.

Agenesis of the appendix is rare and is sometimes associated with cecal hypoplasia. True double appendix and congenital diverticula are very rare but may be the site of acute inflammation.

The appendix is lined by columnar epithelium of the colonic type. Circular and longitudinal muscle layers are often deficient in some areas, allowing contiguity of submucosa and serosa—a fact of importance in appendiceal disease.

The appendix in youth is characterized by a large concentration of lymphoid follicles which appear 2 weeks after birth and number about 200 or more at age 15 years. Thereafter, there is progressive atrophy of lymphoid tissue, concomitant with fibrosis of the wall and partial or total obliteration of the lumen.

The function of the appendix is not known, but there is no justification for the notion that the human appendix is vestigial. Most of the lymphoid follicles of the large intestine are aggregated in the cecum in warm-blooded animals, and in a few vertebrates (including anthropoid apes and man) the lymphoid content of the colon is concentrated in the true cecal apex, the vermiform appendix.

If the appendix has a physiologic function, it is probably related to the presence of lymphoid follicles.

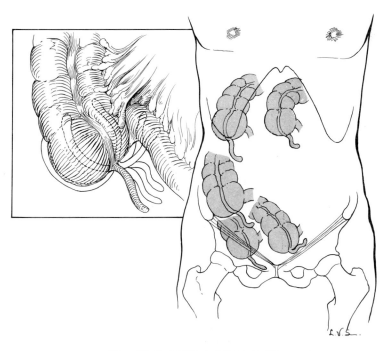

Figure 32–1. Positions of the appendix.

The avian bursa of Fabricius controls the development of peripheral lymphoid tissues such as spleen and lymph nodes, and defective immunoglobulin production results from destruction of the bursa of Fabricius in young fowl. The rabbit appendix histologically resembles the avian bursa, and neonatal appendectomy in rabbits impairs their later capacity to produce antibody to various antigens. However, reports of a statistical relationship between appendectomy and subsequent carcinoma of the colon and other neoplasms in man are not supported by controlled studies.

Berry JA: The true caecal apex, or the vermiform appendix: Its minute and comparative anatomy. J Anat Physiol 35:83, 1900.

Cooper MD & others: A mammalian equivalent of the avian bursa of Fabricius. Lancet 1:1388, 1966.

DeGaris CF: Topography and development of the cecum-appendix. Ann Surg 113:540, 1941.

Moertel CG & others: A prospective study of appendectomy and predisposition to cancer. Surg Gynecol Obstet 138:549, 1974.

ACUTE APPENDICITIS

Essentials of Diagnosis

- Abdominal pain.
- Anorexia, nausea and vomiting.
- Localized abdominal tenderness.
- Low-grade fever.
- Leukocytosis.

General Considerations

Approximately 7% of individuals in western countries develop appendicitis at some time during their lives, and about 200,000 appendectomies for acute appendicitis are performed annually in the USA. Acute appendicitis is uncommon in parts of Africa and Asia, perhaps because of the high-residue diet ingested by inhabitants of some less well developed countries. The ingestion of cellulose-depleted foods in affluent nations alters bacterial flora, slows fecal transit, and results in smaller, firmer, and more tenacious stools which require higher intraluminal pressures. These consequences of highly refined diets may contribute to the development of various colonic diseases, including appendicitis.

The word appendicitis was introduced by Reginald Fitz in 1886; previously, the cecum was thought to be the offending part, and the disorder was called typhlitis or perityphlitis.

According to the classic concept, the pathogenesis of acute appendicitis involves bacterial infection distal to obstruction of the lumen. In approximately 70% of acutely inflamed appendices, obstruction of the proximal lumen by fibrous bands, fecaliths, tumors, parasites, or foreign bodies can be demonstrated; in others, lymphoid hyperplasia in response to viral disease (eg, measles) may be the cause of obstruction. Intraluminal obstruction is not found in one-third of specimens, however, and external compression by bands or kinks has been postulated to explain these cases. Another possibility is that high intraluminal pressure in the cecum—again related to the low-residue diet of western man—might functionally obstruct the appendix and allow bacterial infection to develop. It has also been suggested that acute appendicitis may begin with mucosal ulceration, perhaps viral, followed by secondary bacterial invasion, ie, that obstruction is not always a factor in the pathogenesis of appendicitis.

As appendicitis progresses, the blood supply is impaired by bacterial infection in the wall and distention of the lumen by pus; gangrene and perforation occur at about 24 hours, although the timing is highly variable. Gangrene implies microscopic perforation and bacterial peritonitis (which may be localized by adhesions from nearby viscera).

Clinical Findings

Acute appendicitis has protean manifestations. It may simulate almost any other acute abdominal illness, and in turn may be mimicked by a variety of conditions. The surest route to accurate diagnosis is a careful history and a thorough, systematic physical examination as described in Chapter 24. Positive findings may be absent or minimal in the early stages, particularly in retrocecal, pelvic, and bizarre forms of appendicitis, and repeated physical examinations must be performed. Progression of symptoms and signs is the rule—in contrast to the fluctuating course of some other diseases in the differential diagnosis. Localized tenderness is the one essential physical finding that must be sought by precise one-finger palpation. Even in the very young and the elderly, sharply localized tenderness is the single most valuable finding.

A. Symptoms and Signs:

1. Classic appendicitis—Typically, the patient is awakened in the early morning by vague abdominal discomfort followed by slight nausea, anorexia, and indigestion. The pain is persistent and continuous, but not severe, with occasional mild epigastric cramps. There may be an episode of vomiting, and within several hours the pain shifts to the right lower quadrant, becoming rather sharply localized and causing discomfort on moving, walking, or coughing. The patient has a sense of being constipated and may feel that he should take a cathartic or an enema, but if he does he experiences no relief ("gas stoppage sign").

Examination at this point will show cough tenderness, sharply localized to the right lower quadrant. There will be well-localized tenderness to one-finger palpation and possibly very slight muscular rigidity. Rebound tenderness is classically referred to the same area. Peristalsis is normal or slightly reduced. Rectal and pelvic examinations are likely to be negative.

2. Retrocecal appendicitis—Poorly localized epigastric pain heralds the onset of this form of appendicitis also. "Gas stoppage" may be the dominant symptom. The patient is convinced he has eaten something that has disagreed with him and is apt to take a cathartic. Nausea and vomiting are mild. Because the retrocecal appendix is protected from the anterior abdominal wall, the pain remains poorly localized and the shift to the right lower quadrant may not occur. For similar reasons, the patient does not experience discomfort on walking or coughing. There may be mild diarrhea, and a retrocecal appendix lying adjacent to the ureter may cause urinary frequency or even hematuria.

Examination is deceptively unimpressive unless one-finger palpation is carried carefully into the flank, where tenderness is detected.

3. Pelvic appendicitis—Pelvic appendicitis simulates acute gastroenteritis. Pain is poorly localized. Nausea, vomiting, and diarrhea tend to be more prominent than in other forms of appendicitis. When the disease occurs during an epidemic of gastroenteritis, both the family and the physician are apt to assume that this is the diagnosis. Diarrhea is apt to continue because the inflamed appendix may lie against the pelvic colon.

Abdominal examination is essentially negative, and in the early phases both rectal and pelvic examinations may be negative. Fever is apt to be high—another misleading feature of this form of the disease. The key to diagnosis is the detection of tenderness by repeated examination of the rectum and pelvis.

If the diagnosis is not established early, signs of peritonitis ultimately supervene, with lower abdominal rigidity, distention, and diminished to absent peristalsis.

4. Retroileal appendicitis—If the appendix lies behind the ileum, symptoms and signs are similar to those of retrocecal appendicitis. Because of difficulty in making the diagnosis, retroileal appendicitis frequently proceeds to perforation and abscess formation with appearance of a mass before the nature of the illness is appreciated.

5. Obstructive appendicitis—Obstructive appendicitis is a clinical entity characterized by severe colicky pain. Complete obstruction and invasive infection lead to vascular occlusion. Gangrene develops rapidly, and appendiceal perforation occurs early in the course of the disease. The pain may be so severe that mesenteric vascular occlusion or small bowel obstruction is suspected.

6. Bizarre forms of appendicitis—The cecum may lie on the left side of the abdomen due to malrotation of the colon, and appendicitis may be mistaken for sigmoid diverticulitis. An inflamed appendix in the right upper quadrant may mimic acute cholecystitis or perforated ulcer. Even when the cecum is normally situated, a long appendix may reach to other parts of the abdomen, and acute appendicitis in these circumstances may be very confusing indeed.

7. Chronic appendicitis—Chronic recurrent abdominal pain is a significant clinical problem, and when the complaints are confined to the right lower quadrant the question of chronic appendicitis is usually raised. Occasionally it is clear that the patient has recurrent acute appendicitis. Barium x-rays are sometimes helpful, particularly in children. In many patients the diagnosis is not obvious. Appendectomy in these circumstances relieves symptoms occasionally, but, in general, laparotomy for chronic abdominal pain is unproductive in the absence of objective findings (eg, localized tenderness, palpable mass, leukocytosis).

B. Laboratory Findings: Moderate leukocytosis is characteristic of appendicitis. The leukocyte count is 14,000/μl on the average and is greater than 10,000/μl in 90% of patients. In three-fourths of patients, more than 75% neutrophils are found on differential white counts. It must be emphasized, however, that one patient in 10 with acute appendicitis has a leukocyte count indistinguishable from normal, and many have a normal differential cell count.

The urine is usually normal, but a few leukocytes and erythrocytes and occasionally even gross hematuria may be noted, particularly in retrocecal or pelvic appendicitis.

C. X-Ray Findings: Although acute appendicitis may be diagnosed without radiographic studies in most young patients, plain films of the abdomen may be of value in atypical cases or in very young or very old patients.

Localized air-fluid levels, localized ileus, or increased soft tissue density in the right lower quadrant is present in 50% of patients with early acute appendicitis. Positive radiologic signs become more frequent as appendicitis progresses. Less common findings are fecaliths, an altered right psoas shadow, or an abnormal right flank stripe.

Radiologic examination may be helpful in obscure cases by disclosing evidence of other diseases which may be mistaken for appendicitis, eg, perforated peptic ulcer. Abnormal position of the cecum is an important clue which is detected in abdominal films.

Differential Diagnosis

The diagnosis of acute appendicitis is particularly difficult in the very young and in the elderly. Infants manifest only lethargy, irritability, and anorexia in the early stages, but vomiting, fever, and pain are apparent as the disease progresses. Classic symptoms are seldom elicited in aged patients, and the diagnosis is often not considered by the examining physician. The course of appendicitis is more virulent in the elderly, and perforation occurs at an earlier stage. Other types of individuals presenting diagnostic problems include muscular males (in whom the only symptom may be the "gas stoppage sensation"), pregnant women, and patients recovering from recent abdominal operations. For these reasons, appendicitis should never be lower than second in the differential diagnosis of any acute abdominal condition.

The condition that is perhaps most commonly confused with appendicitis is vague gastrointestinal upset; in many cases, a specific diagnosis is never established.

A. Gastroenteritis: Gastroenteritis often simulates acute appendicitis. The differential diagnosis is especially challenging if gastroenteritis initiates inflammatory changes in appendiceal lymphoid follicles and evolves into true acute appendicitis. It is common to see a few cases of acute appendicitis in a college population in the midst of an epidemic of gastroenteritis. The history is important in differentiating these 2 conditions: In gastroenteritis, nausea, vomiting, or diarrhea often precedes the onset of pain, whereas pain is virtually always the initial symptom in acute appendicitis. Diffuse myalgias, photophobia, headache, etc may suggest a viral illness. On physical examination, tenderness is less sharply localized than in acute appendicitis.

Mesenteric lymphadenitis in children and young adults is often a diagnostic problem (see Chapter 33).

Enterocolitis caused by salmonella or yersinia may simulate appendicitis as with gastroenteritis. The history and physical signs provide the best guide to a correct diagnosis.

B. Female Pelvic Disorders:

1. A ruptured ovarian follicle in a young woman (mittelschmerz) may mimic acute appendicitis. A careful history usually indicates sudden onset of pain in the middle of the menstrual cycle. The pain is most severe initially and gradually subsides thereafter—a sequence not likely to occur in appendicitis. Gastrointestinal symptoms are less prominent than in appendicitis, but sharply localized right lower quadrant tenderness may be quite misleading. These patients seldom appear ill but at times a differential diagnosis is impossible and operation becomes safer than risking delay.

2. Pelvic inflammatory disease (specifically, acute salpingitis) often masquerades as appendicitis. Fever tends to be higher in salpingitis and abdominal tenderness is more diffuse, but the patient does not appear acutely ill. By the time high fever and diffuse tenderness complicate appendicitis, the disease is far advanced and the patient is in desperate straits. Pelvic examination reveals a tender cervix, and demonstration of intracellular gram-negative diplococci in cervical smears clinches the diagnosis of salpingitis.

3. Twisted ovarian cyst is difficult to distinguish from acute pelvic appendicitis. Pain is severe, abdominal findings may be typical of appendicitis, and the ovarian mass may not be felt on pelvic examination because tenderness is exquisite. The cyst may be palpated by repeating the pelvic examination under anesthesia, and the appropriate incision can then be made for its removal.

4. Ectopic pregnancy may be distinguished from appendicitis by the history of menstrual irregularity, sudden onset of pain, and diffuse pelvic tenderness. Pain may be referred to the shoulder because of free blood in the peritoneal cavity, and on occasion there are signs of hypovolemic shock. Bloody fluid is usually obtained by culdocentesis.

C. Genitourinary Diseases:

1. Ureteral or renal calculi can produce right lower quadrant pain, nausea, and vomiting suggestive of retrocecal or pelvic appendicitis. A history of colicky pain radiating into the groin, findings on urinalysis, and a plain film of the abdomen often clarify the diagnosis, but an intravenous urogram is frequently required.

2. Pyelonephritis, with or without renal calculi, is also confused with appendicitis. High fever and chills are common with renal infection but infrequent in acute appendicitis. Costovertebral angle tenderness and pyuria establish the diagnosis.

D. Other Acute Surgical Emergencies: A variety of acute surgical emergencies such as perforated ulcer, acute cholecystitis, pancreatitis, diverticulitis, intestinal obstruction, Meckel's diverticulitis, and perforated carcinoma of the colon may simulate appendicitis. Differential diagnosis is discussed separately under each of these conditions. Acute regional enteritis, a nonsurgical condition, may be difficult to distinguish from appendicitis (see Chapter 33).

An additional word about Meckel's diverticulitis is appropriate at this point. Whenever right lower quadrant pain simulating appendicitis is associated with signs of mechanical small bowel obstruction, the possibility of Meckel's diverticulitis should be entertained. The point of maximal tenderness is more medial than in classic appendicitis, but the differential diagnosis may be impossible. If the appendix is found to be normal during an operation for appendicitis, the surgeon must search for Meckel's diverticulum.

E. Systemic Diseases: Any condition producing diaphragmatic irritation (eg, pneumonia) may cause right-sided abdominal pain. Connective tissue diseases which have vasculitis as a prominent feature may present with abdominal pain, and some of these patients require abdominal operation. Nonsurgical disorders associated with abdominal pain and peritoneal signs are discussed in the section on peritonitis (Chapter 25).

Complications

The complications of acute appendicitis include perforation, peritonitis, abscess, and pylephlebitis.

A. Perforation: It is unusual for the acutely inflamed appendix to perforate within the first 12 hours, although cathartics or enemas may cause perforation at an earlier stage. Perforation may relieve pain temporarily, but the signs of advancing peritonitis are soon apparent.

The consequences of perforation vary from generalized peritonitis to formation of a tiny abscess which may not appreciably alter the symptoms and signs of appendicitis.

B. Peritonitis: Localized peritonitis results from microscopic perforation of a gangrenous appendix, while spreading or generalized peritonitis usually implies gross perforation into the free peritoneal cavity. Increasing tenderness and rigidity, abdominal distention, and adynamic ileus are obvious in patients with peritonitis. High fever and severe toxicity mark progression of this catastrophic illness in untreated patients. Peritonitis is discussed in Chapter 25.

C. Abscess: Localized perforation of the appendix leads to formation of an appendiceal abscess which is protected from the free peritoneal cavity by omentum or loops of small bowel. In retrocecal or retroileal appendicitis, an abscess is walled off by adjacent structures. If perforation is not contained, abscesses may form in any part of the peritoneal cavity.

Fever, pain, ileus, and sometimes a palpable mass are manifestations of an intraperitoneal abscess. When pus collects in the pelvis, diarrhea is a common symptom, and rectal examination discloses tenderness and fullness in the pouch of Douglas. A pelvic abscess may resorb spontaneously, may perforate into the rectum or other neighboring viscus, or may enlarge and require surgical drainage per rectum or vagina.

Subphrenic abscess is most often seen following generalized peritonitis, but retrocecal appendicitis in particular can cause subphrenic abscess in the absence of generalized peritoneal contamination. The management of subphrenic abscess is discussed in Chapter 25.

Postoperative abscesses are a significant problem. Intraperitoneal abscesses may occur anywhere but most commonly are near the surgical incision. Wound abscesses develop in 5% of primarily closed incisions after removal of an acutely inflamed appendix. If the appendix has perforated, the incidence of wound infection is greater than 30%. When skin and subcutaneous tissues are left open and the wound allowed to close by secondary intention, the rate of wound infection can be reduced to 5%. Delayed primary closure has not been effective in preventing wound infection following perforated appendicitis.

D. Pylephlebitis: Pylephlebitis is suppurative thrombophlebitis of the portal venous system. Chills, high fever, low-grade jaundice, and, later, hepatic abscesses are the hallmarks of this grave condition, which fortunately is rare today. The appearance of shaking chills in a patient with acute appendicitis indicates bacteremia and demands vigorous antibiotic therapy to prevent the development of pylephlebitis.

In fulminating pylephlebitis, the portal venous system may be filled with gas from anaerobic organisms, a highly fatal complication. Clinical findings may not reflect the gravity of this condition, but air within the portal venous system demonstrated on x-ray is diagnostic.

Treatment

With few exceptions, the treatment of appendicitis is surgical. Early cases of acute appendicitis occasionally subside spontaneously or with the aid of antibiotics, but nonoperative treatment of acute appendicitis should be reserved for rare instances when adequate anesthesia or a competent surgeon is not available.

Some patients presenting late in the course of appendicitis with a palpable right lower quadrant mass and no signs of spreading peritonitis may be managed expectantly. If the mass is a phlegmon, it may resolve on antibiotic therapy; more often, a clearly defined abscess is ready to be drained after a few days. In some patients with appendiceal abscess, appendectomy is deferred for several weeks after the abscess is drained (interval appendectomy).

A. Preoperative Management: Antibiotics should be withheld in early cases of abdominal pain of uncertain cause lest clinical signs be suppressed and the diagnosis obscured. Furthermore, antibiotic therapy can mask developing complications of appendicitis until the situation becomes critical. Intravenous antibiotics are indicated in patients with known perforation, abscess, or peritonitis.

Analgesics may blunt the physical findings but seldom obscure entirely the signs of progressive peritoneal irritation. When pain is severe and the diagnosis is uncertain, analgesics or sedatives may actually assist in clarifying the issue. This is particularly true when the differential diagnosis lies between appendicitis and renal colic.

Preoperative fluid therapy usually is not required in adults with early acute appendicitis, although infants must be given special attention in this regard. In advanced appendicitis with peritonitis, however, resuscitation of the patient before operation is absolutely mandatory. No matter how skillfully performed, appendectomy in a hypovolemic and hyperpyrexic patient may be fatal. Several hours are needed to replenish a severely dehydrated patient with intravenous crystalloid or colloid solutions; the volumes administered should be titrated to the patient's requirements rather than administered according to some arbitrary formula. Skin turgor, perfusion of peripheral tissues, cardiovascular signs, and urinary output are guides to adequate resuscitation. Hyperpyrexia, particularly in children, must be treated before induction of anesthesia; this is best accomplished by external cooling on a hypothermic blanket.

A nasogastric tube should be inserted upon admission to the emergency ward and before initiation of diagnostic studies if there is any question of peritonitis, ileus, or obstruction. Nasogastric suction decompresses the stomach and prevents further distention.

B. Anesthesia: Spinal anesthesia may be used, but most surgeons prefer general anesthesia.

C. Examination Under Anesthesia: After induction of anesthesia, the surgeon should carefully repeat the abdominal, pelvic, and rectal examinations, particularly if there is doubt about the diagnosis. An ovarian cyst may be palpated in the female, or a mass indicative of carcinoma of the colon may be delineated. Such findings alter placement of the incision.

D. Operation:

1. Incision—In most cases of appendicitis, an oblique muscle-splitting incision of the type shown in Fig 32-2A should be employed. An oblique incision enables the surgeon to deal with lesions in the pelvis, and it can be carried into the flank or across the rectus muscle to permit a more extensive procedure, such as resection of the right colon. A right rectus incision enters the free peritoneal cavity, and the surgeon must work from there into an area of sepsis, resulting in greater morbidity than with the oblique incision.

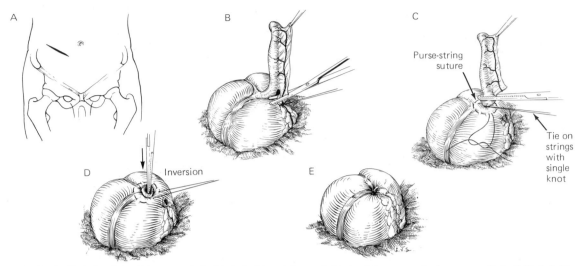

Figure 32–2. Technic of appendectomy. *A:* Incision. *B:* After delivery of the tip of the cecum, the mesoappendix is divided. *C:* The base is clamped and ligated with a simple throw of the knot. *D:* A clamp is placed to hold the knot during inversion with a purse-string suture of fine silk. *E:* The loosely tied inner knot on the stump assures that there is no closed space for the development of a stump abscess.

When the appendix is normal and the acute disease process is located in the upper abdomen, the appendectomy incision should be closed and a separate incision made. Whether the appendix should be removed or not depends upon the circumstances. In the presence of established peritonitis due to some other cause, appendectomy should not be done.

2. Operative approach—The technical approach to the appendix is illustrated in Fig 32–2. The appendix usually can be delivered into the incision. The mesentery is divided between clamps, and the base of the appendix is crushed with a clamp, ligated, and inverted into the cecum. The ligature at the base of the appendix should be of fine, plain catgut and should be tied (as shown) with only one throw on the knot before inversion. With this technic, spillage is avoided but an abscess of the appendiceal stump cannot occur because the loose closure with a fine absorbable ligature permits free communication of the inverted stump with the lumen of the cecum.

If the appendix is retrocecal or retroileal, it is often preferable to divide it, invert the stump, and remove the appendix in a retrograde fashion. Alternatively, the cecum may be mobilized prior to excision of the appendix. Although the initial incision may be kept quite small in favorable cases, the surgeon should never hesitate to enlarge the incision in either direction to provide better exposure.

If the appendix is acutely inflamed and there is local infection of the peritoneal cavity, no attempt is made to explore the rest of the abdomen. If the appendix is normal or the diagnosis is uncertain, the pelvic viscera and the distal small bowel should be inspected.

After removal of the appendix and inversion of the stump, any fluid should be aspirated from the operative field. Extensive contamination warrants the use of peritoneal irrigation with antibiotics such as kanamycin. Before closure, patency of the ileocecal valve should be ascertained, and the mesoappendix should be checked for secure hemostasis.

The peritoneal cavity should be drained if a well-defined abscess is encountered or if there is so much local necrotic material that an abscess seems likely to form. Drainage of the retroperitoneum is advisable in cases of retrocecal appendicitis with gangrene or perforation because the retroperitoneum is more vulnerable to progressive infection than is the peritoneal cavity. Generalized peritonitis or free fluid resembling pus is not an indication for peritoneal drainage.

Closure of the incision should be accomplished in layers. Whenever there is gross contamination—or if the appendix is gangrenous or perforated—the subcutaneous tissue and skin should be left open. Delayed primary closure is not indicated as the small oblique incision closes very rapidly with minimal scarring. Moreover, if there has been gross contamination, delayed primary closure often results in infection. Closure of skin with paper tapes instead of sutures has been shown to cause fewer wound infections in patients with early appendicitis.

E. Postoperative Management: Minimal care is required following appendectomy for simple acute appendicitis. Excessive intravenous fluid administration should be avoided during the first few hours, since bladder distention and catheterization may culminate in chronic urinary tract infection. Bowel function resumes rapidly. Most patients are ready for discharge on the fourth or fifth day.

The postoperative care of patients with advanced appendicitis involves intensive management of peritonitis and ileus. See discussion of complications of peritonitis in Chapter 25 for details of management.

Prognosis

Although a mortality rate of zero is theoretically attainable in acute appendicitis, 40 children per year died of appendicitis in England during the period 1963–1967, and a similar incidence of tragic outcomes is reported in the USA. The mortality rate in simple acute appendicitis is approximately 0.1% and has not changed significantly since 1930. Progress in pre- and postoperative care—particularly the emphasis on fluid resuscitation before operation, has reduced the mortality rate from perforation to about 5%. Despite declining mortality rates, postoperative infections still occur in 30–50% of patients with gangrenous or perforated appendices. Although most of these patients survive, there are many near fatalities which require lengthy hospitalization and exact an enormous toll from the patient and his family.

Further reduction of morbidity and mortality rates from appendicitis clearly rests with prevention of perforation. The greatest need for improvement lies in the diagnosis of appendicitis in young children and the elderly; in both of these groups, the incidence of perforation reaches 75% or higher. Delay by patient or parent may be unavoidable, but failure on the part of physicians to recognize the disease is disturbing. In one series of children with perforated appendices, 40% had been seen by a physician who failed to appreciate the nature of the process before perforation.

In order to minimize the incidence of perforation, it is necessary to remove a certain number of normal appendices in patients with acute illnesses suggesting appendicitis. In early cases in which the diagnosis is in doubt, repeated careful reappraisal of the progress of symptoms and signs will avoid unnecessary operations without increasing the risk of perforation. The incidence of normal appendices removed should be about 15%.

Ackerman NB: The continuing problems of perforated appendicitis. Surg Gynecol Obstet 139:29, 1974.

Bartlett RH & others: Appendicitis in infancy. Surg Gynecol Obstet 130:99, 1970.

Burkitt DP: The aetiology of appendicitis. Br J Surg 58:695, 1971.

Butsch DW & others: Recurrent appendicitis. Postgrad Med 54:132, Oct 1973.

Gilmore OJA: Prevention of wound infection after appendectomy. Lancet 1:220, 1973.

Howie JGR: The place of appendicectomy in the treatment of young adult patients with possible appendicitis. Lancet 1:1365, 1968.

Jona JZ & others: Barium enema as a diagnostic aid in children with abdominal pain. Surg Gynecol Obstet 144:351, 1977.

Law D, Law R, Eiseman B: The continuing challenge of acute and perforated appendicitis. Am J Surg 131:533, 1976.

Lewis FR & others: Appendicitis: A critical review of diagnosis and treatment in 1,000 cases. Arch Surg 110:677, 1975.

Magarey CJ & others: Peritoneal drainage and systemic antibiotics after appendicectomy: A prospective trial. Lancet 2:179, 1971.

Rothman DL: Diagnostic laparotomy for fever or abdominal pain of unknown origin. Am J Surg 133:273, 1977.

Sisson RG & others: Superficial mucosal ulceration and the pathogenesis of acute appendicitis. Am J Surg 122:378, 1971.

Soter CS: The contribution of the radiologist to the diagnosis of acute appendicitis. Semin Roentgenol 8:375, 1973.

Stone HH & others: Perforated appendicitis in children. Surgery 69:673, 1971.

Thomford NR & others: Appendectomy during pregnancy. Surg Gynecol Obstet 129:489, 1969.

TUMORS OF THE APPENDIX

Benign tumors, including carcinoids, were found in 4.6% of 71,000 human appendix specimens examined microscopically. Benign neoplasms may arise from any cellular element and are usually incidental findings. Occasionally, a neoplasm obstructs the appendiceal lumen and produces acute appendicitis. No treatment other than appendectomy is indicated.

Malignant Tumors

Primary malignant tumors were found in 1.4% of appendices in the same large series. Carcinoid and argentaffin tumors comprise the majority of appendiceal malignancies, and the appendix is the commonest location of carcinoid tumors of the gastrointestinal tract. The biologic behavior of carcinoids arising in the appendix is usually benign; tumors greater than 2 cm in diameter are rare, and although local invasion of the appendiceal wall is observed in 25% of cases, only 3% metastasize to lymph nodes and only isolated reports of hepatic metastases and the carcinoid syndrome have appeared. Appendectomy is adequate therapy unless the lymph nodes are obviously involved, the tumor is greater than 2 cm in diameter, or the base of the cecum is invaded. Right hemicolectomy is the treatment of choice for these more advanced lesions.

Adenocarcinoma of the colonic type can arise in the appendix and spread rapidly to regional lymph nodes or implant on ovaries or other peritoneal surfaces. Ten percent of patients have widespread metastases when first seen. Adenocarcinoma is virtually never diagnosed preoperatively; about half present as acute appendicitis, and 15% have formed appendiceal abscesses. Right hemicolectomy should be performed if disease is localized to the appendix and regional lymph nodes. The 5-year survival rate is 63% after right hemicolectomy and only 20% after appendectomy alone, but the latter group includes patients with distant metastases at the time of diagnosis.

Mucocele

Mucocele of the appendix is a cystic, dilated appendix filled with mucin. Simple mucocele is not a neoplasm and results from chronic obstruction of the proximal lumen, usually by fibrous tissue. If the appendiceal contents distally are sterile, mucous cells continue to secrete until distention of the lumen thins the wall and interferes with nutrition of the lining cells; histologically, simple mucocele is lined by flattened, cuboidal epithelium or no epithelium at all. Simple mucocele is cured by appendectomy.

Less commonly, mucocele is caused by a neoplasm—cystadenoma, or adenocarcinoma grade 1 in the older terminology. This lesion may arise de novo or (perhaps) in a preceding simple mucocele. In cystadenoma, the lumen is filled with mucin but the wall is lined by columnar epithelium with papillary projections. Tumor does not infiltrate the appendiceal wall and does not metastasize, although it may recur locally after appendectomy. Cystadenoma is believed to undergo malignant change in some instances. Appendectomy is adequate treatment.

Pseudomyxoma Peritonei

Pseudomyxoma peritonei is a rare disorder characterized by the presence of mucinous material and epithelial cells within the free peritoneal cavity. This lesion usually arises from an ovarian neoplasm, but in some females (and in most men) it originates in the appendix. This disorder is discussed further in Chapter 25.

Bernhardt H, Young JM: Mucocele and pseudomyxoma peritonei of appendiceal origin: Clinicopathologic aspects. Am J Surg 109:235, 1965.

Collins DC: 71,000 human appendix specimens: A final report, summarizing forty years' study. Am J Proctol 14:365, 1963.

Flint FB & others: Adenocarcinoma of the appendix. Am J Surg 120:707, 1970.

Hesketh KT: The management of primary adenocarcinoma of the vermiform appendix. Gut 4:158, 1963.

Melcher DH, Rayan AS: Columnar-cell (non-carcinoid) tumors of the appendix. Br J Surg 55:693, 1968.

Ponka JL: Carcinoid tumors of the appendix. Am J Surg 126:77, 1973.

Wolff M, Ahmed N: Epithelial neoplasms of the vermiform appendix (exclusive of carcinoid). I. Adenocarcinoma of the appendix. II. Cystadenomas, papillary adenomas and adenomatous polyps of the appendix. (2 parts.) Cancer 37:2493, 2511, 1976.

●　　●　　●

General References

Brunn H: Acute pelvic appendicitis. Surg Gynecol Obstet 63:583, 1936.

Fitz RH: Perforating inflammation of the vermiform appendix, with special reference to its early diagnosis and treatment. Am J Med Sci 92:321, 1866.

Law D, Law R, Eiseman B: The continuing challenge of acute and perforated appendicitis. Am J Surg 131:533, 1976.

Lewis FR: Appendicitis: A critical review of diagnosis and treatment in 1000 cases. Arch Surg 110:677, 1975.

Moertel CG & others: A prospective study of appendectomy and predisposition to cancer. Surg Gynecol Obstet 138:549, 1974.

Talbert JL, Zuidema GD: Appendicitis: A reappraisal of an old problem. Surg Clin North Am 46:1101, 1966.

33...
Small Intestine

Theodore R. Schrock, MD

The small intestine is the portion of the alimentary tract extending from the pylorus to the cecum. The structure, function, and diseases of the duodenum are discussed in Chapter 26; the jejunum and ileum are described in the present chapter.

ANATOMY

Macroscopic Anatomy

The length of the small intestine from the ligament of Treitz to the ileocecal valve depends upon the method of measurement. Values obtained during abdominal operations or in autopsy specimens average about 660 cm (22 feet). Indirect measurements in connection with intestinal intubation suggest that the small bowel is only 240 cm (8 feet) long. The greater length is probably more accurate.

The upper two-fifths of the small intestine distal to the duodenum are termed the **jejunum** and the lower three-fifths the **ileum**. There is no sharp demarcation between the jejunum and the ileum; however, as the intestine proceeds distally, the lumen narrows, the mesenteric vascular arcades become more complex, and the circular mucosal folds become shorter and fewer in number (Fig 33–1). In general, the jejunum resides in the left side of the peritoneal cavity and the ileum occupies the pelvis and right lower quadrant.

The small bowel is attached to the posterior abdominal wall by the mesentery, a reflection from the posterior parietal peritoneum. This peritoneal fold arises along a line originating just to the left of the midline and passing obliquely to the right lower quadrant. Although the mesentery joins the intestine along one side, the peritoneal layer of the mesentery envelops the bowel and is called the visceral peritoneum or serosa.

The mesentery contains fat, blood vessels, lymphatics, lymph nodes, and nerves. The arterial blood supply to the jejunum and ileum derives from the superior mesenteric artery. Branches within the mesentery anastomose to form arcades (Fig 33–1), and small straight arteries travel from these arcades to enter the mesenteric border of the gut. It is important to note that the antimesenteric border of the intestinal wall is less richly supplied with arterial blood than the mesenteric side. When blood flow is impaired, the antimesenteric border becomes ischemic first. Venous blood from the small intestine drains into the superior mesenteric vein and then enters the liver through the portal vein.

Submucosal lymphoid aggregates (Peyer's patches) are much more numerous in the ileum than in the jejunum. Lymphatic channels within the mesentery drain through regional lymph nodes at several levels and terminate in the cisterna chyli.

Parasympathetic nerves from the right vagus and sympathetic fibers from the greater and lesser splanch-

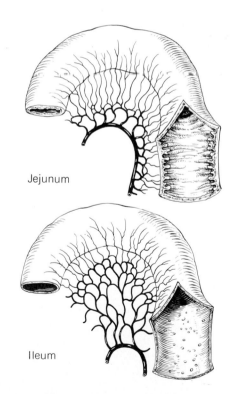

Jejunum

Ileum

Figure 33–1. Blood supply and luminal surface of the small bowel. The arterial arcades of the small intestine increase from 1–2 in the proximal jejunum to 4–5 in the distal ileum, a finding which helps to distinguish proximal from distal bowel at operation. Plicae circulares are more prominent in the jejunum.

nic nerves reach the small intestine through the mesentery. Both types of autonomic nerves contain efferent and afferent fibers, but intestinal pain appears to be mediated by the sympathetic afferents only.

Microscopic Anatomy

The wall of the small intestine consists of 4 layers: mucosa, submucosa, muscularis, and serosa.

A. Mucosa: The absorptive surface of the mucosa is multiplied by convolutions and projections at macroscopic, microscopic, and ultrastructural levels. Visible to the naked eye are circular mucosal folds termed plicae circulares (valvulae conniventes), which project into the lumen; they are taller and more numerous in the proximal jejunum than in the distal ileum (Fig 33–1). On the surface of the plicae circulares are delicate villi less than 1 mm in height, each containing a central lacteal, a small artery and vein, and fibers from the muscularis mucosae which lend contractility to the villus. Villi are in turn covered by columnar epithelial cells which have a brush border consisting of microvilli 1 μm in height (Fig 33–2). The presence of villi multiplies the absorptive surface about 8 times, and microvilli increase it another 14–24 times; the total absorptive area of the small intestine is 200–500 sq m.

The columnar epithelial cells are responsible for absorption; they probably play an important role in digestion as well, since digestive enzymes are present in high concentrations in the brush border. Mucus-secreting goblet cells are also found in villi. The "M" (microfold) cells, which lack microvilli, overlie lymphoid follicles and may have a transport function for antigens or immunoglobulins.

The crypts of Lieberkühn are situated between villi (Fig 33–3). Undifferentiated cells in the crypts are continually proliferating; some of the cells produced remain undifferentiated, but others become columnar cells and migrate to the tips of villi over a 3- to 7-day period, and still others differentiate to form new goblet cells. The mean life span of small intestinal cells in man is 5–6 days. Paneth granular cells and argentaffin (enterochromaffin) cells are present in crypts; Paneth cells may have a phagocytic function.

B. Other Layers: The submucosa is a fibroelastic layer containing blood vessels and nerves. Submucosa is the strongest component of bowel wall and must be included in intestinal sutures. The muscularis consists of an inner circular layer and an outer longitudinal coat of smooth muscle. The serosa is the outermost covering of the intestine.

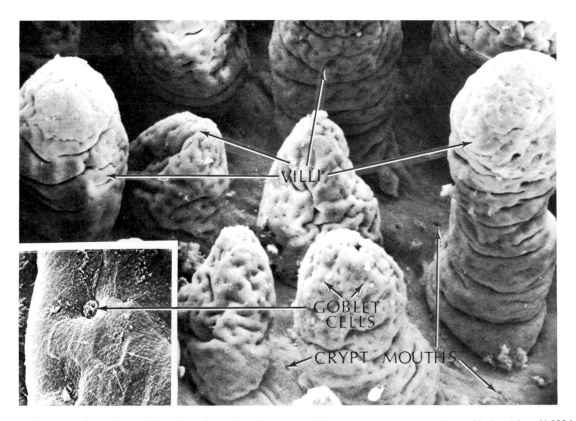

Figure 33–2. Scanning electron microscopic photo of small intestinal villi from the human terminal ileum. (Reduced from × 320.) *Inset:* Detail of a villous surface showing a mucus-filled goblet cell surrounded by polygonal absorptive epithelial cells. (Reduced from × 2100.) Epithelial cell borders are visible (white arrows). The pebbled epithelial cell surface represents closely packed microvilli seen end-on. (Courtesy of Robert L. Owen, MD, and Albert L. Jones, MD.)

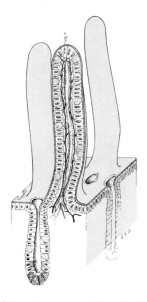

Figure 33—3. Schematic representation of villi and crypts of Lieberkühn. Villus is covered with columnar and goblet cells, and desquamating epithelial cells are seen at the tip. Lamina propria of villus contains an arteriole, a venule, a central lacteal, and muscular fibers. The crypt contains Paneth cells and argentaffin cells at its base and mitotic cells which are responsible for epithelial renewal.

Backman L, Hallberg D: Small-intestinal length: An intraoperative study in obesity. Acta Chir Scand 140:57, 1974.

Marsh MN, Swift JA: A study of the small intestinal mucosa using the scanning electron microscope. Gut 10:940, 1969.

Rodning CB, Wilson ID, Erlandsen SL: Immunoglobulins within human small-intestinal Paneth cells. Lancet 1:984, 1976.

PHYSIOLOGY

The principal function of the small intestine is absorption, and a great many physiologic and biochemical mechanisms are integrated to meet this objective. The endocrine function of the small intestine is discussed in Chapters 26 and 30.

Motility

The most important type of muscular activity is the segmental contraction, which mixes chyme with digestive juices, repeatedly exposes the mixture to the absorptive surface, and moves chyme slowly in an aboral direction. Eccentric contractions are confined to a segment shorter than 2 cm and do not empty the segment completely. Concentric segmental contractions empty portions of intestine longer than 2 cm.

Segmental contractions are controlled by a basic electrical rhythm (BER) arising in cells of the longitudinal muscle layer. Each segment of small intestine has a characteristic BER which is independent of neural influences. The frequency of the BER decreases progressively from duodenum to ileum, but in intact intestine an orally located segment with a higher frequency is partially able to drive an aborally situated neighbor which has a lower frequency. Thus, in man it appears that the controlling BER is located in the duodenum near the ampulla of Vater; segmental contractions occur intermittently, in phase with the BER, at intervals which are some multiple of 3.4 seconds.

Peristalsis in the human small intestine is a short, weak, propulsive movement which travels at about 1 cm/sec for a distance of 10–15 cm before dying out. Peristaltic rushes are powerful waves of contraction which rapidly traverse the entire length of small bowel and are not normally present in man.

Ingestion of food increases muscular activity in the small intestine. Neural and hormonal influences are complex. In general, acetylcholine stimulates and α-adrenergic agents inhibit small bowel motility. Cholecystokinin stimulates motor activity, and secretin, glucagon, and vasoactive intestinal polypeptide (VIP) inhibit it.

Digestion, Secretion, & Absorption

With a few exceptions (eg, iron, calcium), the normal small intestine absorbs indiscriminately without regard to body composition. For example, absorption of fat, carbohydrate, and protein is just as complete in the obese patient as in the slender individual. Body composition is regulated through metabolic processes which dispose of substances after they have been absorbed.

A. Water and Electrolytes: Ingested fluid and salivary, gastric, biliary, pancreatic, and intestinal secretions present a total of 5–9 liters of water to the absorptive surface of the small intestine each day, and 1–2 liters are discharged from the ileum into the colon. Water is absorbed throughout the intestine, but the major site of absorption after a meal is in the upper tract.

The net flow of water and electrolytes across the intestinal mucosa is equal to the difference between 2 opposite unidirectional fluxes: from intestinal lumen to interstitial fluid (absorption), and from interstitial fluid to intestinal lumen (secretion). Water moves passively across the mucosa following osmotic gradients. Hypertonic solutions in the duodenum and upper jejunum are rapidly brought into osmotic equilibrium with blood, and, as the osmotic pressure of luminal contents is increased further by breakdown of large molecules into smaller ones, still more water enters the lumen. Net absorption of water by simple diffusion accompanies active transport of ions and small molecules such as glucose and amino acids. If the lumen contains nonabsorbable solute, water is retained to maintain isotonicity.

Sodium is absorbed in the jejunum and ileum by an active electrogenic transport mechanism. If bicarbonate is present in the luminal contents of the jejunum, as it is normally, sodium absorption is enhanced, perhaps by exchange of sodium for hydrogen. Hexoses stimulate sodium absorption either by promotion of active electrogenic transport or by a phenomenon known as solvent drag, in which sodium is carried with the bulk flow of water accompanying hexose absorption.

Potassium diffuses passively along electrical and concentration gradients. Calcium is actively transported, a process stimulated by vitamin D. Calcium absorption is most efficient in the duodenum, but, because intestinal contents are in the jejunum and ileum longer, most calcium is absorbed in these areas. Magnesium is absorbed by all segments of the intestine, but relatively poorly. Iron is absorbed in the duodenum and jejunum, primarily as the ferrous ion.

The absorption of anions is complex. Some chloride passively follows electrical gradients established by sodium transport, but human intestine is able to absorb chloride against an electrochemical gradient as well. Bicarbonate is absorbed by secretion of hydrogen ions in exchange for sodium ions; one bicarbonate ion is released into the interstitial fluid for every hydrogen ion secreted, and CO_2 is generated in the intestinal lumen. This mechanism is similar to that for acidification of urine in the kidney. Movements of chloride and bicarbonate in opposite directions are closely coupled, especially in the distal ileum, so that chloride concentrations decrease and bicarbonate concentrations increase as chyme passes distally. Phosphate is absorbed in all portions of the small bowel.

Absorption and secretion of water and electrolytes by the small intestine are influenced by bacterial toxins, prostaglandins, polypeptide hormones, and neurohumoral agents. Voluminous net secretion occurs in cholera and in patients with pancreatic tumors that elaborate the hormone vasoactive intestinal polypeptide (VIP). Cholera toxin and VIP activate adenylate cyclase in the membranes of mucosal cells, which raises the intracellular levels of cyclic adenosine monophosphate (cAMP). cAMP causes net secretion of sodium, chloride, and water, and profuse diarrhea results.

B. Carbohydrate: The polysaccharides starch and glycogen and the disaccharides sucrose and lactose comprise about half the calories ingested by man. Digestion of starch is begun by salivary amylase and is completed by pancreatic amylase in the duodenum and upper jejunum. The products of hydrolysis (maltose, maltotriose, and a mixture of dextrins) as well as ingested oligosaccharides are further hydrolyzed by contact with enzymes contained in the brush border of intestinal epithelial cells. The monosaccharides glucose, galactose, and fructose are actively transported against a concentration gradient by a carrier-mediated mechanism. Monosaccharides are delivered directly into portal blood from the intestinal mucosa.

Although the entire small intestine has the capacity for carbohydrate digestion and absorption, the process is so efficient that under normal circumstances complete absorption of monosaccharides occurs in the duodenum and proximal jejunum.

C. Protein: Protein entering the stomach is de-natured by acid and partially digested by pepsin. This mechanism is not essential for protein digestion, and hydrolysis to polypeptides is principally by pancreatic enzymes, chiefly trypsin and chymotrypsin. Polypeptides are attacked by carboxypeptidases and aminopeptidases in or near the brush border, liberating amino acids which are absorbed by means of an active, carrier-mediated transport mechanism. Some oligopeptides enter the intestinal cells intact and are hydrolyzed there. More than 80% of amino acid absorption occurs in the proximal 100 cm of jejunum. Absorption of ingested protein is virtually complete, and the protein excreted in feces is derived from bacteria, desquamated cells, and mucoproteins.

D. Fat: Dietary fat is largely in the form of triglycerides, water-insoluble molecules which must be emulsified in the duodenum in preparation for attack by pancreatic lipase. Fatty acids, monoglycerides, cholesterol, lecithin, lysolecithin, protein, and bile salts are emulsifiers with varying powers. Bile salts by themselves are poor emulsifiers, but when the concentration of bile salts exceeds a certain level (the critical micellar concentration) they spontaneously aggregate with monoglycerides to form micelles. Bile salts in micelles are arranged with the fat-soluble portion of the molecule toward the center of the aggregate and the water-soluble portion at the periphery; this arrangement allows hydrophobic molecules such as free fatty acids, cholesterol, and fat-soluble vitamins to enter the micelles and thus be solubilized in an aqueous environment. Conjugated bile salts have a much lower critical micellar concentration than the unconjugated forms; when bile salts are deconjugated in the intestine (eg, by bacteria, as in blind loop syndrome), monoglycerides and free fatty acids produced by lipolysis precipitate and the efficiency of fat absorption is reduced. Pancreatic lipase is optimally active at the alkaline pH provided by bicarbonate.

Micelles in contact with the microvilli separate into their components, and monoglycerides and fatty acids diffuse through the lipoprotein plasma membrane. Absorption of these substances occurs throughout the intestine, but perhaps to a greater degree in jejunum than in ileum. Within the endoplasmic reticulum of the mucosal cells, triglycerides and phospholipids are resynthesized and delivered to the lymph as aggregates called chylomicrons. Short- and medium-chain fatty acids are absorbed without passing through a micellar phase, and within the epithelial cells triglycerides are hydrolyzed to constituent glycerol and fatty acids which pass directly into portal blood.

Conjugated bile salts are actively absorbed in the distal ileum and returned via portal blood to the liver, where they again are secreted into the bile. Disease or resection of the terminal ileum disrupts this enterohepatic circulation, and bile salts enter the colon in increased amounts where they induce net secretion of water and sodium and cause diarrhea. Malabsorbed fatty acids have an effect on colonic secretion of sodium and water similar to that of castor oil, an effect which probably is mediated by cyclic AMP.

E. Vitamins: Vitamin B_{12} (cyanocobalamin) is a water-soluble cobalt compound which requires a special mechanism for absorption because of its large molecular weight. Dietary vitamin B_{12} complexes with intrinsic factor, a mucoprotein secreted by the gastric parietal cells, and the complex is absorbed in the distal ileum. Other water-soluble vitamins are small enough to be absorbed by passive diffusion, but at least one (ascorbic acid) is actively transported in the human ileum.

Fat-soluble vitamins—notably vitamins A, D, and K—are dissolved in mixed micelles and absorbed as other lipids are. Since they are totally nonpolar lipids, the absence of bile seriously impairs absorption of these substances.

Christensen J: The physiology of gastrointestinal transit. Med Clin North Am 58:1165, 1974.

Field M: Intestinal secretion. Gastroenterology 66:1063, 1974.

Gray G, Cooper HL: Protein digestion and absorption. Gastroenterology 61:535, 1971.

Gray GM: Carbohydrate digestion and absorption: Role of the small intestine. N Engl J Med 292:1225, 1975.

Kimberg DV: Cyclic nucleotides and their role in gastrointestinal secretion. Gastroenterology 67:1023, 1974.

Makhlouf GM: The neuroendocrine design of the gut: The play of chemicals in a chemical playground. Gastroenterology 67:159, 1974.

Schultz SG, Frizzell RA: An overview of intestinal absorptive and secretory processes. Gastroenterology 63:161, 1972.

Westergaard H, Dietschy JM: Normal mechanisms of fat absorption and derangements induced by various gastrointestinal diseases. Med Clin North Am 58:1413, 1974.

BLIND LOOP SYNDROME

Blind loop syndrome (stagnant loop syndrome) is a form of malabsorption due to bacterial proliferation within the lumen of the small intestine. An anatomically blind (poorly emptying) segment of intestine is not required for this syndrome to develop. Bacteria proliferate in static intestinal contents in a variety of situations, including surgical blind loops, side-to-side intestinal bypasses, enteric or enterocolic fistulas, diverticula, inflammatory disease, adhesions, scleroderma, diabetes mellitus, ischemia, and neoplasms.

Steatorrhea, diarrhea, macrocytic anemia, and malnutrition are the hallmarks of the blind loop syndrome. Steatorrhea is the consequence of bacterial deconjugation and dehydroxylation of bile salts in the proximal small bowel. Deconjugated bile salts have a higher critical micellar concentration, and micelle formation is inadequate to solubilize ingested fat in preparation for absorption. Unabsorbed fatty acids enter the colon, where they increase net secretion of water and electrolytes, and diarrhea results. A direct toxic effect of unconjugated bile salts on jejunal mucosa has been demonstrated in animals, but the importance of this mechanism in humans is unknown. Hypocalcemia occurs because calcium is bound to unabsorbed fatty acids in the intestinal lumen. Macrocytic anemia is due to malabsorption of vitamin B_{12}, largely because of bacterial binding of the vitamin. Several mechanisms may account for malnutrition: anorexia, impaired absorption of carbohydrate and amino acids as well as fat, loss of protein from damaged mucosa, and catabolism of nutrients by bacteria.

Laboratory tests for the diagnosis of blind loop syndrome are evolving. Results of conventional studies include high fecal fat content, low absorption of orally administered vitamin B_{12} (Schilling test), and normal or low D-xylose absorption. A trial of oral antibiotics usually improves these values. Quantitative culture of upper intestinal aspirates is sometimes helpful. Bacterial counts of more than 10^5 per milliliter are generally abnormal. Abnormally high concentrations of free bile salts are found in intestinal aspirates. Measurement of plasma and fecal levels of short chain fatty acids, produced by bacterial fermentation, may be a useful test in the future.

The $^{14}CO_2$ breath test is a simple method for the diagnosis of blind loop syndrome. ^{14}C-labeled glycocholate is given orally; in the presence of bacterial overgrowth, the ^{14}C-labeled amino acid is split from the bile salt, metabolized, and appears as $^{14}CO_2$ in the breath during the 4 hours following ingestion. False-negative breath tests occur in patients with increased fecal losses of ^{14}C; this error is avoided by the more cumbersome measurement of $^{14}CO_2$ excretion from the lungs over a 24-hour period.

Treatment is directed toward the underlying disorder whenever possible. Neoplasms, fistulas, blind loops, diverticula, etc can be treated surgically. Conditions not amenable to surgical correction are treated with broad-spectrum antibiotics. It may be necessary to use different antibiotics in sequence.

Arnesjö B & others: Taurocholate metabolism in patients with small intestinal stagnant loops. Scand J Gastroenterol 9:579, 1974.

Broido PW, Gorbach SL, Nyhus LM: Microflora of the gastrointestinal tract and the surgical malabsorption syndromes. Surg Gynecol Obstet 135:449, 1972.

Fromm D: Ileal resection, or disease, and the blind loop syndrome: Current concepts of pathophysiology. Surgery 73:639, 1973.

Hepner GW: Breath analysis: Gastroenterological applications. Gastroenterology 67:1250, 1974.

Rogers AI, Rothman SL: Blind loop syndrome. Postgrad Med 55:99, April 1974.

Wilson FA, Dietschy JM: Differential diagnostic approach to clinical problems of malabsorption. Gastroenterology 61:911, 1971.

SHORT BOWEL SYNDROME

Essentials of Diagnosis

- Extensive small bowel resection.

- Diarrhea.
- Steatorrhea.
- Malnutrition.

General Considerations

The absorptive capacity of the small intestine is normally far in excess of need. However, a complex of deficiencies known as the "short bowel" or "short gut" syndrome may develop after extensive resection of the small intestine for trauma, mesenteric thrombosis, regional enteritis, radiation enteropathy, strangulated small bowel obstruction, neoplasm, or congenital atresia.

The ability of a patient to maintain nutrition after massive small bowel resection depends on the extent and site of resection, the presence of the ileocecal valve and the colon, the absorptive function of the intestinal remnant, adaptation of remaining bowel, and the nature of the underlying disease process and its complications. The nutritional consequences of resecting more than 75% of the small intestine are profound, and survival is unusual if less than 2 feet (60 cm) of jejunum or ileum are present in addition to the duodenum. The site of resection is important also. Normally, most of the dietary fat, carbohydrate, and protein are absorbed in the jejunum, yet loss of the jejunum is less serious than resection of an equivalent length of distal ileum. In the absence of jejunum, the ileum is able to absorb the products of digestion. Because transport of bile salts, vitamin B_{12}, and cholesterol is localized to the ileum, however, resection of this region is poorly tolerated (Fig 33–4). The consequences of bile salt malabsorption have been described in previous sections; in general, steatorrhea occurs if 100 cm or more of distal ileum is resected. Steatorrhea and diarrhea are more pronounced if the ileocecal valve is removed because this sphincter retards transit into the colon and also because it helps prevent reflux of bacteria from the colon. Blind loop syndrome due to bacterial overgrowth in the shortened small bowel (see above) compounds the problems. Patients who have colectomy in addition to extensive small bowel resection are among the most difficult to manage.

Major resection of the midgut results in rapid transit, partly due to the shorter distance chyme must travel, but changes in motility also contribute. There may be insufficient time for digestion of carbohydrates, fats, and proteins, and there may be inadequate absorptive surface to transport the products of digestion as well as water, electrolytes, and vitamins. A solute-type diarrhea occurs if the capacity for salt absorption is exceeded. The normal episodic pattern of eating magnifies these problems.

Calcium oxalate urinary tract calculi form in 7–10% of patients who have extensive ileal resection (or disease) and an intact colon. Unabsorbed fatty acids decrease the amount of intraluminal calcium available for binding with dietary oxalate, and abnormally large quantities of oxalate are absorbed, probably from the colon. Hyperoxaluria and renal calculi result. This condition is called **enteric hyperoxaluria.**

Some patients develop gastric hypersecretion after extensive small bowel resection. It is more marked after proximal resection, and it improves with time. The outpouring of gastric juice may damage the mucosa of the upper intestine, inactivate lipase and trypsin by lowering intraluminal pH, and present an excessive solute load to the intestinal remnant. The increased acid production probably results from loss of inhibitory hormones normally secreted by the small intestine. Although elevated basal and postprandial serum gastrin levels have been detected in some cases, the significance of this finding is not clear.

Clinical Course

During the immediate postoperative period, massive fluid and electrolyte losses from diarrhea are characteristic. The diarrhea lessens in severity after a few weeks, and eventually a reasonably normal existence is possible in most cases. The progression of a patient from strict dependence on intravenous feeding to nutritional maintenance by oral intake is possible because of intestinal **adaptation.** Adaptation is the compensatory increase of absorptive capacity in the intestinal remnant. It is due to villous hypertrophy and epithelial cell hyperplasia.

As a result of adaptation, the bowel dilates,

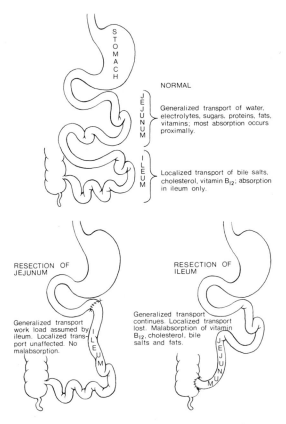

Figure 33–4. The consequences of complete resection of jejunum or ileum are predictable in part from the loss of regionally localized transport processes.

lengthens, and the wall thickens. The mechanisms that regulate adaptation are not understood. Nutritional support is essential for adaptation to occur. Although nutrition must be provided intravenously at first, it is now believed that the physical presence of food in the intestine is required for full adaptation. Dietary bulk is not important, but dextrose and amino acids are. The beneficial effects of intraluminal nutrition on mucosal cells may be direct or indirect via hormonal or neurovascular stimuli. Gastrin, a hormone with known trophic actions on gastric and intestinal cells, probably plays some role in this process.

Treatment

A. General Measures: Treatment of short bowel symptoms may be divided into 3 stages:

1. Stage 1 (intravenous stage)—During this stage, which lasts 1–3 months, patients should receive nothing by mouth. Careful intravenous fluid and electrolyte therapy and intravenous hyperalimentation must be used. Other important measures during this and later stages include control of diarrhea with codeine and protection of perianal skin from irritation.

2. Stage 2 (intravenous fluids and oral feeding)—Oral feedings should not be initiated until diarrhea subsides to less than 2.5 liters/day. Intravenous nutrition should continue as oral isotonic fluids are begun cautiously. Elemental diets require little digestion, but unless they are diluted to isotonicity and administered in small quantities, the absorptive capacity of the gut remnant will be exceeded and diarrhea exacerbated. Recent elemental diet formulas are more palatable than earlier versions, and continuous gavage through a small nasogastric tube may overcome the problem of poor patient acceptance. Diet is slowly advanced, and by trial and error a suitable diet for the individual is determined. Fat is added gradually and should be limited to less than 30 g/day initially. Medium-chain triglycerides, which are absorbed by passive diffusion, are advantageous because they do not require micelle formation for absorption. Milk products may aggravate diarrhea because total intestinal lactase activity is severely reduced after extensive resection.

3. Stage 3 (complete oral feeding)—After about 6 months, complete dependence on oral intake may be expected in patients with resection of 80% of the small bowel, but full adaptation may require up to 2 years. Maintenance of body weight at levels 20% or more below normal, bowel habits acceptable to patients, and return to productive life are reasonable expectations. Chronic intravenous feeding ("artificial gut") should be considered if oral intake is not tolerated.

Patients with extensive ileal resection require parenteral vitamin B_{12} (1000 μg IM every 2–3 months) for life. Hyperoxaluria often can be prevented by a diet low in fat and oxalate; supplementary oral calcium or aluminum, both of which bind oxalate, may be necessary in some patients, and others benefit from oral cholestyramine (4 g 3–4 times a day). Deficiencies in magnesium, vitamins D, A, and K, and water-soluble vitamins should be prevented. Blind loop syndrome may appear and require treatment. Antacids may be needed for gastric hypersecretion.

B. Adjunctive Surgical Procedures: Reversed segments and recirculating loops have been tried in the hope of slowing transit and improving absorption. None of these methods have a clearly established role. By enhancing bacterial growth, damaging additional bowel, and obstructing the intestine, they are likely to make matters worse.

A small number of patients, usually those with peptic ulcer disease before the enterectomy, eventually require operation for gastric hypersecretion. Because gastric operations could have undesirable side-effects, these procedures should not be done prophylactically; they should be limited to patients in whom acid hypersecretion proves to be a significant problem.

Dobbins JW, Binder HJ: Effect of bile salts and fatty acids on the colonic absorption of oxalate. Gastroenterology 70:1096, 1976.

Feldman EJ & others: Effects of oral versus intravenous nutrition on intestinal adaptation after small bowel resection in the dog. Gastroenterology 70:712, 1976.

Johnson LR & others: Action of gastrin on gastrointestinal structure and function. Gastroenterology 68:1184, 1975.

Poley JR, Hofmann AF: Role of fat maldigestion in pathogenesis of steatorrhea in ileal resection: Fat digestion after two sequential test meals with and without cholestyramine. Gastroenterology 71:38, 1976.

Solassol C & others: New techniques for long-term intravenous feeding: An artificial gut in 75 patients. Ann Surg 179:519, 1974.

Straus E, Gerson CD, Yalow RS: Hypersecretion of gastrin associated with the short bowel syndrome. Gastroenterology 66:175, 1974.

Tilson MD, Boyer JL, Wright HK: Jejunal absorption of bile salts after resection of the ileum. Surgery 77:231, 1975.

Weser E: The management of patients after small bowel resection. Gastroenterology 71:146, 1976.

BYPASS PROCEDURES FOR OBESITY OR HYPERLIPIDEMIA

Intestinal Gastric Bypass for Obesity

Massively obese patients—those who weigh 2 or 3 times the calculated ideal—are handicapped physically, emotionally, socially, and economically. This degree of excessive weight has been termed "morbid obesity" to emphasize the life-threatening seriousness of the condition. Complications such as hypertension, diabetes, hyperlipidemia, and Pickwickian syndrome may develop, and the mortality rate for morbidly obese people under age 40 is at least twice that for people of average weight.

The cause of morbid obesity is obscure. Data suggest that obese infants become obese adults, raising the hope of preventing obesity by attention to nutrition early in life. Medical treatment of morbidly obese adults is aimed at reducing caloric intake and increasing caloric expenditure by diet, exercise, and individual or group psychotherapy. Long-term results are discouraging, and patients usually become massively obese again once restrictions are relaxed. The seriousness of the obesity problem and the failure of medical treatment programs are attested to by a variety of drastic therapeutic approaches: in-hospital starvation, destruction of the hypothalamic feeding center, wiring the jaws nearly closed, bypass of 90% of the stomach, and bypass of the small intestine.

Intestinal bypass for refractory obesity aims to dispose of excess adipose tissue but maintain essential nutrition. The original plan was to restore intestinal continuity after ideal weight was achieved. However, because weight was promptly regained, most surgeons now intend the procedure to be permanent although potentially reversible if complications develop.

The original operation was a jejunocolic shunt in which the jejunum was divided close to the ligament of Treitz and the proximal end anastomosed end-to-side to the transverse colon. Serious diarrhea and nutritional depletion led to replacement of this procedure by operations that preserve the ileocecal valve in continuity. The optimal technic has not been determined. In the "14 and 4" operation, the jejunum is divided 14 inches (35 cm) from the ligament of Treitz, the distal stump is oversewn, and the proximal end is anastomosed end-to-side to the ileum 4 inches (10 cm) from the ileocecal valve. Insufficient weight loss in some patients has apparently been due to reflux of ileal contents into the defunctionalized segment. This has prompted some surgeons to turn to an end-to-end jejunoileostomy in which the bypassed gut is joined separately to the colon and is unavailable to intestinal chyme. The overall operative mortality is 3–5% after these procedures—surprisingly low considering the magnitude of obesity and its secondary effects on cardiorespiratory function.

These patients lose weight postoperatively at a rate of about 4.5 kg (10 lb) a month for 6 months and less rapidly thereafter. In most cases, weight stabilizes after 1–1.5 years owing to adaptation of the residual small intestine as in other forms of short bowel syndrome. Both the rate of weight loss and the total amount lost are directly proportionate to the magnitude of obesity before operation. Weight reduction below the calculated ideal apparently does not occur; in fact, the weight may reach a plateau considerably higher than the ideal.

Diarrhea is often severe in the early postoperative period, but later most patients stabilize at 5 or fewer semiformed stools per day. Transit time from stomach to cecum for a barium meal is 5–30 minutes after intestinal bypass. Current operative procedures allow absorption of at least some bile salts by the terminal ileum, and maintenance of the ascending colon in continuity aids in absorption of water and electrolytes.

Most of the weight loss is attributed to malabsorption. Abdominal flatulence, cramping pain, and steatorrhea induced by large meals, particularly food with a high fat content, may condition patients to eat less and contribute to weight loss. Absorption of fat, cholesterol, and vitamins A, D, and K is impaired. Malabsorption of carbohydrate, protein, potassium, calcium, and magnesium depends on the type of operation performed. Vitamin B_{12} is absorbed if some ileum is retained. Immediate and long-term postoperative care must include dietary supplements to prevent electrolyte and vitamin deficiencies; a low-fat diet is recommended.

Studies of body composition following intestinal bypass show that excess body fat is lost in all patients. In about 40% of cases in one study, however, there was also an undesirable loss of body cell mass (lean body mass) and other changes characteristic of protein deficiency. The incidence and severity of protein deficiency are related to the length of small bowel in continuity and the amount of protein consumed in the diet after operation.

Severe, even fatal complications may result from the altered physiology after intestinal bypass. Hepatic steatosis is commonly present in obese people before operation, but it may become worse postoperatively; in a few cases, cirrhosis, liver failure, and death have occurred. Protein malnutrition is one factor believed responsible for hepatic dysfunction, and damage of the liver by endotoxins produced by bacterial overgrowth in the bypassed segment possibly contributes also.

Bacterial proliferation in the bypassed segment may cause "bypass enteropathy," a syndrome characterized by exacerbation of diarrhea, abdominal distention, and sometimes fever and abdominal tenderness; it responds to antibiotics. Oxalate urinary tract calculi, polyarthritis, and colonic dilatation are other complications of this operation. Gastric hypersecretion is seldom a problem.

Dramatic rehabilitation of previously incapacitated patients can result from intestinal bypass, but in 10–20% of cases one or more problems require reoperation to revise or take down the bypass. The operation should only be performed in adult patients who are at least twice ideal weight. Intestinal bypass is best undertaken by a team consisting of a surgeon, an internist, and a psychiatrist. Careful selection of patients and close follow-up for many years are mandatory.

Gastric bypass is technically more difficult in the massively obese but is subject to fewer metabolic complications postoperatively. The stomach is transected high on the body, producing a small (10%) remnant, which is anastomosed end-to-side to a loop of jejunum. The larger distal remnant is left in place. The gastrojejunostomy must not be made too large (< 2 cm) or the patient may be able to tolerate continued huge caloric intake which the operation is intended to prevent. Because acid-secreting mucosa remains in the bypassed portion, its luminal pH is low and hypersecretion of gastrin and stomal ulceration are avoided. The rate and amount of weight loss following gastric bypass appears to compare favorably with intestinal bypass, but there has been insufficient experience with this procedure to know if it might be preferable to intestinal bypass in the average morbidly obese patient.

Benfield JR & others: Experience with jejunoileal bypass for obesity. Surg Gynecol Obstet 143:401, 1976.

Charney E & others: Childhood antecedents of adult obesity: Do chubby infants become obese adults? N Engl J Med 295:6, 1976.

Hermreck AS & others: Gastric bypass for morbid obesity. Surgery 80:498, 1976.

Mason EE & others: Optimizing results of gastric bypass. Ann Surg 182:405, 1975.

Moxley RT, Pozefsky T, Lockwood DH: Protein nutrition and liver disease after jejunoileal bypass in morbid obesity. N Engl J Med 290:921, 1974.

Passaro E Jr, Drenick E, Wilson SE: Bypass enteritis: A new complication of jejunoileal bypass for obesity. Am J Surg 131:169, 1976.

Scott HW Jr, Brill AB, Price RR: Body composition in morbidly obese patients treated by jejunoileal bypass. Ann Surg 182:395, 1975.

Scott HW Jr & others: Changes in hyperlipidemia and hyperlipoproteinemia in morbidly obese patients treated by jejunoileal bypass. Surg Gynecol Obstet 138:353, 1974.

Solow C, Silberfarb PM, Swift K: Psychosocial effects of intestinal bypass surgery for severe obesity. N Engl J Med 290:300, 1974.

Soyer MT, Ceballos R, Aldrete JS: Reversibility of severe hepatic damage caused by jejunoileal bypass after re-establishment of normal intestinal continuity. Surgery 79:601, 1976.

Spanier AH & others: Alterations in body composition following intestinal bypass for morbid obesity. Surgery 80:171, 1976.

Wands JR & others: Arthritis associated with intestinal-bypass procedure for morbid obesity: Complement activation and characterization of circulating cryoproteins. N Engl J Med 294:121, 1976.

Wise L, Vaughan R, Stein T: Studies on the effect of small bowel bypass for massive obesity on gastric secretory function. Ann Surg 183:259, 1976.

Intestinal Bypass for Hyperlipidemia

High circulating levels of cholesterol and probably triglycerides are associated with premature coronary atherosclerosis and myocardial infarction. Although it has not been proved that lowering blood lipid levels will reduce these risks, it is a reasonable expectation, and therapy is directed to that end. Diet and various drugs are only moderately effective in the familial hyperlipidemias, and the rare homozygous familial hypercholesterolemia is particularly refractory to current medical treatment.

Selected patients with hyperlipidemia may be considered for intestinal bypass. This operation, unlike the one performed for obesity, bypasses only the distal one-third or 200 cm (whichever is longer) of the small intestine measured from the ileocecal valve. Postoperatively, circulating cholesterol levels are lowered about 50%, and the total body pool of cholesterol decreases by one-third. Plasma triglycerides decline 50% in primary hypertriglyceridemic patients. Serum cholesterol is lowered by at least 2 mechanisms: reduced absorption by the gut, and increased hepatic synthesis of bile salts from cholesterol to compensate for fecal losses of bile salts.

Consequences of intestinal bypass for obesity such as diarrhea, weight loss, hepatic steatosis, and nephrolithiasis apparently do not occur after partial ileal bypass for hyperlipidemia. There is improvement or total remission of preoperative angina pectoris in 67% of patients with this symptom, and angiograms suggest that coronary atherosclerotic lesions regress also. Despite these encouraging results, this operation is still experimental and should be performed only under rigidly controlled conditions.

Buchwald H, Moore RB, Varco RL: Ten years clinical experience with partial ileal bypass in management of the hyperlipidemias. Ann Surg 180:384, 1974.

Buchwald H & others: Intestinal bypass procedures: Partial ileal bypass for hyperlipidemia and jejunoileal bypass for obesity. Curr Probl Surg, April 1975.

Motulsky AG: Current concepts in genetics: The genetic hyperlipidemias. N Engl J Med 294:823, 1976.

Surgery for hyperlipidaemia. (Leading article.) Br Med J 4:180, 1974.

OBSTRUCTION OF THE SMALL INTESTINE

Essentials of Diagnosis

Complete proximal obstruction
- Vomiting.
- Abdominal discomfort.
- X-ray findings.

Complete mid or distal obstruction
- Colicky abdominal pain.
- Vomiting.
- Abdominal distention.
- Constipation-obstipation.
- Peristaltic rushes.
- Dilated small bowel on x-ray.

General Considerations

Obstruction is the most common surgical disorder of the small intestine.

Mechanical obstruction implies a physical barrier which impedes aboral progress of intestinal contents; it may be complete or partial. If there is one point of obstruction, it is termed simple, and if the lumen is obstructed in at least 2 points, it is a closed loop. **Strangulation** denotes necrosis of the intestinal wall when the blood supply is impaired; most strangulation obstructions are of the closed loop variety, but a few are simple before infarction supervenes. Ileus is a term whose definition includes mechanical obstruction, but in the USA it usually refers to **paralytic ileus** (adynamic ileus), a disorder in which there is failure of peristalsis to propel intestinal contents without mechanical obstruction.

A variety of lesions intrinsic or extrinsic to the intestine may obstruct the lumen (Table 33–1).

A. Etiology:

1. Adhesions—Adhesions are the most common

Table 33–1. Causes of obstruction (in %) of
the small intestine in adults.

Cause		Relative Incidence
Adhesions		60
External hernia		20
Neoplasm		10
Intrinsic	3	
Extrinsic	7	
Miscellaneous		10

cause of mechanical small bowel obstruction. Congenital bands are seen in children, but adhesions acquired from abdominal operations or inflammation are much more frequent in adults.

2. Hernia—Incarceration of an external hernia is the second most common cause of intestinal obstruction. Inguinal, femoral, or umbilical hernias may have been present for years, or the patient may be unaware of the defect before the onset of obstructive symptoms. An incarcerated hernia may be overlooked by the examining surgeon, particularly if the patient is obese or if the hernia is the femoral type, and a careful search for external hernias must be made during evaluation of every patient with acute abdominal illness. Internal hernias into the obturator foramen, foramen epiploicum (Winslow), or other anatomic defects are rare, but internal herniation is one of several mechanisms by which acquired adhesions produce obstruction. Surgical defects—lateral to an ileostomy, for example—also provide sites for internal herniation of small bowel loops.

3. Intussusception—Invagination of one loop of intestine into another is rarely encountered in adults and is usually caused by a polyp or other intraluminal lesion. Intussusception is more often seen in children; an organic lesion is not required, and the syndrome of colicky pain, passage of blood per rectum, and a palpable mass (the intussuscepted segment) is characteristic.

4. Volvulus—Volvulus results from rotation of bowel loops about a fixed point, often the consequence of congenital anomalies or acquired adhesions. Onset of obstruction is abrupt, and strangulation develops rapidly. Malrotation of the intestine is a cause of volvulus in infants.

5. Foreign bodies—Foreign bodies ingested by children or emotionally disturbed adults or bezoars which form in the stomach after gastrectomy may pass into the intestine and impact the lumen.

6. Neoplasms—Intrinsic small bowel neoplasms can progressively occlude the lumen or serve as a leading point in intussusception. Symptoms may be intermittent, onset of obstruction is slow, and signs of chronic anemia are present. Neoplasms extrinsic to small bowel may entrap loops, and strategically situated lesions of the colon—particularly those near the ileocecal valve—may present as small bowel obstruction.

7. Gallstone ileus—Passage of a large gallstone into the intestine through a cholecystoenteric fistula may produce obstruction of the small bowel. Gallstone ileus is considered in detail in Chapter 29.

8. Inflammatory bowel disease often causes obstruction when the lumen is narrowed by inflammation or fibrosis of the wall.

9. Stricture due to ischemia or radiation injury can result in mechanical obstruction.

B. Pathophysiology: The small bowel proximal to a point of obstruction distends with gas and fluid. Swallowed air is the major source of gaseous distention, at least in the early stages, because its principal component (nitrogen) is not well absorbed by mucosa. When bacterial fermentation occurs later on, other gases are produced; the partial pressure of nitrogen within the lumen is lowered, and a gradient for diffusion of nitrogen from blood to lumen is established.

Enormous quantities of isotonic fluid are lost from plasma and interstitial spaces in patients with obstruction. Fluid fills the lumen of the gut proximal to the obstruction because the bidirectional flux of salt and water is disrupted: the flux from blood to lumen is increased, and the flux from lumen to blood is normal or decreased. As the bowel distends with gas and secretions, intraluminal pressure may rise sufficiently high to impair venous drainage; this contributes to edema of the bowel wall and loss of fluid from the serosal surface into the peritoneal cavity. Reflexly induced vomiting accentuates the fluid and electrolyte deficit. Profound hypovolemia is the cause of death in untreated patients with nonstrangulating obstruction.

Audible peristaltic rushes are manifestations of attempts by the small bowel to propel its contents past the obstruction. Eventually, the smooth muscle becomes fatigued, especially when the intestine is greatly distended, and bowel sounds may diminish in prolonged obstruction. Bacteria proliferate as a result of stasis of the luminal contents, and the vomitus becomes feculent as obstruction progresses. Abdominal distention elevates the diaphragm and impairs respiration so that pulmonary complications are frequent.

Strangulation is a threat early in the course of closed loop obstruction but must be feared in any mechanical obstruction. Incarcerated inguinal hernia and volvulus are examples of obstructing mechanisms which occlude the vascular supply as well as the intestinal lumen. If the obstruction is simple, volvulus of the fluid-laden bowel may occur or strangulation may result simply from progressive distention. Venous drainage is more apt to be interrupted than arterial inflow. The gangrenous intestine bleeds into the lumen and into the peritoneal cavity, and eventually it perforates. The luminal contents of strangulated intestine are a potentially lethal mixture of bacteria, bacterial products, necrotic tissue, and blood. Some of this toxic fluid may enter the circulation by way of intestinal lymphatics or by absorption from the peritoneal cavity; septic shock is the result.

Clinical Findings

A. Nonstrangulating Obstruction:

1. Symptoms and Signs—(Fig 33–5.) Proximal

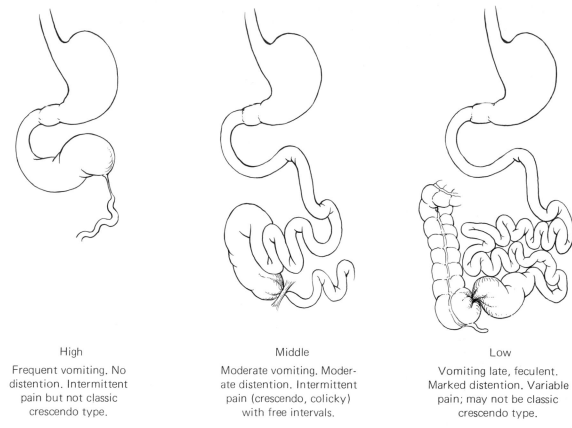

High	Middle	Low
Frequent vomiting. No distention. Intermittent pain but not classic crescendo type.	Moderate vomiting. Moderate distention. Intermittent pain (crescendo, colicky) with free intervals.	Vomiting late, feculent. Marked distention. Variable pain; may not be classic crescendo type.

Figure 33—5. Small bowel obstruction. Variable manifestations of obstruction depend upon the level of blockage of the small bowel.

(high) small bowel obstruction usually presents as profuse vomiting which seldom becomes feculent even in prolonged obstruction. Abdominal pain is variable and often is described as upper abdominal discomfort rather than cramping pain.

Obstruction of the mid or distal small intestine causes cramping periumbilical or poorly localized abdominal pain. Each episode of cramps has a crescendo-decrescendo pattern, lasts for a few seconds to a few minutes, and recurs every few minutes. Between cramps, the patient is entirely free of pain. Vomiting follows the onset of pain after an interval which varies with the level of obstruction; it may not occur until several hours later. The more distal the obstruction, the more likely it is that vomitus will become feculent with the passage of time. Gas and feces present in the colon may be expelled after the onset of pain, but obstipation always occurs eventually in complete obstruction.

Vital signs may be normal in the early stages, but dehydration is noted with continued loss of fluid and electrolytes. Temperature is normal or mildly elevated. Abdominal distention is minimal to absent in proximal obstruction but is pronounced in more distal obstruction. Peristalsis in dilated loops of small bowel may be visible beneath the abdominal wall in thin patients. Mild tenderness may be elicited. Peristaltic rushes, gur-gles, and high-pitched tinkles are audible in coordination with attacks of cramping pain in distal obstruction. Incarcerated hernias should be sought. Rectal examination is usually normal.

2. Laboratory findings—In the early stages, laboratory findings may be normal; with progression of disease, there are hemoconcentration, leukocytosis, and electrolyte abnormalities which depend on the level of obstruction and the severity of dehydration. Serum amylase is often elevated.

3. X-ray findings—Supine and upright plain abdominal films reveal a ladder-like pattern of dilated small bowel loops with air-fluid levels. These features may be minimal or absent in early obstruction, proximal obstruction, closed loop obstruction, or in some cases when fluid-filled loops contain little gas. The colon is often devoid of gas unless the patient has been given an enema or has undergone sigmoidoscopy. Opaque gallstones and air in the biliary tree should be looked for routinely. Contrast media administered orally or through a nasogastric tube may be needed to establish the diagnosis, especially in cases of proximal obstruction.

B. Strangulation Obstruction: Although certain clinical features should make the surgeon suspicious of strangulation, there are no historical, physical, or laboratory findings which exclude the possibility of strangulation in complete small bowel obstruction. At least one-third of strangulating obstructions are unsuspected before operation, a fact which underscores the unreliability of clinical assessment and the need for early operation when obstruction is complete.

1. Symptoms and signs—Shock which appears early in the course of obstruction suggests a strangulated closed loop. When strangulation supervenes in simple obstruction, high fever may develop, previously cramping abdominal pain may become a severe continuous ache, vomitus may contain gross or occult blood, and abdominal tenderness and rigidity may appear.

2. Laboratory findings—Marked leukocytosis not accounted for by hemoconcentration alone should suggest strangulation.

3. X-ray findings—Intraperitoneal fluid is seen as a widened space between adjacent loops of dilated bowel and is often found in simple obstruction as well as in strangulation. Thumbprinting, loss of mucosal pattern, and gas within the bowel wall or within intrahepatic branches of the portal vein may be seen in strangulation. Air-fluid levels outside the bowel indicate perforation.

Differential Diagnosis

Paralytic (adynamic) ileus accompanies inflammatory conditions in the abdomen, intestinal ischemia, ureteral colic, and back injuries; most importantly, it occurs almost routinely following abdominal surgery. Pain is usually constant and diffuse, and the abdomen is distended and mildly tender. If ileus has resulted from an acute intraperitoneal inflammatory process (eg, acute appendicitis), there should be symptoms and signs of the primary problem as well as the ileus. Plain films show uniform distribution of gas throughout the stomach, small bowel, and colon. Radiographic contrast studies (small bowel series) may be required to distinguish ileus from mechanical obstruction, particularly in the postoperative period.

Obstruction of the large intestine is characterized by obstipation and abdominal distention; pain is less often colicky, and vomiting is an inconstant symptom. X-rays usually make the diagnosis by demonstrating colonic dilatation proximal to the obstructing lesion. If the ileocecal valve is incompetent, the distal small bowel will be dilated, and a barium enema may be needed to determine the level of obstruction. This subject is covered in detail in Chapter 34.

Acute gastroenteritis, acute appendicitis, and acute pancreatitis can mimic simple intestinal obstruction. Serum amylase levels are generally higher in acute pancreatitis than in obstruction, but modest elevations are seen in the latter condition. Strangulation obstruction may be confused with acute hemorrhagic pancreatitis or mesenteric vascular occlusion.

Pseudo-obstruction occurs in 2 forms: (1) distention of the colon in elderly patients or those with systemic diseases, sometimes related to fecal impaction in the left colon or rectum; and (2) chronic abdominal pain and small bowel dilatation due to abnormal motility. Pseudo-obstruction of the small intestine has been seen in mesenteric disease with disruption of extrinsic nerve supply to the gut, with collagen diseases, and with diabetes mellitus. In the colon it has been associated with myxedema, hypokalemia, and the use of ganglionic blocking agents, but most cases have no definitely established cause.

Colonic pseudo-obstruction may require decompression of the cecum to avoid perforation. The small bowel variety often requires operation to exclude mechanical obstruction. Radical resection has been reported with improvement of the pain and steatorrhea, but this approach will not be successful if the motility disorder involves the entire gastrointestinal tract, as it often does.

Treatment

Complete obstruction of the small intestine is treated by operation after a period of careful preparation. The compelling reason for operation is that strangulation cannot be excluded with certainty as long as obstruction persists, and strangulation is associated with high morbidity and mortality. The surgeon must avoid being lulled into a false sense of security by the nearly universal improvement in symptoms and signs after resuscitative measures are instituted. There are exceptions to the general rule that operation be performed promptly; postoperative obstruction, a history of numerous previous operations for obstruction, and abdominal carcinomatosis are situations demanding mature judgment, and judicious nonoperative management may occasionally be in the patient's best interests. A long intestinal tube may be passed in these cases to decompress the bowel below the stomach. There are several varieties of such tubes.

A. Preparation: In general, the longer the duration of obstruction, the longer the period of preparation required. The risk of strangulation must be weighed against the severity of fluid and electrolyte abnormalities and the need for evaluation and treatment of associated systemic diseases. Proper timing of the operation, therefore, is determined by the needs of individual patients.

1. Nasogastric suction—A nasogastric tube should be inserted immediately upon admission to the emergency ward in order to relieve vomiting, avoid aspiration, and reduce the contribution of further swallowed air to the abdominal distention. Some surgeons routinely attempt to pass a long intestinal tube.

2. Fluid and electrolyte resuscitation—Depending upon the level and duration of obstruction, fluid and electrolyte deficits are mild to severe. A serious error is to assume that hemoconcentration induced by long-standing obstruction can be corrected by dextrose solutions alone. Fluid losses are isotonic, and resuscitation should begin with infusion of isotonic saline solution. Losses of gastrointestinal fluid also entail acid-base deficits, and, since there is no neuroendocrine mechanism for correcting these deficits, the surgeon must do so. Serum electrolyte concentrations and arterial blood gas determinations are guides to electrolyte therapy; potassium is best withheld until urine output is satisfactory, but patients should not undergo operation until hypokalemia has been treated. The volume of fluid required and its exact electrolyte compensation must be calculated for each patient, and careful monitoring of clinical signs and attention to associated systemic diseases are imperative. Some patients—notably those with strangulation obstruction—require plasma or blood. Antibiotics should be given if strangulation is even remotely suspected.

B. Operation: Operation may commence when the patient has been rehydrated and vital organs are functioning satisfactorily. Occasionally, the toxic effects of strangulation may force operation at an earlier time.

A standard groin incision is used for patients with incarcerated inguinal or femoral hernias, but other types of obstruction require an abdominal incision. Wide exposure is essential, and the position of the incision is partly dictated by the location of scars from previous operations.

Details of the operative procedure vary according to the cause of obstruction. Adhesive bands causing obstruction should be lysed; an obstructing tumor should be resected; and an obstructing foreign body should be removed through an enterotomy. Gangrenous intestine must be resected, but it is often difficult to determine whether obstructed bowel is viable or not. The loop should be wrapped in a warm saline-soaked pack and inspected for color, mesenteric pulsation, and peristalsis several minutes later. If the loop appears nonviable after 15–20 minutes, resection with end-to-end anastomosis is the safest course.

Extirpation of the obstructing lesion is not possible in some patients with carcinoma or radiation injury. Proximal diversion by anastomosing small bowel to colon may be the best procedure in these patients.

Decompression of massively dilated small bowel loops before closure of the abdomen shortens the time for recovery of bowel function postoperatively. Decompression is accomplished by threading a long tube down from above or by needle aspiration through the bowel wall. The needle should be introduced with care to avoid contamination of the peritoneal cavity by bacteria-laden material, and the hole in the intestinal wall should be closed with a suture.

Areas of serosa which have been denuded should be repaired with fine silk sutures or reinforced by suturing an adjacent loop over the denuded portion as a serosal patch. The small bowel should be arranged in regular patterns in the hope that new adhesions will fix the bowel or mesentery to prevent recurrence. Attempts to prevent uncontrolled adhesion formation by surgically fixing the loops of bowel in a suitable relation to one another (plication procedure) have met with limited success.

Prognosis

Nonstrangulating obstruction has a mortality rate of about 5%; most of these deaths occur in the elderly. Strangulation obstruction has a mortality rate of ap-

proximately 8% if operation is performed within 36 hours of the onset of symptoms and 25% if operation is delayed beyond 36 hours. Clearly, early diagnosis and prompt surgical correction of intestinal obstruction are essential to avoid the excessive mortality rate associated with strangulation.

Barnett WO, Petro AB, Williamson JW: A current appraisal of problems with gangrenous bowel. Ann Surg 183:653, 1976.

Bussemaker JB, Lindeman J: Comparison of methods to determine viability of small intestine. Ann Surg 176:97, 1972.

Gans H, Matsumoto K: The escape of enterotoxin from the intestine. Surg Gynecol Obstet 139:395, 1974.

Giuffré JC: Intestinal obstruction: Ten-year experience. Dis Colon Rectum 15:426, 1972.

Maldenado JE & others: Chronic idiopathic intestinal pseudo-obstruction. Am J Med 49:203, 1970.

Nadrowski LF: Pathophysiology and current treatment of intestinal obstruction. Rev Surg 31:381, 1974.

Rosato EF: Intestinal obstruction. Pages 286–297 in: *Gastrointestinal Pathophysiology.* Brooks FP (editor). Oxford Univ Press, 1974.

Shively E & others: Post-traumatic intestinal obstruction. Surgery 79:612, 1976.

Sufian S, Matsumoto T: Intestinal obstruction. Am J Surg 130:9, 1975.

Wangensteen OH: Historical aspects of the management of acute intestinal obstruction. Surgery 65:363, 1969.

Wickstrom P, Haglin JJ, Hitchcock CR: Intraoperative decompression of the obstructed small bowel. Surgery 73:212, 1973.

Wright HK, O'Brien JJ, Tilson MD: Water absorption in experimental closed segment obstruction of the ileum in man. Am J Surg 121:96, 1971.

DIVERTICULAR DISEASE OF THE SMALL INTESTINE

1. MECKEL'S DIVERTICULUM

Meckel's diverticulum occurs in approximately 2% of infants and is the most common congenital anomaly of the gastrointestinal tract. It is due to total or partial persistence of the omphalomesenteric duct.

Meckel's diverticulum is a pouch 1–12 cm long arising on the antimesenteric border of the ileum; 90% are within 100 cm of the ileocecal valve. A fibrous vitello-umbilical cord anchors the tip of the diverticulum to the undersurface of the umbilicus in 10% of cases, and in the remainder the apex is freely mobile.

Meckel's diverticulum is a true diverticulum made up of all layers of intestinal wall. Heterotopic tissue is found in approximately 50% of symptomatic Meckel's diverticula. Gastric mucosa with parietal cells is the most common heterotopic tissue and comprises 80% of cases; pancreas and mucosa of the colonic, duodenal, or jejunal type are encountered with lesser frequency.

Clinical Findings

It was once believed that 25% of Meckel's diverticula become symptomatic, but recent evidence suggests that only 4% cause problems during a lifetime. At least half of patients are less than 10 years old when symptoms develop, and 80% are under age 30.

A. Symptoms and Signs:

1. Bleeding—About 25% of patients with symptomatic Meckel's diverticula have lower gastrointestinal hemorrhage from peptic ulceration related to heterotopic gastric tissue. This complication usually arises before age 2 and rarely after age 10. It is the most common cause of severe intestinal bleeding in childhood.

2. Intestinal obstruction—Approximately 30% of cases of symptomatic Meckel's diverticula present as small bowel obstruction, and 50% have progressed to strangulation by the time operation is performed. Several mechanisms are responsible for obstruction: volvulus around a persistent vitello-umbilical cord, intussusception of the diverticulum, and entrapment of a loop of bowel beneath a mesodiverticular band.

3. Acute diverticulitis—Most Meckel's diverticula are broad-based, but a narrow neck can be obstructed by healing peptic ulcers, external bands, torsion, diverticuloliths, food particles, or tumors. The resulting abdominal pain, anorexia, nausea and vomiting, abdominal tenderness, fever, and leukocytosis mimic acute appendicitis. Perforation is common in acute diverticulitis.

4. Chronic abdominal pain—A few cases of chronic abdominal pain due to peptic ulceration of Meckel's diverticula have been reported.

B. Laboratory Findings: Laboratory studies reflect the mode of clinical presentation. Meckel's diverticula are sometimes seen with radiographic contrast studies. Heterotopic gastric mucosa concentrates ^{99m}Tc sodium pertechnetate, and diverticula containing such tissue may be demonstrated by abdominal scan. False positives have been observed.

Treatment

Symptomatic Meckel's diverticula should be removed. Tangential excision and suture closure of the defect is usually satisfactory, but segmental resection of ileum is required for diverticula with wide bases or acute inflammation of adjacent ileum. Diverticula discovered incidentally during laparotomy for unrelated disease should not be excised as a matter of routine.

Prognosis

About 6% of patients with symptomatic Meckel's diverticula die of their disease. Death is related to erroneous diagnosis and delayed operation.

DeBartolo HM Jr, van Heerden JA: Meckel's diverticulum. Ann Surg 183:30, 1976.

Ho JE, Konieczny KM: The sodium pertechnetate Tc 99m scan: An aid in the evaluation of gastrointestinal bleeding. Pediatrics 56:34, 1975.

Meguid M, Canty T, Fraklis AJ: Complications of Meckel's diverticulum in infants. Surg Gynecol Obstet 139:541, 1974.

Soltero MJ, Bill AH: The natural history of Meckel's diverticulum and its relation to incidental removal: A study of 202 cases of diseased Meckel's diverticulum found in King County, Washington, over a fifteen-year period. Am J Surg 132:168, 1976.

2. ACQUIRED DIVERTICULA

Congenital true diverticula of jejunum and ileum (excluding Meckel's) are rare, but false diverticula are found in 1.3% of radiographic studies or autopsy series when specifically sought. These lesions are wide-mouthed sacs measuring 1–25 cm in diameter, consisting of mucosa and submucosa herniated between the mesenteric leaves at sites of vascular penetration through the wall. False diverticula are often multiple; they diminish in frequency from the ligament of Treitz to the ileocecal valve and are associated with diverticulosis of the duodenum or colon in 30% of cases. The majority of symptomatic patients are in the over 60 age group.

Acute intestinal bleeding and diverticulitis susceptible to perforation are the chief modes of presentation. A few patients with multiple diverticula have developed malabsorption from the blind loop syndrome. Barium x-rays may outline the diverticula (Fig 33–6).

Treatment requires resection of involved portions of intestine.

Altemeier WA & others: The surgical significance of jejunal diverticulosis. Arch Surg 86:732, 1963.

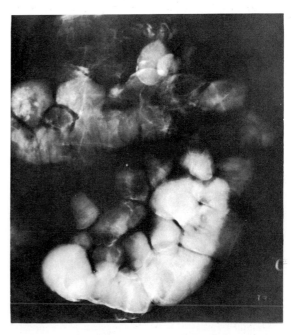

Figure 33–6. Jejunal diverticula.

Goldstein F & others: Diverticulosis of the small intestine: Clinical, bacteriologic, and metabolic observations in a group of seven patients. Am J Dig Dis 14:170, 1969.

Kraus M, Sampson D, Wilson SD: Perforation of diverticulum of terminal ileum presenting as acute appendicitis. Surgery 79:724, 1976.

Localio SA, Stahl WM: Diverticular disease of the alimentary tract. 2. The esophagus, stomach, duodenum and small intestine. Curr Probl Surg, Jan 1968.

Nobles ER Jr: Jejunal diverticula. Arch Surg 102:172, 1971.

CROHN'S DISEASE*
(Regional Enteritis)

Essentials of Diagnosis

- Diarrhea.
- Abdominal pain and palpable mass.
- Low-grade fever, lassitude, weight loss.
- Anemia.
- Radiographic findings of thickened, stenotic bowel with ulceration and internal fistulas.

General Considerations

Crohn's disease is a chronic inflammatory disorder affecting the gastrointestinal tract. Three to 5 new cases per 100,000 population are detected annually in Europe and the USA, and the incidence is apparently rising. The prevalence is 20–40 per 100,000 population. Males are affected slightly more often than females. Only 25% of patients first manifest the disease after the age of 50; the peak incidence occurs between ages 15–20.

A. Etiology: Crohn's disease probably results from the interaction of environmental factors and genetic predisposition. A polygenic genetic influence is suggested by a family history of this disease (or ulcerative colitis) in 15–20% of patients. A transmissible agent, apparently a virus, has been isolated from diseased human ileum, but whether this or some other infectious organism is responsible for Crohn's disease has not been proved. Many immunologic abnormalities have been described in association with Crohn's disease (and ulcerative colitis): antibodies to colonic epithelial cells, antibodies to cross-reacting enterobacterial antigens, circulating lymphocytes which are cytotoxic for colonic epithelial cells, disordered immunoglobulin and complement patterns, circulating antigen-antibody complexes, and others. One attractive hypothesis is that Crohn's disease is the consequence of a lymphocyte-mediated hypersensitivity reaction to bacterial or viral antigens. Older theories holding that Crohn's disease is caused by bovine milk products or is the result of psychophysiologic factors are now generally disregarded.

B. Pathology: Crohn's disease may affect any part of the gastrointestinal tract from the lips to the anus. The distal ileum is the most frequent site of involvement, eventually becoming diseased in about three-fourths of patients. The small bowel alone is involved in 30%, both the distal ileum and the colon in 40%, and the large bowel alone in 30%. Discontinuous areas of disease with segments of normal bowel between ("skip lesions") occur in 15% of patients. It has always been thought that the mucosa away from affected areas is macroscopically and microscopically normal, but the recent identification of subtle histologic changes in "normal" intestine of patients with Crohn's disease raises the disturbing possibility that the mucosa of the entire bowel is abnormal in this disorder.

There are no specific microscopic features of Crohn's disease. Granulomas are seen in the bowel wall in 50–70% and in mesenteric lymph nodes in 25% of patients. The earliest lesion is thought to be hyperplasia of lymphoid follicles and Peyer's patches with later ulceration of overlying mucosa. These lesions appear grossly as tiny (pinpoint) hemorrhagic spots or clearly delimited shallow ulcers with white bases. The next stage is development of fissures, knife-like clefts beginning in mucosa over lymphoid aggregates and extending deeply into the wall. These fissures and the serpiginous or linear ulcers surrounding islands of intact mucosa overlying edematous submucosa give a cobblestone appearance to the luminal surface. Crohn's disease ultimately becomes a transmural inflammatory process with thickening of the bowel wall, and it often progresses to stricture formation. The bowel and its mesentery are foreshortened in advanced cases, and on gross inspection mesenteric fat seems to have advanced over the surface of the bowel toward the antimesenteric border.

Clinical Findings

A. Symptoms and Signs: Crohn's disease has protean modes of presentation:

1. Diarrhea—Continuous or episodic diarrhea is the cardinal clinical feature of Crohn's disease and is noted in about 90% of patients. Stools are liquid or semisolid and characteristically contain no blood if small bowel alone is diseased. One-third of patients with colonic involvement pass blood, however, and a few individuals present with bloody diarrhea resembling that seen in ulcerative colitis.

2. Recurrent abdominal pain—Mild colicky pain initiated by meals, centered in the lower abdomen, and relieved by defecation is common. These symptoms are due to chronic partial obstruction of the small bowel, colon, or both. Some patients progress to complete obstruction and present with severe cramping pain, vomiting, and abdominal distention.

3. Abdominal symptoms and constitutional effects—Episodic attacks of abdominal pain and diarrhea accompanied by lassitude, malaise, weight loss, fever, and anemia are a common symptom complex. A mass is often palpable in the right lower quadrant in these patients. Occasionally, fever of unknown origin is the only clinical finding.

4. Anorectal lesions—Chronic anal fissures, large ulcers, complex fistulas-in-ano, or pararectal abscesses

---

*Crohn's disease of the colon is discussed in Chapter 34.

are seen in 15% of patients with Crohn's disease confined to small bowel and in 40% of those with colonic involvement. These problems may appear many years before the intestinal disease. Histologic features of Crohn's disease, including granulomas, are often found in biopsies of anorectal lesions even when the only other identifiable disease is located much higher in the gastrointestinal tract. Perforations of the ileum may dissect retroperitoneally and present as fistulas in the vagina or perineum.

5. Anemia—Iron deficiency anemia or macrocytic anemia due to vitamin B_{12} or folate deficiency may occur in the absence of abdominal symptoms.

6. Malnutrition—Protein-losing enteropathy, steatorrhea, and diminished dietary intake from chronic illness contribute to malnutrition and weight loss. Children afflicted with extensive Crohn's disease fail to grow and may have severely retarded sexual maturation. Reversal of growth arrest by parenteral feeding and failure to respond to human growth hormone alone emphasize the importance of malnutrition in the cause of growth failure in Crohn's disease.

7. Acute onset—Acute abdominal pain and right lower quadrant tenderness mimicking acute appendicitis may be found at operation to be due to acute inflammation of the distal ileum. Only 15% of such cases eventually develop chronic Crohn's disease, suggesting that most patients with acute ileitis have an infectious process unrelated to Crohn's disease. This condition is discussed further in the section on mesenteric lymphadenitis-enteritis.

8. Systemic complications—Any of the systemic complications described below may prompt the patient to seek medical advice.

9. Psychologic disturbances—When abdominal manifestations are absent or slight and the emotional effects are pronounced, patients may be erroneously diagnosed as suffering only from psychoneurosis.

B. Laboratory Findings: The results of laboratory tests are nonspecific and vary greatly according to the site of intestinal involvement, the severity of disease, and the presence of complications such as abscess or fistula. Hypoalbuminemia, anemia, and steatorrhea are common. Abnormal D-xylose absorption suggests extensive disease or fistula formation, since carbohydrate is normally absorbed in the upper jejunum. High serum lysozyme levels have been reported in association with Crohn's disease, and some investigators believe this test reflects the degree of activity of the inflammatory process.

C. X-Ray Findings: Radiographic studies contribute substantially to the diagnosis of Crohn's disease, although occasionally a patient with Crohn's disease may have normal bowel radiographically. The appearance of small bowel during a barium study is a composite of proliferative and destructive changes. The principal findings include thickened bowel wall with stricture ("string sign"), longitudinal ulceration which is shallow at first but becomes deep and undermining, deep transverse fissures which look like spicules, and cobblestone formation (Fig 33–7). Deformity of the

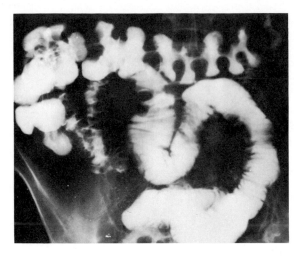

Figure 33–7. Barium x-ray showing spicules, edema, and ulcers in Crohn's disease.

cecum, fistulas, abscesses, and skip lesions are additional findings of importance.

Differential Diagnosis

A. Ulcerative Colitis: Crohn's disease of the colon may be difficult to distinguish from ulcerative colitis. This topic is covered in detail in Chapter 34.

B. Appendicitis: Acute ileitis may be the presenting manifestation, and differentiation from appendicitis may be impossible without operation.

C. Tuberculosis: Tuberculosis may affect any part of the gastrointestinal tract but is uncommon distal to the cecum. Small bowel tuberculosis is discussed elsewhere in this chapter.

D. Lymphoma: Radiographic findings help differentiate lymphoma from Crohn's disease, but histologic examination of the tissue is occasionally required before the diagnosis is certain.

E. Other Diseases: Carcinoma, amebiasis, ischemia, and various inflammatory conditions simulate Crohn's disease at times.

Complications

A. Intestinal: Some intestinal complications, such as obstruction, abscess, fistula, and anorectal lesions, are so common that they are regarded as part of the characteristic clinical picture. Free perforation and massive hemorrhage are rare. Carcinoma may occur in segments of small or large bowel which are involved with Crohn's disease.

B. Systemic: Systemic complications such as hepatobiliary disease, uveitis, arthritis, ankylosing spondylitis, aphthous ulcers, and erythema nodosum are found both in Crohn's disease and in ulcerative colitis. These manifestations are described more fully in Chapter 34.

Treatment

The initial treatment of Crohn's disease is nonoperative. Physical rest, relief of stress, and a confiding patient-doctor relationship have favorable effects. A low-residue, milk-free, high-protein diet is prescribed to reduce excessive stimulation of the bowel and to provide adequate nutrition. An elemental diet may be useful, and, in some cases, total parenteral nutrition may be necessary to nutritionally replete severely ill patients.

There is no specific drug treatment for Crohn's disease. Prednisone (0.25–0.75 mg/kg body weight daily) and sulfasalazine (1 g/15 kg body weight daily) are each superior to placebo in the control of actively symptomatic disease over the short term. Azathioprine, an immunosuppressive agent, in doses of 2.5 mg/kg body weight daily, is no better than placebo in this regard. Possible benefits from various other drugs, notably broad-spectrum antibiotics, have not been scrutinized objectively. Whether any drugs, singly or in combination, are able to prevent relapse of quiescent disease is still an unanswered question. An important advance has been the development of a numerical Crohn's Disease Activity Index which allows objective evaluation of response to various therapeutic regimens.

The indication for operation in Crohn's disease of the small bowel is obstruction in about half of the cases; internal fistula, abscess, and perianal disease are other reasons for operation. Conservative resection of diseased bowel with end-to-end anastomosis is the preferred surgical procedure. If an inflammatory mass adheres to vital structures, however, it may be necessary to bypass rather than resect the involved segment. Extensive involvement of small bowel, either diffusely or by skip lesions, is unfavorable for curative resection. Resection is usually limited to the area responsible for the complications which prompted operation.

Prognosis

Crohn's disease is a chronic, progressive condition. Disease limited to the colon may extend to the small bowel, and Crohn's disease of the small intestine may later involve the colon. The outlook is particularly discouraging for young patients and those with small bowel involvement. Remissions do occur, and in a few fortunate individuals the disease seems to burn itself out spontaneously. Whether medical therapy has any long-term beneficial effect on the course of Crohn's disease is debated.

Recurrence rates after surgical treatment depend on the method of analysis. In a recent study employing actuarial methods, the cumulative reoperation rate 15 years after the initial operation was 89%. The chance of recurrence rises after each operation, and the interval between operations shortens with increasing length of follow-up observation. Despite these dismal statistics, 80–85% of patients operated on are able to lead satisfying, productive lives.

Best WR & others: Development of a Crohn's disease activity index: National cooperative Crohn's disease study. Gastroenterology 70:439, 1976.

Brahme F, Lindström C, Wenckert A: Crohn's disease in a defined population: An epidemiological study of incidence, prevalence, mortality, and secular trends in the city of Malmö, Sweden. Gastroenterology 69:342, 1975.

Falchuk KR, Perrotto JL, Isselbacher KJ: Serum lysozyme in Crohn's disease: A useful index of disease activity. Gastroenterology 69:893, 1975.

Farmer RG, Hawk WA, Turnbull RB Jr: Indications for surgery in Crohn's disease: Analysis of 500 cases. Gastroenterology 71:245, 1976.

Gitnick GL, Rosen VJ: Electron microscopic studies of viral agents in Crohn's disease. Lancet 2:217, 1976.

Goode A & others: Use of an elemental diet for long-term nutritional support in Crohn's disease. Lancet 1:122, 1976.

Goodman MJ, Skinner JM, Truelove SC: Abnormalities in the apparently normal bowel mucosa in Crohn's disease. Lancet 1:275, 1976.

Greenstein AJ & others: Reoperation and recurrence in Crohn's colitis and ileocolitis: Crude and cumulative rates. N Engl J Med 293:685, 1975.

Kirsner JB, Shorter RG (editors): *Inflammatory Bowel Disease.* Lea & Febiger, 1975.

Koudahl G, Kristensen M, Lenz K: Bypass compared with resection for ileal Crohn's disease. Scand J Gastroenterol 9:203, 1974.

Layden T & others: Reversal of growth arrest in adolescents with Crohn's disease after parenteral alimentation. Gastroenterology 70:1017, 1976.

Marshak RH: Granulomatous disease of the intestinal tract (Crohn's disease). Radiology 114:3, 1975.

Reilly J & others: Hyperalimentation in inflammatory bowel disease. Am J Surg 131:192, 1976.

Rosenberg JL, Kraft SC, Kirsner JB: Inflammatory bowel disease in all three members of one family. Gastroenterology 70:759, 1976.

Singleton JW: The National Cooperative Crohn's Disease Study (NCCDS). Preliminary results of Part I. A cooperative study. Paper presented to American Gastroenterological Association, 1976.

Steigmann F: Can regional enteritis resolve completely? Am J Gastroenterol 63:464, 1975.

OTHER INFLAMMATORY & ULCERATIVE DISEASES OF THE SMALL INTESTINE

Acute Mesenteric Lymphadenitis-Enteritis

Acute mesenteric lymphadenitis usually occurs in children. Symptoms include fever, abdominal pain (which may be localized to the right lower quadrant), diarrhea, and vomiting. Some patients have pharyngitis and headache. Abdominal tenderness is more diffuse and fever is higher than in acute appendicitis, but it may not be possible to exclude appendicitis without operation. Large, inflamed lymph nodes are found in the mesentery of the distal ileum, and the bowel itself may be grossly inflamed. In these circumstances, appendectomy is usually performed.

About 75% of operated cases of mesenteric lymphadenitis are due to infection with bacteria of the genus Yersinia (formerly Pasteurella). *Y enterocolitica* was responsible for 60% and *Y pseudotuberculosis* for 15% of infections in one series. Either organism, but especially *Y enterocolitica,* may produce acute regional enteritis. No patient with *Y enterocolitica* enteritis has progressed to classical Crohn's disease. Organisms can be cultured from appendiceal contents or stool, and serologic tests establish that yersiniae caused the infection. A few cases of fatal yersinia septicemia have been reported. The organisms usually are sensitive to chloramphenicol, streptomycin, kanamycin, or tetracycline.

Bradford WE, Noce PS, Gutman LT: Pathologic features of enteric infection with *Yersinia enterocolitica.* Arch Pathol 98:17, 1974.

Gurry JF: Acute terminal ileitis and yersinia infection. Br Med J 2:264, 1974.

Kewenter J, Hultén L, Kock NG: The relationship and epidemiology of acute terminal ileitis and Crohn's disease. Gut 15:801, 1974.

Pseudomembranous Enterocolitis

Pseudomembranous enterocolitis is an inflammatory disease of the small bowel or colon (or both) and has even been found in the stomach. The pathologic findings include focal areas of mucosal necrosis which coalesce and deepen with formation of a characteristic yellow pseudomembrane consisting of necrotic mucosa, cellular debris, fibrin, and bacteria.

In many cases there is a history of antibiotic therapy just prior to the appearance of pseudomembranous enterocolitis. Various antibiotics have been implicated, including neomycin, lincomycin, clindamycin, tetracycline, ampicillin, cephalosporins, and penicillin. The inflammation appears limited to the colon in the case of clindamycin, but with other drugs both small and large bowel may be affected. Inflammation is attributed to overgrowth of *Staphylococcus aureus* in patients receiving large doses of oral neomycin for several days, a method of preparing the colon for surgery seldom used now. *S aureus* does not seem to be responsible for pseudomembranous enterocolitis associated with other antibiotics, however, and possible pathogenetic mechanisms include direct toxic effects of antibiotics on intestinal mucosa, overgrowth of enterotoxin-producing strains of klebsiella or enterobacter, viral infection, or diminished splanchnic blood flow by a variety of mechanisms.

Lethargy, weakness, fever, nausea and vomiting, diarrhea, abdominal pain and distention, and systemic toxicity are the hallmarks of the fully developed syndrome, but sudden circulatory collapse due to abrupt loss of gastrointestinal fluids may be the first manifestation.

Treatment must be instituted promptly. The precipitating factor (usually an antibiotic) must be discontinued. Massive fluid and electrolyte resuscitation and nasogastric decompression are mandatory. Specific antibiotic treatment is given if pathogenic bacteria are present in the stool. Gentamicin is useful in cases where no predominant fecal organism is identified. The mortality rate in severe cases is 66–90%. Adherence to strictly rational indications for the ordering of broad-spectrum antibiotics is the best means of prevention.

Marr JJ, Sans MD, Tedesco FJ: Bacterial studies of clindamycin-associated colitis: A preliminary report. Gastroenterology 69:352, 1975.

Slagle GW, Boggs HW Jr: Drug-induced pseudomembranous enterocolitis: A new etiologic agent. Dis Colon Rectum 19:253, 1976.

Steer HW: The pseudomembranous colitis associated with clindamycin therapy: A viral colitis. Gut 16:695, 1975.

Tully TE, Feinberg SB: A reappearance of antibiotic-induced pseudomembranous enterocolitis. Radiology 110:563, 1974.

Tuberculosis

Primary tuberculous infection of the intestine, caused by ingestion of the bovine strain of *Mycobacterium tuberculosis,* is rare in the USA, probably because milk is pasteurized. Secondary infection, due to swallowing the human tubercle bacillus, is much less common now than formerly, affecting about 1% of patients with pulmonary tuberculosis.

The distal ileum is the most common site of involvement. The bacillus localizes in the mucosal glands and spreads to Peyer's patches, where inflammation, sloughing of tissue, and local attempts at walling off give rise to symptoms. The pathologic reaction is either hypertrophic or, more commonly, ulcerative. Hypertrophic tuberculous enteritis results in stenosis, and the symptoms and signs are those of obstruction. The ulcerative form causes abdominal pain, alternating constipation and diarrhea, and, occasionally, progressive inanition. Free perforation, fistula formation, or hemorrhage may be seen in severe untreated cases of the disease.

Antituberculosis chemotherapy is the mainstay of management, but carcinoma and regional enteritis may be difficult to exclude. Surgery is required if the diagnosis is uncertain, if disease is resistant to chemotherapy, or if complications develop. Resection is the preferred surgical procedure, and bypass is done only if abscesses or fistulas are present. The prognosis is good if the patient is operated on in the early stages of the illness.

Fräki O, Peltokallio P: Intestinal and peritoneal tuberculosis: Report of two cases. Dis Colon Rectum 18:685, 1975.

Moss JD, Knauer CM: Tuberculous enteritis: A report of three patients. Gastroenterology 65:959, 1973.

Tabrisky J & others: Tuberculous enteritis: Review of a protean disease. Am J Gastroenterol 63:497, 1975.

Amebiasis

Amebic ulceration of the small bowel is much less common than colonic involvement. Amebiasis is discussed in Chapter 11.

Nonspecific Ulceration

Isolated, discrete, single or multiple ulcerations of undetermined cause may occur in the small bowel. They are often on the antimesenteric border and less commonly are circumferential. The ileum is involved twice as frequently as the jejunum. Abdominal pain, perforation, hemorrhage, or obstruction may bring the condition to medical attention. Treatment is generally by surgical resection.

Alexander HC, Schwartz GF: Nonspecific jejunal ulceration in search of an etiology. Gastroenterology 50:224, 1966.

Ulceration Due to Enteric-Coated Potassium

Circumferential mucosal ulcerations overlying a zone of cicatricial narrowing may be caused by enteric-coated potassium chloride. This disease has become uncommon since the use of enteric-coated potassium chloride was virtually abandoned.

Boley SJ & others: Experimental evaluation of thiazides and potassium as a cause of small-bowel ulcer. JAMA 192:763, 1965.

Radiation Enteropathy

Aggressive radiation therapy for abdominal or pelvic malignancy is associated with some gastrointestinal injury in nearly every case because proliferating intestinal epithelial cells are extremely radiosensitive. Degeneration of cells and edema of bowel wall may produce abdominal pain, nausea and vomiting, and sometimes bloody diarrhea during therapy or a few months later. Symptoms are minor and transient for most patients receiving radiation therapy with modern technics.

Injury to blood vessels in the bowel wall is far more serious than the early mucosal lesion. Endothelial proliferation and endarteritis gradually obliterate the vessel lumen over months or years, producing chronic intestinal ischemia.

The incidence of significant bowel injury is dose-related and varies from 5% after 4500 rads to 30% after 6000 rads. Fixation of small bowel loops in the radiation field by adhesions from previous operations greatly increases the risk of intestinal complications.

Symptoms necessitating operation appear as early as 1 month or as late as 30 years after completion of therapy. Operation is required for obstruction due to stricture or entrapment in pelvic fibrosis, perforation with abscess or fistula formation, or hemorrhage from ulcerated mucosa. Symptoms should not be attributed to malignancy until residual cancer is proved to be present.

The objective of operation is modest: to relieve symptoms. Resection of the involved segment often is not possible, and bypass is performed. It is imperative that normal bowel be used for anastomoses because disruption of suture lines in irradiated bowel is likely. The bowel is friable despite its thickness, and care must be taken in freeing adhesions. If the distal colon and rectum are involved, diverting colostomy is the safest course. Radiation proctitis is discussed in Chapter 35.

The operative mortality rate is 10–15%, and the prognosis thereafter depends on the extent of involvement and the presence of untreatable fistulas, short bowel syndrome, and cancer. Only 33–56% of patients with significant intestinal complications of radiation therapy are alive 5 years after operation.

Bloomer WD, Hellman S: Current concepts: Normal tissue responses to radiation therapy. N Engl J Med 293:80, 1975.
Deveney CW, Lewis FR Jr, Schrock TR: Surgical management of radiation injury of the small and large intestine. Dis Colon Rectum 19:25, 1976.
Swan RW, Fowler WC Jr, Boronow RC: Surgical management of radiation injury to the small intestine. Surg Gynecol Obstet 142:325, 1976.

SMALL BOWEL FISTULAS

Essentials of Diagnosis

- Fever and sepsis.
- Abdominal pain.
- Localized abdominal tenderness.
- External drainage of small bowel contents.
- Dehydration and malnutrition.

General Considerations

External fistulas of the small bowel may form spontaneously as a result of disease, but the vast majority are complications of surgical procedures (anastomotic dehiscence or injury to bowel during dissection). Fistulas are particularly prone to develop when the surgeon encounters extensive adhesions or inflamed intestine.

Clinical Findings

A. Symptoms and Signs: Postoperative fistula formation is heralded by fever and abdominal pain until bowel contents discharge through the abdominal incision. Spontaneous fistulas from neoplasms or inflammatory disease usually develop in a more indolent manner. Most fistulas are associated with one or more abscesses, which often drain incompletely with fistulization so that persistent sepsis is a common feature. Intestinal fluid escaping through the fistula may severely excoriate the skin of the abdominal wall. Fluid and electrolyte losses may be severe, especially if the fistula is large, if it is located in the upper tract, or if there is partial or complete intestinal obstruction distal to the fistula. Persistent sepsis and difficulty in nourishing the patient contribute to rapid weight loss.

B. Laboratory Findings: Routine laboratory tests reflect the severity of deficits in red cell mass, plasma volume, and electrolytes. Leukocytosis due to sepsis and hemoconcentration is common. Disease of other organs such as liver and kidneys may be detected.

C. X-Ray Findings: Abscesses and intestinal obstruction may be evident on plain abdominal films. Contrast medium administered orally, per rectum, or through the fistula (fistulogram) delineates the abnormal anatomy, including intrinsic bowel disease, and demonstrates the location and number of fistulas, the length and course of fistula tracts, associated abscess cavities, and the presence of distal obstruction. Chest films, excretory urograms, and other special studies may be indicated in certain individuals.

Complications

Fluid and electrolyte losses, malnutrition, and sepsis contribute to multiple organ failure and death unless effective therapy is instituted promptly.

Treatment

A systematic approach combining diagnostic, supportive, and operative procedures is essential in the management of patients with fistulas (Table 33–2). In few other conditions is the proper timing of operative intervention more critical.

A. Fluid and Electrolyte Resuscitation: Many fistula patients are profoundly depleted of intravascular and interstitial volume, and replacement of this fluid with isotonic saline solution takes first priority. Central venous pressure, urine output, and skin turgor are guides to the progress of volume resuscitation. Blood is sent to the laboratory for measurement of serum electrolyte concentrations, and in critical situations arterial blood gases should be determined. Results of these studies assist in correcting electrolyte deficits and deranged acid-base balance. Fluid should be collected from fistula output, nasogastric suction, and urine for measurement of volume and electrolyte composition. Body weight is recorded daily. Fluid and electrolyte resuscitation can usually be accomplished within the first few days. Subsequent maintenance of homeostasis depends on accurately measuring fluid and electrolyte losses and replacing them.

B. Control of Fistula: Fistula drainage fluid must be collected to avoid excoriation of skin and abdominal wall tissues and to record volume losses. Temporary ostomy appliances, catheters, karaya gum rings, and at times prone positioning on a Stryker frame have all been used. Ingenuity and improvisation must be

Table 33–2. Treatment of fistulas.

First:
Restore blood volume and begin correction of fluid and electrolyte imbalance.
Drain accessible abscesses.
Control fistula and measure losses.

Second:
Provide intravenous hyperalimentation.

Third:
Delineate anatomy of fistulas by radiographic studies.
Begin alimentary feedings if possible.

Fourth:
Maintain caloric intake of 3000 Cal or more per day.
Drain abscesses as they appear.
Operate if fistula fails to close.

relied on in devising the best technic for the individual patient.

C. Control of Sepsis: Obvious and easily accessible abscesses should be drained surgically as soon as they are diagnosed. The source of sepsis is often obscure, and a continuous diligent search for the abscess or abscesses must be made by repeated physical examinations and radiologic studies until the infection is located and treated. Blind therapy with broad-spectrum antibiotics is not a substitute for surgical drainage of abscesses.

D. Delineation of Fistula: Radiographic contrast studies (see above) should be obtained as soon as practicable.

E. Nutrition: Adequate nutrition and control of sepsis make the difference between survival and demise of these patients. A useful general rule is to avoid all oral intake at the outset. Nasogastric suction may be necessary temporarily. As soon as intravascular fluid and electrolytes are restored, intravenous hyperalimentation should be instituted through a centrally positioned catheter. In order to maintain a patient on hyperalimentation for prolonged periods, a special type of venous catheter is surgically implanted in the subcutaneous tissue.

In the long run, nutrition through the alimentary tract is preferable to parenteral technics. The method depends on the location of the fistula and the associated anatomy. With high fistulas, fluid may be collected proximally through one catheter and instilled distally through another. In others, a small, soft catheter attached to a tiny mercury-weighted balloon may be passed orally and threaded past the fistula. A Baron pump continuously instills blended food or an elemental diet through the tube. Distal fistulas may not require such measures, and regular diets or elemental diets may be given by mouth. The greatest difficulty is presented by mid small bowel fistulas. These patients often cannot be fed by any method other than intravenously. The average patient receives treatment by both routes, with the objective being an intake of 3000 Cal or more per day.

F. Operation: Although most fistulas close spontaneously, others persist despite drainage of abscesses and provision of adequate nutrition. Failure of a fistula to resolve may be caused by distal obstruction, neoplasm or foreign body at the fistula site, epithelization of the fistula tract, intestinal ischemia, or extensive disruption of bowel continuity. If fistula output does not diminish on optimal treatment, operation should be undertaken. The fistulous segment should be resected, associated obstruction relieved, and continuity reestablished by end-to-end anastomosis. Bypass without resection may be indicated in some patients. The various surgical procedures are illustrated in Fig 33–8.

Prognosis

The plan of management outlined above results in 80–90% survival of patients with external fistulas. Uncontrolled sepsis is the chief cause of death.

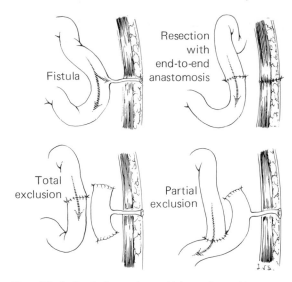

Figure 33—8. Surgical procedures which may be used to remove or defunctionalize small bowel fistulas. Resection with end-to-end anastomosis is the preferred method.

Aguirre A, Fischer JE, Welch CE: The role of surgery and hyperalimentation in therapy of gastrointestinal-cutaneous fistulae. Ann Surg 180:393, 1974.

Fischer JE: The management of high-output intestinal fistulas. Adv Surg 9:139, 1975.

Himal HS & others: The importance of adequate nutrition in closure of small intestinal fistulas. Br J Surg 61:724, 1974.

Sheldon GF & others: Management of gastrointestinal fistulas. Surg Gynecol Obstet 133:385, 1971.

ACUTE VASCULAR LESIONS OF THE SMALL BOWEL & MESENTERY

The blood supply to the gastrointestinal tract derives from the celiac, superior mesenteric, and inferior mesenteric arteries, with collateral connections to other arterial systems at either end. Venous blood from small bowel drains into the portal vein. Lesions producing acute or chronic ischemia or hemorrhage may result from intrinsic vascular disease, systemic illness, pharmacologic agents, and surgical procedures. Chronic occlusion may be amenable to vascular reconstruction and is discussed in Chapter 38.

1. ACUTE MESENTERIC VASCULAR OCCLUSION

Essentials of Diagnosis

- Severe, diffuse abdominal pain.
- Gross or occult intestinal bleeding.
- Minimal physical findings.
- Radiographic findings (sometimes).
- Operative findings.

General Considerations

Sudden occlusion of major small bowel arteries or veins is catastrophic. It is predominantly a disease of the elderly and is highly lethal. Mesenteric **arterial emboli** most commonly originate from mural thrombus in an infarcted left ventricle or clot in a fibrillating left atrium in patients with mitral stenosis. **Thrombosis** of a **mesenteric artery** is the end result of atherosclerotic stenosis, and these patients often relate a history of intestinal angina before the acute thrombosis occurs. Other causes of acute arterial occlusion such as dissecting aortic aneurysm or fusiform aortic aneurysm are rare. Occlusions of smaller mesenteric arteries often are associated with connective tissue or other systemic disorders.

Thrombosis of mesenteric veins is associated with portal hypertension, abdominal sepsis, hypercoagulable states, trauma, or no apparent underlying disease. In recent years, mesenteric venous thrombosis has appeared in women taking oral contraceptives. Some venous occlusions develop peripherally and progress insidiously, causing segmental infarction which resembles strangulation obstruction. Others have acute, severe, rapidly progressive ischemia.

The consequences of major vascular occlusion depend on the vessel involved, the level of occlusion, the status of other visceral vessels, the development of collaterals, and other factors. The principal effect is hemorrhagic necrosis of the mucosa, the layer most sensitive to ischemia. The mucosa ulcerates, sloughs, and bleeds. Bacteria proliferate in the ischemic segment, and infection contributes further to thrombosis of small vessels. Bacterial growth is not essential for a fatal outcome, but absorption of toxic products is an important factor hastening the demise of untreated patients.

Ischemia progresses to full-thickness infarction of bowel wall as early as 6 hours or as long as several days after arterial occlusion. Hemorrhage into the lumen, accumulation of bloody abdominal fluid, diffuse peritonitis, and cardiovascular collapse ensue even in the absence of gross perforation.

Clinical Findings

A. Symptoms and Signs: The most constant symptom is severe, poorly localized abdominal pain which is often unresponsive to narcotics. Nausea, vomiting, diarrhea, and constipation are variable in occurrence.

In the early stages there is a striking paucity of abdominal findings; in fact, pain out of proportion to the objective findings is a hallmark of mesenteric vascular occlusion. Ischemia also can occur with much less severe pain, and serious illness may be recognized only when secondary toxicity develops. Later in the course, abdominal distention and tenderness occur. Shock and generalized peritonitis eventually develop, but by that time the opportunity for salvage has been lost. In some instances—particularly with a high venous occlusion—shock is an early finding. Stool and gastric contents may contain blood. Paracentesis does not help establish the diagnosis in the reversible stages, but later it is positive.

B. Laboratory Findings: Striking leukocytosis and some elevation of serum amylase are present. Significant base deficits may be observed. Hemoconcentration and the effects of hemorrhage into the lumen or mesentery are reflected in laboratory tests in the late stages. Elevated serum levels of the intestinal isomer of alkaline phosphatase may prove to be a useful test.

C. X-Ray Findings: Plain abdominal films allow a presumptive diagnosis of vascular occlusion to be made in about 20% of patients. Absence of intestinal gas, diffuse distention with air-fluid levels, and distention of small bowel and colon up to the splenic flexure are nonspecific but suggestive. Blunt plicae, thickened bowel wall, and small bowel loops that remain unchanged over several hours are seen occasionally. Specific findings of intestinal necrosis, including intramural gas and gas in the portal venous system, occur late. Barium studies reveal "thumbprinting" and disordered motility (either slow or rapid). The primary function of mesenteric arteriography is to determine the presence or absence of occlusion of a major vessel; a normal study does not exclude occlusion of smaller branches.

Differential Diagnosis

Acute pancreatitis and strangulation obstruction of the intestine may be difficult to distinguish from mesenteric vascular occlusion. A very high serum amylase early in the disease suggests pancreatitis. Differentiation from strangulation obstruction is less important since both conditions require operation. Angiography may be definitive. Unfortunately, even surgeons with a special interest in this condition are unable to make an early diagnosis in more than half of cases.

Treatment

Acute occlusion of mesenteric arteries or veins is treated by prompt operation. The clinical picture and angiographic studies may give clues to the cause, but often it is only determined at operation. Acute venous thrombosis is diagnosed by the edematous mesentery and extrusion of clots when mesenteric veins are cut. Resection of all of the involved gut and its mesentery is the treatment of choice; direct mesenteric venous surgery (thrombectomy) is seldom successful. Administration of heparin or dextran postoperatively is recommended.

In arterial occlusion, there is segmental or diffuse ischemia or infarction of small bowel and colon in the distribution of the occluded vessel. Arterial pulsations are absent or reduced, and mesenteric edema is not so striking as in venous occlusion. If reversible ischemia is due to occlusion of the superior mesenteric artery, vascular reconstruction should be attempted. The best

results are achieved in those due to an embolus because the embolus often lodges in the superior mesenteric artery at the origin of the middle colic artery and is accessible for removal. Thromboendarterectomy or bypass of a thrombosed superior mesenteric artery can be attempted, although patency rates are poor.

Infarcted bowel should be resected unless the extent of damage (eg, entire small bowel and right colon) is so great that satisfactory life could not be expected. Ischemic bowel which is not obviously necrotic should be left in, especially if arterial reconstruction was accomplished. Massive volume support and antibiotics are mandatory, and anticoagulants or drugs which inhibit platelet aggregation are given by some surgeons. If resection is performed, it is wise to avoid primary anastomosis unless one is certain that the surgical margins have excellent blood supply. A second look operation is performed 6–12 hours later in most cases to determine patency of arterial reconstructions, assess viability of remaining bowel, and construct an intestinal anastomosis.

Prognosis

Acute mesenteric vascular occlusion is lethal in about 70% of patients because diagnosis and operative treatment are often delayed, infarction is extensive, and arterial reconstruction is technically difficult. Although feasible in only a few cases, prompt embolectomy is associated with a high survival rate if a major bowel resection is averted. Results are less satisfactory in others with emboli or arterial thrombosis. In a few patients, the acute ischemic episode goes unrecognized and the process resolves spontaneously with stricture formation. The prognosis is excellent in this situation. Acute venous thrombosis has a mortality rate of 30%, and the prognosis is determined by the nature of the underlying disease in most cases.

Anane-Sefah JC, Blair E, Reckler S: Primary mesenteric venous occlusive disease. Surg Gynecol Obstet 141:740, 1975.

Barnett SM, Davidson ED, Bradley EL III: Intestinal alkaline phosphatase and base deficit in mesenteric occlusion. J Surg Res 20:243, 1976.

Barnett WO, Petro AB, Williamson JW: A current appraisal of problems with gangrenous bowel. Ann Surg 183:653, 1976.

Bergan JJ & others: Revascularization in treatment of mesenteric infarction. Ann Surg 182:430, 1975.

Gruenberg JC, Smallridge RC, Rosenberg RD: Inherited antithrombin-III deficiency causing mesenteric venous infarction: A new clinical entity. Ann Surg 181:791, 1975.

Singh RP, Shah RC, Lee ST: Acute mesenteric vascular occlusion: A review of thirty-two patients. Surgery 78:613, 1975.

Tjiong B & others: Fluid shifts and metabolic changes during and after occlusion of the superior mesenteric artery. Surg Gynecol Obstet 139:217, 1974.

Tomchik FS & others: The roentgenographic spectrum of bowel infarction. Radiology 96:249, 1970.

2. NONOCCLUSIVE INTESTINAL ISCHEMIA

In about one-third of patients with intestinal ischemia, vascular occlusion does not involve a major artery or vein (although arterial stenosis is usually present) and is confined to smaller vessels, especially arterioles. In the presence of some other acute disease such as a cardiac arrhythmia or sepsis, splanchnic vasoconstriction occurs, and the intestine becomes ischemic because of low perfusion pressure and flow.

The diagnosis is suspected when a potentially susceptible patient develops acute abdominal pain. The clinical picture is similar to that of arterial thrombosis, but the onset is less often sudden. Arteriography documents the absence of major vascular occlusion but is not otherwise diagnostic in most cases.

Direct infusion of vasodilatory agents (glucagon, isoproterenol, phenoxybenzamine) into the superior mesenteric artery is reportedly successful in reversing splanchnic vasoconstriction in selected cases. However, operation is usually required eventually in order to resect infarcted bowel and, very importantly, to exclude other diseases that simulate intestinal ischemia.

Patchy or diffuse ischemia varies in extent and severity. Ischemia is most pronounced on the antimesenteric border, and the mucosa may be extensively involved before abnormalities are visible on the serosal surface. There are often ischemic areas in other organs such as liver and spleen. Vascular reconstruction is ineffective, and surgical procedures are limited to resection of infarcted bowel. Decisions about when to perform a primary anastomosis or second look operation are individualized. The prognosis is poor, mainly because the underlying disease often cannot be corrected.

Athanasoulis CA & others: Vasodilatory drugs in the management of nonocclusive bowel ischemia. Gastroenterology 68:146, 1975.

Habboushe F & others: Nonocclusive mesenteric vascular insufficiency. Ann Surg 180:819, 1974.

Ottinger LW: Nonocclusive mesenteric infarction. Surg Clin North Am 54:689, 1974.

Williams LF Jr: Vascular insufficiency of the intestines. Gastroenterology 61:757, 1971.

3. OTHER VASCULAR LESIONS

Vasculitis

Vascular lesions associated with systemic disorders such as polyarteritis nodosa may cause patchy infarction of the small intestine. Similar lesions have been seen in patients with a history of amphetamine abuse. The presenting manifestation is usually perforation with peritonitis or intraluminal bleeding. The prognosis depends on the underlying pathologic process and the severity of peritoneal contamination. These patients are often on corticosteroid therapy and do not tolerate infection well. Survival is rare.

Mesenteric Apoplexy

Mesenteric apoplexy is an uncommon disorder caused by spontaneous rupture of mesenteric arteries. The more general category of **abdominal apoplexy** includes spontaneous hemorrhage into the peritoneal cavity from tumors (particularly hepatomas), the spleen, or other organs. Arteriosclerotic lesions are the cause of arterial rupture in older individuals; the superior mesenteric, right colic, and branches of the celiac artery are the usual sites. Sudden hemorrhage from congenital aneurysms occurs in younger patients; the splenic artery is most commonly involved and is particularly prone to rupture during pregnancy.

The typical picture is sudden onset of diffuse abdominal pain followed by hypotension. A "double rupture" of splenic artery aneurysms is seen in about half of cases; bleeding initially is confined to the lesser sac, and 1–2 days later this collection breaks into the greater sac with exsanguinating blood loss. These symptoms may be confused with mesenteric vascular occlusion, rupture of an abdominal aortic aneurysm, or perforated viscus. There is diffuse abdominal tenderness and distention due to free blood in the peritoneal cavity. The diagnosis is usually clear from signs of internal blood loss and peritoneal irritation, but paracentesis is sometimes helpful.

Operation is imperative. The site of bleeding is located, and the involved vessel is ligated. Rarely, the bleeding artery can be reconstructed with autogenous or prosthetic material. If blood supply to portions of the intestinal tract is impaired, segments of bowel may have to be resected. Splenectomy with ligation of the splenic artery is preferred for patients with a ruptured splenic artery aneurysm.

GAS CYSTS
(Pneumatosis Cystoides Intestinalis)

Pneumatosis cystoides intestinalis is a rare condition characterized by gas-filled cysts in the wall of the gut and sometimes in the mesentery. The jejunum, the ileocecal region, and the colon are the areas most often involved (in descending order of frequency). Cysts are submucosal or subserosal, vary in size from microscopic to several centimeters in diameter, and are most common in middle age.

Associated diseases of the gastrointestinal tract such as pyloric stenosis due to peptic ulcer, inflammatory bowel disease, diverticulitis, or scleroderma are present in 85% of cases. The mechanism of cyst formation is obscure. Direct communication of cysts with the intestinal lumen cannot be demonstrated, and the most plausible hypothesis is that gas enters the cysts by diffusion. Obstructive lesions producing high intraluminal pressure may be responsible in some cases.

Symptoms are usually those of the underlying disease, and cysts are incidental findings. Rarely, perforation of a cyst, hemorrhage, obstruction, or malabsorption may bring the condition to medical attention. Infection with gas-forming bacteria can produce a similar picture on x-ray. Such patients are usually toxic and may have underlying impaired immunologic defenses. Gas may also be seen within the intestinal wall late in intestinal infarction.

Treatment is directed first to the underlying disease. Pneumatosis itself requires treatment only if symptomatic, and it often resolves spontaneously or by having the patient breathe 70% oxygen for several days. Surgical procedures are required only in those rare individuals with complications. Some of these cysts contain explosive intestinal gases and therefore should not be opened with the electrocautery.

Yale CE, Balish E: Pneumatosis cystoides intestinalis. Dis Colon Rectum 19:107, 1976.

TUMORS OF THE SMALL INTESTINE

Neoplasms of the jejunum and ileum comprise 1–5% of all tumors of the gastrointestinal tract. The terminal ileum is the favored site, followed by proximal jejunum. Approximately 85% of patients are over age 40. There is a high correlation of small bowel tumors with primary neoplasms elsewhere.

Only 10% of small bowel tumors are symptomatic. Benign lesions are 10 times as common as malignant ones, but at least 75% of symptomatic neoplasms are malignant. Bleeding and obstruction, sometimes due to intussusception, are the most frequent symptoms.

1. BENIGN TUMORS

Polyps

Adenomatous or villous polyps of the type seen in the colon are rare in the small bowel; they are usually solitary and cause symptoms by intussusception or bleeding.

Polypoid **hamartomas** are developmental abnormalities rather than neoplasms and therefore have no malignant potential. Patients with solitary lesions are free of associated anomalies. Hamartomas are multiple in 50% of cases, and 10% of these have a familial disorder characterized by diffuse gastrointestinal polyposis and mucocutaneous pigmentation (**Peutz-Jeghers syndrome**). Operation is only indicated for symptoms (eg, obstruction, bleeding), at which time all polyps greater than about 1 cm should be removed.

Gardner's syndrome is another familial disease characterized by multiple intestinal and colonic polyps, osteomas, and subcutaneous cysts or fibromas. The polyps in Gardner's syndrome are true neoplasms, and malignant degeneration is common.

Juvenile (retention) polyps may bleed or obstruct. They are more common in the colon than the small bowel and usually autoamputate before adolescence.

Welch CE, Hedberg SE: *Polypoid Lesions of the Gastrointestinal Tract,* 2nd ed. Saunders, 1975.

Vascular Tumors

Vascular tumors are multicentric in the small bowel in 55% of cases and may involve the intestine diffusely. Hemangiomas may bleed or intussuscept in children and young adults. **Hereditary hemorrhagic telangiectasia** (Rendu-Osler-Weber syndrome) is an inborn progressive tendency toward formation of dilated endothelial spaces in small bowel and other sites. Vascular malformations are not true neoplasms.

It may be difficult to locate the bleeding point. Arteriography may help if performed during active hemorrhage, and calcified lesions may be evident on plain films. If a patient is known to have diffuse vascular lesions and the bleeding site is unknown, it is best to avoid operation if possible. If operation must be performed without knowledge of the bleeding site, transillumination or compression of the bowel between 2 glass slides and intraoperative endoscopy may help in the search. Blind resection is often followed by recurrent episodes of hemorrhage.

Bruusgaard A, Juhl E: Hereditary hemorrhagic telangiectasis (Rendu-Weber-Osler's disease) with intestinal involvement successfully treated by surgery. Gastroenterology 67:1001, 1974.

Other Tumors

Leiomyomas, lipomas, neurofibromas, and fibromas may cause symptoms that require operation.

Wilson JM & others: Benign small bowel tumor. Ann Surg 181:247, 1975.

2. MALIGNANT TUMORS

Primary

Adenocarcinoma usually arises in the proximal jejunum, often causing no or minimal symptoms for prolonged periods. Metastases are present in 80% at the time of operation. Segmental resection of bowel and adjacent mesentery is done when possible, but metastases near the superior mesenteric artery may make the procedure difficult. Five-year survival is 25% in patients undergoing intestinal resection.

Primary malignant lymphoma arising in the ileum may diffusely infiltrate the submucosa, producing a long rigid segment. Some patients present with fever of unknown origin, and up to one-third present with malabsorption syndrome. Sprue-like villous atrophy is often associated with lymphoma, but it is not clear whether this is cause, effect, or coincidence. Wide segmental resection is the treatment of choice. Splenectomy, liver biopsy, and biopsy of retroperitoneal lymph nodes are recommended to determine the stage of the disease and help plan further therapy. **Leiomyosarcoma** in small bowel tends to ulcerate centrally and bleed. Other types of primary malignant neoplasm are rare.

Metastatic

Small bowel metastases are found in 50% of patients dying of malignant melanoma. Carcinomas of the cervix, kidney, breast, etc may also spread to bowel. Obstruction or hemorrhage may require operation if life expectancy is reasonably good. Significant palliation may be achieved, particularly in patients with solitary metastatic lesions.

Kahn LB & others: Primary gastrointestinal lymphoma: A clinicopathologic study of fifty-seven cases. Am J Dig Dis 17:219, 1972.

Wilson JM & others: Primary malignancies of the small bowel: A report of 96 cases and review of the literature. Ann Surg 180:175, 1974.

3. CARCINOID TUMORS & CARCINOID SYNDROME

The small bowel is the second most common site (after the appendix) of carcinoid tumors. About 10 times as many originate in the ileum as in the jejunum. Carcinoids occur in patients 25–45 years of age, and occasionally they are associated with primary neoplasms of other enterochromaffin tissues (medullary carcinoma of the thyroid and pheochromocytoma).

Carcinoid tumors arise from argentaffin (Kulchitsky) cells in the crypts of Lieberkühn and form yellowish, firm nodules in the submucosa; special stains may demonstrate argentaffin granules. Multiple tumors are present in 50% of cases.

Carcinoid of the small bowel should be regarded as "a malignant neoplasm in slow motion." At the time of surgical diagnosis, 40% of tumors have invaded the muscularis and 33% have metastasized to lymph nodes or liver. Fewer than 2% of primary tumors less than 1 cm in diameter metastasize, but 80% of those larger than 2 cm have spread at the time of operation. Huge metastatic deposits emanating from a minute primary are sometimes encountered.

Clinical Findings

A. Symptoms and Signs: Small tumors are usually asymptomatic. Overall, 30% of small bowel carcinoids cause symptoms of obstruction, pain, bleeding, or the carcinoid syndrome. Obstruction due to sclerosis and kinking of the bowel may be related to elaboration of vasoactive materials by metastases in the mesentery.

About 10% of patients with small bowel carcinoids present with **carcinoid syndrome,** and others develop it later. The syndrome consists of cutaneous flushing, diarrhea, bronchoconstriction, and right-sided cardiac valvular disease due to collagen deposition. Biologically active substances secreted by carcinoids are usually inactivated in the liver, but hepatic metastases or primary ovarian or bronchial carcinoids release these compounds directly into the systemic circulation where they produce symptoms. No single substance is believed to be responsible for the entire spectrum of symptoms, and a host of active materials has been implicated, including serotonin, catecholamines, histamine, 5-hydroxytryptophan, bradykinin, prostaglandins, ACTH, and calcitonin.

B. Laboratory Findings: Some carcinoid tumors are detected by radiographic methods. Urinary levels of 5-hydroxyindoleacetic acid (5-HIAA) can be measured, but a negative qualitative or low quantitative test does not rule out carcinoid syndrome because 5-HIAA is a metabolite of serotonin, which is only one of many mediators of the syndrome. Provocative tests can be used, but full laboratory investigation of these patients is a research effort.

Treatment

All accessible carcinoid tumor in small bowel mesentery and the peritoneal cavity should be removed, and repeated operations may be required. Palliative resection of liver metastases has benefited some patients. The tumor responds poorly to fluorouracil and other cytotoxic drugs.

Carcinoid syndrome can be treated by various pharmacologic agents designed to block the effects of active substances; this form of therapy requires definition of the responsible mediators in individual patients. Among the agents sometimes used are phenothiazines, methysergide, methyldopa, and corticosteroids.

Prognosis

Carcinoid tumors grow slowly over months and years. The overall 5-year survival after resection of small bowel carcinoid is 70%; 40% of patients with inoperable metastases and 20% of those with hepatic metastases survive 5 years or longer.

Advanced carcinoid may produce intestinal infarction due to occlusion of the superior mesenteric artery by sclerotic deposits in the mesentery.

Graham-Smith DG: *The Carcinoid Syndrome.* Heinemann, 1972.

Morgan JG, Marks C, Hearn D: Carcinoid tumors of the gastrointestinal tract. Ann Surg 180:720, 1974.

●   ●   ●

General References

Colcock BP, Braasch JW: *Surgery of the Small Intestine in the Adult.* Saunders, 1968.

Sleisenger MH, Fordtran JS: *Gastrointestinal Disease.* Saunders, 1973.

Sleisenger MH, Brandborg LL: *Malabsorption.* Saunders, 1977.

34 . . .
Large Intestine

Theodore R. Schrock, MD, & Walter Birnbaum, MD

ANATOMY

The colon extends from the end of the ileum to the rectum. The cecum, ascending colon, hepatic flexure, and proximal transverse colon comprise the **right colon**. The distal transverse colon, splenic flexure, descending colon, sigmoid colon, and rectosigmoid comprise the **left colon** (Fig 34–1). The ascending and descending portions are fixed in the retroperitoneal space, and the transverse colon and sigmoid colon are suspended in the peritoneal cavity by their mesenteries. The caliber of the lumen is greatest at the cecum and diminishes distally. The wall of the colon has 4 layers: mucosa, submucosa, muscularis, and serosa (Fig 34–2). The muscularis consists of a complete inner

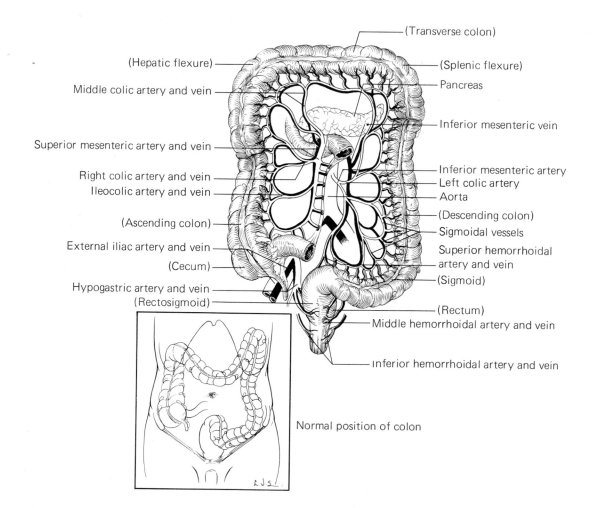

(Transverse colon)

(Hepatic flexure)

(Splenic flexure)

Middle colic artery and vein

Pancreas

Inferior mesenteric vein

Superior mesenteric artery and vein

Inferior mesenteric artery

Left colic artery

Right colic artery and vein

Aorta

Ileocolic artery and vein

(Descending colon)

(Ascending colon)

Sigmoidal vessels

External iliac artery and vein

Superior hemorrhoidal artery and vein

(Cecum)

(Sigmoid)

Hypogastric artery and vein

(Rectosigmoid)

(Rectum)

Middle hemorrhoidal artery and vein

Inferior hemorrhoidal artery and vein

Normal position of colon

Figure 34–1. The large intestine: anatomic divisions and blood supply. The veins are shown in black. The insert shows the usual configuration of the colon.

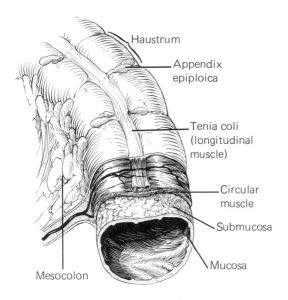

Figure 34-2. Cross-section of colon.

circular layer and an outer longitudinal layer which is gathered into 3 bands (teniae). Sacculations, termed haustra, are formed by shortening of the colon by the teniae as well as by contractions of the circular muscle. The haustra are not fixed anatomic structures and may be observed to move longitudinally. There are fatty appendages (the appendices epiploicae) on the serosal surface. The wall of the colon is so thin that it becomes markedly distended when obstructed.

The rectum is 12–15 cm in length. The teniae spread at the rectosigmoid junction and form a longitudinal muscular layer which completely encircles the rectum. The upper rectum is invested by peritoneum anteriorly and laterally, but posteriorly it is retroperitoneal up to the rectosigmoid. The anterior peritoneal reflection dips low into the pelvis approximately 7 cm above the anal verge—a fact to be noted when rectal lesions are biopsied or fulgurated; perforation into the peritoneal cavity can occur at a much lower level anteriorly than posteriorly. The anterior peritoneal reflection lies behind the bladder in males and behind the uterus (the rectouterine pouch of Douglas) in females. Tumor masses or abscesses in this location are readily palpated on digital rectal or pelvic examination.

The rectum is normally capacious and distensible. When its capacity to distend is lost or impaired by surgery or disease, normal bowel habits are interfered with. Habitual use of laxatives—especially mineral oil—causes constant filling of the ampulla with a resulting vicious cycle of constipation and catharsis. Perception of the urge to defecate requires an intact rectal mucosa. Sacrifice of this portion of the rectum—as in some operations for malignancy—results in incontinence even though the sphincteric ring is undamaged.

The rectal valves of Houston are 3 prominent mucosal folds within the rectum, arranged spirally, 2 on the left and one on the right. Normally the valves appear thin, with sharp edges, but they become thickened and blunted when inflammation occurs. A rectal valve may hide a small lesion from endoscopic view, and during sigmoidoscopy the valve must be "ironed out" so that its superior surface can be examined. The most difficult level to bypass with the sigmoidoscope is where the intra- and extraperitoneal portions of the bowel meet. Local muscular contraction occurs here, although no true sphincter has been demonstrated.

In males, the prostate gland, the seminal vesicles, and the seminal ducts lie anterior to the rectum. The prostate usually is easily felt, but the seminal vesicles are not palpable unless distended because the firm, unyielding rectovesical fascia of Denonvilliers intervenes. In the female, the rectovaginal septum and uterus lie anterior and the uterine adnexa anterolateral to the rectum. The structures are easily palpated with one finger in the vagina and one in the rectum.

Blood Supply & Lymphatic Drainage

The arterial supply of the right colon, from the ileocecal juncture to approximately the mid transverse colon, is from the superior mesenteric artery through its ileocolic, right colic, and middle colic branches.

The **inferior mesenteric artery** arises from the abdominal aorta and gives off the left colic and sigmoid branches before it becomes the superior hemorrhoidal artery. The **vasa recta** are the terminal arterial branches to the colon and run directly to the mesenteric wall or through the bowel wall to the antimesocolic border.

The colic arteries bifurcate and form arcades about 2.5 cm (1 inch) from the mesenteric border of the bowel, forming a pathway of communicating vessels called the **marginal artery of Drummond**. The marginal artery thus forms an anastomosis between the superior mesenteric and inferior mesenteric arteries. The configuration of the blood supply, however, varies greatly; the "typical" pattern is present in only 15% of individuals.

The middle hemorrhoidal artery arises on each side from the anterior division of the internal iliac artery or from the internal pudendal artery and runs inward in the lateral ligaments of the rectum. The inferior hemorrhoidal arteries derive from the internal pudendal arteries and pass through Alcock's canal. The anastomoses between the superior hemorrhoidal vessels and branches of the internal iliac arteries provide collateral circulation which is important after surgical interruption or atherosclerotic occlusion of the vascular supply of the left colon.

The **veins** accompany the corresponding arteries and drain into the liver through the portal vein or into the systemic circulation by way of the hypogastric veins. There are continuous **lymphatic plexuses** in the submucous and subserous layers of the bowel wall which drain into the lymphatic channels and lymph nodes that accompany the blood vessels.

Nerve Supply

The **sympathetic nerves** originating in T10–12

travel in the thoracic splanchnic nerves to the celiac plexus and then to the preaortic and superior mesenteric plexuses, from which postganglionic fibers are distributed along the superior mesenteric artery and its branches to the right colon. The left colon is supplied by sympathetic fibers which arise in L1–3, synapse in the paravertebral ganglia, and accompany the inferior mesenteric artery to the colon. The **parasympathetic nerves** to the right colon come from the right vagus and travel with the sympathetic nerves. The parasympathetic supply to the left colon derives from S2–4. These fibers emerge from the spinal cord as the nervi erigentes, which form the pelvic plexus and send branches to the transverse, descending, and pelvic portions of the colon.

Bacon HE, Recio PM: *Surgical Anatomy of the Colon, Rectum and Anal Canal.* Lippincott, 1962.

Goligher JC: *Surgery of the Anus, Rectum and Colon,* 3rd ed. Thomas, 1975.

Meyers MA & others: Haustral anatomy and pathology: A new look. 1. Roentgen identification of normal patterns and relationships. Radiology 108:497, 1973.

Michels MA & others: Routes of collateral circulation of the gastro-intestinal tract as ascertained in a dissection of 500 bodies. Int Surg 49:8, 1968.

PHYSIOLOGY

The small bowel efficiently digests and absorbs nutrients from ingested foods and passes the residue along to the colon for further processing. The solids in the ileal effluent are largely undigested plant materials such as cellulose. The colon extracts electrolytes and water from the ileal fluid, converting it into semisolid feces which are stored until defecation is convenient. Loss of colonic function through disease or surgery results in a continuous discharge of food wastes and increases daily intestinal losses of water and electrolytes, chiefly sodium chloride. Absorption of glucose, amino acids, lipolytic products, or vitamins is not significant in the large intestine.

The volume and composition of intestinal gas vary greatly among normal individuals. The small intestine contains approximately 100 ml of gas and the colon somewhat more. Some gas is absorbed through the mucosa and excreted through the lungs, and the remaining 400–1200 ml/day is emitted as flatus. Nitrogen (N_2) comprises from 30–90% of intestinal gas. It was at one time believed that swallowed air was the only source of intestinal N_2, but it has been proved that N_2 can diffuse across the mucosa from blood to lumen. This phenomenon occurs when other gases are produced in the lumen in sufficient volume to lower the partial pressure of N_2 below that of blood, thus establishing a gradient for diffusion. Other intestinal gases include oxygen (O_2), carbon dioxide (CO_2), hydrogen (H_2), and methane (CH_4). H_2 and CO_2 are generated by fermentation of ingested nonabsorbed carbohydrate, especially carbohydrate present in certain legumes. Lactose in milk provides the substrate in lactase-deficient patients. Only about one-third of the population produce CH_4, which is also a product of colonic bacteria. Stools of CH_4-producers nearly always float, even in the absence of fecal fat. The mixture of colonic gases is potentially explosive, so that caution must be exercised when using the electrocautery to open the lumen of the colon. Patients who complain of "excess gas" usually have normal gas production but are abnormally sensitive to distention of the gut.

Motility

Motor activity of the colon occurs in 3 patterns. **Retrograde peristalsis,** annular contractions moving orad, dominates in the right colon. This kind of activity churns the contents and tends to confine them to the cecum and ascending colon. As ileal effluent continually enters the cecum, some of the column of liquid stool in the right colon is displaced and flows into the transverse colon. **Segmentation** is the most common type of motor activity in the transverse and descending colon. Annular contractions divide the lumen into uniform segments, propelling feces over short distances in both directions. Segmental contractions form, relax, and reform in different locations, seemingly at random. **Mass movement** is a strong ring contraction moving aborad over long distances in the transverse and descending colon. It occurs infrequently, perhaps only a few times daily.

Colonic motility is modified by neural and hormonal stimuli. Relatively little is known about neural control of muscular activity in the colon in humans. The traditional notion is that parasympathetic nerves are excitatory and sympathetics are inhibitory; this may be an inaccurate generalization. Some investigators believe the response of bowel musculature to a given stimulus depends as much on the state of contraction at that time as on the pathway of stimulation.

Eating produces a group of alterations in colonic motility (gastrocolic responses) which include increased ileal emptying through the ileocecal valve, increased mass movements, and an urge to defecate. These changes are mediated by neural impulses and by a hormone or hormones released from the upper small intestine in response to eating. Cholecystokinin seems likely to be involved in producing the gastrocolic responses, but other hormones may participate also. Experimentally, gastrin stimulates and secretin and glucagon inhibit the colon. Emotional factors influence colonic motility, and physical activity such as changes in posture, walking, and lifting are physiologically important stimuli to the movement of colonic contents. Fecal bulk stimulates motility and speeds transit through the colon.

Normal colonic movements are slow, complex, and extremely variable, making it difficult to define altered motility in disease states. Although colonic motility is said to be quiet in patients with diarrhea and hyperactive in constipated subjects, the results of recent studies have cast doubt on this concept.

The fecal stream itself does not move along in anything resembling orderly laminar flow. Some of the material entering the cecum flows past feces remaining from earlier periods. Portions of the stream enter the periphery of haustra, where they may fail to progress for 24 hours or more. In most persons with normal bowel function, residue from a meal reaches the cecum after 4 hours and the rectosigmoid by 24 hours. Mixing of bowel content in the colon results in passage of residue from a single meal in movements for 3–4 days afterwards.

The urge to defecate is perceived when small amounts of feces enter the rectum and stimulate stretch receptors in the rectal wall. The sensation may be temporarily suppressed by voluntarily contracting the sphincter and pelvic diaphragm. Eventually, increased rectal filling may make the urge to defecate impossible to deny. When defecation is performed, it is aided by assuming a position with the thighs flexed so that intra-abdominal pressure can be increased by abdominal wall contraction. The internal and external anal sphincters relax, and the rectal or rectosigmoid contents are extruded by contraction of the colon and by increasing abdominal pressure via a Valsalva maneuver. The pelvic floor relaxes and the rectum loses its curves as the feces are discharged from the anus. Afterward, the sphincters resume their tone and the rectum remains empty until shortly before the next movement, when arrival of more feces from the sigmoid evokes the urge to defecate once again.

Absorption

The colon participates in maintaining the body economy by absorption of water and electrolytes, but the absorptive function of the colon is not essential to life. Although glucose, amino acids, fatty acids, and vitamins can be absorbed slowly from the large bowel, a negligible amount of digestible nutrients reaches the colon normally. Approximately 1000–2000 ml of ileal effluent containing 90% water enter the cecum each day. This material is desiccated during transit through the colon, so that only 100–200 ml of water are excreted in the feces. Table 34–1 gives average values for the electrolyte and water composition of ileal effluent and feces; the differences provide a rough estimate of colonic absorption and secretion. Data are listed also

for the estimated maximal absorptive capacity, which is greater in the right colon than in the left. Normally, formed feces are composed of 70% water and 30% solids. Almost half of these solids are bacteria; the remainder is food waste and desquamated epithelium.

Sodium is absorbed by an active transport mechanism which is enhanced by mineralocorticoids. Normally, sodium absorption is so efficient that a person can remain in balance on as little as 5 mEq in the daily diet, but colectomy increases the minimum daily requirements to 80–100 mEq to offset losses from the ileostomy. Chloride and water absorption is passive along electrical and osmotic gradients established by the sodium pump.

A small amount of bicarbonate is secreted into the colonic lumen in exchange for chloride. Potassium enters feces by passive diffusion and by secretion in mucus. Excessive mucus production may occur in colitis or with certain tumors such as villous adenomas and may lead to substantial potassium losses in the stool.

Bowel Habits

The frequency of defecation is influenced by social and dietary customs. The average interval between bowel movements among the population of Western countries is a little over 24 hours but may vary in normal subjects from 8–12 hours to 2–3 days. Cellulose or other food residue speeds transit through the colon.

A change in bowel habits demands investigation for organic disease. Diarrhea may be debilitating and even fatal because it is associated with loss of large amounts of water and electrolytes. Diarrhea is usually present if stools contain more than 300 ml of fluid daily. Osmotic diarrhea results when excess water-soluble molecules remain in the bowel lumen, causing osmotic retention of water; this is one mechanism by which saline laxatives act. Bile salts, hydroxy fatty acids, and castor oil (ricinoleic acid) are a few of the many substances which stimulate secretion of fluid by the colon by increasing mucosal cyclic AMP. Increased secretion by the small bowel may also cause diarrhea. Rapid transit, decreased absorptive surface (eg, after intestinal resection), and exudative diseases are other reasons for feces to contain excess fluid.

"Constipation" has different meanings to different people and may refer to infrequency, hard consis-

Table 34–1. Mean values for electrolyte and water balance in the normal colon. A plus (+) sign indicates absorption from the colonic lumen; a minus (−) sign indicates secretion into the lumen.

	Ileal Effluent		Fecal Fluid		Colonic Absorption (per 24 hours)	
	Concentration (mEq/liter)	Quantity (per 24 hours)	Concentration (mEq/liter)	Quantity (per 24 hours)	Normal	Maximal Capacity
Na^+	120	180 mEq	30	2 mEq	+178 mEq	+400 mEq
K^+	6	10 mEq	67	5 mEq	+5 mEq	−45 mEq
Cl^-	67	100 mEq	20	1.5 mEq	+98 mEq	+500 mEq
HCO_3^-	40	60 mEq	50	4 mEq	+56 mEq	
H_2O		1500 ml		100 ml	+1400 ml	+5000 ml

tency, or difficult expulsion of stools. Bowel-conscious Americans spend 200 million dollars on laxatives annually. This stems in part from the discredited notion that "toxic substances" are absorbed from the colon if defecation does not occur on some prescribed schedule. The colons of patients with functional constipation have abnormal motility, but whether disordered motility is a cause or consequence has not been determined. Anxious patients with no organic disease should be discouraged from habitual ingestion of potent laxatives which disrupt intestinal function.

Avery Jones F, Godding EW: *Management of Constipation.* Blackwell, 1972.

Binder HJ, Donowitz M: A new look at laxative action. Gastroenterology 69:1001, 1975.

Binder HJ, Filburn C, Volpe BT: Bile salt alteration of colonic electrolyte transport: Role of cyclic adenosine monophosphate. Gastroenterology 68:503, 1975.

Christensen J: Myoelectric control of the colon. Gastroenterology 68:601, 1975.

Cummings JH: Absorption and secretion by the colon. Gut 16:323, 1975.

Devroede G, Lamarche J: Functional importance of extrinsic parasympathetic innervation to the distal colon and rectum in man. Gastroenterology 66:273, 1974.

Kimberg DV: Cyclic nucleotides and their role in gastrointestinal secretion. Gastroenterology 67:1023, 1974.

Lasser RB, Bond JH, Levitt MD: The role of intestinal gas in functional abdominal pain. N Engl J Med 293:524, 1975.

Levitt MD: Volume and composition of human intestinal gas determined by means of an intestinal washout technique. N Engl J Med 284:1394, 1971.

Phillips SF: Diarrhea: A current view of the pathophysiology. Gastroenterology 63:495, 1972.

Schuster MM: The riddle of the sphincters. Gastroenterology 69:249, 1975.

MICROBIOLOGY

The colon of the fetus is sterile, and the bacterial flora is established soon after birth. The type of bacteria present in the colon depends in part on dietary and environmental factors. The quantity and type of colonic bacteria present are not completely defined because of the limitations of the culture technics now available.

Over 99% of the normal fecal flora is anaerobic. *Bacteroides fragilis* is most prevalent and counts average 10^{10}/g of wet feces. *Lactobacillus bifidus,* clostridia, and cocci of various types are other common anaerobes. Aerobic fecal bacteria are mainly coliforms and enterococci. *Escherichia coli* is the predominant coliform and is present in counts of 10^7/g of feces; *Streptococcus faecalis,* the principal enterococcus, is present in similar numbers.

The fecal flora participates in numerous physiologic processes. Bacteria degrade bile pigments to give the stool its brown color, and the characteristic fecal odor is due to the amines indole and skatole produced by bacterial action. Fecal organisms deconjugate bile salts (only free bile salts are found in feces) and alter the steroid nucleus so that cholate becomes deoxycholate and chenodeoxycholate is converted to lithocholate. Deoxycholate is absorbed from the colon, but lithocholate is excreted in feces. Bacteria influence colonic motility and absorption, supply vitamin K to the host, and may be important in the defense against infection. Intestinal bacteria participate in the pathophysiology of a variety of disease processes.

Donaldson RM Jr: Normal bacterial populations of the intestine and their relation to intestinal function. (2 parts.) N Engl J Med 270:938, 994, 1964.

Dubos RJ, Savage DC, Schaedler RW: The indigenous flora of the gastrointestinal tract. Dis Colon Rectum 10:23, 1967.

Finegold SM: Intestinal bacteria. Calif Med 110:455, 1969.

ROENTGENOLOGIC EXAMINATION

Plain films of the abdomen depict the distribution of gas in the intestines, calcifications, tumor masses, and the size and position of the liver, spleen, and kidneys. In the presence of acute intra-abdominal disease, erect, lateral, and oblique projections and lateral decubitus views are helpful.

The lumen of the colon can be visualized radiographically by instilling a suspension of barium sulfate through the anus (barium enema) (Fig 34—3). Ade-

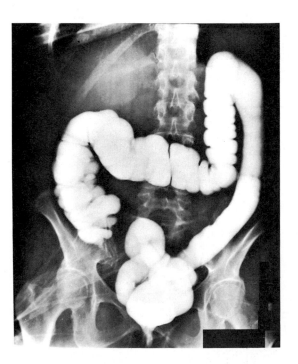

Figure 34—3. Roentgenogram of normal colon. The colon has been rendered radiopaque by a barium enema.

quate preparation of the bowel is imperative before barium enema examination so that the colon will be as free as possible of fecal material and gas. Although many rectal lesions can be visualized by barium enema, x-rays are not as accurate here as with lesions above the rectosigmoid. Proctosigmoidoscopy is the best method for inspecting the rectum. Postevacuation films reveal the mucosal pattern and small lesions. Double contrast (pneumocolon, air contrast) studies are useful to demonstrate small intraluminal lesions such as polyps. This is accomplished by allowing a coat of radiopaque barium to remain on the mucosa and filling the lumen with radiolucent air. The peroral double contrast enema, in which barium is given by mouth and air injected through the anus, is of value to identify abnormalities of the cecum and ascending colon. Arteriography is useful to detect bleeding sites and is discussed in the section on massive hemorrhage.

Margulis AR, Goldberg HI: The current status of radiologic technique in the examination of the colon: A survey. Radiol Clin North Am 7:27, 1969.

Martel W, Robins JM: The barium enema: Technique, value, and limitations. Cancer 28:137, 1971.

Seaman WB: Diseases of the colon: New concepts, old problems. Radiology 100:251, 1971.

FIBEROPTIC COLONOSCOPY

The fiberoptic colonoscope (coloscope) is a flexible instrument which is inserted per rectum and advanced proximally by manipulating controls on the handle. It is an outpatient procedure which is tolerated with little more discomfort than routine sigmoidoscopy. The lumen of the entire colon can be examined endoscopically in most individuals, and biopsies or cytologic material can be obtained under direct vision.

Fiberoptic colonoscopy may be decisive in establishing a correct diagnosis in patients with any of the following: (1) equivocal barium enema; (2) unexplained colonic symptoms; (3) lower gastrointestinal bleeding; (4) radiographic abnormalities in postoperative colons; (5) suspected inflammatory bowel disease. Endoscopic excision is an important aspect of the management of colonic polyps; this application is discussed in the section on polyps. Colonoscopy is contraindicated in fulminant inflammatory or ischemic bowel disease, in acute diverticulitis, and in patients with suspected colonic perforation.

Fiberoptic colonoscopy is a specialized procedure which requires skill, experience, and good judgment. Complications (perforation, bleeding, and cardiopulmonary problems) occur in 0.35% of diagnostic colonoscopy procedures. Success may be limited by technical difficulties such as diverticular disease, strictures, sharp flexures, redundant colon, or previous pelvic surgery.

Kronborg O, Østergaard A: Evaluation of the barium-enema examination and colonoscopy in diagnosis of colonic cancer. Dis Colon Rectum 18:674, 1975.

Overholt BF: Colonoscopy: A review. Gastroenterology 68:1308, 1975.

Schmitt MG Jr & others: Diagnostic colonoscopy: An assessment of the clinical indications. Gastroenterology 69:765, 1975.

Silvis SE & others: Endoscopic complications: Results of the 1974 American Society for Gastrointestinal Endoscopy survey. JAMA 235:928, 1976.

Wolff WI & others: Comparison of colonoscopy and the contrast enema in five hundred patients with colorectal disease. Am J Surg 129:181, 1975.

DISEASES OF THE COLON & RECTUM

COLONIC OBSTRUCTION

Essentials of Diagnosis

- Constipation or obstipation.
- Abdominal distention and sometimes tenderness.
- Abdominal pain.
- Nausea and vomiting (late).
- Characteristic x-ray findings.

General Considerations

Approximately 15% of intestinal obstructions in adults occur in the large bowel. The obstruction may be in any portion of the colon but most commonly is in the sigmoid. Complete colonic obstruction is most often due to carcinoma; volvulus, diverticular disease, inflammatory disorders, benign tumors, and fecal impaction account for the remainder (Table 34–2). Adhesive bands rarely obstruct the colon, and intussusception is uncommon in adults.

Obstruction by a lesion at the ileocecal valve produces the symptoms and signs of small bowel obstruction. The pathophysiology of more distal colonic obstruction depends on the competence of the ileocecal valve (Fig 34–4). In 10–20% of patients, the ileocecal valve is incompetent, and colonic pressure is relieved by reflux into the ileum. If the colon is not decom-

Table 34–2. Causes of colonic obstruction in adults.

Cause	Relative Incidence (%)*
Carcinoma of colon	65
Diverticulitis	20
Volvulus	5
Miscellaneous	10

*Obstruction due to diverticulitis is usually incomplete; volvulus is second to carcinoma as a cause of complete obstruction.

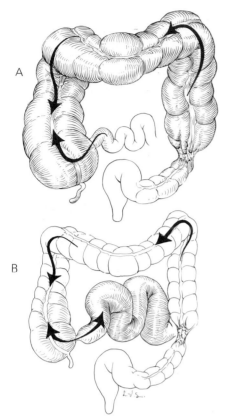

Figure 34—4. The role of the ileocecal valve in obstruction of the colon. The obstruction is in the upper sigmoid. *A:* The ileocecal valve is competent, creating a "closed loop" between the obstruction and the valve. Tension in the closed loop is increased further by emptying of gas and fluid from the ileum into the colon. *B:* The ileocecal valve is incompetent. Reflux into the ileum is permitted. The colon is relieved of some of its distention and the small bowel has become distended.

pressed through the ileocecal valve, a "closed loop" is formed between the valve and the obstructing point. The colon distends progressively because the ileum continues to empty gas and fluid into the obstructed segment. If luminal pressure becomes very high, circulation is impaired and gangrene and perforation can result. The wall of the right colon is thinner than that of the left colon and its luminal caliber is larger, so that the cecum is at greatest risk of perforation in these circumstances (law of Laplace). In general, if the cecum reaches a diameter of 10 cm (4 inches), the risk of perforation is great.

Clinical Findings

A. Symptoms and Signs: Simple mechanical obstruction of the colon may develop insidiously. Deep, visceral, cramping pain from obstruction of the colon is usually referred to the hypogastrium. Lesions of the fixed portions of the colon (cecum, hepatic flexure, splenic flexure) may cause pain which is felt immediately anteriorly. Pain originating from the sigmoid is often located to the left in the lower abdomen. Severe,

continuous abdominal pain suggests strangulation or peritonitis. Borborygmus may be loud and coincident with cramps. Constipation or obstipation is a universal feature of complete obstruction although the colon distal to the obstruction may empty after the initial symptoms begin. Vomiting is a late finding and may not occur at all if the ileocecal valve prevents reflux. If reflux decompresses the cecal contents into the small intestine, the symptoms of small bowel as well as large bowel obstruction appear. Feculent vomiting is a late manifestation.

Physical examination discloses abdominal distention and tympany, and peristaltic waves may be seen if the abdominal wall is thin. High-pitched, metallic tinkles associated with rushes and gurgles may be heard on auscultation. Localized tenderness or a tender, palpable mass may indicate a strangulated closed loop. Signs of localized or generalized peritonitis suggest gangrene or rupture of the bowel wall. Fresh blood may be found in the rectum in intussusception and in carcinoma of the rectum or colon. Sigmoidoscopy may disclose a neoplasm.

B. X-Ray Findings: The distended colon frequently creates a "picture frame" outline of the abdominal cavity. The colon can be distinguished from the small intestine by its haustral markings, which do not cross the entire lumen of the distended colon. Barium enema will confirm the diagnosis of colonic obstruction and identify its exact location. However, barium enema may be dangerous if the vascular supply is compromised, and the increased risk associated with perforation of the colon by the barium is such that the procedure should be omitted if strangulation is suspected or if the cecum is 10 cm (4 inches) in diameter or larger. Barium must not be given orally in the presence of suspected colonic obstruction.

Differential Diagnosis

A. Small Versus Large Bowel Obstruction: X-ray may be required to make the differential diagnosis. Large bowel obstruction is frequently slow in onset, causes less pain, and does not cause vomiting in spite of considerable distention. Elderly patients with no history of abdominal surgery or prior attacks of obstruction will most frequently have carcinoma of the large bowel.

B. Paralytic Ileus: The distinguishing features of paralytic ileus are signs of peritonitis or a history of trauma to the back or pelvis. The abdomen is silent and without cramps. There may be tenderness. Plain films show dilated bowel (see Chapter 25).

C. Pseudo-obstruction: Massive colonic distention in the absence of a mechanically obstructing lesion is important to recognize. Most patients have associated serious illness of some system other than the intestinal tract—acute alcoholism, vertebral fracture, cardiac disease, etc. Abdominal distention without pain or tenderness is the earliest manifestation, but later symptoms mimic those of true obstruction. Plain x-rays of the abdomen show marked gaseous distention of the colon. Although the entire colon may contain gas, typically the distention is localized to the right colon with a cutoff at the hepatic or splenic flexure. Barium enema excludes an obstructing lesion but is hazardous to perform if the cecum is grossly dilated. The risk of cecal perforation is high in this situation, and surgical decompression of the cecum is mandatory if the distention does not subside with enemas.

Complications

Cecal perforation, described above, is a potentially lethal complication. Partially obstructive lesions of the colon may be complicated by acute colitis in the bowel proximal to the obstruction; it is probably a form of ischemic colitis secondary to impaired mucosal blood flow in the distended segment.

Treatment

The primary goal of treatment is decompression of the obstructed segment in order to avoid perforation; an operation is almost always required. The obstructing lesion can be removed at the initial operation in some cases, but often this step is best deferred until the patient is in better condition, the colon is empty, and the edema in the obstructed bowel has subsided.

Obstructing lesions of the cecum are resected in one stage, with ileotransverse colostomy, provided that the patient's condition is good and the small bowel has been adequately decompressed preoperatively. If the ileum is edematous, the cecum is resected and a temporary ileostomy is constructed; anastomosis is performed in a second stage a few weeks later. Nonresectable lesions may be bypassed. Loop ileostomy should be avoided if possible.

Obstructions of the ascending colon, the hepatic flexure, and the right half of the transverse colon are best decompressed by cecostomy. When the ileocecal valve is competent and neither the terminal ileum proximal to the obstruction nor the transverse colon distal to the obstruction is dilated or edematous, an emergency right hemicolectomy and anastomosis of the ileum to the transverse colon may be performed.

In the case of **obstructing lesions distal to the splenic flexure,** either cecostomy or transverse colostomy will provide decompression.

Cecostomy (Fig 34–5) can be done under local anesthesia and is the operation of choice in aged, poor-risk patients with marked distention. It gives adequate decompression if the distal colon is not packed with feces and complete diversion of the fecal stream is not necessary. Cecostomy has the advantage that it does not interfere with subsequent extensive resection of the left colon. **Transverse colostomy,** on the other hand, completely diverts the fecal stream and produces more adequate decompression. Transverse colostomy is preferable to cecostomy (1) in obstruction due to diverticulitis, (2) for removal of impacted barium or feces proximal to the obstruction, or (3) in case of failure of a cecostomy to provide decompression.

Prognosis

The prognosis depends upon the age and general

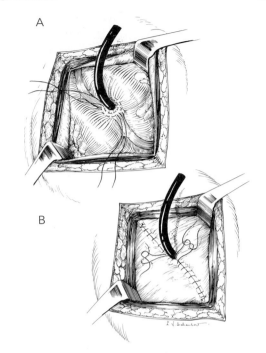

Figure 34–5. Cecostomy. *A:* Through a small incision overlying the cecum, a tube has been inserted through the wall of the cecum into its lumen and secured with a purse-string suture. *B:* Peritoneal closure. The cecum is fixed to the peritoneum. *Note:* A useful modification is to suture the peritoneum to the cecum circumferentially around the proposed cecostomy *before* the bowel is opened; this maneuver excludes the cecum from the peritoneal cavity and avoids the risk of fecal contamination of the abdomen.

condition of the patient, the extent of vascular impairment of the bowel, the presence or absence of perforation, the cause of obstruction, and the promptness of surgical management. Overall mortality rates of 15–30% have been reported.

Clark J, Hall AW, Moossa AR: Treatment of obstructing cancer of the colon and rectum. Surg Gynecol Obstet 141:541, 1975.

Dutton JW, Hreno A, Hampson LG: Mortality and prognosis of obstructing carcinoma of the large bowel. Am J Surg 131:36, 1976.

Feldman PS: Ulcerative disease of the colon proximal to partially obstructive lesions: Report of two cases and review of the literature. Dis Colon Rectum 18:601, 1975.

Fielding LP, Wells BW: Survival after primary and staged resection for large bowel obstruction caused by cancer. Br J Surg 61:16, 1974.

Gurll N, Steer M: Diagnostic and therapeutic considerations for fecal impaction. Dis Colon Rectum 18:507, 1975.

Norton L, Young D, Scribner R: Management of pseudo-obstruction of the colon. Surg Gynecol Obstet 138:595, 1974.

CANCER OF THE COLON & RECTUM

Essentials of Diagnosis

Right colon
- Unexplained weakness or anemia.
- Occult blood in feces.
- Dyspeptic symptoms.
- Persistent right abdominal discomfort.
- Palpable abdominal mass.
- Characteristic x-ray findings.

Left colon
- Change in bowel habits.
- Gross blood in stool.
- Obstructive symptoms.
- Characteristic sigmoidoscopic findings.
- Characteristic x-ray findings.

Rectum
- Rectal bleeding.
- Alteration in bowel habits.
- Sensation of incomplete evacuation.
- Intrarectal palpable tumor.
- Sigmoidoscopic findings.

General Considerations

The colon and rectum account for more cases of cancer in the population of Western countries than any other anatomic site except the skin. Approximately 100,000 new cases are diagnosed and about 49,000 people die of this disease each year in the USA. Cancer of the colon and rectum is the most frequent cause of death among visceral malignancies which affect both sexes. The incidence increases with age, beginning to rise at age 40 and reaching a peak at 60–75 years. Carcinoma of the colon is more common in females, and carcinoma of the rectum is more common in males. The distribution of cancers of the colon and rectum is shown in Fig 34–6. Multiple synchronous colonic cancers—ie, 2 or more carcinomas which occur simultaneously—are found in 5% of patients. Meta-

chronous cancer—a new primary lesion in a patient who has had a previous resection for cancer—has an incidence of 2.5%. Ninety-five percent of malignant tumors of the colon and rectum are adenocarcinomas.

Genetic predisposition to cancer of the large bowel is well recognized in persons with familial polyposis, and in a few other families cancer of the colon is transmitted as a dominant trait. In general, however, the increased risk in the immediate relatives of patients with colonic cancer is relatively low—about 2–3 times normal—and this increased risk may be due as much to familial environmental factors as to genetic factors. Immunologic deficiency states can lead to malignancy in various organs, including the colon, and it has been suggested that defective immune surveillance is characteristic of patients who develop colonic cancer. Other predisposing factors include chronic ulcerative colitis and granulomatous colitis. Benign mucosal neoplasms are manifestations of a neoplastic stimulus already at work and are not predisposing factors in the same sense that ulcerative colitis is.

Variations in the incidence of colonic cancer in different geographic areas have focussed attention on environmental factors, particularly diet, in the etiology of this tumor. Populations with a high incidence of colorectal carcinoma consume diets containing less fiber and more animal protein, fat, and refined carbohydrate than populations with a low incidence of this disease. People whose diets are deficient in fiber have smaller fecal bulk and slower transit time through the colon than those with high fiber intakes. Smaller fecal mass would result in higher concentrations of any carcinogens present, and slower transit would allow a longer time for contact of the carcinogen with the mucosa.

Carcinogenic compounds may be ingested in the diet, but there is no direct evidence to support that possibility, and it seems more likely that carcinogens are produced endogenously from dietary substances or intestinal secretions. Bacterial dehydrogenation of bile salts is one mechanism by which carcinogens might be produced endogenously. Bacteroides and clostridia are particularly able to degrade bile salts in this manner, and some of the derivatives are structurally similar to known potent carcinogens. These anaerobic bacteria are more prevalent in the feces of populations who eat Western diets and have a high incidence of colonic cancer. The hypothesis that colorectal carcinoma is caused by altered bacterial flora in response to diet is under active study.

Cancer of the colon and rectum spreads in the following ways:

A. Colon:

1. Direct extension—Carcinoma grows circumferentially and may completely encircle the bowel before it is diagnosed; this is especially true in the left colon, which has a smaller caliber than the right. It takes about 1 year for a tumor to encircle three-fourths of the circumference of the bowel. Longitudinal submucosal extension occurs with invasion of the intramural lymphatic network, but it rarely goes beyond 5

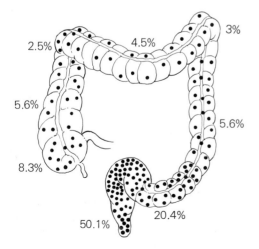

Figure 34–6. Distribution of cancer of the colon and rectum.

cm (2 inches) from the edge of the tumor. As the lesion penetrates the outer layers of the bowel wall, it may extend by contiguity into neighboring structures: the liver, the greater curvature of the stomach, the duodenum, the small bowel, the pancreas, the spleen, the bladder, the vagina, the kidneys and ureters, and the abdominal wall. Subacute perforation with inflammatory attachment of bowel to an adjacent viscus may be indistinguishable from actual invasion on gross examination.

2. Hematogenous metastasis—The tumor may invade colonic veins and be carried via portal venous blood to the liver to establish hepatic metastases. Tumor embolization also occurs through lumbar and vertebral veins to the lungs and elsewhere. Venous invasion occurs in 15–35% of cases even though it does not always cause distant metastases. An attempt is made to avoid producing hematogenous metastases during operation by ligating the major veins before manipulating the tumor.

3. Regional lymph node metastasis—This is the most common form of tumor spread (Fig 34–7). The lymphatic drainage of the tumor must be removed in curative operations. Fifty to 60 lymph nodes can usually be identified in the average specimen, and some nodal involvement will be found in over half of the specimens. Regional nodes are not necessarily involved in a progressive or orderly fashion: positive nodes may be found at some distance from the primary site with normal nodes intervening. The size of the lesion bears

little relationship to the degree of nodal involvement. The more anaplastic the lesion, the more likely that lymph node metastasis will occur.

4. Gravitational metastasis—"Seeding" may occur when the tumor has extended through the serosa and tumor cells are carried to distant points of the peritoneal cavity, eventually producing generalized abdominal carcinomatosis. The rectovesical or rectouterine pouches are usually involved in such patients, and on digital rectal examination these metastases can be felt as a hard shelf (Blumer's shelf) and, later, as a "frozen pelvis." Because metastasis to the ovaries occurs in 3–4% of cases, bilateral oophorectomy should be performed when the bowel is resected in postmenopausal patients.

5. Perineural spread—Invasion of the perineural space permits tumor to spread along nerves which supply the colon. This finding is associated with a poor prognosis.

6. Intraluminal metastasis—Malignant cells which are shed from the surface of the tumor can be swept along in the fecal current and implant more distally in the colon. This mode of spread is extremely rare unless there is a recent surgical suture line, in which case cells do implant and cause "anastomotic recurrence."

B. Rectum:

1. Direct extension—Longitudinal extension usually does not exceed 6 cm. Lateral extension into contiguous viscera occurs when the growth has penetrated through the bowel wall. Cancer of the rectum may invade the vaginal wall, bladder, prostate, or sacrum, and it may extend along the levators.

2. Lymphatic spread—Cancer first involves the lymph nodes adjacent to the tumor and then spreads successively to the more proximal lymph nodes; occasionally it spreads to nodes outside the normal continuity. The lymphatic chain from the rectum is along the superior hemorrhoidal, iliac, and inferior mesenteric arteries and the aorta.

3. Hematogenous metastases—In 10–15% of cases, rectal cancer will have spread through the portal veins to the liver when first diagnosed. Metastasis to the lungs occurs less frequently, and the brain and spine may also be involved.

4. Perineural spread—Cancer may spread by perineural invasion. When it does so, the rate of local recurrence is high.

Clinical Findings

A. Symptoms and Signs: Adenocarcinoma of the colon and rectum has a relatively slow rate of growth. The mean doubling time (the time required for the volume of tumor to double in size) of primary colon cancers has been estimated to be 620 days, suggesting that many years of silent growth might be required before a cancer reaches symptom-producing size. During this asymptomatic phase, diagnosis depends on routine examination. Symptoms which develop eventually depend upon the anatomic location of the lesion, its type and extent, and upon complications, including perforation, obstruction, and hemorrhage. Marked

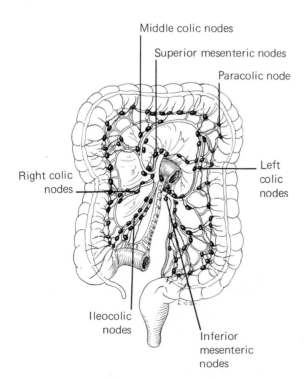

Middle colic nodes

Superior mesenteric nodes

Paracolic node

Right colic nodes

Left colic nodes

Ileocolic nodes

Inferior mesenteric nodes

Figure 34–7. Lymphatic drainage of the colon. The lymph nodes (black) are distributed along the blood vessels to the bowel.

systemic manifestations such as cachexia are indications of advanced disease.

The **right colon** has a large caliber, a thin and distensible wall, and the fecal content is fluid. Because of these anatomic features and because carcinoma of the right colon tends to grow in a fungating fashion, these lesions may attain large size before they are diagnosed. Patients often see a physician for complaints of fatigability and weakness due to severe anemia. Unexplained microcytic hypochromic anemia should always raise the question of carcinoma of the ascending colon. Gross blood may not be visible in the stool, but occult blood may be detected. Patients may complain of vague right abdominal discomfort which is often postprandial and may be mistakenly attributed to gallbladder or gastroduodenal disease. Alterations in bowel habits are not characteristic of carcinoma of the right colon, and obstruction is uncommon. In about 10% of cases, the first evidence of the disease is discovery of a mass by the patient or physician.

The **left colon** has a smaller lumen than the right and the feces are semisolid. Tumors of the left colon tend to encircle the bowel, causing changes in bowel habits with alternating constipation and increased frequency of defecation (not true watery diarrhea). Partial obstruction with colicky abdominal pain or complete obstruction may be the presenting picture. Complete obstruction may occur without previous symptoms, or there may be an antecedent history of increasing constipation, diminution of stool caliber, and increasing abdominal distention with pain or discomfort. Bleeding is common but is rarely massive. The stool may be streaked or mixed with bright red or dark blood, and mucus is often passed together with blood or blood clots.

In **cancer of the rectum**, the most common presenting symptom is the passage of blood with bowel movement. Whenever rectal bleeding occurs, even in the presence of an obviously benign lesion such as hemorrhoids, coexisting cancer must be ruled out. Bleeding is usually persistent; it may be slight or (rarely) copious. Blood may or may not be mixed with stool or with mucus. There may be tenesmus without diarrhea, and the patient may have a feeling of incomplete defecation. Pain is noticeably absent except in advanced stages of the disease or when the carcinoma involves the anal canal.

General physical examination is important to determine the extent of the local disease, to reveal distant metastases, and to detect diseases of other organ systems which may influence treatment. The groin and supraclavicular areas should be carefully palpated for metastatic nodules, and enlarged, firm nodes should be biopsied. Examination of the abdomen may disclose a mass, enlargement of the liver, ascites, or enlargement of the abdominal wall veins if there is portal obstruction. If a mass is palpated, its location and the extent of fixation are important.

Approximately two-thirds of cancers of the colon and rectum are within reach of the examining finger or the sigmoidoscope. Most rectal cancers can be felt as a flat, hard, oval or encircling tumor, which may be nodular on the surface. Its extent, the size of the lumen at the site of the tumor, and the degree of fixation should be noted. Blood may be found on the examining finger. Vaginal and rectovaginal examination will yield additional information on the extent of the tumor.

B. Laboratory Findings: Urinalysis, leukocyte count, and hemoglobin determination should be done. Serum proteins, calcium, bilirubin, alkaline phosphatase, creatinine, and prothrombin time should be measured.

Carcinoembryonic antigen (CEA) is a glycoprotein found in fetal and neoplastic tissues of the gastrointestinal tract. Some of this antigen enters the circulation and is detected by radioimmunoassay of serum. Elevated serum CEA is not specifically associated with colorectal cancer; abnormally high levels of CEA are also found in sera of patients with other gastrointestinal cancers, nonalimentary malignancies, and various benign diseases. CEA levels are high in 70% of patients with cancer of the large intestine, but less than half of patients with localized disease (Dukes A) are CEA-positive. CEA does not, therefore, serve as a useful screening procedure in the general population, nor is it an accurate diagnostic test for colorectal malignancy in a curable stage. CEA is helpful in detecting recurrence after curative surgical resection; if high CEA levels return to normal after operation and then rise progressively during the follow-up period, recurrence of cancer is likely. An isomeric species of CEA (CEA-S) has been identified recently; it may be more specific for gastrointestinal neoplasia.

C. X-Ray Findings: Chest films should be obtained routinely. Barium enema examination is the most important means of diagnosing cancer of the colon above the reach of the examining finger and the sigmoidoscope. It should be obtained even if a rectal cancer is palpable or visible endoscopically in order to exclude synchronous lesions. Carcinoma appears as a fixed filling defect, usually 2–6 cm long, with an annular or "apple core" configuration (Fig 34–8). The bowel wall is inflexible at the site of the lesion, and the mucosal pattern is destroyed. It is important to remember that this is the typical picture of locally advanced carcinoma. Earlier stages of the disease produce less characteristic filling defects which should be investigated with another barium enema or with the colonoscope. Colonoscopy is also indicated if the barium enema shows nothing abnormal in patients whose symptoms are suggestive of malignancy. Artifacts can resemble carcinoma, particularly in the cecum, and colonoscopy or repeat barium enema should be obtained in these circumstances. Localized spasm can mimic carcinoma; glucagon administered intravenously usually relaxes the spastic area. Barium should not be administered by mouth if there is evidence of carcinoma of the colon, especially on the left side, since it may precipitate acute large bowel obstruction.

X-rays are unreliable to detect cancer of the rectum. Such growths are more accurately diagnosed by palpation and endoscopy.

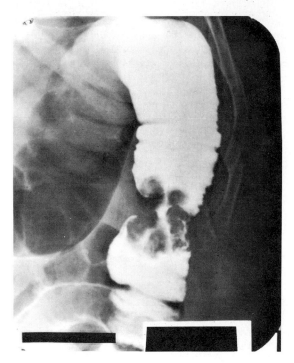

Figure 34—8. Barium enema roentgenogram of an encircling carcinoma of the descending colon presenting an "apple core" appearance. Note the loss of mucosal pattern, the "hooks" at the margins of the lesion due to undermining by the growth, the relatively short (6 cm) length of the lesion, and its abrupt ends.

Intravenous urography should be done before operation in patients with colorectal cancer to determine the number and position of the kidneys and to determine whether ureteral obstruction or displacement has occurred.

The value of radioactive scans of the liver in the diagnosis of hepatic metastases is discussed in Chapters 8 and 27.

D. Special Examinations:

1. Proctosigmoidoscopy—This examination should be performed in every patient with suspected cancer of any portion of the large bowel. If the lesion is above the reach of the proctosigmoidoscope, a bloody discharge may be seen coming from above. Patients with carcinoma of the proximal colon may have associated polyps or even synchronous carcinomas in the rectum or sigmoid. The typical rectal cancer is raised, red, centrally ulcerated, and bleeding slightly. Mobility of the lesion can be determined by manipulation with the tip of the instrument. The size of the rectal lumen should be noted, and the sigmoidoscope should be passed beyond the lesion to inspect the proximal bowel if possible. The tumor should be biopsied.

2. Colonoscopy—Lesions can be inspected at any level in the colon with the fiberoptic instrument, and biopsies or cytologic washings can be obtained. This examination need only be performed when x-ray diag-

nosis is inconclusive. It is especially useful when barium enema films do not exclude lesions in the left colon in patients with obvious carcinoma of the right or transverse colon.

3. Cystoscopy—Cystoscopy may be indicated if symptoms or physical findings suggest invasion of the bladder.

Differential Diagnosis

An initial erroneous diagnosis is made in as many as 25% of patients with cancer of the colon and rectum after gastrointestinal symptoms appear. Symptoms may be attributed mistakenly to disease of the upper gastrointestinal tract, particularly gallstones or peptic ulcer. Chronic anemia may be attributed to a primary hematologic disorder if a specimen of stool is not examined for occult blood. Acute pain in the right side of the abdomen due to carcinoma can simulate appendicitis.

Most errors are made when the clinical findings are ascribed to benign disease, and patients may even be operated upon for benign anorectal conditions in the presence of undetected cancer. Cancer must be searched for in every patient with rectal bleeding, even if he has obvious bleeding hemorrhoids.

Carcinoma may be difficult to distinguish from diverticular disease, and colonoscopy has proved useful in some of these cases. Other colonic diseases, including ulcerative colitis, granulomatous colitis, ischemic colitis, and amebiasis, usually can be diagnosed by sigmoidoscopy, barium enema, and colonoscopy if necessary. Functional bowel disease (irritable colon) should be diagnosed only after organic lesions have been ruled out.

Treatment

A. Cancer of the Colon: Treatment of the colon consists of wide surgical resection of the lesion and its regional lymphatic drainage after preparation of the bowel. The primary tumor usually is resected even if distant metastases have occurred since prevention of obstruction or bleeding may offer palliation for several years. Radiation therapy and chemotherapy are used in selected patients with unresectable or metastatic cancer of the colon.

The abdomen is explored to determine resectability of the tumor and to search for multiple primary carcinomas of the colon, distant metastases, and associated abdominal disease. A "no-touch" technic of colonic resection is preferred on theoretical grounds. Care is taken not to contribute to spread of the tumor by unnecessary palpation, and the blood vessels that supply the involved segment are divided and ligated early in the operation to avoid dissemination of tumor cells into the portal circulation or the lymphatics. Next, the bowel is tied tightly with an encircling tape on either side of the lesion to contain exfoliated cancer cells within the segment to be resected. The cancer-bearing portion of colon is then mobilized and removed. Some surgeons irrigate the 2 ends of bowel before anastomosis with distilled water, 1:500 bichloride of mercury, or Dakin's solution (0.25% sodium hypochlorite) in the hope that tumor cells in the lumen will be destroyed. The extent of resection of the colon and mesentery for cancers in various locations and the methods for restoration of continuity are shown in Fig 34—9.

B. Cancer of the Rectum: For cancer of the rectum, the choice of operation depends on the height of the lesion above the anal verge, the configuration (whether polypoid or infiltrative), the gross extent of the tumor, and the general condition of the patient. Although preservation of the anal sphincter and avoidance of colostomy are desirable, these considerations are secondary to the need to ablate the malignancy.

The principal procedures for rectal tumors are as follows:

1. Abdominoperineal resection of the rectum— The distal sigmoid, rectosigmoid, and rectum are re-moved through a combined abdominal and perineal approach. A permanent end sigmoid colostomy is required. The procedure is contraindicated in the presence of peritoneal seeding or if the tumor is fixed to the bony pelvis.

2. Low anterior resection of the rectum—This operation, performed through an abdominal incision, is the curative procedure of choice provided a margin of 5 cm of normal bowel, as estimated at operation, can be resected below the lesion. At least 10 cm of normal bowel proximal to the growth should also be removed along with the lymph node-bearing tissue. The descending or sigmoid colon is anastomosed to the rectum, thus avoiding a colostomy. This type of resection is contraindicated for extensive carcinoma with local spread.

3. Other "sphincter-preserving" procedures— Anastomosis low in the pelvis is difficult to perform

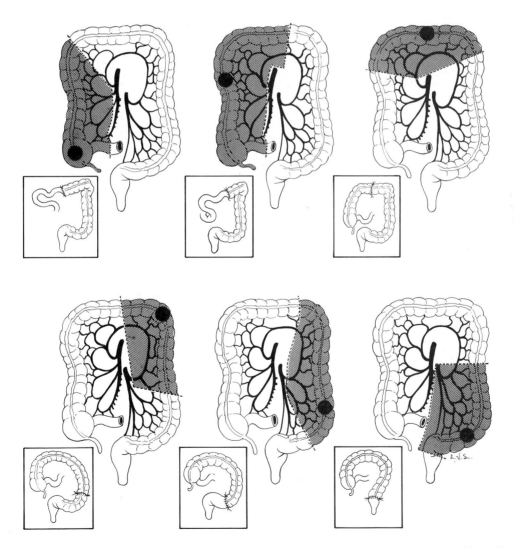

Figure 34—9. Extent of surgical resection for cancer of the colon at various sites. The cancer is represented by a black disk. Anastomosis of the bowel remaining after resection is shown in the small insets. The extent of resection is determined by the distribution of the regional lymph nodes along the blood supply. The lymph nodes may contain metastatic cancer.

from the abdominal approach in obese people and in males because the pelvis is narrow. In certain patients, the anastomosis can be constructed posteriorly by making an incision through the sphincter muscles. The anastomosis can also be done through the dilated anus. "Pull-through" operations, in which the anorectal stump is everted to facilitate low anastomosis, are not recommended because of complications and unsatisfactory bowel function afterward.

4. Palliative procedures—Other (more limited) operations are indicated at times. One palliative operation is the Hartmann procedure, in which the bowel with its contained malignancy is removed through the abdomen with permanent colostomy but without excision of the distal rectum, which is sutured closed.

5. Fulguration—Some tumors can be controlled locally by fulguration (electrocoagulation). This procedure is more than superficial cautery; it is an aggressive technic requiring hospitalization, general anesthesia, and usually several fulguration sessions at intervals. It is suitable only for lesions below the pelvic peritoneal reflection. Because the lymph nodes are not evaluated or treated in this approach, the role of fulguration in the management of rectal cancer has not been precisely defined. The hypothesis that fulguration evokes an immune response to the tumor has not been proved in humans. Fulguration is the treatment of choice in most elderly or poor-risk patients.

6. Radiation therapy—Intracavitary or external radiation therapy is used for definitive treatment only in patients who are poor risks for major operation. Adjunctive radiation therapy may be given prior to curative resection in the hope that long-term survival rates will be increased; the value of this method is under investigation.

Treatment of Complications

A. Obstruction: Standard treatment for obstructing cancer of the left colon is surgical decompression followed later by elective resection. Immediate resection of the obstructed colon (without anastomosis) has been recommended recently; a controlled trial is necessary to determine which course of action has lower morbidity and mortality. Obstructing carcinomas of the right colon can be resected and anastomosed in a single stage in most cases.

B. Perforation: An aggressive approach to perforated cancer of the colon is advisable: the involved segment is resected if possible, the proximal end is exteriorized as a colostomy, and the distal end is exteriorized or closed. Secondary anastomosis is performed after inflammation subsides. If the tumor-bearing bowel cannot be removed initially because a large abscess has formed, the abscess should be drained and a diverting colostomy established proximally. Elective resection is performed subsequently.

C. Direct Extension: When carcinoma of the colon has spread by contiguity to adjacent viscera such as the small intestine, spleen, uterus, or urinary bladder, the involved viscus—or a portion of it—should be resected en bloc with the colon.

Prognosis

The survival rate after surgical resection of large bowel cancer correlates with the extent of disease; results are slightly better for cancer of the colon than for cancer of the rectum. The Dukes classification (Table 34—3) is widely used to describe the extent of disease. Various modifications of the Dukes classification have been proposed, but lack of uniform acceptance of any modification makes it preferable to use the original.

Approximately 10% of lesions are not resectable at the time of operation, and an additional 20% of patients have liver or other distant metastases. Hence, operation for cure can be performed on only about 70% of patients. The operative mortality rate is 2—4%. The survival rate of patients resected for cure is about 65%; the overall survival rate (all stages) about 40%.

The prognosis is adversely affected by complications such as obstruction or perforation. The histologic features—including the degree of differentiation of the tumor, intravascular tumor cells, or malignant cells in the perineural space—also have a bearing on prognosis.

The average delay between the onset of symptoms and definitive therapy of cancer of the colon and rectum is about 10 months; both patients and physicians are partially responsible. The resectability rate has not improved significantly over the past 20 years. Routine screening procedures (eg, testing of stool for occult blood) may lead to earlier detection.

Adjuvant therapy after curative surgical resection is the subject of intense study at present. Postoperative radiation therapy, chemotherapy, and immunotherapy are being investigated in this regard; some of the preliminary results are promising.

Edgington TS, Astarita RW, Plow EF: Association of an isomeric species of carcinoembryonic antigen with neoplasia of the gastrointestinal tract. N Engl J Med 293:103, 1975.

Ekelund GR, Pihl B: Multiple carcinomas of the colon and rectum. Cancer 33:1630, 1974.

Fielding LP, Wells BW: Survival after primary and after staged resection for large bowel obstruction caused by cancer. Br J Surg 61:16, 1974.

Herrera MA, Chu TM, Holyoke ED: Carcinoembryonic antigen (CEA) as a prognostic and monitoring test in clinically complete resection of colorectal carcinoma. Ann Surg 183:5, 1976.

Table 34—3. Dukes classification of cancer of the colon and rectum.

Dukes Stage	Extent	5-Year Survival (%)*
A	Limited to bowel wall.	90
B	Through entire bowel wall; nodes negative.	65
C	Positive nodes.	30
D	Distant metastases or extensive local spread which cannot be removed surgically.	5

*Survival rates differ considerably in various reported series. Actuarial methods yield higher values than the crude survival rates shown here.

Higgins GA & others: Preoperative radiotherapy for colorectal cancer. Ann Surg 181:624, 1975.

Hill MJ & others: Faecal bile-acids and clostridia in patients with cancer of the large bowel. Lancet 1:535, 1975.

Lawrence W & others: Chemotherapy as an adjuvant to surgery for colorectal cancer. Ann Surg 181:616, 1975.

Li MC, Ross ST: Chemoprophylaxis for patients with colorectal cancer: Prospective study with five-year follow-up. JAMA 235:2825, 1976.

Manson PN & others: Anterior resection for adenocarcinoma: Lahey Clinic experience from 1963 through 1969. Am J Surg 131:434, 1976.

Mavligit GM & others: Prolongation of postoperative disease-free interval and survival in human colorectal cancer by B.C.G. or B.C.G. plus 5-fluorouracil. Lancet 1:871, 1976.

Miller DR, Allbritten FF Jr: Carcinoma of the colon and rectum: A review of results of surgical treatment in 164 patients. Arch Surg 111:692, 1976.

Neuhauser D, Lewicki AM: What do we gain from the sixth stool guaiac? N Engl J Med 293:226, 1975.

Wallack MK & others: The treatment of cancer of the large intestine. Surg Gynecol Obstet 142:97, 1976.

Welch JP, Donaldson GA: Perforative carcinoma of colon and rectum. Ann Surg 180:734, 1974.

Whittaker M, Goligher JC: The prognosis after surgical treatment for carcinoma of the rectum. Br J Surg 63:384, 1976.

Wilson SM, Beahrs OH: The curative treatment of carcinoma of the sigmoid, rectosigmoid, and rectum. Ann Surg 183:556, 1976.

Winawer SJ & others: Screening for colon cancer. Gastroenterology 70:783, 1976.

POLYPS OF THE COLON & RECTUM

Essentials of Diagnosis

- Passage of blood per rectum.
- Possible family history.
- Sigmoidoscopic, colonoscopic, or radiologic discovery of polyps.

General Considerations

Colorectal polyps are masses of tissue which project into the lumen. They are a heterogeneous group of sessile or pedunculated, benign or malignant, mucosal, submucosal, or muscular lesions. "Polyp" is a morphologic term, and no histologic diagnosis is implied (Table 34–4).

Estimates of incidence range from 7–50%; the higher figure includes small polyps found at autopsy. Polyps are detected in routine barium enema in about 5% of patients. After age 20, the incidence of adenomatous polyps increases with each decade. Polyps are frequently multiple; in order of decreasing frequency, they are found in the rectum and sigmoid, the descending colon, the splenic flexure, the transverse colon, the hepatic flexure, and the ascending colon.

Adenomatous polyps, papillary adenomas, villoglandular polyps, and adenocarcinomas are all the result of neoplastic epithelial proliferation. Papillary

Table 34—4. Polypoid lesions of the large intestine.

Histologic Diagnosis	Relative Incidence (%)*
Adenomatous polyp (tubular adenoma)	60
Papillary (villous) adenoma	10
Villoglandular (mixed) polyp	15
Cancer arising in adenoma	6
Polypoid adenocarcinoma	2
Pseudopolyp	2
Juvenile polyp	1
Lymphoid polyp	1
Hyperplastic polyp	1
Lipoma	0.5
Hamartoma	0.5
Miscellaneous others	1

*Relative incidence varies according to the patient population, the pathologist, and the method of obtaining the specimens, ie, surgery, colonoscopy, or autopsy.

adenomas become malignant in about one-third of cases. Premalignancy of adenomatous polyps, on the other hand, has been the subject of controversy for 2 decades. Some of the evidence that benign adenomatous polyps become cancer may be summarized as follows: (1) One-fourth of patients with cancer of the colon also have adenomatous polyps. (2) The distribution of polyps and cancer in the large intestine is similar. (3) Patients with familial polyposis die of cancer before age 40 unless the colon is removed. (4) Benign polyps seen through the sigmoidoscope have, at a later date, become typical carcinomas. (5) Cancers smaller than 0.5 cm in diameter are extremely rare, but foci of cancer in adenomatous polyps of that size are seen occasionally. (6) Chemical carcinogens produce adenomas and cancers indiscriminately in the colons of experimental animals. (7) Routine removal of benign polyps from the rectum reduces the incidence of rectal cancer later.

There are contrary arguments to some of these points, but the weight of evidence favors the view that adenomatous polyps can become malignant. In the light of present knowledge, the polyp-cancer relationship may be stated as follows: approximately one-third of papillary adenomas and 2–5% of adenomatous polyps become malignant; villoglandular polyps have an intermediate incidence of cancerous transformation; the great majority of adenocarcinomas evolve from a benign polypoid lesion.

Clinical Findings

A. Symptoms and Signs: Many polyps are asymptomatic; the larger the lesion, the more likely it is to cause symptoms. Rectal bleeding is by far the most frequent complaint. Blood is bright red or dark red depending on the location of the polyp, and bleeding is usually intermittent. Profuse hemorrhage from polyps is rare.

Alterations in bowel habits are more common in the presence of frank carcinoma, but large benign tumors may produce tenesmus, constipation, or increased frequency of bowel movements. Some polyps, notably large villous adenomas, may secrete copious amounts of mucus which are evacuated per rectum. Polypoid tumors may induce peristaltic cramps or varying degrees of intussusception, but most often obstructive symptoms are due to associated diverticular disease or irritable colon syndrome and persist after polypectomy. Occasionally, a polyp on a very long pedicle will prolapse through the anus; this is most apt to occur with juvenile polyps.

General physical examination yields little information about the colonic polyps themselves, although other manifestations of diseases such as Peutz-Jeghers or Gardner's syndrome may be found. A polyp may be palpable by digital rectal examination, and proctosigmoidoscopy may disclose polyps of the rectum, a polyp prolapsing from above, or evidence of bleeding beyond the reach of the instrument. Blood-tinged mucus strongly suggests the presence of a neoplasm situated farther proximally. Since polyps are often multiple and may occur synchronously with cancer, further investigation of the colon is mandatory even if a lesion is found by sigmoidoscopy.

B. X-Ray Findings (Barium Enema): A polyp appears as a rounded filling defect with smooth, sharply defined margins. It may be sessile or pedunculated. The postevacuation film is important since a thin layer of barium usually remains on the polyp. Double contrast (pneumocolon) examination is of great value; in this study, the polyp, coated by barium, forms a positive shadow as it projects into the lumen filled with radiolucent air. Thorough cleansing of the colon, thin barium, high voltage technics, and a skilled radiologist are essential if small polyps are to be demonstrated; even so, polyps smaller than 0.5 cm in diameter often cannot be detected on x-ray.

C. Fiberoptic Colonoscopy: This technic, if performed skillfully, is the most reliable method of diagnosing colonic polyps. The entire colon should be examined, because lesions too small to be seen by x-ray are often detected in the proximal colon.

Differential Diagnosis

Many artifacts seen on barium enema x-ray examination may be confused with polyps. These include bits of feces, oil and air bubbles, diverticula, indenting appendices epiploicae, calcified lymph nodes, and others. Colonoscopy is essential in doubtful situations.

Polyps of various histologic types can be differentiated only by microscopic examination of the entire lesion, although clues may be gained from clinical and radiographic features.

Treatment

Polyps of the colon and rectum are treated because they produce symptoms, because they may be malignant when first discovered, or because they may become malignant later. The risk of treatment must be weighed against the likelihood of malignancy or the severity of symptoms in making a decision about management.

Pedunculated or small sessile polyps within the reach of the proctosigmoidoscope should be removed completely with the electrocautery snare or destroyed by fulguration. The risk of this procedure is negligible. Large, sessile, soft, velvety lesions in the rectum are usually villous adenomas; these tumors have a high malignant potential and must be excised completely. With the patient anesthetized this can be accomplished through the dilated anus or by various perineal operative approaches. Only if histologic sections show invasive cancer is further therapy necessary, usually abdominoperineal resection. Small biopsies of these lesions taken with a forceps are misleading since malignancy may be present in some other part of the growth.

Pedunculated polyps and small sessile lesions in the sigmoid and above should be removed with an electrocautery snare passed through the fiberoptic colonoscope. Colonoscopic polypectomy is usually successful, especially with polyps in the left colon, but occasionally technical obstacles will be insurmountable. It is probably unwise to attempt colonoscopic removal of large sessile lesions because the risk of perforation is greater if there is no pedicle about which to secure the snare. If good judgment is exercised, colonoscopic polypectomy is safer than laparotomy; the combined incidence of perforation and hemorrhage is 2%. The endoscopic approach is less expensive and incurs much less postoperative disability than laparotomy.

Laparotomy should be considered if colonoscopy is unsuccessful, if the lesion is large and sessile, or if there are many polyps. The incidence of cancer in polyps smaller than 1 cm in diameter is less than 1%, and the likelihood of cancer rises in proportion to increasing size of the tumor. The overall operative mortality rate in transabdominal removal of colonic polyps is about 2%, and the incidence of cancer in polyps 1–1.5 cm in diameter is also about 2%. Sessile lesions are more likely to be malignant than pedunculated ones. Operation is indicated, therefore, when a polyp is greater than 1.5 cm in diameter. Operation for large sessile tumors usually consists of resection of the segment of colon containing the lesion. In the occasional patient operated on for a pedunculated polyp, colotomy and polypectomy may be performed. If multiple polyps are present in different anatomic parts of the colon, however, total abdominal colectomy with ileorectal anastomosis may be advisable in good-risk patients.

If a pedunculated polyp removed with the colonoscope contains cancer, the surgeon must decide whether to resect that segment of colon or simply follow the patient. Colonic resection is probably advisable if cancer invades through the muscularis mucosae into the stroma of the polyp, if lymphatics in the head of the polyp contain tumor cells, or if the malignant changes extend close to the site of transection of the pedicle. This decision must be individualized.

Familial polyposis of the colon is a rare disease but an important one because malignancy develops before age 40 in nearly all untreated patients. The trait is heterozygous and autosomal dominant, and the sex incidence is equal. Multiple polyps of varying size and configuration carpet the colon and rectum. Total proctocolectomy eliminates the risk of cancer, but rectal polyps often regress after abdominal colectomy and ileorectal anastomosis, and that operation is favored initially. These patients must be followed very closely, and new polyps which appear in the rectum must be fulgurated. If polyps do not regress or if new ones develop rapidly and in large numbers, the rectum should be excised and a permanent ileostomy established.

Gardner's syndrome is a variant of familial polyposis associated with desmoid tumors, osteomas of the skull or mandible, and sebaceous cysts. The risk of colonic cancer—and therefore the treatment—is the same as for familial polyposis.

Juvenile polyps occur in children; a lesion with the same histologic appearance in an adult is termed a "retention polyp." This lesion has a fibrous stroma with scattered cystic spaces and an infiltrate of acute and chronic inflammatory cells. Juvenile polyps are probably not neoplasms, have no malignant potential, and often autoamputate at puberty; therefore, treatment is required only if bleeding or intussusception occurs. Colonoscopic polypectomy is usually successful. Juvenile polyposis has been reported to have a familial incidence. Juvenile polyposis which occupies the entire gastrointestinal tract is rare, but it can prove fatal in infants.

Peutz-Jeghers syndrome is an uncommon autosomal dominant congenital disease in which multiple polyps appear in the stomach, small bowel, and colon. Affected individuals have melanotic pigmentation of the skin and mucous membranes, especially about the lips and gums. Histologically, these polyps are hamartomas. Although carcinoma has been reported in association with Peutz-Jeghers syndrome, most authorities believe the polyps have no malignant potential and should be removed only if symptomatic.

Pseudopolyps which occur in chronic ulcerative colitis require no treatment, but care must be exercised not to overlook development of true neoplasms in long-standing inflammatory disease of the colon.

Other rare syndromes have been reported in which polyps of the bowel were associated with endocrine adenomatosis, brain tumors, or epidermal abnormalities.

Prognosis

Villous adenomas recur in about 15% of cases after local excision. Adenomatous polyps seldom recur, but new ones may develop, and a patient who has had a villous or adenomatous polyp has a greater likelihood of developing adenocarcinoma than the general population. Periodic examination is essential to detect new benign or malignant neoplasms. A test for occult blood in the stool, sigmoidoscopy, and barium enema should be performed every 1–3 years up to about age 75. The role of routine fiberoptic colonoscopy in follow-up of these patients has not been established.

Behringer GE: Polypoid lesions of the colon: Which should be removed? Surg Clin North Am 54:699, 1974.

Coller JA, Corman ML, Veidenheimer MC: Colonic polypoid disease: Need for total colonoscopy. Am J Surg 131:490, 1976.

Erbe RW: Current concepts in genetics: Inherited gastrointestinal-polyposis syndromes. N Engl J Med 294:1101, 1976.

Gilbertsen VA: Proctosigmoidoscopy and polypectomy in reducing the incidence of rectal cancer. Cancer 34 (Suppl 3): 936, 1974.

Henry LG & others: Risk of recurrence of colon polyps. Ann Surg 182:511, 1975.

Knutson CO, Schrock LG, Polk HC Jr: Polypoid lesions of the proximal colon: Comparison of experiences with removal at laparotomy and by colonoscopy. Ann Surg 179:657, 1974.

Muto T, Bussey HJR, Morson BC: The evolution of cancer of the colon and rectum. Cancer 36:2251, 1975.

Reid JD: Intestinal carcinoma in the Peutz-Jeghers syndrome. JAMA 229:833, 1974.

Shatney CH & others: Management of focally malignant pedunculated adenomatous colorectal polyps. Dis Colon Rectum 19:334, 1976.

Watne AL, Core SK, Carrier JM: Gardner's syndrome. Surg Gynecol Obstet 141:53, 1975.

Welch CE, Hedberg SE: *Polypoid Lesions of the Gastrointestinal Tract,* 2nd ed. Saunders, 1975.

Welch JP, Welch CE: Villous adenomas of the colorectum. Am J Surg 131:185, 1976.

Williams CB & others: Colonoscopy in the management of colon polyps. Br J Surg 61:673, 1974.

Wolff WI, Shinya H: Definitive treatment of "malignant" polyps of the colon. Ann Surg 182:516, 1975.

OTHER TUMORS OF THE COLON & RECTUM

Carcinoids of the large bowel are uncommon, and most of them occur in the rectum. Lesions less than 2 cm in diameter usually are asymptomatic, behave benignly, and can be managed by local excision. Larger rectal carcinoids often are accompanied by metastases and require more extensive resection. Carcinoid syndrome from metastases arising in a rectal primary is extremely rare.

Lymphosarcomas are the most common of the noncarcinomatous malignant tumors of the large bowel.

Benign lymphomas (lymphoid hyperplasia) are the most frequently encountered nonepithelial tumors of the colon and rectum. They are sessile, solitary (occasionally multiple) polypoid lesions.

Lipomas may be difficult to distinguish radiographically from mucosal neoplasms. They are usually asymptomatic but can cause intussusception or obstruction if they occur at the ileocecal valve.

Leiomyomas are much less common in the colon than in the stomach or small intestine. Colonic tumors are less apt to cause significant hemorrhage than those of the upper bowel. Some leiomyomas become malignant.

Hemangiomas are usually multiple and can bleed massively. Selective mesenteric arteriography may localize the bleeding site.

Endometriomas are masses of endometrial tissue which implant on the surface of the rectum, sigmoid colon, appendix, cecum, or distal ileum and may invade locally into the muscularis or submucosa. The ectopic tissue responds to cyclic hormonal stimulation, causing inflammation and fibrosis. Intestinal symptoms of endometriosis include altered bowel habits and occasionally rectal bleeding during menstruation. Tender nodularities are palpable in the pelvis in 90% of cases. Sigmoidoscopy, fiberoptic colonoscopy, and barium enema x-rays may make the diagnosis. Operation is performed only if symptoms are not controlled by endocrine therapy or if malignancy cannot be excluded. Operation in severe cases usually requires hysterectomy and oophorectomy; intestinal lesions are excised or the diseased segment is resected.

Other benign colorectal tumors include neurofibromas associated with Recklinghausen's disease, teratomas, and enterocystomas (duplication of rectum).

Allred HW Jr, Spencer RJ: Hemangiomas of the colon, rectum, and anus. Mayo Clin Proc 49:739, 1974.

Castro EB, Stearns MW: Lipoma of the large intestine: A review of 45 cases. Dis Colon Rectum 15:441, 1972.

Gray LA: Endometriosis of the bowel: Role of bowel resection, superficial excision and oophorectomy in treatment. Ann Surg 177:580, 1973.

Ponka JL, Walke L: Carcinoid tumors of the rectum. Dis Colon Rectum 14:46, 1971.

Wychulis AR, Beahrs OH, Woolner LB: Malignant lymphoma of the colon: A study of 69 cases. Arch Surg 93:215, 1966.

DIVERTICULAR DISEASE OF THE COLON

Diverticula occur more often in the colon than elsewhere in the gastrointestinal tract. True diverticula containing all layers of the bowel wall are rare; false diverticula—herniations of mucosa and submucosa through the muscular coats—are much more common (Fig 34–10). They often develop at points where blood vessels penetrate the muscle to supply the mucosa. Diverticula vary from a few millimeters to several centimeters in diameter; the necks may be narrow or wide; and some contain inspissated fecal matter. Approximately 95% of patients with diverticula have involvement of the sigmoid colon. The descending, transverse, and ascending portions of the colon are involved in decreasing order of frequency.

Diverticular disease becomes more frequent with advancing age. In the USA, diverticula are found in about 10% of individuals at age 40 and in 65% at age 80. Diverticula are somewhat more common in women than in men. The incidence is higher in North America and Europe than in Africa and the Orient, although diverticula confined to the right colon are relatively common in Orientals. An unusually high incidence of

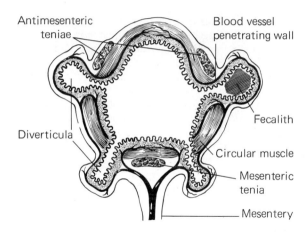

Figure 34—10. Cross-section of the colon depicting the sites where diverticula form. Note that the antimesenteric portion is spared.

the disease occurs in some families.

Although it is possible that the pathogenesis is not the same in all patients, current concepts hold that diverticula develop when abnormally high intraluminal pressures push mucosa and submucosa outward through defects in the circular muscle layer. The colon which contains diverticula is shortened, the circular muscle and teniae are thickened ("myochosis"), and the mucosal infoldings are unusually prominent. Manometric recordings in patients with diverticula show higher pressure than normal (up to 90 mm Hg) in response to meals and pharmacologic stimulants. The propensity for diverticula to develop in the sigmoid is explained by the law of Laplace, which states that pressure within a tube is inversely proportionate to the radius. Therefore, herniation through a weak spot in its wall would more likely develop in the portion of colon with the smallest caliber, ie, the sigmoid. The small radius of the sigmoid also makes it easier for circular muscle contractions to obliterate the lumen completely and create intervening closed compartments in which high pressures are generated.

The weight of evidence suggests that diverticular disease is acquired in response to dietary factors. Diverticular disease is common in North America and Europe, where diets are deficient in residue, rich in refined carbohydrate, and high in fat compared with the diets of populations with a low incidence of diverticula. Although there is some disagreement on this point, the content of indigestible fiber in the diet is probably the important feature. Low-residue diets are associated with slow transit time through the colon, desiccated, scybalous stools, high colonic pressures, and diverticula. High-residue diets have the opposite effects. It is believed that a diet deficient in fiber causes thickening of the colonic musculature over a period of years; in addition, the small fecal bulk allows the lumen to compartmentalize to form pockets of high pressure from which diverticula project.

Some experts consider diverticula to be late sequelae of the "irritable colon" syndrome, a common disorder characterized by abdominal pain and complaints of constipation, diarrhea, or both. Since many patients with diverticula have absolutely no symptoms of bowel disease, the exact relationship to irritable colon syndrome remains unclear.

Diverticulosis is defined as diverticular disease without inflammation; diverticulitis is diverticular disease with (peridiverticular) inflammation. It may be difficult to determine if an individual with abdominal pain, altered bowel habit, and abdominal tenderness has peridiverticular inflammation or not, so the more general term diverticular disease is often preferred.

1. DIVERTICULOSIS

Clinical Findings

A. Symptoms and Signs: Diverticulosis is often asymptomatic and may be found incidentally on barium enema x-rays obtained for suspected polyp or carcinoma. Bleeding may occur, sometimes massively. Some patients with diverticulosis complain of cramping lower abdominal pain and constipation or diarrhea or both. Physical examination may disclose mild tenderness in the left lower quadrant, and the left colon is sometimes palpable as a firm tubular structure. Fever and leukocytosis are absent in patients with painful diverticular disease without inflammation. The pain in these cases is believed to be caused by spastic contraction of the colonic musculature, and the diverticula themselves are asymptomatic.

B. X-Ray Findings: In addition to diverticula, barium enema films may show segmental spasm and muscular thickening which narrow the lumen and give a sawtooth appearance to the colon. In some patients, signs of spasm are present without diverticula, and the condition probably represents a variant of the irritable colon syndrome. If diverticula are present, they may affect only one area, usually the sigmoid, or they may be scattered throughout the colon.

Differential Diagnosis

Painful diverticulosis can be difficult to differentiate from diverticulitis. The presence or absence of systemic signs of inflammation is the chief differential point, but the natural history of the acute episode may be the only way to make the distinction. Diverticulosis with bleeding must be differentiated from other causes of rectal bleeding. Fiberoptic colonoscopy may help in this respect.

Complications

Diverticulitis and massive hemorrhage are complications of diverticulosis. These problems are discussed below.

Treatment

A. Medical Treatment: Diverticular disease with-

out inflammation or massive hemorrhage should be managed medically. Acutely painful episodes may require hospitalization, but most patients are managed as outpatients. A diet high in bulk is recommended, and unprocessed bran (20 g/day) or hemicellulose (1 rounded teaspoon in a full glass of cold water twice a day) may be helpful. Antispasmodics may be used, but the use of sedatives, tranquilizers, and antidepressives should be restricted. Education, reassurance, and a warm personal relationship between physician and patient are important to successful management.

B. Surgical Treatment: Operation is necessary for massive hemorrhage or to rule out carcinoma in some patients, but fiberoptic colonoscopy usually resolves the question of malignancy. Sigmoid myotomy (incision of the thickened circular muscle layer) and transverse teniamyotomy (incision of the thickened teniae coli in the affected segment) are 2 operative approaches designed to interrupt the underlying muscular abnormality. Both procedures are experimental and should not be used until more information becomes available. There is no indication for resection of the colon in patients with uncomplicated diverticulosis.

Prognosis

The natural history of diverticulosis has not been defined. Fifteen to 40% of patients with diverticulosis diagnosed by barium enema x-ray develop diverticulitis or hemorrhage when followed for many years. These patients comprise a selected population, however, and the incidence of complications of diverticulosis in the population at large cannot be estimated at present.

See references at end of next section.

2. DIVERTICULITIS

Essentials of Diagnosis

- Acute abdominal pain.
- Constipation or frequent defecation.
- Left lower quadrant tenderness and mass.
- Fever and leukocytosis.
- Characteristic radiologic signs.

General Considerations

Acute colonic diverticulitis results from rupture of a diverticulum and is more accurately termed peridiverticulitis. The notion that diverticulitis represents infection within an unruptured diverticulum is no longer given much credence. Colonic leakage from the diverticulum may spread throughout the peritoneal cavity but more commonly is localized to the colonic wall, paracolic tissues, and adjacent viscera. Inflammation may progress to form abscesses or fistulas, and partial colonic obstruction is often present.

Clinical Findings

A. Symptoms and Signs: About 50% of patients

with acute diverticulitis have no prior colonic symptoms. The acute attack consists of localized abdominal pain which is mild to severe, aching, and either persistent or cramping; it resembles acute appendicitis except that the findings are situated in the left lower quadrant. Occasionally, pain is suprapubic, in the right lower quadrant, or throughout the lower abdomen. Constipation or increased frequency of defecation (or both in the same patient) is common, and passage of flatus may give some relief of pain. Inflammation adjacent to the bladder may produce dysuria. Nausea and vomiting depend on the location and severity of the inflammation. Physical findings characteristically include low-grade fever, mild abdominal distention, left lower quadrant tenderness, and a left lower quadrant or pelvic mass. Occult or, less commonly, gross blood is present in stools; massive hemorrhage is rare in the presence of peridiverticular inflammation. Leukocytosis is mild to moderate.

The clinical picture described above is typical, but acute diverticulitis has other modes of presentation. Free perforation of a diverticulum produces generalized peritonitis rather than localized inflammation. An acute attack of diverticulitis may go unnoticed until a complication develops, and the complication may be the reason for the patient to seek help. The course of diverticulitis may be so insidious, particularly in advanced age groups, that vague abdominal pain associated with an abscess in the groin or a colovesical fistula is the initial presentation. In some cases, pain and inflammatory signs are not marked, but a palpable mass and signs of large bowel obstruction are present, so that carcinoma of the left colon seems the more likely diagnosis.

B. X-Ray Findings: Plain abdominal films may show free abdominal air if a diverticulum has perforated into the general peritoneal cavity. If inflammation is localized, there will be a picture of ileus, partial colonic obstruction, or left lower quadrant mass.

Barium enema is contraindicated during the initial stages of an acute attack of diverticulitis lest barium leak into the peritoneal cavity. The reliable radiographic signs of active diverticulitis include (1) an abscess cavity or sinus tract outside the colonic wall communicating with the lumen; (2) an intramural abscess producing indentation of the barium column; (3) extrinsic compression by a paracolic mass; (4) intramural sinuses; and (5) fistulas. (See Fig 34–11.)

Intravenous urography may reveal distortion or partial obstruction of the ureter or compression of the bladder by the inflammatory mass.

C. Special Examinations: Sigmoidoscopy is sometimes helpful. The instrument usually cannot be passed beyond the rectosigmoid junction because of acute angulation and fixation at that level with a decrease in size of the lumen. Erythema, edema, and spasm may be noted. A purulent discharge can sometimes be seen coming from above. Cystoscopy may reveal bullous edema of the bladder wall; occasionally, the entrance of a fistula can be visualized. Fiberoptic colonoscopy should be avoided during an acute attack.

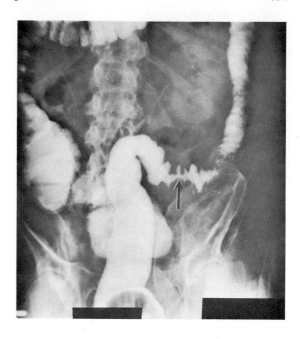

Figure 34—11. Barium enema roentgenogram showing upper sigmoid colon involved with diverticulitis. Note the long segment of narrowing, the spasm, and the deformity (arrow) produced by an intramural abscess.

Differential Diagnosis

Free perforation of a diverticulum with generalized peritonitis often cannot be differentiated from the other causes of perforated viscus. Acute diverticulitis with localized perforation may simulate appendicitis, salpingitis, endometriosis, ovarian tumors, intestinal ischemia, infarction of an epiploic appendage, ulcerative colitis, Crohn's disease, cystitis, and retroperitoneal tumors. Differentiation from appendicitis is especially difficult when a redundant sigmoid colon lies in the right lower quadrant. A history of colonic symptoms on prior occasions and palpation of a mass are sometimes helpful in differentiating these conditions. Sigmoidoscopy may detect carcinoma, vascular insufficiency, or inflammatory disease of the colon. A difficult differential diagnosis lies between diverticulitis and carcinoma of the colon, particularly in the more silent forms of diverticulitis which present with a mass or fistula. Although barium enema, sigmoidoscopy, and fiberoptic colonoscopy may clarify the issue, often the diagnosis is not known until the surgical specimen is examined by the pathologist. Persistent bleeding should not be attributed to diverticular disease until the problem has been investigated thoroughly.

Complications

The clinical spectrum of diverticulitis includes such complications as free perforation, abscess formation, fistulization, and partial obstruction. Colonic obstruction is usually slow in onset and incomplete; small bowel obstruction may result from the attachment of a loop of small intestine to the inflamed sigmoid.

Fistulas in males usually involve the bladder. Urinary frequency, dysuria, pneumaturia, and fecaluria are symptoms of colovesical fistula. Fistulas may also occur to the ureter, urethra, vagina, uterus, cecum, small bowel, perineum, and abdominal wall.

If a patient survives acute diverticulitis without operation, the disease may become chronic with episodes of exacerbation and remission.

Treatment

A. Expectant Treatment: Patients with acute diverticulitis should be hospitalized. Details of management vary with the severity of the attack; generally, nothing is given by mouth, nasogastric suction is instituted, intravenous fluids are given, and systemic broad-spectrum antibiotics are administered. Oral nonabsorbable antibacterial drugs are not thought to be of value. Morphine increases colonic muscular spasm and should not be given for pain; meperidine has less of this side-effect. As acute manifestations subside, oral feeding is resumed gradually and bulk-forming agents such as hemicellulose are prescribed.

B. Surgical Treatment: Surgical treatment should be considered if the patient fails to improve or worsens on the above regimen or if complications occur.

1. Abscess—Abscesses may form within the colonic wall, adjacent to the colon, or in the mesentery. The surgeon must choose one of 3 methods:

a. Primary resection—Resection of the diseased colon, together with the abscess, and performance of colonic anastomosis at the same time have the advantage of solving the entire problem in one operation. Unfortunately, it is seldom possible to anastomose the colon safely in this situation because the bowel is edematous and there is gross infection in the surgical field. The risk of anastomotic leakage is very great.

b. Hartmann procedure—The diseased bowel and the abscess are removed, the proximal end of the colon is brought out as a temporary colostomy, and the distal colonic stump is closed (Fig 34—12). Occasionally, the distal stump can be exteriorized as a mucous fistula. Intestinal continuity is restored in a second operation after the inflammation subsides. This approach is preferred by most surgeons today.

c. Three-stage procedure—If the abscess is large or if the patient is in poor condition, the abscess should be drained through a small incision in the left lower quadrant and the fecal stream diverted by transverse colostomy (Fig 34—13). In a second operation, the diseased area is resected and anastomosis is performed, and in the third stage the colostomy is closed.

There are variations of these basic methods of management which may be applicable in certain instances. Selection of the best operation for an individual patient requires mature judgment. Definitive resection of the diverticula-bearing colon should be performed at the same time in nearly all cases. Ordinarily, only the sigmoid and distal descending colon need be removed even if the entire colon contains diverticula, because more proximal diverticula rarely cause symptoms later.

2. Obstruction—Colonic obstruction is best treated by proximal colostomy with or without simultaneous resection of the involved colon as indicated above. Primary anastomosis after resection for obstruction is not recommended.

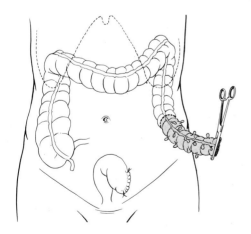

Figure 34—12. Two-stage (Hartmann) resection for diverticulitis of the colon. *Stage I:* The affected segment (shaded) has been divided at its distal end and brought out through the abdominal wall. It will then be removed by transection at its proximal margin (dotted line), leaving a healthy colostomy stoma on the surface of the abdomen. The upper end of the rectosigmoid stump has been sutured closed. Alternatively, it could have been exteriorized as a mucous fistula without closing it. *Stage II:* The divided ends of the bowel will be mobilized and anastomosed.

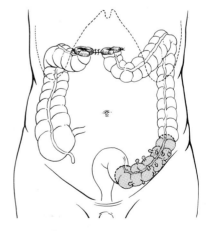

Figure 34—13. Three-stage procedure for resection of a segment of the colon involved by diverticulitis. *Stage I:* Transverse colostomy and external drainage of the abscess. *Stage II:* Resection of the involved segment (shaded) (lines of resection indicated by dotted lines) and anastomosis of healthy ends. *Stage III:* Closure of transverse colostomy.

3. Fistula—Fistula into the bladder, vagina, or other viscus is treated by staged operations if a large abscess is present. Chronic fistulas usually can be managed in one operation; the diseased colon is resected, the fistulous opening in the other structure is closed, and colonic anastomosis is performed.

4. Perforation—In this serious emergency, operation should be performed as soon as the patient can be resuscitated. The perforated segment is exteriorized or resected, but anastomosis should be deferred until later.

5. Diverticulitis of the right colon—About 1% of surgically treated diverticula occur in the cecum. The most common preoperative diagnosis is appendicitis. At operation the extensive indurated mass often cannot be differentiated from carcinoma and a right colectomy is required.

Prognosis

About 25% of patients hospitalized with acute diverticulitis require surgical treatment, and the overall mortality rate for the first attack is about 4%. The natural history of diverticular disease after the first attack of diverticulitis is not clear, and for this reason the indications for interval elective operation to resect the involved colon can be stated only in general terms. Interval operation should be considered for (1) persistent or recurrent left lower quadrant pain; (2) persistent left lower quadrant tender mass; (3) dysuria; (4) if differentiation between diverticulitis and carcinoma cannot be made by x-ray or colonoscopy; and (5) after one attack in a young patient (under 50). When these criteria for elective operation are employed, approximately 25% of nonoperated survivors of the first attack eventually undergo sigmoid resection. The operative mortality rate for these interval procedures is 3–5%, about half of the reported mortality rate for second acute attacks of diverticulitis. Patients who experience 2 or more attacks, especially after only short symptom-free intervals, are obviously candidates for resection.

Alexander-Williams J: Management of the acute complications of diverticular disease: The dangers of colostomy. Dis Colon Rectum 19:289, 1976.

Byrne JJ, Garick EI: Surgical treatment of diverticulitis. Am J Surg 121:379, 1974.

Findlay JM & others: Effects of unprocessed bran on colon function in normal subjects and in diverticular disease. Lancet 1:146, 1974.

Fleischner FG: Diverticular disease of the colon. Curr Clin Concepts 60:316, 1971.

Hodgson J: Colonic diverticular disease: Transverse taeniamyotomy. Dis Colon Rectum 18:555, 1975.

Magness LJ & others: Diverticular disease of the right colon. Surg Gynecol Obstet 140:30, 1975.

Painter NS: Colonic diverticular disease: Miller's bran in management. Dis Colon Rectum 18:549, 1975.

Parks TG: Natural history of diverticular disease of the colon: A review of 521 cases. Br Med J 4:639, 1969.

Parks TG & others: Limitations of radiology in the differentiation of diverticulitis and diverticulosis of the colon. Br Med J 2:136, 1970.

Pheils MT: Colonic diverticular disease: Colovesical fistula. Dis Colon Rectum 18:560, 1975.

Rodkey GV, Welch CE: Colonic diverticular disease with surgical treatment: A study of 338 cases. Surg Clin North Am 54:655, 1974.

Søltoft J & others: A double-blind trial of the effect of wheat bran on symptoms of irritable bowel syndrome. Lancet 1:270, 1976.

MASSIVE LOWER GASTROINTESTINAL HEMORRHAGE

Massive hemorrhage per rectum can originate from lesions in the gastroduodenum, small bowel, colon, or anorectum. A colonic source is suggested by the passage of dark to bright-red blood, but the color of evacuated blood is a function of the length of time it resided in the intestinal tract, and bright-red blood may come from a duodenal ulcer or hemorrhoids as well as any point in between. If a patient passing bright-red blood is not in shock, the bleeding site is probably colonic.

Exsanguinating hemorrhage from the colon in adults is caused by diverticular disease, vascular malformation, solitary ulcer, ulcerative colitis, or ischemic colitis in most cases. Benign or malignant neoplasms rarely cause massive bleeding. The relative incidence of these causes is changing as vascular malformations (arteriovenous communications, vascular ectasias) are being discovered in increasing numbers of patients.

Management of copious rectal bleeding involves intravenous fluid, whole blood, and diagnostic measures. A nasogastric tube should be inserted to determine if blood is present in the stomach. Some patients with bleeding duodenal ulcers do not reflux blood into the stomach, and consideration should be given to gastroduodenoscopy. Anoscopy and sigmoidoscopy should be performed to detect hemorrhoidal bleeding and to exclude ulcerative colitis, distal sigmoid or rectal neoplasms, and distal ischemia.

In about 75% of patients, bleeding stops spontaneously shortly after admission to the hospital. These patients should undergo a barium enema examination. If the barium enema fails to show a lesion, abdominal angiography may be helpful, especially if the patient has had repeated episodes of bleeding without an identifiable source. Fiberoptic colonoscopy may reveal a lesion not disclosed by radiographic studies. If the bleeding site cannot be found, operation is not indicated.

Selective mesenteric angiography is indicated for patients who continue to bleed massively after entering the hospital. The site of bleeding is identified in 60–80% of patients. Massive bleeding is at least as common in the right colon as in the left even though diverticulosis is preponderantly left-sided. Vascular ectasias and superficial mucosal ulcerations are common in the right colon.

In addition to locating the source of hemorrhage, vasoconstrictor drugs (vasopressin or epinephrine) can be infused selectively into the vessels feeding the bleeding segment, and this often stops the bleeding. If angiographic control is successful, if bleeding does not recur, and if the lesion is not neoplastic, operation should not be done. Approximately 25% of patients who stop bleeding initially will rebleed and need an operation.

Emergency operation is required for persistent hemorrhage if angiography is not available, if angiography fails to identify the bleeding site, or if hemorrhage continues or recurs after efforts to control it by arterial infusion of vasoconstrictors. If the bleeding site is unknown, the duodenum, small bowel, and stomach should be examined at operation. Often the surgeon is confronted with a colon massively dilated with blood coming from an unknown site. Various intraoperative maneuvers to locate the source such as endoscopy, isolation of segments between clamps, and temporary transverse colostomy are time-consuming and usually futile. Subtotal colectomy (total abdominal colectomy) with ileoproctostomy is the operation of choice in this situation. The operative mortality rate is 10%—less than that of other treatment strategies.

Athanasoulis CA & others: Mesenteric arterial infusions of vasopressin for hemorrhage from colonic diverticulosis. Am J Surg 129:212, 1975.

Blaisdell FW: Management of the acute complications of diverticular disease: Hemorrhage. Dis Colon Rectum 19:287, 1976.

Casarella WJ & others: "Lower" gastrointestinal tract hemorrhage: New concepts based on arteriography. Am J Roentgenol Radium Ther Nucl Med 121:357, 1974.

Drapanas T & others: Emergency subtotal colectomy: Preferred approach to management of massively bleeding diverticular disease. Ann Surg 177:519, 1973.

VOLVULUS

Essentials of Diagnosis

- Colicky abdominal pain, usually with persistence of pain between spasms.
- Abdominal distention.
- Vomiting sometimes.
- Usually older age groups.
- Characteristic x-ray findings.

General Considerations

Rotation of a segment of the intestine on an axis formed by its mesentery may result in partial or complete obstruction of the lumen and may be followed by circulatory impairment of the bowel (Fig 34–14). In the colon, volvulus usually occurs in the sigmoid or cecum; the transverse colon or splenic flexure is involved in rare instances. Volvulus of the colon accounts for 5–10% of cases of large bowel obstruction in the USA and is the second most common cause of complete colonic obstruction. In populations which consume high-residue diets, volvulus is the most frequent cause of large bowel obstruction.

Elongation of the sigmoid is a predisposing factor in sigmoid volvulus; 50% of patients are over 70 years of age, and the disease is frequently encountered in mentally ill or bedridden persons who do not evacuate stool with regularity. Chagas' disease of the colon is an important cause of sigmoid volvulus in South America. Formation of cecal volvulus requires a hypermobile cecum due to incomplete embryologic fixation of the ascending colon. The bowel twists about the mesentery, forming a closed loop obstruction as the entry and exit points of the twist engage; obstruction usually occurs when the rotation is 180 degrees. When the twist is 360 degrees, the veins are obstructed, and the impaired circulation leads to gangrene and perforation if treatment is not instituted promptly.

Clinical Findings

A. Cecal Volvulus:

1. Symptoms and signs—Not only the cecum but also the terminal ileum are involved in the rotation, so that the symptoms generally include distal small bowel obstruction. Severe, intermittent, colicky pain begins in the right abdomen. Pain eventually becomes continuous, vomiting ensues, and passage of gas and feces per rectum decreases to the point of obstipation. Ab-

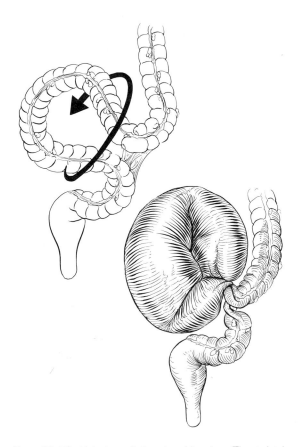

Figure 34–14. Volvulus of the sigmoid colon. The twist is counterclockwise in most cases of sigmoid volvulus.

dominal distention is variable; occasionally, a bulging tympanitic mass may be detected. There may be a history of similar but milder attacks.

2. X-ray findings—The diagnosis is seldom made without x-ray examination. Plain films show a dilated ovoid cecum which may change position but favors the epigastrium or left upper quadrant. In the early stages, there is a single fluid level resembling gastric dilatation, but large amounts of gas or fluid cannot be aspirated from the stomach, and the x-ray picture is not changed by this maneuver. Later, the radiologic findings of small bowel obstruction are superimposed on the cecal volvulus.

B. Sigmoid Volvulus:

1. Symptoms and signs—In volvulus of the sigmoid there are intermittent cramp-like pains, increasing in severity as obstipation becomes complete. Abdominal distention may be marked. There may be a history of transient attacks in which spontaneous reduction of the volvulus has occurred.

2. X-ray findings—On a plain film of the abdomen a single greatly distended loop of bowel which has lost its haustral markings is usually seen rising up out of the pelvis, frequently as high as the diaphragm. The distended loop may assume a "coffee bean" shape. In cecal volvulus, the concavity of the "coffee bean" points toward the right lower abdominal quadrant and in sigmoid volvulus it points toward the left lower quadrant. On barium enema a "bird's beak" or "ace of spades" deformity with spiral narrowing of the upper end of the lower segment is pathognomonic (Fig 34–15). Between attacks, barium enema may reveal sigmoid megacolon.

Differential Diagnosis

Cecal volvulus must be differentiated from other causes of small bowel and colonic obstruction, and sigmoid volvulus mimics other types of large bowel obstruction. Alertness to the possibility and correct interpretation of x-rays are the essentials of diagnosis.

Complications

Early diagnosis and treatment are imperative because perforation may occur if circulation to the bowel is impaired. Delay may be due to incorrect diagnosis or to futile attempts at proximal decompression by gastric intubation.

Treatment

In **cecal volvulus,** operation is required as soon as the patient can be prepared by replacing fluid and electrolyte deficits. In aged, poor-risk patients with a viable colon, the volvulus can be untwisted and the ascending colon fixed to the abdominal wall by cecostomy. Because this method often is followed by recurrence of volvulus, the preferred treatment, if the patient's condition permits, is right hemicolectomy with anastomosis of the ileum to transverse colon. Gangrenous colon must be removed (or exteriorized), but if the patient is critically ill it is wise to defer anastomosis until a more favorable time.

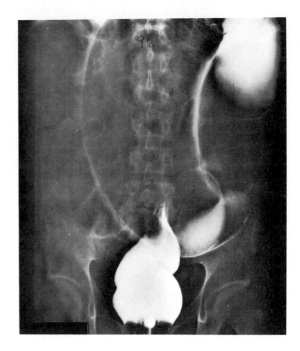

Figure 34–15. Volvulus of the sigmoid colon. Roentgenogram with barium enema taken with the patient in the supine position. Note the massively dilated sigmoid colon. The distinct vertical crease, which represents juxtaposition of adjacent walls of the dilated loop, points toward the site of torsion. The barium column resembles a bird's beak or ace of spades because of the way in which the lumen tapers toward the volvulus.

In **sigmoid volvulus,** the distended sigmoid may be deflated by gently passing a soft rectal tube through a sigmoidoscope into the twisted loop. The patient is placed in the knee-chest position for insertion of the tube; occasionally, spontaneous detorsion occurs in this position. This maneuver is contraindicated if there are signs of strangulation or perforation. If tube decompression is successful, the tube should be left in place and secured by tape or sutures to the perianal skin. Good-risk, young patients should be scheduled for elective resection as soon as the colon can be prepared because the recurrence rate after decompression alone is 50%. No operation is indicated after the first episode of sigmoid volvulus in elderly patients or those with severe disease of other organ systems. If emergency operation is performed for strangulation, resection without anastomosis is the procedure of choice. A recurrent episode is managed by insertion of a rectal tube, and then all patients but those with very severe associated disease should have resection.

Prognosis

The mortality rate during the first episode of sigmoid volvulus is about 25%; death is due to perforation (50% mortality rate) or severe associated disease in most cases. The operative mortality rate for elective resection in young, good-risk patients is low, and recurrent volvulus later is rare. The mortality rate from cecal volvulus is 30%; death is usually ascribed to delay in diagnosis with resultant gangrene. Cecal volvulus does not recur after right hemicolectomy.

Andersson A, Bergdahl L, Van der Linden W: Volvulus of the cecum. Ann Surg 181:876, 1975.

Gama AH & others: Volvulus of the sigmoid colon in Brazil: A report of 230 cases. Dis Colon Rectum 19:314, 1976.

Nemer FD & others: Volvulus of the colon: A continuing surgical problem. Dis Colon Rectum 19:321, 1976.

COLITIS

Colitis is a nonspecific term. Patients have diarrhea, abdominal pain, systemic symptoms, and abnormal endoscopic, radiographic, and laboratory tests. The task of the clinician is to differentiate among the various causes of colitis. If amebiasis, bacillary dysentery, ischemia, and pseudomembranous colitis can be ruled out, one of the 2 forms of nonspecific colitis is likely, ie, idiopathic mucosal ulcerative colitis or granulomatous colitis (Crohn's disease).

1. IDIOPATHIC MUCOSAL ULCERATIVE COLITIS

Essentials of Diagnosis

- Diarrhea, usually bloody.
- Abdominal cramps.
- Fever, weight loss, anemia.
- Absence of specific fecal pathogens.
- Sigmoidoscopic and radiographic abnormalities.

General Considerations

The age at onset of ulcerative colitis has a bimodal distribution, with the first peak between the ages of 15–20 years and a second, much lower peak in the sixth decade. Females are affected slightly more often than males. The annual incidence varies from 6–12 per 100,000 population, and the prevalence is 76–150 per 100,000 population. The disease is found worldwide but is more common in Western Countries. In about 15% of cases, there is a family history of ulcerative colitis or Crohn's disease. In the USA, Jews are more commonly affected than non-Jews, but the incidence in Jewish residents of Israel is relatively low.

The cause of ulcerative colitis is not known. The discussion of the etiology of Crohn's disease in Chapter 33 applies to ulcerative colitis as well. Although authorities disagree about whether Crohn's disease and ulcerative colitis are different diseases or variations of a single disease, most of the immunologic and genetic abnormalities occur in both conditions. A transmissible agent has been tentatively identified in ulcerative colitis tissue as well as Crohn's disease.

Ulcerative colitis is a diffuse inflammatory disease confined to the mucosa initially. Abscesses form in the crypts of Lieberkühn, penetrate the superficial submucosa, and by spreading horizontally cause the overlying mucosa to slough. Vascular congestion and hemorrhage are prominent. The margins of the ulcers are raised as mucosal tags which project into the lumen (pseudopolyps or inflammatory polyps). Except in the most severe forms, the muscular layers are spared; the serosal surface usually shows only dilated congested blood vessels. Strictures are generally due to spastic muscular contraction or neoplasms instead of fibrosis. In fulminant disease, when the full thickness is involved, the colon may dilate or perforate. The colon is shortened, but the mesentery remains thin—in contrast to Crohn's disease.

Ulcerative colitis involves the rectum in nearly all patients. If confined to the rectum, as it is in one-half of cases, it is termed ulcerative proctitis. Inflammation may spread proximally to affect the left colon, and in about one-third of patients the entire colon becomes involved (pancolitis). A few centimeters of distal ileum are ulcerated in 10% of patients with pancolitis (backwash ileitis). The diseased areas are contiguous, ie, segmental disease or skip lesions are rare.

Clinical Findings

A. Symptoms and Signs: The cardinal symptoms are rectal bleeding and diarrhea: frequent discharges of watery stool mixed with blood, pus and mucus accompanied by tenesmus, rectal urgency, and even anal incontinence. Nearly two-thirds of patients have cramping abdominal pain and variable degrees of fever, vomiting, weight loss, and dehydration. The onset may be insidious or acute and fulminating, and the clinical findings differ accordingly. Mild disease may be manifested only by loose or frequent stools, and a few patients complain paradoxically of constipation. In isolated instances, the only symptoms may be from systemic complications such as arthropathy or pyoderma. Dairy products may aggravate diarrhea.

If the disease is mild, physical examination may be normal, but in severe disease the abdomen is tender, especially in the left lower quadrant, and the colon may be distended. The anus is often fissured, tender, and spastic, and the rectal mucosa feels gritty. The examining gloved finger may be covered with blood, mucus, or pus.

Sigmoidoscopy is essential. An enema should not be given before the examination. The rectal mucosa is granular, dull, hyperemic, and friable, so that the touch of a cotton swab causes oozing of blood. The submucosal vascular pattern is lost because of edema. It is rare to see gross ulcers in the rectum in ulcerative colitis because of the superficial nature of these lesions. In more advanced disease, the mucosa is purplish-red, velvety, and extremely friable. Blood mixed with pus and mucus is evident in the lumen. The disease is uniform in the affected bowel, and patches of normal mucosa are not seen. If the mucosa is not diseased grossly, biopsy may be helpful to confirm the diagnosis. In the recovery phase, mucosal hyperemia and edema subside and inflammatory polyps may be seen. The healing mucosa is typically dull, granular, and has a neovascular pattern of telangiectatic vessels which differs from the normal pink mucosa.

B. Laboratory Findings: Anemia, leukocytosis, and elevated sedimentation rate are usually present. Severe disease leads to hypoalbuminemia, depletion of water, electrolytes, and vitamins, and laboratory evidence of steatorrhea.

C. X-Ray Findings: Barium enema examination should not be preceded by catharsis in acute cases and should not be performed at all in severely ill patients because it may precipitate acute colonic dilatation. Plain films of the abdomen should be obtained serially during fulminant attacks in order to detect colonic dilatation (megacolon) if it occurs.

Barium x-rays in acute ulcerative colitis show mucosal irregularity which varies from fine serrations to rough, ragged undermined ulcers. As the disease progresses, haustrations are gradually effaced, and the colon narrows and shortens because of muscular rigidity (Fig 34–16). Pseudopolyposis signifies severe ulceration. Widening of the space between the sacrum and rectum is due either to periproctitis or to shortening of the bowel. The presence of a stricture should always arouse suspicion of malignancy, although some strictures are due to muscular contraction.

D. Colonoscopic Findings: Fiberoptic colonoscopy may be performed if sigmoidoscopic and radiographic findings are not diagnostic, and it may substitute for the barium enema in some situations. The instrument need be inserted only into the sigmoid in order to make the diagnosis in most cases. Colonoscopy should be performed with great care if the disease is active because of the danger of perforation and should not be done in the presence of colonic dilatation. In chronic disease, colonoscopy is valuable in detecting cancer which often is not shown by x-ray examination.

Differential Diagnosis

Malignant neoplasms of the colon and diverticular disease must be considered in the differential diagnosis. Cultures of stool and rectal swabs will detect bacillary dysentery and gonococcal proctitis. Parasitic infection (notably amebiasis; see Chapter 11) is diagnosed by examination of stool for ova and parasites, microscopic study of rectal swabbings, and serologic tests. Rare cases of histoplasmosis, cytomegalic inclusion disease, or schistosomiasis may be very difficult to diagnose. Rectal strictures from lymphogranuloma venereum are recognized by the history and the results of Frei or complement fixation tests. Colitis caused by antibiotics is discussed separately below; the history is important. Ischemic colitis has a segmental pattern of involvement quite unlike the usual distribution of ulcerative colitis. Functional diarrhea can mimic colitis, but organic disease must be excluded before it can be concluded that the diarrhea is functional.

The most difficult differential diagnosis is between mucosal ulcerative colitis and granulomatous colitis (Crohn's disease). Distinguishing features are listed in Table 34–5. None of these features is specific for one or the other disease, and often the differentiation can be made only after all the data have been assembled. About 10% of cases cannot be classified. Serum lysozyme levels have been suggested as an aid to differential diagnosis. Although lysozyme concentrations in the blood are higher in Crohn's disease than in ulcerative colitis, there is too much overlap for the test to be useful at present.

Complications

The following **extracolonic manifestations** may occur in association with ulcerative colitis. There is an inexact relationship between the severity of the colitis and these complications: (1) lesions of the skin and mucous membranes, eg, erythema nodosum, erythema multiforme, pyoderma gangrenosum, pustular dermatitis, and aphthous stomatitis; (2) uveitis; (3) bone and joint lesions, eg, arthralgia, arthritis, and ankylosing spondylitis; (4) hepatobiliary lesions, eg, fatty infiltration, pericholangitis, cirrhosis, sclerosing cholangitis, bile duct carcinoma, and gallstones; (5) anemia, usually due to iron deficiency; (6) malnutrition and growth retardation; and (7) pericarditis. Skin and joint lesions are the most common extracolonic manifestations associated with ulcerative colitis.

Anorectal complications are less frequent than in granulomatous colitis and include anal fissure, pararec-

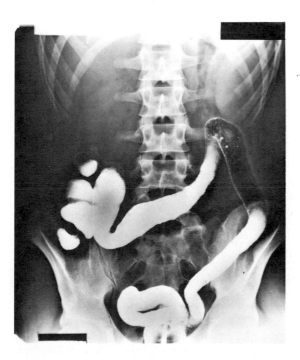

Figure 34–16. Ulcerative colitis. Barium enema roentgenogram of colon. Note shortening of colon, loss of haustral markings ("lead pipe" appearance) and fine serrations at the edges of the bowel wall which represent multiple small ulcers.

Table 34—5. Comparison of various features of ulcerative colitis with those of granulomatous colitis.

	Ulcerative (Mucosal) Colitis	Granulomatous (Transmural) Colitis
Signs and symptoms		
Diarrhea	Marked.	Present; less severe.
Gross bleeding	Characteristic.	Infrequent.
Perianal lesions	Infrequent, mild.	Frequent, complex; may precede diagnosis of intestinal disease.
Toxic dilatation	Yes (3—20%).	Less common.
Carcinoma	Greatly increased incidence.	Increased incidence.
Systemic manifestations (arthritis, uveitis, pyoderma, hepatitis)	Common.	Common.
X-ray studies	Confluent, diffuse.	Skip areas.
	Tiny serrations (crypt abscess), coarse mucosa, mucosal tags.	Longitudinal ulcers, transverse ridges, "cobblestone" appearance.
	Concentric involvement.	Eccentric involvement ("fingerprinting").
	Internal fistulas very rare.	Internal fistulas common.
	Colon only involved; may be limited to left side.	Any portion of intestinal tract may be involved; may be limited to ileum and right colon.
Morphology		
Gross	Confluent involvement.	Segmental involvement with or without skip areas.
	Rectum usually involved.	Rectum often not involved.
	Mesentery not involved; nodes enlarged.	Thickened mesentery; pronounced lymph node enlargement.
	Widespread ragged superficial ulceration.	Large longitudinal ulcers or transverse fissures.
	Inflammatory polyps (pseudopolyps) common.	Inflammatory polyps not prominent.
	No thickening of bowel wall.	Thickened bowel wall.
Microscopic	Inflammatory reaction usually limited to mucosa and submucosa; only in severe disease are muscle coats involved; no fibrosis.	Chronic inflammation of all layers of bowel wall; damage to muscle layers usual; submucosal fibrosis.
	Granulomas rare.	Granulomas frequent.
Natural history	Exacerbations, remissions; may be explosive, lethal.	Indolent, crippling.
Treatment		
Response to medical treatment	Good response in 85% of cases.	Difficult to evaluate; seldom controlled over long term.
Type of surgical treatment and response	Proctocolectomy with ileostomy; rectum can be preserved in some cases.	Partial or complete colectomy with ileostomy or anastomosis; rectum can be preserved in some patients; recurrence common.

tal abscess, fistula-in-ano, and rectovaginal fistula. Rectal strictures are either confined to the mucosa or, if full-thickness, are due to muscular spasm or neoplasm.

Perforation of the colon, which affects about 3% of patients, is responsible for more deaths than any other complication of ulcerative colitis. The risk of perforation is highest in the initial attack of the disease and correlates well with its extent and severity. It occurs most commonly in the sigmoid or splenic flexure and may result in a localized abscess or generalized fecal peritonitis. Any severely diseased colon may perforate, but patients with toxic dilatation (megacolon) are especially vulnerable. Systemic therapy (corticosteroids and antibiotics) may mask the development of this complication.

Acute colonic dilatation (toxic megacolon) occurs in approximately 3% of patients and in about 9% of patients coming to emergency operation. The patients are severely ill (toxic) and usually exhibit one or more of the following contributory factors: inflammation involving the muscular coats, hypokalemia, opiates, anticholinergics, and barium enema examinations. Toxic megacolon is diagnosed by plain abdominal x-rays which show a thickened bowel wall and dilated lumen (greater than 6 cm in the transverse colon); often, the luminal air outlines irregular nodular pseudopolyps (Fig 34—17).

Massive hemorrhage is an uncommon but life-threatening complication.

Carcinoma of the colon develops in less than 5% of patients with ulcerative colitis. Life-table methods give these estimates: cancer occurs in 3% of patients during the first 10 years after the onset of ulcerative colitis; in every decade thereafter, 20% of patients still at risk will develop carcinoma of the colon. It is apparent that not all patients with ulcerative colitis share equally in the risk of cancer. It is most likely to appear in patients who have (1) onset of ulcerative colitis at an early age (15 years or younger); (2) a severe first attack; (3) total colonic involvement; and (4) continu-

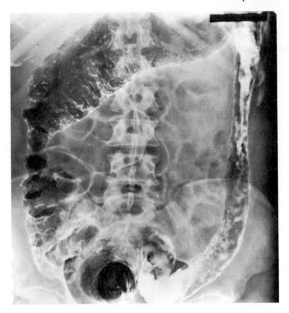

Figure 34—17. Roentgenogram of ulcerative colitis. Note dilatation of the transverse colon, the multiple irregular densities in the lumen which represent pseudopolyps, the thickening of the wall of the descending colon and the loss of haustral markings.

ous symptoms. Cancer is infrequent in mild or controlled disease or disease confined to the distal colon. The sigmoid is the most frequent site, although any portion of the colon may be affected, and tumors may be multicentric. Development of carcinoma is insidious, often difficult to diagnose, and requires vigilance in follow-up care. Attempts at early detection by closely following the patient have been disappointing because the tumor has so often spread when first discovered. There is some hope that serial mucosal biopsies may reveal premalignant changes and permit selection of patients in need of prophylactic colectomy. Cancer in these patients is aggressive, and survival rates are poor.

Treatment

A. Conservative Measures: The goals of conservative therapy are to terminate the acute attack as rapidly as possible and to prevent relapse. Management depends on the severity of the attack and the age group; children and the elderly present special problems.

1. Mild attack—Mild or insidious disease limited to the rectum and sigmoid usually can be checked with outpatient management. Reduced physical activity, even bed rest, is advisable. Diet should be free of bovine milk products and any other food which exacerbates diarrhea in the individual patient. Sulfonamides are effective in controlling acute attacks and may be prescribed as (1) sulfasalazine (Azulfidine), 2–8 g/day orally; or (2) sulfisoxazole (Gantrisin), 2 g/day orally. Topical corticosteroids are indicated in

many cases, and hydrocortisone hemisuccinate may be self-administered nightly as an oil retention enema. It can be prepared inexpensively at home by mixing 1.6 g of hydrocortisone powder in 1 quart of vegetable oil; 60 ml (100 mg) of the mixture are instilled into the rectum with a bulb syringe, preferably with the patient lying on his left side and with the buttocks elevated. If these measures fail to relieve symptoms within 2 weeks, the patient should be admitted to the hospital for more intensive therapy in order to avoid progression to severe disease.

2. Severe attack—Severe or fulminating ulcerative colitis is a medical emergency and requires hospitalization. Depending on the patient's condition, nothing should be given by mouth or a high-protein diet may be allowed; nasogastric suction is required in patients with colonic dilatation or those at risk of developing this complication.

Corticosteroids are given intravenously initially as hydrocortisone (100–300 mg/day) or prednisolone (20–80 mg/day). Alternatively, corticotropin (ACTH) may be administered as an intravenous drip (20–40 units/8 hours); ACTH may have some advantages in patients suffering second attacks. Corticosteroids are given orally when diet is resumed, and doses are tapered gradually over a period of 1–3 months. Topical corticosteroids are instituted when the diarrhea abates.

Hypokalemia is common and should be corrected. Transfusions of blood may be needed. Caution should be exercised in administering anticholinergics and opiates because they may precipitate acute dilatation of the colon. Sulfasalazine should be given orally if the patient is allowed to eat, but the most severely ill require intravenous broad-spectrum antibiotics.

3. Maintenance—Controlled trials have shown that chronic administration of sulfonamides (2 g/day orally) reduces relapse rates. Oral corticosteroids in doses small enough to avoid side-effects are ineffective in preventing relapse, but topical corticosteroids given daily as an enema should be prescribed routinely after an acute attack has resolved. Steroids by enema should be continued for at least 2 years if the patient is in remission or indefinitely if resolution is incomplete. The role of azathioprine (Imuran) is problematic since the available studies show only marginal benefit; it may permit reduction of steroid dosage.

B. Surgical Treatment:

1. Indications—

a. Acute attack—Operation should be performed in patients with severe attacks who do not improve with intensive medical therapy. Operation is required after 2–3 days in severe cases or longer in others with a more indolent course. Emergency operation is indicated for (1) proved or suspected perforation of the colon; (2) persistent massive hemorrhage from the bowel; or (3) acute dilatation of the colon unresponsive to 48–72 hours of treatment.

b. Chronic disease—Operation is required for frequent attacks or for chronic continuous symptoms. Patients so afflicted become bowel cripples, unable to maintain nutrition and incapable of employment. Children with severe chronic disease may have impaired growth and development. Disabling side-effects of chronic high-dose steroid treatment should be avoided, and colectomy may be necessary for this purpose.

c. **Carcinoma**—Operation is performed to treat carcinoma or to prevent it if the patient is in the category of high risk for malignancy: long-standing, continuously symptomatic pancolitis with onset in childhood or adolescence.

d. **Extracolonic manifestations**—Severe arthritis, uveitis, or skin lesions may be an indication for surgery. Ankylosing spondylitis does not appear to respond to colectomy, and it is not clear whether hepatic manifestations improve after radical surgical therapy.

2. Surgical procedures—Total proctocolectomy with permanent ileostomy is the procedure of choice in the majority of patients operated on electively. The role of rectal preservation with immediate or subsequent ileorectal anastomosis is controversial. Some surgeons claim that two-thirds of patients are satisfied with this arrangement, while others believe that very few patients have an acceptable bowel habit after ileoproctostomy. The rate of success correlates well with the presence and severity of rectal disease, although differences in patient populations, surgical technics, and evaluation of patient satisfaction undoubtedly contribute to conflicting reports.

In emergency operations, it may be wise to preserve the rectum in the hope of minimizing operative mortality and morbidity rates, but patients operated on for massive hemorrhage may continue to bleed from the defunctionalized rectum. If the colon is markedly dilated, ileostomy (to divert the fecal stream) and one or more colostomies (for decompression) may be a lifesaving temporary approach.

Prognosis

The prognosis of an acute attack is related to the age of the patient and to the severity and extent of disease. The overall mortality rate of first attacks is 4–15%; it is 17% in patients over 60 years. The mortality rate is related to the severity of the attack as shown by the following figures: severe attack, 10–34% mortality rate; moderate, 2–20%; and mild, 0–2%. Acute ulcerative proctitis has a mortality rate of almost zero, and 26% of patients with pancolitis succumb to the first attack. Sepsis is the predominant cause of death in acute attacks.

Following the initial attack, about 80% of patients have a second attack within 1 year and over 90% have a second attack within 15 years. The long-term risk to life in those who survive the initial attack is disputed; an annual fatality rate of 2.8% (in patients with pancolitis) was recorded in one study, but another report claimed no excess mortality rate after the first year when data were analyzed by actuarial methods. Authorities agree that disease limited to the rectum has an excellent prognosis.

Approximately 15% of patients with ulcerative colitis undergo colectomy at some time. Emergency colectomy has a mortality rate of 5–10%; most of these deaths are due to perforation, a complication which has a fatal outcome in 42% of cases. The operative death rate is 3% for elective colectomy. In an estimated 90% of survivors, colectomy with ileostomy is consistent with a satisfying, productive life but a few patients experience problems such as small bowel obstruction and ileostomy dysfunction. Impotence after properly performed proctectomy occurs in 10–15% of men overall but is limited almost exclusively to those over 50 years of age.

Akwari OE & others: Cancer of the bile ducts associated with ulcerative colitis. Ann Surg 181:303, 1975.

Binder SC, Miller HH, Deterling RA Jr: Emergency and urgent operations for ulcerative colitis: The procedure of choice. Arch Surg 110:284, 1975.

Binder SC, Miller HH, Deterling RA Jr: Fate of the retained rectum after subtotal colectomy for inflammatory disease of the colon. Am J Surg 131:201, 1976.

Bonnevie O & others: The prognosis of ulcerative colitis. Scand J Gastroenterol 9:81, 1974.

Cave DR, Mitchell DN, Brooke BN: Evidence of an agent transmissible from ulcerative colitis tissue. Lancet 1:1311, 1976.

Cook MG, Goligher JC: Carcinoma and epithelial dysplasia complicating ulcerative colitis. Gastroenterology 68:1127, 1975.

Devroede GJ & others: Cancer risk and life expectancy of children with ulcerative colitis. N Engl J Med 285:17, 1971.

Edwards FC, Truelove SC: The course and prognosis of ulcerative colitis. Gut 4:299, 1963.

Farmer RG, Brown CH: Course and prognosis of ulcerative proctosigmoiditis. Am J Gastroenterol 56:227, 1971.

Fry PD, Atkinson KG: Current surgical approach to toxic megacolon. Surg Gynecol Obstet 143:26, 1976.

Gilat T & others: Ulcerative colitis in the Jewish population of Tel-Aviv Yafo. 3. Clinical course. Gastroenterology 70:14, 1976.

Jewell DP, Truelove SC: Azathioprine in ulcerative colitis: Final report on controlled therapeutic trial. Br Med J 4:627, 1974.

Kaplan HP & others: A controlled evaluation of intravenous adrenocorticotropic hormone and hydrocortisone in the treatment of acute colitis. Gastroenterology 69:91, 1975.

Kirsner JB, Shorter RG (editors): *Inflammatory Bowel Disease.* Lea & Febiger, 1975.

Kristensen M & others: High dose prednisone treatment in severe ulcerative colitis. Scand J Gastroenterol 9:177, 1974.

Lennard-Jones JE & others: Prospective study of outpatients with extensive colitis. Lancet 1:1065, 1974.

Mungas JE, Moossa AR, Block GE: Treatment of toxic megacolon. Surg Clin North Am 56:95, 1976.

Myrvold HE, Kock NG, Åhrén C: Rectal biopsy and precancer in ulcerative colitis. Gut 15:301, 1974.

Newton CR, Baker WNW: Comparison of bowel function after ileorectal anastomosis for ulcerative colitis and colonic polyposis. Gut 16:785, 1975.

Nugent FW & others: Serum lysozyme in inflammatory bowel disease. Gastroenterology 70:1014, 1976.

Rosenberg JL & others: A controlled trial of azathioprine in the management of chronic ulcerative colitis. Gastroenterology 69:96, 1975.

Schachter H, Kirsner JB: Definitions of inflammatory bowel disease of unknown etiology. Gastroenterology 68:591, 1975.

Steinberg DM & others: Sequelae of colectomy and ileostomy: Comparison between Crohn's colitis and ulcerative colitis. Gastroenterology 68:33, 1975.

Truelove SC, Jewell DP: Intensive intravenous regimen for severe attacks of ulcerative colitis. Lancet 1:1067, 1974.

2. GRANULOMATOUS COLITIS
(Crohn's Disease)

The general features of Crohn's disease (regional enteritis, granulomatous colitis, transmural colitis) are described in Chapter 33. Approximately 40% of patients with Crohn's disease have both small and large bowel involvement, 27% have colonic disease alone, and another 3% have anorectal involvement only. Diarrhea, cramping abdominal pain, constitutional effects, and extraintestinal manifestations are approximately the same in colonic and enteric disease. Internal fistulas and abscesses and intestinal obstruction are usually complications of small bowel disease. Anorectal complications (perianal fistula, abscess, and rectal stricture) and hemorrhage are more common when the large bowel is affected, and toxic dilatation is limited to patients with inflammation of the colon.

Proctosigmoidoscopy discloses a normal rectum in 50% of patients with granulomatous colitis. Diseased mucosa is patchily involved, with irregular ulcerations separated by edematous or even normal-appearing mucosa. Biopsy may confirm the diagnosis. Radiographic features include sparing of the rectum, right colonic and ileal involvement, skip areas, transverse fissures, longitudinal ulcers, strictures, and fistulas. Features differentiating granulomatous from ulcerative colitis are summarized in Table 34–5. Ischemic colitis is another disease which can be confused with granulomatous colitis, and the differential diagnosis is discussed below.

Frank blood in the stools is observed in about one-third of patients with granulomatous colitis, but massive hemorrhage is unusual. Acute colonic dilatation (toxic megacolon) occurs in 5–8%; it responds to nonoperative treatment more often than it does in ulcerative colitis. Actuarial methods suggest that the risk of colonic cancer in granulomatous colitis patients is 20 times that of the general population.

Medical management is described in Chapter 33. The efficacy of medical treatment of granulomatous colitis over the long term is difficult to judge for lack of objective data. Radiographic resolution associated with clinical improvement is noted in some cases, but it is not clear what percentage of patients come under control and how lasting the benefits are.

Surgical treatment is reserved for the complications of Crohn's disease; because it is typically segmental, limited resection with primary anastomosis often can be done. Total abdominal colectomy with ileorectal anastomosis is done more frequently in granulomatous than in ulcerative colitis. Total proctocolectomy with ileostomy is needed in some cases. Bypass of severe disease is useful mainly as a temporary measure if large abscesses or dense adherence of bowel to adjacent structures makes resection hazardous. Diverting ileostomy improves the clinical status of patients, but in some the disease progresses despite diversion and in others the disease recurs when intestinal continuity is reestablished. The long-term effectiveness of ileostomy in preserving the colon involved with Crohn's disease is questionable.

Recurrence rates after surgical resection of diseased colon are a matter of debate at present. Differences in patient populations, surgical technics, criteria for recurrence, and methods of analysis are responsible for the disparity in published figures. There is a high rate of recurrence at or just proximal to intestinal suture lines; disease reappears in 50–90% of patients after resection and anastomosis. Recurrence is less common following total proctocolectomy and ileostomy. With a combination of medical and surgical therapy, 80–85% of patients lead productive lives, although many live with chronic disease.

Bercovitz ZT & others (editors): *Ulcerative and Granulomatous Colitis.* Thomas, 1973.

Burman JH & others: The effects of diversion of intestinal contents on the progress of Crohn's disease of the large bowel. Gut 12:11, 1971.

DeDombal FT & others: Short-term course and prognosis of Crohn's disease. Gut 15:435, 1974.

Farmer RG, Hawk WA, Turnbull RB Jr: Clinical patterns in Crohn's disease: A statistical study of 615 cases. Gastroenterology 68:627, 1975.

Farmer RG, Hawk WA, Turnbull RB Jr: Indications for surgery in Crohn's disease: Analysis of 500 cases. Gastroenterology 71:245, 1976.

Greenstein AJ, Kark AE, Dreiling DA: Crohn's disease of the colon. 2. Controversial aspects of hemorrhage, anemia and rectal involvement in granulomatous disease involving the colon. Am J Gastroenterol 63:40, 1975.

Greenstein AJ & others: Reoperation and recurrence in Crohn's colitis and ileocolitis: Crude and cumulative rates. N Engl J Med 293:685, 1975.

Korelitz BI & others: Recurrent regional ileitis after ileostomy and colectomy for granulomatous colitis. N Engl J Med 287:110, 1972.

Lefton HB, Farmer RG, Fazio V: Ileorectal anastomosis for Crohn's disease of the colon. Gastroenterology 69:612, 1975.

Lightdale CJ & others: Carcinoma complicating Crohn's disease: Report of seven cases and review of the literature. Am J Med 59:262, 1975.

Nugent FW & others: Prognosis after colonic resection for Crohn's disease of the colon. Gastroenterology 65:308, 1973.

Steinberg DM & others: Excisional surgery with ileostomy for Crohn's colitis with particular reference to factors affecting recurrence. Gut 15:845, 1974.

Weedon DD & others: Crohn's disease and cancer. N Engl J Med 289:1099, 1973.

3. PSEUDOMEMBRANOUS COLITIS

Pseudomembranous colitis is an acute inflammatory disease of the large intestine. Many cases are associated with the use of broad-spectrum antibiotics. The history and sigmoidoscopic findings of grayish-white plaques on the mucosal surface usually differentiate pseudomembranous colitis from ulcerative colitis. This disease is discussed more fully in the section on pseudomembranous enterocolitis in Chapter 33.

Tedesco FJ, Stanley RJ, Alpers DH: Diagnostic features of clindamycin-associated pseudomembranous colitis. N Engl J Med 290:841, 1974.
Viteri AL, Howard PH, Dyck WP: The spectrum of lincomycin-clindamycin colitis. Gastroenterology 66:1137, 1974.

4. ISCHEMIC COLITIS

Ischemic colitis is an acute illness caused by mesenteric vascular occlusion or a variety of nonocclusive diseases (see Chapter 33). The average age is 70 years.

Ischemic colitis is arbitrarily categorized as mild or severe. The mild form is transient and heals rapidly on nonoperative treatment, sometimes with stricture formation. The severe form is fulminant from onset or may pursue an indolent course without resolution for weeks. Both of the severe forms require operation.

Patients with ischemic colitis have an abrupt onset of variable degrees of abdominal pain, diarrhea (commonly bloody), and systemic symptoms. The abdomen may be tender diffusely, in a localized area (eg, left lower quadrant), or not at all. Blood is seen coming from above at sigmoidoscopy; if the rectum itself is ischemic—an unusual occurrence—the mucosa is edematous and ulcerated and a grayish membrane may be present. The same abnormalities are seen in the ischemic segment examined with the fiberoptic colonoscope. Plain abdominal x-rays are nonspecific. Barium enema x-rays show "thumbprints" or pseudotumors, typically limited to a 6–20 cm segment; 75% have involvement of the left colon. Mesenteric arteriography may show major arterial occlusion or no abnormalities.

Differentiating ischemic colitis from carcinoma, ulcerative colitis, and diverticulitis should not be difficult. Crohn's disease presents a greater problem in differential diagnosis. Rectal bleeding—especially gross hemorrhage—is uncommon in Crohn's disease, and the rapid onset of ischemic colitis is also different from Crohn's disease. Radiographic findings and, in some cases, the colonoscopic appearance may be helpful, but often the natural history of the acute attack is the only way to make the distinction. Ischemic colitis usually resolves rapidly or progresses to gangrene or to stricture.

Therapy for mild ischemic colitis consists of intravenous fluids, antibiotics, and observation. Severe disease, whether fulminant from the beginning, becoming fulminant over several days, or just failing to resolve after 2 weeks of treatment, should be treated by operation. The diseased colon is resected, but anastomosis is not performed. The prognosis is excellent for mild disease and fair in patients with severe disease.

McNeill C & others: Ischemic colitis diagnosed by early colonoscopy. Gastrointest Endosc 20:124, 1974.
O'Connell TX, Kadell B, Tompkins RK: Ischemia of the colon. Surg Gynecol Obstet 142:337, 1976.
Williams LF Jr, Wittenberg J: Ischemic colitis: A useful clinical diagnosis, but is it ischemic? Ann Surg 182:439, 1975.
Wittenberg J & others: Ischemic colitis: Radiology and pathophysiology. Am J Roentgenol Radium Ther Nucl Med 123:287, 1975.

COLITIS CYSTICA PROFUNDA

Colitis cystica profunda is a rare benign disease characterized by mucus-containing cysts in the wall of the colon or rectum. Most commonly it is localized to the anterior wall of the rectum, but it may also occur in the colon, either diffusely or confined to a segment. It is probably an acquired condition related to inflammation, eg, ulcerative colitis. The most common symptoms are rectal bleeding, passage of mucus, and diarrhea. The lesion is plaque-like or nodular, and in some cases the center is ulcerated. Microscopically, it can be mistakenly diagnosed as malignant if the pathologist is not alert to the condition. Treatment consists of local excision or limited resection; radical procedures such as abdominoperineal resection are not indicated.

Green GI & others: Colitis cystica profunda. Am J Surg 127:749, 1974.

DISEASES OF THE APPENDICES EPIPLOICAE

The appendices epiploicae are tabs of fat attached to the teniae and are most numerous in the cecum and the sigmoid colon. Each contains an artery which loops through the appendage and continues into the antimesenteric border of the bowel. Colonic diverticula may be hidden in these structures.

Acute epiploic appendagitis is an uncommon condition which may simulate acute appendicitis. The cause of this disease, at least in some cases, is torsion and infarction. Patients, usually obese, note the sudden onset of abdominal pain localized to the involved area. Moderate fever, leukocytosis, and physical findings of localized peritoneal irritation are typical. A mass may be palpable. X-ray examination is nonspecific. Treatment is invariably surgical because of the uncertain diagnosis, and the offending epiploica is amputated.

Chronic and recurrent cases have been reported. Infarction and separation of epiploicae account for some of the free fibrous or calcified intraperitoneal bodies seen on x-ray or at operation. Indentation of the bowel wall by an appendix epiploica may simulate a sessile polypoid tumor.

Thomas JH, Rosato FE, Patterson LT: Epiploic appendagitis. Surg Gynecol Obstet 138:23, 1974.

· · ·

INTESTINAL STOMAS
(Ileostomy & Colostomy)

An intestinal stoma is an opening of the bowel onto the surface of the abdomen. It may be temporary or permanent. Esophagostomy, gastrostomy, jejunostomy, and cecostomy are usually temporary, but ileostomy, colostomy, and some urinary tract stomas arc often permanent. Ileostomy and colostomy are by far the most common stomas. Although "stoma" is the preferred medical term, "ostomy" is used by lay organizations devoted to the rehabilitation of these patients.

Few surgical alterations of anatomy are surrounded by as much misunderstanding as intestinal stomas, and few pronouncements by surgeons are as horrifying to patients as the indication that a stoma will be necessary. For these and other reasons, a paramedical profession, **enterostomy therapy**, has developed. The enterostomal therapist (ET) is usually a registered nurse who has taken specialized training and is certified in the field; many therapists have a stoma themselves. The enterostomal therapist provides the following services: (1) preoperative education and counseling of patient and family; (2) immediate postoperative care of the stoma; (3) training in the use of equipment and supervision of self-care; (4) fitting of a permanent appliance; (5) advice on day-to-day living with a stoma; (6) management of skin problems, odor control, and other minor problems; (7) recognition of major stoma problems; (8) long-term emotional, moral, and physical support; and (9) information about the United Ostomy Association, an organization with chapters in many localities.

1. ILEOSTOMY

Permanent ileostomy is performed most commonly after proctocolectomy for ulcerative colitis; patients with Crohn's disease, familial polyposis, and other conditions may also require ileostomy. An ileostomy discharges small quantities of liquid material continuously; it does not require irrigation; and an appliance must be worn at all times.

Technical details of ileostomy construction essential for a satisfactory stoma are beyond the scope of this text. The optimal position of the stoma is in the right lower quadrant (Fig 34–18). The ileum is brought through the rectus abdominis muscle, everted upon itself, and the mucosa is sutured to the skin (surgically matured). A temporary appliance consisting of a disposable plastic bag attached to a karaya gum ring is placed on the stoma. Karaya gum (sterculia gum) prevents skin irritation, or, if skin irritation has developed, epithelization can occur beneath karaya. After a week or more, postoperative edema subsides and a permanent appliance can be fitted. Modern appliances lie flat against the abdomen, adhere to the skin without cement, are inconspicuous and odor-proof, and need be changed only every 3–5 days in most cases. They are drained at intervals during the day through an opening in the bottom of the pouch.

A **continent ileostomy** is a relatively recent technical innovation designed to avoid the continual discharge of ileal effluent which necessitates wearing an appliance at all times. A reservoir is constructed out of the distal ileum, and the outlet from the reservoir is so arranged that fluid cannot escape onto the abdominal wall. The reservoir is emptied several times a day by inserting a catheter into the stoma. The popularity of the procedure is becoming more widespread, but it is too early to know if continent ileostomy should be performed in preference to standard ileostomy in patients with ulcerative colitis. It is a hazardous operation in patients with regional enteritis because of the risk of recurrent disease.

Physiologic changes after ileostomy are due to the loss of the water- and salt-absorbing capacity of the colon. If the small bowel is free of disease and extensive resection has not been done, an ileostomy puts out 1–2 liters of fluid per day initially. The volume of effluent diminishes to between 500 and 800 ml/day after a month or two (Table 34–1). This loss of fluid is obligatory and is not reduced by manipulations of diet. Obligatory sodium losses are about 50 mEq/day greater than in patients with an intact colon, but potassium losses usually are not significantly increased. These physiologic alterations render the patient with ileostomy susceptible to acute or subacute salt and water depletion manifested by fatigue, anorexia, irritability, headache, drowsiness, muscle cramps, and thirst. Gastroenteritis or diarrhea from any cause and exposure to hot weather or vigorous exercise are situations which patients must be cautioned against; salt and water intake must be increased in these circumstances. Ileostomy patients must never be in a position where salt and water are unavailable, eg, on long hikes in the desert. Low-salt diets and diuretics may induce salt depletion or dehydration also. Patients should be counseled to salt food liberally, but salt tablets will not be required in usual circumstances. Patients with unusually high ileostomy outputs may need supplemental potassium in the form of bananas or orange juice. Water intake in response to thirst may underestimate

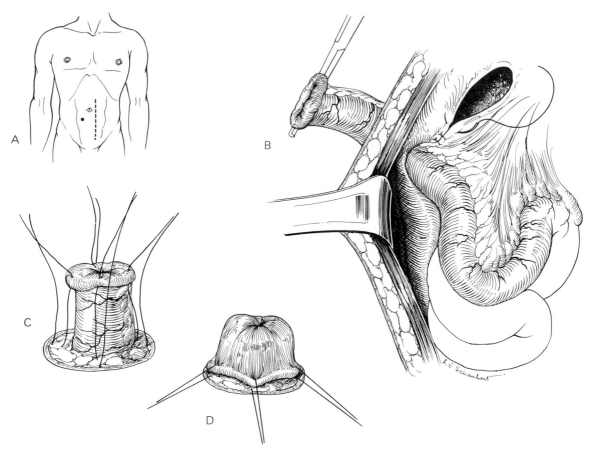

Figure 34—18. Ileostomy after colectomy. *A:* Abdominal incision for colectomy indicated by the dotted line and the site of the ileostomy by the black dot. *B:* The ileum has been brought through the abdominal wall. *C and D:* The ileostomy stoma has been everted and its margins sutured to the edges of the wound.

the optimal amount, and patients should consume sufficient water to keep the urine pale or to maintain a urine output of at least 1 liter per day.

Patients must be informed about these physiologic alterations and measures to compensate for them. Otherwise, instructions are simple, and patients should live normally. No special diet is required, although some discover that certain foods (eg, fish, eggs) may cause excessive odor or gas. Ordinary physical activity, employment, and social activities are encouraged. Bathing, swimming, sexual intercourse, and pregnancy and delivery are unrestricted, although there is a higher incidence of cesarean deliveries, mainly because of the intestinal disease or operations which led to the stoma rather than the stoma itself.

Complications are reported in 30–75% of ileostomy patients; about 25% require operative correction, usually minor. Complications include the following:

(1) Ileostomy dysfunction: Profuse watery discharge from the ileostomy associated with cramping abdominal pain is due to partial obstruction of the ileum. Before ileostomies were surgically matured, this syndrome was routine early in the postoperative period due to serositis on the surface of the exteriorized

ileum. This is rarely a problem now, but a similar syndrome may develop months or years after operation owing to stenosis or recurrent disease at or proximal to the stoma. Early postoperative dysfunction is treated by intravenous fluids and electrolytes, and gentle insertion of a catheter into the ileostomy improves egress of the luminal contents. Treatment of late dysfunction is directed toward the underlying cause.

(2) Intestinal obstruction: Obstruction may be due to adhesive bands, volvulus, or paraileostomy herniation of bowel.

(3) Stenosis: Circumferential scar formation at the skin or subcutaneous level is usually at fault; rarely, the stenosis is at the fascial level. Treatment requires a minor local plastic procedure.

(4) Retraction: The stoma should protrude 2–3 cm above the skin level to avoid leakage beneath the ileostomy pouch. A flush or retracted stoma functions poorly and should be revised.

(5) Prolapse: This is uncommon if the mesentery has been sutured to the parietal peritoneum.

(6) Peri-ileostomy abscess and fistula: Perforation of the ileum by sutures, pressure necrosis from an ill-fitted appliance, or recurrent disease may cause abscess and fistula.

(7) Skin irritation: This is the single most common complication of ileostomy and is due to leakage of ileal effluent onto the peristomal skin; it is usually minor but can be very severe if neglected. Treatment is directed toward the cause of leakage, usually an ill-fitting pouch. Protection of the skin by karaya and a variety of other products will resolve the problem. Enterostomal therapists manage these problems expertly.

(8) Offensive odors: Odor-proof appliances, commercial deodorants placed in the appliance, and attention to diet usually control the problem. Bismuth subgallate (two 200 mg capsules orally before each meal) may be useful.

(9) Diarrhea: Excessive output should be reported to the physician promptly and supplemental water, salt, and potassium should be given.

(10) Urinary tract calculi: Uric acid stones occur in about 5–10% of patients after ileostomy and are probably the result of chronic dehydration due to inadequate fluid intake.

(11) Prestomal ileitis: Patients who develop inflammation of the ileum just proximal to the ileostomy usually have recurrence of their original inflammatory bowel disease. A few patients are reported to have nonspecific inflammation which may be due to mechanical or functional obstruction of the stoma.

In a long-term follow-up of ileostomy patients, 96% returned to their previous occupation, 89% considered their health good or excellent, and 84% did not consider management of the ileostomy a major problem.

2. COLOSTOMY

Colostomies are made for the following purposes: (1) for decompression of an obstructed colon; (2) for diversion of the fecal stream in preparation for resection of an inflammatory or obstructive lesion or following traumatic injury; (3) to serve as the point of evacuation of stool when the distal colon or rectum is removed; and (4) to protect a distal anastomosis following resection. The colostomy may be temporary, in which event it is subsequently closed, or it may be permanent. Colostomies can be constructed by making an opening in a loop of colon (**loop colostomy**) or by dividing the colon and bringing out one end (**end** or **terminal colostomy**). A colostomy is double-barreled if a loop or both ends of the colon are exteriorized, and it is single-barreled if only one end is brought out.

The most common permanent colostomy is a **sigmoid colostomy** made at the time of abdominoperineal resection for cancer of the rectum (Fig 34—19). Such a colostomy is compatible with a normal life except for the route of fecal evacuation. A sigmoid colostomy expels stool approximately once a day, but the frequency varies among individuals just as bowel habits vary in the general population. An appliance is not required, although many patients find that wearing a light pouch is reassuring. Some patients achieve a regular pattern of evacuation on their own; others require irrigation daily or every other day. Irrigation is performed by inserting a catheter into the stoma and instilling water, 500 ml at a time, by gravity flow from a reservoir held at shoulder height. A plastic olive-shaped (Laird) tip on the catheter fits snugly into the stoma and greatly reduces the risk of perforation. Diet is individualized; generally, patients are able to eat the same foods they enjoyed preoperatively. Fresh fruits, fruit juices, and other foods may cause diarrhea. A properly functioning colostomy need not be dilated.

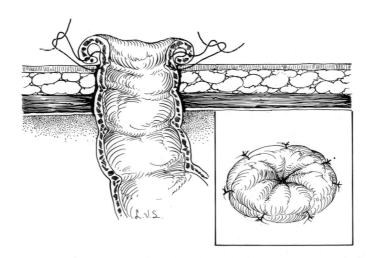

Figure 34—19. Single-barreled end colostomy. The margins of the stoma are fixed to the skin with sutures.

Transverse colostomy should not be constructed as a permanent stoma if it can be avoided. Unlike sigmoid colostomy, transverse colostomy is "wet"—ie, it discharges semiliquid waste frequently—and usually requires an appliance. These stomas are bulky, foul-smelling, and extremely difficult to manage. They are prone to leak under the appliance, and prolapse is common. Most patients who require a permanent stoma are better served by an ileostomy than by a transverse colostomy.

The overall complication rate of colostomies is 20%, and 15% of these require operative correction. Stenosis is largely avoided by maturing the colostomy at the operating table as with ileostomy. Prolapse, necrosis, retraction, and paracolostomy hernia are due to technical errors in constructing the stoma. Perforation is avoided by the Laird tip and by maintaining the irrigation reservoir at no greater than shoulder height. Less serious complications include diarrhea, fecal impaction, and skin irritation.

Beahrs OH & others: Ileostomy with ileal reservoir rather than ileostomy alone. Ann Surg 179:634, 1974.

Goligher JC, Lintott D: Experience with 26 reservoir ileostomies. Br J Surg 62:893, 1975.

Hill GL: *Ileostomy: Surgery, Physiology, & Management.* Grune & Stratton, 1976.

Hill GL, Mair WSJ, Goligher JC: Cause and management of high volume output salt-depleting ileostomy. Br J Surg 62:720, 1975.

Mazier WP & others: Effective colostomy irrigation. Surg Gynecol Obstet 142:905, 1976.

Morton JH, Kinsella EM: The colostomy. JAMA 232:185, 1975.

Roy PH & others: Experience with ileostomies: Evaluation of long-term rehabilitation in 497 patients. Am J Surg 119:77, 1970.

Thow GB & others: Present status of the continent ileostomy. Dis Colon Rectum 19:189, 1976.

PREOPERATIVE PREPARATION OF THE COLON

Complications of colonic surgery such as wound infection and anastomotic dehiscence are partially related to the high bacterial content of the large bowel. It is advisable to eliminate the fecal mass and reduce the numbers of bacteria as much as possible prior to operation. Measures taken to achieve this purpose are known as the "bowel prep."

The fecal mass is reduced by allowing the patient only clear liquids orally for 1–2 days before operation.

Elemental diets also leave a small fecal residue; because of their nutritional advantages, they are useful in patients whose colons are especially difficult to cleanse and require prolonged periods of preparation (eg, children with Hirschsprung's disease). Elemental diets have little or no effect on fecal flora.

Mechanical measures (cathartics and enemas) are employed universally except in patients with obstructing lesions or severe inflammatory bowel disease. Saline lavage or "whole gut irrigation" involves ingestion of large quantities of isotonic saline solution which overwhelms the absorptive capacity of the small bowel and causes diarrhea, thus clearing the colon of fecal matter. This method is new and must be used with caution in patients in tenuous fluid and electrolyte balance.

Direct attack on the bacteria of the large bowel may be undertaken with systemic antibiotics (see Chapter 11) or oral nonabsorbable antibiotics. The latter method has been controversial for many years, but recent controlled clinical trials confirm that wound infections (and perhaps anastomotic complications) are reduced by a short course of a combination of antibiotics plus mechanical cleansing. Although several regimens have been studied, one schedule of antibiotic administration is 1 g each of neomycin and erythromycin base by mouth at 1:00 p.m., 2:00 p.m., and 11:00 p.m. the day before operation. If the bowel cannot be prepared adequately before operation and if colonic resection is necessary, 10% povidone-iodine solution may be injected into the lumen of the part to be removed. This measure seems effective but needs further study.

Bornside GH, Cohn I Jr: Stability of normal human fecal flora during a chemically defined, low residue liquid diet. Ann Surg 181:58, 1975.

Farmer RG: Preoperative preparation of the patient with carcinoma of the colon. Surg Clin North Am 55:1335, 1975.

Goldring J & others: Prophylactic oral antimicrobial agents in elective colonic surgery: A controlled trial. Lancet 2:997, 1975.

Jones FE, DeCosse JJ, Condon RE: Evaluation of "instant" preparation of the colon with povidone-iodine. Ann Surg 184:74, 1976.

Levy AG & others: Saline lavage: A rapid, effective, and acceptable method for cleansing the gastrointestinal tract. Gastroenterology 70:157, 1976.

Nichols RL & others: Effect of preoperative neomycin-erythromycin intestinal preparation on the incidence of infectious complications following colon surgery. Ann Surg 178:453, 1973.

Washington JA II & others: Effect of preoperative antibiotic regimen on development of infection after intestinal surgery: Prospective, randomized, double-blind study. Ann Surg 180:567, 1974.

•   •   •

General References

Bacon HE, Recio PM: *Surgical Anatomy of the Colon, Rectum, and Anal Canal.* Lippincott, 1962.

Bockus HL: *Gastroenterology,* 3rd ed. Saunders, 1974.

Brooks FB (editor): *Gastrointestinal Pathophysiology.* Oxford Univ Press, 1974.

Goligher JC & others: *Surgery of the Anus, Rectum and Colon,* 3rd ed. Thomas, 1975.

Morson BC, Dawson IMP: *Gastrointestinal Pathology.* Blackwell, 1972.

Ottinger LW: *Fundamentals of Colon Surgery.* Little, Brown, 1974.

Sleisenger M, Fordtran J: *Gastrointestinal Disease.* Saunders, 1973.

Truelove SC, Reynell PC: *Diseases of the Digestive System,* 2nd ed. Davis, 1972.

Turell R: *Diseases of the Colon & Anorectum,* 2nd ed. Saunders, 1969.

35...
Anorectum

Walter Birnbaum, MD

SURGICAL ANATOMY & PHYSIOLOGY

The anal canal is derived from the proctodeum, an invagination of the ectoderm. The rectum is of entodermal origin. Because of the difference in their origins, the arterial and nerve supply and the venous and lymphatic drainage differ in the 2 structures, as do their linings also. Thus, the rectum is lined with glandular mucosa and the anal canal with anoderm, a continuation of the external stratified epithelium. It is incorrect to speak of anal "mucosa." The marginal zone between the rectum and the anal canal contains transitional cells. The anal canal and adjacent external skin are generously supplied with somatic sensory nerves and are highly susceptible to painful stimuli; the rectal mucosa has an autonomic nerve supply and is relatively insensitive to pain. Pain is not an early symptom in patients with rectal neoplasm.

Venous drainage above the anorectal juncture is through the portal system; drainage of the anal canal is through the caval system. This distribution is important in understanding the modes of spread of malignant disease and infection and the formation of hemorrhoids. The lymphatic return from the rectum is along the superior hemorrhoidal vascular pedicle to the inferior mesenteric and aortic nodes, but the lymphatics from the anal canal pass through Alcock's canal to the internal iliac nodes, to the posterior vaginal wall, and ventrally to the inguinal nodes.

The **anal canal** is about 3 cm long (Fig 35–1). It points toward the umbilicus and forms a distinct angle with the rectum in its resting state. During defecation, the angle straightens out. At the superior boundary of

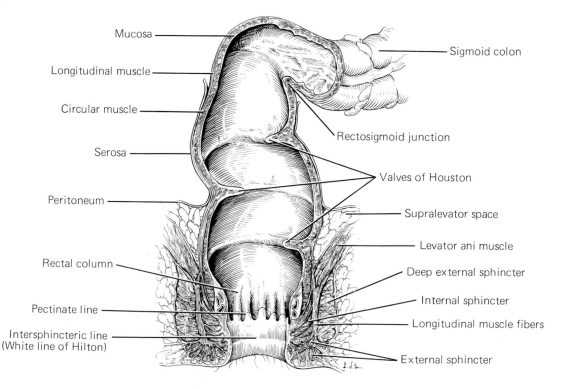

Figure 35–1. Anatomy of the anorectal canal.

the anal canal is the **anorectal juncture** (pectinate line, mucocutaneous juncture or dentate line). Here there are 8–12 **anal crypts** whose openings face cephalad. From each of the crypts a tubular duct extends distally; at the distal end of the duct is a small glandular structure. Anorectal fistulas originate in the crypts. Adjacent to the crypts are 5–8 tiny anal papillae. They become enlarged in inflammatory conditions. The rectal mucosa is red and glistening. The modified skin of the anal canal closely resembles the external skin but is thinner and contains no hair follicles. The white line of Hilton runs around the circumference of the anal canal and represents the intersphincteric line. It is easily palpable.

The **anorectal sphincteric ring** encircles the anal canal. Posteriorly and laterally it is composed of the fusion of the internal sphincter, longitudinal muscle, the central portion of the levators (puborectalis), and components of the external sphincter. Anteriorly it is more vulnerable to trauma because the puborectalis muscle passes directly ventrally and takes no part in the formation of the ring. Thus, the anorectal ring is more distinctly palpated anteriorly. Knowledge of the detailed anatomy of these structures is important in treating rectal abscesses and fistulas since complete surgical division may result in incontinence. The subcutaneous portion of the external sphincter acts as a corrugator of the perianal skin. The internal sphincter is composed of smooth involuntary muscles; the remaining muscles are striated voluntary ones.

Supporting Structures

The **puborectalis** forms a muscular sling around the rectum to give it support and to act synergistically in defecation. The rectum is supported by the **fascia of Waldeyer,** a heavy, avascular layer of the parietal pelvic fascia, the **lateral ligaments,** through which pass the middle hemorrhoidal vessels, and the posterior **mesorectum.** The ligaments and mesorectum fix the rectum to the anterior surface of the sacrum (see Rectal Prolapse).

Arteries

The **superior hemorrhoidal artery** is a direct continuation of the inferior mesenteric artery. It divides into 2 main branches, left and right. The right branch again bifurcates. These 3 terminal divisions probably account for the characteristic location of internal hemorrhoids, ie, 2 in each of the right quadrants and one in the left lateral quadrant.

The **middle hemorrhoidal artery** arises on each side from the anterior division of the internal iliac artery or from the internal pudic artery and runs inward in the lateral ligaments of the rectum. The **inferior hemorrhoidal arteries** are branches of the internal pudic arteries and pass through Alcock's canal. The anastomoses between the superior and inferior vascular arcades provide collateral circulation which is of importance after surgical interruption or atherosclerotic occlusion of the vascular supply of the left colon.

Veins

The **superior hemorrhoidal veins** originate in the internal hemorrhoidal venous plexus and pass cephalad to the inferior mesenteric veins and thence to the portal venous system. They have no valves. Rectal cancer may be disseminated by venous embolism to the liver, and septic emboli may cause pylephlebitis. The inferior hemorrhoidal veins drain into the internal pudic veins and so to the internal iliac and caval system. Varices of the hemorrhoidal veins produce hemorrhoids.

Lymphatics

The **lymphatics** of the anal canal form a fine plexus draining into larger collecting vessels leading to the inguinal lymph nodes, whose efferents lead to the external iliac or common iliac lymph nodes. Infections and cancer in the region of the anus may result in inguinal lymphadenopathy. The lymphatics of the rectum above the level of the anorectal line accompany the veins to the superior hemorrhoidal vascular pedicle and thence to the inferior mesenteric and aortic lymph nodes. Posterior to the rectum lie the nodes of Gerota. Radical operations for eradication of cancer of the rectum and anus are based upon lymphatic anatomy.

Nerves

The nerve supply of the rectum is derived from the sympathetic and parasympathetic systems. The sympathetic fibers are derived from the inferior mesenteric plexus and the hypogastric (presacral) nerve, which arises by 3 roots from the second, third, and fourth lumbar sympathetic ganglia. The parasympathetic supply (nervi erigentes) is derived from the second, third, and fourth sacral nerves. Injury to these nerves during operation may cause bladder dysfunction and sexual impotence.

Devroede G, Lamarche J: Functional importance of extrinsic parasympathetic innervation of the distal colon and rectum in man. Gastroenterology 66:273, 1974.

Hagihara PF, Griffen WO Jr: Physiology of the colon and rectum. Surg Clin North Am 52:797, 1972.

Lawson JON: Pelvic anatomy. 2. Anal canal and associated sphincters. Ann R Coll Surg Engl 54:288, 1974.

McColl I: The comparative anatomy and pathology of the anal glands. Ann R Coll Surg Engl 40:36, 1967.

Oh C, Kark AE: Anatomy of the external anal sphincter. Br J Surg 59:717, 1972.

Oh C, Kark AE: Anatomy of the perineal body. Dis Colon Rectum 16:444, 1973.

Waylonis GW, Powers JJ: Clinical application of anal sphincter electromyography. Surg Clin North Am 52:807, 1972.

DISEASES OF THE RECTUM & ANUS

PRURITUS ANI

The perianal skin has a "maximum readiness to itch." Pruritus ani is due to a wide variety of causes and is not in itself a clinical entity.

Etiology

Note: Contrary to popular belief, hemorrhoids are not a cause of pruritus ani.

A. Dermatologic: Psoriasis, seborrheic dermatitis, atopic eczema, lichen planus, etc.

B. Contact Dermatitis: Due to the use of local anesthetics (all "-caine" preparations must be suspected), topical antihistamines, various ointments, suppositories, douches, aromatic and other chemical substances used in soap.

C. Fungal: Dermatophytosis, candidiasis, etc.

D. Bacterial: Secondary infection due to scratching.

E. Parasitic: Pinworms (*Enterobius vermicularis*) and, less commonly, scabies or pediculosis.

F. After Oral Antibiotic Therapy: Especially tetracyclines.

G. Systemic Diseases: Diabetes (usually candidiasis), liver disease, etc.

H. Proctologic Disorders: Skin tags, cryptitis, draining fistulas or sinuses, etc.

I. Neoplasms: Intradermal carcinoma (Bowen's disease), extramammary Paget's disease, etc.

J. Hygiene: Poor hygiene with residual irritating feces or overmeticulous hygiene with excessive use of soap and rubbing.

K. Warmth and Hyperhidrosis: Due to a tight girdle, jockey shorts, warm bedclothing, obesity, climate.

L. Occupational: Exposure to constant high temperatures.

M. Allergy: Although pruritus may occur following the ingestion of certain foods, it is doubtful that a true allergy is a causative agent.

N. Psychogenic: The importance of the anxiety-itch-anxiety cycle varies from trivial to overwhelming. The significance of this area as an erotic zone in its relation to pruritus ani is not firmly established.

O. Idiopathic.

Clinical Findings

A. Symptoms and Signs: Itching of the anogenital area may be related to sleeping, defecation, warmth, emotional stress, activity, or ingestion of certain foods. It may vary from intermittent and mild to constant and severe. The clinical manifestations are consistent with the underlying cause. Skin changes may be minimal. Characteristic changes may be masked by excoriation caused by scratching and secondary infection.

There may be erythema, fissuring, maceration, lichenification, thickening and fibrosis of the skin, changes suggestive of fungal infection, the presence of pinworms (seen with the endoscope), and lesions elsewhere on the body.

The etiologic diagnosis is based upon a careful history and physical examination and appropriate laboratory tests. Characteristic lesions must be searched for elsewhere on the body. The use of oral or topical medication and the patient's hygienic habits should be determined.

B. Laboratory Findings: Urinalysis may reveal diabetes mellitus. Direct microscopic examination or culture of tissue scrapings may reveal yeasts, other fungi, or parasites. The Scotch Tape test may be used to disclose pinworm ova. In the case of persistent pruritus which does not respond to treatment, a biopsy must be taken to detect unusual but important malignant or premalignant lesions.

Complications

Complications include local secondary infection, dermatitis medicamentosa, and those associated with loss of sleep and persistent severe discomfort.

Prevention

The use of any kind of soap directly applied to the perianal area during bath or shower is interdicted. Self-medication with anesthetic or antihistamine ointments must be avoided. Scratching leads to secondary infection and should be inhibited, as should vigorous rubbing with harsh toilet tissue. Clothing should be loose. For men, the boxer type of underpants is preferred. Women should avoid elastic girdles or body stockings which press the buttocks together. Bedclothing should be light. Systemic causes should be treated. Spices (especially peppers) and citrus fruits (especially grapefruit) should be avoided.

Treatment

Soft, moistened paper tissue or cotton or soft cloth impregnated with glycerin and witch hazel should be used to clean thoroughly after bowel movements. Instruct the patient regarding the harmful effects of scratching, rubbing, and the use of soap. Hydrocortisone acetate, 1% in Emulsion Base applied sparingly 4 times daily, is usually most effective. Iodochlorhydroxyquin (Vioform), 3%, may be added as a fungicide. Moisture may be combated by liberal and frequent dusting with nonmedicated talcum powder. Acute inflammation may be alleviated by the use of 1:20 aluminum acetate solution. A protective ointment of aluminum hydroxide (Protegel) as a protective coating is helpful when there is anal seepage. Surgical correction of anal infection should be performed only when indicated. Specific dermatologic conditions are often best managed by dermatologists. Parasitic infestations must be treated specifically.

X-ray treatment, surgical operations, or injections designed to create permanent local anesthesia are rarely if ever indicated.

Prognosis

The prognosis depends upon the underlying cause. In most cases dramatic relief can be achieved, but some cases are persistent and recurrent.

Anogenital itching. Med Lett Drugs Ther 8:30, 1966.
Gallagher DM: Pruritus ani. Mod Treat 8:963, 1971.
Granet E: Pruritus ani. GP 36:89, 1967.
Lochridge E Jr: Pruritus ani-perianal psoriasis. South Med J 62:450, 1969.
Marks MM: The influence of the intestinal pH on anal pruritus. South Med J 61:1005, 1968.

FECAL IMPACTION

Hardened or putty-like stool in the rectum or colon becomes progressively more dehydrated as it fails to pass. If not removed, it can cause partial or complete intestinal obstruction. It may result from painful anorectal disease, the abuse of bulk laxatives, residual barium from x-ray study, low-residue diet, starvation, drug-induced stasis (especially codeine and anticholinergic drugs), prolonged bed rest, and muscular hypotonicity (especially in senility), and may occur postoperatively in patients in whom the colon and rectum were not evacuated before operation.

Clinical Findings

The manifestations of fecal impaction are a history of small or absent bowel movements for several days, constant bearing down sensations, bowel urgency, and lower abdominal cramps. There may be signs of bowel obstruction. The impacted feces can be palpated.

Paradoxic diarrhea consists of the passage of small amounts of watery stool forced around the impaction by spasm.

Differential Diagnosis

Unless the molded mass is identified by the examining finger, a misdiagnosis of rectal abscess or tumor may be made. After the impaction has been relieved, endoscopic examination of the rectum should always be made to ensure that an inflammatory or neoplastic process has not been missed.

Complications

Neglected impaction may rarely result in complete bowel obstruction, erosion of the impaction through the bowel wall, peritonitis, ulceration, and even death.

Prevention

In patients in whom an impaction is likely to occur, careful attention should be given to the regularity of their bowel habits. Mild laxatives or enemas are ordered when indicated. This is particularly true in postobstetric, postoperative, and cardiac patients; patients confined to bed for long periods; and elderly and mental patients.

Treatment

The impaction must be broken up as thoroughly as possible by placing the finger in the rectum anteriorly and breaking up the mass by pressing it against the sacrum. This is followed by an oil retention enema or by 5 ml of 1% dioctyl sodium sulfosuccinate (Doxinate) in 30 ml of mineral oil. The oil should be allowed to remain in the rectum for 8 hours, preferably overnight. The next morning this should be followed by a sodium phosphate or plain water enema, repeated if necessary. (Hydrogen peroxide enemas should never be used.) At the same time, a magnesium or sodium phosphate cathartic should be given by mouth.

If these methods fail, the impaction should be removed under anesthesia in the hospital.

Abella ME, Fernandez AT: Large fecalomas. Dis Colon Rectum 10:401, 1967.
Braasch JW: Fecal impaction of the colon. Lahey Clin Found Bull 13:60, 1963.
Heffernon EW: Medical management of chronic constipation. Mod Treat 8:870, 1971.
Lal S: Some unusual complications of fecal impaction. Am J Proctol 18:226, 1967.

COCCYGODYNIA

Fracture or deformity of the coccyx is caused by falling to a sitting position or by striking the coccyx against a hard object. This may result in persistent pain and tenderness. However, pain referred to the tailbone or coccygeal area is most frequently related to chronic anal infection, parturition, poor sitting posture, osteoarthritis, or anxiety states. The discomfort is greatest after sitting for long periods on a soft seat such as after a long automobile ride or watching television. Proctalgia fugax consists of a sudden severe lancinating or cramplike pain of brief duration in the rectal or coccygeal region. It may occur at any time and often awakens the patient at night. Examination discloses tenderness and spasm of the coccygeus and levator muscles.

Persistent coccygodynia is often the basis of workers' compensation or legal claims based on personal injury.

Clinical Findings

When actual fracture or displacement of the coccyx has occurred, the coccyx will be tender when it is palpated externally. With the examining index finger in the rectum and the coccyx grasped between it and the external thumb, displacement, deformity, and pain on motion (particularly acute anterior angulation) can be demonstrated. Radiographic studies should also be diagnostic.

In cases not due to trauma, there is no localized tenderness of the coccyx and movement of it is not painful. However, as the intrarectal examining finger is swept laterally from the coccyx and lower sacrum, the coccygeus, levator, and piriformis muscles can be felt to be spastic and tender, usually more so on the left than on the right. Intrarectal digital pressure upon the involved muscle will reproduce the symptoms.

Differential Diagnosis

Anal fissure causes pain during bowel movement, but coccygodynia is not related to defecation. With fissure, tenderness and spasm on examination are localized to the anal canal rather than to the retrorectal musculature. Rectal abscess is identified by the signs of an inflammatory mass and more acute symptoms.

Treatment

When there is no demonstrable bony injury, the sitting posture should be corrected so that the patient sits erect and on a firm, flat surface. A firm seat should be used when driving an automobile. Soft cushions should be avoided.

Intrarectal digital stretching or massage of the involved muscles is often dramatically helpful. When there has been actual injury to the coccyx, warm baths, diathermy, sedation, local anesthetic injections, and special cut-out seat pads may be helpful.

Coccygectomy for intra-articular fracture or deformity is only rarely indicated and may be followed by persistence of symptoms due to chronic spasm of the involved muscles.

Prognosis

Coccygodynia is characteristically a condition of long standing and may persist for periods up to many months, or, rarely, years when appropriate therapy is not undertaken.

Grant SR, Salvati EP, Rubin RJ: Levator syndrome. Dis Colon Rectum 18:161, 1975.
Paradis H, Marganoff H: Rectal pain of extrarectal origin. Dis Colon Rectum 12:306, 1969.
Peilling LF, Swenson WM, Hill JR: The psychologic aspects of proctalgia fugax. Dis Colon Rectum 8:372, 1965.
Thiele GH: Coccygodynia: Cause and treatment. Dis Colon Rectum 6:422, 1963.

ANAL FISSURE
(Fissure-in-Ano, Anal Ulcer)

Essentials of Diagnosis

- Rectal pain related to defecation.
- Bleeding.
- Constipation.
- Spasm of sphincters.
- Anal tenderness.
- Ulceration of anal canal.
- Stenosis.
- Hypertrophic anal papilla.
- Sentinel pile.

General Considerations

Acute fissures of the anal canal are longitudinal tears. Most lesions called anal fissures are actually chronic elliptic or round ulcers which, when examined upon partial eversion of the anus, appear to be longitudinal cracks. They may be extremely painful.

Anal ulcers are usually single and occur in the posterior midline or, less commonly, in the anterior midline. They may occur first in the lower portion of the anal canal or may involve its entire length. Ulcers tend to occur in the posterior midline position because of the acute angulation between the anal canal and the rectum and the lack of support of the subcutaneous portion of the external sphincter.

Infection of the adjacent crypt results in chronic inflammation and then fibrosis of these structures. Edema of the anal papilla adjacent to the crypt occurs with enlargement and fibrosis of the papilla so that it becomes a firm, whitish, finger-like or rounded, polypoid, smooth structure. It is then called a hypertrophic papilla. Hypertrophic papillae are not neoplastic but are often confused with adenomatous polyps. External to the anal ulcer, the adjacent skin likewise is involved in chronic inflammatory changes and interference with its lymphatic drainage. A fibrotic nubbin of skin forms at the anal verge. This is termed a sentinel pile because it stands as a sentinel just below the ulcer. Thus, the fissure triad has been formed: (1) the ulcer itself, (2) the hypertrophic papilla, and (3) the sentinel pile (Fig 35–2).

Although infants normally may pass stools of surprisingly large caliber without pain, they may develop acute linear fissures with diarrhea or as a result of passing hard feces. Fissures may occur as a result of excessive straining at stool, habitual use of cathartics (especially mineral oil), chronic diarrhea, avulsion of an anal valve, childbirth trauma, laceration by a sharp foreign body, or iatrogenic trauma such as the passage of a large speculum or prostatic massage. Usually no cause can be definitely identified.

Fissures of the perianal skin may be associated with pruritus ani and are the result of chronic dermatitis.

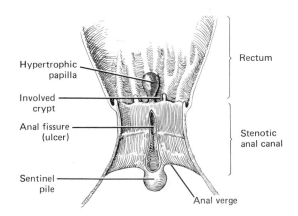

Figure 35–2. Diagram of the anorectum showing the fissure or ulcer triad.

Clinical Findings

A. Symptoms and Signs: Pain may be severe and is described as tearing, burning, or cutting. It occurs during passage of stool, then usually subsides somewhat and becomes more severe when secondary sphincteric spasm occurs. Fissures are characterized by their chronicity, with periods of exacerbation and remission, often over a number of years. Bleeding is bright red, not mixed with the stool, usually noted on the toilet tissue, and small in amount. Constipation develops as a result of fear of defecation, which is so frequently postponed that regular bowel habits become disrupted. During periods of healing, pruritus may occur.

The sentinel pile can be observed externally. Gentle eversion of the anus may reveal the inferior portion of the ulcer. Application of a topical anesthetic should precede a very gentle digital examination to ascertain the site of the ulcer, the degree of induration and stenosis, etc. There is often marked spasm of the sphincters.

B. Special Examinations: A small caliber anoscope can be introduced with pressure on the side of the anal canal opposite the lesion. The hypertrophic papilla, ulcer, and associated lesions can then be seen. Sigmoidoscopic examination should be deferred (but not omitted) until it can be done painlessly.

Differential Diagnosis

Other anal ulcerations which must be differentiated from fissure include the primary lesion of syphilis, malignant epithelioma, tuberculous ulceration, and ulceration associated with blood dyscrasias and granulomatous enteritis higher in the intestinal tract. Each of these lesions has its own characteristics, but any lesion not in the midline nor displaying the typical findings outlined above should be investigated by means of further diagnostic tests. Anal fissure often occurs concomitantly with internal hemorrhoids and may be overlooked. Internal hemorrhoids are not painful; when pain occurs, fissure must be suspected. The persistence of pain following hemorrhoidectomy is frequently due to a missed fissure.

Treatment

A. Medical Treatment: Warm sitz baths for 10 or 15 minutes after each bowel movement or as often as necessary for discomfort will give temporary relief. The water should be comfortably warm, not hot, and just deep enough to sit in. Deep, hot, frequent sitz baths may be enervating. Topical application of anesthetic ointments injected sparingly with a "pile pipe" on the end of an ointment tube is helpful. Suppositories are of no value unless they are inserted into the anal canal and held by the fingers until they have melted. Otherwise, the suppository slips into the rectal ampulla or higher and is ineffective in coating the ulcer in the anal canal.

Topical application of 50% phenol in oil is anesthetic, produces a coating of protein coagulum, and may interrupt the pain-spasm-pain cycle until healing occurs. Mild silver nitrate solution is also used.

Diarrhea or constipation must be corrected. Mineral oil is to be avoided. Stool softeners are of value only when the feces are desiccated and hard. Proper diet and regular bowel habits usually suffice to correct constipation.

B. Surgical Treatment: When conservative measures fail, surgical correction is in order. Operation consists of (1) block excision of the crypt, the hypertrophic papilla, the ulcer and its margins, the sentinel pile, and an adjacent segment of skin for drainage; (2) superficial division of the underlying fibrotic sphincter; and (3) covering of the orad portion of the wound with normal mucosa. Postoperatively, the surgical wound must be followed closely to ensure healing from within outward. Alternative methods favored by many surgeons are (1) subcutaneous division of the stenotic internal sphincter in a lateral quadrant of the anal canal, with removal of a hypertrophic papilla and sentinel pile but without removal of the fissure itself; and (2) divulsion of the canal under anesthesia so as to disrupt the sphincteric fibers.

Prognosis

Anal ulcers tend to become chronic with alternate periods of healing and exacerbation. They do not become malignant. Surgical treatment is highly successful.

Georgoulis B: Pain caused by anal fissure. Proc R Soc Med 62:260, 1969.

Lochridge E Jr: Fissure-in-ano—to operate or not. South Med J 64:240, 1971.

Millar DM: Subcutaneous lateral internal anal sphincterotomy for anal fissure. Br J Surg 58.737, 1971.

Nothman BJ, Schuster MM: Internal anal sphincter derangement with anal fissures. Gastroenterology 67:216, 1974.

Ray JE & others: Lateral subcutaneous internal anal sphincterotomy for anal fissure. Dis Colon Rectum 17:139, 1974.

ANORECTAL ABSCESS

Essentials of Diagnosis

- Persistent throbbing rectal pain.
- External evidence of abscess such as palpable induration and tenderness may or may not be present.
- Systemic evidence of infection.

General Considerations

Anorectal abscess results from the invasion of the pararectal spaces by pathogenic microorganisms. A mixed infection usually occurs, with *Escherichia coli, Proteus vulgaris,* streptococci, staphylococci, and bacteroides predominating. Anaerobes are often present.

The incidence is much higher in men. The most common cause is infection extending from an anal crypt into one of the pararectal spaces. Less commonly, abscesses superficial to the corrugator muscle may result from infection of hair follicles,

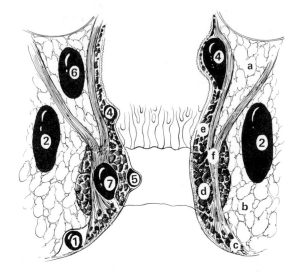

Figure 35—3. Composite diagram of acute anorectal abscesses and spaces. (a) Pelvirectal or supralevator space. (b) Ischiorectal space. (c) Perianal or subcutaneous space. (d) Marginal or mucocutaneous space. (e) Submucous space. (f) Intermuscular space. Numbers designate abscesses as enumerated in text below. (Retrorectal abscess is not shown.)

sebaceous and sweat glands of the skin, abrasions due to scratching, infection of a perianal hematoma, as a complication of deep anal fissure, infection of a prolapsed internal hemorrhoid, or following sclerosing injection of hemorrhoids. Deeper abscesses usually arise in the crypts but may also result from trauma, foreign bodies, etc. (See Anorectal Fistulas, below.)

Abscesses are classified according to the anatomic spaces they occupy (Fig 35—3): (1) Perianal abscess lies immediately beneath the skin of the anus and the lowermost part of the anal canal. (2) Ischiorectal abscess occupies the ischiorectal fossa and is actually uncommon, although the term is often improperly used to describe most anorectal abscesses. (3) Retrorectal (deep postanal) abscess is situated in the retrorectal space. (4) Submucous abscess is situated in the submucosa immediately above the anal canal. (5) Marginal abscess is situated in the anal canal beneath the anoderm. (6) Pelvirectal (supralevator) abscess lies above the levator ani muscle and below the peritoneum. (7) Intermuscular abscess lies between the layers of the sphincter muscles. A lateral abscess may extend through the triangle just posterior to the anal canal and pass around to the opposite side to form a horseshoe abscess. Abscesses may extend from the supralevator space down through the levator into the ischiorectal fossa to form an hourglass abscess.

Rectal abscesses frequently contain a large quantity of foul-smelling pus.

Two-thirds of abscesses will result in fistulas.

Clinical Findings

Superficial abscesses are the most painful, with pain related to sitting and walking but not necessarily to bowel movement. Inspection discloses the characteristic evidence of external swelling with redness, induration, and tenderness. Deeper abscesses will cause toxic symptoms, but localized pain may not be severe. External inspection shows no swelling. Digital rectal examination reveals the tender swelling and, on bidigital examination with the index finger in the rectum and the thumb external, the abscess may be readily felt. High pelvirectal abscesses may cause minimal or no rectal symptoms and may be associated with lower abdominal pain and fever of undetermined origin.

Complications

Unless the abscess is evacuated promptly by surgery or ruptures spontaneously, it will extend into other adjacent anatomic spaces. Rarely, an anaerobic infection will spread extensively without respect for anatomic planes of cleavage.

Treatment

The treatment of pararectal abscesses is prompt incision and adequate drainage. Suppuration will almost always have occurred when the diagnosis is first made. One should not await pointing of the abscess externally. Antibiotics are of limited value, may only serve to mask the infection temporarily, and may result in the outgrowth of resistant organisms. Warm sitz baths and analgesics are palliative.

Prior to operation, the patient should be advised that after the abscess is drained he may have a persistent fistula. The operation for drainage may be a one-stage or 2-stage procedure. If, under anesthesia, the primary origin of the abscess can be found and if the tract connecting it to the abscess can be incised without division of a significant portion of the sphincteric ring, the abscess can be adequately drained externally and fistulotomy performed at the same time. A second operation for fistula will then be avoided. If the fistulous tract is deep, only the abscess should be drained and fistulectomy performed after the cavity completely heals and support is provided for the sphincteric ring. The wound should not be packed since this may result in a broad scar which may interfere with sphincteric closure of the anal canal, resulting in leakage or partial incontinence.

The wound should be inspected at frequent intervals to make certain that it heals from the bottom up so that bridging of the wound will not occur.

Prognosis

Abscesses that rupture spontaneously or are drained surgically without removal of the offending fistulous connection will frequently recur until the underlying cause is removed.

Adams JD, Haisten AS: Perianal hidradenitis suppurativa. Surg Clin North Am 52:467, 1972.

Brightmore T: Perianal gas-producing infections of non-clostridial origin. Br J Surg 59:109, 1972.

Ferguson JA & others: Symposium: Anorectal problems. Dis Colon Rectum 18:641, 1975.

Goligher JC, Ellis M, Pissidis AG: A critique of anal glandular infection in the etiology and treatment of idiopathic anorectal abscesses and fistulas. Br J Surg 54:977, 1967.

Scoma JA, Salvati EP, Rubin RJ: Incidence of fistula subsequent to anal abscesses. Dis Colon Rectum 17:357, 1974.

Waggener HV: Immediate fistulotomy in the treatment of perianal abscess. Surg Clin North Am 49:1227, 1969.

ANORECTAL FISTULAS

Essentials of Diagnosis

- Chronic purulent discharge from a para-anal opening.
- Tract which may be palpated or probed leading to rectum.

General Considerations

By definition, a fistula must have at least 2 openings connected by a hollow tract—as opposed to a sinus, which is a tract with but one opening. Most anorectal fistulas originate in the anal crypts at the anorectal juncture. The crypt becomes injured or infected (cryptitis), the infection extends along one of several well-defined planes, and an abscess occurs. When the abscess is opened or ruptures, a fistula is formed. The fistula may be subcutaneous, submucosal, intramuscular, or submuscular. It may be anterior or posterior, single, complex, or horseshoe.

Fistulas are usually due to pyogenic infection or, less commonly, due to granulomatous disease of the intestine or tuberculosis. Those that do not originate in the crypts may result from diverticulitis, neoplasm, or trauma. Cryptogenic fistulas which have their secondary (external) opening posterior to an imaginary line passing transversely through the center of the anal orifice usually have their primary (internal) opening in a crypt in the posterior midline. When the secondary (external) opening is anterior to the transverse line, the primary (internal) opening is usually in a crypt immediately opposite the secondary opening (Salmon-Goodsall rule; Fig 35–4).

Clinical Findings

A. Symptoms and Signs: The chief complaint is intermittent or constant drainage or discharge. There is usually a history of a recurrent abscess which ruptured spontaneously or was incised surgically. On inspection, one or more secondary openings can be seen. There may be a pink or red elevation exuding purulent material, or it may have healed over. In granulomatous disease or tuberculosis, the margins may be violaceous and the discharge watery. On palpation, the cord-like tract can be felt and its course, both in relation to the sphincters and to its primary orifice, can often be determined. A probe can be inserted into the tract to determine its depth and direction. However, this maneuver should be terminated if it is painful; under these circumstances it is best completed under anes-

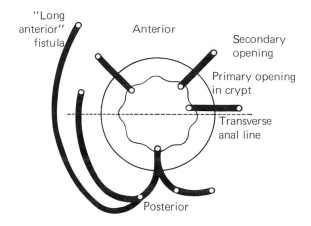

Figure 35—4. Salmon-Goodsall rule. The usual relation of the primary and secondary openings of fistulas. When there is an anterior and also a posterior opening of the same fistula, the rule for the posterior opening applies; the "long anterior" fistula is an exception to the rule.

thesia at the time of operation. Bidigital examination is helpful.

Anorectal fistulas in infants are congenital, may cause abscesses, are more common in boys, and are anterior, straight, and superficial. The treatment is the same as in adult fistulas. Rectovaginal fistulas may be congenital, may follow radiotherapy, pelvic surgery or vaginal repair, obstetric delivery, or may occur in association with malignancy. The most common complaint is the passage of flatus or feces per vagina. The lesion can usually be seen by vaginal inspection, but the aperture may be so small or so well concealed in folds of mucosa that it is not easily discovered. In these instances, a vaginal pack saturated with methylene blue solution may allow the dye to be detected in the rectum.

B. Special Examinations: Anoscopic inspection of the crypts may reveal the primary opening, which at times will discharge pus. Gentle probing of the primary opening with a short crypt hook may be confirmatory. Associated lesions must also be noted. Sigmoidoscopic examination must be done. Roentgen fistulography in fistulas which are suspected of being noncryptogenic or extensive is a valuable diagnostic adjunct. A thin, radiopaque liquid such as diatrizoate (Hypaque) is injected through the external opening, and stereoscopic or multiplane x-ray films are taken. A radiopaque marker may be inserted into the anal canal to localize the inner limit of the sphincters and the position of the anal orifice. A barium enema x-ray study is indicated if the fistula is thought to arise in the sigmoid colon, and an upper gastrointestinal study is done if regional enteritis is suspected.

Differential Diagnosis

Hidradenitis suppurativa is a disease of the apocrine sweat glands characterized by the formation of multiple, deep perianal sinuses. Other sites of predilection are the axillas and the inguinal and pubic areas. There may be scrotal or labial involvement.

Pilonidal sinus with a tract leading into the perianal area may resemble a fistula. The direction of the tract on palpation or probing, the presence of another opening in the sacrococcygeal area, and the possible presence of tufts of hair in the sinus may establish the diagnosis, although the differentiation may be difficult.

Granulomatous disease (regional enteritis) of the small or large bowel is associated with anorectal fistulas in a high percentage of cases. The fistula is often the first manifestation of proximal disease and may precede it by months or even years. Such fistulas are indolent in appearance and have pale granulations and characteristic microscopic findings.

Tuberculous fistulas are now rare. They too have an indolent appearance and are usually associated with pulmonary, glandular, or osseous tuberculosis elsewhere in the body.

Infected comedones, infected sebaceous cysts, chronic folliculitis, and **bartholinitis** are other dermal sources of draining sinuses. The history, the location of the sinus in relation to the anus or vulva, and the absence of an anorectal source are helpful in the diagnosis. Examination under anesthesia may be necessary.

Rectorectal dermoid cysts, more common in females, form chronic perianal sinuses.

Coloperineal fistulas may occur in diverticulitis of the sigmoid colon. Whenever a probe can be passed deeply into a perianal fistula and sigmoidal diverticular disease coexists, the intracolonic origin of the fistula should be suspected and checked by fistulography.

Sinuses from trauma and foreign bodies may occur. The foreign body may gain entrance from the outside by penetration or from within the canal from the ingestion of a sharp piece of bone, etc. An unabsorbed suture remaining from perineorrhaphy or episiotomy or a piece of drainage tubing may act as a foreign body.

Urethroperineal fistulas are often traumatic in origin, resulting from urethral instrumentation or direct external trauma. Rectourethral fistulas may be congenital or may follow urethral instrumentation or prostatectomy. The chief complaint is pneumaturia or fecaluria. Small, recent fistulas may close spontaneously, or urinary diversion by cystostomy and repair may be required.

Less common causes of perianal sinuses and fistulas are **tubo-ovarian abscess, actinomycosis, osteomyelitis,** and **carcinoma.** In these instances the history, physical findings, x-ray examination, and laboratory studies will provide the differential diagnosis.

Complications

Without treatment, chronically infected fistulas may be the source of systemic infection. Although carcinoma develops rarely in a chronic, untreated anorectal fistula, many such cases have been reported, and effective removal of the fistula is a prophylactic measure against such an eventuality.

Treatment

Small acute fistulas may heal spontaneously, but in most cases the only effective treatment is by fistulotomy (commonly termed fistulectomy). The following principles must be observed: (1) The primary opening must be found. (2) The fistulous tract or tracts must be identified completely. (3) The tract must be unroofed throughout its entire length so that the fistulous tunnel is converted into an open "ditch" throughout its entire course. (4) The wound must be constructed so as to make certain that the cavity will heal from within outward. Fistulotomy should never be performed in the presence of chronic diarrhea, active ulcerative colitis, or active granulomatous enterocolitis since delayed wound healing may present a severe problem. When the clinical manifestations of the enteric disease appear to be under control, operation may be performed although prolonged wound healing is to be expected.

A 2-stage operation is indicated only when the fistula passes deep to the entire anorectal ring so that all the muscles must be divided in order to extirpate the tract. This need rarely be done. If the deeper portions of the sphincteric ring and the levator ani muscles are left intact, incontinence will not occur.

Frequent follow-up examination of the wound following fistulotomy is of great importance to make certain that bridging and re-formation of the fistula do not occur.

Prognosis

The recurrence rate following fistulotomy is high for the following reasons: (1) The primary opening of the fistula is not removed; (2) collateral tracts are missed; (3) the operation is inadequate for fear of creating incontinence; (4) there is a mistaken diagnosis; and (5) postoperative care is inadequate.

Dunphy JE, Pikula J: Fact and fancy about fistula-in-ano. Surg Clin North Am 35:1469, 1954.

Heaton JR, Cohen RS: Complicated para-anal fistulas of obscure origin. Dis Colon Rectum 8:437, 1965.

Jackman RJ: Anorectal fistulas: Current concepts. Dis Colon Rectum 11:247, 1968.

Lockhart-Mummery HE: Crohn's disease: Anal lesions. Dis Colon Rectum 18:200, 1975.

Mazier WP: The treatment and care of anal fistulas: A study of 1000 patients. Dis Colon Rectum 14:134, 1971.

Parks AG, Gordon PH, Hardcastle JD: A classification of fistula-in-ano. Br J Surg 63:1, 1976.

CONDYLOMATA ACUMINATA
(Anal Warts)

Condylomata acuminata (anal warts) are verrucous excrescences which grow in the perianal area or in the anal canal. They may be small and discrete but are usually multiple and coalesce to form large, cauliflower masses. Malignant change occurs rarely. They are thought to be caused by a virus similar to or identical with the virus of verruca vulgaris. In males, they are usually associated with homosexual rectal intercourse. Smaller lesions can be removed by application of 10% podophyllum resin in tincture of benzoin or trichloroacetic acid, or by electrofulgeration with local infiltration anesthesia. Large lesions must be excised. Recurrences are frequent.

Fitzgerald DM, Hamit HF: The variable significance of condylomata acuminata. Ann Surg 179:328, 1974.

Samenius B, Hansson HP: Venereal diseases of the anorectum. Mod Treat 8:875, 1971.

Swerdlow DB, Salvati EP: Condyloma acuminatum. Dis Colon Rectum 14:226, 1971.

HEMORRHOIDS*

Essentials of Diagnosis

- Rectal bleeding, protrusion, and vague discomfort.
- Mucoid discharge from rectum.
- Possible secondary anemia.
- Characteristic findings on external anal inspection or anoscopic examination.

General Considerations

Hemorrhoids are varicose dilatations of the veins of the superior or inferior hemorrhoidal venous plexuses, or both. Dilated, chronically infected veins of the superior hemorrhoidal plexus are called internal hemorrhoids and originate above the level of the anorectal juncture immediately above the anal canal. They are covered by redundant mucous membrane and lie in a bed of loose areolar tissue. Those of the inferior hemorrhoidal plexus are termed external hemorrhoids, are situated below the anorectal juncture, and are covered by anal epithelium or external skin. The 2 plexuses anastomose freely, forming internal and external hemorrhoids in continuity known as internoexternal hemorrhoids or mixed hemorrhoids. They contain the terminations of the superior hemorrhoidal arteries. They occur in 3 primary or "cardinal" positions—right anterior, right posterior, and left lateral posterior—depending upon how the artery divides and terminates. Smaller, secondary "satellite" hemorrhoids may develop between the primary hemorrhoids (Fig 35–5).

Since the superior hemorrhoidal venous plexus drains into the portal venous system, which contains no valves, the erect position of man greatly increases the pressure within the hemorrhoidal veins and thus predisposes to hemorrhoidal disease. Hemodynamic studies, clinical features, and the rarity of the disease in quadrupeds support this hypothesis. The importance of heredity as a predisposing cause of hemorrhoids is

*See also Thrombosed External Hemorrhoid (next section).

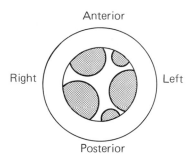

Figure 35—5. The usual arrangement of primary and secondary internal hemorrhoids. The anal canal as seen with the patient in the lithotomy position.

difficult to evaluate accurately because of the high incidence of the disease. However, when severe hemorrhoidal disease is found in young patients, there is frequently a strong family history, suggesting a hereditary background. Abnormalities of the microcirculation with demonstrable arteriovenous communication have also been implicated as causes of hemorrhoids.

Pregnancy is by far the most common cause of hemorrhoids in young women. The increased incidence of hemorrhoids during pregnancy is thought to be due to the steadily increasing pressure exerted on the iliac veins by the enlarged, gravid uterus, causing increased venous pressure within the middle and inferior hemorrhoidal veins, which are tributaries of the internal iliac (hypogastric) veins. These hemorrhoids are not to be confused with the thrombosed external hemorrhoids (see below) occurring in pregnancy. After pregnancy, the hemorrhoids tend to subside, although they may become progressively worse with subsequent pregnancies or with advancing age.

Although the hemorrhoidal vessels do constitute one of the avenues of collateral circulation from the portal venous system, true hemorrhoids rarely if ever are a result of portal hypertension or obstruction due to hepatic cirrhosis. Large, bleeding rectal varices do occur in hepatic cirrhosis, but these are not hemorrhoids.

The question of the pathogenesis of hemorrhoidal disease often arises in medicolegal, health insurance, workers' compensation, and military matters. Hemorrhoidal disease which is already present may be responsible for constipation or, indeed, may reflexly alter bowel habits, but hemorrhoids are not produced by constipation. Sedentary occupations, sitting on hard cold surfaces, straining at work or play, prolonged standing, catharsis, diarrhea, and climate or psychic factors are no longer believed to cause hemorrhoids. Such factors may, however, produce thrombosed external hemorrhoids (see below).

Clinical Findings

A. Symptoms and Signs: Patients will frequently complain of "hemorrhoids" regardless of what their rectal symptoms may be.

Bleeding is usually the first symptom. It is bright

red, unmixed with the stool, and may vary in quantity from streaks on the toilet tissue to amounts sufficient to be noticed in the bowl water. It may actually spurt or, when prolapse occurs, stain the underclothing. Protracted hemorrhoidal bleeding may result in marked secondary anemia. Prolapse occurs at first only with defecation and spontaneously reduces itself. At a later stage, the hemorrhoids must be reduced manually by the patient after defecation. Still later, they protrude with walking, prolonged standing, or other exertion, and, finally become permanently prolapsed. Mucoid discharge is most marked when the piles are permanently prolapsed and soiling of the clothing is noted. Irritation of the perianal skin may occur as a result of the constant leakage of mucus. However, persistent pruritus ani is not a symptom of hemorrhoidal disease. Pain occurs only when there is an acute attack of prolapse with inflammation, congestion, and edema or when there is a coexisting painful lesion.

On external inspection the subcutaneous external varices may be seen in their characteristic distribution. If the internal hemorrhoids are prolapsed, the redundant covering of red, moist mucosa will be observed. The 3 major masses with sulci in between can be noted. Whitish epithelium often extends up onto the mucosa of the internal hemorrhoid in an irregular fashion ("creeping epithelium") owing to chronic trauma of the mucosa.

Internal hemorrhoids are not palpable unless they are inflamed or thrombosed. However, digital examination must be done to detect tenderness or spasm from a concomitant painful lesion and to rule out the presence of a palpable tumor.

B. Special Examinations: Internal hemorrhoids, unless prolapsed, can be seen only with the anoscope. The anoscope is introduced for its full length, and the hemorrhoids will bulge into its lumen as it is slowly withdrawn. If the patient is then instructed to bear down, the hemorrhoids will follow the instrument to the outside if they are prolapsible. Other abnormalities at this level should likewise be noted. It is imperative that proctosigmoidoscopic examination also be carried out to detect the presence of inflammatory or malignant disease at a higher level which may have been responsible for symptoms attributed to the hemorrhoids.

Differential Diagnosis

Rectal bleeding, the most common symptom of internal hemorrhoids, also occurs with carcinoma of the colon and rectum, diverticular disease, adenomatous polyps, ulcerative colitis, and other less common diseases of the colon and rectum. Sigmoidoscopic examination must therefore constitute a part of the routine examination for hemorrhoids. Barium enema x-ray studies must be done in all patients over 40 years of age with rectal bleeding even when the source of the hemorrhage appears to be obviously of hemorrhoidal origin.

Mucosal rectal prolapse (common in children) presents as a circle of mucosa around the entire circumference marked by radial furrows and without varices.

In its later stages, procidentia of the rectum also forms a circle of protruding bowel, greater anteriorly, with the lumen pointing posteriorly, with concentric mucosal folds and without the characteristic cardinal positions of hemorrhoids with intervening sulci. The double, full thickness of the protruding wall can be felt upon bidigital palpation. When the procidentia is reduced, it can usually be prevented from redescending with straining by light pressure of the examining finger on the anterior wall of the rectum. Hemorrhoids and procidentia may coexist.

Perianal and intra-anal condylomas and anorectal tumors are so characteristic in their appearance that differentiation should not be difficult. Thrombosed external hemorrhoid (perianal hematoma) is described below. External skin tabs or tags which are the result of previous marginal thromboses, pregnancy, rectal surgery, or perianal dermatitis are not true hemorrhoids. The sentinel pile usually seen in the midline signifies an adjacent fissure (see above).

Complications

The hemorrhoids may become prolapsed and irreducible (incarcerated) as a result of inflammation, intravascular thrombosis, congestion, and edema. This condition is sometimes erroneously termed "strangulation" on the assumption that the irreducibility is due to the constriction of the hemorrhoids by the sphincteric ring. However, digital examination will show that there is actually some relaxation of the anal canal in this condition. Although the hemorrhoids may appear dark because of the underlying thrombosis, the mucosa is still viable. Ulceration and secondary infection may supervene.

Gangrene occurs following occlusion of the terminal nutrient artery supplying the hemorrhoid. The mucosa becomes black, finely wrinkled, loses its sheen, and appears dead. Sloughing occurs following hemorrhoidal ischemia.

Septic embolism via the portal system to form liver abscess has occurred but is rare. Severe secondary anemia may occur due to intermittent large hemorrhages or the persistent loss of small amounts of blood.

Treatment

Asymptomatic hemorrhoids require no treatment. Pruritus and pain are not symptoms of uncomplicated hemorrhoids. Straining at stool or diarrhea should be avoided to minimize bleeding and prolapse.

Prolapsed, irreducible, thrombosed, inflamed, or gangrenous hemorrhoids may be treated either conservatively or by immediate operation. Surgery offers the most rapid relief of symptoms and the shortest convalescence. Internal hemorrhoids requiring operative removal during pregnancy should be removed during the second trimester. Hemorrhoids appearing at delivery or immediately postpartum should not be treated surgically until sufficient time has elapsed to determine whether they will persist.

A. Medical Treatment: Suppositories and rectal ointment are of limited value in the treatment of uncomplicated internal hemorrhoids except for their transient anesthetic and astringent effects. If prolapsed hemorrhoids are reducible, they should be replaced within the rectum by gentle pressure. The patient is then instructed to lie down and reduce the protrusion whenever necessary. Following reduction, the associated external edema will soon subside. When the piles have been replaced, they may be kept in position by firm compresses and the patient should be confined to bed for a few days. In the acute stage, the patient should be put to bed and cold compresses of either water or witch hazel are applied. After the acute reaction has subsided, warm compresses or warm (not hot) sitz baths are in order. Sedation should be given as required.

In some instances, a spontaneous "cure" will be caused by fibrosis.

B. Injection Treatment: Injection treatment is a form of sclerotherapy in which an irritating chemical solution is injected submucosally into the areolar tissue surrounding the internal hemorrhoidal varices. The scarring which results from the inflammatory reaction effects, in varying degrees, obliteration of the hemorrhoidal varices. Recurrences are reported in about 50% of cases of early hemorrhoids and with increasing frequency in the more advanced stages of hemorrhoidal disease.

The advantages of the injection method are that it will control bleeding due to minor internal hemorrhoids which are not severe enough to require operation; it may be used as a therapeutic test to rule out another, higher source of bleeding in the presence of hemorrhoids; it is useful in the palliative treatment of hemorrhoids in persons who refuse surgery or are poor surgical risks; and it avoids surgery in patients who are cured by this means.

To be suitable for sclerotherapy, hemorrhoids must be early, uncomplicated, and internal.

Several types of sclerosing agents are used; 5% phenol in sesame oil is a satisfactory choice. Quinine urea hydrochloride, 5% aqueous solution, is also an effective agent. The injection is made with a 10 ml Luer-Lok syringe to which is attached a special long angulated hemorrhoidal needle. Through the anoscope, the needle is inserted into the upper pole of the hemorrhoid into the submucosal space. Aspiration is attempted to ensure that the needle is not within the lumen of a vessel. Enough of the solution (usually 1–5 ml) is then injected so that the hemorrhoid is distended but not blanched. One hemorrhoid at a time is usually injected, with subsequent injections of other hemorrhoids at intervals of 3 or 4 days.

Complications of injection treatment include sloughing, infection, acute prostatitis, and sensitivity to the injected material. If the procedure is properly done, however, such complications are rare.

C. Rubber Band Method: Using a special "gun," a rubber band may be placed so as to encircle the base of the hemorrhoid and strangulate it. This method has limited popularity.

D. Cryosurgery: Hemorrhoids may be destroyed by freezing. Liquid nitrogen or carbon dioxide is used to create an extremely low (−190 C) temperature in a probe which is applied to the hemorrhoid. The method has the advantages of usually not requiring either anesthesia or hospitalization; the disadvantages are that it is cumbersome, less accurate in application than surgical operation, and often produces copious, prolonged drainage and delayed healing.

E. Surgical Treatment: Surgical excision of all redundant mucosa and hemorrhoidal tissue produces an excellent long-term result. There are several methods of accomplishing this objective. For explanations of the technical procedure, the reader should consult texts on operative technic.

Prognosis

Recurrence is extremely rare after a properly executed hemorrhoidectomy.

Ferguson JA & others: The closed technique of hemorrhoidectomy. Surgery 70:480, 1971.

Lewis MI: Cryosurgical hemorrhoidectomy: A follow-up report. Dis Colon Rectum 15:128, 1972.

Rowe RJ: Symposium: Management of hemorrhoidal disease. Dis Colon Rectum 11:127, 1968.

Steinberg DM, Liegois H, Alexander-Williams J: Long term review of the results of rubber band ligation of hemorrhoids. Br J Surg 62:144, 1975.

Terrell R (moderator): Symposium: Diverse methods of managing hemorrhoids. Dis Colon Rectum 16:171, 1973.

THROMBOSED EXTERNAL HEMORRHOID

This common lesion is not a true hemorrhoid but rather a thrombosis of one of the subcutaneous external hemorrhoidal veins—either external to the anal verge or in the anal canal. It is characterized by a painful, tense, smooth, bluish, sessile elevation beneath the skin. Varying in size from a few millimeters to several centimeters in diameter, it may be multilobular, and there may be several such lesions. Although rupture may occur through the vein wall, it is usually not complete, so that a thin layer of adventitia covers the clot. Recurrence is frequent. The thrombosis follows a sudden increase in the intravenous pressure and usually occurs after episodes of heavy lifting, coughing, sneezing, athletics, straining at stool, or parturition. The disorder occurs most frequently in otherwise healthy young persons and is not related to internal hemorrhoidal disease.

Pain is greatest at the onset and gradually subsides in 2–3 days as the acute edema subsides. Spontaneous rupture frequently occurs, with disgorgement of the thrombus and considerable bleeding. Spontaneous resolution will occur without treatment.

Symptoms may be alleviated by warm sitz baths, applications of petrolatum to minimize friction on walking, and mild sedation. If examined within the first 48 hours, the course may be shortened and immediate relief obtained by either evacuation of the thrombus or by complete excision ("external hemorrhoidectomy") under local anesthesia. When evacuating the thrombus, an ellipse of skin should be removed to prevent agglutination of the skin edges and re-formation of an underlying clot. After the clot has begun to organize it cannot be evacuated, so that it is best, when the lesion is first seen 48 hours or more after onset, to employ conservative measures. No attempt should be made to reduce the thrombosed external hemorrhoid since it belongs in an external position.

It is important to differentiate this lesion from a prolapsed internal hemorrhoid. The pathology and methods of treatment are entirely different in the 2 conditions.

ANAL STENOSIS

Stenosis or narrowing of the anal canal may be a postoperative event (particularly following hemorrhoidectomy), a congenital variation, a senile change, or due to the habitual use of laxatives (particularly mineral oil). It may also result from chronic inflammatory disease such as fissure-in-ano. It is characteristically caused by an annular subepithelial fibrosis. The most common symptom is increased straining at defecation associated with a small caliber stool and a sense of incomplete evacuation. There may be pain and bleeding due to simple fissuring. Examination reveals an unyielding narrowing of the anal canal.

Anal stenosis must be differentiated from strictures of the rectum due to lymphogranuloma venereum, malignancy, ulcerative colitis, Crohn's disease, and congenital stricture.

Definitive treatment is invariably surgical; digital or instrumental dilatations are of no avail and may even worsen the condition because of trauma. The operation consists of division of the stenotic bundle followed by mobilization, advancement, interposition, and transverse suture of the proximal rectal mucosa. The results are good.

Greenstein AJ, Sachar DB, Kark AE: Stricture of the anorectum in Crohn's disease involving the colon. Ann Surg 181:207, 1975.

Laird DR & others: Symposium: Anoplasty: What, when, how, why. Dis Colon Rectum 12:179, 1969.

Marganoff H, Paradis H: Internal anal sphincterotomy in the correction of anal contracture. Dis Colon Rectum 15:201, 1972.

Turell R: Postoperative anal stenosis. Surg Gynecol Obstet 90:231, 1950.

PILONIDAL DISEASE

Essentials of Diagnosis

- Acute abscess or chronic draining sinuses in the sacrococcygeal area.
- Pain, tenderness, induration.

General Considerations

Pilonidal disease is characterized by a pit or sinus of variable depth lined by epithelium or granulation tissue which may lead to a cavity, often containing hair, which is liable to form abscesses and secondary sinuses. It is usually caused by trauma and the penetration of hair into the subcutaneous tissues. The hair acts as a foreign body and nidus for the development of infection.

In about 10% of cases, pilonidal disease is of congenital origin. It also occurs in the finger webs of barbers as a result of implanted hair and in the umbilical region as result of improper hygiene. The male/female sex incidence is 3:1, usually in hirsute white individuals of dark complexion. In hirsute young men with pilonidal disease the hair of the eyebrows frequently meets above the bridge of the nose.

Pilonidal disease is rare in blacks and is unknown among Orientals and American Indians. It becomes clinically manifest coincident with the increase of hair growth and activity of the sebaceous glands at puberty. In most cases symptoms are first noticed at age 20–25. It is commonly seen in military personnel and has been called "jeep disease" because of its frequent relationship to riding in mechanized vehicles.

Clinical Findings

The lesion is usually asymptomatic until it becomes acutely infected. The symptoms and findings of acute suppuration are similar to those of acute abscesses in other locations. The inflammatory process may spontaneously subside or progress until relief is obtained by spontaneous rupture or surgical drainage. After drainage has occurred, the purulent discharge may cease completely or, more commonly, may recur intermittently with drainage from one or many sinus openings, each communicating with the parent sinus or cyst. On examination, one or several midline or eccentric cutaneous openings in the skin of the sacral region are found. One or several hairs can often be seen projecting from the openings. A probe may be passed into the sinuses for distances of several millimeters to many centimeters.

Pilonidal disease rarely may extend anterior to the coccyx or sacrum.

Differential Diagnosis

The midline postanal dimple commonly noted in infants is rarely the precursor of pilonidal disease. The external openings of anal fistulas are usually closer to the anus, not necessarily in the midline, have a palpable tract extending toward the rectum, and may have a demonstrable internal opening at the anorectal juncture and a history of rectal abscess. Passage of a probe in the tract may indicate its course. Occasionally, however, the differentiation may be difficult.

X-ray fistulograms made by injecting a radiopaque substance in the external opening may be helpful in delineating the extent of the pathology.

Osteomyelitis can be demonstrated by x-ray study.

Furuncle or carbuncle may be associated with similar lesions elsewhere on the skin and presents a rounded, mound-like appearance surrounded by a whitish-yellow head whereas the infected pilonidal cyst is more flattened and blends into the surrounding tissues.

Complications

Untreated pilonidal infection may result in the formation of multiple, sometimes long, draining sinuses. Rarely, malignant degeneration has occurred.

Treatment

Treatment of the acute abscess is by incision and drainage. This may often be accomplished under local anesthesia. If the abscess cavity is small and superficial, unroofing and packing it open may result in complete healing. As a rule, however, a chronic draining sinus persists which must be surgically extirpated by excision and primary closure or, preferably, by an open technic and marsupialization. The variety of closed methods which have been described testifies to their unacceptable recurrence rate and to superiority of the open technic. Two open methods may be described briefly as follows:

(1) The sinuses and all of their ramifications are opened over a grooved director. The sinus tracts are then completely exteriorized by circumcising the overhanging skin edges. Finally, the intact skin edge is sutured to the edge of the sinus tract and a pressure dressing is applied until the following day.

(2) The area involved by the disease is excised with an elliptical skin incision carried down through the subcutaneous tissue to the posterior sacrococcygeal fascia and the block of tissue is dissected from the fascia. The edges of the wound are then sutured to the fascia and a pressure dressing is applied.

The pressure dressing may be removed on the second postoperative day and the sutures in a week. Daily warm sitz baths are then begun. The wound is inspected every 5–7 days so that bridging-over may be prevented.

Healing time depends upon the size of the defect, but is usually 3–6 weeks. The patient is entirely ambulatory throughout the treatment.

Prognosis

The recurrence rate following surgical correction varies with the method and after-care. With the open method, the recurrence rate is 5–10%.

Broadrick GL, Ehrlich FE, Kramer SG: Simplified treatment of pilonidal disease on an outpatient basis. Surgery 70:635, 1971.

Casten DF, Tan BY, Ayuyao A: A technique of radical excision of pilonidal disease with primary closure. Surgery 73:109, 1973.

Miller RJ: Pilonidal disease: A logical approach. Postgrad Med 41:382, 1967.

Sebrechts PH, Anderson JP Jr: Common sense in the treatment of pilonidal disease. Dis Colon Rectum 14:57, 1971.

Zimmerman K: Pilonidal disease. Dis Colon Rectum 13:330, 1970.

FOREIGN BODIES IN THE RECTUM

Swallowed foreign bodies such as chicken or fish bones, toothpicks, false teeth, pins, etc may become lodged at the anorectal juncture. Psychotic persons may swallow all manner of objects. Foreign bodies are swallowed sometimes for the purpose of concealment. Foreign bodies such as gallstones, fecaliths, urinary calculi, vaginal pessaries, orthopedic appliances, or surgical sponges or instruments may erode into the rectum. Foreign bodies may be introduced intentionally into the rectum for purposes of concealment, sexual stimulation, as a prank, for self-therapy, or from impalement. Enema tips and thermometers, broken or intact, are among the most common. The list of foreign bodies so introduced is long and often bizarre.

Clinical manifestations will depend upon the size and shape of the foreign body, its duration in situ, and the presence of infection or perforation. The occurrence of sudden excruciating rectal pain during defecation should arouse suspicion of a penetrating foreign body which is usually lodged at the anorectal juncture. Constant pain and tenesmus are almost invariably present. Bleeding will occur if there is concomitant trauma. There may be severe sphincteric spasm and tenderness. Digital rectal and proctoscopic examinations are usually diagnostic, although very small foreign bodies may be difficult to palpate. X-ray examination is helpful only when the foreign body is radiopaque.

The diagnosis may be missed if, as is often the case, the patient does not admit to insertion of the foreign body. Sharp small foreign bodies which lodge in or tear the anal crypts and cause marked pain and spasm may be missed, leading to an erroneous diagnosis of fissure, cryptitis, or proctitis. Fecal impaction must be differentiated.

Complications include pararectal infection, intra- or extraperitoneal rupture of the bowel, injury to the sphincters, and fistulization to adjacent viscera.

Removal of foreign bodies which have been inserted into the rectum is often difficult because they tend to slip through the tight sphincteric ring into the commodious ampulla and are then difficult to grasp and to extract. Special procedures include the use of gauze coverage, rubber tubing, a corkscrew for soft objects, a tonsil-type snare, etc. The ingenuity and skill of the operator are often taxed. A hole may be bored through the foreign body in order to overcome the suction which opposes withdrawal. Such procedures are best done under the complete relaxation of spinal anesthesia. Sphincterotomy may be necessary. Simultaneous external pressure upon the abdomen is sometimes helpful.

Small foreign bodies may be extracted with a speculum under regional anesthetic. Foreign bodies eroding into the rectum from the uterus, vagina, bladder, prostate, or bowel are best removed and subsequent treatment of the residual fistula delayed until after the acute inflammatory reaction has subsided. If perforation of the bowel has occurred, closure and complementary colostomy must be done. Foreign bodies may be passed spontaneously in the purulent material of a pararectal abscess. Enemas should not be used with the hope of flushing out the object.

In neglected cases, extensive necrosis and gangrene of the buttocks and perirectal tissues may develop. Radical debridement then becomes a life-saving procedure.

Haft JS, Benjamin HB: Foreign bodies in the rectum: Some psychosexual aspects. Med Aspects Hum Sexual 8:74, Aug 1973.

Jansen AAJ: Foreign body in the rectum. NZ Med J 70:174, 1969.

Maleki M, Evans WE: Foreign body perforation of the intestinal tract: Report of 12 cases and review of the literature. Arch Surg 101:475, 1970.

Stone HH, Martin JDJ: Synergistic necrotizing cellulitis. Ann Surg 175:702, 1972.

RECTAL PROLAPSE

Essentials of Diagnosis

- Protrusion of the rectum through the anus.
- Partial or complete fecal incontinence.
- Bleeding and discharge.

General Considerations

The causes of rectal prolapse are often obscure. It is far more common in women than in men and is common in mentally ill patients—perhaps as a result of their tendency to strain excessively at stool. Extensive injury to or weakening of the supporting musculature due to surgery, trauma, neurologic defects, senility, wasting diseases, or nutritional deficiency may be responsible. Secondary muscular weakness is produced by the prolapse itself.

Errors in diagnosis and treatment are partially due to failure to differentiate the 3 types:

(1) Mucosal prolapse: Transient, minor prolapse of just the rectal mucosa frequently occurs in otherwise normal infants and may be alarming to the parents. In adults, however, mucosal prolapse is persistent and may grow progressively worse.

(2) Procidentia: This consists of complete prolapse of the entire thickness of the rectum along with the peritoneum as a sliding hernia. In children, it is thought to be due to the flatness of the sacrum (so that the rectum forms a vertical straight tube), the reduction of the supporting fat of the ischiorectal fossa, and weakness of the supporting ligaments of the rectum. It may be associated with other congenital anomalies such as exstrophy of the bladder. In adults, procidentia associated with a deep cul-de-sac represents a sliding hernia in which the anterior rectal wall and the peritoneal sac attached to it first protrude externally. As the muscular supports become weaker, there is complete procidentia of the entire circumference. The lateral suspensory ligaments of the rectum are attenuated or absent. The levators ani are separated, and the rectovaginal septum is shortened or absent. Prolapse of the uterus with cystocele may be present. The anterior hernial sac may contain omentum or small bowel. Abnormal anterior displacement of the rectum due to elongation of the mesorectum is probably the primary cause. In its early development there may be an internal intussusception of the rectum before the external protrusion becomes evident.

(3) Prolapse of a colonic intussusception: This rare type consists of a protrusion of the intra-abdominal colon through the anus while the rectum remains in its normal position.

Clinical Findings

A. Symptoms and Signs: In internal intussusception of the rectum there may be a sensation of incomplete evacuation of stool and perineal pain with sciatic or obturator radiation. On endoscopic examination the mucosa is seen to be engorged and thickened with a mucous discharge in the lumen. The intussusception is found by colonoscopy or cineradiography with the patient in the sitting position.

When the prolapse becomes external, a mass protrudes from the rectum during defecation or even during walking. At first the mass reduces spontaneously, but with time it becomes more difficult to reduce. Soiling of the clothing occurs from discharge, bleeding, and fecal incontinence. The musculature becomes progressively weaker until it is completely atonic and complete fecal incontinence results.

It is essential that the prolapse be demonstrated. Examination in either a standing or squatting position with the patient straining is required if the full extent of the prolapse is to be demonstrated. The extent of weakness of the pelvic musculature and sphincteric ring should be evaluated by observation of their tonus and their ability to contract voluntarily, by palpation, and by electromyography.

B. Special Examinations: Sigmoidoscopy and barium enema x-ray examination of the colon must be done to search for intrinsic disease. A lateral x-ray or cineradiography may disclose the anterior displacement of the rectum away from the sacrum.

Neurologic examination is necessary to rule out primary neurologic disorders.

Differential Diagnosis

In mucosal prolapse, the protrusion is relatively

small and symmetric about the circumference; the mucosal folds are arranged in a radial fashion; and, by palpating the thickness of the protrusion between the thumb and index finger, the 2 apposed thicknesses of mucosa can be recognized. With procidentia of the sliding hernia type, the protrusion may reach a considerable length. The anterior wall will be larger than the rest of the circumference because of its contained hernial sac; the lumen will be directed posteriorly and will be off center; the mucosal folds will be arranged in a circular fashion; and palpation of the thickness of the protrusion anteriorly will disclose the double full thickness of the bowel wall and its hernial sac. Intussusception is recognized by the deep sulcus between the intussusceptum and the rectal wall.

Prolapsing internal hemorrhoids are recognizable by their varicose appearance and separation into discrete masses. They may be associated with some degree of mucosal prolapse as well. Large hypertrophic anal papillae, fibromas, and rectal polyps are solitary, circumscribed, and of firmer consistency.

Complications

The prolapsing mucosa frequently shows signs of superficial infection, ulceration, and edema. Irreducibility is uncommon. Gangrene or rupture of the anterior wall of the rectum with extrusion of the small bowel is rare and now occurs only in places remote from medical aid.

Treatment

A. Medical Treatment: In children, conservative treatment is most satisfactory; recurrences in adult life occur only rarely. When there is underlying mental deficiency, neurologic disorder, or incurable chronic disease, surgical correction may be required. Underlying nutritional or febrile disorders should be corrected and the causes of straining eliminated. Defecation in a recumbent position is recommended, and the buttocks should be strapped firmly together between bowel movements. Stool softeners and enemas may be necessary.

B. Surgical Treatment: In adults, conservative measures are rarely sufficient, and operative treatment is nearly always required. At least 50 procedures have been described, which testifies to the imperfection of all of them.

The operation must be properly chosen for the particular type of prolapse present.

The most effective operations in current use are as follows:

(1) For simple mucosal prolapse: The operation consists of excision of diamond-shaped segments of mucosa in each of the 4 quadrants, with apposition by suture of the apexes of the diamonds so as to foreshorten the protruding mucosa.

(2) For complete procidentia: There are 3 types of procedures: (a) Abdominal operation with elevation and posterior fixation of the rectum to the sacrum to correct its anterior displacement, either by direct suture or by the use of a Teflon mesh sling. The sigmoid colon may be shortened if it is redundant by

resection and anastomosis. (b) Perineal operation or proctosigmoidectomy, in which the outer layer of the intussusception is circumcised and the intussuscipiens, including the intraperitoneal sigmoid colon, is drawn externally until it is taut up to its point of fixation at its juncture with the descending colon. The anterior hernial sac is then sutured closed in a high position. The diastasis of the puborectalis is repaired. The redundant bowel is amputated, and an anastomosis is made between the walls of the bowel. (c) In patients who are very old or in poor general condition, a Thiersch-Jackman wire may be used. This consists of a stainless steel braided cable which encircles the sphincteric ring.

The muscles supporting the rectum can be strengthened to some degree by exercising the sphincteric mechanism or by electric stimulation.

Prognosis

Success rates are highest when the operation has been properly chosen for the particular type of prolapse. In general, the recurrence rate is high, although individual surgeons who have properly performed an appropriate operation have reported from 75–100% success. When muscle deficiency is great, improvement following postoperative exercising of the sphincter is insignificant. There are conflicting reports concerning the effectiveness of electrical stimulation.

Altmeier WA & others: Nineteen years' experience with the one-stage perineal repair of rectal prolapse. Ann Surg 173:383, 1971.

Goldberg SM & others: Symposium: Procidentia of the rectum. Dis Colon Rectum 18:457, 1975.

Ripstein CB: A simple, effective operation for rectal prolapse. Postgrad Med 45:201, March 1969.

Ripstein CB, Lanter B: Etiology and surgical therapy of massive prolapse of the rectum. Ann Surg 157:259, 1963.

Swinton NW Sr: Management of patients with complete rectal prolapse or procidentia. Surg Clin North Am 51:825, 1971.

Theuerkauf FJ Jr, Beahrs OH, Hill JR: Rectal prolapse: Causation and surgical treatment. Ann Surg 171:819, 1970.

FECAL INCONTINENCE

Essentials of Diagnosis

- Loss of voluntary control of passage of feces through anus.
- Fecal soiling of clothing.

General Considerations

Anal incontinence may result from injuries or diseases of the spinal cord, congenital abnormalities, accidental injuries to the rectum and anus, procidentia, senility, fecal impaction, extensive inflammatory processes, lymphogranuloma venereum, malignant tumors, stricture, and deformities following obstetric, dilatational, and operative procedures. The extent to which gas, liquid feces, or semisolid feces can be controlled may be used as a measure of the severity of the lesion. Postobstetric or postoperative incontinence may not become manifest until many years after the causative incident, when senile hypotonicity of the pelvic musculature occurs.

An understanding of the detailed anatomy and physiology of the anorectum is essential for a proper approach to the prevention and repair of anal incontinence. Rectal incontinence is more than "a simple affair of a purse-string pulled by the cerebral cortex." The rectum is a capacious, distensible organ which forms a (usually empty) reservoir. The anal ring is a composite muscle consisting of the various bundles of the external sphincter, the internal sphincter, the prolongation of the longitudinal layer of the rectum, and the puborectalis portion of the levator ani muscles. The levators support the anal canal only posteriorly and laterally, leaving an area of comparative weakness anteriorly, where it is more vulnerable to injury. The central portion of the levator acts as a sphincter. Maintenance of the acute angulation of the anorectal juncture is also important in effecting normal evacuation.

There is a cerebral inhibitory control over the spinal cord reflex for both defecation and micturition. Destruction of the second, third, and fourth sacral segments or cauda equina results in loss of reflex evacuation. Sensory incontinence may result after removal of the lowermost portion of the rectum, as in some types of operations for cancer.

Clinical Findings

In neurogenic incontinence there is atony of the pelvic musculature with laxity of the anal canal, insensibility to tactile stimulation, inability to contract the anorectal musculature voluntarily, and absence of the anal reflexes. In traumatic or postoperative incontinence, the actual defect in the circumference of the anorectal ring with scarring can be seen and palpated. A clue to the site of the defect is the loss of corrugation or wrinkling of the perianal skin due to the defect in the underlying subcutaneous corrugator cutis ani muscle. Functional ability of the sphincteric musculature can be determined by electromyography. With extensive inflammatory or malignant disease, rigidity of the rectal outlet is readily identifiable. There may be some degree of rectal prolapse.

Prevention

At the time of surgical operation on the anorectum, forceful dilatation and inadvertent division of the sphincters must be avoided. In operations for fistula, a sufficient portion of the anorectal ring must remain to allow control. Postoperative packing must be avoided. Obstetric injuries to the sphincters must be immediately recognized and promptly repaired.

Treatment

A. Medical Measures. For mild degrees of incontinence, nonsurgical measures may suffice. These include a low-residue, bland diet and anticholinergic drugs to reduce intestinal motility; daily enemas with a device to allow for retention of the irrigating fluid; and daily exercises of sphincteric contraction. Patients with neurogenic incontinence may be trained to initiate defecation by digital stimulation of the anal canal. If not immediately corrected, repair of obstetric tears should be delayed for 6 months or more after parturition.

An apparatus for continuous electrical stimulation of the sphincters by an electronic device is available.

B. Surgical Treatment: When anal incontinence is associated with rectocele and cystocele, colpoperineoplasty is essential. Methods of surgical repair of defects in the sphincteric ring include reefing operations; fascial slings using fascia lata or transplantation of the gracilis muscle from the medial side of the thigh; pullout wire reapposition; encircling the anus with a silver or stainless steel wire; and the classical method in which the divided ends of the muscles are reapposed.

Prognosis

Conservative measures as outlined above are frequently all that is required. Operative results are good if surgery is performed before atony of the muscle occurs. Concomitant irritability of the bowel, neurogenic, inflammatory, or neoplastic disease, or other anatomic defects make for a poor prognosis.

Birnbaum WD: Fecal incontinence. In: *Diseases of the Colon and Anorectum.* Turell R (editor). Saunders, 1969.

Duthie HL: Progress report: Anal continence. Gut 12:844, 1971.

Parks AG, McPartlin JF: Late repair of injuries of the anal sphincter. Proc R Soc Med 64:1187, 1971.

Scharli AF, Kieswetter WB: Defecation and continence: Some new concepts. Dis Colon Rectum 13:81, 1970.

MALIGNANT TUMORS OF THE ANAL CANAL & PERINEUM

Basal cell epithelioma is uncommon, usually arises at the anal verge, occurs 3 times as frequently in males as in females, and is similar to the more frequent "rodent ulcer" seen on exposed skin surfaces. All chronic, indurated growths at the anal margin should be suspect. A wide excisional biopsy of the suspicious area should be done which will not only allow a diagnosis but will effect a cure if adequate normal tissue margins are obtained. Local excision is the treatment of choice for anal basal cell epithelioma because of its nonmetastasizing nature. Irradiation therapy can also be used as the primary treatment, but surgical excision is preferable because of the undesirable side-effects of radiation in the anal region.

Perianal Bowen's disease (intraepidermal carcinoma, carcinoma in situ) is a rare, chronic, slowly maturing tumor. Two or 3% of the growths will become infiltrative and metastasize. Other malignant tumors are often present elsewhere in the body. The disease is manifested as a dull red, spreading, irregular, plaque-like, eczematoid, weeping lesion of the skin which is usually pruritic. It must be considered in the differential diagnosis of pruritus ani. The diagnosis is made by biopsy, and the distinguishing histopathologic feature is the presence of intraepidermal, haloed, multinucleated giant Bowen cells. Treatment is by local excision with adequate margins of normal skin.

Extramammary Paget's disease of the anus (epidermotrophic carcinoma) is a rare mucinous carcinoma involving the external anogenital area that occurs most commonly in women over age 50. It probably arises in the apocrine glands with secondary intradermal metastases. It is a malignant, extremely slowly growing tumor that may metastasize late. It must be differentiated from neurodermatitis, psoriasis, Bowen's disease, basal cell cancer, squamous cell cancer, and unpigmented melanoma. Treatment consists of wide excision with microscopic control since the margins of excision may appear to be grossly normal.

Cloacogenic cancer of the anorectal junction (transitional cell, basaloid, basosquamous carcinoma) arises from embryologic remnants that have persisted in the cloacogenic zone just above the dentate line where the glandular mucosa of the rectum meets the stratified epithelium of the anal canal. It occurs twice as frequently in females as in males. The history of discomfort and possibly of bleeding is often a short one. The growth is usually of an "iceberg" type, with the bulk of the tumor in the deeper tissues and only the surface presenting in the anal canal. Early, rapid metastatic spread is common. Microscopically, the appearance is strikingly similar to that of papillary transitional cell tumors seen at the vesical neck and posterior urethra. Treatment consists of early, radical abdominoperineal resection of the rectum.

Anorectal malignant melanoma is rare. Growth is dynamic, with a tendency for early spread, rapid metastasis, and a very high rate of recurrence even after radical surgery. This is the most lethal of the tumors occurring at the anorectal juncture. Most are pigmented, but about a third are amelanotic. When pigmented, the lesion can simulate a thrombosed or strangulated hemorrhoid; when amelanotic, it can resemble a mucosal rectal polyp or internal hemorrhoid. The current treatment of choice is radical abdominoperineal resection of the rectum. Additional dissection of aorto-ileopelvic and bilateral inguinal lymph nodes has not materially improved the survival rate. Primary irradiation has proved ineffective. Perfusion chemotherapy may possibly improve the survival rate.

Epidermoid carcinoma of the anorectum (squamous cell carcinoma) comprises 3–5% of cancers of the rectum and anus. It occurs twice as frequently in females as in males. Leukoplakia, lymphogranuloma venereum, chronic fistulas, and irradiated anal skin are potential predisposing causes. Most of these tumors are histologically moderately well differentiated, but occasional ones are poorly differentiated. The degree of differentiation is inversely proportionate to the rate of growth, infiltration, and metastasis. Direct extension into the perianal tissues and sphincter muscles is frequent. Epidermoid carcinomas arising in the anal canal metastasize along the lymphatics of the rectum to the perirectal and mesenteric lymph nodes as well as to the inguinal lymph nodes. Hepatic metastases via the portal venous system occur in about 10% of cases. Carcinomas arising external to the anus metastasize to the inguinal lymph nodes either across the perineum to the superficial inguinal lymph nodes or along the middle hemorrhoidal lymphatics to the hypogastric and obturator lymph nodes and from there to the external iliac and inguinal lymph nodes. Unsuspected epidermoid carcinoma is occasionally discovered in the specimens from hemorrhoidectomy. When hemorrhoids are removed surgically, they should be marked to show their position in the circumference of the rectum and must always be examined microscopically.

Rectal bleeding is the most common presenting symptom. Local pain, change of bowel habits, sensation of a lump, tenesmus, soilage, perianal itching, or a feeling of moisture also may occur.

Surgery is the treatment of choice. The type of operation indicated is dependent upon evaluation of the clinical features of the tumor. Wide local excision may be done for small superficial lesions which are located at or below the mucocutaneous juncture. Large tumors which penetrate the anal sphincters or which originate above the mucocutaneous line and involve the rectum should have a combined abdominoperineal resection of the rectum with a wide perineal phase of excision to include the levator muscles as well as the contents of the ischiorectal fossae. In the female patient, posterior vaginectomy may also be indicated. Extramesenteric pelvic lymph node dissection is indicated whenever it can be done with little difficulty in good-risk patients as part of combined abdominoperineal resection.

The simultaneous appearance of an inguinal metastasis in a patient whose primary tumor is as yet untreated is an ominous sign. Subsequent appearance of an inguinal metastasis portends a somewhat better outlook. When inguinal lymph nodes are not clinically involved on initial examination, bilateral radical groin dissection should not be done as a prophylactic measure. The poor salvage rate of this procedure must be weighed against the significant morbidity usually attended with bilateral radical groin dissection. Frequent, careful follow-up examination of the inguinal lymph nodes with prompt therapeutic groin dissection when indicated is preferable.

The prognosis of squamous cell carcinoma of the anorectum has improved markedly in recent years. An overall 5-year nonrecurrence rate of greater than 50% can now be anticipated.

Bensaude A, Parturier-Albot M: Anal localization of Bowen's disease. Proc R Soc Med 64:1190, 1971.

Golden GT, Horsley JS: Surgical management of epidermoid carcinoma of the anus. Am J Surg 131:275, 1976.

Hickey RC & others: Anal cancer, with special reference to the cloacogenic variety. Surg Clin North Am 52:543, 1972.

Kheir S & others: Cloacogenic carcinoma of the anal canal. Arch Surg 104:407, 1972.

Newman HK, Quan SHQ: Multi-modality therapy for epidermoid carcinoma of the anus. Cancer 37:12, 1976.

Paradis P & others: The clinical implications of a staging system for carcinoma of the anus. Surg Gynecol Obstet 141:411, 1975.

Williams SL, Rogers LW, Quan SH: Perianal Paget's disease. Dis Colon Rectum 19:30, 1976.

RADIATION (FACTITIAL) PROCTITIS

Exposure to radium, ^{60}Co, and x-ray employed in the treatment of malignant lesions of the pelvis, especially cancer of the cervix, uterus, bladder, and prostate, often causes reaction to the adjacent bowel. With the advent of high-voltage x-ray and ^{60}Co irradiation, skin effects are minimal and no longer limit the depth dose as was the case with 200–400 kv x-ray therapy.

The rectal mucosa is much more sensitive to irradiation than normal vaginal mucosa.

There may be no demonstrable external abnormalities or areas of skin change at the site of the x-ray exposure. On digital rectal examination, the anal canal may be tender and spastic. Induration of the rectal mucosa may be palpable, and the crater of an ulcer may be felt.

Proctosigmoidoscopy in the first few weeks after exposure shows the mucosa to be red and edematous and to bleed easily with slight trauma. It later becomes indurated and then flat, pale, and atrophic, and develops persistent telangiectasis. When ulcers occur, they are grayish, well defined, and oval or circular. Barium enema x-ray examination is helpful in the study of mucosal abnormalities and possible fistulas. It may reveal an annular filling defect due to stricture.

The rectosigmoid may be involved, resulting in a stenosing ulcerative lesion closely resembling cancer. Stenosis may not develop for months or years after treatment.

Small increments of radiation therapy to multiple fields, megavoltage doses, and cobalt therapy reduce the incidence of injury to the rectum and sigmoid colon when irradiation treatment is required. Direct exposure of bladder, bowel, and ureters must be avoided where possible. Special shield applicators for radium insertion and positioning of the patient should be used.

A low-residue diet, rectal instillations of warm oil, antispasmodics, and sedatives are indicated, as well as bed rest if necessary. Rectal instillation of hydrocortisone as in the treatment of ulcerative colitis may be helpful. Hydrocortisone (alcohol), 1.6 g in 1 liter of sesame oil, is shaken well and 60 ml of the mixture are injected into the rectum at bedtime with a rubber syringe. Bleeding often demands iron therapy or blood replacement. Colostomy may be indicated for patients with severe hemorrhage, intractable pain, or fistulas. Resection of the affected portion of the intraperitoneal bowel may be performed when the lesion is very localized and there is obstruction. Healing of irradiated tissue, including bowel, is notoriously poor. Rectal strictures should not be dilated since they often retrogress spontaneously.

It may take 1–2 years for the reaction in the bowel to reach a plateau, during which time bleeding continues. A stricture with partial obstruction may occur during healing. If the neoplastic disease has been eradicated, most patients will recover in time.

Nance FC, Persson AV, Piker JF: Radiation injuries to the lower gastrointestinal tract. Am Surg 34:21, 1968.

Quan SHQ: Factitial proctitis due to irradiation for cancer of the cervix uteri. Surg Gynecol Obstet 126:70, 1968.

Reece NW: Management of bowel complications of radiotherapy. Proc R Soc Med 67:60, 1974.

●   ●   ●

General References

Bacon HE: Office proctology, diagnosis and treatment. Postgrad Med 53:93, Feb 1973.

Beck AR, Turell R: Pediatric proctology. Surg Clin North Am 52:1055, 1972.

Goligher JC: *Surgery of the Anus, Rectum and Colon,* 3rd ed. Thomas, 1975.

Morson BC, Dawson IMP: *Gastrointestinal Pathology.* Blackwell, 1972.

Ross ST (editor): Symposium on anorectal diseases. Mod Treat 8:861, 1971.

Turell R: *Diseases of the Colon and Anorectum,* 2nd ed. 2 vols. Saunders, 1969.

Waite VC & others: Symposium: Complications of colonic and rectal surgery. Dis Colon Rectum 16:1, 1973.

36 . . .
Hernias of the Abdominal Wall*

Albert D. Hall, MD, Harold H. Lindner, MD, & J. Englebert Dunphy, MD

An external hernia is an abnormal protrusion of intra-abdominal tissue or the whole or part of a viscus through an opening or fascial defect in the abdominal wall. About 75% of hernias occur in the groin (indirect inguinal, direct inguinal, femoral). Incisional and ventral hernias comprise about 10%; femoral, 6%; umbilical, 3%; and others, about 3%. Generally, a hernial mass is composed of covering tissues (skin, subcutaneous tissues, etc), a peritoneal sac, and any contained viscera. Frequently, the neck of the sac is narrow where it emerges from the abdomen. This produces a potentially dangerous condition because bowel protruding into the hernia may become obstructed or strangulated. With time, progressive attenuation of normal tissues by the protruding mass weakens the area, causes discomfort, and makes operative repair more complicated. The definitive treatment of hernia is early operative repair.

A **reducible hernia** is one in which the contents of the sac return to the abdomen spontaneously when the patient is recumbent, or with manual pressure.

An **irreducible** or **incarcerated hernia** is one whose contents cannot be returned to the abdomen, usually because they are trapped by the narrow neck. The term incarceration does not imply obstruction, inflammation, or ischemia of the herniated organs.

The lumen of a segment of bowel within the hernia sac may become **obstructed**. Initially, there may be no interference with blood supply.

A **strangulated hernia** denotes compromise to the blood supply of the contents of the sac (eg, omentum or intestine). Gangrene of the sac and its contents may then ensue. The incidence of strangulation is higher in femoral than in inguinal hernias.

Richter's hernia occurs when only a part of the circumference of the bowel becomes incarcerated or strangulated in the fascial defect. This is more frequent in femoral hernias but may occur in inguinal hernias. A strangulated Richter's hernia may spontaneously reduce and the gangrenous piece of intestine be overlooked at operation. The bowel may subsequently perforate with resultant peritonitis. Richter's hernias complicate about 0.65% of all groin hernias, 0.7% of all femoral hernias, and 14% of all strangulated femoral hernias.

*See Chapter 48 for further discussion of hernias in the pediatric age group.

ANATOMY OF THE GROIN

The superficial fascia of the ventrolateral abdominal wall (Scarpa's fascia) attains its greatest thickness in the ilioinguinal region. It fuses laterally with the crest of the ilium and passes ventral to the inguinal ligament to fuse with the deep fascia of the upper thigh about 2.5 cm below and parallel to the inguinal ligament.

The musculature of the ilioinguinal region is composed of 3 flat, thin muscles: the external oblique, the internal oblique, and the transverse abdominal.

The **external oblique,** the most superficial of the ilioinguinal muscles, arises from the lower 8 ribs and runs vertically and medially from cephalad to caudad. The muscle is fleshy until it approaches a line drawn from the anterior superior spine of the ilium to the umbilicus, at which point it forms the aponeurosis of the external oblique which covers the ilioinguinal region deep to Scarpa's fascia. The aponeurosis is a strong, thin membranous structure whose fibers are directed inferiorly and medially.

The **subcutaneous** or **external inguinal ring** is a roughly triangular opening, 2.5 × 1.25 cm, in the aponeurosis of the external oblique just cephalad and lateral to the pubic tubercle. The ring provides egress to the spermatic cord and the ilioinguinal nerve in the male and to the round ligament and ilioinguinal nerve in the female.

The **inguinal ligament** forms the lateral inferior border of the aponeurosis of the external oblique, extending from the anterior superior iliac spine to the pubic tubercle. It is formed as the lateral edge of the aponeurosis rolls upon itself and thickens into a cord. The lower end of the inguinal ligament is reflected dorsally and laterally from the pubic tubercle back along the iliopectineal line of the pubis as the **lacunar (Gimbernat) ligament**. The lacunar ligament is about 1.25 cm long and triangular in shape, with the base directed laterally. The sharp, crescentic lateral border of this ligament is the unyielding noose for the strangulation of a femoral hernia.

Cooper's ligament is a strong fibrous band which extends laterally for about 2.5 cm along the iliopectineal line on the superior aspect of the superior pubic ramus, starting at the lateral base of the lacunar ligament.

The **internal oblique muscle** is thinner and smaller than the external oblique beneath which it lies. Its fibers run predominantly in a transverse direction. In the ilioinguinal region, its fibers arise from the lateral half of the inguinal ligament, arching superiorly and medially across the spermatic cord just below the level of the internal inguinal ring. These fibers then fuse with the lowermost arching fibers of the transverse muscle of the abdomen and insert with them into the pubic tubercle, forming the **conjoined tendon** of the 2 muscles.

The **cremaster muscle** is a thin, attenuated muscle derived from the lowermost, superiorly arching fibers of the internal oblique. The cremaster muscle and fascia form one of the spermatic cord coverings and serve to pull the testis superiorly. This layer must be routinely identified and opened to properly identify an indirect inguinal hernia sac.

The **transverse abdominal** muscle is the deepest of the flat muscles and arises in part by fleshy fibers from the lateral portion of the iliopubic tract, from the inner lip of the iliac crest, and the lumbodorsal fascia to pass medially and transversely around the lateral aspect of the abdomen onto the anterior abdominal wall. Lateral to the rectus sheath its muscular fibers are replaced by tendinous aponeuroses which fuse with the internal oblique aponeurosis to form the rectus sheath. A lower free margin of the **transversus abdominal aponeurosis** forms an arch over the internal ring above the inguinal canal medial to the ring. When this fuses with the arch of the internal oblique aponeurosis, it is called the conjoined tendon or falx inguinalis. The arch itself forms a basic component of the anatomic repair of inguinal hernias.

The **transversalis fascia** is a well-developed aponeurotic extension of the endoabdominal fascia which in the ilioinguinal region lies just superficial to the peritoneum. It is usually thickest and best developed over the ilioinguinal region, and in this area has an opening in it, the **internal inguinal ring**, formed by the embryologic herniation of the processus vaginalis peritonei through the ventrolateral abdominal wall.

The **internal inguinal ring** lies midway between the anterior superior iliac spine and the pubic tubercle, halfway up the inguinal ligament and 1.25 cm medial to it. The ring is bounded superiorly by the arching fibers of the internal oblique muscle and below and medially by the inferior epigastric vessels. Along the medial third of the inguinal ligament, the transversalis fascia passes deep to the ligament onto the medial upper surface of the thigh. In so doing, it forms a triangular covering ventral to the femoral artery, femoral vein, and femoral canal. The **iliopubic tract** of the transversalis fascia is the thickest portion of this fascia in the inguinal region. It parallels and lies just medial to the inguinal ligament and at the level of the pubic spine is reflected along the inner surface of the lacunar ligament to form the medial surface of the femoral ring.

The **inguinal canal** is formed by the passage of the processus vaginalis and the gubernaculum; the testis and the spermatic cord pass through it from the abdomen to the scrotum. In both males and females, the canal also contains the ilioinguinal nerve, which lies between the internal oblique and the external oblique aponeurosis anterior to the spermatic canal; in the female it contains the round ligament of the uterus passing to the labia majora. Ventral to the canal is the external oblique aponeurosis; dorsally, the transversalis fascia.

Hesselbach's triangle is bounded by the inguinal ligament, the inferior epigastric vessels, and the conjoined tendon. Its floor, consisting of transversalis fascia, is the spot where direct inguinal hernias occur.

The **spermatic cord** begins in the properitoneal space at the level of the internal inguinal ring and passes through the internal inguinal ring, down through the inguinal canal, out through the external inguinal ring, and down over the pubis and through the scrotal neck beyond which it is attached to the testis. The cord is composed of arteries, veins, lymphatics, nerves, fatty tissue, and the excretory duct of the testis (vas deferens). The coverings of the spermatic cord are as follows: (1) The internal spermatic fascia, derived from the transversalis fascia, covers the cord from the internal inguinal ring to the testis. (2) The cremasteric muscle and fascia form the middle layer of cord covering. (3) The outermost cord covering is the external spermatic fascia, derived from the external oblique aponeurosis and covering the cord only from the external inguinal ring to the testis.

The **femoral triangle** is bounded superiorly by the inguinal ligament, laterally and inferiorly by the sartorius muscle, and medially by the pectineus and adductor magnus muscles. The superficial fascia of the upper thigh is continuous with Camper's fascia of the lower abdomen and consists of fatty areolar tissue. It covers the fossa ovalis femoralis, being perforated here by numerous blood and lymphatic vessels—hence the name **fascia cribrosa**.

The **femoral canal** lies just medial to the femoral vein on the ventral superior surface of the thigh, beginning at the level of the inguinal ligament and ending just dorsal to the superior border of the fossa ovalis femoris. It is bounded ventrally by the inguinal ligament and transversalis fascia and dorsally by the iliacus fascia and terminates as a result of the fusion of these fasciae.

CAUSES OF HERNIA

Indirect inguinal hernias occur in a congenitally present preformed sac, the processus vaginalis peritonei. The sac may exist as a small peritoneal dimple at the internal ring, or it may extend as a complete saccular diverticulum of the peritoneum to the base of the scrotum. The latter is called a **complete hernia.** These congenital sacs are often only potential hernias until they present with herniation of abdominal contents.

The hernia may be clinically evident during the first year of life or may not appear until late in life. In contrast, **direct inguinal hernias** are acquired as the result of a developed weakness of the transversalis fascia in Hesselbach's area. There is some evidence that direct inguinal hernias may be related to hereditary or acquired defects in collagen synthesis or turnover. **Femoral hernias** involve an acquired protrusion of a peritoneal sac through the femoral ring. In women the ring may become dilated in relation to the physical and biochemical changes during pregnancy.

Any condition that increases intra-abdominal pressure may contribute to the appearance and progression of a hernia. Marked obesity, acute and chronic abdominal strain as found with heavy exercise or lifting, chronic cough or sneezing, chronic constipation with straining at stool, and prostatism with straining on micturition are often implicated. Cirrhosis with ascites, pregnancy, and chronically enlarged pelvic organs may also contribute. Loss of tissue turgor in Hesselbach's area, associated with a weakening of the transversalis fascia, occurs with advancing age and in chronic debilitating disease.

HERNIAS OF THE GROIN

1. INDIRECT & DIRECT INGUINAL HERNIAS

An **indirect inguinal hernia** passes through the internal inguinal ring and descends along the inguinal canal within the spermatic cord. It is due to failure of fusion of the processus vaginalis peritonei after the testis has descended into the scrotum. The highest incidence is in the first year of life. Nearly all inguinal hernias in infants, children, and young adults are indirect. Indirect hernias may appear from infancy to advanced old age, but the majority occur before age 50. Although "congenital," the first clinical evidence of hernia may not appear until middle or old age when increased intra-abdominal pressure and dilatation of the internal inguinal ring allow abdominal contents to enter the previously empty peritoneal diverticulum. An untreated indirect hernia will inevitably dilate the internal ring and displace or attenuate the inguinal floor. The peritoneum may pouch out on either side of the inferior epigastric vessels to give a combined direct and indirect hernia, called a **pantaloon hernia**.

An undescended testis or a testis in the inguinal canal always has an associated persistent processus vaginalis (ie, a potential indirect inguinal hernia). There is a high association of testicular or cord hydroceles with indirect inguinal hernias.

A **direct inguinal hernia** protrudes through Hesselbach's area, lateral to the border of the rectus muscle and inferomedial to the inferior epigastric vessels. A direct inguinal hernia usually occurs as a diffuse bulge owing to a weakness in the transversalis fascia comprising the floor of the inguinal canal. An important variant is the funicular type of direct hernia, which protrudes through a small defect in the transversalis fascia. The funicular type is more prone to incarceration and strangulation. Direct inguinal hernias are rare in women, children, and young adults. Hernias in older men, especially if bilateral, are likely to be direct. Direct inguinal hernias are frequently discovered as an incidental finding on physical examination and become symptomatic only when they are somewhat larger. The usual complaint is a feeling of fullness or a visible bulge. Direct hernias rarely strangulate; however, the funicular type with a narrow neck may do so.

A **femoral hernia** descends through the femoral canal beneath the inguinal ligament. It typically is deflected anteriorly through the fossa ovalis femoris to present as a visible or palpable mass at or above the inguinal ligament, so it can be confused with an inguinal hernia (Fig 36–1). Because of its narrow neck, it is prone to incarceration and strangulation. Femoral hernia is much more common in women than in men, but in both sexes femoral hernia is less common than inguinal hernia. Femoral hernias comprise about one-third of groin hernias in women and about 2% of hernias in men.

Clinical Findings

A. Symptoms: Most hernias produce minimal or no symptoms until the patient notices a lump or swelling in the groin. Frequently, hernias are detected in the course of routine physical examinations such as preemployment examinations.

Occasionally the patient will complain of a dragging sensation and, particularly with indirect inguinal hernias, radiation into the scrotum. As a hernia enlarges it is likely to produce a sense of discomfort or aching pain, and the patient feels it necessary to lie down to manually reduce the hernia.

In general, direct hernias produce less symptoms than indirect inguinal hernias.

Femoral hernias are notoriously asymptomatic until incarceration or strangulation occurs. Even with obstruction or strangulation, the patient may feel discomfort more in the abdomen than in the femoral area. Thus, colicky abdominal pain and signs of intestinal obstruction frequently are the presenting manifestations of a strangulated femoral hernia with no reference to discomfort or pain in the femoral region, and, particularly in obese patients, physical examination may reveal no significant tenderness.

B. Signs: A typical manifestation of a hernia is swelling and a reducible or irreducible mass. The bulge of an indirect hernia tends to be somewhat more elliptical than that of a direct hernia, which is more circular. Only large femoral hernias are readily detected by inspection.

The paucity of symptoms and findings makes it imperative that in all cases of apparent intestinal obstruction, the most precise and careful examination of the inguinal and femoral canals be performed to ex-

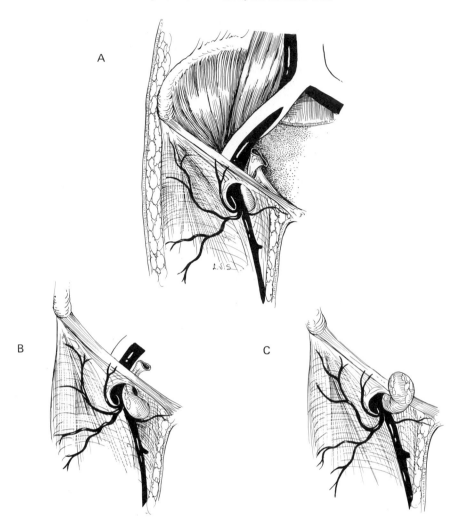

Figure 36—1. Migration of femoral hernia. *A:* Femoral hernia has passed the femoral ring and lies deep to the fossa ovalis femoris beneath the transversalis fascia. *B:* Femoral hernia has broken through the transversalis fascia and the fossa ovalis femoris. *C:* The sharp superior edge of the fossa ovalis femoris has turned the hernia sac superiorly to lie ventral to the inguinal ligament and the lower abdominal wall.

clude hernia, the second most common cause of obstruction of the small intestine.

The differentiation between direct and indirect hernia depends upon careful physical examination. The age of the patient when the hernia develops is suggestive, but indirect hernias may appear in the aged and direct ones in the young. A hernia that descends into the scrotum is almost certainly indirect, although rarely a direct hernia can dissect there through fascial planes.

On inspection with the patient erect and straining, a direct hernia appears as a symmetric swelling at the external ring. It promptly disappears when the patient lies down. An indirect hernia appears as an elliptical swelling coming down the canal and frequently entering the scrotum. It may or may not reduce easily. The patient should be examined in both the supine and standing positions. Invaginating the

scrotum and locating the pubic tubercle readily identify the anatomic landmarks and the external ring (Fig 36—2). The external ring may be so small that the examiner's finger cannot enter, or it may be widely patent.

On palpation, the posterior wall of the inguinal canal is firm and resistant in an indirect hernia but relaxed or absent in a direct hernia. When the patient coughs or strains, a direct hernia protrudes directly forward at the examining finger, whereas an indirect hernia comes down the canal against the side of the finger unless the finger is directed laterally and upward into the canal. If the external ring permits, the sac of both direct and indirect hernias may be felt in the canal. Reduction of an indirect hernia can be maintained by external compression over the internal ring until pressure is released. When the patient increases the intra-abdominal pressure, tissue can be felt de-

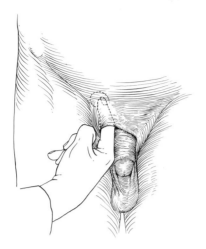

Figure 36—2. Insertion of finger through upper scrotum into external inguinal ring.

scending along the inguinal canal. This may be hernia contents in a sac or properitoneal fat (lipoma of the cord) in the presence of a hernia.

Compression over the internal ring when the patient strains will also help to differentiate between indirect and direct hernias. A direct hernia will bulge forward through Hesselbach's triangle while the thumb or opposite hand is covering the exit of an indirect hernia at the internal ring.

In children the only evidence of a hernia may be increased thickness of the processus vaginalis, which gives a sensation of silk sliding beneath the examining finger as it is rolled across the area of the pubic tubercle (silk purse sign).

Differential Diagnosis

Herniation of properitoneal fat through the inguinal ring into the spermatic cord is commonly misinterpreted as a hernia sac. Its true nature may only be confirmed at operation. Occasionally, a femoral hernia that has extended above the inguinal ligament after passing through the fossa ovalis femoris may be confused with an inguinal hernia. If the examining finger is placed on the pubic spine, the neck of the sac of a femoral hernia lies lateral and below, while that of an inguinal hernia is medial and above.

Indirect inguinal hernia must be differentiated from hydrocele of the spermatic cord, lymphadenopathy or abscesses of the groin, varicocele, and residual hematoma following trauma or spontaneous hemorrhage in patients taking anticoagulants. Undescended testis in the inguinal canal must also be considered when the testis cannot be felt in the scrotum.

Treatment

Indirect inguinal hernias should always be repaired unless there are specific contraindications. The same advice applies to patients of all ages; the complications of incarceration, obstruction, and strangulation are greater threats than are the risks of operation.

Small asymptomatic direct hernias do not require treatment because they rarely incarcerate or strangulate. However, the funicular type of direct hernia, which comes through a small defect in the transversalis fascia, has the same risks as an indirect hernia and should be repaired. Usually it is difficult or impossible to differentiate a funicular type of direct hernia from an indirect hernia until it is exposed at operation. Symptomatic or progressively enlarging direct hernias should be repaired.

Because of the possibility of strangulation, an incarcerated painful or tender hernia usually requires an emergency operation. In certain patients who have serious concomitant disease, nonoperative reduction of the incarcerated hernia may be attempted under carefully controlled conditions. The patient may be placed with hips elevated and given analgesics and sedation sufficient to promote muscle relaxation. If the hernia mass reduces with gentle manipulation, repair of the hernia may be deferred if there is no clinical evidence of strangulated bowel. If strangulation has occurred, it is usually clinically evident. However, there is always the possibility that gangrenous tissue has been reduced into the abdomen by manual or spontaneous reduction of a Richter hernia.

A. Major Principles of Operative Treatment of Inguinal Hernia:

1. An indirect hernia sac should be anatomically isolated and dissected to its origin from the peritoneum, at which point it is ligated (Fig 36—3). In infants and young adults, the inguinal anatomy is normal

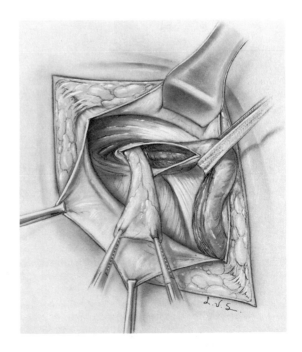

Figure 36—3. Indirect inguinal hernia. Inguinal canal opened showing spermatic cord retracted medially and indirect hernia peritoneal sac dissected free to above the level of the internal inguinal ring.

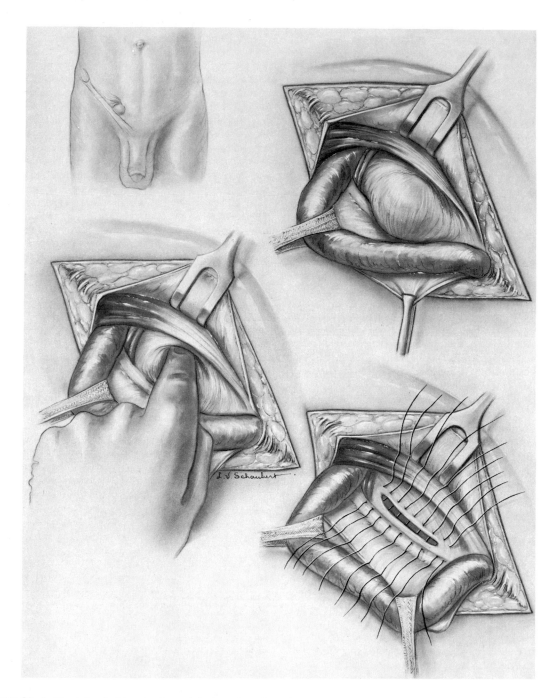

Figure 36—4. Direct inguinal hernia. *Upper left:* Location of hernia above inguinal ligament. *Upper right:* Bulging direct hernia covered with transversalis fascia and just below external oblique aponeurosis. *Lower left:* Direct hernia depressed. *Lower right:* Closure in direct hernia repair, suturing sound transversalis fascia medially to iliopubic band and to shelving edge of inguinal ligament laterally.

and repair can usually be limited to high ligation and removal of the sac and reduction of the internal ring to an appropriate size. For most adult hernias, it is necessary to reconstruct the inguinal floor. The internal ring should be reduced to a size just adequate to allow egress of the cord structures. In women, nothing important passes through the internal ring, so it can be totally closed, eliminating the chance of recurrence through that site. To construct a solid inguinal floor in men with recurrent hernias, it may occasionally be necessary to divide the cord and completely close the internal ring. The testicle may be removed or left in the scrotum.

2. If an incarcerated hernia has reduced spontaneously, one must decide whether to explore the abdomen to make certain that the intestine is viable. If dark or bloody fluid is present in the hernia sac or if clinical signs of peritonitis or leukocytosis are present, the abdomen should be explored. This may be performed through a separate vertical incision or through a muscle-splitting incision, high in the upper portion of the oblique inguinal incision.

3. The operative repair of a direct hernia requires judgment and experience since it involves reconstruction of an attenuated inguinal floor using nearby tissues. In direct inguinal hernia, the sac is usually not opened but instead is invaginated beneath the plane of the transversalis fascia with a series of sutures preliminary to reconstruction of that layer (Fig 36–4). A reconstruction limited to simple medial-to-lateral approximation of the edges of the transversalis fascia defect is more likely to disrupt than a repair that includes medial-to-lateral approximation of aponeurotic tissues. The latter is facilitated by a **relaxing incision** made vertically in the anterior rectus sheath adjacent to the reflection of the aponeurosis of the external oblique and extending upward from the pubic crest for about 6–7 cm. With the resulting increased mobility, the firm, fibrous lateral edge of the rectus muscle and sheath composed of fused portions of the internal oblique and transverse abdominal aponeurosis together with the underlying transversalis fascia can then be anchored without tension to Poupart's or Cooper's ligament. Critical to the success of the repair is the recognition that anatomic variations and changes secondary to attenuation of these structures require a careful assessment of the integrity of the tissues. Each case is slightly different from all others. The spermatic cord must be examined for the concomitant presence of an asymptomatic indirect inguinal hernia; a "recurrent" hernia may be nothing more than a previously overlooked indirect inguinal hernia.

4. When conventional repairs would involve reapproximating tissues under tension, alternative technics involving use of adjacent tissues or of implantation of prosthetic material can be used. Many materials have been used, either from the patient's own body (fascia lata) or of synthetic origin. At present the most commonly used material is Marlex mesh (polypropylene), which is sutured to the margins of available substantial aponeurotic tissue. Such foreign body implantation should be used in the first attempt at hernia repair only for very large direct hernias with marked attenuation of tissue. Marlex mesh implantation has been effectively utilized in the properitoneal type of hernia repair since the mesh avoids approximation of tissues under tension. In occasional older patients, the spermatic cord may be divided or resected to more effectively close Hesselbach's area and the internal ring.

5. In obese adults or those over 45–50 years of age, bilateral repair of indirect inguinal hernias should not usually be performed as one procedure since greater tension in the repairs increases the recurrence rate and surgical morbidity. The repair of direct hernias should also usually be staged. In children, bilateral hernia repair is the procedure of choice and spares the child a second anesthetic.

6. **Recurrent hernia** within a few months or a year of operation usually indicates an inadequate repair, such as overlooking an indirect sac or failure to close the transversalis fascia. Any repair completed under tension is subject to early recurrence. Recurrences 2 or more years after repair are more likely to be due to progressive weakening of the patient's fascia. Repeated recurrence after careful repair by an experienced surgeon suggests a defect in collagen synthesis. Because the fascial defect is so often small, firm, and unyielding, recurrent hernias are much more likely to develop incarceration or strangulation than unoperated inguinal hernias, and they should nearly always be repaired again.

If recurrence is due to an overlooked indirect sac, the posterior wall is often solid and removal of the sac may be all that is required. Occasionally, a recurrence is discovered to consist of a small, sharply circumscribed defect in the previous hernioplasty, in which case closure of the defect suffices. When recurrence involves failure of a previous hernioplasty, reconstruction by the Cooper's ligament technic sometimes gives the most solid repair. More diffuse weakness of the posterior inguinal wall or repeated recurrences often indicate the need for a more elaborate repair using fascia or polypropylene (Marlex) mesh.

B. Types of Operations for Inguinal Hernia: Successful repair requires that any correctable aggravating factors be identified and treated (chronic cough, prostatic obstruction, colonic tumor, ascites, etc) and that the defect be reconstructed with the best available tissues that can be approximated without tension. Different technics are designed to deal with variations in the size and location of a hernia and the extent of associated tissue weakness.

1. **Simple high ligation of the sac**—This is the procedure of choice for infants and children with an indirect hernia. Occasionally a large internal ring may need to be narrowed by suturing, but the cord and the conjoined tendon are not disturbed.

2. **Bassini repair**—The incision is made through a transverse skin crease or parallel to and above the inguinal ligament. The external oblique aponeurosis is incised in the direction of its fibers through the external ring to expose the underlying cord. The sensory

nerves (ilioinguinal and iliohypogastric) are protected, and the spermatic cord is dissected free from the inguinal floor up to the level of the internal ring. At that point the external spermatic vessels can be seen emerging from the inferior epigastric artery and vein where they branch out into the cremasteric muscle of the cord. If the internal ring is enlarged, its reconstruction can be facilitated by dividing and ligating the external spermatic vessels. The layers of the spermatic cord are opened through an anteromedial longitudinal incision to expose the underlying hernia sac. The latter is carefully dissected away from the adjacent vas deferens and internal spermatic vessels up to the neck of the sac and is then closed with a heavy suture. The redundant sac is removed. Transversalis fascia is sutured beneath the cord to the edge of the inguinal ligament, and the edges of the external oblique are reapproximated anterior to the cord. No weakness should be left in the area just superior to the pubic tubercle, so a direct hernia will not develop at this level.

3. Halsted repair—The Halsted repair utilizes the same principles of reconstruction of the inguinal floor as described above and differs from the Bassini repair in that the external oblique aponeurosis is sutured beneath the spermatic cord, placing the latter in a subcutaneous position. This repair has been advocated as especially suitable for certain direct hernias. The lower edges of the cremaster muscle and transversalis fascia are sutured to firm transversalis fascia, which must be mobilized beneath the conjoined tendon. Careful closure of any defect in the transversalis fascia is an essential feature of the repair of direct inguinal hernias.

4. Cooper's ligament (Lotheissen-McVay) repair—This operation is used by some surgeons to repair inguinal and femoral hernias. Transversalis fascia is approximated to Cooper's ligament on the iliopectineal line of the pubis. Mobility of these tissues is obtained with a relaxing incision in the anterior rectus sheath. The procedure effectively reconstructs Hesselbach's triangle and closes the femoral canal. At the medial border of the femoral vein a transition suture is placed, the medial tissues being sutured to the iliopubic band of the transversalis fascia and to the shelving edge of the inguinal ligament superficial to the superficial vein and artery; this suture is then continued laterally to restore the internal ring to an appropriate size in a manner comparable to that described for the Bassini repair. This operation requires the utmost care in protecting the femoral vein from compression or direct injury. Cooper's ligament is not elastic or resilient; thus, if sutures are placed under tension they are prone to tear or break. The Cooper ligament repair has been criticized as less functional than the Halsted or Bassini repair because tissues are sutured to a rigid and inelastic structure.

5. Shouldice repair—The Shouldice repair is similar to the Halsted-Bassini repair except in the method of closure of the transversalis fascia. The transversalis fascia, whether weak or strong, is divided longitudinally and the 2 flaps imbricated to Poupart's ligament. Then the conjoined tendon and internal oblique muscle are sutured in a double layer to the external oblique fascia just above the first suture line. The Shouldice repair assures a sound closure of the transversalis fascia. This method may be used for either direct or indirect hernias. The reported rates of recurrence are low.

6. Properitoneal (preperitoneal) repair—This operation is performed by an approach that exposes the hernial defect from behind. The properitoneal space is opened through a transverse lower abdominal incision about 4 cm above the inguinal ligament. The rectus sheath is incised at its lateral border, and the muscle is retracted medially so that the properitoneal space is visible. The transversalis fascia is incised transversely without entering the peritoneal cavity. This exposes the posterior wall of the inguinal canal and the area of herniation. Direct, indirect, and femoral hernia sacs can be seen and reduced by traction via this exposure. The hernial defects are then closed by approximating the margins of the defect with interrupted nonabsorbable sutures. This approach has the advantage of gaining direct access to the deepest layer of the hernial defect, particularly in recurrent hernias. The usual relaxing incision of the rectus sheath is not possible from this approach, and tension on the suture line may thus be excessive. The incidence of recurrence is substantially higher with the properitoneal method, and this method is rarely used today.

C. Nonsurgical Management (Use of a Truss): The surgeon is occasionally called upon to prescribe a truss when a patient refuses operative repair or when there are absolute contraindications to operation. A truss should be fitted and applied to provide adequate external compression over the defect in the abdominal wall. It should be taken off at night and put on again in the morning before the patient arises. The use of a truss does not preclude later repair of a hernia, although it may cause adherence and fibrosis of the anatomic structures so that operation may become more difficult.

Pre- & Postoperative Course

The preoperative evaluation is usually completed before hospitalization. The patient usually enters the hospital the night before the operation, is given a light evening meal, and the colon is evacuated either by enema or suppository. The choice of anesthetic is usually based upon the surgeon's and patient's preference and may be general, spinal, or local anesthesia. Local anesthetic is effective for most patients when supplemented by analgesia and enables the patient to strain on request during the procedure to facilitate evaluation of the tissues during the hernia repair. The incidence of urinary retention and pulmonary complications is lowest with local anesthesia. Recurrent hernias are more readily repaired under spinal or general anesthesia. The patient is usually discharged from the hospital as soon as he can walk comfortably (2–5 days). Advice regarding activity is based upon recognition that during the period of wound maturation the wound should be protected from sudden straining such as occurs with coughing or lifting. Patients who have attenuated tissues in the inguinal area are subject to early or late recurrence. The variables are too great to assume that every patient can resume early unlimited activity. A sedentary worker may return to work within a few days; one who must perform heavy manual labor should not work for up to 4–6 weeks.

Prognosis

The following conditions predispose to recurrence after any type of hernia repair, but most particularly in repairs of the plastic type: chronic cough, prostatism, poor tissue turgor (in particular, poor transversalis fascia), constipation, errors in operative technic (eg, use of absorbable suture material), and postoperative wound infection with or without wound dehiscence. The recurrence rate after hernioplasty can be minimized by preventing and treating these conditions. Recurrent inguinal hernias are always more difficult to repair than previously unoperated hernias, and they recur more frequently (10–20%).

A. Indirect Inguinal Hernia: The recurrence rate in adults following operative repair of indirect inguinal hernia should be less than 2–3%. In infants, children, and young adults the recurrence rate is negligible. Recurrence of indirect inguinal hernia is usually related to inadequate isolation and high ligation of the hernia sac or failure to reduce the internal inguinal ring to a small enough size. A direct or femoral hernia may develop following repair of an indirect inguinal hernia or may have been missed at the original operation (femoral hernia). Recurrence may also be due to inadequate strengthening of the inguinal floor during the original repair.

B. Direct Inguinal Hernia: The recurrence rate is higher for direct inguinal hernia than indirect hernia. It should be less than 10%. Recurrences of less than 1% have been reported following Shouldice repair. Recurrences of direct inguinal hernia are most often related to inadequate repair of the defect in the transversalis fascia. Incomplete operation for early asymptomatic direct hernias also leads to a high rate of recurrence. The recurrence rate following properitoneal repair is about 30%. The recurrence rate increases with each successive attempt; second operations for direct inguinal hernia have recurrence rates as high as 25% in some series. This is principally due to the extensive attenuation of available tissues that can no longer be approximated without tension.

Cerise EJ & others: The use of Mersilene mesh in repair of abdominal wall hernias. Ann Surg 181:728, 1975.

Condon RE, Nyhus LM: Complications of groin hernia and of hernial repair. Surg Clin North Am 51:1325, 1971.

Conner WT, Peacock EE Jr: Some studies on the etiology of inguinal hernia. Am J Surg 126:732, 1973.

Gibbon NOK, Choudhury A: Inguinal herniorrhaphy reduced to basic principles. Ann R Coll Surg Edinb 14:316, 1969.

Glassow F: Inguinal hernia repair: A comparison of the Shouldice and Cooper ligament repair of the posterior inguinal wall. Am J Surg 131:306, 1976.

Halverson K, McVay CB: Inguinal and femoral hernioplasty: A

22-year study of the authors' methods. Arch Surg 101:127, 1970.

Kauffman HM Jr, O'Brien DP: Selective reduction of incarcerated inguinal hernia. Am J Surg 119:660, 1970.

Licktenstein IL, Shore JM: Exploding the myths of hernia repair. Am J Surg 132:307, 1976.

Lyall D, Doumanen R: Richter's hernia. Am J Surg 75:828, 1948.

Lytle WJ: The deep inguinal ring: Development, function and repair. Br J Surg 57:531, 1970.

Madden JL, Hakim S, Agorogiannis AB: The anatomy and repair of inguinal hernias. Surg Clin North Am 51:1269, 1971.

McVay CB: The anatomic basis for inguinal and femoral hernioplasty. Surg Gynecol Obstet 139:931, 1974.

McVay CB: Inguinal hernioplasty: Common mistakes and pitfalls. Surg Clin North Am 46:1089, 1966.

Morris D & others: Early discharge after hernia repair. Lancet 1:681, 1968.

Myers RN, Shearbom EW: The problem of the recurrent inguinal hernia. Surg Clin North Am 53:555, 1973.

Palumbo LT, Sharpe WS: Primary inguinal hernioplasty in the adult. Surg Clin North Am 51:1293, 1971.

Ponka JL: Seven steps to local anesthesia for ilioinguinal hernia repair. Surg Gynecol Obstet 117:115, 1963.

Postlethwait RW: Causes of recurrence after inguinal herniorrhaphy. Surgery 69:772, 1971.

Rostad H: Inguinal hernia in adults. Recurrence rate related to suture material, recumbency period and anesthesia. Acta Chir Scand 134:49, 1968.

Scandalakis JE & others: The surgical anatomy of hernial rings. Surg Clin North Am 54:1227, 1974.

Shearburn EW, Myers RN: Shouldice repair for inguinal hernia. Surgery 66:450, 1969.

Smith RS: The use of prosthetic materials in the repair of herniae. Surg Clin North Am 51:1387, 1971.

Urbach KF & others: Spinal or general anesthesia for inguinal hernia repair? JAMA 190:137, 1974.

Wagh PV & others: Direct inguinal herniation in men: A disease of collagen. J Surg Res 17:425, 1974.

Williams JS, Hale HW: The advisability of inguinal herniorrhaphy in the elderly. Surg Gynecol Obstet 12:100, 1966.

Zimmerman LM: Recurrent inguinal hernia. Surg Clin North Am 51:1317, 1971.

2. SLIDING INGUINAL HERNIA
(Figs 36–5 and 36–6)

A sliding inguinal hernia is one in which the wall of a viscus forms a portion of the wall of the hernia sac. On the right side the cecum is most commonly involved, and on the left side the sigmoid colon. It is seen more commonly in men than in women and is more common on the left side than the right. The development of a sliding hernia is related to the variable degree of posterior fixation of the large bowel or other sliding components (eg, bladder, ovary) and their proximity to the internal inguinal ring. In effect, these structures can herniate through the internal ring without being completely covered by peritoneum.

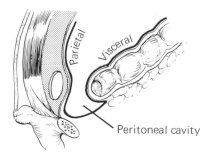

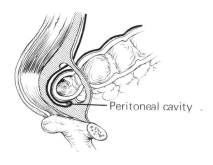

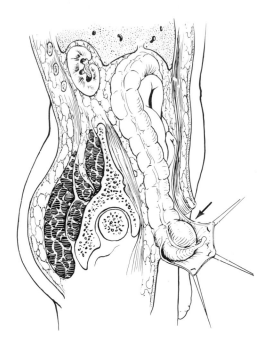

Figure 36—5. Right-sided sliding hernia. *Top:* Note cecum and ascending colon sliding on fascia of posterior abdominal wall. *Bottom:* Hernia has entered internal inguinal ring. Note that one-fourth of the hernia is not related to the peritoneal sac.

Figure 36—6. Right-sided sliding hernia seen in sagittal section. (After Linden in Thorek.) At arrow, the wall of the cecum forms a portion of the hernia sac.

Clinical Findings

Sliding hernias have no special signs that distinguish them from other inguinal hernias. However, they should be suspected whenever a large scrotal hernia is seen in an elderly man or with any large chronically incarcerated hernia. Finding a segment of colon in the scrotum on barium enema strongly suggests a sliding hernia. Recognition of this variation of hernia is of great importance at operation to avoid inadvertently entering the lumen of the bowel or bladder.

Treatment

The most important factor in treatment is recognition of the entity as one proceeds into the inguinal canal and opens the cremasteric fascia over the spermatic cord. As is true of all indirect inguinal hernias, the sac will lie anteriorly, but the posterior wall of the sac will be formed to a greater or lesser degree by colon.

The hernia is approached through the usual oblique inguinal approach. The inguinal canal is opened longitudinally, and the cord coverings are dissected free from the hernia sac. The Bevan technic is the best way to protect the blood supply to the viscus and to adequately eliminate the sac and the enlarged inguinal ring. An incision is made in the sac on either side of the sliding viscus up to the level of the internal ring. The cut edges of the peritonum attached to the viscus are then sutured together, and the viscus is returned to the abdomen. Next, the longitudinal defect

in the sac is sutured closed to recreate a complete sac free of viscus which is suture ligated at the level of the internal ring. The redundant sac distal to the ligature is excised, and one of the standard types of inguinal hernia repairs is performed.

A combined abdominal-inguinal approach (La Roque) has been described for sliding hernia but is more complex and rarely useful. With this method, the peritoneal cavity is entered through a separate incision and the sliding bowel is pulled back into the abdomen and fixed to the posterior abdominal wall. The hernia is then repaired in the usual fashion.

Prognosis

Sliding hernias have a higher recurrence rate than uncomplicated indirect hernias.

The surgical complications most often encountered following sliding hernia repair are encroachment on the circulation to the large bowel with bowel necrosis and actual strangulation of a portion of the large bowel when attempting a high ligation of the hernial sac.

Piedad OH & others: Sliding inguinal hernia. Am J Surg 126:106, 1973.
Ryan EA: An analysis of 313 consecutive cases of indirect sliding inguinal hernias. Surg Gynecol Obstet 102:45, 1956.

FEMORAL HERNIA

Clinical Findings

A femoral hernia may present in a variety of ways. If it is small and uncomplicated, it usually appears as a small bulge in the upper medial thigh just below the level of the inguinal ligament. Because the femoral hernia or its preceding properitoneal fat often takes a J course, the terminal end of the hernia may be found lying above the inguinal ligament where it may be mistakenly thought to be an inguinal hernia or a lymph node. If a femoral hernia incarcerates or strangulates, it is always irreducible. Strangulation of small bowel in a small femoral hernia frequently involves only part of the circumference of the bowel and does not completely obstruct its lumen (Richter hernia).

Differential Diagnosis

Femoral hernia must be distinguished from an inguinal hernia, a saphenous varix, and femoral adenopathy. A saphenous varix transmits a distinct thrill when the patient coughs, and it appears and disappears instantly when the patient stands or lies down—in contrast to femoral hernias, which are either irreducible or reduce gradually on pressure.

Complications

Femoral hernias are extremely prone to incarcerate and strangulate. In many cases pain is not referred to the groin, and on palpation there may be no local tenderness. Signs of small bowel obstruction in an elderly woman should always arouse suspicion of a strangulated femoral hernia even without localized pain or tenderness in the groin. A palpable mass in the inguinofemoral area with signs of obstruction of the small bowel makes laparotomy necessary.

Treatment

A. Principles: The principles of femoral hernia repair are as follows: (1) complete excision of the hernia sac, (2) the use of nonabsorbable sutures, (3) repair of the defect in the transversalis fascia which is responsible for the hernia, and (4) frequent use of Cooper's ligament since it gives a firm support for sutures and is at at the proper level for repair, forming the natural line for the attachment of the transversalis fascia.

B. Simple Repair: Through an inguinal incision, the aponeurosis of the external oblique is incised and the neck of the sac identified. The sac can sometimes be teased out of the canal after the investing layer of transversalis fascia is divided. However, in most cases it is best to open the peritoneum to examine the contents of the sac before manipulating it. The hernia may also have to be freed from adhesive attachments below the inguinal ligament. After reduction, the excess sac is cut away and the neck of the sac is closed well away from the femoral canal. The femoral ring can be closed by sutures that include the inguinal ligament and pectineus muscle, but most surgeons prefer to do a Cooper's ligament (Lothiessen-McVay) repair.

C. Complicated Repair: When the hernia is complicated by obstruction at the femoral ring and cannot be reduced back into the abdomen, the iliopubic tract and the lateral edge of Gimbernat's ligament must be incised cautiously to free up and reduce the hernia. If this is not enough to enlarge the neck of the femoral ring, the inguinal ligament may be divided over the neck of the sac. This is usually sufficient to allow reduction of the hernia mass back into the abdomen. It may be necessary to make an incision in the thigh in addition to the inguinal incision.

If the hernia sac and mass reduce when the patient is given opiates or anesthesia, and if bloody fluid appears in the hernia sac when it is exposed and opened, one must strongly suspect the possibility of nonviable bowel in the peritoneal cavity. In such cases it is mandatory to open and explore the abdomen, usually through a separate midline incision.

The possibility of the presence of an aberrant obturator artery (a branch of the external iliac rather than the internal iliac artery) running on the abdominal surface of Gimbernat's ligament near its sharp lateral edge is one of the reasons why great care must be exercised in cutting this ligament in order to release a femoral hernia strangulated at this level.

Prognosis

Recurrence rates are about the same as for direct inguinal hernia, ie, about 7–12%. The closing of the femoral ring by suture of the transversalis fascia to Cooper's ligament is the main factor in diminishing the number of recurrences.

Dunphy JE: The diagnosis and surgical management of strangulated femoral hernia. JAMA 114:354, 1940.

Lytle WJ: Femoral hernia. Ann R Coll Surg Engl 21:244, 1957.

McVay CB: Inguinal and femoral hernioplasty. Surgery 57:615, 1965.

McVay CB, Savage LE: Etiology of femoral hernia. Ann Surg 154:25, 1961.

OTHER TYPES OF HERNIAS

UMBILICAL HERNIAS IN ADULTS

The umbilical region occupies the most central area of the anterolateral abdominal wall. The area is of great interest because of the occurrence not only of umbilical hernias of various types but also of omphalocele and gastroschisis. A number of congenital anomalies related to fetal circulation, the fetal vitellointestinal duct, and the urachus present in this area.

Umbilical hernia in adults occurs long after closure of the umbilical ring and is due to a gradual yielding of the cicatricial tissue closing the ring. The hernia usually presents at the superior arc of the ring, its weakest area. It occurs in females about 10 times as often as in males.

Predisposing factors include (1) multiple pregnancies with prolonged labor, (2) the ascites of liver cirrhosis, (3) obesity, and (4) the presence, over a long period, of large intra-abdominal tumor masses.

Clinical Findings

In adults, umbilical hernia does not tend toward spontaneous reduction but usually increases steadily in size. The hernia may be covered with a very thin peritoneal sac, but in long-standing hernias the sac may thicken considerably. Its outer coverings are usually so stretched as to make the hernia appear to lie in a subcutaneous position. The hernia is often lobulated in appearance. The hernia sac frequently has multiple loculations. The chief content of umbilical hernias is usually an omental mass, but small and large bowel may be present. This hernia frequently becomes strangulated, and emergency operative procedures on it are common. The necks of the sacs of umbilical hernias are usually quite narrow when compared to the size of the herniated mass.

Umbilical hernias with tight rings and much herniated bowel often lead to chronic constipation and the recurrent cramping and nausea of subacute, incomplete bowel obstruction. Incarceration and strangulation are common. Very large umbilical hernias give a marked feeling of abdominal heaviness and frequently lead to backache.

Treatment

Umbilical hernia in an adult should be repaired as soon as possible after the diagnosis is made in order to avoid the necessity for emergency procedures for strangulation and incarceration. Surgical repair calls for preservation of the umbilical dimple (if possible) and a simple through-and-through fascial and peritoneal one-layer approximation.

Actually, the umbilical defect seldom involves the compartments of the rectus sheath but is a herniation through the attenuated linea alba. The best results in closure of the aponeurotic defect seem to follow suture in a transverse direction. Since the fibers of the sheaths of the 3 flat muscles of the abdominal wall run in a transverse direction as they make up the rectus sheath, transverse closure places sutures at right angles to the direction of the sheath fibers, which then are under less tension during increases in intra-abdominal pressure with respiration, defecation, etc.

Large umbilical hernia defects which cannot be closed without undue tension may be closed with an inlay of Marlex mesh.

Prognosis

Large size of the hernia, old age, debility of the patient, and the presence of any related intra-abdominal disease are factors which may forecast a high mortality and morbidity rate after surgical repair. In healthy individuals, surgical repair of the umbilical defects gives good results with a low rate of recurrence.

EPIGASTRIC HERNIA
(Fig 36–7)

An epigastric hernia is one that protrudes through the linea alba (the midline of the anterior abdominal wall) above the level of the umbilicus. The linea alba is formed by the midline interlacing of the anterior and posterior sheaths of the rectus abdominis muscles. It runs from the xiphoid process of the sternum to the symphysis pubica. In the upper third of the abdomen it is 1.25–3 cm wide and is fibrous, but as it approaches the umbilicus it narrows. Below the level of the umbilicus, it persists simply as a narrow fibrous cord. Deep to the linea alba are the transversalis fascia, some preperitoneal fat, and the peritoneum. Paired small blood vessels and nerves pierce the linea alba on either side of the midline.

There are 2 theories regarding the cause of epigastric hernia: (1) that the hernia develops through one of the foramens of egress of the small paramidline nerves and vessels and (2) that it develops through an area of congenital weakness in the linea alba. The latter view is supported by the observation that epigastric hernia occurs also in infants.

About 3–5% of the population have epigastric hernias. They are 3 times more common in men than in women and most common between the ages of 20–50. About 20% of epigastric hernias are multiple, and about 80% occur just to the left of the midline.

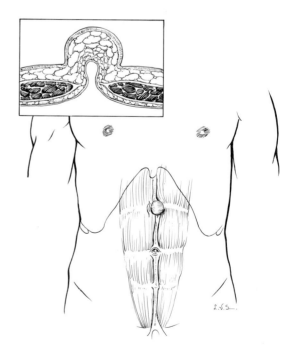

Figure 36–7. Epigastric hernia. Note closeness to midline and presence in upper abdomen. The herniation is through the linea alba.

Clinical Findings

The most common finding is a subcutaneous mass in the midline above the level of the umbilicus. Most are painless and unsuspected by the patient and are frequently found on routine abdominal examination. The smaller masses most frequently contain properitoneal fat only and are especially prone to incarceration and strangulation. These smaller hernias are therefore often tender. Larger hernias seldom strangulate and may contain, in addition to properitoneal fat, a portion of the nearby omentum and occasionally a loop of small or large bowel.

Symptoms of epigastric hernia are many and varied and present difficult problems in diagnosis. They may range from mild epigastric pain and tenderness to deep burning epigastric pain with radiation to the back or the lower abdominal quadrants. The pain may be accompanied by abdominal bloating, nausea, or vomiting. The symptoms are usually apt to occur after a large meal and on occasion may be relieved by reclining, probably because the supine position causes the herniated mass to drop away from the anterior abdominal wall.

The diagnosis is difficult to make in the presence of an obese abdomen, since in such circumstances the presenting epigastric mass is hard to palpate. If the mass is palpable, diagnosis can often be confirmed by any maneuver that will increase intra-abdominal pressure, thus causing the mass to bulge anteriorly. Lower esophageal and upper gastrointestinal x-rays as well as cholecystography may be needed to rule out disease in these organs.

If the upper abdominal diagnostic work-up is negative but the patient has persistent pain of the sort encountered with epigastric hernia, surgical exploration of the linea alba for a possible epigastric hernia may be warranted.

Differential Diagnosis

In differential diagnosis, one must consider peptic ulcer with possible penetration or perforation, gallbladder disease, hiatal hernia, pancreatitis, and upper small bowel obstruction. On occasion it may be impossible to distinguish the hernial mass from a subcutaneous lipoma, fibroma, or neurofibroma.

Treatment

If the epigastric hernia is symptomatic or if it is larger than 0.5 cm in diameter, surgical treatment is indicated. Repair may be done through a transverse incision with direct fascial closure to eliminate the defect. Herniated fat contents are usually dissected free and removed. Intraperitoneal herniating structures are reduced, but no attempt is made to close the peritoneal sac.

Many authors feel that a liberal vertical incision is preferable since it allows the surgeon to search for multiple epigastric hernias, which are occasionally present. The fascia is then closed in a vertical fascia-to-fascia manner. The vertical incision also allows for easy intra-abdominal exploration if indicated.

The operation is best performed under general anesthesia, and postoperative nasogastric suction is usually employed as paralytic ileus is a frequent postoperative complication. This may lead to a breakdown of the fascial repair as a result of pressure of the distended abdomen against the closure.

Prognosis

The recurrence rate is 15–20%. This is a higher incidence than with the routine inguinal or femoral hernia repair.

INCISIONAL HERNIA
(Ventral Hernia)

About 10% of all hernioplasties performed in large general hospitals are for repair of incisional hernias. Despite significant advances in operative technic, improved suture materials, better pre- and postoperative care, the use of reinforcing and "bridging" materials, antibiotics, etc, this iatrogenic type of hernia does not seem to be significantly decreasing in frequency. This may be partly because people are living longer so that geriatric surgery, with its high incidence of postoperative complications of all sorts, has become more frequent.

Causes & Prevention

A. Causes: Many factors contribute to the development of an incisional hernia. Any one may be the only factor responsible for the herniation, but when these causative factors are combined, the likelihood of postoperative wound weakness is greatly increased. The factors most often responsible for incisional hernia are as follows:

1. Age of the patient. Wound healing is usually slower and less solid in geriatric patients.

2. General debility of the patient. Cirrhosis, carcinoma, and chronic wasting diseases are major adverse factors that affect wound healing.

3. Obesity. Fat patients frequently have increased intra-abdominal pressure. The presence of fat in the abdominal wound masks tissue layers and makes for a high incidence of seromas and hematomas in wounds.

4. Postoperative wound infection.

5. Type of incision used. There is much argument concerning the placement of incisions. Many surgeons feel that transverse and oblique wounds are more apt to heal well than vertical ones.

6. Postoperative pulmonary complications that stress the repair from vigorous coughing, etc. These may be secondary to chronic pulmonary disease or anesthesia or may occur as a result of lying on the operating table or on the postoperative bed for long periods.

7. Placement of drains or colostomy or ileostomy openings in the primary operative wound.

8. Failure to use nonabsorbable suture material whenever possible and suitable.

9. Failure to observe the principles of proper preoperative and postoperative nutrition. Proper attention to protein nutrition and vitamin C is of particular importance.

10. Catabolism due to sepsis tends to slow wound healing.

B. Prevention: The major factors in prevention of incisional hernia are as follows:

1. Use transverse or oblique incisions when feasible.

2. Use nonabsorbable suture material in all clean wounds and in a large number of infected wounds as well.

3. Avoid undue tissue tension in wound closure.

4. Avoid dead space in wounds.

5. Ensure meticulous hemostasis.

6. Encourage weight reduction, if possible, before surgery.

7. Treat pulmonary disease before surgery and use positive pressure breathing apparatus after surgery.

8. Maintain fluid, electrolyte, and blood balance before surgery and during the postoperative period.

9. Place wound drains and colostomies and ileostomies away from the main incision whenever possible.

10. Protect wound edges, prepare the skin properly, and use prophylactic antibiotics judiciously if indicated (particularly in bowel surgery) to avoid wound infection.

11. Give cleansing enemas before surgery and initiate nasogastric intestinal suction postoperatively when indicated.

12. Use catheter drainage of bladder when indicated.

13. Use wire, heavy silk, or Dermalon retention sutures when indicated (elderly or debilitated patients, those with carcinoma, those with poor fascial and peritoneal tissues). These retention sutures should be placed 2–3 cm apart and should be tied loosely over bolsters.

14. Insist on early graded ambulation.

Early Dehiscence

Nearly all wound dehiscence is preceded by a period of serosanguineous wound drainage. This may vary in duration from a few hours to several days, but its presence is nearly always a sign of impending dehiscence and possible evisceration and the need for prompt reoperation (see Chapter 10).

In contrast to the above, a surgical wound may show no postoperative indications of discomfort or drainage but (suddenly or gradually) weakens either along its entire length or in a specific area. This is due to complete or partial failure of peritoneal or fascial closure. Clinically, this wound will bulge outward with or without pain during intervals of increased intra-abdominal pressure. This hernia nearly always gradually increases in size and may become painful or show signs of partial bowel obstruction. The incidence of incarceration and strangulation of intraperitoneal con-

tents in the wound is relatively high. These wounds often have one or 2 lengths of bowel or an area of omentum stuck to the peritoneal edge of the weakened area or areas.

Treatment

Incisional hernia should be treated by early repair. In addition to its unsightliness and the pain it causes, it is frequently the cause of bowel obstruction and is sometimes associated with chronic constipation. If the patient is unwilling to undergo surgery or is a poor surgical risk, the hernia should be supported by an elastic abdominal corset.

A. Small Hernias: Small incisional hernias usually present no difficulty in surgical repair. Many surgeons consider a direct fascia-to-fascia repair as sufficient for a satisfactory closure; others insist upon a separate peritoneal layer closure as an integral step in the repair.

B. Large Hernias:

1. Preparation before repair—The closure of a large incisional hernia defect may be difficult and painstaking. Many large ventral hernias cannot be returned to the abdominal cavity because the intraperitoneal space has decreased in size. The repair may be preceded by a series of injections of air into the peritoneal cavity (pneumoperitoneum) to elevate the diaphragm and generally increase the intraperitoneal space. A nasogastric tube placed before surgery is of assistance in closure.

2. Repair technic—Spinal anesthesia, because of its relaxant properties, is frequently used, although general anesthesia with the addition of muscle relaxants also gives excellent results. Excess and scarred skin and subcutaneous tissues over the hernia are removed. The hernia sac is then carefully dissected free from the underlying muscles and fascial tissues. The sac may be opened, particularly if there is incarceration or adhesion of intraperitoneal contents, in which case the abdominal contents are dissected free from the sac and dropped back into the abdomen. The excess sac is trimmed or, if there are no adherent intraperitoneal structures, it may be inverted (as in direct inguinal hernia) and the repair done over the inverted sac. As is true also of adult umbilical hernias of long standing, chronic ventral hernia tends to become loculated. It is essential to thoroughly clean the fascial layers about the defect to be repaired so that the closure will be a direct fascia-to-fascia repair.

Repair may be accomplished by directly approximating the fascial edges or by overlapping the fascia either in a transverse or lateral direction. The direct edge-to-edge approximation with strong nonabsorbable suture is probably strongest.

Nonabsorbable suture material (silk, cotton, or wire) should be used in all closures, and meticulous care should be given to hemostasis and the obliteration of dead space. Where a large dead space persists, a Hemovac type of drain should be employed. The patient's own tissue should always be used if the wound can be closed without tension. If the patient's own fascial tissues are not strong enough to guarantee a good closure—or if they may only be closed under tension—the use of Marlex mesh may be of help. This material may be placed directly over the peritoneal layer in a closure and serves as a bridge between good fascia on either side of the closure. The use of fascial relaxing incisions on either side of the main defect is occasionally of assistance in closure.

Defects too large to close easily are often better left without surgical repair if they are asymptomatic. The use of an abdominal support for 3–6 months after surgery may reduce the recurrence rate in ventral hernia repair.

Prognosis

The recurrence rate for incisional hernia repairs varies directly with the size of the defect to be closed. Small hernias have a recurrence rate of 2–5%; medium-sized hernias recur in 5–15% of cases; and large hernias, too often closed under tension, have a recurrence rate as high as 15–20%.

Ravitch MM: Ventral hernia. Surg Clin North Am 51:1341, 1971.

VARIOUS RARE HERNIATIONS THROUGH THE ABDOMINAL WALLS

Littré's Hernia

This consists of a herniation through one of the weak areas of the abdominal wall with a Meckel's diverticulum as the sole occupant of the hernial sac. It occurs more often on the right side, more often in femoral hernia, and more often in men.

Treatment consists of repair of the hernia (inguinal or femoral) plus, if possible, excision of the diverticulum. If acute Meckel's diverticulitis is present, the acute inflammatory mass may have to be treated through a separate abdominal incision.

Zuniga D, Zupanec R: Littré hernia. JAMA 237:1599, 1977.

Spigelian Hernia

This is a spontaneous ventral hernia through the linea semilunaris, the line where the sheaths of the lateral abdominal muscles fuse to form the lateral rectus sheath. Spigelian hernias are nearly always found above the level of the inferior epigastric vessels and caudal to the fold of Douglas. They usually occur where the semicircular fold of Douglas crosses the linea semilunaris, a weak point which may be further weakened by the passage of the inferior epigastric vessels.

Diagnosis is often difficult since the symptoms simulate those of lower quadrant abdominal disease and the hernia tends to migrate laterally between deep tissue layers. A cutaneous presentation of the mass may be indistinct or in some cases quite distant from the linea semilunaris. Strangulation is frequent.

Symptoms of Spigelian hernia are difficult to elicit. There is usually discomfort at the area of hernia protrusion. The pain is usually aggravated by exertion or by elevations of intra-abdominal pressure. Recumbency will often alleviate the pain. Nausea and vomiting are occasionally associated with the pain, and the overall picture may mimic lower gastrointestinal disease, gallbladder disease, ureteral disease, or disease of the pelvic organs. The diagnosis is most easily made with the patient standing and straining; a bulge then presents in the lower abdominal area which disappears on pressure with a gurgling sound. Following reduction of the mass, the hernial orifice can usually be palpated.

These hernias are quite easily cured by adequate aponeurotic repair. The inferior epigastric vessels may be ligated without adverse effects if they interfere with the closure.

Houlihan TJ: A review of Spigelian hernias. Am J Surg 131:734, 1976.

Lumbar or Dorsal Hernia (Fig 36–8)

These are hernias through the posterior abdominal wall at some level in the lumbar region. They may occur spontaneously or following trauma or a local inflammatory process. The most common sites (95%) are the superior and inferior (Petit's) lumbar triangles. The superior triangle of Grynfeltt-Lesshaft is larger and more often involved. A "lump in the flank" is the common complaint, associated with a dull, heavy, pulling feeling. With the patient erect, the presence of a reducible, often tympanitic mass in the flank usually makes the diagnosis. Incarceration and strangulation occur in about 10% of cases. They must be differentiated from abscesses, hematomas, soft tissue tumors, renal tumors, and muscle strain.

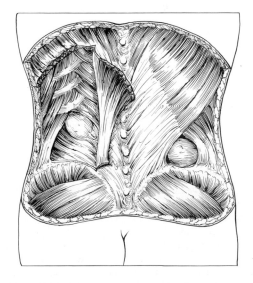

Figure 36–8. Anatomic relationships of lumbar or dorsal hernia. (Adapted from Netter.) On the left, lumbar or dorsal hernia into space of Grynfeltt. On the right, hernia into Petit's triangle (inferior lumbar space).

Acquired hernias may be traumatic or nontraumatic. Severe direct trauma, penetrating wounds, abscesses, and poor healing of flank incisions are the usual causes. Congenital hernias (rare) occur in infants and are not often associated with other congenital defects. They are due to a defect that weakens the dorsolateral abdominal walls and are usually unilateral.

Lumbar hernias increase in size and should be repaired when found. Repair is by mobilization of the nearby fascia and obliteration of the hernia defect by precise fascia-to-fascia closure.

Obturator Hernia

Herniation through the obturator canal at the upper border of the obturator membrane is more frequent in women and debilitated persons and is difficult to diagnose preoperatively. These hernias present as small bowel obstruction with cramping abdominal pain followed by nausea and vomiting. Pain or paresthesias caused by pressure on the obturator nerve may radiate to the anteromedial surface of the thigh.

The abdominal approach gives the best exposure, and these hernias should not be repaired from the thigh approach. The Cheatle-Henry approach (retropubic) gives excellent exposure. After a transverse suprapubic incision, the sheaths of the recti are split transversely, exposing the rectus abdominis and the pyramidalis muscles. The recti are separated and retracted laterally. The peritoneum is stripped off the ventrolateral abdominal wall, and the bladder is retracted dorsally to give direct visualization of the obturator foramen.

Gray SW & others: Strangulated obturator hernia. Surgery 75:20, 1974.
Jenner RE: Strangulated obturator hernia. Ann R Coll Surg Engl 56:266, 1975.

Perineal Hernia

Perineal hernia protrudes through the muscles and fascia of the perineal floor. It may be primary or acquired following perineal prostatectomy, abdominoperineal resection of the rectum, or pelvic exenteration.

These hernias are anterior or posterior to the transverse perineal muscle. They present as easily reducible perineal bulges and cause few symptoms. The anterior ones may cause dysuria; the posterior ones may cause difficulty in sitting. The perineal skin over the hernia may ulcerate.

Repair is usually done by a combined abdominal and perineal approach, with an adequate fascial and muscular perineal repair.

Interparietal Hernia

Interparietal hernias, in which the sac insinuates itself between the layers of the abdominal wall, are usually of an indirect inguinal type but rarely may be direct or ventral hernias. There are 3 anatomic groups, depending upon the location of the sac in the abdominal wall: (1) properitoneal, in which the sac lies between the peritoneum and the transversalis fascia; (2) inguinal-interstitial, in which the sac passes through the internal ring and becomes lodged between any of the muscle layers of the abdominal wall; and (3) inguinal-superficial, in which the sac passes through the external ring but dissects subcutaneously. Sometimes there are 2 sacs which are hourglass in shape: One occupies the usual position of an indirect hernia in the inguinal canal and the other extends laterally between the layers of the abdominal wall. There is always a common opening at the internal ring.

Although interparietal hernias are rare, it is essential to recognize them because strangulation is common and the mass is easily mistaken for a tumor or abscess. The lesion usually can be suspected on the basis of the physical examination provided it is kept in mind. In most cases, extensive studies for intra-abdominal tumors have preceded diagnosis. A lateral film of the abdomen will usually show bowel within the layers of the abdominal wall in cases with intestinal incarceration or strangulation.

As soon as the diagnosis is established, operation should be performed, usually through the standard inguinal approach.

Altman B: Interparietal hernia. In: *Hernia.* Nyhus LM, Harkins HN (editors). Lippincott, 1964.
Dunphy JE: Strangulated hernia. N Engl J Med 220:819, 1939.

Sciatic Hernia

This rarest of abdominal hernias consists of an outpouching of intra-abdominal contents through the greater sciatic foramen. The diagnosis is made after incarceration or strangulation of the bowel occurs. The repair is usually made through the abdominal approach. The hernia sac and contents are reduced, and the weak area is closed by making a fascial flap of the piriformis muscle.

INTERNAL HERNIAS

Internal hernias occur into a large fossa, fovea, or foramen. The 4 major internal hernias, all extremely rare, are (1) paraduodenal hernias, (2) hernias into the foramen of Winslow, (3) mesenteric hernias, and (4) omental hernias.

These hernias may cause chronic digestive complaints and acute or chronic intestinal obstruction.

Treatment is as follows: Attempt to reduce the hernia without opening the hernia sac, or open the anterior wall of the sac and divide any adhesions present. Perform needle decompression of dilated bowel if necessary. Reduce herniated bowel by pressure from within and traction from without. Close the hernial defect or resect the wall of the hernia area.

Great care should be taken not to injure major arteries or veins.

37 . . .
Adrenals

Thomas K. Hunt, MD

Operations on the adrenal glands are performed for hyperadrenocorticism (Cushing's disease or Cushing's syndrome), ectopic ACTH-producing tumors, primary hyperaldosteronism, pheochromocytoma, and, less commonly, other adrenocortical tumors. These conditions are usually characterized by hypersecretion of one or more of the adrenal hormones. Adrenalectomy is also sometimes useful in the management of metastatic breast and prostatic carcinoma.

Anatomy & Surgical Principles

The normal combined weight of the adrenals is 7–12 g. The right gland lies posterior and lateral to the vena cava and superior to the kidney (Fig 37–1). The left gland lies medial to the superior pole of the kidney, just lateral to the aorta, and immediately posterior to the superior border of the pancreas. An important surgical feature is the remarkable constancy of the adrenal veins. The right adrenal vein, 2–5 mm long and several millimeters wide, joins the anterior aspect of the adrenal gland to the posterolateral aspect of the vena cava. The left adrenal vein is several centimeters long and travels inferiorly from the lower pole of the gland, joining the left renal vein after receiving the inferior phrenic vein. The adrenal arteries are small, multiple, and inconstant.

The major principles of adrenal surgery are as follows:

(1) The diagnosis must be certain before operation is undertaken. The surgeon must be so confident of the preoperative diagnosis that he will conduct an exhaustive search if the expected pathologic picture is not found in the adrenal area. He must be prepared to take definitive action based on the preoperative diagnosis even if no visible lesion is found.

(2) Since the gross pathologic changes are often subtle, the surgeon must work with complete hemostasis and must be able to recognize even minor variations from normal.

(3) The patient must be carefully prepared so that he will be able to withstand the metabolic problems caused by his disease and the operation.

(4) The surgeon and his consultants must be able to detect and treat any metabolic crisis occurring during operation or afterward.

The anterior or transperitoneal approach through a long vertical midline incision or a bilateral subcostal incision is used for pheochromocytoma and is the approach of choice for most potentially bilateral diseases of the adrenals. This approach permits adequate exposure of most of the retroperitoneum. Unfortunately, the postoperative period is painful. Ileus is a problem, and the patient is exposed to the risks of poor healing such as evisceration. Poor wound healing is fairly common in patients with Cushing's syndrome (Table 37–1).

The posterior approach, performed through incisions on each side of the spine with the patient lying prone, is somewhat better tolerated postoperatively but gives only limited exposure. In this retroperitoneal operation, poor healing does not have the potential of evisceration. The posterior approach can be made through many incisions varying from transpleural to those through the bed of the 11th or 12th rib. The 12th rib incision is best tolerated by the patient and is best for small lesions whose location is known in advance. A lateral approach through the bed of the 12th rib, exposing the adrenals retroperitoneally, is useful for known unilateral conditions or for bilateral conditions in obese or very poor risk patients.

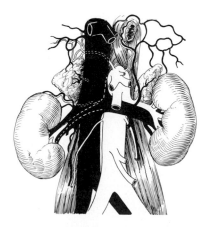

Figure 37–1. Anatomy of the adrenals showing venous return.

DISEASES OF THE ADRENALS

PRIMARY HYPERALDOSTERONISM

Essentials of Diagnosis

- Hypertension, polyuria, polydipsia, muscular weakness, tetany.
- Hypokalemia, alkalosis, renal damage.
- Elevated autonomous urine and plasma aldosterone levels and low plasma renin level.
- Tumors are usually too small to be seen by x-ray but can often be demonstrated by adrenal scan.

General Considerations

Primary hyperaldosteronism is renin-independent aldosterone hypersecretion in hypertensive, nonedematous patients. The syndrome was first recognized in the early 1950s by Conn, who found that it was usually caused by an adrenal tumor and could be cured by excision of the tumor. Almost all adenomas are unilateral, and most are 1–2 cm in diameter. They have a characteristic chromate-yellow color when sectioned. Adrenal adenoma is the cause in about 85% of cases. The other 15% are caused by bilateral nodular hyperplasia.

On examination by light microscopy, most adenomas appear to arise from the zona fasciculata, although the electron microscopic characteristics of the cells more closely resemble the zona glomerulosa. A few adenomas are multiple, occurring in the same gland or in both glands. About 15% of patients—particularly those with atypical clinical syndromes—have bilateral adrenal hyperplasia.

Aldosterone is the most potent mineralocorticoid hormone secreted by the adrenal cortex. Its major functions are to regulate the electrolyte composition of the body, the fluid volume, and the blood pressure. In contrast to other adrenal steroids, its major control is by the renin-angiotensin system.

Hyperaldosteronism can be classified as (1) primary hyperaldosteronism due to adrenal disease, usually tumor; (2) secondary hyperaldosteronism, usually in the hypertensive nonedematous patient; and (3) hyperaldosteronism in the edematous patient. Only primary hyperaldosteronism will be discussed here.

Clinical Findings

Hypertension and hypokalemia are the findings which most often lead to investigation of hyperaldosteronism.

A. Symptoms and Signs: The usual clinical symptoms are muscle weakness, polydipsia, nocturia, and headache. Carpopedal spasm and paresthesias sometimes occur from hypokalemic alkalosis. Hypertension is usually moderate and rarely malignant. The patient may have signs of advanced hypertension but rarely has severe retinopathy. Although extracellular fluid volume is usually larger than normal, edema is almost never seen until severe renal failure occurs. There are no other characteristic physical findings.

B. Laboratory Findings: One of the major sites of aldosterone action is in the distal nephron, where it facilitates the exchange of sodium for potassium and hydrogen ions whereby sodium is retained and potassium is lost. Therefore, when aldosterone secretion is chronically elevated, body potassium and hydrogen ion concentration fall (alkalosis), total body sodium rises, and hypertension eventually results. Thus, the most expedient way to identify patients with primary hyperaldosteronism is to demonstrate hypokalemia. This can be accomplished by salt-loading patients who are not taking diuretics or potassium with 2 g of sodium chloride during each meal for 4 days. If hypokalemia is provoked or if spontaneous hypokalemia occurs, measurement of urinary or plasma aldosterone is indicated.

In primary hyperaldosteronism, the plasma renin level is low. The diagnostic value of this finding, taken by itself, is somewhat limited because of the high incidence (25%) of reduced plasma renin activity in patients with essential hypertension. However, a high renin measurement, characteristic of hyperaldosteronism secondary to liver or renal disease, is of great value in eliminating the possibility of primary aldosteronism. In aldosteronism due to adrenal hyperplasia (as opposed to adrenal adenoma), renin values often are in an intermediate range.

Aldosterone secretion rates are high and autonomous, ie, they are not suppressed by fludrocortisone, desoxycorticosterone acetate (DOCA), or plasma volume expansion. Plasma aldosterone varies diurnally from a high at about 6 am to a low in the afternoon. The pattern is the same for cortisol. Normally, renin rises when the patient assumes the erect posture. The patient with adenoma will usually demonstrate a normal diurnal fall of plasma aldosterone between 6 am and 12 noon despite assuming the erect posture because the adenoma has gained autonomy from renin stimulation.

Differential Diagnosis

Secondary hyperaldosteronism in hypertensive patients can be caused by a number of disorders, particularly malignant hypertension, renovascular hypertension, and the recent use of diuretics or birth control pills. Consequently, patients who are taking estrogens (particularly birth control pills) must cease taking the medication for at least 2 months before valid measurements of renin or aldosterone can be made. Increased plasma renin activity also occurs with stress, pregnancy, diabetes, and alcohol intoxication.

Complications

Progressive cardiorenal failure secondary to hypertension is the most common complication. In rare cases, almost complete muscular paralysis occurs when serum potassium becomes very low. Patients with heart disease may have arrhythmias from hypokalemia, especially if they are taking digitalis. Stroke is a common and serious complication.

Treatment

A. Medical Treatment: The only cure for this disease is excision of hyperfunctioning adrenal tissue. Even so, unless hypokalemia or hypertension is unusually severe, there is little urgency about operation. Patients with mild disease can be managed with spironolactone and methyldopa, but the side-effects, particularly impotence, gynecomastia, and postural hypotension, are relatively severe. Escape from treatment is common.

B. Preoperative Care: Preoperative preparation is important since hypokalemic, alkalotic patients tend to develop serious cardiac arrhythmias under anesthesia. Antihypertensive medication should be discontinued for about 7 days unless hypertension is severe. Sodium is restricted, and potassium chloride (up to 120 mEq/liter/day in addition to regular diet) is administered in the immediate preoperative period until serum potassium is normal. If hypertension is severe, spironolactone or methyldopa can be continued.

C. Surgical Treatment: Operation is usually reserved for patients with adrenal adenoma. Patients with bilateral nodular hyperplasia are rarely cured by operation and sometimes are not even significantly benefited. Therefore, the preoperative distinction between hyperplasia and adenoma is important.

Hyperplasia usually does not produce a fully developed syndrome of hyperaldosteronism; one or more features are usually absent or present to only a minor degree. Furthermore, the normal circadian rhythm of aldosterone secretion is lost, ie, serum aldosterone is usually about the same throughout the day, and plasma aldosterone is renin-dependent and rises from 6 am to noon when the patient assumes the erect posture at 6 am and remains erect until noon (see Laboratory Findings).

The patient should be treated medically as long as less than about 150 mg of spironolactone daily controls the hypertension. If larger doses are required, an attempt should be made to localize the adenoma so that a unilateral exploration will be sufficient. However, bilateral exploration is often required. This procedure can be done through an anterior transabdominal approach, using a bilateral subcostal incision, or through a posterior retroperitoneal approach, using separate incisions to expose each adrenal. Most adenomas are found on the left side.

Localization of adenomas can often be accomplished by determining the plasma aldosterone levels in the right and left adrenal vein. A clear difference between the 2 sides is a reliable diagnostic finding, but a negative study does not necessarily rule out unilateral adenoma. Adrenal venography can be helpful but is difficult and relatively hazardous. [131]I-19 iodocholesterol scans can localize by a positive image adenomas which are larger than 7 mm in diameter. The small but appreciable incidence of multiple adenomas and the 10–20% incidence of hyperplasia often make bilateral adrenal exploration desirable if preoperative localization is not absolutely certain. The alternative is to risk the need of another operation to achieve cure.

Only 2 cases of aldosterone-producing heterotopic adrenocortical adenoma have been described; one was in the kidney and the other in the ovary.

Patients with carcinoma usually have very high or chaotic aldosterone levels, and carcinomas usually give no image on [131]I-19 iodocholesterol scan.

When hyperplasia is found at operation, bilateral total or subtotal adrenalectomy can be performed, leaving only a small remnant (about 30%) of the left gland. The right gland usually is totally removed; reoperations on the right adrenal gland are particularly hazardous because the gland remnant adheres to the vena cava. In a few patients, the glands will appear grossly normal on close inspection. Signs of hyperplasia are subtle and consist of a mealy appearance of the cortex and a rounded rather than sharp adrenal edge. The experienced surgeon can usually recognize hyperplasia and small adenomas before any tissue is removed. If both adrenals appear normal, subtotal or total adrenalectomy must be done. Obviously, the surgeon must be absolutely confident of the diagnosis before undertaking this operation.

D. Postoperative Care: Unilateral adrenalectomy does not require administration of corticosteroids pre- or postoperatively. The patient generally comes to operation with increased total body salt and hypervolemia. Blood losses are small; therefore, no more than normal water needs must be given in the postoperative period, and saline is not usually necessary. Large amounts of saline may cause bladder decompensation and atelectasis. Potassium is also rarely indicated.

Rarely, glucocorticoid deficiency has followed unilateral adrenalectomy. A few patients have temporary aldosterone deficiency because the normal adrenal gland has been suppressed by the hyperfunctioning adenoma. The signs of hypoaldosteronism are continuing weight loss, undue fall in blood pressure, and hyperkalemia. In these cases it is usually necessary to give fludrocortisone, 0.1 mg/day orally, until the other adrenal gland has regained its ability to secrete aldosterone. The problem arises about a week after operation. The patient can usually be weaned from this drug within a month after operation.

For adrenocortical steroid maintenance therapy after total adrenalectomy, see Hyperadrenocorticism.

Prognosis

In some cases, blood pressure does not fall until 1–6 months after resection of an adenoma. However, if an obvious adenoma was removed, the response is usually excellent. When hyperplasia is the cause, a drop in blood pressure may occur but the patient usually retains some hypertension and may need medical treatment. The response usually parallels the preoperative response to spironolactone.

Weakness from hypokalemia is sometimes so severe and intractable that operation is desirable for relief of symptoms.

Pure hyperaldosteronism is almost always due to a benign adenoma, and the prognosis is excellent. The uncommon adrenal malignancies are rarely curable.

Hyperaldosteronism usually follows a prolonged and subtly changing course. In untreated cases, death may result from stroke and cardiac and renal failure.

Ferriss JB & others: Results of adrenal surgery in patients with hypertension, aldosterone excess, and low plasma renin concentration. Br Med J 1:135, 1976.

Hogan MJ & others: Location of aldosterone-producing adenomas with [131]I-19-iodocholesterol. N Engl J Med 294: 410, 1976.

Hunt TK & others: Selection of patients and operative approach in primary aldosteronism. Ann Surg 182:353, 1975.

Mills IH: Primary hyperaldosteronism. Clin Endocrinol Metabol 3:593, 1974.

Morris DJ, Davis RP: Aldosterone: Current concepts. Metabolism 23:473, 1974.

Schambelan M & others: Circadian rhythm and effect of posture on plasma aldosterone concentration in primary aldosteronism. J Clin Endocrinol Metab 43:115, 1976.

Yune HY & others: Radiology in primary hyperaldosteronism. Am J Roentgenol Radium Ther Nucl Med 127:761, 1976.

PHEOCHROMOCYTOMA

Essentials of Diagnosis

- Episodic headache, visual blurring, severe sweats, vasomotor changes in a young adult, weight loss.
- Hypertension, often paroxysmal but frequently sustained; cardiac enlargement.
- Postural tachycardia and hypotension.
- Elevated urinary catecholamines or their metabolites.

General Considerations

Pheochromocytomas are tumors of the adrenal medulla and related chromaffin tissues elsewhere in the body which release epinephrine or norepinephrine (or both), resulting in sustained or episodic hypertension and other symptoms of excessive catecholamine secretion.

Pheochromocytomas may occur sporadically in patients with no other disease or in patients with Sipple's syndrome (MEA II). In the latter case, pheochromocytomas are often bilateral and associated with medullary carcinoma of the thyroid, hyperparathyroidism, neurofibromatosis, and ganglioneuromatosis.

On pathologic examination, these tumors are quite uniform. They are reddish-brown and vascular. They feel firm but may be multicystic. Cells in any single tumor vary in size and shape. The cytoplasm is finely granular. Nuclei are round or oval, with prominent nucleoli. Mitoses are frequent, and necrotic areas are common. Ganglion-like cells are often seen. Veins and capsules may be invaded, even in clinically benign tumors. Size varies widely from a few grams to 3600 g, more than twice the size of the normal adult liver. The average is about 100 g. The only reliable signs of malig-

nancy are the presence of metastases and infiltrative invasion of surrounding tissues.

Clinical Findings

A. Symptoms and Signs: The clinical findings of pheochromocytoma are so variable that some recommend investigation for pheochromocytoma in all patients with newly discovered hypertension regardless of symptoms. Nevertheless, pheochromocytoma is a rare disease, making up perhaps 0.5% of all hypertensives. The classic symptoms are episodic hypertension associated with pallor and subsequent flushing, palpitations, headache, excessive perspiration, nervousness, and anxiety. An important feature is the triad of palpitations, headache, and sweating occurring simultaneously. The symptoms are what one would expect from an injection of epinephrine. The physical examination is usually unremarkable unless the patient is observed during an attack.

Pheochromocytomas can, and usually do, cause *sustained* hypertension with or without obvious manifestations of excessive catecholamine secretion. In this case, the usual signs are tachycardia, retinopathy, signs of hypermetabolism, emotional lability, and weight loss. Clinical findings may mimic hyperthyroidism even to the point of exophthalmos. Excess secretion of epinephrine raises blood glucose and therefore may mimic diabetes mellitus.

Pheochromocytomas in adults are usually benign. Multiple tumors are present in about 10% of cases. In children, hypertension is less prominent, and about 50% of children have multiple or extra-adrenal tumors. Malignancy is also a more common occurrence in children than in adults.

B. Laboratory Findings: The laboratory plays a very important part in the diagnosis. Urinary 3-methoxy-4-hydroxymandelic acid (VMA) and metanephrine determinations are useful for screening. If these are positive, urinary assay for the individual catecholamines, epinephrine and norepinephrine, is indicated. Direct measurement of elevated epinephrine and norepinephrine in the urine or blood is the key to diagnosis.

"Normal" values for catecholamines are difficult to define. Minor degrees of stress will considerably elevate catecholamines in a normal person, even to the levels seen in some patients with intermittently secreting tumors.

Suppression or excitation tests are rarely necessary. *All excitation or suppression tests are hazardous and should be used only if essential for diagnosis.* If they must be done because of equivocal laboratory findings, the glucagon test is the safest method of stimulation and phentolamine (Regitine) the safest and most definitive method of suppression. In a sustained hypertensive crisis, cautiously used phentolamine can be both diagnostic and therapeutic.

As soon as the diagnosis is made, medical treatment of hypertension should be started before further diagnostic tests are performed.

C. X-Ray Findings: X-ray findings include a solid

tumor or displacement of a kidney shadow, both of which are often detectable on plain films of the abdomen. Nephrotomograms obtained during an intravenous urogram may show displacement of a kidney and an adrenal mass. Arteriograms are indicated in most patients and show prominent feeding vessels and a tumor blush. Since the procedure can precipitate a hypertensive crisis, arteriography should not be done until good medical control of the blood pressure has been achieved.

Differential Diagnosis

The differential diagnosis includes all causes of hypertension. Hyperthyroidism and pheochromocytoma have many features in common. The differential diagnosis is easier if episodic hypertension is present. Acute anxiety attacks mimic the symptoms, but anxiety rarely produces severe hypertension. Labile essential hypertension is ruled out when clearly elevated catecholamine levels are detected.

Carcinoid syndrome may be mistaken for pheochromocytoma. In taking the history and making the differential diagnosis, remember that the pheochromocytoma attack mimics the symptoms of an injection of epinephrine.

Mild cases may be very difficult to diagnose. In labile hypertension, blood or urinary catecholamine levels should be checked several times during episodes of hypertension before the possibility of pheochromocytoma is discarded.

Hypertension in pregnancy is usually ascribed to preeclampsia-eclampsia. Unfortunately, a number of cases of pheochromocytoma, some of them fatal, have occurred in pregnant women.

Complications

Complications of pheochromocytoma are usually the sequelae of hypertension, ie, stroke, renal failure, myocardial infarction, and cardiac decompensation. Sudden ventricular arrhythmia from catecholamines is probably responsible for many deaths. The patient with pheochromocytoma usually has a blood volume deficit due to sustained vasoconstriction which is not clinically manifest as long as the vasoconstriction is maintained. When the excess catecholamines are removed, as during an operation, the blood volume can suddenly be inadequate. In patients not treated preoperatively with alpha-adrenergic blocking agents, postoperative hypotension is common, requiring catecholamine infusion or blood volume expansion to maintain tissue perfusion.

The major complication of pheochromocytoma—and one of considerable significance to the surgeon—is multifocal myocardial lesions, which can be duplicated experimentally by infusion of catecholamines. This cardiac damage produces a cardiomyopathy which can easily complicate operation.

Treatment

A. Medical Treatment: *Treatment with alpha-adrenergic blocking agents should be started as soon as the biochemical diagnosis is established.* The aims of preoperative therapy are (1) to restore the blood volume, which has been depleted by excessive catecholamines, and (2) to relieve the patient of the danger of a severe attack with its potential complications. Blood volume is characteristically decreased about 15% in pheochromocytoma. Close control of hypertension is necessary in order to keep blood volume normal. Even 15 minutes of hypertension due to release of catecholamines can significantly reduce blood volume.

Phentolamine (Regitine) and phenoxybenzamine (Dibenzyline) are the most frequently used drugs. Phentolamine has been effective in doses up to 600 mg/day orally, but it must be given every few hours. Because of its longer action, phenoxybenzamine, 20–50 mg orally once daily, is now preferred. These drugs have complex actions and may be dangerous.

Propranolol (Inderal), a beta-adrenergic blocking agent, is often useful when cardiac arrhythmias and severe tachycardia are prominent features of the disease but should only be given after the patient has received an alpha-blocker. Otherwise, a hypertensive crisis may occur. Sedatives and tranquilizers are also useful in treating the very real anxiety that often accompanies pheochromocytoma.

Once treatment is established, localization by angiography is safe and useful. Tumors are located by the characteristic enlargement of feeding vessels and tumor blush. Tomography in conjunction with intravenous urography will localize large tumors. Extra-adrenal tumors lack the methylating enzyme needed to convert norepinephrine to epinephrine. Hence, they often secrete norepinephrine (Fig 37–2). When epinephrine levels are elevated, the tumor is almost always in or near the adrenal area. In any case, 90% of pheochromocytomas in adults are in the adrenal areas. Thus, if the tumor secretes epinephrine, aggressive attempts to localize it preoperatively are not required. However, all patients should have a chest x-ray and neck palpation to rule out an extra-abdominal tumor.

B. Surgical Treatment: The definitive treatment

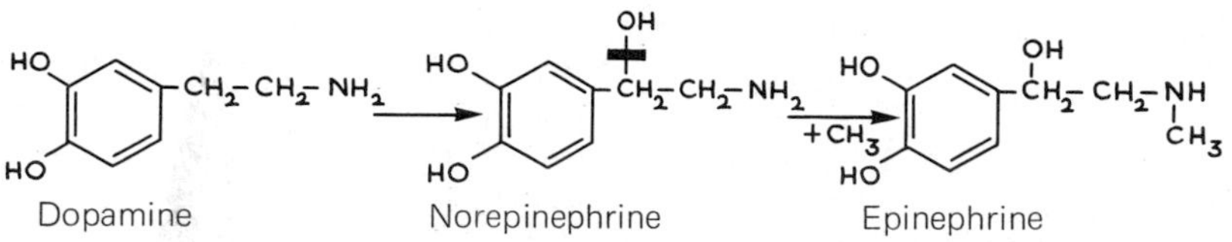

Figure 37–2. Sequence of catecholamine synthesis from dopamine. The more primitive extra-adrenal pheochromocytomas lack the methylating enzyme necessary to convert norepinephrine to epinephrine. Thus, when norepinephrine levels are high and epinephrine levels are normal or low, extra-adrenal tumor becomes a good possibility.

of pheochromocytoma is excision. In most cases, the tumor is relatively small and is confined to the adrenal area. The transabdominal approach is almost always used unless the tumor has been localized elsewhere. If multiple tumors are present, they are more likely to be found by the transabdominal approach.

The anesthesiologist should use an arterial catheter and ECG for constant monitoring of arterial pressure and heart action. Phentolamine and propranolol should be immediately available to treat sudden hypertension or cardiac arrhythmias which often occur when the tumor is manipulated. The surgeon usually tries early in the procedure to divide the major veins draining the tumor to avoid these crises. Most anesthesiologists use nitrous oxide and muscle relaxants for anesthesia, although many other agents have been recommended.

The major surgical problems arise in excising large malignant tumors and in detecting multiple and ectopic tumors. Both adrenals should be explored thoroughly before the operation is concluded. About 10% of tumors will be multiple or bilateral (a larger percentage in children). About 7% will be malignant. Extra-adrenal pheochrome tumors are usually found along the abdominal aorta and in the organ of Zuckerkandl. However, tumors have been reported in widely scattered sites such as the genital organs, the mediastinum, the neck, and even the skull.

The well-prepared patient seldom needs treatment with drugs during surgery, and the well-prepared surgeon seldom fails to find all the functioning tumor. It is best to pretreat the patient in such a way that he still develops a pressor reaction to manipulation of the tumor at surgery since this facilitates detection of ectopic and multiple tumors. Blood pressure will almost always fall when all functioning tissue has been removed. If the patient has been properly prepared with alpha-blockers, the pressure fall will not be severe.

Prognosis

The outlook for patients with untreated pheochromocytoma is grim. The operative mortality rate has dropped to less than 5% since the introduction of drug therapy, but it is higher for malignant tumors. Second tumors in the remaining adrenal have been reported to occur years after excision of the primary pheochromocytoma. The results of surgery for benign disease are most gratifying.

The outlook for the few patients with malignant tumors is variable. Some have had long symptom-free intervals after the tumor was excised. X-ray therapy will sometimes control symptoms caused by metastases. Blocking agents can give good palliation, but death usually occurs a short time after the appearance of metastases.

ReMine WH & others: Current management of pheochromocytoma. Ann Surg 179.740, 1974.

Scott HW Jr & others: Pheochromocytoma. Ann Surg 183:587, 1976.

Sebel EF & others: Responses to glucagon in hypertensive pa-

tients with and without pheochromocytoma. Am J Med Sci 267:337, 1974.

Sturman MF & others: Radiocholesterol adrenal images for the localization of pheochromocytoma. Surg Gynecol Obstet 138:177, 1974.

Van Way CW & others: Pheochromocytoma. Curr Probl Surg, June 1974.

Wolf RL: Phaeochromocytoma. Clin Endocrinol Metabol 3:609,' 1974.

HYPERADRENOCORTICISM
(Cushing's Disease & Cushing's Syndrome)

Essentials of Diagnosis

- Buffalo hump, obesity, easy bruisability, psychosis, hirsutism, purple striae, acne, impotence or amenorrhea, and moon facies.
- Osteoporosis, hypertension, glycosuria.
- Elevated, autonomous 17-hydroxycorticosteroids, low serum potassium and chloride, low total eosinophils, and lymphopenia.
- Special x-ray studies and scans may reveal a tumor or hyperplasia of the adrenals.

General Considerations

Cushing's syndrome is due to an excess of cortisol and corticosterone. It may be caused by bilateral adrenal hyperplasia from increased stimulation by ACTH (corticotropin) or ACTH-independent adrenocortical tumors. Excess ACTH may be produced by pituitary overactivity, pituitary tumors (Cushing's disease), or extrapituitary ACTH-producing tumors. Cushing's syndrome not dependent on ACTH may be caused by an autonomous adrenocortical adenoma or carcinoma.

Table 37—1. Estimated frequency of manifestations of hyperadrenocorticism.

	Percentage
Obesity	90
Hypertension	80
Evidence of diabetes with normal fasting blood glucose	80
Centripetal distribution of fat	80
Weakness	80
Muscle atrophy in upper and lower extremities	70
Hirsutism	70
Menstrual disturbance or impotence	70
Purple striae	70
Plethoric facies	60
Osteoporosis	50
Easy bruisability	50
Acne or skin pigmentation	50
Mental changes	50
Edema	50
Headache	40
Poor wound healing	40
Leukocytosis with lymphopenia	Frequent

Females predominate by a ratio of 10:1. The peak incidence is in the third and fourth decades, although the span ranges from infancy to the eighth decade. The natural history varies widely from a mild, indolent disease to rapid progression and death. The diagnosis is complex, and the choice of treatment often depends on a precise clinical and biochemical appraisal.

Clinical Findings

A. Symptoms and Signs: (Table 37–1 and Fig 37–3.) The classic description of Cushing's syndrome includes truncal obesity, hirsutism, moon facies, acne, buffalo hump, purple striae, hypertension, and diabetes, but other signs and symptoms are common. The most striking single feature is weakness. Weakness and the other features are also seen after prolonged and excessive administration of adrenocortical steroids or ACTH. Pituitary tumors and tumors producing ectopic ACTH usually secrete melanotropins (MSH) as well as ACTH. Therefore, increased skin pigmentation is an important feature of Cushing's syndrome due to excess ACTH.

As in other diseases of the adrenals, the syndrome is somewhat different in children, the most consistent finding being cessation of growth. The most common cause in children is malignant adrenal tumor, but benign tumors and bilateral hyperplasia have been described.

For the surgeon, some of the important findings are obesity (which only rarely surpasses 90 kg [200 lb]) and muscular weakness, both of which have predictive value in relation to the likelihood of postoperative pulmonary difficulties. Other important fea-

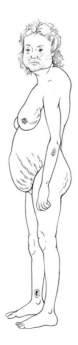

Figure 37–3. Major clinical features of Cushing's syndrome. The masculinization is not always present.

tures are acne and diabetes, which indicate susceptibility to infection; and atrophic skin and easy bruisability, which forecast a difficult operation and poor wound healing.

B. Pathologic Examination: The pathologic features of the adrenal gland vary widely. The gross changes in adrenal hyperplasia may be subtle. Adrenal weights vary from normal (7–12 g combined weight) to as much as 70 g for both glands combined; the usual combined adrenal weight in hyperadrenocorticism is below 25 g.

The pituitary tumors responsible for many cases of adrenal hyperplasia are usually benign and may be basophilic, acidophilic, or chromophobic.

Adrenal adenomas in Cushing's syndrome range in weight from a few grams to over 100 g and are usually larger than aldosterone-producing adenomas. The typical cells usually resemble those of the zona fasciculata. Variable degrees of anaplasia are seen, and differentiation of benign from malignant tumors is often difficult. They are very rare in males.

Adrenal malignancies are frequently highly undifferentiated and spread by direct invasion or via the blood stream. When they invade surrounding structures, they are technically difficult to remove.

In a few cases, ectopic adrenal tissue has been the source of excessive cortisol secretion. This tissue has been found in a wide variety of locations, but most commonly is near the abdominal aorta.

Occasionally, the disease is caused by a nonendocrine, ACTH-secreting neoplasm. By far the most common example is cancer of the lung, but it has also been associated with tumors of the pancreas, thymus, thyroid, prostate, esophagus, colon, and other organs.

Cushing's syndrome sometimes results from ovarian tumors. These are usually malignant and are associated with adrenal hyperplasia and consequently represent a form of ectopic ACTH syndrome.

C. Laboratory Findings: The diagnosis is difficult. Since no one test is specific, a combination of facts must be assembled. Normal subjects have a daily rhythmic variation of plasma ACTH which is paralleled by cortisol secretion. Levels are highest in the morning and decline during the day to their lowest in the evening. Normal variation is responsible for the inexactness of many of the tests. Taking circadian rhythms into account increases the precision of analysis. In Cushing's disease, the circadian rhythm is abolished and total secretion of cortisol is increased. In mild cases, the plasma cortisol and ACTH levels may be within the generally accepted limits of normal during much of the day, but if serial tests are done, levels will be seen to be abnormally high during at least part of the day. The excessive cortisol production elevates plasma and urinary free cortisol, 17-hydroxycorticosteroids, and 17-ketogenic steroids. Therefore, the 24-hour urine free cortisol is one of the most discriminating tests available.

When Cushing's syndrome is suspected, the first objective is to establish the diagnosis—the second is to establish the cause. An algorithm for the diagnosis is

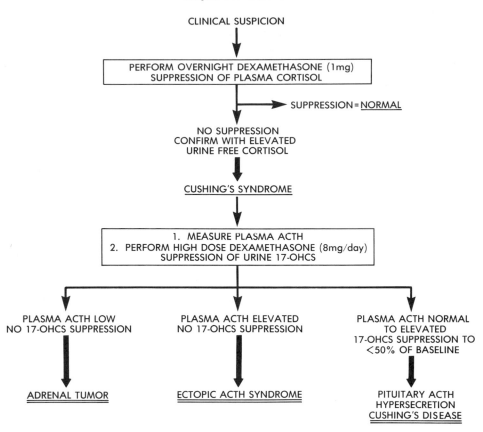

Figure 37—4. Cushing's syndrome: diagnosis and differential diagnosis.

presented in Fig 37—4. When hyperadrenocorticism is suspected, an overnight **dexamethasone suppression test** is the best first diagnostic step. Unstressed normal subjects produce about 30 mg of cortisol a day. Dexamethasone, 1 mg orally (equivalent to about 30 mg of cortisol), will suppress ACTH secretion, and cortisol production will cease in normal subjects. This amount of dexamethasone, however, will not suppress excessive cortisol production from autonomous adrenocortical tumors or adrenals which are being driven by excess of ACTH secretion. Since 1 mg of dexamethasone contributes almost nothing to the plasma cortisol level, suppression of endogenous circulating cortisol is easily demonstrated. The test is done as follows: At exactly 11:00 pm, the patient is given 1 mg of dexamethasone and 100 mg of pentobarbital by mouth. The sedation ensures an unstressed night's rest. A fasting plasma sample for cortisol determination is drawn the following morning. A basal plasma sample (drawn previously) is required for evaluating suppression if the patient is receiving estrogen therapy. Normal women receiving estrogen (birth control pills, etc) will have increased cortisol-binding globulin and thus will have a high basal plasma cortisol level. In normal and obese subjects, the morning plasma cortisol level will be suppressed to less than 5 μg/100 ml by dexamethasone. Normal individuals who are taking estrogens will suppress more than 50% below basal. Patients with Cushing's syn-

drome will not suppress below 12 μg/100 ml. Absence of suppression indicates fixed production of ACTH or cortisol, ie, Cushing's syndrome. Partial suppression may occur in patients with thyrotoxicosis or acromegaly, chemically suppressed patients, and patients who are chronically ill or under chronic physical stress. These conditions are almost always clinically obvious.

The results of the dexamethasone test can be confirmed with a measurement of 24-hour urinary excretion of free cortisol. It directly measures the physiologically active form of circulating cortisol, integrates the daily variations of cortisol production, and is the most sensitive and reliable means of diagnosing Cushing's syndrome. Free urinary cortisol excretion will exceed 120 μg/24 hours only in hyperadrenocorticism.

If the plasma cortisol level does not suppress and the urinary free cortisol is elevated, the patient has Cushing's syndrome. The next step is to determine the cause. **Plasma ACTH** measurement by radioimmunoassay is the most direct method. A very high ACTH level is diagnostic of hypercortisolism due to pituitary adenoma or ectopic ACTH secretion. The adrenal lesion will then be bilateral nodular hyperplasia. Very low ACTH levels are diagnostic of hypercortisolism due to adrenal adenoma or carcinoma. Unfortunately, the state of plasma ACTH radioimmunoassay is such that only very high and very low levels can be reliably determined. Therefore, another test may be required.

The **24-hour dexamethasone suppression test** is the one most likely to clarify the problem. It is useful for noncushingoid patients suspected of having Cushing's disease when cortisol suppression is incomplete. Eight milligrams of dexamethasone are given over 24 hours. After the suppression period, 24-hour urine collection for urinary 17-hydroxycorticosteroids is done. In normal persons, 17-hydroxycorticosteroid output will be suppressed to below 4 mg/24 hours. In patients with Cushing's disease, there is no suppression.

The algorithm shown in Fig 37–4 is now complete. Hypercortisolism and nonsuppressibility to a low dose of dexamethasone diagnose Cushing's syndrome. High ACTH and partial suppressibility by high doses of dexamethasone indicate Cushing's disease. Lack of suppressibility and low ACTH levels indicate primary adrenal disease, adenoma, or carcinoma. Carcinoma becomes more likely as 17-ketogenic steroid levels rise, although adenomas usually secrete some 17-ketogenic steroids as well. As 11-deoxycortisol (compound S) and aldosterone appear in excess (and as serum potassium falls), the chance of carcinoma increases still further. The **metyrapone test** is occasionally useful since it helps detect bilateral hyperplasia due to overproduction of pituitary ACTH. In this case, following metyrapone administration there will be at least a doubling of urinary 17-hydroxycorticosteroid output.

Localization of unilateral adrenal disease: There are 3 methods for localizing adrenal disease. They are (1) ^{131}I-19 iodocholesterol scan, (2) tomograms by means of urography, and (3) angiograms. In some cases a tomogram of the suprarenal area is all that is necessary to disclose a unilateral adrenocortical tumor with typical contralateral adrenal atrophy.

^{131}I-19 iodocholesterol scanning is useful in localizing adenomas and demonstrating greatly enlarged glands. However, it is not entirely reliable in detecting small adenomas. Hyperplastic glands usually give an enlarged image. Atrophic glands usually give no image. Adenomas in Cushing's syndrome give very large images and are usually unmistakable. Carcinomas show no image, which is often a useful diagnostic feature.

Rarely, an angiogram is necessary to find an ectopic source of cortisol.

Complications

The severe or terminal complications are most often those of hypertension (renal failure, strokes, etc), diabetes (hyperglycemia, insulin reactions, infections), or severe, debilitating muscular wasting and weakness. Cancer of the adrenals and pituitary tumors also have their characteristic complications.

Nelson's syndrome occurs in about 20% of cases following adrenalectomy. It is due to pituitary oversecretion. It includes hyperpigmentation, headaches, exophthalmos, and heightened sex hormone effects. Findings of pituitary enlargement are usually present, and blindness may result.

Treatment

Cushing's syndrome can be treated by surgery or irradiation of the pituitary, adrenals, or both; or by attempts to modify the synthesis of adrenal hormones.

A. Medical Treatment: Temporary control of Cushing's disease is possible with metyrapone (see above) and aminoglutethimide, both of which inhibit steps in steroid biosynthesis. Eventual escape from control is the rule in ACTH-dependent Cushing's syndrome, but temporary control (usually for months) may be advantageous in preoperative preparation. This treatment is often effective for prolonged periods in patients with benign adrenocortical tumors when immediate surgery is contraindicated—eg, in patients with myocardial infarction.

Mitotane (o,p'DDD, Lysodren) is a DDT derivative which is toxic to the adrenal cortex. It has been used with modest success in treatment of adrenal hypersecretory states, especially adrenal cancer. Unfortunately, serious side-effects are common at effective doses.

B. Pituitary Ablation or Excision of Adenoma: The pituitary can be excised (rarely done for Cushing's syndrome) or irradiated. Irradiation is effective; however, it takes 8–18 months or even longer before significant effects are achieved—too long for patients with rapidly progressive disease. Recurrences after radiotherapy are common.

Currently, most patients who have adrenal hyperplasia are being treated by means of microsurgical excision of pituitary adenomas. Relief of symptoms is rapid, and the prognosis for adequate residual pituitary-adrenal function is good. However, the long-term results are not yet established.

C. Adrenalectomy: Even though operation is the treatment of choice, patients with severe Cushing's syndrome are poor candidates for operation. Postoperative complications are common, with wound infection, hemorrhage, peptic ulceration, and pulmonary problems heading the list.

Total bilateral adrenalectomy is the surest treatment of Cushing's syndrome due to bilateral hyperplasia. Various surgical approaches can be used: transabdominal, bilateral flank, or transpleural. The manifestations of excessive cortisol secretion subside rapidly after surgery. Total extirpation necessitates total adrenal replacement therapy, but if patients are chosen properly this is a small price to pay for relief of Cushing's syndrome.

Subtotal resection is still preferred by a few surgeons, but the results are unpredictable. We do not recommend it because it leaves inadequate adrenocortical reserve, often with a fixed high output of cortisol secretion. Furthermore, Cushing's disease recurs in about 40% of patients after partial resections.

In rare cases, for very poor risk patients, the surgeon may elect to do adrenalectomy in 2 stages through flank incisions.

For malignant tumors, resection is the treatment of choice. Unilateral adrenalectomy is the method of treatment of benign adenomas, which are rarely bilateral.

D. Postoperative Maintenance Therapy: After

total adrenalectomy, lifelong corticosteroid maintenance therapy becomes necessary. The following schedule is commonly used: No cortisol is given until the adrenals are removed during surgery. On the first day, give 100 mg IM of cortisol phosphate or hemisuccinate every 8 hours. (If the patient is not doing well and is in shock, give the drug intravenously.) In the next 24 hours after surgery, give 50 mg IM every 8 hours. Thereafter, the dose should be tapered downward as tolerated. The higher doses are sometimes maintained if the patient had extremely high levels preoperatively. The same tapering process is used after excision of adenoma because the remaining adrenal rarely functions normally again for weeks or months.

As the hydrocortisone dose is reduced below 50 mg/day, it is wise to add fludrocortisone, 0.1 mg daily orally, to avoid excessive urinary electrolyte losses. The usual maintenance doses are about 20–30 mg of hydrocortisone and 0.1 mg of fludrocortisone daily. More than half the dose is given in the morning.

The above schedule can be used for maintaining the addisonian patient through any operation. If shock or hypovolemia occurs despite cortisol, some saline or blood must be given. If salt losses are increased (eg, diarrhea or gastric losses), salt intake must be maintained and an increase in steroids should be considered. Fever, hyperkalemia, and abdominal pain are the 3 most common indications of adrenal insufficiency.

Prognosis

The prognosis for patients with benign Cushing's syndrome is quite good after adrenalectomy or removal of pituitary adenoma. The clinical manifestations begin to subside in several weeks, and complete cure is the rule. The major long-term problems are recurrence due to retained adrenal or adenoma tissue (about 10%) and Nelson's syndrome, which occurs in about 20% of patients with hyperplasia of the pituitary associated with an ACTH-producing pituitary tumor.

When the syndrome is due to malignant disease, the prognosis is grave. Unfortunately, by the time Cushing's syndrome occurs secondary to ectopic ACTH-producing cancers, the tumor is almost always beyond surgical curability. Palliation can occasionally be achieved by adrenalectomy when Cushing's syndrome is the principal clinical problem.

Eddy RL & others: Cushing's syndrome: A prospective study of diagnostic methods. Am J Med 55:621, 1973.

Lieberman LM & others: Diagnosis of adrenal disease by visualization of human adrenal glands with [131]I-19 iodocholesterol. N Engl J Med 285:1387, 1971.

Orth DN, Liddle GW: Results of treating Cushing's syndrome. N Engl J Med 285:243, 1971.

Raux MC & others: Studies of ACTH secretion control in 116 cases of Cushing's syndrome. J Clin Endocrinol Metab 40:186, 1975.

Welbourn RB, Montgomery DAD, Kennedy TL: The natural history of treated Cushing's syndrome. Br J Surg 58:1, 1971.

VIRILIZING & FEMINIZING TUMORS OF THE ADRENAL GLANDS

Congenital adrenal hyperplasia is the most common cause of virilization. Virilizing adrenal tumors are rare. These conditions must be distinguished from virilization due to ovarian tumors, testicular tumors, and adrenal carcinoma.

ACTH stimulates the adrenal cortex to secrete a number of weakly androgenic hormones which contribute several milligrams to the total 24-hour urinary output of 17-ketosteroids. Virilization of adrenal origin is caused by overproduction of these androgens and their subsequent partial conversion to testosterone and is associated with marked increases in urinary excretion of 17-ketosteroids. Testosterone, the most potent androgen, is not a 17-ketosteroid. Thus, marked virilization with normal or only slightly elevated urinary 17-ketosteroid excretion suggests that the excess testosterone is not from the adrenal but rather from the ovary or testis. Virilization may also be caused by specific deficiency of one or more of the enzymes necessary for normal formation of cortisol and mineralocorticoids. It may be associated with Cushing's syndrome, as in adrenocortical carcinoma, or may be due to excess testosterone production—a condition occurring only in females.

The 3 major patterns of congenital virilizing adrenal hyperplasia are simple virilism, virilism with renal sodium loss, and virilism with hypertension. Simple virilism is caused by a partial defect in synthesis of 21-hydroxycorticosteroids. As a result, a precursor of cortisol, 17-hydroxyprogesterone, accumulates and its metabolites pregnanetriol and 11-ketopregnanetriol appear in large amounts in the urine. When the defect in 21-hydroxylation becomes more severe, synthesis of aldosterone is impaired and renal sodium loss occurs. In the third type, 11-hydroxylation is incomplete, DOC concentration increases, and renal sodium conservation and hypertension occur. Virilization in these cases occurs because of oversecretion of androgens—principally testosterone—which is due to excessive ACTH secretion in response to the block in hydrocortisone synthesis. Amelioration is easily achieved by administration of small quantities of hydrocortisone.

Virilization caused by tumor is distinguished by the following: (1) It does not occur early in life, (2) there is no increase of pregnanetriol or of DOC in the urine and no salt wasting, and (3) treatment with hydrocortisone or ACTH has no effect on androgen excretion or secretion. Therefore, excision is necessary.

Feminization as a result of adrenal disease is almost always due to adrenal tumors, most of which are malignant. The only known treatment is excision.

Clinical Findings

A. Symptoms and Signs: (Fig 37–5.) The clinical findings are the usual ones of virilization: sexual precocity, acne, increased hirsutism, male physique, male hair pattern and baldness, and, in males, increased

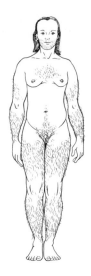

Figure 37—5. Woman with adrenogenital syndrome.

or decreased libido. In females, the principal manifestations are atrophy of secondary sex characteristics, decreased libido, hirsutism, and acne. Rapid growth may occur in prepubertal females. Hypertension may accompany tumor-induced virilization.

These tumors are frequently large and are often palpable.

Feminization due to estrogen-secreting tumors also follows standard patterns as outlined above.

B. Laboratory Findings:

1. ACTH stimulation test—17-Ketosteroid, pregnanetriol (or 17-KGS), and 17-hydroxycorticosteroids are estimated in 24-hour urine samples collected in the basal state and after stimulation with ACTH given intravenously for 8 hours. With reduced cortisol and mineralocorticoid formation from an enzymatic defect in the adrenal cortex, there is no suppression of ACTH production by the pituitary. This increases various cortisol and aldosterone precursors, which is reflected in elevated urinary 17-ketosteroid and pregnanetriol (or 17-KGS) levels. Basally, in an adult with adrenogenital syndrome due to 21-hydroxylase deficiency, the urinary 17-hydroxycorticosteroid output is low or normal, 17-ketosteroids are moderately elevated, and the pregnanetriol characteristically exceeds the upper normal limit of 2 mg/day. ACTH stimulation markedly accentuates these differences: pregnanetriol levels increase several times, 17-ketosteroid levels usually more than double, and the 17-hydroxycorticosteroid remains the same or increases minimally.

2. Dexamethasone suppression test—Dexamethasone suppression differentiates androgenic adrenal hyperplasia from adrenocortical carcinoma (characterized by very high levels of 17-ketosteroids and pregnanetriol in the basal state). 17-Ketosteroids, pregnanetriol, and 17-hydroxycorticosteroids are estimated in 24-hour urine samples collected in the basal state and after dexamethasone, 2 mg orally every 6 hours for 8 doses (2 days). In the absence of carcinoma, excretion drops to very low levels on the second day of suppression.

In cases of marked androgenicity with normal or only slightly elevated urinary 17-ketosteroids, a search must be made for the origin of the excess testosterone. In normal women, plasma testosterone should not exceed 0.06 μg/100 ml. If the basal level is higher than this, it should be suppressed more than 50% by dexamethasone unless it comes from the ovary or an independent tumor of the adrenal cortex.

Differentiation of adrenal tumors from those that arise in the ovary or testis is based on physical examination and culdoscopy or may require laparotomy.

The diagnosis of feminizing tumors of the adrenal depends on recognition of the syndrome, identification of increased urinary or plasma estrogens, and exclusion of ovarian or testicular feminizing neoplasms.

C. X-Ray Findings: Adrenal tumors can often be localized by nephrotomography or arteriography since they are usually large.

Differential Diagnosis

The differential diagnosis includes testicular and ovarian tumors and other causes of ovarian dysfunction such as Stein-Leventhal syndrome, Cushing's syndrome, adrenal hyperplasia with virilization, and exogenous sex steroid administration.

Treatment

Treatment consists of excision of the tumor. Complications of the operation are relatively uncommon. Tumors are rarely bilateral or ectopic.

Prognosis

The prognosis is generally good after operation for virilizing tumors. Feminizing tumors are usually large and malignant, and the prognosis is guarded.

Glenn F, Peterson RE, Mannix H Jr: *Surgery of the Adrenal Gland.* Macmillan, 1968.

Solomon SS & others: Feminizing adrenocortical carcinoma with hypertension. J Clin Endocrinol 28:608, 1968.

NONENDOCRINE TUMORS OF THE ADRENAL GLANDS

The most common nonendocrine adrenal tumor is neuroblastoma. It occurs only in children and is discussed in Chapter 48.

Nonfunctioning cancers of the adrenal cortex in the adult present as malignant masses. Fewer than 100 have been reported.

About 200 adrenal cysts have been reported. They may become quite large but are rarely malignant. They can usually be decompressed and removed by the abdominal route.

Hajjar RA & others: Adrenal cortical carcinoma. Cancer 35:549, 1975.

PALLIATIVE ADRENALECTOMY
FOR BREAST & PROSTATIC CANCER

Bilateral adrenalectomy is a recognized (though infrequently applicable) palliative treatment for metastatic breast carcinoma in both sexes. It is also effective in some patients with metastatic cancer of the prostate gland. The criteria for selection of patients are somewhat uncertain and the subject of considerable controversy. In general, the best candidates for bilateral adrenalectomy are patients who have responded to previous endocrine manipulation, usually castration. Patients who respond to adrenalectomy usually have had at least a 2-year tumor-free interval after the original mastectomy, and the first recurrence is in the area of the mastectomy or in bone.

About 30% of all premenopausal patients with breast cancer will have an objective remission following oophorectomy. About half of this group will have an objective remission after adrenalectomy. Only about 20% of patients who have not responded to oophorectomy will respond to adrenalectomy. Attempts to base the selection of patients for adrenalectomy on measurements of endocrine function have not yet proved successful enough for widespread use.

In terms of tumor response, adrenalectomy and hypophysectomy are about equally effective, but the side-effects of bilateral adrenalectomy are usually more tolerable. However, new surgical technics have made hypophysectomy more acceptable.

The rationale of endocrine ablation is to decrease circulating estrogen levels. Oophorectomy in premenopausal women or in women no more than 1 year past the menopause usually reduces estrogen levels by about 50%. The remaining estrogen is produced by the adrenals. Therefore, adrenalectomy can entirely eliminate circulating estrogens if oophorectomy has already been done. If estrogen excretion tests are available, it is wise to measure urinary estrogens before adrenalectomy to determine (1) whether total oophorectomy has in fact been done, and (2) that estrogen levels are high enough so that regression of the tumor can be expected if estrogen levels are reduced to zero.

High doses of cortisone will also lower estrogen levels. However, they also produce Cushing's syndrome and cause complications.

For palliation of cancer, the posterior surgical approach is generally considered preferable. Tumor implants in the abdomen can make the anterior approach very difficult, and the posterior approach is better tolerated by debilitated patients.

Postoperative complications are usually due to metastatic breast cancer. Pathologic fractures may occur during manipulation under anesthesia; pleural effusion secondary to tumor implants is common.

If patients are selected properly, about half can be expected to respond with objective improvement that lasts several months or more. Corticosteroid replacement therapy is easy and safe, and the patient is no more difficult to manage than the diabetic who takes insulin.

Prognosis is also a function of the preoperative state of the patient. Adrenalectomy done in desperation for a patient with terminal disease is often fatal. Patients with pleural effusion, restricted pulmonary function, and extensive soft tissue metastases are poor operative risks.

Bhanalaph TM, Varkarakis GP, Murphy GP: Current status of bilateral adrenalectomy for advanced prostatic carcinoma. Ann Surg 79:17, 1974.

Chamberlain A: Efficacy of adrenalectomy in treatment of patients with carcinoma of the breast. Surg Gynecol Obstet 138:891, 1974.

Moseley HS & others: Predictive criteria for the selection of breast cancer patients for adrenalectomy. Am J Surg 128:143, 1974.

●   ●   ●

General References

Bledsoe T: Surgery and the adrenal cortex. Surg Clin North Am 54:449, 1974.

Edis AJ, Ayala LA, Egdahl RH: Manual of Endocrine Surgery. Springer-Verlag, 1975.

Ganong WF & others: ACTH and the regulation of adrenocortical secretion. N Engl J Med 290:1006, 1974.

Harrison JH & others: Tumors of the adrenal cortex. Cancer 32:1227, 1973.

Harrison TS & others: Surgical Disorders of the Adrenal Gland: Physiologic Background and Treatment. Grune & Stratton, New York, 1975.

Kaplan NN: Adrenal causes of hypertension. Arch Intern Med 133:1001, 1974.

Laragy JH: Vasoconstriction-volume analysis for understanding and treating hypertension: The use of renin and aldosterone profiles. Am J Med 55:261, 1973.

Lecky JW: Current concepts of adrenal angiography. Radiol Clin North Am 14:309, 1976.

Montgomery DAD, Welbourn RB: Medical and Surgical Endocrinology. Arnold, 1975.

Steinbeck AW, Theile HM: The adrenal cortex. Clin Endocrinol Metabol 3:557, 1974.

Williams RH: Textbook of Endocrinology, 5th ed. Saunders, 1974.

38 . . .
Arteries

Edwin J. Wylie, MD, William K. Ehrenfeld, MD, & Wesley S. Moore, MD

This chapter deals with acute and chronic arterial occlusive disease, vasoconstrictive disorders, and arterial aneurysms. Operative treatment must usually be considered in the management of most patients with any of these conditions.

CHRONIC OCCLUSIVE DISEASES OF LARGE ARTERIES; ATHEROSCLEROSIS

The degenerative processes that characterize atherosclerosis appear in 2 forms. One consists of diffuse destruction and weakening of the arterial media, which may cause dilatation and elongation of any of the major arteries of the body. The process may be exaggerated in places, with the production of focal aneurysms. The other degenerative process principally involves the intima without weakening the media. The degeneration is diffuse but in some areas may be apparent only on microscopic examination, and grossly visible disease may be localized to short segments. Intimal atheromas produce focal arterial narrowing which may progress to total occlusion of the lumen. The obstructive lesions have a predilection for the arterial wall adjacent to arterial bifurcations. In extremities there is often symmetry in the distribution of lesions between the 2 sides.

Progressive narrowing of the arterial lumen at any given site stimulates the development of collateral circulation about the obstructed segment. Stenosis of more than 50% of the lumen reduces arterial pressure beyond the stenotic zone. This creates a pressure gradient compared with the proximal branches and causes blood in nearby branches to return to the parent artery beyond the stenotic zone. With time, the sizes of the collateral vessels expand to accommodate greater flow.

When the stenosis approaches total occlusion, the sharply reduced blood flow eventually leads to thrombosis. The clot propagates in the stagnant column of blood both proximally and distally to the first major tributary. Persistent flow at these sites halts the propa-

gation of clot. The end result is a totally occluded segment bypassed by a collateral system (Fig 38–1). Since resistance to flow in the collaterals is greater than that in the normal primary system, total collateral flow may be less than normal and unresponsive to increased distal demand. Clinical ischemia is related to the overall effectiveness of the collateral system. The development of additional occlusions further reduces blood flow. Severe chronic ischemia is nearly always accompanied by multiple sites of occlusion of the major vessels proximal to the affected tissues.

PERIPHERAL ATHEROSCLEROTIC OCCLUSIVE DISEASE

Essentials of Diagnosis
- Intermittent claudication; rest pain.
- Impotence.

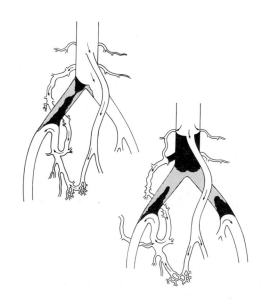

Figure 38–1. Development of collateral channels in response to occlusion of the right common iliac artery and the terminal aortic bifurcation.

- Bruit over constriction.
- Decreased pulsation, thickening of arteries.
- Pallor, cyanosis, and coldness.
- Necrosis and atrophy.

General Considerations

Peripheral occlusive atherosclerosis is predominantly a disease of the lower extremities. In the arms, arterial lesions are largely confined to the subclavian and axillary arteries, and symptoms, if present at all, are limited to fatigue of the forearms with extremes of exertion. In the lower extremities, obstructive lesions are usually confined to segments of the arterial system from the infrarenal aorta to a few centimeters beyond the origins of the terminal branches of the popliteal artery (Fig 38–2). The symptoms are related to the location and number of obstructed arterial segments.

Clinical Findings

A. Symptoms:

1. Intermittent claudication–Intermittent claudication is muscular pain or fatigue in muscles of the lower extremity caused by exertion (eg, walking) and relieved by rest. The pain is a deep-seated ache which gradually progresses to a degree that halts further exertion. It is completely relieved after 2–5 minutes of inactivity. It is distinguished from other pains in the extremities in that some exertion is always required before it appears, it does not occur at rest, and it is relieved in the standing position. The pain appears first in the dominant muscle group in the ischemic zone but may spread to other muscle groups in the same zone. The distance a patient can walk varies with the rate of walking, the level of incline, and the degree of arterial obstruction. The average patient with obstruction in a single arterial segment can walk 90–180 meters (100–200 yards) on a level terrain at an average pace

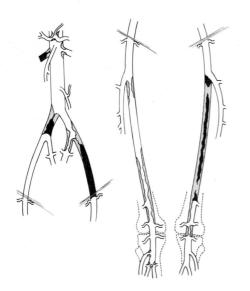

Figure 38–2. Common sites of stenosis and occlusion of the visceral and peripheral arterial systems.

before pain appears. The presence of additional lesions may reduce his walking tolerance to less than 18 meters (20 yards).

Claudication produced by obstruction in the superficial femoral-popliteal arterial segment is localized to the calf muscles. Occlusions proximal to the origin of the profunda femoris extend the pain to involve the thigh. Gluteal pain is added by lesions in or proximal to the hypogastric arteries. When obstruction occurs in this more proximal level, claudication is often described as extreme fatigability of the entire lower extremity. Similar symptoms, but involving both lower extremities, may be caused by occlusion of the distal aorta. An occasional patient may describe transient numbness of the extremity accompanying the pain and fatigue of claudication.

Muscular fatigue or pain may also occur from arterial lesions in the arms, but the disability is minor except in persons whose occupations require prolonged muscular activity of the arms, ie, carpenters. The term claudication is not strictly appropriate since this word derives from Latin *claudicare,* meaning to limp.

2. Impotence–Inability to attain or maintain a penile erection is produced by lesions which obstruct blood flow through both hypogastric arteries and is most commonly found in association with obstruction of the terminal aorta.

3. Rest pain–Ischemic rest pain is a continuous burning pain usually confined to the forefoot. In accord with the gravitational influence on blood flow, it is aggravated by elevation of the extremity or even by bringing the leg to the horizontal position. Thus it appears at bed rest and if severe may prevent sleep. The patient obtains relief by returning the foot to the dependent position. It occasionally may extend to involve the entire foot but never to a level proximal to the ankle. In its extreme form, narcotics may be required for relief. Rest pain indicates an advanced stage of ischemia.

4. Sensation–Although the patient may experience subjective numbness in the extremity, except when actual tissue necrosis has developed, sensory abnormalities are generally not present on examination. If decreased sensation is found in the foot, one should suspect a peripheral neuropathy, often of diabetic origin.

B. Signs: The physical findings of peripheral atherosclerosis are related to changes in the peripheral arteries and to tissue ischemia.

1. Bruits–A bruit is the sound produced by the turbulence of blood flowing through an irregular arterial lumen and is usually due to stenosis. It is heard only during systole and is transmitted distally along the course of the artery. Thus, when a bruit is heard through a stethoscope placed over a peripheral artery, stenosis is present at or proximal to that level. The pitch of the bruit rises as the stenosis becomes more marked

2. Arterial palpation–Thickening and rubbery firmness of the arterial wall are easily palpable in vessels near the surface of the extremity, ie, the brachial, common femoral, and superficial femoral arteries. Decreased amplitude of the pulse denotes proximal stenosis. Occasionally, collateral flow is sufficient to produce a pulse distally even when an artery is completely occluded. The differentiation between stenosis and occlusion, in this circumstance, is made by the presence of a bruit in the former.

3. **Pallor**—Pallor of the foot (or of the hand in cases of upper extremity disease) on elevation of the extremity uniformly accompanies clinically significant arterial obstruction. Lesser degrees of elevation are necessary to produce pallor in patients with advanced lesions. The rate of return of color when the extremity is returned to a dependent position is proportionate to the efficiency of the collateral circulation.

Exercise in a normal individual increases the pulse rate or amplitude without producing arterial bruits or peripheral color change. Exercise will sometimes produce peripheral pallor, an audible bruit, and decrease in pulse strength in an individual who complains of claudication but has no abnormal findings at rest. The findings indicate an otherwise inapparent stenosis. A typical example is seen in the patient with mild claudication of the entire lower extremity from minimal iliac stenosis who has normal peripheral pulses without bruits while at rest. If the patient is made to walk briskly and is reexamined after claudication appears, a bruit will be heard over the femoral triangle and the foot will be pale, with decreased or absent pulses.

4. **Cyanosis**—In advanced stages of atherosclerotic occlusion, the skin of the foot displays a peculiar ruborous cyanosis on dependency. During the delay while blood reaches the foot, hemoglobin is deoxygenated and the color of the blood when it reaches the capillary circulation is similar to that usually found in the venous side of the circuit. The concurrent vasodilatation due to ischemia causes blood to suffuse the cutaneous plexus, imparting a particularly livid appearance to the skin.

5. **Temperature**—With chronic ischemia, the temperature of the skin of the foot approaches that of its surroundings. The examiner can best detect a fall in skin temperature by palpating with the back of his hand against the sole of the foot.

6. **Necrosis**—Tissue necrosis first becomes apparent in the most distal portions of the extremity, often at a site where pressure from a shoe or position in bed causes additional ischemia. Necrosis often is the sequel to mechanical trauma or local infection which increases the local metabolic needs of tissues. Necrosis halts proximally at a line where the blood supply is adequate to maintain viability.

7. **Atrophy**—Moderate to severe degrees of chronic ischemia produce gradual muscle atrophy and loss of strength in the ischemic zone. A frequently associated complaint is reduction of joint mobility in the forefeet.

C. **X-Ray Findings:** Calcification in the walls of atherosclerotic arteries is often visible by standard x-ray technics. Calcification in the arterial wall may occur, however, without narrowing of the arterial lumen; for this reason, it is not an index of the functional status of the artery.

Arteriography supplements the physical findings by defining precisely the degree and site of arterial occlusion and the status of the arteries in the collateral circulation and of the primary arterial tree both proximal and distal to the diseased segment. Investigation of occlusive disease in the lower extremities can be accomplished by injection of contrast media into the abdominal aorta by the translumbar route or through a catheter threaded into the aorta from a peripheral artery followed by exposure of successive films to opacify the arteries of the abdomen and lower extremities.

Treatment & Prognosis

A. **Upper Extremities:** Symptoms are rarely severe enough to require operations on the arteries for vascular insufficiency in the upper extremities. Cervicothoracic sympathectomy usually relieves fatigability or coldness, and the viability of fingers or hands is rarely in question.

B. **Lower Extremities:** The objectives of management of atherosclerotic occlusive disease in the lower extremities are the relief of disability and the prevention of leg loss. Vasodilating or anticoagulant drugs are generally of no value. When disability is minimal (claudication well tolerated) and arteriography demonstrates one or more isolated lesions with unimpaired, well-functioning collateral channels, expectant treatment is all that is required. Under these circumstances, the patient is counseled on foot care and the need for avoiding infection or mechanical and thermal trauma.

Severe disability or impending gangrene requires surgical revascularization if anatomically feasible. The method selected depends upon the location and distribution of arterial lesions and is influenced by associated pulmonary or cardiothoracic disease.

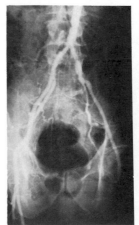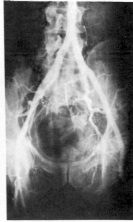

Figure 38—3. *Left:* Aortogram showing atherosclerotic occlusive disease of the infrarenal aorta and iliac arteries. *Right:* Postoperative aortogram showing wide patency after aortoiliac endarterectomy.

1. **Arterial reconstruction**—Direct revascularization operations are applicable for patients with obstructive lesions located anywhere from the abdominal aorta to the terminal branches of the popliteal artery providing there is demonstrable patency of the arteries immediately distal to the segment to be revascularized. The favored operations for occlusion in the aortoiliac-common femoral segments are (1) endarterectomy or (2) arterial bypass grafts of knitted Dacron (Fig 38—3). Long-term success can be expected provided the patient is left with a widely patent arterial tree to and including the profunda femoris artery. In most clinical situations, revascularization to the common femoral artery is generally adequate even when additional occlusive lesions are present in the femoropopliteal segment.

The most successful operation for occlusive disease in the femoropopliteal segment is bypass grafting using a reversed segment of the saphenous vein. If a saphenous vein of adequate size (diameter exceeding 3—4 mm) is not available, the cephalic vein from the arm may be used. The immediate results with endarterectomy are nearly comparable, but the frequency of late occlusion is higher (Fig 39—4). The frequency of late closure with synthetic grafts is even higher. In general, the durability of reconstructive operations in the femoral and popliteal segments is considerably less than for similar operations in the aortoiliac segment. The reasons are the lesser volume of blood flow through the femoral artery, the smaller caliber of the arteries at this level, and the higher incidence of advanced atherosclerosis in the outflow arteries. For these reasons, many surgeons limit direct operation at this level to situations where leg salvage is the principal objective.

Bypass operations, in which grafts are brought to arteries beyond the popliteal artery, are occasionally successful. Information on the long-term patency of these grafts is not yet available.

2. **Lumbar sympathectomy**—Lumbar sympathectomy is seldom indicated as the only method of treatment for patients with occlusion of major arteries in the lower extremities. This approach is reserved for circumstances in which revascularization operations are not technically applicable and where experience indicates that it would benefit the patient. Sympathectomy is of greatest value (1) for patients in the early stage of advanced ischemia whose primary complaint is mild nocturnal rest pain and (2) for the treatment of chronic ulceration of the leg due to arterial insufficiency. Sympathectomy is ineffective in the management of gangrene of the toes or foot and does not lower the required level for amputation.

Many surgeons routinely combine lumbar sympathectomy with arterial reconstructive operations which entail a laparotomy. Sympathectomy causes dilatation of the peripheral arteries, decreasing peripheral resistance. This increases flow through the reconstructed segment and perhaps decreases postoperative thrombosis.

3. **Amputation**—Amputation is required for the

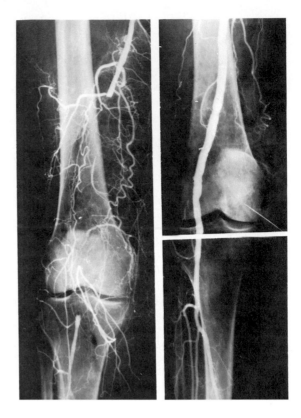

Figure 38—4. *Left:* Femoral arteriogram showing occlusion of the superficial femoral and proximal popliteal arteries. *Right:* Femoral arteriogram showing patency of the femoral and popliteal arteries after endarterectomy. (Reproduced, with permission, from Morton DL, Ehrenfeld WK, Wylie EJ: Significance of outflow obstruction after femoropopliteal endarterectomy. Arch Surg 94:592, 1967.)

management of peripheral gangrene and intractable rest pain whenever arterial reconstruction cannot be successfully performed. Amputation of the toes or the forefoot at the transmetatarsal level is successful in the rare circumstance of distal gangrene where there is adequate blood supply in the remainder of the foot.

Barker WF & others: Current status of femoropopliteal bypass for arteriosclerotic occlusive disease. (Panel discussion.) Surgery 79:30, 1976.

Cutler BS & others: Autologous saphenous vein femoropopliteal bypass: Analysis of 298 cases. Surgery 79:325, 1976.

Duncan WC, Linton RR, Darling RC: Aortoiliofemoral atherosclerotic occlusive disease: Comparative results of endarterectomy and Dacron bypass grafts. Surgery 70:794, 1971.

Imparato AM & others: Intermittent claudication: Its natural course. Surgery 78:795, 1975.

Inahara T: Endarterectomy for occlusive disease of the aortoiliac and common femoral arteries. Am J Surg 124:234, 1972.

Martin P, Crawford J: The rationale for and measurement after profundaplasty. Surg Clin North Am 54:95, 1974.

Reichle RA, Tyson RR: Comparison of long term results of 364 femoropopliteal or femorotibial bypasses for revascularization of severely ischemic lower extremities. Ann Surg 182:449, 1975.

Ross R, Glomet JA: The pathogenesis of atherosclerosis. (2 parts.) N Engl J Med 295:369, 420, 1976.

Starrett RW, Stoney RJ: Juxtarenal aortic occlusion. Surgery 78:890, 1974.

Szilagyi DE & others: Biologic fate of autogenous vein implants as arterial substitutes: Clinical, angiographic and histopathologic observations in femoropopliteal operations for atherosclerosis. Ann Surg 178:232, 1973.

POPLITEAL ARTERY ENTRAPMENT SYNDROME

A rare cause of popliteal artery stenosis or occlusion occurs as a result of an anomalous course of the popliteal artery. The popliteal artery normally passes between the 2 heads of the gastrocnemius muscle as it enters the lower leg. In the entrapment syndrome, the artery passes medial to the medial head of the gastrocnemius, causing compression of the popliteal artery when the knee is extended. Fibrous thickening of the intima occurs at the site of compression and gradually progresses to total occlusion.

Symptoms vary from simple calf claudication to those of more severe ischemia depending upon the adequacy of collateral channels and the extent of distal or proximal clot propagation. Until the artery becomes occluded, the only finding is a decrease in strength of the pedal pulses, most evident with the knee in extension. Arteriograms, in addition to revealing a zone of stenosis or occlusion in the distal third of the popliteal artery, show medial deviation of the popliteal artery beginning in the middle third. Treatment consists of sympathectomy, division of the medial head of the gastrocnemius muscle, and resection and graft replacement of the diseased arterial segment where possible.

Darling RC & others: Intermittent claudication in young athletes: Popliteal artery entrapment syndrome. J Trauma 14:543, 1974.

Delaney TA, Gonzalez LL: Occlusion of popliteal artery due to muscular entrapment. Surgery 69:97, 1971.

Insua JA, Young JR, Humphries AW: Popliteal artery entrapment syndrome. Arch Surg 101:771, 1970.

Love JW, Whelan TJ: Popliteal artery entrapment syndrome. Am J Surg 109:620, 1965.

Schlenker JD, Johnston K, Wolkoff JS: Occlusion of popliteal artery caused by popliteal cysts. Surgery 67:833, 1974.

Wolfe RD, Colloff B: Popliteal cysts: An arthrographic study and review of the literature. J Bone Joint Surg 54A:1057, 1972.

CYSTIC DEGENERATION OF THE POPLITEAL ARTERY

This is another rare disorder involving the popliteal artery. Arterial stenosis is produced by a mucoid cyst in the adventitia usually located in the middle third of the artery. Calf claudication is the most common symptom, and the only finding is decrease in the strength of the peripheral pulses. Arteriography shows a sharply localized zone of popliteal stenosis. Evacuation of the cyst may relieve the stenosis, but, because of the possibility of recurrence, local arterial excision and graft replacement is the preferred therapy.

Hildreth DH: Cystic adventitial disease of the common femoral artery. Am J Surg 130:92, 1975.

ACUTE PERIPHERAL ARTERIAL OCCLUSION

Essentials of Diagnosis

- Abrupt onset of ischemia with coldness, numbness, and occasionally pain.
- Late pain (12–18 hours later).

General Considerations

Sudden total occlusion of a previously patent artery supplying an extremity is usually a dramatic event characterized by abrupt and severe distal ischemia. Tissue viability depends on the extent to which flow is maintained by collateral circuits or surgical intervention. The clinical manifestations are those of ischemia of nerves, muscle, and skin. When ischemia persists, motor and sensory paralysis, muscle infarction, and cutaneous gangrene become irreversible in a matter of hours. A line of demarcation develops between viable and nonviable tissue. Flow in the distal arteries is reduced progressively by propagating intraluminal thrombus, and surgical restoration of blood flow to the ischemic portion of the extremity eventually becomes impossible.

Ischemia after occlusion of the superficial femoral or brachial arteries beyond their respective profunda branches is often followed by progressive recovery. Recovery after brachial occlusion reaches its maximum within 2–4 days; from femoral occlusion, within 2–4 months. The terminal aorta and common femoral artery are 2 sites where collaterals are inadequate to supply distal needs. Sudden occlusion of these arteries is generally followed by severe, progressive ischemia culminating in gangrene.

Acute arterial occlusion may be caused by an embolus, thrombosis, or trauma. Embolic occlusion results from dislodgement of a blood clot or a tumor fragment into the blood stream. The former usually originates from the left atrium in patients with atrial fibrillation or from an intraventricular mural thrombus in patients with recent myocardial infarction. Tumor emboli are rare, the most common being fragments of a cardiac myxoma.

Sudden thrombosis of an atherosclerotic peripheral artery may be difficult to differentiate clinically from embolic occlusion. The usual mechanism is hemorrhagic dissection beneath an atherosclerotic plaque.

Traumatic occlusion may be due to numerous causes, eg, contusion or laceration by a bone after a fracture or dislocation, penetrating injuries, and—commonly in recent years—as a complication of arterial catheterization.

Clinical Findings

Coldness, numbness, and occasionally pain in the ischemic zone are the first complaints and are followed by loss of motor function. Late pain, appearing after 12–18 hours, is the result of swelling of infarcted muscle confined in fascial compartments.

Pallor appears first but is replaced by mottled cyanosis after a few hours as deoxygenated blood gradually suffuses the extremity. Cutaneous hypesthesia slowly progresses to anesthesia, and function is lost in muscles supplied by the ischemic nerves. When these changes persist beyond 12 hours, gangrene is inevitable. If collateral flow increases, it becomes evident by return of warmth and pinkness of the skin and a lessening of the sensory deficit. When collateral flow has reached its maximum, the signs and symptoms are those of chronic occlusion of the involved artery. When reversible ischemia has been severe and protracted at the onset, normal sensory function may not return for 6 months.

Tense swelling and acute tenderness of a muscle belly—a common occurrence in the gastrocnemius following superficial femoral artery occlusion—generally denotes irreversible muscle infarction.

The level of demarcation of ischemic changes suggests the site of arterial occlusion. Since collaterals always supply the tissues just beyond the occlusion, the demarcation is as follows:

Site of Occlusion	Line of Demarcation
Infrarenal aorta	Mid abdomen
Aortic bifurcation and common iliac arteries	Groin
External iliacs	Proximal thigh
Common femoral	Lower third of thigh
Superficial femoral	Upper third of calf
Popliteal	Lower third of calf

Treatment & Prognosis

Immediate anticoagulation by intravenous heparin slows the development of distal thrombosis and allows time for assessment of adequacy of collateral flow and preparation for operation if indicated. Nonoperative management is best for many emboli to major arteries in the upper extremities and for some in the lower extremities but only when skin color improves or neural function returns within 3 hours after occlusion. If the initial ischemia recedes, the decision

for removal of the embolus is based upon an estimate of the disability that will be produced by chronic occlusion of the involved artery. Chronic occlusion of the axillary or brachial arteries is usually well tolerated, whereas chronic occlusion of lower extremity vessels causes claudication at best.

If advanced ischemia persists, the embolus must be removed within 8–12 hours after the occlusion. Successful embolectomy requires removal of the embolus and the "tail" of thrombus which extends distally or proximally from it. If operation is not performed within the first 8–12 hours, the ramifications of this thrombus into arterial branches usually cannot be extracted and revascularization is impossible. Late thrombectomy (after 18 hours) is successful only when propagation of thrombus has been arrested by collateral blood flow reentering the vessel distal to the embolus.

Embolectomy may be performed through an arteriotomy at the site of the embolus or, most commonly, by extraction with a balloon (Fogarty) catheter inserted through a proximal arteriotomy.

Traumatic arterial occlusion (see also Chapter 16) must also be corrected within a few hours to avoid gangrene. Management of the arterial injury is often only one part of an operation which includes repair of other traumatized structures. The general principles in treatment of the arterial injury are as follows:

(1) Restore patency of the distal arterial tree (remove distal thrombus by retrograde "milking" of the extremity or passage of a balloon catheter).

(2) Suture simple arterial lacerations or anastomose cleanly transected arteries.

(3) Replace extensively damaged arterial segments by grafting: Use synthetic fabric for replacing large vessels in uncontaminated wounds; use autologous tissue (vein or artery) to replace small vessels or if the wound is contaminated.

Fogarty TJ, Cranley JJ: Catheter technic for arterial embolectomy. Ann Surg 161:325, 1965.

Hight DW, Tilrey NL, Couch NP: Changing clinical trends in patients with peripheral arterial emboli. Surgery 79:172, 1976.

Thompson JE: Current concepts: Acute peripheral arterial occlusions. N Engl J Med 290:950, 1974.

Thompson JE & others: Arterial embolectomy: A 20-year experience with 163 cases. Surgery 67:212, 1970.

SMALL ARTERY OCCLUSIVE DISEASE

This section deals with occlusive diseases involving the small (< 3 mm diameter) arteries in the extremities. As a group, their clinical manifestations are similar, but they can usually be distinguished without difficulty from conditions involving larger arteries.

Induced reactive hyperemia is a particularly useful technic for the localization of occluded arterial segments and for differentiating occlusive diseases from vasoconstrictive disorders. This is accomplished by first rendering the extremity ischemic by proximal arterial compression. In the arm, the brachial artery is compressed above the elbow; the forearm is elevated above the head; and the patient is made to open and close his hand until it becomes white. In the leg, the femoral artery is compressed in the groin while the leg is supported in 45 degrees of elevation. After 1 minute of total ischemia, the hand or foot is returned to a dependent position and arterial compression is released.

Acute ischemia is a profound stimulus for vasodilatation. In a patient with undiseased arteries and normal sympathetic tone, sudden restoration of arterial patency is followed by an immediate vivid flush of the hand or foot with color seemingly returning simultaneously in all areas. When small artery occlusion is present, there will be a delay in color return to the cutaneous areas supplied by the occluded arteries.

PERIPHERAL EMBOLI

Recurrent emboli to the small arteries in the extremities can arise from clots on prosthetic cardiac valves, from mural thrombi lining the walls of peripheral aneurysms, and from ulcerative atheromatous deposits in the proximal arteries. The peripheral aneurysms most commonly involved are in the popliteal and subclavian arteries. The popliteal aneurysms are atherosclerotic, and the mural thrombus in the wall is particularly susceptible to fragmentation with flexion of the knee joint. The subclavian aneurysms are almost always associated with an anomalous cervical rib which compresses the artery and develops as an extension of the poststenotic dilatation.

The source of atheromatous embolization is almost always lesions in the aorto-iliac-femoral portions of the arterial tree.

When an embolus occludes a digital artery, the patient experiences sudden pain, cyanosis, and coldness or numbness in the affected digit. Those changes characteristically improve over several days, only to reappear perhaps in a different area of the hand or foot. With each succeeding episode, recovery is slower and less complete.

There are no other lesions which acutely occlude small peripheral arteries in this manner. Pregangrenous changes may develop in one toe as a result of proximal lesions in more major arteries. When this occurs, the adjacent toes show changes of advanced ischemia. With embolic occlusion of distal arteries, one customarily finds a normal blood supply in adjacent tissue segments. Unless this difference is recognized and the lesion of origin corrected, survival of the foot or hand may be in peril from recurrent emboli which progressively occlude additional arteries.

Once discovered, the source of emboli must be removed by appropriate valvular or arterial reconstruction. Sympathectomy aids in recovery from ischemia. Chronic anticoagulation may be necessary, particularly with valvular disease.

Crane C: Atheromatous embolism to lower extremities in arteriosclerosis. Arch Surg 94:96, 1967.

Hoye SJ & others: Atheromatous embolization: A factor in peripheral gangrene. N Engl J Med 261:128, 1959.

Karmody AM & others: "Blue toe" syndrome: An indication for limb salvage surgery. Arch Surg 111:1263, 1976.

Perdue GD Jr, Smith RB: Atheromatous microemboli. Ann Surg 169:954, 1969.

THROMBOANGIITIS OBLITERANS

Thromboangiitis obliterans (Buerger's disease) is characterized by multiple segmental occlusions of small arteries in the extremities distal to the brachial and popliteal arteries. Migratory phlebitis is frequently present. The disease occurs almost exclusively in young adult cigarette-smoking males and is believed to represent an allergic response to nicotine. Contrary to former belief, it is not confined to Jews.

Symptoms consist of slowly developing digital pain, cyanosis, and coldness, progressing eventually to necrosis and gangrene. Claudication in the muscles of the foot may be the first symptom.

Examination shows an irregular pattern of digital ischemia. The induced hyperemia test (see above) demonstrates delayed filling of affected digital arteries and rapid filling in adjacent vessels.

Arteriography, although rarely necessary to confirm the diagnosis, shows discrete zones of total arterial occlusion in one or more arteries combined with apparently uninvolved arterial segments.

It is essential that the patient stop smoking to avoid progression of the disease. Sympathectomy dramatically improves collateral blood flow and is advisable in all but the least symptomatic patients. Consideration of amputation should be postponed until the effect of sympathectomy has been observed since advanced lesions often heal completely. Amputation is indicated for persisting pain or gangrene and can be performed adjacent to the line of demarcation with satisfactory primary healing.

The disease may become dormant if the patient can stop smoking, but this is unfortunately difficult to achieve in many who ultimately develop gangrene of additional digits.

Brown H & others: Thromboangiitis obliterans. Br J Surg 56:59, 1969.

McKusick VA & others: Buerger's disease: A distinct clinical and pathologic entity. JAMA 181:5, 1962.

Szilagyi DE, DeRusso FJ, Elliott JP: Thromboangiitis obliterans: Clinico-angiographic correlations. Arch Surg 88:824, 1964.

Wessler S & others: A critical evaluation of thromboangiitis obliterans: The case against Buerger's disease. N Engl J Med 262:1149, 1960.

SCLERODERMA

Scleroderma is a connective tissue disease characterized pathologically by fibrosis due to increase and swelling of collagenous tissue, fragmentation and swelling of the elastic fibers in the cutis, and arterial and intimal thickening. It may present as a multisystem disease with changes in the lung, kidney, gastrointestinal tract, muscle, and CNS. It occurs more frequently in women, and its first manifestations usually appear between the ages of 25 and 50.

Its most common form involves first the skin and vasculature of the fingers, hands, and forearms. The skin becomes thickened and taut. Flexion of the fingers is limited by the tightness of the overlying skin. The muscles in the forearm develop woody induration.

Similar skin changes may occur in the face and restrict ability to open the mouth. Fibrosis of the esophagus may interfere with solid food ingestion in advanced stages of the disease. Ischemic symptoms and findings are usually limited to the hands and fingers but occasionally involve the feet as well. These are the result of both arteriolar thickening and chronic vasoconstriction. Vasomotor phenomena often precede organic tissue changes, and an erroneous diagnosis of primary Raynaud's disease may be made.

Symptoms in the early stages consist of progressive coldness and occasional numbness of the fingers. Intermittent episodic blanching of one or more fingers is frequent. With increasing ischemia, one or more of the terminal phalanges become painful and tender. Atrophy and ulceration of the fingertips with exquisite tenderness follow. At this stage, cutaneous fibrosis of the hands and fingers is usually far-advanced.

Gangrene of the ends of the fingers is the terminal ischemic event.

Vascular examination in the early phases may show only chronic cyanosis and coldness of the hands and fingers. Coincident with the development of skin changes, pallor and atrophy of the fingertips appear. Attempts at finger flexion cause blanching of the knuckles. The induced hyperemia test shows slow return of color starting in the proximal hand and progressing in an uneven fashion into the fingers.

Treatment is palliative at best since there is no way to halt the progression of pathologic change. Sympathectomy is occasionally of value for ischemic symptoms, and fingertip ulcerations will occasionally heal temporarily. Eventual recurrence should be anticipated. Systemic corticosteroid therapy occasionally slows progression. Finger amputation is necessary once gangrene has developed.

Norton WL, Nardo JM: Vascular disease in progressive systemic sclerosis (scleroderma). Ann Intern Med 73:317, 1970.

ERGOTISM

Ergotism was once common as a result of consumption of rye containing the fungus ergot. At present, the condition appears only rarely as an idiosyncratic reaction to ergotamine tartrate taken for migraine. Vascular changes are the result of profound vasoconstriction, almost always limited to the lower extremities. This causes mottled cyanosis of the skin of the thighs and lower legs and diffuse cyanosis of the feet. It can be differentiated from the vasoconstriction of acrocyanosis by the rapidity of onset, which varies from a week to as little as 24 hours. Prolonged vasospasm may produce intimal damage and eventual thrombosis distally. Gangrene and ulceration are, however, uncommon.

Findings include reticular cyanosis, coldness, and absence of pedal and occasionally popliteal pulses.

Prompt withdrawal of ergotamine medication is usually followed by a slow return to normal circulation. If cyanosis fails to clear within 1–2 days, lumbar sympathectomy is indicated.

Spittell JA Jr: Chap 19 in: *Allen-Barker-Hines Peripheral Vascular Diseases,* 4th ed. Fairbairn JF II, Juergens JL, Spittell JA Jr (editors). Saunders, 1972.

VASOCONSTRICTIVE DISORDERS

Vasoconstrictive disorders are characterized by abnormal lability of the sympathetic nervous system which affects the arterial and venous side of the capillary bed to reduce cutaneous blood flow. Sluggish flow of deoxygenated blood causes cutaneous cyanosis, coldness, numbness, and pain.

Raynaud's phenomenon can be precipitated by exposure to cold. It consists of sequential pallor, cyanosis, and rubor after a cold stimulus and is the visible manifestation of vasoconstriction, sluggish flow, and reflex vasodilatation. The term **Raynaud's disease** has been applied to disorders associated with the above findings but in which no specific cause, such as scleroderma, is discovered. Digital gangrene may appear as small vessel occlusion is added to the vasoconstrictive process.

ACROCYANOSIS

Acrocyanosis is a common chronic, benign vaso-constrictive disorder which is largely restricted to young females. It is characterized by persistent cyanosis of the hands and feet. Numbness and pain accompany its more severe form. The changes disappear with exposure to a warm environment. Examination in a cool room shows diffuse symmetric cyanosis, coldness, and occasionally hyperhidrosis of hands and feet. Cyanosis of the skin of the calf, thigh, or forearm usually displays a reticulated pattern and has been called **livedo reticularis** and **cutis marmorata**. The peripheral pulses may diminish in the cold but return to normal with rewarming. The induced hyperemia test may show a normal response, but in patients with particularly intense vasoconstriction, color return will be slow but even (as compared to the uneven return in patients with scleroderma and thromboangiitis obliterans).

The patient usually benefits by wearing warm gloves or socks when exposed to extremes of cold. When genuine disability from chronic pain or coldness results, sympathectomy gives dramatic relief. Vaso-dilating drugs are of little benefit.

The pattern of reticular cyanosis of the leg and diffuse cyanosis of the foot can appear as an idiosyncratic response to the drug amantadine (Symmetrel) used in the treatment of Parkinson's disease. There are no reports in the medical literature regarding long-term prognosis, but from the authors' personal experience of this condition it can be considered favorable.

Porter JM & others: The clinical significance of Raynaud's syndrome. Surgery 80:756, 1976.

POSTPOLIOMYELITIS VASOCONSTRICTION

Chronic vasoconstriction confined to an extremity affected by poliomyelitis may develop many years later. Pain and coldness are often severe, and cutaneous ulcers may develop, particularly in the skin of the lower legs. Sympathectomy for the more severe forms gives excellent symptomatic relief and causes rapid healing of cutaneous ulceration.

Holmes TW Jr, Gilfillan RS, Cuthbertson EM: Sympathectomy in the release of vasoconstriction: Similarities of response in cerebral palsy and poliomyelitis. Surgery 61:129, 1967.

POSTTRAUMATIC VASOMOTOR DYSTROPHY

Contusing injuries to the distal arms or legs—often complicated by bony fracture—are occasionally the precipitating incident to a prolonged and often intractable pain syndrome. When accompanied by chronic cyanosis or coldness due to vasoconstriction, the term **posttraumatic vasomotor dystrophy** is applied. The syndrome is more common in the lower extremities and frequently follows ankle fractures. Diffuse pain and tenderness through the foot and ankle develop out of proportion to the degree of injury. Mild edema is common. The patient's resistance to weight-bearing or movement of the foot and ankle leads to bony atrophy and joint fixation. When x-ray shows additional punched-out areas of bony rarefaction, the term **Sudeck's atrophy** is applied.

Management requires vigorous physical therapy. Sympathectomy is occasionally useful in overcoming the vasomotor symptoms.

CAUSALGIA

Causalgia is a unique pain syndrome largely confined to the upper extremities. The original description was by Weir Mitchell & others in 1864, based upon his Civil War experiences. His observations and most of the subsequent reports describe the cause when the upper extremity is involved as a contusing injury of the median nerve. Some have reported partial or even total transection of the nerve. It is described in this section on vascular disease because of the associated vasomotor phenomena.

The most distinctive and dramatic feature of the syndrome is the almost unendurable pain that occurs. It is a burning pain involving the entire hand. The slightest stimuli can produce sudden increase in the severity of pain (eg, a breeze from an open window, the touch of clothing, or a step on the stair).

Vasomotor changes in the foot or hand are prominent and may present either as vasodilatation or vasoconstriction. The latter tends to dominate the longer the syndrome has been established, with the result that the extremity becomes cold, cyanotic, and moist.

The treatment is sympathectomy of the involved extremity. Relief of pain is complete.

Baker AG, Wineganer FG: Causalgia. Am J Surg 117:690, 1969.
Mayfield FH: *Causalgia.* Thomas, 1951.
Mitchell SW, Morehouse GR, Keen WW: *Gunshot Wounds and Other Injuries of Nerves.* Lippincott, 1864.

. . .

SYMPATHECTOMY

The sympathetic nervous system consists of 2 ganglionated chains of neurons coursing longitudinally along each side of the spinal column. Fibers are sent to the prevertebral ganglia and the mixed plexuses. The ganglia are divided into cervical, thoracic, lumbar, and sacral paravertebral components. The first 3 or 4 ganglia comprise the superior cervical ganglion; the fifth and sixth represent the middle cervical ganglion; and the seventh and eighth combine into the first thoracic to form the "stellate ganglion."

The thoracic is the most regular component with regard to representation by separate segments. There are 12 separate ganglia. In the lumbar segment, 3–5 ganglia may be present. The sacral-paravertebral portion is a continuation of the lumbar segment into the pelvis. The splanchnic nerves are derived from the thoracic sympathetic trunk.

The postganglionic fibers in the extremities supply smooth muscle of small vessel walls, sweat glands, and piloerector muscles. The sympathetic innervation is vasoconstrictor. Its functions include the regulation of the economy of body heat. Sympathetic denervation is then confirmed if increased warmth and redness, dryness of skin, and inability to have "gooseflesh" occur.

Indications for Sympathectomy

A. Nonarterial Disease: Sympathectomy may be of benefit in numerous nonarterial disease states, eg, hyperhidrosis, acrocyanosis, posttraumatic dystrophy, and some cases of frostbite and causalgia.

B. Arterial Disease: Sympathectomy is of benefit in Raynaud's disease, Buerger's disease, and connective tissue diseases that cause Raynaud's phenomenon. It has fallen into disrepute for the therapy of hypertension. Sympathectomy is occasionally helpful in occlusive disease due to atherosclerosis. Many surgeons perform lumbar sympathectomy as an adjunct to aortoiliac and femoral and popliteal artery reconstructive operations.

The operation removes vasoconstrictor tone and increases skin blood flow. Higher flow rates are thought to increase the chances of arterial patency and help sustain a collateral circulation. In addition, drying of the skin diminishes the chance for infection.

Types of Sympathectomy

A. Cervical Sympathectomy: Denervation of the upper extremity is achieved by division and resection of the cervicothoracic ganglia and trunks. If resection does not include the inferior cervical ganglion, sympathetic innervation to the eye is preserved.

B. Lumbar Sympathectomy: Denervation of the lower extremity is achieved by division and resection of the lumbar ganglia and trunks. Resection of the L4 ganglion alone is usually adequate, and extensive sympathetic resection is rarely worthwhile.

Results of Sympathectomy

Sympathectomy lowers peripheral resistance by reducing tone in the arterioles, venules, and capillaries to the skin and subcutaneous tissues. Whether sympathectomy increases blood flow to muscle is disputed. Unilateral cervicothoracic or lumbar sympathectomy in a normal resting subject increases blood flow to the extremity by 400%, and even greater increases occur when excessive vasomotor tone was present preoperatively. Smaller responses may occur (1) if the peripheral vessels are incapable of vasodilatation (scleroderma), (2) if an "auto-sympathectomy" already exists as a result of profound chronic ischemia, or (3) if arterial occlusion prevents greater flow. Lumbar sympathectomy only affects the vessels distal to the knee.

Claudication caused by obstructive arterial lesions in the aorto-popliteal segments responds variably to sympathectomy. Walking tolerances may be slightly increased, and pain usually subsides more rapidly after cessation of walking. The relatively slight effect of sympathectomy on claudication is explained by the theory that muscular ischemia during exercise produces maximal vasodilatation in the muscular arterial branches and that sympathectomy does not increase it further.

Sympathectomy is rarely effective for severe chronic rest pain or for toe or forefoot gangrene due to extensive proximal arterial disease. In both situations, sympathectomy cannot increase blood supply sufficiently to relieve pain or to promote healing of gangrene. Gangrenous ulcers proximal to the ankle generally respond favorably.

When digital gangrene is the result of segmental small artery occlusion (as with peripheral emboli or Buerger's disease), sympathectomy often provides dramatic relief. As might be expected, syndromes associated with profound cutaneous vasoconstriction without occlusion are often markedly improved by sympathectomy.

Palumbo LT, Lulu DJ: Anterior transthoracic upper dorsal sympathectomy. Arch Surg 92:247, 1966.

Ruberti U, Edwards EA, Ottinger L: Changes in the peripheral pulses after sympathectomy for arteriosclerosis. Surgery 47:105, 1960.

Shackelford RT: Henry's anterior, transthoracic extrapleural upper dorsal sympathectomy. Am Surg 32:853, 1966.

Szilagyi DE & others: Lumbar sympathectomy: Current role in the treatment of arteriosclerotic occlusive disease. Arch Surg 95:753, 1967.

ATHEROSCLEROTIC ANEURYSM

An atherosclerotic aneurysm is a true aneurysm appearing as a focal fusiform arterial dilatation. It is found, in descending order of frequency, in the distal abdominal aorta, the popliteal artery (Fig 38–5), the common femoral artery, the arch and descending portions of the thoracic aorta, the carotid arteries, and other peripheral arteries. As the aneurysm enlarges, mural thrombus is deposited on its interior surface owing to eddy currents and stagnant flow. The functional lumen of the artery may remain unchanged and may appear relatively normal on arteriograms—a factor which limits their usefulness in diagnosis.

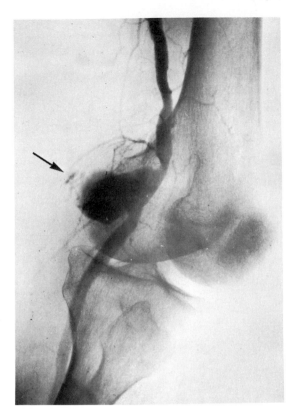

Figure 38—5. Arteriogram showing aneurysm of the popliteal artery (arrow).

1. INFRARENAL ABDOMINAL ANEURYSM

Over 99% of aneurysms of the abdominal aorta are caused by atherosclerosis. Most of these involve the segment of the aorta between the takeoff of the renal arteries and the aortic bifurcation but may include variable portions of the common iliac arteries. Rupture and exsanguination are the major complications.

Clinical Findings

A. Symptoms and Signs: An intact abdominal aneurysm rarely produces more than minimal symptoms. The patient is usually aware of little more than a painless, throbbing mass. Severe pain in the absence of rupture characterizes the rare inflammatory aneurysm which is surrounded by 2—4 cm of perianeurysmal inflammatory reaction.

The sole physical finding is usually a palpable fusiform or globular pulsatile abdominal mass. With smaller aneurysms, this mass is centered in the upper abdomen just above the umbilicus, the normal location of the infrarenal portion of the abdominal aorta. Larger aneurysms bulge distally into the abdomen below the umbilicus and proximally into the space behind the rib cage. The aneurysm may be slightly tender to palpation. Severe tenderness is found only in inflammatory aneurysms or after rupture has occurred.

B. X-Ray Findings: Plain films of the abdomen in anteroposterior, lateral, and oblique projections reveal calcification in the outer layers of over 90% of atherosclerotic abdominal aneurysms. This allows assessment of its size and proximal extent. Aortography is indicated whenever suprarenal involvement of the aorta or associated visceral artery occlusion is suspected. Suprarenal aneurysms are usually associated with dilatation of the descending thoracic aorta, detectable on posteroanterior and right posterior oblique chest x-rays.

Treatment

Since most uncomplicated abdominal aneurysms are asymptomatic, the principal indication for elective operation is to prevent rupture. Rupture rarely occurs until the diameter of the aneurysm exceeds 6 cm; operation for aneurysms smaller than 6 cm is advised only in young patients with a long life expectancy.

Operation consists of replacing the aneurysmal segment with a synthetic fabric graft. Tubular or bifurcation grafts of knitted Dacron are preferred. The proximal anastomosis is usually made to the transected aorta proximal to the aneurysm, 3—6 cm distal to the origin of the renal arteries. The site of the distal anastomosis is determined by the extent of aneurysmal involvement of the iliac arteries. In most circumstances, the iliac arms of a bifurcated graft are anastomosed to the distal ends of the transected common iliac arteries. The graft is generally placed in the lumen of the incised and isolated aneurysm, the outer layers of which are sutured around the graft after the anastomoses are completed (Figs 38—6 and 38—7).

2. SUPRARENAL AORTIC ANEURYSMS

Aneurysms of the segment of aorta between the diaphragm and the renal arteries are rare and are usually associated with similar changes in the thoracic and infrarenal aorta. When they do occur, the 3—6 cm segment at the level of the renal arteries is frequently less dilated, and a dumbbell-shaped aneurysm results. The risk of rupture of the suprarenal segment is not appreciable until its diameter exceeds 7—9 cm. Symptoms are rare unless rupture occurs.

Aneurysms proximal to the renal arteries cannot be palpated. They should be suspected when chest films show dilatation of the descending thoracic aorta. Translumbar aortography performed by injection of contrast medium through needles inserted into the aorta at the level of the diaphragm accurately delineates the entire abdominal aorta.

Resection and graft replacement of the upper abdominal aorta is an operation of far greater magnitude and risk than operations on the infrarenal aorta. A thoracoabdominal approach is necessary, and provision must be made for reimplantation of the celiac axis and the superior mesenteric and renal arteries. At this time, the risks of operation for asymptomatic aneu-

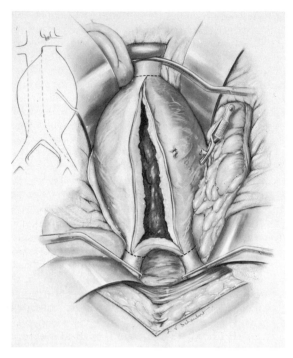

Figure 38–6. Exposure of an infrarenal abdominal aortic aneurysm. Arterial clamps are placed at the neck of the aneurysm below the left renal vein and on the common iliac arteries.

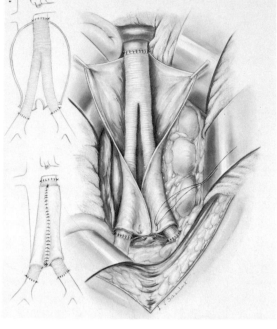

Figure 38–7. Replacement of an aortic aneurysm with a synthetic bifurcation graft. The laminated clot within the aneurysm has been removed and the outer wall is closed over the graft.

rysms at this level less than 7–9 cm in diameter are probably greater than the risk of rupture.

3. RUPTURED AORTIC ANEURYSM

With increasing size, lateral pressure within the aneurysm may eventually lead to spontaneous rupture of the aneurysmal wall. Although immediate exsanguination may ensue, there is usually an interval of several hours between the first episode of bleeding, consisting of a self-limited extravasation into the subadventitia or periaortic tissue, and later retroperitoneal rupture.

Clinical Findings

A. Symptoms and Signs: Most aortic aneurysms are asymptomatic until rupture begins with sudden severe abdominal pain which occasionally radiates into the back. Faintness or syncope results from blood loss. Pain may lessen or faintness may disappear after the first hemorrhage, only to reappear and progress to shock if bleeding continues.

When bleeding remains contained in the periaortic tissue, a discrete, pulsatile abdominal mass can be felt. In contrast with an intact aneurysm, the ruptured aneurysm at this stage is exquisitely tender. As bleeding continues—usually into the retroperitoneum—the discrete mass is replaced by a poorly defined mid-

abdominal fullness, often extending toward the left flank. Shock becomes profound, manifested by peripheral vasoconstriction, hypotension, and anuria.

B. X-Ray Findings: Immediate operation should be performed without pausing to obtain x-rays.

Treatment & Prognosis

Immediate laparotomy is mandatory whenever aortic rupture is suspected. If operation can be performed during the first phase, the mortality rate is only slightly greater than for elective aneurysmectomy. When massive bleeding has produced shock, the operative mortality exceeds 50%. Without operation, however, the outcome is uniformly fatal.

The operation is identical to that for unruptured aneurysms except for the necessity of gaining immediate control of the aorta proximal to the aneurysm to halt bleeding.

The early local complications of abdominal aortic aneurysmectomy are those of any arterial reconstructive operation, ie, arterial thrombosis and hemorrhage. In experienced hands, these are negligible. Disruption of arterial suture lines with false aneurysm formation is a rare late complication. The use of synthetic suture material instead of silk has resulted in a sharp decrease in the incidence of false aneurysms.

Crawford ES: Thoraco-abdominal and abdominal aortic aneurysms involving renal, superior mesenteric and celiac arteries. Ann Surg 179:763, 1974.

Hicks GC & others: Survival improvement following aortic aneurysm resection. Ann Surg 181:863, 1975.

Stoney RJ, Wylie EJ: Surgical treatment of ruptured abdominal aneurysms: Factors influencing outcome. Calif Med 111:1, 1969.

Thompson JE & others: Surgical management of abdominal aortic aneurysms: Factors influencing mortality and morbidity—a 20-year experience. Ann Surg 181:654, 1975.

Walker DI & others: Inflammatory aneurysms of abdominal aorta. Br J Surg 59:609, 1972.

4. FEMORAL & POPLITEAL ANEURYSMS

Atherosclerotic aneurysms of the common femoral and popliteal arteries tend to thrombose and produce distal ischemia. Unlike aortic aneurysms, rupture is rare. Occlusion results from fragmentation of the mural thrombus lining the aneurysmal sac, an event which may partly be due to the mobility of the adjacent hip or knee. Thrombus may occlude the lumen at the aneurysm or embolize downstream into smaller arteries in the leg or foot.

Clinical Findings

A. Symptoms and Signs: Until thrombosis occurs, symptoms are usually minimal or absent. The patient is aware of a throbbing mass when the aneurysm is in the groin, but popliteal aneurysms are usually undetected by the patient. Rarely, popliteal aneurysms will produce symptoms by compressing the popliteal vein or tibial nerve. In most patients, the first symptom is produced by the ischemia of acute arterial occlusion. The pathologic findings range from rapidly developing gangrene to only moderate ischemia which slowly lessens as collateral circulation develops. Symptoms from recurrent embolization to the leg are often transient; sudden ischemia may appear in a toe or part of the foot, followed by slow resolution, and the true diagnosis may be elusive. Recurrent ischemic episodes due to occlusion of small arteries in the leg in patients over age 50 are almost always embolic in origin.

Palpation of local arterial enlargement is generally adequate for diagnosis. Since popliteal aneurysms are usually bilateral, the diagnosis of thrombosis of a popliteal aneurysm is often aided by the palpation of a pulsatile aneurysm in the contralateral popliteal space.

B. X-Ray Findings: Arteriography may not demonstrate the aneurysm accurately because mural thrombus reduces the apparent diameter of the lumen. Nevertheless, arteriography is advised—especially when operation is considered—to define the status of the arteries distal to the aneurysm.

Treatment

Immediate operation is indicated when acute thrombosis has caused pregangrenous ischemia. Operation may not be necessary if ischemic changes are reversible and lessening. Early operation is indicated

for recurrent peripheral embolization. The evidence is unclear regarding the advisability of routine operation in the absence of symptoms, but operation is usually recommended if the external diameter of the aneurysm exceeds 3 times the normal arterial diameter at that site.

The standard surgical treatment for both femoral and popliteal aneurysms has been resection with graft replacement. Recently, however, popliteal aneurysms have been more satisfactorily managed by exclusion and bypass graft. In this procedure, the popliteal artery distal to the aneurysm is transected and the proximal end oversewn. A graft is then interposed from the side of the distal superficial femoral artery to the transected distal end of the popliteal artery. The undissected aneurysm is left in place. As with other arterial grafting operations in the extremities, the saphenous vein or an autologous artery is preferred for the graft to one of synthetic material.

Prognosis

The long-term patency of bypass grafts for femoral and popliteal aneurysms depends on the adequacy of the outflow tract. Late graft occlusion is less common than in similar operations for occlusive disease.

Buda JA & others: The results of treatment of popliteal artery aneurysms: A follow-up study of 86 aneurysms. J Cardiovasc Surg 15:615, 1974.

Edwards WJ: Exclusion and saphenous vein bypass of popliteal aneurysms. Surg Gynecol Obstet 128:829, 1969.

Towne JB & others: Progression of popliteal aneurysmal disease following popliteal aneurysm resection with graft: A twenty-year experience. Surgery 80:426, 1976.

Wychulis AR, Spittel JA Jr, Wallace RB: Popliteal aneurysms. Surgery 68:942, 1970.

OCCLUSIVE
CEREBROVASCULAR DISEASE

Essentials of Diagnosis

- Episodic ataxia, diplopia, blurring of vision.
- Stroke.
- Bruits over common carotids or subclavians.

General Considerations

The origin of symptoms in about 80% of patients with occlusive cerebrovascular disease is an atherosclerotic lesion in a surgically accessible artery in the neck or mediastinum (Figs 38—8 and 38—9). Less common causes are arterial emboli, fibromuscular dysplasia, dissecting aneurysm, and Takayasu's arteritis. The syndromes are sometimes associated with cerebral infarction through either of 2 mechanisms.

Cerebral infarction can be produced by a sudden decrease in blood supply which, if it drops below a critical level, causes cellular death within minutes. This

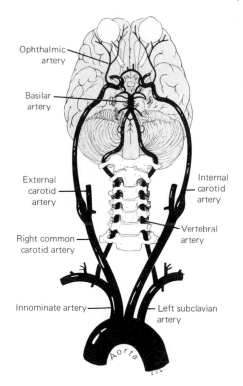

Figure 38—8. Diagram of arterial blood supply to the eyes and brain. (Reproduced, with permission, from Wylie EJ, Ehrenfeld WK: *Extracranial Occlusive Cerebrovascular Disease: Diagnosis and Management.* Saunders, 1970.)

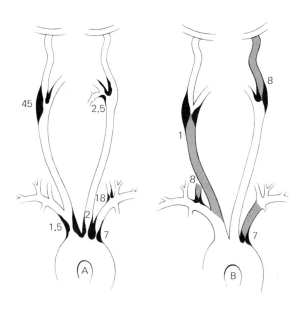

Figure 38—9. Diagram showing common sites of stenosis and occlusion of the extracranial cerebral vasculature. (Reproduced, with permission, from Wylie EJ, Ehrenfeld WK: *Extracranial Occlusive Cerebrovascular Disease: Diagnosis and Management.* Saunders, 1970.)

event is manifested by a fixed or advancing neurologic deficit. It can result from local arterial thrombosis, cerebral embolization, or sudden decrease in cardiac output, all of which are complications of stenosis of the internal carotid artery.

Except for the internal carotid, isolated occlusion of an extracranial artery does not produce infarction or a neurologic deficit since collateral flow is usually adequate. When occlusion occurs in the internal carotid, the usual cause is an atherosclerotic lesion just distal to the common carotid bifurcation. Contralateral hemiplegia often results.

Embolization is the second mechanism of cerebral infarction from carotid lesions. The atherosclerotic plaque ulcerates, and atheromatous debris and blood clot accumulates on its surface and may dislodge to produce cerebral infarction when they reach the brain. Most lesions of this sort occur at the origin of the internal carotid, but the innominate artery and ascending aorta are sometimes implicated.

Neurologic dysfunction without infarction may be produced in 2 ways: (1) Cerebral embolization by small (microembolic) fragments which only temporarily impede arterial flow; and (2) transient reduction in cerebral perfusion short of that required to give irreversible ischemia.

Since most microemboli originate from an ulcerative lesion in the internal carotid artery, neurologic dysfunction is confined to the carotid territory and appears as momentary paresis or numbness of the contralateral arm or leg. This is called a **transient ischemic attack (TIA)**. A TIA from microembolization to the retinal artery may consist of temporary loss of vision (amaurosis fugax) in all or part of the visual field in the ipsilateral eye. Emboli may be visible in the retinas of some patients as small bright flecks of cholesterol. The diagnosis of TIA rests on the transient dysfunction and is supported by finding a bruit at the bifurcation of the common carotid artery on the appropriate side. In the absence of surgical treatment, many patients with TIAs will eventually develop permanent neurologic or visual impairment either from dislodgement of a macroembolus or thrombotic occlusion of the internal carotid artery.

Cerebral ischemia sufficient to produce neurologic dysfunction is usually caused by lesions in the extracranial arteries which are amenable to surgery (Fig 38—10), but episodic symptoms may sometimes be precipitated by maneuvers which impair blood flow in otherwise unobstructed collateral arteries—eg, rising from a supine to an upright position (producing momentary postural hypotension) or hyperextension or rotation of the neck.

Clinical Findings

A. Symptoms: Obstruction of the proximal subclavian or vertebral artery may produce episodic ataxia, diplopia, bilateral blurring of vision, and drop attacks, symptoms caused by reduction of blood flow in the basilar artery. Internal carotid stenosis may cause only recurrent faintness or "lightheadedness"

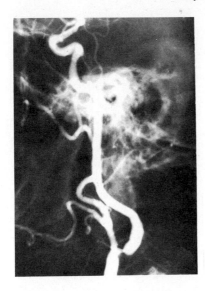 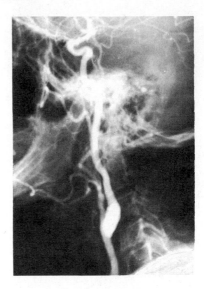

Figure 38—10. *Left:* Preoperative carotid arteriogram showing stenosis of the proximal internal carotid artery. *Right:* Postoperative carotid arteriogram showing restoration of normal luminal size following endarterectomy. (Reproduced, with permission, from Wylie EJ, Ehrenfeld WK: *Extracranial Occlusive Cerebrovascular Disease: Diagnosis and Management.* Saunders, 1970.)

without motor or sensory changes unless hypotension is unusually severe. Innominate artery obstruction may cause symptoms in either the vertebrobasilar or carotid territories or both.

Persistent (but reversible) symptoms may occur with any of the lesions just described. Notable are subtle mentation or memory deficits and chronic decrease of vision. The former are frequently seen in patients with bilateral internal carotid lesions—the latter as a unilateral complaint in patients with common carotid occlusion.

Since many hemodynamic symptoms are mild and infrequent, the decision to surgically relieve arterial obstruction often depends upon the surgeon's assessment of the natural history of the specific lesion. In this regard, occlusion or stenosis of the innominate, subclavian, or vertebral arteries can be considered benign, whereas occlusion of the common or internal carotid artery poses a much greater threat.

B. Signs: Reduced pulses, audible bruits, and asymmetry of pressure in the brachial arteries reveal the presence of most clinically important lesions in the extracranial arteries. The following may exist without clinical signs: occlusion of the internal carotid artery, occlusion and (frequently) stenosis of the vertebral arteries, and ulceration without stenosis in any artery.

1. Palpation—Of the cerebral vessels, only the pulse of the common carotid artery can be felt with certainty. The internal carotid artery is not palpable, either externally or from within the oropharynx. Although the subclavian pulse cannot be reliably evaluated, a weakened axillary pulse usually indicates a subclavian artery lesion.

2. Bruits—Bruits over both subclavian and common carotid arteries generally denote stenosis of the aortic valve. A bruit localized to one artery indicates a stenosis at or proximal to the point where it can be heard. A bruit with maximal intensity high in the neck indicates stenosis at the common carotid bifurcation. Bruits caused by stenosis at the origin of the vertebral artery, if heard at all, are most prominent over the lower portion of the trapezius muscle at the back of the neck. Bruits due to proximal subclavian stenosis are most audible above the midpoint of the clavicle and are transmitted into the axilla. Innominate artery stenosis produces a bruit heard along the full length of the right common carotid and right subclavian arteries.

3. Brachial blood pressures—A discrepancy between the blood pressures in the 2 arms indicates arterial stenosis or occlusion proximal to the brachial artery on the side of reduced pressure.

C. X-Ray Findings: Cerebral arteriography is indicated whenever a lesion is suspected which might require operation. The procedure provides valuable ancillary information about collateral blood supply, other unsuspected stenoses, and occasionally a CNS lesion. The ideal study visualizes both the vertebral-basilar and carotid systems and their intracranial branches.

Treatment

The objectives of operative treatment are to prevent stroke or relieve an existing disability, and these may be accomplished by improving blood flow or removing a source of microemboli. There is no effective medical treatment in most cases.

Surgery is only performed for syndromes not involving cerebral infarction because restoration of normal blood flow and arterial pressures to an infarcted area often causes hemorrhage into the infarct. Most surgical candidates have an accessible lesion in the neck or mediastinum, either causing transient cere-

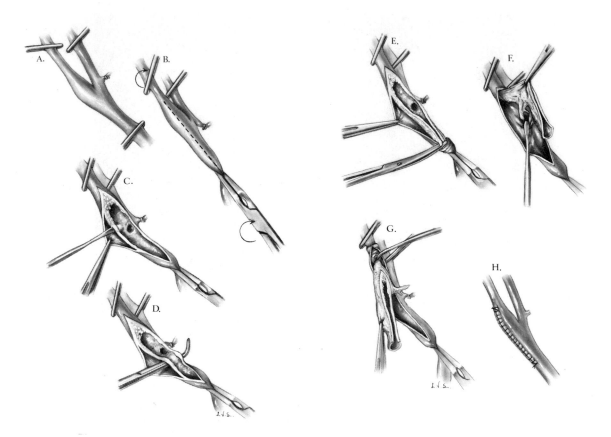

Figure 38–11. Technic of carotid endarterectomy. (Reproduced, with permission, from Wylie EJ, Ehrenfeld WK: *Extracranial Occlusive Cerebrovascular Disease: Diagnosis and Management.* Saunders, 1970.)

bral ischemia or threatening to cause a stroke. Carotid lesions found in patients who have had a previous stroke should be considered for correction. Asymptomatic healthy patients are candidates for surgery when severe stenosis is present and life expectancy is long.

Endarterectomy is the preferred technic for the removal of atherosclerotic lesions at the common carotid bifurcation, in the orifices of the right vertebral and subclavian arteries, and in the innominate artery (sternum splitting approach) (Fig 38–11). The left vertebral artery is difficult to approach through the neck, and obstruction at its orifice is more easily managed by transplanting the vertebral artery to the side of the adjacent left common carotid artery. Obstruction at the origins of the left common carotid artery and left subclavian artery would require an open thoracotomy for endarterectomy. However, thoracotomy and its risks can be avoided by dividing the common carotid low in the neck and transplanting it to the distal cervical portion of the left subclavian artery. Lesions in the proximal subclavian artery causing the "subclavian steal" syndrome can be managed by inserting a bypass graft from the left common carotid to the subclavian artery distal to the lesion (Fig 38–12).

Variations of Occlusive Cerebrovascular Disease

Primary disease in the extracranial arteries other than atherosclerosis is rare. **Takayasu's arteritis** is an obliterative arteriopathy principally involving the aortic arch vessels which often affects young females. Surgery may be necessary to alleviate symptoms due to low cerebral perfusion. Bypass grafts may occasionally be adaptable to overcome the obstructive process.

Dissecting aneurysms of the aorta may extend into the arch branches, producing obstruction and cerebral symptoms. These are discussed in Chapter 22.

Internal carotid dissection. Dissection originating in the internal carotid artery and localized to its extracranial segment occurs as an acute event which may severely narrow or obliterate the internal carotid lumen. The primary lesion is an intimal tear at the distal end of the carotid bulb. It may follow contusion of the neck or, more commonly, severe hyperextension or rotation of the neck. Dissection may also develop spontaneously, most frequently in young adults.

Cerebral symptoms, if they appear, are the result of ischemia in the ipsilateral hemisphere. Localized cervical tenderness adjacent to the angle of the mandible is a frequent finding.

Arteriography shows a characteristic pattern of tapered narrowing at or just beyond the distal portion

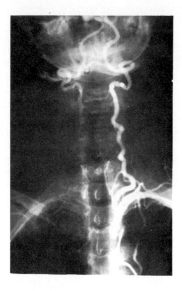 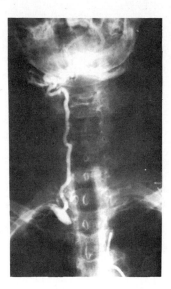

Figure 38—12. *Left:* Arteriogram showing selective injection of the left subclavian artery. There is antegrade flow in the ipsilateral vertebral artery and retrograde flow in the contralateral vetebral artery. *Right:* A later film in this sequence shows filling of the right subclavian artery by retrograde flow in the right vertebral artery. There is proximal occlusion of the right subclavian artery causing the "subclavian steal" syndrome. (Reproduced, with permission, from Wylie EJ, Ehrenfeld WK: *Extracranial Occlusive Cerebrovascular Disease: Diagnosis and Management.* Saunders, 1970.)

of the carotid bulb. The lumen beyond this point may be obliterated or may persist as a barely visible narrow shadow. In the latter case, the lumen resumes a normal caliber beyond the bony foramen.

Operation is indicated only for patients with recurrent TIA's. In the rare case in which the dissection is confined to the surgically accessible proximal third, this segment may be resected and replaced with a graft (usually a segment of the saphenous vein). If the involvement is longer and the TIAs are believed to result from embolization (and if the carotid back pressure exceeds 65 mm Hg), proximal ligation is indicated. In many patients the intramural clot will be resorbed, restoring a normal lumen.

Fibromuscular dysplasia of the internal carotid arteries is a recently recognized cause of cerebral ischemic syndromes. It is usually bilateral and involves primarily the middle and distal thirds of the extracranial portions of the internal carotid artery. Several pathologic variants of the disease have been described, but in most of them the primary lesion is overgrowth of the media in a segmental distribution, producing irregular zones of arterial narrowing. The most common result is a series of concentric rings, producing the radiologic appearance of a "string of beads." The disorder is largely confined to women between the ages of 25 and 55.

The most frequent complaint is awareness of an abnormal noise in the ear synchronous with the heartbeat. Transient ischemic attacks and completed strokes are not uncommon.

An uncommonly loud bruit high in the neck is the only physical finding on vascular examination. Bruits at this location in young adult women are almost always caused by fibromuscular dysplasia.

Because of the high incidence of eventual neurologic disability, the lesion should be corrected surgically whenever possible. Surgery was originally limited to patients with accessible lesions in the proximal half of the internal carotid artery and consisted of resection and graft replacement. More recently, graduated arterial dilatation with arterial dilators has given excellent results and is currently the procedure of choice.

Acute embolic obstruction of the extracranial arteries usually involves the carotid bifurcation and produces hemiplegia due to cerebral infarction. As with other conditions causing cerebral infarction, surgical removal of the obstructing lesion is contraindicated.

Prognosis

Postoperatively, late restenosis or occlusion is rare. The morbidity from operation consists mainly of neurologic deficits and occurs in less than 2%. The operative mortality for all extracranial cerebrovascular operations in our personal experience is less than 1%.

Ehrenfeld WK, Hoyt WF, Wylie EJ: Embolization and transient blindness from carotid atheroma. Arch Surg 93:787, 1966.

Ehrenfeld WK, Wylie EJ: Fibromuscular dysplasia of the internal carotid artery: Surgical management. Arch Surg 109:676, 1974.

Ehrenfeld WK, Wylie EJ: Spontaneous dissection of internal carotid artery. Arch Surg 111:1294, 1976.

Javid H & others: Natural history of carotid bifurcation atheroma. Surgery 67:80, 1970.

Stoney RJ, String ST: Recurrent carotid stenosis. Surgery 80:705, 1976.

Thompson JE, Talkington CM: Carotid endarterectomy. Ann

Surg 184:1, 1976.

Wylie EJ, Ehrenfeld WK: *Extracranial Occlusive Cerebrovascular Disease: Diagnosis and Management.* Saunders, 1970.

RENOVASCULAR HYPERTENSION

Essentials of Diagnosis

- Hypertension.
- Suspicion of renal artery involvement.

General Considerations

Hypertension may result from any process which causes prolonged ischemia of one or both kidneys. Ischemia presumably causes an increase in numbers and activity of juxtaglomerular cells which leads to increased renin production. Assay of renal vein plasma for renin is used in the selection of patients for operation since a large difference in plasma renin levels between one or both kidneys and the vena caval plasma supports a renal cause for the hypertension.

The most common causes of renovascular hypertension are stenosis or occlusion of the renal arteries by atherosclerosis or fibromuscular dysplasia. Less common causes are emboli, dissecting aneurysm, hypoplasia of the renal arteries, and stenosis of the suprarenal artery. Atherosclerosis characteristically produces stenosis at the orifice of a main renal artery and is more prominent in males over age 45. The process is bilateral in over 35% of cases.

Fibromuscular dysplasia usually involves the middle and distal thirds of the main renal artery (Fig 38–13). It often extends into the renal artery branches and involves both renal arteries in 50% of cases. Arterial stenosis is caused by one or more concentric rings of medial hyperplasia which project into the arterial lumen as a perforated diaphragm. The disease is largely confined to women, and the onset of hypertension is usually before age 45.

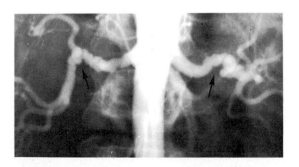

Figure 38–13. Renal arteriogram showing bilateral fibromuscular hyperplasia of the renal arteries (arrows).

Clinical Findings

A. Symptoms and Signs: Most patients are asymptomatic, but irritability, headache, and emotional depression are seen in a few. Persistent elevation of the diastolic pressure is usually the only abnormal physical finding. A bruit is frequently audible to one or both sides of the midline in the upper abdomen. Other signs of atherosclerosis may be present when this is the cause of the renal artery disease.

B. Diagnostic Studies: At one time, divided urinary excretion studies were used to indicate which of the 2 kidneys was the cause of hypertension. These have largely been discarded because of the high morbidity rate of retrograde ureteral catheterization and the frequency of false-negative results when both renal arteries are equally diseased. Selective renin determinations from renal vein blood samples are suggestive of the diagnosis if the ratio of the renin from the involved kidney to the uninvolved one exceeds 1.5. At this time, the arteriographic demonstration of stenosing lesions in one or more renal arteries continues to be the most reliable method for the diagnosis of renovascular hypertension.

Comparative measurements of renal blood flow are considered by some to be a more specific test for renovascular hypertension than measurements of urinary excretion. The most commonly used methods employ radioactive iodohippurate sodium or technetium 99m pertechnetate and are described in Chapter 8.

C. X-Ray Findings: Intravenous urography with rapid injection and rapid sequence exposure is a common screening test which also depends upon comparison of the 2 kidneys. The ischemic kidney has delayed appearance of dye in the calyces and hyperconcentration in the later films as water is extracted by the tubules. The nephrogram phase may show a small kidney on the affected side.

Renal arteriography is the only method that delineates the occlusive lesion. The Seldinger technic, with retrograde passage of a catheter from the femoral arteries, is preferred. Renal arteriography should be performed if the diastolic blood pressure exceeds 110 mm Hg, other clinical criteria are consistent with renovascular hypertension, and long life is otherwise expected.

Treatment

Surgical treatment consists of nephrectomy or revascularization of the renal artery. The indications for arterial reconstruction are influenced by the extent of disease in the renal arteries, the degree of associated arterial disease, the response to medical control of hypertension, the patient's life expectancy, and the anticipated morbidity of the operation. Nephrectomy should be considered when arterial repair is impossible or especially hazardous and the disease is unilateral.

Endarterectomy is effective in the management of atherosclerotic lesions and is most easily accomplished by a transaortic approach. When there is extensive intimal degeneration in the aorta (eg, associated aneu-

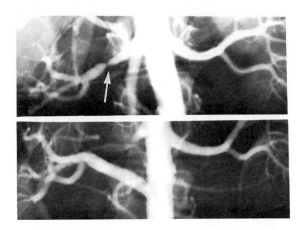

Figure 38—14. *Top:* Preoperative renal arteriogram of a patient with stenosis of the midportion of the right renal artery (arrow). *Bottom:* Postoperative renal arteriogram after renal artery bypass with an autograft of the hypogastric artery. (Reproduced, with permission, from Wylie EJ, Perloff DL, Stoney RJ: Autogenous tissue revascularization technics in surgery for renovascular hypertension. Ann Surg 170:416, 1969.)

rysmal disease in the aorta), a fabric bypass graft may be used as a sidearm from the aortic prosthesis.

By pass grafting is the preferred method in patients with fibromuscular dysplasia of the renal artery. Autologous grafts using a segment of saphenous vein or hypogastric artery are advised (Fig 38—14). Instrumental dilatation of the diseased renal artery may be effective in relieving stenosis in selected patients.

Obstructive lesions in the secondary branches of the renal artery due to fibromuscular dysplasia were originally considered to be inoperable. Technics have recently been developed which appear in most instances to overcome the technical difficulties. These require removal of the kidney from the abdomen, continuous cold perfusion of its vascular tree by cryoprecipated plasma, and microvascular technics for arterial replacement. The kidney is then either returned to a site near its original position or transplanted to the ipsilateral iliac fossa.

Prognosis

Operations for revascularization of the renal artery are successful in lowering blood pressure in over 90% of patients with fibromuscular hyperplasia. Operation for atherosclerotic stenosis results in improvement or cure in about 60%.

Belzer FO & others: Surgical correction of advanced fibromuscular dysplasia of the renal artery. Surgery 75:31, 1974.

Kaufman JJ: Symposium on the management of renovascular hypertension. Urol Clin North Am 2:215, 1975.

Lye CR & others: Aortorenal arterial autografts: Late observations. Arch Surg 110:1321, 1975.

Stanley JC, Ernst CB, Fry WS: Rate of 100 aortorenal vein grafts: Characteristics of late graft expansion, aneurysmal dilatation and stenosis. Surgery 74:931, 1973.

Wylie EJ, Perloff D, Wellington JS: Fibromuscular hyperplasia of the renal arteries. Ann Surg 156:592, 1962.

GASTROINTESTINAL ISCHEMIA SYNDROMES

The celiac axis, the superior and inferior mesenteric arteries, and the 2 internal iliac arteries are the principal sources of blood supply to the stomach and intestines. The anatomic collateral interconnections between these arteries are numerous and may become quite large. Single or even multiple occlusions are generally well tolerated because collateral flow is readily available (Fig 38—15). With the exception of the superior mesenteric artery, even acute occlusion of any one of them rarely causes significant visceral ischemia. This section only deals with the diagnosis and management of the syndromes that are produced by chronic obstruction of these visceral arteries. The syndromes of bowel ischemia caused by acute occlusion are described in Chapter 33.

CHRONIC OCCLUSION

Chronic occlusion of either the celiac or superior mesenteric arteries is caused by atherosclerosis or external compression by ligamentous or neural bands. When atherosclerosis is the cause, the usual lesion is a collar of thickened intima in the orifice of the visceral

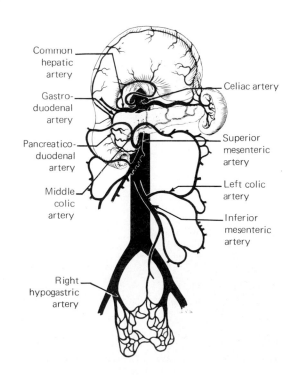

Common hepatic artery

Gastroduodenal artery

Pancreaticoduodenal artery

Middle colic artery

Right hypogastric artery

Celiac artery

Superior mesenteric artery

Left colic artery

Inferior mesenteric artery

Figure 38—15. Visceral arterial circulation and interconnections.

artery. Associated atherosclerosis in the aorta and its other branches is frequent.

Visceral ischemia due to external compression of visceral arteries is a syndrome that has only recently been described. The celiac artery is customarily involved where compression is by the median arcuate ligament of the diaphragm. Women 25–50 years of age are most commonly affected.

Clinical Findings

The principal complaint is postprandial abdominal pain, which has been labeled abdominal or visceral angina. Pain characteristically appears 15–30 minutes after the beginning of a meal and lasts for an hour or longer. It occasionally is so severe and prolonged that opiates are required for relief. It is a deep-seated steady ache in the epigastrium, occasionally radiating to the right or left upper quadrant. Weight loss results from reluctance to eat. Diarrhea and vomiting have been described but in our experience are rare. An upper abdominal bruit may be heard in over 80% of patients.

Arteriography (by retrograde catheter injection whenever possible) in the anteroposterior and lateral projections demonstrates both the arterial lesion and the patterns of collateral blood flow (Fig 38–16).

Treatment

When the obstruction is atherosclerotic, surgical revascularization of the superior mesenteric or the celiac axis (or both) may be performed either by endarterectomy or graft replacement (Fig 38–16). The most effective technic for endarterectomy is one in which a sleeve of aortic intima and the orifice lesions in the celiac or superior mesenteric arteries are removed as a single specimen. The operation is performed by a retroperitoneal approach through a left thoracoabdominal incision carried through the 8th intercostal space. External compression of the celiac

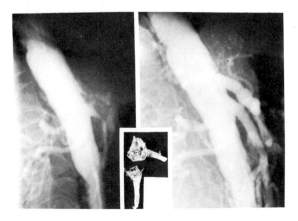

Figure 38–16. *Left:* Preoperative visceral arteriogram showing severe stenosis of the celiac and superior mesenteric arteries. *Right:* The postoperative visceral arteriogram shows wide patency of the celiac and superior mesenteric arteries after transaortic endarterectomy. The inset shows the atherosclerotic stenotic lesions removed by endarterectomy.

artery by the median arcuate ligament may be relieved by simple division of the ligament in 50% of cases. In the remainder, residual stenosis may persist and must be relieved by instrumental arterial dilatation or by resection of the stenotic segment and graft replacement.

Prognosis

Surgery for atherosclerotic visceral artery insufficiency almost always results in relief of symptoms if a technically adequate operation is accomplished. If operation in these patients is not performed, death will often occur from inanition or massive bowel infarction.

Patients with median arcuate ligament compression respond favorably to operation in the majority of instances. Because of the greater difficulty of clinical diagnosis, some of these patients may not improve even though a technically adequate operation is accomplished.

Marable SA & others: Celiac compression syndrome. Am J Surg 115:97, 1968.

Rob D: Surgical diseases of the celiac and mesenteric arteries. Arch Surg 93:21, 1966.

Stoney RJ, Wylie EJ: Recognition and surgical treatment of visceral ischemic syndromes. Ann Surg 164:714, 1966.

THORACIC OUTLET SYNDROME

The term thoracic outlet syndrome refers to the variety of disorders caused by abnormal compression of arterial, venous, or neural structures in the base of the neck. Numerous mechanisms for compression have been described, including cervical rib, anomalous ligaments, hypertrophy of the scalenus anticus muscle, and positional changes which alter the normal relation of the first rib to the structures that pass over it. This has prompted the confusing assortment of names related to the assumed mechanism, ie, **cervical rib, scalenus anticus, costoclavicular,** and **hyperabduction syndromes.** The term **shoulder-hand syndrome** developed from the observation that the hand and forearm are the usual site of symptoms from compression at the base of the neck and shoulder.

Symptoms rarely develop until adulthood. For this reason, it has been assumed that an alteration of normal structural relationships which occurs with advancing years is the primary factor. Even anomalous cervical ribs seem well tolerated during childhood and adolescence.

Inclusion of these syndromes in discussions of vascular disease originates from a former view that many of the symptoms were the result of intermittent compression of the subclavian or axillary arteries. This assumption was reinforced by the frequent finding that certain postural manipulations could produce depression of the radial pulse. The present view holds that whereas transient circulatory changes may indeed occur, the primary cause of symptoms in most patients is intermittent compression of one or more trunks of the brachial plexus. Thus, neurologic symptoms predominate over those of ischemia or venous compression.

Most patients associate their symptoms with certain positions of the shoulder girdle. These may occur from prolonged hyperabduction, as in house painters, hairdressers, and truck drivers. Others may relate their symptoms to the downward traction of the shoulder girdle produced by carrying heavy objects. Numbness of the hands often wakes the patient from sleep.

Clinical Findings

A. Symptoms and Signs: Symptoms consist of pain, paresthesias, or numbness in the distribution of one or more trunks of the brachial plexus (usually in the ulnar distribution). These symptoms can be elicited by specific positions of the arm. Peripheral sensory or motor deficits are rare and usually indicate severe compression of long duration. Muscular atrophy may be present in the hand. The radial pulse can be weakened by abduction of the arm with the head rotated to the opposite side (**Adson's test**), though pulse reduction by this maneuver often occurs in completely asymptomatic persons. A bruit is commonly heard over the subclavian artery above the center of the clavicle with abduction of the arm. Dilatation of the superficial veins of the arm usually indicates axillary vein thrombosis, a complication of chronic venous compression. Peripheral cyanosis and coldness from vasoconstriction occur rarely.

B. X-Ray Findings: X-rays of the neck are of value only in the diagnosis of cervical rib or an elongated transverse process at C5 or C6. The demonstration of subclavian or axillary artery stenosis by arteriograms with the arm in abduction has minimal usefulness since similar changes may be produced in asymptomatic patients.

Treatment

Most patients benefit from postural correction and a physical therapy program directed toward restoring the normal relation and strengthening the structures in the shoulder girdle. Surgical technics for decompression of the thoracic outlet are reserved for patients who have not responded after 3–6 months of conservative treatment. Resection of an anomalous cervical rib may give dramatic relief. Resection of the first rib is the best method for decompressing the space at the thoracic outlet. The transaxillary approach is preferred.

Prognosis

When the correct diagnosis is made, resection of the first rib gives dramatic relief of symptoms.

Judy KL, Heymann RL: Vascular complications of thoracic outlet syndrome. Am J Surg 123:521, 1972.

Roos DB: Experience with first rib resection for thoracic outlet syndrome. Ann Surg 173:429, 1971.

Urschel JC Jr, Razzuk MA: Management of the thoracic-outlet syndrome. N Engl J Med 286:1140, 1972.

ARTERIOVENOUS FISTULAS

Arteriovenous fistulas may be congenital or acquired. Abnormal communications between arteries and veins occur in many diseases and may affect vessels of all sizes. Their effects depend upon the degree of communication present. In congenital fistulas, the systemic effect is often not great because the degree of communication, though diffuse, is small. Larger acquired fistulas enlarge rapidly and may ultimately produce cardiac failure. Cardiac dilatation and heart failure may result when shunting is excessive, prolonged, or untreated. Overloading of the venous side of the circulation may ultimately cause venous insufficiency.

Congenital fistulas are often noted in infancy or childhood. When a limb is involved, muscle mass or bone length may be increased. Arteriovenous malformations frequently involve the brain, visceral organs, or lungs. Gastrointestinal hemorrhage may occur. Pulmonary lesions cause polycythemia, clubbing, and cyanosis.

Acquired fistulas result from injuries that produce artificial connections between adjacent arteries and veins and may be the result of trauma or disease. Penetrating injuries are the most common cause, but fistulas are sometimes seen after blunt trauma. Connective tissue disorders (eg, Ehlers-Danlos syndrome), erosion of an atherosclerotic or mycotic arterial aneurysm into adjacent veins, communication with an arterial prosthetic graft, and neoplastic invasion are other causes. A rare but dramatic cause of atraumatic arteriovenous fistula is combined injury to the left common iliac artery and vein during surgical excision of a herniated nucleus pulposus by the dorsal approach.

Clinical Findings

A. Symptoms and Signs: The time of onset and the presence or absence of associated disease should be determined. A typical continuous machinery murmur can be heard over most fistulas and is often associated with a palpable thrill and locally increased skin temperature. Proximally, the arteries and veins dilate and the pulse distal to the lesion diminishes. There may be signs of venous insufficiency and coolness distal to the communication on the involved extremity.

B. X-Ray Findings: Precise delineation of arteriovenous fistulas can only be done with appropriate arteriograms. The use of selective catheter injection technics has permitted accurate radiologic diagnosis.

Treatment

Not all arteriovenous connections require operation. Small peripheral fistulas may be observed and frequently will never cause difficulties. Some fistulas close spontaneously, often as a result of venous thrombosis. Some are surgically inaccessible.

The indications for surgery include hemorrhage, expanding false aneurysm, severe venous or arterial insufficiency, cosmetic deformity, and heart failure.

Numerous technics are available. These include the classic quadruple ligation, amputation, en bloc excision, and repair of the fistula with reconstruction of the involved arteries and veins. Iatrogenic embolization with beads or muscle has recently been recommended for inaccessible or inoperable fistulas. Quadruple ligation of both proximal and distal artery and vein ensures obliteration of the fistula. This technic depends upon collateral blood flow to compensate for the arterial ligation and preserve tissue viability.

Since the introduction of refined vascular surgical technics in recent years, primary repair is being attempted more often. The arterial repair is most important since venous ligation can usually be done with impunity.

En bloc resection is reserved for diffuse arteriovenous malformations, though hemostasis may be difficult. Congenital arteriovenous fistulas are amenable to surgical management only when en bloc resection of all tissue involved in the fistula can be accomplished. When the fistulous connections involve substantial portions of an extremity, local arterial ligation is invariably followed by recurrence, and only temporary palliation can be expected. Amputation may be a last resort to control unmanageable peripheral fistulas.

Prognosis

The results of surgery vary according to the extent, location, and type of fistula. In general, traumatic fistulas have the most favorable prognosis. Congenital fistulas are more difficult to eradicate because of the numerous arteriovenous connections usually present. These fistulas have a high propensity for recurrence, and most surgeons are reluctant to operate unless the surgical indications are urgent.

Holman E: *Arteriovenous Aneurysms.* Macmillan, 1937.

Olcott C & others: Intra-arterial embolization in the management of arteriovenous malformations. Surgery 79:3, 1976.

Rich NM, Hobson RW, Collins GS: Traumatic arteriovenous fistulas and false aneurysms: Review of 558 lesions. Surgery 78:817, 1975.

Szilagyi DE & others: Congenital arteriovenous anomalies of the limbs. Arch Surg 111:423, 1976.

Szilagyi DE & others: Peripheral congenital arteriovenous fistulas. Surgery 57:61, 1965.

AMPUTATION OF THE LOWER EXTREMITY IN ARTERIAL OCCLUSIVE DISEASE
Wesley S. Moore, MD

Arterial reconstruction is the preferred treatment for reversible ischemic lesions of the lower extremity. However, when the arterial disease is not amenable to reconstruction—or when the ischemic changes are irreversible—amputation of the lower extremity must be done. The indications for amputation are gangrene, uncontrolled infection, or rest pain.

General Principles

(1) The goal of amputation is to treat the lower extremity ischemia and to rehabilitate the patient to his preischemic ambulatory status.

(2) The amputation should be designed to remove the least amount of viable tissue but should be done at a level which has a blood supply sufficient to ensure a reasonable chance of primary healing.

Preoperative Preparation

A. Control of Infection: When a patient has wet gangrene or acute bacterial infection of the foot, infection should be treated before elective amputation. Culture and sensitivity data should be obtained and the patient started on appropriate antibiotic therapy. If cellulitis and lymphangitis are treated successfully, elective amputation with primary closure can be safely performed. If infection cannot be controlled by local measures and antibiotics, major debridement of the infected tissue may be necessary. Effective debridement may require supramalleolar open guillotine amputation of the foot. This is an effective method of preparing for below-the-knee amputation. Guillotine debridement above the level of lymphangitis is not necessary because open supramalleolar amputation removes the source of infection and provides drainage through the open end of the stump. This form of radical debridement, combined with antibiotic therapy, will effectively prepare the patient for below-the-knee amputation within 2 or 3 days.

B. Vascular Supply: One method of making certain that amputation can be successfully carried out at the most distal level possible is to establish good inflow to the profunda femoris artery. Diminution of the femoral pulse on the affected side is evidence of reduced profunda femoris blood flow. However, a good pulse does not in itself guarantee adequate inflow to the profunda femoris since a high-grade obstruction of the iliac system in conjunction with a tandem stenotic lesion of the orifice of the profunda femoris artery can produce a femoral pulse of normal quality. Therefore, when time permits, angiography should be performed before amputation to determine the adequacy of arterial inflow to the profunda femoris artery. If inflow disease of the vessel is found and corrected, the amputation may be successfully performed at a more distal level.

C. **Sympathectomy:** It has been suggested that lumbar sympathectomy will improve blood supply to the skin of the lower extremity and facilitate primary healing at a distal amputation level. This contention has not been proved and at the present time cannot be recommended.

Determination of Amputation Level

The selection of amputation level depends upon the extent of tissue necrosis and the quantity of skin blood flow immediately proximal to the infected or gangrenous part. Evaluation of the circulatory status at a proposed level for amputation has been classically done by determining the presence and quality of peripheral pulses, the level to which dependent rubor reaches, and the capillary refill time. The condition of the skin and skin appendages should be examined for distribution of hair, ischemic nail changes, thickness of skin, and the amount of subcutaneous tissue at the level of proposed amputation. Angiography of the distal aorta and its branches down to and including the tibial vessels is helpful in establishing the location of major arterial occlusions and delineating the patterns of collateral circulation. The temperature of the skin at the level of proposed amputation may also be helpful in evaluating the quality of circulation. All of these methods, however, are relatively inexact, and only when combined with the experience of the surgeon do they result in selection of an appropriate level with a relatively good chance of healing. More recently, a method has been proposed of quantitatively determining skin blood flow at the level of proposed amputation, and a preliminary report suggests that this technic may result in a more objective means of determining the chances of healing at the level selected. The method utilizes an intradermal injection of xenon-133 with monitoring of its rate of removal by a radioactive detector combined with a strip chart recorder. Xenon-133 has been shown to be an accurate means of measuring capillary blood flow in the skin. Since it is the capillary component that represents the nutritional contribution of blood flow to tissues, it appears possible to establish a quantitative minimum requirement for blood flow that correlates positively with the ability of a skin incision to heal.

Moore WS: Determination of amputation level: Measurement of skin blood flow with xenon Xe 133. Arch Surg 107:798, 1973.

Amputation for Acute Arterial Occlusion

Amputation of the acutely ischemic limb deserves special attention. The timing of amputation will be determined partly by the success or failure of arterial reconstruction. Also influencing this decision will be the duration of arterial occlusion before reconstruction and evidence of massive limb swelling after reestablishment of arterial blood flow. In general, if only a slight amount of ischemic or necrotic tissue results from acute arterial occlusion, amputation should be deferred until there is a clear demarcation between viable and nonviable skin. This also permits the development of collateral blood supply to viable tissue. However, if extensive tissue is involved, delayed amputation runs the risk of systemic toxicity from ischemic by-products in marginally vascularized tissue. The anticipation of systemic toxicity—or its actual manifestations as evidenced by deterioration of vital signs, confused mentation, hemoglobinuria, or failing renal function—is an indication for emergency amputation. Emergency amputation after acute arterial occlusion must be carried out at a higher level than if collateral circulation and demarcation were allowed to develop. However, the disadvantage of amputation at a higher level must be balanced against the life-threatening danger of delayed amputation if a large amount of ischemic tissue is present.

Committee on Prosthetic-Orthotic Education: *The Geriatric Amputee: Principles of Management.* National Academy of Sciences, 1971.

Prosthetic and Sensory Aids Service: *The Management of Lower-Extremity Amputations.* Publication No. TR 10–6. Veterans Administration, Aug 1969.

Sarmiento A, Warren WD: A re-evaluation of lower extremity amputations. Surg Gynecol Obstet 129:799, 1969.

Warren R, Kihn RB: A survey of lower extremity amputations for ischemia. Surgery 63:107, 1968.

TOE AMPUTATION

Indications

Toe amputation is indicated for infection or gangrene limited to the distal or middle phalanx of one or more toes, associated with sharp demarcation and good circulation in the proximal skin.

Contraindications

(1) Gangrene or infection extending toward the metatarsal crease with an indistinct line of demarcation.

(2) Extensive ischemic disease of the foot involving the tissue through which the incision for toe amputation would be made. This includes rest pain, atrophy of the skin and subcutaneous tissue, or dependent rubor.

Procedure

Toe amputation can be accomplished by surgical excision or autoamputation. If there is dry gangrene with distinct demarcation and no evidence of infection, the safest method is to allow autoamputation of the gangrenous toe (or toes) to take place. The patient must be instructed regarding care of the ischemic foot, eg, separation of the toes, hygiene, avoidance of hot water, and meticulous drying between the toes following washing. With time, epithelization will take place under the ischemic eschar. When epithelization is complete, the gangrenous phalanx will autoamputate, leaving a well-healed epithelized stump. This process usually takes several months.

In toe amputation, a circular incision is made proximal to the line of demarcation, down to bone. The bone is divided and rongeured back far enough to permit transverse closure of the skin with careful coaptation of the skin edges.

Advantages Over Amputation at a Higher Level

The operative procedure is simple and produces no major deformity or interference with the patient's gait.

Disadvantages

Failure to heal may produce a spreading space infection which may require amputation at a considerably higher level.

Results & Postoperative Considerations

The functional result is excellent. No prosthesis, specific gait training, or rehabilitation is required.

TRANSMETATARSAL AMPUTATION
(Fig 38–17)

Indication

(1) Gangrenous changes in 3 or more toes.

(2) Gangrene extending past the metatarsal crease on the anterior aspect of the foot but sparing plantar skin.

(3) Contiguous osteomyelitis of the metatarsal head with good plantar skin and good circulation.

This amputation is most successfully applied to diabetic patients with gangrene due to necrotizing infection but with good peripheral circulation confirmed by the presence of pedal pulses.

Contraindications

(1) Neuropathy of plantar skin, resulting in anesthesia.

(2) Dependent rubor of the forefoot involving the area of proposed skin incision.

(3) Rest pain of the forefoot, suggesting more extensive ischemia.

(4) Infection extending into the metatarsal spaces.

(5) The absence of pedal pulses is a relative contraindication for amputation, but this contraindication can be negated by evidence of good collateral circulation as manifested by absence of skin atrophy, the presence of hair, and a normal amount of subcutaneous tissue.

Procedure

The forefoot is amputated at the midmetatarsal level. A long, full thickness, posterior skin flap is brought up over the divided surface of the metatarsals and sutured to the anterior skin. The anterior skin is incised at the same level as metatarsal bone division. The plantar skin flap can be thinned by excision of tendon and fascial structures, but the plantar muscles and subcutaneous tissues are left intact so that blood supply to the skin flap is undisturbed. Edge-to-edge coaptation is obtained between posterior skin and anterior skin using interrupted vertical mattress sutures. Particular care is taken to avoid trauma to the skin edges. Handling of skin edges with forceps is not permitted.

Advantages Over Amputation at a Higher Level

Amputation at this level does not require a prosthesis. The gait will be reasonably normal, and walking will not require unusual (or additional) effort.

Disadvantages

Amputation at this level often fails in the absence of pedal pulses.

Results & Postoperative Considerations

The functional result is excellent. The only prosthetic requirement is a shoe insert consisting of a spring steel plantar shank with an attached piece of wood or plastic simulating the forefoot, which will fill out the tip of the shoe. Minimal gait training is required.

Wheelock FC: Transmetatarsal amputations and arterial surgery in diabetic patients. N Engl J Med 264:316, 1961.

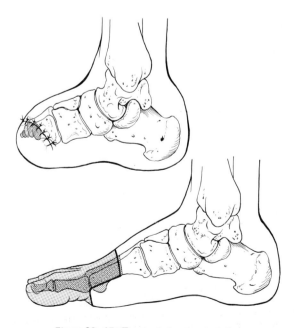

Figure 38–17. Transmetatarsal amputation.

SYME'S AMPUTATION
(Fig 38—18)

Indications

The indications for the Syme amputation are gangrene or infection (or both) that involves the forefoot but spares the heel. This amputation is most successfully used in patients with diabetes mellitus and gangrene caused by necrotizing infection but who have a good peripheral blood supply as manifested by the presence of one or both pedal pulses.

Contraindications

(1) Neuropathy of the skin of the heel, manifested by anesthesia.

(2) Evidence of inadequate blood supply, demonstrated by rubor of the entire foot, ulceration about the ankle or heel, or atrophic skin changes extending to the area of proposed incision.

Procedure

The foot is disarticulated at the ankle mortise by dividing the collateral ligaments and carefully filleting the calcaneus from the heel pad to avoid damage to the blood supply from the posterior tibial artery. The weight-bearing surface is prepared by cutting off the tips of both malleoli so that the distal portions of the tibia and fibula become a continuously flat surface in the same plane as the articular surface of the tibiofibular synostosis. The heel pad is brought up and sutured to the anterior skin by a single-layer closure with vertical mattress sutures to obtain perfect edge-to-edge skin closure. The heel pad must be stabilized to prevent medial or lateral dislocation. This is best accomplished by a carefully applied plaster cast to achieve immobilization.

Advantages Over Amputation at a Higher Level

(1) A Syme amputation produces an end weight-bearing stump, giving greater stability during ambulation.

(2) The patient can use a simple cup slipper as a prosthesis to wear around the house. This is easily and quickly applied, and a definitive prosthesis is not needed except for cosmetic effect.

Disadvantages

(1) The cosmetic prosthesis is more difficult to fit than a below-the-knee prosthesis. The Syme prosthesis is less cosmetic in appearance than the below-the-knee prosthesis because of increased width of the ankle required to accommodate the amputation stump.

(2) Amputation at this level often fails to heal in the absence of pedal pulses.

Results of Postoperative Considerations

The functional result is excellent. A cup slipper is used for wear around the house. The formal prosthesis consists of a foot attached to a laminated plastic shell that fits around the calf and stump. Minimal gait training is required.

BELOW-THE-KNEE AMPUTATION
(Fig 38—19)

Indications

Amputation below the knee is the method most frequently used for ischemic disease in major amputation centers. Gangrene or infection of the foot in conjunction with a good blood inflow to the profunda

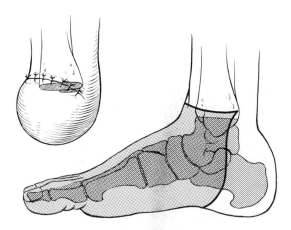

Figure 38—18. Syme's amputation.

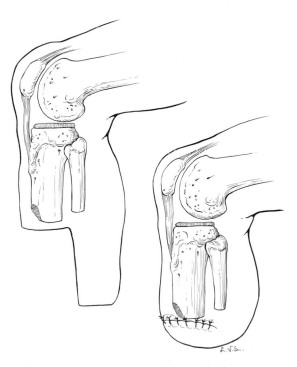

Figure 38—19. Below-the-knee amputation.

femoris artery will result in a high rate of primary healing. A popliteal pulse is desirable (but not necessary) for satisfactory healing.

Contraindications

(1) Gangrene or ulceration at the level of proposed skin incision.

(2) Hemiparesis on the side of the amputation. Below-the-knee amputation on the side of a hemiparesis causes spastic flexion contracture of the stump, preventing satisfactory prosthetic rehabilitation.

(3) A knee flexion contracture greater than 20 degrees that cannot be improved by physical therapy.

Procedure

Below-the-knee amputation is best performed by using a long posterior skin flap. The posterior skin is thicker and has a better blood supply than the corresponding anterior skin at the calf level. The optimum length of the tibia is 10 cm measured from the tibial tuberosity. The fibula is divided 6 mm shorter than the tibia. The fascia is closed with interrupted absorbable sutures, and the skin is meticulously approximated with vertical mattress sutures to obtain exact edge-to-edge coaptation.

In patients with a satisfactory blood supply (evidenced by bleeding at operation), there may be an advantage to stabilizing the anterior and posterior muscle groups. This is accomplished by suturing the anterior tibial and gastrocnemius-soleus muscles to bone through holes drilled in the anterolateral and posterior aspects of the tibia. The sutured muscles are then amputated flush with the end of the bone. A tourniquet should never be used in amputations for ischemic disease.

Advantages Over Amputation at a Higher Level

(1) Below-the-knee amputation will result in a higher rate of prosthetic rehabilitation, and less energy is required to walk than with an above-the-knee amputation. This is of particular importance to elderly patients. The presence of a knee joint will assure prosthetic rehabilitation if the patient was ambulatory before amputation. This includes patients who may ultimately require bilateral below-the-knee amputation.

(2) The mortality rate for below-the-knee amputation is considerably less than that for above-the-knee amputation in geriatric patients.

Results & Postoperative Considerations

The functional result is excellent. Ambulation and prosthetic rehabilitation have been made possible by advances in prosthetic technology. Some younger patients can even engage in sports with a below-the-knee prosthesis. Elderly patients confined to bed who are not suitable candidates for ambulation find that the presence of a knee joint helps them to turn and to transfer their weight.

The artificial leg for the below-the-knee amputee is a patellar tendon weight-bearing prosthesis. This has

an excellent design and mechanical capability. The prosthesis is lightweight and is easily managed by the elderly patient with limited strength.

Prosthetic rehabilitation with below-the-knee amputation is quite successful. Patients easily achieve a good gait pattern after proper training.

Lim RC Jr & others: Below-knee amputation for ischemic gangrene. Surg Gynecol Obstet 125:493, 1967.

Moore WS, Hall AD, Lim RC Jr: Below knee amputation for ischemic gangrene: Comparative results of conventional operation and immediate postoperative fitting technic. Am J Surg 124:127, 1972.

Moore WS, Hall AD, Wylie EJ: Below knee amputation for vascular insufficiency. Arch Surg 97:886, 1968.

KNEE DISARTICULATION
(Fig 38–20)

Indications

Knee disarticulation is indicated for ulceration, infection, or gangrene at a level that precludes a high below-the-knee amputation in patients with good arterial inflow to the profunda femoris artery and adequate viable skin to cross over the disarticulated femur.

Contraindications

Ulceration of anterior skin over the tibial tuberosity.

Procedure

A knee disarticulation operation is most easily performed with the patient prone and the knee flexed. A long, total anterior flap is used because of the better quality of the prepatellar skin in this area. The patella

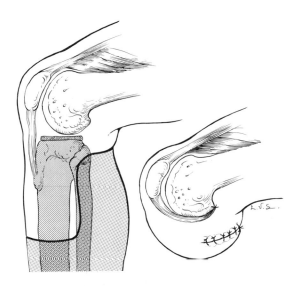

Figure 38–20. Knee disarticulation.

is not excised but is pulled into an articulated position of flexion over the femoral condyles and fixed in that position by suturing the patellar tendon to the posterior capsule of the knee joint. Disarticulation is accomplished by division of the collateral ligaments and joint capsule after separation of the attachment of the patellar tendon to the tibial tuberosity. The anterior skin flap is brought over the end of the stump and sutured to the posterior skin with interrupted vertical mattress sutures.

Advantages Over Amputation at a Higher Level

(1) The knee disarticulation amputation produces an end weight-bearing stump which provides greater stability during ambulation.

(2) The knee disarticulation prosthesis is lighter and easier to handle than the prosthesis used for above-the-knee amputation. Gait training—particularly for the geriatric amputee—is considerably easier than gait training with above-the-knee amputation.

(3) More patients will obtain prosthetic ambulatory rehabilitation on a knee disarticulation prosthesis than with an above-the-knee prosthesis.

Results & Postoperative Considerations

The ambulatory result of the knee disarticulation is almost as good as that of the below-the-knee amputation. The knee disarticulation prosthesis consists of an artificial distal leg and foot combined with a leather thigh lacer that is articulated with the use of external hinges to simulate knee joint motion.

Rehabilitation is excellent. The training period for ambulation and the gait obtained with a knee disarticulation are almost comparable to those of the below-the-knee amputation.

ABOVE-THE-KNEE AMPUTATION

Until recently, lower extremity amputation for ischemia was usually performed above the knee; below-the-knee amputation was rare. This practice was reversed when it was recognized that most patients with vascular disease can heal at the below-the-knee level and benefit from a superior functional result and lower immediate morbidity and mortality.

Indications

The indications for above-the-knee amputation include healing failure of below-the-knee or disarticulation amputation and extensive ischemic damage from an acute embolus or thrombus, resulting in destruction of tissue distal to the knee joint.

Contraindications

The principal contraindication to above-the-knee amputation is the possibility of obtaining a better functional result with a more distal amputation.

Procedure

The site of amputation is usually in the mid or distal thigh. Either a circular skin incision or equal anterior or posterior flaps are developed. Bone division is performed at a level proximal enough to permit a transverse fascial and skin closure.

Advantages Over Amputation at a Higher Level

(1) The operation is easy to perform.

(2) Primary healing is the rule.

(3) Hip disarticulation is rarely required for ischemic disease.

Disadvantages

(1) Above-the-knee amputation has a higher mortality rate than amputation at the lower level.

(2) The energy required for ambulation on an above-the-knee prosthesis is considerably greater than with amputation at the lower level.

(3) The ability to achieve prosthetic rehabilitation in the elderly debilitated patient is less likely with an above-the-knee amputation than with an amputation at the lower level.

Results & Postoperative Considerations

The functional result is fair. Ambulation on a prosthesis is possible after extended training provided the patient is in reasonably good health and has adequate strength. If prosthetic rehabilitation is not possible, crutches or a wheelchair must be used.

The artificial limb used for the above-the-knee amputee is an ischial weight-bearing prosthesis with a mechanical knee joint.

Rehabilitation after above-the-knee amputation is much less satisfactory than is the case with amputation at a lower level, particularly in geriatric patients. In relatively healthy patients, after a period of extensive physical therapy and gait training, a suitable gait—often supplemented with a cane or a crutch—can be achieved.

•   •   •

COMPLICATIONS OF AMPUTATION

The early complications of amputation are necrosis of the stump, infection, and hematoma formation. Later complications include flexion contracture of the next proximal joint, edema of the stump, or the development of a painful neuroma due to improper handling of the nerve or nerves at the time of amputation. Morbidity and mortality after amputation are often due to pulmonary complications such as pneumonia and pulmonary embolization due to venous thromboembolic disease. Myocardial infarction is also a major cause of morbidity and mortality. These complications are seen more frequently after amputations above the knee than after those at a more distal level.

Thompson RC, Del Blanco TL, McAllister FF: Complications following lower extremity amputation. Surg Gynecol Obstet 120:301, 1965.

IMMEDIATE POSTOPERATIVE PROSTHESIS

This relatively new technic has been used as an adjunct to amputation in an attempt to facilitate early ambulation, improve healing, decrease the morbidity and mortality, and shorten the period of prosthetic rehabilitation. Immediate application of a prosthesis can be achieved at any amputation level but has been most frequently used in below-the-knee amputation.

A plaster of Paris cast is applied to the stump in the operating room after the amputation is completed. A pylon device and prosthetic foot are incorporated into the cast, which enables the patient to ambulate. Prosthetic gait training begins on the first or second postoperative day and continues during the healing phase of amputation.

Advocates of this technic claim that it has several advantages over conventional amputation with a soft dressing:

(1) Prevention of edema. With the stump in a rigid dressing, the external support prevents edema, thus promoting healing in marginally vascularized tissue. Prevention of edema also accelerates rehabilitation by eliminating the need to wait for stump maturation and shrinkage before fitting a permanent prosthesis.

(2) Reduction of postoperative pain by wound immobilization.

(3) Prevention of knee flexion deformity by knee immobilization.

(4) Protection of the wound from external trauma.

The method also leads to earlier ambulation, with the following advantages:

(1) Fewer pulmonary complications. Pulmonary embolism and pneumonia—major causes of morbidity and mortality following amputation—are the result of prolonged immobilization. Immediate ambulation apparently reduces the incidence of these complications.

(2) Weight-bearing with limited stump compression contributes to control of edema.

(3) Rehabilitation is accelerated by gait training in the early postoperative period. Since there is no prolonged period of bed rest, the patient does not forget how to walk. He is able to maintain strength and muscle tone by continuing to be ambulatory immediately after operation.

(4) Immediate ambulation provides psychologic benefits to the patient adjusting to amputation. When the amputee realizes that he is able to walk on the day following operation, his attitude toward amputation changes. He begins to think positively and starts to work toward rehabilitation on an artificial limb.

The immediate postoperative prosthesis appears to have several advantages in the management of patients following amputation. However, because a prosthetist trained in immediate fitting technics is necessary, this procedure may have to be reserved for centers that perform a large number of amputations.

Burgess EM, Romano RL: The management of lower extremity amputees using immediate postsurgical prostheses. Clin Orthop 57:137, 1968.

• • •

General References

Barker WF: *Peripheral Arterial Disease,* 2nd ed. Saunders, 1975.

Cranley JJ: *Vascular Surgery.* Vol 1. *Peripheral Arterial Diseases.* Harper & Row, 1972.

DeBakey M (editor): Symposium on vascular surgery. Surg Clin North Am 46:823, 1966.

Fairbairn JF II, Juergens JL, Spitell JA (editors): *Allen-Barker-Hines Peripheral Vascular Diseases,* 4th ed. Saunders, 1972.

Holling HE (editor): *Peripheral Vascular Diseases.* Lippincott, 1972.

Kappert A, Winsor T: *Diagnosis of Peripheral Vascular Disease.* Davis, 1972.

39...
Veins & Lymphatics

Jerry Goldstone, MD

THE VEINS

Functional & Surgical Anatomy of the Venous System

There are 3 anatomically and functionally distinct sets of veins draining the lower extremities.

A. Superficial Veins: The subcutaneous veins, superficial to the muscular fascia, consist of the greater and lesser saphenous veins on the anteromedial and posterior aspects of the legs, respectively. The 2 systems communicate freely with each other as well as with the deep veins, and each ends by joining the deep system. The greater saphenous vein is constant in its position at the ankle, just anterior to the medial malleolus, where it is quickly and easily exposed for emergency intravenous cannulation. The anatomy of the other veins is quite variable.

B. Deep Veins: These are the intra and intermuscular veins, which accompany the named arteries within the musculofascial compartments of the lower extremity and usually are given the same name. They usually run as paired venae comitantes below the knee. About 90% of the venous return from the lower extremities normally flows in these veins.

C. Communicating Veins: The communicating veins perforate the deep muscular fascia to connect the superficial and deep venous systems. The valves in the perforating veins direct the flow of blood from the superficial to the deep veins. These veins are more numerous in the distal portion of the leg and ankle in a plane just posterior to the tibia.

The valves are the most distinctive and important feature of the venous capacitance system. They first appear in venules of about 1 mm in diameter, particularly in the limbs. These valves permit the flow of blood only toward the heart. They are more prominent in the veins of the legs than in those of the arms and are found in both the deep and superficial venous systems of the legs. They are also prominent in the communicating vessels that connect the superficial and deep leg veins. These bicuspid valves direct blood flow from distal to proximal and from superficial to deep, except in the perforating veins of the hands, feet, and forearms, in which flow is from deep to superficial. Some veins have no valves or possess only functionally incompetent intimal folds. These include the venae

cavae and the hepatic, portal, splenic, renal, pulmonary, mesenteric, cerebral, and superficial head and neck veins.

Vein walls are much thinner (with less elastic tissue and smooth muscle) than those of arteries of similar size, and, because of the low transmural pressure, they collapse easily, changing from a circular to an elliptical profile. This change in geometric configuration is of considerable importance to venous capacitance and venous resistance to flow. Normally, the venous contribution to total vascular resistance is insignificant.

The capacitance function of the venous system plays an important role in cardiovascular regulation. Thus, marked increases in venous volume produce only slight to moderate increases in venous pressure. Characteristically, the thin-walled veins collapse when the transmural pressure falls and become distended when pressure rises. Consequently, the veins below the level of the heart can increase in volume during standing by 500 ml or more, and it is this venous pooling which may cause dizziness or fainting during prolonged standing.

In humans, when the body is erect, the effective zero level of venous pressure is in the right atrium. The hydrostatic pressure in a vein on the dorsum of the foot is equal to the distance from the right atrium to the foot—about 100 cm water. The more dependent a vein, the higher the hydrostatic pressure and the thicker the vein wall. This is why the greater saphenous vein can be used so readily as an arterial substitute. The valves in the veins of the leg do not by themselves dissipate the hydrostatic pressure of the column of blood between heart and foot. But muscular action, by compressing the deep veins, forces blood toward the heart since the valves prevent backflow. With muscular relaxation, the pressure in the deep veins drops and they again fill with blood. The more frequent and powerful the muscular movements, the more efficient is this venous pump. With walking, the pressure in the veins on the dorsum of the foot falls to 30–40 cm water from the resting venous pressure of approximately 100–120 cm water (Fig 39–1). The fall in venous pressure is maintained until the exercise is halted and pressure returns slowly to the preexercise level (Fig 39–2).

Knowledge of the above anatomic and physio-

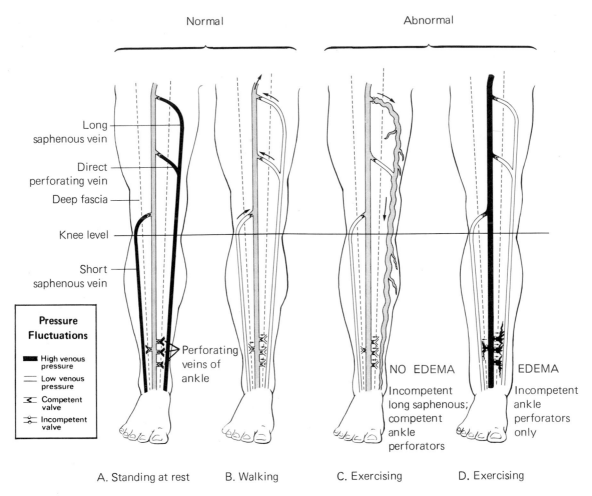

Figure 39–1. Normal venous physiology during standing *(A)* and walking *(B)* and abnormalities during exercise *(C, D)*. Pressure in the superficial veins is diminished (if the valves are competent) by the pumping action of the muscles, which facilitates venous return to the heart *(B)*. When the proximal valves are incompetent, the superficial veins become varicose, but competence of the valves in the distal communicators maintains the integrity of the muscle pump, and pressure remains high in the superficial veins even during exercise *(C)*. If the valves of the leg communicators are incompetent, the muscle pump is ineffective even when the valves in the thigh are competent, and the venous pressure at the ankle remains high even during exercise *(D)*. This produces edema, diapedesis of red cells, poor tissue nutrition, and, ultimately, ulceration (postphlebitic syndrome).

logic facts allows for a better understanding of the disturbances produced by the venous diseases described below. For example, the basic pathophysiologic mechanism responsible for the postphlebitic state is walking venous hypertension.

DISEASES OF THE VENOUS SYSTEM

VARICOSE VEINS

Essentials of Diagnosis

- Dilated, tortuous superficial veins in the lower extremities.
- Symptoms may be absent or may consist only of fatigue, aching discomfort, and slight swelling.
- Symptoms relieved by leg elevation.
- Pigmentation, ulceration, and edema of the lower leg suggest secondary varicose veins.

General Considerations

It is estimated that 10–20% of the world's population have varicose veins in the lower extremities. Although varicose means dilated, varicose veins are elongated and tortuous as well. They are most common in the lower extremities but also occur in other areas, such as the spermatic cord (varicocele), esophagus (esophageal varices), and anorectum (hemorrhoids).

On the basis of predisposing causes, varicose veins

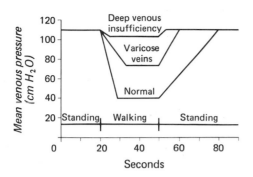

Figure 39–2. Ambulatory venous pressure. Responses of venous pressure measured in a vein on dorsum of foot during standing and walking. While standing, venous pressure is that of a hydrostatic column extending from the right atrium to the foot. With contraction of calf muscles, venous pressure falls rapidly and returns to normal slowly after exercise stops. The postphlebitic state is characterized by little if any fall in pressure with exercise and a rapid return to normal (walking venous hypertension). Patients with primary varicose veins show a response between these 2 extremes. (See text for details.)

are divided into 2 classes: primary and secondary. **Primary varicose veins** are associated with normal deep veins. **Secondary varicose veins**, on the other hand, are complications of deep venous occlusive disease or arteriovenous fistula.

The cause of primary or simple varicose veins remains obscure. There are 2 major theories, neither of which satisfactorily explains all cases. Because venous valvular incompetence is the dominant clinical finding in saphenous varicosity and the factor that largely determines the clinical course and rate of progression, it has been postulated that the fundamental abnormality is sequential incompetence of the valves, either in the main saphenous trunks or in the communicating veins. Incompetent valves cause higher pressure at the subjacent valve and localized dilatation of the affected venous segment. The alternative "weak wall" theory assumes an inherited weakness of the vein wall, producing venous dilatation even with normal pressures and secondary failure of valvular competence. Although there is often a positive family history, the weakness is probably not inherited but due to postnatal factors.

Varicose veins are more common in patients with diverticular disease of the colon and correlate well with the low-roughage diet consumed in "developed" countries. The presumed etiologic link is obscure. Aggravating factors associated with an increased incidence of varicose veins are female sex, parity, constricting clothing, prolonged standing, marked obesity, and consumption of estrogens (oral contraceptives).

Secondary varicosities are those that develop following damage or obstruction to the deep veins. Recanalization of the thrombosed deep veins leaves the valves incompetent, and this loss of valve sufficiency

places an unusual strain on the superficial veins, which have little external support because of their location relative to the deep fascia of the leg. Secondary varicosities thus progressively develop because of the increased venous pressure and flow transmitted from the deep to the superficial veins via incompetent perforating veins. Obstruction of the inferior vena cava or iliac veins can result in secondary varicosities in the lower extremities. An example of this is suprapubic varicosities, which represent residual collateral veins that develop with iliofemoral thrombosis. An arteriovenous fistula may lead to regional varicose veins.

Clinical Findings

A. Symptoms and Signs: Some patients have extremely severe varicose veins and no symptoms, whereas others have severe symptoms from small varices. The commonest symptoms are aching, swelling, heaviness, cramps, itching, and cosmetic disfigurement. Aching, usually described as a dull, heavy, bursting sensation, is particularly apt to occur after prolonged standing and is relieved by elevation of the leg or by the use of an elastic stocking. Symptoms usually become more severe as the day progresses. The swelling that occurs with primary varicose veins is mild and usually involves the feet and ankles only. It resolves completely on elevation of the leg in bed overnight. In women, symptoms are often more severe in the few days just prior to menses. The symptoms of simple, primary varicose veins are rarely severe, and most patients seek medical advice for cosmetic reasons or because they are concerned about the future of the leg.

Secondary varicose veins due to chronic deep venous insufficiency often cause more severe symptoms. Progression to ankle ulcers is relatively common, whereas this complication is almost unheard of with primary varicosities. Hemorrhage, sometimes of serious magnitude, may be induced by traumatic rupture of a varix or may be spontaneous. In 1971 there were 21 reported deaths in Great Britain from this problem. Dryness and scaling dermatitis with pruritus may be seen over prominent varices, especially at the ankle. Although varicose veins may be tender, it must be emphasized that severe pain or disability should never be ascribed to primary varicose veins but should stimulate a search for primary musculoskeletal or arterial disease.

The general physical examination may reveal predisposing causes of varicosities or conditions which would modify treatment. With the patient standing, inspection readily reveals dilated, elongated, and tortuous subcutaneous veins of the thigh and leg. If they are less obvious because of edema or obesity, palpation and percussion along the course of the greater saphenous vein (Schwartz test) is a useful diagnostic maneuver. Mild pitting edema of the ankles and slight pigmentation of the skin are common, especially just above the medial malleolus.

The Brodie-Trendelenburg test should then be performed to test the valvular competence of the perforating veins and those in the greater saphenous system

(Fig 39–3): With the patient supine, the leg is elevated until all the blood is drained from the superficial veins. The saphenous vein is then compressed in the thigh and the patient stands up; the varices are observed for 30 seconds, and the tourniquet is then removed. Normally, gradual filling of the superficial veins occurs from below after the patient stands, and when the tourniquet is removed filling continues to be gradual. If the veins fill rapidly from below, the valves in the perforating veins are incompetent and the varices are being filled from the deep system. The location of the incompetent communicating veins can be determined by placing multiple tourniquets around the leg and thigh and observing which venous segment fills. To determine competency of the valve at the saphenofemoral junction, the tourniquet around the thigh is removed after 30 seconds. If blood refluxes rapidly into the greater saphenous system, the valves above this level are incompetent. The short saphenous vein can be tested in a similar manner by compressing it in the popliteal fossa with a tourniquet, but the long saphenous system should be occluded as well to facilitate interpretation.

Careful palpation along the superficial dilated veins will often identify perforating veins by defects in the fascia through which they traverse. In general, they are more frequent in the lower leg just posterior to the tibia.

Differential Diagnosis

When ulceration, brawny induration, and marked hyperpigmentation are present, one can be reasonably certain that deep venous insufficiency exists and that the varicose veins are secondary. Otherwise, they are usually primary. A thrill and bruit over the extremity suggest that an arteriovenous fistula is the cause. If present, sources of extrinsic venous compression are usually obvious in the inguinal and retroperitoneal areas.

Complications

Complications from varicose veins are much more frequent and severe with the secondary type. They result from the venous stasis and venous hypertension present in the subcutaneous veins. The elevated pressure bursts small blood vessels, and skin hyperpigmentation results from the accumulation of hemosiderin in macrophages. The skin, especially at the distal leg and ankle, may become atrophic and thin, allowing the underlying varices to become eroded either spontaneously or after trauma. Surprisingly brisk hemorrhage can occur, but it is readily controlled by means of direct compression and elevation of the leg. Dermatitis and skin irritation can cause itching and severe excoriation from scratching. The affected skin is quite susceptible to cellulitis. Superficial thrombophlebitis, a frequent complication of varicose veins, is discussed further below.

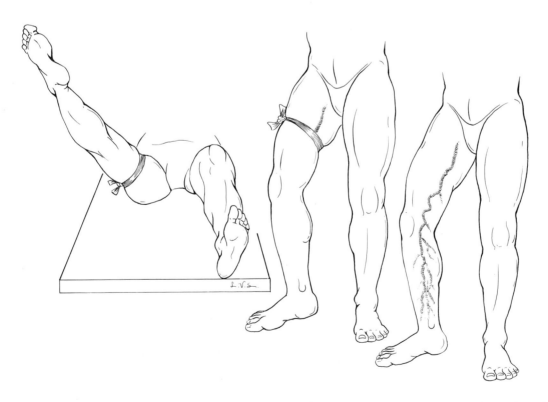

Figure 39–3. Positive Brodie-Trendelenburg test. Blood refluxes into the varicosities through incompetent valves at the saphenofemoral junction when the tourniquet is released. Absence of distal filling while the tourniquet is in place for 30 seconds indicates that the valves of the communicating veins between the superficial and the deep systems are competent (Fig 39–1C).

Treatment

Treatment of varicose veins should relieve discomfort, prevent or ameliorate the complications of venous stasis, improve the appearance of the extremity, and, if possible, eliminate the cause of the varicosities to prevent progression of the disease. The severity and cause of the venous insufficiency determine the type of therapy recommended. About one-third of patients with simple varicose veins require no therapy at all or only common sense advice about taking care of their legs.

A. Nonoperative Management: Nonoperative management can improve venous return and reduce pressure in varicose superficial veins. Walking should be encouraged, and prolonged sitting and standing should be forbidden. The patient should be instructed to elevate the leg as frequently as possible to reduce venous pressure. Properly fitted elastic stockings will compress the superficial veins and prevent reflux of blood from the deep to the superficial veins via incompetent perforators, prevent edema, and assist the muscular pumping action of the calf. The stockings should extend from the distal metatarsals to just below the knee because this is where the varicosities are most severe and because stockings which include the thigh always slip downward unless supported by a garter. Ace bandages can also be used for compression but must be applied carefully to avoid a tourniquet effect.

Elastic support combined with periodic elevation and exercise is the treatment of choice for most patients with uncomplicated varicose veins and gives excellent relief of symptoms when the varicosities are mild or when the patient is elderly or refuses surgery.

B. Compression Sclerotherapy: Sclerotherapy, as now used, obliterates and produces permanent fibrosis of collapsed veins—unlike earlier injection procedures, which attempted to induce thrombosis of the varices. With the patient recumbent and the vein collapsed, small amounts (0.5 ml) of sclerosing solution (3% sodium tetradecyl sulfate) are injected into each varix with a fine-gauge needle. Isolation of the injected segment is maintained by digital pressure; thereafter, continuous pressure on the veins is maintained for 6 weeks with elastic bandages. This prevents thrombosis and allows a fibrous union to form between the 2 walls of the collapsed vein. Multiple sites can be injected at the initial visit and others subsequently. This method of treatment is generally performed as an outpatient procedure. Complications are few, and when injection is successful it offers the best cosmetic result of any available method. The short-term results of injection-sclerotherapy are as good as operation, but long-term follow-up favors surgery. Injection-sclerotherapy is best reserved for small unsightly veins, dilated superficial veins, lower leg perforators, and recurrent or persistent veins after operation. Sclerotherapy at or above the knee tends to be unsatisfactory. Where there is long or short saphenous incompetence, the best initial treatment is surgery.

C. Surgical Therapy: A minority of patients will require surgical therapy for one of the following indications: (1) severe symptoms; (2) very large varices, even if asymptomatic; (3) attacks of superficial phlebitis; (4) hemorrhage from ruptured varix; (5) ulceration from venous stasis (usually in conjunction with deep venous insufficiency); or (6) for cosmetic reasons. Surgical treatment entails removal of the varicose veins and ligation of incompetent perforating branches. No reconstructive procedures have been developed which successfully repair the abnormal valves and veins. For secondary varicosities with deep venous insufficiency, surgical removal is usually only an adjunct to the conservative measures outlined above.

The results of vein stripping depend upon the thoroughness of the procedure. Incompetent superficial and perforating veins must all be identified and marked preoperatively. This is best done the evening before operation, using an ink or dye that will not wash off during the surgical scrub. The operation, performed under general or regional anesthesia, involves ligation of the greater saphenous vein and its tributaries at its junction with the common femoral vein in the groin. The entire saphenous vein is then removed by passing an intraluminal stripper from the exposed saphenous vein at the ankle to the divided end in the groin and avulsing the entire vein. Since most of the visible varicosities are actually tributaries of the main trunk, they should be eliminated either through multiple small incisions or by later sclerotherapy. Once the main channels have been removed, however, most of the tributaries will thrombose. Subfascial ligation of the incompetent perforating branches via separate small incisions is important since they often communicate with tributaries of the main trunk rather than the main trunk itself. Varicosities of the lesser saphenous system are removed through incisions behind the lateral malleolus and just below the popliteal fossa.

Postoperatively, the legs are supported with elastic bandages for approximately 6 weeks. Elevation of the legs in bed minimizes postoperative swelling. Walking is encouraged, but sitting and standing are forbidden.

Results & Prognosis

After surgical treatment, recurrent varicosities occur in about 10% of patients. The most common causes of recurrence are failure to ligate all the tributaries of the greater saphenous system at the saphenofemoral junction and failure to ligate the incompetent perforators. Some recurrences may be due to progression of the initial pathologic process. Symptomatic relief can be expected in nearly all cases if the symptoms were in fact due to the varicose veins. Cosmetic results can be similarly gratifying.

Alexander CJ: The theoretical basis of varicose vein formation. Med J Aust 1:258, 1972.

Burkitt DP: Veins, deep vein thrombosis, and hemorrhoids: Epidemiology and suggested etiology. Br Med J 2:556, 1972.

Fegan WG: Conservative treatment of varicose veins. Prog Surg 11:37, 1973.

Hobbs JT: Surgery and sclerotherapy in the treatment of varicose veins: A random trial. Arch Surg 109:793, 1974.

Larson HL & others: Long-term results after vein surgery: Study of 1000 cases after 10 years. Mayo Clin Proc 49:114, 1974.

Meyers TT: Results and technique of stripping operation for varicose veins. JAMA 163:87, 1957.

Seddon J: The management of varicose veins. Br J Surg 60:345, 1973.

Somerville JJF, Byrne PJ, Fegan WG: Analysis of flow patterns in venous insufficiency. Br J Surg 61:40, 1974.

VENOUS THROMBOSIS & THROMBOPHLEBITIS

Essentials of Diagnosis

- Clinical manifestations may be absent.
- Swelling, pain, erythema, warmth, discomfort, calf tenderness, and a positive Homans sign may be present.
- Fever, tachycardia, elevated sedimentation rate.
- Pulmonary embolism, usually without signs or symptoms in the leg.

General Considerations

Thrombophlebitis and pulmonary embolism are common, frequently fatal complications of venous thrombosis in surgical patients and appear to be increasing in frequency.

With insight that has withstood the test of many experiments, Virchow postulated in 1856 that venous thrombosis was related to 3 factors (Virchow's triad): (1) abnormalities in the vein wall (inflammation), (2) alterations in blood flow (stasis), and (3) alterations in the blood (hypercoagulability) (Table 39–1). Although much still remains to be learned, it is useful in evaluating patients to think of thrombosis as a response of blood to injury and then attempt to identify the injurious agents.

Some understanding of primary hemostasis, coagulation, and the functions of the venous wall is required to appreciate the pathophysiology and treatment of this disease (Fig 39–4). Venous thrombi (red thrombi) are composed principally of erythrocytes trapped in a fine fibrin mesh with few platelets. Arterial thrombi, on the other hand, are composed of large aggregates of platelets trapped in fibrin strands with very few red cells (white thrombi), suggesting a different mechanism of formation.

A. Flow Stasis: It is generally assumed that stasis of blood flow and pooling of blood in the veins of the lower extremities predispose to venous thrombosis. For example, postoperative bed rest and inactivity are associated with decreased velocity of flow in the femoral vein. Experimentally, however, stasis alone does not

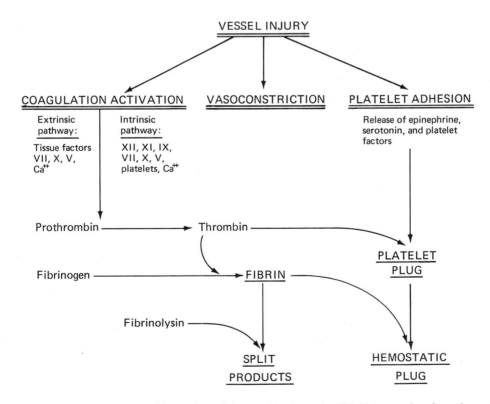

Figure 39–4. Factors involved in arrest of hemorrhage. Injury to blood vessel wall initiates a series of reactions which arrest hemorrhage. The exposed subendothelial collagen initiates formation of the platelet plug (primary hemostasis). The coagulation system is activated, leading to production of fibrin, which interacts with the platelet plug to form a hemostatic plug. These relationships are also involved in spontaneous thrombus formation, although the inciting event is usually not identifiable.

Table 39—1. Pathogenesis of venous thrombosis.

Abnormal vein wall
  Varicose veins
  Previous thrombophlebitis
  Trauma to vein wall (intravenous cannulations)
  Inflammatory process around veins (especially pelvic)
Venous stasis
  Bed rest
  Prolonged positions of dependency of legs
  Restriction of leg motion (casts, debility, postoperative pain)
  Congestive heart failure
  Compression of veins by tumor
  Pressure from pillows under knees
  Decreased arterial flow (shock)
Hypercoagulability of blood
  Trauma (surgery, childbirth, injury)
  Hyperviscosity (polycythemia)
  Malignancy
  Use of oral contraceptives

produce thrombosis although, by protecting activated procoagulants from circulating inhibitors and fibrinolysins and from clearance by the liver, it predisposes to spontaneous venous thrombosis.

B. Hypercoagulability: Thrombophlebitis is rare among patients with congenital coagulation deficiencies. In postoperative patients, the plasma concentrations of clotting factors rise, and the peak corresponds in time to the peak incidence of thromboembolism. These 2 observations tend to implicate hypercoagulability, a state in which activated coagulation factors, normally absent, are present intravascularly. Hypercoagulability remains difficult to define and detect in the laboratory, although most physicians accept that it has a role in the genesis of thromboembolic disease (Table 39—2). The postpartum state, for example, is associated with increased plasma levels of fibrinogen, prothrombin, and other coagulation factors and decreased fibrinolysin. Use of oral contraceptives also appears to cause hypercoagulation, and thromboembolic complications are several times more common in women taking these hormones than in those who do not. Circulatory shock is another condition in which thromboembolic complications are increased in association with hypercoagulability.

Table 39—2. Risk factors for development of venous thrombosis.

  Malignancy
  Oral contraceptive use
  Operations on hips or pelvis
  High blood viscosity (polycythemia)
  Obesity
  Varicose veins
  Obstructed venous return
  Lack of movement
  Childbirth
  Previous history of deep vein thrombosis
  Old age (over 60)

C. Changes in the Vessel Wall: Damage to the intima explains certain forms of venous thrombosis such as those due to catheters, infection, and external compression, but there has been no conclusive evidence of an abnormal intima preceding the majority of deep venous thromboses. The possibility cannot be excluded, however, that minor breaches in the endothelium expose underlying collagen and lead to platelet aggregation, degranulation, and thrombus formation. It seems certain that most venous thromboses develop in the absence of inflammation of the vein wall (phlebothrombosis) and that the thrombotic process itself initiates the inflammatory reaction recognized clinically as thrombophlebitis.

Pathogenesis of Venous Thrombosis (Table 39—1)

In a given patient the cause of venous thrombosis may be difficult to pinpoint, but the following general factors in pathogenesis are accepted: Venous thrombi may develop on normal endothelium. The process usually begins in the venous sinuses in the muscles of the legs and in the valve cusps, both localized areas of relative stasis which allow accumulation of activated clotting factors. Platelets play an important role in the early phases of thrombus formation and trigger the coagulation process. As the platelet aggregate grows, procoagulants are released, the venous lumen becomes compromised, and local stasis and hypercoagulability sustain the process. In addition, the platelet nidus creates turbulent flow which augments platelet aggregation. Once initiated, however, coagulation is the dominant process and produces retrograde thrombosis.

Clinical Findings

A. Symptoms and Signs: The clinical spectrum varies greatly from no symptoms to severe pain and systemic signs of inflammation. Most patients complain of aching discomfort and tightness in the involved calf or thigh. The pain is aggravated by muscular exercise, and the involved leg may feel stiff. Swelling varies from minimal to massive. In some cases the onset is rapid and associated with tachycardia, anxiety, and fever.

The location of the thrombus determines the location of the physical findings. The most frequent site is the calf, especially the venous sinuses of the soleus muscle, and the posterior tibial and peroneal veins (Fig 39—5). Swelling in these cases involves the foot and ankle but is usually slight or even absent. Calf pain and tenderness are usually prominent but may be absent.

Femoral vein thrombosis, which is frequently associated with calf thrombosis, produces pain and tenderness in the distal thigh and popliteal region. Swelling is more prominent than with calf vein thrombosis alone and extends to the level of the knee. Thrombi involving the iliofemoral venous segment produce the most dramatic manifestations, often with massive swelling, pain, and tenderness of the entire lower extremity. **Phlegmasia cerulea dolens** is a severe form of iliofemoral thrombosis which causes such

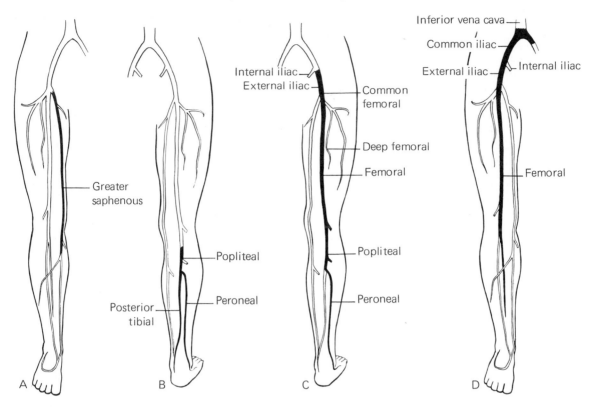

Figure 39—5. Common patterns of venous thrombosis. *A:* Superficial thrombophlebitis. *B:* The most common form of deep thrombophlebitis. *C* and *D:* Deep thrombophlebitis from the calf to the iliac veins. These patterns produce phlegmasia alba dolens or, if more complete, phlegmasia cerulea dolens. The usual locations of thrombosis in milk leg are shown in *C.* (Reproduced, with permission, from Haller JA Jr: *Deep Thrombophlebitis: Pathophysiology and Treatment.* Saunders, 1967.)

marked obstruction of venous outflow that cyanosis develops. It can progress to venous gangrene. **Phlegmasia alba dolens** is another variant characterized by arterial spasm and a pale cool leg with diminished pulses.

There may be tenderness to palpation along any of the involved veins. With deep venous thrombosis in the calf, active dorsiflexion of the foot often produces calf pain (Homans' sign), but diagnostically this is an unreliable test. Tenderness of the calf when the muscles are compressed against the tibia indicates inflammation of the deep veins and therefore thrombosis. This test is also unreliable but may be the first clue to deep venous thrombosis.

Differences in the circumference of the affected extremity compared to the unaffected one are often detectable only with a measuring tape; this is one of the most reliable diagnostic signs. The superficial veins are sometimes visibly dilated, and, if the inflammatory component is significant, there may be increased local warmth and erythema.

B. Diagnostic Tests: The diagnosis of deep venous thrombosis by clinical examination is incorrect in about half of cases, principally because about half of patients with this condition have no physical signs. This has stimulated the development of other objective means of assessment.

1. Ascending phlebography—With the patient semi-upright but not bearing weight on the extremity being examined, radiopaque contrast medium is injected into a vein on the dorsum of the foot. Fluoroscopy and serial x-rays can opacify calf, popliteal, femoral, and iliac veins in one or more views. The 4 cardinal signs of thrombosis are constant filling defects, abrupt termination of the dye column, nonfilling of the entire deep venous system or portions thereof, and diversion of flow. Not all veins in the lower extremities can be visualized by this method—notably the sinuses of the calf muscles, which are common places for thrombosis to begin. Even so, phlebography demonstrates over 90% of thrombi and is probably the most accurate method of detection. A properly performed negative venogram essentially rules out venous thrombosis of the lower extremities. Because it is impractical to repeat phlebography at frequent intervals, the procedure is unsatisfactory for screening. Venography using radioisotopes instead of contrast medium is a simpler method which appears to be accurate and reliable and may become more widely used in the future.

2. Ultrasound—The Doppler ultrasound probe can distinguish between flow and stasis in a major vein and indicate whether the vein is patent or obstructed.

Small thrombi are not revealed since they produce insignificant obstruction. One method involves vigorously squeezing the calf or thigh and looking for the augmented flow in the femoral vein which usually follows. Theoretically, a thrombus might be broken loose if the leg is squeezed too vigorously. When the iliofemoral veins are thrombosed, normal respiratory fluctuations in flow are abolished. This can be detected by ultrasound technics. False-negative results occur with the ultrasound flowmeter, but it is a simple and rapid method of searching for large occlusive thrombi. The examination is inexpensive and noninvasive and can be repeated frequently, but it is insensitive to isolated calf vein thrombosis and cannot be relied upon as a screening method to detect early disease in this area.

3. Plethysmography—Deep inspiration slows venous flow so that if the leg veins are patent the volume and pressure of their blood rise during inspiration and fall during expiration. Plethysmography measures changes in volume of the extremity resulting from obstruction of venous outflow. Electrical impedance plethysmography involves calculation of the amount of blood in the leg based upon changes in conductivity and electrical resistance. This technic can detect iliac, femoral, and popliteal thrombi, the most important sources of pulmonary emboli. As with ultrasound, impedance plethysmography is less accurate for examining the calf and is insensitive to partially occluding thrombi. Cooperation of the patient is essential for the respiratory maneuvers and may be difficult to obtain in the immediate postoperative period. Cranley has recently introduced a sophisticated instrument called a **phleborrheograph** consisting of multiple strain gauge plethysmographs which appears to be very accurate in detecting venous obstruction (thrombosis) in the calf, thigh, and pelvis.

4. Radioactive fibrinogen—Since circulating fibrinogen becomes incorporated into newly forming thrombi, if it is labeled with radioactive material, such as ^{125}I, the thrombi can be detected by external scanning over the veins. Routine screening with this method has shown that deep venous thrombosis occurs in as many as 30–60% of patients following general surgical procedures and in 50% of patients undergoing orthopedic or neurosurgical operations. Clinical signs of venous thrombosis are present in only 5–10% of cases. The thrombosis appears to begin during the operation. About 90% of postoperative thrombi detected by this method are confined to the calf and are probably not dangerous, but about 20% of these calf thrombi extend into the popliteal or femoral veins where they produce clinical signs and potentially significant emboli. Radioactive fibrinogen seems sensitive enough to detect small thrombi in venous sinuses of the soleus muscle or the posterior tibial and peroneal veins. At present, this is the most sensitive test for venous thrombosis and is therefore the best screening method, but it will not detect preexisting thrombi which are not actively incorporating fibrinogen and it cannot detect iliac or pelvic thromboses. There is a potential risk of hepatitis transmitted in the pooled fibrinogen. The results with radioactive fibrinogen correlate closely with phlebography, and false-positive and false-negative tests are rare. By this method, about 90% of postoperative thrombi are in the calf and about 20% of the calf thrombi extend into the popliteal or femoral veins, where they produce clinical signs. One of the advantages of the radioactive fibrinogen test is that it can be repeated daily and the progress of the thrombi followed. Radioactive fibrinogen is now commercially available in the USA under the trade name Sensor.

5. Venous pressure measurements—The physiology of the deep veins has been discussed earlier in this chapter. With deep venous thrombosis, the walking venous pressure in the veins on the dorsum of the foot is abnormally elevated. Pressure measurement, however, will not distinguish acute from chronic deep venous thrombosis and therefore has relatively little clinical usefulness.

Differential Diagnosis

As already noted, the frequency of clinical diagnosis of deep venous thrombosis is much lower than the true incidence of this disorder. Leg swelling could be due to lymphatic obstruction, but the process is usually chronic and the edema nonpitting. It may be more acute if cellulitis is superimposed, but in this case inflammation is more prominent and a wound is often present.

Contusion of a calf muscle or rupture of the plantaris tendon can produce a swollen, painful calf and may be difficult to differentiate from deep venous occlusion. Acute onset of symptoms during exercise and ecchymosis in the calf would point to muscle injury. In some cases, phlebography or ^{125}I-fibrinogen scanning may be required to establish a true diagnosis. Bilateral swelling of the lower extremities, while sometimes seen in deep venous thrombosis, is usually of cardiac or renal origin. Occasionally it is difficult to distinguish an arterial from a venous occlusion. In arterial occlusion, there is generally more pain and no swelling, the superficial veins are not distended, and they fill very slowly when emptied. In venous thrombosis, the superficial veins are full and dilated. Sensation in the extremity usually disappears promptly in acute arterial occlusion, whereas it usually persists in acute thrombophlebitis. The greatest usefulness of phlebography is to demonstrate a patent venous system when venous thrombosis cannot be differentiated from other entities, thus avoiding unnecessary anticoagulation and hospitalization.

Complications

A. Chronic Venous Insufficiency: This complication, discussed in detail later, usually follows iliofemoral thrombophlebitis but not thrombosis confined to the leg.

B. Varicose Veins: Secondary varicose veins may develop as collaterals when the deep venous system is occluded.

C. Venous Gangrene: Gangrene due to massive venous thrombosis may occur in phlegmasia cerulea dolens without associated arterial thrombosis. This is a rare condition but is often fatal when it does occur. Venous thrombectomy in phlegmasia cerulea dolens is strongly indicated since it may prevent gangrene.

D. Pulmonary Embolism: Pulmonary embolism occurs when a thrombus becomes dislodged from its attachment to the venous wall and is carried into the pulmonary arteries. The mortality rate of 10% is caused by massive embolism with occlusion of two-thirds or more of the pulmonary blood flow. The incidence is highest in elderly patients (85% are above 50 years) and is increased 7- to 10-fold in young women taking oral contraceptives.

Table 39–3. Classification of chronic leg ulcers.

Vascular
  Arterial
    Atherosclerosis obliterans
    Thromboangiitis obliterans
    Arteriovenous fistula
    Collagen vascular disease (polyarteritis nodosa)
    Hypertension
    Raynaud's disease
  Venous
    Chronic deep venous insufficiency
    Varicose veins
    Postinjection reaction
  Lymphatic: Chronic lymphedema
Infective
  Bone
    Chronic osteomyelitis
    Adherent fracture site
  Pyogenic
  Synergistic gangrene (Meleney's ulcer)
  Miscellaneous
    Syphilis
    Tuberculosis
    Tropical diseases (leishmaniasis)
    Fungal diseases
Systemic-metabolic
  Ulcerative colitis
  Diabetes mellitus
  Sickle cell anemia
  Avitaminosis
Neoplastic
  Primary skin tumor
    Kaposi's sarcoma
    Melanoma
    Squamous cell carcinoma
  Leukemia
  Metastatic
Traumatic
  Radiation
  Thermal burns
  Decubitus
  Insect bites
Neurotrophic
  Cord lesions
  Peripheral neuropathies
    Trauma
    Diabetes
    Tabes dorsalis
    Alcoholism

About 70% of pulmonary emboli originate from thrombi in lower extremity veins, 20% from pelvic veins, and 5% from the upper extremities and right atrium. It is not clear why some thrombi become detached and others do not, but bed rest with elevation of an affected extremity has been shown to help prevent embolism. Emboli arise principally when the clot extends into the major femoral veins, and, because most remain localized in tributaries, the majority of calf thrombi revealed by radioactive fibrinogen are unimportant clinically. Most fatal emboli arise from iliac, femoral, and pelvic veins.

About half of patients with clinical findings of deep thrombophlebitis develop pulmonary emboli. However, most patients with pulmonary emboli do not have clinical phlebitis even though the clots are known to originate in the legs. It has also been shown that in patients with clinical signs of phlebitis, emboli frequently come from the opposite, clinically silent leg.

Both the initial and recurrent episodes are largely preventable. Untreated, the recurrence rate is 30% and the mortality rate 20%; heparin treatment reduces the recurrence rate to 5% or less.

Prevention

Patients with predisposing factors (Table 39–2) comprise a high-risk group in whom the following preventive measures should be considered:

A. Physical Measures to Reduce Venous Stasis: Active leg exercises (quadriceps, plantar flexion), leg elevation, and the use of elastic support improve femoral venous blood flow and reduce the incidence of deep venous thrombosis, especially in elderly patients. Early ambulation after surgery and avoidance of prolonged bed rest also promote venous return. Prolonged sitting and standing should be avoided because they cause venous stasis. During operative procedures, galvanic stimulation to produce contraction of calf muscles, intermittent external calf compression with a pneumatic sleeve, and the use of motorized foot maneuvers all diminish the incidence of formation of calf thrombi. Passive measures which promote venous drainage, such as elevating the foot of the bed 15–20 degrees, should also be employed. Brief regular periods of walking during long automobile or airplane trips should be encouraged, for venous thrombosis may occur in such settings even in active healthy adults.

B. Anticoagulation: Controlled trials have proved that prophylactic anticoagulation in high-risk patients markedly reduces the incidence of postoperative deep venous thrombosis and pulmonary thromboembolism. The following agents have been studied:

1. Prothrombin depressants—Warfarin or phenindione derivatives are effective prophylactic agents when anticoagulation is initiated before and maintained for several days after operation. They are associated with a slightly increased incidence of bleeding complications following surgery, and for this reason their use has not become popular.

2. Platelet function suppressants—The use of

these agents has been fostered because platelet thrombi in the valve cusps are the first step in venous thrombosis and because platelet aggregation is relatively unaffected by conventional anticoagulants. Infusions of dextran 40 or dextran 70 during and after surgery reduce the incidence of thromboembolism. The mechanism of action of dextran is complex but includes plasma volume expansion, reduced platelet adhesiveness, and coating of platelet and red cell surfaces (increased electronegativity). Among the side-effects of dextran infusions are congestive heart failure, acute renal failure, and allergic reactions. The bleeding complications can be avoided if the dose is limited to less than 1 liter per day. Other antiplatelet drugs such as dipyridamole and aspirin fail to lower the incidence of thromboembolic complications and cannot be recommended for prophylaxis.

3. Heparin—A number of good clinical trials using ^{125}I-fibrinogen scanning have demonstrated the efficacy and safety of low-dose (mini) heparin in preventing deep venous thrombosis. The usual regimen is 5000 units subcut 2 hours preoperatively and every 8–12 hours postoperatively for several days. This dose of heparin does not significantly prolong the coagulation time as measured by the standard laboratory tests (APTT, Lee-White). The beneficial effect is thought to be through enhancement of a natural inhibitor of activated factor X. Since bleeding complications and transfusion requirements are only slightly increased with this regimen, it is being used more often for prophylaxis in patients at high risk of developing venous thromboembolism (Table 39–2). In general, heparin is easier to control than the prothrombin depressants.

Treatment of Deep Venous Thrombosis

The objectives of treatment are to prevent growth of the thrombus, embolization, and formation of additional thrombi.

A. Bed Rest and Elevation: The patient should be confined to bed with the feet elevated 15–20 degrees above the level of his heart. Since it takes 7–8 days for experimental thrombi to become firmly adherent to vein walls, it is common practice to continue bed rest for about this long after the onset of symptoms. Elevation reduces the edema and pain, and the resulting increased venous flow inhibits formation of new thrombus. Application of elastic bandages to the leg is indicated because they increase the velocity of venous flow. Bed rest should be continued until the swelling, pain, and tenderness have resolved. Graduated ambulation with elastic support is then permitted, but standing and sitting are forbidden because the accompanying rise in venous pressure aggravates edema and discomfort. The use of elastic support and limitations on sitting and standing are required for 3–6 months until recanalization and collaterization develop. Continuous warm moist dressings on the involved leg provide symptomatic relief in the acute phase.

B. Drug Treatment: Unless there are specific contraindications, anticoagulants are indicated. The goals are to prevent propagation of the original throm-

bus, the development of new sites of thrombosis, and pulmonary embolization of thrombi. By allowing the natural fibrinolysis to operate unopposed, anticoagulation also hastens dissolution of the thrombus.

1. Heparin—Heparin, an acid mucopolysaccharide, inhibits thrombus formation by neutralizing thrombin, by blocking the formation of thromboplastin, and by inhibiting the platelet release reaction. It is of proved benefit in the treatment of deep venous thrombosis and in the prevention of pulmonary embolism. Heparin therapy should be started as soon as the diagnosis of deep venous thrombosis has been confirmed. Since it is not absorbed from the gastrointestinal tract, it must be given either intravenously or subcutaneously. Bleeding complications are reduced if dosage is regulated according to one of the coagulation tests such as the whole blood clotting time (Lee and White), activated partial thromboplastin time, or activated clotting time. Since the amount of heparin required may vary from day to day, the degree of anticoagulation should be monitored daily by one of these tests. Bleeding complications are lowest if the heparin is given by continuous intravenous infusion. An initial dose of 100 units/kg body weight should be given IV and subsequent doses determined by laboratory tests. The anticoagulant effects of heparin are immediate. If bolus therapy is selected, the drug should be given every 4 or 6 hours and the test of coagulation performed 1 hour before the next scheduled dose. For acute thrombophlebitis, heparin should be continued for 7–10 days, the time required for thrombi to become firmly adherent to the vein walls. If at the end of this time leg pain and tenderness persist, heparin should be continued until they resolve. If pulmonary embolism has occurred, heparin should be continued for an additional 7–10 days (total of 2–3 weeks). Bleeding, the major complication, is most likely to occur in fresh surgical wounds or in the gastrointestinal tract and usually indicates that too much heparin has been administered. Protamine sulfate, a heparin inhibitor, should be given if hemorrhage is significant. Excess protamine does not produce anticoagulation, as was formerly believed. Drugs such as aspirin that inhibit platelet aggregation should not be given to heparinized patients because the combination seriously interferes with primary hemostasis as well as coagulation. Intramuscular injections should be avoided because of the danger of local hemorrhage at the injection site.

2. Oral anticoagulants—Coumarin derivatives block synthesis in the liver of at least 4 clotting factors and reduce the prothrombin time. Therapy should aim for a prothrombin time about 2–2½ times the control value (20–25% of normal), a level which is reached only 3–4 days after treatment is instituted. Further prolongation of the prothrombin time is associated with an unacceptably high incidence of bleeding complications.

Since oral anticoagulants are not as effective as heparin and their onset of action is slow, they are best reserved for prophylaxis (see above) of deep venous thrombosis or for long-term anticoagulation after heparin treatment has been discontinued. For acute deep venous thrombosis, anticoagulation should be continued for the 3–6 months required for development of venous collaterals. The oral agent should be started and heparin then discontinued several days later when the prothrombin time has reached the therapeutic level. Because interaction occurs between the coumarin derivatives and many other drugs (eg, barbiturates), patients on oral anticoagulants must be carefully monitored. Excessive prolongation of the prothrombin time can be treated by administration of vitamin K.

3. Other medications—Fibrinolytic activators (urokinase, streptokinase) lyse intravascular thrombi, but bleeding complications are more common than with conventional anticoagulants, especially in fresh surgical wounds. In some studies, fibrinolytic agents not only produced rapid clearance of the occluded vein but preserved competency and function of the valves. Because streptokinase is antigenic, most recent studies have been performed with nonantigenic urokinase, a natural product of human urine. A coagulant fraction (Ancrod) prepared from the venom of the Malayan pit viper attacks fibrinogen and produces intravascular defibrination. It seems effective for deep venous thrombosis but is not superior to heparin. Fibrinolytic and defibrinating agents will undoubtedly receive much attention in the future as they have several theoretic advantages over conventional anticoagulants.

C. Operative Procedures: The vast majority of patients with acute venous thrombosis are satisfactorily managed medically. In a small percentage, however, operation is necessary.

1. Venous thrombectomy—This operation involves incising the common femoral vein in the groin and extracting the clots. The goals are (1) to prevent the postphlebitic syndrome, (2) to prevent pulmonary embolism, (3) to decrease hospital morbidity, and (4) in phlegmasia cerulea dolens, to save the limb. It is most likely to be successful if performed within the first 24 hours after onset of symptoms. In iliofemoral venous thrombosis, successful thrombectomy will rapidly relieve acute venous stasis and the inflammatory reaction and may save the limb when impending venous gangrene exists. In about two-thirds of patients, postoperative phlebograms reveal reocclusion of the involved segments, so that the ultimate value of this procedure remains unproved. Except for the treatment of phlegmasia cerulea dolens, most surgeons are unenthusiastic about this procedure.

2. Venous interruption—The rationale of venous interruption is the prevention of pulmonary embolism by trapping the thrombus in the peripheral venous segment. Ligation of the superficial femoral vein just before its junction with the common femoral vein prevents embolization from distal muscular and deep veins and rarely is followed by chronic venous insufficiency. Obviously, it does not protect against emboli arising central to the point of ligation. Ligation of the common femoral vein is almost always followed by chronic venous insufficiency. With the realization that many (if not most) fatal pulmonary emboli arise from iliac or pelvic veins, venous interruption in the extremities has given way to technics which trap emboli in the inferior vena cava. Ligation of the inferior vena cava prevents fatal pulmonary embolism, and the operative mortality rate is low. The incidence of significant venous insufficiency of the legs following vena caval ligation varies greatly and is probably more closely related to the extent of preexisting venous disease than to the caval interruption itself. The lower extremity sequelae are minimized by procedures such as plication or clipping which only partially occlude the lumen and create a sieve through which blood flows unimpeded but which prevents passage of clot. Ligation of the left ovarian or spermatic vein should be performed concomitantly, particularly when there is pelvic vein thrombosis. More recently, small filters have been developed which can be inserted into the cava transvenously under local anesthesia (Fig 39–6).

The indications for venous interruption are prevention of recurrent embolism in patients who cannot be safely anticoagulated or in patients who have emboli while adequately anticoagulated. Some surgeons advocate partial caval interruption as prophylaxis in high-risk patients undergoing abdominal operations. When emboli arise from septic pelvic thrombophlebitis, the cava should be ligated, not compartmentalized. After caval ligation, as many as 5–10% of patients

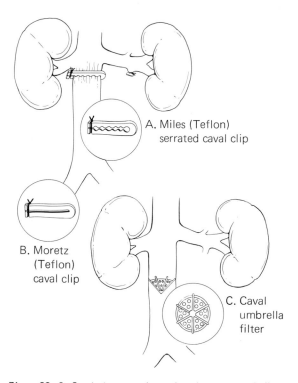

Figure 39–6. Surgical prevention of pulmonary embolism. Large emboli can be trapped by partial interruption of the inferior vena cava. *A:* Serrated Teflon (Miles) clip. *B:* Smooth Teflon (Moretz) clip. These should be placed just distal to the renal veins and the gonadal veins ligated. *C:* Caval umbrella filter, which is inserted transvenously through a jugular cutdown. Many surgeons prefer to simply ligate the cava.

develop recurrent emboli transported in collateral veins around the caval ligature or arising in the venous cul-de-sac between the caval ligature and renal veins. Other possible additional sources are the right atrium and upper extremities.

Adams JT, Feingold BE, DeWeese JA: Comparative evaluation of ligation and partial interruption of the inferior vena cava. Arch Surg 103:272, 1971.

Alexander RH & others: Thrombophlebitis and thromboembolism: Results of a prospective study. Ann Surg 180:883, 1974.

Bertelsen S, Anker W: Phlegmasia coerulea dolens: Pathophysiology, clinical features, treatment, and prognosis. Acta Chir Scand 134:107, 1968.

Bettmann MA, Paulin S: Leg phlebography: The incidence, nature, and modification of undesirable side-effects. Radiology 122:101, 1977.

Bülow S, Sager P: Venous gangrene. Acta Chir Scand 141:272, 1975.

Clagett GP, Salzman EW: Prevention of venous thromboembolism in surgical patients. N Engl J Med 290:93, 1974.

Cranley JJ, Canos AJ, Sull WJ: The diagnosis of deep venous thrombosis: Fallibility of clinical symptoms and signs. Arch Surg 111:34, 1976.

Fogarty TJ, Dennis D, Krippaehne WW: Surgical management of ilio-femoral venous thrombosis. Am J Surg 112:211, 1966.

Gallus AS & others: Small subcutaneous doses of heparin in prevention of venous thrombosis. N Engl J Med 288:545, 1973.

Handin RI: Thromboembolic complications of pregnancy and oral contraceptives. Prog Cardiovasc Dis 16:395, 1974.

Hirsh J, Gallus AS: ^{125}I-labeled fibrinogen scanning: Use in the diagnosis of venous thrombosis. JAMA 233:970, 1975.

Hjelmstedt A: The pressure in the veins of the dorsum of the foot in quiet standing and during exercise in limbs without signs of venous disorder. Acta Chir Scand 134:235, 1968.

Kakkar VV & others: Efficacy of low doses of heparin in prevention of deep-vein thrombosis after major surgery: A double-blind, randomized trial. Lancet 2:101, 1972.

Kakkar VV & others: Prevention of fatal postoperative pulmonary embolism by low doses of heparin: An international multicentre trial. Lancet 2:45, 1975.

Kistner RL & others: Incidence of pulmonary embolism in the course of thrombophlebitis of the lower extremities. Am J Surg 124:169, 1972.

Lambie JM & others: Diagnostic accuracy in venous thrombosis. Br Med J 2:142, 1970.

LeQuesne LP: Relation between deep vein thrombosis and pulmonary embolism in surgical patients. N Engl J Med 291:1292, 1974.

Mavor GE, Galloway JMD: Ilio-femoral venous thrombosis. Br J Surg 56:45, 1969.

Mavor GE & others: Streptokinase therapy in deep-vein thrombosis. Br J Surg 60:468, 1973.

Mustard JF, Packham MD: Thromboembolism: A manifestation of the response of blood to injury. Circulation 42:1, 1970.

Rabinov K, Paulin S: Roentgen diagnosis of venous thrombosis in the leg. Arch Surg 104:134, 1972.

Sagar S & others: Oral contraceptives, antithrombin III activity, and postoperative deep-vein thrombosis. Lancet 1:509, 1976.

Salzman EW & others: Management of heparin therapy: Controlled prospective trial. N Engl J Med 292:1046, 1975.

Sigel B, Ipsen J, Felix WR Jr: The epidemiology of lower extremity deep venous thrombosis in surgical patients. Ann Surg 179:278, 1974.

Skillman JJ: Postoperative deep vein thrombosis and pulmonary embolism: A selective review and personal viewpoint. Surgery 75:114, 1974.

Strandness DE Jr, Sumner DS: Acute venous thrombosis: A case of progress and confusion. JAMA 233:46, 1975.

Wessler S, Yin TE: Theory and practice of minidose heparin in surgical patients: A status report. Circulation 47:671, 1973.

SUPERFICIAL THROMBOPHLEBITIS

Essentials of Diagnosis

- Pain, tenderness, and induration along course of a superficial vein.
- Palpable "cord" corresponding to course of vein.
- Absence of significant extremity swelling.
- Identifiable source of infection often present in proximity.

General Considerations

Because of their subcutaneous position, thromboses of superficial veins are usually easily recognized. In the upper extremities, intravenous infusions are the most common cause. In the lower extremities, thrombosis may be associated with varicose veins, thromboangiitis obliterans, or a neighboring bacterial infection. There is often a history of trauma. Recurrent or migratory superficial thrombophlebitis may be an early manifestation of abdominal malignancy (Trousseau's sign) or other systemic illness.

Clinical Findings

Superficial venous thrombosis is almost always accompanied by pain, induration, heat, tenderness, and erythema along the course of the involved vein. The patient may be febrile and have leukocytosis. The involved veins may feel like cords or ovoid nodules. The process most commonly involves the long saphenous vein and its tributaries and tends to remain localized. The inflammatory reaction may take 2–3 weeks to subside, and the thrombosed vein may be palpable for a much longer time. There is no associated edema of the extremity as a whole unless the process is extensive and the patient ambulatory.

Differential Diagnosis

This lesion can be confused with acute bacterial cellulitis, lymphangitis, and other acute inflammatory lesions. The distribution of the process along the course of the superficial veins should help in making this distinction. It is frequently confused with deep thrombophlebitis, but the edema associated with the latter condition is not present and indurated superficial venous cords are not present in deep venous thrombosis. Rarely, the 2 may coexist when the superficial phlebitis extends into the deep system via the communicating veins or at the saphenofemoral junction. When chills and high fever are present, suppuration has most likely developed in the involved vein (septic thrombophlebitis). *Staphylococcus aureus* is the most frequently cultured organism.

Treatment

In the absence of associated deep venous involvement, treatment is symptomatic and includes analgesics for pain, local heat, elastic compression bandages, and continued ambulation. Bed rest and anticoagulation are not necessary. When inflammation in the saphenous vein is progressing toward the saphenofemoral junction, pulmonary embolism is possible and ligation and division of the saphenous vein is indicated. It can be done under local anesthesia. If the vein is varicosed, many would recommend that it be removed. Resolution of the process is usually prompt following surgical therapy. If there is concomitant deep venous involvement, anticoagulation and bed rest should be instituted. When the involved vein is infected (septic thrombophlebitis), high doses of antibiotics should be given and the involved segment should be excised to avoid persistent bacterial seeding of the blood stream.

Prognosis

The course is ordinarily short and uncomplicated. Pulmonary emboli are rare because the inflammation produces firm adherence of the clot to the vein wall. Recurrent superficial phlebitis is an indication for venous stripping.

Collin J & others: Infusion thrombophlebitis and infection with various cannulas. Lancet 2:150, 1975.

Munster AM: Septic thrombophlebitis: A surgical disorder. JAMA 230:1010, 1974.

Stein JM, Pruitt BA Jr: Suppurative thrombophlebitis. N Engl J Med 282:1452, 1970.

Zinner MJ, Zuidema ED, Lowery BD: Septic nonsuppurative thrombophlebitis. Arch Surg 111:122, 1976.

AXILLARY-SUBCLAVIAN VENOUS THROMBOSIS

Essentials of Diagnosis

- History of repetitive or unusual muscular activity of upper extremity.
- Swelling of entire upper extremity.
- Collateral venous pattern over anterior chest wall.
- Swelling and pain made worse by exercise.
- Obstruction of vein at thoracic outlet by phlebography.

General Considerations

Thrombosis of the axillary and subclavian veins accounts for only 2–3% of all cases of deep venous thrombosis. This low incidence is thought to be due to the shorter course that the blood travels in the upper extremity and to the absence of venous stasis because of the frequent movements of the arms.

When axillary vein thrombosis does occur, it frequently is in association with predisposing factors such as congestive heart failure, metastatic tumor in the axilla, indwelling venous catheters, or external trauma. Many cases are spontaneous but preceded by exercise of the extremity during sports participation or occupational activities which produce direct or indirect injury to the vein (effort thrombosis). Injury is thought to result at the thoracic outlet, where the axillary and subclavian veins may be compressed by nearby structures, most often in the costoclavicular space between the clavicle and the first rib.

Clinical Findings

Pain and swelling appear within 24 hours of the inciting event. The swelling usually involves the entire arm and is nonpitting. The pain is usually described as an aching sensation with a feeling of tightness, often most severe in the axilla. A prominent collateral venous pattern is usually visible over the shoulder and anterior chest wall, and the breast may be enlarged on the side of involvement. The extremity may be cyanotic. Only one-third of patients have a palpable tender cord in the axilla.

Diagnosis

In most cases the diagnosis can be made on the basis of the signs and symptoms alone. Dilated superficial veins on the anterior chest wall may be shown best by infrared photography. Pressure in the antecubital veins is high and rises further with muscular exercise (normally, venous pressure drops with exercise). Final confirmation can be made only with phlebographic demonstration of thrombotic occlusion of the deep veins. Obstruction is most frequently seen in the region where the vein crosses the first rib, and a collateral venous network bypassing this obstruction can usually be visualized. This supports the etiologic theory of compression of the vein in the costoclavicular space between the clavicle and the first rib.

Complications

Complications of axillary vein thrombosis are few, but prolonged disability is not rare. Venous gangrene, the counterpart of phlegmasia cerulea dolens in the lower extremity, develops rarely. Pulmonary embolism is seen in 12% of patients—more than has generally been thought.

Treatment

Most patients with primary axillary or subclavian venous thrombosis recover rapidly from the acute symptoms with no therapy other than rest and elevation of the arm. Anticoagulation should be instituted to prevent progression of the thrombus and embolization and to foster development of collaterals. The anticoagulation regimen is the same as described earlier for deep leg vein thrombosis. When peripheral vasospasm is an important part of the clinical picture, stellate ganglion block may be useful.

Venous thrombectomy is performed occasionally with the goal of relieving the venous obstruction and preserving valvular integrity. The operation is seldom used because prompt rethrombosis is the rule postoperatively. However, if it is possible to simultaneously remove a predisposing extraluminal obstruction, long-term patency may be achieved by thrombectomy.

Serious consideration should be given to relieving the cause of the venous compression to prevent recurrence even if thrombectomy is not performed. Since the site of the most severe compression is invariably in the costoclavicular space, it should be enlarged either by resection of the clavicle or the first rib. In general, transaxillary resection of the first rib has produced the best results.

Prognosis

Although rapid recovery from the initial symptoms occurs in most patients, residual symptoms occur in 60–85% of those treated conservatively. Even though the acute swelling and pain subside within a few days to weeks, most patients have persistent or recurrent swelling, numbness, tingling, easy fatigability, and episodes of recurrent superficial phlebitis. Symptoms tend to be precipitated by exercise. Some have claimed that the incidence of late symptoms is markedly reduced by early thrombectomy.

Adams JT & others: Intermittent subclavian vein obstruction without thrombosis. Surgery 63:147, 1968.

Coon WW, Willis PW: Thrombosis of axillary and subclavian veins. Arch Surg 94:557, 1967.

DeWeese JA, Adams JT, Gaiser DL: Subclavian venous thrombectomy. Circulation 16 (Suppl 2):168, 1972.

Mahorner H: Results of surgical operations for venous thrombosis. Surg Gynecol Obstet 129:66, 1969.

Swinton NW Jr, Edgett JW Jr, Hall RJ: Primary subclavian-axillary vein thrombosis. Circulation 38:727, 1968.

Tilney NL, Griffiths HJG, Edwards EA: Natural history of major venous thrombosis of upper extremity. Arch Surg 101:792, 1970.

CHRONIC DEEP VENOUS INSUFFICIENCY

Essentials of Diagnosis

- History of previous deep vein thrombosis may be absent.
- Edema, hyperpigmentation, brawny induration, and dermatitis of distal leg and ankle.
- Ulceration, especially above the medial malleolus.
- Secondary superficial varicose veins.
- Positive Trendelenburg test.

General Considerations

The principal late complication of deep vein thrombosis is chronic venous stasis, and most patients with serious problems have originally had iliofemoral thrombophlebitis. There is persistent obstruction from incomplete recanalization of the thrombosed veins, destruction of the venous valves, and reflux of blood through incompetent perforator veins—and, thereby, a high pressure in the superficial veins. When the patient is standing at rest, pressure in a dorsal foot vein is normal in the postphlebitic leg, but with exercise the pressure fails to drop because the valves are incompetent. The sustained high pressure results in the **postphlebitic syndrome,** which consists of edema, stasis dermatitis, and ulceration of the distal leg (Fig 39–1).

Clinical Findings

A. Edema: Subcutaneous edema primarily involving the distal leg and ankle is usually the first manifestation of chronic venous insufficiency. At first, it accumulates during the day and disappears at night during recumbency. Orthostatic edema is usually present for some time before the more serious manifestations of the syndrome appear, and the increased tissue pressure resulting from the accumulation of edema fluid is one of the main factors in the evolution of the syndrome.

B. Dermatitis and Hyperpigmentation: The brownish pigmentation occurs at the ankle, consisting of hemosiderin in macrophages, which represents destroyed blood pigment from extravasated red blood cells. Melanocytic reaction also contributes to pigmentary changes. A pruritic eczematous reaction (stasis dermatitis) is common and may lead to neurodermatitis from prolonged scratching.

C. Induration: With long-standing edema, fibrosis develops in the subcutaneous tissues and reduces elasticity of the skin. Low-grade, often clinically insignificant bacterial infection may contribute to these changes which ultimately make the swelling refractory to recumbency.

D. Ulceration: Ulceration is the major complication which stimulates the patient to seek medical attention. Approximately half of venous ulcers are associated with incompetent perforating veins in the region of the ankle. It is rarely a manifestation of primary varicose veins. Stasis ulcers are most often just proximal or distal to the medial malleolus and often develop at sites of minor trauma or skin infections. Induration, scarring, and secondary bacterial infection all impair healing and make recurrences common if healing does occur. The natural history of venous ulceration is cyclic healing and recurrence unless something definitive is done to correct the high venous pressure at the ankle.

E. Pain: Whether there is ulceration or just swelling, the dull pain is relieved by recumbency and elevation of the foot. In general, arterial ischemic ulcers are more painful than venous ulcers; the pain is made worse by elevation of the foot; and they are less often located at the medial malleolus. Arterial ulcers may extend to or through the fascia, whereas venous ulcers are shallow.

Treatment

The primary goal of therapy is control of the persistent venous hypertension and avoidance of edema. This is readily accomplished in most patients with custom-fitted, heavy duty, knee-length elastic stockings. Intermittent periods of leg elevation and avoidance of prolonged sitting and standing should be advised. There is no need for elastic support above the knee because the complications of venous insufficiency practically never extend this high. The support must be used indefinitely.

Of primary importance to healing of venous stasis ulcers is the elimination of edema. If the ulcers are small and recent and edema has been controlled, treatment can be instituted on an outpatient basis by providing support to the tissues with a well-fitted, semirigid, bootlike dressing (Gelocast, Unna paste boot, or Gauztex). The boot is reapplied at intervals of 1–2 weeks. After the ulcer has healed, the boot is discarded in favor of heavy duty elastic stockings. Large ulcers usually require hospitalization for bed rest, elevation of the leg, and local wound care, but healing may be slow. Local treatment of the ulcer consists of moist dressings, which should be changed several times daily. Granulation tissue develops and exudate decreases as the surface infection is controlled. Antibiotics are usually unnecessary except in rare cases when infection is spreading and the patient is febrile.

If the ulcers cannot be controlled by conservative management or if they are large, surgery is indicated. Split thickness skin grafts may be applied directly to a clean granulating ulcer, or the ulcer may be excised and a skin graft applied primarily. Recurrences are common if nothing is done to remove the diseased veins. The initial operation should include ligation and stripping of the greater saphenous vein and ligation of incompetent perforators in the region of the ulcer. If the lesser saphenous system is involved, it should be removed as well. Contrary to what has been taught in the past, removal of secondary varicosities of the saphenous system, except in rare instances, does not impair venous return from the extremity.

When ulceration recurs in spite of these measures, more radical surgical procedures are indicated. The most successful of these is ligation of all of the perforating veins. The perforators which are invariably associated with recurrent ulceration are more easily located and more readily ligated in the subfascial plane than by attempts at individual ligation in the scarred, indurated subcutaneous tissue. They are best approached through a simple long posterior midline incision which extends through the fascia, creating 2 full thickness flaps. The exposed perforating veins are ligated as they pass from the muscle to penetrate the fascia. Even after this procedure, recurrent ulceration occurs in as many as 10% of patients. As no operation eliminates the venous hypertension, elastic support is required indefinitely after all these procedures.

Rarely, after many years, a chronic ulcer may undergo malignant transformation (**Marjolin's ulcer**), a change that is not always easy to recognize. Therefore,

intractable ulcers should be biopsied to check for tumor.

Bypass of an obstructed iliac or femoral vein (or both) with a vein graft has resulted in prolonged patency of the graft and symptomatic relief in a number of patients. The procedure is most applicable for localized venous obstruction due to extrinsic compression of the vein.

Prognosis

Recurrent thrombophlebitis is frequent and requires prophylactic measures such as elastic support, periodic elevation of the legs, and avoidance of stasis-producing activities.

Abramowitz MD: The postphlebitic syndrome: A critical assessment of diagnostic parameters. S Afr J Surg 10:153, 1972.

Arnoldi CC, Linderholm H: On the pathogenesis of the venous leg ulcer. Acta Chir Scand 134:427, 1968.

Barnes RW & others: Noninvasive quantitations of venous hemodynamics in the postphlebitic syndrome. Arch Surg 107:807, 1973.

Corrigan TP, Kakkar VV: Early changes in the postphlebitic limb: Their clinical significance. Br J Surg 60:808, 1973.

Haller JA Jr: Pathophysiology and management of postphlebitic venous insufficiency. South Med J 63:177, 1970.

Lim RC & others: Subfascial ligation of perforating veins in recurrent stasis ulceration. Am J Surg 119:246, 1970.

THE SWOLLEN LEG

Edema consists of increased interstitial fluid which results from an imbalance between the filtration pressure in proximal capillaries and the absorptive osmotic pressure at the venous end of the capillaries. Venous, lymphatic, or systemic causes can produce chronic edema of the lower extremity. The peripheral lymphatics serve as the major route whereby large protein molecules which have escaped from the vascular compartment are removed and returned to the circulation. Failure to remove interstitial proteins, the major pathophysiologic abnormality in lymphedema, produces an osmotic force which perpetuates water retention (edema). In chronic venous insufficiency, edema is principally a consequence of abnormally high net fluid filtration from elevated venular pressure. The lymphatics still remove extracellular protein, so venous edema is characteristically low in protein. In either case, edema means that lymph formation has exceeded lymph resorption. Whatever the cause, long-standing edema produces similar patterns of secondary inflammation and fibrosis.

The causes of chronic leg edema are listed in Table 39–4. If systemic causes can be excluded or if the swelling is unilateral, the disease must be local, and the major diagnostic problem is to decide between a venous and lymphatic origin. The distinction can be based on clinical findings in most cases, but special

Table 39—4. Etiology of the swollen leg.

Venous
    Postphlebitic syndrome
    Extrinsic compression
        Tumor
        Retroperitoneal fibrosis
        Compression by iliac artery
    Trauma
        Surgical ligation, plication, clip
        Wound
    Arteriovenous fistula
Lymphatic
    Primary lymphedema
        Congenital lymphedema
        Lymphedema praecox
        Lymphedema tarda
    Secondary lymphedema
        Infection (filariasis)
        Neoplasia
        Radiation
        Insect bites
        Surgical excision
        Motor paralysis (disuse)
Systemic
    Congestive heart failure
    Cirrhosis
    Nephrosis
    Myxedema
    Drugs, hormones
    Hypoproteinemia

procedures such as venography and lymphangiography are occasionally required.

Dale WA: The swollen leg. Curr Probl Surg, Sept 1973.
Gill JR Jr: Edema. Annu Rev Med 21:269, 1970.

THE LYMPHATICS

Surgical Anatomy

Phylogenetically, the lymph vessels are modified veins. Histologically, the lymphatic capillaries are blind endothelial tubes which differ from vascular capillaries mainly in that they are highly permeable to macromolecules. The larger lymphatics have smooth muscle walls and endothelial valves which permit flow only in a central direction. Lymph nodes are interspersed in the course of larger lymphatics and serve a filtrative, phagocytic, and immunologic function. Total lymph flow entering the subclavian veins in humans is 2—4 liters daily and contains 75—200 g of protein. Venous obstruction, vasodilatation, muscular exercise, and increased capillary permeability all increase the rate of lymph flow.

The lymphatic capillaries form a superficial plexus in the superficial dermis, a deep plexus in the deeper dermis, and, in the extremities, a subfascial plexus within the muscular compartments. The larger lymph channels tend to travel with the major blood vessels. As with the veins, active or passive contraction of skeletal muscles plays an important role in the movement of lymph, and the lymphatic valves determine its direction.

Lymphangiography

Organic dyes injected into the skin are rapidly picked up by the subdermal or superficial dermal lymphatics, which can then easily be recognized by their color. This allows cannulation of the lymphatics and injection of radiopaque contrast media. X-rays (lymphangiograms) reveal normal lymphatics as slender vessels of uniform diameter which branch as they proceed centrally. Lymphangiography is not practiced as widely as arteriography or venography because the technic is difficult and the complication rates relatively high. It is nevertheless often helpful in identifying the cause of a chronically swollen lower extremity. Lymphangiography can also be used to detect abnormal lymph nodes in the retroperitoneum or mediastinum in the evaluation of patients with lymphomas. Since the contrast medium used for lymphangiography may produce a temporary diffusion barrier when it reaches the lungs, preliminary pulmonary function testing is advisable so that the test can be avoided in patients with significant pulmonary disability.

LYMPHEDEMA

Essentials of Diagnosis

- Progressive swelling of one or both lower extremities, often without antecedent history.
- Nonpitting edema.
- Recurrent episodes of lymphangitis and cellulitis.
- Edema does not respond to leg elevation.

General Considerations

Lymphedema has multiple causes (Table 39—4), but the pathophysiologic mechanism—obstruction of lymphatics—is similar in all.

Clinical Findings

Primary lymphedema may be present at birth **(congenital lymphedema)** but more often becomes manifest in the teens or twenties **(lymphedema praecox)**. In a small percentage of cases, it develops after age 35 **(lymphedema tarda)**. It is caused by developmental abnormalities of the lymphatics, either hypoplasia (55%), varicose dilatation (24%), or aplasia (14%). Whatever the anatomic cause, the functional result is lymphatic obstruction and increased pressure. The lymph vessels dilate, and their valves become incompetent. Since the valves are essential to maintaining the central direction of flow, incompetency aggravates lymph stasis. The resulting inability to remove subcutaneous protein stimulates fibrosis and further obstruction. The protein-rich fluid is also prone to bacterial infection.

Lymphedema praecox, predominantly a disease of females, begins at puberty or during adolescence. The first symptom, spontaneous swelling, starts as a puffiness about the foot or ankle made worse by long periods of activity. It may be unilateral or bilateral. The edema usually progresses up the leg slowly, with the entire limb becoming involved over a period of months or years. Gradually, the swelling becomes more marked, and elevation and bed rest become less effective for its control. Originally soft and pitting, the edema gradually becomes resistant to pressure, subcutaneous tissue hypertrophies, and the limb becomes permanently enlarged, unsightly, and uncomfortable. The patient experiences a dull, heavy sensation but no actual pain unless infection occurs. About half of patients with primary lymphedema eventually develop bilateral involvement.

Secondary lymphedema, in contrast to primary idiopathic lymphedema, is due to some definable extralymphatic process. Neoplastic obstruction of lymph vessels is the most frequent cause and is usually a result of prostatic carcinoma in men and lymphoma in women. Surgical removal of lymphatics—eg, after radical mastectomy or radical groin dissection—is also a common cause. In some cases, recurrent lymphangitis and cellulitis with progressive obliteration of the lymphatic vessels are the presumed causes. Subsequent attacks tend to occur with increasing frequency, producing more severe degrees of edema. In some parts of the world, filiariasis is the most common cause of lymphedema. In this group of patients, lymphangiograms will demonstrate the point of lymphatic obstruction.

Complications

Recurrent cellulitis and lymphangitis are the most frequent complications and usually follow minor injuries to the affected extremity. The patient experiences swelling, erythema, pain, and systemic signs and symptoms. The infection tends to spread rapidly up the involved lymphatics, producing visible red streaks in the skin from the foot to the groin. Streptococcus is the most frequent causative organism.

Another late complication is **lymphangiosarcoma,** an uncommon neoplasm which arises from lymphatic endothelium. It is almost always associated with lymphedema, most commonly postmastectomy lymphedema of the upper extremity. The tumor appears as multiple blue, red, or purple macular or papular lesions in the skin or subcutaneous tissue which may coalesce to form a large ulcerating mass. Lymphangiosarcoma spreads rapidly and has an extremely poor prognosis.

Differential Diagnosis

Because it is soft, pitting, and bilateral, lower

extremity edema from systemic diseases such as congestive heart failure, cirrhosis, or nephrosis is relatively easy to differentiate from lymphedema. The major difficulty in differential diagnosis is to distinguish between lymphedema and the edema of chronic deep venous insufficiency. Lymphedema is firm, rubbery, and nonpitting and decreases little if at all with overnight elevation. The edema of chronic deep venous insufficiency is soft and pitting initially but later may become firm, and is associated with secondary pigmentation, dermatitis, ulceration, and varicosities. Recurrent cellulitis and lymphangitis are much more common in lymphedema. However, lymphedema may exist in the postphlebitic limb, and so differentiation on clinical grounds is not always possible. Phlebograms or lymphangiograms are occasionally useful in such cases.

Treatment

The objectives of treatment are to control edema and prevent recurrent infection. The best results are obtained when treatment is instituted early in the course of the disease, before fibrosis develops and the health of the skin and subcutaneous tissues becomes impaired.

A. Nonoperative Management: Most patients with early lymphedema can be managed adequately without operation. The main objective of treatment is to rid the limbs of as much edema as possible and maintain the reduction permanently. Measures to reduce lymph formation are important. These include elevation of the foot of the bed by 6 inches and elevation of the feet and ankles at intervals during the day. External compression should be provided with custom fitted, heavy duty elastic stockings worn from the moment of arising until retiring at night. The patient should not be measured for the stockings until maximal reduction of swelling has been accomplished. If compression of the thigh is required, the stocking should be supported by a waist belt and garter or a leotard. Alternating air compression devices (Jobst Co.) which milk edema fluid from the extremity are quite helpful in some patients. Dietary sodium must be restricted and diuretics occasionally prescribed when actively treating the edema. It is essential that the patient be instructed regarding hygiene to prevent minor foot injuries or infections, which are prone to cause severe cellulitis. If recurrent lymphangitis and cellulitis are otherwise not preventable, long-term prophylactic antibiotics are indicated using a drug effective against the most prevalent invasive organism, usually streptococcus.

B. Surgical Treatment: Surgery should be considered only in severe cases that are unresponsive to aggressive medical management. Thus, only a few patients with lymphedema require operative therapy, either for a large, intractably swollen limb which impairs ambulation or for recurrent infections. Cosmetic reasons alone should rarely be the sole basis for surgical treatment, since the result is not a cosmetically normal appearing extremity. The excisional procedures which remove skin and edematous subcutaneous tissue (eg, Kondoleon operation) have proved cosmetically unsatisfactory. Recently developed procedures designed to improve lymph drainage involve transfer of normal lymphatic channels from a healthy area into the lymphedematous one. The operation described by Thompson in 1962 consists of folding a longitudinal flap of dermis beneath the muscles along the medial and lateral aspects of the leg, thereby allowing connections to form between blocked superficial dermal lymphatics and the normal deep lymphatic system. The available reports indicate that clinical and cosmetic results are good, but lymphangiographic evidence of new lymphatic connections is scarce. The Thompson operation is probably the most satisfactory one now available.

In 1967, Goldsmith and De los Santos described a procedure in which a pedicle of omentum was laid on thigh muscles denuded of fascia with the expectation that new lymphatic connections would develop. Good results are reported in about 40% of cases, and patent lymphatic communications between the thigh and omentum have been demonstrated by lymphangiography. Like the Thompson procedure, this one can be applied to the upper as well as the lower extremity.

Elastic support and physical measures to reduce the formation of edema are required indefinitely following any of these surgical procedures.

Prognosis

The natural history of lymphedema is one of gradual but steady progression of swelling, progressive disability imposed on the patient by the heavy, clumsy extremity, and recurrent episodes of infection. Some limbs become so large that specially made trousers and shoes are required. Fortunately, most patients can be greatly benefited by strict adherence to the therapeutic program. In severe cases the cosmetic deformity may produce psychologic problems which interfere with therapy. Insufficient experience with the currently used operations makes it impossible to predict their long-term efficacy.

Goldsmith HS: Long-term evaluation of omental transposition for chronic lymphedema. Ann Surg 180:847, 1974.

Gough MH: Primary lymphedema: Clinical and lymphangiographic studies. Br J Surg 53:917, 1966.

Herrmann JB: Lymphangiosarcoma of the chronically edematous extremity. Surg Gynecol Obstet 121:1107, 1965.

Kinmouth JB & others: Primary lymphoedema: Clinical and lymphangiographic studies of a series of 107 patients in which the lower limbs were affected. Br J Surg 45:1, 1958.

Pflug JJ, Calnan JS: The normal anatomy of the lymphatic system of the human leg. Br J Surg 58:925, 1971.

Taylor GW: New aspects of lymphatic surgery. In: *Modern Trends in Vascular Surgery I.* Gillespie JA (editor). Butterworths, 1970.

Thompson N: The surgical treatment of chronic lymphoedema of the extremity. Surg Clin North Am 47:445, 1967.

Treves N: Evaluation of the etiological factors in lymphedema following radical mastectomy: Analysis of 1,007 cases. Cancer 10:444, 1957.

Vitek J, Kaspar Z: The radiology of the deep lymphatic system of the leg. Br J Radiol 46:120, 1973.

Woodward AH, Ivins JC, Sowle EH: Lymphangiosarcoma arising in chronic lymphedematous extremities. Cancer 30:562, 1972.

• • •

General References

Biggs R (editor): *Human Blood Coagulation, Haemostasis, and Thrombosis.* Blackwell, 1972.

Dodd DH, Cockett FB: *The Pathology and Surgery of the Veins of the Lower Limb.* Livingstone, 1956.

Fairbairn JF II & others: *Peripheral Vascular Diseases.* Saunders, 1972.

Foldi M: *Diseases of Lymphatics and Lymph Circulation.* Thomas, 1969.

Greenfield LJ: Pulmonary embolism: Diagnosis and management. Curr Probl Surg 13:1, April 1976.

Haller JA Jr: *Deep Thrombophlebitis: Pathophysiology and Treatment.* Saunders, 1967.

Hume M, Sevitts S, Thomas DP: *Venous Thrombosis and Pulmonary Embolism.* Harvard Univ Press, 1970.

Kakkar VV, Jouhar AJ: *Thromboembolism: Diagnosis and Treatment.* Williams & Wilkins, 1972.

Kinmonth JB: *The Lymphatics: Diseases, Lymphography, and Surgery.* Williams & Wilkins, 1972.

McLachlin D: Venous disease of the lower extremities. Curr Probl Surg, Jan 1967.

Shepard JT, Vanhoutte PM: *Veins and Their Control.* Saunders, 1975.

Standness DE, Sumner DS: *Hemodynamics for Surgeons.* Grune & Stratton, 1975.

Swan KG (editor): *Venous Surgery in the Lower Extremities.* Warren H Green, 1975.

40 . . .
Neurosurgery & Surgery of the Pituitary

DIAGNOSIS & MANAGEMENT OF DEPRESSED STATES OF CONSCIOUSNESS
Julian T. Hoff, MD, & Charles B. Wilson, MD

Definitions

The clinical definition of consciousness ranges from alert wakefulness to deep coma. An **alert**, wakeful patient responds immediately and appropriately to all stimuli. A **stuporous** patient responds only when aroused by vigorous stimulation. **Coma** implies failure to respond to stimulation. Most patients with depressed states of consciousness lie within the extremes of this spectrum and are best categorized by accurate descriptions of their responses to specific stimuli—eg, auditory, visual, and tactile (touch or pain).

The Neurologic Examination

The most reliable index for assessing the level of consciousness at any moment is the patient's response to external stimuli, ie, How quickly and how accurately does he respond to questions, to touch, to pain, etc? Brain stem reflexes also allow an accurate estimate of the level of consciousness—pupillary responses to light, corneal reflexes, oculocephalic and caloric responses, cough and gag reflexes, pattern of breathing, etc. Motor activity of the extremities, either spontaneous or induced by the examiner's stimulus, provides assessment of the entire neuraxis. Does the patient move the extremities purposefully, equally, and briskly? Does he fail to move at all? Which extremities do not move? Nonpurposeful or reflex movement of the arms and legs may also establish the level of neuraxis function, though less reliably (eg, decorticate or decerebrate posturing).

Depressed consciousness may occur abruptly (eg, cerebral concussion) or gradually (eg, barbiturate overdose), often with fluctuations in the level of consciousness (eg, waxing-waning consciousness associated with subdural hematoma). Accurate and repeated examinations will establish not only the level of consciousness but also its changing course. The urgency of diagnosis largely depends upon the rate of change in the patient's course as determined by repeated examinations.

Diagnostic Possibilities

Depressed states of consciousness may be due to many causes. **Trauma** is usually obvious, both by history and by examination of the patient. **Metabolic disorders** (eg, diabetes mellitus, uremia, poisoning, electrolyte imbalance, hypoxia) may similarly alter the state of consciousness. In addition to an accurate history and physical examination, laboratory investigations are required to establish a diagnosis of metabolic coma.

Patients with **intracranial neoplasms** may be alert, comatose, or at any level of consciousness in between. A progressive, unrelenting history is a valuable criterion of this initial diagnosis. **CNS infections** (eg, encephalitis, meningitis) are usually accompanied by systemic signs of infection and a progressively worsening course. Cerebral abscess, on the other hand, behaves more like an expanding neoplasm than a fulminating infection.

Vascular occlusions (emboli, thrombosis) usually cause abrupt neurologic deficits without grossly impaired consciousness, whereas cerebral hemorrhage typically causes abrupt coma with profound neurologic deficits. Conversely, subarachnoid hemorrhage may occur without any alteration of wakefulness. **Degenerative diseases** are usually slowly progressive, dementing illnesses that dull consciousness but characteristically do not produce coma.

Diagnostic Tools

Laboratory and radiographic tests help to establish the clinical diagnosis. Routine examinations should include a complete blood count, urinalysis, plasma glucose, BUN, and serum electrolytes.

Urine and blood for toxicologic study are essential if poisoning is a possibility. Skull and cervical spine films and a chest x-ray are obvious aids after trauma. CSF analysis is an essential step toward diagnosis of meningitis or subarachnoid hemorrhage. Lumbar puncture is rarely helpful in the assessment of head trauma and probably is contraindicated during the initial work-up after injury.

While most patients are unconscious for a single reason, some may have combined or additive reasons. A severe head injury may have been caused by abrupt coma induced by cerebral hemorrhage in a hypertensive patient, or a diabetic patient with glioblastoma multiforme may be in coma from an insulin overdose and not from the expanding neoplasm. The physician must be aware of these possible—though uncommon—complexities.

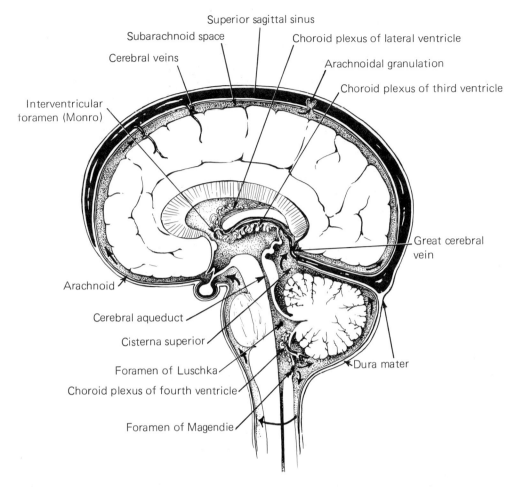

Figure 40–1. Circulation of CSF. (Redrawn from original drawings by Frank H. Netter, MD, which first appeared in Ciba Clinical Symposia, © 1950. Reproduced with permission.)

The administration of intravenous hypertonic glucose (50%, 50 ml) is occasionally diagnostic but should be done only after blood has been taken for glucose measurement and before an intravenous glucose drip has been started.

Management

Protection of the airway and control of shock are fundamental principles of management of patients with depressed consciousness. Most complications of coma can be attributed to failure to follow these basic rules. The responsive patient with a good cough reflex can often protect his own airway. Other patients, usually stuporous or comatose, require endotracheal intubation or tracheostomy in order to (1) reduce the likelihood of aspiration of gastric contents and (2) ensure unrestricted gas exchange (P_{O_2}, P_{CO_2}).

Adequate tracheal suctioning, frequent position change, pulmonary physiotherapy, and intermittent positive pressure breathing help maintain good pulmonary function once the airway is secure.

Shock must be controlled. If it is due to hypovolemia, blood and fluids must be given intravenously.

In the absence of trauma, other causes of hypotension must be sought and treated specifically (eg, gram-negative sepsis).

A nasogastric tube (to sample ingested drugs, to remove gastric contents that might be aspirated into the lungs, etc), intravenous cannulas to administer drugs and fluids, and an indwelling bladder catheter to assess fluid balance are necessary steps in the early management of comatose patients.

ELEVATED INTRACRANIAL PRESSURE (ICP)

The skull contains brain, CSF, and blood (Fig 40–1). At normal ICP 10–15 mm Hg (120–180 mm water), these 3 components maintain volumetric equilibrium. Increased volume of one component will elevate ICP unless the volume of the other 2 components decreases proportionately (Monro-Kellie hypothesis). Because compensatory volumetric changes have physical and physiologic limits, the ability of the skull's

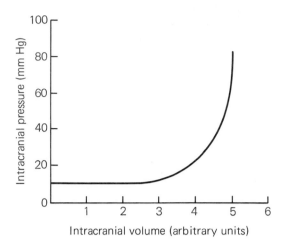

Figure 40–2. Change in ICP with changes in intracranial compartment volume. The figures along the abscissa represent units of volume.

contents to maintain normal pressure can be exceeded by a change of volume that is either too fast or too great.

The compensatory properties of the intracranial contents follow a pressure-volume exponential curve (Fig 40–2). Increased volume of any of the 3 components can be accommodated to a certain point without change in ICP. Once that critical volume is reached, however, additional volume increase produces an increase in intracranial pressure.

Increased ICP exerts its deleterious effect (1) by distorting and shifting the brain as pressure gradients develop, and (2) by reducing the effective perfusion pressure of the brain (cerebral perfusion pressure [CPP] = blood pressure [BP] minus intracranial pressure [ICP]). Common examples of a significant volumetric change in one or more of the 3 normal intracranial components are cerebral edema (brain), hydrocephalus (CSF), and cerebral venous occlusion (blood).

An intracranial mass (eg, tumor, hematoma) represents a fourth component, and its presence initiates compensatory adjustments of the other three: (1) Intracranial vessels are compressed, reducing the amount of intracranial blood; (2) CSF volume is reduced by increased absorption or reduced production (at high ICP); and (3) intracranial bulk is reduced by brain seeping out of adjacent foramens (eg, transtentorial herniation, tonsillar herniation). Children with expandable skulls have an additional compensatory mechanism to accommodate expanding intracranial volume and are thereby partially protected from extreme rises of ICP.

Clinical Findings

Most brain insults, whether from trauma, ischemia, poisoning, or other sources, are accompanied by raised intracranial pressure. Following head trauma, ICP may rise quickly to very high levels as a result of

vascular congestion, extravasation, and cerebral edema. ICP may also rise substantially when a neoplasm occupies the intracranial cavity. Intracranial hypertension may occur after cerebrovascular occlusions (stroke), during CNS infections, and following cerebral hypoxia. ICP is rarely a clinical problem alone when coma is the result of a metabolic disorder (eg, uremia, hepatic coma).

A. Specific Signs of Raised ICP: While any of the following clinical signs may result from causes other than raised ICP, most will appear during raised ICP if the elevation is severe or prolonged.

1. Cardiovascular—Blood pressure elevation accompanied by bradycardia and respiratory slowing classically results from raised ICP. This "Cushing response," however, usually appears only when intracranial hypertension is severe.

2. Gastrointestinal—Hemorrhage from gastric ulcerations (Cushing's ulcer) may accompany raised ICP.

3. Pulmonary—Hemorrhagic pulmonary edema may result from severe elevation of intracranial pressure as well as from other brain insults. The lung lesion is the end product of a pathophysiologic sequence mediated by the sympathetic nervous system (see Ducker reference, below). Few patients survive this hemodynamic storm of neurogenic origin unless intracranial pressure is reduced.

4. Neurologic—Papilledema, abducens nerve paresis (unilateral occasionally; bilateral often), and depressed consciousness are the most common signs associated with generalized ICP elevations. Loss of visual acuity may appear late due to optic nerve atrophy.

B. Specific Syndromes: Specific syndromes may appear when ICP is raised as a consequence of the presence of an intracranial mass.

1. Transtentorial herniation—A laterally placed supratentorial mass may push the uncus and hippocampus medially into the tentorial incisure. The oculomotor nerves, the cerebral peduncles, the cerebral aqueduct, and the midbrain (containing the reticular formation) are vulnerable to compression from the displaced temporal lobe. Transtentorial herniation may then appear clinically (Table 40–1).

2. Tonsillar herniation—Herniation of the cerebellar tonsils into the foramen magnum causes compression of the medulla. The hallmark of medullary compression is respiratory failure: slow and irregular breathing followed by apnea. Earlier signs of herniation are nuchal rigidity, intermittent opisthotonos, and depressed gag and cough reflexes. Consciousness is often retained.

Whereas raised ICP usually becomes obvious clinically, it may go undetected for months. Patients with benign intracranial hypertension (pseudotumor cerebri) often have no symptoms despite severe papilledema and intracranial hypertension. Similarly, patients with obstruction of CSF pathways may tolerate ICP elevation for weeks or months without developing overt clinical signs. Failing mentation may provide the only clue to progressive hydrocephalus in the latter circumstance.

Table 40-1. Clinical manifestations of tentorial herniation.

Compressed Structure	Clinical Manifestation
Cranial nerve III	Ipsilateral mydriasis
Midbrain: physiologic (functional) transection	Decerebrate rigidity
Reticular formation	Coma
Ipsilateral cerebral peduncle	Contralateral hemiparesis
Contralateral cerebral peduncle	Ipsilateral hemiparesis (false localizing sign)*
Cerebral aqueduct (of Sylvius)	Headache and vomiting due to acute hydrocephalus
Posterior cerebral artery	Contralateral hemianopsia (false localizing sign)*

*This sign is the consequence of herniation and does not indicate the localization of the primary process; in this sense, the sign falsely localizes the primary lesion.

Treatment

A. Specific Treatment: If a specific cause of raised ICP can be found, its treatment will effectively treat the ICP. Removal of intracranial masses, shunting of obstructed CSF, and removal of toxins (eg, lead, in lead encephalopathy) are examples of specific forms of treatment.

B. Nonspecific Treatment: When raised ICP as such must also be managed, the following nonspecific measures are useful:

1. Control of respiration—Accumulation of CO_2 ($Pa_{CO_2} > 40$ mm Hg) will increase cerebral blood flow and raise ICP. A therapeutic goal is maintenance of Pa_{CO_2} in the range of 30-40 mm Hg.

2. Control of body temperature—Hypothermia reduces cerebral metabolism and lowers ICP. Hyperthermia increases ICP. Thus, fever must be controlled.

3. Osmotic diuretics—Mannitol, urea, or glycerin can reduce ICP by cerebral dehydration.

4. Steroids—These agents reduce or prevent cerebral edema, thereby helping to control ICP.

5. Bony decompression—This nonspecific method of reducing ICP may be employed when other treatments fail.

Brock M, Dietz H: *Intracranial Pressure.* Springer, 1972.

Ducker TB: Increased intracranial pressure and pulmonary edema. J Neurosurg 28:112, 1968.

Jennett WB, Stern WE: Tentorial herniation, the midbrain, and the pupil. J Neurosurg 17:598, 1960.

Lundberg N, Ponten N: *Intracranial Pressure II.* Springer-Verlag, 1974.

Miller JD: Induced changes of cerebro-spinal fluid volume. Arch Neurol 28:265, 1973.

Plum F, Posner JB: *Diagnosis of Stupor and Coma,* 2nd ed. Davis, 1972.

Posner JB: The comatose patient. JAMA 233:1313, 1975.

NEUROSURGICAL DIAGNOSTIC PROCEDURES
Philip R. Weinstein, MD

RADIOGRAPHIC STUDIES

Although plain x-rays of the skull and spine are valuable when calcification is present or bone changes have occurred, they often provide only preliminary information. The examiner should then consider using one or more isotope or contrast studies in order to visualize nonradiopaque CNS structures. Skull or spinal tomography may identify or confirm subtle or suspected erosion or fracture in the sella turcica or vertebral pedicles.

ECHOENCEPHALOGRAPHY

By passing an electric current through a crystal, a beam of ultrasound can be produced which is then directed from one side of the skull to the other. Some of the sound waves are deflected by midline structures in the area of the third ventricle, and a characteristic response is produced on the recording apparatus. This is a rapid, safe, and noninvasive method of detecting a shift of midline structures—information that is particularly helpful in acute head injuries, especially when a calcified pineal gland cannot be visualized on plain skull x-rays.

ISOTOPE STUDIES

Isotopes of arsenic, copper, mercury, and other elements have been used for brain scanning, but technetium Tc 99m pertechnetate has the most desirable characteristics. The intravenously injected isotope is preferentially taken up in the brain where the blood-brain barrier has been disturbed, and this area of isotope concentration shows up as a "hot spot" on the scan readout. With high-speed repetitive scanning, it is also possible to determine intracranial vascular flow patterns.

The flow characteristics of CSF can be studied by isotope cisternography, which involves the lumbar or upper cervical injection of radioiodinated serum albumin (RISA) and scanning during its course through the subarachnoid space. Such a study provides useful information in certain cases of hydrocephalus.

Regional cerebral blood flow can be quantitatively measured by injecting xenon Xe 133 into the carotid artery. Such information may be helpful in the diagnosis and management of cerebrovascular disease and other conditions such as trauma, tumor, and hemorrhage which indirectly cause cerebral hypoxia. Since puncture or catheterization of the carotid artery and computerized calculations are required, widespread application is not expected until newer intravenous isotope injection technics are perfected.

COMPUTERIZED AXIAL TOMOGRAPHY (CT)

A recently developed method of recording relative intracranial tissue densities by transmission through the head of x-ray photons focussed from a rotating source provides a noninvasive technic for visualization of the brain, skull, and ventricles. Using a continuously scanning narrow collimated x-ray beam and a system of crystal detectors, 28,000 computer-analyzed density readings are obtained. The matrix can be displayed and photographed as a series of transverse axial sections of the cranium either 2.6 or 1.6 cm thick. This detailed anatomic representation often eliminates the need for angiography or pneumoencephalography. Since many lesions such as edema, infarct, hematoma, abscess, cyst, and tumor—especially if calcified—have abnormal densities, information can be obtained about the nature and location of intracranial mass lesions. Repeat scanning after intravenous iodinated contrast injection can provide additional information if a blood-brain barrier defect is present. Ventricular size and position can be determined in the diagnosis of hydrocephalus or cerebral atrophy.

MYELOGRAPHY

Myelography is useful principally in the study of the spinal canal, although injection of a contrast medium such as iophendylate (Pantopaque) into the subarachnoid space has been used to delineate the cerebellopontine angle and the internal auditory meatus in the posterior fossa. By this technic, contrast medium is introduced into the subarachnoid space via lumbar or cervical puncture. The patient is tilted at various angles, the contrast medium (heavier than CSF) flows by gravity, and x-rays are obtained in desired projections at the appropriate level. The defects produced in the dye column by the various pathologic entities such as fracture, tumor, cyst, or herniated disk can be characterized, in general, as extradural, intradural-intramedullary, or intradural-extramedullary. Unless a complete block is present, the contrast medium should be removed (if feasible) at the completion of the study. Water soluble contrast materials which are absorbed without removal will soon be available. Air may be used instead of contrast medium but is generally helpful only when hydromyelia is suspected. Contrast medium myelography should not be done in the presence of a bloody spinal tap because of the reported increased risk of aseptic arachnoiditis.

ANGIOGRAPHY
(Fig 40–3)

The arterial and venous systems of the brain and spinal cord can be imaged by the intra-arterial injection of a water-soluble iodinated contrast medium. If angiography is indicated, it is generally performed before other contrast studies. The contrast material may be injected via a femoral catheter introduced through the aortic arch by the Seldinger technic. All of the extracranial cerebral vessels may be studied separately, including the external and internal carotid and vertebral arteries. Such a study may demonstrate displacement or enlargement of vessels, anomalous vessels, occlusion of vessels, abnormality of the vessel wall,

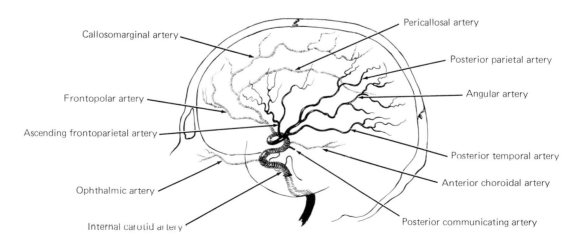

Figure 40–3. Schematic drawing of normal arteriograms of the internal carotid artery. Lateral projection. (Redrawn and reproduced, with permission, from List, Burge, & Hodges: Intracranial angiography. Radiology 45:1, 1945.)

aneurysms, or avascular areas. The risk of neurologic sequelae following angiography has been reduced by the newer contrast media and technics but has not been eliminated, particularly in elderly patients with cerebrovascular disease.

PNEUMOENCEPHALOGRAPHY
(Fig 40–4)

In performing pneumoencephalography, the basal subarachnoid cisterns and the ventricular system of the brain are gradually filled with increments of air introduced via a lumbar puncture needle as CSF is with-

drawn. The study is hazardous in patients with increased intracranial pressure and may precipitate respiratory arrest. Such an occurrence is rare if, after the initial injection of a small volume of air, tomograms are taken to demonstrate the position of the cerebellar tonsils. If the tonsils are herniated through the foramen magnum, the procedure should be terminated.

Pneumoencephalograms are particularly helpful in the study of posterior fossa lesions, sellar and suprasellar lesions, hydrocephalus, and atrophic processes. When tomography is done during this study, the value of the study is greatly enhanced. Pneumoencephalography may produce transient fever, headache, nausea, vomiting, and vertigo.

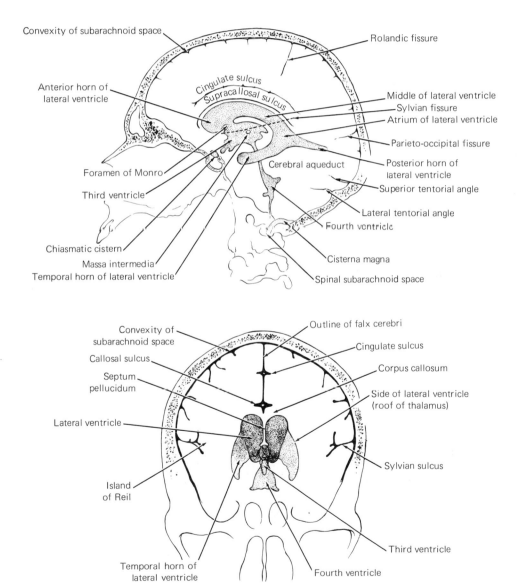

Figure 40–4. *Above:* Lateral encephalogram. *Below:* Anteroposterior encephalogram. (Reproduced, with permission, from Chusid JG: *Correlative Neuroanatomy & Functional Neurology,* 16th ed. Lange, 1976.)

VENTRICULOGRAPHY

In the presence of papilledema as a sign of increased intracranial pressure or cerebellar tonsillar herniation, direct study of the ventricular system with air or contrast material may be necessary in place of pneumoencephalography. Such a study is carried out via a bur hole made off the midline at the coronal or lambdoidal suture. Air may then be introduced by ventricular puncture in exchange for CSF. The lateral ventricles and the third ventricle can usually be filled quite satisfactorily by this technic, but visualization of the cerebral aqueduct and the fourth ventricle may be inadequate unless a positive contrast agent is used instead of air. As a rule, the basal cisterns and the subarachnoid space over the hemispheres are not satisfactorily visualized. Definitive surgical treatment nearly always follows ventriculography, since a patient with a demonstrable lesion deteriorates rapidly from the effects of injected air on the dynamics of the intracranial fluid. Ventricular puncture can produce cerebral hemorrhage, porencephalic cysts, seizures, or infection and should be done only when clearly necessary. Occasionally, such taps are done for emergency decompression, for inserting ventricular shunts, for obtaining ventricular fluid for analysis, for introducing an antibiotic agent, or for establishing continuous monitoring and drainage to control intracranial pressure.

ELECTRICAL STUDIES

Nervous system function can be evaluated by recording the electrical potentials generated in brain, nerve, and muscle.

ELECTROMYOGRAPHY (EMG)

EMG records muscle and nerve action potentials through needle or skin electrodes. It is helpful in the diagnosis of neuromuscular disorders, particularly in determining the anatomic site of a lesion on an individual peripheral nerve or in separating a diffuse peripheral neuropathy from a single root or nerve lesion. It is sometimes useful in identifying the specific nerve, root, or cord segment involved. In conjunction with muscle biopsy, it is frequently helpful in the diagnosis of muscle diseases. In peripheral nerve lesions it can be used to identify nerve compression, to determine whether injury has caused complete or partial loss of conduction, and to document the occurrence of regeneration. Muscle denervation potentials may not appear for up to two weeks after nerve or neuronal injury. EMG studies should be normal if muscle weakness is due to an upper motor neuron lesion.

ELECTROENCEPHALOGRAPHY (EEG)

EEG records the electrical activity of the cerebral cortex with electrodes placed on the scalp. It is perhaps most useful in identifying and localizing seizure disorders, but diffusely abnormal or localizing patterns may also be seen in brain abscess, subdural hematomas, brain tumors, metabolic disorders, and degenerative diseases of the CNS. Although it is a diagnostic procedure without risk, it is useful to the neurosurgeon only as a screening procedure.

Alexander E: Lumbar puncture. JAMA 201:316, 1967.
Ambrose J: Computerized x-ray scanning of the brain. J Neurosurg 40:679, 1974.
Brinker RA, King DL, Taveras JM: Echoencephalography. Am J Roentgenol Radium Ther Nucl Med 93:781, 1965.
Cohen HL, Brumlik J: *A Manual of Electroneuromyography.* Harper & Row, 1968.
Kiloh LG, McComas AJ, Osselton JM: *Clinical Electroencephalography.* Butterworth, 1972.
Smoak WM III, Gilson AJ: The central nervous system. Chap 4, pp 23–37, in: *Practical Nuclear Medicine.* Ashkar FS (editor). Medcom Press, 1974.
Taveras JM, Wood EH: *Diagnostic Neuroradiology.* Williams & Wilkins, 1976.

CRANIOCEREBRAL TRAUMA
Roland K. Perkins, MD, & Lawrence Pitts, MD

Most head injuries seen in the emergency room are closed injuries, ie, the brain and its coverings have not been penetrated. The major diagnostic difficulties, then, are recognizing, localizing, and determining the extent of intracranial damage.

Head injuries may be induced by many forces, the most common being low-velocity impacts (such as those received in a car accident), direct blows from a solid object, and high-velocity wounds from missiles. In civilian practice, low-velocity impacts are most frequent. About 60% of all injuries due to traffic accidents involve the head, and in fatal accidents the percentage rises to 70%. In two-thirds of these fatal cases, the injuries to the head are the cause of death. At autopsy following head injury, about 35–50% of patients have intracranial hemorrhage. If an individual is comatose after an accident, there is an estimated 50% chance of intracranial hemorrhage with or without brain damage.

Sudden acceleration or deceleration of the brain may cause injuries due to compression (pushing material together), tension (tearing material apart), or shearing (sliding portions of material over other portions). These may occur singly or in any combination.

With a localized head injury, the forces spent upon local areas of the skull and its underlying brain may give rise to complications, including those of hemorrhage and infection, but the mortality rate is low. With generalized head injuries, large forces can move or deform the entire skull, accelerate and compress the entire brain, and transmit this distortion to vital central core and brain stem structures.

Pathology

Injuries may be limited to the scalp, the skull, or the brain; they may involve only 2 of these or all 3.

A. Scalp: The scalp consists of 5 layers: epidermis, dermis, fat, galea, and the subareolar area. From a practical standpoint, it consists of the epidermis and galea. The rigidity of these 2 layers holds open the many blood vessels in the fatty layer between them. Because it is unyielding, blunt injuries tend to burst rather than crush the scalp.

B. Skull: Skull fractures can be classified as simple (linear or depressed) or compound. A skull fracture does not necessarily provide an index to the severity of head injuries, since fatal damage to the brain may follow a closed head injury without evidence of fracture. However, skull fracture does indicate that a severe blow to the head has been sustained.

1. Simple skull fractures—If the fracture overlies the groove of the middle meningeal artery or one of the dural venous sinuses, extradural or subdural hemorrhage must be suspected and the patient must be followed carefully for signs that may suggest the need for operative intervention.

2. Basilar skull fractures—These are often not seen on x-rays. A linear fracture that extends into an accessory nasal sinus or into mastoid air cells is really a compound fracture since it is in communication with the external surfaces of the body.

3. Depressed skull fractures and compound skull fractures—These are often obvious clinically, but x-ray confirmation is essential. Palpation of the intact scalp is often misleading because of subgaleal edema and hematoma.

C. Brain: Brain injuries are commonly designated as concussion, contusion, or laceration. These may occur singly but are more commonly seen in various combinations. With contusion and laceration or subsequent pressure from a hematoma, the brain often becomes edematous. Although the mechanism of brain swelling is not clearly understood, it is related to increased vascular permeability; in severe head injuries at least, superimposed hypoxia plays a role.

1. Concussion—Concussion is a clinical syndrome characterized by immediate and transient impairment of neural function due to a blow to the head. The term was formerly restricted to an injury resulting in loss of consciousness. At present, an injury which has caused no loss of consciousness but only a brief period of mental confusion is referred to as a mild concussion. The terms moderate and severe concussion imply a longer period of unconsciousness. Amnesia for the events preceding the injury is termed retrograde amnesia. In cerebral concussion, there is little or no demonstrable permanent pathologic change in the brain.

2. Cerebral contusion (bruise)—This term implies a structural alteration of the brain. A localized external or cortical blow usually produces slight direct cortical injury. Contusions frequently occur along the base of the posterior frontal lobes and at the tips of adjacent temporal lobes. Trauma to the underlying neuroglia may produce local edema. Injuries to surface vessels usually produce only local hematoma, although there may be some ischemia. Subcortical and deep injuries are more devastating and involve larger masses of brain.

3. Brain laceration—Laceration of the brain usually occurs at the point of application of substantial force to the head or directly opposite that point ("contrecoup").

Clinical Findings

The treatment of head injury is emergency medicine, and early therapy of trauma is stereotyped. First, an adequate airway must be guaranteed, using an endotracheal tube if necessary. Second, adequate perfusion must be maintained. If the patient is in shock, look for sources of bleeding. Although scalp lacerations may cause hemorrhagic hypotension, shock is rarely secondary to head injury alone. Third, evaluate possible injuries outside the nervous system to prevent further damage during CNS evaluation.

A. Symptoms and Signs: A rapid nervous system examination is mandatory to establish a valid baseline against which to measure improvement or deterioration and thereby dictate therapy. The following features of the examination are especially useful because they are repeatable at different times and by different observers.

1. Eye opening—This in part replaces "level of consciousness" and is graded by the required stimulus: (1) spontaneous eye opening, (2) eye opening on command, (3) eye opening to shaking, (4) eye opening to painful stimulus, (5) no eye opening.

2. Best motor response—This describes the patient's movement ability and is graded as (1) follows commands, (2) localizes painful stimulus, (3) responds with abnormal flexion to painful stimulus (flexion of one or both upper extremities, formerly "decorticate"), (4) responds with abnormal extension to pain (formerly "decerebrate"), and (5) gives no motor response.

3. Best verbal response—This documents the patient's ability to speak as well as his speech content: (1) answers appropriately, (2) gives confused answers, (3) makes unintelligible noises, (4) makes no verbal response. In each case the *best* response is recorded even if a painful stimulus is required to elicit the response.

These 3 functions give a sensitive and reproducible measure of the patient's state and should be supplemented by noting the following features, which sometimes accompany head injury:

4. Headache—Severe unilateral headache may indicate an expanding intracranial hematoma. Severe occipital headache may be caused by an odontoid fracture.

5. Amnesia—A significant period of retrograde amnesia indicates a definite cerebral injury. A long amnestic period suggests a moderately severe head injury. Absence of amnesia suggests that little or no brain damage occurred at the time of injury but does not exclude the possibility of later development of an intracranial hematoma.

6. Cranial abnormalities—Lacerations must be carefully noted. Even very small scalp defects may represent stab wounds to the brain. Skull fractures sometimes may be palpated at the depth of a laceration, but a laceration of the pericranium (skull periosteum) often is misinterpreted as a fracture. Blood in the mastoid region (Battle's sign) indicates a temporal bone fracture, but it commonly is not apparent for 12–18 hours after injury.

7. Eye signs—Pupillary size (in millimeters) and reaction to light (direct and consensual responses) should be documented. Funduscopic examination may reveal retinal hemorrhage, but even with markedly increased intracranial pressure papilledema does not become evident for 12–24 hours.

Third nerve paresis (including pupillary dilatation and loss of medial rectus function) associated with head injury usually signifies compression of the third nerve against the brain stem by an expanding intracranial mass which requires immediate diagnosis and treatment. This emergency is accompanied by progressive obtundation and by a lesser motor response (see ¶2, above). In an awake patient, a third nerve paresis usually signifies direct trauma in the cavernous sinus or superior orbital fissure.

Eye movement can be evaluated by either cold water caloric testing or the doll's head maneuver (rapid lateral rotation of the head while observing eye motion); the latter test should be done only after a lateral cervical spine x-ray has excluded a neck fracture.

Conjugate deviation of both eyes usually indicates a lesion of the opposite frontal lobe (adversive fields). Spontaneous nystagmus indicates damage to the cerebellum or vestibular connections. Skew deviation of the eyes occurs in injuries to the brain stem; local damage to the orbit or to the ocular muscles can also produce deviation of the eyes.

8. Muscle examination—Facial weakness may be evaluated by exerting pressure over the supraorbital ridge. In alert patients it is possible to estimate the strength of muscles in the extremities; in drowsy or semicomatose patients, this is often possible only by administering painful stimuli. The most common motor sign of craniocerebral trauma is hemiparesis or hemiplegia. Abnormal posturing also occurs—most frequently a stereotyped flexion of one or both arms at the elbows and an extension of the lower extremities, either spontaneously or evoked by painful stimuli. Abnormal posturing immediately after injury generally indicates direct injury to the brain stem, although a rapidly expanding intracranial hematoma can cause early brain stem injury by compression of the midbrain.

B. Lumbar Puncture: The only absolute indication for lumbar puncture is a suspicion of meningitis. Lumbar puncture **should never be done** when intracranial pressure is thought to be increased or when there is evidence of brain herniation at the tentorial notch or the foramen magnum. A normal lumbar puncture does not exclude intracranial trauma or disease, and an abnormal lumbar puncture does not give a specific diagnosis. Leakage of CSF from the needle hole in the arachnoid following lumbar puncture may increase brain shift if an intracranial mass is present and hasten the patient's deterioration. Therefore, *lumbar puncture has no role in the management of head injury.*

C. Special Diagnostic Studies: A number of diagnostic studies are useful in evaluating acute head injury and defining intracranial complications. The patient's clinical state determines what diagnostic studies can and should be performed. For example, with a rapidly expanding hematoma, deterioration may be too rapid to permit special studies. In such instances, surgical bur holes allow rapid diagnosis of extracerebral hematomas and can be coupled with craniotomy for evacuation of these hematomas.

1. Skull x-rays—X-rays should be obtained as soon as the patient's general condition permits. They may show a depressed fracture or a fracture line crossing one of the major vascular structures, with the possibility of an extradural hematoma. A fracture extending into a sinus warns of the danger of ascending intracranial infection. A shift of the pineal gland (which is calcified and radiopaque in 70% of persons after age 20) 3 mm or more to either side of the midline suggests an expanding intracranial lesion. Lateral cervical spine x-rays should be taken to evaluate possible concomitant fractures.

2. Echoencephalography—An echoencephalogram may demonstrate midline shifts, indicating the presence of an extracerebral or an intracerebral mass. Bilateral lesions, however, may not shift midline structures.

3. Brain scan—Radioactive brain scan is becoming increasingly useful in the diagnosis of intracranial injuries such as cerebral contusion and extra- or intracerebral hematoma but is rarely used acutely.

4. Cerebral angiography—Angiography has the distinct value of accurately localizing intra- and extracerebral hematomas. The venous phase of the angiogram may show obstruction of the venous sinuses by fracture fragments, and the arterial phase may reveal partial or complete occlusion of the carotid artery or one of its branches.

5. Air contrast studies—In some centers, the lateral ventricle is tapped by passing a catheter through a small drill hole in the skull. Air or water-soluble contrast material is then injected and will demonstrate shifts in the ventricles. Intracranial pressure can also be determined.

6. Computerized tomographic scan (CT scan)—This new device will demonstrate intracranial masses without patient hazard or discomfort. It is very accurate, but its availability is limited at present. Since it requires patient immobility, its use is restricted.

Differential Diagnosis

The history of a blow to the head usually makes evident the cause of the unconsciousness, although a concomitant pathologic state may exist. Without a history of head trauma, other causes of unconsciousness must be kept in mind, including cardiac conditions, cerebrovascular accidents, and diabetic, hepatic, alcoholic, or drug-induced coma. An expanding intracranial tumor may have been responsible for a seizure with subsequent fall and head injury.

Cerebral fat embolism, which may follow fracture of a long bone, may mimic extradural hemorrhage, subdural hematoma, or midbrain injury. With cerebral fat embolism, fat globules usually appear in the urine 2–6 days after the fracture. The optic fundi should be examined for emboli, small hemorrhages, white exudates, and edema. Petechiae may arise in the conjunctiva and on the skin of the chest and arms. A sudden rise in temperature without evidence of pneumonia suggests the possibility of cerebral fat embolism.

Following a blow to the neck the progressive deterioration after traumatic internal carotid artery thrombosis may suggest an expanding intracranial lesion. The diagnosis is made by angiography; palpation of the vessels of the neck is of little aid.

Complications

The complications of trauma to the head include vascular lesions (hemorrhage, thrombosis, fistula formation), infections (meningitis, abscess, osteomyelitis), rhinorrhea, otorrhea, pneumatocele, leptomeningeal cysts, cranial nerve injuries, and focal brain lesions.

A. Hemorrhage: Intracranial hemorrhage may occur within the extradural, subdural, or subarachnoid spaces, or within the brain. Extradural and subdural hemorrhage are discussed below as separate entities.

1. Subarachnoid hemorrhage—Blood in the spinal fluid is a common finding with head injuries. The bleeding usually arises from the superficial cortical vessels, particularly veins draining the cerebral cortex into the dural venous sinuses. Large amounts of blood within the subarachnoid space may be tolerated well and require no specific treatment. Initially, the patient may have severe headache, restlessness, nuchal rigidity, fever, and a positive Kernig sign.

Acute subarachnoid hemorrhage is not a surgical lesion, and spinal fluid drainage is rarely of benefit. If the hemorrhage has been massive, arachnoiditis may later interfere with absorption of CSF, and this may require surgery for shunting CSF to another site where it can be reabsorbed.

2. Subdural hygroma—Subdural hygroma is an accumulation of spinal fluid in the subdural space, usually through a fine tear in the arachnoid created by a craniocerebral injury. The spinal fluid is trapped in the subdural space and is poorly absorbed. Patients with subdural hygromas are usually suspected of having subdural hematomas; the fluid is identified and removed by surgical exploration.

3. Intracerebral hemorrhage—Intracerebral hematomas may result from injury to a cerebral vessel with major hemorrhage or from a coalescence of smaller subcortical hemorrhages. These hematomas produce no clear-cut clinical picture but may present as an expanding intracranial lesion. They are often associated with cortical lacerations and contusion, and the patient's condition either becomes stable after a few days or deteriorates. The most common sites are in the anterior temporal lobe and the frontal lobe. CT scan establishes the diagnosis.

Hematomas large enough to cause symptoms and signs should be evacuated.

B. Carotid Cavernous Fistula: A carotid cavernous fistula is a channel which shunts blood from the internal carotid artery into the cavernous sinus. The traumatic carotid cavernous fistula results from a tear in one of the small intracavernous carotid branches. The symptoms usually arise within a month following injury and include headache, retro-orbital pain, blurred vision, diplopia, and often a bruit. The eye becomes proptotic, and the conjunctiva and eye muscles are extremely edematous. The eye is often immobile. Papilledema and engorgement of the retinal veins are usually present.

The fistula is demonstrated by cerebral angiography. Digital pressure upon the carotid artery in the neck often abolishes or diminishes the bruit. Treatment is directed toward reducing the arterial supply to the fistula; it often involves a combination of cervical and intracranial carotid ligations. More recently, technics to create thrombosis within the cavernous sinus have also been used.

C. CSF Leak: CSF rhinorrhea and otorrhea indicate a fistulous communication between the subarachnoid space (or ventricular system) and the nose or ear, respectively. This fistulous connection can serve as a path for spreading infection; the longer the leak persists, the greater the risk of infection. This can lead to meningitis, brain abscess, or both.

A persistent, clear, watery discharge from the ears or nose should suggest a CSF leak. The fluid contains glucose while nasal mucus usually does not.

CSF rhinorrhea can result from a fracture which communicates with any of the paranasal sinuses. The most common site is a fracture through the cribriform plate extending into an ethmoid sinus. If the leak persists beyond 2 weeks, intracranial repair is indicated. Occasionally, early infection is encountered, and antibiotic therapy may cure both the infection and the leak. However, months later, the patient may abruptly develop meningitis, usually pneumococcal. Surgical repair should be done after antibiotic treatment.

CSF otorrhea or otorrhagia occurs often in association with fractures through the petrous portion of the temporal bone with a dural tear in the middle or posterior fossa. In most cases, the leak seals off spontaneously; if it does not, surgical repair is necessary.

D. Cranial Nerve Palsies: The olfactory nerves are often torn at the cribriform plate, and loss of smell after trauma is seldom recovered. The prognosis is generally poor in an optic nerve lesion where there has been immediate complete blindness. Partial lesions may be followed by recovery of visual function as edema subsides. Palsies of the third, fourth, and sixth cranial nerves usually improve following trauma, although they may remain complete. Recovery, if it occurs, may take 6–9 months. Facial palsies may occur immediately or several days after trauma. Recovery of a delayed facial palsy is generally the rule; the prognosis is not as good if the palsy occurs at the moment of injury. If there has been no return of function within 6–8 weeks, intratemporal decompression of the facial nerve should be considered. If the nerve has been irreversibly damaged, a facial nerve anastomosis can be done, utilizing either the hypoglossal or the spinal accessory nerve. If deafness occurs following auditory nerve damage, improvement is usually slight.

E. Posttraumatic Cerebral Syndrome: The posttraumatic cerebral syndrome is more common after serious head injuries but may be produced by relatively mild ones. The patient complains of headache, difficulty in concentration, dizziness, memory defects, giddiness, and fatigability. Auditory evoked potentials may be abnormal for months, giving some physiologic basis for the complaints. In most instances, these symptoms clear within a few months and rarely last more than a year.

F. Posttraumatic Epilepsy: Patients may develop seizures during the initial phase of a head injury. This may be due to an expanding intracranial hematoma as well as to brain swelling. These seizures do not mean, however, that the patient will develop posttraumatic epilepsy. The incidence of seizures following closed head injuries is reported to be 3–6%. The incidence following penetrating injuries is much higher (20–50%). In most cases, the epileptic seizures begin within 2 years after injury, and most of these patients are still subject to seizures after 5 years.

Treatment

A. Emergency Measures: The first requirement is to ensure an adequate airway, with tracheal intubation and respiratory assistance if necessary. Hypoxia and hypercapnia can further damage injured brain.

Any external hemorrhage should be controlled, and shock must be treated. Intravenous fluids and blood should be given as required.

The patient's clinical situation should be assessed—particularly his state of consciousness. The type and severity of the nervous system injury should be determined as accurately as possible. In addition, a general examination should be done to identify any associated injuries.

B. General Measures: If the patient's condition is rapidly deteriorating and there is a possibility that an expanding intracranial hematoma is present, bur hole exploration should be done without delay.

A prominent factor in most severe head injuries is cerebral swelling or edema, occurring as a consequence of increased vascular permeability. Hypoxia due to decreased respiratory exchange also contributes to cerebral swelling. In general, this should be treated by intravenous urea or mannitol, and corticosteroid injec-tions. Intravenous hyperosmolar agents will temporarily decrease intracranial pressure. *Caution:* The use of any of these agents before a definitive diagnosis has been established could allow further expansion of an intracranial hematoma.

Antibiotic treatment should be instituted in contaminated compound wounds and with CSF leak but are not indicated in basal skull fracture without CSF leak.

Anticonvulsant medication is given if seizures occur. However, it must be remembered that seizures may be the sign of a rapidly expanding intracranial lesion that requires immediate treatment by operation.

Progressive deterioration of the patient's condition is an indication for exploratory bur holes or for angiography, depending upon the rate of progression and the patient's overall condition. This deterioration may be manifested by progressive impairment of the state of consciousness, progression of neurologic signs, or evidence of increased intracranial pressure. Compound fractures of the skull and penetrating wounds of the brain are clear-cut indications for operation.

C. Specific Measures:

1. Scalp wounds—Bleeding can usually be controlled with a simple pressure dressing or, in the case of arterial bleeding, by means of firm finger pressure along the edges of the wound or by a hemostat attached to the galea. The hemostat is allowed to hang down over the skin to hold the galea firmly against the skin and compress the bleeding vessels. With simple wounds, debridement and control of hemorrhage are the important considerations. These wounds should be closed as soon as possible unless they overlie a depressed fracture or a wound that penetrates the skull.

Scalp hair must be shaved with a generous margin about the wound. The wound should be thoroughly cleansed and the edges approximated either with buried galeal sutures and removable superficial sutures or with a vertical mattress suture utilizing stainless steel wire. Buried sutures should not be used for infected wounds.

2. Depressed skull fractures—Depressed bone fragments beneath intact scalp usually require elevation, depending upon the anatomic area and the degree of depression. As a general rule, depressions of 4 mm or more over the motor and speech areas should be elevated. Unless there are untoward neurologic signs, however, elevation can be delayed until optimal surgical facilities are available.

3. Compound skull fractures—To prevent infection, debridement and repair should be undertaken as soon as possible after injury. The patient with a depressed compound skull fracture should be taken to a hospital with complete neurosurgical facilities and treated by a surgeon with adequate neurosurgical training.

Emergency treatment consists of applying a sterile compression dressing. The wound should not be closed, and no attempt should be made to remove any foreign body protruding from the wound until the patient is in the operating room and all preparations have been made for craniotomy. If the fragments are depressed into the transverse or sagittal sinus, their removal may cause alarming hemorrhage at the edge of the bone opening. Thus, adequate access to control the sinus distally and proximally must be made before such a depressed fragment is elevated. Mature judgment is required in deciding whether bone fragments should be removed or realigned.

If the dura is torn, the opening is enlarged to allow inspection and debridement of the brain. The brain substance may contain foreign bodies such as bone or hair which must be removed.

4. **Linear or stellate undepressed fractures**—These can be treated by simple closure of the skin wound after a thorough cleansing. If there is suspicion of a coexistent intracranial hemorrhage, the epidural and subdural spaces may need to be explored concurrently.

Prognosis

The prognosis and course are related to the severity and site of cranial injury. The longer the period of unconsciousness, the poorer the prognosis—although in children recovery from a severe injury may be quite gratifying. The early development of a decerebrate state implies a poor prognosis. The prognosis is very poor in an adult who presents in coma with dilated fixed pupils and signs of brain stem injury.

Improvement following head injury can continue for 6 months or more, but the greatest improvement occurs in the first 3 months. Late disability often includes both physical handicaps (weakness, dysphasia, blindness, etc) and psychosocial abnormalities.

See references on pp 760–761.

EXTRADURAL HEMORRHAGE

The most common cause of extradural hematoma is laceration of a branch of the middle meningeal artery after skull fracture. This artery is liable to injury where it lies within a groove in the inner table of the temporal bone. Extradural bleeding may also result from laceration of the dural sinuses; fractures that cross the superior sagittal sinus or the transverse sinus are most likely to cause extradural bleeding.

Extradural hemorrhage may be produced by a minor blow to the head, and there may have been no period of unconsciousness. An initially unconscious patient may have a "lucid interval"—ie, he may become more alert and then progressively less so—but this classic sign is not invariably present. The hematoma rapidly increases in size and compresses the cerebral cortex, producing contralateral hemiparesis or hemiplegia. As the hemisphere is further compressed, the medial portion of the temporal lobe is forced through the tentorial incisure (compressing the third cranial nerve and producing dilatation of the pupil on

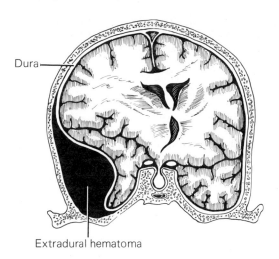

Figure 40–5. Extradural hemorrhage. (Reprinted from Hosp Med 1:9, Oct 1965, by permission of the authors and Wallace Laboratories.)

the same side) and the brain stem is shifted to the opposite side of the tentorial notch. If compression of the brain stem becomes severe enough, venous hemorrhages into the stem will lead to irreversible neurologic deficit or death (Fig 40–5).

Extradural hematoma carries a mortality rate of approximately 50%, principally because it often is not recognized until irreversible changes have occurred within the brain. Thus, it is important to realize that a serious hemorrhage may develop even though the blow to the head was minor. The patient with a history of blow to the head leading to unconsciousness for even a brief interval should have a thorough neurologic examination and skull x-rays. If the x-rays show a fracture, careful monitoring of the level of consciousness and the vital signs is indicated. If the patient is admitted in deep coma with findings—dilated pupils, decerebrate rigidity, hemiplegia—indicating the possibility of an extradural clot, immediate placement of bur holes is justified. Since most extradural clots occur in the temporal area, this should be the site of initial exploration.

Extradural hematomas may also be seen in the posterior fossa. Trephination over the posterior fossa is justified in a patient with an occipital contusion or laceration plus a fracture traversing the transverse sinus or entering the foramen magnum with further impairment of consciousness and no signs of a supratentorial lesion that would account for the symptoms.

SUBDURAL HEMATOMA

The symptoms that develop from subdural bleeding depend in large measure on the speed and the magnitude of the initial hemorrhage. A subdural hematoma may be acute, subacute, or chronic depending on the type and size of the blood vessel torn. The latter factors determine the rapidity of the bleeding.

Acute Subdural Hematoma

In general, the symptoms and signs of acute subdural hematoma may be those of rapid and massive compression of the brain. The term acute is usually reserved for a hematoma that develops within 24 hours. The hemorrhage can result from lacerations of the pia with arterial bleeding as well as from laceration of the veins that bridge from the cortex to the sagittal sinus. An acute subdural hematoma is often accompanied by diffuse cerebral swelling, which further increases intracranial pressure.

The mortality rate in patients with acute subdural hematoma is approximately 80–90%. Treatment consists of removal of the hematoma. Unfortunately, this often does not produce significant improvement because the major neurologic deficit is produced by extensive cerebral contusion, laceration, or both.

Subacute Subdural Hematoma

Subdural hematomas that are detected within 1–10 days after injury are termed subacute. They may be associated with contusion and laceration of the brain. The majority of these hematomas result from laceration of veins that traverse the subdural space. Their neurologic signs develop more gradually than those of acute subdural hematomas, and in many cases are masked by the signs of contusion and laceration of the brain.

Evacuation of the clot may improve the patient's condition, but the degree of ultimate recovery depends upon the extent of underlying brain damage.

Chronic Subdural Hematoma

Chronic subdural hematomas become symptomatic from 10 days to 3 months after injury—an interval of 6 weeks is common. The symptomatology may be very insidious and may occur after a seemingly minor traumatic incident has been forgotten. The history is usually one of progressive mental or personality changes with or without focal signs and symptoms.

The hemorrhage usually results from trauma to the veins that bridge from the cortex to the sagittal sinus. Since venous bleeding is under low pressure, it arrests spontaneously before becoming large enough to compress the brain. A membrane forms around the clot, and, as the protein molecules disintegrate, osmotic pressure increases so that blood serum or CSF is drawn through the semipermeable membranes, causing further expansion of the encapsulated hematoma (Fig 40–6).

Chronic subdural hematomas are most common in infants and in adults past middle age. Because of the slow and insidious development of symptoms, the patient's behavior may be attributed to a psychiatric rather than a physical cause. Skull x-rays often show a shift of the pineal gland, although 20% of hematomas

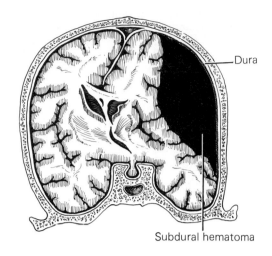

Figure 40–6. Subdural hemorrhage. (Reprinted from Hosp Med 1:9, Oct 1965, by permission of the authors and Wallace Laboratories.)

are bilateral and may be unassociated with a shift in midline structures. The spinal fluid pressure may or may not be elevated. EEG may show slowing on the side of the hematoma and depressed voltage. An echoencephalogram will often disclose a shift of midline structures. A definitive diagnosis is made by angiography also. The brain scan of a chronic subdural hematoma is usually diagnostic.

Chronic subdural hematomas are usually found in the frontoparietal region. This lesion must be strongly suspected in the middle-aged person with a history of head injury who has shown a progressive personality change, headache, and mental dulling. Treatment consists of evacuation of the hematoma via bur holes.

Brock S: *Injuries of the Brain and Spinal Cord and Their Coverings,* 4th ed. Springer, 1960.

Clare FB, Bell HS: Extradural hematomas. JAMA 177:887, 1961.

Craigmile TK: Operative treatment of acute craniocerebral injuries. Surg Clin North Am 49:1425, 1969.

Ducker TB & others: Emergency care of patients with cerebral injuries. Postgrad Med 55:102, Jan 1974.

Evans JP: *Acute Head Injury,* 2nd ed. Thomas, 1963.

Evans JP & others: A summary of current concepts of the dynamics of head injury. Trans Am Neurol Assoc 94:256, 1969.

Finney LA, Walker AE: *Transtentorial Herniation.* Thomas, 1962.

Gurdjian ES: Recent advances in the study of the mechanism of impact injury of the head: A summary. Clin Neurosurg 19:1, 1972.

Gurdjian ES: Webster JE: *Head Injuries.* Little, Brown, 1958.

Jennett B: Prognosis after severe head injury. Clin Neurosurg 19:200, 1972.

McKissock W, Richardson A, Bloom WH: Subdural haematoma: A review of 389 cases. Lancet 1:1365, 1960.

Morley TP, Hetherington RF: Traumatic cerebrospinal fluid rhinorrhea and otorrhea, pneumocephalus, and meningitis. Surg Gynecol Obstet 104:88, 1957.

Paul FJ & others: Computerized axial tomography with the EMI scanner. Radiology 110:109, 1974.

Rowbotham GF: *Acute Injuries of the Head,* 4th ed. Williams & Wilkins, 1964.

Schneider RC: Craniocerebral trauma. In: *Correlative Neurosurgery,* 2nd ed. Kahn EA & others. Thomas, 1969.

Shulman K, Ransohoff J: Subdural hematoma in children. J Neurosurg 18:175, 1961.

Teasdale G, Jennett B: Assessment of coma and impaired consciousness. Lancet 2:81, 1974.

Yaragaray F: Craniocerebral trauma in children. Surg Clin North Am 53:59, 1973.

Zulch KJ: Neuropathology of intracranial hemorrhage. Prog Brain Res 30:151, 1968.

. . .

SPINAL TRAUMA
Charles B. Wilson, MD, & Julian T. Hoff, MD

The spine supports the head and trunk, allows a wide range of mobility, and protects neural structures contained within it. Impairment of spinal stability and mobility is an orthopedic problem and is discussed in Chapter 45; this section is concerned only with the neurologic aspects of spinal injuries. All spinal injuries, however, should be managed by the neurosurgeon and the orthopedist in collaboration.

Spinal injuries damage neural structures by encroaching upon the spinal canal and intervertebral foramens. The injuries to be considered here are fractures of the vertebral body and neural arch; dislocations, partial or complete, unilateral or bilateral, with or without x-ray fracture; and lateral or posterior herniation of intervertebral disk fragments. Neurologic involvement ranges from mild and transient to severe and permanent. Injuries of the cervical and thoracic spine may involve spinal cord and local nerve roots; injuries from T11 through L1 involve the conus, local nerve roots, and nerve roots of the cauda equina; and injuries below L1 involve nerve roots only (Fig 40—7).

Clinical Findings

Spinal injury may be unsuspected, particularly in the patient sustaining other more obvious injuries—eg, cerebral concussion, blunt abdominal trauma, facial fractures. Spinal injury should be considered in the presence of the following findings: (1) all acute injuries to the head and jaw; (2) pain in occiput, spine, or limbs; (3) weakness of one or more limbs; (4) spinal deformity; (5) paralysis of accessory muscles of respiration, with diaphragmatic breathing; and (6) manifestations of "spinal shock" such as ileus, priapism, hyper- or hypothermia, and low blood pressure.

Caution: Extreme care must be exercised in transporting or examining a patient with a suspected spine injury.

A. Symptoms and Signs: Isolated injury of the spinal nerve roots causes motor and sensory loss in corresponding myotomes and dermatomes. The characteristic pain of nerve root injuries may be intensified by the slightest movement.

1. Total loss of spinal cord function—There are 3 types of manifestations: (1) **motor** (immediate areflexia and flaccid paralysis; in time, reflexes return and spasticity replaces flaccidity); (2) **sensory** (absence of sensation below the injured segment; sacral sensation must be examined because in otherwise complete transection it may be spared); and (3) **autonomic** (urinary retention due to detrusor paralysis, paralytic ileus, anhidrosis below the injury, mild hypotension secondary to vasomotor paralysis, and, with high injuries, fever caused by failure to dissipate body heat). The early depression of motor and autonomic function goes by the unfortunate term "spinal shock."

2. Regional injury—

a. Cervical—

(1) C1—2—Because spinal cord injury at this level causes fatal respiratory paralysis, patients reaching a hospital alive have either no or minimal neurologic damage. Dislocation at C1—2 (almost always associated with odontoid fracture) causes pain in the neck and occiput, rigidity or rotation of the neck, and abnormal prominence of the C2 spine. The signs and symptoms of "hangman's fracture," a bilateral pedicle fracture of C2 with C2—3 dislocation, are similar.

(2) C4—T1—Quadriparesis or quadriplegia occurs in varying degrees, the extent being determined by the severity of injury and the level involved. Lesions at C4 involve the entire upper limb; lower injuries spare the proximal muscles.

(3) Hyperextension—Extreme hyperextension of the neck narrows the anteroposterior diameter of the spinal canal. If intraspinal osteophytes are present, the cord may be injured. Because most damage occurs centrally within the cord, the posterior and lateral columns are relatively spared. Good motor function of the legs with impaired motor function of the arms is then characteristic.

b. Thoracolumbar—Except for simple compression fractures of the vertebral body without neurologic impairment, high and mid thoracic injuries are uncommon. In the less common but more serious thoracolumbar injuries, paralysis due to lesions of lower motor neurons is immediately and permanently flaccid. The extent of lower limb involvement is determined by the level of injury, but all thoracolumbar injuries cause paralysis of bowel and bladder.

B. X-Ray Examination: Although invaluable in diagnosis, x-ray examination of a spinal injury may cause further damage (perhaps fatal) if care is not taken. Any patient with a suspected or known spinal injury should be moved onto the x-ray table by 2 or more persons standing *on one side,* their arms beneath his body. Moving in unison, they should lift him onto the table while 2 more persons (one at his head and one at his feet) exert gentle traction to maintain alignment. The patient should not be turned to a lateral position; lateral views are taken across the x-ray table. When injury to the cervical spine is suspected, the head

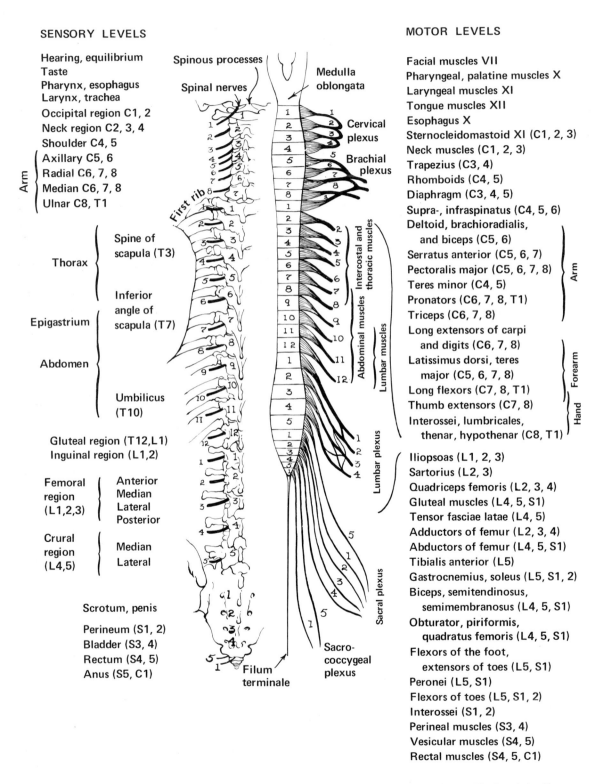

SENSORY LEVELS

Hearing, equilibrium
Taste
Pharynx, esophagus
Larynx, trachea
Occipital region C1, 2
Neck region C2, 3, 4
Shoulder C4, 5
Axillary C5, 6
Radial C6, 7, 8
Median C6, 7, 8
Ulnar C8, T1

Arm

Spinous processes
Spinal nerves
First rib

Thorax
Spine of
scapula (T3)

Inferior
angle of
scapula (T7)

Epigastrium

Abdomen

Umbilicus
(T10)

Gluteal region (T12,L1)
Inguinal region (L1,2)

Femoral
region
(L1,2,3)

Anterior
Median
Lateral
Posterior

Crural
region
(L4,5)

Median
Lateral

Scrotum, penis

Perineum (S1, 2)
Bladder (S3, 4)
Rectum (S4, 5)
Anus (S5, C1)

Medulla
oblongata

Cervical
plexus

Brachial
plexus

Intercostal and
thoracic muscles

Abdominal muscles
Lumbar muscles

Lumbar plexus

Sacral plexus

Filum
terminale

Sacro-
coccygeal
plexus

MOTOR LEVELS

Facial muscles VII
Pharyngeal, palatine muscles X
Laryngeal muscles XI
Tongue muscles XII
Esophagus X
Sternocleidomastoid XI (C1, 2, 3)
Neck muscles (C1, 2, 3)
Trapezius (C3, 4)
Rhomboids (C4, 5)
Diaphragm (C3, 4, 5)
Supra-, infraspinatus (C4, 5, 6)
Deltoid, brachioradialis,
    and biceps (C5, 6)
Serratus anterior (C5, 6, 7)
Pectoralis major (C5, 6, 7, 8)
Teres minor (C4, 5)
Pronators (C6, 7, 8, T1)
Triceps (C6, 7, 8)
Long extensors of carpi
    and digits (C6, 7, 8)
Latissimus dorsi, teres
    major (C5, 6, 7, 8)
Long flexors (C7, 8, T1)
Thumb extensors (C7, 8)
Interossei, lumbricales,
    thenar, hypothenar (C8, T1)

Arm
Forearm
Hand

Iliopsoas (L1, 2, 3)
Sartorius (L2, 3)
Quadriceps femoris (L2, 3, 4)
Gluteal muscles (L4, 5, S1)
Tensor fasciae latae (L4, 5)
Adductors of femur (L2, 3, 4)
Abductors of femur (L4, 5, S1)
Tibialis anterior (L5)
Gastrocnemius, soleus (L5, S1, 2)
Biceps, semitendinosus,
    semimembranosus (L4, 5, S1)
Obturator, piriformis,
    quadratus femoris (L4, 5, S1)
Flexors of the foot,
    extensors of toes (L5, S1)
Peronei (L5, S1)
Flexors of toes (L5, S1, 2)
Interossei (S1, 2)
Perineal muscles (S3, 4)
Vesicular muscles (S4, 5)
Rectal muscles (S4, 5, C1)

Figure 40–7. Motor and sensory levels of the spinal cord. (Reproduced, with permission, from Chusid JG: *Correlative Neuroanatomy & Functional Neurology,* 16th ed. Lange, 1976.)

and neck should be immobilized in the neutral position before x-rays are taken. This can be done by placing sandbags alongside the head, strapping the head to a spine board with a forehead strap, applying an adjustable cervical collar, or by cervical halter traction. The C7–T1 junction must be visualized, which may require pulling the supine patient's arms directly downward or taking a "swimmer's view" exposure. The patient with a thoracolumbar injury is easily immobilized on a board.

Myelography may be indicated when neurologic changes are present but the spine films are normal. Acute rupture of an intervertebral disk may injure the spinal cord, nerve roots, or both, without fracture or dislocation of the spine. Acute disk rupture is suspected when plain spine x-rays do not explain observed neurologic deficits, and in this circumstance myelographic verification of a ruptured disk precedes its surgical removal.

Complications

Quadriplegic patients have an ineffective cough and reduced tidal volume secondary to paralysis of accessory muscles of respiration, so that tracheostomy is indicated in selected cases. Frequent but less threatening early complications involve the skin (pressure sores), bladder (urinary tract infection), and paralyzed muscles (contractures and deformity).

Prevention

Inexpert handling at the scene of the accident and during transportation to the emergency department may cause or aggravate neurologic damage, and movement of the victim with known or suspected spinal injury should await arrival of trained personnel. Prevention of further injury during x-ray examination is discussed above.

Training leading to certification of ambulance personnel and standardization of ambulance vehicles and equipment will prevent many serious and permanent sequelae of spine injuries.

Treatment

The objectives of treatment are to protect undamaged neural structures, to restore function to reversibly damaged structures, to correct spinal alignment, and to achieve permanent spinal stability. Early supportive care is of great importance. This includes attention to the skin, bladder, paralyzed and paretic muscles, and nutrition. The quality of early care determines the speed with which active rehabilitative measures can be started.

A. Immediate Care: An adequate airway must be established and maintained. The injured spinal segment must be immobilized while a search for associated injuries—particularly injuries involving anesthetic areas—is carried out.

1. Care of the skin—Pressure sores (decubitus ulcers) may develop with astonishing rapidity. As soon as a diagnosis of cord transection is made, it is essential to change the position of paralyzed parts at least every 2 hours. Stabilization of cervical spine injury by traction is a critical component of early change in position (see Chapter 10).

2. Vesical paralysis and ileus—These require insertion of a urethral catheter and a nasogastric tube.

3. Cervical—All cervical injuries with fracture or dislocation of vertebrae are managed by skeletal traction, usually by means of tongs placed in line with the mastoid tips. Dislocations are reduced gradually with up to 16 kg (35 lb) of traction. Nonoperative management requires 6 weeks of continuous traction followed by 12 weeks of external support (by brace or plaster cast); fractures of C1 and C2 require traction for twice as long.

Three surgical procedures have been applied to cervical fractures: (1) Laminectomy for decompression of the spinal cord and nerve roots, the accepted indication being progression of neurologic deficit. (2) Posterior fusion, either at the time of laminectomy or later, because of spinal instability. (3) Anterior removal of intervertebral disk and involved bone, exploration of the spinal canal, and interbody fusion. This should be considered for cervical injuries below C2 with or without neurologic deficit. It permits early activity, allows removal of intraspinal disk and bone fragments, and assures a stable undeformed spine. Hyperextension injuries without fracture require neither traction nor operation.

4. Thoracolumbar—Immediate, complete paraplegia rarely improves with or without operative management. Reduction of the fracture, whether by traction or operation, does offer maximum potential for recovery of function, however. Conus injuries seldom improve following decompression, but the injured cauda equina may regain function eventually.

5. Disk rupture—Operative removal of a ruptured disk at any level should follow localization of the lesion by myelography.

B. Special Care of Missile Injuries: High velocity missiles can damage the spinal cord without entering the spinal canal. Missiles that enter or traverse the spinal canal produce open wounds of the spinal cord and cauda equina that should be debrided. The prognosis for missile injuries of the spinal cord is poor with or without operation. However, elective removal of the missile may be helpful in lesions of the cauda equina.

C. Long-Term Care (Rehabilitation): A critical part of rehabilitation is bladder training, the goal being a catheter-free patient with sterile urine. Repeated bouts of pyelonephritis and dilatation of the collecting system are indications for urinary diversion. Vocational training is essential in paraplegic patients and must offer emotional as well as physical adaptation to the neurologic deficit.

Prognosis

Although physiologic transection of the cord (total paralysis and anesthesia below the site of damage) is indistinguishable from anatomic transection immediately after injury, a thorough neurologic examination 24 hours after injury permits an accurate prognosis. There is early return of some function following concussion of the cord. If total interruption of cord function is documented 24 hours after injury, the spinal cord has been irreversibly damaged and any slight recovery will be functionally insignificant. Any evidence of voluntary motor or sensory function below the level of injury indicates an incomplete injury with the potential for incomplete to near-complete recovery. Testing of sacral sensation is particularly important because of the prognostic implications of sacral sparing as an indication of incomplete transection.

The long-term prognosis in severe spinal injury is intimately related to renal function because uremia is the major cause of death.

Alexander E Jr, Davis CH Jr, Forsyth HF: Reduction and fusion of fracture dislocation of the cervical spine. J Neurosurg 27:588, 1967.

Aufranc OE, Jones WN, Harris WH: Thoracic spine fracture with paralysis. JAMA 189: 1018, 1964.

Bailey RW: Fractures and dislocations of the cervical spine: Orthopedic and neurosurgical aspects. Postgrad Med 35:588, 1964.

Bertrand G: Management of spinal injuries with associated cord damage. Postgrad Med 37:249, 1965.

Bray EA, Miller JA, Bouzard WC: Traumatic dislocation of the cervical spine. J Trauma 3:569, 1963.

Guttmann L: *Spinal Cord Injuries.* Blackwell, 1973.

Jane JA, Evans JP, Fisher LE: An investigation concerning the restitution of motor function following injury to the spinal cord. J Neurosurg 21:167, 1964.

Kaufer H, Hayes JT: Lumbar fracture-dislocation. J Bone Joint Surg 48A: 712, 1966.

Norrell H, Wilson CB: Early anterior cervical fusion for injuries of the cervical spine. JAMA 214:525, 1970.

Nyquist RH, Bors E: Mortality and survival in traumatic myelopathy during nineteen years, from 1946 to 1965. Paraplegia 5:22, 1967.

TRAUMATIC PERIPHERAL NERVE LESIONS
Barton A. Brown, MD

Regardless of cause, peripheral nerve injuries fall into 3 categories: neurotmesis, in which both the axons and the investing sheaths are disrupted; axonotmesis, in which the axons are interrupted but the sheath remains intact; and axonapraxia, in which both axons and nerve sheaths are intact but there is a failure of conduction. The types of injuries may be compression (from casts, tourniquets, bandages, entrapment), lacerations (by sharp objects, missiles, fractures), contusions (by blunt trauma, either chronic or acute), stretch, ischemia, and injection.

The peripheral nerves contain sensory and motor fibers, most of which are myelinated. Each axon is surrounded by an endoneurial connective tissue tube; groups of axons are bound together by perineurium, and the resultant fascicles are enmeshed in the epineurium, which is bounded by the external nerve sheath.

Depending upon its severity, trauma may produce edema, swelling, and variable disruption of the axonal and connective tissue elements, and distal wallerian degeneration. Resolution of the acute process results in scar formation within the nerve and for variable distances above and below the site of injury. If the nerve has been completely divided, no immediate prediction can be made of the extent of scarring.

In a divided nerve, the proximal end will develop a neuroma composed of connective tissue and tangled axons. The distal free end will have an end bulb of connective tissue. If the injured nerve retains its continuity, scar tissue may develop within the nerve and cause constriction of the axons with resultant dysfunction.

Clinical Findings

Sensory, motor, and reflex changes will depend upon the peripheral nerve involved and the level of involvement. A standard neuroanatomy textbook should be available for review of specific motor and sensory innervation and possible anatomic variations.

A history of remote as well as recent trauma should be elicited. In neurologic diagnosis, the history suggests the type of pathology while the neurologic examination localizes the lesion. A complete neurologic examination must be done, with emphasis on the nerves involved. Motor, sensory, and reflex deficits must be correlated to determine severity and distribution of involvement. Electromyography and nerve conduction studies establish a baseline for monitoring subsequent recovery but will not be helpful until 2–3 weeks after an acute injury.

Differential Diagnosis

An accurate history and a meticulous examination are the key elements. The history will help differentiate traumatic neuropathies from those of infectious origin (diphtheria, mumps, influenza, pneumonia, meningitis, malaria, syphilis, typhoid, typhus, dysentery, tuberculosis, gonorrhea) or toxic or metabolic origin (diabetes, rheumatic fever, gout, leukemia, vitamin deficiency, polyarteritis nodosa, drug reaction, heavy metals, carbon monoxide).

Complications

Causalgia is a dysesthetic, severe burning pain in the distribution of a nerve with a partial lesion. Hyperpathia, trophic changes, and vasomotor hyperactivity are characteristic. (Minor stimuli may produce severe pain.) Although spontaneous remissions may occur, sympathetic blocks and sympathectomy are specific diagnostic and therapeutic procedures.

"Reflex sympathetic dystrophy" or "minor causalgia" sometimes occurs, usually in relation to painful osteoporosis or Sudeck's atrophy. The major complaint is hyperesthesia. Treatment consists of sympathetic blocks and active physical therapy.

Treatment

When a peripheral nerve has been severed, reanastomosis by suture is the appropriate treatment. Primary suture should be attempted only in wounds that are clean, seen immediately, caused by knife or razor, and devoid of adjacent tissue damage. In the remainder of cases, the nerve ends should be tagged and secondary suture undertaken when the wound has completely healed, adjacent tissue reaction has subsided, and infection has cleared. After a delay of 3 weeks or more, the extent of intraneural scarring can be determined at the time of secondary suture, and the nerve ends should be resected until normal tissue is reached. Delayed repair greatly enhances the chances for functional recovery. If removal of scarred ends leaves a gap that is too large to be bridged, the limb can be flexed until the gap is closed. After healing, the sutured nerve can be stretched over a period of months by placing the limb in a series of gradually straightened casts. Frozen irradiated homografts offer a means of bridging extensive nerve defects, but all the problems of rejection have not yet been solved and chance of success is limited. Interfascicular sural autografts have had some success and can be used to bridge large defects.

Nerve injuries in continuity—whether loss of function is complete or incomplete—should be explored if they do not improve within 6 weeks after injury. Intra- and extraneural scar tissue at the site of the lesion often causes axonopraxia or prevents axonal regrowth by virtue of its constricting effects. External and internal neurolyses via microsurgical technics are indicated. Some of these lesions would improve spontaneously if left alone for more than 6 weeks, but the disadvantage of continued denervation outweighs the risk of surgical exploration.

Some lesions resulting from contusion or compression are improved by neurolysis. The same is true of some injection neuropathies (depending upon the substance injected).

Prompt institution of physical therapy for improvement of muscle function and maintenance of joint range of motion is indicated. The denervated portion of the limb is subject to muscle atrophy and fibrosis, joint stiffness, motor end plate atrophy, and trophic skin changes. The longer the denervation persists, the less likely it is that a good functional result will be achieved. Physical therapy is the best means of minimizing the complications of denervation.

Prognosis

Grading of sensorimotor function from 0–5 is helpful in documenting progress. Most improvement occurs during the first year, but the maximum may not be reached for 3–4 years. The younger the patient, the better the prognosis; injuries with minimal adjacent tissue damage have a better prognosis than those with widespread tissue damage such as war wounds. Proximal lesions recover less well than distal ones. Intraoperative factors such as axial orientation of the nerve, proper coaptation, suture material, hemostasis, and suture line tension are important determinants of the end result. Electromyography and nerve conduction studies are helpful guides during the recovery period.

Healing in a damaged peripheral nerve is slow (approximately 1 mm/day), and the patient must be prepared for this. He must understand that his role in treatment is an active one, and his motivation must be maintained.

Brown BA: Internal neurolysis in treatment of traumatic peripheral nerve lesions. Calif Med 110:460, 1969.

Brown HA, Brown BA: Treatment of peripheral nerve injuries. Rev Surg 24:1, 1967.

Campbell JB: Peripheral nerve repair. Clin Neurosurg 17:77, 1969.

Chusid JG: *Correlative Neuroanatomy & Functional Neurology,* 16th ed. Lange, 1976.

Millesi H, Meissl G, Berger A: The interfascicular nerve-grafting of the median and ulnar nerves. J Bone Joint Surg 54A:727, 1972.

Simeone FA (editor): Symposium on operative nerve injuries and their repair. Surg Clin North Am 52:1097, 1972. [Entire issue.]

Sunderland S: *Nerves and Nerve Injuries.* Williams & Wilkins, 1968.

BRAIN TUMORS
Charles B. Wilson, MD

Essentials of Diagnosis
- Headache.
- Progressive neurologic deficit.
- Convulsions, focal or generalized.
- Increased intracranial pressure.
- Organic mental changes.

General Considerations

Although by custom tumors are considered either benign or malignant, *all* brain tumors are malignant in the sense that they may lead to death if not treated. By compression or invasion of neighboring structures, brain tumors cause specific signs of localizing value. Most brain tumors, either by virtue of their bulk or by obstructing the flow of CSF, eventually produce increased intracranial pressure which may have no localizing value.

Among adults, 70% of brain tumors originate above the tentorium cerebelli; the remainder occupy the infratentorial compartment (posterior fossa). In children, the majority of tumors are infratentorial. Age and site are correlated with tumor type in Table 40–2. The frequency of major tumor types is indicated in Table 40–3.

Meningiomas and nerve sheath tumors are more common in females than in males; most glial tumors—particularly medulloblastomas—have a predilection for males, and pineal tumors occur almost exclusively in young males. Other primary tumors attack the sexes equally.

Classification

A. Gliomas: Tumors composed of glial cells con-

Table 40—2. Frequency of brain tumor types according to age and site.

Age	Cerebral Hemisphere	Intrasellar and Parasellar	Posterior Fossa
Childhood and adolescence	Ependymomas; less commonly, astrocytomas.	Astrocytomas, mixed gliomas, ependymomas.	Astrocytomas, medulloblastomas, ependymomas.
Age 20—40	Meningiomas, astrocytomas; less commonly, metastatic tumors.	Pituitary adenomas; less commonly, meningiomas.	Acoustic neuromas, meningiomas, hemangioblastomas; less commonly, metastatic tumors.
Over age 40	Glioblastoma multiforme, meningiomas, metastatic tumors.	Pituitary adenomas; less commonly, meningiomas.	Metastatic tumors, acoustic neuromas, meningiomas.

stitute 50% of intracranial neoplasms. The neuroglia, once thought to serve only as a supporting structure, contains complex cellular elements involved with important functions such as the blood-brain barrier, myelin metabolism, and neuronal metabolism. Astrocytes and oligodendroglia are present throughout the CNS, whereas ependymal cells are confined to the ventricular cavities and the central canal. Medulloblastomas are included among gliomas, although a medulloblast is a theoretically bipotential cell (neuroglial and neuronal).

1. Astrocytomas—These slowly invasive tumors are widely distributed throughout the brain at all ages. Among younger patients, they involve predominantly 3 sites—optic nerves and hypothalamus, brain stem, and cerebellar hemispheres—typically as a cyst containing a relatively small neoplastic mural nodule.

2. Oligodendrogliomas—These slowly growing tumors rarely arise outside the cerebral hemispheres. They are tumors of adult life, and calcification within the tumor is often seen on x-ray.

3. Ependymomas—Ependymomas are uncommon

in adults. In the cerebral hemispheres, they may extend intracerebrally, whereas in the fourth ventricle they show less tendency to invade deeply into adjacent neural tissue. Papillomas of the choroid plexus may be considered to be a special type of ependymoma; their ability to overproduce CSF is no longer questioned.

4. Glioblastoma multiforme—Biologically and histologically, these are malignant astrocytomas (and are sometimes classified as astrocytoma grade III—IV). Mean survival from the date of diagnosis is slightly over 6 months—in contrast to 2—5 years for the tumors described above. Most occupy the cerebral hemisphere in adults, and the remainder occur in the brain stems of children. Characteristic features include tumor tissue with necrosis, new vessel formation, spontaneous hemorrhage, and associated cerebral edema.

5. Medulloblastomas—Predominantly tumors of infancy and childhood, medulloblastomas are highly malignant tumors arising in the cerebellar vermis. Distinctive features are their extreme radiosensitivity and their tendency to seed down the spine in the CSF.

B. Nonglial Tumors: These tumors arise from various tissues. They are biologically benign and compress rather than invade adjacent brain.

1. Meningiomas—These are firm, generally globular tumors readily separable from compressed neural tissues. Because of their slow rate of growth, meningiomas often attain massive proportions. Believed to originate from arachnoid granulations, they have a broad base along the dura (including the dural partitions, the falx cerebri, and the tentorium cerebelli), often extend into bone, and derive a portion of their blood supply from extracerebral arteries, eg, external carotid branches. Preferred sites are along the length of the superior sagittal sinus (parasagittal; Fig 40—8), over the cerebral convexities, beneath the frontal lobe (olfactory groove and tuberculum sellae; Fig 40—9), along the sphenoid wing, and within the posterior fossa (cerebellopontine angle and clivus). The tendency of meningiomas to involve the orbit explains the frequent occurrence of exophthalmos (sphenoid wing; Fig 40—10).

Table 40—3. Frequency of major types of brain tumors.

Intracranial Tumors*		Frequency of Occurrence
Gliomas		50%
Glioblastoma multiforme	50%	
Astrocytoma	20%	
Ependymoma	10%	
Medulloblastoma	10%	
Oligodendroglioma	5%	
Mixed	5%	
Meningiomas		20%
Nerve sheath tumors		10%
Metastatic tumors		10%
Congenital tumors		5%
Miscellaneous tumors		5%

*Exclusive of pituitary tumors.

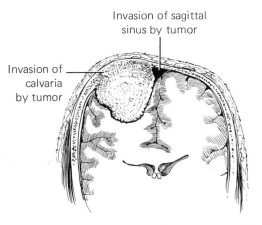

Figure 40—8. Parasagittal meningioma. Disturbances of cerebral function, depending on localization. Focal hyperplasia and hypervascularization of the overlying bones.

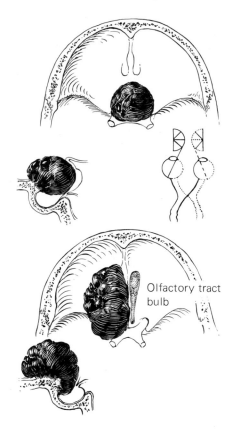

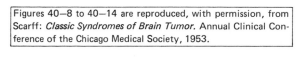

Figures 40—8 to 40—14 are reproduced, with permission, from Scarff: *Classic Syndromes of Brain Tumor.* Annual Clinical Conference of the Chicago Medical Society, 1953.

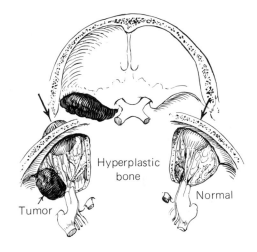

Figure 40—9. *Top:* Meningioma of tuberculum sellae. Failing vision, primary optic atrophy, bitemporal hemianopsia, but no endocrine disturbance and no enlargement of the sella turcica in middle-aged persons. *Bottom:* Olfactory groove meningioma. Ipsilateral anosmia and primary optic atrophy; contralateral papilledema.

Figure 40—10. Retro-orbital meningioma. *Early stage:* Unilateral exophthalmos, slowly progressing (months to years). Increased density (in x-rays): retro-orbital plate, ipsilateral side.

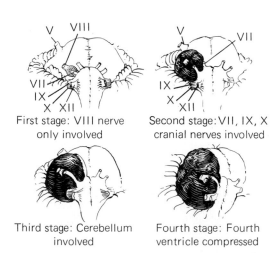

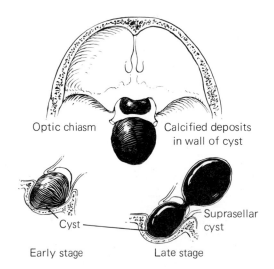

Figure 40—11. Acoustic neurinoma. *First stage:* Tinnitus; later, deafness and disturbances of equilibrium. *Second stage:* Subtle weakness of facial muscles, facial numbness, dysphagia, and dysarthria. *Third stage:* Ataxia and incoordination. *Fourth stage:* Evidence of increased intracranial pressure.

Figure 40—12. Craniopharyngioma. *Early stage:* Failing vision, primary optic atrophy, bitemporal field defects, endocrine disturbances (hypopituitarism), suprasellar calcification (80%) in children and adolescents. *Late stage:* Headache, nausea, and vomiting.

2. Nerve sheath tumors—(Fig 40–11.) These tumors are termed acoustic neurinomas because they originate almost exclusively in the eighth cranial nerve. From its point of origin within the internal auditory canal, this slowly growing tumor expands the auditory meatus as it extends into the angle formed by the cerebellum and pons. At the time of diagnosis it typically compresses the fifth cranial nerve, the pons, the cerebellum, and the fourth ventricle. The seventh cranial nerve is stretched remarkably, but its function is usually little affected. Patients with multiple neurofibromatosis are liable to develop sheath tumors of the eighth nerve, but the vast majority of patients harboring acoustic tumors have no stigmas of this disease.

3. Craniopharyngiomas—(Fig 40–12.) Arising from remnants of Rathke's pouch, this typically cystic tumor extends from the sella turcica to involve the optic nerves, the hypothalamus, and the third ventricle. Fluid within this tumor resembles motor oil in appearance. Most craniopharyngiomas contain calcified areas which can be seen on x-ray and become symptomatic in childhood. Some, however, first appear in mid and late adult life.

4. Congenital tumors—

a. Epidermoid tumors—These consist of a mass of desquamated epithelium produced by a simple epithelium-lined cyst. Intracranially, they occur most frequently in the parasellar region and at the cerebellopontine angle.

b. Intracranial dermoids—These tumors are rare. Most occupy the posterior fossa.

c. Teratomas—These tumors (also rare) arise most commonly in the pineal gland.

d. Chordomas—These tumors originate from notochordal remnants along the clivus. Like the more common sacrococcygeal chordomas, they grow slowly.

e. Pineal tumors—(Fig 40–13.) Almost all pineal tumors are either true teratomas or atypical teratomas. The latter are germinomas identical with testicular seminomas and ovarian dysgerminomas. Germinomas

may originate in the hypothalamus, where they have been termed (incorrectly) "ectopic pinealomas."

5. Metastatic tumors—Carcinoma of the lung in males and carcinoma of the breast in females account for almost 70% of all metastases within the skull; other primary tumors are other supradiaphragmatic tumors (eg, thyroid), renal carcinoma, and malignant melanoma. The distribution of metastatic tumors is determined by blood flow in different areas, and the frequency in a particular site is roughly proportionate to its mass. One-third of brain metastases are solitary. Metastatic tumors provoke varying degrees of surrounding brain edema.

Clinical Findings

Brain tumors may produce general and focal signs either singly or together. General signs relate to increased intracranial pressure. Local signs may be irritative (convulsive) or destructive (paralytic). The temporal evolution (rate of progression) of neurologic signs correlates with each tumor's rate of growth.

The manifestations of intrinsic supratentorial tumors are related to the site involved. Frontal tumors may cause personality changes, with loss of interest, facetiousness, and moral laxity. Tumors involving the posterior frontal region may produce contralateral mono- or hemiparesis. Temporal lobe tumors may cause behavior disorders, often accompanied by superior quadrantanopsia or uncinate seizures. Parietal lobe tumors may cause contralateral hemisensory disturbances and homonymous hemianopia. Occipital tumors may produce homonymous visual field defects characteristically consisting of unformed visual hallucinations. Tumors in the dominant hemisphere may cause disorders of communication (aphasia); nondominant cerebral hemispheric lesions may cause apraxia. Extrinsic supratentorial tumors cause similar disturbances appropriate to their location. Frontal meningiomas unsuspected during life may be discovered on postmortem examination of inmates of state mental institutions. Subfrontal meningiomas should be suspected in the presence of mental deterioration accompanied by anosmia and optic atrophy. Tumors in the region of the sella turcica may involve the optic chiasm (visual loss), hypothalamus (endocrine abnormalities), or foramen interventriculare (hydrocephalus). Intraventricular tumors usually present with signs of intracranial hypertension.

Posterior fossa tumors have characteristic patterns. Brain stem tumors cause multiple cranial nerve palsies (usually fifth through seventh) and later involve motor and sensory long tracts. Tumors in the cerebellar vermis produce truncal ataxia and those in the cerebellar hemisphere an ipsilateral limb ataxia and hypotonia. Tumors originating within the fourth ventricle often produce hydrocephalus without involvement of neighboring structures; and extrinsic tumors occupying the cerebellopontine angle may involve the fifth, seventh, and eighth cranial nerves in association with cerebellar deficits and, in later stages, hydrocephalus through deformity of the fourth ventricle.

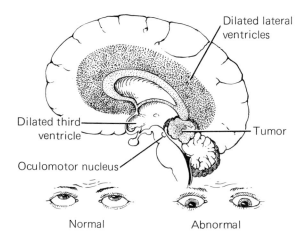

Figure 40–13. Pinealoma. Symptoms and signs of increased intracranial pressure, without lateralizing signs. Limitation of upward gaze. Abnormal pupillary reactions.

Differential Diagnosis

Because brain tumors can cause focal neurologic signs and increased intracranial pressure, many conditions may be simulated by a brain tumor.

During infancy and childhood, an unexplained convulsion usually indicates the onset of idiopathic epilepsy, whereas in later life a convulsion is often the initial manifestation of a brain tumor. Neurologic examination, skull x-rays, EEG, and radioisotopic brain scan will serve to select patients for more definitive radiologic procedures such as angiography and pneumography.

Brain tumors may mimic cerebrovascular disease, and glioblastomas and metastatic tumors in particular cause confusion in this regard. A careful inquiry into antecedent symptoms may disclose evidence suggestive of tumor, but the diagnosis is often not suspected until the patient's course indicates deterioration rather than improvement.

Chronic subdural hematomas and brain abscesses may pursue a course similar to that of a tumor. Without a history of head injury or a source of infection, the diagnosis may be unsuspected until disclosed by angiography or operation.

Increased intracranial pressure has many causes. In the pediatric age group, the list includes lead encephalopathy, acute glomerulonephritis, administration of antibiotics to infants predisposed to increased intracranial pressure, and downward adjustment of dosage in patients being given long-term corticosteroid therapy. The history usually makes the diagnosis.

Pseudotumor cerebri (idiopathic brain swelling, benign intracranial hypertension) typically affects adolescent and young adult females, and the cause is probably an endocrine imbalance. A similar "benign brain edema" occurs in women receiving oral contraceptives and in certain patients with Addison's disease and hyperparathyroidism. Again, the history, neurologic examination, and special neuroradiologic tests such as angiography should distinguish these patients from those with increased intracranial pressure caused by brain tumor.

Complications

Missed or late diagnosis may lead to irreversible brain damage, which is all the more tragic in the case of a favorably situated benign tumor. Injudicious lumbar puncture may precipitate fatal temporal lobe or tonsillar herniation.

Treatment

Total removal is the surgeon's goal in the treatment of most extrinsic tumors (meningiomas, nerve sheath tumors, craniopharyngiomas, colloid cysts, and epidermoids) and cerebellar hemangioblastomas. If the location, size, and vascularity of the tumor preclude safe extirpation, subtotal removal may be all that can be done. With the exception of cystic cerebellar astrocytomas containing a mural tumor nodule, glial tumors in the cerebral hemispheres and cerebellum are rarely curable by operation alone, and the surgeon's objective becomes radical subtotal removal within the limits determined by the tumor's location—eg, dominant hemisphere, motor area. Postoperative radiation therapy in the range of 5000 rads over the course of 5–6 weeks is then delivered to the residual tumor. In patients with medulloblastoma, the spinal axis is also irradiated because this tumor frequently seeds throughout the CSF.

Tumors of the brain stem and pineal regions are usually treated by irradiation alone on the basis of clinical and x-ray diagnosis. Although pineal tumors can be removed, their marked radiosensitivity and the high risk of operation argue for radiotherapy, usually preceded by placement of a CSF shunt for hydrocephalus.

Under certain circumstances, solitary metastatic tumors are suitable for surgical extirpation. Their radiosensitivity varies.

Chemotherapy has been used with variable and modest success for recurrent glioblastomas and medulloblastomas.

A recently concluded national cooperative study of patients harboring malignant gliomas (anaplastic astrocytomas and glioblastomas) established the value of postoperative radiotherapy and the added benefit (measured by survival) of combined radiotherapy and chemotherapy (carmustine [BCNU]).

Prognosis

Surgically removable tumors can be cured, and this group includes the majority of meningiomas and nerve sheath tumors, epidermoids, colloid cysts, small craniopharyngiomas, and many cerebellar astrocytomas and hemangioblastomas. Although low-grade gliomas are not highly radiosensitive, long survival is possible when operation and irradiation are combined. Some glioblastomas appear to be radiosensitive, but survival beyond 18 months is uncommon. For medulloblastomas treated by operation and irradiation, the 5-year survival rate is 40%.

Cushing H, Eisenhardt L: *Meningiomas: Their Classification, Regional Behaviour, Life History, and Surgical End Results.* Thomas, 1938.

Matson DD: *Neurosurgery of Infancy and Childhood,* 2nd ed. Thomas, 1969.

Russell DS, Rubinstein LJ: *Pathology of Tumours of the Nervous System,* 2nd ed. Williams & Wilkins, 1963.

Wilson CB, Hoff JT: Tumors of the brain. Chap 11 in: *Practice of Surgery.* Harper & Row, 1973.

TUMORS OF THE SPINAL CANAL
Kenneth Tuerk, MD

Neoplasms of the spinal canal are generally divided into 3 types: extradural, intradural-extramedullary, and intramedullary. The extradural tumors are usually malignant, often metastatic, and account for

30—50% of all spinal canal tumors. Most intradural-extramedullary tumors are benign meningiomas or neurofibromas. About 60% of the intramedullary tumors are astrocytomas or ependymomas, with both kinds occurring with equal frequency. Thus, about 60—70% of all intradural spinal cord tumors are benign, and, with proper treatment, long-term palliation can often be obtained for the remaining 40%.

Pathophysiology

Pressure of the tumor against the spinal cord and its roots as well as interference with the spinal cord's vascular supply produce dysfunction. Intramedullary tumors, which grow in the center of the spinal cord, interfere with the long tracts bilaterally, producing loss of sensation and weakness distal to the level of the tumor. "Sacral sparing" of sensation is a prominent feature of these tumors because the long tracts which subserve the lowest spinal segments travel in the most superficial areas of the spinal cord. Some pain may be present at times, but it is not as prominent a feature as in extramedullary tumors.

Intradural-extramedullary tumors often grow from the lateral aspect of the spinal canal, between the dura and the cord, causing pressure on both the roots and the spinal cord and often affecting one side of the spinal cord more than the other. Common symptoms are spinal cord dysfunction, with motor loss often prominent ipsilaterally to the side of the tumor, loss of pain sensation in the spinal cord often prominent contralaterally to the tumor, and pain related to the roots at the tumor level.

Extradural tumors involve the extradural space, the roots, and the surrounding bony structures. Because the nerve roots, dura, bone, and periosteum are involved, the pain, frequently a prominent symptom, may either be localized to the area of the tumor or radicular in nature. At times this pain may be present for weeks to months before the onset of neurologic signs and symptoms. The pain may heighten during the night and increase with bed rest. Once noticeable neurologic symptoms begin developing, they may intensify over a 48- to 72-hour period, leading to paraplegia or quadriplegia. This rapid progression is thought to be due to interference with the spinal cord's vascular supply.

One symptom common to all 3 tumor types is difficulty with urination—an indication for urgent evaluation and treatment. Complete urinary incontinence is usually irreversible if it lasts for 48—72 hours. As in all patients, a complete history and physical examination are imperative. One may find a primary neoplasm denoting a probable metastatic epidural spinal cord tumor, or café au lait spots, and peripheral neuromas indicating neurofibromatosis.

Laboratory & X-Ray Examination

Spinal fluid examination usually shows a high protein content with normal glucose concentration and cell count. X-ray examinations of the spine are the most important diagnostic tests. Plain x-rays of the suspected area should include films of the foramens as well as anteroposterior and lateral views. Tomography may be useful. Destruction of bone is often seen in malignant epidural tumors. Widening of the intervertebral foramens is sometimes noted in neurofibromas. Broadening of the interpedicular distance of the spinal canal's sagittal plane with scalloping of the body is often seen in slow-growing intradural tumors. Lumbar puncture should be done at the time of myelography; if that is not possible, positive contrast material (usually iophendylate [Pantopaque]) should be available in case a complete block is found by manometric examination. Neither myelography nor lumbar puncture should be performed unless arrangements have been made to proceed with surgery should the symptoms increase rapidly during or immediately after the studies.

Only a small amount of contrast material (3 ml of iophendylate) should be injected initially if the procedure reveals a high-grade spinal cord block. A formal myelogram is used in low-grade block. If the block appears to be complete or almost complete after adequate radiographs are taken, the contrast material is left in place, preventing a rapid progression of symptoms by withdrawal of the material. It is helpful to demonstrate not only the lower level of the tumor but the upper level as well. At times it is necessary to insert positive contrast material from above (cisternal puncture or C2 puncture) to accomplish this.

Myelography provides an accurate diagnosis of spinal cord tumors and can usually differentiate between extradural, intradural, and intermedullary tumors. Occasionally, spinal cord angiography may provide further useful information.

Differential Diagnosis

Differential diagnosis includes inflammatory transverse myelopathy, multiple sclerosis, arteriovenous malformations of the spinal cord, cervical spondylosis, and thoracic disk disease.

Treatment

Treatment consists of surgical removal of the tumor. The more rapid and more severe the onset of symptoms, the more urgent the need for treatment. Recovery of spinal cord function is limited after severe compression and particularly after acute compression. Symptoms of acute compression are characteristic of metastatic epidural tumors, and early decompression may give useful palliation. Even when death is expected within a few months, a patient with terminal cancer who is ambulatory and continent is still better off than one who is paraplegic.

The affected area is approached by laminectomy. Recent advances in surgical technic, including the use of the microscope and bipolar coagulation, have made it possible to totally remove and cure most meningiomas, neurofibromas, and ependymomas; these account for 65% of all intradural tumors. Patients with other types of intradural tumors may receive long-term palliation from surgery, at times lasting over 10 years.

After decompression, metastatic tumors as well as incompletely removed intradural tumors should be treated by the method appropriate to the neoplasm: radiation, chemotherapy, or hormonal therapy.

In seriously incapacitated patients, appropriate supportive care must be given to the tissue below the level of involvement to avoid pressure sores, and adequate urinary drainage must be assured. Complications in these areas may retard postsurgical improvement. An active rehabilitation program must be started early.

Prognosis

In general, the more acute and severe the symptoms are before treatment, the less favorable the prognosis. The earlier the diagnosis can be made and therapy started, the better the outlook for improvement and prevention of further neurologic deterioration.

Greenwood J Jr: Spinal cord tumors. Page 1514 in: *Neurological Surgery.* Youmans JR (editor). Saunders, 1973.

Pool JL: The surgery of spinal cord tumors. Clin Neurosurg 17:310, 1969.

Sloof JL, Kernohan JW, McCarty CS: *Primary Intramedullary Tumors of the Spinal Cord and Filum Terminale.* Saunders, 1964.

TUMORS OF PERIPHERAL NERVES
Edwin B. Boldrey, MD

Essentials of Diagnosis

- A mass along the course of a peripheral nerve.
- Evidence of motor or sensory dysfunction confined to a single peripheral nerve.
- Pain in the distribution of a single peripheral nerve.

General Considerations

Peripheral nerve tumors may be benign or malignant. The most common benign tumor is the nerve sheath tumor, variously called perineurial fibroblastoma, neurilemmoma, schwannoma, or neurofibroma. These tumors displace the major portion of the nerve to one side and often can be totally or almost totally excised. Nerve sheath tumors are more common in patients with Recklinghausen's disease than in the general population. With *chronic* trauma—particularly in patients with Recklinghausen's disease at puberty—these tumors may become malignant, metastasizing to other portions of the body and invading surrounding tissues.

The true schwannoma—a tumor of verifiable Schwann cells (fortunately rare)—has a high potential for malignancy, particularly in patients with Recklinghausen's disease.

When a neurofibroma is present, the neoplastic activity in the sheath is generalized; in any histologic preparation, a wide spectrum of connective tissue, endoneurial cells, and axonal fibers will be seen. These are diffuse growths and usually cannot be excised; at times they may spread in a plexiform fashion along all of a nerve's branches. Neurofibromas are almost invariably a part of the Recklinghausen disease complex.

Nerve sheath tumors may be less than 1 mm in diameter, and these usually occur on the smaller nerves. They may be quite painful. In deeper structures, these tumors may grow to substantial size—eg, as extensive as the entire sciatic nerve in the thigh, extending from the ischium to the popliteal space.

Clinical Findings

The symptoms and signs are those of peripheral nerve dysfunction, either irritative or paralytic. The nature and distribution of this dysfunction show that it is related to a specific nerve rather than to a root, tracts in the cord, or cerebral disease. The diagnostic problem is determining the final common pathway. Nerve conduction tests may be of assistance.

Differential Diagnosis

Peripheral neuropathies may mimic peripheral nerve tumors, but a tumor that produces symptoms ordinarily is large enough to be palpated. Generalized sensitivity along the nerve pathway is more common in neuritis than in dysfunction secondary to tumor mass.

Treatment

If possible, sheath tumors—aside from the true neurofibromas—should be removed. Some response to radiation therapy has been reported for certain types of nonremovable sheath tumors, but on the whole they must be regarded as resistant to irradiation and other forms of nonsurgical therapy. When an invasive malignant sheath tumor exists in an extremity, amputation of the extremity may be advisable unless the malignancy is so advanced that the likelihood of long-term survival is slight under any circumstances.

In Recklinghausen's disease, removal of peripheral nerve tumors is confined to those that cause clinical signs and symptoms such as pain or sensorimotor loss. Tumors that do not cause apparent clinical dysfunction should usually be left alone unless they cause exceptional cosmetic deformity or when they are subject to repeated trauma or irritation, eg, at the beltline.

Prognosis

The prognosis for life is good with most peripheral tumors. Multiplicity and recurrence plus a tendency to produce motor or sensory deficits usually result in moderate morbidity.

PITUITARY TUMORS
Robert J. Seymour, MD, & Charles B. Wilson, MD

Essentials of Diagnosis

- Signs and symptoms referable to abnormal endocrine function and compression of the optic chiasm.

- Headache, easy fatigability, and diminished libido; sweating and paresthesias in acromegalic patients.
- Visual field changes are usual with nonsecreting adenomas; acral and facial changes are usual with growth hormone-producing tumors.
- Hypopituitarism is usual with nonsecreting adenomas; elevated serum growth hormone and abnormal glucose tolerance test in acromegalic patients. Cushing's disease may be seen with ACTH-secreting tumors.
- Sella turcica enlarged on skull x-rays.

General Considerations

Classically, on the basis of light microscopy, the cells in the adenohypophysis have been divided into (1) granular chromophils, which are either acidophilic (35%) or basophilic (15%); and (2) agranular chromophobes (50%). Recent studies indicate a more diverse cell population, and a specific cell type for each hormone can be designated on the basis of granule size and special histochemical reactions. Pituitary tumors are still being classified as chromophobe, acidophilic, or basophilic adenomas based on tinctorial characteristics, although these terms are now obsolete and meaningless since current knowledge permits more specific designation according to secretion: tumors composed of nonsecreting cells should be termed nonsecreting.

All of these types of pituitary tumors taken together account for 10–15% of intracranial tumors. By routine light microscopy, about 80% are chromophobes and most of the remainder are acidophils. Basophilic adenomas are rare.

Clinical Findings

Nonsecreting tumors of the pituitary cause symptoms by compressing adjacent structures, by impairing pituitary function, or by doing both (Fig 40–14). Suprasellar extension causes visual field changes, first in the upper temporal quadrants and progressing to bitemporal hemianopsia. As the tumor grows, visual acuity diminishes and optic disk pallor develops. Occasionally, the tumor grows laterally to produce a cavernous sinus syndrome with facial numbness and extraocular muscle palsies. Rarely, the tumor may extend into the temporal lobe or hypothalamus.

Pituitary tumors commonly produce hypopituitarism manifested by amenorrhea, sterility, loss of libido, easy fatigability, loss of body hair, and fineness of the skin. On rare occasions, sudden bleeding occurs in a pituitary tumor, producing "pituitary apoplexy" and precipitous rather than slowly evolving clinical signs. The patient suddenly becomes blind and hypotensive and develops acute fluid and electrolyte imbalances.

Cushing's disease is the initial indication of an ACTH-secreting pituitary adenoma. Following adrenalectomy, the sella enlarges and skin pigmentation is striking (Nelson's syndrome).

The clinical manifestations of HGH-producing adenomas result from the systemic effects of elevated serum growth hormone. Headache, typical facial and acral changes, easy fatigability, paresthesias of the extremities, increased sweating, and decreased sexual function occur in acromegaly. Gigantism is added when the tumor appears before epiphyseal closure. Occasionally there are ophthalmologic findings, signs of hypopituitarism, or both. As with all pituitary tumors, the sella is often enlarged.

Prolactin-secreting tumors may cause no distinctive clinical syndrome, but characteristically they produce amenorrhea and galactorrhea in young women. When recognized, many of these tumors are microadenomas (< 1 cm in diameter).

Pituitary, adrenal, thyroid, and gonadal function are depressed in patients with large adenomas. In acromegaly, plasma serum growth hormone is elevated and cannot be suppressed by glucose. In Cushing's disease, plasma cortisol is elevated and ACTH levels are in the high normal range or elevated; the disease must be differentiated from the syndrome caused by adrenal tumors and certain nonadrenal cancers, eg, lung. In the amenorrhea-galactorrhea syndrome, plasma prolactin is elevated.

Differential Diagnosis

The characteristic appearance of the acromegalic patient makes the diagnosis a simple one. It is confirmed by assaying the serum growth hormone. Although patients with nonsecreting adenomas usually present a fairly characteristic clinical picture, several pathologic entities can present similarly: craniopharyngiomas, aneurysms of the internal carotid artery, suprasellar meningiomas, optic chiasm gliomas, dilatation of the third ventricle in hydrocephalus, mucoceles of the sphenoid sinus, and encephaloceles.

Without histologic verification, a tentative diagnosis can be established by tomograms of the sella, angiography, and pneumoencephalography with tomography. All patients suspected of harboring a pitui-

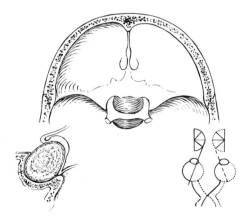

Figure 40–14. Pituitary adenoma (chromophobe type). Failing vision, primary optic atrophy, bitemporal hemianopsia, endocrine disturbances, and enlargement of sella turcica.

tary tumor should be investigated by means of contrast studies and evaluations of endocrine function. CT scans are helpful in evaluating lesions in the pituitary region and should be obtained prior to angiography and pneumoencephalography.

Treatment

Nonsecreting adenomas must be treated. If there is pressure on contiguous structures, decompression is indicated followed by postoperative irradiation since tumor removal is seldom complete. In many cases, a microscopic transsphenoidal surgical approach rather than a craniotomy is the treatment of choice. If the presumptive diagnosis is a nonsecreting adenoma—ie, an abnormal sella associated with endocrine abnormalities but without evidence of pressure on contiguous structures—a transsphenoidal surgical approach is indicated for diagnostic and therapeutic purposes. Such a procedure can be performed stereotactically or by open microsurgical methods. Irradiation alone is not predictable because a significant number of pituitary tumors are cystic, and even after extensive study the responsible lesion may prove to be something other than a tumor. Furthermore, the effects of radiation are delayed and cannot produce the prompt decompression that is necessary if vision is to be preserved. In at least two-thirds of patients, vision will be improved by decompression alone; in about one-third, it will be unchanged. A recurrence rate of 5—15% is reported.

Acromegaly must be treated because the cardiovascular effects of excess growth hormone shorten the life span. Transsphenoidal cryohypophysectomy is a highly satisfactory method of treatment. Both conventional and supervoltage irradiation have given inferior results. Heavy particle irradiation offers an alternative to the surgical procedure but is not widely available. The open transsphenoidal approach usually preserves pituitary and adrenal function.

Adams JE & others: Transsphenoidal cryohypophysectomy in acromegaly: Clinical and endocrinological evaluation. J Neurosurg 28:100, 1968.

Chamlin M, Davidoff LM: Ophthalmologic criteria in diagnosis and management of pituitary tumors. J Neurosurg 19:9, 1962.

Chang RJ & others: Detection, evaluation and treatment of pituitary microadenomas in patients with galactorrhea and amenorrhea. N Engl J Med, 1977. (In press.)

Cushing H: *Pituitary Body and Hypothalamus.* Thomas, 1932.

Cushing H: Surgical experience with pituitary disorders. JAMA 63:115, 1914.

Davidoff L: Studies in acromegaly. Endocrinology 10:453, 1926.

Kahn EA: Forty-five years' experience with the craniopharyngioma. Surg Neurol 1:5, 1973.

Kolodny HD & others: Laboratory aids in the diagnosis of pituitary tumors. Ann Clin Lab Sci 4:67, 1974.

Lawrence JH & others: Successful treatment of acromegaly. J Clin Endocrinol Metab 31:180, 1970.

Rovit RL, Berry R: Cushing's syndrome and the hypophysis. J Neurosurg 23:270, 1965.

Russell DS, Rubinstein LJ: *Pathology of Tumours of the Nervous System.* Williams & Wilkins, 1963.

Schechter J: Electron microscopic studies of known pituitary tumors. Am J Anat 138:371, 1973.

Sheline GE: Diagnosis of non-functioning chromophobe adenomas of the pituitary. Am J Roentgenol Radium Ther Nucl Med 120:553, 1974.

Svien HJ, Colby M: *Treatment for Chromophobe Adenoma.* Thomas, 1967.

U HS, Wilson CB, Tyrrell JB: Transsphenoidal microhypophysectomy in acromegaly. J Neurosurg, 1977. (In press.)

Wilson CB, Dempsey LC: Transsphenoidal microsurgical removal of pituitary adenomas. J Neurosurg, 1977. (In press.)

Wilson CB & others: Surgical experience with microscopic transsphenoidal approach to pituitary tumors and non-neoplastic parasellar conditions. Calif Med 117:1, Nov 1972.

CERVICAL DISK DISEASE
Edward S. Connolly, MD

Essentials of Diagnosis

Subjective
- Pain in the suboccipital, cervical, interscapular, thoracic, and shoulder areas and in the upper extremities.
- Discomfort aggravated by neck movements and Valsalva's maneuver.
- Paresthesias and dysesthesias in the cervical dermatomes.

Objective
- Lower motor neuron signs in the upper extremities manifested by weakness, fasciculations, depression of deep tendon reflexes, and dermatome sensory changes.
- Upper motor neuron signs in the lower extremities manifested by spasticity, weakness, and a positive plantar extensor sign.
- Spastic neurogenic bladder.
- Straightening of cervical curve, limitation of cervical movements, and paraspinous muscle spasm.
- Radiologic evidence of collapsed disk spaces and formation of osteophytes.
- Myelographic evidence of extradural cervical mass.

General Considerations

Cervical intervertebral disk disease is a general term used to describe degeneration of the cervical intervertebral disk that may develop into 3 separate clinical and pathologic entities. Perhaps the most common is the "hard disk," in which osteophytes arising from the anterior margin of the intervertebral foramen narrow the foramen and compress a cervical nerve root. The second most common is the "soft disk," in which herniation of the nucleus pulposus through a rupture in the posterior or posterolateral aspect of the annulus fibrosus compresses the spinal cord, the nerve root, or both. The third type is cervical spondylosis, characterized by bony spurs that form on the superior and inferior aspects of the posterior surface of the vertebral bodies to produce a washboard effect or so-called bar disk. These compress the spinal cord, causing spasticity in the lower segments but frequently without pain or discomfort in the neck.

Clinical Findings

A. Symptoms and Signs: The onset of symptoms and signs of "soft disk" may be acute or insidious. Acute symptoms may follow trauma or may be unrelated to trauma. Neck and radicular discomfort occur simultaneously; spinal cord symptoms are rare. There is usually limitation of neck motion with tenderness over the brachial plexus and straightening of the normal cervical lordosis. Decrease in a deep tendon reflex is common with or without weakness in the muscles supplied by the compressed root. There is also hypesthesia or hyperesthesia in the dermatome pattern of the affected root. With "hard disks," episodes of cervical discomfort recur over many months or years before radicular symptoms occur. Interscapular aching and suboccipital headaches are common complaints. Following the onset of radicular symptoms, the signs of a "hard disk" are indistinguishable from those of a "soft disk." The signs and symptoms of cervical spondylosis are those of progressive spastic paraparesis with some limitation of neck motion, mild to moderate sensory changes in the lower extremities, and a cervical dermatome pattern.

B. X-Ray Findings: Plain x-rays of "soft disks" may be within normal limits (except for straightening of the cervical lordosis) or may demonstrate narrowing of a disk space. X-rays of "hard disks" show osteophytic formation at the appropriate neural foramen with disk narrowing. This is usually best seen on oblique views. In cervical spondylosis there is usually x-ray evidence of osteophytes and disk narrowing at multiple levels, and in most cases the sagittal diameter of the cervical spinal canal is congenitally narrow.

Myelography in "soft disks" may show no abnormality, but more commonly, there is a small ventral extradural defect obliterating a nerve root cuff. In "hard disks" the myelogram usually demonstrates a root cuff defect. In cervical spondylosis, the myelogram shows bar-like ventral defects at the disk space, usually occurring at multiple levels and sometimes associated with apparent widening of the cord shadow on the anteroposterior projection.

Differential Diagnosis

Cervical disk disease must be differentiated from inflammatory diseases affecting the soft tissues and joints of the pectoral girdle, such as subdeltoid and subacromial bursitis, Tietze's syndrome, and cervical sprains; cervical rib and scalenus anticus syndrome, nerve entrapment syndromes in the upper extremities such as carpal tunnel syndrome and tardy ulnar palsy; coronary insufficiency and angina pectoris; neoplasms of the pulmonary apex, eg, Pancoast tumors; neoplasms of the brachial plexus; neoplasms of the cervical cord and medullocervical junction; fractures, dislocations, or subluxations of the cervical spine; and inflammatory disease of the cervical theca such as arachnoiditis, sarcoidosis, and Pott's disease.

Complications

Permanent damage to the nerve roots and spinal cord may occur, with loss of motor and sensory function. This is particularly true in cervical spondylosis, in which both direct pressure on the spinal cord and compression of its vascular supply may produce a severe irreversible myelopathy with spastic paraplegia or quadriplegia and loss of sphincteric control.

Treatment

A. Conservative Measures: Initially, cervical disk disease should be treated conservatively unless there is evidence of spinal cord compression or severe motor loss in an extremity secondary to root compression. In these situations, prompt surgical decompression is indicated.

Adequate conservative therapy for patients suffering from radiculitis involves immobilization of the neck with mild traction exerted on the neck in a neutral position. This is usually best achieved with continuous or interrupted (2 hours in and 1 hour out) halter cervical traction. Salicylates, other analgesics, tranquilizers with muscle-relaxing properties, and local heat are frequently used in combination with traction. *Caution:* Since improper traction may produce increased discomfort and additional muscle spasm, cervical traction must be applied correctly and be checked repeatedly by the physician with daily counseling of the patient about the importance of proper alignment of the traction to provide a neutral pull. Cervical traction may be applied so that the neck is held neutral in both the sitting and supine positions. The weight used generally ranges from 2–5 kg (5–10 lb) depending on the size of the patient.

B. Surgical Treatment: There are 2 methods of treating cervical disk disease surgically: (1) posterior decompression of the nerve roots, spinal cord, or both; and (2) anterior decompression of nerve roots, spinal cord (or both) with or without fusion. Neither can be designated as *the* correct procedure. The choice is based on consideration of a particular patient's anatomic lesions. It may occasionally be necessary to use both an anterior and a posterior approach.

Prognosis

Seventy-five percent of patients will recover following an adequate trial (10–14 days) of conservative therapy even though some will continue to have cervical or interscapular discomfort or mild paresthesias and some will have recurrence of their radicular symptoms on return to full activity status. In some cases, these patients can be managed for years with intervals of cervical traction and a cervical collar, but many will require surgical therapy. For the 25% who do not respond to conservative therapy, operation is required.

Improvement follows operative treatment of hard and soft cervical disks in approximately 80% of patients. Surgical treatment of cervical spondylosis with myelopathy results in improvement in 65% of cases and arrest of progression in most of the remainder.

Cloward RD: New method of diagnosis and treatment of cervical disc disease. Clin Neurosurg 8:93, 1962.

Connolly ES, Seymour RJ, Adams JE: Clinical evaluation of anterior cervical fusion for degenerative cervical disc disease. J Neurosurg 23:431, 1965.

Foger CA: Results of adequate posterior decompression in the relief of spondylotic cervical myelopathy. J Neurosurg 38:684, 1973.

Guidetti B, Fortuna A: Long-term results of surgical treatment of myelopathy due to cervical spondylosis. J Neurosurg 30:714, 1969.

Haft A, Shenkin HA: Surgical end results of cervical ridge and disk problems. JAMA 186:312, 1963.

Hankinson HL, Wilson CB: Use of the operating microscope in anterior discectomy without fusion. J Neurosurg 43:452, 1975.

Murphey F, Simmons JC, Brunson B: Surgical treatment of laterally ruptured cervical disc: Review of 648 cases, 1939–1972. J Neurosurg 38:679, 1973.

Odom GL, Finney W, Woodhall B: Cervical disk lesions. JAMA 166:23, 1958.

Roaf JE: Surgical treatment of patients with cervical disk lesions. J Trauma 9:327, 1969.

Robinson RA: The results of anterior interbody fusion of the cervical spine. J Bone Joint Surg 44A:1569, 1962.

Spurling RG: *Lesions of the Cervical Intervertebral Disc.* American Lecture Series. Thomas, 1956.

LUMBAR DISK DISEASE
Norman L. Chater, MD

Essentials of Diagnosis

- History of back injury (common).
- Low back pain (usual).
- Signs of root compression, eg, sciatica.
- Pain aggravated by activity and relieved by bed rest.
- Abnormal straight leg raising test.
- Neurologic findings are variable and usually mild.

General Considerations

Intervertebral disk disease takes 3 forms: (1) degeneration of the nucleus pulposus without demonstrable protrusion; (2) degeneration and protrusion or bulging behind a weakened annulus fibrosus which, if posterior or posterolateral, may cause pressure on adjacent nerve roots; or (3) extrusion or herniation of the nucleus pulposus through a rent in the annulus, again commonly associated with nerve root compression. The predominant precipitating factor in all is acute or repeated trauma.

Clinical Findings

Over 90% of problems arise from the L4–5 and L5–S1 intervertebral areas and most of the remainder at L3–4. Lumbar disk disease rarely involves higher levels.

A. Symptoms and Signs: Pain is usually chronic and of long standing, but the onset may be acute when associated with frank herniation. There may be back pain, leg pain, or both. The radiation of low back pain into the buttock, posterior thigh, and calf is usually the same with disease at the L4–5 or L5–S1 interspaces. This radiating pain may be aggravated by coughing, sneezing, or the Valsalva maneuver. Bending or sitting accentuates the discomfort, whereas lying down characteristically relieves it. Most commonly, the pain is described as aching, but it frequently has a sharp or shooting element.

Numbness of the legs is present in fewer than one-third of patients. Rarely, bowel and bladder sphincteric disturbances are noted.

Palpation over the buttock (less frequently, over the vertebral spines) usually reveals tenderness over the sciatic notch or nerve. The paravertebral musculature may be in spasm. Straight leg raising produces back or leg pain that may be accentuated by further stretching of the sciatic nerve (by foot dorsiflexion or palpation in the popliteal fossa). Pain produced when the leg opposite the affected side is raised is highly suggestive of disk herniation.

Weakness of the anterior leg (with the extensor hallucis longus being the first affected) is a common finding, especially with L4–5 disease. Weakness of the gastrocnemius when testing strength in the standing position is difficult to evaluate because of pain. Weakness of the quadriceps may occur with L3–4 herniation. Atrophy may be present in long-standing cases.

Sensory patterns are extremely variable. Hypesthesia on the dorsum of the foot is common; sensory deficit on the outside of the foot is more frequent with L5–S1 disease, and deficit on the medial aspect of the foot is more frequent with L4–5 disease.

Comparison of knee and ankle reflexes is important. Depression of the ankle jerk is common with L5–S1 disease but is also present in a significant number of cases of L4–5 disease. The knee jerk may be depressed in L3–4 disease.

B. X Ray Findings: Plain films of the lumbosacral spine should be taken to identify congenital or acquired bony changes. The common narrowing of the disk spaces occurs in asymptomatic patients with the same frequency as in symptomatic patients and therefore has no diagnostic value.

Myelography is diagnostic in 70–80% of cases and is important in localizing the disease and ruling out intraspinal tumors. Sufficient iodized oil to cover the lower disk spaces in the semi-upright position is injected into the subarachnoid space, and posteroanterior, lateral, and oblique pictures are then taken. It must be remembered that both false-positive and false-negative findings occur.

Contrast material may be injected directly into the disk space with the diffusion monitored radiographically (diskography). A normal disk will usually accept less than 0.5 ml, whereas a degenerated disk will accept 2–3 ml. Diskography is used infrequently because the finding of disk degeneration has no consistent relationship to symptoms.

C. Special Examinations: Electromyography may demonstrate denervation of the muscles in the appropriate nerve root distribution and can be used as an adjunct to difficult diagnosis. Electromyography alone is not diagnostic.

Some physicians use segmental epidural block with local anesthetics as an aid in identifying single or multiple root irritations and in distinguishing between a peripheral or a central source of pain.

Differential Diagnosis

Back pain with radiation to the leg has many causes: (1) bony abnormalities such as spondylolisthesis, spondylosis, or the "narrowed" lumbar canal; (2) primary and metastatic tumors of the cauda equina or the intrapelvic region; (3) inflammatory disorders, including abscess, arachnoiditis, and rheumatoid spondylitis; (4) degenerative lesions of the spinal cord and peripheral neuropathies; and (5) peripheral vascular occlusive disease.

Treatment

A. Conservative Measures: A trial of conservative treatment is indicated in all patients who do not demonstrate progressive weakness or sphincteric disturbance. This consists of bed rest with local heat; analgesics and skeletal muscle relaxants; pelvic traction, partially immobilizing the patient, which helps relieve muscle spasm; physical therapy and graded exercise in chronic cases or after an acute episode subsides; corset or back brace to act as an immobilizer and to allow patients with a musculoskeletal component to return earlier to activity, or a body cast or plastic jacket in cases where chronic pain is relieved by immobilization.

B. Surgical Treatment: Surgical treatment is indicated in patients with progressive neurologic deficits and chronic disabling pain. Acute onset of symptoms associated with weakness or sphincteric disturbance must be treated with all expediency to curtail or reverse permanent deficit.

A simple laminotomy is made at the appropriate interspace, with care being taken to protect the nerve root and dura. If actual herniation has occurred, the surgeon should attempt to remove this in one piece and should diligently search for other extruded portions. In the absence of herniation, the surgeon makes a window in the ligamentous annulus and removes all degenerated material from the interspace. Some surgeons recommend that a fusion be done primarily or as a secondary procedure in chronic cases where immobilization has relieved symptoms.

Prognosis

Surgical results vary greatly. The best results are obtained in the patient with true extrusion of disk material where compensation for injury is not a factor.

Emotional factors play a great part in the results and must be carefully evaluated before operation is undertaken.

Brown HA, Pont MD: Disease of lumbar discs: Ten years of surgical treatment. J Neurosurg 20:410, 1963.

Gurdjian ES & others: Herniated lumbar intervertebral discs: An analysis of 1776 operated cases. J Trauma 1:158, 1961.

Mixter WJ, Barr JS: Rupture of the intervertebral disc with involvement of the spinal canal. N Engl J Med 211:210, 1934.

Parkinson D, Shields C: Treatment of protruded lumbar intervertebral discs with chymopapain (Discase). J Neurosurg 39:203, 1973.

Raaf J: Removal of protruded lumbar intervertebral discs. J Neurosurg 32:604, 1970.

Raaf J: Some observations regarding 905 patients operated upon for protruded lumbar intervertebral disc. Am J Surg 97:388, 1959.

Spurling RG: *Lesions of the Lumbar Intervertebral Disc With Special Reference to Rupture of the Annulus Fibrosus With Herniation of the Nucleus Pulposus.* Thomas, 1953.

PEDIATRIC NEUROSURGICAL PROBLEMS
Byron C. Pevehouse, MD

Most neurosurgical problems in infancy and childhood are due to 4 causes: congenital malformation, neoplasm, infection, and trauma. Infection and trauma are adequately discussed in other sections of this chapter and will not be considered in this section.

Congenital malformations occur in the nervous system more frequently than in any other organ system and are exceeded only by prematurity as a cause of death in infants. In most cases, no specific cause can be demonstrated, although a number of teratogenic factors have been recognized:

(1) Maternal infections such as rubella, toxoplasmosis, cytomegalic inclusion disease, and syphilis.

(2) Drugs ingested by the mother during a critical period of gestation, eg, thalidomide, LSD, methotrexate.

(3) Ionizing radiation (x-rays, radioisotopes) to the mother.

(4) Maternal anesthesia.

(5) Systemic disease, electrolyte imbalance, and dietary deficiencies.

Even the "genetic" anomalies such as spina bifida, anencephaly, and Down's syndrome probably result from a complicated interplay of genetic predisposition and various intrauterine factors.

The gross structural neonatal abnormalities that can be repaired surgically include the following: (1) malformations of the skull or spine, (2) incomplete formation of the neural tube, (3) disturbances of CSF circulation and absorption, and (4) vascular malformations.

1. MALFORMATIONS OF THE SKULL OR SPINE

Craniosynostosis is defined as premature closure of one or more cranial sutures, producing deformity of the skull. Primary craniosynostosis, which is always present at birth, must be differentiated from the secondary approximation and fusion of sutures in microcephaly and that which sometimes follows operative procedures on the skull or treatment to reduce increased intracranial pressure.

Compensatory growth of the craniosynostotic skull occurs parallel to the plane of the fused suture. When the process involves 2 or more sutures, growth and development of the brain are affected, particularly during the first year of life when the brain ordinarily triples its weight.

In order of diminishing incidence, the following malformations occur: fusion of the sagittal suture results in a long, narrow head (scaphocephaly); of a coronal suture, a broad, shortened head with flattened forehead (brachycephaly); of both sagittal and coronal sutures, a high, pointed head (oxycephaly); and of the metopic suture, a vertical midline prominence of the forehead (trigonocephaly).

Treatment consists of excision of the fused suture and insertion of a polyethylene film barrier to prevent rapid reclosure. This should be done as early as possible (before significant cranial deformity is present) and is probably ineffective after the patient is 2 years old.

Numerous other skeletal anomalies involve the base of the skull and cervical spine with various signs related to compression of the cerebellum, medulla, spinal cord, or adjacent nerves:

Basilar impression—upward displacement of the cervical spine into the base of the skull—results in reduced capacity of the posterior fossa and stenosis of the foramen magnum.

Arnold-Chiari malformation—caudal displacement of the cerebellum and medulla through the foramen magnum into the cervical canal—is often associated with hydrocephalus or myelomeningocele.

Klippel-Feil deformity—improper segmentation and fusion of elements of the cervical spine—is associated with abnormalities of the spinal cord.

Atlanto-occipital fusion—fusion of the atlas to the foramen magnum.

Diastematomyelia—bony spicule projecting through the middle of the spinal canal to divide the meninges and spinal cord into 2 compartments; other skeletal anomalies are usually present.

2. INCOMPLETE FORMATION OF THE NEURAL TUBE

Such defects originate during the third and fourth week of fetal life; they may be small and concealed or may be exposed and involve large areas of spinal cord, meninges, spine, overlying muscles, and skin. The most frequently involved anatomic level is the lumbosacral area; the least frequently involved is the thoracic area.

Spina bifida occulta is a defect in fusion of the spinous processes and laminas which is present in about 25% of all children. It usually has no clinical significance.

Meningocele consists of herniation of meninges through a spina bifida without abnormality of the spinal cord or nerve roots.

Myelomeningocele is protrusion of nerve roots or cord elements along with the meninges. It occurs about 7 times more often than simple meningocele and always causes some degree of neurologic deficit. Findings range from mild weakness and slight sphincteric disturbance to complete sensory and motor paralysis below the lesion and no control of bowel or bladder function. Hydrocephalus is associated with at least 80% of lumbosacral myelomeningoceles; Arnold-Chiari malformation is typically present.

Encephalocele with cranium bifidum is a much less common midline protrusion of meninges through the skull. It is usually occipital or at the base of the nose.

Treatment of all such defects includes early repair of the meningeal lesion to prevent meningitis, to preserve maximal neurologic function, and to facilitate nursing care. Supportive appliances should be provided if paralysis is present. Early recognition and control of hydrocephalus are essential.

Improved means of treating such problems have increased the number of children who survive and have greatly improved their condition. Musculoskeletal abnormalities require close attention to prevent contractures, joint dislocation, and deformities and to provide as much physical independence as the neurologic deficit and intelligence permit. Urologic problems, also either congenital or paralytic, represent the greatest threat to life after the second year of age, usually from chronic pyelonephritis.

3. DISTURBANCES OF CSF CIRCULATION & ABSORPTION

A considerable portion of CSF originates in the choroid plexus of the lateral and fourth ventricles, passes through the internal channels, and out the foramens of the fourth ventricle into the subarachnoid spaces and thence over the cerebral hemispheres to be absorbed through the arachnoidal villi into the venous circulation. Hydrocephalus, the "backing up" of flow and dilatation of the ventricles, can result from any of the 3 following disturbances in this normal pattern of flow: (1) excess production of CSF, as by a papilloma of the choroid plexus; (2) obstruction of pathways of flow, either internal or external to the brain; and (3) inadequate absorption of CSF through the arachnoidal villi.

Obstruction of the internal channels—ie, the foramen interventriculare, the third ventricle, the cerebral aqueduct, the fourth ventricle, or the outlet foramens —produces a noncommunicating hydrocephalus, so-named because dye injected into the lateral ventricle cannot be recovered 20 minutes later by lumbar subarachnoid puncture. Internal or noncommunicating hydrocephalus is commonly congenital, with atresia or "forking" of the aqueduct or inadequate opening of the fourth ventricle foramens with massive enlargement of the fourth ventricle (Dandy-Walker syndrome). Other causes include neoplasms that obstruct the channels at any level and ependymal reaction subsequent to ventricular hemorrhage or infection.

Obstruction of the external pathways or diminished absorption of CSF will produce a communicating hydrocephalus, in which dye can be recovered from the lumbar caudal sac after ventricular injection but CSF flow into the venous circulation is retarded, resulting in an excess volume of CSF within the skull. External or communicating hydrocephalus usually results from arachnoiditis involving the basal cisterns and subarachnoid spaces over the cerebrum, subsequent to meningitis, hemorrhage, or occasionally a tumor at the tentorium.

Hydrocephalus is treated by removal of the obstruction or opening of the channel for normal flow, excision of a choroid plexus papilloma, or bypass of CSF around the obstruction via a shunt of silicone rubber tubing. A lumbar subarachnoid-peritoneal shunt is usually effective in communicating hydrocephalus; in noncommunicating hydrocephalus, ventriculoatrial or ventriculoperitoneal shunt is necessary, usually with a valve mechanism to control the rate of CSF flow. Complications are frequent, including obstruction of the tubing, displacement by growth, intravenous or cardiac thrombus, acute or chronic septicemia, and pulmonary hypertension.

4. VASCULAR MALFORMATIONS

Collections of abnormal blood vessels, ranging in size from a large mass to a microscopic crypt, usually provide a direct arteriovenous shunt. The involved vessels have thin walls with defective muscular and elastic layers and thus frequently bleed. The hemorrhage may be minimal or massive. It is usually not fatal in children but is often repeated during later life. Other symptoms include epileptic seizures and intellectual deterioration due to ischemia of the cortex. A loud bruit can be heard over the cranium in many cases. The diagnosis is suggested by the history and confirmed by bloody spinal fluid, skull x-rays, and cerebral angiography. Treatment depends on the patient's symptoms, his age and condition, and the size and location of the malformation. If feasible, total excision is preferred, but not if it would produce a severe neurologic deficit.

A saccular aneurysm at the bifurcation of the arteries that form the circle of Willis is a frequent cause of subarachnoid hemorrhage in the young adult but is rarely symptomatic in childhood or infancy. Aneurysm of the great cerebral vein (of Galen) is more common in the pediatric patient, with obstruction of the aqueduct causing hydrocephalus, a loud cranial bruit, and signs of high-output cardiac failure.

•　•　•

NEOPLASMS

Neoplasms of the CNS are the most common solid tumors of childhood, exceeded only by neoplastic disease of the hematopoietic system. Twenty percent of pediatric neural tumors are located in the spinal cord and 80% in the brain. Of the latter, 60% are in the posterior fossa and 40% in the supratentorial area (Table 40–4).

Brain Tumors

Brain tumors produce symptoms (1) by occupying space, obstructing spinal fluid pathways, or both, thereby increasing intracranial pressure; and (2) by direct invasion or compression of neural tissues.

In infants and children, the symptoms and signs of increased intracranial pressure are vomiting, headache, papilledema, mental dysfunction, personality changes, and abducens nerve palsy. Symptoms and signs of direct brain involvement are ataxia, incoordination, nystagmus, weakness of extremities, seizures, and head tilt to the side of the lesion (cerebellar). (See section on brain tumors for details.)

The object of treatment is always total removal of the neoplasm, but in childhood this is possible in only a few types (cerebellar astrocytoma, hemangioblastoma, dermoid cyst, craniopharyngioma, unilateral optic nerve glioma). The remaining types are partially resected, CSF pathways are reopened or bypassed, and radiation therapy or chemotherapy is given postoperatively.

Spinal Cord Tumors

Spinal cord tumors are uncommon, and early

Table 40–4. Types of CNS tumors in children.

Cell Type	Incidence	Supratentorial	Posterior Fossa
Medulloblastoma	30%	. . .	Midline cerebellum
Astrocytoma	30%	Occasional	Cerebellar hemisphere
Ependymoma	10%	Rare	Fourth ventricle
Pontine glioma	10%	. . .	Pons
Craniopharyngioma	4%	Suprasellar	. . .
Dermoid tumors and teratoma	3%	Rare	Rare
Other gliomas	8%	Uncommon	Uncommon

diagnosis is most important. Spinal tumors comprise congenital tumors such as dermoids, lipomas, teratomas, and neurofibromas; gliomas such as astrocytomas and ependymomas; medulloblastomas which seed from primary brain tumors; and extradural metastatic tumors such as neuroblastomas and lymphosarcomas.

The manifestations of spinal cord tumors usually include pain in the spine, weakness of the legs or disturbances of gait, torticollis or scoliosis, impairment of bowel or bladder function, numbness of one or more limbs, local tenderness, and paravertebral muscle spasm.

Plain films of the spine are abnormal in 65% of children with spinal cord tumor. Electromyography will differentiate diffuse peripheral nerve and muscle disorders. Contrast myelography is the definitive test to confirm and localize an intraspinal mass lesion.

Treatment begins with operative biopsy followed by removal if possible. For those tumors that are radiosensitive and clearly cannot be excised—or those that are obviously metastatic—radiation therapy is the treatment of choice.

American Academy of Orthopaedic Surgeons: *Symposium on Myelomeningocele.* Mosby, 1972.

Bray PF: *Neurology in Pediatrics.* Year Book, 1969.

Carter S, Gold AP: *Neurology of Infancy and Childhood.* Appleton-Century-Crofts, 1974.

Foltz EL, Shurtleff DB: Five-year comparative study of hydrocephalus in children with and without operation. J Neurosurg 20:1064, 1963.

Gardner JW: Myelocele: Rupture of the neural tube. Clin Neurosurg 15:57, 1967.

James CCM, Lassman LP: *Spinal Dysraphism.* Appleton-Century-Crofts, 1972.

Nellhaus G: Head circumference from birth to eighteen years. Pediatrics 41:106, 1968.

Russell DS: *Observations on the Pathology of Hydrocephalus.* Her Majesty's Stationery Office, London, 1949.

Smith ED: *Spina Bifida and the Total Care of Myelomeningocele.* Thomas, 1965.

INTRACRANIAL ANEURYSMS
Edwin B. Boldrey, MD

Essentials of Diagnosis

- Evidence of intracranial hemorrhage (headache, stiff neck, etc).
- Evidence of progressive involvement of cranial nerves, or of fiber pathways or major ganglionic centers of the cerebrum, cerebellum, or brain stem.
- Angiographic demonstration of aneurysmal sac.

General Considerations

There are 5 types of intracranial aneurysm: congenital, most commonly involving the vessels of the circle of Willis (Fig 40–15); arteriosclerotic, mycotic, traumatic, and dissecting. Congenital aneurysms vary in size from a few millimeters to 4–5 cm in diameter, and they are smoothly or irregularly globoid. The others are markedly variable in size and configuration; fortunately, they are less common.

Above the age of 40 years, the incidence of intracranial aneurysm is greater in females by a ratio of 3:2; below the age of 40, the incidence is greater in males.

The location of congenital aneurysm leading to intracranial hemorrhage is, in order of frequency (Fig 40–16): (1) anterior cerebral-anterior communicating arteries, (2) internal carotid-posterior communicating arteries, (3) middle cerebral artery, (4) terminal bifurcation of internal carotid artery, (5) vertebral-basilar system, and (6) distal anterior cerebral artery. Multiple aneurysms occur in 14–20% of patients and may be scattered widely or clustered.

Ruptured intracranial aneurysm is the most common single cause of subarachnoid intracranial hemorrhage after the third decade of life (51%). One-third of hemorrhages from aneurysm occur during periods of rest, and another third during general activity. A variety of acutely stressful activities, such as lifting, bending, straining at stool, etc account for the remainder.

When an intracranial aneurysm of any type ruptures, the severity of clinical symptoms will usually be directly related to the amount of bleeding. Major hemorrhage may be followed by impairment of consciousness, coma, respiratory paralysis, and death. Minimal bleeding may produce only a sudden, severe headache, often with neck stiffness and usually with nausea and vomiting.

Clinical Findings

A. Symptoms and Signs: The classic history is that of sudden, severe headache with nausea, vomiting, and often prostration. The process may advance to coma, respiratory paralysis, and death within minutes or within the first few days. With less serious bleeding, there is stiffness of the neck, pain in the back, and photophobia.

Hemorrhage from the internal carotid artery may cause paralysis of function of the second through sixth cranial nerves. Ruptured aneurysms from the middle cerebral artery may be followed by contralateral hemiparesis. Ruptured aneurysms of the posterior circulation may produce brain stem as well as cerebellar signs and paralysis of the adjacent cranial nerves. Aneurysms of the anterior communicating arteries frequently bleed into the cerebral tissue and the ventricles, the latter usually being fatal. Middle cerebral aneurysms frequently bleed into the temporal and frontal lobes.

In approximately 10% of ruptured intracranial aneurysms, blood in a significant amount does not reach the subarachnoid space. Subhyaloid ocular hemorrhages may be found in association with intracranial hemorrhage.

Intracranial aneurysms can manifest themselves

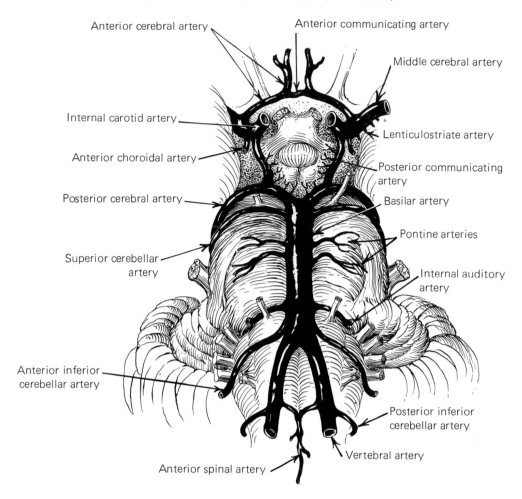

Figure 40–15. Circle of Willis and principal arteries of the brain. (Reproduced, with permission, from Chusid JG: *Correlative Neuroanatomy & Functional Neurology,* 16th ed. Lange, 1976.)

by virtue of their size. Enlargement of an aneurysm without hemorrhage may produce only cranial nerve palsies, or intrinsic nuclear or fiber tract dysfunction. The problem of identification is that of any intracranial space-occupying mass.

B. Lumbar Puncture: Proof of subarachnoid intracranial hemorrhage is the demonstration of blood in the CSF by lumbar puncture. The spinal fluid is uniformly bloody, and, within hours, the supernatant will be xanthochromic. With the passage of time, white blood cells increase in the fluid—a sign of meningeal irritation. *Caution:* Withdrawal of spinal fluid in the presence of spontaneous subarachnoid hemorrhage should be done with great care since the abrupt removal of large amounts may precipitate secondary bleeding. On the other hand, repeated controlled puncture may help to identify or confirm suspected secondary bleeding.

C. Cerebral Angiography: Cerebral angiography is a most important diagnostic procedure and must be done in all cases of spontaneous subarachnoid hemorrhage unless there is an obvious compelling contraindication. It should be done as soon as the patient's

condition permits and the necessary equipment and personnel are available. Ideally, the angiogram should show both carotid arteries and the vertebral-basilar system. At times, the intracranial portion of both vertebral arteries can be demonstrated following injection of one vertebral artery in which case direct injection of the second artery may not be necessary. If the initial angiogram is within normal limits, it may be repeated in 4–6 weeks; about one-fifth of these second arteriograms will demonstrate an aneurysm.

Differential Diagnosis

Although there is seldom serious question about the diagnosis when the clinical symptoms and signs are as described above, intracranial neoplasms will occasionally bleed into the subarachnoid space. There are also other vascular sources of hemorrhage such as vascular hypertension, intracranial arteriovenous malformations, and inflammatory intracranial vascular disease. Occasionally, acute meningitis will mimic the clinical signs of spontaneous subarachnoid hemorrhage, but examination of the spinal fluid will clarify the issue.

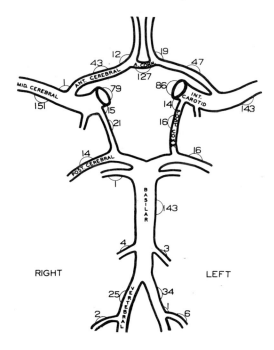

Figure 40—16. Location of intracranial aneurysms in 1023 cases. (Reproduced, with permission, from McDonald & Korb: Arch Neurol Psychiat 42:298, 1939.)

is successfully treated, the patient's long-term outlook depends upon the damage caused by initial and subsequent hemorrhage and on whether complications of surgical treatment develop.

The accumulated mortality from ruptured intracranial aneurysm is reported to be approximately 10% during the first 24 hours, 20% within the first 5 days, 30% within the first 9 days, 40% within the first 16 days, and 50% within 29 days. Secondary subarachnoid hemorrhage occurs most frequently between days 3—11, with a peak on the seventh day. The mortality rate during second episodes of subarachnoid hemorrhage is approximately 42%. With ruptured aneurysms of the posterior (ie, vertebral-basilar) circulation, secondary bleeding is less frequent during the first 2 weeks after initial hemorrhage.

Cooperative study of intracranial aneurysms and subarachnoid hemorrhage: Report on a randomized treatment study. Stroke 5:550, 1974.

Forbus WD: On origin of miliary aneurysms of superficial cerebral arteries. Bull Johns Hopkins Hosp 47:239, 1930.

Sahs AL: *Intracranial Aneurysms and Subarachnoid Hemorrhage: A Cooperative Study.* Lippincott, 1969.

Treatment

A. Medical Treatment: Nonoperative treatment consists of absolute bed rest with or without the use of hypotensive agents. This is usually continued for 4—6 weeks, with subsequent gradual resumption of activity over a similar period of time.

B. Surgical Treatment: Surgical treatment consists of a direct attack upon the aneurysm by clipping the base, wrapping the aneurysm with foreign materials to reinforce the wall, isolating the aneurysm by proximal and distal clipping of the parent vessel, or, for certain carotid aneurysms, by ligating the cervical carotid artery. The location and size of the aneurysm, the condition of the patient, and the preference of the surgeon will determine which procedure is used.

In general, most neurosurgeons advocate a direct intracranial approach to ruptured aneurysms. Other factors being equal (eg, location of aneurysm), the results depend upon the patient's condition at the time of operation. Except for the removal of intracerebral and subdural hematomas, aneurysm surgery is preventive, ie, aimed at the prevention of further bleeding.

There is compelling evidence that the results of operation can be materially improved by a delay of 14 days, during which time lysis of the clot is inhibited by agents such as aminocaproic acid (EACA, Amicar). There is enhancement of this drug's effect by reduced fluid intake (1200 ml in 24 hours).

Prognosis

Irreversible damage occurring at the time of initial rupture will remain as a fixed deficit. If the aneurysm

CONGENITAL ARTERIOVENOUS MALFORMATIONS OF THE BRAIN
Robert F. Palmer, MD

Essentials of Diagnosis

- Spontaneous subarachnoid or intracerebral hemorrhages (bloody, xanthochromic spinal fluid and subhyaloid hemorrhages).
- Convulsive seizures.
- Progressive signs of cerebral, cerebellar, or brain stem dysfunction.
- Subjective or objective bruits (cranial and retrobulbar).
- Cerebral angiography.
- CT scanning.

General Considerations

Arteriovenous malformations vary greatly in size. They may be smaller than 1 cm in diameter or may involve an entire cerebral hemisphere. They may be supplied by a single small artery or by all vessels entering the cranium.

Arteriovenous malformations and congenital aneurysms may occur in the same patient, and there is increasing evidence that the 2 occur simultaneously more often than previously realized. Bilateral malformations are not rare, particularly in the deeper structures of the brain, including the basal ganglia.

The intracranial hemorrhage secondary to arteriovenous malformation usually occurs during the first 3 decades of life and is seldom encountered after the fourth decade. The mortality rate from the first intracranial hemorrhage is about 10%, which is less than that from intracranial aneurysm; but the mortality rate is higher from arteriovenous malformation of the choroid plexus. Second episodes occur in approximately 23% of patients, and the mortality rate in this group is about 12%. The time between the first and second hemorrhages may be days or years; in the latter case, convulsive seizures commonly intervene.

Arteriovenous malformations may enlarge by dilatation of connecting vessels, producing the signs and symptoms of an intracranial space-occupying mass.

Clinical Findings

The clinical findings of intracranial hemorrhage due to arteriovenous malformations are the same as those of subarachnoid or intracerebral hemorrhage due to other causes.

A bruit over the cranium or eye strongly suggests an angioma but is not pathognomonic of angioma. Subhyaloid hemorrhage is probably pathognomonic of subarachnoid hemorrhage. Occasionally, brain scans may be helpful in identifying large arteriovenous angiomas. EEG may show focal changes in the affected cerebral hemisphere.

Computerized tomography is becoming of more value in the preangiographic diagnosis of arteriovenous malformations, particularly if there is calcification or an adjacent blood clot, and it will show cerebral atrophy and shift and dilatation of the ventricles as well as other coincidental lesions such as tumors.

Differential Diagnosis

See section on Intracranial Aneurysms. If arteriography is negative, spinal arteriovenous malformations must be considered.

Treatment

The key to good surgical results is extensive preoperative angiographic study to locate the feeding arteries. CT scanning may add to the evaluation.

When possible, arteriovenous angiomas are excised; ligation of extracranial vessels has proved to have very limited value. In some instances, however (eg, interhemispheric angiomas), the likelihood of secondary hemorrhage may be reduced if the main feeding vessel is clipped even though the lesion cannot be extirpated. This should be done as close to the lesion as possible.

No matter what is or is not done, the possibility always exists that a convulsive state will develop.

If surgery is indicated, the timing depends upon the condition and the desires of the patient, the location of the lesion, and the size of the malformation.

Microsurgical technic and bipolar coagulation have added to the ease of surgical treatment, and patients once considered "inoperable" are being successfully treated. Successful treatment by embolization and stereotactic clipping has been reported.

Prognosis

When the lesion is surgically extirpated, the prognosis for life is good but the morbidity rate (especially the development of seizures) is significant. The operative mortality rate is directly related to the size and location of the malformation. Symptoms due to shunting of arterial blood may be reversed by surgical excision of the malformation.

Spontaneous regression without treatment has been reported also.

Carter LP, Morgan M, Lirrea D: Psychological improvement following arteriovenous malformation excision. J Neurosurg 42:452, 1975.

Drake CG: Surgical removal of arteriovenous malformations from the brain stem and cerebellopontine angle. J Neurosurg 43:661, 1975.

Hansen JH, Søgaard I: Spontaneous regression of an extra- and intracranial arteriovenous malformation. J Neurosurg 45: 338, 1976.

Hilal SK, Michelsen JW: Therapeutic embolization for extra-axial vascular lesions of the head, neck, and spine. J Neurosurg 43:275, 1975.

Hodge CJ Jr, King RB: Arteriovenous malformation of choroid plexus. J Neurosurg 42:457, 1975.

Luessenhop AJ, Presper JH: Surgical embolization of cerebral arteriovenous malformations through internal carotid and vertebral arteries. J Neurosurg 42:443, 1975.

Sahs AL: *Intracranial Aneurysms and Subarachnoid Hemorrhage: A Cooperative Study,* Lippincott, 1969.

Spetzler RF, Wilson CB: Enlargement of an arteriovenous malformation documented by angiography. J Neurosurg 43:767, 1975.

SURGICAL INFECTIONS OF THE CNS

Edward S. Connolly, MD

BRAIN ABSCESS

Essentials of Diagnosis

- History of sinusitis, otitis, systemic pulmonary infection, or congenital heart defect.
- Headache, localized neurologic signs.
- High-voltage, slow-wave focus on EEG.
- Angiographic evidence of a mass lesion creating a vascular halo.
- Positive brain scan.

General Considerations

Brain abscesses usually occur secondary to a focus of infection outside the CNS, chronic middle ear infection with mastoiditis being the most common source. Infections of the nasal cavity and its accessory sinuses, chronic suppurative diseases of the lungs and pleura, congenital heart disease, acquired valvular heart disease, and retained foreign objects from trauma are other sources. The organisms most commonly responsible are staphylococci, streptococci, and pneumococci, although abscesses have been reported as a result of infection with almost every known bacterium.

Abscesses arising from sinusitis usually occur in the frontal lobes, whereas those arising from middle ear disease occur in the posterior temporal lobe or cerebellum. Hematogenous abscesses are usually found in the distribution of the middle cerebral arteries.

Clinical Findings

A. Symptoms and Signs: The usual presenting symptom is headache followed (in order of frequency) by decrease in sensorium, drowsiness, confusion and stupor, generalized or focal seizures, nausea and vomiting, and focal motor, sensory, or speech disorders. There is usually a low-grade fever (38–39 C [100.4–102.2 F]).

B. Laboratory Findings: Blood and CSF studies may be within normal limits, but more commonly there is a mild polymorphonuclear leukocytosis, mildly increased CSF pressure with an occasional neutrophil, and mildly elevated CSF protein.

C. X-Ray Findings: Skull films may show evidence of mastoiditis, sinusitis, or a pineal shift.

D. Special Examinations: EEG may show a high-voltage, slow-wave focus. Brain scans are usually positive. Angiography demonstrates a mass lesion with a circular halo blush. CT scan shows a discrete mass with a high uptake ring and low density center.

Differential Diagnosis

Brain abscess must be differentiated from brain tumor, cerebral infarction, intracranial thrombophlebitis, subdural empyema, extradural abscess, and encephalitis.

Complications

The major complication of brain abscess is rupture, usually into the ventricles, leading to acute ventriculitis and meningitis. Other complications may include obstruction of CSF pathways, transtentorial herniation, seizures, hemiparesis, and mental deficiency.

Prevention

Correct management of otitis media, mastoiditis, sinusitis, and other systemic infections usually prevents brain abscesses.

Treatment

The most desirable method of treatment of brain abscess is systemic administration of specific antibiotics and total surgical extirpation if the abscess is in an accessible location. Drainage and secondary excision or marsupialization are sometimes necessary. While sensitivity tests on the organisms that caused the abscess are being completed, the patient should be treated with an antibiotic that is effective against the suspected organism, eg, the ear flora if the patient has mastoiditis. Anticonvulsants should be used supportively, and eradication of the primary source of infection is essential. If the abscess is tapped, specific antibiotics and a radiopaque substance are instilled, the latter allowing visualization of the contraction and migration of the abscess.

Prognosis

The mortality rate of brain abscess remains between 25–50% despite antibiotic therapy.

LESS COMMON PYOGENIC INFECTIONS

Epidural Abscess

Epidural abscess in the cranial or spinal epidural space produces focal neurologic deficit by pressure on the underlying neural tissues. In the cranium, it is usually secondary to adjacent osteomyelitis; in the spine, it is usually metastatic from a remote infection in the pelvis or lower extremities.

Treatment consists of immediate drainage of the pus followed by appropriate treatment of the primary infection with antibiotics and operation.

Subdural Abscess

Subdural abscess or empyema, a serious complication of (usually) frontal sinusitis, progresses rapidly and has a high mortality rate. Immediate surgical drainage and antibiotic therapy are indicated. There is a significant incidence of hydrocephalus among survivors, necessitating a shunt procedure following eradication of the infection.

Cerebral Thrombophlebitis

Cerebral thrombophlebitis is a complication of meningitis, epidural and subdural abscesses, and thrombophlebitis of facial veins. The lateral, cavernous, and superior sagittal sinuses are most commonly involved, producing neurologic deficit by venous infarction. Treatment is with specific antibiotics. If marked cerebral edema is associated, treatment with glucocorticoids and diuretics as well as operative decompression should be considered.

CLOSED DISK SPACE INFECTIONS FOLLOWING REMOVAL OF LUMBAR INTERVERTEBRAL DISK

Closed disk space infection is seen in approximately 1–3% of patients following lumbar laminectomy with diskectomy and is thought to be due to pyogenic infection confined to the disk space. Symptoms usually occur 1–2 weeks or longer after operation. Preoperative sciatica has usually resolved when the patient complains of severe pain localized in the back and thighs, aggravated by any motion. The patient may run a low-grade fever or be afebrile; the white count may be normal or slightly elevated. The erythrocyte sedimentation rate is usually over 50 mm/hour. Radiographic signs usually appear in 4 weeks and consist of destruction of the vertebral end plates and narrowing and eventual bony fusion of the disk space.

Treatment consists of immobilization and analgesics. Antibiotics do not enhance therapy.

TUBERCULOSIS OF THE SPINE
(Pott's Disease)

The spinal cord dysfunction usually seen with far-advanced vertebral tuberculous lesions progresses rapidly to paraplegia or quadriplegia within a few weeks. The thoracic cord is most commonly involved, followed by the cervical cord and the lumbar cord segments. Radiographically, there is usually destruction of one or more intervertebral disks, apposition of the adjacent vertebral bodies, and destruction of one or more vertebral bodies. Soft tissue swelling is usually evident around the affected area, and a soft tissue mass of varying size is commonly present. A total extradural type block may be seen myelographically 1–2 levels below the obvious bony changes.

Treatment consists of (1) streptomycin, 1 g IM 4 times a day; aminosalicylic acid, 3 g orally 4 times a day; and isoniazid, 100 mg orally 3 times a day; (2) surgical drainage of the abscess via an anterior or lateral approach; and (3) immobilization of the affected area, eg, with skeletal tongs if in the cervical area, with Circoelectric bed or Stryker frame if in the thoracic or lumbar area. Posterior laminectomy has no place in the treatment of Pott's disease.

HERPES ZOSTER (SHINGLES)
& HERPES SIMPLEX ENCEPHALITIS

Herpes zoster is caused by a virus that has a predilection for the posterior root ganglia, posterior roots, and posterior gray horns of the spinal cord. The ganglion most often involved is the fifth thoracic ganglion; of the cranial nerves, the gasserian and geniculate ganglia are most commonly affected. The most significant complications are postherpetic pain, corneal ulceration and scarring, and persistent facial palsy.

Surgical treatment of postherpetic pain has included undercutting of the affected cutaneous distribution, posterior rhizotomy, cordotomy, medullary tractotomy, thalamotomy, and leukotomy. None of these procedures are particularly effective.

Herpes simplex encephalitis produces an acute necrotizing hemorrhagic leukoencephalitis. It has an abrupt onset characterized by fever, headache, drowsiness, and convulsions. Temporal lobe signs such as dysphasia, olfactory hallucinations, and psychomotor activity are common. X-ray contrast studies, brain scans, and EEG may demonstrate a mass in one temporal lobe. CSF studies usually show increased pressure and pleocytosis; routine cultures of CSF are negative. When a temporal lobe mass is present, surgical exploration of the lobe is indicated with brain biopsy and external decompression. A portion of the brain tissue should be cultured. The characteristic Cowdry type A intranuclear inclusion bodies may be seen histologically, and herpes simplex virus may be isolated in the culture.

Carpenter RR, Petersdorf RG: The clinical spectrum of bacterial meningitis. Am J Med 33:262, 1962.

Farmer TW, Wise GR: Subdural empyema in infants, children and adults. Neurology 23:254, 1973.

Fetter BF, Klintworth GK, Hendry WS: Pages 74–88 in: *Mycoses of the Central Nervous System.* Williams & Wilkins, 1967.

Garfield J: Management of supratentorial intracranial abscesses: A review of 200 cases. Br Med J 2:7, 1969.

Hoffman HJ, Hendrick EB, Hiscox JL: Cerebral abscesses in early infancy. J Neurosurg 33:172, 1970.

Kiser JL, Kendig JH: Intracranial suppuration: A review of 139 consecutive cases with electromicroscopic observations on three. J Neurosurg 20:494, 1963.

Krayenbühl HA: Abscess of the brain. Clin Neurosurg 14:25, 1966.

MacGee EE, Cauthen JC, Brackett CE: Meningitis following acute traumatic cerebrospinal fluid fistula. J Neurosurg 33:312, 1970.

Morgan H, Wood MW, Murphey F: Experience with 88 consecutive cases of brain abscess. J Neurosurg 38:698, 1973.

New PFJ, Scott WR: Page 362 in: *Computed Tomography of the Brain and Orbit.* Williams & Wilkins, 1975.

Page LK, Tyler HR, Shillito J: Neurosurgical experience with herpes simplex encephalitis. J Neurosurg 27:346, 1967.

Pilgaard S: Discitis (closed space infection) following removal of lumbar intervertebral disk. J Bone Joint Surg 51A: 713, 1969.

Sullivan CR: Diagnosis and treatment of pyogenic infection of the intervertebral disk. Surg Clin North Am 41:1077, 1961.

Swartz MN, Dodge PR: Bacterial meningitis: A review of select aspects. (6 parts.) N Engl J Med 272:725, 779, 842, 898, 954, 1003, 1965.

Te Beau J & others: Surgical treatment of brain abscesses and subdural empyema. J Neurosurg 38:198, 1973.

Tuli SM: Treatment of neurological complications in tuberculosis of the spine. J Bone Joint Surg 51A:680, 1969.

Victor M, Banker BQ: Brain abscess. Med Clin North Am 47:1355, 1963.

Wilkinson HA & others: Central nervous system tuberculosis: A persistent disease. J Neurosurg 34:15, 1971.

Witorsch P & others: Intraventricular administration of amphotericin B. JAMA 194:699, 1965.

ZOSTER

PROTAMIDE

MOVEMENT & PSYCHOPATHOLOGIC DISORDERS RESPONSIVE TO SURGERY
John E. Adams, MD

PARKINSON'S DISEASE

Parkinson's disease is the most common of the various disorders of movement and posture. However, such disorders are not clear-cut entities but constitute a spectrum of abnormal postures, states of muscle tone, and movements varying from hypotonic flaccidity to extreme muscular contraction and from akinesia (inability to initiate movement) to relentless violent movements capable of producing exhaustion and death. The extremes of such a spectrum would be from the severe akinesia of advanced Parkinson's disease—rendering the patient incapable of voluntary movement and thereby preventing any degree of self-care—to the wild, uncontrollable movements of Huntington's chorea.

Clinical Findings

Parkinson's disease is characterized by 3 main disturbances in movement and posture: tremor, rigidity, and bradykinesia or akinesia. The tremor is characteristically of the pill-rolling type that begins in the distal upper extremities and progresses proximally as time passes. It is usually abolished by voluntary movement. Rigidity involves both the agonist and antagonist muscles of the extremity and, when severe, literally immobilizes the arm or leg. The bradykinesia or akinesia is represented by a gradually worsening stooped posture, shuffling gait, festination, or a tendency to fall forward; poverty of speech to the point where the voice becomes only a whisper; difficulty in swallowing, etc.

Treatment

In its early stages, parkinsonism is treated medically and is primarily the concern of the internist or neurologist. The treatment of tremor in medically unresponsive patients is surgical and the operation should be done relatively early before the tremor becomes incapacitating.

Stereotaxic surgery is a technic for reaching subcortical or deeper intracerebral structures via electrodes or probes that are guided to the site by a 3-dimensional coordinate system attached to the skull. This technic allows creation of subcortical lesions with minimal trauma to overlying cortex. In patients with Parkinson's disease, the lesion is made by most surgeons in the ventrolateral nucleus of the thalamus, but some surgeons prefer to place the lesion in the ansa lenticularis (campotomy). Elimination of tremor can be anticipated in 80—85% of cases. At present, most surgeons make a small lesion (5 mm in diameter) in the ventrolateral nucleus just posterior to the posterior ventrolateral nucleus of the thalamus. If correctly placed, this lesion will effectively stop a tremor in the contralateral hand and arm in well over 80% of cases. Rigidity is likewise improved. The disabling hypokinetic symptoms of parkinsonism are not benefited by such a thalamotomy, and at times may even be made worse.

Levodopa (Larodopa, Dopar) is very effective in the treatment of the akinetic aspects of the disease, although it may have little effect on tremor. A combination of surgical thalamotomy and levodopa would seem to provide the most effective approach to therapy at the present time.

Other movement disorders that will respond to a lesion in the same thalamic area are dystonia musculorum deformans, essential cerebellar tremors, hemiballismus, chorea, etc. Stereotaxic destruction of the dentate nucleus has recently been used effectively in the treatment of such disabling conditions as choreoathetosis.

EPILEPSY

Epilepsy may be defined as an uncontrolled paroxysmal discharge of an aggregate of neurons within the brain. These neurons are most frequently within the cerebral cortex but may be subcortical. The unrestrained discharge may remain focal, or it may spread to adjacent areas of cortex and may ultimately involve both hemispheres as well as diencephalic and brain stem structures. Loss of consciousness during or at the onset of the seizure indicates involvement of diencephalic structures in the abnormal electrical discharge. A discharging focus in the motor area will produce a seizure initiated by clonic contractions of the appropriate portion of the body (face, hand, arm, etc). It is obvious, therefore, that the clinical manifestations of seizure discharges are greatly variable and may involve essentially all body systems. For practical purposes, however, all epilepsy may be considered focal in origin, and this constitutes the basis for the surgical treatment of the disease.

Only intractable cases are treated surgically. About 15—20% of all epileptic patients cannot be controlled by medical therapy and are candidates for surgical excision of the epileptogenic focus if it can be localized and is accessible. Stereotaxic placement of depth electrodes is a new technic for recording from and possibly locating subcortical epileptogenic foci.

PSYCHIATRIC DISORDERS

Small, carefully placed stereotaxic lesions have replaced the much more disabling and destructive frontal lobotomy in the treatment of certain psychiatric disturbances. Patients with obsessive compulsive behavior can be dramatically improved by small lesions in the cingulum. In rare instances, a severe anxiety neurosis that cannot be managed by more conservative methods will be improved by small lesions placed in the white matter just anterior to the dorsal medial thalamic nucleus or more anteriorly in the frontal orbital white matter.

Criticism of this form of surgical treatment of severe behavior disorder is based upon the misconception that these procedures are analogous to the now discredited prefrontal lobotomy with the attendant often severe alteration in the patient's human character. Such alterations do not result from the more restricted and precise stereotaxic surgical lesion.

Brazier MAB: *Epilepsy—Its Phenomena in Man.* UCLA Forum in Medical Sciences No. 17. Academic Press, 1973.

Cooper IS: *Involuntary Movement Disorders.* Harper, 1969.

Spiegel EA, Wycis HT (editors): *Advances in Stereoencephalotomy.* Part 1. *Methodology and Extrapyramidal Systems.* Part 2: *Pain, Convulsive Disorders, Behavioral and Other Effects of Stereoencephalotomy.* Karger (New York), 1965, 1966.

Sykes MK, Tredgold RF: Restricted orbital undercutting: A study of its effects on 350 patients over the ten years 1951–1960. Br J Psychiatry 110:609, 1964.

Van Manew J: *Stereotactic Methods and Their Applications in Disorders of the Motor System.* Thomas, 1967.

PAIN
Yoshio Hosobuchi, MD

Pain is a symptom resulting from the stimulation of specialized nerve endings. The psychologic effect of pain varies according to individual factors and the patient's cultural and ethnic background.

Pain may serve as a warning of some disease or abnormal condition in the body, eg, ureteral colic or angina pectoris, or it may be a pathologic derangement of the pain conduction system itself, eg, thalamic pain following a vascular accident in that area.

Pain is the major cause of suffering in the terminal stage of malignancy. Terminal cancer pain usually originates from malignant invasion of the intercostal nerves, brachial and lumbosacral plexuses, or osseous structures. Pain may be particularly severe if the malignancy is situated at the orifices of the body, where it is increased by ingestion or excretion.

Useful pain warns of abnormal body function and aids in diagnosis of that dysfunction. Useless pain is triggered by diseases, mostly neoplastic or degenerative, about which little can be done. Many neurosurgical procedures are available to alleviate severe forms of useless pain by interruption of pain conduction pathways.

In the not too distant future, surgical procedures for relief of pain will be relegated to the annals of medical history. However, until this urgently desired goal is achieved, the neurosurgeon must assume responsibility for relief of pain in many patients. The extent to which our operative technics (eg, stereotactic surgery) should be used for the treatment of pain is no longer limited by technical factors as much as by our incomplete understanding cf the mechanisms and central representations of pain.

Surgery is indicated in the management of pain when the cause defies more direct treatment and when the severity of the pain justifies a major operative procedure. Experience has shown that operation should be considered when a patient requires more than codeine by mouth (or its equivalent) for relief of chronic pain. Patients with a life expectancy shorter than 2 months should rarely be subjected to a neurosurgical pain-relieving operation. While not an absolute contraindication to operation, established narcotic addiction complicates surgical management and reduces the chances of obtaining a satisfactory result. Emotional instability—more often a lifelong pattern than the response to illness—constitutes a relative contraindication to operation on pain pathways.

SURGICAL ANATOMY

Because the peripheral nerves usually have mixed components, distal division of a peripheral nerve for control of pain is a poor procedure unless the nerve is purely sensory. At the level of the spinal roots, however, the peripheral nerves are clearly divided into motor and sensory components, and the posterior (sensory) root can be sectioned without loss of motor strength. Because of sensory overlap, several adjacent posterior roots must be divided to control a small area of pain. Posterior rhizotomy must be done carefully at the cervical and lumbar levels to preserve proprioceptive fibers; a limb without proprioception is quite useless despite its intact muscle strength.

Within the spinal cord, pain and proprioceptive fibers diverge, the proprioceptive fibers ascending the posterior column. The pain fibers synapse in the posterior horn of the cord and then decussate to the opposite anterolateral region to form the lateral spinothalamic tract. Since the motor fibers traverse the corticospinal tracts, it is possible to divide the lateral spinothalamic tract without losing motor or proprioceptive function. Such a division in the upper thoracic (T2–3) or upper cervical (C2–3) areas is known as cordotomy. Previously a procedure requiring laminectomy, it is now easily performed, especially in the cervical area, by a simple percutaneous stereotaxic approach with local anesthesia. Percutaneous cervical cordotomy is of particular value in providing pain relief to severely ill patients who are not good candidates for open surgical cordotomy. If the pain is located bilaterally or in the midline, as is often the case with neoplasm of the rectum, bladder, and uterus, bilateral cordotomy may be required.

In the medulla, the descending sensory tract of the trigeminal nerve and the spinothalamic tract are located superficially and are accessible for surgical ablation. Because of their proximity to each other, it is difficult to make a lesion in one tract without affecting the other. In addition, if the restiform body is damaged during the procedure, ipsilateral ataxia will result.

Enthusiasm for mesencephalic tractotomy has increased with the recent advances in stereotactic procedures. With this technic, extremely discrete lesions can be made in the still superficially located spinothalamic tract, in the quintothalamic tract, or in both, after stimulation studies via chronically implanted electrodes have determined the appropriate area. This procedure is quite effective for the control of pain involving the face or upper half of the body, although it is often followed by transient abnormal oculomotor activity. Another approach to pain in this area of the head—eg, pain from carcinoma of the mouth, pharynx, and larynx—involves denervation of pertinent cranial nerves. Complete denervation of the fifth nerve, the nervus intermedius of the seventh nerve, the ninth nerve, and the upper part of the tenth nerve is often required to assure good results.

Chronic intractable pain or pain originating from a thalamic disorder can be treated stereotactically. Lesions placed in the main sensory thalamic nuclei, although producing complete analgesia and anesthesia of the contralateral half of the body, do not always relieve pain. Carefully placed lesions in the nucleus centrum medianum and the parafascicularis of the thalamus (the nonspecific midline projection nuclei) usually do relieve pain although they fail to produce any sensory disturbance. Lesions placed in the postero-median portion of the thalamus encompassing the probable terminations of the multisynaptic spino-thalamic pain pathways are effective in relieving pain, as are similar lesions placed in the tegmentum of the mesencephalon. In general, however, these operations are best reserved for patients with a short life expectancy since the pain pattern frequently recurs after a few months or a few years.

Psychosurgery (eg, frontal lobectomy or leukot-omy, cingulotomy) has been used in relief of intractable pain, although the results are unpredictable. Frontal lobectomy especially is losing support among neurosurgeons.

CEPHALIC NEURALGIA

Trigeminal Neuralgia

Trigeminal neuralgia is characterized by parox-ysmal attacks of severe stabbing pain in the distribu-tion of one or more branches of the trigeminal nerve. The maxillary and mandibular divisions are most often affected. The pain lasts for only a few seconds and may be triggered by talking, eating, or merely touching the affected area of the face. It is usually unilateral and occurs in the middle-aged and especially the elderly patient. Trigeminal neuralgia in patients under age 30 is quite unusual. Most patients respond well to medical management by carbamazepine (Tegretol). For those who cannot tolerate the medication or who do not respond to it, surgery is the ultimate method of treat-ment. Peripheral nerve block can be accomplished with alcohol or other substances injected at the foramen ovale or in the pterygopalatine fossa; the immediate effect of alcohol block is good, but it is usually only temporary. The overall results of supraorbital or infraorbital nerve avulsion are unsatisfactory. Probably the most satisfactory neurosurgical treatments of trigeminal neuralgia are intracranial decompression or massage of the trigeminal ganglion or trigeminal rhizot-omy in either the middle or posterior fossa.

Glossopharyngeal Neuralgia

Sharp stabbing pain similar to that of trigeminal neuralgia may occur at the root of the tongue, radi-ating down the throat and to the ear. The pain can be triggered by swallowing or by touching the pharynx. Cocainization of the area temporarily blocks the pain and serves as a diagnostic test. Section of the glosso-pharyngeal nerve and the upper vagal fibers in the pos-terior fossa will alleviate the pain.

Nervus Intermedius Neuralgia

The postero-inferior margin of the external auditory meatus is thought to be innervated by the nervus intermedius of the facial nerve. Characteristic paroxysmal pain occurring in this area can be relieved by section of the nerve at the cerebellopontine angle.

POSTINFECTION PAIN

Postherpetic Neuralgia

Vesicular eruption of herpes zoster infection along the distribution of the cutaneous nerves is often followed by a continuous, intense burning pain in the area that is also hyperesthetic to touch. Undercutting of the involved skin or posterior rhizotomy is practi-cally always unsatisfactory. Anterolateral cordotomy or quintothalamic medullary tractotomy for facial postherpetic neuralgia is successful in less than 70% of cases. The failure of these procedures is thought to be due to the involvement of secondary and tertiary sensory neurons by herpesvirus.

Pain of Tabes Dorsalis

The lancinating pain of tabes dorsalis frequently seen in the lower extremities responds well to carbamazepine (Tegretol). If the patient cannot toler-ate the medication, anterolateral cordotomy is the pro-cedure of choice.

PAIN FOLLOWING INJURIES TO PERIPHERAL NERVES

Long-standing severe pain after laceration or contusion of the peripheral nerves is associated with the formation of perineuronal or intraneuronal scarring. Simple excision of neuromas in areas of traumatic or postoperative fibrosis has consistently failed to abolish such pain. Neurolysis rarely helps except in cases of compression of the median nerve by the carpal ligament, but in these cases the results are excellent.

Proximal neurotomy is likely to be rewarding when the nerve can be divided high enough to include all the branches that enter the scar below. Posterior rhizotomy is often successful provided a sufficient number of roots can be sacrificed to prevent sensory overlap. For pain in the extremities, this operation has been limited to the roots of the ulnar, lateral femoral, cutaneous, and either the fifth lumbar or first sacral nerves, in order to retain proprioception.

Anterolateral cordotomy has been followed by early success in nearly all cases, but more than a third of cases have failed to maintain permanent analgesia.

PAIN FOLLOWING AMPUTATION

At the time of amputation, chemical injection of the severed nerve ends has proved useless in preventing postamputation pain. Most general surgeons and orthopedists agree that the best routine procedure is to cut the nerve trunks high and let their ends retract into a deep bed of healthy muscle. In the case of painful bulbs, a single resection is recommended. If the more simple procedures fail to produce relief, anterolateral cordotomy is the only alternative.

In the more difficult problem of phantom limbs, effective analgesia by cordotomy has seldom eliminated awareness of the ghost extremity, and pain often recurs when the effect of cordotomy wears off. Postcentral resection of the sensory cortex has usually failed, but extensive undercutting of the parietal lobe is worthy of trial if it can be done in the nondominant hemisphere. Frontal lobotomy has also been ineffectual unless carried out to the extent that it produces psychologic deterioration. The value of thalamotomy is too premature to be assessed, but this may well prove to be the procedure of choice.

White JC, Sweet WH: *Pain and the Neurosurgeon.* Thomas, 1969.

ELECTROANALGESIA

It has been demonstrated physiologically that all pain information travels to the spinal cord via gamma, delta, or C fibers. Stimulation of the larger A-beta fibers is never painful. Activity in beta fibers inhibits, at the first spinal synapse, immediate subsequent activity from the smallest fibers considered essential to pain conduction. Melzack and Wall suggested that this mechanism normally acts as a gate to balance pain and nonpain input. Wall and Sweet used this theory in demonstrating control of pain by low-voltage electrical stimulation of peripheral nerves. Since the dorsal columns contain almost pure and concentrated beta fibers, Shealy hypothesized that the dorsal columns offered the best sites for selective stimulation of beta fibers. Experimentally, Shealy & others demonstrated more than 12-fold increases in pain threshold during dorsal column stimulation. This technic has subsequently been applied to human patients with chronic intractable pain.

In response to dorsal column stimulation, patients develop a buzzing or tingling sensation that radiates downward through much of the body below the electrode. Clinical results to date reveal that good pain relief usually occurs only in areas where the buzzing is felt.

Normal sensory function is not significantly altered during dorsal column stimulation except in patients with preexisting spinal cord damage or deficits due to cordotomy. Dorsal cord stimulation may potentiate neurologic deficiencies in these patients. Pinprick leads to a slightly hyperalgesic response in the skin of the legs, but deep pressure is less painful than normal. Muscle power, motor function, and bladder and bowel control have not been altered during dorsal cord stimulation except in patients with preexisting problems due to spinal cord damage or cordotomy. Patients have had no difficulty in walking during stimulation.

Melzack R, Wall PD: Pain mechanism: A new theory. Science 150:971, 1965.

Nielson KD, Adams JE, Hosobuchi Y: Experience with dorsal column stimulation for relief of chronic intractable pain 1968–1973. Surg Neurol 4:148, 1975.

Shealy CN: The physiological substrate of pain. Headache 6:101, 1966.

Shealy CN & others: Dorsal column electroanalgesia. J Neurosurg 32:560, 1970.

Wall PD, Sweet WH: Temporary abolition of pain in man. Science 155:108, 1967.

White JC, Sweet WH: *Pain and the Neurosurgeon.* Thomas, 1969.

• • •

General References

Jennett WB: *An Introduction to Neurosurgery.* Mosby, 1970.

Kahn EA & others: *Correlative Neurosurgery,* 2nd ed. Thomas, 1969.

Mullan S: *Essentials of Neurosurgery for Students and Practitioners.* Springer-Verlag, 1961.

Youmans JR: *Neurological Surgery.* Saunders, 1973.

41 . . .
Otolaryngology

Herbert H. Dedo, MD, & Francis A. Sooy, MD

THE EAR

EAR INFECTIONS

1. PERICHONDRITIS & CHONDRITIS OF THE PINNA

Perichondritis or chondritis of the pinna may occur spontaneously or following trauma, ear surgery, or frostbite. It is manifested by swelling, pain, tenderness, and discoloration (redness) of the pinna.

Treatment consists of systemic antibiotics, incision and drainage to release any blood or pus, and insertion of cotton packing in the crevices of the pinna to suppress fluid collection in the subcutaneous space. The antibiotic most often used is penicillin. A mastoid dressing is then applied so as to exert moderate pressure on the cotton. If blood or pus is allowed to collect adjacent to the cartilage and is not removed, infection can destroy the cartilage, produce fibrosis, and leave a severely deformed "cauliflower" ear.

2. EXTERNAL OTITIS

External otitis—superficial infection of the skin of the ear canal—causes itching or pain and is usually due to local trauma from water, cotton swabs, or other foreign bodies. Hearing is not impaired unless the ear canal has swelled shut. There may be minimal discharge.

Treatment consists of cleaning the ear canal with suction and administering antibiotic-corticosteroid ear drops for 5–7 days. If the skin of the ear canal is severely swollen, a cotton wick saturated with antibiotic corticosteroid ointment should be placed in the ear canal for 48 hours to squeeze out the edema before the ear drops are administered.

Systemic antibiotics and analgesics may be neces-

sary for acute pain (cellulitis). Tetracycline, penicillin, or erythromycin is preferred unless the patient is allergic.

McDonald TJ, Neel HB III: External otitis. Postgrad Med 57:95, May 1975.

3. ACUTE SUPPURATIVE OTITIS MEDIA

The presenting complaint is usually pain—except in infants, in whom the first symptom may be fever. This disease is more common in children than adults and is usually caused by obstruction of the eustachian tube by an upper respiratory infection, which causes the adenoid to enlarge. Allergy and hypoimmune states are occasionally causative factors. Conductive hearing loss is usually present because pus has collected behind the eardrum. Examination of the ear shows a reddened and, in the later stages, bulging tympanic membrane. If the tympanic membrane has ruptured (Fig 41–1),

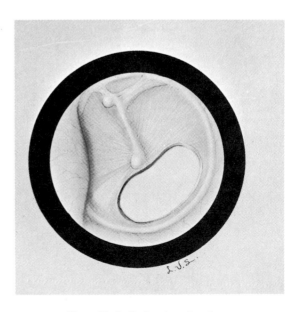

Figure 41–1. Perforation of eardrum.

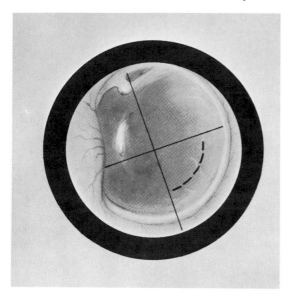

Figure 41—2. Site of myringotomy.

serosanguineous to thick, purulent discharge will be found in the external ear canal.

Treatment is with oral penicillin G, erythromycin, or tetracycline. Oral decongestants should be given to shrink the nasal and eustachian tube membranes.

If there is significant pain from the bulging eardrum, myringotomy should be done (Fig 41—2), both for immediate pain relief and to release the pus before it erodes a hole in the eardrum that is too large to heal. The incision should be made in the posterior-inferior quadrant of the drum, midway between the umbo and the rim, to avoid injury to the incus and stapes, which are in the posterior-superior quadrant.

In children, if acute otitis media recurs 2 or 3 times a year, tonsillectomy and adenoidectomy (or adenoidectomy alone) should be done to improve the function of the eustachian tube and thus decrease or prevent future ear infections.

4. SEROUS OTITIS MEDIA

Serous otitis media is characterized by serous fluid in the middle ear. The patient is aware of a stuffy feeling in his ear, occasionally accompanied by gurgling when he moves his head, and has a conductive hearing loss. Pneumatic otoscopy demonstrates either that the middle ear is completely filled with fluid (manifested by a dull and immobile tympanic membrane) or that there is a fluid level behind the tympanic membrane. In adults with unilateral serous otitis media—especially if they are Chinese—cancer of the nasopharynx must be ruled out by nasopharyngeal examination.

Serous otitis media is treated with antibiotics and decongestants. Allergy, if present, is treated.

If the fluid persists for more than 4 weeks in a patient between the ages of 12 months and puberty, tonsillectomy and adenoidectomy (or adenoidectomy alone) and myringotomy (Fig 41—2), with suction removal of the middle ear fluid, should be done. In infants under 1 year and in adults, myringotomy, suction removal, and placement of Teflon collar button tubes should be done. Nasal allergy and sinusitis should be treated if present. If the fluid recurs after tonsillectomy and adenoidectomy, myringotomy should be done and the collar button tubes placed. The tubes are ordinarily extruded by the body after 1—18 months, but if the serous otitis media recurs they may be replaced in infants.

5. CHRONIC OTITIS MEDIA

The presenting symptoms of chronic otitis media are chronic or recurrent ear discharge and pain. Examination shows a perforation in the eardrum with purulent yellow or white mucoid discharge in the external canal. Chronic infection of the middle ear is usually the result of chronic mastoid infection or abnormal function of the eustachian tube. The latter cause can be eliminated in some children by tonsillectomy and adenoidectomy and by control of sinus infection, if present, with antibiotics and decongestants. Allergy of the respiratory system should be treated if present.

Local treatment of chronic otitis media includes administration of ear drops (1% boric acid in 80% ethyl alcohol), or antibiotic solutions or powders and frequent suction cleansing of the ear canal and middle ear.

If the infection cannot be controlled or if complications such as meningitis, brain abscess, lateral sinus thrombosis, seventh nerve paralysis, or labyrinthitis develop, modified radical or radical mastoidectomy is required. Once the infection is controlled and the ear remains clean and dry for 3—6 months, myringoplasty may be done to close the perforation in the eardrum. Successful closure is possible in 80% of patients, and reconstruction technics now available for the eardrum and ossicular chain improve hearing in 50% of patients—ie, each patient has a 80% chance of closure and a 50% chance of hearing again.

Birrell JF: Otitis media. Br Med J 1:443, 1976.

Coates HL, McDonald TJ: Serous otitis media. Postgrad Med 57:87, May 1975.

Nickerson HJ & others: How dependable is diagnosis and management of earache by telephone? Clin Pediatr 14:920, 1975.

Rowe DS: Acute suppurative otitis media. Pediatrics 56:285, 1975.

6. MASTOIDITIS

The presenting complaints are ordinarily pain and tenderness behind the ear, occasionally a swelling on the mastoid, discharge from the middle ear, sagging of the posterior-superior ear canal, fever, or any of the complications of chronic otitis media mentioned previously. Ear examination shows mastoid tenderness, ear discharge, a protuberant pinna, or mastoid swelling (from a subperiosteal abscess). In chronic cases, x-rays of the mastoid may show breakdown of the septa (from osteomyelitis) and cloudiness (from pus).

Acute mastoiditis is a complication of infection of the middle ear since the mucous membrane of the mastoid is always infected when the middle ear is infected. If untreated, osteomyelitis may result. Antibiotics are effective, and emergency mastoidectomy is only occasionally necessary to remove the pus and infected bone.

Chronic mastoiditis may follow acute mastoiditis and otitis media. The chronic drainage of pus from the ear can often be controlled by mastoidectomy to remove the diseased bone. If a cholesteatoma (a squamous epithelial sac that has grown inward from the skin of the ear canal or drum) develops, it will gradually erode the bone surrounding the antrum. Cholesteatomas can drain intermittently for years as they gradually enlarge until a complication such as meningitis, brain abscess, seventh nerve paralysis, labyrinthitis, or lateral sinus thrombosis occurs. Mastoidectomy should be done and the cholesteatoma removed or the sac opened to the surface whenever a cholesteatoma has been demonstrated (by keratin debris in the attic or middle ear space or by bony erosion on roentgeno-grams), whenever one of the above complications of chronic ear discharge appears, or whenever a fistula test is positive.

EIGHTH NERVE DISORDERS

1. HEARING LOSS

Differentiation between conductive hearing loss and sensorineural hearing loss is essential because each is treated differently. The patient with a significant conductive hearing loss will hear the 512 Hz tuning fork more clearly when it is vibrating on his mastoid bone than when it is moved 5 cm (2 inches) in front of the ear on the same side (**Rinne's test**). When it is placed on his forehead immediately above his nose or on his upper incisors (**Weber's test**), he will hear it best in the ear with the greater conductive hearing loss. Conversely, the patient with a sensorineural hearing loss will hear the tuning fork better during the Rinne test when it is vibrating in front of his ear and will hear the tuning fork better in the Weber test with his better ear. For any patient with a clinically significant hearing loss, an audiogram, including tests for pure tone and speech, should be obtained (1) to confirm the diagnosis, (2) to measure the amount of hearing loss in decibels at the different frequencies, and (3) to determine the amount of distortion (loss of discrimination or understanding of words). A normal audiogram is shown in Fig 41–3.

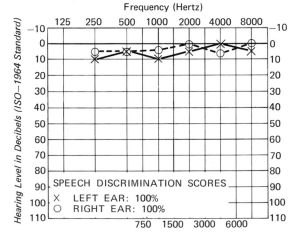

To convert the above readings based on the 1964 ISO reference thresholds to readings based on the 1951 ASA reference thresholds, subtract the following (rounded) difference in dB:

125	250	500	1000	2000	4000	8000
10	15	15	10	10	5	10

Figure 41–3. Normal hearing.

CONDUCTIVE HEARING LOSS

Perforation of the Eardrum

Diagnosis is made by examination with an ear speculum and a pneumatic otoscope. If discharge is present, it must be controlled (see Chronic Otitis Media) for 3 months with suction, cleaning, and ear drops (or, if necessary, with mastoidectomy) before the hole in the eardrum is closed by myringoplasty. Several tissues have been used successfully in closing tympanic perforations; a favored one at present is a pedicle graft of canal wall skin, usually supplemented by a temporalis fascia graft for large or anterior perforations. Initial reports of results from homograft eardrum and ossicle transplants have been encouraging.

Otosclerosis

Otosclerosis is manifested by a progressive conductive hearing loss that begins at or after puberty without evidence of eardrum or middle ear disease (Fig 41—4). The eardrum is intact and mobile when tested with pneumatic otoscopy, and there is no evidence of previous infection that might have resulted in necrosis of the ossicular chain.

Treatment is by stapedectomy. After a flap of posterior canal wall skin is elevated in continuity with the posterior-superior eardrum, the stapes can be seen fixed in the oval window by formation of otosclerotic bone around the edges of the footplate. The stapes is removed in fragments and the ossicular chain is reconstituted—eg, by placing a piece of vein from the patient's hand over the oval window as a diaphragm and then placing a stainless steel wire prosthesis, approximately 4.5—5 mm long, crimped around the long process of the incus and reaching down to the surface of the vein. This procedure can dramatically reduce or eliminate the conductive hearing loss in properly selected patients.

Ossicular Chain Disruption

A diagnosis of ossicular chain disruption is made when a patient has a conductive hearing loss and a history of significant chronic infection, head trauma, or ear trauma. The most common disruptions are disarticulation, necrosis of the long process of the incus, and absent stapes crura. The hearing loss is usually in the range of 45—55 dB unless a partial connection with fibrous tissue or a cholesteatoma has occurred.

Treatment consists of reconstruction of the ossicular mechanism with one of a variety of natural and artificial prostheses through an exploratory tympanotomy approach to the middle ear.

Adhesions in the Middle Ear

Middle ear adhesions are common in a patient with conductive hearing loss and a retracted and immobile tympanic membrane as demonstrated by pneumatic otoscopy. The diagnosis can be confirmed by exploratory tympanotomy, using the stapedectomy approach described above. If any air space exists in the anterior-superior middle ear, a layer of Silastic sheeting can be placed between the drum and the promontory in an attempt to reestablish the middle ear space. The results vary depending on the disease process.

SENSORINEURAL HEARING LOSS

The most common causes of significant sensorineural hearing loss are advancing age, trauma from prolonged exposure to sound above 90 dB, viral or bacterial infections, labyrinthine hydrops, **Ménière's syndrome** (sensorineural hearing loss, tinnitus, and vertigo), vascular obstruction, diabetes, or prediabetes. Typical audiograms are shown in Figs 41—5 and 41—6.

The only treatment is preventive since, with the

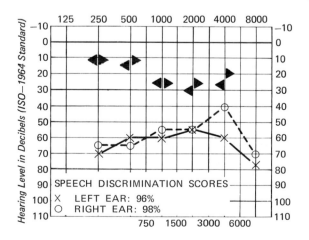

Figure 41—4. Bilateral severe conductive hearing loss due to otosclerosis.

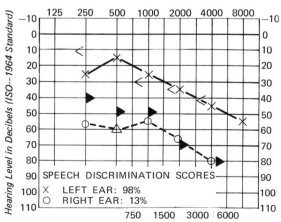

Figure 41—5. Mild left high-frequency and severe right sensorineural hearing loss (latter due to internal auditory meatus tumor).

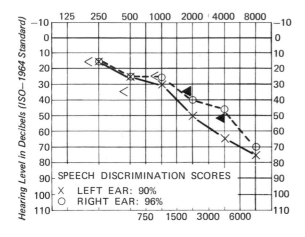

Figure 41—6. Bilateral high-frequency sensorineural hearing loss.

exception of those accompanying Ménière's syndrome, these hearing losses are irreversible and some tend to be progressive. Rehabilitation can be achieved with a hearing aid if necessary. The ear should be examined to rule out correctable diseases such as chronic infection and otosclerosis.

Rose DE: Hearing aids and hearing loss. Postgrad Med 57:67, May 1975.
Shea JJ: Fluctuant hearing loss (symposium). Otolaryngol Clin North Am 8:259, June 1975. [Entire issue.]

2. VERTIGO

Because the patient with vertigo ordinarily complains of "dizziness," the physician must be careful to distinguish between true vertigo, faintness (which is more apt to signify orthostatic hypotension), and a floating sensation (more apt to signify hyperventilation syndrome). True vertigo (a sensation of rolling or spinning in relationship to the environment) is evaluated on the basis of (1) the history, (2) audiograms—including special audiologic studies (Békésy and SISI [small increment sensitivity index] tests) to ascertain whether the lesion is cochlear or retrocochlear, (3) tests of vestibular function (caloric or electronystagmographic), and (4) roentgenograms of the internal auditory meatus to detect any erosion by an eighth nerve tumor. If a defect of the labyrinthine system is diagnosed, it is treated medically (low-salt diet; no caffeine, tobacco, or alcohol; and an antihistamine such as chlorpheniramine maleate). The patient with acute vertigo (as well as the patient with severe sudden unilateral sensorineural hearing loss) should be hospitalized and given an intravenous histamine drip twice daily for 5 days. (This consists of giving histamine phosphate, 2.75 mg in 250 ml of 5% dextrose in water. Administer twice daily at a rate that achieves flushing.) If the pa-

tient is still incapacitated by the vertigo after 3 months, surgical decompression or section of the vestibular nerve (if useful hearing persists) or destruction of the labyrinth is done.

Facer GW, Maragos NE: The dizzy patient. Postgrad Med 57:73, May 1975.
Ruben RJ: Persistent vertigo. Otolaryngol Clin North Am 7:23, 1974.
Stahle J: Advanced Ménière's disease. Acta Otolaryngol 81:113, 1976.
Wolfson RJ (editor): Symposium on vertigo. Otolaryngol Clin North Am 6:3, Feb 1973. [Entire issue.]

3. TINNITUS

The patient with tinnitus hears a constant or intermittent ringing, humming, or buzzing sound not caused by a source external to the ear. The cause is not known. It frequently accompanies otosclerosis and diminishes in 80% of patients after stapedectomy. In other patients, the tinnitus may disappear with the treatment regimen outlined above for vertigo. If tinnitus persists for more than 6 months in spite of treatment, the patient must learn to live with it. He can minimize it at bedtime by placing a noisy clock or radio near his bed.

Systemic contributing causes such as early diabetes, anemia, and carotid atherosclerosis should be eliminated.

BENIGN TUMORS & FOREIGN BODIES OF THE EAR

Osteomas & Exostoses

Osteomas and exostoses are rounded, bony-hard protuberances that develop under the skin of the ear canal adjacent to the drum. They are usually asymptomatic and are detected during routine ear examination. They should be removed if they obstruct 75—90% of the ear canal since further growth will cause hearing loss and infection from obstruction.

Granulomas & Polyps of the Ear Canal

These growths, ordinarily the result of chronic otitis media, are soft, pink, friable masses usually projecting through a perforation in the eardrum. They require surgical removal via a tympanotomy or mastoidectomy incision.

Internal Auditory Meatus Tumor (Schwannoma)

This is a benign tumor of the sheath of the eighth nerve which tends to erode bone and may eventually create enough pressure on the seventh and eighth nerves to cause complete loss of function. As it enlarges, compression of the fifth and seventh nerve is common. Early diagnosis and surgical removal may avoid late complications such as involvement of the brain stem.

Foreign Bodies in the Ear Canal

Most foreign bodies in the ear canal can be removed with a ring curet, a 90 degree angle hook, or an alligator forceps. If the object is firmly fixed, it should be removed under local or general anesthesia since the patient's movements in response to pain can result in injury to the eardrum and the ossicular chain. Vegetable foreign bodies (eg, beans) should not be irrigated.

MALIGNANT TUMORS
OF THE EXTERNAL EAR

Basal cell carcinoma, squamous cell carcinoma, and occasionally melanoma can occur in the pinna, external ear canal, or middle ear. They should be suspected in the presence of a lesion that persists for over 2 weeks. They should be removed surgically if that can be done. If the eardrum or the mastoid has been invaded, mastoidectomy or total resection of the temporal bone may be necessary. If the tumor cannot be removed completely, radiation therapy is required.

MALIGNANT TUMORS OF
THE MIDDLE EAR

Squamous Cell Carcinoma

Squamous cell carcinoma, although rare, should be suspected in any patient with ear discharge and unexplained ear pain or ear pain more severe than the physical findings would seem to justify. It may appear as a mass in the ear canal or middle ear. Roentgenograms may show erosion. The diagnosis is made by tympanotomy and biopsy. Treatment consists of temporal bone resection if feasible or radiation therapy (or both). The 5-year cure rate is very low.

GLOMUS JUGULARE TUMOR

Glomus jugulare is a vascular tumor that usually arises from the jugular bulb and spreads upward into the middle ear space and posteriorly into the mastoid bone. If it is not controlled, it will progressively paralyze the nerves of the jugular foramen (cranial nerves IX, X, and XI) and then nerves VII, VIII, and XII. The diagnosis is based on the appearance of a pink mass behind the eardrum which compresses with pneumatic otoscopy and then pulsates back to full size when the

air pressure is released. In some cases, the diagnosis is based on the occurrence of pulsating tinnitus or signs of cranial nerve defects with roentgenographic enlargement of the jugular foramen and, in more advanced cases, erosion of the temporal bone. Carotid arteriography and retrograde jugular venography are used to outline the extent of the tumor and to evaluate the patency of the contralateral sigmoid sinus. The tumor, which can resemble an inflammatory polyp, will bleed profusely if biopsied.

Surgical removal of glomus jugulare may be feasible, but complete removal is quite difficult. Postoperative radiation is helpful in controlling symptoms.

Moore GR & others: Chemodectomas of the middle ear. Arch Otolaryngol 98:330, 1973.

Spector GJ & others: A comparison of therapeutic modalities of glomus tumors in the temporal bone. Laryngoscope 86:690, 1976.

Spector GJ & others: Glomus tumors in the middle ear. Laryngoscope 83:1652, 1973.

CONGENITAL DEFECTS OF THE EAR

Atresia of the External Ear & Ear Canal

This disfiguring congenital defect is uncommon. Since the results of surgical correction to improve hearing are modest, unilateral defects should not be so treated. The external ear can be reconstructed with plastic surgery or with an adhesive prosthesis if the patient desires. If the defect is bilateral and roentgenograms of the mastoid show an air-filled middle ear space with some pneumatization of the mastoid, surgical reconstruction of the ear canal can be achieved by mastoidectomy and skin graft. If hearing is thus improved and the ear can be kept dry, a hearing aid can be placed in the reconstructed ear canal. If this is not feasible, a bone conduction hearing aid can be placed on the mastoid bone behind the ear. Normal hearing will not be achieved, but significant improvement often results. The best surgical results are obtained when the external auricular deformity is minimal.

Preauricular Sinus or Cyst

The sinus (measuring 1 mm in diameter and 5–10 mm or more in depth) or cyst is located just anterior to the upper helix. Excision is indicated to stop discharge.

SEVENTH NERVE PALSY

Paralysis of the facial (seventh) nerve immobilizes the muscles of expression on that side of the face. There is loss of both voluntary and involuntary contraction; the eye fails to close; the forehead cannot be wrinkled; and that side of the mouth droops. Paralysis can result from trauma that injures or fractures the base of the skull or from surgical procedures on the parotid gland, the middle ear, the mastoid, or in the area of the brain stem in the posterior fossa. It can also be caused by viral infections (Ramsay Hunt syndrome with herpes zoster or other neurotropic viral infections), pressure on the seventh nerve in the posterior fossa by tumors of the cerebellopontine angle or internal auditory meatus, or diabetes or prediabetes. When the cause is not known, it is called **Bell's palsy.** Some cases of Bell's palsy may be the result of vascular spasm causing nerve edema, most often in the vertical portion near the stylomastoid foramen.

The diagnostic work-up includes a careful history; ear, nose, and throat examination; pure tone, speech, and special audiograms; roentgenograms of the mastoid to detect any erosion of the internal auditory meatus or in the area of the antrum or attic; a 5-hour glucose tolerance test to exclude diabetes and prediabetes; and an electronystagmography (caloric) test. Electromyographic or nerve conduction studies (or both) may be done but are of limited value in predicting the outcome of facial nerve paralysis. Loss of voluntary muscle potentials immediately and response to external electrical stimulation 3—7 days later occur after both anatomic (surgical or traumatic) or physiologic interruption of the nerve. This does not mean that facial nerve function will not return spontaneously in 1—16 weeks; spontaneous recovery occurs in approximately 80% of cases of Bell's palsy.

Treatment consists of removing identifiable causes such as cholesteatoma or tumors of the internal auditory meatus, or of treating the infection or diabetes. The treatment of Bell's palsy is still controversial; statistical data support the effectiveness of early treatment with corticosteroids to reduce edema in the nerve, eg, dexamethasone, 1.5 mg 4 times daily for 2 weeks. Surgical decompression (through the mastoid) is frequently done if function has not returned within 3—4 months after the onset of Bell's palsy. Immediate decompression is indicated if the nerve is paralyzed after head trauma with roentgenographic evidence of a fracture in the area of the nerve or if the nerve is damaged during a mastoid or middle ear operation. If a damaged segment of the nerve must be removed, a section of the great auricular or sural nerve may be grafted in its place. If function has not returned by 12 months after decompression or grafting, the facial nerve may be anastomosed to the hypoglossal nerve. This latter procedure will not result in return of involuntary function, but the patient will have better tone in the facial muscles at rest and, with practice, will be able to move his face. He does this by pressing his tongue against his teeth to send impulses along the 12th nerve into the face through the anastomosis and the seventh nerve.

Graham MD (editor): Disease and injury of the facial nerve. Otolaryngol Clin North Am 7:289, June 1974.
May M & others: Natural history of Bell's palsy. Laryngoscope 86:704, 1976.

CEREBROSPINAL FLUID OTORRHEA & ENDAURAL ENCEPHALOCELE

CSF leakage or brain herniation into the temporal bone occurs most commonly after mastoidectomy. It is usually manifested by clear watery discharge from the ear; a polyp or a pink, pulsating, enlarging mass in a mastoid bowl; or meningitis. The diagnosis is confirmed by analysis of the fluid for protein and sugar and by dye tests (indigo carmine or 5% fluorescein injected via lumbar puncture to see if it appears in the discharge). If it does not close spontaneously within 2 weeks of onset, the dural defect needs to be closed surgically from below via the mastoid with a muscle graft or via craniotomy with fascia. *Note:* Methylene blue should never be injected into the spinal canal; severe paralysis can result.

Dedo HH, Sooy FA: Endaural brain hernia (encephalocele): Diagnosis and treatment. Laryngoscope 80:1090, 1970.
Saunders WH, Paparella MM: *Atlas of Ear Surgery.* Mosby, 1968.

NOSE, PARANASAL SINUSES, & FACE

INFECTIONS OF THE NOSE, PARANASAL SINUSES, & FACE

1. SINUSITIS

Sinusitis is usually preceded by nasal allergy or by a bacterial or viral upper respiratory infection. In the acute stage, there is severe pain in the maxilla or forehead. The diagnosis is based on an aching facial pain aggravated by stooping or straining and associated with or preceded by purulent nasal drainage or upper respiratory tract infection and the appearance of mucopus in the nose. Sinus x-rays frequently show fluid partially or completely filling one or more of the sinuses (Fig 41—7). This is probably pus and should be treated with antibiotics and a decongestant.

Maxillary Sinusitis

When pus is demonstrated in the maxillary sinus, it should be washed out by antral irrigation—passing a trocar either through the lateral wall of the inferior nasal meatus or through the canine fossa and anterior wall into the maxillary sinus and running water or saline through the needle, into the sinus, and out the ostium. This should be done only after a trial of medical treatment, eg, antibiotics for 48—72 hours. Care

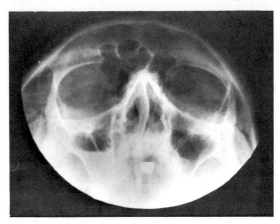

Figure 41–7. Sinus x-ray showing air-fluid (pus) level in maxillary sinuses (20% on left; 50% on right).

must be taken to avoid advancing the trocar into the orbital space. If nasal polyps are present, they should be removed when the acute (pain) phase has passed (see below). If antral irrigations 4–7 days apart do not control the infection in 2–3 months, a Caldwell-Luc operation (Fig 41–10) should be done to remove the diseased membrane from the sinus and to create a permanent opening for drainage from the antrum into the nose.

Acute or Chronic Ethmoidal, Sphenoidal, or Frontal Sinusitis

This infection is suggested by chronic postnasal purulent discharge or pain and tenderness between and above the eyes. An underlying cause should be sought (trauma, allergy, polyps, foreign body, neoplasm, etc). It is diagnosed by x-ray and can often be cured by treating the concurrent maxillary sinusitis and by antibiotics, decongestants, and Proetz displacements (displacement of air in the sinus with a topical vasoconstrictor). If these fail and no maxillary sinusitis exists, treatment is by exenteration of the ethmoid or sphenoid sinuses (or both), either via the antrum (Caldwell-Luc operation; Fig 41–10) or via an external Lynch incision between the medial canthus of the eye and the bridge of the nose. If anything is obstructing drainage of the frontal sinus, a large nasofrontal duct should be created with a flap of mucosa from the nasal septum to prevent future accumulations of pus in the frontal sinus (Sewall operation). If drainage cannot be established, all mucous membrane must be removed from the frontal sinus and the space obliterated either with fat or by removing its anterior wall.

Baron SH, Dedo HH, Henry CR: Mucoperiosteal flap in frontal sinus surgery (Sewall-Boyden-McNaught operation). Laryngoscope 83:1266, 1973.

Bell RD & others: Conservative surgical procedures in inflammatory disease of the maxillary sinus. Otolaryngol Clin North Am 9:175, 1976.

Chapnik JS, Bach MC: Bacterial and fungal infections of the maxillary sinus. Otolaryngol Clin North Am 9:43, 1976.

Evans FO Jr & others: Sinusitis of the maxillary antrum. N Engl J Med 293:735, 1975.

Goodman WS: The Caldwell-Luc procedure. Otolaryngol Clin North Am 9:187, 1976.

2. FOLLICULITIS

Folliculitis, an infection of a hair follicle at the anterior nasal choana, is characterized by pain, swelling, redness, and tenderness of the anterior nose. Treatment is with local warm compresses and local applications of antibiotic and corticosteroid ointment. Systemic antibiotics are given for significant swelling or spreading cellulitis. Incision and drainage are done if an abscess appears. Folliculitis should be treated vigorously as soon as it is detected because cavernous sinus thrombosis has been known to result from infection in the face between the mouth and the eyes.

EPISTAXIS

Spontaneous nosebleed most commonly occurs from Kiesselbach's triangle on the septum just inside the anterior nares. The patient himself can usually control a minor nosebleed by pinching his nostrils together or by placing a cotton plug in the bleeding nostril. If this is not successful, apply a cotton pressure pack soaked with a mild vasoconstrictor such as phenylephrine, 0.25%, to the bleeding area for 5 minutes and then cauterize the bleeding vessel with silver nitrate or a chromic acid bead (Fig 41–8). Cautery should not be used in patients taking anticoagulants or in patients with leukemia, thrombocytopenic purpura, or other bleeding problems. The best treatment in patients with bleeding problems is petrolatum packing or insertion of a wedge of salt pork in the nostril for 4 or 5 days.

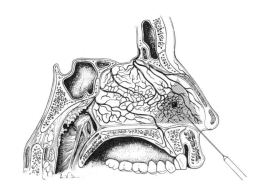

Figure 41–8. Cauterization to control bleeding in Kiesselbach's area.

(Start with a piece 2 × 2 × 4 cm and carve off just enough so it can be inserted.) When the pork is removed, it does not stick to the nasal membrane, thereby breaking loose the newly formed clot.

Bleeding from the middle portion of the nose that cannot be controlled by cautery requires treatment with an anterior nasal pack left in place for 6—9 days.

Bleeding from the posterior part of the nose usually requires both a posterior and an anterior pack, placed after local anesthesia and shrinkage of the nasal membranes with tetracaine, 2%, and epinephrine, 1:1000, applied with cotton swabs. The posterior pack is installed by passing a catheter posteriorly along the floor of the nose and out the posterior choana into the pharynx where it can be grasped through the mouth with a hemostat (Fig 41—9). Two of the 3 strings on the posterior pack are tied to the pharyngeal end of the catheter, and both are brought back out through one anterior naris and tied over a bolster. The anterior nose is then packed with half-inch gauze.

Note: A posterior pack must always have a third string attached to it extending downward along the posterior pharyngeal wall. When the pack is removed (after 4—7 days), the third string should be grasped with a locked hemostat to prevent the pack from falling into the larynx and asphyxiating the patient when the 2 anterior strings have been cut.

If anterior and posterior packing still fails to arrest bleeding in the posterior or superior part of the nose, ligation of the anterior ethmoid, internal maxillary, or external carotid arteries—singly or in any combination—is required. An alternative is arterial plugging under fluoroscopic control.

Pearson BW: Epistaxis. Postgrad Med 57:117, May 1975.

Sessions RB: Nasal hemorrhage. Otolaryngol Clin North Am 6:727, 1973.

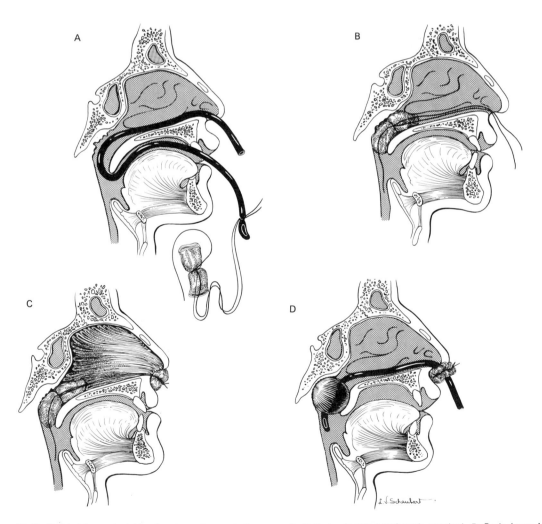

Figure 41—9. Packing to control bleeding from the posterior nose. *A:* Catheter inserted and pack attached. *B:* Pack drawn into position as catheter is removed. *C:* Strip tied over a bolster to hold pack in place with anterior pack installed "accordion pleating" style. *D:* Alternative method using balloon catheter instead of gauze pack.

DEVIATED SEPTUM

Deviated nasal septum can result from trauma during birth or later or from progressive, differential growth of the septum and the rest of the nose. It is corrected by straightening the deformed portions and removing the permanently deformed cartilage and bone of the septum through an incision in the anterior septal mucosa (nasal septoplasty).

BENIGN TUMORS & FOREIGN BODIES OF THE NOSE, PARANASAL SINUSES, & FACE

Rhinophyma

Rhinophyma is a swelling of the tip of the nose caused by proliferation of the connective tissue and glands in the skin. Treatment is by excision of the affected skin down to the basal layer.

Nasal Polyps

Nasal polyps can cause nasal and sinus obstruction. They are usually associated with allergy, although intensive therapy for nasal allergy, including the use of corticosteroids, does not abolish them and rarely prevents their recurrence. Nasal polyps should be removed surgically. If infection has resulted from their obstruction of sinuses, drainage procedures such as a Caldwell-Luc operation (Fig 41–10) or a fronto-ethmoidectomy are required.

Mucocele of the Sinus

Mucocele is usually manifested by pain or swelling over a paranasal sinus. If a paranasal sinus is chronically and totally obstructed, mucous secretion gradually accumulates under sufficient pressure to erode the surrounding bone. In the frontal sinus, such erosion can expose the dura and lead to meningitis and brain abscess, especially if the mucocele becomes infected (mucopyocele). The pain results from progressive pressure and irritation of surrounding structures.

Treatment consists of surgical removal of the mucocele and reestablishment of drainage from the involved sinuses as described above for acute sinusitis.

Juvenile Angiofibroma of the Nasopharynx

Recurrent nasal bleeding or chronic nasal obstruction is the usual sign of this locally invasive but usually nonmetastasizing tumor, which occurs most frequently in teen-age boys. It arises from the periosteal layer of the basilar process of the occipital bone (the posterior superior nasopharynx) and progressively erodes into the sphenoid sinus, the posterior nose, the pterygomaxillary fossa, the maxillary sinus, and rarely, into the brain.

Polytome x-rays and arteriograms are used to evaluate the extent of involvement. The tumor should be removed via a transpalatal route. Radiation is used for inoperable tumors (eg, intracranial extension) or recurrences.

Nasal Foreign Bodies

A foreign body must be suspected in any patient with unilateral nasal secretion or unilateral reduction in the nasal airway. The object should be removed with appropriate forceps or hooks. Vegetable material such as a bean should be removed as early as possible because of swelling.

CHRONIC NASAL CONGESTION & DISCHARGE

Vasomotor Rhinitis

This diagnosis is made in a patient with no evidence of infection who has recurrent episodes of copious, thin nasal drainage precipitated by cold air or by eating hot or cold foods and whose sinus roentgenograms show no significant abnormalities. Decongestants and reassurance are used for treatment but are not entirely satisfactory.

Cerebrospinal Fluid Rhinorrhea

Unilateral, clear, watery nasal discharge which increases during the Valsalva maneuver must be regarded as CSF until proved otherwise. The most common cause of CSF leakage is head trauma. Chemical tests for glucose and protein (to identify the fluid) and dye studies (to indicate the site of a bony and dural defect) may be useful. The defect must be closed surgically if it does not close spontaneously within 2 weeks after onset. Frontal and sphenoid leaks are best approached from below by the otolaryngologist.

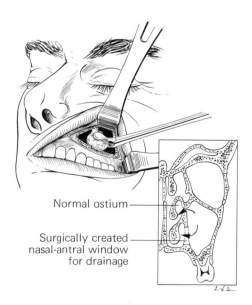

Normal ostium

Surgically created
nasal-antral window
for drainage

Figure 41–10. Caldwell-Luc nasal polypectomy.

Ethmoid defects are best closed via craniotomy by the neurosurgeon.

McCoy G: Cerebrospinal rhinorrhea: A comprehensive review. Laryngoscope 73:1125, 1963.

Chemical Rhinitis

The chronic use of nasal drops or sprays causes the nasal membranes to swell severely and drain continuously. Treatment consists of stopping the local nasal medication and administering oral decongestants for 2—3 weeks to allow the membranes to return to normal.

CONGENITAL ABNORMALITIES OF THE NOSE

Anterior choanal atresia is rare but is obvious when it occurs. Posterior choanal atresia should be suspected in any newborn who has difficulty breathing. The diagnosis is made by holding the baby's mouth closed and seeing if a piece of cotton held in front of each nostril moves. If there is still doubt, the inability to pass a catheter through each nostril into the pharynx will substantiate the diagnosis. If both posterior nares appear to be closed, the baby's respiration should be assured by holding his mouth open with an oral airway or, if necessary, by inserting an endotracheal tube. Definitive diagnosis is made by placing a few drops of radiopaque material in each anterior naris while the baby is supine and taking a lateral roentgenogram of the skull to see if the material has entered the nasopharynx.

To establish an immediate airway, a temporary opening is made with a mastoid curet through the mucosal—often bony—membrane that extends from the posterior end of the hard palate to the sphenoid basiocciput. This opening is kept patent by placing a segment of No. 16 or No. 18F Portex endotracheal tube through it. When the baby's general condition permits, transnasal resection of the obstruction and resection of the posterior end of the nasal septum should be done under general anesthesia using the operating microscope. If this fails—and in older children or in adults with unilateral posterior choanal atresia—surgical repair is best done via the transpalatal route. This route permits the surgeon to use the nasal septal mucosa on the uninvolved side to epithelize part of the raw portion left after removal of the unilateral posterior choanal atresia, thereby minimizing the chances of stenosis.

MOUTH, PHARYNX, & SALIVARY GLANDS

INFECTIONS OF THE MOUTH, PHARYNX, & SALIVARY GLANDS

Glossitis & Pharyngitis

The presenting symptom is mouth or throat pain. The membranes of the mouth or pharynx are injected and may have a white coating. Bacterial glossitis or pharyngitis is treated with systemic antibiotics; candida infections (thrush) are treated with topical nystatin (1%).

Tonsillitis

Acute tonsillitis is diagnosed on the basis of sore throat and fever in a patient with injected, enlarged tonsils—often with an exudate or white crypts on their surfaces. Tonsillitis is differentiated from diphtheria by the absence (in tonsillitis) of extension of this surface coating onto the soft palate and anterior pillars and by culture of a throat smear. Treatment is with antibiotics and, if necessary, analgesics. The tonsils should be removed if tonsillitis recurs more than 3 or 4 times a year in a child or more than once or twice a year in an adult. In children, the adenoids should also be removed at this time since they become infected whenever the tonsils do.

Other indications for tonsillectomy and adenoidectomy in children include recurrent otitis media, chronic otitis media, obstruction of the nasopharynx by enlarged adenoids, and subacute bacterial endocarditis or chronic glomerulonephritis resulting from recurrent or chronic streptococcal infections of the pharynx or tonsils.

Sprinkle PM, Veltri RW: The tonsil and adenoid dilemma: Medical or surgical treatment? Otolaryngol Clin North Am 7:909, 1974.

Sialitis (Infection of the Salivary Glands)

The swelling and pain of acute infection of the parotid or submandibular (submaxillary) glands usually respond rapidly to treatment with antibiotics and warm compresses. Secretions from Stensen's duct should be cultured. Staphylococci are often the cause of parotid gland infection, especially in elderly or severely debilitated people. If a gram-stained smear or culture shows coagulase-positive *Staphylococcus aureus,* methicillin should be given. If the infection does not respond to antibiotic therapy, incision and drainage should be carried out. Multiple incisions made parallel to the course of the facial nerve and its branches may be required.

Infection can often be prevented by the maintenance of good hydration, so that there is an adequate salivary flow to prevent retrograde infection via Stensen's duct. When the parotid gland must be removed—as in cases of chronic recurrent infection, often associated with calculi—care must be taken to preserve the facial nerve.

Abscesses

Abscesses of the floor of the mouth or of the peritonsillar, pharyngeal, or parapharyngeal spaces are usually the result of tooth or tonsillar infection and are manifested by swelling and pain. While still in the cellulitis stage, they may be controlled by antibiotics and warm compresses. If rapid resolution does not occur, incision and drainage should be done.

BENIGN TUMORS OF THE MOUTH & PHARYNX

Papilloma

Small papillomas resembling warts can occur anywhere in the mucosa of the pharynx but are most common on the soft palate. They do not ordinarily become malignant.

Alveolar Ridge Tumors

These tumors (embryonic rests of teeth) appear as mandibular or maxillary lumps and are diagnosed by biopsy. Treatment is usually by surgical excision after the extent of the tumor has been delineated radiographically and after biopsy has proved it not to be a carcinoma.

Leukoplakia

Localized "white spots" less than 5–10 mm in diameter which persist longer than 2 weeks should be biopsied. Extensive oral leukoplakias should be observed and, if ulcers or piled up areas develop, these should be biopsied.

Hemangioma & Lymphangioma

Hemangiomas and lymphangiomas can occur anywhere in the buccal or pharyngeal mucosa. In the tongue, they can be so large at birth that they interfere with breathing and swallowing. Hemangiomas are purplish; lymphangiomas tend to be the color of the overlying mucous membrane. Diagnosis should be by biopsy since a sarcoma or lymphoma may resemble these tumors. Surgical treatment is by excision if feasible, although extensive hemangiomas and lymphangiomas often cannot be removed completely since they do not remain encapsulated.

Palatal Exostosis (Torus Palatinus)

Palatal exostosis is a malformation composed of knobby, bony, submucosal nodules projecting downward from the midline of the hard palate. It results from the overriding of the 2 palatal bones when they come together in the midline in the embryo. It does not become malignant and need not be removed unless it interferes with the fitting of an upper dental plate.

TRAUMA TO THE MOUTH, PHARYNX, & SALIVARY GLANDS

Perforation of the soft palate often occurs when a child falls on an object, such as a pencil, that he is carrying in his mouth. It should not be sutured. If cellulitis develops, it should be treated with antibiotics. A small laceration of the tongue should not be closed with sutures, but more extensive lacerations should be closed with interrupted 3–0 chromic gut sutures to minimize scarring.

Perforations of the hard palate or around the eyes may be intracranial as well. The penetrating object should not be removed until the depth of penetration has been ascertained—with roentgenograms if possible—and until neurosurgical assistance is available.

The location, number, and extent of mandibular fractures should be determined by x-ray. Any teeth in the fracture line should be removed to help prevent infection. After the fracture has been reduced, fixation can be achieved by intraoral wiring, an external prosthesis, or wiring at the side of the fracture through an external incision.

Mathog RH, Rosenberg Z: Complications in the treatment of facial fractures: Symposium on maxillofacial trauma. Otolaryngol Clin North Am 9:533, 1976.

LARYNX, HYPOPHARYNX, & TRACHEA

INFECTION

Infection of the epiglottis, larynx, or trachea (acute epiglottitis or laryngotracheobronchitis, ie, "croup") causes airway obstruction in children but only hoarseness in adults because the adult airway at the glottic level is so much larger than the minimum space required for breathing. Cultures have usually shown gram-positive organisms or *Haemophilus influenzae*. Treatment is with ampicillin, corticosteroids, and cold mist. In children, close observation in the hospital for 72 hours is necessary so that endotracheal intubation and tracheostomy can be done immediately if the airway obstruction becomes too severe or if the effort of breathing tires the child too much.

BENIGN TUMORS & FOREIGN BODIES OF THE LARYNX, HYPOPHARYNX, & TRACHEA

All tumors and foreign bodies of these structures cause hoarseness and occasionally airway obstruction.

Singer's Nodules

Singer's nodules are small projections from the free edge of the cord, each resembling a grain of sand. They usually occur at the junction of the anterior and middle thirds of the true vocal cords and are caused by singing or shouting, especially during an episode of laryngitis. The patient should avoid shouting, singing, smoking, and drinking alcohol. Removal of the nodule, if required, is by direct laryngoscopy with the newer types of large-opening fiberoptic laryngoscopes such as the Jako-Dedo, which utilize the operating microscope to improve visualization and facilitate precise removal.

Laryngoscopy is illustrated in Fig 41–11.

Granulomas

Granulomas appear on the posterior third of the vocal cord, usually as a result of injury to the mucosa over the arytenoid cartilage. The most common causes of injury are endotracheal intubation and excessive shouting, singing, or throat clearing. Granulomas appear as pink or purple (and later white) rough masses. Early, when they are sessile, they should not be removed because they will return and grow larger than before. Treatment is by avoidance of further vocal trauma and removal of the tumor when its base has become pinched into a narrow stalk.

Polyps of the Vocal Cord

Polyps usually occur as a late stage in granuloma of the arytenoid portion of the cord. Like granulomas, they should be removed only when they have a narrow stalk. The term "polypoid cords" refers to cords that are thickened in the membranous portion and, in extreme cases, resemble floppy elephant ears. Some polyps may be due to vocal abuse, excessive use of tobacco or alcohol, diabetes, or hypothyroidism.

Treatment consists of resting the voice and eliminating the underlying problem. If the polypoid cord persists, the mucous membrane should be stripped from the vocal cord, care being taken not to remove tissue deeper than Rinke's space to avoid injuring the thyroarytenoid muscle fibers themselves.

Papilloma of the Larynx

Laryngeal papilloma occurs more commonly in children than in adults. Treatment is by surgical removal after placement of a low-pressure balloon-cuffed tracheostomy tube to protect the airway, simplify anesthesia, and prevent blood from reaching the lower trachea during the operation. Because they keep returning, removal should be repeated at 6-week intervals. Removal should be thorough each time but not so deep that the underlying normal tissue is injured. The surgical instruments should not be passed into the lower trachea or bronchi below the point where the airway can be protected by a tracheostomy tube.

Laryngeal Web

This thin membrane, usually formed between the true cords, can occur as a congenital deformity or after laryngeal trauma. It is diagnosed by inspection via

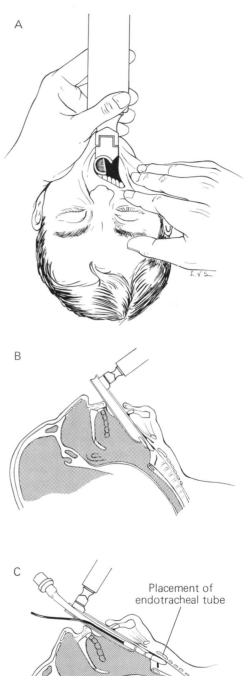

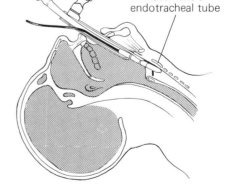

Figure 41–11. Technic of laryngoscopy. *A:* The blade is passed behind the tongue and under the tip of the epiglottis. *B:* Lateral view showing laryngoscope blade under tip of epiglottis exposing glottic opening. *C:* Insertion of endotracheal tube to establish airway during obstruction or general anesthesia.

direct laryngoscopy. It is treated by division and placement of a tantalum keel by the laryngofissure (McNaught) or endolaryngeal (Haslinger) technic.

Hemangioma

Subglottic hemangioma is a pink or purple mass which usually occurs in infants and causes airway obstruction which increases dramatically during crying (because the Valsalva effect causes venous obstruction and distention). Diagnosis is made by direct laryngoscopy under general anesthesia, using inspection and palpation but not biopsy. Tracheostomy may be necessary to maintain the airway until spontaneous regression occurs, usually about age 6–12 months. Radiation therapy is not given because of the high incidence of subsequent thyroid carcinoma.

Chondroma

These hard, white, submucosal, subglottic masses cause airway obstruction in infants which, like other fixed obstructions, increases with crying. The diagnosis is based on inspection via direct laryngoscopy under general anesthesia. Trachcostomy may be necessary to maintain an adequate airway until differential growth or surgical resection via laryngofissure provides an adequate laryngeal breathing space.

Foreign Bodies

Foreign bodies of the hypopharynx or trachea usually require removal with a bronchoscope and special instruments under general anesthesia. When the foreign body is in the upper trachea, the bronchoscope should be introduced quickly through the larynx and used to push the foreign body into the right main stem bronchus to reestablish the airway. The best treatment is prevention, and this is best done in children by keeping them away from tiny toys or toys that can be separated into tiny parts and by not letting them eat nuts or hard candies until their molar teeth have appeared.

MALIGNANT TUMORS OF THE LARYNX, HYPOPHARYNX, & TRACHEA

Malignant tumors of the throat structures are manifested by hoarseness, pain, and, in later stages, obstruction of the airway. Ninety-five percent of carcinomas of the larynx are squamous cell. The diagnosis is made by means of indirect laryngoscopy, direct laryngoscopy, and palpation of the neck to determine the extent of the lesion, plus biopsy of the lesion via direct laryngoscopy for microscopic diagnosis. *Note:* Squamous cell carcinoma should be suspected in any patient with hoarseness that lasts for over 2 weeks. Evaluation of these patients includes general physical examination, routine laboratory studies of blood and urine, ECG, and evaluation of other major systems. A chest x-ray is necessary to rule out metastasis to the lung. Early diagnosis permits conservation of the voice with removal of the tumor by partial laryngectomy.

Radiation treatment with 4500 rads over a 5-week period and supraglottic laryngectomy 3–4 weeks later (sparing the vocal cords and hence the voice) is feasible for tumors in the upper larynx and hypopharynx (1) if they are in the vallecula, epiglottis, false cord, or piriform sinus; (2) if they do not reach more than 5 mm above the vallecula, do not involve the true cord, and do not extend within 1 cm of the apex of the piriform sinus and 1 cm of the apex of the interarytenoid notch; and (3) if they stop 5 mm above the anterior commissure. If they extend lower than this, treatment is with full-course radiation therapy (6500 rads over 6–7 weeks).

If a tumor persists or recurs and the patient's general condition permits, treatment is by total laryngectomy and radical neck dissection under the following circumstances: (1) if the tumor does not extend more than 5 mm up the base of the tongue, into the posterior pharyngeal wall, or below the upper edge of the cricopharyngeus muscle; and (2) if there is no evidence of distant metastases.

Carcinoma limited to the true vocal cord is treated by full-course radiation therapy (6000–6500 rads over 6–7 weeks), with vertical hemilaryngectomy or laryngectomy and radical neck dissection being reserved for persistence or recurrence.

Radiation therapy plus surgery is indicated for the following: (1) transglottic (false and true cord) lesions; (2) subglottic lesions (ie, those that extend more than 1 cm below the free edge of the cord); and (3) large lesions involving the piriform sinus or the base of the tongue in the midline. The dosage is 5500 rads in 6 weeks. Laryngectomy and radical neck dissection are done 4–6 weeks later.

Laryngectomy and radical neck dissection is used for large laryngeal cancers with fixation.

Bryce DP, Rider WD: Pre-operative irradiation in the treatment of advanced laryngeal carcinoma. Laryngoscope 81:1481, 1971.

Cocke EW Jr, Wang CC: Cancer of the larynx. CA 26:194, 1976.

Dedo HH: Supraglottic laryngectomy, indications and techniques. Laryngoscope 78:1183, 1968.

DeSanto LW & others: Surgical salvage after irradiation for laryngeal cancer. Laryngoscope 86:649, 1976.

Fletcher GH & others: Reasons for radiation failure in squamous cell carcinoma of the larynx. Laryngoscope 85:987, 1975.

Strong MS: Diagnosis of carcinoma of the larynx: A review of current methods. Laryngoscope 85:516, 1975.

Till JE & others: A preliminary analysis of end results for cancer of the larynx. Laryngoscope 85:259, 1975.

LARYNGEAL PARALYSIS

Vocal cord paralysis can occur as a result of surgical or external trauma; malignancy in the base of the skull, neck, or chest; or infection. In 30% of cases, the cause is not known. Work-up should include esophagography and roentgenograms of the chest and the base of the skull to check for malignancy if the cause is uncertain.

If the vocal cord is paralyzed as a result of malignancy or operation, immediate Teflon injection may be performed under topical anesthesia to move the paralyzed cord to the midline. This will improve the voice and minimize or stop aspiration during swallowing. If the cause is not clear, Teflon injection to improve the voice or swallowing should be deferred for 6 months because function may return spontaneously.

STENOSIS OF THE LARYNX & TRACHEA

Stenosis of the larynx and trachea is usually due to infection, external trauma such as a blow to the neck, or internal trauma from balloon cuffs of the tracheostomy tubes. If there has been severe trauma to the neck, the possibility that the larynx has been fractured or that the trachea has been transected should be considered even though the skin remains intact. The airway obstruction from such an injury may not become apparent until 3–4 days after the trauma. Suspicion that such a severe injury has occurred is heightened if there is hoarseness, hemoptysis, significant soreness in the anterior neck, or any suggestion of airway obstruction. When airway obstruction is abrupt and severe, an endotracheal tube should be placed and the trachea and larynx explored through an anterior neck incision. If the trachea has been transected, it should be anastomosed with interrupted 3–0 Tefdek sutures. Fracture of the thyroid cartilage should be reduced and the segments fixed with 2–0 chromic gut sutures. If the mucosa of the interior of the larynx has been lacerated, a laryngofissure should be done and the lacerations closed with interrupted 4–0 plain gut sutures. If the airway is not so severely occluded that it requires a tracheostomy, laryngeal edema and infection should be treated with systemic corticosteroids and antibiotics. Follow-up examination by indirect laryngoscopy after 24–72 hours should then permit more precise evaluation of the extent of the injuries in the larynx.

Laryngeal Stenosis

Stenosis of the larynx requires repair via a laryngofissure using tantalum keel or skin graft and stent or mucosal advancement flaps.

Dedo HH, Sooy FA: Surgical repair of late glottic stenosis. Ann Otol Rhinol Laryngol 77:435, 1968.

Tracheal Stenosis

Internal trauma to the trachea can occur from endotracheal tubes; removal of large windows to insert tracheostomy tubes; and overinflation of balloon cuffs on endotracheal and tracheostomy tubes. Treatment is by dilatation for up to 6 dilatations. Stenoses such as those caused by balloon cuffs can occasionally be successfully treated with prolonged stenting or a skin graft plus stenting, but often require segmental resection of the trachea with (1) release of the superior attachments of the larynx to permit it to drop downward and (2) upward mobilization of the mediastinal trachea to permit primary anastomosis of the tracheal stumps.

Dedo HH, Fishman NH: Laryngeal release and sleeve resection for tracheal stenosis. Ann Otol Rhinol Laryngol 78:285, 1969.

●   ●   ●

General References

Ballenger JJ (editor): *Diseases of the Nose, Throat and Ear,* 12th ed. Lea & Febiger, 1976.

Block GE (editor): Symposium on head and neck surgery. Surg Clin North Am 53:1, 1973.

Boles R: Larynx. Chapter 28 in: *Differential Diagnosis in Pediatric Otolaryngology.* Strome M (editor). Little, Brown, 1976.

Cotton R, Fearon B: Esophageal strictures in infants and children. Can J Otolaryngol 1:224, 1972.

DeWeese DD, Saunders WH: *Textbook of Otolaryngology,* 4th ed. Mosby, 1973.

Herzon FS (editor): Symposium on infectious diseases of the head and neck. Otolaryngol Clin North Am 9:561, 1976. [Entire issue.]

Jazbi B (editor): Symposium on pediatric otorhinolaryngology. Otolaryngol Clin North Am 10:3, 1977. [Entire issue.]

Loré JM Jr: *An Atlas of Head and Neck Surgery,* 2nd ed. Saunders, 1973.

Montgomery WW: *Surgery of the Upper Respiratory System.* 2 vols. Lea & Febiger, 1971, 1973.

Northern JL: *Hearing Disorders.* Little, Brown, 1976.

Ryan RE & others: *Synopsis of Ear, Nose, and Throat Diseases,* 3rd ed. Mosby, 1970.

42...
Ophthalmology

Daniel G. Vaughan, MD

OCULAR EMERGENCIES

It is not necessary to refer every patient with an eye disease to an ophthalmologist for treatment. In general, sties, bacterial conjunctivitis, superficial trauma to the lids, corneas, and conjunctivas, and superficial corneal foreign bodies can be treated just as effectively by the surgeon or primary physician as by the ophthalmologist. More serious eye disease such as the following should be referred as soon as possible for specialized care: iritis, acute glaucoma, retinal detachment, strabismus, contusion of the globe, and severe corneal trauma or infection.

In the management of acute ocular disorders it is most important to establish a definitive diagnosis before prescribing treatment. The maxim, "All red eyes are not pink-eye," is a useful one; and the physician must be alert for the more serious iritis, keratitis, or glaucoma (Table 42–1). The common practice of prescribing "shotgun" topical antibiotic combinations containing corticosteroids is to be discouraged, because inappropriate use of steroids can lead to complications (see p 815).

This chapter attempts to summarize the basic principles and technics of diagnosis and management of common ocular problems, with special emphasis on emergencies, particularly those caused by trauma.

Ocular emergencies may be classified as true emergencies and urgent cases. A true emergency is defined as one in which a few hours' delay in treatment can lead to permanent ocular damage or extreme discomfort to the patient. An urgent case is one in which treatment should be started as soon as possible but in which a delay of a few days can be tolerated.

FOREIGN BODIES

If a patient complains of "something in my eye" and gives a consistent history, he usually has a foreign body even though it may not be readily visible. Almost all foreign bodies, however, can be seen under oblique illumination with the aid of a hand flashlight and loupe or other magnifying device.

Note the time, place, and other circumstances of the accident. Test visual acuity before treatment is instituted as a basis for comparison in the event of complications.

Conjunctival Foreign Body

A foreign body of the upper tarsal conjunctiva is

Table 42–1. Differential diagnosis of common causes of inflamed eye.

	Acute Conjunctivitis	Acute Iritis*	Acute Glaucoma†	Corneal Trauma or Infection
Incidence	Extremely common	Common	Uncommon	Common
Discharge	Moderate to copious	None	None	Watery or purulent
Vision	No effect on vision	Slightly blurred	Markedly blurred	Usually blurred
Pain	None	Moderate	Severe	Moderate to severe
Conjunctival injection	Diffuse; more toward fornices	Mainly circumcorneal	Diffuse	Diffuse
Cornea	Clear	Usually clear	Steamy	Change in clarity related to cause
Pupil size	Normal	Small	Moderately dilated and fixed	Normal
Pupillary light response	Normal	Poor	None	Normal
Intraocular pressure	Normal	Normal	Elevated	Normal
Smear	Causative organisms	No organisms	No organisms	Organisms found only in corneal ulcers due to infection

*Acute anterior uveitis.
†Angle-closure glaucoma.

suggested by pain and blepharospasm of sudden onset in the presence of a clear cornea. After instilling a local anesthetic, evert the lid by grasping the lashes gently and exerting pressure on the midportion of the outer surface of the upper lid with an applicator. If a foreign body is present, it can be easily removed by passing a sterile wet cotton applicator across the conjunctival surface.

Corneal Foreign Body

When a corneal foreign body is suspected but is not apparent on simple inspection, instill *sterile* sodium fluorescein into the conjunctival sac and examine the cornea with the aid of a magnifying device and strong illumination. The foreign body may then be removed with a sterile wet cotton applicator. An antibiotic should be instilled, eg, polymyxin B-bacitracin (Polysporin) ointment. It is not necessary to patch the eye, but the patient must be examined in 24 hours for secondary infection of the crater. If the nonspecialist cannot remove the corneal foreign body in this manner, it should be removed by an ophthalmologist. If there is no infection, a layer of corneal epithelial cells will line the crater within 24 hours. It should be emphasized that the intact corneal epithelium forms an effective barrier to infection. Once the corneal epithelium is disturbed, the cornea becomes extremely susceptible to infection.

Early infection is manifested by a white necrotic area around the crater and a small amount of gray exudate. These patients should be referred immediately to an ophthalmologist. Untreated corneal infection may lead to severe corneal ulceration, panophthalmitis, and loss of the eye.

Intraocular Foreign Bodies

Foreign bodies which have become lodged within the eye should be identified and localized as soon as possible. They usually cause extensive damage to the eye upon entry, and the degree of ocular injury is increased by leaving the foreign body in place.

In unusual cases, a metallic foreign body can enter the eye, cause minimal initial damage, and be overlooked by the physician. A patient using a hammer and chisel may be struck by a metallic splinter from either tool which enters his eye at high speed and with minimal symptoms. Complications arising weeks to years later may lead to loss of the eye. The important diagnostic points are to obtain a history of pounding "steel on steel" and to order an x-ray. The anterior portion of the eye, including the cornea, iris, lens, and sclera should be inspected with a loupe or slitlamp in an attempt to localize the entry wound. Direct ophthalmoscopic visualization of an intraocular foreign body may be possible. An orbital x-ray must be taken to verify the presence of a radiopaque foreign body.

An intraocular foreign body should be removed as soon as possible, preferably through the wound of entry. Foreign bodies with magnetic properties can be quickly and dramatically removed by holding the tip of a sterilized magnet in the wound of entry.

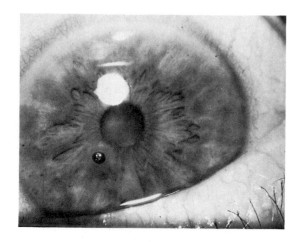

Figure 42–1. Metallic corneal foreign body. (Courtesy of A. Rosenberg.)

TRAUMATIC CATARACT

Traumatic cataract (Fig 42–2) is most commonly due to a metallic intraocular foreign body striking the lens. BB shot is a frequent cause; less frequent causes include arrows, rocks, overexposure to heat ("glassblower's cataract"), x-rays, and radioactive materials. Most traumatic cataracts are preventable. In industry, the best safety measure is a good pair of safety goggles.

The lens becomes white soon after the entry of the foreign body since the puncture of the lens capsule allows aqueous and sometimes vitreous to penetrate

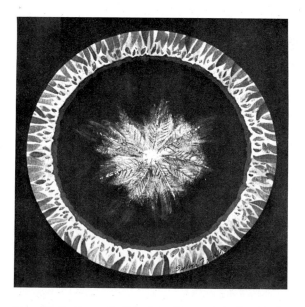

Figure 42–2. Traumatic "star-shaped" cataract in the posterior lens. This is usually due to ocular contusion and is only detectable through a well-dilated pupil. (From Cordes F. *Cataract Types*, 3rd ed. American Academy of Ophthalmology and Otolaryngology, 1954.)

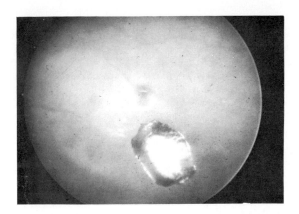

Figure 42–3. Ophthalmoscopic view of intraocular metallic (iron) foreign body in vitreous. (Actual size 1 × 3 mm.)

into the lens structure. The patient is often an industrial worker who gives a history of striking steel upon steel. A minute fragment of a steel hammer, for example, may pass through the cornea and lens at high speed and lodge in the vitreous, where it can usually be seen with the ophthalmoscope (Fig 42–3).

The patient complains immediately of blurred vision. The eye becomes red, the lens opaque, and there may be intraocular hemorrhage. If aqueous or vitreous escapes from the eye, the eye becomes extremely soft. Complications include infection, uveitis, retinal detachment, and glaucoma.

The cataractous lens should be removed after the inflammation subsides and it is certain that no further absorption of lens material is taking place. In persons under the age of 25 or 30, the lens material in a traumatic cataract will often absorb almost completely over a period of months without surgery. A thin membrane may remain, in which case discission (needling) may be necessary to improve vision.

The lens material may clog the anterior chamber angle, interfering with aqueous outflow and causing glaucoma. If glaucoma occurs and cannot be controlled medically, the lens must be removed without delay. Most eye surgeons are now using a combination of irrigation and aspiration for traumatic cataract in younger people. Alternative procedures are (1) phacoemulsification and aspiration and (2) phacofragmentation and irrigation.

LACERATIONS

Note: Tetanus prophylaxis is indicated whenever penetrating eye or lid injury occurs.

Lacerations are usually caused by sharp objects (knives, scissors, a projecting portion of the dashboard of an automobile, etc). Such injuries are treated in different ways depending upon whether there is prolapse of tissue.

Lacerations Without Prolapse of Tissue

If the eyeball has been penetrated anteriorly without gross evidence of prolapse of intraocular contents, and if the wound is clean and grossly free from contamination, it can usually be repaired by direct interrupted sutures of fine silk, catgut, or nylon.

Lacerations With Prolapse

If only a small portion of the iris prolapses through the wound, it should be grasped with a forceps and excised at the level of the wound lip. In any type of uveal tissue injury, the possibility of sympathetic ophthalmia must be kept in mind during the period of recovery.

If the wound has been extensive and loss of contents has been great enough that the prognosis for useful function is hopeless, evisceration or enucleation is indicated as the primary surgical procedure.

Lacerations of the Lids

Many lacerations of the lids do not involve the margins and may be sutured in the same way as other lacerations of the skin. If the margin of the eyelid is involved, special technics are required to prevent notching of the lid margin.

Rarely, extreme edema of the tissues prevents apposition of the wound for primary closure and the repair must be delayed (secondary repair) until the edema has subsided. Local debridement and irrigation, with use of antibiotics, should be carried out until it is possible to approximate the edges of the wound.

Lacerations of the lids near the inner canthus frequently involve the canaliculi (Fig 42–4). If these are not repaired, permanent strictures with epiphora will result. Small polyethylene tubes are usually placed in the canaliculi at the time of repair and left in place until healing occurs.

Canaliculus repair should be performed immediately since later repair is much more difficult.

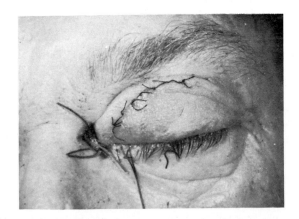

Figure 42–4. Complete laceration of upper lid and upper and lower canaliculi. Large sutures used in repair of severed canaliculi and medial canthal tendon.

NONPENETRATING INJURIES
OF THE EYEBALL

Corneal Abrasions

Abrasions of the cornea do not require surgical treatment. The wound should be cleansed of imbedded foreign material. To facilitate the examination, pain can be relieved by instillation of a local anesthetic such as 0.5% tetracaine (Pontocaine) solution, but routine instillation of a local anesthetic by the patient must not be permitted since it may delay the diagnosis of complications and is conducive to further injury. Antibiotic ointment, eg, polymyxin B-bacitracin (Polysporin), helps prevent bacterial infection. An eye bandage applied with firm pressure lessens discomfort and promotes healing (in 48–72 hours) by preventing movement of the lids over the involved area. The dressing should be changed daily until healing is complete.

Corneal abrasions cause pain severe enough to require strong analgesics. If not treated properly they may lead to recurrent corneal erosion.

Contusions

Contusions of the eyeball and its surrounding tissues are commonly produced by blunt trauma. The results of such injury are variable and are often not obvious upon superficial examination. Careful study and adequate follow-up are indicated. The possible results of contusion injury are hemorrhage and swelling of the eyelids (ecchymosis, "black eye"), subconjunctival hemorrhages, edema or rupture of the cornea, hemorrhage into the anterior chamber (hyphema), rupture of the root of the iris (iridodialysis), traumatic paralysis of the pupil (mydriasis), paralysis or spasm of the muscles of accommodation, traumatic cataract, dislocation of the lens (subluxation and luxation), vitreous hemorrhage, retinal hemorrhage and retinal edema (most common in the macular area, called commotio retinae, or Berlin's traumatic edema), detachment of the retina, rupture of the choroid posteriorly, and optic nerve injury.

Many of these injuries cannot be seen on casual external observation, and some may not develop for many days or weeks following the injury.

Except for those cases involving rupture of the eyeball, intraocular hemorrhage, or retinal detachment, most ocular contusions do not require immediate definitive treatment.

Rupture of the Eyeball

Rupture of the eyeball may be direct, at the site of injury, or may occur indirectly as a result of sudden increase in intraocular pressure, causing the wall of the eyeball to tear at one of the weaker points. Common sites of rupture are the limbus and the area around the optic nerve. Anterior ruptures can be repaired surgically by interrupted sutures if the intraocular contents have not become deranged in a manner that will prohibit useful function of the eye. If this is the case, evisceration or enucleation is indicated. If either of

these procedures is required, implantation of a plastic sphere is useful as a space-filler and to aid in movement of an artificial eye.

CHEMICAL CONJUNCTIVITIS
& KERATITIS

Chemical burns are best treated by thorough irrigation of the eyes with saline solution or water immediately after exposure. It is wise not to try to neutralize an acid or alkali by using its chemical counterpart, as the heat generated by the reaction may cause further damage. If the chemical irritant is an alkali, the irrigation should be continued longer since alkalies are not precipitated by the proteins of the eye, as acids are, but tend to linger in the tissues, producing further damage long after exposure. A local anesthetic solution is instilled before the irrigation in order to relieve pain. The pupil should be dilated with sterile 2% atropine or 0.25% scopolamine solution to prevent synechia formation.

Corticosteroid ointment is placed in the affected eye often enough to relieve pain and irritation. The frequency of instillation depends upon the severity of the burn. The patient must be watched carefully for such complications as symblepharon, corneal scarring, closure of the puncta, and secondary infection.

ULTRAVIOLET KERATITIS
(Actinic Keratitis)

Ultraviolet burns of the cornea are usually caused by exposure to a welding arc or to the sun and snow when skiing ("snow blindness"). There are no immediate symptoms, but about 12 hours later the patient complains of agonizing pain and severe photophobia. Slitlamp examination after instillation of sterile fluorescein shows diffuse punctate staining of both corneas in the exposed areas.

Treatment consists of topical corticosteroids, systemic analgesics, and sedatives as indicated. All patients recover within 24–48 hours without complications.

ORBITAL INJURY

There are many types of injury to the bony orbit. Only blowout fracture will be considered here.

Blowout Fracture

Isolated orbital floor or "blowout" fracture, without concurrent orbital rim fracture, may follow blunt injury to the eye. Orbital contents herniate into the maxillary sinus, and the inferior rectus or inferior oblique muscle may become incarcerated at the fracture site.

Signs and symptoms are pain and nausea at the time of injury and diplopia on looking up or down. Diplopia may occur immediately or within a few days. Enophthalmos may not be present until the orbital reaction clears. The fracture site is best demonstrated by antral roof deformation on Waters' view x-rays or laminograms. There is limited movement of the eye even with forced ductions.

If the fracture is large or the muscle imbalance is great, prompt surgical reduction is imperative. If the vertical imbalance is small, surgery can be delayed a few days or weeks as long as steady improvement is noted. The orbital floor fracture is most commonly repaired using the Caldwell-Luc approach.

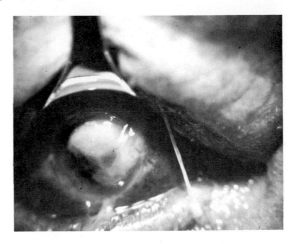

Figure 42–5. Pseudomonas corneal ulcer of right eye. Evisceration was done.

INFECTIONS OF THE EYE

1. BACTERIAL CORNEAL ULCER

Corneal ulcers constitute a medical emergency. The typical gray, necrotic corneal ulcer is preceded by trauma, usually a corneal foreign body. The eye is red with lacrimation and conjunctival discharge, and the patient complains of blurred vision, pain, and photophobia.

Prompt treatment is essential to prevent complications. Otherwise, visual impairment may occur as a result of corneal scarring or intraocular infection.

Corneal ulcers may result from many causes including bacterial, viral, fungal, and allergic. Only the most serious types will be discussed here.

Pneumococcal ("Acute Serpiginous") Ulcer

Streptococcus pneumoniae is the commonest bacterial cause of corneal ulcer. The early ulcer is gray and fairly well circumscribed.

Since the pneumococcus is sensitive to both sulfonamides and antibiotics, local therapy is usually effective. If untreated, the cornea may perforate. Concurrent dacryocystitis, if present, should also be treated.

Pseudomonas Ulcer

A less common but much more virulent cause of corneal ulcer is *Pseudomonas aeruginosa* (Fig 42–5). The ulceration characteristically starts in a traumatized area and spreads rapidly, frequently causing perforation of the cornea and loss of the eye within 48 hours. *Ps aeruginosa* usually produces a pathognomonic bluish-green pigment.

Early diagnosis and vigorous treatment with topical polymyxin and gentamicin are essential if the eye is to be saved.

2. HERPES SIMPLEX KERATITIS

Corneal ulceration caused by herpes simplex virus is more common than any type of bacterial corneal ulcer. It is almost always unilateral and may affect any age group of either sex. It is often preceded by facial "cold sores" and upper respiratory tract infection with fever.

The commonest finding is of one or more dendritic ulcers (superficial branching gray areas) on the corneal surface (Fig 42–6). These are composed of clear vesicles in the corneal epithelium; when the vesicles rupture, the area stains green with fluorescein. Although the dendritic figure is its most characteristic manifestation, herpes simplex keratitis may appear in a number of other configurations.

Treatment consists of mechanical removal of the virus-containing corneal epithelium without disturbing Bowman's membrane or the corneal stroma. This is best done by an ophthalmologist.

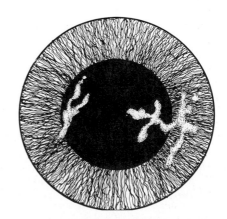

Figure 42–6. Herpes simplex keratitis with dendritic figures.

Frequent instillation of idoxuridine drops is used by many ophthalmologists in preference to removing the corneal epithelium.

3. ACUTE IRITIS
(Nongranulomatous Uveitis, Endogenous)

Nongranulomatous uveitis is primarily an anterior autoimmune noninfectious disease, but it may occasionally be associated with ankylosing spondylitis or Crohn's disease. The iris and ciliary body are primarily affected, but occasional foci are found in the choroid.

The onset is acute, with marked pain, redness, photophobia, and blurred vision. A circumcorneal flush, caused by dilated limbal blood vessels, is present. Fine white keratic precipitates (KPs) on the posterior surface of the cornea can be seen with the slitlamp or with a loupe. The pupil is small, and there may be a collection of fibrin with cells in the anterior chamber. If posterior synechias are present, the pupil will be irregular and the light reflex will be absent.

Local corticosteroid therapy tends to shorten the course. Warm compresses will decrease pain. Atropine, 2%, 2 drops in the affected eye, will prevent posterior synechia formation and alleviate photophobia. The frequency of instillation will depend upon the severity of the symptoms and may vary from once a day to several times a day. Recurrences are common, but the prognosis is good.

4. ORBITAL CELLULITIS

Orbital cellulitis is manifested by an abrupt onset of swelling and redness of the lids, often accompanied by proptosis (Fig 42–7). Fever is common. It is usu-

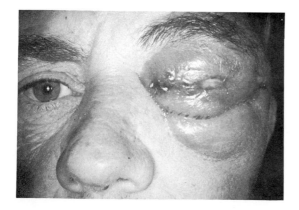

Figure 42–7. Orbital cellulitis. Abscess draining through upper eyelid.

ally caused by a pyogenic organism. Immediate treatment with systemic antibiotics is indicated to prevent brain abscess or rapid increase in the orbital pressure, causing subsequent embarrassment of the blood supply to the eye. The response to antibiotics is usually excellent.

DIPLOPIA

Double vision is due to muscle imbalance or to paralysis of an extraocular muscle as a result of inflammation, hemorrhage, trauma, tumefaction, congenital defect, or infection of the third, fourth, or sixth nerves. The sixth nerve is most commonly affected.

ANGLE-CLOSURE (ACUTE) GLAUCOMA

Acute glaucoma can occur only with the closure of a preexisting narrow anterior chamber angle. If the pupil dilates spontaneously or is dilated with a mydriatic or cycloplegic, the angle will close and an attack of acute glaucoma is precipitated; for this reason, it is a wise precaution to estimate the depth of the anterior chamber angle before instilling these drugs (Fig 42–8). About 1% of people over age 35 have narrow anterior chamber angles, but many of these never develop acute glaucoma.

A quiet eye with a narrow anterior chamber angle may convert spontaneously to angle-closure glaucoma. The process can be precipitated by anything that will dilate the pupil, eg, indiscriminate use of mydriatics or cycloplegics by the patient or the physician. The cycloplegic (anticholinergic) can be administered in the form of eyedrops or systemically, eg, by the anesthesiologist ordering scopolamine or atropine before a general surgical procedure. Increased circulating epinephrine in times of stress can also dilate the pupil and cause acute glaucoma. Sitting in a darkened movie theater can have the same effect.

It should be emphasized that about 95% of patients with glaucoma have the open angle (chronic) type and are in no danger of converting to angle-closure glaucoma. This is particularly important to understand when doing a general surgical procedure on a patient with open angle glaucoma. It is quite safe to premedicate with scopolamine, atropine, or other anticholinergic drugs. Acute glaucoma is usually precipitated by these drugs in patients with narrow anterior chamber angles without a history of glaucoma.

Patients with acute glaucoma seek treatment immediately because of extreme pain and blurring of vision. The eye is red, the cornea is steamy, and the pupil is moderately dilated and does not react to light. Intraocular pressure is elevated.

Acute glaucoma must be differentiated from conjunctivitis and acute iritis.

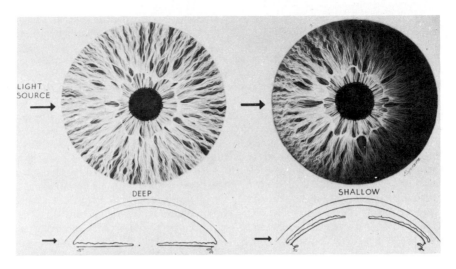

Figure 42–8. Estimation of depth of the anterior chamber by oblique illumination (diagram). (Courtesy of R. Shaffer.)

Peripheral iridectomy within 12–48 hours after onset of symptoms will usually result in a permanent cure. Untreated acute glaucoma results in complete and permanent blindness within 2–5 days after onset of symptoms. Before surgery, the intraocular pressure must be lowered by miotics instilled locally and osmotic agents and carbonic anhydrase inhibitors administered systemically.

OCCLUSION OF THE CENTRAL RETINAL ARTERY

This uncommon unilateral disorder (the ocular equivalent of coronary thrombosis) occurs only in older people. Occlusion may be the result of thrombin formation on a preexisting plaque or may be due to subintimal hemorrhage with resultant displacement of the plaque. Spasm of the artery is often a complicating factor. Emboli may occur. There is a sudden, painless, complete loss of vision in the affected eye. Ophthalmoscopic examination soon after onset reveals segmentation of the blood in the veins and arterioles as a result of the absence of retinal blood flow. The disk is pale, and there is marked retinal edema in the posterior pole associated with a cherry-red spot in the macula (Fig 42–9). If the occlusion is complete, total light perception is permanently lost and the pupil will not react directly to light (although the consensual pupillary light reflex is normal).

If the patient is seen within 30–60 minutes after onset, an effort should be made to restore blood flow through the obstructed artery by vigorous massage of the eyeball or paracentesis of the anterior chamber followed by systemic administration of a rapid-acting vasodilator, eg, tolazoline (Priscoline), 75 mg IV.

Because the retina can survive hypoxia longer than brain tissue, the prognosis is not hopeless if treatment is instituted promptly. If treatment is delayed for over 30–60 minutes, the visual prognosis is all but hopeless and the value of any type of treatment is questionable.

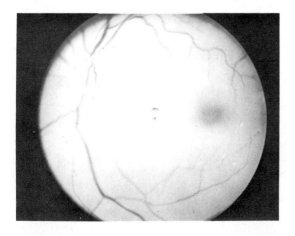

Figure 42–9. Twenty-four hours after closure of the central retinal artery, left eye. The disk is pale; the macula is edematous and ischemic. The fovea appears as a cherry-red spot because of its choroidal blood supply showing through.

RETINAL DETACHMENT

Essentials of Diagnosis
- Blurred vision in one eye becoming progressively worse. ("A curtain came down over my eye.")
- No pain or redness.
- Visible detachment ophthalmoscopically.

General Considerations

Detachment of the retina is usually spontaneous but may be secondary to trauma. Spontaneous detachment occurs most frequently in persons over 50 years old. Predisposing causes such as aphakia and myopia are commonly present.

Clinical Findings

As soon as the retina is torn, a transudate from the choroidal vessels, mixed with vitreous, combines with abnormal vitreous traction on the retina and the force of gravity to strip the retina from the choroid. The superior temporal area is the most common site of detachment. The area of detachment rapidly increases, causing correspondingly progressive visual loss (Fig 42—10). Central vision remains intact until the macula becomes detached.

On ophthalmoscopic examination, the retina is seen hanging in the vitreous like a gray cloud. One or more retinal tears, usually crescent-shaped and red or orange, are always present and can be seen by an experienced examiner.

Differential Diagnosis

Sudden partial loss of vision in one eye may also be due to vitreous hemorrhage or thrombosis of the central retinal vein or one of its branches.

Treatment

All cases of retinal detachment should be referred immediately to an ophthalmologist. If the patient must be transported a long distance, his head should be positioned so that the detached portion of the retina will recede with the aid of gravity. For example, a patient with a superior temporal retinal detachment in the right eye should lie on his back with his head turned to the right. Position is less important for a short trip.

Retinal detachment is a true emergency if the macula is threatened. If the macula is detached, permanent loss of central vision usually occurs even though the retina is eventually successfully reattached by surgery.

Treatment consists of drainage of the subretinal fluid and closure of the retinal tears by diathermy or scleral buckling (or both). This produces an inflammatory reaction which causes the retina to adhere to the choroid. Photocoagulation is of value in a limited number of cases of minimal detachment. It consists of focusing a strong light from various sources through the pupil to create an inflammatory adhesion between the choroid and the retina.

The main use of the photocoagulator and laser is in the prevention of detachment by sealing small retinal tears before detachment occurs.

Cryosurgery is also being used effectively in the treatment of retinal detachment. A supercooled probe is applied to the sclera to cause a chorioretinal scar with minimal scleral damage. This decreased scleral damage (as compared with diathermy) makes the operation less hazardous and, because scar formation is minimal, greatly facilitates reoperation. Cryosurgery may eventually replace diathermy completely.

Prognosis

About 85% of uncomplicated cases can be cured with one operation; an additional 10% will need repeated operations; the remainder never reattach. The prognosis is worse if the macula is detached, if there are many vitreous strands, or if the detachment is of long duration. Without treatment, retinal detachment almost always becomes total in 1—6 months. Spontaneous detachments are ultimately bilateral in 20—25% of cases.

VITREOUS HEMORRHAGE

Hemorrhage into the vitreous is an uncommon but serious disorder. It is usually due to traumatic rupture of a retinal vessel but may be related to diabetes mellitus, hypertension, perivasculitis, blood dyscrasia, or retinal detachment. One or both eyes may be affected, depending on the cause.

There is a sudden loss of vision in the affected eye. The fundus reflection is absent, but the anterior chamber, cornea, and lens are clear.

The prognosis for vision is guarded no matter what the cause, since the blood often remains in the vitreous for months. *Note:* These patients should be observed periodically, as the hemorrhage occasionally clears dramatically in a few days or weeks to reveal a retinal detachment. If this happens, vision may be restored by surgical reattachment of the retina.

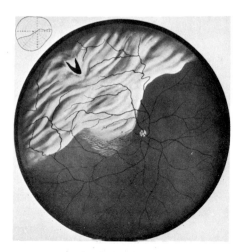

Figure 42—10. Retinal detachment and retinal tear 6 days after onset. (From Arruga: *Detachment of Retina.* Salvat, 1936.)

HORDEOLUM

Hordeolum is a common staphylococcal abscess which is characterized by a localized red, swollen, acutely tender area on the upper or lower lid. Internal hordeolum is a meibomian gland abscess which points to the skin or to the conjunctival side of the lid; external hordeolum or sty (infection of the glands of Moll or Zeis) is smaller and on the margin.

The primary symptom is pain. The severity of the pain is directly related to the amount of swelling.

Warm compresses are helpful. Incision is indicated if resolution does not begin within 48 hours. An antibiotic or sulfonamide instilled into the conjunctival sac every 3 hours is beneficial during the acute stage. Without treatment, internal hordeolum may lead to generalized cellulitis of the lid.

CHALAZION

Chalazion is a common granulomatous inflammation of a meibomian gland characterized by a hard, nontender swelling on the upper or lower lid. It may be preceded by a sty. The majority point toward the conjunctival side.

If the chalazion is large enough to impress the cornea, vision will be distorted. The conjunctiva in the region of the chalazion is red and elevated.

Treatment consists of excision by an ophthalmologist.

DACRYOCYSTITIS

Dacryocystitis is a common infection of the lacrimal sac. It may be acute or chronic and occurs most often in infants and in persons over 40. It is usually unilateral and is always secondary to obstruction of the nasolacrimal duct.

Adult Dacryocystitis

The cause of obstruction is usually unknown, but a history of trauma to the nose may be obtained. In acute dacryocystitis, the usual infectious organism is *Staphylococcus aureus* or the beta-hemolytic streptococcus; in chronic dacryocystitis, *Streptococcus pneumoniae. Haemophilus influenzae* is not a cause of dacryocystitis in adults. Mixed infections do not occur.

Acute dacryocystitis is characterized by pain, swelling, tenderness, and redness in the tear sac area; pus may be expressed. In chronic dacryocystitis, tearing and discharge are the principal signs. Mucus or pus may be expressed from the tear sac.

Acute dacryocystitis responds well to antibiotic therapy, but recurrences are common if the obstruction is not surgically removed. The chronic form may

be kept latent by using antibiotic eye drops, but relief of the obstruction is the only cure.

Infantile Dacryocystitis

H influenzae is the only organism that causes infantile dacryocystitis.

Normally the nasolacrimal ducts open spontaneously during the first month of life. Occasionally, one of the ducts fails to canalize and a secondary pneumococcal dacryocystitis develops. When this happens, forceful massage of the tear sac is indicated, and antibiotic or sulfonamide drops should be instilled in the conjunctival sac 4–5 times daily. If this is not successful after a few weeks, probing of the nasolacrimal duct is indicated regardless of the infant's age. When probing the nasolacrimal duct, the probe should be passed through the upper canaliculus; it is easier to do and avoids possible trauma to the lower canaliculus, the more important tear drainage canal.

STRABISMUS

Any child under age 7 with strabismus should be seen without delay to prevent or to treat the beginning of amblyopia. In adults, the sudden onset of strabismus usually follows head trauma, intracranial hemorrhage, or brain tumor.

About 5% of children are born with or develop a malfunction of binocular coordination known as strabismus. In descending order of frequency, the eyes may deviate inward (esotropia), outward (exotropia), upward (hypertropia), or downward (hypotropia). The cause is not known, but fusion is lacking in almost all cases. If a child is born with straight eyes but has inherited "weak fusion," he may develop strabismus.

Clinical Findings

Children with frank strabismus first develop diplopia. They soon learn to suppress the image from the deviating eye and the vision in that eye therefore fails to develop. This is the first stage of amblyopia ex anopsia.

Most cases of strabismus are obvious, but if the angle of deviation is small or if the strabismus is intermittent, the diagnosis may be obscure. The best method for detecting strabismus is to direct a light toward each pupil from a distance of 1–2 feet. If the corneal reflection is seen in the center of each pupil, the eyes can be presumed to be straight at that moment.

As a further diagnostic test ("cover test"), cover the right eye with an opaque object ("cover") and instruct the patient to fix his gaze on the examining light with the left eye. If fusion is weak, covering the right eye will disturb the fusion process sufficiently to allow the right eye to deviate, and this can be observed behind the cover. The right eye may swing back into alignment when the cover is removed (phoria). In obvious strabismus, the covered eye will maintain the deviated position after the cover is removed (tropia). Ask the patient to follow the examining light with both eyes to the right, left, up, and down to rule out extraocular muscle paralysis. If there is a history of deviation but it cannot be demonstrated, the patient should be reexamined in a few months.

Prevention

Amblyopia due to strabismus can be detected by routine visual acuity examination of all preschool children. Visual acuity testing is best done with an illiterate E card close to the fourth birthday by the child's mother, but is often performed in the physician's office as a routine procedure. Treatment by occlusion of the good eye is simple and effective.

The prevention of blindness by these simple diagnostic and treatment procedures is one of the most rewarding experiences in medical practice.

Treatment

The objectives in the treatment of strabismus are (1) good visual acuity in each eye; (2) straight eyes, for cosmetic purposes; and (3) coordinate function of both eyes.

The best time to initiate treatment is around the age of 6 months. If treatment is delayed beyond this time, the child will favor the straight eye and suppress the image in the other eye; this results in failure of visual development (amblyopia ex anopsia) in the deviating eye.

If the child is under 7 years of age and has an amblyopic eye, the amblyopia can be cured by occluding the good eye. At 1 year of age, patching may be successful within 1 week; at 6 years it may take a year to achieve the same result, ie, to equalize the visual acuity in both eyes. Prolonged patching seldom impairs vision in the good eye. Surgery is usually performed after the visual acuity has been equalized.

Prognosis

The prognosis is more favorable for strabismus which has its onset at age 1–4 than for strabismus which is present at birth; better for divergent (outward deviation) than for convergent strabismus; and better for intermittent than for constant strabismus.

OTHER DISEASES OF THE EYE

OCULAR TUMORS

Many tumors of the ocular adnexa can be completely excised if they are diagnosed in an early stage.

Malignant intraocular tumors (except of the iris) nearly always require enucleation. The 2 most common intraocular tumors are retinoblastoma and malignant melanoma.

OPTIC NERVE PATHOLOGY

Optic nerve disorders such as optic neuritis, optic atrophy, and papilledema are very serious and may indicate accompanying intracranial or systemic disease. The patient should be examined from a neurologic as well as an ophthalmologic standpoint.

SYMPATHETIC OPHTHALMIA
(Sympathetic Uveitis)

Sympathetic ophthalmia is a rare, severe bilateral granulomatous uveitis. The cause is not known, but the disease may occur at any time from 1 week to many years after a penetrating injury near the ciliary body. The injured (exciting) eye becomes inflamed first and the fellow (sympathizing) eye second. Symptoms and signs include blurred vision with light sensitivity and redness.

The best treatment of sympathetic ophthalmia is prevention by removing the damaged eye. Any severely injured eye (eg, one with perforation of the sclera and ciliary body, with loss of vitreous and retinal damage) should be enucleated within 1 week after the injury. Every effort should be made to secure the patient's reasoned consent to the operation. In established cases of sympathetic ophthalmia, systemic corticosteroid therapy may be helpful. Without treatment, the disease progresses gradually to bilateral blindness.

CHRONIC GLAUCOMA

Antiglaucoma therapy should be instituted without delay in order to decrease the intraocular pressure and preserve the remaining visual field.

UNILATERAL EXOPHTHALMOS OF RECENT ORIGIN

The most common cause of bilateral exophthalmos is hyperthyroidism, although it may also appear after thyroidectomy. Unilateral exophthalmos may be due to an orbital tumor, cavernous sinus thrombosis, or atrioventricular shunt from the internal carotid artery to the cavernous sinus. Some of these disorders are treatable.

·   ·   ·

TECHNICS USED IN THE TREATMENT OF OCULAR DISORDERS

Instilling Medications

Place the patient in a chair with his head tilted back, both eyes open, and looking up. Retract the lower lid slightly and instill 2 drops of liquid into the lower cul-de-sac. Have the patient look down while finger contact on the lower lid is maintained for a few seconds. Do not let him squeeze his eye shut.

Ointments are instilled in the same general manner.

Self-Medication

The same technics are used as described above, except that drops should usually be instilled with the patient lying down.

Eye Bandage

Most eye bandages should be applied firmly enough to hold the lid securely against the cornea. An ordinary patch consisting of gauze-covered cotton is usually sufficient. Tape is applied from the cheek to the forehead. If more pressure is desired, use 2 or 3 bandages. A black eye patch is difficult to sterilize and therefore is seldom used in modern medical practice.

Water Compresses

A clean towel or washcloth soaked in warm tap water is applied to the affected eye 2–4 times a day for 10–15 minutes.

Removal of a Superficial Corneal Foreign Body

Record the patient's visual acuity, if possible, and instill sterile local anesthetic drops. With the patient sitting or lying down, an assistant should direct a strong light into the eye so that the rays strike the cornea obliquely. Using either a loupe or a slitlamp, the physician locates the foreign body on the corneal surface. He may remove it with a sterile wet cotton applicator or, if this fails, with a spud, holding the lids apart with the other hand to prevent blinking. An antibacterial ointment (eg, Polysporin) is instilled after the foreign body has been removed. It is preferable not to patch the eye, but the patient must be seen on the following day to make certain healing is under way.

PRECAUTIONS IN THE MANAGEMENT OF OCULAR DISORDERS

Use of Local Anesthetics

Unsupervised self-administration of local anesthetics is dangerous because they delay healing and because the patient may further injure an anesthetized eye without knowing it.

Pupillary Dilation

Cycloplegics and mydriatics should be used with caution. Dilating the pupil can precipitate an attack of acute glaucoma if the patient has a narrow anterior chamber angle.

Local Corticosteroid Therapy

Repeated use of local corticosteroids presents several serious hazards: herpes simplex (dendritic) keratitis, fungal overgrowth, open angle glaucoma, and cataract. Furthermore, perforation of the cornea may occur when the corticosteroids are used for herpes simplex keratitis.

Contaminated Eye Medications

Ophthalmic solutions must be prepared with the same degree of care as fluids intended for intravenous administration.

Tetracaine (Pontocaine), proparacaine (Ophthaine, Ophthetic), physostigmine, and fluorescein are most likely to become contaminated. The most dangerous is fluorescein, as this solution is frequently contaminated with *Pseudomonas aeruginosa,* an organism which can rapidly destroy the eye. Sterile fluorescein filter paper strips are now available and are recommended in place of fluorescein solutions.

Plastic dropper bottles are becoming more popular each year. Solutions from these bottles are safe to use in uninjured eyes. Whether in plastic or glass containers, eye solutions should not be used for more than about 2 weeks after the bottle is first opened.

If the eye has been injured accidentally or by surgical trauma, it is critical to use sterile medications supplied in sterile, disposable, single use eye-dropper units.

Fungal Overgrowth

Since antibiotics, like corticosteroids, when used over a prolonged time in bacterial corneal ulcers, favor the development of secondary fungal corneal infection, the sulfonamides should be used whenever they are adequate for the purpose.

Sensitization

A significant portion of a soluble substance instilled in the eye may pass into the blood stream. An antibiotic instilled into the eye can sensitize the patient to that drug and cause a hypersensitivity reaction upon subsequent systemic administration.

·   ·   ·

General References

Allen JH: *May's Manual of Diseases of the Eye,* 24th ed. Williams & Wilkins, 1968.

Arruga HM: *Ocular Surgery,* 3rd English ed. McGraw-Hill, 1962. [Translated from the Spanish by Hogan and Chapparo.]

Beard C, Quickert MH: *Anatomy of the Orbit: A Dissection Manual.* Aesculapius, 1969.

Blodi FC (editor): *Current Concepts in Ophthalmology.* Vol 4. Mosby, 1974.

Duke-Elder WS: *Parson's Diseases of the Eye,* 15th ed. Churchill, 1970.

Ellis PP, Smith DL: *Handbook of Ocular Therapeutics and Pharmacology,* 4th ed. Mosby, 1973.

Havener WH: *Atlas of Cataract Surgery.* Mosby, 1972.

Havener WH: *Ocular Pharmacology,* 3rd ed. Mosby, 1974.

Hogan MJ, Zimmermann LE: *Ophthalmic Pathology: An Atlas and Textbook,* 2nd ed. Saunders, 1962.

Hughes WF (editor): *Year Book of Ophthalmology.* Year Book, 1976.

Keeney AH: *Ocular Examination: Basis and Technique,* 2nd ed. Mosby, 1976.

King JH, Wadsworth JAC: *An Atlas of Ophthalmic Surgery,* 2nd ed. Lippincott, 1970.

Kolker AE, Hetherington J: *Becker-Shaffer's Diagnosis and Therapy of the Glaucomas,* 4th ed. Mosby, 1976.

Leopold IH (editor): *Symposium on Ocular Therapy.* Vol 7. Mosby, 1974.

Martin-Doyle JLC: *A Synopsis of Ophthalmology,* 4th ed. Williams & Wilkins, 1971.

Moses RA: *Adler's Physiology of the Eye: Clinical Application,* 6th ed. Mosby, 1975.

Newell FW, Ernest JT: *Ophthalmology: Principles and Concepts,* 3rd ed. Mosby, 1974.

Scheie HG, Albert DM: *Adler's Textbook of Ophthalmology,* 8th ed. Saunders, 1969.

Trevor-Roper PD: *Lecture Notes on Ophthalmology,* 5th ed. Blackwell, 1975.

Vaughan D, Asbury T: *General Ophthalmology,* 8th ed. Lange, 1977.

Von Noorden GK, Maumenee AE: *Atlas of Strabismus,* 2nd ed. Mosby, 1973.

Walsh FB, Hoyt WF: *Clinical Neuro-ophthalmology,* 3rd ed. Williams & Wilkins, 1969.

43...
Urology

Emil A. Tanagho, MD, & Donald R. Smith, MD

DEVELOPMENT OF THE GENITOURINARY TRACT & ANOMALIES OF DEVELOPMENT

Embryologically, the genital and urinary systems are intimately related. Associated anomalies are commonly encountered.

THE KIDNEYS

The kidneys pass through 3 embryonic phases (Fig 43–1): (1) The **pronephros** is a vestigial structure that disappears completely by the fourth week except for its primary duct. (2) The primary duct gains connection to the **mesonephros** tubules and becomes the mesonephric duct. While most of the mesonephric tubules degenerate, the mesonephric duct persists; where it bends to open into the cloaca, the ureteric bud develops, starts to grow cranially, and meets the metanephric blastema. (3) This forms the **metanephros**, which is the final phase. During cephalad migration and rotation, the metanephric tissue progressively enlarges, with rapid internal differentiation into small vesicular masses that will later differentiate into uriniferous tubules. Simultaneously, the cephalad end of the ureteric bud expands within the metanephros to form the renal pelvis. Numerous outgrowths from the renal pelvic dilatation develop, branch and rebranch, and finally connect to the differentiating metanephric vesicular masses, establishing continuity of the secreting and collecting ducts.

Failure of the metanephros to ascend leads to ectopic kidney; failure to rotate during ascent causes a malrotated kidney. Horseshoe kidney results from fusion of the 2 metanephric masses.

Bifurcation of the ureteric bud results in a bifid ureter. Development of an accessory bud leads to a duplicated ureter, commonly meeting the same nephric mass; rarely, each bud has a separate metanephric

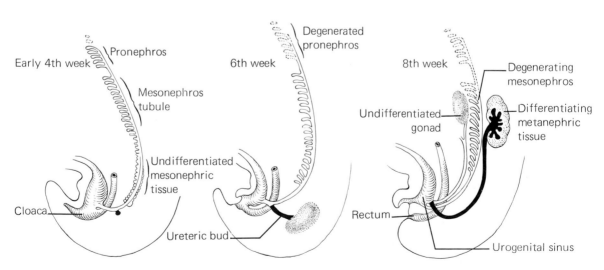

Figure 43–1. Schematic representation of the development of the nephric system. Only a few of the tubules of the pronephros are seen early in the fourth week, while the mesonephric tissue differentiates into mesonephric tubules that progressively join the mesonephric duct. The first sign of the ureteric bud from the mesonephric duct is seen. At 6 weeks, the pronephros has completely degenerated and the mesonephric tubules start to do so. The ureteric bud grows dorsocranially and has met the metanephrogenic cap. At the eighth week there is cranial migration of the differentiating metanephros. The cranial end of the ureteric bud expands and starts to show multiple successive outgrowths.

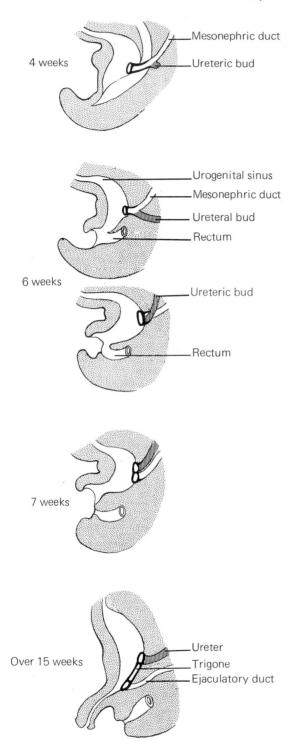

4 weeks — Mesonephric duct
— Ureteric bud

6 weeks — Urogenital sinus
— Mesonephric duct
— Ureteral bud
— Rectum

— Ureteric bud
— Rectum

7 weeks

Over 15 weeks — Ureter
— Trigone
— Ejaculatory duct

Figure 43—2. The development of the ureteric bud from the mesonephric duct and their relationship to the urogenital sinus. The ureteric bud appears at the fourth week. The mesonephric duct distal to this ureteric bud will be gradually absorbed into the urogenital sinus, resulting in separate endings for the ureter and the mesonephric duct. The mesonephric tissue that is incorporated into the urogenital sinus will expand and form the trigonal tissue.

mass, resulting in supernumerary kidneys. Failure of a ureteric bud to develop results in a solitary kidney and a hemitrigone.

BLADDER & URETHRA

Subdivision of the cloaca (the blind end of the hindgut) into a ventral (urogenital sinus) and a dorsal (rectum) segment is completed during the seventh week and initiates the early differentiation of the urinary bladder and urethra. The urogenital sinus receives the mesonephric duct and gradually absorbs its caudal end so that by the end of the seventh week the ureteric bud and mesonephric duct have independent openings. The former migrates upward and laterally. The latter moves downward and medially, and the structure in between (the trigone) is formed by the absorbed mesodermal tissue, which maintains direct continuity between the 2 tubes (Fig 43–2).

The fused müllerian ducts also meet the urogenital sinus at Müller's tubercle. The urogenital sinus above Müller's tubercle differentiates to form the bladder and part of the urethra in the male (supramontanal part of the prostatic urethra) or the bladder and the whole urethra in the female. Below it, the urogenital sinus differentiates into the inframontanal part of the prostatic urethra and the membranous urethra in the male or the distal vagina and vaginal vestibule in the female. The rest of the male urethra is formed by fusion of the urethral folds on the ventral surface of the genital tubercle. In the female, the genital folds remain separate and form the labia minora.

Failure of cloacal division results in persistent cloaca. Incomplete division is more frequent and results in rectovesical, rectourethral, or rectovestibular fistulas (usually with imperforate anus or anal atresia). Development of genital primordia in an area more caudal than normal results in complete or incomplete epispadias. A more extensive defect results in vesical exstrophy. Failure of the urethral folds to fuse leads to various grades of hypospadias.

The prostate develops at the end of the 11th week as 5 groups of outgrowths of urethral epithelium both above and below the entrance of the mesonephric duct. These form the 5 lobes of the prostate. The developing glandular element incorporates within it the differentiating mesenchymal cells surrounding that segment of the urogenital sinus. These form the muscular stroma and capsule of the prostate.

THE GONADS

Each embryo is at first morphologically bisexual; the development of one set of sex primordia and the gradual involution of the other are determined by the sex type of the gonad, which starts to be differentiated during the seventh week (Fig 43—3). If the gonad develops into a testis, the germinal epithelium grows into radially arranged, cord-like masses that differentiate later into seminiferous tubules. If it develops into an ovary, it becomes differentiated into a cortex and a medulla; the cortex later differentiates into ovarian follicles containing ova.

The testis remains at the abdominal end of the inguinal canal until the seventh month. It then passes through the inguinal canal to the scrotum, guided by the primary attachment of the gubernaculum. The ovary undergoes internal descent to enter the pelvis.

Lack of complete testicular descent is known as cryptorchidism; descent to an abnormal site is known as testicular ectopia. In the male, the genital duct system develops from the wolffian duct, which differentiates into epididymis, vas deferens, seminal vesicles, and ejaculatory ducts. In the female, the genital duct system develops from the müllerian ducts, which

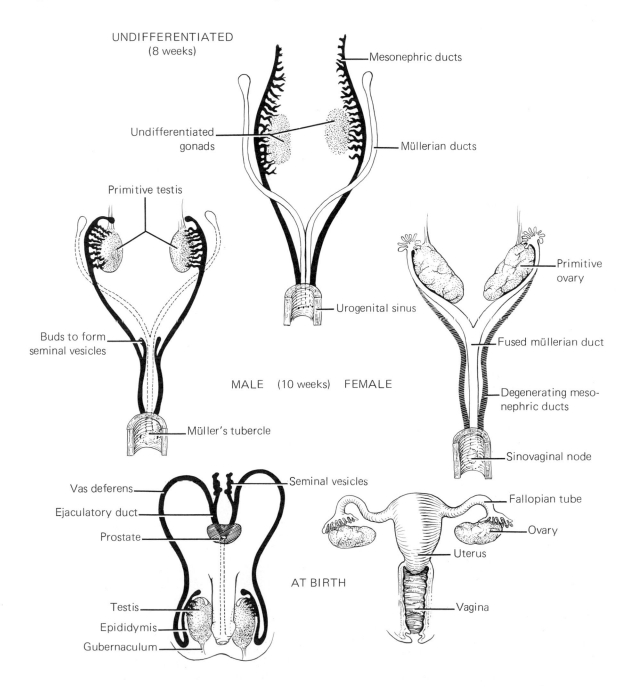

Figure 43—3. Transformation of the undifferentiated genital system into the definitive male and female systems.

fuse at their caudal ends and differentiate into the fallopian tubes, uterus, and most of the vagina.

The external genitalia start to differentiate by the eighth week. The genital tubercle and the genital swellings develop into the penis and scrotum in the male and the clitoris and labia majora in the female.

With the breakdown of the urogenital membrane in the seventh week, the urogenital sinus achieves a separate opening on the undersurface of the genital tubercle. The expansion of the infratubercular part of the urogenital sinus will form the vaginal vestibule and distal part of the vagina. The 2 folds on the undersurface of the genital tubercle unite in the male to form the penile urethra; in the female, they remain separate to form the labia minora. Their failure to fuse in the male leads to hypospadias, which is usually associated with incomplete formation of the prepuce with a dorsal hood and a ventral penile curvature. It is never proximal to the bulbous urethra, and continence is always preserved. Epispadias is a milder form of bladder exstrophy. If extensive, epispadias can extend to the bladder neck and is frequently associated with incontinence. A rudimentary penis or a hypertrophied clitoris is seen with pseudohermaphroditism.

·   ·   ·

Ambrose SS, O'Brien DP III: Surgical embryology of the exstrophy-epispadias complex. Surg Clin North Am 54:1379, 1974.

Gray SW, Skandalakis JE: *Embryology for Surgeons.* Saunders, 1972.

Mackie GG, Stephens FD: Duplex kidneys: A correlation of renal dysplasia with position of ureteral orifice. J Urol 114:274, 1975.

Schulman CC: The single ectopic ureter. Eur Urol 2:69, 1976.

Stephens FD: *Congenital Malformations of the Rectum, Anus and Genitourinary Tracts.* Livingstone, 1963.

Tanagho EA: Embryologic basis of lower ureteral anomalies. Urology 5:451, 1976.

APPLIED ANATOMY OF THE GENITOURINARY TRACT: GROSS & MICROSCOPIC

The Kidneys

The kidneys are paired organs lying retroperitoneally in the posterior abdomen and separated from the surrounding renal fascia by perinephric fat. The renal vascular pedicle enters the renal sinus; the vein is anterior to the artery, and both are anterior to the renal pelvis. The renal artery divides in the renal sinus into anterior and posterior branches that undergo further subdivisions with variable extents of distribution. They are end arteries. The venous tributaries anastomose freely and usually drain into one renal vein. Accessory vessels are not uncommon.

The Renal Parenchyma

The renal parenchyma consists of over 1 million functioning units (nephrons) and is divided into a peripheral cortex containing secretory elements and a central medulla containing excretory elements. The nephron starts as Bowman's capsule, which surrounds the glomeruli and leads to a long tubular structure consisting of proximal and distal convoluted tubules with the loop of Henle in between; it ends in a collecting duct that opens at the tip of a papilla into a minor calyx.

The Renal Pelvis & Calyces

The renal pelvis and calyces are within the renal sinus and function as the main collecting reservoir. The pelvis, which is partly extrarenal and partly intrarenal (but could be totally extra- or intrarenal), branches into 3 major calyces that in turn branch into several minor calyces. These calyces are directly related to the renal parenchyma; they receive the tips of the medullary pyramids (the papillae) and act as a receiving cup to the collecting tubules. The pelvicalyceal system is a highly muscular structure; the musculature runs in every direction and is directly continuous between the pelvis and the various calyces, helping to synchronize their contractile activity.

The Ureter

The ureter connects the renal pelvis to the urinary bladder. It is a small, muscularized tube; its muscle fibers lie in an irregular helical arrangement and are meant primarily for peristaltic activity. Ureteral musculature is directly continuous with the renal pelvis cranially and with the vesical trigone distally.

The pelvic and ureteric blood supply is segmental, arising from the renal, spermatic or ovarian, and vesical arteries—with rich subadventitial anastomosis.

The Bladder

The bladder is primarily a reservoir with a meshwork of muscle bundles that not only change from one plane to the other but also branch and join each other to constitute a synchronized organ. Its musculature is directly continuous with the urethral musculature, and this functions as a urethral sphincteric mechanism in spite of the lack of a true circular sphincter.

The ureters enter the bladder posteroinferiorly through the ureteral hiatus; after a short intravesical submucosal course, they lose their lumen and become continuous with the trigone, which is superimposed on the bladder base though deeply connected to it.

The Urethra

The adult female urethra is about 4 cm long and is muscular in its proximal four-fifths. This musculature is arranged in an inner longitudinal coat which is continuous with the inner longitudinal fibers of the bladder, and an outer circular coat which is continuous with the outer longitudinal coat of the bladder. These outer circular fibers comprise the sphincteric mechanism. The striated external sphincter surrounds the middle third of the urethra.

In the male, the prostatic urethra is heavily muscular and sphincteric. The membranous urethra is within the urogenital diaphragm and is surrounded by the striated external sphincter. The penile urethra is poorly muscularized and traverses the corpus spongiosum to open at the tip of the glans.

The Prostate

The prostate surrounds the proximal portion of the male urethra; it is a fibromuscular, glandular, cone-shaped structure about 2.5 cm long and weighing about 20 g. It is traversed from base to apex by the urethra and is pierced posterolaterally by the ejaculatory ducts that converge to open at the verumontanum on the floor of the urethra.

The prostatic glandular elements drain through about 12 paired excretory ducts that open into the floor of the urethra above the verumontanum. The prostate is surrounded by a thin capsule, derived from its stroma, which is rich in musculature, and part of the urethral musculature and the sphincteric mechanism. A rich venous plexus surrounds the prostate, especially anteriorly and laterally. Its arterial blood supply is from the inferior vesical, internal pudendal, and middle hemorrhoidal arteries. Its lymphatic drainage is into the hypogastric, sacral, vesical, and external iliac lymph nodes.

The Testis

The testis is a paired organ surrounded by the tunica albuginea and subdivided into numerous lobules by fibrous septa. The extremely convoluted seminiferous tubules gather to open into the rete testis, where they join the efferent duct to drain into the epididymis.

Arterial supply is via the internal spermatic artery; venous drainage is through the pampiniform plexus, which drains into the spermatic veins. The right joins the vena cava and the left joins the renal vein.

The lymphatics drain into the lumbar lymph nodes.

Cussen LJ: The structure of the normal human ureter in infancy and childhood. Invest Urol 5:179, 1967.
Hutch JA, Rambo ON Jr: A study of the anatomy of the prostate, prostatic urethra and the urinary sphincter system. J Urol 104:443, 1970.
Osathanondh V, Potter EL: Development of human kidney shown by microdissection. 4. Development of tubular portions of nephrons. 5. Development of vascular pattern of glomerulus. (2 parts.) Arch Pathol 82:391, 403, 1966.
Tanagho EA, Meyers FH, Smith DR: The trigone: Anatomical and physiological considerations. (2 parts.) J Urol 100:623, 633, 1968.

PHYSIOLOGY OF THE URINARY SYSTEM

The Kidneys

The kidneys maintain and regulate homeostasis of body fluids by the following mechanisms:

A. Glomerular Filtration: This is dependent on glomerular capillary arterial pressure minus plasma colloid osmotic pressure plus capsular resistance. The resultant glomerular filtration pressure (about 10–15 mm Hg) forces protein-free plasma through the capillary filtering surface into Bowman's capsule. Normally, about 130 ml of plasma are filtered every minute through the extremely rich renal circulation; every drop of plasma recirculates through the kidney and is subjected to the filtration process once every 27 minutes.

B. Tubular Reabsorption: About 99% of the filtered volume will be reabsorbed through the tubules, together with all the valuable constituents of the filtrate (chlorides, glucose, sodium, potassium, calcium, and amino acids). Urea, uric acid, phosphates, and sulfates are also reabsorbed to varying degrees. The process of reabsorption is partly passive (by diffusion) and partly active. Reabsorption of water and electrolytes is under control of adrenal, pituitary, and parathyroid hormonal influence.

C. Tubular Secretion: This helps (1) to eliminate and thus maintain plasma levels of certain substances, or (2) to exchange valuable ions from the filtrate for less desirable ions in the plasma (eg, sodium ion from the urine for a hydrogen ion in the plasma). Failure of adequate secretory function leads to the acidosis commonly encountered in chronic renal disease.

The Uretero-pelvicalyceal System

This system is one continuous tubular structure with adequate musculature which is imperceptibly moving from one segment to the other to maintain anatomic continuity and physiologic synchrony at various levels. Waves of contraction starting from the renal pelvis or occasionally from the calyces usually proceed in antegrade (anterograde) fashion toward the urinary bladder. These peristaltic waves occur at a rate of about 5–8 per minute, involve 2–3 cm segments at a time, and usually proceed at the velocity of 3 cm/second. Frequency, amplitude, and velocity are influenced by urine output and flow rate. Ureteral filling is primarily passive; ureteral emptying is primarily active. Ureteral peristaltic activity is essential in order to transport urine across points of resistance (eg, ureterovesical junction) and to prevent retrograde flow.

The Ureterovesical Junction

The ureterovesical junction allows free flow of urine from the ureter to the bladder and at the same time prevents retrograde flow. The continuity and the specific muscular arrangement of the intravesical ureter and the trigone provide a muscularly active valvular mechanism that can efficiently adapt itself to the variable phases of bladder activity during filling and voiding.

Progressive bladder filling leads to firm occlusion of the intravesical ureter against retrograde flow and increased resistance to antegrade urine flow due to trigonal stretching. During voiding, trigonal contraction completely seals the intravesical ureter against any antegrade flow of urine and definitely against any retrograde flow.

The Urinary Bladder

The urinary bladder functions primarily as a reservoir that can accommodate variable volumes without increasing its intraluminal pressure. When the bladder reaches full capacity voluntarily, the detrusor muscle contracts uniformly and maintains its contraction until the bladder is completely empty. Funneling of the bladder outlet with progressive downward movement of the dome ensures complete emptying.

The vesical sphincteric mechanism is primarily a smooth muscle sphincter in the male prostatic urethra and in the proximal four-fifths of the female urethra. There is no purely circular sphincteric entity, but there are abundant circularly oriented muscle fibers which are directly continuous with the outer coat of the detrusor muscles. The sphincter has the same nerve supply as, and reacts simultaneously with, the detrusor. It maintains urethral closure by its passive tone, yet when it shares detrusor contraction it does not hinder voiding.

There is another voluntary striated sphincter which is part of the urogenital diaphragm and surrounds the midurethra in the female and the membranous urethra in the male. It is not essential for continence, though it adds to urethral resistance. Its pathologic irritability or spasticity can lead to obstructive manifestations.

Harper HA, Rodwell V, Mayes PA: *Review of Physiological Chemistry,* 16th ed. Lange, 1977.

Maxwell MH, Kleeman CR (editors): *Clinical Disorders of Fluid and Electrolyte Metabolism,* 2nd ed. Blakiston-McGraw, 1972.

Pitts RF: *Physiology of the Kidney and Body Fluids,* 3rd ed. Year Book, 1974.

Vander AJ: *Renal Physiology,* McGraw-Hill, 1975.

Welt L: *Clinical Disorders of Hydration and Acid-Base Equilibrium,* 3rd ed. Little, Brown, 1971.

Wesson LG Jr: *Physiology of the Human Kidney.* Grune & Stratton, 1969.

Windhager EE: Kidney, water and electrolytes. Annu Rev Physiol 31:198, 1969.

VESICOURETERAL REFLUX

The main function of the ureterovesical junction is to offer free drainage from the ureter to the bladder and at the same time to prevent urine that passes through from refluxing back. Anatomically, the ureterovesical junction is well equipped for this function. Although the ureter seemingly ends at the ureteral orifice, all of its musculature actually continues uninterrupted into the base of the bladder to form the superficial trigone. The intravesical ureter is of purely longitudinal muscle fibers. The roof fibers split at the ureteral orifice and sweep on either side to meet the floor fibers and continue as one sheet, the superficial trigone. The terminal 4–5 cm of ureter are surrounded by a musculofascial sheath (Waldeyer's sheath) which follows the ureter through the ureteral hiatus; after its fibers split on the roof of the ureter, they sweep to the sides and continue in the base of the bladder as the deep trigone (Fig 43–4).

Both the superficial and the deep trigones are superimposed on the detrusor muscle. The deep trigone, which is closely adherent to the detrusor, forms the link between the ureteral mesodermal structures and the detrusor endodermal structure through interchange of a few muscle fibers. Direct continuity between the ureter and the trigone offers an efficient, muscularly active, valvular function. Any stretch of the trigone (with bladder filling) or any trigonal contraction (with voiding) leads to firm occlusion of the intravesical ureter, thus increasing resistance to flow from

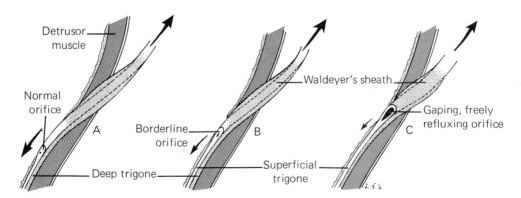

Figure 43–4. Vesicoureteral reflux. The length and fixation of the intravesical ureter and the appearance of the ureteral orifice depend upon the muscular development and efficiency of the lower ureter and its trigone. The normal appearance is shown in *A.* Moderate muscular deficiency leads to the appearance shown in *B.* Marked deficiency results in a golf hole distortion of the submucosal ureter as shown in *C.*

above downward and perfectly sealing the intravesical ureter against any retrograde flow (Fig 43—5).

Etiology & Classification

Vesicoureteral reflux may be classified according to cause as follows:

(1) Primary reflux (developmental ureterotrigonal weakness).

(2) Reflux secondary to infravesical obstruction, neurogenic dysfunction, iatrogenic causes, and inflammation, especially specific infection (eg, tuberculosis).

(3) Reflux due to congenital ureteral anomalies—ectopic orifices, duplicated ureters, or ureterocele.

Primary reflux is by far the most common type and is consistently associated with some degree of developmental muscular deficiency in the trigone and terminal ureter. The severity of reflux is proportionate to the degree of this muscular deficiency.

Secondary reflux and congenital types are relatively rare. In most such cases there is also an underlying muscular deficiency, especially in cases of inflammation. Aside from specific infections (tuberculosis, schistosomiasis), nonspecific infections can never lead to reflux unless there is an underlying muscular deficiency in a marginally competent valve.

Reflux is harmful to the upper urinary tract for the following reasons: (1) It leads to postvoiding residual urine that encourages infection. (2) It carries infection from the bladder to the kidney. (3) It permits the relatively high intravesical pressure to be transmitted to the renal papillae and calyceal fornices leading to interstitial extravasation of sterile or infected urine. (4) It has serious hydrodynamic effects since it increases the load of urine to be transported by the ureter and also subjects the weak pelviureteral musculature to high intravesical pressures, leading to stasis, dilatation, and tortuosity. (5) It can encourage stone formation, papillary necrosis, or secondary ureteropelvic junction obstruction.

Reflux is the commonest cause of pyelonephritis and is found in about 50% of children presenting with urinary tract infection. It is present in over 75% of patients with radiologic evidence of chronic pyelonephritis. Inability to demonstrate reflux does not exclude its presence.

In primary reflux, the patient usually presents

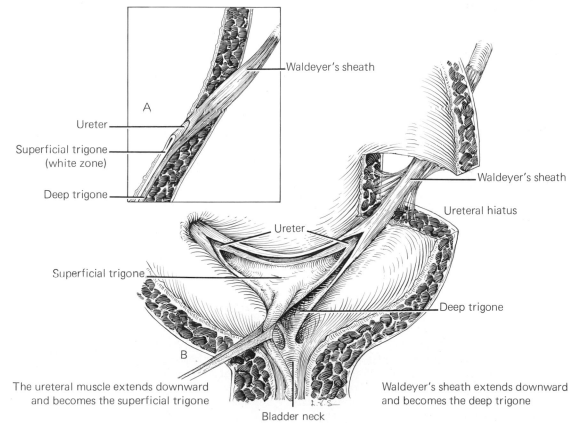

Figure 43—5. Normal ureterotrigonal complex. *A:* Side view of ureterovesical junction. Waldeyer's muscular sheath invests the juxtavesical ureter and continues downward as the deep trigone, which extends to the bladder neck. The ureteral musculature becomes the superficial trigone, which extends to the verumontanum in the male and stops just short of the external meatus in the female. *B:* Waldeyer's sheath is connected by a few fibers to the detrusor muscle in the ureteral hiatus. This muscular sheath, inferior to the ureteral orifices, becomes the deep trigone. The musculature of the ureters continues downward as the superficial trigone. (Adapted from Tanagho EA, Pugh RCB: Br J Urol 35:151, 1963.)

with symptoms of pyelonephritis or cystitis. Vague abdominal pain is not uncommon. Renal pain and pain with voiding are relatively rare. Pyelonephritis is not uncommonly asymptomatic and the patient may present with azotemia and advanced renal failure due to bilateral renal parenchymal damage with pyelonephritic or hydronephrotic changes. In males, who are relatively protected from infection, reflux is frequently detected late as an incidental finding with a variable degree of renal parenchymal damage.

In secondary reflux, manifestations of the primary disease (neurogenic, obstructive, etc) are usually the presenting symptoms.

Clinical Findings

A. Symptoms and Signs: With acute pyelonephritis, fever, chills, and costovertebral angle tenderness may be present. In cases of obstruction or neurogenic deficit, palpable hydronephrotic kidney or a distended bladder may be found.

B. Laboratory Findings: Urinalysis reveals evidence of infection. The intravenous phenolsulfonphthalein (PSP) renal function test may be depressed if vesical or renal residual urine is present or if renal function is depressed. The PSP excretion will be low in the face of renal damage in which case serum creatinine levels will be elevated.

C. X-Ray Findings: The intravenous urogram may be normal but usually reveals pyelonephritic changes or ureteropyelectasis. Dilatation of the lower ureters is commonly seen in mild cases.

Voiding cystourethrography gives conclusive evidence of reflux and should be done in every case of recurrent urinary tract infection. It may also reveal distal obstruction as with posterior urethral valves or spastic external sphincter syndrome in girls (commonly seen with distal urethral stenosis).

Endoscopic examination and evaluation of the trigonal development and the position and configuration of the ureteral orifice are the most helpful means not only of diagnosis but also of assessing prognosis and reversibility. Cineradiography, chromocystoscopy, lipoidal cystography, and radioisotope studies are adjunctive diagnostic measures.

Differential Diagnosis

Ureteral stasis and dilatation due to trigonal hypertrophy are seen in infravesical obstruction or neurogenic lesions.

Functional ureteral obstruction is due to abundance of circularly oriented muscle fibers. It is commonly seen in the lower end, where the muscle fibers act as a partially obstructive sphincteric segment.

Spastic striated external sphincter syndrome can also perpetuate urinary tract infection.

Treatment

In primary reflux, treatment of infection, dilatation of any distal urethral stenosis, and proper evaluation for degree of trigonal ureteral muscular deficiency and the chances of reversibility are the essential preliminary management steps. Not every refluxing orifice requires surgical repair. The improvement in voiding dynamics achieved by conservative management may be all that is needed in borderline valve incompetence. If infection is kept suppressed, reflux may never recur. One-third of cases of reflux are cured in this way. In another third of cases, advanced ureteral or pyelonephritic changes have occurred together with severe ureteral orifice deformity, indicating immediate surgical intervention.

Most of the cases in the remaining third will come to surgical repair after repeated conservative trials to control urinary tract infection and to stop progression of the renal damage have proved inadequate.

Spontaneous reversal of ureteral orifice incompetence occurs only in marginally incompetent valves due to the relief of an existing insult—commonly urinary tract infection or abnormal voiding dynamics.

In obstructive secondary reflux (eg, posterior urethral valves) release of obstruction may cure reflux. Occasionally, reimplantation is still required. In neurogenic reflux, urinary diversion usually is the wisest choice. In congenital reflux, ectopic orifices, duplication with ureterocele, and other congenital malformations, nothing short of reimplantation will cure the reflux.

The aim of surgery is to excise the muscularly weak terminal ureter, provide proper ureterotrigonal fixation, and give adequate posterior support to an intravesical ureter about 2.5 cm long. There are 3 main approaches to achieve this repair:

A. Suprahiatal Repair: (Politano-Leadbetter, Paquin.) A new ureteral hiatus is developed about 2.5 cm above the original one, and the ureter, after passing through a submucosal tunnel, is sutured to the cut edge of the trigone at the level of the original orifice.

B. Infrahiatal Repair: The original hiatus is maintained and, after discarding the weak terminal ureter, the ureter is advanced through a 2.5 cm submucosal tunnel to end closer to the internal meatus.

C. Supra-infrahiatal Repair: A combination of the above.

Prognosis

The prognosis is good both for those who are treated conservatively and for those requiring surgery. The success rate of surgical repair (no reflux, clearance of infection, and no obstruction) is about 95%.

The ultimate prognosis depends on the severity of kidney damage and the degree of ureteral decompensation and atony. In advanced cases, where neither one is reversible, the prognosis is not favorable. These cases constitute about 30% of cases now coming to kidney transplant.

Amar AD: Vesicoureteral reflux in adults: A 12-year study of 122 patients. Urology 3:184, 1974.

Hutch JA, Amar AD: *Vesicoureteral Reflux and Pyelonephritis.* Appleton-Century-Crofts, 1972.

Lenaghan D & others: Natural history of reflux and long-term effects of reflux on kidney. J Urol 115:728, 1976.

Lyon RP, Marshall S, Tanagho EA: The ureteral orifice: Its configuration and competency. J Urol 102:504, 1969.

Rose J, Glassberg K, Waterhouse K: Intrarenal reflux and its relation to renal scarring. Trans Am Assoc Genitourin Surg 66:94, 1974.

Siegel SR, Sokoloff B, Siegel B: Asymptomatic and symptomatic urinary tract infection in infancy. Am J Dis Child 125:45, 1973.

Tanagho EA: Surgical revision of the incompetent ureterovesical junction: A critical analysis of techniques and requirements. Br J Urol 42:410, 1970.

OBSTRUCTIVE UROPATHY

Obstruction is one of the most important pathologic entities affecting the urinary tract, since it eventually leads to decompensation of the muscular conduits and reservoirs, back pressure, and atrophy of renal parenchyma; it also invites infection and stone formation, which cause additional damage to the organ involved and can ultimately end in complete unilateral or bilateral destruction of the kidneys.

Both the level at which the obstruction occurs and the degree of obstruction are important to an understanding of the pathologic consequences of this group of disorders.

(1) **Level of obstruction:** Any obstruction at or distal to the internal meatus leads to back pressure effects on both kidneys. Obstruction at or proximal to the ureteral orifice leads to unilateral damage unless the lesion involves both ureters simultaneously.

(2) **Degree of obstruction:** Complete obstruction leads to rapid decompensation of the system proximal to the site of obstruction with immediate muscular failure. For example, acute retention occurs if the obstruction is distal to the bladder, and anuria occurs if obstruction involves both ureters. Partial obstruction leads to gradual progressive muscular hypertrophy followed by gradual dilatation, decompensation, and hydronephrotic changes.

Etiology

Urinary tract obstruction may be congenital or acquired.

A. **Congenital:**

1. Meatal stenosis, urethral strictures, posterior urethral valves; ureterovesical and ureteropelvic junction obstruction (various causes).

2. Neurologic deficits.

B. **Acquired:**

1. Urethral strictures, inflammatory or traumatic.

2. Bladder outlet obstruction (benign prostatic hypertrophy or cancer of the prostate).

3. Vesical tumors.

4. Neurogenic bladder.

5. Extrinsic ureteral compression (tumor, retroperitoneal fibrosis, enlarged lymph nodes).

6. Ureteral or pelvic stones.

7. Ureteral strictures.

8. Ureteral or pelvic tumors.

Pathogenesis

Regardless of its cause, acquired obstruction leads to the same changes in the various segments in the urinary tract, depending on its severity and duration. Congenital obstruction, though basically similar to the acquired type, produces its effect while the system is still in the phase of differentiation and development; its effect may go beyond simple obstruction, leading to other anomalous renal development or kidney dysplasia.

A. **Urethral Changes:** Proximal to the obstruction, the urethra dilates and balloons. A urethral diverticulum may develop, and dilatation and gaping of the prostatic and ejaculatory ducts may occur.

B. **Vesical Changes:** Early, the detrusor and trigonal thickening and hypertrophy compensate for the outlet obstruction and lead to complete bladder emptying. This change leads to progressive development of bladder trabeculation, cellules, saccules, then diverticula. Beyond a certain phase, bladder decompensation occurs and is characterized by the above changes, plus variable amounts of residual urine. Trigonal hypertrophy leads to secondary ureteral obstruction due to increased resistance to flow through the intravesical ureter. With the detrusor decompensation and residual urine accumulation, there is stretching of the hypertrophied trigone, which appreciably increases ureteral obstruction. This is the mechanism of back pressure on the kidney in the presence of vesical outlet obstruction (while the ureterovesical junction maintains its competence). Catheter drainage of the bladder relieves trigonal stretch and improves drainage from the upper tract.

A very late change with persistent obstruction (more frequently encountered with neurogenic dysfunction) is decompensation of the ureterovesical junction, leading to reflux, which aggravates the back pressure effect on the upper tract by exposing it to abnormally high intravesical pressures—in addition to favoring the onset or persistence of urinary tract infection. Should ureteral obstruction be unilateral, compensatory hypertrophy of the contralateral kidney will develop. Total renal function, therefore, remains normal.

C. **Ureteral Changes:** The first noted change is a gradually progressive increase in ureteral distention. This increases ureteral wall stretch, which in turn increases contractile power, and ureteral hyperactivity and hypertrophy develop. Because the ureteral musculature runs in an irregular helical pattern, stretching of its muscular elements leads to lengthening as well as widening. This is the start of ureteral decompensation, where tortuosity and dilatation become apparent. These changes can progress, leading to marked ureteral dilatation and lengthening, and the ureter becomes atonic with infrequent or completely absent peristalsis.

D. **Pelvicalyceal Changes:** The renal pelvis and calyces, being subjected to progressively increasing volumes of retained urine, progressively distend. The pelvis first shows evidence of hyperactivity and hypertrophy and then progressive dilatation and atony. The calyces show the same changes to a variable degree depending on whether the renal pelvis is intra- or extrarenal. In the latter, the calyceal dilatation may be minimal in spite of marked pelvic dilatation. In the intrarenal pelvis, calyceal dilatation and renal parenchymal damage are maximum. The successive phases seen with obstruction are rounding of the fornices, followed by flattening of the papillae and finally clubbing of the minor calyces.

E. Renal Parenchymal Changes: With progressive pelvicalyceal distention, there is parenchymal compression against the renal capsule. This, plus the more important factor of compression of the arcuate vessels as a result of the expanding distended calyces, results in a marked drop in renal blood flow. This phenomenon leads to progressive parenchymal compression and ischemic atrophy. Lateral groups of nephrons are affected more than central ones, leading to patchy atrophy with variable degree of severity. The glomeruli and proximal convoluted tubules suffer most of this ischemia. Associated with the increased intrapelvic pressure there is progressive dilatation of the collecting and distal tubules with compression and atrophy of tubular cells.

Clinical Findings

A. Symptoms and Signs: These vary according to the site of obstruction:

1. Infravesical obstruction—Infravesical obstruction leads to difficulty in initiation of voiding, a weak stream, and a diminished flow rate with terminal dribbling. Burning and frequency are common associated symptoms. A distended or thickened bladder wall may be palpable. Urethral induration of a stricture, benign prostatic hypertrophy, or cancer of the prostate may be noted on rectal examination. Meatal stenosis and impacted urethral stones are readily diagnosed.

2. Supravesical obstruction—Renal pain or renal colic and gastrointestinal symptoms are commonly associated. Supravesical obstruction may be completely asymptomatic when it develops very gradually over a period of several weeks or months. An enlarged kidney may be palpable. Costovertebral angle tenderness may be present.

B. Laboratory Findings: Evidence of urinary infection, hematuria, or crystalluria may be seen. Impaired kidney function is noted by diminished PSP excretion and elevated BUN and serum creatinine, with the ratio well above the normal 10:1 relationship because of significant urea reabsorption.

C. X-Ray Findings: Radiologic examination is usually diagnostic in cases of stasis, tumors, and strictures. Dilatation and anatomic changes occur above the level of obstruction, whereas distal to the obstruction the configuration is usually normal. This helps in localizing the site of obstruction. Combined antegrade visualization by intravenous urograms and retrograde visualization by ureterograms or urethrograms, depend-

ing on the site of obstruction, is sometimes needed to demonstrate the extent of the obstructed segment. In supravesical obstruction, demonstration of stasis and delayed drainage are essential to establish and measure the severity of obstruction.

D. Special Examinations: Instrumental calibration of sites of obstruction is also valuable.

Complications

The most important complication of urinary tract obstruction is renal parenchymal atrophy as a result of the back pressure effect.

Urinary tract obstruction predisposes to infection and stone formation, and infection added to obstruction leads to rapid kidney destruction.

Treatment

The aim of therapy is relief of the obstruction—eg, in acute urinary retention, treatment consists of bladder drainage by a catheter. Surgery is often necessary. Simple urethral stricture may be managed conservatively by dilatation. Urethrotomy or urethroplasty may be required. Urethral valves must be ruptured. Benign prostatic hypertrophy and obstructing bladder tumors require surgical removal.

Impacted stones must be either removed or bypassed by a catheter to be surgically removed later or given a chance to pass spontaneously.

Ureteral or ureteropelvic obstruction requires surgical revision and plastic repair, either by ureterovesicoplasty, ureterolithotomy, ureteroureteral anastomosis, bladder flaps to bridge a gap in the lower ureter, transureteroureteral anastomosis, or ureteropyeloplasty.

Preliminary drainage above the obstruction is sometimes needed to improve kidney function. Occasionally, permanent drainage and diversion by cutaneous ureterostomy, ileal or colonic loop diversion, or permanent nephrostomy are required.

Prognosis

The prognosis depends on the cause, site, duration, and degree of kidney damage and renal decompensation. In general, relief of obstruction leads to improvement in kidney function except in seriously damaged kidneys, especially those destroyed by inflammatory scarring.

Hendren H: Urinary tract reconstitution after prior diversion in children. Ann Surg 180:496, 1974.

Johnston JH: The presentation and management of neonatal obstructive uropathies. Postgrad Med J 48:486, 1972.

Kornitzer AD, Olson CM: Methods of urinary diversion. Geriatrics 29:85, 1974.

Pedersen JF: Percutaneous nephrostomy guided by ultrasound. J Urol 112:157, 1974.

Perlmutter AD, Patil J: Loop cutaneous ureterostomy in infants and young children: Late results in 32 cases. J Urol 107:655, 1972.

Pitts WR, Muecke E: Congenital megaloureter: Review of 80 patients. J Urol 111:468, 1974.

Rose J, Gillenwater J: Effect of chronic ureteral obstruction and infection on ureteral function. Invest Urol 11:471, 1974.

Stephens FD: Idiopathic dilatation of the urinary tract. J Urol 112:819, 1974.

Tanagho EA, Smith DR, Guthrie TH: Pathophysiology of functional ureteral obstruction. J Urol 104:73, 1970.

Tsingoglou S, Dickson JAS: Lower urinary obstruction in infancy: A review of lesions in 165 cases. Arch Dis Child 47:215, 1972.

Zinke H, Kelalis PV, Culp A: Ureteropelvic obstruction in children. Surg Gynecol Obstet 139:873, 1974.

GENITOURINARY TRACT TUBERCULOSIS

Specific infections of the urinary tract are those (tuberculosis, actinomycosis, and syphilis) that cause a specific pathologic tissue reaction and usually have a distinctive clinical course. Only tuberculosis will be discussed here.

Tuberculosis is the most important and the most commonly missed type of specific genitourinary infection. It should always be considered in any case of pyuria without bacteriuria or in any resistant urinary tract infection that does not respond to treatment.

Genitourinary tuberculosis is always secondary to pulmonary infection though in many cases the primary focus has already healed or is in a subclinical form. Infection occurs via the hematogenous route. The kidneys and (less commonly) the prostate are the principal sites of urinary tract involvement, though all other segments of the genitourinary system can be affected.

Pathology

Renal tuberculosis usually starts as a tuberculoma that gradually enlarges, then caseates, and later ulcerates and breaks through the pelvicalyceal system. Caseation and scarring are the principal pathologic features of renal tuberculosis. In the ureter, tuberculosis usually leads to stricture, periureteritis, and mural fibrosis.

In the bladder, the infection is characterized by areas of hyperemia and a coalescent group of tubercles followed by ulcerations around the involved ureteral orifice. Bladder wall fibrosis and contracted bladder are the end results.

Urethral involvement in the male (uncommon) leads to urethral stricture, usually in the bulbous portion. Periurethral abscess and fistula are common complications.

Genital tuberculosis involves the prostate, seminal vesicles, and epididymides, either separately or in association with renal involvement. Tubercle formation with later caseation and fibrosis is the basic pathologic feature, leading to enlargement, nodulation, and irregular consistency of the prostate and to fibrosis and distention of the seminal vesicles. Induration, thickening of the epididymis, and beading of the vas deferens are characteristic findings.

Clinical Findings

A. Symptoms and Signs: The patient commonly presents with lower urinary tract irritation, usually with pyuria. Less common manifestations are hematuria, renal pain, and renal colic.

B. Laboratory Findings: Sterile pyuria is the rule. The organism can be identified on an acid-fast stain of the centrifuged sediment of a 24-hour urine specimen, by culture, or by guinea pig inoculation.

C. X-Ray Findings: Radiologic findings of moth-eaten, caseous cavities or bizarre irregular calyces, strictures in straight, rigid, moderately dilated ureters, and a contracted bladder with vesicoureteral reflux are all suggestive evidence.

D. Special Examinations: Cystoscopy will show typical findings of tuberculous cystitis.

Treatment

A. Medical Treatment: Tuberculosis must be treated as a generalized disease. Once the diagnosis is established, medical treatment for at least 2 years is indicated whether or not surgery is required also. Whenever possible, medical treatment should be continued for at least 3 months before surgery.

Specific triple drug therapy should be given to eradicate the infecting organism. This might include sodium aminosalicylic acid (PAS), 15 g/day orally in divided doses; isoniazid (INH), 5 mg/kg in divided doses, and rifampin, 600 mg/day as a single dose. Pyridoxine, 100 mg/day in divided doses, will counteract the vitamin B_6 depletion effect of INH. This regimen should be followed for at least 2 years.

B. Surgical Measures: In unilateral renal lesions, nephrectomy is indicated. In bilateral disease that has seriously damaged one kidney and is in an early stage in the other, unilateral nephrectomy still should be considered; in localized polar lesions, partial nephrectomy may be done.

In unilateral epididymal involvement, epididymectomy plus contralateral vasectomy is indicated to prevent descent of the infection from the prostate to that organ; bilateral epididymectomy should be done if both sides are involved.

Prognosis

Tuberculous involvement of other structures in the genitourinary tract must be treated medically.

Ehrlich RM, Lattimer JK: Urogenital tuberculosis in children. J Urol 105:461, 1971.

Gow FG: Genitourinary tuberculosis: Study of short course regimens. J Urol 115:707, 1976.

Teklu B, Ostrow JH: Urinary tuberculosis: Review of 44 cases treated since 1963. J Urol 115:507, 1976.

NONSPECIFIC URINARY TRACT INFECTIONS

General Considerations

Nonspecific urinary tract infection is the second most common type of infection in humans and is encountered in about 75% of patients seen by urologists.

These infections are caused by a variety of pyogenic bacteria, and the pathologic tissue response is not specific to the offending organism. The commonest organisms are gram-negative bacteria, particularly *Escherichia coli.* Less common are *Enterobacter aerogenes, Proteus vulgaris* and *P mirabilis, Pseudomonas aeruginosa,* and *Streptococcus faecalis.*

The ascending route of infection is by far the most common. Infection by this route is a common occurrence encountered in young girls and in women during active sexual life. It is related to the short length of the female urethra and the perineal bacterial flora. In males, ascending infection is usually a consequence of urethral instrumentation. Infection may be contained in the bladder if there is a competent ureterovesical junction. Otherwise, ascending infection can reach the kidney, leading to pyelonephritis (see below).

Descending or hematogenous infection is relatively uncommon. When it occurs, it is usually in association with local urinary tract disorders—most commonly, obstruction and stasis; less commonly, trauma, foreign bodies, or tumors.

Lymphatic spread occasionally occurs from the large bowel or from the cervix and adnexa in the female through the perivesical and periureteral lymphatics.

Direct extension to the urinary bladder of nearby inflammatory processes—eg, appendiceal abscess or a pelvic abscess—may occur.

Predisposing Factors

Urinary tract infection is usually initiated or maintained because of certain predisposing factors, including the following:

A. General Systemic Factors: Examples include diabetes, debilitation, and prolonged illness. These disorders probably favor urinary tract infection by interfering with normal bladder and body defense mechanisms.

B. Local Factors: Any of the following local conditions predisposes to a urinary tract infection: obstruction, organic or functional; stasis (residual urine); vesicoureteral reflux; foreign bodies, especially catheters and stones; tumors or any necrotic tissue; and trauma, especially to the kidneys.

Classification of Nonspecific Urinary Tract Infection

A. Upper Urinary Tract Infection: Acute or chronic pyelonephritis, papillary necrosis, and renal carbuncle are the most common types.

B. Lower Urinary Tract Infection: Cystitis and urethritis, including gonorrheal urethritis.

C. Genital Infection: Prostatitis, epididymitis, seminal vesiculitis, and orchitis.

Kunin CM, McCormack RC: Prevention of catheter-induced urinary tract infections by sterile closed drainage. N Engl J Med 274:1155, 1966.

Kunin CM & others: Detection of urinary tract infection in 3- to 5-year-old girls by mothers using a nitrite indicator strip. Pediatrics 57:829, 1976.

Stamey TA, Howell JJ: Studies of introital colonization in women with recurrent urinary infections. 4. The role of local vaginal antibodies. J Urol 115:413, 1976.

Stamey TA, Mihara G: Studies of introital colonization in women with recurrent urinary infections. 5. The inhibitory activity of normal vaginal fluid on *Proteus mirabilis* and *Pseudomonas aeruginosa.* J Urol 115:416, 1976.

Stamey TA, Pfau A: Urinary infections: A selective review and some observations. Calif Med 113:16, Dec 1970.

Stamey TA, Timothy MM: Studies of introital colonization in women with recurrent urinary infections. 3. Vaginal glycogen concentration. J Urol 114:268, 1975.

Stamey TA & others: Recurrent urinary infections and nothing else. J Urol 106:441, 1971.

1. ACUTE & CHRONIC PYELONEPHRITIS

Except in the presence of stasis, foreign bodies, or trauma, pyelonephritis is an ascending type of infection. Pathogenic organisms usually reach the kidney from the bladder via an incompetent ureterovesical junction.

Clinical Findings

A. Symptoms and Signs: In the acute attack, pain is present in one or both loins. Young children commonly present with ill-localized abdominal pain. Irritative lower urinary tract symptoms may be associated. Chills and fever are common. In chronic pyelonephritis, dull aching pain in the loins may be present; however, there are usually no symptoms.

B. Laboratory Findings: Pyuria and bacteria on stained smear are consistent findings. In acute attacks, the sedimentation rate is elevated. Urine culture identifies the organism.

C. X-Ray Findings: In acute attacks, only minimal changes such as delayed function and poorer concentration are usually noted. In chronic cases, typical calyceal deformities with evidence of peripheral scarring can usually be seen. Evidence of stasis may be apparent. Cystography usually reveals reflux.

Complications

If the diagnosis is missed in the acute stage, the infection may become chronic. Both acute and chronic pyelonephritis lead to progressive renal scarring and destruction and may result in a small, atrophic, scarred, nonfunctioning kidney.

Treatment

Specific therapy should be given to eradicate the

infecting organism after proper identification and sensitivity testing. Symptomatic treatment is indicated for pain and bladder irritability. Rest and adequate urinary output are required. Failure to simultaneously identify and treat predisposing factors is the principal cause of failure of therapy or chronicity and ultimate renal failure.

Prognosis

The prognosis is good with adequate treatment of both the infection and its predisposing cause, depending on the degree of preexisting renal parenchymal damage.

Davidson AJ, Talner LB: Urographic and angiographic abnormalities in adult-onset acute bacterial nephritis. Radiology 106:249, 1973.

Palmer JM: Differential antibiotic excretion in unilateral structural pyelonephritis. West J Med 120:363, 1974.

Saunders CD, Corriere JN Jr: The inability to diagnose chronic pyelonephritis on the excretory urogram in adults. J Urol 111:560, 1974.

Stephens SD: Urologic aspects of recurrent urinary tract infection in children. J Pediatr 80:725, 1972.

Strong DW & others: Experimentally induced chronic pyelonephritis using bacterial antigens and its prevention with immunosuppression. Invest Urol 11:479, 1974.

Zinner SH, Kass EH: Long-term (10–14 years) follow-up of bacteriuria of pregnancy. N Engl J Med 285:820, 1971.

2. PAPILLARY NECROSIS

This disorder consists of ischemic necrosis of the renal papillae or of the entire pyramid. Excessive ingestion of analgesics, sickle cell trait, diabetes, obstruction with infection, and vesicoureteral reflux with infection are common predisposing factors.

The symptoms are usually those of chronic cystitis with recurring exacerbation of pyelonephritis. Renal pain or renal colic may be present. Azotemic manifestations may be the presenting symptoms. In acute attacks, localized loin tenderness and generalized toxemia may occur. Laboratory findings consist of pyuria, occasionally glycosuria, and acidosis. Impaired kidney function is shown by diminished PSP excretion and elevated serum creatinine and BUN. X-ray usually shows impaired function and poor visualization in advanced cases; evidence of ulceration, cavitation, or linear breaks in the base of the papillae and negative shadows due to sloughed papillae may be seen. Retrograde urograms may be needed for proper visualization if kidney function is markedly impaired.

Preventive measures consist of proper management of diabetic patients with recurrent infection and avoidance of chronic use of analgesic compounds containing phenacetin and aspirin.

Intensive antibacterial therapy may be needed, yet it is commonly unsuccessful in eradicating infection. Little can be done surgically except to remove obstructing papillae and correct predisposing factors (reflux, obstruction) if identified.

In severe cases, the prognosis is poor. Kidney transplant might be considered.

Flanter S, Lome LG, Presman D: Urologic complications of renal papillary necrosis. Urology 5:331, 1975.

Flint LD, Libertino JA, Desai SG: Renal papillary necrosis: Unusual patterns and treatment. J Urol 111:321, 1974.

Husband P, Howlett KA: Renal papillary necrosis in infancy. Arch Dis Child 48:116, 1973.

Jameson RM, Heal MR: The surgical management of acute renal papillary necrosis. Br J Surg 60:428, 1973.

Macklon AF & others: Aspirin and analgesic nephropathy. Br Med J 1:597, 1974.

3. RENAL CARBUNCLE

Renal carbuncle is usually due to a hemolytic staphylococcal infection which spreads to the kidney by the hematogenous route from a pyogenic skin lesion. The onset may be acute, with high fever and definite localization. In occasional cases, low-grade fever and general malaise are the presenting symptoms. Localized costovertebral angle tenderness and a palpable kidney mass may be present. The mass may be evident on intravenous urograms or renal angiograms. The urine is not infected until the abscess breaks into the pelvicalyceal system.

If organism sensitivity can be established by appropriate tests (blood and urine cultures and sensitivity tests), treat with the proper antibiotic. Local drainage or even heminephrectomy may be indicated.

Lyons RW & others: Arteriographic and antibiotic therapy of a renal carbuncle. J Urol 107:524, 1972.

Moore CA, Gangai MP: Renal cortical abscess. J Urol 89:303, 1967.

Rabinowitz JG & others: Acute renal carbuncle: The roentgenographic clarification of a medical enigma. Am J Roentgenol 116:740, 1972.

Renal carbuncle. (Editorial.) Br Med J 3:63, 1973.

4. CYSTITIS

Cystitis is more common in females and is usually an ascending infection. In the male, it usually occurs in association with obstruction, prostatitis, foreign bodies, or tumors. The urinary bladder is normally capable of clearing itself of infection unless an underlying pathologic process interferes with its defensive mechanisms.

In the acute phase, the principal symptoms of cystitis are burning on urination, frequency, urgency, and hematuria; low-grade fever and suprapubic, perineal, and low back pain may be present. In chronic cystitis, irritative symptoms are usually milder.

Evidence of prostatitis, urethritis, and vaginitis may be present. Laboratory findings, in addition to hematuria, consist of bacteriuria and pyuria. Urine culture identifies the organism. Cystoscopy is not advisable in the acute phase. In chronic cystitis, evidence of mucosal irritation may be present.

In any recurrent lower urinary tract infection, a complete urologic work-up is indicated. Instrumentation is contraindicated in the acute phase but essential in chronic or recurrent cases to identify the predisposing factor.

Specific antibacterial therapy is given according to the results of sensitivity testing of recovered organisms. Sterilization of urine is preferably followed by a variable period of suppressive medication depending upon the predisposing factor or the chronicity and recurrence of the disease.

In children with cystitis due to distal urethral stenosis, dilatation is required. Prolonged suppressive medication is usually indicated in cases associated with voiding dysfunction.

In women with recurrent postcoital cystitis, prosuppressive medication (eg, sulfonamides) on the night of intercourse and the following day and immediate postcoital voiding usually help in preventing recurrences.

Bailey RR & others: Urinary-tract infection in non-pregnant women. Lancet 2:275, 1973.

Mufson MA & others: Cause of acute hemorrhagic cystitis in children. Am J Dis Child 126:605, 1973.

Vosti KL: Recurrent urinary tract infection: Prevention by prophylactic antibiotics after sexual intercourse. JAMA 231:934, 1975.

5. URETHRITIS

Nonspecific urethritis is not uncommon in both men and women. It usually occurs as an ascending bacterial infection in women and is associated with prostatitis in men. Viral and chemical urethritis may also be encountered.

Urethral discharge and a burning sensation with urination are commonly the presenting symptoms. The onset of symptoms is usually related to intercourse. Examination reveals meatal congestion and tenderness along the urethra. The first glass of urine usually shows urethral discharge, bacteriuria, and pyuria. The midstream urine is clean unless there is associated cystitis or prostatitis.

Treatment consists of giving specific antimicrobial therapy. The best combination is one of the tetracyclines and a sulfonamide.

If prostatitis is the underlying factor, prostatic massage is indicated after the acute phase has subsided. Urethral stricture should be treated. Empirical urethral dilatation may help in the female with urethritis. Infected periurethral glands may have to be properly drained or fulgurated.

Gonorrheal Urethritis

Gonorrhea is usually transmitted through sexual contact. *Neisseria gonorrhoeae* is a gram-negative organism commonly seen as intracellular diplococci. It can be identified on a stained smear of discharge or urine sediment or, if necessary, by culture.

A purulent yellow or brown urethral discharge starting 3–4 days after sexual contact is the first symptom. Burning and pain along the urethra and meatal inflammation are common. The first glass of urine is cloudy but midstream urine is clear.

Penicillin and tetracycline cure over 90% of cases each. A combination of the 2 is more effective. Simultaneous treatment of the partner is essential. Prolonged therapy is indicated in the presence of gonorrheal prostatitis, seminal vesiculitis, epididymitis, or cystitis. Inadequate treatment can lead to periurethritis, periurethral abscess, and urethral strictures.

McChesney JA & others: Acute urethritis in male college students. JAMA 226:37, 1973.

McCormack WM & others: The genital mycoplasmas. N Engl J Med 288:78, 1973.

6. PROSTATITIS

Prostatitis commonly follows ascending urethral infection and inadequately treated urethritis. Occasionally it is due to hematogenous infection. It is most commonly seen in young adults but also occurs in young children and more frequently in association with benign prostatic hyperplasia.

Symptoms of acute prostatitis consist of perineal pain, urethral discharge, marked irritative urinary symptoms, and fever. The prostate is tender, enlarged, and usually firm. Fluctuation may be elicited if there is abscess formation. In chronic prostatitis, mild perineal pain, low backache, or mild irritative symptoms are common. The prostate is usually enlarged, firm, and irregular. Prostatic massage (contraindicated in the acute phase) leads to copious discharge. Laboratory findings consist of bacteria and pus in the urethral discharge, the prostatic smear, or the first glass of urine. Leukocytosis is present in the acute phase.

Specific antibacterial therapy should be given according to culture and sensitivity testing. The response is usually good in the acute phase but not so gratifying in chronic cases. Diffusion of antibiotics in prostatic acini is very poor. There is some evidence that trimethoprim is active in the prostate. Give 2 tablets of sulfamethoxazole-trimethoprim twice daily for 10 days.

Prostatic massage is helpful in chronic cases. Regular sexual intercourse is advisable.

Drach GW: Problems in diagnosis of bacterial prostatis: Gram-negative, gram-positive and mixed infections. J Urol 111:630, 1974.

Eykyn S & others: Prostatic calculi as source of recurrent bacteriuria in the male. Br J Urol 46:527, 1974.

Meares EM Jr, Stamey TA: The diagnosis and management of bacterial prostatitis. Br J Urol 44:175, 1972.

Nielsen ML, Justesen T: Studies on the pathology of prostatitis. Scand J Urol Nephrol 8:1, 1974.

Pai MG, Bhat HS: Prostatic abscess. J Urol 108:599, 1972.

7. EPIDIDYMITIS

Common causes of epididymitis include urethral instrumentation, chronic prostatitis, and reflux of sterile urine into the ejaculatory ducts. Epididymitis is a rare complication of vasectomy. In acute cases there is usually a history of preceding instrumentation, catheterization, chronic prostatitis, or severe straining. The symptoms are sudden pain in the scrotum, rapid unilateral scrotal enlargement, and marked tenderness that extends over the spermatic cord and is relieved by lifting the testis. In the chronic phase there is usually minimal local tenderness and pain, with irregular nodular enlargement of the epididymis. Hydrocele may be associated. Laboratory findings reveal pyuria, bacteriuria, and marked leukocytosis.

Nonspecific epididymitis must be differentiated from torsion of the testis, testicular tumor, and tuberculous epididymitis. If torsion of the spermatic cord cannot be ruled out, immediate surgical exploration should be done.

In the acute phase, treatment consists of infiltrating the spermatic cord with 20 ml of 1% procaine hydrochloride. Pain, fever, and swelling usually subside gradually. Antibiotics (tetracycline) are helpful. Scrotal support, rest, and hot sitz baths and sedation are indicated. Chronic prostatitis should be treated if present.

Acute attacks usually resolve in 2—3 weeks with treatment; exacerbations can be controlled by treating the predisposing factor. Chronic epididymitis usually never resolves completely; it has no consequences except, occasionally, sterility in bilateral cases.

Furness G & others: Relationship of epididymitis to gonorrhea. Invest Urol 11:313, 1974.

Kiviat MD, Shurtleff D, Ansell JS: Urinary reflux via the vas deferens: Unusual cause of epididymitis in infancy. J Pediatr 80:476, 1972.

Lyon RP, Bruyn HB: Treatment of mumps epididymo-orchitis. JAMA 196:736, 1966.

CALCULOUS DISEASE

1. RENAL STONE

Essentials of Diagnosis
- Flank pain, hematuria, pyelonephritis, previous stone passage; high vitamin D, milk, and alkaline intake.
- Renal tenderness.
- Urinalysis shows red cells and sometimes white cells and bacteria in the urine.
- Stone visualized on urography.

General Considerations

Most stones are composed of calcium salts (oxalate, phosphate, magnesium-ammonium phosphate —the latter secondary to urea-splitting organisms). Most calcium stones are idiopathic (idiopathic hypercalciuria), and hypercalciuria encourages stone formation in hyperparathyroidism, immobilization, high calcium or vitamin D intake, and dehydration. An alkaline urine increases the insolubility of calcium.

The less common metabolic stones, cystine and uric acid, usually form secondary to hypersecretion of these substances. Uric acid stones are radiolucent. Stones that obstruct the ureteropelvic junction lead to hydronephrosis and infection.

Clinical Findings

A. Symptoms and Signs: If the stone obstructs the ureteropelvic junction or a calyx, moderate to severe renal pain will be noted, often accompanied by nausea, vomiting, and ileus. Hematuria is common. Symptoms of infection, if present, will be exacerbated. Nonobstructive calculi are usually painless. This includes staghorn calculus, which may form a cast of all calyces and the pelvis. In the symptomatic patient, there may be costovertebral angle tenderness and a quiet abdomen. Infection secondary to obstruction may lead to high fever, prostration, and abdominal muscle rigidity.

B. Laboratory Findings: With acute infection, leukocytosis is to be expected. With renal insufficiency, anemia may be noted. Urinalysis may reveal red and white blood cells and bacteria. A pH of 7.6 or higher implies the presence of urea-splitting organisms. A pH consistently below 5.5 is compatible with the formation of uric acid or cystine stones. Crystals of uric acid or cystine in the urine are suggestive. A Sulkowitch test may reveal evidence of hypercalciuria, which is observed with hyperparathyroidism, essential hypercalciuria, and disseminated osseous metastases.

Determination of serum calcium and phosphorus may afford evidence of hyperparathyroidism, in which the tubular reabsorption of phosphate is diminished. An elevated serum uric acid is compatible with uric acid lithiasis. Significant cystinuria may be found. Hyperchloremic acidosis suggests renal tubular acidosis

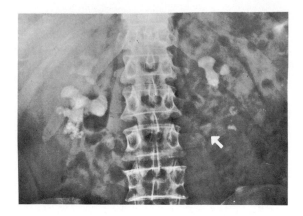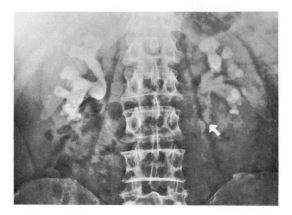

Figure 43–6. Bilateral staghorn calculi and left upper ureteral stone. *Left:* Plain film. Arrow points to ureteral stone. *Right:* Excretory urogram showing bilateral impaired function.

with secondary renal calcifications. Total renal function will be impaired only if the stones are bilateral, and particularly if infection is a complication.

C. X-Ray Findings: About 90% of calculi are radiopaque (calcium, cystine). Excretory urography is necessary to place them in the excretory tract and also affords a measure of renal function (Fig 43–6). An acutely obstructed kidney may only show increasing density of the renal shadow without significant radiopaque material in the calyces. A nonopaque stone (uric acid) will show as a "negative" shadow since it displaces the contrast medium.

Bone disease due to metastatic carcinoma or Paget's disease may account for hypercalciuria.

D. Stone Analysis: If a stone has previously been passed or the present one is recovered, its chemical nature should be analyzed. Such knowledge may be significant when planning a regimen of prevention.

Differential Diagnosis

Acute pyelonephritis may start with acute renal pain, thus mimicking a renal stone. Urinalysis reveals infection, and urograms fail to reveal a calculus.

Renal tumor may bleed into its own substance, causing acute pain simulating obstructing stone. Urograms make the differentiation.

Renal tuberculosis is complicated by stone in 10% of cases. Pyuria without bacteriuria is suggestive. Urography reveals the motheaten calyces typical of tuberculosis.

Papillary necrosis may cause renal colic if a sloughed papilla obstructs the ureteropelvic junction. Excretory urography will settle the issue.

Renal infarction may cause renal pain and hematuria. Evidence of a cardiac lesion, nonfunction of the kidney on urography, and absence of evidence of calculus help in differentiation. Infarction may be established by angiography.

Complications

The presence of a stone lowers the resistance of the kidney to infection, although in many instances

the infection is primary. A stone lodged in the ureteropelvic junction leads to progressive hydronephrosis. A staghorn calculus, as it grows, may destroy renal tissue by pressure, although the infection that is usually present also contributes to renal damage.

Prevention

An effective preventive regimen depends upon stone analysis and chemical studies of the serum and urine.

A. General Measures: Ensure a high fluid intake to keep solutes well diluted. Combat infection, relieve stasis or obstruction, and advise the patient to avoid prolonged recumbency. For calcium stone formers, stop vitamin supplements (vitamin D) and medications containing calcium salts. Eliminate alkalies from the diet (by reducing the intake of fruit and vegetables) to produce an acid urine in which calcium is most soluble.

B. Specific Measures:

1. Calcium stones—Remove parathyroid tumor, if present. Eliminate dairy products (milk, cheese) from the diet. Calcium is most soluble in acid urine (below pH 6.0). Give cranberry juice, 200 ml 4 times a day; ascorbic acid, 1 g 4 times a day; and potassium acid phosphate (see below). In renal tubular acidosis, however, give alkali to reduce urinary calcium excretion.

To convert "stone-forming" to "non-stone-forming" urine, give 2.5 g of neutral sodium (or potassium) phosphate daily in divided doses. Potassium acid phosphate, 4–6 g/day, is also effective. These drugs, however, are contraindicated if the kidney is infected.

Thiazide diuretics such as hydrochlorothiazide (HydroDiuril), 50 mg twice a day, decrease the calcium content in the urine.

2. Oxalate stones (calcium oxalate)—Prescribe phosphate or a thiazide diuretic (see above) and limit calcium intake.

3. Metabolic stones (uric acid, cystine)—These substances are most soluble at a pH of 7.0 or higher. Give 50% citrate solution, 4–8 ml 4 times a day; check urine pH with paper indicator. For uric acid stone formers, limit purines in the diet and give allopurinol

(Zyloprim), 300 mg every 12 hours. Patients with mild cystinuria should receive a low-methionine diet. For severe cystinurics, give penicillamine (Cuprimine), 30 mg/kg/day orally in divided doses. This regimen should reduce urinary cystine to safe levels. Penicillamine should be supplemented with pyridoxine, 50 mg/day orally.

Treatment

A. Conservative Measures: No intervention is indicated for a small, asymptomatic stone trapped in a calyx. A conservative approach should be utilized for coralliform (staghorn) stones—particularly if bilateral—in an older individual with impaired renal function since function is not apt to improve after their removal, the recurrence rate is significant, and infection is difficult to eradicate. Stones secondary to renal tubular acidosis should be treated with alkalies. Give 50% solution of sodium (or potassium) citrate, 4–8 ml 4 times a day. Secondary stones are apt to be small and may pass spontaneously.

Combat infection. Urea-splitting organisms significantly contribute to development and growth of stones (triple phosphate).

Metabolic stones may cease to grow or even dissolve on specific medication.

B. Surgical Measures: Removal of the stone is indicated for disabling pain, progressive hydronephrosis, or infection that resists chemotherapy. If the kidney is badly damaged and its mate is normal, nephrectomy may be indicated.

Prognosis

The recurrence rate of renal stone is high unless sufficient attention is paid to measures for prevention of stone formation. The danger of recurrent stone is the progressive destruction of the kidney that results from obstruction and infection.

Blandy JP, Singh M: Case for a more aggressive approach to staghorn stones. J Urol 115:505, 1976.

Boyce WH, Elkins IB: Reconstructive renal surgery following anatrophic nephrolithotomy: Follow-up of 100 consecutive cases. J Urol 111:307, 1974.

Burdette DC, Thomas WC Jr, Finlayson B: Urinary supersaturation with calcium oxalate before and during orthophosphate therapy. J Urol 115:418, 1976.

Coe FL, Raisen L: Allopurinol treatment of uric-acid disorders in calcium-stone formers. Lancet 1:129, 1973.

Kolb F: Medical management of the patient with renal stones. Primary Care 2:317, 1975.

Malek RS, Kelalis PP: Urologic manifestations of hyperparathyroidism in childhood. J Urol 115:717, 1976.

Malek RS, Wilkiemeyer RM, Boyce WH: Stone-forming kidney: Study of functional differences between individual kidneys in idiopathic renal lithiasis. J Urol 116:11, 1976.

Scholten HG, Bakker NJ, Cornil C: Urolithiasis in childhood. J Urol 109:744, 1973.

Thompson RB, Stamey TA: Bacteriology of infected stones. Urology 2:627, 1973.

Williams HE: Nephrolithiasis. N Engl J Med 290:33, 1974.

2. URETERAL STONE

Essentials of Diagnosis

- Severe ureterorenal colic.
- Hematuria.
- Nausea, vomiting, and ileus.
- Stone, usually obstructive, on excretory urography.

General Considerations

Stones passing down the ureter originate in the kidney. They are ordinarily obstructive and are therefore a threat to renal function. Complicating infection may occur. Most stones entering the ureter will pass spontaneously.

Clinical Findings

A. Symptoms and Signs: The pain usually comes on abruptly and is felt in the costovertebral angle; it tends to radiate into the ipsilateral lower abdominal quadrant. Nausea, vomiting, and abdominal distention are common. Gross hematuria is usual. When the stone approaches the bladder, symptoms resembling those of cystitis are experienced. Should the kidney be infected, the resulting obstruction will lead to its exacerbation.

The patient is usually in such agony that only the intravenous injection of an opiate will give relief. There is tenderness in the costovertebral angle. Spasm of the ipsilateral abdominal muscles is present. Peristalsis is minimal; abdominal distention is usual. Fever indicates a complicating renal infection.

B. Laboratory Findings: Same as for renal stone.

C. X-Ray Findings: Excretory urograms are essential. The plain film may reveal an opacity in the region of the ureter, but proof that it is indeed a stone depends on seeing it within the ureteral lumen (Fig 43–7). This procedure depicts the degree of obstruction and the size and position of the stone, observations that permit judgment as to treatment. If the stone is nonopaque, it will show as a negative shadow in the ureter, which is dilated above it; ureteral tumor or a blood clot will give a similar finding. If the diagnosis is still in doubt, cystoscopy, ureteral catheterization, and retrograde urography may be indicated.

Differential Diagnosis

Passage of crystals down the ureter may cause colic. Urograms are usually normal. The presence of many crystals in the urine may be significant.

A tumor of the kidney or renal pelvis may bleed. Passage of a blood clot will cause symptoms typical of stone. Urograms may reveal a radiolucent area in the ureter surrounded by the radiopaque urine.

Primary tumor of the ureter may become obstructive and cause pain and hematuria. The urogram will reveal the ureteral filling defect, often with secondary obstruction. Urinary cytology will reveal malignant transitional cells.

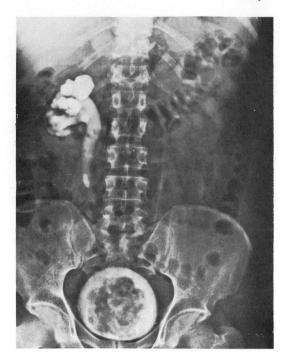

Figure 43–7. Excretory urogram showing right ureteral stone causing hydronephrosis. Large irregular filling defect from unsuspected vesical neoplasm.

Acute pyelonephritis may be associated with pain as acute as that seen with stone. Pyuria and bacteriuria are found. Stone is absent on urography.

A sloughed papilla coursing down the ureter may cause colic and will afford a urogram compatible with uric acid stone. Evidence of papillary sloughs, however, will be noted.

Complications

If obstruction from the ureteral stone is prolonged, progressive renal damage may ensue. Bilateral stones may cause anuria, requiring immediate establishment of drainage with indwelling ureteral catheters or removal of the stones.

Infection may supervene, but most renal infections are iatrogenic, ie, introduced at the time of stone manipulation.

Prevention

See section on renal stone.

Treatment

A. General Measures: Most ureteral stones will pass spontaneously—particularly those 0.5 cm in diameter or less. Once the diagnosis has been established, pain should be relieved by suitable opiates given intravenously, eg, morphine, 8 mg.

B. Specific Measures: Should the stone cause intractable pain, lead to progressive hydronephrosis, or be complicated by acute infection, removal is indicated. Cystoscopic manipulation is highly successful

for stones in the lower ureter. Surgical removal is at times necessary.

Prognosis

About 80% of ureteral stones pass spontaneously. Periodic plain films of the abdomen or excretory urograms will portray progress of the stone and any renal damage that might develop.

Mahon FB Jr, Waters RF: A critical review of stone manipulation: A 5-year study. J Urol 110:387, 1973.
Raney AM: Electrohydraulic lithotripsy: Experimental study and case reports with stone disintegration. J Urol 113:345, 1975.
Skolnick AM, Lome LG, Presman D: Spontaneous urinary extravasation secondary to acute ureteral obstruction. J Urol 110:391, 1973.
Walsh A: An aggressive approach to stones in the lower ureter. Br J Urol 46:11, 1974.

3. VESICAL STONE

Primary vesical calculi are rare in the USA but are common in Southeast Asia. The cause is probably dietary. Secondary stones usually complicate vesical outlet obstruction with residual urine and infection; 90% of those affected are men. They are common in vesical schistosomiasis or in association with radiation cystitis. Foreign bodies in the bladder may act as nuclei for the precipitation of urinary salts. Most stones are calcific; some are composed of uric acid.

Clinical Findings

A. Symptoms and Signs: Symptoms typical of obstruction distal to the bladder are elicited. There may be sudden interruption of the stream, associated with urethral pain if a stone occludes the bladder neck during voiding. Hematuria is not uncommon. Vesical distention may be noted; evidence of urethral stricture or an enlarged prostate is usually found.

B. Laboratory Findings: Pyuria and bacteriuria are almost always present; hematuria is usual. The PSP excretion is depressed because of residual vesical urine.

C. X-Ray Findings: Vesical calculi are usually radiopaque. Excretory urograms will reveal that the stones are indeed intravesical; residual urine is usually depicted on the postvoiding film.

D. Instrumental Examination: Arrest of a sound or endoscope may lead to the diagnosis of urethral stricture. The catheter may uncover residual urine. Cystoscopy will visualize the stones and, in addition, reveal an obstructing prostate.

Differential Diagnosis

A pedunculated vesical tumor may suddenly occlude the vesical neck during voiding. Cystoscopy leads to definitive diagnosis.

Extravesical opacifications may simulate stones on a plain film. Cystoscopy will make the differentiation.

Complications

Vesical infection is worsened by the presence of a stone, which defeats attempts at sterilization of the urine. A small stone may lodge in the urethra, causing complete urinary obstruction. It must be removed.

Prevention

Prevention requires relief of the primary obstruction, removal of the stones, and sterilization of the urine.

Treatment

A. Specific Measures: Small stones can be removed or crushed transurethrally. Large stones will require suprapubic transvesical removal. The obstructive lesion must also be corrected.

Chemical dissolution is feasible, but it fails to attack the cause. Frequent instillation of hemiacidrin (Renacidin), with the catheter clamped off for 1 hour, may prove successful.

B. General Measures: Analgesics for pain and antimicrobials for control of infection can be utilized until the stones can be removed.

Prognosis

The recurrence rate of vesical stone is low if the obstruction and infection are treated.

Amin SA: Urethral calculi. Br J Urol 45:192, 1973.

Aurora AL, Taneja OP, Gupta DN: Bladder stone disease of childhood. 1. An epidemiologic study. 2. A clinicopathologic study. Acta Paediatr Scand 59:117, 385, 1970.

Reuter HJ, Jones LW: Trocar lithotripsy: A new perspective. J Urol 110:197, 1973.

4. NEPHROCALCINOSIS

Nephrocalcinosis is a precipitation of calcium in the tubules, parenchyma, and, occasionally, the glomeruli. Its presence implies some renal functional impairment, often severe. Stones may be found in the calyces and pelvis. The common causes are primary hyperparathyroidism, high milk-alkali ingestion, high vitamin D intake, and secondary hyperparathyroidism which develops secondary to severe renal damage associated with hyperchloremic acidosis. Calcifications may also be seen in the skin, lungs, stomach, spleen, corneas, and around the joints.

There are no specific symptoms. If the patient is a child, he may merely fail to thrive. Stones or sand may be passed. The complaints are usually those of the primary disease. Physical examination may reveal an enlarged parathyroid gland, corneal calcifications, and pseudorickets.

The urine may be infected. In renal tubular acidosis, the pH is fixed between 6.0–7.0. The Sulkowitch test is strongly positive in hyperparathyroidism, both primary and secondary. Tests of renal function are depressed; uremia is common. Hypercalcemia and hypophosphatemia are seen with primary hyperparathyroidism; secondary hyperparathyroidism may be associated with a low serum calcium and an elevated serum phosphate. Hyperchloremic acidosis and hypokalemia accompany renal tubular acidosis.

A plain x-ray will reveal punctate calcifications in the papillae of the kidneys. Calyceal or pelvic stones may also be noted. This calcification may have to be differentiated from renal tuberculosis and medullary sponge kidney.

The complications include renal damage caused by the calcifications and renal and ureteral calculi. Chronic renal infection may complicate the primary disease.

The primary cause should be treated, if possible (eg, parathyroidectomy). Discontinue vitamin D, give a low-calcium diet, and force fluids. With hyperchloremic acidosis, replace base to decrease hypercalciuria; give a 50% solution of potassium citrate, 4–8 ml 4 times a day, in order to alkalinize the urine.

If nephrocalcinosis is secondary to primary renal disease, the outlook is poor. If the cause is correctable and renal function is fairly good, the prognosis is more favorable.

Buckalew VM & others: Hereditary renal tubular acidosis. Medicine 53:229, 1974.

Courey WR, Pfister RC: The radiographic findings in renal tubular acidosis: Analysis of 21 cases. Radiology 105:497, 1972.

Farrell RM, Horwith M, Muecke EC: Renal tubular acidosis and nephrocalcinosis: Diagnosis and clinical management. J Urol 111:429, 1974.

TRAUMA

1. INJURIES TO THE KIDNEY

Essentials of Diagnosis

- History or evidence of trauma, usually local.
- Hematuria.
- Mass in the flank.
- Failure of visualization of kidney or urinary extravasation on excretory urography.

General Considerations

Renal injury is not common, but it is potentially serious and is often accompanied by injury to other organs or structures. The most common causes are athletics and industrial or automobile accidents. The degree of injury may range from mere bruising to complete laceration of the parenchyma or even rupture of the renal pedicle.

Clinical Findings

A. Symptoms and Signs: Gross hematuria following trauma means injury to the urinary tract. Pain and tenderness over the renal area may be significant, but they could be due to injury to osseous or muscular structures. Shock is common with multiple injuries or brisk bleeding from a lacerated kidney. It is accompanied by oliguria. Nausea, vomiting, and abdominal distention (ileus) are the rule. Bruising may be noted over the costovertebral area. A mass in the flank may represent extravasation of blood, urine, or both. This is best judged by percussion. Other injuries should be sought.

B. Laboratory Findings: Serial hematocrit determinations will give clues to persistent bleeding. Hematuria is to be expected.

C. X-Ray Findings: A plain film may reveal a large area of grayness in the region of the injured organ and obliteration of the psoas shadow. These findings imply the presence of a hematoma or urinary extravasation. Bowel gas may be displaced from that area. Evidence of fractures may be noted. Excretory urograms (high dose of radiopaque medium in the face of hypotension) may show a reasonably normal kidney if mildly contused, or extensive extravasation of the radiopaque material with laceration. Nonfunction suggests the possibility of injury to the vascular pedicle. The greatest value of excretory urograms lies in demonstrating that the contralateral kidney is normal; emergency removal of the injured kidney would then be feasible. Retrograde urograms are seldom necessary. Angiography may prove useful in selected cases depending on the findings on excretory urography. If significant renal damage is suspected, renal angiography should be done. This procedure will contribute to preoperative planning of renal reconstruction. Bleeding from a localized source in the kidney can often be controlled by injecting 0.5–1 ml of autologous clot through the selectively positioned arterial catheter.

Differential Diagnosis

Bony fractures or contusion of soft tissues in the region of the kidney may cause confusion. Hematuria might be secondary to vesical injury. The absence of a perirenal mass and normal urograms and radioisotope scans would rule out renal trauma.

Complications

A. Early: The most important complication is continuing perirenal hemorrhage, which can reach the stage of exsanguination. Serial hematocrit, blood pressure, and pulse determinations are essential. Evidence of an enlarging mass in the flank implies persistent bleeding. In the majority of cases, bleeding stops spontaneously, probably as a result of the tamponade effect of the perirenal fascia. Secondary bleeding 1 or 2 weeks later is occasionally observed. Spontaneous infection of the perirenal hematoma may occur.

B. Late: Excretory urograms should be obtained 3–6 months after surgery to observe for progressive hydronephrosis from ureteral obstruction or progressive atrophy due to vascular injury; this may cause hypertension.

Treatment

A. Emergency Measures: Treat shock and hemorrhage with blood transfusions. Bed rest is indicated until hematuria stops.

B. Surgical Measures: Most injured kidneys cease to bleed and heal without surgical intervention. Persistent bleeding requires exploration. A laceration may be sutured; nephrectomy or partial nephrectomy may be indicated.

C. Complications: Perinephric infection requires drainage. Nephrectomy or repair of secondary ureteral obstruction may be necessary.

Prognosis

Most injured kidneys heal spontaneously, although the patient must be examined at intervals for the onset of hypertension (renal ischemia) or progressive hydronephrosis due to secondary ureteral stricture.

Krahn HP, Axenrod H: The management of severe renal lacerations. J Urol 109:11, 1973.

Radwin HM, Fitch WP, Robison JR: Unified concept of renal trauma. J Urol 116:20, 1976.

Richter MW & others: Radiology of genitourinary trauma. Radiol Clin North Am 11:593, 1973.

Silber SJ, Collins E, Clark R: Treatment of hemorrhage from renal trauma by angiographic injection of clot. J Urol 116:15, 1976.

Spenle FR, Berg S: Renal trauma and hypertension. Arch Intern Med 136:1097, 1976.

2. INJURIES TO THE URETER

Essentials of Diagnosis

- Anuria or oliguria; prolonged ileus or flank pain following pelvic operation.
- Onset of urinary drainage through wound or vagina.
- Demonstration of urinary extravasation or ureteral obstruction by urography.

General Considerations

Most ureteral injuries follow extensive operations in the pelvis, eg, gynecologic procedures. A few follow cystoscopic ureteral manipulation. One ureter may inadvertently be sutured without evident complications, although progressive hydronephrosis develops. Division of the ureter will cause urinary extravasation, which usually results in a urinary fistula.

Clinical Findings

A. Symptoms and Signs: If the accident is not recognized at surgery, the patient may complain of flank and lower abdominal pain on the injured side. Ileus may be marked. Pyelonephritis may develop. Later, urine may drain through the wound or vagina. Anuria following pelvic surgery means bilateral ureteral ligation until proved otherwise. Rebound tenderness may be found if urine leaks into the peritoneal cavity. Leakage of urine into the deep vagina may be noted.

B. Laboratory Findings: Tests of renal function will be normal unless both ureters are occluded.

C. X-Ray Findings: Excretory urograms may show evidence of ureteral occlusion. Extravasation of radiopaque fluid may be seen in the region of the ureter. Retrograde urography will depict the site and nature of the injury.

Differential Diagnosis

Peritonitis may be mimicked if urine leaks into the peritoneal cavity. Excretory urography will reveal the ureteral involvement.

Oliguria may be due to dehydration, transfusion reaction, or bilateral incomplete ureteral injury. A survey of fluid and electrolyte intake and output, including serial body weights, should prove definitive. Total anuria implies bilateral ureteral injury and indicates the need for urologic investigation.

Vesicovaginal and ureterovaginal fistulas may be confused. Methylene blue solution instilled into the bladder will stain the vaginal urine in the former. Cystoscopy will visualize the vesical defect. Retrograde urography should reveal the ureteral fistula.

Complications

These include urinary fistula, ureteral stenosis with hydronephrosis, renal infection, peritonitis, and uremia (with bilateral injury).

Prevention

In the presence of large pelvic masses wherein the ureters may be dislocated, preoperative indwelling ureteral catheters should be placed for easy identification at surgery.

Treatment

A. Accident Recognized at Surgery:

1. Ureteral division—Repair of a ureter inadvertently cut during surgery consists of anastomosis of the ends over an indwelling T tube or 2 catheters; reimplanting the ureter into the bladder if the injury is juxtavesical; or implanting the end of the injured ureter into the side of the other ureter. The area must be drained.

2. Ureteral ligation—Remove the suture. To prevent late necrosis, excise the injured segment and anastomose the ureteral ends over a splint. Drain the area.

B. Accident Discovered After Surgery: Early intervention is recommended. Depending on the findings, the following procedures may be utilized: end-to-end anastomosis, reimplantation into the bladder, transureteroureterostomy, and replacement of a long ureteral segment with an isolated ileal segment. Nephrectomy may be indicated if the contralateral kidney is normal.

Prognosis

The results are best if the injury is recognized at the time of surgery. Late repair, if severe periureteral fibrosis has developed, is less likely to afford a good outcome.

Gangai MD, Agee RE, Spence CE: Surgical injury to the ureter. Urology 8:22, 1976.

Lee RA, Symmonds RE: Ureterovaginal fistula. Am J Obstet Gynecol 109:1032, 1971.

Reznichek RC, Brosman SA, Rhodes DB: Ureteral avulsion from blunt trauma. J Urol 109:812, 1973.

Thompson IM, Ross G Jr: Long-term results of bladder flap repair of ureteral injuries. J Urol 111:483, 1974.

3. INJURIES TO THE BLADDER

Essentials of Diagnosis

- History of trauma (including surgical and endoscopic).
- Fracture of the pelvis.
- Suprapubic pain and muscle rigidity.
- Hematuria.

General Considerations

The most common cause of vesical injury is external force over a full bladder. Rupture of the organ is seen in 15% of patients with pelvic fracture. The bladder may be inadvertently opened during pelvic surgery or injured by cystoscopic maneuvers, eg, transurethral resection of vesical tumor. If intraperitoneal, free extravasation of blood and urine will supervene, leading to signs of peritonitis. If extravesical, a mass will develop in the pelvis.

Clinical Findings

A. Symptoms and Signs: There is usually a history of local trauma. Hematuria is to be expected. Low abdominal pain is the rule. With severe trauma, the patient may be in shock. There is suprapubic tenderness and muscle rigidity. With intraperitoneal extravasation, rebound tenderness may be elicited. With extraperitoneal injury, a mass may be felt or percussed in the suprapubic area.

B. Laboratory Findings: Progressive bleeding may be reflected by a falling hematocrit. Hematuria is to be expected if the patient can void at all.

C. X-Ray Findings: A plain film may reveal fracture of the pelvis. An extraperitoneal collection of blood and urine may be revealed by a large gray area in the vesical area. Excretory urograms will survey the kidneys for damage. Extravasation of radiopaque fluid may be noted in the extravesical space or peritoneal cavity. The bladder may be compressed by a surrounding mass. A cystogram will almost always reveal escape of the fluid outside the bladder (Fig 43–8).

Differential Diagnosis

Renal injury is also associated with trauma and usually presents with hematuria. Excretory urograms show changes compatible with trauma; the cystogram is negative.

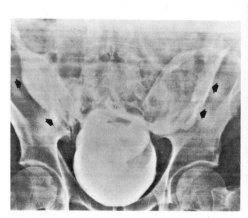
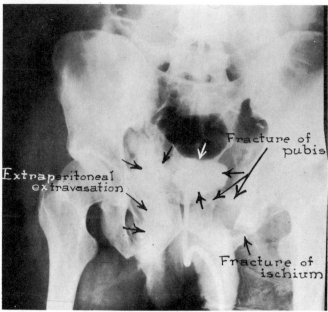

Figure 43—8. Vesical injuries. *Left:* Retrograde cystogram showing intraperitoneal extravasation. Note radiopaque material in both lumbar gutters. *Right:* Retrograde cystogram showing extraperitoneal rupture of the bladder secondary to fracture of the pelvis.

Injury to the membranous urethra can mimic extraperitoneal rupture of the bladder. With avulsion of the urethra, a catheter will be arrested in its passage. A urethrogram will reveal the site of injury.

Treatment

A. Emergency Measures: Treat shock and hemorrhage.

B. Specific Measures: For extraperitoneal rupture, drain the site of injury and insert a cystostomy tube. For intraperitoneal rupture, close the rent transperitoneally and drain the bladder by cystostomy.

Injury to other organs should be sought.

Prognosis

Early diagnosis and treatment lead to low morbidity and mortality rates.

Brosman SA, Fay R: Diagnosis and management of bladder trauma. J Trauma 13:687, 1973.

Cass AS: Bladder trauma in multiple injury patient. J Urol 115:667, 1976.

Holcroft JW, Trunkey DD: Renal trauma and retroperitoneal hematomas: Indications for exploration. J Trauma 15:1045, 1975.

Kerr WS Jr & others: Arteriography in pelvic fractures with massive hemorrhage. J Urol 109:479, 1973.

Lipsky H, Petritsch P, Schreyer H: Role of angiography in diagnosis and management of blunt renal trauma. Br J Urol 47:711, 1975.

4. INJURIES TO THE URETHRA

Membranous Urethra

This injury is commonly associated with pelvic fracture. Urinary extravasation and bleeding are periprostatic and perivesical. Urethral bleeding may be noted. With complete avulsion, voiding will lead to urinary extravasation. A suprapubic mass may develop. Rectal examination may reveal upward dislocation of the prostate.

The degree of bleeding may lower the hematocrit. If the patient can void, the urine will be found to contain red cells. A plain x-ray film usually reveals a fractured pelvis. A retrograde urethrogram will show extravasation at the site of injury. If a catheter can be passed to the bladder, the injury is minor.

Differentiation from vesical injury is made by urethrography and cystography. Injury to the bulbous urethra leads to perineal extravasation; injury to the membranous portion causes extravasation above the urogenital diaphragm (Fig 43—9).

Bleeding may be severe, requiring prompt replacement. Late complications include urethral stricture at the site of healing and impotence as a result of damage to local nerves or blood vessels.

If a catheter passes readily to the bladder, it should be left in for 10—14 days. If the urethra is completely avulsed, the area should be exposed surgically and the ends of the urethra anastomosed over a catheter. Postoperative urethrograms should be made in search of evidence of late stricture. There is no treatment for the impotence. Implantation of a plastic prosthesis may be considered.

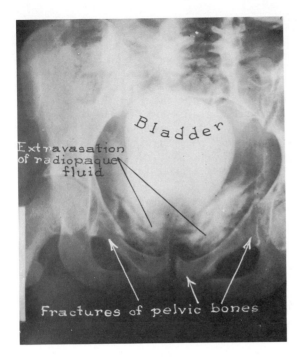
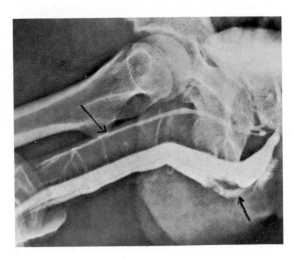

Figure 43—9. Injury to the membranous urethra. *Left:* Retrograde cystogram showing periprostatic extravasation; laceration of membranous urethra with fracture of pelvis. *Right:* Oblique urethrogram showing extravasation in region of bulbous urethra. Pressure injection caused radiopaque solution to enter venous system. (This is the mechanism for emboli if oily lubricants are injected into the urethra.)

The prognosis must be guarded because of the frequent occurrence of late stricture, which will require appropriate therapy.

Bulbous Urethra

Injuries to the bulbous urethra may occur as a result of instrumentation or, more commonly, falling astride an object. Urethral contusion may merely cause a perineal hematoma without injury to the urethral wall. Laceration will lead to urinary extravasation.

A history of perineal injury can usually be obtained. Local pain and some urethral bleeding are to be expected. Sudden swelling in the perineum may develop on attempt at urination. Examination reveals a perineal mass; extravasation of blood and urine involves the penis and scrotum and may spread onto the abdominal wall.

A catheter may pass to the bladder if the injury is minor but not if a severe laceration is present. The latter can be demonstrated by urethrography (Fig 43–9).

If the patient can void well and the perineal hematoma is small, no treatment is necessary. If the caliber of the urinary stream diminishes later, the urethra should be explored for stricture. If the injury is more severe and a catheter can be passed to the bladder, it should be left in for 10 days. Drainage of a large hematoma may be indicated.

If a catheter cannot be passed, surgical repair over an indwelling catheter will be necessary. If urinary extravasation is extensive, drainage will be required. If infected, appropriate antibiotics should be administered. If the patient has suffered multiple injuries and is in a state of shock, suprapubic cystotomy should be considered. Later, repair can be accomplished.

The only serious complication is stricture, which will require urethral dilatations.

Pendulous Urethra

External injury to this portion of the urethra is not common since the penis tends to "ride with the blow." The erect organ, however, is not so protected. Most trauma to this area is secondary to instrumentation. As a rule these injuries are mild, although a few may be complicated by stricture.

Some urethral bleeding and penile swelling are to be expected. The history of local injury is clear. A urethrogram may reveal the site and degree of injury.

If voiding is normal, no treatment is required. A large hematoma may be an indication for drainage. If a catheter cannot be passed, surgical repair over an indwelling catheter should be done.

Allison RC: Urethrography in pelvic trauma. J Urol 111:778, 1974.

Blumberg N: Anterior urethral injuries. J Urol 102:210, 1969.

Clark SS, Prudencio RF: Lower urinary tract injuries associated with pelvic fractures: Diagnosis and management. Surg Clin North Am 52:183, 1972.

Gibson GR: Urological management and complications of fractured pelvis and ruptured urethra. J Urol 111:353, 1974.

Jankegt RA: Management of complete disruption of the posterior urethra. Br J Urol 47:305, 1975.

Pierce JM Jr: Management of dismemberment of the prostatic-membranous urethra and ensuing stricture disease. J Urol 107:259, 1972.

5. INJURIES TO THE PENIS

The penis may be injured by a penetrating object or by a blow when the organ is erect. A constricting steel washer or rubber band can lead to gangrene. The skin of the penis may be avulsed if caught in machinery. The corpora cavernosa may be ruptured, leading to considerable extravasation of blood which can spread to the penis, scrotum, perineum, and abdominal wall. Occasionally, the urethra may be injured as well.

Constricting bodies must be removed. Avulsion of skin may require grafting. If a corpus cavernosum has been ruptured, suture of its tunica albuginea will be necessary.

Meares EM Jr: Traumatic rupture of the corpus cavernosum. J Urol 105:407, 1971.

Mendez R, Kiely WF, Morrow JW: Self-emasculation. J Urol 107:981, 1972.

Tuerk M, Weir WH Jr: Successful replantation of a traumatically amputated glans penis. Plast Reconstr Surg 48:499, 1971.

6. INJURIES TO THE TESTIS

Because of their mobility, the testes are seldom injured. If traumatized, pain is severe and there may be nausea and vomiting. Shock may result. The organ may be merely contused but can undergo complete rupture, in which case bleeding into the tunica vaginalis occurs, leading to marked swelling. In case of doubt, exploration should be done and lacerations closed. A few testes, seriously injured, may later undergo atrophy.

Schulman CC: Traumatic rupture of the testicle: An underestimated pathology. Urol Int 29:31, 1974.

TUMORS OF THE GENITOURINARY TRACT

1. TUMORS OF THE KIDNEY*

Essentials of Diagnosis
- Painless gross hematuria.
- Enlarged, firm kidney.
- Urographic evidence of vascular renal tumor.

*Wilms's tumor is discussed in Chapter 48, Pediatric Surgery.

General Considerations

Benign renal tumors are rare. Although lymphomatous or metastatic tumors occasionally involve the kidneys, by far the most common malignant neoplasm is adenocarcinoma. Adenocarcinoma arises from renal tubular cells, and as it expands it displaces calyces, blood vessels, and the renal pelvis. It is these characteristics that lead to urographic diagnosis. Later, the renal vein and even the vena cava may be occluded by tumor cells. Intraperitoneal organs may be displaced or invaded by the tumor.

The tumor has a pseudocapsule, and its cells resemble tubular cells. This tumor most commonly metastasizes to the liver, lungs, long bones, and regional lymph nodes.

Clinical Findings

A. Symptoms and Signs: Painless gross hematuria is the most common symptom. Pain is a late manifestation and is apt to be caused by hemorrhage into the tumor. The patient may discover a flank mass. Symptoms from metastasis may be the primary complaint, eg, loss of weight, anemia, bone pain (at times with spontaneous fracture), and pulmonary difficulties.

If the tumor is large, it may be easily palpable. It is nontender, firm, and may be nodular. With local invasion, it is fixed on respiration. Swelling over a bone may represent a metastasis. The liver may be enlarged and nodular.

B. Laboratory Findings: Gross or microscopic hematuria is usual. Erythrocytosis is seen in a few patients, and anemia is usually present in advanced disease. Total renal function is usually normal. The sedimentation rate is elevated in most cases. Hypercalcemia is at times observed.

C. X-Ray Findings: A plain abdominal film may reveal an enlarged kidney or a definite bulge of one portion. Osseous metastases may be seen on a skeletal series or discovered on bone scan. Excretory urograms show evidence of a space-occupying lesion typified by bending and displacement of calyces, and possibly an indentation of the renal pelvis (Fig 43–10). Visualization may be poor if most of the kidney is involved or if the renal vein is occluded by tumor. In the latter instance, retrograde urograms may be needed to afford necessary calyceal detail.

Nephrotomography may reveal increased density of the mass because of its vascularity. A cyst, from which tumor must be differentiated, will be revealed by lack of opacification. Angiography, particularly by the selective technic, will reveal typical tumor vessels in the capillary phase and increased opacification in the venous phase (Fig 43–11). Venacavography and selective renal phlebography will portray invasion of these structures.

A chest film is essential since pulmonary metastases are common.

D. Isotope Scanning: The ^{203}Hg scan will portray a tumor as a "cold" area but does not differentiate from cyst. The gamma camera, however, will reveal the

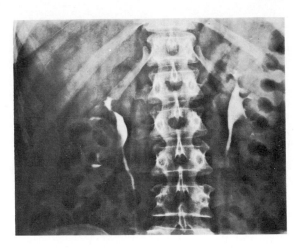

Figure 43—10. Adenocarcinoma of the kidney. Excretory urogram. Distortion of the pelvis and the middle and lower calyces of the right kidney. The left kidney is normal.

vascularity of the mass with ^{99m}Tc infusion.

E. Instrumental Examination: If the patient has gross hematuria when seen, immediate cystoscopy should be performed to identify the source of bleeding (renal or vesical).

Differential Diagnosis

Other renal lesions may present as a mass in the flank, including hydronephrosis and polycystic disease. Radiographic technics afford differentiation.

Renal cyst causes urographic changes similar to tumor, but steps taken to reveal vascularity of the mass (nephrotomography, sonography, angiography) lead to the proper diagnosis. In case of doubt, the cyst can be aspirated, then filled with radiopaque fluid. If the fluid is bloody, tumor should be expected. If clear, it should be subjected to cytologic study.

Lesions that also cause hematuria are stone; renal pelvic, ureteral, and vesical neoplasm; and tuberculosis. Excretory urograms should differentiate these from renal parenchymal tumor. In the case of vesical tumor, cystoscopy will be definitive.

Complications

These are usually related to local invasion or metastases. A few patients develop hydronephrosis from ureteral compression or hypertension from interference with renal blood supply. Occlusion of the renal vein may cause findings compatible with the nephrotic syndrome.

Treatment

A. Nephrectomy: In the absence of demonstrable metastases, radical nephrectomy is indicated.

B. X-Ray Therapy: These tumors are ordinarily radioresistant, but radiotherapy may have value in the palliative treatment of osseous metastases.

C. Chemotherapy: The administration of medroxyprogesterone (Depo-Provera), 1000 mg/week IM, may have some palliative effect, but in general chemotherapy has been disappointing.

Prognosis

About 35% of nephrectomized patients are alive at 5 years, but metastases may become evident 10—15 years later. The prognosis is poor if the renal vein is involved by tumor. A solitary metastasis should be surgically excised.

Blath RA, Mancilla-Jimenez R, Stanley RJ: Clinical comparison between vascular and avascular renal cell carcinoma. J Urol 115:514, 1976.

Bloom HJG: Adjuvant therapy for adenocarcinoma of the kidney: Present position and prospects. Br J Urol 45:237, 1973.

Dorr RP, Cerny JC, Hoskins PA: Inferior venacavagrams and renal venograms in the management of renal tumors. J Urol 110:280, 1973.

Doust VL, Doust BD, Redman HC: Evaluation of ultrasonic B-mode scanning in the diagnosis of renal masses. Am J Roentgenol 117:112, 1973.

Gehring GG: Coexisting avascular lesions and renal cell carcinoma. Urology 8:183, 1976.

Morales A, Eidinger D: Immune reactivity in renal cancer: Sequential study. J Urol 115:510, 1976.

Nygaard KK, Simon HB: Hypernephroma in children. Arch Surg 108:97, 1974.

Puigvert A: Partial nephrectomy for renal tumours: 21 cases. Eur Urol 2:70, 1976.

Tveter KJ: Unusual manifestations of renal carcinoma: A review of the literature. Acta Chir Scand 139:401, 1973.

Wagh DG, Murphy GP: Hormonal therapy in advanced renal cell carcinoma. Cancer 28:318, 1971.

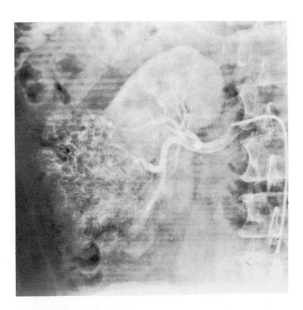

Figure 43—11. Adenocarcinoma of the kidney. Selective renal angiogram showing marked vascularity of mass in lower portion of right kidney typical of malignant tumor.

2. TUMORS OF THE RENAL PELVIS

Histologically, these tumors are similar to those seen in the ureter and bladder. They comprise about 10% of renal neoplasms. Benign tumors are very rare. Satellite tumors may involve the ureter. The rare epidermoid carcinoma is associated with chronic infection, and often with calculi. Such tumors may obstruct the ureteropelvic junction. The more malignant types may invade the renal parenchyma. These tumors metastasize to regional lymph nodes. Almost all are transitional cell carcinomas. The metabolites of tryptophan are suspect as carcinogenic agents.

Clinical Findings

A. Symptoms and Signs: Gross painless hematuria is the usual initial symptom. There may be flank pain if the tumor is obstructive.

B. Laboratory Findings: Hematuria is to be expected. Cytologic study discloses malignant cells in the urine in a high percentage of cases.

C. X-Ray Findings: Excretory or retrograde urograms will show a space-occupying lesion in the pelvis displacing the radiopaque medium (Fig 43–12). Secondary ureteral growths may be seen.

D. Instrumental Examination: Cystoscopy must be done immediately if there is gross hematuria so that its source can be identified. Such examination may reveal satellite tumors near the ureteral orifice.

Differential Diagnosis

Adenocarcinoma of the kidney usually presents with hematuria also, but urography should show the intrarenal position of the mass.

A nonopaque renal stone (ie, uric acid) may simulate renal pelvic tumor on urograms. Cytology is negative. The differential diagnosis may be made only at the operating table.

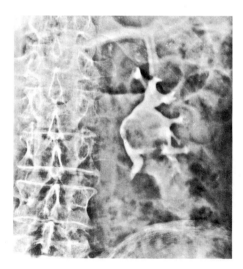

Figure 43–12. Excretory urogram showing space-occupying lesion of left renal pelvis. Transitional cell carcinoma.

Renal tuberculosis may show an obliterated calyx, thus simulating an invasive pelvic neoplasm. Other calyces, however, may show ulceration. Sterile pyuria and a positive urine culture for tubercle bacilli will make the differentiation.

Complications

Rarely, hemorrhage may be so severe as to require immediate nephrectomy. Obstruction may lead to secondary infection.

Treatment

Nephroureterectomy plus removal of a cuff of bladder mucosa around the ureteral orifice should be done, for satellite tumors in the ureter and bladder may develop later. These tumors are somewhat resistant to radiotherapy.

Prognosis

With low-grade malignancies, the cure rate is about 75%. The outlook is poor with the more anaplastic neoplasms.

Cummings KB & others: Renal pelvic tumours. J Urol 113:158, 1975.

Johansson S & others: Uroepithelial tumors of the renal pelvis associated with abuse of phenacetin-containing analgesics. Cancer 33:743, 1974.

Poole-Wilson DS: Occupational tumours of the renal pelvis and ureter arising in the dye-making industry. Proc R Soc Med 62:93, 1969.

Ulagle DC & others: Primary carcinoma of renal pelvis. Cancer 33:1642, 1974.

3. TUMORS OF THE URETER

Tumors of the ureter are seldom benign. They may be found in association with transitional cell tumors of the renal pelvis or bladder. Carcinogens are suspect as the etiologic factor (see Tumors of the Bladder, General Considerations). Transitional cell carcinomas range from a low to a high grade of malignancy. The latter are invasive and most commonly metastasize to regional lymph nodes, lungs, and liver.

Clinical Findings

A. Symptoms and Signs: Micro- or macrohematuria is the most common symptom. Should the tumor produce obstruction, renal pain may be noted. Local examination is usually unrewarding; a large hydronephrotic kidney might be palpable.

B. Laboratory Findings: Hematuria is usually found. Anemia may be noted if bleeding has been severe or if metastases are widespread. Tests of renal function are normal if the disease is unilateral.

C. X-Ray Findings: Excretory urograms portray a space-occupying lesion in the ureter (Fig 43–13). The ureter may be dilated proximal to that point. Evidence of tumor of the renal pelvis should also be sought. A

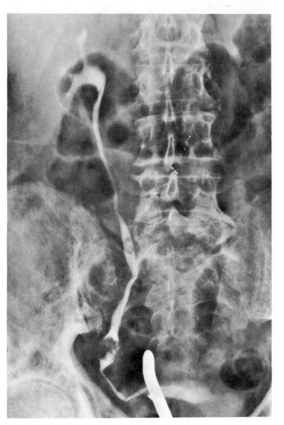

Figure 43–13. Retrograde urogram showing "negative" shadow caused by transitional cell carcinoma of the lower right ureter without evidence of obstruction.

chest film should be examined for evidence of metastasis. If the kidney is nonfunctioning, a retrograde ureterogram is essential to delineate the lesion.

D. Instrumental Examination: Any patient who presents with gross hematuria should immediately undergo cystoscopy to identify the source of bleeding. Bloody efflux from a ureteral orifice requires further study of the upper urinary tract. Occasionally, the tumor can be seen protruding from the ureteral orifice. Applying a special brush, one can scrape epithelial cells from the surface for histologic examination.

E. Urinary Cytology: Cytologic examination of urine sediment shows cancer cells in well over 90% of patients with transitional cell tumors (renal pelvis, ureter, bladder).

Differential Diagnosis

A radiolucent ureteral stone can mimic the signs and symptoms of ureteral tumor. The excretory (or retrograde) urogram will reveal a "negative" shadow in each. Cytology is negative with stone. At times, the definitive diagnosis is made only at the operating table.

Ureteral stenosis—usually due to external compression by a blood vessel or lymph nodes involved by cancer—may cause similar symptoms, signs, and x-ray findings. Negative cytology and evidence of a primary site of metastases should lead to the differentiation.

Complications

Hydronephrosis may develop secondary to an obstructing tumor. The stasis that results may lead to infection.

Treatment

In the absence of metastases, complete nephroureterectomy plus removal of the periureteral vesical area is indicated in order to prevent "seeding" of the ureter below the lesion and in the bladder. Nephroureterectomy may be needed even in advanced cases if pain or severe hematuria becomes disabling. Benign lesions may lend themselves to local excision.

Prognosis

The outlook for the patient with a tumor of lowgrade malignancy is good. Those with highly malignant tumors seldom live 2 years after definitive surgery.

Cancelmo JJ Jr & others: Tumors of the ureter: Problems in diagnosis. Am J Roentgenol 117:132, 1973.
Colgan JR III, Skaist L, Morrow JW: Benign ureteral tumors in childhood: A case report and a plea for conservative management. J Urol 109:308, 1973.
Petković SD: A plea for conservative operation for ureteral tumors. J Urol 107:220, 1972.
Williams CB, Mitchell JP: Carcinoma of the ureter: A review of 54 cases. Br J Urol 45:377, 1973.

4. TUMORS OF THE BLADDER

Essentials of Diagnosis

- Hematuria.
- Symptoms of cystitis.
- Renal pain.
- Positive urinary cytology.
- Cystoscopic visualization and positive biopsy.

General Considerations

Most vesical neoplasms are transitional cell in type. Both the prognosis and the type of treatment indicated depend upon the degree of differentiation of the cells and the depth of penetration of the tumor in the bladder. Low-grade tumors (I and II) tend to be superficial, whereas grade III and IV tumors are more invasive and are usually found in the muscle layer. The higher the grade and the more invasive, the poorer the prognosis. Low-grade superficial tumors respond well to transurethral technics; high-grade invasive tumors require radiotherapy or radical surgery or both.

Most vesical tumors develop in the posterior half of the bladder (trigonal region). Occlusion of a ureteral orifice, leading to hydronephrosis, is therefore not uncommon. An ulcerated tumor not only tends to bleed but may become secondarily infected. Multifocal tumors are common.

Rarer tumors include squamous cell carcinoma, adenocarcinoma (in a urachal remnant), and rhabdomyosarcoma (mostly in children).

It has long been established that prolonged exposure to certain industrial aromatic amines is associated with a high incidence of vesical neoplasia. Recent work suggests that multiple transitional cell tumors are probably caused by carcinogens, particularly tryptophan, which is changed in the urinary tract to orthophenols which have proved to be carcinogenic in dogs and mice. Smoking increases the amount of these substances in the urine. On cessation of smoking, the levels return to normal.

Clinical Findings

A. Symptoms and Signs: Gross hematuria is the most common complaint. Secondary infection leads to symptoms of cystitis. Should the tumor involve the vesical neck, symptoms of urinary obstruction may supervene. Extravesical extension may cause constant suprapubic pain. If the tumor occludes a ureteral orifice, renal pain may develop; if both are overgrown, uremia results.

In most cases, nothing abnormal is found on physical examination. An extensive tumor may be palpable suprapubically, vaginally, or rectally. Bimanual palpation (abdominovaginal or rectal) may reveal a palpable mass and evidence of fixation (invasion). This is best done under anesthesia.

B. Laboratory Findings: Anemia (secondary to uremia or hemorrhage) may be present. Red cells are usually found in the urine. Pyuria and bacteriuria are

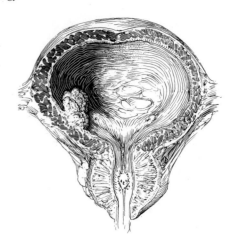

Figure 43–15. Transitional cell (papillary) carcinoma of the bladder with minimal invasion of the bladder wall.

common. Renal function tests are normal unless bilateral ureteral obstruction has developed.

C. X-Ray Findings: Excretory urograms are usually normal, but the tumor may be depicted as a "negative" shadow (Fig 43–14). Ureteral occlusion will be reflected by the presence of hydroureteronephrosis. Vesical angiography may prove helpful in judging the presence of invasion of the extravesical tissues.

D. Instrumental Examination: Cystoscopy is the definitive test since the tumor is readily visualized (Fig 43–15). Biopsy is mandatory.

E. Cytology: Papanicolaou preparations are almost diagnostic.

F. Staging: Staging of bladder tumors is dependent on the depth of invasion and the presence or absence of metastasis. Staging usually relates to the grade of the tumor. A commonly used classification of staging and the basic principles of treatment and prognosis are shown in Table 43–1.

Differential Diagnosis

Vesical neoplasm is differentiated from other causes of hematuria by cystoscopy, urography, and cytologic examination.

Complications

Secondary vesical infection is common when the tumor becomes ulcerated. Hydroureteronephrosis is the product of invasion of the intravesical ureter. The degree of hemorrhage may become a problem.

Prevention

Contact with analine dyes should be limited to 3 years, during which time urinary cytologic studies and periodic cystoscopy are indicated.

Treatment

A. Surgical Measures: Most single or multiple superficial tumors can be cured by deep saucerization

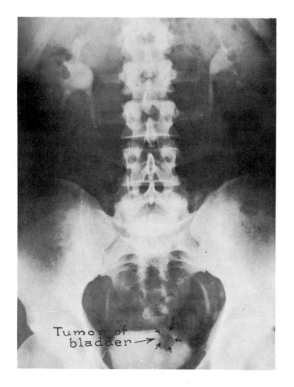

Figure 43–14. Excretory urogram showing space-occupying lesion (transitional cell carcinoma) on the left side of the bladder; the upper tracts are normal.

Table 43–1. Treatment and prognosis of bladder tumors related to stage of disease.

Stage		Treatment	Five-Year Survival Rate
0	Mucosa only	Transurethral resection	90%
A	Submucosal invasion	Transurethral resection, partial cystectomy,	60–80%
B_1	Superficial muscle invasion	total cystectomy	
B_2	Deep muscle invasion	(1) Radical cystectomy	30–50%
C	Perivesical fat invasion	(2) Preoperative radiation followed by radical cystectomy	30–50%
D_1	Regional lymph nodes	(3) Radiation therapy	5–30%
D_2	Distant metastases	Radiation and chemotherapy	nil

of the vesical wall with the resectoscope. However, this method will fail if the tumor has invaded deeply. Wide partial cystectomy may be utilized for tumors involving the dome. Total cystectomy (with removal of the prostate) may be indicated for papillomatosis and for high-grade invasive tumors. Urinary diversion is then necessary, eg, ureteroileal cutaneous conduit or ureterosigmoidostomy. The former is complicated by renal stone formation and stomal stenosis. In the latter, hyperchloremic acidosis and hypokalemia may be noted. This is usually controlled with $NaHCO_3$ or sodium or potassium citrate. Added potassium is essential. A rectal tube, worn at night, will lessen electrolyte absorption. Pyelonephritis or ureteral stenosis at the sigmoid level may develop.

B. Radiation Therapy: The more undifferentiated the tumor, the more radiosensitive it is. Radiotherapy is particularly useful for high-grade invasive neoplasms. A dosage of 6000 rads given over 6 weeks preserves vesical function. If recurrence of the tumor is discovered 3 months after therapy, total cystectomy is feasible.

C. Chemotherapy: The effects of parenterally administered chemotherapeutic agents have been disappointing. Superficial low-grade tumors may be controlled or even disappear with thiotepa instillations. Sixty mg are dissolved in 30–60 ml of normal saline. Instillations by catheter are made weekly for 4–6 weeks. Monthly treatment should then be given for 6–10 months. Before each instillation, a white cell and platelet count should be obtained. If the white count is less than $4000/\mu l$ or the platelets below $100,000/\mu l$, treatment should be deferred until the hemogram improves.

Prognosis

Superficial, well-differentiated tumors may recur or new papillomas may appear. Periodic urinary cytologic examination and cystoscopy should be done for at least 3 years. The low-grade tumors afford the best prognosis. The more undifferentiated invasive tumors are controlled by cystectomy or radiation therapy in 15–20% of cases.

Dretler SP, Ragsdale BD, Leadbetter WF: The value of pelvic lymphadenectomy with surgical treatment of bladder cancer. J Urol 104:414, 1973.

Goffinet DR & others: Bladder cancer: Result of radiation therapy in 384 patients. Radiology 117:149, 1975.

Johnson DE & others: Squamous cell carcinoma of the bladder. J Urol 115:542, 1976.

Prout GR Jr: Surgical management of bladder cancer. Urol Clin North Am 3:149, 1976.

Ray B & others: Bladder tumors in children. Urology 2:426, 1973.

Redman JF, Tranum BT: Late recurrence of transitional cell carcinoma of the bladder. Urology 8:51, 1976.

Resnick MI, O'Conor VJ Jr: Segmental resection for carcinoma of the bladder: Review of 102 patients. J Urol 109:1007, 1973.

Richie JP & others: Squamous carcinoma of the bladder: Treatment by radical cystectomy. J Urol 115:670, 1976.

Riddle PR: The management of superficial bladder tumours with intravesical Epodyl. Br J Urol 45:84, 1973.

Stams UK, Gursel EO, Veenema RJ: Prophylactic urethrectomy in male patients with bladder cancer. J Urol 111:177, 1974.

Tank ES & others: Treatment of urogenital tract rhabdomyosarcoma in infants and children. J Urol 107:324, 1972.

Trott PA, Edwards L: Comparison of bladder washings and urine cytology in the diagnosis of bladder cancer. J Urol 110:664, 1973.

5. BENIGN PROSTATIC HYPERPLASIA

Essentials of Diagnosis

- Prostatism: hesitancy, slow stream, terminal dribbling, frequency.
- Residual urine.
- Acute urinary retention.
- Uremia in advanced cases.

General Considerations

The cause of benign prostatic enlargement is not known, but it is probably related to estrogen-androgen imbalance. Hyperplasia of the prostatic lobes causes increased outflow resistance, largely by upsetting the mechanism for opening and funneling the vesical neck at the time of voiding. This creates a need for a higher intravesical voiding pressure to accomplish voiding, which in turn causes hypertrophy of the vesical and trigonal muscles. This may lead to the development of vesical diverticula, which represent outpocketings of vesical mucosa through the detrusor muscle bundles. Hypertrophy of the trigone causes an abnormal degree

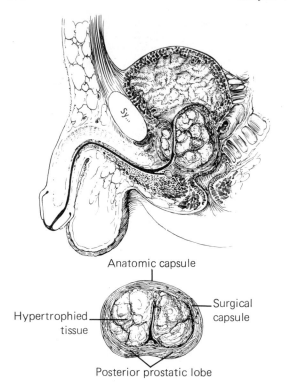

Anatomic capsule

Hypertrophied
tissue

Surgical
capsule

Posterior prostatic lobe

Figure 43—16. Pathogenesis of benign prostatic hyperplasia. Enlarged prostate enclosed by relatively thick "surgical" capsule which is composed of the posterior prostatic lobe.

of traction upon the intravesical ureter, leading to its functional obstruction and resulting in hydroureteronephrosis. In late cases, ureterovesical reflux may develop.

Stagnation of urine leads to the complication of infection; the onset of cystitis will exacerbate the obstructive symptoms. Pyelonephritis will only occur if there is reflux of infected urine from the bladder.

The lobes that most commonly undergo enlargement are the 2 lateral lobes and the subcervical lobe.

The prostate of the young adult has an anatomic capsule like an apple peel. In the man with prostatic enlargement, there is a thick "surgical" capsule similar to an orange peel composed of peripherally compressed prostatic tissue (posterior lobe). This permits intracapsular enucleation of the enlarged lobes (Fig 43–16).

Clinical Findings

A. Symptoms and Signs: Typically, the patient notices hesitancy and loss of force and caliber of the stream. Terminal dribbling is particularly disturbing. The complication of infection increases the degree of obstructive symptoms and is often associated with burning on urination. Acute urinary retention may supervene. This is associated with severe urgency, suprapubic pain, and a palpable bladder.

The size of the prostate is not of diagnostic importance since the correlation between the size of

the gland and the degree of symptoms and amount of residual urine is poor.

B. Laboratory Findings: Urinalysis may reveal evidence of infection. The PSP test may show an excretion curve compatible with residual urine or impaired renal function. The serum creatinine may be elevated in cases with prolonged severe obstruction.

C. X-Ray Findings: Excretory urograms are usually normal but may show hydroureteronephrosis if significant obstruction is present. This is usually due to an abnormal pull on the intravesical ureters by the hypertrophied trigonal muscle; these changes usually revert to normal after prostatectomy. An indentation into the inferior surface of the bladder from the enlarged gland may be seen.

D. Instrumental Examination: The presence of residual urine may be discovered if the patient is catheterized immediately after voiding. Endoscopy will reveal secondary vesical changes (eg, trabeculation) and enlargement of prostatic lobes.

Differential Diagnosis

Neurogenic bladder may offer a similar syndrome. A history suggesting a neurogenic difficulty may be obtained. Neurologic deficit involving S2–4 is particularly significant.

Cancer of the prostate also causes symptoms of vesical neck obstruction. Such a patient may have, in addition, symptoms and signs of osseous metastases. Typically, the cancerous gland is stony hard. Serum and bone marrow acid phosphatase are elevated in advanced cases. Serum alkaline phosphatase is usually increased if the tumor has spread to bone.

Acute prostatitis may cause symptoms of obstruction, but the patient is septic and has infected urine. The prostate is hot and exquisitely tender.

Urethral stricture diminishes the caliber of the urinary stream. There is usually a history of complicated gonorrhea or local trauma. A retrograde urethrogram will show the stenotic area. A stricture arrests the passage of an instrument.

Complications

Obstruction and residual urine lead to vesical and prostatic infection which may be difficult to eradicate. In the few patients with vesicoureteral reflux, pyelonephritis may ensue.

The obstruction may lead to the development of vesical diverticula. Infected residual urine may contribute to the formation of calculi.

Functional obstruction of the intravesical ureter, caused by the hypertrophic trigone, may lead to hydroureteronephrosis.

Treatment

The criteria for operative intervention are impairment of or threat to renal function and symptoms disturbing enough so that the patient demands relief. Because the degree of obstruction progresses slowly if at all in most patients, conservative treatment is usually adequate.

A. Conservative Measures: Regular intercourse or masturbation is the best means of relieving prostatic congestion. If this is not feasible, periodic prostatic massage (3 or 4 times at 2-week intervals) will relieve the congestion and cause some alleviation of symptoms. Should symptoms increase, another series of massages can be given. Treatment of prostatitis may reduce prostatic edema. The resolution of a complicating cystitis will usually afford some relief. In order to protect vesical tone, the patient should be cautioned to void as soon as the urge develops. Forcing fluids over a short period of time, leading to rapid vesical filling, decreases vesical tone and is a common cause of sudden acute urinary retention.

Catheterization is mandatory for acute urinary retention. In most cases, spontaneous voiding will result. If it does not, a catheter should be left indwelling for 3 days while detrusor tone returns to maximum. If this fails, surgery is indicated. If the patient is a very poor operative risk, cryosurgery or a permanent catheter may be necessary.

B. Surgery: Four methods of prostatectomy are available to the surgeon: transurethral, retropubic, suprapubic, and perineal. The type of approach should be left to the judgment of the urologist. The mortality rate is low for all (1–4%). Sexual potency is threatened only when the perineal route is used.

Cryosurgery has its proponents in the poor-risk patient. The place for this procedure in the treatment of the obstructing prostatic hypertrophy remains to be evaluated.

Prognosis

Most patients receive considerable relief following conservative treatment. If, on follow-up, symptoms increase or renal function begins to diminish, surgery is warranted.

Marshall A & others: An assessment of cryosurgery in the treatment of prostatic obstruction. J Urol 109:1026, 1973.

Nicoll GA: Suprapubic prostatectomy: A comparative analysis of 525 consecutive cases. J Urol 111:213, 1974.

Singh M, Tresidder GC, Blandy JP: The evaluation of transurethral resection for benign enlargement of the prostate. Br J Urol 45:93, 1973.

Turner-Warwick R & others: A urodynamic view of prostatic obstruction and the results of prostatectomy. Br J Urol 45:631, 1973.

Watanabe H & others: Diagnostic application of ultrasonotomography to the prostate. Invest Urol 8:548, 1971.

6. CARCINOMA OF THE PROSTATE

Essentials of Diagnosis

- Symptoms of vesical neck obstruction.
- Stony hard prostate.
- Osteoblastic osseous metastases.
- Anemia.
- Elevated serum and bone marrow acid phosphatase in advanced cases.

General Considerations

Prostatic cancer is rare before age 60. The cause is not known. Androgens stimulate its growth; estrogens retard it. Most malignancies arise in the posterior lobe, which does not undergo benign enlargement. The early hard lesion is usually found in the lateral sulcus of one lobe. As it progresses, it involves the entire gland and the seminal vesicles (Fig 43–17). Metastasis to the pelvic lymph nodes and the bones of the pelvis is common.

Clinical Findings

A. Symptoms and Signs: The presenting symptoms in 95% of men with prostatic malignancy are due to obstruction, infection, or both. (See Benign Prostatic Hyperplasia, above.) Some patients have symptoms due to metastases also when first seen—eg, low back pain radiating down one or both legs. In a few cases, only the latter symptoms are present at onset.

Rectal examination may reveal an isolated hard nodule in the prostate, usually in one of the lateral margins. In advanced cases, the entire gland may be stony hard and fixed. The seminal vesicles may be involved. Signs of metastases include a nodular liver, pathologic fracture, and paraplegia due to sudden collapse of a vertebral body.

B. Laboratory Findings: Anemia may be found in patients whose bone marrow has been replaced by tumor or those with uremia. Urinalysis may reveal infection. In the early stages, renal function is normal, but if ureteral occlusion develops or if there is residual urine, the PSP will be depressed. Serum creatinine may be elevated. Serum acid phosphatase levels are usually increased when the tumor has extended outside its capsule. In the presence of osseous metastases, the alkaline phosphatase is elevated, reflecting osteogenic activity.

C. X-Ray Findings: A chest film may show evidence of metastases to hilar nodes, lungs, or ribs. A plain film of the abdomen may reveal osseous spread.

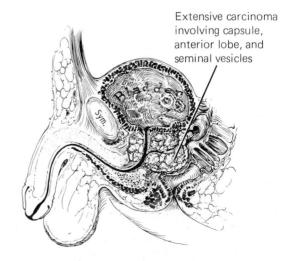

Extensive carcinoma involving capsule, anterior lobe, and seminal vesicles

Figure 43–17. Advanced carcinoma of prostate; trabeculation of bladder wall.

The common sites include the pelvic bones, lumbar spine, and femoral heads. Excretory urograms may show hydroureteronephrosis from vesical neck or ureteral obstruction.

D. Isotope Studies: A total body scan may show increased uptake of the isotope in areas of bony metastases even before the osteograms reveal such evidence.

E. Instrumental Examination: Passage of a catheter will measure the amount of residual urine. Cystoscopy will reveal the degree of prostatic encroachment and secondary vesical changes, eg, trabeculation. Invasion of the trigone is a late sign.

F. Biopsy: The diagnosis in advanced cases may be established on tissue removed by transurethral resection or needle biopsy. With small localized lesions, these methods may fail. Aspiration of marrow from the iliac crest may reveal tumor cells and increased levels of acid phosphatase even though osteograms are normal.

Differential Diagnosis

Benign prostatic hyperplasia lacks the hard areas exhibited by cancer. Bone films and serum phosphatase levels are normal.

Hard nodules may be caused by scarring secondary to chronic infection, tuberculosis, or calculi. Evidence of tuberculosis, or stones seen in an x-ray of the prostatic area, may be of help. Needle biopsy, perineal or transrectal, should be definitive.

Complications

Significant vesical neck or ureteral obstruction may lead to uremia. Edema of a leg may develop from compression of the iliac vein by metastases to regional lymph nodes. Spontaneous fractures may occur.

Treatment

A. Curative Measures: In the patient with an isolated nodule, and in the absence of demonstrable metastases, radical prostatectomy may lead to cure. Radiation therapy has proved to be effective in eradicating localized disease.

B. Palliative Measures: Antiandrogen therapy has an excellent palliative effect on advanced prostatic cancer, but it has been suggested that estrogens are apt to increase the incidence of thromboembolic phenomena. It is probably best to reserve it for the most advanced cases, eg, urinary retention, osseous metastases. Bilateral orchiectomy (which can be combined with estrogen therapy) is an excellent palliative procedure.

In late cases, medical adrenalectomy—accomplished by the administration of corticosteroids—may afford temporary relief from the pain of metastatic bone lesions. Destruction of the pituitary by the local injection of ^{90}yttrium or by cryotherapy may afford a remission.

Transurethral prostatic resection may be necessary to relieve prostatic obstruction. Cryosurgery has its advocates. Radiation therapy to the gland is being accepted with increasing enthusiasm. In the absence of metastasis to lymph nodes, possibly 20% of patients can be cured. The prostate is apt to shrink, thus relieving obstructive symptoms. X-ray therapy to painful osseous metastases may relieve pain. Table 43–2 outlines the various stages, methods of treatment, and survival rates.

Prognosis

Radical prostatectomy cures more than 70% of the patients suitable for this operation, but it should be limited to men with a reasonable life expectancy. After age 70, palliative therapy will afford as good a result as radical surgery. This means that only about 5% of patients with prostatic malignancy are curable. Careful rectal examination, seeking suspicious areas of induration, in all men over age 50 is mandatory if this cure rate is to be improved.

Barnes R, Hirst A, Rosenquist R: Early carcinoma of the prostate: Comparison of stages A and B. J Urol 115:404, 1976.

Barnes RW, Ninan CA: Carcinoma of the prostate: Biopsy and conservative therapy. J Urol 108:897, 1972.

Bhanalaph T, Varkarakis MJ, Murphy GP: Current status of bilateral adrenalectomy for advanced prostatic carcinoma. Ann Surg 179:17, 1974.

Blackard CE, Byar DP, Jordan WP Jr: Orchiectomy for advanced prostatic carcinoma. Urology 1:553, 1973.

Carlton CE & others: Radiotherapy in the management of stage C carcinoma of the prostate. J Urol 116:206, 1976.

Table 43–2. Treatment and prognosis of prostatic cancer related to stage of disease.

Stage	Clinical Findings	Treatment	Ten-Year Survival Rate
A	No palpable lesion; incidental histologic findings.	Observation.	50–70%
B$_1$	Localized nodule 1–1.5 cm in diameter surrounded by normal prostate.	Radical prostatectomy with or without pelvic lymphadenectomy.	50–70%
B$_2$	Larger nodule; more diffuse induration.	Radiation, with or without pelvic lymphadenectomy for staging, with or without hormonal therapy.	25–30%
C	Periprostatic extension.		
D	Distant metastases.	Hormonal therapy, with or without radiotherapy, with or without transurethral resection for relief of obstruction.	0–5%

Castellino RA & others: Lymphangiography in prostatic carcinoma. JAMA 223:877, 1973.

Fossa DS, Miller A: Treatment of advanced carcinoma of the prostate with estramustine phosphate. J Urol 115:406, 1976.

Gill WB & others: Radical retropubic prostatectomy and retroperitoneal lymphadenectomy following radiotherapy conversion of stage C to stage B carcinoma of the prostate. J Urol 111:656, 1974.

Ray GR, Cassady JR, Bagshaw MA: Definitive radiation therapy of carcinoma of the prostate: A report on 15 years of experience. Radiology 106:407, 1973.

Scott WW & others: Continued evaluation of the effects of chemotherapy in patients with advanced carcinoma of the prostate. J Urol 116:211, 1976.

Tong ECK, Finkelstein P: The treatment of prostatic bone metastases with parathormone and radioactive phosphorus. J Urol 109:71, 1973.

7. SARCOMA OF THE PROSTATE

Sarcoma of the prostate is rare. Half of cases occur in boys under age 5. The tumor is highly malignant and metastasizes to the pelvic and lumbar lymph nodes, lungs, liver, and bone. Symptoms are those of obstruction to urination. The prostate is found to be enlarged. Cystography or excretory urography may show superior displacement of the bladder or encroachment of the tumor into the bladder. Endoscopy will reveal the growth and allows biopsy.

Total prostatocystectomy has cured a few cases. The neoplasm is relatively radioresistant.

Smith BH, Dehner LP: Sarcoma of the prostate gland. Am J Clin Pathol 58:43, 1972.

8. TUMORS OF THE URETHRA

Malignant tumors of the urethra are uncommon. They occur most often in women. Those arising distally are squamous epitheliomas which metastasize to the inguinal nodes. The deeper tumors are transitional cell in type and spread to the lymph nodes in the pelvis. Bleeding on urination or bloody spotting is noted. The growth may be visible at the meatus. The more proximal tumors may cause obstructive symptoms as well. The diagnosis is established by biopsy.

In the female, distal tumors will require resection. In men, penile amputation is necessary. For the most proximal neoplasms, urethrocystectomy is indicated. In general, these tumors are radioresistant.

The prognosis is fair to poor.

Bracken RB & others: Primary carcinoma of the female urethra. J Urol 116:188, 1976.

Chu AM: Female urethral carcinoma. Radiology 107:627, 1973.

Grabstald H: Tumors of the urethra in men and women. Cancer 32:1236, 1973.

9. TUMORS OF THE TESTIS

Essentials of Diagnosis

- Painless, enlarged, firm testis developing between the ages of 18–35.
- Midline abdominal mass (lymph nodes).
- Gynecomastia.

General Considerations

With rare exceptions, all tumors of the testis are malignant. Most are observed between the ages of 18–35. Those containing trophoblastic cells are highly malignant and are associated with gynecomastia and increased levels of urinary chorionic gonadotropins. Most arise from germ cells; seminomas, embryonal carcinomas, and malignant teratomas are the most common. Choriocarcinoma is rare. Testicular tumors metastasize to the lumbar, mediastinal, and supraclavicular lymph nodes and lungs. Probably 30–40% of patients will have metastases when first seen.

The rarest testicular tumors are Sertoli cell and interstitial cell tumors, and most of these are benign.

Clinical Findings

A. Symptoms and Signs: These tumors usually

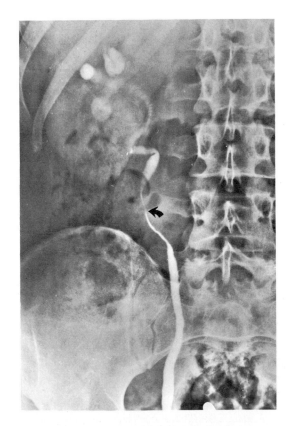

Figure 43–18. Carcinoma of the testis. Retrograde bulb ureterogram showing hydronephrosis and ureteral deviation at L4 secondary to metastases in right lumbar lymph nodes.

present as a painless enlargement, although the onset may be painful if spontaneous bleeding occurs. With endocrine-functioning tumors, gynecomastia may be the initial complaint. Symptoms due to metastases include a supraclavicular or upper midline abdominal mass (lymph nodes) or loss of weight and anorexia.

Examination usually reveals a symmetrically enlarged, firm, nontender organ, though occasionally an isolated nodule may be noted. Secondary hydrocele is present in 10% of cases. Gynecomastia may be present. A midline abdominal mass or enlarged Virchow's nodes are evidence of metastases.

B. Laboratory Findings: Analysis of a preoperative sample of urine for chorionic gonadotropins is essential since their elevation reflects a poor prognosis (choriocarcinoma).

C. X-Ray Findings: A chest film may reveal pulmonary or hilar node metastases. Excretory urograms are indicated in all cases to note whether the upper ureter is deviated by the presence of metastases to the lumbar lymph nodes (Fig 43-18). Lymphangiography will reveal evidence of metastases to these nodes.

Differential Diagnosis

Hydrocele presents as a scrotal enlargement. The mass feels cystic and transilluminates. Some tumors, however, are associated with secondary hydrocele. This should be aspirated if the testicle cannot be properly palpated.

Spermatocele is a small cystic mass lying free above the testis. Aspiration will reveal dead sperms.

Should the tumor bleed spontaneously, it may present as a painful swelling, thus being confused with acute epididymitis. The latter usually presents with fever and pyuria. In the early stages, the enlarged, tender epididymis can be delineated from the normal testis. Confusion in this differentiation is a common cause of delayed diagnosis.

Complications

These arise from metastasis. A ureter may be occluded by involved lumbar nodes, leading to hydronephrosis.

Treatment

A. Surgery: If tumor cannot be ruled out, the testis should be removed. Orchiectomy is performed through an inguinal incision and the spermatic cord divided at the internal ring. The testicle is then delivered from the scrotum and removed. Radical resection of the retroperitoneal lymph nodes is indicated in all cases of embryonal carcinomas, teratocarcinomas, and, possibly, choriocarcinomas. In some, inoperability is discovered.

B. X-Ray Therapy: Radiotherapy is indicated in all cases. Seminomas are highly radiosensitive. For the other types of tumors, radiotherapy is given following lymph node resection. Some surgeons give half the radiation before node dissection and the rest after surgery. X-ray to the mediastinum and neck for prophylactic reasons is essential.

C. Chemotherapy: Antitumor chemotherapy is utilized in the palliation of metastatic cancer with demonstrable benefit. Triple drug therapy is favored. This usually consists of an alkylating agent (eg, chlorambucil), an antimetabolite (eg, methotrexate), and the antitumor antibiotic dactinomycin. (See Chapter 49.)

Prognosis

Except in the case of seminomas, which are the least malignant and the most radiosensitive testicular tumors, the presence of metastases implies a poor prognosis. In teratocarcinoma or embryonal carcinoma, the 5-year survival rate is 75-80%. With few exceptions, patients with choriocarcinoma are dead at 2 years despite intensive therapy.

Biswamay R & others: Distribution of retroperitoneal lymph node metastases in testicular germinal tumors. Cancer 33:340, 1974.

Bradfield JS, Hagen RO, Ytredal DO: Carcinoma of the testis: An analysis of 104 patients with germinal tumors of the testes other than seminoma. Cancer 31:633, 1973.

Earle JD, Bagshaw MA, Kaplan HS: Supervoltage radiation therapy of the testicular tumors. Am J Roentgenol 117:653, 1973.

Giebink GS, Ruymann FB: Testicular tumors in children. Am J Dis Child 127:433, 1974.

Jonsson K, Ingemansson S, Ling L: Lymphangiography in patients with testicular tumor. Br J Urol 45:548, 1973.

Keorgh B & others: Urinary gonadotropins in the management and prognosis of testicular tumors. Urology 5:496, 1975.

Smith JP: Testicular tumors in infants and children. Urology 2:353, 1973.

Smithers DW: Chemotherapy for metastatic teratomas of the testis. Br J Urol 44:217, 1972.

Staubitz WJ & others: Surgical management of testis tumor. J Urol 111:205, 1974.

10. TUMORS OF THE PENIS

Almost all penile tumors are malignant and usually involve the prepuce and glans. The incidence is higher in the uncircumcised. With rare exceptions, these are squamous cell epitheliomas. They metastasize to the inguinal lymph nodes; the iliac nodes may then become involved.

A nodular or warty growth is noted on the inner side of the foreskin or on the glans. Ulceration and secondary infections are common. If the foreskin cannot be retracted, a dorsal slit of the prepuce is essential for diagnosis and biopsy. Matted enlarged inguinal nodes may represent either metastasis or secondary infection from the tumor. Biopsy is necessary for the establishment of the diagnosis.

In differential diagnosis, syphilitic chancre must be considered. The demonstration of the specific organism (and biopsy) should settle the issue. Chancroid may present as an ulcerating lesion. The demonstration of *Haemophilus ducreyi* is diagnostic. Condylomata acuminata are soft warty growths of viral origin. If doubt exists, biopsy is indicated.

After establishing the diagnosis by biopsy, amputation of the penis at least 2 cm proximal to the lesion must be done, though very small tumors may be curable with radiotherapy. In the presence of inguinal lymph node involvement, node dissection should be considered, for these are radioresistant.

The prognosis is fairly good in the absence of metastases.

Alexander LL & others: Radium management of tumors of the penis. NY State J Med 71:1946, 1971.

Almgård LE, Edsmyr F: Radiotherapy in treatment of patients with carcinoma of the penis. Scand J Urol Nephrol 7:1, 1973.

Das Gupta TK: Radical groin dissection. Surg Gynecol Obstet 129:1275, 1969.

Dehner LP, Smith BH: Soft tissue tumors of the penis. Cancer 25:1431, 1970.

deKernion JB & others: Carcinoma of the penis. Cancer 32:1256, 1973.

Kossow JH, Hotchkiss RS, Morales PA: Carcinoma of penis treated surgically: Analysis of 100 cases. Urology 2:169, 1973.

NEUROGENIC BLADDER

Myoneural Anatomy

The urinary bladder and its involuntary sphincter develop and differentiate from the tubular urogenital sinus. The differentiation of the encasing mesenchymal cells forms the musculature of the detrusor and urethral sphincter. They are one and the same continuous structure with the same innervation.

Innervation

The innervation of the bladder and its involuntary sphincter is through the autonomic nervous system. The motor supply to the bladder and the sphincter is parasympathetic via the pelvic nerves, which arise from S2–4. These fibers carry also the stretch sensory receptors to the same spinal cord center (S2–4).

The sensory supply for pain, touch, and temperature is carried via the sympathetic fibers arising from the thoracolumbar segments (T11–L2).

Motor and sensory supply of the trigone is via the thoracolumbar sympathetic fibers.

The striated external sphincter as well as the entire urogenital diaphragm receive their motor and sensory innervation from the somatic fibers arising from S2–4 (via the pudendal nerve).

It is clear that S2–4 are the origin of the motor supply to the bladder musculature, to the involuntary sphincter, and to the striated external sphincter. The trigone is the only structure that is partly independent in its innervation. This is why segment S2–4 is called the spinal cord center for micturition. It is located at the level of the T12 and L1 vertebral bodies. There is

connection between the spinal cord center and the midbrain and cerebral cortex. Through these connections, inhibition and control of the spinal cord reflexes can be maintained. Any injury above the level of the T12 vertebral body will leave the spinal cord center intact, leading to an upper motor neuron lesion; injuries at the spinal cord center or below will lead to a lower motor neuron lesion.

Myoneurophysiology

The primary functions of the urinary bladder are to act as a reservoir, maintain urinary continence, and prevent vesicoureteral reflux. Intact myoneural elements are essential for these functions. The primary reservoir function is possible through the particular detrusor muscular arrangement and because of the accommodation phenomenon. The normal bladder can accommodate variable volumes (up to 400 ml) without increasing intravesical pressure. We perceive bladder fullness through increases in intravesical pressure. Until this happens, we have no perception of the actual volume in the bladder.

Overdistention and stretch initiate detrusor activity that can be controlled and inhibited by the high cortical centers or can be allowed to progress to active detrusor contraction associated with voiding. Normally, voiding detrusor contraction is maintained until the bladder is completely empty unless voluntarily interrupted or inhibited.

Normally, before voiding starts, there is relaxation of the pelvic floor and the striated external sphincter. This leads to a drop in the bladder base, funneling of the bladder outlet, and appreciable lowering of urethral resistance. This is shortly followed by active detrusor contraction, generating a rise in intravesical pressure to about 20–40 cm water and resulting in a flow rate of about 15–25 ml/second. The detrusor contraction is maintained until the bladder is completely empty, when the pelvic floor and striated external sphincter contract, elevating the bladder base and increasing urethral closure pressure, and terminating voiding. Intact nerve pathways are essential for these synchronized activities to occur.

Cystometry

Cystometry is a simple method for testing the above functions and gives information about the following: residual urine, bladder capacity, the accommodation phenomenon and its extent, sensation of fullness, and effective detrusor contraction. A simple water cystometer and a normal cystometrogram are shown in Fig 43–19.

Classification & Clinical Findings

Neurogenic bladder can be divided into 2 main groups depending on the site of the lesion in relation to the spinal cord center (S2–4): upper motor neuron lesions (above the spinal cord center) and lower motor neuron lesions (at or below the spinal cord center).

A. Upper Motor Neuron Lesions (Spastic): Lesions above the voiding reflex arc are most com-

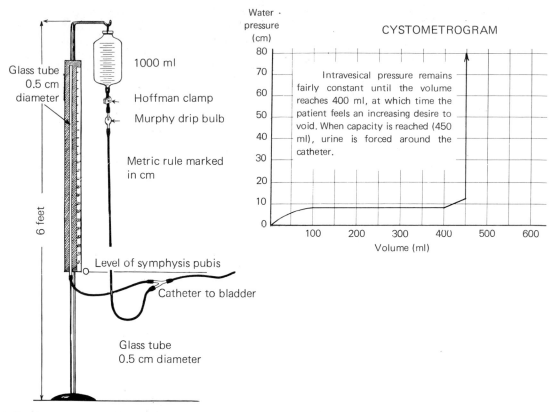

Figure 43–19. Cystometry. *Left:* A simple water manometer. *Right:* Normal cystometrogram. As fluid is slowly introduced into the bladder, the detrusor gradually relaxes to accept increasing amounts of fluid without change in intravesical pressure. At a volume of 400 ml, the patient felt an urge to void. Shortly thereafter, an involuntary contraction of the detrusor occurred which was reflected in a sharp increase in intravesical pressure.

monly due to trauma. Although the reflex arc is intact, it has lost the inhibitory control of the higher centers. Both motor and sensory fibers are commonly involved. There is loss of accommodation and, frequently, uninhibited detrusor contraction. The bladder outlet is usually funneled. The striated external sphincter and pelvic floor are spastic. Detrusor contractions, though they can generate abnormally high intravesical pressure, are not effective in producing adequate urine flow (because of the spastic external sphincter) and are incapable of maintaining the contraction, so that there is always some residual urine. Bladder capacity is reduced. Detrusor contraction and mass reflexes can be initiated from certain trigger areas.

There is marked detrusor thickening and hypertrophy, together with trigonal hypertrophy, that initially leads to functional obstruction at the ureterovesical junction. Later, decompensation of the ureterovesical valve and reflux accentuates renal back pressure and pyelonephritic damage.

Fig 43–20 is a typical cystometrogram of a spastic upper motor neuron lesion.

B. Lower Motor Neuron Lesions (Flaccid): Any lesion involving the spinal cord center (S2–4), cauda equina, sacral roots, or peripheral nerves leads to atonic or flaccid lower motor neuron involvement.

Trauma is the most common cause, but tumors, ruptured intervertebral disks, and meningomyelocele may cause this type of neurogenic bladder also. Again, both motor and sensory fibers are usually affected. Damage of stretch receptors results in loss of sense of fullness. Accordingly, bladder capacity progressively increases.

Detrusor contractions are primarily on a myogenic basis, as the bladder has lost its connection to the spinal cord center (Fig 43–21). They are usually weak and unsustained. In spite of diminished outflow resistance (funneled bladder neck and flaccid external sphincter), flow rates are inadequate and bladder emptying is incomplete, resulting in relatively large amounts of residual urine. Bladder thickening and trabeculation and trigonal hypertrophy develop but are less apparent because of the overstretching. Trigonal hypertrophy, augmented by the stretch caused by the large amounts of residual urine, leads to functional obstruction of the ureterovesical junction. Decompensation and reflux occur relatively late in comparison to spastic upper motor neuron lesions.

Differential Diagnosis

Cystitis, interstitial cystitis, and organic obstruction are occasionally confused with neurogenic bladder, but associated neurologic lesions usually make the

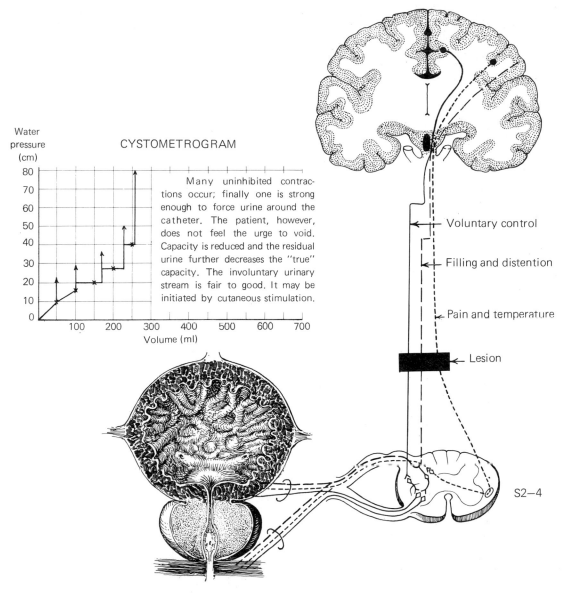

CYSTOMETROGRAM

Many uninhibited contractions occur; finally one is strong enough to force urine around the catheter. The patient, however, does not feel the urge to void. Capacity is reduced and the residual urine further decreases the "true" capacity. The involuntary urinary stream is fair to good. It may be initiated by cutaneous stimulation.

Figure 43—20. Complete spastic neurogenic bladder. Caused by a more or less complete transection of the spinal cord above S2. Cystometric study of a typical case shows function after recovery from spinal shock. (Modified after Nesbit, Lapides, & Baum: *Fundamentals of Urology.* Edwards, 1953.)

diagnosis of neurogenic bladder easy. However, psychosomatic disturbances such as spastic external sphincter, incomplete voiding, retention, or incontinence should always be considered.

Complications

Common complications include urinary tract infection, stone formation, and incontinence. The most serious consequences of these lesions are the hydrodynamic back pressure on the kidneys, causing hydronephrosis with or without infection and resulting ultimately in trigonal hypertrophy—aggravated by stretch if there is residual urine—and decompensation of the ureterovesical junctions.

Treatment

Immediately following spinal cord injury there is a shock phase which may last a few weeks to 2–3 years. The average time is 2–3 months. The bladder is completely dissociated from any nervous control and thus has no sensation and is completely inactive.

Treatment is aimed at avoiding the aforementioned complications in the hope of partial or complete recovery or intermittent (every 4–6 hours) aseptic catheterization. During the shock phase, continuous closed drainage should be instituted until bladder activity resumes.

Control of infection and maintenance of a high fluid intake are important. Dietary measures (low-cal-

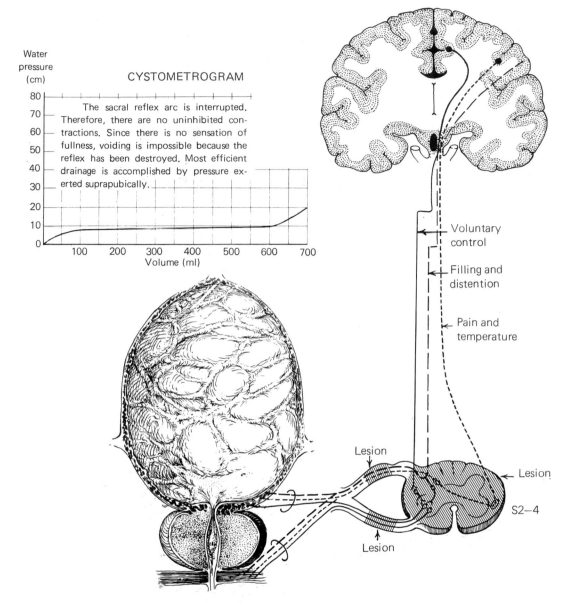

Figure 43–21. Flaccid neurogenic bladder. Caused by a lesion of the sacral portion of the cord or of the cauda equina. Cystometric study of a typical case shows function after recovery from spinal shock. (Modified after Nesbit, Lapides, & Baum: *Fundamentals of Urology.* Edwards, 1953.)

cium diet, increased fluid intake, etc) and early ambulation are helpful in prevention of stone formation.

Urinary incontinence alone is occasionally an indication for diversion in the female. In the male, the use of external penile collecting devices is helpful.

A. Spastic Neurogenic Bladder: In the spastic neurogenic lesions, bladder rehabilitation is the aim. Residual urine should be minimized by diminishing urethral resistance by means of transurethral resection of the prostate or incision of the spastic external sphincter, or by unilateral or bilateral blocking or excision of the pudendal nerves.

Functional capacity can be increased by eliminating infection. Anticholinergics—eg, methantheline

bromide (Banthine), 50–100 mg 4 times daily, or propantheline bromide (Pro-Banthine), 15–30 mg 4 times daily—increase functional capacity. Trigger areas should be used to initiate voiding. Conversion to a flaccid lower motor neuron lesion can be achieved by subarachnoid injection of absolute alcohol or by anterior and posterior rhizotomy. If decompensation of the ureterovesical junction and deterioration of the upper urinary tract occur, urinary diversion is indicated.

B. Flaccid Neurogenic Bladder: In the flaccid neurogenic bladder, functional capacity can be improved by manual compression (Credé) and by diminishing resistance of the bladder outlet (transurethral resections of the bladder neck). The patient should be instructed to void on a time schedule to avoid wetness. Continuous drainage by a urethral catheter or a suprapubic cystostomy should be employed when necessary. Decompensation of the ureterovesical junction and deterioration of the upper urinary tract require urinary diversion.

Prognosis

Decompensation of the ureterovesical junction and persistence of infection are the most serious consequences of neurogenic bladder. Spastic neurogenic bladders deteriorate more rapidly than lower motor neuron lesions. Proper timing of operation is essential for preservation of kidney function.

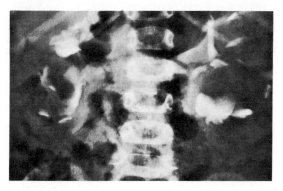

Figure 43–22. Polycystic kidneys. Excretory urogram in a child showing elongation, broadening, and bending of the calyces around cysts. Good renal function.

Cass AS, Spence BR: Urinary incontinence in myelomeningocele. J Urol 110:136, 1973.

Conan AE: Urologic management of traumatic cord bladder. Clin Orthop 112:53, 1975.

Engel RME, Schirmer H: Pudendal neurectomy in neurogenic bladder. J Urol 112:57, 1974.

Hackler RH: Spinal cord injuries: Urologic care. Urology 2:13, 1973.

Jones DL, Moore T: The types of neuropathic bladder dysfunction associated with prolapsed lumbar intervertebral discs. Br J Urol 45:39, 1973.

Kontturi M, Larmi TKI, Tuononen S: Bladder dysfunction and its manifestations following abdominoperineal extirpation of the rectum. Ann Surg 179:179, 1974.

McCrae WH: External sphincterotomy for the obstructed neurogenic bladder. Can J Surg 16:132, 1973.

Merrill DC: Clinical experience with the Mentor bladder stimulator. 2. Meningomyelocele patients. J Urol 112:823, 1976.

Perkash I: Intermittent catheterization: The urologist's point of view. J Urol 111:356, 1974.

Rossier AB, Ott R: Bladder and urethral recordings in acute and chronic spinal cord injury patients. Urol Int 31:49, 1976.

Rudy SM, Tanagho EA: Transient neurogenic bladder secondary to presacral abscess: Association with regional ileitis. Urology 4:593, 1974.

Yalla SV, Rossier AB, Fam B: Dyssynergic vesicourethral responses during bladder rehabilitation in spinal cord injury patients: Effects of suprapubic percussion, Credé method, and bethanechol chloride. J Urol 115:575, 1976.

Zinke H & others: Neurovesical vesical dysfunction in diabetes mellitus: Another look at vesical neck resection. J Urol 111:488, 1974.

DISORDERS OF THE KIDNEYS

POLYCYSTIC KIDNEYS

Polycystic kidney disease is a familial disorder that involves not only the kidneys but sometimes the liver and pancreas as well. A few cases are seen in infancy and early childhood. The renal cysts are thought to be due to failure of union of the collecting and convoluted tubules. As the cysts enlarge, pressure

is exerted on normal tissue, leading to its gradual destruction. The diagnosis is usually made during investigation for the cause of hypertension or uremia discovered in the third or fourth decade. The sex incidence is about equal. Flank pain may be noticed if bleeding occurs into a cyst; hematuria may then occur. Examination reveals bilateral nodular enlargement of the kidneys.

The urine often shows red blood cells and evidence of infection. Serum creatinine or BUN measures the degree of renal insufficiency. Urograms reveal the enlarged kidneys, with marked bending and elongation of the calyces that are bent around large cysts (Fig 43–22).

Surgery is not warranted unless a large extrarenal cyst obstructs the upper ureter. Therapy is medical.

When manifested in infancy the prognosis is poor. In the adult type, death usually occurs 5–10 years after the onset of clinical symptoms. In the stage of significant uremia, renal transplantation should be considered.

Lufkin EG & others: Polycystic kidney disease: Earlier diagnosis using ultrasound. Urology 4:5, 1974.

Salvatierra O Jr, Kountz SL, Belzer FO: Polycystic renal disease treated by renal transplantation. Surg Gynecol Obstet 137:431, 1973.

Vuthibhagdee A, Singleton EB: Infantile polycystic disease of the kidney. Am J Dis Child 125:167, 1973.

Wallack HI, Kandel G, Presman DC: Polycystic kidneys: Indication for surgical intervention. Urology 3:552, 1974.

SIMPLE RENAL CYST

Simple cyst of the kidney is usually unilateral and single, but it may be multiple and bilateral. Whether this disorder is congenital or acquired is not clear. By compression, the cysts can destroy adjacent parenchyma. They contain fluid that resembles (but is not) urine. A very few harbor cancer on their walls. Most cysts are diagnosed after the age of 40 years.

Flank pain may be the presenting symptom, though most renal cysts are found incidentally on urography done for other purposes. A mass may be felt in the renal area and must be differentiated from tumor. Urinalysis and tests of renal function are normal. Excretory urograms reveal a mass in the kidney that distorts adjacent calyces. Nephrotomography may show that the mass is avascular (in contradistinction to tumor). If renal sonography is compatible with cyst, a needle should be passed into the lesion. The recovery of clear fluid implies a cyst; it should be subjected to cytologic study. If no fluid can be aspirated, angiography should be done. This shows similar findings, including the absence of capillaries in the area of the mass. A technetium gamma camera scan will also demonstrate the absence of blood vessels in the cyst.

Simple cyst must be differentiated from adenocarcinoma of the kidney. Nephrotomography, angiography, and the technetium scan usually make the differentiation. If the presumptive diagnosis is cyst, a needle can be introduced into the mass. Clear fluid implies a cyst; it should be subjected to cytologic study. In polycystic disease the cysts are multiple and bilateral and renal insufficiency is to be expected.

Complications are rare, but bleeding into the cyst or infection of a cyst may occur.

The diagnosis can be positively made in most instances. If not, renal exploration should be done.

Firstater M, Farkas A: Simple renal cyst in a newborn. Br J Urol 45:366, 1973.

Pollack HM, Goldberg BB, Bogash M: Changing concepts in the diagnosis and management of renal cysts. J Urol 111:326, 1974.

Romeiser RS, Walls WJ, Valk WL: B-scan ultrasound in the evaluation of renal mass lesions. J Urol 112:8, 1974.

MEDULLARY SPONGE KIDNEY

Cystic dilatation of the renal collecting tubules is occasionally seen. It represents a congenital ectasia of these tubules, which may be complicated by the development of microcalculi. The lesion is often bilateral and may involve all calyces.

There is an increased incidence of infection in such kidneys. Symptoms include those of pyelonephritis or stone. Hematuria is not uncommon. Excretory urograms reveal dilated distal tubules as a "blush."

There is no specific treatment. Infection must be combated. In the presence of calculi, a prophylactic regimen should be prescribed.

Hayt DB & others: Direct magnification intravenous pyelography in the evaluation of medullary sponge kidney. Am J Roentgenol 119:701, 1973.

Spence HM, Singleton R: What is sponge kidney disease and where does it fit in the spectrum of cystic disorders? J Urol 107:176, 1972.

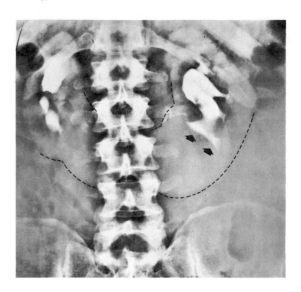

Figure 43—23. Excretory urogram showing horseshoe kidney with expansion of left side of isthmus and compression of lower left calyceal system. Surgical diagnosis: adenocarcinoma.

RENAL FUSION

The metanephric tissue may form one renal mass occupying one flank, or it may lie ectopically in the pelvis. The most common anomaly, however, is horseshoe kidney with the renal poles joined inferiorly. These anomalous kidneys are fed by many aberrant arteries, one of which is apt to compress the upper ureter and lead to hydronephrosis. Complicating infection is not uncommon.

There are usually no symptoms unless complications arise, in which case pain from obstruction or symptoms of infection may appear. An enlarged renal mass may be felt, and the isthmus of a horseshoe kidney may be palpable. Urography establishes the diagnosis (Fig 43—23). In the case of a "cake" kidney, both ureters will be shown to arise from their own calyceal system in the renal mass. The renal masses of a horseshoe kidney lie on the psoas muscles, and their inferior calyces point medially into the isthmus.

No treatment is necessary unless there is evidence of obstruction or infection.

Kvarstein B, Mathisen W: Surgical treatment of horseshoe kidney: A follow-up study. Scand J Urol Nephrol 8:10, 1974.

Segura JW, Kelalis PP, Burke EC: Horseshoe kidney in children. J Urol 108:333, 1972.

ANEURYSM OF THE RENAL ARTERY

Aneurysm of the renal artery is relatively rare. It results from weakening of its wall by arteriosclerosis,

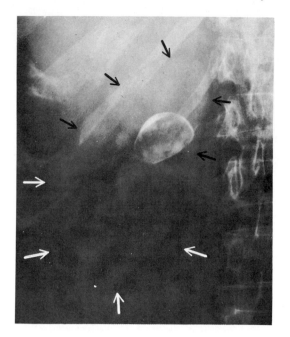

Figure 43—24. Intrarenal aneurysm of renal artery. Plain film showing calcified structure over the right renal shadow.

polyarteritis nodosa, or trauma. Some are congenital. If the aneurysm causes stenosis of the artery, hypertension may ensue secondary to ischemia. A plain abdominal x-ray may reveal a ring-like calcification in its wall (Fig 43—24). Angiography is diagnostic.

Because there is a significant incidence of spontaneous rupture of these lesions, their repair or removal by heminephrectomy must be considered. Nephrectomy may be necessary, particularly if emergency intervention for bleeding is necessary. A few of these patients will become normotensive after definitive surgery.

Canon J & others: Renal artery aneurysm in polyaneurysmal lesion of the kidney. Urology 5:1, 1975.

Cerny JC, Chang C-Y, Fry WJ: Renal artery aneurisms. Arch Surg 96:653, 1968.

RENAL INFARCTION

The common causes of occlusion of the renal artery are subacute bacterial endocarditis, atrial or ventricular thrombi, arteriosclerosis, polyarteritis nodosa, and trauma. Multiple emboli are common and lead to patchy renal ischemia. Occlusion of a main renal artery will cause atrophy of a portion or all of the kidney.

The patient may suffer from flank pain, or the lesion may be silent. Hematuria is common. Excretory urograms may reveal no excretion of radiopaque material or may only opacify a portion of the kidney.

With complete occlusion of the main renal artery, a ureteral catheter will drain no urine, yet the retrograde urogram will reveal normal anatomy. Renal angiography makes the diagnosis by revealing occlusion of the artery or arterioles; a renal scan will show similar findings. This disease may be mimicked by ureteral stone, but urograms and angiograms will differentiate them. Following renal infarction, hypertension may develop secondary to renal ischemia; it may later resolve spontaneously.

If the diagnosis is made promptly, endarterectomy should be considered. Otherwise, anticoagulation therapy should be instituted. If permanent hypertension develops, definitive treatment of the arterial occlusion or nephrectomy should be performed.

Fay R & others: Renal artery thrombosis: A successful revascularization by autotransplantation. J Urol 111:572, 1974.

Mounger EJ: Hypertension resulting from segmental renal artery infarction. Urology 1:189, 1973.

Moyer JD & others: Conservative management of renal artery embolus. J Urol 109:138, 1973.

THROMBOSIS OF THE RENAL VEIN

Thrombosis of the renal vein affects both infants and adults. In infants, it is apt to complicate ileocolitis. In the adult, it may be secondary to renal infection or ascending thrombosis of the vena cava. There is usually flank pain and a palpable kidney. If secondary to infection, the patient is septic and urinalysis reveals pus

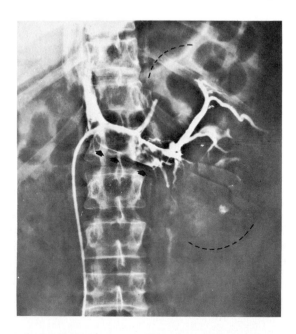

Figure 43—25. Thrombosis of renal vein. Selective left renal venogram showing almost complete occlusion of vein. Veins to lower pole failed to fill. Note large size of kidney.

cells and bacteria. The patient with bilateral involvement is found to have renal insufficiency. Nephrotic syndrome may develop. Excretory urograms show delayed and impaired opacification in an enlarged kidney. The calyces are elongated. Later, the kidney may become atrophic. Renal angiography reveals stretching and bowing of arterioles. Selective renal venography will demonstrate the thrombus (Fig 43–25).

If the diagnosis of unilateral infected renal vein thrombosis can be established, nephrectomy should be done. In bilateral disease, anticoagulant therapy is required. A few cases of successful thrombectomy have been reported.

Duffy JL & others: Renal vein thrombosis and the nephrotic syndrome: Report of two cases with successful treatment in one. Am J Med 54:663, 1973.

McDonald P & others: Some radiologic observations on renal vein thrombosis. Am J Roentgenol 120:368, 1974.

Miller RA, Tremann JA, Ansell JS: The conservative management of renal vein thrombosis. J Urol 111:568, 1974.

Weiner PL & others: Retrograde pyelography in renal vein thrombosis. Radiology 111:77, 1974.

DISEASES OF THE RETROPERITONEUM

RETROPERITONEAL FIBROSIS

One or both ureters may be compressed by a chronic inflammatory process, usually of unknown cause, which involves the retroperitoneal tissues of the lumbosacral area. Patients treated for migraine with methysergide (Sansert) may develop this fibrosis. Sclerosing Hodgkin's disease has been found to be an occasional cause. The symptoms include renal pain, low backache, and the syndrome of uremia. Some patients present with complete anuria. Urinary infection is unusual. If both ureters are obstructed, the serum creatinine will be elevated.

Excretory urograms show hydronephrosis and a dilated ureter down to the point of obstruction. The ureters are displaced medially in the lumbar area. Retrograde ureterograms show a long segment of ureteral stenosis, although a catheter passes easily through it. If anuric, indwelling ureteral catheters should be placed as a temporary measure. Definitive treatment consists of lysis of the ureters and implantation into the peritoneal cavity. Those caused by the ingestion of methysergide may resolve on cessation of the drug. Resolution of the lesion has been reported following the administration of corticosteroids.

Arger PH, Stolz JL, Miller WT: Retroperitoneal fibrosis: An analysis of the clinical spectrum and roentgenographic signs. Am J Roentgenol 119:812, 1973.

Robertson JA: Retroperitoneal fibrosis. Urology 3:741, 1974.

Skeel DA & others: Retroperitoneal fibrosis with intrinsic ureteral involvement. J Urol 113:166, 1975.

PERINEPHRIC ABSCESS

Perinephric abscess can arise secondary to a staphylococcal infection of the kidney, but in most cases it is a complication of advanced chronic renal infection. The abscess is enclosed within the perirenal fascia. There may be a long history of repeated attacks of urinary infection. In the rare staphylococcal type, a history of an antecedent skin infection may be elicited. Most patients with abscess are septic, but a few may present with no more than mild flank pain. Tenderness over the kidney is to be expected. A flank mass may be palpable. The diaphragm on the affected side may be elevated and fixed. Urograms show obliteration of the psoas shadow and scoliosis of the spine with its concavity on the side of the abscess. Calculous pyonephrosis may be noted. The lower pole of the kidney may be displaced laterally.

The history and physical findings may be consistent with infected hydronephrosis. Excretory urograms should make the differentiation. Considerable compression of the abscess upon the ureter may lead to hydronephrosis. Later, after definitive treatment retroperitoneal scarring may cause ureteral stenosis.

If seen early, those cases secondary to staphylococcal infection of the kidney may resolve with appropriate antimicrobial therapy. When a frank abscess is present, surgical drainage is indicated. If the kidney is badly damaged, nephrectomy should be done. If the kidney is not removed, serial urograms should be obtained in search of secondary ureteral stenosis that might require repair.

Meyers MA & others: Radiologic features of extraperitoneal effusions. Radiology 104:249, 1972.

Simpkins KC, Barraclough NC: Renal cortical abscess, perinephritis and perinephric abscess in diabetes. Br J Radiol 46:433, 1973.

DISEASES OF THE URETERS

DUPLICATION

Complete or incomplete (Y-type) duplication of the ureters is not uncommon. It presupposes 2 renal pelves in the renal mass. Most are observed in females. The Y-type ureter seldom causes trouble. With complete duplication, the ureter from the upper renal pole

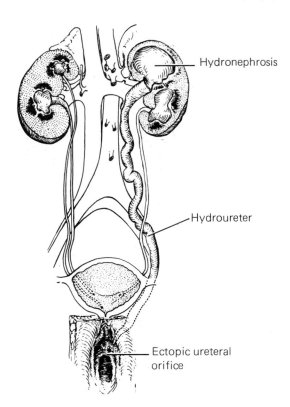

Figure 43—26. Duplication of ureters and ectopic ureteral orifice. Complete duplication with obstruction to one ureter with ectopic orifice on left. The ureter with the ectopic opening always drains the upper pole of the kidney.

opens closest to the bladder neck (Fig 43—26). The ureter to the lower pole thus has a relatively short intravesical segment and is therefore prone to reflux. Most ureteroceles in children involve the ureter from the superior pelvis, leading to hydroureteronephrosis. This ureter may open ectopically at the bladder neck or in the urethra and frequently exhibits reflux. If it opens at the vestibule, it is obstructed. Duplication is significant only if it leads to pyelonephritis or hydronephrosis, evidence of which is found on excretory urograms. Vesicoureteral reflux may require repair of the incompetent ureterovesical junction. Obstruction to the upper pole ureter often indicates the need for heminephroureterectomy.

Amar AD, Chabra K: Reflux in duplicated ureters: Treatment in children. J Pediatr Surg 5:419, 1970.

Lundin E, Riggs W: Upper urinary tract duplication associated with ectopic ureterocele in childhood and infancy. Acta Radiol 7:13, 1968.

Mackie GG, Stephens FD: Duplex kidneys: A correlation of renal dysplasia with position of ureteral orifice. J Urol 114:274, 1975.

Schulman CC: The single ectopic ureter. Eur Urol 2:64, 1976.

Tanagho EA: Embryologic basis for lower ureteral anomalies: A hypothesis. Urology 5:451, 1976.

URETEROCELE

A ureterocele is a ballooning of the submucosal ureter into the bladder. This cyst-like structure has a pinpoint orifice and is therefore obstructive, leading to hydronephrosis. If large enough, it may obstruct the vesical neck. It is most common in little girls with ureteral duplication and always involves the ureter draining the upper renal pole. Because of its position and size, it may cause the ipsilateral ureterovesical junction to become incompetent (reflux).

Symptoms are usually those of pyelonephritis or obstruction. Excretory urograms may show a negative shadow in the bladder cast by the ureterocele (Fig 43—27). The ureter and renal pole so obstructed reveal marked dilatation or no function at all. A cystogram may show reflux into the second ureter going to the lower pole of the kidney.

Small, mildly obstructive ureteroceles can be destroyed transurethrally. The large ones seen in childhood require transvesical excision and, usually, reimplantation of both ureters into the bladder to prevent reflux. If the kidney tissue obstructed by this cyst is badly damaged, nephroureterectomy (or heminephrectomy with ureteral duplication) is necessary.

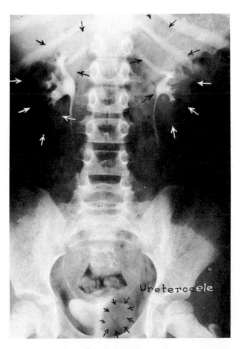

Figure 43—27. Ureterocele. Excretory urogram in a girl 8 years old, showing a space-occupying lesion on the left side of the bladder caused by ureterocele. Absence of calyceal system in the upper portion of the left kidney implies duplication of the ureters and pelves and nonfunction (advanced hydronephrosis) of the upper pole; its dilated ureter drains into the obstructing ureterocele and displaces the visualized ureter laterally just below the kidney.

Newman LB, McAlister WH, Kissane J: Segmental renal dysplasia associated with ectopic ureteroceles in children. Urology 3:23, 1974.

Shaw RE: Ureterocele. Br J Surg 60:337, 1973.

Tanagho EA: Anatomy and management of ureteroceles. J Urol 107:729, 1972.

Weiss RM, Spackman TJ: Everting ectopic ureterocele. J Urol 111:538, 1974.

ECTOPIC URETERAL ORIFICE

In rare instances, the ureter may drain into the urethra, vestibule, seminal vesicle, or vagina. If the orifice lies proximal to the external urinary sphincter, no incontinence ensues, but vesicoureteral reflux is common. Should it drain into the vagina or at the vestibule, there is continuous leakage of urine apart from voiding. Most ectopic orifices involve the ureter draining the upper pole of a duplicated system, and most are observed in the female. Hydroureteronephrosis of the involved segment is to be expected.

Symptoms are those of infection or obstruction. If the orifice is distal to the external sphincter, constant wetness is noticed. Such an orifice may be seen beside the urethral orifice or in the roof of the vagina on endoscopy. Excretory urograms will reveal hydroureteronephrosis, usually involving the upper renal segment. Cystography may show reflux into the ectopic orifice. If the hydronephrotic segment is only moderately damaged, the ureter can be divided and reimplanted into the bladder. Usually, however, heminephroureterectomy is necessary.

Brannan W, Henry HH Jr: Ureteral ectopia: Report of 39 cases. J Urol 109:192, 1973.

Mogg RA: The single ectopic ureter. Br J Urol 46:3, 1974.

CONGENITAL STENOSIS OF THE URETER

The common sites of congenital ureteral stricture are the ureteropelvic and ureterovesical junctions. Ureteral dilatation down to the bladder level is most often caused by vesicoureteral reflux. True stenosis at this point is uncommon. Functional obstruction does occur, however, as a result of a sphincter-like muscle bundle found in the juxtavesical ureter. The common symptoms are renal pain from obstruction and symptoms due to pyelonephritis. Excretory urograms depict the dilatation above the ureterovesical junction. There is no reflux on cystography. Treatment consists of division of the ureter just proximal to the obstruction with reimplantation of the ureter into the bladder.

Ureteropelvic obstruction is much more common than stricture at the ureterovesical level. Urographic studies in patients with vesicoureteral reflux are apt to reveal pseudostenosis at the ureteropelvic junction.

Some of these become truly obstructive. Symptoms include renal pain and those of renal infection. Excretory urograms show varying degrees of hydrocalycosis with a ureter of normal caliber below the site of obstruction. (If the ureter is dilated below the ureteropelvic junction, such changes suggest reflux as the cause.) Even on late films, much of the contrast medium is retained in the kidney. Cystography should also be done in order to rule out reflux, since repair of the ureterovesical junction usually causes the pseudostenosis to disappear.

If the kidney appears to have functional potential, surgical repair of the stenotic area should be accomplished. Nephrectomy may be indicated if damage is severe.

Allen TD: Congenital ureteral strictures. J Urol 104:196, 1970.

Smart WR: Surgical correction of hydronephrosis. Pages 2198–2239 in: *Urology,* 3rd ed. Campbell MT, Harrison JH (editors). Saunders, 1970.

Tanagho EA, Smith DR, Guthrie TH: Pathophysiology of functional ureteral obstruction. J Urol 104:73, 1970.

ACQUIRED STENOSIS OF THE URETER

Acquired ureteral stenosis is not so common as the congenital types. Causes include (1) ureteral injury (surgical, traumatic, radiation therapy), (2) compression of the ureter by lymph nodes harboring cancer, (3) prolonged pressure by an aberrant blood vessel, (4) tuberculous or bilharzial ureteritis, (5) retroperitoneal fibrosis, (6) aneurysm of the aorta or following aortofemoral bypass grafts, (7) ureteropelvic obstruction secondary to reflux, (8) occlusion of the ureterovesical junction by infiltrating cancer of the bladder, and (9) functional obstruction of the ureterovesical junction secondary to hypertrophy of the trigone developing from obstruction distal to the bladder neck.

Symptoms are usually those of obstruction to urine flow from the kidney, though many are silent. An unsuspected lesion is often discovered on excretory urography.

Therapy consists of treatment of the cause, eg, prostatectomy or resection of the stenosed segment with end-to-end anastomosis.

Bagby RJ & others: Genitourinary complications of granulomatous bowel disease. Am J Roentgenol 117:297, 1973.

Graham JB, Abad RS: Ureteral obstruction due to radiation. Am J Obstet Gynecol 99:409, 1967.

Kaplan JH, Kudish HG: Endometrial obstruction of ureter. Urology 3:327, 1974.

Kerr WS Jr & others: Idiopathic retroperitoneal fibrosis: Clinical experiences with 15 cases, 1957–1967. J Urol 99:575, 1968.

Lang EK, Nourse M: The roentgenographic diagnosis of obstructive lesions of the ureter. J Urol 101:812, 1969.

Lang EK & others: Complications in the urinary tract related to treatment of carcinoma of the cervix. South Med J 66:228, 1973.

Petrone AF, Dudzinski PJ, Maniatis W: Ureteral obstruction secondary to aortic femoral bypass. Ann Surg 179:192, 1974.

Tanagho EA, Meyers FH: Trigonal hypertrophy: A cause of ureteral obstruction. J Urol 93:678, 1965.

DISORDERS OF THE URINARY BLADDER*

VESICAL FISTULAS

Vesical fistulas may be congenital or acquired. Congenital fistulas usually involve the urachus. Acquired fistulas may be secondary to trauma (physical, surgical, or obstetric), malignant tumors, or inflammatory lesions. The most common types of vesical fistulas are vesicovaginal, vesicointestinal, and vesicocutaneous. Vesicovaginal fistulas are commonly secondary to obstetric or gynecologic trauma. They occur rarely as a complication of tumor infiltration from the cervix of the bladder. Vesicointestinal fistulas are commonly due to malignant lesions of the bowel or the bladder. They also occur secondary to inflammatory pelvic lesions in association with diverticulitis, pelvic abscess, or appendiceal abscess. Vesicocutaneous fistulas are common after cystostomy in the presence of bladder outlet obstruction, bladder malignancy, or foreign bodies.

Vesicovaginal fistulas must be differentiated from ureterovaginal fistulas, vesicorectal fistulas from urethrorectal fistulas, and vesicocutaneous fistulas from either ureterocutaneous or urethrocutaneous fistulas.

Therapy for vesicovaginal fistula requires surgical closure with drainage by cystostomy tube. For vesicointestinal fistula, the primary intestinal lesion must be resected and the hole in the bladder closed. An indwelling urethral catheter is necessary during the healing period.

Aldrete JS, ReMine WH: Vesicocolic fistula: A complication of colonic cancer. Arch Surg 94:627, 1967.

Baumrucker GO: Ball repair of vesicovaginal fistula. Urology 3:333, 1974.

Moir JC: Vesico-vaginal fistulae as seen in Britain. J Obstet Gynaecol Br Commonw 80:598, 1973.

Morse FP III, Dretler SP: Diagnosis and treatment of colovesical fistula. J Urol 111:22, 1974.

O'Conor VJ Jr & others: Suprapubic closure of vesicovaginal fistula. J Urol 109:51, 1973.

Vargas AD, Quattlebaum RB Jr, Scardino PL: Vesicoenteric fistula. Urology 3:200, 1974.

---

*Urinary stress incontinence in women is discussed in Chapter 44.

DISORDERS OF THE SCROTUM, TESTIS, & SPERMATIC CORD*

SCROTAL LESIONS

Congenital scrotal lesions include congenital (unilateral or bilateral) hypoplasia of the scrotum in association with cryptorchidism (see below) and bifid scrotum with extensive hypospadias. Acquired lesions may consist of scrotal abscess, sebaceous cysts, lymphedema (parasitic, traumatic, idiopathic), or gangrene. These are not specific for the scrotum, and each follows general rules of clinical course and management for similar disorders elsewhere.

SPERMATOCELE

Spermatocele is a retention cyst of an aberrant tubule of the rete testis or head of the epididymis. The cyst is distended with a whitish milky fluid that contains sperm. Cysts are usually at the superior pole of the testis or between it and the epididymis. They are usually soft, with the feeling of not being fully distended.

No therapy is needed unless the patient is concerned, in which case aspiration or surgical excision may be done.

VARICOCELE

Varicocele is due to an impediment in the deep venous drainage of the scrotal contents, leading to dilatation, tortuosity, and distention of the pampiniform plexus. It is more common on the left side since on that side the testicular vein is more subject to venous stasis because of its right angle drainage into the renal vein, absent or incompetent valves, or compression by the pelvic colon.

Mild degrees are commonly asymptomatic, but a dragging scrotal sensation and occasionally sexual neurosis may be associated. Varicocele may lead to low fertility in some men.

Asymptomatic varicocele is best left alone unless its possible effect on fertility is a matter of concern. Symptomatic varicocele can be corrected surgically, either by ligating the external spermatic vein at the level of the internal inguinal ring or by a direct scrotal approach and isolation and ligation of individual vessels.

---

*Cryptorchidism, hydrocele, and inguinal hernias are covered in Chapter 48.

Clarke BG: Incidence of varicocele in normal men and among men of different age groups. JAMA 198:1121, 1966.

Kiska EF, Cowart GT: Treatment of varicocele by high ligation. J Urol 83:713, 1960.

McGowan AJ, Howley TF: Experiences with the extrusion operation for hydrocele. J Urol 101:366, 1969.

TORSION OF THE SPERMATIC CORD

Torsion of the spermatic cord is most common in adolescent boys. A twist in the spermatic cord interferes with testicular blood supply. If torsion is complete, testicular gangrene may occur. The cause is unknown, but an underlying anatomic abnormality (spacious tunica vaginalis, loose epididymotesticular connection, undescended testis) is usually present.

Clinical findings consist of lower abdominal and scrotal pain and scrotal swelling of sudden onset. There may be a history of previous attacks in young adolescents. These findings warrant a diagnosis of torsion until it can be disproved on examination. The testis is swollen, tender, and retracted. The pain is not relieved by testicular support. The cord above the swelling is normal.

Torsion must be differentiated from orchitis, epididymitis, and pain due to testicular trauma. If the diagnosis cannot be established by examination and history, exploration is required.

Torsion of the spermatic cord is a surgical emergency. Unless the testis is definitely gangrenous and there is a long history of neglected exploration, try to conserve the testis. Orchiopexy on the other side is always necessary because of the common incidence of bilateral congenital anomaly and the possibility that torsion will occur on that side at a later time.

Korbel EI: Torsion of the testis. J Urol 111:521, 1974.

Lyon RP: Torsion of the testicle in childhood: A painless emergency requiring contralateral orchiopexy. JAMA 178:702, 1961.

Nadel NS & others: Preoperative diagnosis of testicular torsion. Urology 1:478, 1973.

Skoglund RW, McRoberts JW, Ragde H: Torsion of the spermatic cord: A review of the literature and an analysis of 70 new cases. J Urol 104:604, 1970.

PENILE & URETHRAL LESIONS

HYPOSPADIAS

The hypospadiac penis presents with a urethral orifice proximal to the usual site. It may be coronal, midshaft, penoscrotal, or midscrotal. In the case of the

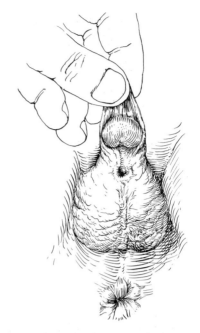

Figure 43—28. Hypospadias, penoscrotal type. Redundant dorsal foreskin which is deficient ventrally; ventral chordee.

latter, the scrotum is bifid. The penis is bent ventrally distal to the ectopic meatus (Fig 43—28). In many cases, this may preclude intercourse. The midscrotal hypospadiac penis may resemble female external genitalia with an enlarged clitoris and labia. Buccal smears are indicated in this group, a few of which may be found to have a rudimentary uterus and vagina (pseudohermaphroditism). The urinary sphincters are normal. The incidence of cryptorchidism is high.

If it is obvious that the degree of hypospadias will make intercourse difficult or impossible (due to the degree of chordee) and that the position of the urethral orifice will not allow the boy to stand to urinate or to deposit semen deep in the vagina in adulthood, surgical correction of the chordee and, later, urethroplasty are indicated. These operations are highly successful and should be completed before school age.

Fallon B, Devine CJ Jr, Horton CE: Congenital anomalies associated with hypospadias. J Urol 116:585, 1976.

Horton CE, Devine CJ Jr: A one-stage repair for hypospadias cripples. Plast Reconstr Surg 45:425, 1970.

Kelami A, Fiedler U, Richter-Reichelm M: One-stage correction of distal hypospadias: Modification of Allen-Spence-Hoffman-Hall procedure. Urology 8:496, 1976.

Ross G, Thompson IM, Montie JE: Hypospadias: Results of surgical treatment of and perspectives in management. Urology 8:143, 1976.

Wettlaufer JU: Cutaneous chordee: Fact or fancy? Urology 4:293, 1974.

EPISPADIAS

Epispadias is a rare congenital anomaly which is also always present in association with bladder exstrophy; it is considered a milder degree of the latter.

The urethra opens on the dorsum of the penis with deficient corpus spongiosum and loosely attached corpora cavernosa. If the defect is extensive, it can reach up to the bladder neck and is associated with complete incontinence. The pubic bones are separated, as in exstrophy. Marked dorsiflexion of the penis is usually present.

Treatment consists of correction of penile encurvature, reconstruction of the urethra, and reconstruction of bladder neck in incontinent cases. If these measures fail, urinary diversion may be indicated.

Bredin HC, Muecke EC: Surgical correction of male epispadias with total incontinence. J Urol 109:904, 1973.

Klauber GT, Williams DI: Epispadias with incontinence. J Urol 111:110, 1974.

Tanagho EA: Male epispadias: Surgical repair of urethropenile deformity. Br J Urol 48:127, 1976.

URETHRAL FISTULAS

Urethral fistulas may be urethrovaginal, urethrorectal, or urethrocutaneous. The first and second types are commonly traumatic (obstetric or surgical); rarely, congenital or due to malignant infiltration. Urethrocutaneous fistulas commonly complicate urethral trauma, stricture, periurethral abscesses, and surgery. Urethral tumor is a rare cause.

Treatment consists of correction of any underlying disease (if feasible), and excision of all fistulous tracts and proximal diversions.

Blandy JP, Singh M: Fistulae involving the adult male urethra. Br J Urol 44:632, 1972.

POSTERIOR URETHRAL VALVES

Posterior urethral valves are folds of mucosa, seen only in males, which originate at or are attached at some point to the verumontanum. The embryologic bases are indefinite. They are partially obstructive and thus lead to variable degrees of back pressure damage to the urinary bladder and upper urinary tract. Progressive renal damage may occur as a result of hypertrophy, trabeculation, diverticula formation, bilateral hydroureter, or hydronephrosis, with early obstruction at the ureterovesical junction because of trigonal hypertrophy and later development of reflux. Dilatation and obstruction of the prostatic urethra are always present.

Manifestations consist of difficult voiding, a weak urinary stream, an abdominal mass that represents a distended or hypertrophied bladder, and in some cases palpable kidneys. Urinary incontinence and urinary tract infection may occur in young boys. Laboratory findings include elevated BUN and serum creatinine, diminished PSP excretion, and evidence of urinary infection. Urograms show evidence of bladder thickening and trabeculation, hydroureter, hydronephrosis, and reflux. Demonstration of urethral valves on retrograde urethrograms or, preferably, voiding cystourethrograms establishes the diagnosis. Endoscopic visualization of valves and evidence of bladder changes are also usually seen.

Posterior urethral valves must be differentiated from neurogenic dysfunction, tumors, and meatal stenosis. If meatal stenosis and phimosis are excluded, any lower urinary tract obstructive disorder in a newborn or young boy should be considered posterior urethral valves until proved otherwise.

Treatment consists of destruction of the valves by overstretching, either by means of dilators through a perineal urethrotomy or by endoscopic fulguration or resection. Supravesical drainage (bilateral nephrostomy or bilateral loop ureterostomy) may be required to improve markedly impaired kidney function. Bilateral ureterovesicoplasty may be needed for a persistently obstructed or refluxing ureterovesical junction. Permanent urinary diversion is sometimes required.

The prognosis depends upon the original degree of kidney damage and the success of efforts to prevent or treat infection. In early cases, the prognosis is quite favorable.

Schoenberg HW, Miyai K, Gregory JG: Posterior urethral valves. Urology 7:611, 1976.

Scott TW: Urinary ascites secondary to posterior urethral valves. J Urol 116:1, 1976.

URETHRAL STRICTURE

Congenital urethral strictures are common at the meatus, rare in the penile urethra. Acquired strictures may be due to external trauma and rupture, or to instrumentation; may be inflammatory, due to gonorrhea (most common), tuberculous urethritis, or schistosomiasis; or, rarely, may be a complication of malignancy. The common presenting symptoms are dysuria, weak stream, bifurcation of the urinary stream, urinary retention, and urinary tract infection. Evidence of scarring due to trauma or induration and perineal fistula may be seen. Urethral calibration reveals the degree of narrowing. A retrograde urethrogram will delineate the site and degree of stricture. A voiding cystourethrogram may show its proximal extension.

Urethral stricture must be differentiated from bladder outlet obstruction due to prostatism, impacted urethral stones, urethral foreign bodies, and tumors.

Treatment consists of repeated dilatation, internal urethrotomy for limited annular strictures, and urethroplasty for extensive stricture.

Helmstein K: Internal urethrotomy: Modifications in the operative technique. Acta Chir Scand (Suppl):340, 1965.

Jessen C: Resection of urethral stricture and end-to-end anastomosis. Scand J Urol Nephrol 4:87, 1970.

Katz AS, Waterhouse K: Treatment of urethral stricture in man by internal urethrotomy: A study of 61 patients. J Urol 105:807, 1971.

Turner-Warwick R: The repair of urethral strictures in the region of the membranous urethra. J Urol 100:303, 1968.

PRIAPISM

Priapism is a rare disorder that consists of prolonged erection, usually painful, which is unassociated with sexual stimulation. The blood in the corpora cavernosa becomes sludge-like rather than clotted. About 25% of cases are associated with leukemia, metastatic carcinoma, or sickle cell anemia. In most cases the cause is unclear.

If the erection does not subside in a few hours, ice water enemas may lead to resolution. If not, evacuation of the sludged blood of the corpora with a needle and syringe, followed by lavage with an anticoagulant, or controlled hypotension and systemic anticoagulation should be tried. If these methods fail, anastomosis of the saphenous vein to the ipsilateral corpus cavernosum or spongiosum cavernosum shunt should be done, and the earlier the better.

Even though one of these methods relieves the erection, inability to achieve an erection thereafter is a common sequence.

Harrow BR: Simple technique for treating priapism. J Urol 101:71, 1969.

Howe GE & others: Priapism: A surgical emergency. J Urol 101:576, 1969.

Seeler RA: Priapism in children with sickle cell anemia: Successful management with liberal red cell transfusions. Clin Pediatr 10:418, 1971.

DISORDERS OF THE FEMALE URETHRA

DISTAL URETHRAL STENOSIS

The female urethra is muscular in its entire length except for the terminal 0.5 cm, where there is a dense collagen deposition which probably acts as a point of fixation for the urethral musculature. This collagenous ring is a normal histologic finding in the female urethra. Abnormal abundance of this collagenous tissue may encroach on the urethral lumen. This tissue seems to be under the influence of female hormones and becomes quite soft at puberty. This distal urethral segment receives its sensory supply from the pudendal nerve; any irritation to this area (commonly by infection) leads to reflex spasm of the striated external sphincter, which in turn leads to variable symptoms of irritative, obstructive voiding with urethrovesical reflux, washing urethral bacteria into the bladder and thus initiating or perpetuating lower urinary tract infection.

Urethral dilatation (up to 36F), rupture of the distal urethral ring, and clearance of infection relieve the urethral spasm. Normal voiding dynamics are restored, and urinary tract infection is cleared in most of these cases.

A marginally competent ureterovesical junction might become incompetent in the face of the abnormally high voiding pressure caused by the sphincter spasm. Where the latter is relieved, reflux may spontaneously disappear.

Hendry WF, Stanton SL, Williams DI: Recurrent urinary infections in girls: Effects of urethral dilatation. Br J Urol 45:72, 1973.

Hradec E & others: Significance of urethral obstruction in girls. Urol Int 28:440, 1973.

Kaplan GW, Sammons TA, King LR: A blind comparison of dilatation, urethrotomy and medication alone in the treatment of urinary tract infection in girls. J Urol 109:917, 1973.

Lyon RP, Marshall S: Urinary tract infections and difficult urination in girls: Long-term follow-up. J Urol 105:314, 1971.

Tanagho EA & others: Spastic striated external sphincter and urinary tract infection in girls. Br J Urol 43:69, 1971.

URETHRITIS & PERIURETHRITIS

Urethritis in the female may be acute or chronic. Acute urethritis is commonly gonorrheal in origin. Chemical urethritis is occasionally acquired from exposure to bubble bath crystals. Chronic urethritis is a common problem in females because the female urethra is always exposed to pathogenic bacteria due to its anatomic location; the distal part of the urethra is always infected. Urethral trauma, instrumentation, and increase in the number of pathogenic organisms lead to flare-up of infection and overt, manifest urethritis. Urethritis usually precedes cystitis.

Hormonal changes associated with menopause cause vaginal and urethral mucosal changes which lead to irritative symptoms and increased susceptibility to inflammatory flare-ups. Repeated labor and coital trauma can lead to periurethral fibrosis, which again can lead to irritative lower urinary tract symptoms even in the absence of any bacterial infection.

Urethritis usually causes irritative lower urinary tract symptoms similar to those of cystitis and, occasionally, functional obstructive symptoms. Examination may reveal urethral discharge, marked tenderness, or congested everted mucosa at the external meatus. Thickening and induration along the urethra, associated vaginal mucosal changes, and evidence of cervicitis and vaginitis may be present. Endoscopic examination may reveal obstruction, congested mucous membranes, infected urethral glands with pus exuding from their ducts, or inflammatory polyps around the internal meatus. Urethral calibration rarely reveals obstruction. Resistance of the spastic external sphincter may be noted.

Treatment consists of removal of the underlying cause, if possible. Estrogen cream or diethylstilbestrol suppositories are indicated for senile urethritis. Surgical treatment consists of urethral dilatation and opening and draining of infected periurethral ducts. Correction of vaginitis, cervicitis, and cervical erosions helps in ameliorating symptoms.

Bruce AW & others: Recurrent urethritis in women. Can Med Assoc J 108:973, 1973.

Marshall S, Lyon RP, Schieble J: Nonspecific urethritis in females. Calif Med 112:9, June 1970.

Smith P: Age changes in the female urethra. Br J Urol 44:667, 1972.

URETHRAL CARUNCLE

Urethral caruncle, commonly seen after menopause, represents granulomatous overgrowth of the posterior lip of the external meatus. It is usually painful to touch, during intercourse, and with urination. The most important consideration is to exclude malignancy.

Treatment is local excision.

Marshall FC, Uson AC, Melicow MM: Neoplasms and caruncles of the female urethra. Surg Gynecol Obstet 110:723, 1960.

URETHRAL DIVERTICULUM

Urethral diverticulum in the female commonly presents as recurrent lower urinary tract infection. It should be suspected whenever urinary infection fails to resolve with treatment. Symptoms are urinary dribbling and cystic swelling in the anterior vaginal wall during voiding. If diverticulum is suspected, it can usually be seen during panendoscopy and visualized radiographically on a voiding cystourethrogram with the external meatus occluded, or by using special catheters.

Treatment consists of transvaginal surgical excision, taking care not to injure the urethral sphincter during dissection.

Benjamin J & others: Urethral diverticulum in adult female: Clinical aspects, operative procedure, and pathology. Urology 3:1, 1974.

Golimbu M, Al-Askari S: High pressure voiding urethrography: Principle and technique. Urology 3:717, 1974.

Houser LM II, VonEschenbach AC: Diverticula of female urethra: Diagnostic importance of postvoiding film. Urology 3:453, 1974.

Widholm O, Rynänen VA: Diverticulum of the female urethra. Acta Obstet Gynecol Scand 46:107, 1967.

MALE INFERTILITY

A couple can be judged infertile if conception does not occur after 12 months of adequate cohabitation. About 10% of marriages are barren, and spermatogenic deficiencies are responsible in at least 40% of cases. The common causes are (1) deficiencies in maturation of germ cells (the most common), (2) obstruction to the conduction system, (3) hypothyroidism, (4) hyperadrenalism, (5) the formation of sperm antibodies, and (6) varicocele.

A history of mumps, cryptorchidism, testicular trauma, varicocele, or epididymitis may prove significant. Evidence of endocrinologic abnormality should be sought. The scrotal contents should be carefully examined for testicular size and consistency, scarring of the epididymides, and the presence of intact vasa deferentia. The finding of varicocele is of the greatest importance, for its treatment offers the best hope for reversal of infertility.

Analysis of the semen is the most important laboratory test. The specimen should be obtained after at least 4 days of abstinence from intercourse. Most fertile men have at least 40 million sperms/ml, 70% of which are motile. A differential count, judging morphology, should be done; at least 70% of the sperms in most fertile men are normally formed.

A test of thyroid function and an estimate of urinary pituitary gonadotropins and 17-ketosteroids or plasma testosterone level should be obtained. A buccal smear should be taken for nuclear chromatin analysis. If chromatin mass is positive, the patient has Klinefelter's syndrome. In the face of azoospermia, testicular biopsy will differentiate between deficiency of maturation and obstruction of the conduction system.

Treatment

A. Hormonal Therapy: Appropriate therapy should be instituted for hypothyroidism. Hyperadrenocorticism should be suppressed with corticosteroids, which will lead to increase in the number of sperms and a higher percentage of normal forms. There is some evidence that the administration of human gonadotropins may be of value in hypopituitarism.

Small doses of androgen (eg, 5–10 mg/day) may improve motility if the sperm count is high. Androgens may also be helpful if the count is normal but the volume of ejaculate is low. If the quality of the semen is very poor, testosterone, 50 mg IM 3 times a week, should be given for 3 months; this will result in complete azoospermia. On cessation of the drug, a "rebound" phenomenon may occur.

B. General Measures: The patient should abstain from intercourse for a few days before his wife's fertile period. Obesity should be treated.

C. Surgical Measures: Vasovasostomy is indicated for men who have had previous vasoligation. Epididymovasostomy should be done for epididymal occlusion. Ligation of the spermatic vein is indicated in the presence of varicocele; fertility will be restored in half of this group.

Prognosis

The poorer the quality of the semen, the poorer the outlook. When the count is under 1 million/ml, there is little room for optimism.

Amelar RD, Dubin L: Male infertility: Current diagnosis and treatment. Urology 1:1, 1973.

Amelar RD, Dubin L, Schoenfeld C: Semen analysis: An office technique. Urology 2:605, 1973.

Furuhjelm M, Carlström K, Jonson B: Endocrinological aspects of male infertility. Acta Obstet Gynecol Scand 53:181, 1974.

Halim A & others: Investigation and treatment of the infertile male. Proc R Soc Med 66:737, 1973.

Halim A & others: The significance of antibodies to sperm in infertile men and their wives. Br J Urol 46:65, 1974.

Hendry WF & others: Investigation and treatment of the subfertile male. Br J Urol 45:684, 1973.

Meinhard E, McRae CU, Chisholm GD: Testicular biopsy in evaluation of male infertility. Br Med J 3:577, 1973.

Stewart BH: Varicocele in infertility: Incidence and results of surgical therapy. J Urol 112:222, 1974.

Stewart BH, Montie JE: Male infertility: An optimistic report. J Urol 110:216, 1973.

● ● ●

General References

Black DAK: *Renal Disease,* 3rd ed. Lippincott, 1973.

Boyarsky S, Labay P: *Ureteral Dynamics.* Williams & Wilkins, 1972.

Campbell MF, Harrison JH (editors): *Urology,* 3rd ed. Saunders, 1970.

Dodson AI Jr: *Urological Surgery,* 4th ed. Mosby, 1970.

Emmett JL, Witten DM (editors): *Clinical Urography: An Atlas and Textbook of Roentgenologic Diagnosis,* 3rd ed. Saunders, 1971.

Federman DD (editor): *Abnormal Sexual Development.* Saunders, 1967.

Glenn JF, Boyce WH: *Urologic Surgery,* 2nd ed. Harper & Row, 1975.

Graves FT (editor): *The Arterial Anatomy of the Kidney.* Williams & Wilkins, 1971.

Hinman F Jr (editor): *Hydrodynamics of Micturition.* Thomas, 1971.

Kossow JH (editor): Proceedings of the American Cancer Society's National Conference on Urologic Cancer. Cancer 32:1017, 1973.

Nowinski W, Goss RJ: *Compensatory Renal Hypertrophy.* Academic Press, 1970.

Pitts RF (editor): *Physiology of the Kidney and Body Fluids,* 3rd ed. Year Book, 1974.

Potter EL: *Normal and Abnormal Development of the Kidney.* Year Book, 1973.

Smith DR: *General Urology,* 8th ed. Lange, 1975.

Stamey TA: *Urinary Infections.* Williams & Wilkins, 1972.

Strauss MB, Welt LG: *Diseases of the Kidney,* 2nd ed. Little, Brown, 1971.

44 . . .
Gynecology

Edward C. Hill, MD

CONGENITAL ANOMALIES OF THE FEMALE REPRODUCTIVE SYSTEM

Congenital defects of the female reproductive system arise as a result of abnormal embryologic development of the müllerian ducts and urogenital sinus. The most common defects are imperforate hymen, septate or double vagina, transverse septum of the vagina, congenital absence of the vagina, and duplication defects of the uterus.

An adequate physical examination will detect or at least arouse a suspicion of defective development. Examination under anesthesia and exploration of the uterus with a sound will often provide additional valuable information. An intravenous urogram should be done in all cases because one-third to one-half of cases are associated with anomalies of the urinary tract such as absent kidney, horseshoe kidney, and duplication of the collecting system. Injury to the urinary tract can result from failure to recognize associated urinary tract anomalies during corrective surgery.

Congenital anomalies of the genitourinary tract must be distinguished from primary amenorrhea due to endocrine disorders, leiomyomas of the uterus, and ovarian tumors. Errors in diagnosis have resulted in unnecessary surgery, particularly when a preoperative diagnosis of leiomyoma uteri is made in a case of uterus didelphys or bicornuate uterus. Laparoscopic examination may be of considerable value in an evaluation of the patient with a suspected anomaly of the genitourinary tract.

Minor anomalies of the reproductive tract require only explanation and reassurance. For example, a small vaginal septum, bicornuate uterus, or even a complete uterus didelphys usually will not interfere with coital or reproductive function and will cause no significant symptoms.

Imperforate Hymen

Imperforate hymen is often not recognized until puberty, when, despite the appearance of menstrual symptoms, bleeding fails to occur. Examination at this time will reveal a bulging, imperforate hymen. Rectal examination may demonstrate a large, cystic pelvic mass representing a distended vagina (hematocolpos) and even a cystically enlarged uterus (hematometra).

Urinary obstruction has been reported due to a large hematocolpos resulting from menstruation behind an imperforate hymen.

Imperforate hymen is treated by cruciate incisions of the mucous membrane (hymenotomy), releasing the trapped menstrual discharges and correcting the hematocolpos and hematometra. Antibiotics should be given when there is a significant hematocolpos and hematometra in order to prevent secondary infection.

Duplication of the Vagina

Duplication of the vagina may occur with or without a single or a double uterus. There may be a double vagina, a double cervix, and a single uterus. The duplication may be only partial and take the form of a longitudinal septum, in which case excision may be required in the event that there is soft tissue dystocia in labor. Complete duplication of the vagina usually requires no treatment.

Occasionally, the duplication takes the form of a rudimentary vagina which fails to communicate with the second vagina or the outside. This may result in the formation of a hematocolpos at the time of menarche, with an apparent paravaginal cystic mass as a presenting sign. The finding of old blood upon incising such a tumor should lead to the correct diagnosis. A separate cervix and corpus will be found at the top of this space. Marsupialization of the rudimentary vagina with the primary vagina is the usual method of management.

Transverse Septum of the Vagina

A transverse vaginal septum usually is incomplete. If imperforate, it may be mistaken for congenital absence of the vagina.

Transverse vaginal septa are treated by excision.

Absence of the Vagina

Absence of the vagina usually is associated with absence of the uterus. Often there is a very small lower vagina, representing that portion that develops from the urogenital sinus. The condition is commonly not recognized until the physician is consulted because of primary amenorrhea in a teen-ager.

Congenital absence of the vagina is managed by construction of an artificial vagina. This should be deferred until the patient has a desire and a need for a functioning vagina. A variety of technics have been described, but those utilizing skin grafts placed in an artificially created channel between the bladder and the rectum have been the most widely used. Artificial vaginas can be constructed from the labia majora or by using isolated segments of the large intestine.

Construction of an artificial vagina will allow girls to develop satisfactory social and sexual relationships with members of the opposite sex. The psychologic benefits are as important as the physical ones.

Duplication Defects of the Uterus

Duplication defects of the uterus are most often detected in the course of investigation for habitual abortion or for repeated premature labor. They may vary from a simple midline septum in a single uterus to a complete duplication of the corpus and cervix. Uterine anomalies of this type can often be detected during the third trimester of pregnancy because of the characteristic abdominal outlines of the uterine fundus and persistent malpresentations of the fetus. Manual exploration of the uterine cavity immediately post-partum will demonstrate a uterine septum or a double horn. Hysterosalpingography is essential to an accurate diagnosis.

If there is a history of repeated fetal loss due to abortions or premature labor, the surgical correction of uterine anomalies is warranted in the hope of improving the patient's fertility. The classic operation for bicornuate uterus is that described by Strassman in which the horns are incised transversely anterior to the insertion of the fallopian tubes and then closed in a longitudinal direction. The septate uterus is corrected either by excising a midline wedge, removing the septum, or merely incising the septum and suturing the margins, thus constructing a single cavity. Subsequent pregnancies after operations for such uterine anomalies should be delivered by cesarean section in order to avoid the risk of uterine rupture in labor. This ideally is done approximately 10 days prior to the expected date of confinement as the risk of rupture increases with approaching term and with labor.

When uterine anomalies are responsible for a poor obstetric history with high fetal wastage, one can expect significant improvement following surgical correction. Fortunately, most patients with abnormalities of the uterus have no significant obstetric problems and require no therapy.

Beasley JM: Congenital malformations of the genital tract. Clin Obstet Gynaecol 1:571, 1974.
Capraro VJ, Gallego MB: Vaginal agenesis. Am J Obstet Gynecol 124:98, 1976.
David A & others: Congenital absence of the vagina: Clinical and psychologic aspects. Obstet Gynecol 46:407, 1975.
Fore SR & others: Urologic and genital anomalies in patients with congenital absence of the vagina. Obstet Gynecol 46:410, 1975.

Cervical & Vaginal Abnormalities Associated With Prenatal Exposure to Diethylstilbestrol (DES)

Since 1971 it has been recognized that women exposed in utero to stilbestrol and other related non-steroidal estrogens have characteristic changes in the cervix and vagina which are essentially pathognomonic of such exposure. Careful inspection and palpation will reveal these changes. The cervical anomalies may present as circular sulci on the exocervix or recessed areas around the external os. There may be a complete covering of the exocervix by columnar epithelium, giving it the so-called "eroded" appearance, or it may present as a "pseudopolyp." Often there is an anterior cervical protuberance which has been described as a "cock's comb."

The vaginal changes take the form of surface or cystic adenosis, fibrous bands, mucosal membranes or elevations, narrowing at the apices, and obliteration of the fornices.

Over two-thirds of the patients thus exposed will show one or more of these changes. There is a relationship between exposure to nonsteroidal estrogens in utero and the subsequent development of clear cell carcinoma of the vagina or cervix, but thus far the risk of malignancy seems to be small—in the range of less than 1:1000.

Careful follow-up examinations of the DES-exposed female population is indicated, with examinations and Papanicolaou smears annually for those in whom pelvic examination reveals no abnormalities and 2 or 3 times a year if vaginal or cervical anomalies such as those described above are found.

Robboy SJ & others: Pathology of vaginal and cervical abnormalities associated with prenatal exposure to diethylstilbestrol. J Reprod Med 15:13, 1975.
Sandberg EC: Benign cervical and vaginal changes associated with exposure to stilbestrol in utero. Am J Obstet Gynecol 125:777, 1976.

BACTERIAL & SPIROCHETAL INFECTIONS OF THE FEMALE REPRODUCTIVE SYSTEM

Chancroid

Chancroid is an acute ulcerative (soft chancre) lesion of the vulva with secondary involvement of the inguinal and femoral lymph nodes caused by *Haemophilus ducreyi*. It is transmitted through coitus and has an incubation period of 2–14 days. The lesion first appears as a papule which rapidly becomes a large pustule. This breaks down, ulcerates, and forms satellite lesions. The regional nodes become enlarged and painful, and chills, fever, and malaise develop. Leukocytosis is usually present. The diagnosis is confirmed by finding the organism in a smear of the exudate, although a culture may be required.

The skin test for chancroid (suspension of the organism) becomes positive within 3–5 weeks of an acute infection and remains positive for life. It is, therefore, of limited value.

The sulfonamides are the drugs of choice, eg, sulfadiazine, 1 g 4 times daily for 7 days. Streptomycin, 1–2 g daily IM for 7 days, may be used as an alternative.

Large, painful, fluctuant buboes may be aspirated, but prompt antibiotic therapy usually allows prompt regression.

Syphilis

The primary lesion of syphilis in women is often a transient, painless, small ulcer on the cervix or the labia. Because this lesion does not take the usual classic form of a chancre, it is often overlooked. The disease usually is transmitted by coitus and is due to the spirochete *Treponema pallidum,* which can be recognized in a darkfield examination of serum obtained from the lesion. Most often, however, the diagnosis is made on the basis of a positive serologic test. The fluorescent treponema antibody absorption test may be helpful in identifying the false-positive VDRL reaction.

Penicillin is the antibiotic of choice. Primary syphilis is treated with benzathine penicillin G, 2 million units IM. Secondary and latent syphilis should receive more vigorous antibiotic therapy by repetition of the injection after 1 week. Tetracycline or erythromycin can be used in the patient allergic to penicillin.

Gonorrhea

Neisseria gonorrhoeae is transmitted by sexual intercourse. It may involve the lower genital tract as a suppurative process involving the Bartholin glands, Skene's ducts, or the cervix. Only in prepubertal girls does it involve the vaginal mucosa since cornified squamous epithelium of the adult vagina resists infection. After infection of the lower tract it may spread via the endometrial surface, following a menstrual period, to the fallopian tubes, where it produces an acute salpingitis, sometimes leading to pelvic peritonitis, tubo-ovarian abscess, chronic salpingitis, and tubal obstruction with bilateral hydrosalpinx. The incidence of subsequent sterility is very high.

If the infection involves only the lower tract, there may be no or few symptoms unless a Bartholin abscess develops, in which case there is a large, painful swelling in the posterior aspect of the labium majus. Acute gonorrheal cervicitis is seen as a mucopurulent exudate from an inflamed cervix. With tubal involvement, which is almost always bilateral, there is lower abdominal pain of a colicky nature, malaise, and fever. There may be signs of acute peritonitis with tenderness, rigidity, rebound tenderness, and ileus. The white blood cell count and the sedimentation rate are moderately elevated.

Pain in the right upper quadrant of the abdomen is an unusual manifestation due to spread of infection in a cephalad direction up the right "peritoneal gutter." Violin string adhesions between the liver and parietal peritoneum may result. Pain and tenderness may closely simulate the findings in acute cholecystitis (Fitz-Hugh and Curtis syndrome).

The diagnosis of gonorrhea is made by finding the typical gram-negative intracellular diplococci in smears or in anaerobic culture (Thayer-Martin V.C.N. media). Disease of the upper tract and the pelvic peritoneum must be distinguished from acute appendicitis, ovarian cysts, tubal pregnancy, endometriosis, diverticulitis, tuberculous salpingitis, and pedunculated leiomyomas of the uterus.

Penicillin is the antibiotic of choice. Acute lower tract infection is effectively treated with aqueous procaine penicillin G, 4.8 million units IM at one time in divided sites. One gram of probenecid should be given orally at least 30 minutes before the injection.

Spectinomycin dihydrochloride pentahydrate may be used in the patient who is allergic to penicillin or ampicillin. Tetracycline is recommended if oral rather than parenteral therapy is desired.

Mild gonorrheal salpingitis can be treated on an outpatient basis with the same regimen described above for lower tract disease. Hospitalization is recommended for those patients in whom the diagnosis is unclear, and surgical emergencies such as ectopic pregnancy must be excluded if there is suspicion of pelvic abscess, if the patient with salpingitis is pregnant, or if the patient is unable to follow an outpatient regimen. Hospitalized patients with proved gonorrheal salpingitis should be given aqueous crystalline penicillin G, 20 million units IV daily, until improvement occurs. This should be followed by 500 mg of ampicillin orally 4 times daily to complete 10 days of treatment.

Anaerobic infection with *Bacteroides fragilis* should be strongly suspected in the patient who fails to respond. With appropriate anaerobic culture technics, these organisms can frequently be recovered from soft-tissue infection sites. *B fragilis* is not susceptible to penicillin at easily maintained therapeutic levels and is insensitive to the cephalosporins and aminoglycosides. The current drugs of choice are chloramphenicol and clindamycin.

Bartholin abscess should be incised and drained. Marsupialization or excision of Bartholin cysts may be required if the duct remains obstructed and the cyst is large or symptomatic. Tubo-ovarian abscesses require incision and drainage. This can usually be accomplished through the vagina via the cul-de-sac. Tuboplastic procedures are done for the relief of sterility in chronic tubal obstruction. Chronic salpingo-oophoritis often requires a total abdominal hysterectomy and bilateral salpingo-oophorectomy.

Barrett-Connor E: Current status of the treatment of syphilis. West J Med 122:7, 1975.

Gaisin A, Heaton CL: Chancroid—alias the soft chancre. Int J Dermatol 14:188, 1975.

Gonorrhea: Recommended treatment schedules—1974. (2 parts.) Obstet Gynecol 45:596, 691, 1975.

Ledger WJ: Anaerobic infections. Am J Obstet Gynecol 123:111, 1975.

Mead PB: Practical applications of antibiotics in prevention and treatment of pelvic infections. J Reprod Med 13:135, 1974.

Sweet RL: Anaerobic infections of female genital tract. Am J Obstet Gynecol 122:891, 1975.

Tuberculosis

Tuberculous infection of the fallopian tubes with secondary involvement of the endometrium (and, rarely, the cervix) is an uncommon disease in the USA, accounting for 5–10% of cases of salpingitis. It is usually secondary to tuberculous infections elsewhere, such as the lung or the urinary tract.

The process may be asymptomatic, with infertility the only complaint. Symptoms, when they occur, are those of low-grade fever, weight loss, fatigue, and menstrual irregularities. There may be palpable adnexal masses.

The diagnosis may be made upon finding a granulomatous lesion in the endometrium at the time of dilatation and curettage for menstrual irregularity. The acid-fast organisms are difficult to demonstrate in histologic sections, and culture of endometrial tissue or the menstrual discharge often is necessary. Chest x-ray, sputum studies, and acid-fast smears and cultures of the urine should be done as well.

Treatment of advanced genital tuberculosis consists of medical therapy with isoniazid, streptomycin, and ethambutol for at least 6 months followed by total abdominal hysterectomy and bilateral salpingo-oophorectomy. Mild cases may be treated medically in the hope of relieving infertility, but close follow-up is mandatory.

Rico LR, Garcia-Valdecasas R: Current status of female genital tuberculosis. Acta Ginec (Madrid) 23:635, 1972.
Schaefer G: Diagnosis and treatment of female genital tuberculosis. Int Surg 48:240, 1967.
Sutherland A: Diagnosis and treatment of female genital tuberculosis. Gynäkologe 5:208, 1972.

Granuloma Inguinale

Infection with *Calymmatobacterium (Donovania) granulomatis* is seen in the USA most often in the southern states. It is transmitted through sexual intercourse and begins as a small vulval papule which then becomes a small area of beefy-red granulomatous tissue. This process spreads superficially and eventually involves the entire perineum, extending into the inguinal areas. Secondary infection is a common complication.

The symptoms are pain, burning, itching, and discharge from the involved area. Smears or biopsies stained with Wright's stain or hematoxylin-eosin stain will show the characteristic Donovan inclusion bodies within large mononuclear cells.

Treatment is with tetracycline, 500 mg orally 4 times daily for 1 week and then 250 mg 4 times daily for an additional 2 weeks.

Lymphogranuloma (Lymphopathia) Venereum

Lymphogranuloma venereum (LGV) is caused by infection with one of the chlamydia group of gram-negative, obligately intracellular bacteria (not by a "large virus," as formerly believed). It is transmitted by coitus and is manifested initially as a small vulval vesicle which appears 1–3 weeks after exposure. This soon disappears but is followed in another 2–3 weeks by an inguinal lymphadenitis which progresses to bubo formation, ulceration, and breakdown. The perirectal lymphatics frequently are similarly involved. Healing often leads to inguinal scarring, rectal stricture, and vulval elephantiasis.

The Frei skin test has been used to confirm the diagnosis and becomes positive about 1 week after the enlargement of the inguinal lymph nodes. It is nonspecific for LGV infection and will be positive in individuals previously infected with other members of the psittacosis group. Therefore, it is diagnostic only if it is negative in the acute phase of the disease and then becomes positive. A positive complement fixation test with a rising titer is also diagnostic.

Treatment is with sulfadiazine, 1 g orally 4 times daily for 3 weeks, or tetracycline, 500 mg orally 4 times daily for 1 week followed by 250 mg 4 times daily for an additional 2 weeks.

VIRAL INFECTIONS OF THE FEMALE REPRODUCTIVE SYSTEM

Condylomata Acuminata (Venereal Warts)

These are usually multiple papules seen on the skin of the vulva and the mucous membranes of the vagina and cervix. They are of viral origin and are usually associated with a vaginal discharge and irritation.

Treatment is with podophyllum resin applied topically in a 25% solution of compound tincture of benzoin, or by electrocoagulation.

The topical application of fluorouracil (5-FU) ointment, 5%, has been found to be effective in the treatment of extensive perianal condylomas.

Graber EA & others: Simple surgical treatment for condyloma acuminatum of the vulva. Obstet Gynecol 29:247, 1967.
Nel WS, Fourie ED: Immunotherapy and 5% topical 5-fluouracil ointment in treatment of condylomata acuminata. S Afr Med J 47:45, 1973.

Herpes Genitalis

Herpes genitalis is caused by herpesvirus hominis type 2 and is venereally transmitted. It is characterized by the appearance of clusters of small, painful, erythematous vesicular lesions on the vulva. Examination may also demonstrate these in the vagina and on the portio vaginalis of the cervix. The vesicles often proceed to ulceration; with coalescence, large, painful ulcers of the vulva, vagina, and cervix may develop.

The diagnosis can be made cytologically by finding characteristic "ground glass" inclusions in mono- or multinucleated giant cells from the squamous epithelium.

There appears to be a relationship between herpes progenitalis and carcinoma of the cervix, as antibodies to herpesvirus type 2 have been found significantly more often in women with cervical cancer than in matched control groups. Whether this is merely a coincidental factor transmitted sexually or an etiologic relationship has not yet been established.

Some viruses can be inactivated if exposed to one of several dyes and then irradiated with ordinary white light. Heterotricyclic dyes such as neutral red or proflavine have an affinity for the guanine base portions of DNA and are bound firmly to the DNA of some viruses. Exposure to light then leads to inactivation of the virus by producing breaks in the viral DNA. Application of 0.1% aqueous proflavine dye to the lesion, followed by a 15-minute exposure to fluorescent light, is effective treatment. However, recent reports of the possibility of premalignant change resulting from this method of treatment have led some clinicians to abandon its use pending further study.

Idoxuridine, 5% in DMSO (not available in the USA), is reported to be effective topically.

Because of the risk of severe systemic disease in infants delivered vaginally, a patient with an acute infection near term in pregnancy should be delivered by cesarean section.

Josey WE & others: Genital herpes simplex infection in the female. Am J Obstet Gynecol 96:493, 1966.

Naili ZM & others: Genital herpetic infection: Association with cervical dysplasia and carcinoma. Cancer 23:940, 1969.

Rawles WE & others: Herpesvirus type 2: Association with carcinoma of cervix. Science 161:1255, 1968.

Yen SSC, Reagen JW, Rosenthal MS: Herpes simplex infection in the female genital tract. Obstet Gynecol 25:479, 1965.

TRICHOMONAS VAGINALIS VAGINITIS

Trichomonas vaginalis vaginitis is caused by a motile flagellated protozoon which produces a vaginal inflammation characterized by a profuse, thin, foamy, yellowish discharge, local burning, and itching. The diagnosis is made by finding the organism in a wet mount smear from the vagina.

Treatment with metronidazole (Flagyl), 250 mg orally 3 times daily for 7 days, is usually successful. It may be necessary to treat the patient's sexual partner concomitantly in order to prevent recurrent infections. Numerous topical agents are available for use in the vagina, and until the teratogenicity of metronidazole has been ruled out the drug should not be used in the pregnant patient.

CANDIDIASIS
(Moniliasis)

Candida albicans, a yeast organism, is the cause of candidal vaginitis, seen often in diabetics, pregnant patients, and women using oral contraceptives. Candidal infections also occur as a complication of antibiotic therapy, with suppression of the normal bacterial flora and overgrowth by yeast organisms. Candidal vaginitis and vulvitis are characterized by intense itching and inflamed skin and mucosa. Frequently there is a clinging, cheesy-white exudate, although this finding may be absent. Intense pruritus is the primary symptom. The diagnosis is made by finding spores or mycelia on a wet mount smear preparation to which a few drops of 10% potassium hydroxide are added or by culturing the organism on Nickerson's medium.

Office treatment consists of cleansing the vagina of the curd-like exudate and applying a 2% aqueous solution of gentian violet. Nystatin (Mycostatin) vaginal tablets are used by the patient each night at bedtime for 2–3 weeks. Nystatin cream is also available for use on the irritated vulval skin.

A newer effective fungicide is 2% miconazole nitrate cream (Monistat), which can be applied to the vagina as well as to the vulvar skin and mucous membranes daily for 14 days.

Culbertson C: Monistat: A new fungicide for treatment of vulvovaginal candidiasis. Am J Obstet Gynecol 120:973, 1974.

MENSTRUAL DISORDERS

AMENORRHEA

Amenorrhea may be primary (a delay of the menarche beyond age 17) or secondary (a cessation of menstrual function of several months' or years' duration occurring after the development of normal, cyclic menstruation). True primary amenorrhea may be due to an abnormality in function or disease of the ovary, pituitary, or hypothalamus. Congenital anomalies of the uterus and vagina as a cause of primary amenorrhea are discussed above.

Clinical Findings
  A. Primary Amenorrhea:
    1. Congenital anomalies
    2. Ovarian agenesis and dysgenesis—
      a. Short stature.
      b. Webbing of neck.
      c. Cubitus valgus.
      d. Infantile external genitalia.
      e. Absent sex chromatin on buccal smear.
      f. Most have a chromosomal karyotype of 45,X, but mosaic patterns (45,X/46,XX or 45,X/46,XX/47,XXX) are encountered.
    3. Hermaphroditism—
      a. Ambiguous external genitalia with en-

larged clitoris and urogenital sinus into
which vagina and urethra open.
  b. Normal breast development.
  c. Menstruation may occur.
  d. Sex chromatin present in buccal smear.
  e. Chromosomal karyotype usually 46,XX.
  f. Ovarian and testicular tissue combined in
     a single gonad (ovotestis).
  4. **Testicular feminization syndrome—**
     a. Female habitus with relatively large hands
        and feet.
     b. Normal breast development.
     c. Scant or absent pubic and axillary hair.
     d. Normal external genitalia.
     e. Hypoplastic vagina ending in a short,
        blind pouch.
     f. Absent or rudimentary uterus and tubes.
     g. Sex chromatin absent in buccal smear.
     h. Chromosomal karyotype is 46,XY.
     i. Gonads are testes which lie in abdomen,
        pelvis, or inguinal canal.
B. Secondary Amenorrhea:
  1. **Pregnancy—**
     a. Signs and symptoms of pregnancy.
     b. Positive chorionic gonadotropin test.
  2. **Menopause—**
     a. Hot flashes.
     b. Familial history of early menopause.
     c. Elevated pituitary gonadotropin.
  3. **Psychogenic—**
     a. Traumatic experience or psychologic dis-
        turbance.
     b. Usually temporary (less than 6 months).
  4. **Following oral contraceptives.**
  5. **Stein-Leventhal syndrome—**
     a. Obesity.
     b. Hirsutism.
     c. Bilaterally enlarged ovaries.
  6. **Pituitary insufficiency or failure (depressed
     pituitary gonadotropins)—**
     a. Following traumatic labor or delivery
        (Sheehan's syndrome).
     b. Pituitary tumors (headache and visual dis-
        turbances).

Treatment
A. Primary Amenorrhea:
  1. **Congenital anomalies**
  2. **Ovarian agenesis and dysgenesis—**
     a. Cyclic estrogen-progestin therapy to sim-
        ulate normal menstrual cycle and develop
        secondary sex characteristics.
     b. Plastic surgery if webbing of neck is
        severe.
  3. **Hermaphroditism—**Surgical removal of con-
     tradictory sex organs and reconstruction of
     those compatible with sex in which patient
     has been reared.
  4. **Testicular feminization syndrome—**
     a. Excision of gonads.
     b. Cyclic estrogen therapy.

B. **Secondary Amenorrhea:**
  1. **Pregnancy**—Obstetrical care.
  2. **Menopause**—Replacement estrogen therapy
     given cyclically to relieve menopausal
     symptoms.
  3. **Psychogenic—**
     a. Usually self-limited.
     b. Cyclic estrogen-progestin therapy in the
        anxious patient.
  4. **Following oral contraceptives**—Same as for
     psychogenic amenorrhea.
  5. **Stein-Leventhal syndrome—**
     a. Clomiphene citrate (Clomid).
     b. Human gonadotropin therapy.
     c. Bilateral wedge resection of ovaries if fail-
        ure to respond to above.
  6. **Pituitary insufficiency or failure—**
     a. Replacement therapy (corticosteroids,
        thyroid, estrogens).
     b. Treatment of pituitary tumors.

ABNORMAL UTERINE BLEEDING

Abnormal uterine bleeding may occur at any age.
In the newborn it is frequently related to removal of
the infant at birth from the influence of maternal
estrogen which has produced endometrial proliferation
in the baby's uterus. During the reproductive years, it
may occur as **hypermenorrhea,** excessive or prolonged
bleeding at the normal time of menstruation; **polymenorrhea,** bleeding which occurs more frequently
than every 3 weeks; or **intermenstrual bleeding,** which
occurs during the interval between normal menstrual
periods.

Hypermenorrhea may be due to such organic conditions as uterine leiomyoma, endometrial polyps, and
blood dyscrasias, or it may be related to a functional
disturbance such as irregular shedding of the endometrium, presumably due to faulty regression of the
corpus luteum of the ovary. Polymenorrhea may be
related to early ovulation with a shortened proliferative phase, which frequently is secondary to hypothyroidism. One of the most frequently encountered
problems is the completely acyclic and sometimes
heavy and prolonged bleeding of the anovulatory
patient, leading to so-called **dysfunctional uterine
bleeding.** This condition is seen most often in adolescents and in premenopausal women and is due to a
failure in regular ovulatory function by the ovaries.
The endometrium is proliferative in type at a time in
the menstrual cycle when it would show secretory
changes had ovulation occurred. In many instances
there is, after a period of time, the development of
endometrial hyperplasia, either of the cystic glandular
or adenomatous pattern, due to the prolonged stimulus
of estrogen on the endometrium without the modify-
ing influence of progesterone. Intermenstrual bleeding
may be due to the slight drop in estrogen titer asso-

ciated with ovulation, in which event it occurs quite regularly at about midcycle. Other causes of intermenstrual bleeding which occurs at any time during the cycle are polyps, submucous leiomyomas, blood dyscrasias, genital tuberculosis, and cancer of the cervix, uterine corpus, or fallopian tube. Complications of pregnancy should not be overlooked as a cause of abnormal bleeding in women of the reproductive age.

Postmenopausal bleeding (vaginal bleeding which occurs a year or more following the menopause) is due to cancer in about 40% of cases. The exogenous administration of estrogenic substances, including their use in cosmetic preparations, is another important cause of this type of abnormal bleeding. Atrophic changes, polyps, trauma, blood dyscrasias, hypertensive cardiovascular disease, and estrogen-producing tumors of the ovary are less frequent causes. The bleeding may be represented by a scant brownish vaginal discharge, or it may be frank, profuse, bright-red bleeding. Because it looms so large in the etiology of postmenopausal bleeding, cancer should be considered the cause until proved otherwise.

Clinical Findings

In the assessment of any type of menstrual disorder, the following points should be considered:

(1) Careful documentation of the menstrual history and an accurate record of the temporal relationship of the abnormal bleeding to the menstrual cycle are necessary. A special menstrual calendar kept by the patient or a basal body temperature graph can be very helpful in this regard.

(2) A history of hormonal medication or cosmetics containing hormones.

(3) A general medical history and physical examination may lead to the correct diagnosis of hypothyroidism, blood dyscrasia, genital tuberculosis, etc.

(4) A carefully performed pelvic examination often will reveal vaginal, cervical, uterine, or adnexal pathology.

(5) Cytologic examination is essential in all patients, and the specimen should be collected prior to the introduction of lubricating jelly into the vagina.

(6) A complete blood count and measurement of red cell indices will reflect the degree of iron deficiency secondary to acute or chronic blood loss. Additional blood studies may be necessary when blood dyscrasias are suspected.

(7) Thyroid function studies may be indicated.

(8) Dilatation and curettage of the uterus with biopsies of the cervix often are required to establish the cause of abnormal menstrual bleeding. This should be done at an appropriate time in the menstrual cycle—eg, after the 16th day of the cycle if anovulatory bleeding is suspected, or on the fourth or fifth day if the working diagnosis is irregular shedding of the endometrium. Curettage will reveal unsuspected endometrial polyps or submucous myomas. Fractional curettage and cervical biopsies are recommended if malignancy is suspected.

Treatment

Acute, massive blood loss should be treated by recording the central venous pressure, placing the patient in the Trendelenburg position, and replenishing the circulating blood volume with intravenous fluids and whole blood transfusions.

Dilatation and curettage is the most effective method of controlling uterine bleeding.

In chronic blood loss due to hypermenorrhea produced by leiomyomas, total menstrual suppression may be achieved by the continuous administration of an estrogen-progestin preparation (see section on endometriosis). The oral administration of iron may obviate blood transfusion in the preparation of the patient for a definitive surgical procedure.

After organic causes have been excluded, the dysfunctional bleeding of the teen-ager and the premenopausal woman is treated with cyclic progestin therapy (aqueous progesterone, 50 mg IM on the 25th day, or norethindrone acetate, 5 mg orally daily from the 20th to the 25th days of the cycle).

Severe, intractable bleeding of a dysfunctional nature may require hysterectomy, but this is rare.

Postmenopausal bleeding of nonneoplastic cause may require estrogen therapy if due to atrophic changes. Curettage is curative if the bleeding is due to endometrial polyps. Endometrial carcinoma is a contraindication to estrogen therapy and is treated by total abdominal hysterectomy and bilateral salpingo-oophorectomy with or without preoperative radiation therapy.

DeCosta EJ: Menstrual problems: Dysfunctional uterine bleeding. JAMA 193:950, 1965.

Greenblatt RB & others: Spectrum of gonadal dysgenesis: Clinical, cytogenetic, and pathologic study. Am J Obstet Gynecol 98:151, 1967.

Jones GS: Endocrine problems of the adolescent. Md State Med J 16:45, 1967.

Kletzky OA & others: Clinical categorization of patients with secondary amenorrhea using progesterone-induced uterine bleeding and measurement of serum gonadotropin levels. Am J Obstet Gynecol 121:695, 1975.

Lang W & others: Pediatric and adolescent gynecology. Ann NY Acad Sci 142:547, 1967.

Lorencz AB: Managing gynecologic problems in the adolescent. GP 36:83, Dec 1967.

•   •   •

CERVICITIS

Essentials of Diagnosis

- Leukorrhea.
- Intermenstrual bleeding may occur.
- Sense of pelvic heaviness and backache.
- Dyspareunia.
- Cervix may show old, healed obstetric lacerations and appear elongated and enlarged.
- Cervical eversion or ectopy is common.

General Considerations

Acute cervicitis is caused by acute gonorrheal infection or occurs in association with trichomonal or candidal vaginitis. Chronic cervicitis (very common) is usually the aftermath of pregnancy and vaginal delivery. After the trauma of cervical effacement and dilatation, the cervix often heals with islands of ectopic, mucus-secreting columnar epithelium on the portio vaginalis of the cervix. This cervical "ectopy" or "eversion" without the healed lacerations and deformities of the cervix is also common in young nulligravidas (15–20%) and is related to a dislocation of the squamocolumnar junction onto the portio vaginalis; it is often asymptomatic and is of no clinical significance except in the occasional instance of excessive mucus production.

Clinical Findings

A. Symptoms and Signs: In acute cases the cervix is acutely inflamed and there is a purulent exudate; gonorrhea should be suspected. Chronic cervicitis may be mild and asymptomatic. In symptomatic cases, a copious vaginal discharge is the most common presenting complaint. In severe, deep-seated infections, there may be a low-grade pelvic cellulitis (parametritis) with a sense of heaviness in the pelvis, low backache, and dyspareunia. Postcoital bleeding may be present. The cervix appears distorted by old, healed obstetric lacerations and is reddened, boggy, and edematous. Nabothian cysts are frequently seen and are due to obstruction of the cervical tunnels, clefts, and crypts lined by mucus-secreting columnar epithelium. Endocervical and ectocervical polyps are commonly present.

B. Laboratory Findings: Cytologic smears demonstrate numerous pus cells and may show epithelial dysplasia. Cervical biopsy shows a leukocytic infiltrate in the subepithelial stroma and often squamous metaplasia and cystic dilatation of the glandular spaces. A gram-stained smear from a patient with acute gonorrheal cervicitis will often show the typical diplococci. Anaerobic cultures are often required for diagnosis in chronic cases.

Differential Diagnosis

Early cervical cancer may present similar symptoms and signs and must be excluded before proceeding with treatment. A negative cytologic smear does not rule out malignant disease. Multiple, representative punch biopsies from the "transformation zone" of the cervix are required.

Complications

Infertility may result from chronic cervical inflammation, which produces an environment unfavorable to penetration of the cervical mucus by spermatozoa.

Treatment

Acute gonorrheal cervicitis is best treated with penicillin. Tetracycline or kanamycin may be used in penicillin-resistant cases or in individuals who are aller-

gic to penicillin. Treatment of nonspecific cervicitis is indicated even in asymptomatic cases because of the possible relationship between chronic cervicitis and carcinoma of the cervix. Mild degrees of cervicitis can be treated effectively with office cauterization, either chemically, with 20% silver nitrate solution on cotton-tipped applicators, or by light radial cauterization with the nasal-tipped thermal cautery or electrocautery. For the deeply involved, deformed cervix, hospitalization is required for electroconization of the cervix under anesthesia. Trachelorrhaphy (plastic repair) of the obstetrically deformed cervix may be necessary in an occasional patient with secondary infertility due to chronic cervicitis. Cryosurgery (freezing) of chronic cervicitis has been used recently with good results.

Cervical polyps usually can be removed in the office. These should be examined by a pathologist for evidence of malignancy.

Prognosis

Cure of acute cervicitis can usually be accomplished within a few days. Chronic cervicitis usually is more resistant and may require several weeks or months of treatment.

Keys TF & others: Single-dose treatment of gonorrhea with selected antibiotic agents. JAMA 210:857, 1969.

Ostergard DR, Townsend DE, Herose FM: The treatment of chronic cervicitis by cryotherapy. Am J Obstet Gynecol 102:426, 1968.

Saylor LF: The physician's role in venereal disease control. California Med 114:114, May 1971.

Singer A: Uterine cervix from adolescence to menopause. Br J Obstet Gynaecol 82:81, 1975.

ADENOMYOSIS

Essentials of Diagnosis

- Multiparous patient 35–50 years of age.
- Hypermenorrhea, polymenorrhea, or intermenstrual bleeding with dysmenorrhea or dyspareunia.
- Uterus slightly to moderately enlarged, symmetric and globular.
- May be tender to palpation, particularly in premenstrual phase of cycle.

General Considerations

Adenomyosis—formerly called "internal endometriosis"—occurs when fingers of endometrium extend into the myometrium to a depth greater than 2 low-power microscopic fields. It may be a focal or a diffuse process and not infrequently involves the entire thickness of the myometrium. The pathogenesis is not known, but the theory of direct growth of the basal layer of endometrium into the myometrium is widely accepted. Estrogen has been implicated as a stimulus to the development of adenomyosis, and the symptomatic improvement which occurs with the menopause supports this concept. The disease is seen most often in the decade which precedes the menopause.

Clinical Findings

A. Symptoms and Signs: The preoperative diagnosis of adenomyosis is very difficult, and the diagnosis is usually not made until pathologic examination of a uterus which has been removed because of hypermenorrhea, polymenorrhea, or intermenstrual bleeding occurring just prior to menses. Because it may be associated with endometriosis (see next section), there may be an acquired dysmenorrhea and dyspareunia. The condition should be suspected if one or more of these symptoms occurs in a multiparous woman age 35–50. Examination will reveal a slightly to moderately enlarged, symmetric, mobile uterus with a finely granular external surface.

B. Special Examinations: Hysterography may be helpful in confirming the clinical diagnosis.

Differential Diagnosis

Adenomyosis must be distinguished principally from leiomyomas of the uterus. The symptoms may be quite similar, but the palpatory findings should enable a careful observer to make the correct diagnosis. Hysterography is necessary in doubtful cases.

An analogous condition, endolymphatic stromal myosis (stromal endometriosis), although histologically benign, clinically behaves as a low-grade malignancy. In this condition, connective tissue cells resembling those of the endometrial stroma infiltrate the lymphatic and venous spaces of the myometrium. This process may extend into the vessels of the broad ligament, in which event local recurrence is possible following hysterectomy. Metastases to the ovary, peritoneal surfaces, and lung have been reported, but only rarely. This disease, usually of the postmenopausal years, is very rare and should not be confused with adenomyosis.

Other disorders which may be confused with adenomyosis are chronic subinvolution of the uterus (benign, idiopathic uterine hypertrophy), endometriosis, chronic salpingitis, and cancer of the endometrium.

Treatment

Total hysterectomy with or without bilateral salpingo-oophrectomy is curative. Hormonal therapy—estrogen alone, progesterone alone, or estrogen-progesterone combinations—has not been successful and has actually caused exacerbations of symptoms. If the symptoms are not severe and more serious conditions such as endometrial carcinoma or submucous leiomyomas have been excluded, symptomatic treatment in anticipation of the menopause constitutes rational therapy.

Prognosis

Adenomyosis is a self-limited process that undergoes spontaneous regression, becoming asymptomatic after the menopause.

ENDOMETRIOSIS

Essentials of Diagnosis

- History of progressive dysmenorrhea and dyspareunia.
- Patient (often nulligravid and infertile) 20–40 years of age.
- Symptoms of rectal or bladder pain at menses, rarely with blood in feces or urine at the time of menstruation.
- Tender, shotty nodules in cul-de-sac.
- Enlarged, adherent ovary.
- Constricting lesion of large intestine on barium enema.
- Typical findings at peritoneoscopy (laparoscopy or culdoscopy).

General Considerations

In endometriosis, functioning endometrial tissue is present in ectopic sites other than the myometrium (see Adenomyosis, above). The areas most often involved are the ovaries, the cul-de-sac peritoneum, the uterosacral ligaments and rectovaginal septum, the sigmoid colon, the pelvic peritoneum, and the small intestine (Fig 44–1). Malignancy may develop in areas of ovarian endometriosis. Ectopic endometrium has

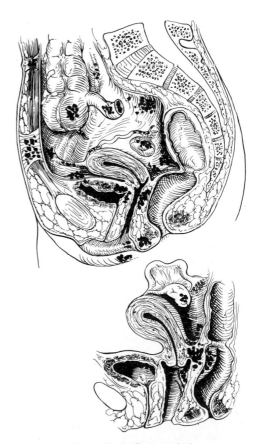

Figure 44–1. Endometriosis.

been found in the umbilicus, in abdominal scars, and (rarely) in the breasts, the extremities, the pleural cavity, and the lungs.

The histogenesis of endometriosis involves 3 different mechanisms: (1) Sampson's theory of retrograde menstruation and implantation; (2) müllerian metaplasia of coelomic epithelium; and (3) lymphatic and venous dissemination. Most cases of endometriosis probably develop as a result of the retrograde passage of bits of menstrual endometrium through the lumens of the fallopian tubes into the peritoneal cavity. Here they implant on the surface of the ovaries and fall by gravity into the cul-de-sac (pouch of Douglas), where they implant and respond to the cyclic hormonal influences of the menstrual cycle, shedding and bleeding at the time of menstruation. Conditions which favor retrograde passage of menstrual discharge, eg, cervical stenosis, uterine retroflexion, congenital anomalies such as vaginal atresia and bicornuate uterus, and uterotubal insufflation—particularly in the menstrual or premenstrual phase of the cycle—predispose to endometriosis.

Endometriosis is primarily a disease of women in the higher socioeconomic levels and is uncommon in black women. It occurs only after the onset of regular menstruation, sometimes in teenage girls, but is rarely encountered in patients with anovulatory cycles.

Endometriosis is commonly associated with infertility, but it is not known which comes first. It becomes quiescent during pregnancy and hormonally induced pseudopregnancy. Multiparity—particularly if childbearing starts early in menstrual life—appears to protect against the development of endometriosis.

Clinical Findings

A. Symptoms and Signs: Endometriosis has protean manifestations. Some patients with extensive disease with large, bilateral ovarian endometriomas may remain essentially asymptomatic, whereas others with small peritoneal implants may be incapacitated with pain. Characteristically, the disease is first manifest as dysmenorrhea developing in the 20s or 30s. This progresses, with increasing severity, to pain that occurs not only with menstruation but also during several days preceding menses, often accompanied by dyspareunia and rectal tenesmus. There may be a continuous, vague sense of lower abdominal and pelvic discomfort throughout the menstrual cycle which is markedly exaggerated during menstruation. Some women complain of low back pain and of painful defecation associated with the menstrual period. This symptom is quite characteristic of cul-de-sac and rectovaginal septum involvement.

Menstrual aberrations are reported in fewer than 50% of patients with endometriosis, and these are probably related to associated conditions such as endometrial polyps or leiomyomas as much as to interference with ovarian function by the endometriotic process.

Bladder involvement may be signified by a suprapubic bearing-down type of pain with or without dysuria and hematuria at the time of menstruation. Involvement of the bladder mucosa is quite rare. If an endometriotic implant involves the peritoneum overlying the ureter, the resulting tissue reaction may produce hydroureter and hydronephrosis with flank and lower abdominal pain.

Implants on the sigmoid colon or rectum may produce signs of partial obstruction of the large bowel, recurring with the menstrual periods.

Occasionally, rupture of a large ovarian endometrial cyst presents symptoms of an acute abdominal emergency with all the signs and symptoms of peritonitis.

B. Pelvic Examination: Rectovaginal bimanual pelvic examination is vital to the detection of pelvic endometriosis since this is the only way the cul-de-sac, the area of the uterosacral ligaments, and the posterior wall of the uterine corpus can be adequately palpated. Moreover, the ovaries, when they are involved, frequently are prolapsed and adherent to the posterior leaf of the broad ligament lateral to the cul-de-sac and are best felt by the rectal finger. An examination performed during the days just preceding the menstrual period is most likely to provide the best opportunity for palpation of the characteristic shotty nodules in the pouch of Douglas, since this is the stage of the menstrual cycle when they are under the full stimulus of the ovarian hormones.

Bilateral, tender, fixed ovarian cystic masses 5–10 cm in diameter are significant findings.

C. Special Examinations: Laparoscopic examination is often quite helpful in establishing a diagnosis of endometriosis in a patient in whom the symptoms are suggestive but the signs are minimal or absent. A finding of characteristic raspberry or blueberry implants or of the powder-burn marks of scarred endometriosis is most valuable. Biopsy of such lesions will establish the diagnosis. Laparotomy is occasionally necessary.

Differential Diagnosis

Endometriosis may mimic chronic salpingitis with bilateral tubo-ovarian masses, ovarian carcinoma, twisted ovarian cyst, appendicitis, ectopic pregnancy, diverticulitis, and carcinoma of the rectosigmoid colon. A detailed history, a carefully performed physical examination, and the use of diagnostic x-ray and laparoscopy or culdoscopy will be helpful in the differential diagnosis. Biopsy of suspicious lesions of the intestine prior to resection will be helpful in avoiding needless bowel resections when endometriosis simulates carcinoma of the gastrointestinal tract.

Complications

Infertility is a common problem in patients with endometriosis and occurs in about three-fourths of women with this disease.

Bowel obstruction does not develop often, but it may occur when there is intestinal involvement by endometrial implantation involving either the small or large bowel. A mechanical ileus may result from the numerous dense adhesions which form as a result of the inflammatory reaction in response to cyclical bleeding from peritoneal implants.

Rupture of a large endometrial cyst of the ovary usually produces an acute, widespread peritoneal reaction with signs and symptoms of an acute surgical emergency.

Scarring around the ureter may cause obstruction, with the development of hydroureter and hydronephrosis, and this may explain many cases of idiopathic hydronephrosis seen in women during the reproductive years.

Ovarian carcinoma has been known to develop in endometriomas and usually takes the form of adenocarcinoma resembling serous cystadenocarcinoma of the ovary. Adenoacanthomas and endometrial stromal sarcomas have been reported, but these are rare.

Prevention

Early, repeated pregnancy appears to prevent the development of endometriosis.

Assuming that retrograde passage of endometrial tissue through the fallopian tubes is the primary method of implantation, one should avoid repeated injections into the endometrial cavity such as gas insufflation for determination of tubal patency or the introduction of radiopaque media for the purpose of x-ray delineation of the uterine cavity and tubal lumen (hysterosalpingography), particularly at or near the menstrual period.

The early diagnosis and treatment of menstrual obstruction (dilatation of the cervix, hymenotomy, metroplasty, and the correction of fixed retroversion) may help to prevent or delay the development of endometriosis.

There is suggestive evidence that long-term contraceptive pill users are less likely to develop endometriosis, particularly if the pill contains a small amount of estrogen in combination with a potent progestin.

Treatment

Therapy may be medical, surgical, or a combination of both methods. Treatment should be tailored to fit the circumstances with respect to the age of the patient, her symptoms, her desire for children, and the extent of the disease. Therapy may vary, therefore, from mere observation, reassurance, and analgesia if necessary, to complete surgical removal of the uterus, tubes, and ovaries.

A conservative approach is recommended for the patient who is symptom-free or only mildly symptomatic with minimal pelvic findings such as slightly tender cul-de-sac nodules. Regular examinations should be carried out at intervals of not more than 6 months. Evidence of progression of the disease—either in the form of increasing symptomatology, infertility, or the development of pelvic masses—requires more specific treatment.

A. Hormonal Treatment: The induction of anovulation and amenorrhea has been successful in bringing about regression in a high percentage of patients with endometriosis. This may be accomplished in several ways:

1. Estrogens alone—Give diethylstilbestrol in increasing doses, beginning on the first day of the menstrual period with 1 mg/day orally and increasing every 3 days by 1 mg until 5 mg/day are being given. The patient is then instructed to take one-fourth of a 25 mg tablet, increasing this by one-fourth tablet every 3 days to 100 mg/day. This method has the side-effects of nausea early in the course of treatment, breast tenderness, and occasional breakthrough bleeding with endometrial hyperplasia.

2. Androgens alone—Methyltestosterone, 5–10 mg sublingually daily, will be effective in some patients, but side-effects such as acne, voice changes, and hirsutism in sensitive patients are drawbacks. Doses in excess of 300 mg/month are not recommended. In the therapeutic dose range, ovulation and menstruation are not inhibited by androgens; their effect is probably a direct one on the endometrial implants rather than a suppression of the anterior pituitary.

3. Progestins—Norethynodrel, norethindrone, hydroxyprogesterone caproate, and medroxyprogesterone are the agents most commonly used. They are most often used in combination with an estrogen (to prevent breakthrough bleeding). One such combination—norethynodrel, 2.5 mg, with mestranol, 0.1 mg (Enovid-E), may be given in the following schedule: 2.5 mg/day for 1 week, 5 mg/day for 1 week, and 10 mg/day for 2 weeks, increasing by 2.5 mg *each time there is breakthrough bleeding*. The production of a pseudopregnancy state through hormonal therapy is maintained for 6–12 months and is effective in about 80% of patients. It is useful as a preoperative adjunct for 6 weeks to soften areas of scarred endometriosis and to make the surgical procedure somewhat easier. The most frequent indication for the prolonged use of these compounds is recurrent endometriosis following a conservative operation. Side-effects are nausea, breast tenderness, fluid retention, and breakthrough bleeding.

Hormonal therapy is not indicated in patients with unproved endometriosis or uterine leiomyomas or in individuals with a history of breast cancer, thrombophlebitis, pulmonary embolus, or liver disease.

B. Surgical Treatment: The surgical approach to endometriosis may be designed to improve fertility, to prevent further progression of the disease with preservation of the ovaries, or to cure the disease by removal of the uterus and the adnexal structures.

1. Conservative surgery—Preservation of childbearing function by removal or cauterization of implants, freeing up of tubal adhesions, presacral neurectomy for the relief of pain, and uterine suspension is indicated in the young woman who desires to have children. It is not recommended in the patient with extensive endometriosis involving the intestines.

2. Modified radical surgery—This involves the removal of the uterus, excision or fulguration of endometrial implants, and preservation of the ovaries. This approach may be considered in the younger woman who has no desire to retain her childbearing function but is not near the menopause. It carries the risk of recurrence, but without the uterus the risk is small.

3. **Definitive surgery**—This requires the removal not only of the uterus but of the tubes and ovaries as well. Since endometriosis is dependent upon ovarian function for its continued growth and development, total hysterectomy and bilateral salpingo-oophorectomy should be done in patients with extensive disease, particularly those with bowel involvement. It is critically important not to mistake bowel implants for cancer. Unnecessary abdominoperineal resections have been performed in young women for unrecognized endometriosis.

Oral estrogen replacement therapy in the form of diethylstilbestrol, 0.25–0.5 mg/day, ethinyl estradiol, 0.02–0.05 mg/day, or conjugated estrogens, 0.625–1.25 mg/day, interrupting the cycle for 5–7 days each month, may be given without danger of exacerbating the endometriotic process. The use of estrogen-progestin combinations is not recommended.

Kistner RW: Management of endometriosis in the infertile patient. Fertil Steril 26:1151, 1975.

Molitor JJ: Adenomyosis: A clinical and pathologic appraisal. Am J Obstet Gynecol 110:275, 1971.

Ranney B: Prevention, inhibition, palliation, and treatment of endometriosis. Am J Obstet Gynecol 123:778, 1975.

Schifrin BS, Erez S, Moore JG: Teenage endometriosis. Am J Obstet Gynecol 116:973, 1973.

Williams TJ: The role of surgery in the management of endometriosis. Mayo Clin Proc 50:198, 1975.

TUBAL PREGNANCY

Essentials of Diagnosis

- Cramping, colicky, or steady lower abdominal pain.
- Missed period or menstrual irregularity.
- Vaginal bleeding.
- Tender adnexal mass.
- Signs of intraperitoneal bleeding (culdocentesis).
- Slight uterine enlargement.

General Considerations

Ectopic pregnancy occurs once in every 150–200 pregnancies. The fallopian tube is the most frequent site of an ectopic pregnancy (95%), and the ampulla or isthmic portion of the tube is the section usually involved. Interstitial (cornual) pregnancies are infrequent but significant because profuse, exsanguinating intraperitoneal bleeding occurs at the time of rupture. Ectopic pregnancies are seen also in the peritoneal cavity (abdominal pregnancy), ovary, and cervix; because they are extremely rare, only tubal pregnancy will be discussed here.

Tubal pregnancy is the result of implantation of the fertilized ovum into the wall of the fallopian tube,

an event probably related to a delay in the transfer of the egg through the tubal lumen. Preexisting disease affecting the tubes (salpingitis, appendicitis, endometriosis, and pelvic operations, particularly tuboplastic procedures and partial salpingectomy for sterilization) predisposes to tubal pregnancy, but tubal pregnancy is not infrequent in patients with no such history.

With implantation of the ovum, there is vascular engorgement and trophoblastic invasion with resultant weakening of the wall of the fallopian tube. Rupture of the tube frequently follows, often with massive bleeding into the peritoneal cavity. The pregnancy, on the other hand, may separate from the implantation site into the lumen of the tube and then be extruded through the fimbriated extremity into the peritoneal cavity together with a considerable amount of blood (tubal abortion). In either event there may be sufficient acute blood loss to produce the clinical picture of hypovolemic shock.

Regardless of the implantation site in the fallopian tube, uterine enlargement with decidual change in the endometrium occurs because of the influence on the uterus of pregnancy levels of estrogen and progesterone.

Clinical Findings

The symptoms and signs of tubal pregnancy are extremely variable, and this disease is not infrequently overlooked or misdiagnosed because of the atypical clinical picture.

A. "Classical" Findings: Classically, in a ruptured tubal pregnancy the history is of 1–2 missed menstrual periods with accompanying presumptive symptoms of pregnancy (tender breasts, urinary frequency, nausea). Mild to moderate vaginal bleeding then ensues, followed, after an interval of a few days, by the onset of unilateral lower abdominal pain—at first cramping or colicky and then steady, becoming generalized through the lower abdomen. Referred shoulder pain results from irritation of the diaphragm by the intraperitoneal blood. Syncope often occurs due to hypotension.

Examination reveals a pale, cold, clammy, apprehensive patient with a rapid, thready pulse and hypotension. The abdomen is tender throughout, with rigidity and rebound tenderness. These findings are often more pronounced on the affected side. Rarely, there is a bluish discoloration around the umbilicus (Cullen's sign). Dark blood is often present in the vagina, issuing from the cervical canal. Marked tenderness throughout the entire abdomen can be elicited, and displacement of the cervix digitally produces considerable discomfort in the abdomen. The uterus is slightly to moderately enlarged and soft. A tender adnexal mass may be palpated, and there is often a feeling of fullness in the cul-de-sac. Culdocentesis reveals nonclotting blood in the peritoneal cavity.

Hemoglobin and hematocrit are below normal values, and a moderate leukocytosis is present. The pregnancy test may or may not be positive.

B. "Atypical" Findings: The majority of tubal

pregnancies (60–85%) do not fit this typical picture and manifest themselves in more subtle ways. There may be no history of menstrual irregularity or presumptive symptoms of pregnancy. The abdominal pain may be mild and vague. Physical findings often are confusing with some pelvic tenderness but no palpable adnexal mass. The uterus may or may not be enlarged and softened. Slow hemorrhage into the peritoneal cavity may circumvent the clinical picture of surgical shock. A gradually falling hematocrit may be the only real clue to bleeding. For these reasons, tubal pregnancy often is a diagnostic enigma, and it is necessary to be alert to the possibility and to properly investigate suspected cases in order to avoid a tragic outcome.

Culdocentesis is particularly helpful in proving the presence of free blood in the peritoneal cavity, but it may be negative in an unruptured tubal pregnancy or if a blood clot obstructs the lumen of the needle.

A decidual cast from the uterus passed through the vagina or curettings which demonstrate decidua but no evidence of trophoblast on careful pathologic examination are suggestive of ectopic pregnancy. Laparoscopy may help establish the correct diagnosis.

Differential Diagnosis

Early intrauterine pregnancy with or without threatened abortion and pelvic inflammatory disease are the conditions most often confused with ectopic pregnancy. The cramping pain of a threatened or inevitable intrauterine abortion is usually suprapubic rather than unilateral. There is no adnexal structure suggestive of tubal pregnancy; little pain is present in the adnexal area or on cervical motion; and culdocentesis shows no blood in the peritoneal cavity. Laparoscopy reveals normal adnexal structures. Acute appendicitis may simulate a tubal pregnancy on the right side. A diagnosis of appendicitis is suggested by nausea and vomiting of acute onset, absence of a significant menstrual history or vaginal bleeding, a higher white blood count, and culdocentesis negative for blood but perhaps productive of a small amount of fluid which has a high white blood count. Acute salpingitis, particularly when the symptoms and signs are more pronounced on one side, may be confused with ectopic pregnancy. In this condition, there is usually some evidence of bilateral disease. There are no symptoms or signs of pregnancy, and culdocentesis may show inflammatory elements rather than blood in the peritoneal cavity. A corpus luteum cyst of the ovary with rupture and bleeding into the peritoneal cavity may closely simulate a ruptured tubal pregnancy and often requires laparotomy for the differential diagnosis. Laparoscopy may be diagnostic.

Complications

The complications of tubal pregnancy are those of shock due to hemorrhage, infection, and sterility.

Prevention

Prompt diagnosis and treatment of unruptured ectopic pregnancy will prevent the often massive intra-peritoneal hemorrhage associated with rupture. Unruptured ectopic pregnancy must be considered whenever a patient is presumed to be pregnant and an adnexal mass is palpated which is thought to be separate from the ovary on that side. Only prompt investigation regarding the nature of the mass will circumvent the possibility of a ruptured tubal pregnancy.

Treatment

Ideally, treatment is surgical, with excision of the implant and preservation of the fallopian tube before rupture occurs.

Ruptured tubal pregnancy is a surgical emergency. Immediate transfusion and operation are imperative. The surgical procedure usually performed is unilateral salpingectomy or salpingo-oophorectomy, although it may be possible to preserve the fallopian tube in unruptured pregnancies and in cases of tubal abortion. Hysterectomy should be considered in patients with a known recent benign cervical smear whose vital signs are stable and who have obvious inflammatory destruction of both fallopian tubes or surgical loss of both tubes.

Prognosis

The prognosis is good if the diagnosis is made promptly and appropriate therapy given. Death may result from hemorrhage or infection in neglected cases.

Breen JL: A 21-year survey of 654 ectopic pregnancies. Am J Obstet Gynecol 106:1004, 1970.
Capraro VJ & others: Cul-de-sac aspiration and other diagnostic aids for ectopic pregnancy: 22-year analysis. Int Surg 53:245, 1970.
Harralson JD & others: Operative management of ruptured tubal pregnancy. Am J Obstet Gynecol 115:995, 1973.
Samuelsson S, Sjövell A: Laparoscopy in suspected ectopic pregnancy. Acta Obstet Gynecol Scand 51:31, 1972.
Stromme WB: Conservative surgery for ectopic pregnancy: Twenty-year review. Obstet Gynecol 41:215, 1973.

INCOMPETENCE OF PELVIC SUPPORT
(Uterine Prolapse, Cystourethrocele, Rectocele, Enterocele, Prolapse of Vagina After Hysterectomy)

Essentials of Diagnosis

- Parous woman.
- Complaints of "bearing down" or "falling out" sensation in the pelvis, mass protruding from vaginal introitus, stress incontinence of urine, and difficulty in evacuating rectum.
- Physical findings of defective perineal body, bulge of anterior vaginal wall with loss of urethrovesical angle, bulge of posterior vaginal wall due to defect in rectovaginal septum or hernia sac between rectum and vagina (enterocele), descent of uterus in pelvis, and protrusion of vagina (following hysterectomy).

General Considerations

An understanding of pelvic floor relaxation with its sequelae of cystourethrocele, rectocele, enterocele, and uterine (or vaginal) prolapse requires a thorough knowledge of the anatomic relationships of the pelvic viscera and their supporting tissues. Almost invariably, these conditions result initially from stretching and tearing of the connective tissues of the pelvis during delivery. The supporting structures are weakened, and this is followed by the slow, insidious additional loss of strength brought about by the gravitational forces of the erect position over the years and the sudden, intermittent increases of pressure from above (intraabdominal pressure) associated with lifting, coughing, straining, sneezing, etc. Finally comes the additional insult of loss of tone due to the hormonal withdrawal associated with the menopause.

These conditions are rarely seen in nulligravidas, in whom they are thought to be related to congenital anomalies (spina bifida occulta).

The levator ani muscle forms the basic portion of the floor of the pelvis. It is trough-shaped and perforated in its thickened, central portion (pubococcygeus) by the urethra, vagina, and rectum. The fascia covering the superior surface of this muscle is continuous with the endopelvic fascia as well as the cardinal and uterosacral ligaments supporting the uterus. The fascia covering the inferior surface of the levator ani muscle is in continuity with that of the obturator internus and the urogenital diaphragm (Fig 44–2). The urogenital diaphragm (triangular ligament) bridges that portion of the perineum anterior to the ischial tuberosities, between the descending rami of the pubis. It is composed of the deep transverse perineal muscle and its

investing superficial and deep fascia and is penetrated by the urethra and the vagina. It forms a secondary but less important support for these structures.

In obstetric injuries to the pelvic floor there is often damage to the investing endopelvic fascia and the supporting ligaments of the uterus as well as to the levator sling, so that combinations of anatomic defects often are encountered rather than a single one—ie, prolapse of the uterus in combination with cystourethrocele, rectocele, and enterocele.

Stress incontinence represents the involuntary loss of urine from the urethra with increases in intraabdominal pressure such as that which occurs with coughing, straining, sneezing, laughing, etc. It can be demonstrated clinically during pelvic examination by asking the patient to cough. Stress incontinence should be carefully distinguished from another common type of involuntary loss of urine, ie, urgency incontinence. The latter condition usually is related to inflammatory conditions in and around the bladder trigone, producing bladder irritability, and the patient experiences the loss of urine with bladder filling and the desire to void. The 2 conditions may occur simultaneously. Surgical correction of stress incontinence may produce a temporary urgency incontinence until the postoperative inflammatory reaction subsides. Other types of urinary incontinence such as the overflow type of neurogenic bladder must also be recognized.

Anatomically, the bladder and urethra are supported by the muscles of the pelvic floor and the endopelvic fascia. The intraluminal hydrostatic pressure relationships are all-important to an understanding of the mechanism of stress incontinence and its correction. In the nulliparous woman, the proximal urethra is

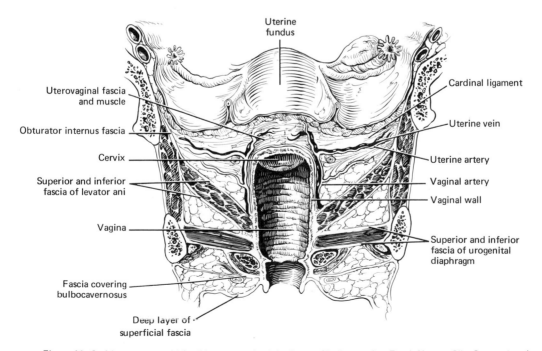

Figure 44–2. Ligamentous and fascial support of pelvic viscera. (Redrawn after Frank Netter: Ciba Symposium.)

held high and is subjected to the same intra-abdominal pressure changes as those affecting the bladder. Thus, with coughing, straining, sneezing, etc, the greater "closure pressure" of the proximal urethra (50–135 cm water) over that of the intravesical pressure (10–60 cm water) is maintained, and the patient remains continent. In the multipara with pelvic floor relaxation, however, descent of the posterior wall of the bladder neck and urethra produces a funneling effect (loss of the posterior urethrovesical angle). The proximal urethra no longer maintains a higher closing pressure with stress, and incontinence occurs. Most operations for the correction of urinary stress incontinence are designed to reconstruct the posterior urethrovesical angle and prevent funneling of the bladder neck and proximal urethra, restoring the increased "closing pressure" of the urethra over the hydrostatic pressure within the bladder during stress.

A cystocele of significant degree may be present without stress incontinence, and the overzealous surgeon may, in correcting the cystocele, straighten out the posterior angle, produce a funneling of the bladder neck and urethra, and thus cause an iatrogenic stress incontinence.

Clinical Findings

Mild degrees of pelvic floor relaxation are found in many multiparous women without significant symptoms. Prolapse of the uterus varies in degree depending upon the level of the uterus in the pelvis. In a first degree prolapse, the cervix does not protrude through the vaginal introitus. Second degree prolapse is manifest by the presence of the cervix outside the vagina, whereas in third degree prolapse (procidentia) the entire uterus comes through the introitus covered by the everted vagina.

Descent and bulging of the anterior wall of the vagina indicates the presence of a cystocele, urethrocele, or both, whereas a similar anatomic defect in the posterior wall signifies that a rectocele or enterocele (or both) exists. All of these conditions can be demonstrated during examination with the patient in the lithotomy position by asking her to bear down or strain. However, the existence of an enterocele can best be demonstrated by performing a rectovaginal examination with the patient in the standing position. The hernia is felt between the rectal and vaginal fingers.

The symptoms of pelvic floor incompetence are those of a dragging sensation or sense of "falling out" of the pelvic organs, a mass protruding from the vagina (which may be a cystocele, rectocele, cervix, or all 3), stress incontinence, repeated urinary tract infections due to sacculation of the bladder and a high residual urine, and difficulties in defecation, occasionally requiring digital compression of the posterior vaginal wall.

Differential Diagnosis

Prolapse of the uterus must be distinguished from hypertrophy and elongation of the cervix due to chronic inflammation. Sounding of the cervical canal to the level of the internal os will accomplish this.

Urethral diverticula may simulate cystourethrocele, producing a bulge of the anterior vaginal wall. The diverticulum is usually palpable as a discrete mass, and pressure against the mass often expresses purulent material from the urethral meatus. Endoscopic and urethrocystographic examinations confirm the diagnosis.

Treatment

The asymptomatic patient requires no treatment, and it is best to defer therapy in such a patient or one with only mild symptoms until she requests correction for the relief of symptoms.

A. Nonoperative Treatment: The postmenopausal woman with mild to moderate anatomic defects may become symptom-free after the administration of estrogen—either topically, in the form of creams or suppositories, or systemically, by oral tablets or intramuscular injections of a long-acting estrogen preparation. Programmed, active exercises of the pelvic floor musculature (Kegel exercises) may prove helpful in relieving symptoms of mild degree.

Pessary support of the descending pelvic structures will provide temporary relief of symptoms and is useful in the surgical high-risk patient.

B. Surgical Treatment: The operation performed most often for the correction of pelvic floor relaxation with multiple anatomic defects is vaginal hysterectomy with anterior colporrhaphy (urethral suspension, plication of the bladder neck, and cystocele repair) and posterior colporrhaphy (rectocele [and enterocele] repair with perineoplasty).

Retropubic urethral suspension is the operation of choice for severe stress incontinence.

Prognosis

The surgical correction of these conditions results in complete relief of symptoms and no recurrence of the defect in about 85% of patients. Obesity, chronic cough, and straining contribute to recurrences. Overlooking an enterocele at the time of repair is a frequent cause of failure of surgical correction.

Enhorning G & others: Urethral closure studied with cineroentgenography and simultaneous bladder-urethra pressure recording. Surg Gynecol Obstet 118:507, 1964.

Green TH: Urinary stress incontinence: Differential diagnosis, pathophysiology and management. Am J Obstet Gynecol 122:368, 1975.

Greenhill JP: Nonsurgical management of pelvic relaxation. Clin Obstet Gynecol 15:1083, 1974.

Lee RA, Symmonds RE: Repeat Marshall-Marchetti procedure for recurrent stress urinary incontinence. Am J Obstet Gynecol 122:219, 1975.

Morgan JE: Suprapubic approach to primary stress urinary incontinence. Am J Obstet Gynecol 115:316, 1973.

Ullery JC, Villalon R: Urinary tract injuries in obstetrics and gynecology. W Va Med J 64:127, 1968.

URINARY TRACT FISTULAS

Urinary tract fistulas are of several varieties: vesicovaginal (most common), ureterovaginal, and urethrovaginal. They occur most often as a result of accidental injury to the urinary tract at the time of pelvic surgery or because of ischemic necrosis resulting from an impaired blood supply. The latter can occur either following radiation therapy for carcinoma of the reproductive organs (especially the cervix) or as a result of prolonged impaction of the fetal head during labor in obstetrics.

Total abdominal hysterectomy is the operation most often complicated by the development of vesicovaginal fistula, which may also occur as a result of tumor invasion of the vesicovaginal septum.

Clinical Findings

A. Symptoms and Signs: Constant urinary incontinence is the cardinal symptom. Urine can be seen usually coming through an opening in the vagina. In vesicovaginal and ureterovaginal fistulas, the vaginal ostium is at or near the vault closure, whereas the urethrovaginal fistula opens along the anterior wall of the vagina. If the urethrovaginal fistula involves the distal urethra, the patient may remain continent and lose urine into the vagina only at the time of voiding.

A communication between the urinary bladder and the vagina can be demonstrated by instilling sterile milk or a dye (methylene blue or indigo carmine) into the bladder via a catheter and watching it come through into the vagina on speculum examination. If leakage of urine into the vagina cannot be colored in this fashion, the defect probably is ureteral and can be demonstrated by giving the patient methylene blue tablets by mouth and finding a blue stain on a cotton pledget placed in the vagina.

B. Urologic Examination: Cystoscopy and x-ray studies of the urinary tract will localize the urinary tract opening of the fistulous tract. Occasionally, the fistulous tracts are branching or multiple.

Prevention

Close attention to surgical technic, recognition of urinary tract injuries, and their proper repair at the time of surgery will prevent most of the fistulas which are the result of urinary tract injury.

Treatment

Urinary tract fistulas rarely close spontaneously. They must be repaired surgically, but sufficient time should elapse (4–6 months) to allow for resolution of edema and inflammatory reaction. Otherwise, attempts at repair are doomed to failure. The use of cortisone has been recommended as an anti-inflammatory agent to shorten this waiting period. Control of the urine leakage from the vaginal vault pending surgical repair often is possible by introducing a small rubber menstrual cup (Tassette) to which is attached a catheter and a leg bag urinal (Fig 44–3). Urinary tract infec-

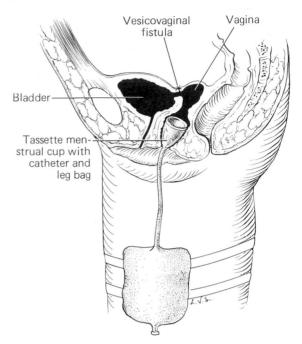

Figure 44–3. Vesicovaginal fistula with menstrual cup and leg bag.

tions should be treated with appropriate urinary antiseptic agents before surgical correction.

Ureterovaginal fistulas are repaired by performing a uretero-ureterostomy or by implanting the severed ureter into the bladder (uretero-neocystostomy).

The abdominal (suprapubic) and vaginal approaches are used to repair vesicovaginal fistulas, and a number of technics are available (layer closure, partial colpocleisis). Regardless of the method used, the principles of repair are the same: meticulous technic, using fine suture material; approximation of broad surfaces without tension; and maintenance of bladder decompression postoperatively until healing can occur.

Falk HC: Prevention of vesicovaginal fistula in total hysterectomy for benign disease. Obstet Gynecol 29:865, 1967.

Higgins CC: Ureteral injuries during surgery. JAMA 199:82, 1967.

Moir JC: Vesicovaginal fistulas as seen in Britain. J Obstet Gynaecol Br Commonw 80:598, 1973.

RECTOVAGINAL FISTULAS

Rectovaginal fistulas are most often a result of obstetric injury, surgical procedures, cervical cancer, or radiation therapy. The symptoms are those of incontinence of flatus or feces through the vagina. The vaginal ostium usually can be demonstrated by speculum examination, and a probe passed through the fistulous tract can be palpated by the rectal finger.

Low rectovaginal fistulas near the vaginal introitus should be repaired after the surrounding inflammatory reaction and edema have subsided. This may require 3—4 months. Those that are found high in the vagina—particularly fistulas resulting from radiation therapy—are often best managed with an initial diverting colostomy which is then closed 2—3 months after a successful repair.

Before surgical repair of a rectovaginal fistula, the bowel should be prepared with a low-residue diet, enteric antibiotics, and cleansing enemas.

Fistulas which occur as a result of malignancy are not amenable to surgical repair. A diverting colostomy may give the patient considerable comfort.

Lescher TC, Pratt JH: Vaginal repair of simple rectovaginal fistula. Surg Gynecol Obstet 124:1317, 1967.

CORRECTION OF INFERTILITY DUE TO TUBAL ABNORMALITIES

A married couple may be considered infertile if a pregnancy does not occur after 1 year of normal coital activity without contraceptives. About 15% of marriages are infertile, and in approximately 40% of these there is a significant male factor (low sperm count, impaired motility, or anomalous forms). Chronic salpingitis is the single most common cause of sterility in women, although endometriosis and peritubal adhesions from previous appendicitis (with rupture) may be causative factors.

Clinical Findings

There may or may not be palpable adnexal pathology. Tubal insufflation with carbon dioxide (Rubin's test) demonstrates some impairment in tubal patency. If several Rubin tests done during the week following menstruation and prior to ovulation reveal nonpatency, a hysterosalpingogram should be obtained. This may reveal an obstruction at the cornu, hydrosalpinx, fimbrial occlusion, or peritubal adhesions. Peritoneoscopy (culdoscopy, laparoscopy) with the passage of a dye through a uterine cannula while the fallopian tubes are under vision is also an excellent diagnostic method.

Treatment

Tuboplasty operations are designed to reestablish tubal patency. These surgical procedures are more successful if the obstruction is localized with little damage to the fallopian tube as a whole (fimbrial adhesions, previous tubal ligation). Reestablishment and maintenance of tubal patency has been more successful with the development of inert plastic materials for splinting and protecting the tube from adhesions during the healing process. Salpingolysis, reimplantation of the tube into the uterus, end-to-end anastomosis, and fimbrial salpingostomy are the operations usually performed. Preoperative, intraoperative, and postoperative administration of dexamethasone and promethazine is useful in prevention of postoperative pelvic adhesions following operations for infertility.

Prognosis

An overall pregnancy incidence of about 20% is reported following tuboplasty, but about one in 10 of these is a tubal pregnancy. The best results (26%) are achieved following cornual reimplantation when the remainder of the tube is anatomically and physiologically normal. Conception rates in excess of 50% can be achieved in the surgical correction of the simpler forms of tubal sterilization.

Gomel V: Laparoscopic tubal surgery in infertility. Obstet Gynecol 46:47, 1975.
Horne HW & others: Prevention of postoperative pelvic adhesions following conservative operative treatment for human infertility: A final 3-year follow-up report. Int J Fertil 18:109, 1973.
Siegler AM: Salpingoplasty: Classification and report of 115 operations. Obstet Gynecol 34:339, 1969.
Siegler AM, Perez RJ: Reconstruction of fallopian tubes in previously sterilized patients. Fertil Steril 26:383, 1975.
Williams GFJ: Fallopian tube surgery for reversal of sterilization. Br Med J 1:599, 1973.

TUMORS OF THE FEMALE GENITAL TRACT

BENIGN TUMORS OF THE VULVA & VAGINA

Hidradenoma

Hidradenomas are small, discrete, firm, mobile structures in the subcutaneous tissues of the labia or perianal region. These sweat gland tumors are benign but may be mistaken for a malignancy because of an adenomatous microscopic pattern.

Treatment consists of local excision.

Sebaceous Cysts

Sebaceous cysts are small, raised, discrete, white, cystic structures in the skin of the labia majora or minora which contain white sebaceous material. They may become infected, producing small abscesses.

Most sebaceous cysts require no therapy. If they cause discomfort, simple excision is indicated.

Bartholin Cyst

Bartholin cysts cause swelling deep in the tissues of the posterior portion of the labium majus. The cysts vary in size from 1 cm in diameter to several centimeters. The larger masses tend to bulge into the vestibule of the vulva and the lower vagina. They may be asymptomatic or may produce local pressure symptoms and dyspareunia. Secondary infection occurs frequently, producing a large, painful abscess.

Bartholin abscesses with surrounding cellulitis should be treated with antibiotic therapy followed by incision and drainage. Symptomatic cysts and low-grade abscesses should be either marsupialized (in order to retain the mucus-secreting gland) or surgically excised.

Gartner Duct Cysts

These occur as small round or fusiform cystic swellings, often bilateral, beneath the mucosa of the anterolateral wall of the vagina. They arise from remnants of the vaginal portion of the mesonephric (wolffian) duct and contain a clear serous fluid. They are usually asymptomatic and discovered in the course of a routine physical examination. Occasionally they reach 5–6 cm in size.

Small asymptomatic cysts require no therapy. Larger masses should be surgically excised.

Endometriosis

Small, bluish, cystic elevations of the vaginal mucosa representing ectopic endometrial tissue are seen most often in the posterior fornix (as an extension of cul-de-sac endometriosis) or in episiotomy scars.

Vaginal endometrial implants are treated by local excision or fulguration. (See Endometriosis, p 875.)

CARCINOMA OF VULVA

Essentials of Diagnosis

- Patient in postmenopausal age group.
- Long history of vulval irritation with pruritus, local discomfort, and slightly bloody discharge.
- Early lesions may appear as chronic vulval dermatitis.
- Late lesions appear as a lump in the labium, a large cauliflower growth, or a hard ulcerative area in the vulva.
- Biopsy is necessary to make the diagnosis.

General Considerations

The vast majority (90–95%) of vulval malignancies are squamous cell carcinomas, and these tumors represent about 5% of all cancers of the female reproductive tract. Other types of vulval malignancy are Bartholin gland carcinoma (adenocarcinoma), Paget's disease of the vulva, basal cell carcinoma, malignant melanoma, and metastatic carcinoma from the cervix, endometrium, ovary, or elsewhere. Rarely, sarcomas are found arising primarily in the vulval soft tissues.

Squamous cell carcinoma is frequently associated with leukoplakia (50–70%), which, in the vulva, is considered a premalignant change only when asso-

Table 44–1. Clinical staging of carcinoma of the vulva.*

Stage 0	Carcinoma in situ, eg, Bowen's disease, noninvasive Paget's disease.
Stage I	Tumor confined to vulva—2 cm or less in larger diameter. Nodes not palpable, or are palpable in either groin, not enlarged, mobile (not clinically suggestive of cancer).
Stage II	Tumor confined to vulva—more than 2 cm in diameter. Nodes not palpable, or are palpable in either groin, not enlarged, mobile (not clinically suggestive of cancer).
Stage III	Tumor of any size with (1) adjacent spread to urethra and any or all of the vagina, the perineum, and the anus, and/or (2) nodes palpable in either or both groins (enlarged, firm, and mobile, not fixed but clinically suggestive of neoplasm).
Stage IV	Tumor of any size with (1) infiltration of the bladder mucosa, or rectal mucosa, or both, including the upper part of the urethral mucosa, and/or (2) fixed to the bone or other distant metastases.

*According to the Clinical Classification of the International Federation of Gynecology and Obstetrics.

ciated with epithelial dysplasia. A history of syphilis with or without associated granuloma inguinale or lymphogranuloma venereum is a frequent finding in vulval cancer.

The area most often involved is the labium majus. The clitoris is the second most often involved.

Metastasis to the regional lymph nodes (inguinal, femoral, iliac, and obturator) occurs in about 35–60% of invasive lesions. Because of bilateral lymph drainage, the nodes on the contralateral side may be involved (Fig 44–4). There is a high incidence of second primary malignancies in these patients, particularly in the cervix, endometrium, and breast. Cancer of the vulva should be classified and clinically staged according to the recommendations of the Cancer Committee of the International Federation of Gynecology and Obstetrics (Table 44–1).

Clinical Findings

In situ carcinoma (Bowen's disease) of the vulva usually is found in areas of "leukoplakia." The early lesion is a small, elevated, superficial papillary or ulcerated lesion with underlying subcutaneous induration. Late cancers present either as large, fungating, infected tumors or as shallow ulcers with indurated margins. The larger the primary lesion, the greater the chance of lymph node involvement; but palpatory evidence is misleading, as regional node enlargement may be related to secondary infection in these tumors. Furthermore, metastatic disease in the lymph nodes may not be palpable. There may be submucosal spread of the tumor cephalad to involve the vagina and urethra, or there may be involvement of the posterior vulva with invasion of the anus and rectum.

All suspicious lesions should be examined frequently by biopsy.

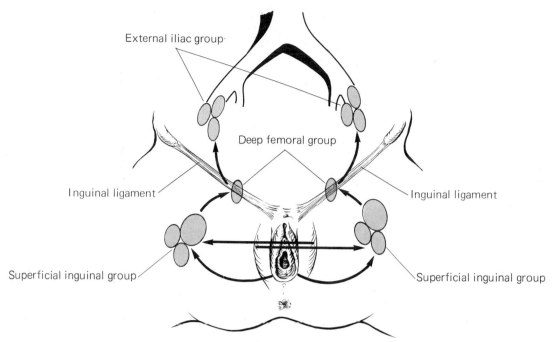

External iliac group

Deep femoral group

Inguinal ligament

Inguinal ligament

Superficial inguinal group

Superficial inguinal group

Figure 44—4. Diagram of lymphatic drainage of vulva, showing capacity for bilateral node involvement. (From Way S: Carcinoma of the vulva. In: *Progress in Gynecology.* Meigs JV, Sturgis SS [editors]. Vol 3. Grune & Stratton, 1957.)

Differential Diagnosis

Chronic hypertrophic and atrophic skin conditions may or may not be associated with vulval malignancy. Multiple biopsies are necessary to establish the correct diagnosis. Granulomatous venereal lesions of the vulva may be clinically suspicious, and biopsy of the involved area is mandatory. The Frei and complement fixation tests may be helpful, but it must be remembered that granulomatous disease and cancer of the vulva may occur simultaneously.

Prevention

Simple vulvectomy in cases of lesions which show epithelial dysplasia will prevent the subsequent development of invasive carcinoma. Likewise, the discovery and removal (by simple vulvectomy) of intraepithelial carcinoma of the vulva is effective prophylaxis for the invasive form of the disease. Toluidine blue in 1% solution applied to the vulval skin and mucosa and then decolorized with 1% acetic acid solution has been effective in determining the extent of the neoplastic epithelial change.

Treatment

Radical vulvectomy with bilateral superficial and deep groin dissection is the most widely accepted form of therapy. Radiation therapy is used in the inoperable lesions.

Prognosis

Adequate surgery is effective in a high percentage of patients, even when there is evidence of spread to the inguinal and femoral nodes. Eighty-six percent

5-year cure rates are reported when the nodes are not involved, and a 50% salvage rate is possible in the presence of lymph node involvement if the surgical procedure has been adequate.

Hunter DJS: Carcinoma of the vulva: A review of 361 patients. Gynecol Oncol 3:117, 1975.
Kaplan AL, Kaufman RH: Management of advanced carcinoma of the vulva. Gynecol Oncol 3:220, 1975.
Krupp PJ & others: Prognostic parameters and clinical staging criteria in epidermoid carcinoma of the vulva. Obstet Gynecol 46:84, 1975.
Parker RT & others: Operative management of early invasive epidermoid carcinoma of vulva. Am J Obstet Gynecol 123:349, 1975.

CARCINOMA OF THE VAGINA

Carcinoma in situ of the vagina occurs either as a direct extension of the process from the portio vaginalis of the cervix or as a separate area in a "neoplastic field." It should be suspected whenever carcinoma in situ or invasive carcinoma of the vulva or cervix is present, and it may appear in the vagina many months or years after successful treatment of either of these 2 conditions. Carcinoma in situ of the vagina is most often diagnosed by cytologic examination and by biopsying Schiller-positive areas* of the vagina.

*After application of Lugol's solution, the area of carcinoma does not take up the iodine stain.

Treatment is by local excision of involved areas when they are few and small. Extensive involvement of the vaginal mucosa may require vaginectomy with complete colpocleisis in the elderly, sexually inactive patient or with skin graft construction of an artificial vagina in the patient who wishes to retain coital function.

Invasive squamous cell carcinoma of the vagina, arising primarily from the vagina, is an unusual lesion, most cancers of the vagina being extensions from an epidermoid carcinoma of the cervix. The lesion is most often ulcerative, with a cauliflower configuration being less common. There is a firm induration surrounding the ulcerative lesion, and these are easily palpated, whereas a small, soft, papillary lesion may be missed. The upper third of the vagina is the site in about 75% of patients. In many cases the only symptom is a bloody vaginal discharge, and the diagnosis is made by biopsy.

Treatment is by radiation therapy or radical surgery. Unfortunately, these tumors grow rapidly and insidiously, and in over 50% of patients they have penetrated the vaginal wall at the time of the initial examination. Involvement of the bladder and rectum is common. As a result, the overall 5-year survival figures are in the range of 20–30%.

Recently, adenocarcinoma of the vagina arising in teen-age girls has been described, apparently arising in areas of vaginal adenosis (probably müllerian duct remnants). There appears to be a relationship between the appearance of this tumor in these young patients and the administration of diethylstilbestrol to their mothers during the fetal life of the patient.

The International Classification of Carcinoma of the Vagina is outlined in Table 44–2.

Metastatic carcinoma of the vagina is much more common than primary carcinoma, the most frequent sources being the cervix, vulva, bladder, urethra, rectum, endometrium, and ovary.

Rare primary tumors of the vagina are sarcoma (mixed mesodermal tumors, including sarcoma botryoides of infants, fibrosarcoma, leiomyosarcoma, hemangiosarcoma), adenocarcinoma arising from mesonephric (Gartner's) duct or müllerian duct remnants, embryonal carcinoma, and malignant melanoma. Radical surgical removal offers the best hope of cure for the majority of these neoplasms.

Table 44–2. Clinical staging of carcinoma of the vagina.*

Stage 0	Carcinoma in situ.
Stage I	Carcinoma is confined to the vaginal wall.
Stage II	Carcinoma involves the subvaginal tissue but not the pelvic wall.
Stage III	Carcinoma extends to the pelvic wall.
Stage IV	Carcinoma extends beyond the true pelvis or involves the mucosa of the bladder or rectum (biopsy proof is required).

*According to the Clinical Classification of the International Federation of Gynecology and Obstetrics.

Herbst AL & others: The significance of adenosis and clear-cell adenocarcinoma of the genital tract in young females. J Reprod Med 15:5, 1975.

Hill EC: Clear cell carcinoma of cervix and vagina in young women: Report of six cases with association of maternal stilbestrol therapy and adenosis of vagina. Am J Obstet Gynecol 116:470, 1973.

Kottmeier HL (editor): *Annual Report on the Results of Treatment in Carcinoma of the Uterus, Vagina and Ovary.* Vol 15. International Federation of Gynecology and Obstetrics (Stockholm), 1973.

Morrow CP, Townsend DE: Management of adenosis and clear-cell adenocarcinoma of vagina and cervix. J Reprod Med 15:25, 1975.

Stafl A: Clinical detection of vaginal adenosis and clear-cell adenocarcinoma. J Reprod Med 15:20, 1975.

Weiss K: Epidemiology of vaginal adenocarcinoma and adenosis: Current status. J Am Med Wom Assoc 30:59, 1975.

TUMORS OF THE FALLOPIAN TUBE (ADENOCARCINOMA)

Benign tumors of the fallopian tubes are very rare. Primary carcinoma of the tube is the most common malignant lesion, but it is rarely encountered, comprising less than 1% of female reproductive cancers.

Postmenopausal vaginal bleeding is the usual presenting complaint. There may be a history of intermittent, profuse, serous, yellow or bloody vaginal discharge (hydrops tubae profluens). An adnexal mass may or may not be palpable.

The diagnosis of primary carcinoma of the fallopian tube is rarely made preoperatively. Total abdominal hysterectomy and bilateral salpingo-oophorectomy is the treatment of choice in operable lesions. Tumors which are inoperable yet confined to the pelvic structures should receive radiation therapy—followed by operation if there is a favorable response as judged by increased mobility and diminution in tumor size. Radical hysterectomy and bilateral pelvic lymph node dissection have been advocated as possibly a more curative procedure than simple hysterectomy and bilateral salpingo-oophorectomy.

If the disease is confined to the tube, the prognosis is quite good. Unfortunately, most of these tumors are advanced at the time of discovery, and the overall 5-year cure rate is in the range of 10–20%.

The early use of the laparoscope or the CT scanner may be of aid in the earlier diagnosis of this disease and should be considered in any postmenopausal woman with a vague adnexal mass, particularly if accompanied by a watery discharge or postmenopausal bleeding.

Boutselis JG, Thompson JN: Clinical aspects of primary carcinoma of the fallopian tube. Am J Obstet Gynecol 111:98, 1971.

Kinzel GE: Primary carcinoma of the fallopian tube. Am J Obstet Gynecol 125:816, 1976.

CANCER OF THE CERVIX

Essentials of Diagnosis

- May be asymptomatic.
- Vaginal discharge.
- Intermenstrual bleeding.
- Suspicious or positive cytologic examination.
- Biopsy diagnosis is essential.

General Considerations

Carcinoma of the cervix is the most common cancer in the female reproductive tract and second only to carcinoma of the breast as the most frequent malignancy in women.

Early sexual activity, promiscuity, parity, and chronic inflammation are predisposing factors. Herpesvirus type 2 has been found to be frequently associated with cervical cancer. However, there is no proof of an etiologic relationship. Dysplasia of the cervical epithelium is probably a precursor.

The majority of cervical cancers are squamous cell (95%); the remainder consist of adenocarcinomas, mixed carcinomas (adenosquamous), and rare sarcomas (mixed mesodermal tumors, lymphosarcomas).

The earliest squamous cell carcinoma is confined to the epithelial layers (carcinoma in situ, intraepithelial carcinoma, preinvasive carcinoma), and it is thought that the disease remains confined to the mucous membrane for several years before invading the subjacent stroma. Carcinoma in situ occurs most frequently during the decade between 30 and 40 years of age, whereas invasive carcinoma is encountered most often in women between 40 and 50.

Following penetration of the basement membrane and involvement of the cervical stroma, the disease spreads by direct contiguity to the vagina and the adjacent parametrium, and via the lymphatic channels (which are abundant in this area) to the regional lymph nodes of the pelvis (iliac and obturator) and to the periaortic lymph nodes.

Estimating the extent of the malignant process is extremely important in determining the mode of therapy and in estimating the prognosis. This is judged clinically and is defined according to the Clinical Classification of the International Federation of Gynecology and Obstetrics as shown in Table 44–3.

It is known from an examination of surgical specimens that the probability of lymph node metastasis increases according to the local extent of the disease, being approximately 15% in stage I, 30% in stage II, and 45% in stage III. About 80% of patients with stage IV cancer have lymph node involvement.

Clinical Findings

A. Carcinoma in Situ: Carcinoma in situ does not cause symptoms. However, the majority of patients with this condition have an area of redness (erythroplakia) on the portio vaginalis of the cervix which is indistinguishable from chronic cervicitis. In fact, the 2

Table 44–3. Clinical staging of carcinoma of the cervix.*

Stage 0	Carcinoma in situ, intraepithelial carcinoma.
Stage I	Carcinoma strictly confined to the cervix (extension to the corpus should be disregarded).
IA	Microinvasive carcinoma (early stromal invasion).
IB	All other cases of stage I. (Occult carcinoma should be marked "occ.")
Stage II	Carcinoma extends beyond the cervix but has not extended onto the pelvic wall. The carcinoma involves the vagina but not the lower third.
IIA	No obvious parametrial involvement.
IIB	Obvious parametrial involvement.
Stage III	Carcinoma has extended onto the pelvic wall. On rectal examination, there is no cancer-free space between the tumor and the pelvic wall. The tumor involves the lower third of the vagina. All cases with hydronephrosis or nonfunctioning kidney.
IIIA	No extension onto the pelvic wall. (Vaginal involvement including the lower third.)
IIIB	Extension onto the pelvic wall and/or hydronephrosis or nonfunctioning kidney.
Stage IV	Carcinoma has extended beyond the true pelvis or clinically involving the mucosa of the bladder or rectum. Do not allow a case of bullous edema as such to be allotted to stage IV.
IVA	Spread of growth to adjacent organs.
IVB	Spread of growth to distant organs.

*According to the Clinical Classification of the International Federation of Gynecology and Obstetrics.

conditions often coexist. Fifteen to 20% of patients with carcinoma in situ have no visible lesion. Cytologic examination (Papanicolaou) of a representative specimen collected from the squamocolumnar junction (transformation zone) of the cervix will demonstrate severely dysplastic or frankly malignant cells in 95% of women with this stage of disease.

The Schiller test, using Lugol's solution (see p 885, *note*), is often helpful in demonstrating areas of abnormal epithelium, even in cervixes which appear normal on gross inspection, because of the lack of glycogen in these cells and their failure to take up the stain. The test is not specific for neoplasm since areas of ectopy, cervicitis, atrophy, and dysplasia are also iodine-negative. A sharply demarcated border of nonstaining is more suggestive of epithelial neoplasia.

Colposcopic examination of the cervix has been useful in detecting areas of dysplasia and carcinoma in situ. This method is based primarily upon changes which occur in the capillary vascular pattern of the cervix associated with epithelial proliferation.

Punch biopsy is required in all cases in which there is a visible area of redness or an iodine-negative area. A knife cone biopsy and curettage of the endometrial cavity should be done in the following circumstances:

1. No visible lesion; no iodine-negative zone; cytologic examination indicates dysplasia or malignant cells.

2. Punch biopsies of a visible lesion (erythroplakia) or an iodine-negative zone demonstrate dysplasia or carcinoma in situ.

3. Punch biopsies and cytologic examination do not agree; eg, biopsy demonstrates chronic cervicitis, cytology indicates dysplasia or carcinoma.

B. Invasive Carcinoma: Invasive carcinoma of the cervix usually produces symptoms. Intermenstrual or postcoital bleeding is often the first symptom. A watery vaginal discharge, occasionally blood-streaked, may be the only symptom. Pain is a manifestation of far-advanced disease. In most patients with invasive cancer, inspection of the cervix reveals an ulcerated or papillary lesion of the cervix which bleeds on contact. The cytologic examination almost always demonstrates exfoliated malignant cells, and biopsy reveals the invasive nature of the lesion. An occasional endocervical, endophytic lesion will produce enlargement of the cervix without becoming evident on the portio vaginalis.

Differential Diagnosis

Chronic cervicitis can be distinguished from cancer of the cervix only by multiple negative cytologic and biopsy examinations. Polyps of the cervix should be examined by a pathologist to exclude malignant change. It may be very difficult to distinguish severe dysplasia of the cervical epithelium from carcinoma in situ. These now are considered different stages of the same basic process. One pathologist's dysplasia will be another's carcinoma in situ, and more rigid pathologic criteria are needed in order to differentiate the 2 conditions. Lesser degrees of dysplasia usually cause no diagnostic problem.

Complications

The complications are those due to the spread of the disease or secondary to treatment. Obstruction of the ureter, resulting in hydroureter, hydronephrosis, and uremia, occurs with advancing disease. Bilateral obstruction of the ureters leads to failure of kidney function and death.

Involvement of the iliac and obturator lymph nodes may lead to lymphatic obstruction with lymphedema of the lower extremity.

The lumbosacral plexus may become infiltrated by tumor, causing pain in the low back, hip, and leg.

Vesicovaginal and rectovaginal fistulas occur as a result of tumor involvement of these structures or as complications of radiation therapy. A cloaca may result from massive slough of necrotic tumor tissue. Widespread metastases to lung, liver, brain, and bone may occur.

Complications of radiation therapy such as cystitis, colitis, and proctitis are not uncommon but are usually only transitory problems in modern treatment centers. Castration is an unavoidable complication of radiation therapy. Severe radiation damage to the bladder and rectum may result in hemorrhage, fistulas, and strictures. Radiation necrosis of the cervix and diffuse radiation pelvic fibrosis are rare complications.

The complications of surgery are hemorrhage, infection, thromboembolism, and fistula (ureterovaginal, vesicovaginal, rectovaginal) formation.

Prevention

Invasive cancer of the cervix can be prevented by detecting and properly treating chronic cervicitis, cervical dysplasia, and carcinoma in situ of the cervix. Annual cytologic and pelvic examinations with appropriate therapy have proved to be effective in the prevention of this disease.

Treatment

The proper treatment of cervical cancer requires individualization of therapy for each patient according to the clinical circumstances. Cervical epithelial dysplasia is destroyed by cauterization or cryosurgery.

A. Carcinoma in Situ: Carcinoma in situ is most often treated by total hysterectomy with an adequate margin of normal adjacent vaginal mucosa. When the lesion is confined to the cervix and can be removed in its entirety, conization of the cervix may be considered definitive therapy in a young woman who desires to retain her childbearing potential. Close cytologic follow-up is necessary in order to ensure that this form of therapy has, indeed, been adequate.

B. Invasive Carcinoma: In general, invasive carcinoma is best treated by irradiation under the cooperative management of a radiotherapist and a gynecologist experienced in the treatment of cancer. Both internal (radium) and external sources (x-ray, cobaltous chloride Co 60, betatron, linear accelerator) should be employed. Radical pelvic surgery (radical hysterectomy, exenteration procedures) may be indicated in certain cases of invasive carcinoma complicating pregnancy, mixed adenosquamous carcinomas, or recurrent or persistent cancer following radiation therapy.

Prognosis

The earlier the disease is treated, the better the prognosis. Carcinoma in situ is almost 100% curable. The prevalence of invasive carcinoma of the cervix is decreasing partly as a result of detection and treatment in the intraepithelial stage of the disease. The best results in stage I cancer of the cervix approach a 90% 5-year survival rate. For stage II, the figure drops to 60%; for stage III, to 30%; and for stage IV, to less than 10%.

Dickinson LE: Control of cancer of the uterine cervix by cytologic screening. Gynecol Oncol 3:1, 1975.

Garcia RL & others: Evaluation of cone biopsy in the management of carcinoma in situ of the cervix. Gynecol Oncol 3:39, 1975.

Gray LA, Christopherson WM: The treatment of cervical dysplasias. Gynecol Oncol 3:149, 1975.

Hilgers RD: Carcinoma of the cervix: Clinical and surgical staging. Minn Med 58:733, 1975.

Nelson JH & others: Detection, diagnostic evaluation and treatment of dysplasia and early carcinoma of the cervix. CA 25:134, 1975.

Newton M: Radical hysterectomy or radiotherapy for stage-1 cervical cancer: Prospective comparison with 5-year and 10-year follow-up. Am J Obstet Gynecol 123:535, 1975.

Piver MS: Invasive carcinoma of uterine cervix: Diagnostic and therapeutic changes. NY State J Med 75:2510, 1975.

Symmonds RE & others: Exenterative operations: Experience with 198 patients. Am J Obstet Gynecol 121:907, 1975.

Welander CE & others: Factors affecting survival in stage I and stage II carcinoma of the cervix. Obstet Gynecol 46:439, 1975.

LEIOMYOMAS OF THE UTERUS

Essentials of Diagnosis

- Often asymptomatic.
- Palpable, irregular enlargements of the corpus uteri.
- Abnormal uterine bleeding (hypermenorrhea or intermenstrual bleeding).
- Vague pelvic discomfort or pressure on neighboring pelvic organs (urinary frequency, constipation).
- Enlargement of uterine cavity (sounding).
- X-rays may demonstrate calcifications within myomas.
- Laparoscopy (peritoneoscopy) may be useful in difficult diagnostic cases.

General Considerations

Leiomyomas of the uterus are found in approximately 20% of all white women and 50% of black women. The cause is not known. Most are asymptomatic. They probably arise from the smooth muscle of the myometrium, and they grow in response to the stimulus of estrogen as evidenced by an increased growth rate during pregnancy and a cessation of growth with the menopause. They are usually multiple and, depending upon the direction of growth, may remain within the myometrium (intramural), distend the external surface of the uterus (subserous), or come to lie beneath the endometrium (submucous). Other types of myomas are intraligamentous (between the leaves of the broad ligament), parasitic (detached from the uterus and deriving blood supply from other abdominal organs), and cervical. Myomas may vary in size from tiny "seedlings" to massive tumors filling the entire abdomen and pelvis.

On cut section, leiomyomas are well circumscribed, solid tumors with a pseudocapsule of compressed myometrium and a pearly-gray whorled appearance.

Leiomyomas are subject to various degenerative changes, probably as a result of interference with the blood supply to various segments of the tumor: hyaline and cystic degeneration, calcification, carneous degeneration (during pregnancy), and, rarely, malignant change (sarcoma).

Clinical Findings

A. Symptoms and Signs: The majority of leiomyomas produce no symptoms and are discovered in the course of a routine pelvic examination. Symptoms, when they occur, are those of an enlarging tumor, causing abdominal distention, discomfort, urinary frequency, constipation, and hypermenorrhea. Submucous myomas may cause intermenstrual bleeding, at times alarmingly profuse. They may also become pedunculated and protrude through the cervix.

Palpation of the uterus reveals an irregularly enlarged structure which, if large enough, may be felt on abdominal examination. They are usually nontender, but they may become painful in the event of carneous degeneration or torsion of the pedicle of a pedunculated subserous myoma.

A rapidly growing myoma suggests the possibility of sarcomatous change within the tumor (leiomyosarcoma).

B. Laboratory Findings: Anemia may result from acute or chronic blood loss.

C. X-Ray Findings: X-rays may demonstrate the typical calcifications. Hysterography or exploration of the uterine cavity with a curet will define submucous tumors.

Differential Diagnosis

Enlargement of the uterus by a large, soft myoma (cystic degeneration) may mimic the pregnant uterus or vice versa. A history of amenorrhea suggests pregnancy, as does the appearance of any of the presumptive signs of pregnancy such as secondary breast changes, Montgomery follicles, and a positive Chadwick or Hegar sign. A pregnancy test should be done in all suspected cases. Pregnancy may occur in a myomatous uterus.

Solid ovarian tumors and pedunculated subserous myomas pose a problem in differential diagnosis. In ovarian neoplasm there is a distinct separation between the adnexal mass and the uterus. If examination (under anesthesia if necessary) does not provide sufficient information to allow differentiation, laparoscopy or culdoscopy may be helpful.

Complications

Hemorrhage from a submucous myoma or prolonged hypermenorrhea often results in secondary iron deficiency anemia. Rapid growth of myomas and degenerative changes may occur in women taking oral contraceptives. Torsion of the pedicle of a pedunculated subserous myoma may result in necrosis and present the picture of an acute abdominal emergency.

Infertility may be secondary to myomas. Abortion, premature labor, prolonged labor, and postpartum hemorrhage due to uterine atony are encountered in pregnancy complicated by myomas. These tumors infrequently obstruct the birth canal, producing a soft tissue dystocia.

Treatment

Small, asymptomatic myomas require no therapy.

Examination every 6 months to observe the rate of growth is recommended. Myomectomy should be done in the young woman who desires preservation of child-bearing function should symptoms or infertility require treatment. Hysterectomy is the treatment of choice in most patients with symptoms or in the asymptomatic woman who harbors a rapidly growing myoma. Myomectomy usually requires laparotomy and, in terms of postoperative morbidity, is a more hazardous operation than hysterectomy.

Prognosis

Myomectomy may not cure the condition, and the risk of recurrence should be accepted by the patient before proceeding with the operation. Hysterectomy is curative.

Miller NF, Ludvici PP: On the origin and development of uterine fibroids. Am J Obstet Gynecol 70:720, 1955.

Parks J, Barter RH: The myomatous uterus complicated by pregnancy. Am J Obstet Gynecol 63:260, 1952.

Wilson JR: Premenopausal pelvic neoplasms. Hosp Med 3:15, Aug 1967.

ENDOMETRIAL CARCINOMA

Essentials of Diagnosis

- Postmenopausal bleeding.
- Uterus frequently not enlarged.
- Uterine enlargement and pain are signs of advanced disease.
- Vaginal cytology fails to detect a high percentage of cases.
- Endometrial biopsy or curettage is required to confirm the diagnosis.

General Considerations

Endometrial carcinoma is primarily a disease of postmenopausal women, with a peak incidence in the decade from 55–65 years of age. It also occurs in pre-menopausal women, particularly those with prolonged anovulation. Evidence suggests that prolonged unopposed (by progesterone) estrogen stimulation of the endometrium may be a predisposing factor in the development of endometrial carcinoma. The coincidence of obesity, hypertension, and diabetes in many patients with this disease is indicative of an underlying endocrine disorder. The peripheral conversion of androstenedione to estrone in relatively large amounts has been implicated as a cause of this disease. Although cancer of the endometrium has been produced in laboratory animals through the continuous administration of estrogen, there is no conclusive evidence that estrogens cause cancer in women.

Benign cystic hyperplasia progressing to adenomatous hyperplasia and then adenomatous hyperplasia with anaplasia and, finally, neoplasia has been demonstrated as a preliminary sequence in a number of patients with endometrial carcinoma.

Carcinoma of the endometrium probably has an in situ (intraepithelial) first stage, followed by invasion of the surrounding endometrial stroma before it involves the underlying myometrium. Fortunately, deep myometrial penetration, extension beyond the corpus of the uterus, lymph node involvement, and distant metastases occur relatively late in the disease, so that most lesions are detected early. This is especially true if the lesion is well differentiated histologically. Anaplastic tumors, on the other hand, are much more aggressive.

The International Classification (clinical staging) of endometrial cancer is shown in the accompanying table (Table 44–4).

Clinical Findings

Postmenopausal bleeding is the primary symptom and should be considered to be caused by malignancy until proved otherwise. About 40% of women with vaginal bleeding following the menopause will have reproductive tract cancer, and in the vast majority of these cases the malignancy is endometrial. Cervical stenosis with pyometra or hematometra is highly suggestive of endometrial carcinoma. Pain is not a common symptom, but there may be mild uterine cramping, particularly if there is any degree of stenosis of the cervix. Vaginal cytology is positive in 40–80% of cases. Endometrial biopsy will almost always detect an endometrial carcinoma, as will cytologic sampling of the endometrial cavity also. Curettage, first of the endocervix and then of the endometrial cavity, with careful examination under anesthesia is considered the most definitive method of diagnosing and clinically staging the disease. Myometrial involvement is suspected if the corpus is enlarged.

Table 44–4. Clinical staging of endometrial carcinoma.*

Stage 0	Carcinoma in situ. Histologic findings suggestive of malignancy.
Stage I	Carcinoma is confined to the corpus.
IA	The length of the uterine cavity is 8 cm or less.
IB	The length of the uterine cavity is more than 8 cm.
	Stage I cases should be subgrouped with regard to the histologic type of adenocarcinoma as follows:
	G1 Highly differentiated adenomatous carcinoma.
	G2 Differentiated adenomatous carcinoma with partly solid areas.
	G3 Predominantly solid or entirely undifferentiated carcinoma.
Stage II	The carcinoma has involved the corpus and the cervix.
Stage III	The carcinoma has extended outside of the uterus but not outside of the true pelvis.
Stage IV	The carcinoma has extended outside the true pelvis or has obviously involved the mucosa of the bladder or rectum. A bullous edema as such does not permit a case to be allotted to stage IV.

*According to the Clinical Classification of the International Federation of Gynecology and Obstetrics.

Differential Diagnosis

Other causes of postmenopausal and intermenstrual bleeding such as vaginitis, cervicitis, polyps, cervical cancer, and hormonal therapy must be considered. (See section on menstrual disorders, above.)

Complications

Endometrial carcinoma which is histologically poorly differentiated may disseminate relatively early in the course of the disease. Metastatic spread to the vagina, regional pelvic and para-aortic lymph nodes, ovaries, lungs, liver, brain, and bone may occur.

The most frequent site of recurrence following treatment for endometrial carcinoma is the vaginal vault.

Prevention

There is presumptive evidence that cyclic progesterone therapy will reduce the possibility of endometrial carcinoma in the anovulatory patient. Detection and adequate therapy of the precursors of the disease (polyps, hyperplasia, and carcinoma in situ of the endometrium) will prevent the subsequent development of endometrial carcinoma.

Treatment

Total hysterectomy and bilateral salpingo-oophorectomy is recommended in the patient with a well-differentiated tumor in a small uterus without cervical involvement.

In less well differentiated tumors or if the disease extends beyond the endometrium, preoperative irradiation therapy, either with intrauterine and intravaginal radium or by full pelvic external radiation, should be given prior to hysterectomy. Radical hysterectomy with bilateral pelvic lymph node dissection can be used in carefully selected patients who are in good general condition in stage II carcinomas.

The application of multiple small dose radium capsules (Heyman packing technic) to the endometrial cavity, supplemented by intravaginal radium and full pelvis external therapy, is the treatment of choice in patients who are considered poor surgical risks.

Disseminated endometrial carcinoma is treated with large dose progestin therapy (hydroxyprogesterone caproate or medroxyprogesterone) which produces satisfactory remission of the metastatic disease in about 35% of cases. Subjective improvement is noted in the majority of patients so treated.

Prognosis

Five-year survival rates in the range of 70–90% are recorded in stage I disease. This drops to 60% in stage II.

Barber HRK & others: Cancer of the endometrium. RI Med J 58:259, 1975.

Brown R: Clinical features associated with endometrial carcinoma. J Obstet Gynaecol Br Commonw 81:933, 1974.

Donovan JF: Nonhormonal chemotherapy of endometrial adenocarcinoma: A review. Cancer 34:1587, 1974.

Fletcher G: Radiation treatment of carcinoma of the endometrium. RI Med J 58:267, 1975.

Gravlee LC Jr: An office procedure for early detection of endometrial carcinoma. Am Fam Physician 10:88, Dec 1974.

Henriksen E: Lymphatic dissemination in endometrial carcinoma: Study of 188 necropsies. Am J Obstet Gynecol 123:570, 1975.

Kelley RM: Medical management of carcinoma of the endometrium. RI Med J 58:271, 1975.

SARCOMAS OF THE UTERUS

Uterine sarcomas are relatively rare. They may arise in preexisting leiomyomas, from the myometrium itself, or from the endometrial stroma. Mixed tumors (carcinosarcoma, mixed mesodermal tumors) containing both epithelial and connective tissue malignant cells are also encountered.

Sarcomas of the uterus metastasize via the blood stream and lymphatics and spread by contiguity. The lungs are a frequent site of metastatic disease.

In patients in whom the tumor is confined to the pelvic organs, treatment consists of total hysterectomy and bilateral salpingo-oophorectomy.

The outlook for patients with uterine sarcoma is variable. Sarcomas arising in preexisting myomas carry a relatively good prognosis, whereas those of mixed mesodermal origin are almost invariably fatal within 2 years.

Radiation therapy and chemotherapy have not been successful in treating uterine sarcomas. Mixed mesodermal tumors with predominantly adenocarcinomatous elements may respond to palliation with large doses of progestins.

Belgrad R & others: Uterine sarcoma. Radiology 114:181, 1975.

Bolitho O: Primary malignant tumours of the body of the uterus. Med J Aust 1:94, 1975.

Gilbert HA & others: The value of radiation therapy of uterine sarcoma. Obstet Gynecol 45:84, 1975.

Norris HJ, Parmley T: Mesenchymal tumors of uterus. Cancer 36:2164, 1975.

OVARIAN TUMORS

Essentials of Diagnosis

- Adnexal mass palpated during pelvic examination.
- Rupture of a cyst or a twisted pedicle may produce symptoms of an acute abdominal emergency.
- Abdominal distention and symptoms of pressure on surrounding organs are manifestations of a large tumor or of ascites due to peritoneal seeding.

- Plain films of the abdomen and pelvic pneumography often are helpful. Because the ovaries are a frequent metastatic site for bowel malignancy, x-ray studies of the small and large intestine are indicated when one suspects ovarian malignancy.
- Peritoneoscopy (laparoscopy or culdoscopy) is often useful.
- Paracentesis with cytologic examination of ascitic fluid.
- Chest x-ray will demonstrate pulmonary disease and pleural fluid.
- Culdocentesis with cytologic examination of a small amount of peritoneal fluid (which is present under normal circumstances) may detect very early lesions.

General Considerations

Because of their complex embryologic and histogenetic development, the ovaries are a source of a greater variety of tumors, both benign and malignant, than any other organ in the body. Ovarian tumors may be frankly benign, frankly malignant, or somewhere in between; they may be solid or cystic, or there may be mixed types; and they may be functional (producing sex steroids) or nonfunctional. Of the greatest clinical significance is the fact that, whether benign or malignant, they are often clinically silent until late in the course of their development.

Benign cysts of the ovary may be functional (follicle or corpus luteum cysts) or proliferative (dermoid, serous, and mucinous cystadenomas). The more frequent solid benign tumors are fibroma-thecomas, fibroadenomas, and the Brenner tumors. Endometriosis is a frequent cause of cystic enlargement of the ovary (see section on endometriosis, above).

The common malignant tumors are serous and mucinous cystadenocarcinoma, endometrioid carcinoma, and undifferentiated solid adenocarcinoma. Less common are the hormone-producing neoplasms: granulosa-theca cell tumors, arrhenoblastomas, and adrenal cell rest tumors. These have variable degrees of malignancy. Rarely encountered are tumors of germ cell origin, ranging from the dysgerminoma, the homologue of the testicular seminoma, to the highly malignant teratocarcinoma. Metastatic carcinoma from the gastrointestinal tract (Krukenberg's tumor), breast, pancreas, and kidney must always be considered as a possible diagnosis whenever there is bilateral malignant disease of the ovaries.

Follicle cysts result from failure of a number of developing ovarian follicles to undergo atresia (regression) during the second half of the menstrual cycle. Usually they appear as multiple cystic structures filled with clear serous fluid, but they may be single. Rarely do they cause the ovary to become larger than 6–7 cm in diameter.

Corpus luteum cysts, likewise, do not become very large; they are single cysts, resulting from failure of the corpus luteum to regress, and they often contain an amber or brown serous fluid or they may be filled with blood.

Dermoid cysts (benign cystic teratomas) are common, comprising about 20% of all ovarian tumors in mature women. Occasionally they are bilateral (8–15%). They may vary from a few millimeters to more than 20 cm in diameter, and the external appearance is one of a smooth, glistening, thick-walled, pearly-gray cyst. When opened, they are found to contain a thick sebaceous material and hair. Occasionally, bone structures and teeth are found. In fact, almost any tissue may be found on microscopic examination. A rare but interesting type is the benign cystic teratoma composed largely of thyroid tissue (struma ovarii) which, if functional, may give rise to hyperthyroidism. Current thinking regarding the histogenesis of these tumors is that they develop from an auto-fertilization of haploid germ cells. Malignant change is rarely encountered in dermoid cysts.

Serous, endometrioid, and mucinous cystic tumors (cystomas, cystadenomas, cystadenocarcinomas) arise from the surface epithelium of the ovary, derived from the primitive coelomic epithelium. Approximately 85–90% of ovarian cancers arise from these cells, and the tumor type depends on the direction of cellular differentiation. The serous variety is the most common (20% of benign tumors and 40% of malignant tumors). They may become very large—particularly those of the mucinous type—and may fill and distend the entire abdomen. They may be unilocular or multilocular. If they contain small papillary excrescences, the likelihood of malignancy is greater. Although mucinous tumors of a benign type are about as frequent as the serous variety, malignant mucinous tumors are less common (10% of ovarian cancers). Endometrioid carcinomas are the second most frequent variety (24% of ovarian cancers).

Granulosa-theca cell tumors and **arrhenoblastomas** arise from the ovarian stroma. They frequently retain the ability to secrete sex hormones (estrogen, androgen), producing the systemic effects associated with these steroids—feminization or masculinization, as the case may be. The granulosa-theca cell tumors are the most frequent of the hormonally active tumors, constituting about 4–6% of ovarian malignancies. About two-thirds are benign in their clinical behavior. Arrhenoblastomas are rare and usually manifest themselves first by producing defeminization (amenorrhea, atrophy of the breasts) and then masculinization (deepening of the voice, hirsutism, clitoral hypertrophy). Like granulosa-theca cell tumors, the majority are benign, the reported incidence of malignancy being about 20%.

The clinical staging of ovarian malignancy recommended by the International Federation of Gynecology and Obstetrics is shown in Table 44–5.

Clinical Findings

Cystic enlargements of one or both ovaries are a frequent finding on routine pelvic examination of young women in the reproductive age group. In gen-

Table 44—5. Clinical staging of ovarian tumors.*

Stage I	Growth limited to the ovaries.
IA	Growth limited to one ovary; no ascites.
	(i) No tumor on external surface; capsule intact.
	(ii) Tumor present on external surface and/or capsule ruptured.
IB	Growth limited to both ovaries; no ascites.
	(i) No tumor on external surface; capsule intact.
	(ii) Tumor present on external surface and/or capsule(s) ruptured.
IC	Tumor either stage IA or stage IB, but with ascites† present or positive peritoneal washings.
Stage II	Growth involving one or both ovaries with pelvic extension.
IIA	Extension and/or metastases to the uterus and/or tubes.
IIB	Extension to other pelvic tissues.
IIC	Tumor either stage IIA or stage IIB, but with ascites† present or positive peritoneal washings.
Stage III	Growth involving one or both ovaries with intraperitoneal metastases outside the pelvis and/or positive retroperitoneal nodes.
	Tumor limited to the true pelvis with histologically proved malignant extension to small bowel or omentum.
Stage IV	Growth involving one or both ovaries with distant metastases. If pleural effusion is present, there must be positive cytology to allot a case to stage IV. Parenchymal liver metastases equal stage IV.
Special category	Unexplored cases which are thought to be ovarian carcinoma.

*According to the Clinical Classification of the International Federation of Gynecology and Obstetrics.
†Ascites is peritoneal effusion which in the opinion of the surgeon is pathologic and/or clearly exceeds normal amounts.

eral, these are nonneoplastic and cause no symptoms. They rarely become larger than 8 cm in diameter and usually regress without treatment. Torsion of the pedicle with consequent strangulation may occur, producing abdominal pain of sudden onset, nausea and vomiting, a tender abdominopelvic mass, peritoneal irritation, slight fever, and moderate leukocytosis. Dermoid cysts are particularly apt to twist in this fashion. Because they are usually filled with sebaceous material and may contain tooth structures, these may be diagnosed by x-ray.

Any enlargement of the ovary in women of menopausal or postmenopausal age should be regarded as malignant until proved otherwise. Nodularity of an ovarian tumor (palpated on pelvic examination) is presumptive evidence of malignancy, as is associated ascites also. It is often impossible to determine the benign or malignant nature of an ovarian tumor until laparotomy. Papillarity of the external surface, adherence to surrounding structures, and peritoneal implants are signs of malignancy. Psammoma bodies seen on x-ray may arouse suspicion of a papillary process. If there is any doubt at the time of surgery, the tumor should be removed without spilling its contents into the peritoneal cavity and submitted to a pathologist in the operating room for gross examination and frozen section microscopic analysis of any suspicious areas. These cystic enlargements may represent simple cysts, serous or mucinous cystadenomas, or cystadenocarcinomas with serous, mucinous, endometrioid, or mesonephric duct epithelium.

Solid enlargements of the ovary may be benign. Fibroma-thecoma tumors of the ovary comprise about 5% of benign ovarian neoplasms. They are smooth, rounded, firm, mobile masses, usually unilateral and relatively small. An infrequent accompaniment of these solid, benign ovarian tumors is the development of ascites and hydrothorax (Meigs' syndrome). The ascites in these benign tumors is believed to be related to fluid seepage from the tumor into the peritoneal cavity with subsequent transfer to the pleural cavity via the diaphragmatic lymphatics.

Tumors with solid as well as cystic areas palpated at the time of pelvic examination are highly suspicious of malignancy, and the diagnosis is virtually certain if there are, in addition, nodulations in the cul-de-sac, an upper abdominal mass (omental cake), and ascites.

Differential Diagnosis

Ovarian enlargements must be distinguished from pedunculated uterine myomas, hydrosalpinx, tubal tuberculosis, diverticulitis, tumors of the colon, pelvic kidney, retroperitoneal tumors, and metastatic disease from distant sites. In most instances the correct diagnosis can be made if an accurate medical history is obtained, a careful physical examination performed, and judicious use made of ancillary diagnostic procedures such as radiology, cytology, and peritoneoscopy.

Prevention

Bilateral salpingo-oophorectomy at the time of hysterectomy for benign uterine disease in women over age 40 is advocated by many to prevent the possible development of ovarian cancer. Estrogen replacement should be given to forestall menopausal symptoms, osteoporosis, and atherosclerosis. The detection and removal of potentially malignant ovarian tumors (serous cystadenoma, granulosa-theca cell tumors, dysgerminomas, arrhenoblastomas) may prevent the subsequent development of ovarian cancer, particularly if both ovaries are removed. Problems arise when one encounters such neoplasms in young women who wish to retain their childbearing potential. In such patients, a conservative approach with very careful follow-up examinations is probably best.

Treatment

Cystic enlargements of the ovary suspected to be physiologic (follicle and corpus luteum cysts) require only repeat examinations at intervals of 4—6 weeks to ascertain that they are regressing.

Many benign neoplasms can be treated by simple

excision, conserving the ovary. Dermoid cysts, endometriomas, simple serous cysts, and para-ovarian cysts (broad ligament cysts arising from mesonephric duct remnants) can be managed in this fashion. The proper management of ovarian neoplasms obviously requires an intimate knowledge of the gross appearance of ovarian tumors.

Cystadenomas and solid tumors of the ovary should, in younger women, be removed by unilateral salpingo-oophorectomy. The tumor should be opened in the operating room, and frozen-section examination of any solid or papillary areas should be done before the incision is closed.

In women approaching the menopause or older, or in whom there is bilateral disease, total hysterectomy and bilateral salpingo-oophorectomy are indicated.

When the disease extends beyond the ovaries into the pelvis or abdomen, abdominal hysterectomy and bilateral salpingo-oophorectomy are done if surgically feasible. The omentum is removed if it contains metastatic deposits. Postoperative radiation therapy is then given. If surgical removal of the uterus, tubes, and ovaries is not possible, a biopsy is taken and radiation therapy is administered. It is not uncommon to find, following irradiation, that surgical removal of the internal genitalia can then be done.

Disseminated disease is best treated with chemotherapy, the polyfunctional alkylating agents—mechlorethamine (Mustargen) and its analogues, thiotepa, chlorambucil (Leukeran), and others—being the drugs of choice. These agents are toxic, and close attention—particularly to the hematopoietic function—must be maintained during treatment. Although these drugs are not curative, long-term remissions have occasionally been achieved with their use.

Small bowel obstruction due to tumor occasionally requires surgical treatment, but this should not be done in a patient in the terminal stage of the disease.

Prognosis

The outlook for patients with benign ovarian neoplasms is excellent. The prognosis for those with malignant disease is poor, primarily because most of them are discovered when the disease is far-advanced. The overall cure rate for ovarian cancer is no more than 30%. For stage IA disease, however, 5-year survival rates of 80–85% can be achieved.

Buchsbaum HJ & others: The use of radioisotopes as adjunct therapy of localized ovarian cancer. Semin Oncol 2:247, 1975.

Day TG Jr, Smith JP: Diagnosis and staging of ovarian carcinoma. Semin Oncol 2:217, 1975.

Depalo GM & others: Melphalan vs adriamycin in treatment of advanced carcinoma of ovary. Surg Gynecol Obstet 141:899, 1975.

Fuks Z, Bagshaw MA: The rationale for curative radiotherapy for ovarian cancer. Int J Radiat Oncol 1:21, 1975.

Julian CG & others: Biologic behavior of primary ovarian malignancy. Obstet Gynecol 44:873, 1974.

Linder D & others: Parthenogenic origin of benign ovarian teratomas. N Engl J Med 292:63, 1974.

Malkasian GD Jr & others: Histology of epithelial tumors of the ovary: Clinical usefulness and prognostic significance of the histologic classification and grading. Semin Oncol 2:191, 1975.

Miller SP & others: Comparative evaluation of combined radiation-chlorambucil treatment of ovarian carcinomatosis. Cancer 36:1625, 1975.

Pantoja E & others: Complications of dermoid tumors of the ovary. Obstet Gynecol 45:89, 1975.

Rosenoff SH & others: Peritoneoscopy: A valuable staging tool in ovarian carcinoma. Ann Intern Med 83:37, 1975.

Samuels BI: Usefulness of ultrasound in patients with ovarian cancer. Semin Oncol 2:229, 1975.

Young RC: Chemotherapy of ovarian cancer: Past and present. Semin Oncol 2:267, 1975.

HYDATIDIFORM MOLE & CHORIOCARCINOMA

Essentials of Diagnosis

- Presumptive symptoms of pregnancy.
- Vaginal bleeding.
- Uterus disproportionately large for duration of pregnancy.
- Absence of fetus.
- Passage of grape-like vesicles.
- High serum or urine levels of chorionic gonadotropin.

General Considerations

Hydatidiform mole represents hydropic changes in the placental villi of a pregnancy which is developing in the absence of an embryo (blighted ovum). The swelling of the villi is related to the absence of a fetal circulation and is often accompanied by varying degrees of trophoblastic proliferation. There is a tendency to myometrial penetration which may progress to frank, deep invasion of the uterine wall (chorioadenoma destruens or invasive mole), and a small percentage (about 5%) of hydatidiform moles are followed by the highly malignant choriocarcinoma.

The frequency of hydatidiform mole is about 1:1500–2000 pregnancies in the USA and about 1:240–650 pregnancies in the Far East. Hydatidiform mole is also more common in women over 40 years of age.

Clinical Findings

The usual picture is one of a presumed threatened abortion with a missed menstrual period, nausea, breast changes, and urinary frequency followed by vaginal bleeding. This may go on for several weeks with little or no abdominal pain. Examination reveals a uterus which is disproportionately large for the duration of the pregnancy. There may be bilateral cystic enlargement of the ovaries (theca lutein cysts). Preeclamptic toxemia may develop in women with large moles, and molar pregnancy should be suspected in any patient who develops hypertension, edema, and proteinuria in the first half of pregnancy.

Serum and urinary chorionic gonadotropin levels are unusually high and persist at high levels beyond the 12th week, when in normal pregnancy there is usually a significant drop. X-ray studies are helpful, and the absence of a fetal skeleton in a pregnancy longer than 16 weeks in duration is suggestive of molar pregnancy. Amniography (transabdominal injection of radiopaque material) has been largely replaced by ultrasound (B-scan), which is diagnostic.

In many cases the diagnosis is not made until the patient spontaneously aborts the molar pregnancy. All therapeutic abortion specimens should be carefully examined for the presence of hydatidiform mole.

Differential Diagnosis

Threatened abortion is the diagnosis most often entertained in the presence of a mole. Multiple pregnancy must be considered because it may produce unusually high levels of chorionic gonadotropin. If a fetal skeleton is visible on x-ray (at 16 weeks) or if a fetal heartbeat can be heard, the patient almost certainly does not have a mole.

Complications

About 15% of moles become locally invasive (chorioadenoma destruens), which carries the danger of hemorrhage due to penetration of the vascular uterine wall or pelvic infection from perforation.

About 5% of moles are followed by choriocarcinoma, a highly malignant tumor. Although this cancer may occur after normal pregnancy, abortion, or ectopic pregnancy, about half of them develop from an antecedent hydatidiform mole. Metastases are found in the lungs, liver, CNS, bone, vagina, and vulva.

Treatment

Once the diagnosis of a molar pregnancy has been established, the uterus should be emptied. This is done by dilatation and curettage if the uterus is smaller than a 12-week pregnancy. Larger moles are better evacuated by suction with the simultaneous administration of oxytocin solution intravenously; this is then followed by careful curettage to ensure complete removal of the molar tissue. All specimens are examined pathologically for evidence of proliferative activity of the trophoblast, which serves as an index to the probability of malignant change.

Lutein cysts of the ovaries, which occur in about a third of molar pregnancies, will regress following removal of the mole and should not be surgically excised.

All patients with hydatidiform mole should be examined weekly following evacuation of the uterus for the possible development of chorioadenoma destruens or choriocarcinoma. They should be given effective contraceptive advice and advised not to become pregnant for at least a year. Weekly gonadotropin levels should be obtained, initially in urine and subsequently in serum, using beta subunit radioimmunoassays of HCG. An elevated gonadotropin level beyond 8

weeks from the evacuation of a molar pregnancy or a rise in titer before this time is evidence of persistent trophoblastic disease. Disappearance of the hormone followed by a later reappearance, particularly with rising titers, is strongly suggestive of choriocarcinoma or invasive mole if pregnancy can be ruled out.

Methotrexate, a chemotherapeutic agent which competes with folic acid in cellular metabolism, has been very effective in controlling not only invasive moles but choriocarcinoma as well. It is given in courses of 15–25 mg/day for 5 days. It is an extremely cytotoxic agent and is preferably given by someone skilled in its use (see Chapter 49). Dactinomycin has been found to be equally effective and less toxic than methotrexate. Other effective chemotherapeutic agents useful in methotrexate- and dactinomycin-resistant tumors are chlorambucil (Leukeran), vinblastine (Velban), and cyclophosphamide.

Prognosis

The prognosis for cure in hydatidiform mole and chorioadenoma destruens is excellent. Before the anticancer drugs became available, the outlook for choriocarcinoma was very poor. Five-year remission rates in the range of 80% or better are now being reported. In fact, if adequate treatment is initiated within 3 months of apparent onset, the figure is close to 100% if metastatic disease is limited to the lungs or pelvis and the initial chorionic gonadotropin titer is less than 100,000 IU/24 hours. A relatively poor prognosis exists in patients with one or more of the following: (1) initial chorionic gonadotropin titer in excess of 1,000,000 IU/24 hours; (2) metastatic disease involving the CNS, liver, or gastrointestinal tract; (3) duration of disease of more than 4 months without treatment; or (4) resistance of the disease to single agent chemotherapy.

Curry SL & others: Hydatidiform mole: Diagnosis, management and long-term followup of 347 patients. Obstet Gynecol 45:1, 1975.

Hilgers RD, Lewis JL Jr: Gestational trophoblastic neoplasms. Gynecol Oncol 2:460, 1974.

Jones WB & others: Monitor of chemotherapy in gestational trophoblastic neoplasm by radioimmunoassay of the B-subunit of human chorionic gonadotropin. Am J Obstet Gynecol 121:669, 1975.

Tsai W: Use of sonar in diagnosis and management of invasive gestational trophoblastic tumors. Int J Fertil 19:227, 1974.

• • •

CELIOSCOPY IN GYNECOLOGY

The development of fiber optics has stimulated the use of 2 technics for the visualization of the internal organs of reproduction: culdoscopy and laparoscopy. The first utilizes the knee-chest position and can be performed with either local or conduction (caudal or spinal) anesthesia. Laparoscopy is usually performed with the patient in the Trendelenburg position or in the dorsal recumbent position under general anesthesia. Both depend upon the introduction of a pneumoperitoneum, atmospheric air usually being used in culdoscopy and either carbon dioxide or nitrous oxide in laparoscopy. In addition to the value of these technics diagnostically, certain operative and manipulative procedures can be carried out. Each method has its advantages and disadvantages and its proponents and opponents.

Culdoscopy can be performed under local anesthesia after preoperative sedation. Although CO_2 or N_2O pneumoperitoneum can be used, air is usually allowed to enter the peritoneal cavity through a posterior vaginal fornix/cul-de-sac puncture. Visualization is carried out transvaginally, and the view of the pelvic organs is somewhat more restricted than that seen through the laparoscope. The procedure is contraindicated whenever a lesion such as endometriosis, chronic salpingitis, or a tumor occupies the cul-de-sac. It cannot be done in the presence of vaginal atresia.

Laparoscopy has the disadvantage of requiring endotracheal anesthesia and operating room facilities. It affords a better view of the pelvic contents and allows a greater variety of manipulative and minor operative procedures than does culdoscopy. Laparo-

scopic cauterization and sectioning of the fallopian tubes has become a widely accepted method of female sterilization. It can be done under local anesthesia in selected patients. The most significant complication is injury to the small intestine. It is contraindicated in patients with cardiac or respiratory insufficiency, abdominal hernias, large abdominal tumors, or advanced pregnancy and in patients with a likelihood of disseminated abdominal malignancy. Previous abdominal surgery is not an absolute contraindication, and the procedure can be done safely in patients with abdominal surgical scars provided certain safeguards are observed in the induction of the pneumoperitoneum and the placement of the trocar through the anterior abdominal wall.

Corson SL, Bolognese RJ: Laparoscopy: Overview and results of a large series. J Reprod Med 9:148, 1972.

Edgerton WD: Experience with laparoscopy in a nonteaching hospital. Am J Obstet Gynecol 116:184, 1973.

Paterson PJ, Grimwade JC: Laparoscopic sterilization: Review of its value and hazards. Aust NZ J Surg 42:167, 1972.

Riva HL & others: Further experience with culdoscopy: An analysis of 2850 cases. JAMA 178:873, 1961.

Steptoe PC: *Laparoscopy in Gynaecology.* Livingstone, 1967.

Thompson BH, Wheeless CR Jr: Gastrointestinal complications of laparoscopy sterilization. Obstet Gynecol 41:669, 1973.

●   ●   ●

General References

Burghardt E: *Early Histological Diagnosis of Cervical Cancer.* Saunders, 1973.

Danforth DN: *Textbook of Obstetrics and Gynecology,* 2nd ed. Harper & Row, 1971.

DiSaia PJ & others: *Synopsis of Gynecologic Oncology.* Wiley, 1975.

Dougherty CM, Rowena S: *Female Sex Anomalies.* Harper & Row, 1972.

Ferin M & others: *Biorhythms and Human Reproduction.* Wiley, 1974.

Gold JJ & others: *Gynecologic Endocrinology,* 2nd ed. Harper & Row, 1975.

Gray SW, Skandalakis JE: *Embryology for Surgeons.* Saunders, 1972.

Green TH: *Gynecology: Essentials of Clinical Practice,* 3rd ed. Little, Brown, 1977.

Greenhill JP: *Office Gynecology,* 9th ed. Year Book, 1971.

Huffman JW: *The Gynecology of Childhood & Adolescence.* Saunders, 1968.

Janovski NA, Douglas C: *Diseases of the Vulva.* Harper & Row, 1972.

Janovski NA, Paramanandhan TL: *Ovarian Tumors.* Saunders, 1973.

Kistner RW: *Gynecology: Principles and Practice,* 2nd ed. Year Book, 1971.

Mukherjee TK: *Modern Concepts of Obstetrics and Gynecology.* Warren H. Green, 1974.

Novak ER & others: *Novak's Textbook of Gynecology.* Williams & Wilkins, 1975.

Rutledge F & others: *Gynecologic Oncology.* Wiley, 1976.

Shearman RP: *Human Reproductive Physiology.* Lippincott, 1972.

45 . . .
Orthopedics

Floyd H. Jergesen, MD

INFECTIONS OF BONES & JOINTS

OSTEOMYELITIS

Osteomyelitis is an acute or chronic infection of bone and is classified according to origin as primary or secondary, according to microbial flora, and according to course as acute, subacute, or chronic.

Primary osteomyelitis is caused by direct implantation of microorganisms into bone and is usually localized to that site. Open (compound) fractures, penetrating wounds (especially those due to firearms), and surgical operations on bone are the most common causes. Operative treatment is usually necessary; treatment with antimicrobial drugs is adjunctive.

Secondary or **acute hematogenous osteomyelitis** is usually due to spread through the blood stream. Occasionally, secondary osteomyelitis may result from direct extension of infection in contiguous soft tissues or from septic arthritis in an adjacent joint.

1. ACUTE PYOGENIC OSTEOMYELITIS
(Secondary or Hematogenous Osteomyelitis)

Essentials of Diagnosis

- Pain, tenderness, swelling, and limitation of joint motion.
- Fever, chills, malaise, and sweating.

General Considerations

About 95% of cases of acute secondary osteomyelitis are caused by pyogenic organisms, usually a single strain. Secondary contamination during treatment may produce a mixed infection.

Acute hematogenous osteomyelitis occurs predominantly during the period of skeletal growth, with the peak incidence during childhood. About 75% of cases in children are due to staphylococci; group A streptococci are the next most common pathogen; and the remainder of cases are caused by a wide variety of organisms. Preexisting infection of another organ system is present in about half of cases. Males are affected about 4 times as frequently as females. The tibia and femur are the most commonly involved of the long bones.

The initial lesion may become progressive or chronic, or the infection may resolve with or without treatment.

If the initial lesion is not controlled, spread of infection causes bony destruction that differs in infancy, childhood, and adulthood due to the vascular supply of bone. During infancy, terminal ramifications of the nutrient artery perforate the growth plate and end in the cartilaginous precursor of the epiphysis. This may explain both the frequency of complicating septic arthritis during infancy and subsequent disturbances of growth. There may also be rapid spread of infection throughout the entire length of the bone, but involucrum formation is not characteristic.

At about 18 months of age, the epiphyseal plate becomes a vascular barrier. The blood flow on the metaphyseal side of the growth plate reverses its direction, forming loops that empty into the large sinusoidal veins where the rate of blood flow is slower. This may explain the frequency of metaphyseal infections in the long bones during childhood. Initial localization of infection in cancellous bone is rapidly followed by edema which causes increased intraosseous pressure. Suppuration follows edema, and the escape of exudate beneath the periosteum causes elevation with disruption of vascular channels. The inflamed periosteum starts to produce a shell-like layer of new bone which can be identified by x-ray. Disturbance of blood supply to the inner surface of the cortex from thrombosed branches of nutrient vessels leads to necrosis of compact bone and sequestration. Because the epiphysis is separated from the metaphysis by the growth plate, it is protected from direct involvement.

In adulthood, metaphyseal and epiphyseal vessels communicate across the scar of the previous growth plate, and microorganisms can enter the epiphysis through the nutrient artery. This permits organisms to reach the subchondral bone of joints and precipitate a complicating septic arthritis. Since the periosteum of adults is rather fibrous and adherent, extensive subperiosteal abscess formation is not a prominent feature. However, periosteal inflammation can be identified by demineralization and absorption of the cortex. Involucrum formation and extensive cortical sequestration are not uncommon in adulthood. Involvement of the diaphysis, chronic infection of the marrow, and abscesses of the soft tissues surrounding bone are more common sequelae in adults.

Clinical Findings

A. Symptoms and Signs: In infants and children, the onset is often sudden, with marked toxicity; an insidious onset may produce more subtle symptoms. Voluntary movement of the extremity is inhibited. Tenderness followed by swelling and redness are the local manifestations.

The onset in adults is likely to be less striking than in infants and children. Generalized symptoms of bacteremia may be absent, and vague, shifting, or evanescent local pain may be the earliest manifestation. Limitation of joint motion may be marked, especially in patients with spine involvement or when lesions are near joints.

B. Laboratory Findings: Identification of the causative organism is often possible by blood culture. The ESR and white count are often elevated.

C. X-Ray Findings: (Fig 45–1.) Significant changes in bone cannot be identified by x-ray before 7–10 days after onset in infants and 2–4 weeks after onset in adults, but extraosseous soft tissue swelling adjacent to the infection may appear within 3–5 days after the onset of symptoms. Xeroradiography may demonstrate subtle changes in extracortical soft tissues that are not apparent on routine x-ray films. If antimicrobial therapy was started early, x-ray changes in bone may not appear for 3–5 weeks. Subperiosteal new bone formation is a late manifestation of healing.

D. Special Examinations: Exudates may be recovered for culture by aspiration of extraosseous tissues in areas of tenderness or directly from the involved bone. In severe infections of more than 2 days' duration, material for culture and smear is usually obtained during open surgical treatment.

Radionuclide imaging may help to localize an occult focus of infection before routine x-ray studies become diagnostic.

Differential Diagnosis

Acute local infections of bone must be differentiated from the prodromal stages of acute exanthems and from traumatic injuries.

Acute hematogenous osteomyelitis must be differentiated from suppurative arthritis, rheumatic fever, cellulitis, tuberculosis, mycotic infections, and Ewing's sarcoma. The pseudoparalysis associated with acute osteomyelitis in infancy may simulate poliomyelitis. When symptoms are mild, osteomyelitis may initially mimic Legg-Perthes disease.

Complications

Delayed diagnosis or inadequate early treatment can lead to chronic osteomyelitis. Other complications include soft tissue abscess formation, septic arthritis, and metastatic infections to other organs. Pathologic fracture may occur at sites of extensive bone destruction.

Treatment

A. General Measures: Toxic patients require intravenous administration of fluid and electrolytes. Accompanying anemia should often be corrected by blood transfusion. Immobilization of the affected extremity by splinting, plaster encasement, or suspension in an orthopedic apparatus is advisable for relief of pain and protection against pathologic fracture.

B. Specific Measures: Although antibiotics are of great benefit, they are not usually curative. The mainstay of therapy is surgery. Treatment must be individualized, and only broad guidelines will be given here.

1. Operative treatment–During the first 2–3 days after the onset of acute infection, open surgical treatment can be avoided in many cases, especially in infants and children. If vigorous general care and appropriate antibiotic therapy are instituted promptly, the progress of the local lesion may be controlled and spread of the infection halted before suppuration and significant tissue destruction have occurred.

If an abscess has formed beneath the periosteum or has extended into the soft tissues of infants and children, it should be drained at least once daily by aspiration. Pain and fever that persist longer than 2–3 days after initiating aspiration and antimicrobial therapy suggest spread. Surgical decompression of the medullary cavity by drilling or limited fenestration should be done promptly with the hope of minimizing

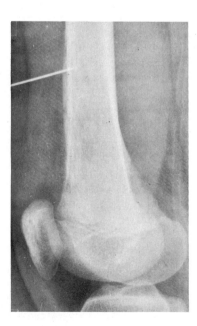

Figure 45–1. Pyogenic osteomyelitis in a 9-year-old girl 5 weeks after onset of symptoms and treatment only by systemic antibiotics. Cortical destruction and subperiosteal new bone formation are apparent anteriorly. The needle tip lies in a subperiosteal abscess.

progression of bone necrosis. Subsequent treatment of the local lesion may be by open or closed technics. Open treatment of the wound by packing requires multiple dressing changes, which are painful and frequently cannot be accomplished except under general anesthesia. Closed wound treatment with intermittent suction drainage provides egress of exudates and minimizes the likelihood of secondary contamination. Antibiotics can be given topically through the drainage tube in concentrations that systemically would be toxic.

Radical surgical technics such as extensive guttering and diaphysectomy should be reserved for the treatment of chronic osteomyelitis.

2. Antibiotics—(See Chapter 11.) Antibiotic therapy is aided by identification of the organism and its antibiotic sensitivities. Since acute infections in children are usually due to staphylococci or β-hemolytic streptococci, appropriate systemic antibiotics for these organisms should be administered without waiting for culture reports. Chemotherapy should be continued for about 2–3 weeks after the patient becomes afebrile or repeated wound cultures fail to show growth.

Course & Prognosis

The mortality rate in treated acute osteomyelitis is about 1%, but morbidity continues to be high. If effective treatment can be instituted within 48 hours after onset, prompt recovery can be expected in about two-thirds of cases. Chronicity and recurrence of infection are likely when treatment is delayed.

Capitanio MA, Kirkpatrick JA: Early roentgen observations in acute osteomyelitis. Am J Roentgenol Radium Ther Nucl Med 108:488, 1970.

Klastersky J & others: Gram-negative infections in cancer: Study of empiric therapy comparing carbenicillin-cephalothin with and without gentamicin. JAMA 227:45, 1974.

Waldvogel FA, Medoff G, Swartz MN: Osteomyelitis: A review of clinical features, therapeutic considerations and unusual aspects. (3 parts.) N Engl J Med 282:198, 260, 316, 1970.

2. CHRONIC PYOGENIC OSTEOMYELITIS

Essentials of Diagnosis

- Pain, tenderness, swelling, edema, and redness of overlying skin.
- Sinus tract formation.

General Considerations

Chronic pyogenic osteomyelitis may occur as a consequence of acute infection or may appear as an indolent, slowly progressive process with no striking symptoms. Recurrent infection is manifested by exacerbation of symptoms with or without drainage after a quiescent period of days, weeks, or years. Chronic osteomyelitis at the site of healed or unhealed fracture is discussed under the treatment of fractures.

Clinical Findings

A. Symptoms and Signs: Symptoms may be so mild and the onset so insidious that there is little or no disability, but recurrent fever, pain, and swelling are common. There may be a history of injury. The infection may communicate through a sinus to the skin surface with periodic or constant discharge of pus.

B. Laboratory Findings: Leukocytosis, anemia, and acceleration of the ESR are inconstant and cannot be relied upon.

C. X-Ray Findings: (Fig 45–2.) Architectural alterations of bone depend upon the stage, extent, and rate of progress of the disease. Destruction of bone may create diffuse areas of radiolucency. Bone necrosis, apparent as areas of increased density, is due in part to increased absorption of calcium from surrounding vascularized bone. Involucrum and new bone formation are healing responses which may be identified beneath the periosteum or within bone. Subperiosteal new bone may be seen as a lamellar pattern. Progressive resorption of sclerotic bone and re-formation of

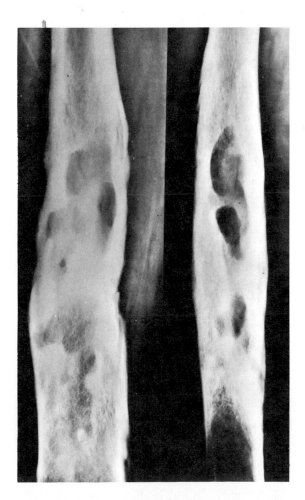

Figure 45–2. Chronic pyogenic osteomyelitis of the lower femur due to *S aureus* in a 38-year-old woman. This patient had numerous clinical exacerbations with 17 operations over a period of 35 years.

the normal trabecular pattern also suggest healing.

Tomography may be helpful in identifying deep areas of bone destruction. Sinograms made with aqueous radiographic media may aid in localization of sequestra or points of persistent infection and will demonstrate the course of sinus tracts. Occasionally, bone scanning with radioisotopes will localize otherwise occult infection.

D. Special Examinations: The causative organisms should be cultured and drug sensitivity studies performed. Culture of exudates from sinus orifices may be misleading because skin contaminants are likely to be present. More reliable specimens can be obtained by taking samples of suspected tissue at operation or by deep aspiration at a distance from sinus tracts.

Differential Diagnosis

Chronic pyogenic osteomyelitis should be differentiated from benign and malignant tumors; from certain forms of osseous dysplasia; from fatigue fracture; and from specific infections discussed later in this section.

Complications

The most common complication is persistence of infection and acute recurrences. Persistent infection may cause anemia, weight loss, weakness, and amyloidosis. Chronic osteomyelitis may disseminate to other organs.

Acute exacerbations can be complicated by serious effusions in adjacent joints or by frank purulent arthritis.

Constant erosion and progressive destruction of bone cause structural weakening which occasionally leads to pathologic fracture.

Before epiphyseal closure, osteomyelitis can produce overgrowth of a long bone from chronic hyperemia of the growth plate. Focal destruction of an epiphyseal plate can create asymmetric growth.

Rarely, after many years of drainage, squamous cell carcinoma or a fibrosarcoma arises in persistently infected tissues.

Treatment

A. General Measures: During the quiescent phase, no treatment is necessary and the patient lives an essentially normal life. Minor exacerbations accompanied by drainage may be managed adequately with dressing changes. More acute episodes may require immobilization, bed rest, local heat, and mild analgesics.

B. Medical Measures: Occasionally, when the drug sensitivities of the causative organism are known, systemic antibiotic therapy without surgical intervention is advantageous. This is especially true during the early phase of a recurrence without external drainage or abscess formation.

Copious drainage and clinical and x-ray evidence of progressive bone destruction and sequestration require more aggressive treatment.

C. Surgical Treatment: Soft tissue abscesses without sequestration can be treated adequately by operation and open or closed drainage. Similar treatment may also suffice for **Brodie's abscess,** a rare, walled-off infection of bone. Removal of a sequestrum with drainage of the abscess cavity often permits rapid healing. With the exception of the fibula, metatarsals, and possibly the metacarpals, diaphysectomy should be avoided if possible because the resected shaft will not regenerate. More extensive and long-standing infections may require more radical surgery such as diaphysectomy or amputation.

Course & Prognosis

Even after vigorous treatment, recurrence of infection is likely. This is usually due to incomplete removal of all areas of infected soft tissue scar or necrotic and unseparated bone.

Gordon SL & others: Recurrent osteomyelitis: Report of four cases culturing L-form variants of staphylococci. J Bone Joint Surg 53A:1150, 1971.

Johnson LL, Kempson RL: Epidermoid carcinoma in osteomyelitis. J Bone Joint Surg 47A:133, 1965.

Kemp HB & others: The role of fluorine-18 and strontium-87m scintigraphy in the management of infective spondylitis. J Bone Joint Surg 55B:301, 1973.

West WF & others: Chronic osteomyelitis. 1. Factors affecting the results of treatment in 186 patients. JAMA 213:1837, 1970.

SPECIFIC INFECTIONS OF BONES & JOINTS

MYCOTIC INFECTIONS OF BONES & JOINTS

Fungal infections of the skeletal system are usually secondary to a primary infection in another organ system, frequently the lower pulmonary tract. Although skeletal lesions have a predilection for the cancellous extremities of long bones and the bodies of vertebrae, the predominant lesion—a granuloma with varying degrees of necrosis and abscess formation—does not produce a characteristic clinical picture.

The principal mycotic infections of the skeletal system are **coccidioidomycosis,** which is usually secondary to a primary pulmonary infection; **histoplasmosis** (rare), which usually represents dissemination from a primary focus in the lungs; **cryptococcosis** (torulosis or European blastomycosis), an uncommon chronic granulomatous pulmonary disease that may be disseminated to the nervous system and rarely to the skeletal system; and **North American blastomycosis** (Gilchrist's disease), which may be disseminated to skeletal structures from the lungs or, less commonly, from a cutaneous lesion.

Treatment is usually with amphotericin B (Fungizone). Surgical debridement and in some cases saucerization are often required.

Bennett JE: Chemotherapy of systemic mycoses. (2 parts.) N Engl J Med 290:30, 320, 1974.
Schwarz J, Salfelder K: Diagnosis of surgical deep mycoses. Surg Gynecol Obstet 128.252, 1969.

SYPHILIS OF BONES & JOINTS

Congenital syphilis causes periostitis and osteoperiostitis in **childhood** and **adolescence**. Bone involvement is frequently symmetric, and periosteal proliferation along the tibial crest causes the classic "saber shin." A painless bilateral effusion of the knees (Clutton's joints) is a rare manifestation.

In **adults**, gumma formation is a tertiary manifestation. This granulomatous process is characterized by localized destruction of bone accompanied by surrounding areas of sclerosis. Extensive destruction with accompanying rarefaction may cause pathologic fracture. Periostitis in the adult is likely to occur in the bones of the thorax and in the shafts of long bones. The x-ray picture of syphilitic osteitis in the adult is not diagnostic, but bone production is generally more pronounced than bone destruction.

Osteoarticular lesions due to other causes must be differentiated from syphilis. Serologic studies will usually provide confirmatory evidence. Biopsy is not necessary to establish a direct diagnosis, but it may differentiate a gumma from other lesions. A favorable response to penicillin treatment supports the diagnosis.

The only local treatment necessary is immobilization to provide comfort or protection from fracture if the bone is seriously weakened. Lesions of bones and joints respond promptly to adequate chemotherapy.

Syphilitic arthritis or osteitis may occur during any stage of congenital or acquired infection. Neurotrophic arthropathy (Charcot's joints) can be caused indirectly by syphilitic disease of the spinal cord.

In **infancy**, congenital syphilis typically causes epiphysitis and metaphysitis. Radiologically, a zone of sclerosis appears adjacent to the growth plate but is separated from another similar zone by one of rarefaction. Partial replacement of the rarefied bone by inflammatory tissue precedes suppuration, which may in turn allow epiphyseal displacement because of structural weakening.

Fleming TC, Bardenstein MB: Congenital syphilis. J Bone Joint Surg 53A:1648, 1971.
Johns D: Syphilitic disorders of the spine. J Bone Joint Surg 52B:724, 1970.

TUBERCULOSIS OF BONES & JOINTS

Essentials of Diagnosis

- Pain, tenderness, swelling, limitation of joint motion.
- Known primary infection in another organ system.

General Considerations

Infection of the musculoskeletal system with *Mycobacterium tuberculosis* is usually caused by hematogenous spread from the respiratory or gastrointestinal tract. Tuberculosis of the thoracic or lumbar spine may be associated with an active lesion of the genitourinary tract.

Clinical Findings

A. Symptoms and Signs: The onset of symptoms is generally insidious. Pain in an involved joint may be mild and accompanied by a sensation of stiffness. It is commonly accentuated at night. Limping and restriction of joint motion are seen. As the disease progresses, the joint becomes fixed by muscle contractures, organic destruction of the joint, and healing in soft tissues and bone.

Local findings during the early stages may be limited to tenderness, soft tissue swelling, joint effusion, and increase in skin temperature about the involved area. As the disease progresses without treatment, muscle atrophy and deformity become apparent. Abscess formation with spontaneous external drainage leads to sinus formation. Progressive destruction of bone in the spine, especially in the thoracolumbar region, may cause a gibbus.

B. Laboratory Findings: The diagnosis rests upon recovery of acid-fast bacilli from joint fluid, tissue exudates, or tissue specimens. Biopsy of the lesion or of a regional lymph node may demonstrate the characteristic histologic picture but does not differentiate tuberculosis from other mycobacterial lesions.

C. X-Ray Findings: The earliest changes of tuberculous arthritis are soft tissue swelling and distention of the capsule by effusion. Subsequently, bone atrophy causes thinning of the trabecular pattern, narrowing of the cortex, and enlargement of the medullary canal. As joint disease progresses, destruction of cartilage causes narrowing of the joint cleft and focal erosion of the articular surface, especially at the margins. Extensive destruction of joint surfaces causes deformity. As healing takes place, osteosclerosis becomes apparent around areas of necrosis and sequestration. Where the lesion is limited to bone, especially in the cancellous portion of the metaphysis, the x-ray picture may be that of single or multilocular cysts surrounded by sclerotic bone. As intraosseous foci expand toward the limiting cortex and erode it, subperiosteal new bone formation takes place.

D. Special Examinations: Exudates for culture may be collected by aspiration, or representative tissues may be removed by percutaneous or open biopsy.

Differential Diagnosis

Tuberculosis of the musculoskeletal system must be differentiated from other subacute and chronic infections, rheumatoid arthritis, gout, and occasionally from osseous dysplasia. Infections caused by nontuberculous mycobacteria can be differentiated only by laboratory procedures.

Complications

Destruction of bones or joints may occur in a few weeks or months if adequate treatment is not provided. Deformity due to joint destruction, abscess formation with spread into adjacent soft tissues, and sinus formation are common. Paraplegia is the most serious complication of spinal tuberculosis. As healing of severe joint lesions takes place, spontaneous fibrous or bony ankylosis follows.

Treatment

A. Surgical Treatment: In acute infections where synovitis is the predominant feature, treatment can be conservative, at least initially; immobilization by splint or plaster, aspiration, and chemotherapy may suffice. A similar approach is used for infections of large joints of the lower extremities in children during an early stage. It may also be used in adults either as definitive treatment of mild infections or before operation. Synovectomy may be valuable for less acute hypertrophic lesions of tendon sheaths, bursas, or joints.

Various types of operative treatment are necessary for chronic or advanced tuberculosis of bones and joints. The advent of effective drug treatment has broadened the indications for synovectomy and debridement at the expense of more radical surgical procedures such as arthrodesis and amputation. Even though the infection is active and all involved tissue cannot be removed, supplementary chemotherapy may permit healing to occur. In general, arthrodesis of weight-bearing joints is preferred when function cannot be salvaged. Reconstructive arthroplasty to restore function has not proved reliable in eradicating disease and is not recommended at present.

B. Chemotherapy: Chemotherapy of osteoarticular tuberculosis is based essentially on the systemic administration of drugs to which the strain of pathogen is likely to be susceptible as indicated by in vitro testing. Resistant strains are likely to emerge during administration of single drugs. Therefore, combinations of antituberculous agents are recommended. Although isoniazid (INH) plus aminosalicylic acid (PAS) with or without streptomycin have been used widely in the past, combinations of isoniazid and ethambutol or rifampin and ethambutol are now employed more frequently. Other useful but more toxic drugs include viomycin, capreomycin, pyrazinamide, cycloserine, and ethionamide.

Kelly PJ & others: Infection of synovial tissues by mycobacteria other than *Mycobacterium tuberculosis.* J Bone Joint Surg 49A:1521, 1967.

Martin NS: Pott's paraplegia: A report on 120 cases. J Bone Joint Surg 53B:596, 1971.
Neville CH Jr & others: Is surgical fusion still desirable in spinal tuberculosis? Clin Orthop 75:179, 1971.
O'Connor BT & others: Disseminated bone tuberculosis. J Bone Joint Surg 52A:537, 1970.
Tuli SM & others: The experimental induction of localised skeletal tuberculous lesions and their accessibility to streptomycin. J Bone Joint Surg 56B:551, 1974.
Wilkinson MC: Tuberculosis of the hip and knee treated by chemotherapy, synovectomy, and debridement. J Bone Joint Surg 51A:1343, 1969.

PYOGENIC ARTHRITIS

Pyogenic arthritis (suppurative, infectious, or septic arthritis) is an acute or chronic inflammation of joints which may be caused by a variety of microorganisms, especially cocci or enteric gram-negative bacilli. Classification can be based on the mechanism of introduction of the pathogen or the microbial etiology.

Primary pyogenic arthritis can be the result of direct implantation of microorganisms into joints through penetrating wounds or can complicate open surgical procedures (eg, arthrocentesis or intra-articular drug therapy). Joint infections that follow open surgical operations are discussed under acute pyogenic arthritis.

Secondary pyogenic arthritis is generally blood-borne; it can also result from direct extension from an adjacent focus of osteomyelitis or from an extra-articular soft tissue infection.

Chronic pyogenic arthritis is usually a sequel to untreated or unsuccessfully treated acute primary or secondary pyogenic arthritis.

1. ACUTE PYOGENIC ARTHRITIS

Essentials of Diagnosis

- Acute onset of pain.
- Restriction of joint motion.
- Local tenderness, swelling, warmth.
- Fever, chills, and malaise.
- Recovery of the pathogen from the joint cavity.

General Considerations

Pyogenic cocci—staphylococci, streptococci, pneumococci, and meningococci—are the most frequent pathogens. Enteric gram-negative bacilli, especially *Escherichia coli,* may produce infection in adults. *Haemophilus influenzae* is a frequent pathogen in children 6 months to 2 years of age.

In acute hematogenous arthritis, the larger joints (knee, hip, elbow, shoulder, and ankle) are more commonly involved. The presence of a nearby acute or chronic infection of bone or soft tissue may secondarily involve a joint. Infections of other organ systems, eg, skin, respiratory tract, and genitourinary tract, are possible sources of blood-borne infections. Although a single joint is generally involved in adults, multiple joints may be involved by hematogenous arthritis in children. Antecedent trauma to the area may be misleading.

The initial reaction is an acute synovitis. The intra-articular fluid during this phase may show a few polymorphonuclear leukocytes. Later, the synovial fluid changes to pus and edema, and cellular infiltration occurs in the subsynovial soft tissues. Destruction of cartilage follows, especially at the point of contact of opposing joint surfaces. Continued infection may produce destruction of synovial and capsular components as well as cartilage and bone. Following successfully treated early infections, there may be no permanent sequelae, but extensive tissue destruction after severe infections can only be partially repaired and fibrous or complete bony ankylosis may result.

Clinical Findings

A. Symptoms and Signs: Systemic disease or another serious infection may distract attention from the infected joint. Migratory polyarthralgia or multiple joint symptoms may be misleading. Systemic symptoms include fever, chills, and malaise. Pain is generally progressive and is usually accentuated by active or passive joint motions. The patient tends to limit motion of the involved joint. Local tenderness and warmth are present over the joint and are often accompanied by soft tissue swelling and joint effusion.

B. Laboratory Findings: Examination of joint fluid is crucial. During the incipient stage of infection, the fluid may be grossly clear or only slightly turbid, but it tends to become purulent as the infection progresses. The white cell count is likely to be greater than $50,000/\mu l$, with more than 90% polymorphonuclear neutrophils. The fasting blood glucose level is usually more than 50 mg/100 ml above that of the synovial fluid. The mucin clot tends to fragment or form a flocculent precipitate (in comparison to its normal ropy consistency) which suggests an inflammatory cause of the effusion. The sedimentation rate is almost invariably accelerated.

The morphologic and staining characteristics of the pathogen on Gram stain alone may suggest the appropriate antibiotic. Culture of the blood and synovial fluid establishes a definitive diagnosis and provides specific information on antibiotic sensitivities.

C. X-Ray Findings: The appearance of significant x-ray findings depends in part on the virulence of the infection. X-ray changes lag behind the clinical and pathologic process. During the first 2 weeks, the joint capsule can be seen on x-ray to be distended by effusion. As the inflammatory reaction spreads, demarcation between capsule and fat becomes obliterated. Increase in intra-articular pressure from effusion may cause widening of the joint cleft in hip infections, especially in infants, where subluxation can occur. Compar-

ative x-rays of the opposite normal joint can aid in the identification of subtle changes. With persistent hyperemia and disuse, demineralization of subchondral bone occurs adjacent to the joint cleft and extends centrifugally. Trabecular detail is progressively lost and the compact subchondral bone appears accentuated. Destruction of cartilage is reflected by narrowing of the width of the joint cleft until subchondral bone is in apposition.

Complications

Joint infections can disseminate to other sites either via the blood stream or directly.

Differential Diagnosis

Acute pyogenic arthritis must be differentiated from other acute arthropathies (eg, rheumatic fever, rheumatoid arthritis, gout and pseudogout, and gonococcal arthritis). Hematogenous osteomyelitis, rheumatic fever, and epiphyseal trauma may mimic acute septic arthritis in childhood.

Acute pyogenic arthritis may complicate other types of preexisting joint disease, notably rheumatoid arthritis or neurotrophic arthropathy. Concomitant or recent systemic treatment with corticosteroids may cloud the diagnosis, especially during the prodromal stage, by modification of physical signs. Polyarthralgia may occur in systemic viral infections or allergic reactions, but other features of pyogenic arthritis are lacking. Acute infections or inflammations of periarticular structures (eg, septic bursitis and tenosynovitis, osteomyelitis, cellulitis, and acute calcific tendinitis) may be difficult to differentiate. Transient synovitis of the hip in infancy and childhood may be especially difficult to distinguish from bacterial infection, and culture of aspirated joint fluid may be the only method of differentiation.

Treatment

A. General Measures: Analgesics and splinting of the involved joint in the position of maximum comfort alleviate pain. Pain caused by increased intra-articular pressure can be relieved by intermittent aspiration or surgical drainage. Bilateral suspension of the lower extremities in abduction with traction may prevent subluxation or dislocation of a septic hip joint, especially in infants and children.

B. Specific Measures: Definitive treatment is based on surgery and effective drug therapy. The specific operation depends in part upon the infecting agent, the stage of the infection, and the response of the patient.

During the first 48–72 hours after onset, open drainage of the joint may be replaced by intermittent aspiration to relieve intra-articular tension and to evacuate exudates. When the infection is due to *Staphylococcus aureus,* open or tube drainage is preferable because of the chondrolytic nature of the altered synovial secretions. If infection is not recognized or not treated effectively within the first 72 hours, immediate drainage by open or closed tube methods is advocated for most cases. Open drainage implies arthrotomy without closure of the surgical wound whereas closed drainage indicates closure of the surgical wound with an indwelling tube or percutaneous insertion of a tube via a small trocar into the joint cavity.

C. Drug Therapy: Antibiotics should be given based on smear and culture determinations.

Course & Prognosis

If effective treatment can be instituted within the first 48–72 hours of onset, a prompt favorable response can be expected in an otherwise healthy patient. Defervescence, disappearance of pain, return of uninhibited joint motion, resorption of joint effusion, and a decreasing sedimentation rate are some of the factors that indicate a favorable response to treatment.

Prompt diagnosis and aggressive treatment can prevent the most serious sequel of acute joint infection: loss of function due to bone and soft tissue destruction during the subacute or chronic stage.

Kelly PJ & others: Bacterial arthritis. J Bone Joint Surg 52A:819, 1970.

Lloyd-Roberts GC: Suppurative arthritis in infancy. J Bone Joint Surg 42B:706, 1960.

Nelson JD, Koontz WC: Septic arthritis in infants and children: Review of 117 cases. Pediatrics 38:965, 1966.

Rimoin DL, Wennberg JE: Acute septic arthritis complicating chronic rheumatoid arthritis. JAMA 196:617, 1966.

2. GONORRHEAL ARTHRITIS

Acute gonorrheal arthritis caused by *Neisseria gonorrhoeae* is almost always secondary to infection of the genitourinary tract. At one time, joint involvement occurred in 2–5% of all gonococcal infections, but it is now seen more frequently in women who have occult genitourinary infections and sometimes in children. Joint symptoms are likely to appear during the third week of an active infection.

Joint infection is via the blood stream. Clinical evidence of involvement of multiple joints is often present at onset, but symptoms are usually transient in all joints but one. Large weight-bearing joints are most often affected. Systemic symptoms may accompany acute arthritis. Initial synovitis with effusion progresses to a purulent exudate with destruction of cartilage which may lead to fibrous or bony ankylosis.

The precise diagnosis is established by recovery of the causative microorganism from the involved joint by culture, which may be successful in only a minority of acute cases.

Gonorrheal arthritis must be differentiated from rheumatoid arthritis, pyogenic arthritis caused by other organisms, acute synovitis, Reiter's disease, and gout.

Nonspecific treatment includes immobilization of the joint, bed rest, and analgesics as necessary for pain.

If the joint fluid is purulent and recurs rapidly, systemic antibiotic treatment can be supplemented by instillation into large joints of 25–50 thousand units of penicillin G in 5 ml saline, repeated once or twice at daily intervals.

The prognosis for preservation of joint function is good if the diagnosis is established promptly and treatment is vigorous.

Cooke CL & others: Gonococcal arthritis. JAMA 217:204, 1971.

Hess EV, Hunter DK, Ziff M: Gonococcal antibodies in acute arthritis. JAMA 191:531, 1965.

Holmes KK & others: Recovery of *Neisseria gonorrhoeae* from "sterile" synovial fluid in gonococcal arthritis. N Engl J Med 284:318, 1974.

3. CHRONIC PYOGENIC ARTHRITIS

Chronic pyogenic arthritis may follow acute primary or secondary pyogenic arthritis. Pyogenic cocci and enteric gram-negative rods are the most common organisms. Although a previously identified pathogen is likely to persist, superinfection can occur, especially after open surgical treatment and antibiotics. The original bacterial strain is sometimes supplanted by another during treatment, or a mixed infection may occur.

The infection can be continuously or intermittently active. Uninterrupted progress from the acute stage is characterized by continued local pain and swelling, restriction of joint motion, sinus formation, and increasing deformity. X-rays show progressive destruction of cartilage manifested by narrowing of the joint cleft, erosion of bone, and even infraction or cavitation. Even though the course is indolent, it is that of continued deterioration. Episodic abatement may follow treatment with antibiotics in the recurrent type. Occult infections may be unrecognized for long periods since they do not produce striking clinical findings. They may occur concomitantly with other joint diseases or may complicate surgical operations on joints, especially after surgical implants or antibiotic prophylaxis of postoperative infection.

Chronic pyogenic arthritis must be differentiated from chronic nonpyogenic microbial infections of joints, gout, rheumatoid arthritis, and symptomatic degenerative arthritis.

The goal of treatment is eradication of infection and restoration of maximum joint function. Bacterial sensitivity tests provide a basis for selection of antimicrobial drugs. Operative destruction of the joint by arthrodesis or resection is often necessary to eliminate chronic infection.

Jergesen F, Jawetz E: Pyogenic infections in orthopaedic surgery: Combined antibiotic and closed wound treatment. Am J Surg 106:152, 1963.

SALMONELLA OSTEOMYELITIS & ARTHRITIS

Infection of bones and joints occurs as a complication in less than 1% of cases of typhoid fever. The precise diagnosis depends upon recovery of *Salmonella typhi* from the osteoarticular focus, and treatment is essentially the same as for other salmonella infections and osteomyelitis in general.

In otherwise healthy patients, the bone lesion of salmonellosis is more likely to be solitary and may exhibit any of the protean gross pathologic manifestations of acute or chronic pyogenic osteomyelitis. In infants and children, it commonly affects the metaphysis of a major long bone, especially the lower femur, proximal humerus, or distal tibia. In the adult, in addition to the shafts of long bones, the lesion may be found in the metaphyses or epiphyses; other probable locations include the ribs and spine.

Infants and children with sickle cell disease complicated by antecedent episodes of marrow thrombosis and bone infarction can present a somewhat different picture since there is a tendency toward diaphyseal involvement, multiple foci, and a propensity toward symmetric localization.

The principles of surgical treatment are the same as for pyogenic osteomyelitis.

Constant E & others: Salmonella osteomyelitis of both hands and the hand-foot syndrome. Arch Surg 102:148, 1971.
Engh CA & others: Osteomyelitis in the patient with sickle-cell disease. J Bone Joint Surg 53A:1, 1971.

BRUCELLA OSTEOMYELITIS & ARTHRITIS

Osteoarticular infection due to brucellae is not common in the USA. The manifestations include chronic osteomyelitis, pyogenic arthritis, synovitis, and bursitis. In the USA, *Brucella abortus* and *B suis* are the usual organisms, but *B melitensis* is more common worldwide. Adult men employed in the meat processing or dairy industries and persons who ingest unpasteurized milk products are most likely to be infected.

The osteoarticular lesions appear histologically as caseating or noncaseating granulomas. The lesion caused by *B suis* is more likely to be suppurative and caseous than those caused by other species; the similarity to sarcoidosis and tuberculosis has also been emphasized.

General treatment measures are those applicable to any chronic pyogenic infection, modified when acute symptoms of septicemia are present. Tetracycline, streptomycin, or chloramphenicol is used systemically, although if the drug is administered solely by this route it will not completely penetrate all foci of bone infection.

Seal PV, Morris CA: Brucellosis of the carpus: Report of a case. J Bone Joint Surg 56B:327, 1974.
Serre H & others: Sacro-iliitis due to brucellosis. Sem Hôp Paris 46:3311, 1970.

TUMORS & TUMOR-LIKE LESIONS OF BONE

Primary tumors of bone are relatively uncommon in comparison with secondary or metastatic neoplasms. They are, however, of great clinical significance because of the possibility of malignancy and because some of them grow rapidly and metastasize widely.

Although tumors of bone have been categorized classically as primary or secondary, there is some disagreement about which tumors are primary to the skeleton. Tumors of mesenchymal origin that reflect skeletal tissues (eg, bone, cartilage, and connective tissue) and tumors developing in bones that are of hematopoietic, nerve, vascular, fat cell, and notochordal origin should be differentiated from secondary malignant tumors that involve bone by direct extension or hematogenous spread.

Persistent skeletal pain, localized tenderness, and an enlarging mass, with or without limitation of motion of adjacent joints or spontaneous fracture, are indications for prompt clinical, x-ray, laboratory, and possible biopsy examination. Routine x-ray examination may reveal the location and extent of the lesion, and certain characteristics may suggest a specific diagnosis. Special examinations—laminagraphy, osteography, scintigraphy, etc—may show occult lesions. Arteriography may help to differentiate a benign from a malignant process.

The possibility of benign developmental skeletal abnormalities, metastatic neoplastic disease, infections (eg, osteomyelitis), collagenoses, or metabolic disease of bone must always be kept in mind. If bone tumors occur in or near the joints, they may be confused with the various types of arthritis, especially monarticular arthritis.

Histologic characteristics generally provide the best information about the nature of the lesion, but they must be correlated with all other related facts. The diagnosis of bone tumors is most precise when it is made in close consultation between the clinician, radiologist, and pathologist.

Although prompt action is essential for optimal treatment of certain bone tumors, accurate diagnosis is required because of the great potential for harm which may result either from temporization or from radical or ablative operations or unnecessary irradiation. If conservative treatment is elected, careful clinical and x-ray follow-up and expert consultation are necessary.

The clinical features, treatment, and prognosis of a few primary bone tumors are summarized in Table 45–1.

Table 45-1. Primary bone tumors.

Name and Source	Age and Sex Incidence	Clinical Features*	X-Ray Findings	Treatment	Prognosis
Osteoid osteoma Osteoblastic connective tissue origin	Older children and adolescents. M 2:1.	Small, painful (especially nocturnal), tender tumor of almost any bone, but more often in the femur and tibia	Dense sclerotic lesion with radiolucent center.	Surgical removal.	Good. Removal is curative.
Osteogenic sarcoma Osteoblastic connective tissue derivation	Peak incidence 20 years. Rare over 40 years. Slight male preponderance.	Gradually progressive pain with variable swelling, local heat, venous engorgement, and tenderness, commonly at metaphyses of major long bones; about 50% involve the knee region. Other sites include pelvis, slender long bones, and flat bones. Weight loss, anemia, and elevation of serum alkaline phosphatase occur later. Histologic examination of biopsy specimen is the most useful laboratory procedure.	Variable, depending upon the osteolytic or sclerosing nature of the tumor. Penetration of cortical bone usually occurs with periosteal elevation and extension into soft tissues. Bone spicules perpendicular to the normal cortical surface—"sunburst" effect—may appear in sclerosing lesions. Chest x-ray may reveal pulmonary metastases.	Amputation if accessible and metastases have not occurred. Preliminary reports of results of multidrug chemotherapy combined with surgery appear to show improved survival in some cases.	Poor. Smallest and most distal lesions offer best prognosis. Prognosis less favorable for large tumors and trunk tumors. Five-year overall survival is 5–20%. Death due to widespread metastases.
Fibrosarcoma Nonosteoblastic connective tissue derivation	Adults 30–70 years, but also seen in second decade. M = F.	Similar to above. Differentiation from osteogenic sarcoma depends upon histologic findings. May be a history (very rare) of irradiation exposure of bone many years previously.	Similar to above.	Amputation if accessible, with or without preliminary irradiation.	Poor, but perhaps slightly better than for osteogenic sarcoma.
Enchondroma Cartilaginous derivation	Adults. Rare before 10 years. M = F.	Mild pain, tenderness, or swelling or spontaneous fracture of bones of hands or feet or of metaphyses of major long bones or flat bones. Lesions may be multiple. Histologic examination confirms diagnosis.	Discrete foci of radiolucency with mottling and compartmentalization. Cortical expansion occurs without extensive erosion.	Curettement of solitary nodules.	Usually good. Pelvic lesions may be malignant.
Chondromyxoid fibroma Cartilaginous derivation	Young adults 10–30 years. Rare before 10 years. M = F.	Pain, swelling, tenderness at metaphyses of major long bones, bones of hands or feet, and flat bones. Histologic examination confirms the diagnosis.	Not characteristic. Ovoid or elongated focus of rarefaction and cortical expansion with erosion. May be multiple foci of osteolysis.	Thorough curettement or excision.	Good.
Chondrosarcoma Cartilaginous derivation	Adults 30–60 years, but also found in childhood and adolescence. M = F.	Slow development of pain and swelling of almost any bone, especially long bones, with delayed tendency to metastasis (compare with osteogenic sarcoma).	Irregularly mottled and calcified interior of long bones with fuzzy localized destruction of cortex. Peripheral lesions present a dense, blotchy peripheral outline.	Radical surgical excision or amputation.	If excision is complete, prognosis is excellent. If incomplete, recurrence and progression.

Giant cell tumor (osteoclastoma) Nonosteoblastic connective tissue derivation	10–50 years. M = F.	Pain and swelling at ends of major long bones, especially near knee and lower radius. Also found in other bones of extremities and spine.	Eccentrically located osteolytic focus with expansion and cortical erosion. Roughly spherical foamlike areas in cancellous ends of femur and tibia or in distal radial metaphyses.	Excision preferred to curettement when feasible.	About half are biologically benign and have a favorable outcome regardless of treatment. About a third are aggressive, recur, and require further treatment. The rest are frankly malignant.
Chondroblastoma (epiphyseal giant cell tumor) Cartilaginous derivation	Almost always under 20 years. Predominantly male.	Pain and swelling in epiphyseal areas of major tubular bones and in flat bones.	Ovoid areas of mottled translucency in epiphyses or adjacent metaphyses with demarcating wall of sclerotic bone.	Thorough curettement usually adequate.	Almost always benign. Instances of malignancy reported.
Ewing's sarcoma Mesenchymal connective tissue derivation	Adolescents and young adults, but may occur in children. Slight male preponderance.	Pain, swelling, and tenderness of single or multiple lesions of shafts of major tubular bones, vertebrae, or flat bones of trunk. Later findings include fever, anemia, leukocytosis, and increased sedimentation rate. Biopsy essential for diagnosis. Course may be slow, with remissions and exacerbations to progression with metastases.	Diffuse osteosclerosis of cortex with fusiform configuration, subperiosteal lamination ("onion peel") and occasionally "sunburst" periosteal reaction and medullary destruction evidenced by diffuse rarefaction or mottling.	Supervoltage radiation and chemotherapy.	Very poor. Treatment is palliative. Mortality rate above 95% despite treatment.
Plasma cell myeloma (multiple myeloma) Hematopoietic origin	Adults over 40 years. M 2:1.	Multifocal skeletal involvement. Local pain, swelling, and tendency to pathologic fractures. Spine involvement can cause kyphosis and decreased stature. Late findings include anemia, hypercalcemia, hypercalciuria, hyperglobulinemia, Bence Jones proteinuria, and hyperuricemia. Marrow aspiration or bone biopsy essential for diagnosis. Course may be slow, with remissions and exacerbations.	Variable. Diffuse osteoporosis. Focal lesions appear as diffuse or circumscribed (punched-out) areas of rarefaction without surrounding sclerosis and sometimes with cortical expansion.	X-ray therapy for relief of pain. Chemotherapy (alkylating agents).	Chemotherapy may relieve symptoms and sometimes prolongs life. Average survival is about 1–2 years but may be much longer.

Chalmers J, Heard BE: A metastasizing chordoma: A further note. J Bone Joint Surg 54B:526, 1972.

Dahlin DC: *Bone Tumors,* 2nd ed. Thomas, 1967.

Eyre-Brook AL, Price CHG: Fibrosarcoma of bone: Review of 50 consecutive cases from the Bristol Bone Tumour Registry. J Bone Joint Surg 51B:20, 1969.

Farr GH, Huvos AG: Juxtacortical osteogenic sarcoma: An analysis of fourteen cases. J Bone Joint Surg 54A:1205, 1972.

Goldenberg RR & others: Giant-cell tumor of bone: An analysis of 218 cases. J Bone Joint Surg 52A:619, 1970.

Jaffe N, Watts HG: Multidrug chemotherapy in primary treatment of osteosarcoma: An editorial commentary. J Bone Joint Surg 58A:634, 1976.

Kendrick JI, Evarts CM: Osteoid-osteoma: A critical analysis of 40 tumors. Clin Orthop 54:51, 1967.

Lichtenstein L: *Bone Tumors,* 5th ed. Mosby, 1972.

Lichtenstein L, Sawyer WB: Benign osteoblastoma. J Bone Joint Surg 46A:755, 1964.

Mainzer F & others: The variable manifestations of multiple enchondromatosis. Radiology 99:377, 1971.

Marcove RC & others: Chondrosarcoma of the pelvis and upper end of the femur: An analysis of factors influencing survival time in 113 cases. J Bone Joint Surg 54A:561, 1972.

Marcove RC & others: Osteogenic sarcoma under the age of 21: A review of 145 operative cases. J Bone Joint Surg 52A:411, 1970.

Morton KS: Bone production in non-osteogenic fibroma. J Bone Joint Surg 46B:233, 1964.

Parrish FF, Murray JA: Surgical treatment for secondary neoplastic fractures. J Bone Joint Surg 52A:665, 1970.

Pritchard DJ, Dahlin DC: Ewing's sarcoma: A clinicopathologic and statistical analysis of patients surviving five years or longer. J Bone Joint Surg 56A:1305, 1974.

Schajowicz F, Gallardo H: Chondromyxoid fibroma (fibromyxoid chondroma) of bone: A clinico-pathologic study of thirty-two cases. J Bone Joint Surg 53B:198, 1971.

Schajowicz F, Gallardo H: Epiphysial chondroblastoma of bone: A clinico-pathological study of sixty-nine cases. J Bone Joint Surg 52B:205, 1970.

Shoji H, Miller TR: Reticulum cell sarcoma of bone. Cancer 28:1234, 1971.

Sutow WW & others: Multidrug chemotherapy in primary treatment of osteosarcoma. J Bone Joint Surg 58A:629, 1976.

Tachdjian MO: *Pediatric Orthopedics.* 2 vols. Saunders, 1972.

Velez-Garcia E, Maldonado N: Long-term follow-up therapy in multiple myeloma. Cancer 27:44, 1971.

INJURIES TO THE SPINE

Traumatic injuries to the spine may vary from comparatively minor soft tissue injuries such as contusions, muscle strains, and sprains to severe fracture-dislocations with extensive neurologic impairment. Disease of the spine (eg, osteoarthritis) that existed before the traumatic injury may modify signs and symptoms and adversely affect the prognosis.

These injuries commonly result from indirect violence such as hyperextension or hyperflexion. They may also be caused by axial compression (eg, a blow on the top of the head) or by lateral flexion, torsion, or shearing, either singly or in combination. Blunt trauma is more likely to fracture a spinous process, rarely the lamina, and occasionally a transverse process in the lumbar region. Open fractures are usually due to penetrating injuries.

In most cases of injury to the spine, neither the spinal cord nor the nerve root is injured, but the possibility of such injury, especially in the cervical region, is always present. The greatest permanent disability caused by injury to the spine is due to associated injury to the spinal cord or the spinal nerves. Injury to the cord or nerves may result from displaced bone fragments, portions of the intervertebral disk, or a segment of an intact but dislocated vertebra. Neurologic injury may be caused by the initial accident or may be the result of subsequent manipulation. Initial x-rays do not necessarily reflect the degree of displacement which may have occurred. Severe neurologic deficit may be present even though only minor fracture or minimal subluxation—or neither—can be demonstrated.

Concomitant injury at multiple levels of the spine may occur as the result of severe trauma. Because of its more dramatic clinical findings, a major injury, especially when it is proximal, may mask a lesser one even in the conscious patient. In addition to physical examination, survey x-rays of the entire spine may be warranted in the unconscious patient.

Careful inquiry should be made concerning any period of unconsciousness which may require interpretation of the mechanism of a spinal injury. A precise history of the time of onset of motor or sensory deficit can provide information of prognostic value.

The physical examination must be complete. Superficial soft tissue lesions such as abrasions, contusions, and lacerations may indicate the direction of applied force and its comparative magnitude. Tenderness may suggest the location of a deep lesion. Palpation may reveal an abnormal prominence suggesting a compression fracture of the body, or an abnormal separation of adjacent processes may indicate tearing of posterior ligaments with dislocation.

A record of the neurologic examination must be kept beginning as soon after injury as possible. A clear distinction must be drawn between damage to the spinal cord and to the nerve roots. The time of onset of paraplegia or quadriplegia—whether immediate or delayed—must be noted.

The comparative anatomic level in the spine of neurologic interruption may be determined by x-rays. Comparison of the x-ray findings with the physical findings—which establish the upper level of the total neurologic lesion—will indicate that part due to cord damage and that due to root damage. Retained muscle or sensory function below the level of the cord lesion during the first 24 hours after injury indicates that it is partial; the presence of reflex activity under similar circumstances indicates that function of the distal segment of the cord is not suppressed by spinal shock, which lasts no longer than 24 hours. The presence of reflex activity within 24 hours after injury or its subsequent return without recovery of any sensation or motor function distal to the level of the cord lesion within 24 hours after injury denotes complete and permanent damage to the cord.

The prevention of decubitus ulcers after spine injury with paraplegia or quadriplegia requires stabilization of the injured skeletal segment to permit turning the patient every 2 hours. This can be accomplished by a combination of padded plaster shells, half of which can be removed for proper skin care, and a turning frame. In this way, encircling plaster casts are avoided.

Injuries of the spine are discussed here according to regional location because the extent of any neurologic deficit resulting from spinal cord or nerve injury depends in part upon the level at which injury occurs.

Holdsworth F: Fractures, dislocations, and fracture-dislocations of the spine. J Bone Joint Surg 45B:6, 1963.

SPRAIN OF THE CERVICAL SPINE

Indirect injury of the cervical spine that does not cause fracture or dislocation or objective neurologic disturbance may involve only the muscles and supporting soft tissues of joints; such injuries are considered here. When the extremes of the accustomed range of movements of the cervical spine are exceeded suddenly, the resulting sprain of joints or strain of neck muscles can be manifested predominantly by subjective symptoms. "Whiplash" is a term used to describe a mechanism of injury—sudden hyperflexion followed by extension recoil—that causes a variety of lesions of the cervical region. The term has been construed—especially by the laity—to denote a nonspecific post-traumatic cervical syndrome consequent to motor vehicle accidents. Accidents involving motor vehicles account for most of these injuries; a lesser number are due to sports mishaps.

The diagnosis of sprain of the cervical spine is based upon critical differentiation of this condition from structural lesions of bones and joints that can be demonstrated by x-ray and from lesions of the brain, spinal cord, and nerve roots that produce objective findings. A detailed history of the accident is necessary to assess the significance of certain symptoms. A period of unconsciousness or transitory amnesia immediately after the accident and the presence of other more serious injuries may cause temporary disregard of less dramatic complaints or findings related to the neck. When motor vehicles are involved, an indirect index of severity of injury to the neck region may be suggested by the extent of injury to other parts of the body and by an estimate of the degree of structural damage to the vehicle.

Clinical Findings

A. Symptoms and Signs: The onset of symptoms may be immediate or late. Delayed onset is more often associated with minor injury. The principal clinical feature is dull, aching pain vaguely distributed to the back of the neck and the trapezius regions; it may radiate into the occipital or interscapular region or down the arm. The pain is accentuated by neck movement, and a sensation of stiffness is common; both are relieved by immobility. Radiation of pain to a dermatome supplied by a cervical root should alert the examiner to the possible presence of a lesion involving the respective anatomic segment of the spine. Similar distribution of paresthesia, especially when accompanied by other sensory disturbances such as hypesthesia or hypalgesia, increases the likelihood that a focal lesion is present. Occipital or frontal headache is a frequent complaint. Persistent headache requires investigation of sources other than the neck. Difficulty in swallowing has been attributed to edema of the pharynx, but this indicates a more serious condition than a sprain of the cervical spine. Continuing ocular symptoms such as blurring of vision or diplopia require investigation by an ophthalmologist. Dizziness and tinnitus suggesting vestibular and auditory dysfunction of the eighth cranial nerve are frequent complaints. Posttraumatic vertigo has been attributed to transient ischemia due to vertebral artery injury and to hemorrhage in the labyrinth. When these complaints persist, their assessment requires diagnostic technics such as electroencephalography and vestibular and auditory testing. Functional complaints such as anxiety, inability to concentrate, loss of memory, depression, sweating, and coldness of the extremities are likely to persist in the emotionally labile patient. There is a greater frequency of prolonged complaints following rear end automobile collisions in comparison with those following front-end collisions.

Physical findings require critical evaluation. Restriction of active neck motion is likely to be symmetric and to involve all components. Persistent asymmetric limitation of motion suggests the possibility of fracture or dislocation. Symmetric limitation may be due to unconscious muscle guarding or conscious inhibition. Bizarrely performed active neck movements through a near-average range in all directions and accompanied by theatrical grimacing suggest malingering. Tenderness, like pain, is frequently diffuse, and the site is poorly defined during sequential examinations. Persistent, localized tenderness may identify the site of an occult fracture or joint derangement. Muscle spasm as determined by palpation is difficult to perceive and quantitate because it is commonly associated with diffuse deep tenderness.

B. X-Ray Examination: X-ray examination of the cervical spine must be thorough because differentiation of sprain from other lesions discussed below may depend entirely upon the reliability of this study. In addition to the routine projections, which include lateral views in flexion and extension, laminagraphy and cineradiography may help to differentiate sprain from fracture or dislocation. Myelography can demonstrate intervertebral disk derangements. Patients with osteoarthritis which antedated the injury may exhibit

Table 45—2. Trauma to the cervical spine.

Disorder and Mechanism	Common Symptoms	Common Signs	Neurologic Findings	Radiologic Findings
Sprain of cervical spine due to sudden movement of neck	Dull aching pain in neck radiating to adjacent areas. Stiffness. Relieved by immobility.	Stiffness with symmetric limitation of movement. Diffuse tenderness.	No objective findings.	None.
Dislocations				
Forward bilateral dislocation due to forced flexion with rotation	Localized tenderness posteriorly. Discomfort increased on extension if facets locked.	Head held in slight flexion without tilting.	Neurologic deficits most marked on complete dislocation and may be severe. Incomplete subluxation may have no cord symptoms.	Oblique views and stereoroentgenography needed to detect locked facets.
Unilateral dislocation due to forward flexion with marked rotation	May be only slight pain.	Head in slight flexion with head tilted toward lesion and chin rotated to opposite side. Tenderness over site of dislocation.	Asymmetric and noted on side of displacement.	Upper articular process displaced forward. Body of vertebra displaced forward less than half its depth. Spinous process rotated to side of dislocation.
Unilateral subluxation due to minimal injury; can occur in sleep	Slight discomfort on neck movements.	Head tilted away from side of subluxation and held immobile. Resistance to movements to affected side.	None.	Dislocation may show on lateral stereoroentgenograms.
Atlantoaxial dislocation (traumatic; after URI in children and in arthritis)	Pain is mild to severe. Tenderness is suboccipital.	Head rotated from affected side and tilted toward it in unilateral subluxation. In bilateral, head is flexed and chin down. Movements restricted.	Can be severe in traumatic type and may cause instant death. Variable in other forms.	Subluxation (incomplete dislocation) will show on lateral stereoroentgenograms.
Extension dislocation due to forced extension with rotation	Pain on head or neck movement.	Head held rigidly. Position depends on presence of dislocation.	Incomplete or extensive cord lesions.	Widening of space of involved disk. Dislocation may or may not be present.
Fractures				
Fracture of atlas due to severe blow to top of head	Pain in suboccipital region. Headache.	Restriction of neck movements.	Usually none.	Fracture clefts seen on special views.
Fracture of odontoid process due to complex stresses and shearing force	Suboccipital pain, headache. May have associated injuries of accident.	Severe restriction of movement.	No neurologic lesion in undisplaced fracture.	Fracture observed usually on standard films; laminagrams may be needed.
Compression fracture of vertebral body due to blow to head	Localized pain.	Restriction of movement.	Usually none unless dislocation occurs.	Wedge-shaped deformity seen in lateral x-rays. Dislocation may occur or may have reduced spontaneously.
Comminuted fracture of vertebral body due to severe blow on head	Localized pain and headache. Unconsciousness.	Severe restriction of movement.	High incidence of neurologic complications.	X-ray shows fragmented body of vertebra. Posteroinferior fragment may be driven into spinal canal.
Fracture of spinous process due to severe flexion (avulsion) or severe extension	Pain in back of neck; localized tenderness.	Restriction and guarding of movements.	None.	Lateral views usually show fracture, but oblique views may be needed.
Fracture of odontoid process of axis and dislocation of atlas due to severe complex forces	Suboccipital pain, headache. May be associated injuries.	Severe restriction of movement.	May have some neurologic findings.	Fracture usually observed in standard films. Special views or technics may be needed.
Fracture-dislocation of axis (rare)	Suboccipital pain.	Restriction of movement.	Usually none.	Dislocation of axis seen on roentgenograms.
Compression fracture of vertebral body with dislocation	Localized pain.	Restriction of movement.	Neurologic complications may occur.	Standard x-rays usually show fracture and displacement.
Lateral flexion fracture-dislocation	Unilateral localized pain.	Restriction of motion with head tilted toward lesion.	Asymmetric lesions of cord or brachial plexus.	Oblique views needed to show facet subluxation. Other technics may be needed.

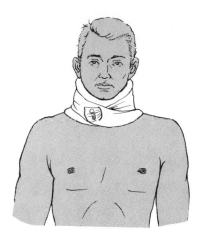

Figure 45–3. Cervical collar.

restriction of motion in the lower cervical segments when the involved joint is more proximal.

Treatment

Immobilization may be accomplished by external cervical support such as a felt collar (Fig 45–3) or by recumbency at bed rest; light cervical traction by means of a head halter can give further relief from discomfort. Analgesics and sedatives for apprehensive patients generally suffice for relief of mild pain. Some observers find that muscle relaxants are helpful. A persistent localized area of pain and tenderness may respond favorably to local anesthetic injections. The application of heat or cold may give temporary relief from pain.

Prognosis

Where litigation or emotional lability is not a factor, symptoms generally respond promptly to conservative measures. Younger patients can be expected to become asymptomatic more rapidly than older ones with osteoarthritis.

Breck LW & others: Medicolegal aspects of cervical spine sprains. Clin Orthop 74:124, 1971.

Burke DC: Hyperextension injuries of the spine. J Bone Joint Surg 53B:3, 1971.

Janes JM, Hooshmand H: Extension-flexion injury of the neck. Mayo Clin Proc 40:353, 1965.

Pang LQ: The otological aspects of whiplash injuries. Laryngoscope 81:1331, 1971.

Williams JS & others: The nature of seat belt injuries. J Trauma 11:207, 1971.

DISLOCATIONS, FRACTURES, & FRACTURE-DISLOCATIONS OF THE CERVICAL REGION

Dislocations, fractures, and fracture-dislocations of the cervical spine comprise fewer than 1% of all cervical spine injuries. Concomitant injury to the cord and nerve roots can be expected in about 25% of severe injuries to the cervical spine. Injuries that reduce the diameter of the spinal canal account for most instances of lesions of the cord or nerve roots. Any neck injury severe enough to cause these lesions also involves the possibility of neurologic damage, and this hazard exists from the moment of the accident until any displacement of anatomic structures has been corrected and permanent stability provided. Extensive damage to the cord may be present without x-ray evidence of fracture or dislocation, and, conversely, dramatic skeletal injury may be present without neurologic deficit.

The diagnosis is suggested by the history and confirmed by physical examination and x-ray studies. Accurate diagnosis of the extent of skeletal and neurologic injury is essential to treatment, which should be started as soon as possible. In addition to the general examination, the patient with neurologic deficit must be evaluated within the first 24 hours to differentiate between complete and partial spinal cord injury.

The fourth cervical cord segment is situated at about the level of the body of the third cervical vertebra. Therefore, a complete lesion at this site or at a more proximal point causes death by respiratory paralysis. An incomplete lesion may be identified by spared perianal sensation and the presence of any voluntary action of the toe flexors. Permanent and complete division of the distal cord segment from the proximal segment can be assumed if these minimal findings are not present within 24 hours after injury. Some improvement of motor, sensory, and reflex function can be anticipated if findings of cord sparing are exhibited within 24 hours after injury. Spinal cord sparing must be distinguished from recovery of function temporarily lost because of root injury. Voluntary bowel and bladder control may be recovered in partial cord lesions when motor and sensory function of the sacral segments is retained. Reflex automatic bowel and bladder function may be recovered after complete cord lesions when anal and bulbocavernosus reflex activity is preserved.

Other mechanisms of injury and other lesions may also cause spinal cord disruption. Forced flexion can cause retropulsion of the nucleus pulposus even though compression fracture of the body or complete dislocation does not occur. This mechanism may cause serious cord damage when associated with minor wedge-shaped compression fracture of the body. Forced extension with or without dislocation may also cause cord damage.

Partial loss of cord function may occur as a result of contusion injuries to the cervical spine without apparent alteration of bony alignment. When this occurs, damage to the posterior columns and the lateral spinothalamic tracts may be either transient or permanent, and the resulting impairment of motor function is greater in the upper extremities than in the lower. Bladder dysfunction and varying degrees of sensory loss below the level of the lesion can also be present.

Return of bladder function follows motor recovery in the lower extremities, and both precede return of muscle function in the upper extremities. Sensory deficit varies from minor to complete and immediate loss, and recovery does not follow any predictable pattern. Vascular insufficiency caused by compression of the vertebral arteries may be an indirect mechanism of damage to the cord which may account for the minimal or absent sensory impairment observed in some patients.

Radiologic Examination

The surgeon should supervise transfer of the patient to the x-ray table for the preliminary examination. Further injury may be avoided by temporary stabilization with an adjustable brace or by light traction applied manually with a head halter. Initial anteroposterior and lateral films of the entire cervical and upper thoracic spines should be taken to determine whether any extensive skeletal lesion is present. If so, the configuration of the fracture, the extent and direction of displacement of bone fragments, and the presence of dislocation will dictate whether to initiate skeletal traction before further manipulation to accomplish definitive x-ray studies. Routine studies should include films prepared in both oblique projections and open-mouth odontoid views. When these studies do not adequately demonstrate suspected lesions, special technics such as laminagraphy and cineradiography may be helpful. Myelography is useful to localize obstruction of the spinal canal and to differentiate complete from incomplete blockage. When evidence of neurologic deficit is lacking and dislocation is not apparent, films may be prepared in the lateral projection with actively assisted but limited flexion and extension to determine whether gross instability exists.

Treatment

A prime objective of treatment is to protect the spinal cord, spinal nerves, and vertebral arteries during transportation of the patient, during diagnostic and x-ray procedures, and throughout definitive treatment.

A. Emergency Treatment: Initially, the patient can be transported on a flat surface in the supine decubitus position with bolsters at the side of the head and neck to prevent rotation. When medical help becomes available, a head halter with 3–4 kg of force directed axially to the spine while maintaining the head in anatomic posture can be substituted for the bolsters.

B. Definitive Treatment: Although the head halter is useful for the application of heavy traction for short periods, it is not suitable for continuous traction because more than 3–4 kg of force causes pain in the regions of the chin and occiput. When halter traction is used continuously for prolonged periods, even with light loads, the submental region and the occiput should be carefully padded to prevent pressure necrosis of skin and ulceration. Skeletal traction applied to the cranial vault or the zygomatic arches will support as much as 30 kg of force over prolonged periods without causing significant discomfort. To effect closed reduc-

tion after application of a skeletal traction apparatus, the initial force of 5–8 kg is gradually increased by increments of 2.5 kg every 30 minutes with the patient awake and with periodic physical examination and x-ray control. Gentle and limited manipulation of the head during this critical period may be necessary to facilitate reduction. Once this has been accomplished, the force is gradually reduced to 4–5 kg, which is usually sufficient to maintain reduction.

Closed reduction by manipulation with concomitant skull traction under general anesthesia can be effective in the hands of experts. Heavy manual traction and forceful manipulation, with or without general anesthesia, are hazardous to the spinal cord and nerves.

Dislocations of Cervical Spine

Braakman R, Vinken PJ: Unilateral facet interlocking in the lower cervical spine. J Bone Joint Surg 49B:249, 1967.

Burke DC: Hyperextension injuries of the spine. J Bone Joint Surg 53B:3, 1971.

Burke DC, Berryman D: The place of closed manipulation in the management of flexion-rotation dislocations of the cervical spine. J Bone Joint Surg 53B:165, 1971.

Holdsworth F: Fractures, dislocations, and fracture-dislocations of the spine. J Bone Joint Surg 52A:1534, 1970.

Schneider RC, Schemm GW: Vertebral artery insufficiency in acute and chronic spinal trauma. J Neurosurg 18:348, 1961.

Stauffer ES & others: Diagnosis and prognosis of acute cervical spinal cord injury. J Bone Joint Surg 53A:1242, 1971.

Fractures of Cervical Spine

Ewald FC: Fracture of the odontoid process in a seventeen-month-old infant treated with a halo. J Bone Joint Surg 53A:1636, 1971.

Holdsworth F: Fractures, dislocations, and fracture-dislocations of the spine. J Bone Joint Surg 52A:1534, 1970.

Schatzker J & others: Fractures of the dens (odontoid process). J Bone Joint Surg 53B:392, 1971.

Sherk HH, Nicholson JT: Fractures of the atlas. J Bone Joint Surg 52A:1017, 1970.

Fracture-Dislocations of Cervical Spine

Cornish BL: Traumatic spondylolisthesis of the axis. J Bone Joint Surg 50B:31, 1968.

Prolo DJ & others: The injured cervical spine: Immediate and long-term immobilization with the halo. JAMA 224:591, 1973.

Roaf R: Lateral flexion injuries of the cervical spine. J Bone Joint Surg 45B:36, 1963.

FRACTURES OF THE THORACIC SPINE

The thoracic spine is comparatively stable. Fracture results either from direct violence, which may involve only a spinous process; or indirect violence, which may result in compression of the body of the vertebra. Occasionally an avulsion fracture of the spinous process of the seventh cervical or first thoracic vertebra is caused by muscle activity ("clay shoveler's fracture").

Compression fractures of the thoracic vertebrae are rare in young children and are caused only by severe trauma in older children. In this age group, therefore, unless there is a positive history of severe trauma, a wedge-shaped deformity in the thoracic spine should suggest pathologic fracture. This must not be confused with Calvé's or Scheuermann's disease or deformity due to traumatic fracture.

Minimal (frequently unrecognized) trauma may cause compression fracture of the body of the thoracic vertebrae in adults with osteoporosis. Disability is not great, and reduction is not indicated. If rest in bed for 3–4 days does not relieve the pain, a surgical corset with shoulder restraints or brace (Taylor or Arnold type) may provide comfort and permit early ambulation.

Compression fractures of the thoracic spine caused by severe trauma are characterized by wedge-shaped deformity of the vertebral body. No adequate method has been devised for the reduction of these injuries. However, because of the inherent stability of the thoracic spine, prolonged immobilization is not necessary. In fracture of the upper thoracic region, if immobilization is required for relief of pain, a long plaster Minerva jacket that includes the iliac crests may be the only adequate method of external support that will provide relief from pain.

Rotational fracture-dislocations near the thoracolumbar junction and shear fractures of the thoracic spine are commonly associated with paraplegia. Rotational fracture-dislocation is inherently unstable because of extensive rupture of supporting ligaments, fracture of the vertebral body in the transverse plane, and disruption of the articular facet joints by fracture or dislocation. These fractures may or may not be stable, and fusion may be necessary to minimize injury to the cord.

Shear fracture is a term used to describe a fracture-dislocation of the thoracic spine whereby dislocation takes place at or near the intervertebral disk with fracture of the articular processes or the pedicles. Forward displacement takes place in the transverse plane.

Holdsworth F: Fractures, dislocations, and fracture-dislocations of the spine. J Bone Joint Surg 52A:1534, 1970.
Roberts JB, Curtiss PH Jr: Stability of the thoracic and lumbar spine in traumatic paraplegia following fracture or fracture-dislocation. J Bone Joint Surg 52A:1115, 1970.

FRACTURES OF THE LUMBAR SPINE

Uncomplicated Compression Fractures

Compression fractures of the vertebral bodies caused by hyperflexion injury are the most common fractures of the lumbar spine and occur most often near the thoracolumbar junction. The widespread use of seat belts in automobiles has been accompanied by an increasing incidence of fractures that occur near the lumbosacral level as the result of accidents. More than one vertebral body is often involved, but deformity may be greatest in one segment. Acute angulation of the spine caused by a compression deformity of the body of a vertebra may be associated with varying degrees of disruption of the facet joints, from sprain to complete dislocation.

Anteroposterior, lateral, and oblique x-rays are required to demonstrate the characteristic lesions such as wedge-shaped deformity of the body and the presence of dislocation of the facets, comminuted fracture of the body, and fracture of the pedicle. Laminagraphy is a useful adjunctive technic for disclosure of lesions that might not be demonstrated by routine x-ray studies.

Treatment depends upon the age of the patient, the presence of preexisting disease, and the severity of injury. In older patients with preexisting degenerative arthritis where there is mild deformity involving no more than one-fourth of the anterior height of the body of the vertebra, the surgeon may elect not to reduce the deformity but merely to place the patient at bed rest for a few days. As soon as acute pain is relieved, the back should be braced and increasing physical activity encouraged within the tolerance of pain. In the more active age group when the compression deformity involves more than one-half of the anterior height of the body of the vertebra, reduction by hyperextension and immobilization in a plaster jacket (Fig 45–4) is the treatment preferred by some surgeons for these uncomplicated fractures.

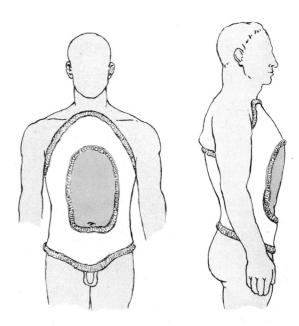

Figure 45–4. Hyperextension plaster for compression fracture of the lumbar spine.

Comminuted Fractures

Comminuted fracture of the vertebral body is characterized by disruption of the adjacent intervertebral disks and varying degrees of displacement of the fragments. The end plates of the body are forced into the centrum together with the disk. The extent of fragmentation (comminution) of the body depends upon the severity of the causative injury. A large fragment of the body may be displaced anteriorly. Posteriorly displaced fragments are apt to cause compression of the cord or cauda equina; and the facet joints may be fractured or dislocated. Therefore, careful physical and x-ray examinations are mandatory before treatment is instituted.

The method of treatment may be dictated by the extent of bone injury and the presence of neurologic complications. When neurologic involvement is absent and comminution is not manifest by extensive fragmentation, reduction may not be necessary. Under these circumstances, immobilization in a plaster jacket may be sufficient. It must be determined whether dislocation has occurred or is likely because of posterior element injury (see below). Mobilization of the patient from recumbency should be controlled by periodic physical and x-ray examinations to determine incipient displacement of fragments which may herald or accompany the onset of neurologic deficit. When the posterior elements are intact and compression of the body has been greater than one-fourth to one-third its former height, reduction by extension of the spine and immobilization in a plaster jacket should be considered in young adults. When cauda equina injury has occurred, laminectomy may be indicated, in which case spine fusion may also be performed. Bone healing is likely to be slow, and immobilization should be prolonged until stabilization has occurred. Cautiously executed biplane bending x-ray studies give helpful guidance in determining the soundness of healing and the extent to which mechanical stability is restored.

Fracture of the Transverse Processes

Fracture of the transverse processes may result from direct violence, such as a crushing injury, or may be incidental to a more serious fracture of the lumbar spine. It may result also from violent muscle contraction alone. One or more segments may be involved. If displacement is minimal, soft tissue injury is likely to be minor. Extensive displacement of the fragments indicates severe soft tissue tearing and hematoma formation.

Treatment depends upon the presence or absence of associated injuries. If fracture of the transverse process is the sole injury, and if pain is not severe upon guarded motions of the back, strapping and prompt ambulation may be sufficient. If displacement and soft tissue injury are extensive, bed rest for a few days followed by prolonged support in a corset or brace may be necessary and slow symptomatic recovery may be anticipated.

FRACTURE-DISLOCATION OF THE LUMBAR SPINE

Severe compression trauma may cause fracture-dislocation with rupture of one disk or, if comminution occurs, rupture of 2 disks. Varying degrees of injury to the posterior elements occur, including unilateral or bilateral dislocation of the facets or fracture of the pedicles or facets. Accompanying fractures of spinous and transverse processes, and tearing of the posterior ligaments and adjacent muscles can add to the complexity of this severe lesion. The dislocation of the upper segment may be solely in the anteroposterior plane, or it may be complex, with additional displacement in the coronal plane with torsion around the longitudinal axis of the spine.

Treatment depends upon the type of injury. If there is no neurologic involvement and dislocation was associated with fracture of the pedicles or facets, reduction may be attempted by cautious extension with traction on the lower extremities under x-ray control without anesthesia. When dislocation has been corrected, immobilization in a plaster body cast with a spica extension to incorporate at least one thigh may be necessary for adequate support. Mobilization of the patient from the recumbent position should be accomplished slowly because displacement of fragments can occur and neurologic complications may result. When reasonable doubt exists, it is preferred to continue recumbency for 8–12 weeks until initial healing has provided mechanical stability. If closed reduction is not successful, or if extension causes neurologic symptoms, the attempt should be abandoned at once in favor of open reduction.

In complete dislocation of one or both facets, reduction can be accomplished by open operation.

Fletcher BD, Brogden BG: Seat-belt fractures of the spine and sternum. JAMA 200:167, 1967.

Holdsworth F: Fractures, dislocations, and fracture-dislocations of the spine. J Bone Joint Surg 52A:1534, 1970.

Rennie W, Mitchell N: Flexion distraction fractures of the thoracolumbar spine. J Bone Joint Surg 55A:386, 1973.

Young MH: Long-term consequences of stable fractures of the thoracic and lumbar vertebral bodies. J Bone Joint Surg 55B:295, 1973.

FRACTURE OF THE SACRUM

Fracture of the sacrum may accompany fracture of the pelvis. It may also appear as an isolated lesion as a result of direct violence. Linear fracture of the sacrum without displacement should be treated symptomatically. Strapping of the buttocks of males and the wearing of a snug girdle by females can provide some comfort during the acutely painful stage. If the fracture extends through a sacral foramen and is associated with displacement, there may be injury to one of the sacral nerves and consequent neurologic deficit. If the sacral fragment is displaced anteriorly, reduction should be attempted by means of bimanual manipulation. Great care should be exercised to prevent injury to the rectal wall by pressure of the palpating finger against a sharp spicule of underlying bone.

FRACTURE OF THE COCCYX

Fracture of the coccyx is usually the result of a blow on the buttock. No specific treatment is required other than protection. Strapping the buttocks together for a few days may minimize pain. Pressure on the coccygeal region can be avoided by selecting a firm chair in which to sit or placing a support beneath the thighs to relieve pressure. The patient should be warned that pain may persist for many weeks. Fracture-dislocation can be reduced by bimanual manipulation, but recurrence of the deformity is likely. Every effort toward conservative management should be made before coccygectomy is considered for treatment of the painful unhealed or malunited fracture.

FRACTURES OF THE PELVIS

AVULSION FRACTURES OF THE PELVIS

Avulsion fractures of the pelvis include those involving the anterior superior and anterior inferior iliac spines, a portion of the iliac crest epiphysis anteriorly, and the apophysis of the ischium. The ischial apophysis may be avulsed indirectly by violent contraction of the hamstring muscles in the older child or adolescent. If displacement is minimal, prompt healing without disability is to be expected. If displacement is marked (ie, more than 1 cm), reattachment by open operation is justifiable.

Barnes ST, Hinds RB: Pseudotumor of the ischium: A late manifestation of avulsion of the ischial epiphysis. J Bone Joint Surg 54A:645, 1972.

Godshal RW, Hansen CA: Incomplete avulsion of a portion of the iliac epiphysis: An injury of young athletes. J Bone Joint Surg 55A:1301, 1973.

FRACTURE OF THE WING OF THE ILIUM

Isolated fracture of the wing of the ilium without involvement of the hip or sacroiliac joints most often occurs as a result of direct trauma. With minor displacement of the free fragment, soft tissue injury is usually minimal and treatment is symptomatic. Wide displacement of the free fragment may be associated with extensive soft tissue injury and hematoma formation. Healing may be accompanied by ossification of the hematoma with exuberant new bone formation.

ISOLATED FRACTURE OF THE OBTURATOR RING

Isolated fracture of the obturator ring, involving either the pubis or ischium with minimal displacement, is associated with little or no injury to the sacroiliac joints. This is also true of minor subluxation of the symphysis pubica. Initial treatment consists of bed rest for a few days followed by ambulation on crutches. A sacroiliac belt or pelvic binder may give additional comfort. As soon as discomfort disappears, unsupported weight-bearing may be permitted.

COMPLEX FRACTURES OF THE PELVIC RING

Complex fractures of the pelvic ring are due either to direct violence or to force transmitted indirectly through the lower extremities. They are characterized by disruption of the pelvic ring at 2 points: (1) anteriorly, near the symphysis pubica, manifested either by dislocation of that joint or by fracture through the body of the pubis, by unilateral or bilateral fracture through the obturator ring, or by fracture through the acetabulum; and (2) disruption of the pelvic ring through or in the vicinity of the sacroiliac joint. The disruption can extend partially through the sacroiliac joint as a dislocation and extend into the sacrum or into the adjacent ilium as a fracture. The magnitude of displacement of the fragments may indicate the severity of soft tissue injury. These complex injuries are often associated with extensive hemorrhage into the soft tissues or injury to the bladder, urethra, or intra-abdominal organs. When anterior and posterior disruptions are ipsilateral, the entire involved hemipelvis and extremity may be displaced proximally. Anterior disruption may occur on one side, and posterior disruption on the opposite side with wide opening of the pelvic ring.

When severe and complex fractures of the pelvic ring are suspected, the extent of associated injuries must be determined at once by physical and x-ray examination. Shock due to blood loss may be present. Treatment of the fracture by reduction should not be instituted until the extent of associated injuries has been determined. Treatment of some of those injuries may be more urgent than that of the fracture lesion. A careful search must be made for possible injury to bowel, bladder, ureters, and major blood vessels (see Chapter 43).

If displacement and soft tissue injury are minimal, a pelvic sling to facilitate nursing care may be all that is required. When the hemipelvis has been displaced proximally, skeletal traction on the distal end of the femur on the affected side with suspension of the extremity may permit reduction.

If the sacroiliac joint has been dislocated and the ilium is rotated posterior to the sacrum, with opening of the anterior fracture, closed reduction can be attempted. Postmanipulation maintenance of reduction is accomplished by a pelvic sling or a short bilateral thigh spica.

Cass AS, Ireland CW: Bladder trauma associated with pelvic fractures in severely injured patients. J Trauma 13:205, 1973.

Margolies MN & others: Arteriography in the management of hemorrhage from pelvic fractures. N Engl J Med 287:317, 1972.

Patterson FP, Morton KS: Neurological complications of fractures and dislocations of the pelvis. J Trauma 12:1013, 1972.

INJURIES OF THE SHOULDER GIRDLE

FRACTURE OF THE CLAVICLE

Fracture of the clavicle may occur as a result of direct trauma or indirect force transmitted through the shoulder. Most fractures of the clavicle are seen in the distal half, commonly at the junction of the middle and distal thirds. About two-thirds of clavicular fractures occur in children. Birth fractures of the clavicle vary from greenstick to complete displacement and must be differentiated from congenital pseudarthrosis.

Because of the relative fixation of the medial fragment and the weight of the arm, the distal fragment is displaced downward and toward the midline. Anteroposterior x-rays should always be taken, but oblique projections are occasionally of more value. Although injury to the brachial plexus or subclavian vessels is not common, such complications can usually be demonstrated on physical examination.

Treatment

Fracture of the outer third of the clavicle distal to the coracoclavicular ligaments is comparable to dislocation of the acromioclavicular joint. If the coracoclavicular ligaments are intact and the fragments are not widely displaced, immobilization in a sling and swathe is adequate. If the coracoclavicular ligaments have been

lacerated and extensive displacement of the main medial fragment is present, treatment is similar to that advocated for acromioclavicular dislocation.

A. Without Displacement: Immobilization of greenstick fractures is not required in children, and healing is rapid. Complete fractures should be immobilized for 10–21 days. A figure-of-eight dressing made of sheet cotton and an elastic bandage is adequate (Fig 45–5). In adolescents and adults, treatment is by immobilization in a sling and swathe for 4–6 weeks.

B. With Displacement: In infants and small children, apply a figure-of-eight dressing of sheet cotton and elastic bandage reinforced with adhesive tape. Healing usually takes 2–4 weeks. Older children and adolescents require reduction by closed manipulation and immobilization with a figure-of-eight dressing reinforced with plaster. Reduction need not be exact, since exuberant callus formation will be partially or completely obliterated by remodeling of bone architecture incidental to the late stage of the fracture reparative process.

C. With Displacement or Comminution (in Adults):

1. Closed reduction—Comminuted fractures of the clavicle with displacement can usually be managed successfully by closed reduction, although in women greater effort must be made to secure accurate realign-

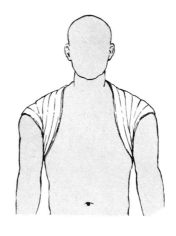

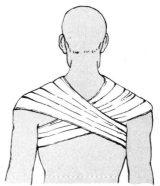

Figure 45–5. Figure-of-eight dressing.

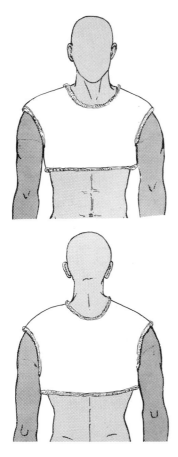

Figure 45—6. Plaster shoulder spica for fracture of clavicle

ment without deformity. Fractured surfaces of displaced fragments which cannot be reduced closed can sometimes be manipulated into apposition by seizing the main fragments percutaneously with large towel clamps. A plaster shoulder spica (Fig 45—6) gives more secure immobilization than the figure-of-eight dressing. Immobilization must be maintained for 6—12 weeks. The patient should remain ambulatory if possible, but in some cases the position of the fragments requires bed rest initially, with skin traction applied to the abducted upper arm and a sandbag between the shoulders to permit the distal fragment to fall into position and to aid in maintaining reduction. Recumbency in this position may be necessary for 5—6 weeks or even longer until stabilization has occurred.

2. Open reduction—Open reduction may be justifiable occasionally to prevent delay of healing where there is interposition of soft tissue.

Gibson DA, Carroll N: Congenital pseudarthrosis of the clavicle. J Bone Joint Surg 52B:629, 1970.

ACROMIOCLAVICULAR DISLOCATION

Dislocation of the acromioclavicular joint may be incomplete or complete. A history of a blow or fall on the tip of the shoulder can often be obtained. The acromial end of the clavicle is displaced upward and backward; the shoulder falls downward and inward. Careful physical examination generally demonstrates this deformity. Anteroposterior x-rays should be taken of both shoulders with the patient erect. Displacement is more likely to be demonstrated when the patient holds a 5—8 kg weight in each hand. An axillary projection will demonstrate backward displacement of the acromial end of the clavicle.

Incomplete dislocation (subluxation) is associated with only minor tearing of the acromioclavicular ligaments, since complete dislocation requires concomitant rupture of the conoid and trapezoid components of the coracoclavicular ligament. These ligaments may be torn within their substance, or they may be avulsed with adjacent periosteum from the acromial end of the clavicle.

Treatment

Unreduced acromioclavicular dislocations usually cause no disability; however, painful posttraumatic arthritis may require excision of the distal 4 cm of the clavicle. In general, reduction is indicated for both complete and incomplete acute dislocations.

A. Incomplete Dislocation: When displacement is minimal, initial treatment may be by sling until acute pain from movement and the weight of the upper extremity has been relieved. Stimson's dressing (Fig 45—7) can be used for injuries of intermediate severity, where displacement is greater but not complete. This dressing must be maintained for at least 4 weeks; frequent adjustment is necessary to maintain immobilization in the correct position. The patient is encouraged to sleep in a semireclining position.

B. Complete Dislocation: It is difficult to maintain reduction and adequate immobilization of com-

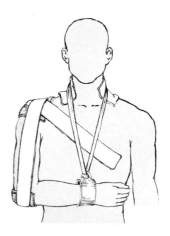

Figure 45—7. Stimson's dressing.

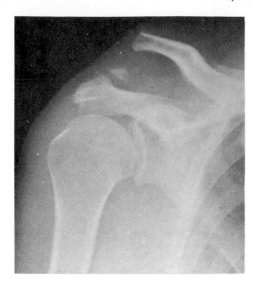

Figure 45–8. Complete dislocation of the acromioclavicular joint in a 41-year-old man. Wide separation of the clavicle from the coracoid process indicates complete tear of the conoid and trapezoid ligaments.

plete acromioclavicular dislocations by closed methods. Stimson's dressing or its modifications may be used successfully only if the patient can be kept under constant observation and frequent x-ray examinations made.

Open operation performed within the first 3 weeks after complete acromioclavicular dislocation offers the best hope of restoring anatomic alignment. If it is deferred longer, the ligaments will have partially healed with elongation and the deformity can be expected to recur when immobilization is discontinued unless the ligaments have been reconstructed. Open reduction, when performed soon after injury, should be supplemented by temporary internal stabilization of either the acromioclavicular joint or the coracoclavicular relationship even though there has been no ligamentous damage. Torn ligaments should be repaired by suture or reconstructive technics.

Old and unreduced dislocations with secondary osteoarthritis can be treated by resection of the segment of the clavicle between the acromioclavicular joint and the conoid and trapezoid ligaments; when gross displacement and marked instability are present, supplementary reconstruction of the damaged coracoclavicular ligament is indicated.

Ahstrom JP: Surgical repair of complete acromioclavicular separation. JAMA 217:785, 1971.
Weaver JK, Dunn HK: Treatment of acromioclavicular injuries, especially complete acromioclavicular separation. J Bone Joint Surg 54A:1187, 1972.

STERNOCLAVICULAR DISLOCATION

Displacement of the sternal end of the clavicle may occur superiorly, anteriorly, or, less commonly, inferiorly. Retrosternal displacement is rare. Complete dislocation can be diagnosed by physical examination. Anteroposterior and oblique x-rays confirm the diagnosis. Laminagraphy may also be helpful.

For incomplete dislocation, a plaster shoulder spica is adequate. Complete dislocations are not difficult to reduce, but external dressings are not adequate to maintain reduction. Open reduction with repair of torn sternoclavicular and costoclavicular ligaments with or without internal fixation are normally required to maintain adequate reduction of complete dislocations. Additional protection by external immobilization should be continued at least while the internal fixation apparatus is in situ.

Painful symptoms caused by posttraumatic degenerative arthritis from anatomically reduced or unreduced sternoclavicular dislocation may be persistent. Extraperiosteal resection of the medial two-thirds of the clavicle may be necessary for relief.

Elting JJ: Retrosternal dislocation of the clavicle. Arch Surg 104:35, 1972.

FRACTURE OF THE SCAPULA

Fracture of the neck of the scapula is most often caused by a blow on the shoulder or by a fall on the outstretched arm. The degree of fragmentation varies from a crack to extensive comminution. The main glenoid fragment may be impacted into the body fragment. The treatment of impacted or undisplaced fractures in patients 40 years of age or older should be directed toward the preservation of shoulder joint function, since stiffness may cause prolonged disability. In young adults especially, unstable fractures require arm traction with the arm at right angles to the trunk for about 4 weeks and protection in a sling and swathe for an additional 2–4 weeks. Open reduction is rarely required even for major displaced fragments except for those involving the articular surface when associated with dislocation of the humeral head. These fractures are likely to involve only a segment of the articular surface and may be impacted. When it is displaced, accurate reposition of the minor fragment is desirable because of the likelihood of secondary glenohumeral osteoarthritis (discussed below).

Fracture of the acromion or spine of the scapula requires reduction only when the displaced fragment is apt to cause interference with abduction of the shoulder. Persistence of an acromial epiphysis should not be confused with fracture.

Fracture of the coracoid process may result from violent muscular contraction or, rarely, may be associated with anterior dislocation of the shoulder joint.

When fracture of the body of the scapula is caused by direct violence, fractures of underlying ribs may be associated. Treatment of uncomplicated fracture should be directed toward the comfort of the patient and the preservation of shoulder joint function.

Aston JW Jr, Gregory CF: Dislocation of the shoulder with significant fracture of the glenoid. J Bone Joint Surg 55A:1531, 1973.

Benton J, Nelson C: Avulsion of the coracoid process in an athlete: Report of a case. J Bone Joint Surg 53A:356, 1971.

FRACTURE OF THE PROXIMAL HUMERUS

Fracture of the proximal humerus occurs most frequently during the sixth decade. It is commonly the result of indirect injury such as a fall on the hand with the arm outstretched. Swelling of the shoulder region with visible or palpable deformity and restriction of motion due to pain are the most prominent clinical features. The precise diagnosis is established by x-rays prepared perpendicular to the plane of the scapula and a lateral view made at a right angle to the former, tangential to the body of the scapula. The transthoracic projection may be inadequate to demonstrate detail because of interference by the ribs and spine. Axillary x-rays are helpful to demonstrate the direction of any displacement of the head of the humerus from the glenoid or infractions involving the articular surfaces of the shoulder joint.

This discussion follows a classification of proximal humeral fractures proposed by Neer which is based on the presence or absence of displacement of the articular surface of the humeral head, greater tuberosity, lesser tuberosity, and shaft.

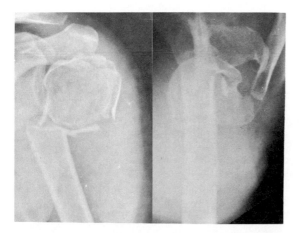

Figure 45—9. Comminuted fracture of the proximal humerus involving the surgical neck and greater tuberosity in a 44-year-old woman. The uninjured lesser tuberosity suggests that the articular fragment retains some blood supply.

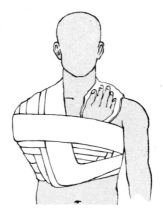

Figure 45—10. Velpeau dressing.

Undisplaced Fractures of the Proximal Humerus

Undisplaced or minimally displaced fractures of the proximal humerus—with the exception of those of the anatomic neck—require little treatment beyond guarding of the shoulder by the use of a sling until discomfort is tolerable and, subsequently, judicious exercise. Restoration of firm bone continuity occurs in about 8—12 weeks.

Single Fractures of the Proximal Humerus

A. Fracture of the Anatomic Neck: Isolated fracture of the anatomic neck of the humerus is uncommon and may be followed by avascular necrosis of the articular fragment even in the absence of displacement. Malhealing of displaced fractures may cause limitation of shoulder motion. When displacement is the determinant of open operation, primary humeral prosthetic arthroplasty is likely to provide a more satisfactory long-term result than anatomic replacement of the devascularized articular fragment.

B. Fracture of the Surgical Neck: The main fracture cleft is distal to the tuberosities. Minor comminution of the proximal segment can be disregarded when displacement of those fragments does not occur. Some angulation is likely to accompany any displacement in the transverse plane of the humerus. The apex of angulation is generally directed anteriorly, but its direction should be accurately determined by biplane x-rays. When angulation greater than 45 degrees occurs in the active person, it should be corrected to avoid subsequent restriction of abduction and elevation. Lesser degrees of deformity do not require manipulation, especially when encountered in elderly persons. Impacted and minimally angulated fractures can be treated by means of a sling.

When displacement at the fracture site is complete, the free end of the distal fragment lies medially, and anteriorly (in relation to the proximal fragment). Neurovascular injury is not a common complication. Closed manipulation is justifiable, but, because persistent instability is a frequent complication, impaction or locking of the fragments is desirable. If reduction is stable, Velpeau's dressing (Fig 45—10) provides reliable

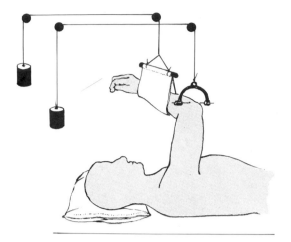

Figure 45–11. Method of suspension of upper extremity with skeletal traction on olecranon.

immobilization after correction of anterior angulation. Redisplacement may occur when reduction is not stable or when the arm is immobilized in abduction. Continuous traction by a Kirschner wire through the proximal ulna with the arm at right angle elevation (Fig 45–11) is advisable when the fracture cannot be maintained in reduction by a dressing such as Velpeau's. Traction must be continued for about 4 weeks before partial healing provides stability. This closed method of traction treatment is commonly required also for comminuted fractures of the surgical neck. When comminution is not extensive, the fracture that has been adequately reduced closed may be stabilized by one or 2 heavy Kirschner wires introduced percutaneously and obliquely in the deltoid region through the distal fragment into the head of the humerus. With the fragments fixed, the arm is then brought to the side and immobilized either by a sling and swathe or by a plaster Velpeau dressing. Open reduction and internal fixation of uncomplicated fractures of the surgical neck are not commonly required to ensure an adequate functional result.

C. Fracture of the Greater Tuberosity: Fracture of the greater tuberosity generally is a component of a complex injury—either comminuted fracture of the proximal humerus or anterior dislocation of the shoulder joint. Fracture of the greater tuberosity with no associated injury is apt to be undisplaced. When isolated and displaced fracture does occur, it is likely to be associated with persistent or spontaneously reduced anterior dislocation of the humeral head and longitudinal tear of the capsulotendinous cuff.

When accurate repositioning of the greater tuberosity fragment does not occur following closed reduction of the dislocated humeral head, open operation is desirable to fix anatomically the avulsed fragment and to repair any capsulotendinous tear.

D. Fracture of the Lesser Tuberosity: Fracture of the lesser tuberosity is generally a part of comminuted fractures of the proximal humerus. Isolated fracture is

rare and is due to avulsion by the subscapularis muscle. Because of the broad insertion of that muscle which extends to the adjacent humeral shaft inferiorly, displacement of the bony fragment is unlikely to be marked.

Treatment consists of immobilization in a sling for about 4 weeks.

Combined & Displaced Fractures of the Proximal Humerus

A. Fracture of the Surgical Neck and Greater Tuberosity: Combined and displaced fractures involving the surgical neck and greater tuberosity are unique because the persistently active subscapularis muscle attached to the intact lesser tuberosity causes the proximal articular fragment to be rotated internally in relation to the shaft. It is difficult to correct this torsional displacement by closed methods. It may be accomplished with the aid of the image intensifier by initially inserting percutaneously and transversely a small Steinmann pin into the proximal segment which is used to derotate that fragment and to stabilize it while completing the reduction. The 2 major fragments are then fixed percutaneously as described for unstable fractures of the surgical neck. If reduction of displacement at both fracture sites is not adequate, open reduction and internal fixation of the bone fragments and repair of any rotator cuff tear is indicated. This combined lesion may be complicated by anterior dislocation of the proximal head fragment from the glenoid.

B. Fracture of the Surgical Neck and Lesser Tuberosity: Combined and displaced fractures of the surgical neck and lesser tuberosity are significant because the external rotators cause the proximal fragment to be externally rotated with reference to the shaft so that the cartilaginous surface of the humeral head is directed anteriorly. Correction of torsional displacement and adequate reduction is difficult by closed methods but may be achieved by appropriate modification of the technic described for combined fracture of the surgical neck and greater tuberosity. If satisfactory reduction cannot be attained, open reduction with fixation of the bone fragments and repair of any coexisting laceration of the capsulotendinous cuff is appropriate. Posterior dislocation of the head fragment from the glenoid may complicate this combined lesion.

C. Fracture of the Surgical Neck and Both Tuberosities: This uncommon but serious lesion is generally complicated by displacement of one or all of the component fragments. Dehiscence of the tuberosities and displacement of the shaft provide a mechanism for subluxation or dislocation of the main articular fragment which may be anterior, posterior, lateral, or inferior. Shattering of the articular segment provides the opportunity for multidirectional displacement of component fragments. Extensive laceration of the rotator cuff is a part of the total lesion.

Because of comminution and displacement of component fragments of the proximal segment, satisfactory functional results are unlikely and delay of bone healing is probable after any type of closed treatment. Avascular necrosis of the articular fragment is an anticipated sequel because of its inherently jeopardized blood supply. Open operation offers the best chance for preservation of some function with tolerable discomfort. Removal of the articular segments and repair of the remaining structures cannot be expected to be as successful in the treatment of recent lesions of this type as replacement arthroplasty of the humeral head and fixation of the tuberosities to each other and to the distal shaft fragment.

A sequel of articular fractures of the proximal humerus is secondary glenohumeral osteoarthritis; its treatment is discussed below.

Separation of Epiphysis of Head of Humerus

When this injury occurs as a result of birth trauma, it is difficult to recognize because of the absence of a bony nucleus in the capital epiphysis. Even though x-ray examination is negative, the injury should be suspected when there is swelling of the shoulder region and limitation of active movements of the arm. Fracture through the epiphyseal plate may be encountered in older children. The principles of treatment are the same as for fracture of the surgical neck of the humerus. Open reduction is rarely desirable, and every effort should be made to obtain reduction by manipulation or traction.

Chaco J, Yosipovitch Z: Fracture of the humerus with delayed subluxation of the shoulder joint. J Trauma 12:728, 1972.

Neer C3 II. Displaced proximal humeral fractures. 1. Classification and evaluation. 2. Treatment of three-part and four-part displacement. J Bone Joint Surg 52A:1077, 1090, 1970.

DISLOCATION OF THE SHOULDER JOINT

Over 95% of all cases of shoulder joint dislocation are anterior or subcoracoid. Subglenoid and posterior dislocations comprise the remainder.

Anterior Dislocation of the Shoulder Joint

Anterior dislocation presents the clinical appearance of flattening of the deltoid region, anterior fullness, and restriction of motion due to pain. Both anteroposterior and axillary x-rays are necessary to determine the site of the head and the presence or absence of complicating fracture which may involve either the head of the humerus or the glenoid. Anterior dislocation may be complicated by (1) injury to major nerves arising from the brachial plexus; (2) fracture of the upper extremity of the humerus, especially the head or greater tuberosity; (3) compression or avulsion of the anterior glenoid; and (4) tears of the capsulotendinous rotator cuff. The most common sequel is recurrent dislocation. Before manipulation, careful examination is necessary to determine the presence or absence of complicating nerve or vascular injury. Under general anesthesia, reduction can usually be accomplished by simple traction on the arm for a few minutes or until the head has been disengaged from the coracoid. If reduction cannot be achieved in this way, the surgeon should apply lateral traction manually to the upper arm, close to the axilla, while the assistant continues to exert axial traction on the extremity. This is a modification of **Hippocrates' manipulation** in which the surgeon exerts traction on the arm while the heel of his unshod foot in the axilla provides countertraction and simultaneously forces the head of the humerus laterally from beneath the acromion.

If neither of the foregoing technics proves successful, **Kocher's method** may be useful. This maneuver, however, must be carried out gently or spiral fracture of the humerus may result. The elbow is flexed to a right angle and the surgeon applies traction and gentle external rotation to the forearm in the axis of the humerus. The surgeon continues traction to the arm while gentle external rotation about the longitudinal axis of the humerus is applied, using the forearm flexed to a right angle at the elbow as a lever. The maneuver can be completed by shifting the elbow across the anterior chest while traction is continuously exerted and, finally, slow internal rotation of the arm until the palm of the affected side rests on the opposite shoulder.

After closed reduction of an initial dislocation the extremity is immobilized in a sling and swathe for 3 weeks before active motion is begun. If a second episode is the result of minor trauma, the lesion is considered permanent and treated accordingly.

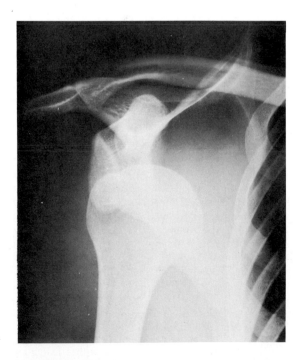

Figure 45–12. Anterior (subcoracoid) dislocation of the shoulder in a 28-year-old man.

Subcoracoid Dislocation of the Shoulder Joint

Uncomplicated subcoracoid dislocation can almost always be reduced by closed manipulation. With associated fracture, or when the dislocation is old, open reduction may be necessary. Even when the dislocation is old, however, closed reduction by skeletal traction should be tried before open reduction is elected.

Posterior Dislocation of the Shoulder Joint

Posterior dislocation is characterized by fullness beneath the spine of the scapula and by restriction of motion in external rotation. An axillary x-ray view demonstrates the position of the head of the humerus in relationship to the glenoid. This uncommon lesion may be reduced by the same combination of coaxial and transverse traction as described for anterior dislocation. Immobilization following an initial episode should be accomplished by plaster spica, with the arm in approximately 30 degrees external rotation and the elbow flexed to a right angle.

Recurrent Dislocation of the Shoulder Joint

Recurrent dislocation of the shoulder is almost always anterior. Various factors can influence recurrent dislocation. Avulsion of the anterior and inferior glenoid labrum or tears in the anterior capsule remove the natural buttress that gives stability to the arm with abduction and external rotation. Other lesions which impair the stability of the shoulder joint are fractures of the posterior and superior surface of the head of the humerus (or of the greater tuberosity) and longitudinal tears of the rotator cuff between the supraspinatus and subscapularis. Reduction of the acute episodic dislocation is by closed manipulation. Immobilization does not prevent subsequent dislocation, and it should be discontinued as soon as acute symptoms subside, usually within a few days.

Adequate curative treatment of recurrent dislocation of the shoulder, so that unrestricted normal use of the joint is possible, almost always requires plastic repair of the anterior capsulotendinous cuff by an operation.

Although reparative operations for recurrent dislocation of the shoulder joint may prove successful in preventing further episodes, a late sequel is secondary osteoarthritis. Complicating fractures of the articular surfaces of either the humeral head or the glenoid (or both) which cause incongruity may hasten the onset and intensify the symptoms of the complication. Other contributing factors include axillary nerve lesions with loss of deltoid muscle function and laxity of the capsulotendinous cuff with episodes of transient subluxation.

Boyd HB, Sisk TD: Recurrent posterior dislocation of the shoulder. J Bone Joint Surg 54A:779, 1972.

Detenbeck LC: Posterior dislocation of the shoulder. J Trauma 12:183, 1972.

Rowe CR: Complicated dislocation of the shoulder. Am J Surg 117:549, 1969.

SECONDARY GLENOHUMERAL OSTEOARTHRITIS

Among the causes of secondary osteoarthritis of the shoulder joint are traumatic injuries that cause tears of the rotator cuff, dislocation of the joint, or fractures of the articular surfaces of the humerus or scapula. Similar to the relatively uncommon primary type, secondary osteoarthritis of the shoulder joint is characterized on x-ray by thinning of the articular cartilage, especially at the site of maximum contact of the apposing surfaces. Osteophytes form at the chondrosynovial junction, especially in the region of the inferior head and the superior glenoid. If the cause was fracture, incongruity of the articular surface of the involved component may be identified on that basis. Subjective symptoms are essentially painful restriction of motion.

Treatment of this sequel is directed primarily toward the relief of pain and secondarily toward preservation or augmentation of motion. Before operative treatment is elected, a thorough test of conservative measures is indicated.

Fusion of the joint (**arthrodesis**) may be necessary because of antecedent or persistent infection, irreparable instability due either to prior destruction of surrounding soft tissues or bone, or denervation of muscles essential for shoulder joint function. This procedure may also be arbitrarily selected by the patient. Bony fusion of the joint eliminates pain from that source but results in disability due to loss of function.

Because of the non-weight-bearing nature of the shoulder joint and other factors, **hemiarthroplasty** by use of a humeral head prosthesis has proved to be a gratifying procedure in the hands of experienced surgeons when the indications are critically observed. Serviceable function and relief of pain to the point of tolerance are likely to be obtained afterward.

More recent investigative studies have been directed toward enlargement of the scope of arthroplasty in cases of simultaneous disease of the humeral head and the glenoid. The concept of total joint replacement has been used as a salvage procedure by employing humeral and glenoidal components which may be stabilized in the respective bone because of peculiarity of design of the implants or with the aid of a plastic grouting substance—currently methyl methacrylate. Because the long-term results of total replacement of the glenohumeral joint are unknown, this procedure should be selected cautiously.

Resection of a portion of the humeral head to create a pseudarthrosis may give relief of pain but leaves restricted function because of disturbed joint mechanics.

Neer CS II: Replacement arthroplasty for glenohumeral osteoarthritis. J Bone Joint Surg 56A:1, 1974.

Rowe CR: Re-evaluation of the position of the arm in arthrodesis of the shoulder in the adult. J Bone Joint Surg 56A:913, 1974.

FRACTURES OF THE SHAFT OF THE HUMERUS

Fracture of the shaft of the humerus is more common in adults than in children. Direct violence is accountable for the majority of such fractures, although spiral fracture of the middle third of the shaft may result from violent muscular activity such as throwing a ball. X-rays in 2 planes are necessary to determine the configuration of the fracture and the direction of displacement of the fragments. Documentation of torsional displacement about the longitudinal axis of the shaft of transverse and comminuted fractures requires inclusion of the shoulder and elbow in the anteroposterior view. Before initiating definitive treatment, a careful neurologic examination should be done (and recorded) to determine the status of the radial nerve. Injury to the brachial vessels is not common.

Fracture of the Upper Third of the Shaft of the Humerus

Fracture through the metaphysis proximal to the insertion of the pectoralis major is classified as fracture of the surgical neck of the humerus.

Fractures between the insertions of the pectoralis major and the deltoid commonly demonstrate adduction of the distal end of the proximal fragment, with lateral and proximal displacement of the distal fragment. Medial displacement occurs with fracture distal to the insertion of the deltoid in the middle third of the shaft.

Treatment depends upon the presence or absence of complicating neurovascular injury, the site and configuration of the fracture, and the magnitude of displacement.

In infants, skin traction for 1–2 weeks will permit sufficient callus to form so that immobilization can be maintained by a sling and swathe or a Velpeau dressing. Open reduction for the sole purpose of accurate positioning of the fragments is rarely justified in children and adolescents, since slight shortening and less than 15 degrees of angulation will be compensated during growth. Torsional displacement, however, will not be compensated and must be corrected initially.

In the adult, an effort should be made to reduce completely displaced transverse or slightly oblique fractures by manipulation. A local anesthetic solution injected directly into the hematoma at the fracture site will provide adequate anesthesia for manipulation. To prevent recurrence of medial convex angulation and maintain proper alignment, it may be necessary to bring the distal fragment into alignment with the proximal by bringing the arm across the chest and immobilizing it with a plaster Velpeau dressing (Fig 45–10). If the ends of the fragments cannot be approximated by manipulative methods, traction on the skin or skeletal traction with a wire through the olecranon is indicated (Fig 45–11). In young patients, the olecranon

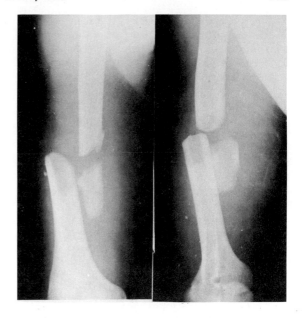

Figure 45–13. Comminuted fracture of the middle third of the humeral shaft complicated by immediate and complete paralysis of the radial nerve in a 20-year-old man.

wire should be placed opposite the coronoid process to avoid injury to the epiphysis. Traction should be continued for 3–4 weeks until stabilization occurs, after which time the patient can be ambulatory with an external immobilization device.

Fracture of the Middle & Lower Thirds of the Shaft of the Humerus

Spiral, oblique, and comminuted fractures of the shaft below the insertion of the pectoralis major may be treated by Caldwell's hanging cast, which consists of a plaster dressing from the axilla to the wrist with the elbow in 90 degrees of flexion and the forearm in midposition (Fig 45–14). The cast is suspended from a bandage around the neck by means of a ring at the wrist. Alignment should be verified on anteroposterior

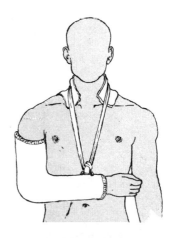

Figure 45–14. Caldwell's hanging cast.

and transthoracic x-rays with the patient standing. Angulation may be corrected by lengthening or shortening the suspension bandage. When lateral convex angulation cannot be corrected by adjustment of the bandage, moving the suspension ring closer to the elbow may be effective. Traction is afforded by the weight of the plaster. The patient is instructed to sleep in the semireclining position. As soon as clinical examination demonstrates stabilization (in about 6–8 weeks), the plaster may be discarded and a sling and swathe substituted.

When fracture of the shaft of the humerus is associated with other injuries which require confinement to bed, initial treatment may be by skin or skeletal traction (Fig 45–11).

Fractures of the shaft of the humerus—especially transverse fractures—may heal slowly. If stabilization has not taken place after 6–8 weeks of traction, more secure immobilization, such as with a plaster shoulder spica (Fig 45–15), must be considered. Immobilization for 6 months or more may be necessary.

When complete loss of radial nerve function is apparent immediately after injury, open operation is indicated to determine the type of nerve lesion or to remove impinging bone fragments. Internal fixation of the fragments can be accomplished at the same time. If partial function of the radial nerve is retained, exploration can be deferred since spontaneous recovery sometimes occurs and may be complete by the time the fracture has healed. Open reduction of closed fractures is indicated also if arterial circulation has been interrupted or (in the adult) if adequate apposition of major fragments cannot be obtained by closed methods, as is likely to be the case with transverse fractures near the middle third of the shaft. When 4–5 months of treatment by closed methods have not resulted in clinical or x-ray evidence of healing, operative treatment should be considered.

Fenyö G: On fractures of the shaft of the humerus. Acta Chir Scand 137:221, 1971.

Sim FH & others: Radial nerve palsy complicating fractures of the humeral shaft. J Bone Joint Surg 53A:1034, 1971.

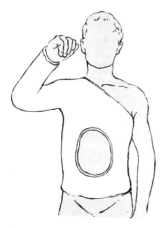

Figure 45–15. Plaster shoulder spica for fracture of humerus.

INJURIES OF THE ELBOW REGION

FRACTURE OF THE DISTAL HUMERUS

Fracture of the distal humerus is most often caused by indirect violence. Therefore, the configuration of the fracture cleft and the direction of displacement of the fragments are likely to be typical. Injuries of major vessels and nerves and elbow joint dislocation are apt to be present.

Clinical findings consist of pain, swelling, and restriction of motion. Minor deformity may not be apparent because swelling usually obliterates landmarks. The type of fracture is determined by x-ray examination. Especially in children, it is advisable to obtain films of the opposite elbow for comparison.

Examination for peripheral nerve and vascular injury must be made and all findings carefully recorded before treatment is instituted.

Supracondylar Fracture of the Humerus

Supracondylar fracture of the humerus occurs proximal to the olecranon fossa; transcondylar (diacondylar) fracture occurs more distally and extends into the olecranon fossa. Neither fracture extends to the articular surface of the humerus. Treatment is the same for both types.

Supracondylar fractures are observed more commonly in children and adolescents, and they may extend into the epiphyseal plates of the capitellum and trochlea. Transcondylar fracture is very rare in children.

The direction of displacement of the distal fragment from the midcoronal plane of the arm serves to differentiate the "extension" from the less common "flexion" type. This differentiation has important implications for treatment.

A. Extension-Type Fractures: In the extension type of supracondylar fracture, the usual direction of displacement of the main distal fragment is posterior and proximal. The distal fragment may also be displaced laterally and, less frequently, medially. The direction of these displacements is identified easily on biplane x-ray films. Internal torsional displacement, however, is more difficult to recognize; and unless torsional displacement is reduced, relative cubitus varus with loss of carrying angle will persist.

Displaced supracondylar fractures are surgical emergencies. Immediate treatment is required to avoid occlusion of the brachial artery and to prevent or to avoid further peripheral nerve injury. If hemorrhage and edema prevent complete reduction of the fracture at the first attempt, a second manipulation will be required after swelling has regressed.

1. Manipulative reduction—Minor angular displacements (tilting) may be reduced by gentle forced flexion of the elbow under local or general anesthesia, weeks, after which time the plaster splint may be discarded and a sling worn for another 2 weeks before active motion is permitted. In adults, healing is less rapid and immobilization must be continued for 8–12 weeks or even longer before active exercise is permitted.

2. Traction and immobilization–In certain instances, supracondylar fractures of the humerus with posterior displacement of the distal fragment should be treated by traction (Figs 45–17 and 45–18): (1) If comminution is marked and stability cannot be obtained by flexion of the elbow, traction is indicated until the fragments have stabilized. (2) If 2 or 3 attempts at manipulative reduction have been unsuccessful, continuous traction under x-ray control for 1–2 days is justifiable before further manipulation. (3) If the radial pulse is absent or weak when the patient is examined initially and does not improve with manipulation, traction may be necessary to prevent displacement of the fracture and further embarrassment of circulation. During the early phase of treatment by continuous traction, flexion of the elbow beyond 90 degrees should be avoided since this may jeopardize circulation.

B. Flexion-Type Fracture: Flexion-type fracture of the humerus is characterized by anterior and sometimes also torsional and lateral displacement of the main distal fragment. Treatment is by closed manipulation. A posterior plaster splint is then applied from the axillary fold to the level of the wrist, with the forearm in supination and the elbow in full extension. Elevation is advisable for at least 24 hours or until soft tissue swelling has reached the maximum, after which time the patient may be ambulatory. Immobilization is then continued for 4–6 weeks. When satisfactory

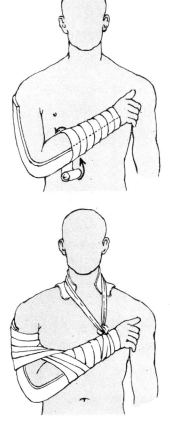

Figure 45–16. Posterior plaster splint for supracondylar fracture.

followed by immobilization in a posterior plaster splint in 45 degrees of flexion (Fig 45–16). If displacement is marked but normal radial pulsation indicates that circulation is not impaired, closed manipulation under general anesthesia should be done as soon as possible. If radial pulses are absent or weak on initial examination and do not improve with manipulation, traction is indicated (see below). Capillary flush in the nail beds cannot be relied on as the sole indication of competency of deep circulation. After reduction and casting the patient should be placed at bed rest, preferably in a hospital, with his elbow elevated on a pillow and the dressing arranged so that the radial pulse is accessible for frequent observation. Swelling can be expected to increase for 24–72 hours. During this critical period continued observation is necessary so that any circulatory embarrassment which may lead to Volkmann's ischemic contracture can be identified at once. The circular bandage must be adjusted frequently to compensate for initial increase and subsequent decrease of swelling. If during manipulation it was necessary to extend the elbow beyond 45 degrees to restore radial pulses, the joint should be flexed to the optimal angle as swelling subsides to prevent loss of the reduction.

In children, stabilization will take place in 4–5

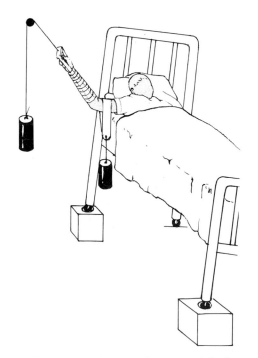

Figure 45–17. Dunlop's traction for supracondylar fracture.

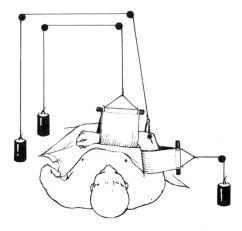

Figure 45—18. Skeletal traction for supracondylar fracture.

reduction cannot be accomplished by closed manipulation, treatment should be by traction with the elbow in full extension until the fragments become stabilized.

Separation of the Distal Humeral Epiphyses

An uncommon variation of supracondylar fracture is separation of the distal humeral epiphyses with or without appreciable displacement. Sprains of the elbow do not commonly occur in children; injury more often involves the distal humeral epiphyses. X-ray comparison of the injured elbow with the uninjured elbow may show no deviation, but careful physical examination may demonstrate posterior tenderness over the lower epiphyses and also swelling. This combination of swelling and tenderness should suggest epiphyseal separation, and warrants protection from further injury by means of a sling worn for about 3 weeks.

The direction of displacement is determined by careful clinical and radiographic examinations. Depending upon the direction of angulation of the osseous nuclei of the capitellum and trochlea (as demonstrated in the lateral x-ray), immobilization is as described for supracondylar fractures.

Intercondylar Fracture of the Humerus

Intercondylar fracture of the humerus is classically described as being of the T or Y type (or both), according to the configuration of the fracture cleft observed on an anteroposterior x-ray. This fracture is usually seen in adults, commonly as the result of a blow over the posterior aspect of the flexed elbow. Open fracture and other injuries to the soft tissues are frequently present. The fracture often extends into the trochlear surface of the elbow joint, and unless the articular surfaces of the distal humerus can be accurately repositioned, restriction of joint motion, pain, instability, and deformity can be expected.

A. Closed Reduction: If the fragments are not widely displaced, closed reduction may be successful. Since comminution is always present, stabilization is difficult to achieve and maintain by manipulation and external immobilization.

1. Anterior displacement may be treated first by a combination of continuous skin traction with the elbow in full extension and closed manipulation of the main fragments. If adequate positioning can be achieved in this manner, traction is continued until stabilization occurs. The extremity may then be immobilized in a tubular plaster cast.

2. Significant posterior displacement requires overhead skeletal traction by means of a Kirschner wire inserted through the olecranon (Fig 45—18). It may be necessary to apply a swathe around the arm and body for simultaneous transverse traction.

B. Open Reduction: Open reduction may be indicated if adequate positioning cannot be obtained by closed methods. A requirement for acceptable results of open reduction and internal fixation is that the fragments be sufficiently large so that they can be fixed to one another. Comminution may be so extensive that satisfactory stabilization cannot be accomplished by current technics of internal fixation. Under such circumstances, it is better either to abandon open operation and to accept the imperfect results of closed treatment, or, if the proximal radius and ulna are intact, to plan subsequent replacement arthroplasty by means of a custom-made lower humeral prosthesis. Total elbow replacement technics are currently in the developmental stage.

Fracture of the Lateral Condyle of the Humerus

The 3 major varieties of fracture of the lateral condyle of the humerus are (1) fracture of a portion of the capitellum in the coronal plane of the humerus, with or without extension into the trochlea (seen only in adults); (2) isolated fracture of the lateral condyle without extension into the trochlea;* and (3) separation of the capitellar epiphysis (in children).

A. Fracture of the Capitellum: This is characterized by proximal displacement of the anterior detached fragment, and probably occurs as one component of a spontaneously reduced incomplete dislocation of the elbow joint. The lesion is most clearly demonstrated on lateral x-rays. Closed reduction should be attempted by forcing the elbow into acute flexion. After reduction the extremity is immobilized in a posterior plaster splint with the elbow in full flexion to prevent displacement of the small distal fragment.

When accurate reduction cannot be accomplished by closed technics, open operation may be desirable to avoid subsequent restriction of elbow movement. If the small distal fragment retains sufficient soft tissue attachment to assure adequate blood supply, it may be temporarily fixed to the main fragment in anatomic position by a Kirschner wire. If the articular fragment lacks significant soft tissue bonds, removal is recommended since avascular necrosis is likely to follow.

*Fracture which involves the entire capitellum and extends into the trochlea is associated with proximal and lateral displacement of the detached fragment and lateral subluxation of the elbow. This lesion is discussed below.

B. Isolated Complete Fracture: Isolated complete fracture of the lateral condyle without extension into the trochlea is uncommon, and is not usually associated with major displacement of the detached fragment. The extremity should be supported by a sling. If tense hemarthrosis is present, aspiration may minimize pain. Guarded active motions of the elbow should be initiated as soon as pain subsides.

C. Separation of the Capitellar Epiphysis: Fracture of the lateral condyle of the humerus in children is essentially separation of the capitellar epiphysis, even though the fracture may extend into the metaphysis and the trochlear epiphysis. If the center of ossification of the capitellum is small, minor displacement may be missed on initial examination; further displacement will then result from unguarded use. The fact that a part of the extensor muscles originates on the fragment is an important factor in displacement.

1. Closed reduction—Minor displacement may be treated by manipulative reduction and external immobilization in a posterior plaster splint which extends from the posterior axillary fold to the level of the heads of the metacarpals. X-rays are taken at least twice a week for the first 3 weeks to determine whether displacement has recurred.

2. Open reduction—When anatomic reduction cannot be achieved by one or 2 manipulations, open reduction is indicated.

Avulsion of the Medial Epicondylar Apophysis

Avulsion of the medial epicondylar apophysis in children may occur without dislocation of the elbow. Minor displacement causing localized tenderness and swelling over the medial aspect of the elbow can be treated by immobilization in a sling and swathe for a few days. More extensive injury should be suspected if tenderness and swelling are diffuse. When separation is greater than 1–2 mm, treatment is similar to that for dislocation of the elbow associated with separation of the apophysis (see p 928).

Bryan RS, Bickel WH: "T" condylar fractures of distal humerus. J Trauma 11:830, 1971.
D'Ambrosia RD: Supracondylar fractures of humerus: Prevention of cubitus varus. J Bone Joint Surg 54A:60, 1972.
Flynn JC & others: Blind pinning of displaced supracondylar fractures of the humerus in children: Sixteen years' experience with long-term follow-up. J Bone Joint Surg 56A:263, 1974.
Fowles JV, Kassab MT: Fracture of the capitulum humeri: Treatment by excision. J Bone Joint Surg 56A:794, 1974.
Hardacre JA & others: Fractures of the lateral condyle of the humerus in children. J Bone Joint Surg 53A:1083, 1971.
Riseborough EJ, Radin EL: Intercondylar T fractures of the humerus in the adult. J Bone Joint Surg 51A:130, 1969.

FRACTURE OF THE PROXIMAL ULNA

Common fractures of the proximal ulna include fracture of the olecranon and fracture of the coronoid process. Fracture of the coronoid process is a complication of posterior dislocation of the elbow joint, and is discussed below.

Fracture of the olecranon which occurs as the result of indirect violence (eg, forced flexion of the forearm against the actively contracted triceps muscle) is typically transverse or slightly oblique. Fracture due to direct violence is usually comminuted and associated with other fracture or anterior dislocation of the joint. Since the major fracture cleft extends into the elbow joint, treatment should be directed toward restoration of anatomic position to afford maximal recovery of range of motion and functional competency of the triceps.

Treatment

The method of treatment depends upon the degree of displacement and the extent of comminution.

A. Closed Reduction: Minimal displacement (1–2 mm) can be treated by closed manipulation with the elbow in full extension, assisted by digital pressure over the proximal fragment, and immobilization in a volar plaster splint which extends from the anterior axillary fold to the wrist. X-rays should be taken twice weekly for 2 weeks after reduction to determine whether reduction has been maintained. Immobilization must be continued for at least 6 weeks before active flexion exercises are begun.

B. Open Reduction and Internal Fixation: Open reduction and internal fixation are indicated if closed methods are not successful in approximating displaced fragments and restoring congruity to articular surfaces. The extremity is then immobilized in 90 degrees of flexion for at least 6–8 weeks before active flexion exercises are instituted.

FRACTURE OF THE PROXIMAL RADIUS

Fracture of the Head & Neck of the Radius

Fracture of the head and neck of the radius may occur in adults as an isolated injury uncomplicated by dislocation of the elbow or the superior radioulnar joint. This fracture is caused by indirect violence, such as a fall on the outstretched hand, when the radial head is driven against the capitellum. Care must be taken to obtain true anteroposterior and lateral x-rays of the proximal radius as well as of the elbow joint, since minor lesions may be obscured by a change in position from midposition to full supination during exposure of the films.

A. Conservative Measures: Fissure fractures and those with minimal displacement can be treated symptomatically, with evacuation of tense hemarthrosis by aspiration to minimize pain. The extremity may be supported by a sling or immobilized in a posterior plaster splint with the elbow in 90 degrees of flexion. Active exercises of the elbow are to be encouraged within a few days. Recovery of function is slow, and slight restriction of motion (especially extension) may persist.

B. Surgical Treatment: When the fracture involves the articular surface and is comminuted, or when displacement is greater than 1–2 mm, excision of the entire head of the radius is generally recommended. However, simple removal of a minor fragment of the head which comprises less than a quarter of the articular surface is compatible with recovery of satisfactory elbow function.

Fracture of the Upper Epiphysis of the Radius

Fracture of the upper radial epiphysis in a child is not a true epiphyseal separation since the fracture cleft commonly extends into the neck of the bone. Because the articular surface of the proximal fragment remains intact, the prominent features of displacement are angulation and impaction. Wide displacement of the minor proximal fragment may mean that the elbow joint was dislocated but has reduced spontaneously since the injury.

A. Closed Reduction: Every effort should be made to reduce these fractures by closed manipulation. Several x-rays taken with the forearm in various degrees of rotation should be examined so that the position can be selected which is best suited for digital pressure on the proximal fragment. Anteroposterior and lateral x-rays with the elbow in flexion are then taken; if angulation has been reduced to less than 45 degrees, the end result is likely to be satisfactory.

B. Open Reduction: If closed reduction is not successful, open reduction and repositioning under direct vision is indicated even in the child.

Jeffery CC: Fractures of the neck of the radius in children. J Bone Joint Surg 54B:717, 1972.

SUBLUXATION & DISLOCATION OF THE ELBOW JOINT

Subluxation of the Head of the Radius

This injury occurs most frequently in infants between the ages of 18 months and 4 years, usually when the child is suddenly lifted by his hands with the forearm in pronation. Because of comparative laxity of the interosseous membrane and other supporting ligamentous structures, the direction of displacement of the radial head is distal in the direction of the longitudinal axis of the shaft. It has been suggested that this permits the proximal part of the annular ligament to become infolded between the radial head and the capitellum. In unreduced subluxations, in addition to tenderness about the radial head and restriction of supination, swelling and tenderness may be present in the region of the ulnar head at the level of the inferior radioulnar joint. The infant holds the forearm semiflexed and pronated. If spontaneous reduction has

occurred, diagnosis is dependent upon finding slightly restricted supination associated with discomfort. X-rays are generally not helpful, but in the older child the distance between the radial head and the capitellum may be increased in comparison to the uninjured side.

Reduction by forced supination of the forearm can usually be accomplished easily without anesthesia. The extremity should be protected in a sling for 1 week. Rarely, in an older child, closed manipulation may be unsuccessful and open release of the annular ligament may be necessary.

Dislocation of the Head of the Radius

Isolated dislocation of the radius at the elbow is a rare lesion which implies dislocation of the proximal radioulnar and radiohumeral joints without fracture. This lesion, which occurs in children older than 5 years or occasionally in adults, should be differentiated from subluxation of the head of the radius. To cause dislocation, the injury must be sufficiently severe to disrupt the capsulotendinous support—especially the annular ligament—of the proximal radius. The direction of displacement of the radial head is usually anterior or lateral, but it may be posterior.

Reduction can usually be accomplished by forced supination of the forearm under anesthesia. The extremity should be immobilized for 3–4 weeks with the elbow in flexion and the forearm in supination.

Dislocation of the Elbow Joint Without Fracture

Dislocation of the elbow joint without major fracture is almost always posterior. It may be encountered at any age but is most common in children. Complete backward dislocation of the ulna and radius implies extensive tearing of the capsuloligamentous structures and injury to the region of insertion of the brachialis muscle. The coronoid process of the ulna is usually displaced posteriorly and proximally into the olecranon fossa, but it may be displaced laterally or medially. Biplane x-rays of the highest quality are necessary

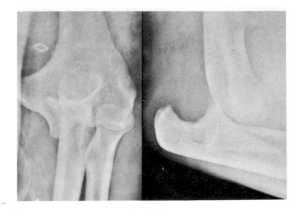

Figure 45–19. Complete posterior dislocation of the elbow joint without fracture or neurovascular injury in a 19-year-old man.

to determine that no fracture is associated.

Peripheral nerve function must be carefully assessed before definitive treatment is instituted. The ulnar nerve is most likely to be injured.

In recent dislocations, closed reduction can be achieved (under general anesthesia) by axial traction on the forearm with the elbow in the position of deformity. Hyperextension is not necessary. Lateral or medial dislocation can be corrected during traction. As soon as proximal displacement is corrected, the elbow should be brought into 90 degrees of flexion and a posterior plaster splint applied which reaches from the posterior axillary fold to the wrist. Active motion is permitted after 3 weeks.

Closed reduction should be attempted even if unreduced dislocation has persisted for 2 months following the injury.

Myositis ossificans of the brachialis anticus muscle is a rare sequel.

Heinrich G, Mordeja J: The so-called Chassaignac's arm paralysis of small children. Arch Klin Chir 309:256, 1965.
Roberts PH: Dislocation of the elbow. Br J Surg 56:806, 1969.
Wiley JJ & others: Traumatic dislocation of the radius at the elbow. J Bone Joint Surg 56B:501, 1974.

FRACTURE-DISLOCATION OF THE ELBOW JOINT

Dislocation of the elbow is frequently associated with fracture. Some fractures are insignificant and require no specific treatment; others demand specialized care.

Fracture of the Coronoid Process of the Ulna

Fracture of the coronoid process of the ulna is the most frequent complication of posterior dislocation of the elbow joint. Treatment is the same as for uncomplicated posterior dislocation of the elbow joint (see above).

Fracture of the Head of the Radius With Posterior Dislocation of the Elbow Joint

This injury is treated as 2 separate lesions. The severity of comminution and the magnitude of displacement of the radial head fragments are first determined by x-ray. If comminution has occurred or the fragments are widely displaced, the dislocation is reduced by closed manipulation; the head of the radius is then excised.

If fracture of the head of the radius is not comminuted and the fragments are not widely displaced, treatment is as for uncomplicated posterior dislocation of the elbow joint.

Fracture of the Olecranon With Anterior Dislocation of the Elbow Joint

This very unstable injury usually occurs from a blow on the dorsum of the flexed forearm. Fracture

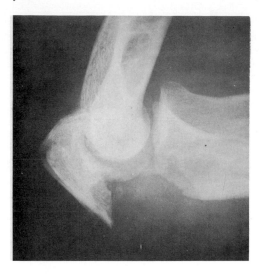

Figure 45–20. Fracture of the olecranon and anterior subluxation of the radius and ulna in a 51-year-old woman.

through the olecranon permits the distal fragment of the ulna and the proximal radius to be displaced anterior to the humerus, and may cause extensive tearing of the capsuloligamentous structures around the elbow joint. The dislocation can be reduced by bringing the elbow into full extension, but anatomic reduction of the olecranon fracture by closed manipulation is not likely to be successful and immediate open reduction is usually indicated. Recovery of function is likely to be delayed and incomplete.

Fracture of the Medial Epicondylar Apophysis With Dislocation of the Elbow Joint

Dislocation of the elbow joint in children may be complicated by avulsion of the medial epicondylar apophysis. The direction of dislocation may have been lateral, posterior, or posterolateral. Physical and x-ray examination may not demonstrate the extent of displacement at the time of injury since partial reduction may have occurred spontaneously. X-rays of the uninjured elbow in similar projections are desirable to compare the exact locations of the 2 apophyses. The free fragment is normally displaced downward by the action of the flexor muscles. If partial spontaneous reduction of the elbow dislocation has occurred, the detached apophysis may be found incarcerated within the elbow joint between the articular surfaces of the trochlea and the olecranon. This may happen also during manual reduction. Ulnar nerve function must be evaluated before definitive treatment is given.

Dislocation of the elbow joint may be reduced by closed manipulation, but accurate repositioning of a widely separated apophysis cannot be achieved by closed methods. Opinion differs concerning the necessity for anatomic reduction of the apophysis if it is not incarcerated within the elbow joint. Some authorities maintain that fibrous healing of the apophysis causes no disability; others anticipate weakness of grasp or subsequent pain as the result of development of a pseudarthrosis between the apophysis and the medial condyle. Exuberant bone formation around the apophysis may cause tardy ulnar paralysis. If it is elected not to reduce displacement of an apophysis outside the elbow joint, the extremity should be immobilized at a right angle for 3 weeks in a tubular plaster cast before active motion is permitted.

If the ulnar nerve has been injured, or if the apophysis cannot be displaced from the elbow joint by closed manipulation, open reduction is advisable.

Fracture of the Lateral Condyle With Lateral Dislocation of the Elbow Joint

Fracture of the lateral condyle of the humerus with lateral dislocation of the elbow joint must be differentiated from fracture of the lateral condyle with or without posterior dislocation of the joint (see below). Neither lesion is common. A complicating feature of fracture of the lateral condyle with lateral dislocation is inclusion not only of the entire capitellum but also extension of the fracture cleft into the trochlea. This creates an unstable mechanism which cannot be reliably immobilized in either flexion or extension even though closed reduction has been successful. If closed methods of treatment are not adequate, open reduction is recommended.

Fracture of the Lateral Condyle With Posterior Dislocation of the Elbow Joint

Treatment should be divided into 2 phases. The dislocation should be reduced first by closed manipulation. This maneuver may also simultaneously accomplish adequate reduction of the condylar fracture. If the condylar fragment cannot be adequately repositioned by closed manipulation, open reduction and internal fixation are justifiable to assure anatomic restoration of the articular surfaces.

INJURIES OF THE SHAFTS OF THE RADIUS & ULNA

FRACTURES OF THE SHAFTS OF THE RADIUS & ULNA

General Considerations

A. Causative Injury: Spiral and oblique fractures are likely to be caused by indirect injury. Greenstick, transverse, and comminuted fractures are commonly the result of direct injury.

B. Radiography:

1. In addition to anteroposterior and lateral films of the entire forearm, including the elbow and wrist joints, oblique views are often desirable.

2. The lateral projection is usually taken with the forearm in midposition (between complete pronation and supination).

3. For the anteroposterior projection care must be taken to prevent any change in relative supination of the radius; if this happens, the distal radius will be the same in both views.

4. Especially in children, films of the uninjured forearm are desirable for comparison of epiphyses and for future reference if growth is impaired.

C. Anatomic Peculiarities: Both the radius and the ulna have biplane curves which permit 180 degrees of rotation in the forearm. If the curves are not preserved by reduction, full rotatory motion of the forearm may not be recovered or derangement of the radioulnar joints may follow.

Torsional displacement by muscle activity has important implications for manipulative treatment of certain fractures of the radial shaft. The direction of torsional displacement of the distal fragment following fracture of the shaft is influenced by the location of the lesion in reference to muscle insertion. If the fracture is in the upper third (above the insertion of the pronator teres), the proximal fragment will be drawn into relative supination by the biceps and supinator and the distal fragment into pronation by the pronator teres and pronator quadratus. The relative position in torsion of the proximal fragment may be determined by comparing the position of the bicipital tubercle on an anteroposterior film with similar projections of the uninjured arm taken in varying degrees of forearm rotation. In fractures below the middle of the radius (below the insertion of the pronator teres), the proximal fragment characteristically remains in midposition and the distal fragment is pronated; this is due to the antagonistic action of the pronator teres on the biceps and supinator.

D. Closed Reduction and Splinting: With fracture and displacement of the shaft of either the radius or the ulna, injury of the proximal or distal radioulnar joints should always be suspected. The presence of swelling and tenderness around the joint may aid in localization of an occult injury when x-rays are not helpful.

In both adults and children, closed reduction of uncomplicated fractures of the radius and ulna should be attempted. The type of manipulative maneuver depends upon the configuration and location of the fracture and the age of the patient. The position of immobilization of the elbow, forearm, and wrist depends upon the location of the fracture and its inherent stability.

Fracture of the Shaft of the Ulna

Isolated fracture of the shaft of the proximal third of the ulna (above the insertion of the pronator teres) with displacement is often associated with dislocation of the head of the radius. Reduction of an undislocated transverse fracture may be achieved by axial traction followed by digital pressure to correct displacement in the transverse plane. With the patient supine, the hand is suspended overhead and countertraction is provided by a sling around the arm above the flexed elbow. After the fragments are distracted, transverse displacement is corrected by digital pressure. With the elbow at a right angle and the forearm in midposition, the extremity is then immobilized in a tubular plaster cast extending from the axilla to the metacarpophalangeal joints. During the first month, weekly examination by x-ray is necessary to determine whether displacement has occurred. Immobilization must be maintained until bone continuity is restored (usually in 8–12 weeks).

Fracture of the shaft of the ulna distal to the insertion of the pronator teres is apt to be complicated by angulation. The proximal end of the distal fragment is displaced toward the radius by the pronator quadratus muscle. Reduction can be achieved by the maneuver described above. To prevent recurrent displacement of the distal fragment, the plaster cast must be carefully molded so as to force the mass of the forearm musculature between the radius and ulna in the anteroposterior plane. Care should be taken to avoid pressure over the subcutaneous surfaces of the radius and ulna around the wrist. Healing is slow, and frequent radiologic examination is necessary to make certain that displacement has not occurred. Stabilization by bone healing may require more than 4 months of immobilization.

An oblique fracture cleft creates an unstable mechanism with a tendency toward displacement, and immobilization in a tubular plaster is not reliable. Open reduction and rigid internal fixation with bone plates or an intramedullary rod are indicated.

Open reduction of uncomplicated fracture of the ulna in children is rarely justifiable because accurate reduction is not imperative; in children under 12 years of age an angular deformity as great as 15 degrees may be corrected by growth. Torsional displacement of uncomplicated fractures of the shaft is not likely to occur. Deformity caused by transverse displacement will be corrected by growth and remodeling.

Fracture of the Shaft of the Radius

Isolated closed fracture of the shaft of the radius can be caused by direct or indirect violence; open fracture usually results from penetrating injury. Closed fracture with displacement is usually associated with other injury (eg, fracture of the ulna or dislocation of the distal radioulnar joint). X-rays may not reveal dislocation, but localized tenderness and swelling suggest injury to the distal radioulnar joint.

If the fracture is proximal to the insertion of the pronator teres, closed reduction is indicated. The extremity should then be immobilized in a tubular plaster cast which extends from the axilla to the metacarpophalangeal joints, with the elbow at a right angle and the forearm in full supination (Fig 45–21).

If the fracture is distal to the insertion of the pronator teres, manipulation and immobilization are as described above except that the forearm should be in midrotation rather than full supination. Since injury to the distal radioulnar joint is apt to be associated with

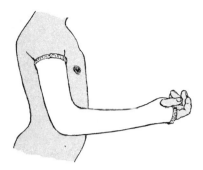

Figure 45–21. Full upper extremity plaster for fracture of both bones of the forearm.

fracture of the radial shaft below the insertion of the pronator teres, weekly anteroposterior and lateral x-ray projections should be taken during the first month to determine the exact status of reduction.

If the configuration of the fracture cleft is transverse rather than oblique, displacement is less apt to take place following anatomic reduction. In the adult, if stability cannot be achieved or if reduction does not approach the anatomic, open reduction and internal fixation are recommended since deformity as a result of displacement of fragments is likely to cause limitation of forearm and hand movements. Children under 12 years of age are likely to recover function provided that torsional displacement has been corrected and angulation does not exceed 15 degrees. Especially if it is convex anteriorly, angulation greater than 15 degrees should be corrected in children even though open reduction is required.

In adults, a snug plaster should be maintained for 8–12 weeks or even longer, since healing may be slow. Healing is rapid in children even though reduction is not anatomic; open reduction to promote bone healing in children is not necessary.

Fracture of the Shafts of Both Bones

The management of fractures of the shafts of both bones of the forearm is essentially a combination of those technics which have been described for the individual bones. If both bones are fractured at the same time, dislocation of either radioulnar joint is not likely to occur. If the configuration of the fracture cleft is approximately transverse, stability can be attained by closed methods provided reduction is anatomic or nearly so. Oblique or comminuted fractures are unstable.

Treatment depends in part upon the degree of displacement, the severity of comminution, and the age of the patient.

A. Without Displacement: In adults, fracture of the shaft of the radius and ulna without displacement can be treated by immobilization in a tubular plaster cast extending from the axilla to the metacarpophalangeal joints with the elbow at a right angle and the forearm in supination (fractures of the upper third) or midposition (fractures of the mid and lower thirds).

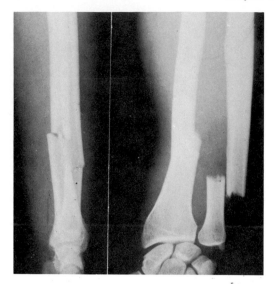

Figure 45—22. Fracture of the lower third of the shafts of the radius and ulna in a 29-year-old man.

Immobilization for 8—12 weeks is generally sufficient for restoration of bone continuity in children; immobilization for a longer time is necessary for adults. To avoid late angulation or refracture, the elbow should be included in the plaster until the callus is well mineralized.

B. Greenstick Fractures: Greenstick fractures of both bones of the forearm are common in children. With fractures of the lower third in children under 12 years of age, if angulation is no more than 15 degrees and convex posteriorly, satisfactory correction of the deformity can be expected to occur spontaneously with growth. If angulation is greater than 15 degrees or if the apex is directed anteriorly, deformity should be corrected and the extremity immobilized in a tubular plaster cast extending from the axilla to the bases of the fingers, the elbow at a right angle, the forearm in pronation, and the wrist in the neutral position. Reduction is maintained by snug anteroposterior molding of the plaster over the distal third of the forearm rather than by placing the wrist in volar flexion.

Greenstick fracture of both bones proximal to the distal third of the shaft can cause a tendency toward increased angular deformity if angulation alone is corrected without completion of the fracture. It is recommended that the fracture be completed by sharply reversing the direction of angulation until a palpable "snap" indicates that intact fibers of bone and periosteum on the convex surface have ruptured. The extremity is then immobilized in a plaster cast similar to that used for lower third fractures, with the forearm in semisupination.

C. With Displacement: Although it is not always possible to correct displaced fractures of both bones of the forearm by closed methods, an attempt should be made to do so both in adults and in children if x-ray studies show a configuration whereby stabilization can

be accomplished without operation. Manipulative reduction is recommended if the patient is treated soon after injury and overriding is less than 1 cm. It is essential that good apposition of the fragments of each bone be obtained. Once adequate reduction has been achieved, and while traction is maintained, a padded tubular plaster cast is applied from the bases of the fingers to the axilla.

If treatment is delayed until hemorrhage and swelling have caused induration by infiltration of the soft tissues, or if overriding is more than 1 cm, sustained traction for 2—3 hours will probably be necessary to overcome shortening. Traction on the skin with countertraction on soft tissues is hazardous in these circumstances because of the possibility of decubiti or vascular injury. Skeletal traction is indicated. When correction of the overriding is demonstrated by x-ray, the fragments are manipulated into position under local or general anesthesia. A plaster cast with wires incorporated is then applied and the tension bows maintained to keep the wires taut.

Persistent overriding without angulation in children is not a problem since 0.5 cm of shortening may be corrected by growth. If overriding of more than 0.5

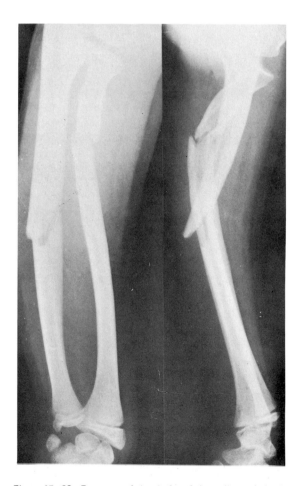

Figure 45—23. Fractures of the shafts of the radius and ulna in an 11-year-old girl.

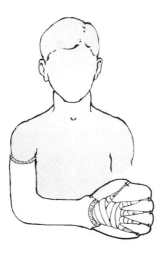

Figure 45—24. Banjo splint and skin traction for fracture of the forearm in children (Blount).

cm is demonstrated, continuous skin traction upon the fingers with elastic bands attached to a banjo loop incorporated into the tubular plaster is indicated (Fig 45—24).

In adults, if accurate apposition of fragments or stability cannot be achieved in fractures of both bones, open reduction and internal fixation are recommended provided that experienced personnel and adequate equipment are available. Persistent displacement of the fragments of one or both bones may be associated with delay of healing, restriction of forearm movements, derangement of the radioulnar joints, and deformity. In those fractures in which open reduction is justifiable in the adult, rigid internal fixation is indicated; a technical pitfall to be avoided is the use of a single wire loop or transfixation screw, a short bone plate attached with unicortical screws, or small intramedullary wires. Even though excellent stability is achieved at operation with internal devices, the extremity should be protected by external fixation until bone healing is well under way.

FRACTURE-DISLOCATIONS OF THE RADIUS & ULNA

Fracture of the Ulna With Dislocation of the Radial Head (Monteggia's Fracture)

Fracture of the ulna, especially when it occurs near the junction of the middle and upper thirds of the shaft, may be complicated by dislocation of the radial head. This unstable fracture-dislocation, the so-called **Monteggia fracture,** is categorized commonly under 3 types. When the radial head is dislocated anteriorly, angulation at the ulnar fracture site is convex in the same direction (type I). In type II, posterior dislocation of the radial head is accompanied by posterior convex angulation at the fracture site of the ulna. The type III lesion—lateral dislocation of the radial head

with fracture of the ulna in its proximal third, distal to the coronoid process—is rare. All 3 types occur both in children and in adults.

A. Closed Reduction:

1. Anterior dislocation of the head of the radius— Although this lesion can be caused by direct violence upon the dorsum of the forearm, it may also be caused by forced pronation. The annular ligament may be torn, or the head may be displaced distally from beneath the annular ligament without causing a significant tear. The injured ligament may be interposed between the articular surface of the head of the radius and the capitellum of the humerus or the adjacent ulna.

Adequate reduction can usually be achieved by closed manipulation in children and sometimes in adults. A posterior plaster splint is applied from the axillary fold to the heads of the metacarpals with the elbow in 110—130 degrees of flexion and the forearm either in midrotation or slight supination (Fig 45—16). If reduction is satisfactory, the extremity is elevated and observed frequently for signs of circulatory embarrassment for at least 72 hours. Bandages must be adjusted at appropriate intervals to accommodate for changes of soft tissue swelling which may embarrass circulation soon after reduction and later may cause displacement of the splint and loss of reduction. X-ray examination should be repeated as soon as the dressings are applied, on the third day, and at least once weekly during the first month. Immobilization is continued until bone continuity of the ulna is restored, usually 10—12 weeks or even longer, since healing is likely to be slow. Acute flexion of the elbow in plaster should not be decreased before the eighth week.

2. Posterior dislocation of the head of the radius— This lesion is caused by direct violence to the volar surface of the forearm. Treatment is by closed reduction. Anteroposterior and lateral x-rays are then taken, and a tubular plaster cast or stout posterior plaster splint is applied from the metacarpal heads to the axilla with the elbow in full extension and the forearm in midposition. Careful postreduction observation as for anterior dislocation (see above) is essential.

B. Open Reduction: If accurate reduction of the fracture and the dislocation cannot be achieved by closed methods, open reduction is indicated. Plaster immobilization is indicated until bone healing is well under way.

Bryan RS: Monteggia fracture of the forearm. J Trauma 11:992, 1971.

Reckling FW, Cordell LD: Unstable fracture-dislocations of the forearm: The Monteggia and Galeazzi lesions. Arch Surg 96:999, 1968.

Tompkins DG: The anterior Monteggia fracture: Observations on etiology and treatment. J Bone Surg 53A:1109, 1971.

Fracture of the Shaft of the Radius With Dislocation of the Ulnar Head

In fracture of the shaft of the radius near the junction of the middle and lower thirds with dislocation of the head of the ulna (Dupuytren's fracture, Galeazzi's fracture), the apex of major angulation is usually directed anteriorly while the ulnar head lies volar to the distal end of the radius. (Convex dorsal angulation with the ulnar head posterior to the lower end of the radius is rare.)

A. Closed Reduction: Anatomic alignment is difficult to obtain by closed manipulation and difficult to maintain in plaster, but these technics should be tried before open reduction is used. After reduction, anteroposterior and lateral x-rays are taken and developed before application of the cast. If reduction is adequate, a tubular plaster cast is applied from the axilla to the knuckles with the elbow at a right angle, the forearm in pronation, and the wrist in neutral position. Weekly x-ray examination is indicated during the first month. Immobilization in a snug tubular plaster cast is continued until healing of the radius is complete.

Immobilization of the rare posterior type is with the forearm in supination.

B. Open Reduction: If anatomic reduction cannot be achieved by closed methods, open reduction of recent fracture of the radius is the recommended method of treatment.

Adler JB & others: Adult forearm fractures: Principles of management. J Trauma 5:319, 1965.

Botting TD: Posttraumatic radio-ulnar cross union. J Trauma 10:16, 1970.

Dodge HS, Cady GW: Treatment of fractures of the radius and ulna with compression plates: A retrospective study of one hundred and nineteen fractures in seventy-eight patients. J Bone Joint Surg 54A:1167, 1972.

Sargent JP, Teipner WA: Treatment of forearm shaft fractures by double-plating. J Bone Joint Surg 47A:1475, 1965.

INJURIES OF THE WRIST REGION

SPRAINS OF THE WRIST

Isolated severe sprain of the ligaments of the wrist joint is not common, and the diagnosis of wrist sprain should not be made until other lesions, eg, injury to the lower radial epiphysis (in children) and carpal fractures and dislocations (in adults), have been ruled out. If symptoms persist for more than 2 weeks, and especially if pain and swelling are present, x-ray examination should be repeated.

Treatment may be by immobilization with a volar splint extending from the palmar flexion crease to the elbow. The splint should be attached with elastic bandages so that it can be removed at least 3 times daily for gentle active exercise and warm soaks.

COLLES' FRACTURE

Abraham Colles described the fracture that bears his name as an impacted fracture of the radius 4 cm above the wrist joint. Modern usage has extended the term Colles' fracture to include a variety of complete fractures of the distal radius characterized by convex volar angulation and by varying degrees of dorsal displacement of the distal fragment.

The fracture is commonly caused by a fall with the hand outstretched, the wrist in dorsiflexion, and the forearm in pronation, so that the force is applied to the palmar surface of the hand. Colles' fracture is most common in middle life and old age.

The fracture cleft may be transverse or oblique, and extends across the distal radius. It may be comminuted, extending into the radiocarpal joint. Displacement is often minimal, with dorsal impaction caused by tilting of the distal fragment and volar convex angulation. As displacement becomes more marked, dorsal and radial tilt of the distal fragment causes increased angulation and torsional displacement in supination of the distal fragment. The normal volar and ulnar inclination of the carpal articular surface of the radius is reduced or reversed.

Avulsion of the styloid process is the usual injury to the distal ulna. Extension of the fracture cleft into the ulnar notch may injure the distal radioulnar articulation. The carpus is displaced with the distal fragment of the radius. Marked displacement at the fracture site causes dislocation of the distal radioulnar and ulnocarpal articulations, and tearing of the triangular fibrocartilage, both radioulnar ligaments, and the volar ulnocarpal ligament. If the ulnar styloid is not fractured, then the collateral ulnar ligament is torn. The head of the ulna lies anterior to the distal fragment of the radius.

Clinical Findings

Clinical findings vary according to the magnitude

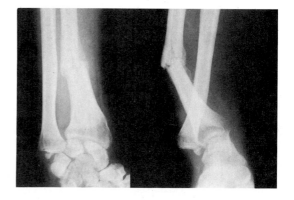

Figure 45—25. Unreduced fractures of the lower shaft of the radius and the ulnar styloid and posterior dislocation of the distal radioulnar joint 5 weeks after injury in a 29-year-old woman.

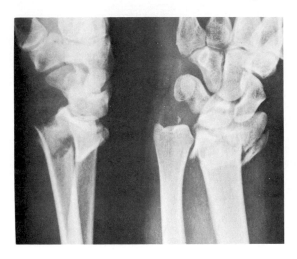

Figure 45—26. Comminuted Colles' fracture in a 58-year-old man. Because of severe comminution, this fracture is unstable.

of injury, the degree of displacement of fragments, and the interval since injury. If the fragments are not displaced, examination soon after injury will demonstrate only slight tenderness and insignificant swelling; pain may be absent. Marked displacement produces the classic "silver fork" or "bayonet" deformity, in which a dorsal prominence caused by displacement of the distal fragment replaces the normal convex curve of the lower radius and the ulnar head is prominent on the anteromedial aspect of the wrist. Later, swelling may extend from the fingertips to the elbow.

Complications

Derangement of the distal radioulnar joint is the most common complicating injury. Direct injury to the median nerve by bone spicules is not common. Compression of the nerve by hemorrhage and edema or by displaced bone fragments is frequent and may cause all gradations of sensory and motor paralysis. Initial treatment of the fracture by immobilization of the wrist in acute flexion can be a significant factor in aggravation of compression. Persistent compression of the nerve creates classic symptoms of the carpal tunnel syndrome, which may require operative division of the volar carpal ligament for relief. Other complicating injuries are fractures involving the carpal navicular, the head of the radius, or the capitellum. Dislocation of the elbow and shoulder and tears of the capsulotendinous cuff of the shoulder may be associated.

Treatment

Complete recovery of function and a pleasing cosmetic result are goals of treatment which cannot always be achieved. The patient's age, sex, and occupation, the presence of complicating injury or disease, the severity of comminution, and the configuration of the fracture cleft govern the selection of treatment.

Open reduction of recent closed Colles' fracture is rarely the treatment of choice. Many technics of closed

reduction and external immobilization have been advocated; the experience and preference of the surgeon determine the selection.

A. Minor Displacement: Colles' fracture with minimal displacement is characterized by absence of comminution and slight dorsal impaction. Deformity is barely perceptible, or may not be visible even to a trained observer. In the elderly patient, treatment is directed toward early recovery of function. In young patients, prevention of further displacement is the first consideration.

Reduction is not necessary. The wrist is immobilized for 3—5 days in a volar plaster splint extending from the distal palmar flexion crease to the elbow. Thereafter the splint may be removed periodically (4—5 times daily) to permit active exercise of the wrist. Soaking the hand and forearm for 15—20 minutes in warm water 2—3 times a day tends to relieve pain and stiffness. The splint can usually be discarded within 2 weeks.

B. Marked Displacement: Early reduction and immobilization are indicated. When reduction has been delayed until preliminary healing is advanced, open reduction may be elected or correction of the deformity can be deferred until healing is sound. The malunion can then be corrected by osteotomy and bone grafting.

In an old person with complicating arthritis, when impaction causes stability, the mild deformity may be accepted in favor of early restoration of function.

1. Stable fractures—Colles' fracture is characterized by comminution of the dorsal cortex. Correction of the deformity creates a wedge-shaped area of fragmented and impacted cancellous bone. The base of the wedge is directed dorsally, and there is no buttress to prevent recurrence of displacement. In part, stability is attained by bringing the volar cortices of the fragments into anatomic apposition.

Muscular relaxation of the extremity can usually be attained more readily under general anesthesia, but local anesthesia is commonly the better choice for the elderly patient.

Reduction is by manipulation. Success of manipulation is determined by clinical examination. Swelling is dissipated by massaging the volar and lateral aspects of the radius until the subcutaneous border can be palpated. Restoration of the normal convex curve of the distal radius implies that transverse displacement and angulation are absent. Proximal displacement has been reduced if the radial styloid process can be palpated 1 cm distal to the ulnar styloid.

A lightly padded tubular cast extending above the elbow or a "sugar tong" splint (Fig 45—27) is preferred. The plaster should extend distally only to the palmar flexion crease, with the forearm in midposition and the wrist in slight volar flexion and ulnar deviation. In obese patients, immobilization is more reliable if the elbow is included in the plaster. After the plaster has been applied, it is molded carefully around the wrist until it has set. X-rays are taken while anesthesia is continued. If x-rays show that reduction is not

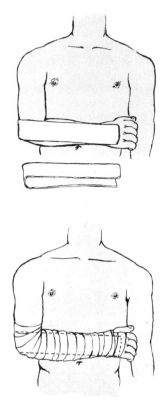

Figure 45–27. "Sugar tong" plaster splint.

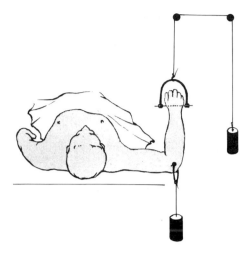

Figure 45–28. Skeletal distraction for closed manipulation of fracture of the forearm or wrist.

adequate, remanipulation is carried out immediately.

X-ray examination is repeated on the third day and thereafter at weekly intervals during the first 3 weeks. The plaster must remain snug; if loosening occurs after absorption of hemorrhagic exudate, a new cast should be applied.

2. Unstable fractures–If x-rays show extensive comminution with intra-articular extension and involvement of the volar cortex, the fracture is likely to be unstable and skeletal distraction is probably indicated by means of traction on Kirschner wires (Fig 45–28). Traction is continued while the plaster is applied. To ensure maximal external support, the extremity is immobilized in a tubular plaster cast extending from the axilla to the palmar flexion crease, with the elbow at a right angle, the forearm in midposition, and the wrist in slight ulnar deviation and volar flexion. The Kirschner wires are incorporated in the plaster, and the bows are maintained to hold the wires taut (Fig 45–29). The wires are left in place for 6 weeks. The fracture is protected for an additional 2 weeks following removal of the wires by a gauntlet or a "sugar tong" splint.

Postreduction Treatment

Frequent observation and careful management can prevent or minimize some of the disabling sequelae of Colles' fracture. The patient's full cooperation in the exercise program is essential. If comminution is

marked, if swelling is severe, or if there is evidence of median nerve deficit, the patient should remain under close observation (preferably in a hospital) for at least 72 hours. The extremity should be elevated to minimize swelling, and the adequacy of circulation determined at frequent intervals. Active exercise of the fingers and shoulder is encouraged. In order that the extremity should be used as much as possible, the plaster should be trimmed in the palm to permit full finger flexion.

As soon as the plaster is removed, the patient is advised to use the extremity for customary daily care but to avoid strenuous activity that might cause refracture.

Complications & Sequelae

Joint stiffness is the most disabling sequel of Colles' fracture. Derangement of the distal radioulnar joint may be caused by the original injury and perpetuated by incomplete reduction; it is characterized by restriction of forearm movements and pain. Late rupture of the extensor pollicis longus tendon is relatively uncommon. Symptoms of median nerve injury due to compression caused by acute swelling alone usually do

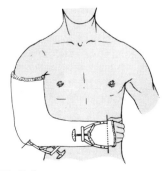

Figure 45–29. Full upper extremity plaster with Kirschner wires incorporated.

not persist more than 6 months. Prolonged symptoms can cause carpal tunnel syndrome. Failure to perform shoulder joint exercises several times daily can result in disabling stiffness.

Colles A: Colles's classic description of fractures of the lower end of the radius: On the fracture of the carpal extremity of the radius. J Bone Joint Surg 55B:454, 1973.

Marsh HO, Teal SW: Treatment of comminuted fractures of the distal radius with self-contained skeletal traction. Am J Surg 124:715, 1972.

Mital MA, Patel UH: Fractures and dislocations about the distal forearm, wrist, and hand: Progress in treatment in the last decade. Am J Surg 124:660, 1972.

Pool C: Colles's fracture: A prospective study of treatment. J Bone Joint Surg 55B:540, 1973.

SMITH'S FRACTURE
("Reversed Colles")

Although Smith did not observe an anatomic preparation of this lesion, his description in 1847 placed the fracture site of the radius ½ inch to 1 inch above the wrist joint. The normal volar concavity of the lower radius is accentuated because the apex of angulation at the fracture site is posterior. The ulnar head is prominent dorsally, and there may be derangement of the inferior radioulnar joint. This lesion should be differentiated from Barton's fracture-dislocation (see below).

The fracture can be reduced by closed manipulation and immobilized with the wrist in dorsiflexion. Unstable fractures may require initial skeletal distraction (see above for unstable Colles' fracture). Those fractures which cannot be reduced adequately by closed methods may require open reduction and bone plating.

Ellis J: Smith's and Barton's fractures. J Bone Joint Surg 47B:724, 1965.

Fuller DJ: The Ellis plate operation for Smith's fracture. J Bone Joint Surg 55B:173, 1973.

FRACTURE OF THE RADIAL STYLOID

Forced radial deviation of the hand at the wrist joint can fracture the radial styloid. A large fragment of the styloid is usually displaced by impingement against the carpal navicular. Avulsion of the tip of the styloid by the radial collateral ligament occurs less frequently, and may be associated with dislocation of the radiocarpal joint. If the fragment is large, it can be displaced farther by the brachioradialis muscle, which inserts into it.

Because the fracture is intra-articular, reduction of large fragments should be anatomic. If the styloid fragment is not displaced, immobilization in a plaster gauntlet for 3 weeks is sufficient. If the fragment is displaced, manipulative reduction should be tried. If the distal, smaller fragment tends to displace but can be apposed by digital pressure, percutaneous fixation can be achieved by a medium Kirschner wire inserted through the proximal anatomic snuffbox so as to transfix both fragments. The wrist is then immobilized in a snugly molded plaster gauntlet for 6 weeks. X-ray examination is repeated every week for at least 3 weeks.

If closed methods fail, open reduction is indicated since persistent displacement is likely to cause post-traumatic degenerative arthritis relatively early.

FRACTURE OF THE DISTAL RADIAL EPIPHYSIS

Fracture through the distal radial epiphyseal plate in children is the counterpart of Colles' fracture in the adult. Wrist sprain is rare in childhood and should be differentiated as early as possible from fracture of the distal epiphysis. Such an injury is usually caused by indirect violence due to a fall on the outstretched hand. The magnitude of displacement of the epiphyseal fragment varies.

In some cases, separation and displacement of the epiphysis cannot be demonstrated by radiologic examination and may be quite difficult to identify on clinical examination. The patient may complain of pain in the region of the wrist joint, and slight swelling may be present. Pressure with a blunt object, eg, the eraser of a lead pencil, may demonstrate maximal tenderness at the epiphyseal plate instead of at the wrist joint. Buckling of the adjacent metaphyseal cortex manifests greater displacement.

Displacement is posterior and to the radial side. Marked displacement may be accompanied by crushing of the epiphyseal plate, tear of the triangular fibrocartilage of the distal radioulnar articulation, displacement of the distal ulnar epiphysis, or avulsion of the ulnar styloid.

Both wrists should be examined by x-ray if injury to the distal radial epiphysis is suspected. Severe injury, crushing the epiphyseal cartilage and fracturing the epiphysis, is likely to impede growth and may even lead to early epiphyseal fusion; continued growth of the distal ulnar epiphysis produces derangement of the distal radioulnar joint.

Open reduction is rarely necessary. The trauma of the operation superimposed on the injury is likely to cause early arrest of epiphyseal growth. Closed reduction by manipulation is usually successful if it can be done within the week following injury. Immobilization is with a plaster gauntlet or "sugar tong" splint. The plaster should be worn for 4—6 weeks. Permanent stiffness due to immobilization of the wrist is not to be feared.

The child should be examined yearly to determine whether there is any growth disturbance.

FRACTURE-DISLOCATIONS OF THE RADIOCARPAL JOINT

Dislocation of the radiocarpal joint without fracture is rare. Dislocation without injury to one of the carpal bones is usually associated with fracture of the anterior surface of the radius or the ulna. Comminuted fracture of the distal radius may involve either the anterior or posterior cortex and extends into the wrist joint. Subluxation of the carpus may occur at the same time. The most common fracture-dislocation of the wrist joint involves the posterior or anterior margin of the articular surface of the radius.

Anterior Fracture-Dislocation of the Radiocarpal Joint (Barton's Fracture)

Anterior fracture-dislocation of the wrist joint is characterized by fracture of the volar margin of the carpal articular surface of the radius. The fracture cleft extends proximally in the coronal plane in an oblique direction, so that the free fragment has a wedge-shaped configuration. The carpus is displaced volar and proximally with the articular fragment. This uncommon injury should be differentiated from Smith's fracture by x-ray examination.

Treatment by closed reduction may be successful, especially in cases in which the free fragment of the radius does not involve a large portion of the articular surface. Immobilization is with a tubular plaster cast extending from the palmar flexion crease to above the elbow with the wrist in volar flexion and the elbow at a right angle. Immediate x-rays are taken in 2 projections. If reduction is not anatomic and the fracture is unstable, skeletal distraction may be necessary. Weekly x-ray examination should be repeated during the first month. Skeletal distraction should be continued for 6 weeks or until preliminary bone healing has stabilized the fracture.

Posterior Fracture-Dislocation of the Radiocarpal Joint

Posterior fracture-dislocation of the wrist joint should be differentiated from Colles' fracture by x-ray. In most cases the marginal fragment is smaller than in anterior injury, and often involves the medial aspect where the extensor pollicis longus crosses the distal radius. If reduction is not anatomic, fraying of the tendon at this level may lead to late rupture.

Treatment is by manipulative reduction as for Colles' fracture and immobilization in a snug plaster gauntlet with the wrist in dorsiflexion.

De Oliveira JC: Barton's fractures. J Bone Joint Surg 55A:586, 1973.

DISLOCATION OF THE DISTAL RADIOULNAR JOINT

The triangular fibrocartilage is the most important structure in preventing dislocation of the distal radioulnar joint. The accessory ligaments and the pronator quadratus muscle play a secondary role. Complete anterior or posterior dislocation implies a tear of the triangular fibrocartilage and disruption of accessory joint ligaments. Tearing of the triangular fibrocartilage in the absence of major injury to the supporting capsular ligaments causes subluxation or abnormal laxity of the joint. Since the ulnar attachment of the triangular fibrocartilage is at the base of the styloid process, x-rays may demonstrate associated fracture. Widening of the cleft in comparison with the opposite radioulnar joint, which is apparent by x-ray examination, demonstrates diastasis of the radius and ulna if frank anterior or posterior displacement is not present.

Complete anterior or posterior dislocation of the distal radioulnar joint is rare. Medial dislocation is associated with fracture of the radius. The direction of dislocation is indicated by the location of the ulnar head in relation to the distal end of the radius.

Levin PD: Fracture of the radial head with dislocation of the distal radio-ulnar joint: Case report. J Bone Joint Surg 55A:837, 1973.

Weseley MS & others: Volar dislocation distal radioulnar joint. J Trauma 12:1083, 1972.

FRACTURES & DISLOCATIONS OF THE CARPUS

Injury to the carpal bones occurs predominantly in men during the most active period of life. Because it is difficult to differentiate these injuries by clinical examination, it is imperative to obtain x-ray films of the best possible quality. The oblique film should be taken in midpronation, the anteroposterior film with the wrist in maximal ulnar deviation. Special views, such as midsupination to demonstrate the pisiform, and carpal tunnel views for the hamate, may be necessary.

Fracture of the Carpal Navicular

The most common injury to the carpus is fracture of the navicular. Fracture of the carpal navicular should be suspected in any injury to the wrist in an adult male unless a specific diagnosis of another type of injury is obvious. If tenderness on the radial aspect of the wrist is present and fracture cannot be demonstrated, initial treatment should be the same as if fracture were present (see below) and should be continued for at least 3 weeks. Further x-ray examination after 3 weeks may demonstrate an occult fracture.

Three types of fracture are distinguished:

(1) Fracture of the tubercle: This fracture usually

is not widely displaced, and healing is generally prompt if immobilization in a plaster gauntlet is maintained for 2–3 weeks.

(2) Fracture through the waist: Fracture through the narrowest portion of the bone is the most common type. The blood supply to the proximal fragment is usually not disturbed, and healing will take place if reduction is adequate and treatment is instituted early. If the nutrient artery to the proximal third is injured, avascular necrosis of that portion of the bone may occur.

X-ray examination in multiple projections is necessary to determine the direction of the fracture cleft and displacement of the proximal fragment. If the proximal fragment is displaced, it can be reduced under local anesthesia by forced dorsiflexion and radial deviation of the wrist. Immobilization in a plaster gauntlet with the wrist in slight dorsiflexion is necessary. The plaster should extend distally to the palmar flexion crease in the hand and to the base of the thumbnail. If reduction has been anatomic and the blood supply to the proximal fragment has not been jeopardized, adequate bone healing can be expected within 10 weeks. However, such healing must be demonstrated by the disappearance of the fracture cleft and restoration of the trabecular pattern between the 2 main fragments. X-ray examination to verify healing should be repeated 3 weeks after removal of the cast.

(3) Fracture through the proximal third: Fracture through the proximal third of the navicular is likely to be associated with injury to the arterial supply of the minor fragment. This can be manifested by avascular necrosis of that fragment. If the lesion is observed soon after injury, reduction and immobilization in a plaster gauntlet will promote healing. The plaster gauntlet should be applied snugly, and must be changed if it becomes loose; it is usually necessary to renew the gauntlet every 4 weeks. X-rays should be taken once a month to determine the progress of bone healing; it may be necessary to prolong immobilization for 4–6 months. The same criteria of radiographic examination as are used for healing of fractures through the waist are used in fractures of the proximal third. It is advisable to make an additional x-ray examination 3–4 weeks after removal of the cast.

If evidence of healing is not apparent after immobilization for 6 months or more, further immobilization will probably not be effective. This is especially true if x-rays show that the fracture cleft has widened and if sclerosis is noted adjacent to the cleft. If the interval between the time of injury and the establishment of a diagnosis is 3 months or more, a trial of immobilization for 2–3 months may be elected. If obliteration of the fracture cleft and evidence of restoration of bone continuity are not visible in x-rays taken after this trial period, some form of operative treatment will be necessary to initiate bone healing. Bone grafting is probably more successful. Prolonged immobilization in a plaster gauntlet is necessary before bony continuity is restored.

If avascular necrosis has occurred in the proximal fragment, bone grafting is less likely to be successful. Although excision of the avascular fragment may relieve painful symptoms for a time, the patient usually notes weakness of grasp and discomfort after prolonged use. Posttraumatic arthritis is apt to develop late.

Prolonged failure of bone healing predisposes to posttraumatic arthritis. Bone grafting operations or other procedures directed toward restoration of bone continuity may be successful, but arthritis causes continued disability. Arthrodesis of the wrist gives the best assurance of relief of pain and a functionally competent extremity.

Fracture of the Lunate

Fracture of the lunate may be manifested by minor avulsion fractures of the posterior or anterior horn. Careful multiplane x-ray examination is necessary to establish the diagnosis. Either of these lesions may be treated by the use of a volar splint for 3 weeks.

Fracture of the body may be manifested by a crack, by comminution, or by impaction. A fissure fracture can be treated by immobilization in plaster for 3 weeks.

One complication of this fracture is persistent pain in the wrist, slight restriction of motion, and tenderness over the lunate. X-ray examination can demonstrate areas of sclerosis and rarefaction. Impaction or collapse can be accompanied by arthritic changes surrounding the lunate. This x-ray appearance is referred to as Kienböck's disease, osteochondrosis of the lunate, or avascular necrosis.

Fracture of the Hamate

Fracture of the hamate may occur through the body and is shown on x-ray as a fissure or compression. Fracture of the base of the hamulus is less common and more difficult to diagnose; special projections are necessary to demonstrate the cleft. If the hamulus is displaced, closed manipulation will not be effective. Prolonged painful symptoms or evidence of irritation of the ulnar nerve may require excision of the loose fragment.

Fracture of the Triquetrum

Fracture of the triquetrum is caused commonly by direct violence and is often associated with fracture of other carpal bones. Treatment is by immobilization in a plaster gauntlet for 4 weeks.

Dislocation of the Lunate

Dislocation of the lunate is the second most common injury of the carpus. Dislocation is caused by forced dorsiflexion of the wrist, and the direction of dislocation is almost always anterior. The diagnosis is usually made by x-ray examination. Dislocation may be manifest by dorsal displacement of the capitate while the lunate retains contact with the radius. A further degree of injury is manifested by complete displacement of the lunate from the radius, so that it comes to lie anterior to the capitate and loses its relationship to the articular surface of the radius. If x-ray examination is adequate, the diagnosis can be established easily.

Reduction may be achieved by closed manipulation. X-rays are then taken to determine the success of treatment. If reduction is adequate, the extremity is immobilized in a plaster gauntlet with the wrist in full volar flexion for about 2 weeks. The plaster is then removed and another applied with the wrist in neutral position for an additional 2 weeks. If x-rays show that this manipulative maneuver has not caused reduction, skeletal distraction by means of Kirschner wires may separate the radiocarpal joint sufficiently to permit manipulative reduction (Fig 45–28). If closed methods are not successful, open reduction should be done promptly.

Dislocation of the Capitate

Dislocation of the capitate is most often associated with other lesions of the carpus and is commonly called transcarpal or midcarpal dislocation. The most frequent accompanying injury is fracture of the carpal navicular, in which case the lunate and the proximal fragment of the navicular retain their relationship to the articular surface of the radius whereas the distal fragment of the navicular, the capitate, and the remainder of the carpus are displaced dorsally. Thus the dislocation is retrolunar.

Subluxation of the navicular is less often associated with dislocation of the lunate. The direction of this dislocation is also retrolunar. Fracture of the radial or ulnar styloid process is likely to be present also.

X-rays of poor technical quality may not demonstrate the lesion satisfactorily; anteroposterior and true lateral projections are necessary.

The comparatively uncommon midcarpal dislocation can be reduced by closed manipulation if the lesion is uncomplicated and recognized within 10–14 days after injury. Immobilization in a plaster gauntlet with the wrist in slight dorsiflexion for 4 weeks is sufficient for stabilization by early ligamentous healing. If fracture complicates the dislocation, treatment is divided into 2 phases. Reduction of the fracture-dislocation is accomplished by closed manipulation. The navicular fracture is then treated as outlined above.

Gordon SL: Scaphoid and lunate dislocation. J Bone Joint Surg 54A:1769, 1972.

Linscheid RL & others: Traumatic instability of the wrist: Diagnosis, classification, and pathomechanics. J Bone Joint Surg 54A:1612, 1972.

Monahan PR, Galasko CS: The scapho-capitate fracture syndrome: A mechanism of injury. J Bone Joint Surg 54B:122, 1972.

Nahigan SH & others: The dorsal flap arthroplasty in the treatment of Kienböck's disease. J Bone Joint Surg 52A:245, 1970.

Sprague B, Justis EJ Jr: Nonunion of the carpal navicular: Modes of treatment. Arch Surg 108:692, 1974.

Weseley MS, Barenfeld PA: Trans-scaphoid, transtriquetral, perilunate fracture-dislocation of the wrist: A case report. J Bone Joint Surg 54A:1073, 1972.

INJURIES OF THE HIP REGION

BIRTH FRACTURE OF THE UPPER FEMORAL EPIPHYSES

Birth injury to the upper femoral epiphyses is rare, and the diagnosis by physical examination alone is difficult because the skeletal structures involved are deeply situated. Swelling of the upper thigh and pseudoparalysis of the extremity following a difficult delivery suggest the injury. X-ray examination may demonstrate outward and proximal displacement of the shaft of the femur. Formation of new bone in the region of the metaphysis may be demonstrated in 7–10 days. If displacement has occurred, treatment for 2–3 weeks by Bryant's traction (Fig 45–39) is recommended. Otherwise, protection by a perineal pillow splint for the same length of time is adequate.

Lindseth RE, Rosene HA Jr: Traumatic separation of the upper femoral epiphysis in a newborn infant. J Bone Joint Surg 53A:1641, 1971.

DISPLACEMENT & SEPARATION OF THE CAPITAL FEMORAL EPIPHYSIS

Displacement of the capital femoral epiphysis due to trauma in the normal child should be differentiated from idiopathic slipped epiphysis (epiphysiolysis, adolescent coxa vara) due possibly to endocrine or metabolic dysfunction. However, between the ages of 10 and 16 years, differentiation may be impossible. Mild injury may cause sudden separation and displacement because of weakening of the plate by antecedent idiopathic disturbance of cartilage growth.

Traumatic separation of the capital femoral epiphysis is rare in normal children, but it may occur as a result of a single episode of severe trauma which otherwise might cause fracture of the femoral neck. The direction of displacement is likely to be the same as in adolescent coxa vara. Although anatomic reduction can be obtained by closed manipulation, immobilization in a plaster spica should not be trusted since redisplacement is possible; internal fixation is more reliable. Traumatic separation of the capital epiphysis associated with dislocation of the hip joint (epiphysis and proximal femur) is a rare lesion with an unfavorable prognosis. Avascular necrosis of the epiphysis is almost certain.

Casey BH & others: Reduction of acutely slipped upper femoral epiphysis. J Bone Joint Surg 54B:607, 1972.

FRACTURE OF THE FEMORAL NECK

Fracture of the femoral neck occurs most commonly in patients over the age of 50. If displacement has occurred, the extremity is in external rotation and adduction. Leg shortening is usually obvious. Motion of the hip joint causes pain. If the fracture is impacted in the valgus position, the injured extremity may be slightly longer than the opposite side and active external rotation may not be possible. If the fragments are not displaced and the fracture is stable, pain at the extremes of passive hip motion may be the only significant finding. The fact that the patient can actively move the extremity often interferes with prompt diagnosis.

Before treatment is instituted, anteroposterior and lateral films of excellent quality must be obtained. Gentle traction and internal rotation of the extremity while the anteroposterior film is exposed may provide a more favorable relation of fragments to demonstrate the fracture cleft.

Fractures of the femoral neck may be classified as abduction or adduction fractures.

Abduction Fracture of the Femoral Neck

Abduction describes the relationship between the neck and shaft fragment and the head, which creates a coxa valga deformity. Abduction fractures occur most often in the proximal femoral neck adjacent to the head. Displacement is apt to be minimal, and impaction is often present. The direction of the fracture cleft approaches the transverse plane of the body, and the angle is 30 degrees or less (Fig 45–30). The anteroposterior x-ray may show a wedge-shaped area of increased density whose base is directed superiorly. A good lateral film will demonstrate both the anterior and posterior cortices of the femoral neck. In this plane the neck and shaft fragment may be angulated slightly, so that only the posterior cortex appears to be impacted and the anterior cortices of the fragments appear to be separated.

Impaction is precarious and undependable as a fixation mechanism; if internal fixation is not used, separation may occur before healing is sound. If firm impaction can be demonstrated in both the anterior and posterior x-rays, some surgeons recommend conservative treatment, ie, bed rest with the extremity in balanced suspension for 4–8 weeks. The patient is

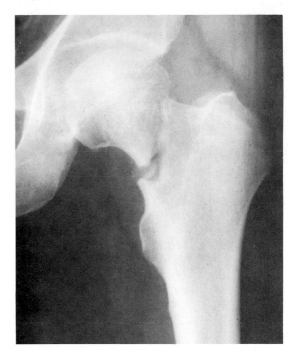

Figure 45–31. Pauwel's type III fracture of the neck of the femur in a 59-year-old man. Interposition of a small intermediate fragment and soft tissues prevented adequate reduction by closed manipulation.

then permitted to be ambulatory with crutches, but full weight-bearing is not permitted until complete healing can be demonstrated by x-rays (usually 4–12 months after injury). Other surgeons prefer internal fixation because it permits the patient to be out of bed soon after the operation even though unsupported weight-bearing is not permitted any sooner than after nonoperative treatment.

If examination in the lateral projection does not show firm impaction of both cortices at the fracture site, closed manipulation and internal fixation are indicated.

Adduction Fracture of the Femoral Neck

Adduction fracture is characterized by coxa vara deformity. The fracture may be at any level of the neck, and the direction of the fracture cleft approaches that of the sagittal plane of the body. Displacement is usually present. The relatively vertical configuration of the fracture cleft favors proximal displacement of the distal fragment by the force of any axial thrust transmitted through the extremity. The fracture should be considered unstable if the angle between the fracture cleft and the transverse plane of the body is greater than 30 degrees (Pauwel) (Fig 45–30).

Adduction fracture of the femoral neck can be a life-endangering injury, especially when it occurs in elderly persons. Treatment is directed toward the preservation of life and restoration of function to the hip joint. In most cases, when the life expectancy of the

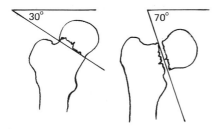

Figure 45–30. Pauwel's angles.

patient is more than a few weeks, open operation is the treatment of choice. Immobilization of this unstable fracture by means of a plaster spica is unreliable. Definitive treatment by skeletal traction requires prolonged recumbency with constant nursing care and is associated with more numerous complications than early mobilization. Some surgeons believe that immediate operative treatment is required after fracture; others reply that 1–2 days of evaluation of the general health status of the patient is rewarded by a lower mortality rate. Operative treatment usually consists of internal fixation or primary arthroplasty.

A. Internal Fixation: The goal of internal fixation is to preserve the capital fragment by providing a setting for bony healing of the fracture. The objective is to allow the patient as much general physical activity during healing as is compatible with the mechanics of fixation. To permit necessary preoperative evaluation of the patient when internal fixation is elected, initial treatment may be by balanced suspension, skeletal traction, and prompt closed reduction of the fracture. Persistent displacement may cause further compromise of the retinacular blood supply to the articular fragment.

Anatomic or near anatomic reduction and firm fixation are desirable to provide optimal circumstances for bone healing. Comminution at the fracture site, injury to the retinacular blood supply of the capital fragment, excessive stressing of the fracture site, and insecure fixation are some of the factors that lead to failure.

The wide variety of surgical technics that make use of the many fixation appliances available testifies to the multiplicity of problems that can be encountered and the variability of opinion concerning treatment. When the fragments are undisplaced or minimally displaced, manipulation is unnecessary. When displacement occurs, reduction may be closed as a preliminary step to fixation or can be accomplished by surgical exposure of the fracture site, especially when determination of competency of blood supply of the proximal fragment is necessary. The fixation apparatus may consist of multiple pins applied percutaneously or more elaborate implants that require open operation. In addition to reduction and internal fixation of the fracture, some surgeons believe that either displacement or valgus osteotomy in the trochanteric region enhances the chances of osseous healing of the fracture and minimizes the incidence of ischemic osteonecrosis of the articular fragment. After operation, the patient may be free in bed and may be mobilized at an early date. To salvage the operative effort if fixation is precarious, traction in balanced suspension or immobilization in a plaster spica for 1–4 months may be necessary until preliminary healing gives additional stability.

Depending upon the relative security of fixation, the extent of early weight-bearing must be regulated until bone continuity is restored to the point where displacement of fragments is unlikely. The agile and cooperative patient may be ambulatory on crutches (but within the limitations of acceptable weight-bear-

ing) within a few days after operative treatment. Crutch walking is hazardous in elderly patients since inadvertent loading may disrupt the fracture relationship.

B. Primary Arthroplasty: In selecting primary arthroplasty, the surgeon realizes that the main proximal fragment must be sacrificed because of injury to the blood supply, preexisting disease, or the intent to permit early unrestricted weight-bearing with stability of the coxofemoral relationship. When the acetabulum is undamaged or is not the site of preexisting disease, the commonly accepted technic is hemiarthroplasty using a femoral component (generally of the intramedullary type) which may or may not be stabilized by a grouting substance such as methyl methacrylate. In the rare circumstance when there is concomitant involvement of the acetabulum, total joint replacement may be justified. Primary head and neck resection may be indicated when there is preexisting infection or local tumor.

The most common sequels of cervical fracture of the femur are redisplacement after reduction and internal fixation, failure of bone healing, and osteonecrosis (avascular, aseptic, or ischemic necrosis) of the head fragment. Secondary osteoarthritis (posttraumatic arthritis) appears somewhat later and may be complicated by any of the common sequels mentioned above. The most serious complication of any open operative treatment is infection. The treatment of sequels and complications is discussed below.

Femoral Neck Fracture in Childhood

Traumatic cervical fracture of the femur in childhood (rare) must be differentiated from congenital coxa vara. Traumatic fracture is usually caused by severe injury. Anatomic reduction by closed manipulation and immobilization in a plaster spica are necessary to prevent deformity. Internal fixation with wires or screws may be necessary. Removal of the fixation apparatus after healing may prevent early fusion of the epiphysis.

Osteonecrosis of the capital epiphysis is a frequent sequel.

Arnold WD & others: Treatment of intracapsular fractures of the femoral neck, with special reference to percutaneous Knowles pinning. J Bone Joint Surg 56A:254, 1974.

Johnson JTH, Crothers O: Nailing versus prosthesis for femoral-neck fractures: A critical review of long-term results in 239 consecutive private patients. J Bone Joint Surg 57A:686, 1975.

Solheim K: Fracture of the femoral neck in children. Acta Orthop Scand 43:523, 1972.

Whittaker RP & others: Fifteen years' experience with metallic endoprosthetic replacement of the femoral head for femoral neck fractures. J Trauma 12:799, 1972.

TROCHANTERIC FRACTURES

Fracture of the Lesser Trochanter

Isolated fracture of the lesser trochanter is quite rare but may develop as a result of the avulsion force of the iliopsoas muscle. It occurs commonly as a component of intertrochanteric fracture.

Fracture of the Greater Trochanter

Isolated fracture of the greater trochanter may be caused by direct injury, or may occur indirectly as a result of the activity of the gluteus medius and gluteus minimus muscles. It occurs most commonly as a component of intertrochanteric fracture.

If displacement is less than 1 cm and there is no tendency to further displacement (determined by repeated x-ray examinations), treatment may be by bed rest with the affected extremity in balanced suspension until acute pain subsides. As rapidly as symptoms permit, activity can increase gradually to protected weight-bearing with crutches. Full weight-bearing is permitted as soon as healing is apparent, usually in 6–8 weeks. If displacement is greater than 1 cm and increases on adduction of the thigh, extensive tearing of surrounding soft tissues may be assumed and open reduction is indicated, followed by internal fixation with 2–3 loops of stainless steel wire.

Intertrochanteric (Including Pertrochanteric) Fractures

These fractures occur most commonly among elderly persons. The cleft of an intertrochanteric fracture extends upward and outward from the medial region of the junction of the neck and lesser trochanter toward the summit of the greater trochanter. Pertrochanteric fracture includes both trochanters, and is likely to be comminuted.

It is important to determine whether comminution has occurred and the magnitude of displacement. These fractures may vary from fissure fracture without significant separation to severe comminution into 4 major fragments: head-neck, greater trochanter, lesser trochanter, and shaft. Displacement may be so marked that the head-neck fragment forms a right angle with the shaft fragment and the distal fragment is rotated externally through an arc of 90 degrees.

Failure of restoration of bone continuity by healing of intertrochanteric fractures is unlikely and, when it occurs, the causes are usually apparent. Of the many factors that influence the rate of healing, those of particular significance are inadequate treatment as manifested by incomplete reduction with unsatisfactory apposition of fragments and unsustained immobilization; comminution; and osteopenia (osteoporosis and disuse atrophy). Healing in malposition (varus and external rotation) is abetted by the major stresses that cause displacement (gravity and muscle activity).

Initial treatment of the fracture in the hospital can be by balanced suspension and, when indicated, by the addition of traction. The selection of definitive

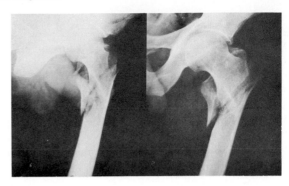

Figure 45–32. Comminuted ("4-part") intertrochanteric fracture of the femur in a 61-year-old man.

treatment—closed or operative technics—depends in part upon the general condition of the patient. Because of the elderly age group in which intertrochanteric fracture is likely to occur, multiple system disease is a determinant of the mortality rate and for that reason the incidence of complications is diminished by the avoidance of prolonged recumbency in bed. Some surgeons are of the opinion that delay in open treatment is hazardous to the life of the patient, and they prefer to operate promptly. Others believe that an evaluation of the general health status of the patient should be made and that preliminary treatment of the fracture—reduction by closed technics—can proceed simultaneously.

Undisplaced fractures can be treated by balanced suspension of the lower extremity until the fragments are stabilized by preliminary bone healing. These fractures can also be treated initially by immobilization in a plaster spica. Sufficient healing generally occurs within 2–3 months to permit the patient to follow a bed and wheelchair existence until partial weight-bearing with crutches can be initiated. Unsupported weight-bearing should not be resumed until the fracture cleft has been obliterated by healing.

If comminution is present and displacement is significant, skin or (preferably) skeletal traction by a Kirschner wire through the tibial tubercle must be added to provide immobilization and to accomplish reduction. Definitive treatment of the fracture can be given in this way or it can be used as a preliminary to open operation.

Open operation may be done electively or may be mandatory for optimal treatment. Reduction of the fracture can be accomplished by closed technics, or it can be an integral part of the open operation. Some surgeons do not prefer to anatomically reduce unstable fractures caused by comminution of the medial femoral cortex. It is maintained that medial displacement of the upper end of the main distal fragment enhances mechanical stability (although it may cause concomitant varus deformity), and this advantageously permits earlier weight-bearing and more prompt healing. The chief intent of open operation is to provide sufficient

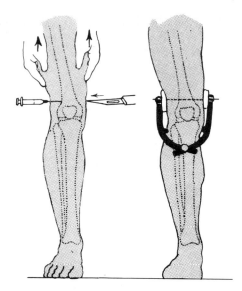

Figure 45—33. Technic of insertion of Kirschner wire in the supracondylar region of the femur.

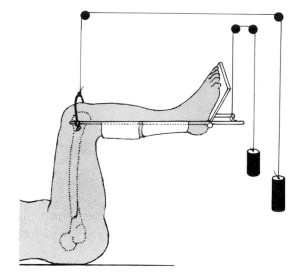

Figure 45—34. Method of suspension of lower extremity with skeletal traction for subtrochanteric fracture.

fixation of the fragments by a metallic surgical implant so that the patient need not be confined to bed during the healing process.

Intertrochanteric fracture during childhood can be treated by skeletal traction with a Kirschner wire inserted through the lower femur above the epiphyseal line (Fig 45—33) or by closed reduction and internal fixation. Varus deformity should be avoided if possible.

Collado F & others: Condylo-cephalic nail fixation for trochanteric fractures of the femur. J Bone Joint Surg 55B:774, 1973.

Laros GS: Intertrochanteric fractures: The role of complications of fixation. Arch Surg 110:37, 1975.

Sarmiento A, Williams EM: The unstable intertrochanteric fracture: Treatment with a valgus osteotomy and I-beam nailplate. J Bone Joint Surg 52A:1309, 1970.

Weiner DS, O'Dell HW: Fractures of the hip in children. J Trauma 9:62, 1969.

SUBTROCHANTERIC FRACTURE

Subtrochanteric fracture due to severe trauma occurs below the level of the lesser trochanter at the junction of cancellous and cortical bone. It is most common in men during the active years of life. Soft tissue damage is extensive. The direction of the fracture cleft may be transverse or oblique. Comminution occurs and the fracture may extend proximally into the intertrochanteric region or distally into the shaft. Muscle is often interposed between the major fragments.

Closed reduction should be attempted by continuous traction to bring the distal fragment into align-

ment with the proximal fragment. If comminution is not extensive and the lesser trochanter is not detached, the proximal fragment is often drawn into relative flexion, external rotation, and abduction by the predominant activity of the iliopsoas, gluteus medius, and gluteus minimus muscles.

Prolonged skeletal traction by means of a Kirschner wire inserted through the supracondylar region of the femur (with the hip and knee flexed to a right angle) is necessary (Fig 45—34). X-ray is repeated every 4—8 hours until reduction has been accomplished. If soft tissue interposition is not a factor, reduction can be achieved within 48 hours. Thereafter the extremity is left in this position with an appropriate amount of traction until stabilization occurs, usually in 8—12 weeks. The angle of flexion is then reduced by gradually bringing the hip and knee into extension. After 2—3 months of continuous traction, the extremity can be immobilized in a plaster spica provided stabilization of the fracture has occurred. Weight-bearing must not be resumed for 6 months or even longer, until bone healing obliterates the fracture cleft.

Interposition of soft tissue between the major fragments may prevent closed reduction. Open reduction of this fracture is difficult and should be undertaken early; if treatment is delayed until the third week following injury, extensive bleeding at the fracture site is likely to be encountered.

After open reduction has been performed, internal fixation is required to prevent redisplacement. If comminution is present, or if it is important to avoid prolonged immobilization, biplane fixation is recommended.

The activity status after operation depends upon the adequacy of internal fixation. If fixation is precarious, skeletal traction in balanced suspension should be continued until healing is well under way. Otherwise, if the patient is agile and cooperative, he may be ambulatory on crutches (but without weight-bearing) a few days after the operation.

Aronoff PN & others: Intramedullary nail fixation as treatment of subtrochanteric fractures of the femur. J Trauma 11:637, 1971.

DiStefano VJ & others: Stable fixation of the difficult subtrochanteric fracture. J Trauma 12:1066, 1972.

Shelton ML: Subtrochanteric fractures of the femur. Arch Surg 110:41, 1975.

TRAUMATIC DISLOCATION OF THE HIP JOINT

Traumatic dislocation of the hip joint may occur with or without fracture of the acetabulum of the proximal end of the femur. It is most common during the active years of life and is usually the result of severe trauma unless there is preexisting disease of the femoral head, acetabulum, or neuromuscular system. The head of the femur cannot be completely displaced from the normal acetabulum unless the ligamentum teres is ruptured or deficient because of some unrelated cause. Traumatic dislocations can be classified according to the direction of displacement of the femoral head from the acetabulum.

Posterior Hip Dislocation

The head of the femur is usually dislocated posterior to the acetabulum while the thigh is flexed, eg, as may occur in a head-on automobile collision when the passenger's knee is driven violently against the dashboard.

The significant clinical findings are shortening, adduction, and internal rotation of the extremity. Anteroposterior, transpelvic, and, if fracture of the acetabulum is demonstrated, oblique projections are required. Common complications are fracture of the acetabulum, injury to the sciatic nerve, and fracture of the head or shaft of the femur. The head of the femur may be displaced through a rent in the posterior hip joint capsule, or the glenoid lip may be avulsed from the acetabulum. The short external rotator muscles of the hip joint are commonly lacerated. Fracture of the posterior margin of the acetabulum can create an unstable mechanism.

If the acetabulum is not fractured or if the fragment is small, reduction by closed manipulation either by Bigelow's or Stimson's method is indicated.

The success of reduction is determined immediately by anteroposterior and lateral x-rays. Interposition of capsule substance will be manifest by widening of the joint cleft. If reduction is adequate the hip will be stable with the extremity in extension and slight external rotation.

Postreduction treatment may be by immobiliza-

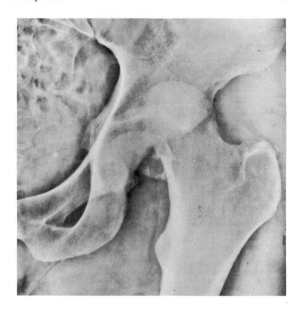

Figure 45–35. Fracture of the head of the femur and posterior dislocation of the hip joint in a 23-year-old man. Closed reduction was unsuccessful because of the head fragment that was retained in the acetabulum.

tion in a plaster spica or by balanced suspension. Since this is primarily a soft tissue injury, sound healing should take place in 4 weeks. Opinion differs on when unsupported weight-bearing should be resumed. Some authors believe that disability caused by ischemic osteonecrosis of the femoral head is less likely when complete weight-bearing is deferred for 6 months after injury; others believe that early loading is not harmful.

If the posterior or superior acetabulum is fractured, dislocation of the hip must be assumed to have occurred even though displacement is not present at the time of examination. Undisplaced fissure fractures may be treated initially by bed rest and avoidance of full weight-bearing for 2 months. Frequent examination is necessary to make certain that the head of the femur has not become displaced from the acetabulum.

Minor fragments of the posterior margin of the acetabulum may be disregarded unless they are in the hip joint cavity. Larger displaced fragments often cannot be reduced adequately by closed methods. If the fragment is large and the hip is unstable following closed manipulation, open operation is indicated. If the sciatic nerve has been injured it should be exposed and treated by appropriate neurosurgical technics when the posterior hip joint is exposed. The fragment is then placed in anatomic position and fixed with 1–2 bone screws.

After the operation the patient is placed in bed with the extremity in balanced suspension (Fig 45–36) under 5–8 kg of skeletal traction on the tibial tubercle for about 6 weeks or until healing of the acetabular fracture is sound. Full weight-bearing is not permitted for 6 months or more.

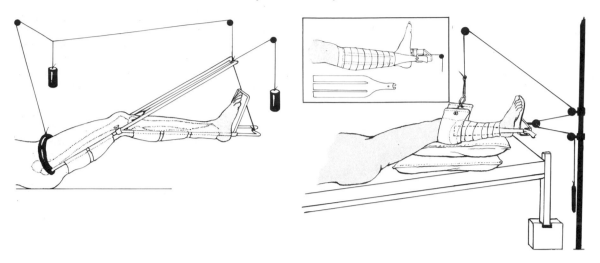

Figure 45—36. Methods of traction for lower extremity fractures. *Left:* Method of suspension of lower extremity with skeletal traction on tibial tubercle. *Right:* Russell's traction. Inset shows method of application of skin traction.

Anterior Hip Dislocation

In anterior hip dislocation the head of the femur may lie medially on the obturator membrane, beneath the obturator externus muscle (obturator or thyroid dislocation), or, in a somewhat more superior direction, beneath the iliopsoas muscle and in contact with the superior ramus of the pubis (pubic dislocation). The thigh is classically in flexion, abduction, and external rotation, and the head of the femur is palpable anteriorly and distal to the inguinal flexion crease. Anteroposterior and lateral films are required; films prepared by transpelvic projection may be helpful.

Closed manipulation with general anesthesia is usually adequate. Postreduction treatment may be by balanced suspension or by immobilization in a plaster spica with the hip in extension and the extremity in neutral rotation. Active hip motion is permitted after 3 weeks.

Central Dislocation of the Hip
With Fracture of the Pelvis

Central dislocation of the head of the femur with fracture of the acetabulum may be caused by crushing injury or by an axial force transmitted through the abducted extremity to the acetabulum. Comminution is commonly present. There are usually 2 fragments: superiorly, the ilium with the roof of the acetabulum; inferiorly and medially, the remainder of the acetabulum and the obturator ring. Fracture occurs near the roof of the acetabulum, and the components of the obturator ring are displaced inward with the head of the femur. Extensive soft tissue injury and massive bleeding into the soft tissues are likely to be present. Intra-abdominal injury must not be overlooked. Initially, stereoanteroposterior and oblique x-rays are required.

In the absence of complicating injury or immediately after such an injury has received priority attention, closed treatment of the fracture-dislocation by skeletal traction should be tried. Open reduction is hazardous and technically difficult; it should not be attempted except by the expert. Bidirectional traction is likely to achieve the most satisfactory results in all but the exceptional case. For the average adult, approximately 10 kg of force are applied axially to the shaft of the femur, in neither abduction nor adduction, through a Kirschner wire placed preferably in the supracondylar region. A second Kirschner wire is inserted in the anteroposterior plane between the greater and lesser trochanters (in substantial cortical bone). Force is applied at a right angle to the direction of axial traction and the magnitude is the same. The extremity is placed in balanced suspension. Progress of reduction is observed by portable x-rays made 3 times a day until adequate positioning is manifested by relocation of the head of the femur beneath the roof of the acetabulum. Bidirectional traction is maintained for 4–6 weeks. Thereafter, the transverse traction component is gradually diminished under appropriate x-ray control until it can be discontinued. Axial traction is maintained until stabilization of the fracture fragments by early bone healing has occurred, usually about 8 weeks after injury. During the next 4–6 weeks, while balanced suspension is continued, gentle active exercises of the knee and hip are encouraged. After discontinuation of balanced suspension, more elaborate exercises designed to aid recovery of maximal hip function are performed frequently during the day. Full and unprotected weight-bearing should not be advised before 6 months.

Sequels are common, and the patient should be warned of their probable occurrence. Anatomic reduction is an unattainable goal in most severely comminuted and widely displaced fractures of this type. Scarring within and around the hip joint, with or without ectopic bone and exuberant callus formation, is incidental to the healing process and can be a significant factor in restriction of motion in varying degrees.

Osteonecrosis of the femoral head and secondary osteoarthritis are common sequels that appear somewhat later.

Dunn AW, Russo CL: Central acetabular fractures. J Trauma 13:695, 1973.

Epstein HC: Posterior fracture-dislocations of the hip: Long-term follow-up. J Bone Joint Surg 56A:1103, 1974.

Schlonsky J, Miller PR: Traumatic hip dislocations in children. J Bone Joint Surg 55A:1057, 1973.

TREATMENT OF SEQUELS OF FRACTURES & DISLOCATIONS OF THE HIP REGION

Sequels of fractures, dislocations, and fracture-dislocations of the hip region may be due to or modified by the nature of the initial lesion, preexisting local or systemic disease, or the type of antecedent treatment. Some sequels are unique to one injury while others are common to the 3 major categories.

Femoral Neck Fractures

Comminution can make precise reduction difficult or impossible by either open or closed technics. When comminution is so severe that intimate approximation of major fragments is impossible, fibrous healing or pseudarthrosis is probable. Further complications result from injury to the retinacular blood supply of the proximal articular fragment of the femur, which enhances the likelihood of ischemic necrosis. Prefractural osteopenia due to osteoporosis or other causes is characterized by a reduced volume of cancellous bone at the fracture site available for endosteal healing. Lack of bone substance offers insecure support to internal fixation apparatus. Infection after the primary surgical procedure may limit or determine the selection of types of reconstructive operations. Excessive physical activity such as unsupported weight-bearing prior to bone healing may cause loosening at the interface between the surgical implant and bone or may cause either episodic or fatigue breakage of the fixation apparatus.

Operations designed to enhance bone healing may be done primarily as prophylaxis or secondarily as corrective procedures. These operations include cancellous or cortical bone grafting, muscle pedicle flap transfers to the fracture site with or without attached bone, supportive or displacement osteotomies with or without internal fixation apparatus, and refixation.

As time passes, either partial or complete ischemic osteonecrosis of the femoral head is likely to complicate or be associated with secondary osteoarthritis. Before infraction or collapse of the superior sector of the head occurs, operations designed to enhance blood supply such as bone grafting or muscle pedicle flap transfers have been performed with varying success. The rationale of osteotomy in the trochanteric region for the treatment of osteonecrosis is to place an uninvolved area of the femoral head in contact with the major weight-bearing surface of the acetabulum. Arthrodesis for this condition was used more frequently in the past. Arthroplasty, which provides both mobility and stability, is currently more popular than head and neck resection, which offers only mobility, or arthrodesis, which gives only stability.

If active infection has been of short duration and apparently has been suppressed, any of the operations mentioned above may be justified if there is reasonable assurance that any reactivation may be controlled. Otherwise, head and neck resection or, possibly, arthrodesis combined with removal of implants and aggressive adjunctive antimicrobial drug therapy are more realistic alternatives. A tertiary reconstructive procedure such as total hip joint replacement may some day be feasible.

Trochanteric Fractures

Undisplaced or anatomically reduced fractures of the trochanteric region that have been firmly fixed with a cervicodiaphyseal apparatus and have not been loaded excessively during the phase of restoration of bone continuity are unlikely to exhibit prolonged delay of healing. Comminution and incomplete reduction are factors that do delay healing. Occasionally, especially in younger persons, extensive comminution and marked displacement may be complicated by ischemic necrosis of the femoral head and secondary osteoarthritis.

If the fracture has no intracapsular extension and infection is limited to the fracture site, treatment is the same as for chronic osteomyelitis. If the internal fixation apparatus is firmly attached and adequately stabilizes an incompletely healed fracture, removal of the implant may be deferred until sound bone healing occurs. The treatment of complicating intra-articular infection is similar to that for cervical fractures with pyogenic arthritis.

Traumatic Dislocation of the Hip Joint

Recurrent posttraumatic dislocation of the hip joint uncomplicated by capital or acetabular fracture or a neurologic lesion is uncommon and may be anterior or posterior; it is likely to be due to extensive soft tissue dehiscence. Treatment is by repair of the soft tissues. Recurrent or persistent subluxation or dislocation is more common to fracture-dislocation. The precise cause must be determined by physical and x-ray examination. If significant secondary osteoarthritis is not a complication, operative replacement and fixation of displaced acetabular fragments or removal of a minor but offending capital fragment can correct articular instability. If it is a complication, arthroplasty or arthrodesis will probably give a more favorable long-term result than repair of the fracture followed by tertiary osteotomy (see below).

Persistent infection of the joint after operation for fracture-dislocation requires treatment similar to that for infection complicating cervical or trochanteric fractures.

OPERATIONS FOR SEQUELS OF FRACTURES & DISLOCATIONS OF THE HIP REGION

Soft Tissue Operations

Denervation and myotomy ("hanging hip") have been performed for relief of pain associated with ischemic osteonecrosis and secondary osteoarthritis. Because of lack of predictability of the result, these procedures have not gained wide acceptance.

Osteotomy

Osteotomy is usually performed in the predominantly cancellous intertrochanteric region, and the bone fragments are generally stabilized by a fixation device. An indication is correction of torsional or varus deformity. Supportive osteotomy is used to minimize displacing stresses at unhealed fracture sites. Abduction or adduction osteotomy has been performed for relief of pain associated with ischemic osteonecrosis of the femoral head or secondary osteoarthritis. Although osteotomy preserves joint motion and provides stability, the prognosis for relief of pain is unpredictable for the individual patient.

Arthrodesis

Arthrodesis may be intra-articular, extra-articular, or a combination of both. Bone grafting to aid fusion and internal fixation to provide rest at the coxofemoral relationship are elective supplemental features. Arthrodesis has been a favored operation as an adjunct in the control of chronic hip joint infection. When arthrodesis is bony—although articular pain is relieved and mechanical stability of the joint is assured—added stress is placed on the lumbar spine and knee joint. Pain is a frequent result. The patient must also accept some disability because of loss of hip joint function.

Head & Neck Resection

The indications for resection of the head and neck of the femur for treatment of fractures, dislocations, and fracture-dislocations have been frequently modified. This operation provides coxofemoral motion, causes comparative shortening of the extremity, and creates instability that usually requires supplemental external support. Currently, its chief application is in the treatment of chronic hip joint infection. It is useful occasionally in the treatment of pathologic fracture of the proximal femur due to primary or metastatic tumors. Rarely is osteopenia or destruction of bone from causes other than those mentioned above so extensive that resection is preferable to prosthetic arthroplasty.

Hemiarthroplasty

Hemiarthroplasty implies surfacing or replacement of either the acetabular or femoral part of the hip joint. Rarely is there an indication for acetabular arthroplasty alone. This requires a normal or nearly normal femoral head and a diseased acetabulum. As a rule, hemiarthroplasty implies substitution of all or part of the cervicocapital segment. When it is feasible to restore joint mechanics by minor sacrifice of bone structure, some surgeons prefer a limited constructive operation by cavitary mold or by attaching a prosthetic device designed to cover the articular surface of the proximal femoral segment. When femoral head involvement is extensive or treatment is selected for unhealed cervical fracture, replacement of the head and a part of the neck is necessary. "Short stem" devices have failed frequently because of breakage or gross loosening and no longer enjoy popularity. The intramedullary type of prosthesis is more reliable. Because even minor movement between the implant and the host's femur may be the source of pain, stabilization of the prosthesis in the femur with a grouting material, methyl methacrylate, may eliminate that source of symptoms. Other causes of failure have been postoperative infection and acetabular deterioration secondary to wear which may accelerate the onset of symptomatic degenerative disease.

Total Hip Joint Replacement

Increasing interest in total hip joint replacement has been generated during the past 10 years both abroad and in the USA. This technic implies substitution of at least the articular surfaces of both the acetabulum and the head of the femur by implants usually made of metal or plastic. The femoral component is usually made of cobalt-chrome alloy, stainless steel, or titanium. The acetabular constituent is usually made of plastic unless the femoral component is made of cobalt-chrome alloy; in the latter case, the acetabular part may be of the same metal. Depending upon the specific design, the implants may be attached to the respective bone by their configuration, or a grouting substance may be used as an intermediary. The Ring prosthesis is a practical example of an all-metal implant pair that is applied without a grouting material. The Charnley apparatus is composed of a metal femoral segment and a polyethylene acetabular component; both are stabilized in bone by self-curing polymethylmethacrylate.

Total hip joint replacement has wider application in the treatment of sequels of fracture and fracture-dislocation of the hip joint in the mature adult than in the primary treatment of those lesions. Total hip joint replacement is useful as a reconstructive procedure in the treatment of failure of hemiarthroplasty or when disease or injury involves both articular components of the joint without infection. Total hip joint replacement is still considered a salvage operation. Because long-term reliability has not been established, the operation should be reserved for patients over 50 years of age unless specific factors warrant its use in younger persons.

Failure of total hip joint replacement can be caused by recurrent dislocation within the prosthesis complex, loosening of the components at the interface between the implant and grouting substance, breakage of the femoral component, and undetermined causes of disabling pain. The long-term effects of wear of the material and the effect of wear debris on the surrounding tissues have not been certainly determined. Infection is the most serious complication; even though it is promptly discovered and vigorously treated, removal of the device complex may be necessary for its ultimate control.

Carnesale PG, Anderson LD: Primary prosthetic replacement for femoral neck fractures. Arch Surg 110:27, 1975.

Coventry MB & others: 2012 total hip arthroplasties: A study of postoperative course and early complications. J Bone Joint Surg 56A:273, 1974.

Stinchfield FE & others: Low friction arthroplasty. Surg Gynecol Obstet 135:1, 1972.

Welch RB & others: Total hip replacement as a salvage in traumatic lesions about the hip. Surg Gynecol Obstet 140:708, 1975.

Whittaker RP & others: Fifteen years' experience with metallic endoprosthetic replacement of the femoral head for femoral neck fractures. J Trauma 12:799, 1972.

Zabahi T & others: A modified Girdlestone operation in the treatment of complications of fractures of the femoral neck. J Bone Joint Surg 55A:129, 1973.

FRACTURE OF THE SHAFT OF THE FEMUR

FRACTURE OF THE SHAFT OF THE FEMUR IN ADULTS

Fracture of the shaft of the femur usually occurs as a result of severe direct trauma. Indirect violence, especially torsional stress, is likely to cause spiral fractures that extend proximally or, more commonly, distally into the metaphyseal regions. These fractures are likely to be encountered in bone that has become atrophic as a result of disuse or senescence. Most are closed fractures; open fracture is often the result of compounding from within. Extensive soft tissue injury, bleeding, and shock are commonly present.

If the fracture is through the upper third of the shaft, the proximal fragment is apt to be in flexion, external rotation, and abduction, with proximal displacement or overriding of the distal fragment. In midshaft fracture the direction of displacement is not constant, but the distal fragment is almost always displaced proximally if the fracture is unstable; and angulation is commonly present with the apex directed anterolaterally. In complete fracture of the lower third of the shaft the distal fragment is often displaced proximally; the upper end of the distal fragment may be displaced posteriorly to the distal end of the upper fragment.

The most significant features are severe pain in the thigh and deformity of the lower extremity. Surgical shock is likely to be present. Careful x-ray examina-

tion in at least 2 planes is necessary to determine the exact site and configuration of the fracture cleft. Splints should be removed either by the surgeon or by a qualified assistant so that manipulation will not cause further damage. The hip and knee should be examined for associated injury.

Injuries to the sciatic nerve and to the superficial femoral artery and vein are not common but must be recognized promptly. Surgical shock and secondary anemia are the most important early complications. Later complications are essentially those of prolonged recumbency, eg, the formation of renal calculi.

Treatment

Treatment depends upon the age of the patient and the site and configuration of the fracture. Displaced, oblique, spiral, and comminuted fractures are unstable, and can rarely be treated successfully by closed manipulation and external plaster fixation. Traction followed by closed manipulation should be tried. Skeletal traction is generally the most effective form of closed treatment.

After preliminary traction, biplane x-rays are made to determine the progress of correction of overriding. If alignment and apposition of fragments are not satisfactory, closed manipulation, preferably under general anesthesia, should be carried out while traction is continued.

If soft tissue interposition prevents reduction by closed methods, open reduction may be required in the adult to avoid delay of bone healing.

A. Fracture of the Upper Third: The treatment of subtrochanteric fracture is discussed above. If a comminuted subtrochanteric fracture extends into the upper third of the femoral shaft, it may be necessary to use skeletal traction through the supracondylar region of the femur and suspend the extremity with the hip and knee at a right angle (Fig 45–34). Otherwise, skeletal traction can be through either the lower femur or the tibial tubercle with the extremity at a less acute angle in balanced suspension. Russell's traction can be used if the patient is small and muscular development is not great. External rotation and abduction of the extremity are usually required to bring the lower fragment into alignment with the proximal fragment.

B. Fracture of the Middle Third: The deformity caused by fracture at this level is not constant. Angulation is commonly present with the apex directed anterolaterally. Treatment may be by skeletal traction through the tibial tubercle or the lower end of the femur (Fig 45–36). Traction in the transverse plane by a swathe around the thigh may be necessary to prevent recurrence of angulation.

C. Fracture of the Lower Third: In transverse and comminuted fractures, the proximal end of the distal fragment is likely to be displaced posterior to the distal end of the proximal fragment. The same displacement is likely to be encountered in supracondylar fracture. Russell's traction should not be used for comminuted or widely displaced fractures since it may injure the

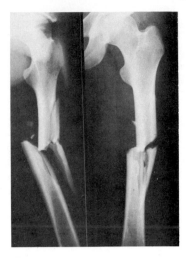

Figure 45–37. Comminuted fracture of the middle third of the femur in a 33-year-old man.

obtain adequate reduction by closed technics and delay of bone healing. The purpose of open reduction is generally to provide anatomic reposition and clinically rigid fixation that will permit the patient to be ambulatory without such external supportive apparatus as casts, splints, or braces. Unprotected weight-bearing without crutches until restoration of bone continuity should not be a goal of open operation of most fractures.

Connolly JF, King P: Closed reduction and early cast-brace ambulation in the treatment of femoral fractures. Part 1. An in vivo quantitative analysis of immobilization in skeletal traction and a cast-brace. Part 2. Results in one hundred and forty-three fractures. J Bone Joint Surg 55A:1559, 1581, 1973.

Rascher JJ & others: Closed nailing of femoral-shaft fractures. J Bone Joint Surg 54A:534, 1972.

Ruoff AC III, Biddulph EC: Dual plating of selected femoral fractures. J Trauma 12:233, 1972.

femoral or popliteal vessels. Simultaneous skeletal traction through the distal femur at right angles to the tibial tubercle can correct displacement of the distal fragment. The same mechanism of traction is used for supracondylar fracture (Fig 45–38).

After reduction has been accomplished by traction, biplane x-ray examination should be repeated at least weekly to determine maintenance of reduction and the progress of healing. When sufficient callus has formed to assure stabilization of the fragments, generally after 12 weeks or more, further immobilization can be given by a one and one half plaster spica. Prior to application of the spica, there should be a period of observation in balanced suspension without traction to determine whether displacement of the fracture fragments by overriding will occur. Angulation can generally be corrected in plaster by appropriate wedging.

Elective indications for open reduction and internal fixation may be based upon the desire to avoid prolonged recumbency in bed and hospitalization. Some mandatory indications include inability to

FRACTURE OF THE SHAFT OF THE FEMUR IN INFANTS & CHILDREN

Femoral fracture at birth occurs most often in the middle third. Comminution is usually not present.

Skin traction and plaster immobilization are adequate, although skeletal traction may be necessary in older children. Open reduction is rarely necessary.

Fracture of the proximal or middle third of the femur in a child under 5 years of age can be treated with Bryant's traction (Fig 45–39). Adhesive strips are applied to both extremities from the upper thirds of the thighs to the supramalleolar regions, and held firm by circular bandages. Both hips are flexed to a right angle, and the knees are maintained in full extension. Sufficient traction force is applied to raise the buttocks free of the bed. Circulatory adequacy must be observed carefully, and another method substituted if swelling, cyanosis or pallor of the foot, or obliteration

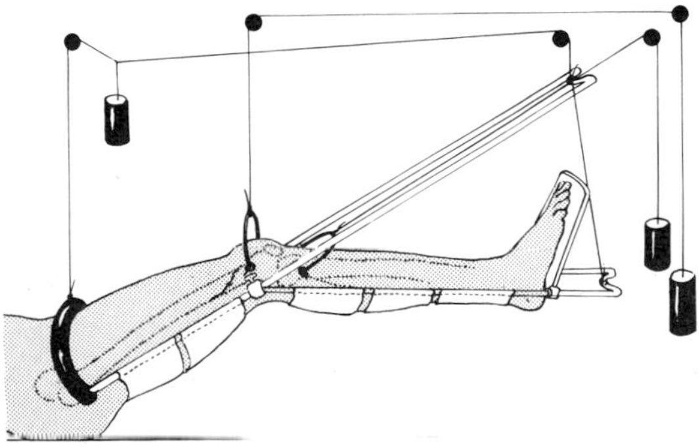

Figure 45–38. Method of suspension of lower extremity with biplane skeletal traction for supracondylar fracture.

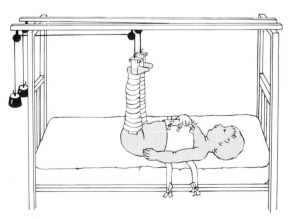

Figure 45–39. Bryant's traction.

of pedal pulsations cannot be managed by adjustment of dressings.

As a rule, sufficient callus is present at the fracture site after 3–4 weeks so that traction can be discontinued. If callus formation is adequate, infants who have not yet begun to walk need no further protection; walking infants may require a single plaster hip spica for an additional 4–6 weeks.

Preliminary treatment of unstable fracture of the femur in children over 5 years of age can be by Russell's traction (Fig 45–36). If the child is uncooperative, or if adequate correction cannot be obtained, it may also be necessary to place the sound extremity in traction. Traction should be continued until the fracture is stabilized; if traction is discontinued before the reparative callus is sufficiently mature, the deformity (especially angulation) may recur even though the extremity is protected by a plaster spica. Correction of angulation and torsional displacement around the long axis of the femur are mandatory. Slight shortening (1–2 cm) can be compensated by growth. Close apposition of fragments is not necessary, since healing will take place in spite of minimal soft tissue interposition.

It is usually necessary to continue traction for 6–8 weeks or until sufficient callus has formed to prevent recurrence of the deformity. Immobilization in a plaster spica should be maintained for another 2 months. Weight-bearing must not be resumed until x-rays show that healing is sound.

Burwell HN: Fracture of the femoral shaft in children. Postgrad Med J 45:617, 1969.

INJURIES OF THE KNEE REGION

FRACTURES OF THE DISTAL FEMUR

Supracondylar Fracture of the Femur

This comparatively uncommon fracture (at the junction of cortical and cancellous bone) may be transverse, oblique, or comminuted. The distal end of the proximal fragment is apt to perforate the overlying vastus intermedius, vastus medialis, or rectus femoris muscles, and may penetrate the suprapatellar pouch of the knee joint to cause hemarthrosis. The proximal end of the distal fragment is usually displaced posteriorly and slightly laterally.

Since the distal fragment may impinge upon the popliteal vessels, circulatory adequacy distal to the fracture site should be verified as soon as possible. Absence of pedal pulsations is an indication for immediate reduction. If pulsation does not return promptly after reduction, immediate exploration and appropriate treatment of the vascular lesion is indicated.

A less frequent complication is injury to the peroneal or tibial nerve.

If the fracture is transverse or nearly so, closed manipulation under general anesthesia will occasionally be successful. Stable fractures with minimal displacement can be immobilized in a single plaster hip spica with the hip and knee in about 30 degrees of flexion. Frequent x-ray examination is necessary to make certain that redisplacement has not occurred.

Stable or unstable uncomplicated supracondylar fracture is best treated with biplane skeletal traction if soft tissue interposition does not interfere with reduction (Fig 45–38). If adequate reduction cannot be obtained, it may be necessary to manipulate the fragments under general anesthesia, using skeletal traction to control the distal fragment.

Traction must be continued for about 6 weeks or until stabilization occurs. The wires can then be removed and the extremity immobilized in a single plaster spica for an additional 2–3 months.

An alternative method of treatment (applicable only to stable fractures) is to incorporate the wires into a plaster spica after reduction.

Supracondylar fracture is likely to be followed by restriction of knee motion due to scarring and adhesion formation in adjacent soft tissues.

Intercondylar Fracture of the Femur

This uncommon comminuted fracture, which occurs only in older patients, is classically described as T or Y according to the x-ray configuration of the fragments. Closed reduction is difficult when the proximal shaft fragment is interposed between the 2 main distal fragments. Maximal recovery of function of the knee joint requires anatomic reduction of the articular components. If alignment is satisfactory and displacement minimal, immobilization for about 4 months in a plaster spica will be sufficient. If displacement is marked, skeletal traction through the tibial tubercle (with the knee in flexion) is required. Manual molding of the distal fragments may be necessary. Open reduc-

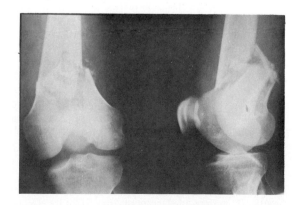

Figure 45–40. Comminuted T fracture of the distal femur in a 30-year-old man. Adequate closed reduction was prevented by interposition of small intermediate fragments between the 2 main condylar fragments.

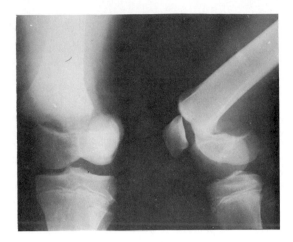

Figure 45—41. Traumatic separation of the distal femoral epiphysis in an 11-year-old boy.

tion and bolt fixation of the distal fragments may be indicated to restore articular congruity. Further treatment is as described for supracondylar fracture.

Condylar Fracture of the Femur

Isolated fracture of the lateral or medial condyle of the femur is rare. Occasionally only the posterior portion of the condyle is separated. The cruciate ligaments or the collateral ligament of the opposite side of the knee are often injured.

The objective of treatment is restoration of anatomic intra-articular relationships. If displacement is minimal, the knee can be manipulated into varus or valgus (opposite the position of deformity). If anatomic reduction cannot be obtained by closed manipulation, open reduction and fixation of the minor fragment with 2–3 bone screws is recommended. The ligaments must be explored, and repaired if found to be injured.

Separation of the Distal Femoral Epiphysis

Traumatic separation of the distal femoral epiphysis in children is the counterpart of supracondylar fracture in the adult. The direction of displacement of the epiphyseal fragment is most commonly anterior. Torsional displacement may occur.

Reduction of anterior displacement can be achieved by closed manipulation. After reduction is complete, the knee is flexed to a right angle and a tubular plaster cast is applied from the inguinal region to the toes. If the thigh is obese, the plaster should be extended proximally to include the pelvis in a single hip spica.

Peripheral circulation must be observed carefully. After 4 weeks the plaster is changed and flexion of the knee reduced to 135 degrees. At the end of the second month the patient may be permitted to be free in bed until he regains complete knee extension.

Mooney V & others: Cast-brace treatment for fractures of the distal part of the femur: A prospective controlled study of one hundred and fifty patients. J Bone Joint Surg 52A:1563, 1970.

Olerud S: Operative treatment of supracondylar-condylar fractures of the femur: Technique and results in fifteen cases. J Bone Joint Surg 54A:1015, 1972.

FRACTURE OF THE PATELLA

Transverse Fracture of the Patella

Transverse fracture of the patella is the result of indirect violence, usually with the knee in semiflexion. Fracture may be due to sudden voluntary contraction of the quadriceps muscles or sudden forced flexion of the leg when these muscles are contracted. The level of fracture is most often in the middle. The extent of tearing of the patellar retinacula depends upon the degree of force of the initiating injury. The activity of the quadriceps muscles causes displacement of the proximal fragment; the magnitude of displacement is dependent upon the extent of the tear of the quadriceps expansion.

Swelling of the anterior knee region is caused by hemarthrosis and hemorrhage into the soft tissues overlying the joint. If displacement is present, the defect in the patella can be palpated and active extension of the knee is lost.

Open reduction is indicated if the fragments are separated more than 2–3 mm. The fragments must be accurately repositioned to prevent early posttraumatic arthritis of the patellofemoral joint. If the minor fragment is small (no more than 1 cm in height), it may be excised and the rectus or patellar tendon (depending upon which pole of the patella is involved) sutured directly to the major fragment. If the fragments are approximately the same size, repair by wire cerclage is preferred.

Removal of 50% of the patella causes incongruity of joint surfaces, and posttraumatic arthritis may occur early.

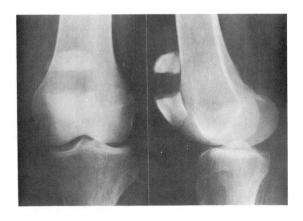

Figure 45—42. Transverse fracture of the patella in a 52-year-old woman.

Comminuted Fracture of the Patella

Comminuted fracture of the patella is caused only by direct violence. Little or no separation of the fragments occurs because the quadriceps expansion is not extensively torn. Severe injury may cause extensive comminution of the articular cartilages of both the patella and the opposing femur. If comminution is not severe and displacement is insignificant, plaster immobilization for 8 weeks in a cylinder extending from the groin to the supramalleolar region is sufficient.

Severe comminution requires excision of the patella and repair of the defect by imbrication of the quadriceps expansion.

Seligo W: Fractures of the patella: Treatment and results. Reconstr Surg Traumatol 12:84, 1971.

TEAR OF THE QUADRICEPS TENDON

Tear of the quadriceps tendon occurs most often in patients over 40 years of age. Preexisting attritional disease of the tendon is apt to be present, and the causative injury may be minor. The tear commonly results from sudden deceleration, such as stumbling, or slipping on a wet surface. A small flake of bone may be avulsed from the superior pole of the patella, or the tear may occur entirely through tendinous and muscle tissue.

Pain may be noted in the anterior knee region. Swelling is due to hemarthrosis and extravasation of blood into the soft tissues. The patient is unable to extend his knee completely. X-rays may show avulsion of a bit of bone from the superior patella.

Operative repair is required for complete tear. If treatment is delayed until partial healing has occurred, the suture line can be reinforced by transplantation of the iliotibial band from the upper extremity of the tibia.

TEAR OF THE PATELLAR LIGAMENT

The same mechanism which causes tears of the quadriceps tendon, transverse fracture of the patella, or avulsion of the tibial tuberosity may also cause tear of the patellar ligament. The characteristic clinical finding is proximal displacement of the patella. A bit of bone may be avulsed from the lower pole of the patella if the tear takes place in the proximal patellar tendon.

Operative treatment is necessary for complete tear. The ligament is resutured to the patella and any tear in the quadriceps expansion is repaired. The extremity should be immobilized for 8 weeks in a tubular plaster cast extending from the inguinal to the supramalleolar region. Guarded exercises may then be started.

DISLOCATION OF THE PATELLA

Traumatic dislocation of the patellofemoral joint may be associated with dislocation of the knee joint. When this injury occurs alone it may be due to direct violence or muscle activity of the quadriceps, and the direction of dislocation of the patella may be lateral. Spontaneous reduction is apt to occur if the knee joint is extended; if so, the clinical findings may consist merely of hemarthrosis and localized tenderness over the medial patellar retinaculum. Gross instability of the patella, which can be demonstrated by physical examination, indicates that injury to the soft tissues of the medial aspect of the knee has been extensive. Recurrent episodes require operative repair for effective treatment.

DISLOCATION OF THE KNEE JOINT

Traumatic dislocation of the knee joint is uncommon in adults and extremely rare in children. It is caused by severe trauma. Displacement may be transverse or torsional. Complete dislocation can occur only after extensive tearing of the supporting ligaments, and is apt to cause injury to the popliteal vessels or the tibial and peroneal nerves.

Signs of neurovascular injury below the site of dislocation are an absolute indication for prompt reduction under general anesthesia, since failure of circulation will undoubtedly result in gangrene of the leg and foot. Axial traction is applied to the leg and a shearing force is exerted over the fragments in the appropriate direction. If pedal pulses do not return promptly, the popliteal fossa should be explored at once for treatment of any vascular injury.

Anatomic reduction of uncomplicated dislocation should be attempted. If impinging soft tissues cannot be removed by closed manipulation, arthrotomy is indicated. After reduction the extremity is immobilized in a tubular plaster cast extending from the inguinal region to the toes with the knee in slight flexion. (In the obese patient, a single hip spica should be applied.) A window should be cut in the plaster over the dorsum of the foot to allow frequent determination of dorsalis pedis pulsation. After 8 weeks' immobilization the knee can be protected by a long leg brace. Intensive quadriceps exercises are necessary to minimize functional loss.

Meyers MH, Harvey JP Jr: Traumatic dislocation of the knee joint: A study of eighteen cases. J Bone Joint Surg 53A:16, 1971.

INTERNAL DERANGEMENTS OF
THE KNEE JOINT

Internal derangements of the knee joint mechanism may be caused by trauma or attritional disease. Although ligamentous and cartilaginous injuries are discussed separately, they commonly occur as combined lesions.

Arthroscopy and newer technics of arthrography using single or double contrast media can be valuable adjuncts in establishing a precise diagnosis when the usual diagnostic methods are inconclusive.

Injury to the Menisci

Injury to the medial meniscus is the most frequent internal derangement of the knee joint. Any portion of the meniscus may be torn. A marginal tear permits displacement of the medial fragment into the intercondylar region ("bucket-handle tear"). A fragment of cartilage displaced between the articular surfaces of the femur and tibia prevents either complete extension or complete flexion.

The significant clinical findings after acute injury are swelling (due to hemarthrosis) and varying degrees of restriction of flexion or extension. Motion may cause pain over the anteromedial or posteromedial joint line. Tenderness can often be elicited at the point of pain. Forcible external rotation of the foot with the knee flexed to a right angle may cause pain over the medial joint line. If symptoms have persisted for 2–3 weeks, weakness and atrophy of the quadriceps femoris may be present.

Injury to the lateral meniscus less often causes mechanical blockage of joint motion. Pain and tenderness may be present over the lateral joint line. Pain can be elicited by forcible rotation of the leg with the knee flexed to a right angle.

Initial treatment may be conservative. Swelling and pain caused by tense hemarthrosis can be relieved by aspiration. If pain is severe, the extremity should be immobilized in a posterior plaster splint with the knee in slight flexion. Younger patients usually prefer to be

ambulatory on crutches, but immediate weight-bearing must not be permitted. As long as acute symptoms persist, isometric quadriceps exercises should be performed frequently throughout the day with the knee in maximum extension (as a "straight leg lift"). Unrestricted activity must not be resumed until complete motion is recovered and healing is complete.

Exploratory arthrotomy is advisable for recurrent "locking," recurrent effusion, or disabling pain. Isometric quadriceps exercises are instituted immediately after the operation and gradually increased in frequency. As soon as the patient is able to perform these exercises comfortably, graded resistance maneuvers should be started. Exercises must be continued until all motion has been recovered and the volume and competency of the quadriceps are equal to those of the uninjured side.

Injury to the Collateral Ligaments

The collateral ligaments prevent excursion of the joint beyond normal limits. When the knee is in full extension, the collateral ligaments are taut; in flexion, only the anterior fibers of the tibial collateral ligament are taut.

A. Tibial Collateral Ligament: Forced abduction of the leg at the knee, which is frequently associated with torsional strain, causes injury varying from tear of a few fibers to complete rupture of the ligament. A bit of bone may be avulsed from its femoral or tibial attachment.

A history of a twisting injury at the knee with valgus strain can usually be obtained. Pain is present over the medial aspect of the knee joint. In severe injury joint effusion may be present. Tenderness can be elicited at the site of the lesion. When only an isolated ligamentous tear is present, x-ray examination may not be helpful unless it is made while valgus stress is applied to the extended knee. Under local or general anesthesia the extremities are bound together in full extension at the knee joint, and an anteroposterior film is made with the legs in forced abduction. Widening of the medial joint cleft suggests complete rupture.

Treatment of incomplete tear consists of protection from further injury while healing progresses. Painful hemarthrosis should be relieved by aspiration. The knee may be immobilized in a posterior plaster splint or a tubular cast extending from the inguinal to the supramalleolar region.

Complete rupture should be surgically repaired immediately so that healing will take place without ligamentous elongation and subsequent instability of the knee joint. Tear of the medial collateral ligament is frequently associated with other lesions, such as tear of the medial meniscus, rupture of the anterior cruciate ligament, or fracture of the lateral condyle of the tibia.

B. Fibular Collateral Ligament: Tear of the fibular collateral ligament is often associated with injury to surrounding structures, eg, the popliteus muscle tendon and the iliotibial band. Avulsion of the apex of the fibular head may occur, and the peroneal nerve may be injured.

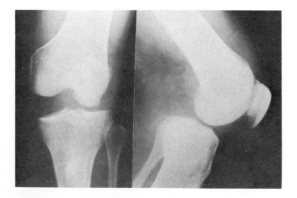

Figure 45–43. Incomplete closed dislocation of the knee joint in a 28-year-old man.

Pain and tenderness are present over the lateral aspect of the knee joint, and hemarthrosis may be present. X-rays may show a bit of bone avulsed from the fibular head. If severe injury is suspected, x-ray examination under stress, using local or general anesthesia, is required. A firm, padded nonopaque object about 20–30 cm in diameter is placed between the knees and the legs are forcibly adducted while an anteroposterior exposure is made. Widening of the lateral joint cleft indicates severe injury.

The treatment of partial tear is similar to that described for partial tear of the medial collateral ligament. If complete tear is suspected, and especially if the peroneal nerve has been injured, exploration is indicated. The extremity is protected for 8 weeks in a plaster cylinder extending from the inguinal region to above the ankle.

Injury to the Cruciate Ligaments

The function of the anterior and posterior cruciate ligaments is to restrict anterior and posterior gliding of the tibia when the knee is flexed. If the tibia is rotated internally on the femur, the ligaments twist around themselves and become taut; if the tibia is rotated externally, they become lax.

A. Anterior Cruciate Ligament: Injury to the anterior cruciate ligament is usually associated with injury to the medial meniscus or the tibial collateral ligament. The cruciate ligament may be avulsed with a part of the medial tibial tubercle or may rupture within the substance of its fibers.

The characteristic clinical sign of tear of either cruciate ligament is a positive "drawer" sign; the knee is flexed at a right angle and pulled forward; if excessive anterior excursion of the proximal tibia (in comparison with the opposite normal side) can be noted, a tear of the anterior ligament is likely.

Complete recent rupture of the anterior cruciate ligament within its substance can occasionally be repaired with stout sutures. When manifest by avulsed tibial bone that is displaced, attachment of the fragment in anatomic position by arthrotomy is necessary. When the fragment of bone is large, displaced, and not treated until 4 weeks or more after injury, excision of the fragment and reinsertion of the ligament may be necessary to eliminate the blocking effect of the bone fragment and to permit recovery of function. Old tears may require reconstructive procedures.

B. Posterior Cruciate Ligament: Tear of the posterior ligament may occur within its substance or may be manifest by avulsion of a fragment of bone of variable size at its tibial attachment. Tear of the posterior cruciate ligament can be diagnosed by the "drawer" sign: the knee is flexed at a right angle and the upper tibia is pushed backward; if excessive posterior excursion of the proximal tibia can be noted, tear of the posterior ligament is likely.

Treatment is directed primarily at the associated injuries and maintenance of the competency of the quadriceps musculature. Primary repair of tears within the fibers is difficult and of dubious value. Open reduc-

tion and fixation of a fragment of tibia with the attached ligament is feasible and is likely to restore functional competency of the ligament.

Hughston JC, Eilers AF: The role of the posterior oblique ligament in repairs of acute medial (collateral) ligament tears of the knee. J Bone Joint Surg 55A:923, 1973.

McIntyre JL: Arthrography of the lateral meniscus. Radiology 105:531, 1972.

McMaster JH & others: Diagnosis and management of isolated anterior cruciate ligament tears: A preliminary report on reconstruction with the gracilis tendon. J Trauma 14:230, 1974.

Nicholas JA: The five-one reconstruction for anteromedial instability of the knee. J Bone Joint Surg 55A:899, 1973.

Nicholas JA & others: Double-contrast arthrography of the knee: Its value in the management of 225 derangements. J Bone Joint Surg 52A:203, 1970.

O'Connor RL: Arthroscopy in the diagnosis and treatment of acute ligament injuries of the knee. J Bone Joint Surg 56A:333, 1974.

O'Donoghue DH: Reconstruction for medial instability of the knee. J Bone Joint Surg 55A:941, 1973.

FRACTURES OF THE PROXIMAL TIBIA

Fracture of the Lateral Tibial Condyle

Fracture of the lateral condyle of the tibia is commonly caused by a blow on the lateral aspect of the knee with the foot in fixed position, producing an abduction strain. Hemarthrosis is always present, as the fracture cleft involves the knee joint. Soft tissue injuries are likely to be present also. The tibial collateral and anterior cruciate ligaments may be torn. A displaced free fragment may tear the overlying lateral

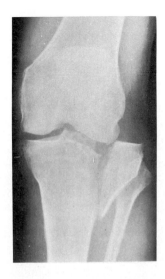

Figure 45–44. Fracture of the lateral condyle of the tibia in a 37-year-old man.

meniscus. If displacement is marked, fracture of the proximal fibula may be present also.

The objective of treatment is to restore the articular surface and normal anatomic relationships, so that torn ligaments can heal without elongation. In cases of minimal displacement where ligaments have not been extensively damaged, treatment may be by immobilization for 6 weeks in a tubular plaster cast extending from the toes to the inguinal region with the knee in slight flexion. Reduction of marked displacement can be achieved by closed manipulation unless comminution is severe. After x-ray verification of reduction, the extremity can be immobilized in a tubular plaster cast extending from the inguinal region to the toes, preferably with the knee in full extension.

Many fractures of the lateral condyle of the tibia, especially comminuted fractures, cannot be reduced adequately by closed methods. Open reduction and stabilization with a bolt or multiple bone screws may be necessary.

Fracture of the Medial Tibial Condyle

Fracture of the medial condyle of the tibia is caused by the adduction strain produced by a blow against the medial aspect of the knee with the foot in fixed position. The medial meniscus and the fibular collateral ligament may be torn. Severe comminution is not usually present, and there is only one major free fragment.

Treatment is by closed reduction to restore the articular surface of the tibia so that ligamentous healing can occur without elongation. After reduction the extremity is immobilized for 10—12 weeks in a tubular plaster cast extending from the inguinal region to the toes with the knee in full extension. Weight-bearing is not permitted for 4 months at least.

Fracture of Both Tibial Condyles

Axial force, such as may result from falling on the foot or sudden deceleration with the knee in full extension (during an automobile accident), can cause simultaneous fracture of both condyles of the tibia. Comminution is apt to be severe. Swelling of the knee due to hemarthrosis is marked. Deformity is either genu varum or genu valgum. X-ray examination should include oblique projections.

Severe comminution makes anatomic reduction difficult to achieve by any means and difficult to maintain following closed manipulation alone. Sustained skeletal traction is usually necessary. When stability has been achieved, the extremity can be immobilized for another 4—6 weeks in a tubular plaster cast extending from the toes to the inguinal region with the knee in full extension. Unassisted weight-bearing is not permitted before the end of the fourth month.

If closed methods are not effective, open reduction must be attempted.

Instability and restriction of motion of the knee are common sequelae of this type of fracture. If reduction is not adequate, posttraumatic arthritis will appear early.

Fracture of the Tibial Tuberosity

Violent contraction of the quadriceps muscle may cause avulsion of the tibial tuberosity. Avulsion of the anterior portion of the upper tibial epiphysis, uncommon in childhood, must be differentiated from Osgood-Schlatter disease (osteochondrosis of the tibial tuberosity).

When avulsion of the tuberosity is complete, active extension of the knee is not possible.

If displacement is minimal, treatment is by immobilization in a tubular plaster cast extending from the inguinal to the supramalleolar region with the knee in full extension. Immobilization is maintained for 8 weeks or until stabilization occurs.

A loose fragment which has been displaced more than 0.5 cm can be treated either by closed reduction and percutaneous fixation, with plaster immobilization, or by open reduction.

Fracture of the Tibial Tubercle

This injury usually occurs in association with comminuted fracture of the condyles. The medial intercondyloid tubercle may be avulsed with adjacent bone attached to the anterior cruciate ligament, and injury to that structure is of greater importance. In addition to avulsion of the anterior cruciate ligament, there may also be injury to the tibial collateral ligament and the medial knee joint capsule. Hemarthrosis is always present.

Isolated and undisplaced fracture may be treated by immobilization of the extremity for 6 weeks in a tubular plaster cast extending from the inguinal region to the toes with the knee in slight flexion. The treatment of displaced fracture is the same as that of rupture of the anterior cruciate ligament (see below).

Separation of the Proximal Tibial Epiphysis

Complete displacement of the proximal tibial epiphysis is rare; partial separation due to forceful hyperextension of the knee is more common. The distal metaphyseal fragment is displaced posteriorly.

If no circulatory or neurologic deficit is present, immediate treatment by closed manipulation is indicated. Reduction can be accomplished by forced flexion of the knee. Anteroposterior films are then exposed by holding the plate against the anterior surface of the leg with the beam directed through the lower thigh. A lateral film is also prepared. If x-rays show that reduction is adequate, a heavy anterior plaster splint is applied from the inguinal region to the bases of the toes, with the knee in acute flexion. The splint is maintained in position with circular bandages around the foot, ankle, and upper thigh. The bandages are wrapped in figure-of-eight fashion around the thigh and leg (as is done for supracondylar fracture of the humerus). Peripheral circulation must be observed frequently for at least 72 hours. After 3 weeks the knee may be brought to a right angle and a tubular plaster cast applied from the inguinal region to the toes for another 3—4 weeks. Even guarded weight-bearing must be avoided until the end of the second month.

Injury to the proximal tibial epiphyseal plate as a result of a blow on the lateral aspect of the knee causes compression but only minor displacement. This lesion, analogous to fracture of the lateral condyle in the adult, is apt to retard or arrest the growth of the lateral aspect of the tibia and thus cause tibia valga, or knock-knee. Surgical arrest of the growth of the medial tibial epiphysis may be necessary to prevent this deformity.

Hand WL & others: Avulsion fractures of the tibial tubercle. J Bone Joint Surg 53A:1579, 1971.

Moore TM, Harvey JP Jr: Roentgenographic measurement of tibial-plateau depression due to fracture. J Bone Joint Surg 56A:155, 1974.

Rasmussen PS: Tibial condylar fractures: Impairment of knee joint stability as an indication for surgical treatment. J Bone Joint Surg 55A:1331, 1973.

FRACTURE OF THE PROXIMAL FIBULA

Isolated fracture of the proximal fibula is uncommon; this fracture is usually associated with fracture of the femur or of the tibia or fracture-dislocation of the ankle joint. The apex of the fibular head may be avulsed by the activity of the biceps femoris muscle or detached with the fibular collateral ligament by an adduction strain of the knee.

The fracture usually requires no treatment, but avulsion of the apex of the head may necessitate operative repair of the ligament or tendon.

Fracture in this region may be associated with paralysis of the common peroneal nerve.

DISLOCATION OF THE PROXIMAL TIBIOFIBULAR JOINT

This extremely rare lesion is caused by the activity of the biceps femoris muscle. Displacement is posterior, and can be reduced by digital pressure over the head of the fibula in the opposite direction.

Ogden JA: Subluxation and dislocation of the proximal tibiofibular joint. J Bone Joint Surg 56A:145, 1974.

FRACTURES OF THE SHAFTS OF THE TIBIA & FIBULA

Fracture of the shaft of the tibia or fibula occurs at any age but is most common during youth and active adulthood. In general, open, transverse, comminuted, and segmental fractures are caused by indirect violence. Fracture of the middle third of the shaft (especially if comminuted) is apt to be complicated by delay of bone healing.

If fracture is complete and displacement is present, clinical diagnosis is not difficult. However, critical local examination is of utmost importance in planning treatment. The nature of the skin wounds which may communicate with the fracture site often suggests the mechanism of compounding, whether it has occurred from within or from without. A small laceration without contused edges suggests that the point of a bone fragment has caused compounding from within. A large wound with contused edges, especially over the subcutaneous surface of the tibia, suggests compounding from without. The presence of abrasions more than 6 hours old, blebs, pyoderma, and preexisting ulcers precludes immediate open treatment of closed fracture. Extensive swelling due to hemorrhagic exudate in closed fascial compartments may prevent complete reduction immediately. Extensive hemorrhagic and edematous infiltration can complicate and make difficult satisfactory closure of the subcutaneous tissue and skin incidental to elective open reduction. Neurovascular integrity below the level of the fracture must be verified before definitive treatment is instituted.

X-rays in the anteroposterior and lateral projection of the entire leg, including both the knee and ankle joints, are always necessary, and oblique projections are often desirable. The surgeon must know the exact site and configuration of the fracture, the severity of comminution, and the direction of displacement of fragments. Inadequate x-ray examination can lead to an incomplete diagnosis.

FRACTURE OF THE SHAFT OF THE FIBULA

Isolated fracture of the shaft of the fibula is uncommon and is usually caused by direct trauma. Fibular shaft fracture is usually associated with other injury of the leg, such as fracture of the tibia or fracture-dislocation of the ankle joint. If no other lesion is present, immobilization for 4 weeks in a plaster boot (equipped with a walking surface) extending from the knee to the toes is sufficient for displaced, painful fractures. Undisplaced fractures require no immobilization, but discomfort can be minimized during the early days after injury by the use of crutches or a cane. Complete healing of uncomplicated fracture can be expected.

FRACTURE OF THE SHAFT OF THE TIBIA

Isolated fracture of the shaft of the tibia is likely to be caused by indirect injury, such as torsional stress.

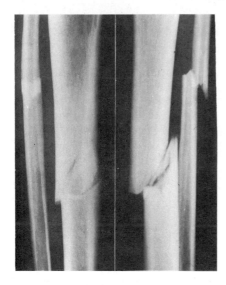

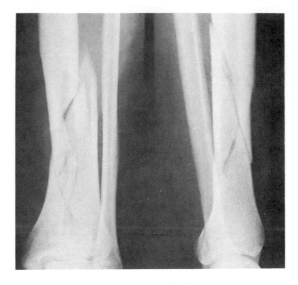

Figure 45–45. Short oblique fracture of the mid diaphysis of the tibia and fracture of the fibular shaft in a 33-year-old man. This fracture is inherently unstable and is likely to become displaced when treated by plaster immobilization alone.

Figure 45–46. Comminuted fracture of the distal diaphysis of the tibia extending into the metaphysis and entering the ankle joint in a 34-year-old man.

Because of mechanical stability provided by the intact fibula, marked displacement is not apt to occur. Marked overriding suggests a lesion of either tibiofibular joint.

If the fragments are not displaced, reliable treatment may be given by immobilization in a tubular plaster cast extending from the inguinal region to the toes with the knee in flexion and the foot in neutral position. The plaster should be changed at appropriate intervals to correct the loosening which will occur as a result of absorption of hemorrhagic exudate and atrophy of the thigh and calf muscles. Immobilization should be continued for at least 10 weeks, or until early bone healing is demonstrated by x-ray.

If the fragments are displaced, manipulation under anesthesia may be necessary. Fractures with a comparative transverse cleft tend to be stable after reduction. Oblique and spiral fractures tend to become displaced unless the fragments are locked.

A tubular plaster cast is applied as for undisplaced fracture. If x-rays do not show satisfactory apposition of fragments, alternative methods of treatment should be used (see below).

FRACTURE OF THE SHAFTS OF BOTH BONES IN ADULTS

Simultaneous fracture of the shafts of the tibia and fibula are unstable lesions which tend to become displaced following reduction. Treatment is directed toward reduction and stabilization of the tibial fracture until healing takes place. For adequate reduction, the fragments must be apposed almost completely, and

angulation and torsional displacement of the tibial fracture must be corrected.

If reduction by closed manipulation is anatomic, transverse fractures tend to be stable. Repeated x-rays are necessary to determine whether displacement has recurred. The plaster must remain snug at all times. Recurrent angular displacement can be corrected by dividing the plaster circumferentially and inserting wedges in the appropriate direction. If apposition is disturbed, another type of treatment must be substituted.

If oblique and spiral fractures are unstable following manipulation and immobilization, internal fixation, percutaneous fixation, or skeletal traction is usually required (Fig 45–47). Percutaneous fixation (osteotaxis) can be accomplished either by incorporation of pins or wires into the cast which transfix the major bone fragments or by the use of an extraskeletal apparatus such as that of Anderson, Stader, or Haynes.

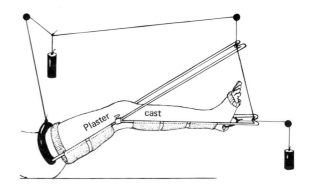

Figure 45–47. Calcaneal skeletal traction and full lower extremity plaster for unstable fracture of the tibia and fibula.

An alternative method is continuous skeletal traction, which must be continued for about 6 weeks or until preliminary healing causes stabilization. The extremity is then immobilized in plaster for at least 12 weeks until bone continuity has been restored.

If adequate apposition and correction of the deformity cannot be achieved by closed methods, open reduction and internal fixation are required.

The blood supply to intermediate fragments is likely to be disturbed in comminuted and segmental fractures. These unstable fractures can usually be treated successfully only by closed reduction and external immobilization. If the patient wishes to remain ambulatory, percutaneous fixation of the major fragments with Steinmann pins or Kirschner wires will maintain reduction and alignment. However, continuous skeletal traction in plaster with a Kirschner wire inserted through the calcaneus is usually preferred until stabilization occurs (Fig 45–47).

Rankin EA, Metz CW Jr: Management of delayed union in early weight-bearing treatment of the fractured tibia. J Trauma 10:751, 1970.

Silva JF: Fractures of the tibia and fibula. J Trauma 12:1029, 1972.

Weissman SL & others: Fractures of the middle two-thirds of the tibial shaft: Results of treatment without internal fixation in one hundred and forty consecutive cases. J Bone Joint Surg 48A:257, 1966.

FRACTURE OF THE SHAFTS OF THE TIBIA & FIBULA IN CHILDREN

Open reduction and internal fixation of closed fractures of the tibia or fibula in children are rarely necessary. If a tibial fracture is stable because of the configuration of the ends of the fragments, or if the fibular shaft is intact, closed reduction of axial displacement (overriding) is desirable; angular and torsional displacement must be corrected also. If proper alignment is secured, 1 cm of overriding is acceptable.

Comminuted or oblique tibial fractures with displacement or fractures of both bones require continuous skeletal traction by means of a Kirschner wire inserted through the calcaneus until early bone healing stabilizes the fragments. Further immobilization in a tubular plaster cast is necessary until bone healing is sufficiently well along to permit weight-bearing.

INJURIES OF THE ANKLE REGION

ANKLE SPRAIN

Sprain of the ankle joint during childhood is rare. In the adult, ankle sprain is most often caused by forced inversion of the foot, as may occur in stumbling on uneven ground. Pain is usually maximal over the anterolateral aspect of the joint; greatest tenderness is apt to be found in the region of the anterior talofibular and talocalcaneal ligaments. Eversion sprain is less common; maximal tenderness and swelling are usually found over the deltoid ligament.

Sprain is differentiated from major partial or complete ligamentous tears by anteroposterior, lateral, and 30 degrees internal oblique x-ray projections; if the joint cleft between either malleolus and the talus is greater than 4 mm, major ligamentous tear is probable. Occult lesions can be demonstrated by x-ray examination under inversion or eversion stress after infiltration of the area of maximal swelling and tenderness with 5 ml of 2% procaine.

If swelling is marked, elevation of the extremity and avoidance of weight-bearing for a few days is advisable. The ankle can be supported with a Gibney strapping (Fig 45–48). Adhesive support for another 2 weeks will relieve pain and swelling. Further treatment may be by warm foot baths and elastic bandages. Continue treatment until muscle strength and full joint motion are recovered. Tears of major ligaments of the ankle joint are discussed below.

Fordyce AJW, Horn CV: Arthrography in recent injuries of the ligaments of the ankle. J Bone Joint Surg 54B:116, 1972.

Heck CC: Sprained ankle. NY State J Med 72:1620, 1972.

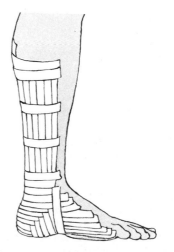

Figure 45—48. Gibney ankle strapping.

FRACTURES & DISLOCATIONS OF
THE ANKLE JOINT

Fractures and dislocations of the ankle joint may be caused by direct injury, in which case they are apt to be comminuted and open; or by indirect violence, which often causes typical lesions (see below).

Pain and swelling are the prominent clinical findings. Deformity may or may not be present. X-rays of excellent technical quality must be prepared in a sufficient variety of projections to demonstrate the extent and configuration of all major fragments. Special oblique projections may be required.

Fracture of the Medial Malleolus

Fracture of the medial malleolus may occur as an isolated lesion of any part of the malleolus (including the tip), or may be associated with (1) fracture of the lateral malleolus with medial or lateral dislocation of the talus, and (2) dislocation of the inferior tibiofibular joint with or without fracture of the fibula. Isolated fracture does not usually cause instability of the ankle joint.

Undisplaced isolated fracture of the medial malleolus should be treated by immobilization in a plaster boot extending from the knee to the toes with the ankle flexed to a right angle and the foot slightly inverted to relax the tension on the deltoid ligament (Fig 45–49). Immobilization must be continued for 6–8 weeks or until bone healing is sound.

Displaced isolated fracture of the medial malleolus may be treated by closed manipulation under general or local anesthesia. The essential maneuver consists of anatomic realignment by digital pressure over the distal fragment, followed by immobilization in a plas-

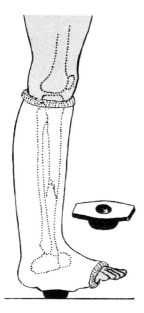

Figure 45–49. Weight-bearing plaster boot.

ter boot (as for undisplaced fracture) until bone healing is sound (Fig 45–49). If anatomic reduction cannot be obtained by closed methods, open reduction and internal fixation with 1–2 bone screws are required.

Fracture of the Lateral Malleolus

Fracture of the lateral malleolus may occur as an isolated lesion, or may be associated with fracture of the medial malleolus, tear of the deltoid or posterior lateral malleolar ligament, or avulsion of the posterior tibial tubercle. If the medial aspect of the ankle is injured, lateral dislocation of the talus is apt to be present. The tip of the lateral malleolus may be avulsed by the calcaneofibular and anterior talofibular ligaments. Transverse or oblique fracture may occur. Oblique fractures commonly extend downward and anteriorly from the posterior and superior aspects.

If swelling and pain are not marked, isolated undisplaced fracture of the lateral malleolus may be treated by Gibney ankle strapping (Fig 45–48). Otherwise, a plaster boot should be applied for 6 weeks and an elastic bandage worn thereafter until full joint motion is recovered and the calf muscles are functioning normally.

Isolated displaced fracture of the lateral malleolus should be treated by closed manipulation. The foot should be immobilized in slight inversion, which tautens the ligaments over the lateral aspect of the ankle joint and tends to prevent displacement.

If anatomic reduction cannot be achieved by closed methods, open reduction is required.

Combined Fracture of the Medial
& Lateral Malleoli

Bimalleolar fractures are commonly accompanied by displacement of the talus, usually in a medial or lateral direction. In conjunction with dislocation in the coronal plane, concurrent displacement may take place in the sagittal plane, either anteriorly or posteriorly, or in torsion about the longitudinal axis of the tibia.

Bimalleolar fracture may be treated by closed manipulation. A tubular plaster cast is then applied from the inguinal region to the toes with the knee in about 45 degrees of flexion and the foot in neutral position. Immediate open reduction must be resorted to if x-rays show that perfect anatomic reduction has not been achieved by closed manipulation.

Fractures of the Distal Tibia

Fracture of the distal tibia is usually associated with other lesions.

A. Fracture of the Posterior Margin: Fracture of the posterior articular margin may involve part or all of the entire posterior half and is apt to be accompanied by fracture of either malleolus and posterior dislocation of the talus. It must be differentiated from fracture of the posterior tibial tubercle, which is usually caused by avulsion with the attached posterior lateral malleolar ligament.

Anatomic reduction by closed manipulation is

required if the fracture involves more than 25% of the articular surface. The extremity is immobilized in a plaster cast extending from the inguinal region to the toes with the knee in about 40 degrees of flexion, the ankle at a right angle, and the foot in neutral position.

Frequent x-ray examination is necessary to make certain that redisplacement does not occur. The plaster should be changed as soon as loosening becomes apparent. Immobilization must be maintained for at least 8 weeks. Weight-bearing must not be resumed until bone healing is sound, usually in about 12 weeks.

B. Fracture of the Anterior Margin: Fracture of the anterior articular margin of the tibia (rare) is likely to be caused by forced dorsiflexion of the foot. If displacement is marked and the talus is dislocated, tear of the collateral ligaments or fractures of the malleoli are likely to be present.

Reduction is by closed manipulation. If comminution is present, the extremity should be immobilized for about 12 weeks. Healing is apt to be slow.

C. Comminuted Fractures: Extensive comminution of the distal tibia ("compression type" fracture) presents a difficult problem of management. The congruity of articular surfaces cannot be restored by closed manipulation, and satisfactory anatomic restoration is usually not possible even by open reduction. The best form of treatment for extensively comminuted and widely displaced fractures is closed manipulation and skeletal traction (Fig 45–47). After traction has been applied and impaction of fragments has been disrupted, displacement in the transverse plane is corrected by manual molding with compression. A tubular plaster cast is applied from the inguinal region to the toes with the knee in 10–15 degrees of flexion and the foot in neutral position. With the extremity immobilized in plaster, continuous skeletal traction can be maintained for 8–12 weeks or until stabilization by early bone healing occurs. An alternative is distraction with a wire or pin in the calcaneus and one or 2 wires or pins in the shaft of the tibia.

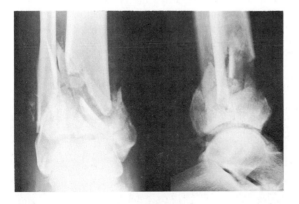

Figure 45–50. Comminuted fracture of the distal tibia and fibula with disruption of the ankle joint in a 45-year-old man. The position achieved by skeletal traction on the calcaneus and closed manipulation is unsatisfactory. Early onset of secondary osteoarthritis is likely.

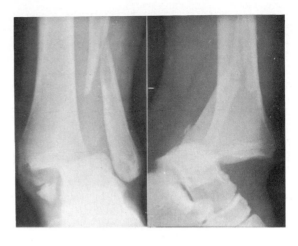

Figure 45–51. Closed fracture of the lower fibular shaft and medial malleolus with dislocation of the inferior tibiofibular and ankle joints in a 35-year-old man. Open reduction and internal fixation are necessary for optimal treatment.

Healing is likely to be slow. If the articular surfaces of the ankle joint have not been properly realigned, disabling posttraumatic arthritis is likely to occur early. Early arthrodesis is indicated to shorten the period of disability.

Dislocation of the Ankle Joint

A. Complete Dislocation: The talus cannot be completely dislocated from the ankle joint unless all ligaments are torn. This lesion is rare.

B. Incomplete Dislocation: Major ligamentous injuries in the region of the ankle joint are usually associated with fracture.

1. Tear of the deltoid ligament—Complete tear of the talotibial portion of the deltoid ligament can permit interposition of the posterior tibial tendon between the medial malleolus and the talus. Associated injury is usually present, especially fracture of the lateral malleolus with lateral dislocation of the talus.

Pain, tenderness, swelling, and ecchymosis in the region of the medial malleolus without fracture suggest partial or complete tear of the deltoid ligament. If fracture of the lateral malleolus or dislocation of the distal tibiofibular joint is present, the cleft between the malleolus and talus is likely to be widened. If significant widening is not apparent, x-ray examination under stress is necessary.

Interposition of the deltoid ligament between the talus and the medial malleolus often cannot be corrected by closed manipulation. If widening persists after closed manipulation, surgical exploration is indicated so that the ligament can be removed and repaired by suture.

Associated fracture of the fibula can be treated by fixation with a coaxial intramedullary standard bone screw or a bone nail to assure maintenance of anatomic reduction.

2. Tear of the talofibular ligament—Isolated tear

of the anterior talofibular ligament is caused by forced inversion of the foot. X-ray examination under stress may be necessary, using local or general anesthesia. Both feet are forcibly inverted and internally rotated about 20 degrees while an anteroposterior film is exposed. If the tear is complete, the talus will be seen to be axially displaced from the tibial articular surface.

Rupture of the anterior talofibular ligament may be associated with tear of the calcaneofibular ligament. Tear of both ligaments may be associated with fracture of the medial malleolus and medial dislocation of the talus.

Instability of the ankle joint, characterized by a history of recurrent sprains, may result from unrecognized tears of the anterior talofibular ligament.

Recent isolated tear of the anterior talofibular ligament or combined tear of the calcaneofibular ligament should be treated by immobilization for 4 weeks in a plaster boot. Associated fracture of the medial malleolus creates an unstable mechanism. Unless anatomic reduction can be achieved and maintained by closed methods, open reduction of the malleolar fragment is indicated, followed by internal fixation of the fracture and repair of the ligamentous injury.

Dislocation of the Distal Tibiofibular Joint

Both the anterior and posterior lateral malleolar ligaments must be torn before dislocation of the distal tibiofibular joint can occur. Lateral dislocation of the talus is also an essential feature, and this cannot occur unless the medial malleolus is fractured or the deltoid ligament is torn. The distal fibula is commonly fractured, but it may remain intact, and dislocation may be caused by a tear of the interosseous ligament.

Anatomic reduction by closed manipulation is difficult to achieve, but should be tried. Under general anesthesia, the foot is forced medially by a shearing maneuver and a snug plaster cast is applied from the inguinal region to the toes. If immediate and repeated x-ray examinations do not demonstrate that anatomic reduction has been achieved and maintained, open reduction and internal fixation should be performed as soon as possible.

Separation of the Distal Tibial & Fibular Epiphyses

The most common injury of the ankle region of children is traumatic separation of the distal tibial and fibular epiphyses. Sprain is rare in children. Separation of the distal fibular epiphysis may occur as an isolated injury, or may be associated with separation of the tibial epiphysis.

If displacement has occurred, treatment is by closed manipulation and plaster immobilization. Open reduction is seldom justifiable. If injury has been severe, disturbance of growth is likely to follow.

Brodie IA, Denham RA: The treatment of unstable ankle fractures. J Bone Joint Surg 56B:256, 1974.

Broock GJ, Greer RB: Traumatic rotation displacements of the distal tibial growth plate: A case report. J Bone Joint Surg 52A:1666, 1970.

Colton CL: The treatment of Dupuytren's fracture-dislocation of the ankle. J Bone Joint Surg 53B:63, 1971.

Joy G & others: Precise evaluation of the reduction of severe ankle fractures. J Bone Joint Surg 56A:979, 1974.

INJURIES OF THE FOOT

FRACTURE & DISLOCATION OF THE TALUS

Dislocation of the Subtalar & Talonavicular Joints

Dislocation of the subtalar and talonavicular joints without fracture occasionally occurs. The talocrural joint is not injured. Displacement of the foot can be either in varus or valgus. Reduction by closed manipulation is usually not difficult. Incarceration of the posterior tibial tendon in the talonavicular joint may prevent reduction by closed manipulation. After reduction, the extremity should be immobilized in a plaster boot for 4 weeks.

Fracture of the Talus

Major fracture of the talus commonly occurs either through the body or through the neck; the uncommon fracture of the head involves essentially a portion of the neck with extension into the head. Indirect injury is usually the cause of closed fracture as well as most open fractures; severe comminution is not commonly present. Compression fracture or infraction of the tibial articular surface may be caused by the initial injury or may occur later in association with complicating avascular necrosis. The proximal or distal fragments may be dislocated.

A. Fracture of the Neck: Forced dorsiflexion of the foot may cause this injury. Undisplaced fracture of the neck can be treated adequately by a non-weight-

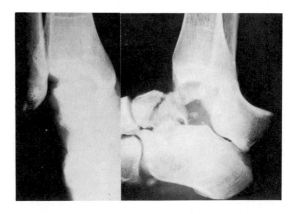

Figure 45–52. Comminuted fracture of the talus with dislocation of the body from the ankle and subtalar joints in a 28-year-old man. Closed reduction is impossible.

bearing plaster boot for 8–12 weeks. Dislocation of the body or the distal neck fragment with the foot may complicate this injury. Fracture of the neck with anterior and frequently medial dislocation of the distal fragment and foot can usually be reduced by closed manipulation. Subsequent treatment is the same as that of undisplaced fracture.

Dislocation of the proximal body fragment may occur separately or may be associated with dislocation of the distal fragment. If dislocation of the body fragment is complete, reduction by closed manipulation may not be possible. If reduction by closed manipulation is not successful, open reduction should be done as soon as possible to prevent or to minimize the extent of the avascular necrosis. Bone healing is likely to be retarded since some degree of avascular necrosis is probable.

Complete dislocation of the neck fragment from the talonavicular and subtalar joints is rare, but if it does happen avascular necrosis of the fragment is to be expected even though anatomic reduction is promptly accomplished. If reduction by closed manipulation is not possible, immediate open operation with reduction of the fragment or its removal is advisable since delay may cause necrosis of overlying soft tissues.

B. Fracture of the Body: Closed uncomminuted fracture of the body of the talus with minimal displacement of fragments is not likely to cause disability if immobilization is continued until bone continuity is restored. If significant displacement occurs, the proximal fragment is apt to be dislocated from the subtalar and ankle joints. Reduction by closed manipulation can be achieved best by traction and forced plantar flexion of the foot. Immobilization in a plaster boot with the foot in equinus for about 8 weeks should be followed by further casting with the foot at a right angle until the fracture cleft has been obliterated by new bone formation as evidenced by x-ray examination. Even though prompt adequate reduction is obtained by either closed manipulation or by open operation, extensive displacement of the proximal body fragment is likely to be followed by avascular necrosis. If reduction is not anatomic, delayed healing of the fracture may follow and posttraumatic arthritis is a likely sequel. If this occurs, arthrodesis of the ankle and subtalar joints may be necessary to relieve painful symptoms.

C. Compression Fracture: Compression fracture or infraction of the dome of the talus from the initial injury (which is likely to have been violent) cannot be reduced. When this lesion occurs as a separate entity or in combination with other fractures of the body, prolonged protection from weight-bearing is the major means of preventing the further collapse that is so likely to occur in the area of healing.

Mukherjee SK, Young AB: Dome fracture of the talus: A report of ten cases. J Bone Joint Surg 55B:319, 1973.
Mukherjee SK & others: Fracture of the lateral process of the talus: A report of thirteen cases. J Bone Joint Surg 56B:263, 1974.

Reckling FW: Early tibiocalcaneal fusion in the treatment of severe injuries of the talus. J Trauma 12:390, 1972.

FRACTURE OF THE CALCANEUS

Fracture of the calcaneus is commonly caused by direct trauma. Since this fracture is likely to occur as a result of a fall from a height, fracture of the spine may also be present. Comminution and impaction are general characteristics. Minor infractions or impactions and fissure fractures are easy to miss on clinical examination, and x-rays must be prepared in multiple projections to demonstrate adequately some fracture clefts. In some instances, minor impactions of articular surfaces will be evident only by tomography.

Various classifications have been advocated. Fractures that are generally comminuted and disrupt the subtalar and calcaneocuboid articulations should be distinguished from those that do not; this differentiation has important implications for treatment and prognosis.

Fracture of the Tuberosity

Isolated fracture of the tuberosity is not common. It may occur in a vertical or a horizontal direction.

A. Horizontal Fracture: Horizontal fracture may be limited to the superior portion of the region of the former apophysis and represents an avulsion by the Achilles tendon. Where the superior minor fragment is widely displaced proximally with the tendon, open reduction and fixation with a stout wire suture may be necessary to obtain the most satisfactory functional result.

Further extension of the fracture cleft toward the subtalar joint in the substance of the tuberosity creates the "beak" fracture. The minor fragment may be displaced proximally by the action of the triceps surae. If displacement is significant, reduction can be achieved by skeletal traction applied to the proximal fragment with the foot in equinus. Immobilization is obtained by incorporation of the traction pin or wire in a full extremity plaster with the knee flexed 30 degrees and the foot in plantar flexion. If adequate reduction cannot be accomplished in this way, open reduction is advised.

B. Vertical Fracture: Vertical fracture occurs near the sagittal plane somewhat medially through the tuberosity. Because the minor medial fragment normally is not widely displaced, plaster immobilization is not required. Comfort can be enhanced by limitation of weight-bearing with the aid of crutches.

Fracture of the Sustentaculum

Isolated fracture of the sustentaculum tali is a rare lesion which may be caused by forced eversion of the foot. Where displacement of the larger body fragment occurs, it is lateral. Incarceration of the tendon of the flexor hallucis longus in the fracture cleft has been reported. Generally this fracture occurs in association with comminution of the body.

Fracture of the Anterior Process

Fracture of the anterior process is caused by forced inversion of the foot. It must be differentiated from midtarsal and ankle joint sprains. The firmly attached bifurcate ligament (calcaneonavicular and calcaneocuboid components) avulses a bit of bone. Maximum tenderness and slight swelling occur midway between the tip of the lateral malleolus and the base of the fifth metatarsal. The lateral x-ray view projected obliquely is the most satisfactory to demonstrate the fracture cleft. Treatment is by a non-weight-bearing plaster boot with the foot in neutral position for 4 weeks.

Fracture of the Body

Fracture of the body may occur posterior to the articular surfaces, in a general vertical but somewhat oblique plane, without disruption of the subtalar joint. Most severe fractures of the calcaneal body are comminuted and extend into the subtalar and frequently the calcaneocuboid joints. Fissure fractures without significant displacement cause minor disability and can be treated simply by protection from weight-bearing, either by crutches alone or in combination with a plaster boot until bone healing is sufficiently sound to justify graded increments of loading.

A. Nonarticular Fracture: Where fracture of the body with comminution occurs posterior to the articular surface, the direction of significant displacement of the fragment attached to the tuberosity is proximal, causing diminution of the tuber joint angle. Since the subtalar joint is not disrupted, symptomatic posttraumatic degenerative arthritis is not an important sequel even though some joint stiffness persists permanently. Marked displacement should be corrected by skeletal traction applied to the main posterior fragment to obtain an optimal cosmetic result, especially in women. Success of reduction can be judged by the adequacy of restoration of the tuber joint angle.

B. Articular Fracture: Articular fractures are of 3 general types:

1. Noncomminuted—Fracture of the body without comminution may involve the posterior articular facet. Where displacement of the posterior fragment of the tuberosity occurs, the direction is lateral. Fractures of this category with more than minimal displacement should be treated by the method advocated for nonarticular fracture of the body.

2. With minor comminution—In fractures with minor comminution, the main cleft occurs vertically, in a somewhat oblique lateral deviation from the sagittal plane. From emergence on the medial surface posterior to the sustentaculum it is directed forward and rather obliquely laterally through the posterior articular facet. The sustentaculum and the medial portion of the posterior articular facet remain undisplaced with relation to the talus. The body below the remaining lateral portion of the posterior articular facet with the tuberosity are impacted into the lateral portion of the posterior articular facet. Since anatomic reduction cannot be achieved by closed technics, Palmer has advocated open reduction and bone grafting. Lack of precise reduction, determined in part by restoration of the normal tuber joint angle, causes derangement of the subtalar joint, and symptomatic posttraumatic arthritis is a frequent sequel.

3. With extensive comminution—Fracture with extensive comminution extending into the subtalar joint may involve the calcaneocuboid joint as well as the tuberosity. The multiple fracture clefts involve the entire posterior articular surface, and the facet is impacted into the substance of the underlying body. There are many variants; the clefts may extend across the calcaneal groove into the medial and anterior articular surfaces, and detachment of the peroneal tubercle may be a feature. This serious injury may cause major disability in spite of the best treatment since the bursting nature of the injury defies anatomic restoration.

Some surgeons advise nonintervention. Displacement of fragments is disregarded. Initially, a compression dressing is applied and the extremity is elevated for a week or so. Warm soaks and active exercises are then started, but weight-bearing is avoided until early bone healing has taken place. In spite of residual deformity of the heel, varying degrees of weakness of the calf, and discomfort in the region of the subtalar joint (which may be intensified by weight-bearing), acceptable functional results can be obtained, especially among vigorous men who are willing to put up with the discomforts involved.

Other surgeons, notably Hermann and Böhler, advocate early closed manipulation which can partially restore the external anatomic configuration of the heel region, a cosmetic goal particularly desirable for women.

Persistent and disabling painful symptoms originating in the deranged subtalar joint may require arthrodesis for adequate relief. Concomitant involvement of the calcaneocuboid joint is an indication for the more extensive triple arthrodesis.

Hazlett JW: Open reduction of fractures of the calcaneum. Can J Surg 12:310, 1969.

Isbister JF StC: Calcaneo-fibular abutment following crush fracture of the calcaneus. J Bone Joint Surg 56B:274, 1974.

FRACTURE OF THE TARSAL NAVICULAR

Minor avulsion fractures of the tarsal navicular may occur as a feature of severe midtarsal sprain and require neither reduction nor elaborate treatment. Avulsion fracture of the tuberosity near the insertion of the posterior tibialis muscle is uncommon and must be differentiated from a persistent, ununited apophysis (accessory scaphoid) and from the supernumerary sesamoid bone, the os tibiale externum.

Major fracture occurs either through the middle in a horizontal or, more rarely, in the vertical plane, or is characterized by impaction of its substance. Only noncomminuted fractures with displacement of the dorsal fragment can be reduced. Closed manipulation by strong traction on the forefoot and simultaneous digital pressure over the displaced fragment can restore it to its normal position. If a tendency to redisplacement is apparent, this can be counteracted by temporary fixation with a percutaneously inserted Kirschner wire. Comminuted and impacted fractures cannot be anatomically reduced. Some authorities offer a pessimistic prognosis for comminuted or impacted fractures. It is their contention that even though partial reduction has been achieved, posttraumatic arthritis supervenes, and that arthrodesis of the talonavicular and cuneonavicular joints will be ultimately necessary to relieve painful symptoms.

FRACTURE OF THE CUNEIFORM & CUBOID BONES

Because of their relatively protected position in the midtarsus, isolated fracture of the cuboid and cuneiform bones is rarely encountered. Minor avulsion fractures occur as a component of severe midtarsal sprains. Extensive fracture usually occurs in association with other injuries of the foot and often is caused by severe crushing. Simple classification is impractical because of the complex character and the multiple combinations of the whole injury.

MIDTARSAL DISLOCATIONS

Midtarsal dislocation through the cuneonavicular and the calcaneocuboid joints or, more proximally, through the talocalcaneonavicular and the calcaneocuboid joints may occur as a result of twisting injury to the forefoot. Fractures of varying extent of adjacent bones are frequent complications. When treatment is given soon after the accident, closed reduction by traction on the forefoot and manipulation is generally effective. If reduction is unstable and displacement tends to recur upon release of traction, stabilization for 4 weeks by percutaneously inserted Kirschner wires is recommended.

FRACTURES & DISLOCATIONS OF THE METATARSALS

Fractures of metatarsals and tarsometatarsal dislocations are likely to be caused by direct crushing or indirect twisting injury to the forefoot. Besides osseous and articular injury, complicating soft tissue lesions are often present. Tense subfascial hematoma of the dorsum of the forefoot, if not relieved, may cause necrosis of overlying skin or may even lead to gangrene of the toes by interruption of the arterial supply.

Tarsometatarsal Dislocations

Possibly because of strong ligamentous support and relative size, dislocation of the first metatarsal at its base occurs less frequently than similar involvement of the lesser bones. If dislocation occurs, fracture of the first cuneiform is likely to be present also. More often, however, tarsometatarsal dislocation involves the lesser metatarsals, and associated fractures are to be expected. Dislocation is more commonly caused by direct injury but may be the result of stress applied indirectly through the forefoot. The direction of displacement is ordinarily dorsal, lateral, or a combination of both.

Attempted closed reduction should not be deferred. Skeletal traction applied to the involved bone by a Kirschner wire or a stout towel clamp can be a valuable aid to manipulation. Even though persistent dislocation may not cause significant disability, the resulting deformity can make shoe fitting difficult for men and the cosmetic effect undesirable to women. Open reduction with evacuation of dorsal subfascial hematoma and Kirschner wire stabilization is a preferred alternative to unsuccessful closed treatment. When effective treatment has been deferred 4 weeks or even longer, early healing will prevent satisfactory reduction of persisting displacement by closed technics. Under such circumstances, it is better to defer open operation and to direct treatment toward recovery of function. Extensive operative procedures and continued immobilization can increase joint stiffness. Reconstructive operation can be planned more suitably after residual disability becomes established.

Wiley JJ: The mechanism of tarso-metatarsal joint injuries. J Bone Joint Surg 53B:474, 1971.

Fractures of the Shafts

Undisplaced fractures of the metatarsal shafts cause no permanent disability unless failure of bone healing is encountered. Displacement is rarely significant where fracture of the middle metatarsals is oblique and the first and fifth are uninjured, since they act as splints. Even fissure fractures should be treated by a stiff-soled shoe (with partial weight-bearing) or, if pain is marked, by a plaster walking boot.

Great care should be taken in displaced fractures to correct angulation in the longitudinal axis of the shaft. Persistent convex dorsal angulation causes prominence of the head of the involved metatarsal on the plantar aspect with the implication of concentrated local pressure and production of painful skin callosities. Deformity of the shaft of the first metatarsal due to convex plantar angulation can transfer weight-bearing stress to the region of the head of the third metatarsal. After correction of angular displacement, the plaster casing should be molded well to the plantar aspect of the foot to minimize recurrence of deformity and to support the longitudinal and transverse arches.

If reduction is not reasonably accurate, fractures through the shafts near the heads (the "neck") may cause great discomfort from concentrated pressure beneath the head on the plantar surface and reactive skin callus formation. Every effort should be made to correct convex dorsal angulation by disrupting impaction and appropriate manipulation. Unstable fracture can be treated by sustained skeletal traction using a Kirschner wire inserted through the distal phalanx and traction supplied by an elastic band attached to a "banjo" bow. The efficacy of closed treatment should be determined without delay, and, where it is lacking, open operation should be substituted.

Fatigue Fracture of the Shafts

Fatigue fracture of the shafts of the metatarsals has been described by various terms, eg, march, stress, and insufficiency fracture, and by a variety of other terms in the French and German literature. Its protean clinical manifestations cause difficulty in precise recognition, even to the point of confusion with osteogenic sarcoma. Commonly, it occurs in active young adults, such as military recruits, who are unaccustomed to vigorous and excessive walking. A history of a single significant injury is lacking. Incipient pain of varying intensity in the forefoot which is accentuated by walking, swelling, and localized tenderness of the involved metatarsal are cardinal manifestations. Depending upon the stage of progress, x-rays may not demonstrate the fracture cleft and extracortical callus formation may ultimately be the only clue. More striking findings may vary from an incomplete fissure to an evident transverse cleft. Persistent unprotected weight-bearing may cause arrest of bone healing and even displacement of the distal fragment. The second and third metatarsals are most frequently involved near the junction of the middle and distal thirds. The lesion can occur more proximally and in other lesser metatarsals. Since weight-bearing is likely to prolong and aggravate symptoms, treatment is by protection in either a plaster walking boot or a heavy shoe with the sole reinforced by a steel strut. Weight-bearing should be restricted until painful symptoms subside and restoration of bone continuity has been demonstrated by x-ray examination.

Fracture of the Tuberosity of the Fifth Metatarsal

Forced adduction of the forefoot may cause avulsion fracture of the tuberosity of the fifth metatarsal, and, where supporting soft tissues have been torn,

activity of the peroneus brevis muscle may increase displacement of the avulsed proximal fragment. If displacement of the minor fragment is minimal, adhesive strapping or a stiff-soled shoe is adequate treatment. If displacement is significant, treatment should be by a walking boot until bone healing occurs (Fig 45-49). Rarely does healing fail to occur. Fracture should be differentiated from a separate ossific center of the tuberosity in adolescence and the supernumerary os vesalianum pedis in adulthood.

FRACTURES & DISLOCATIONS OF THE PHALANGES OF THE TOES

Fractures of the phalanges of the toes are caused most commonly by direct violence such as crushing or stubbing. Spiral or oblique fractures of the shafts of the proximal phalanges of the lesser toes may occur as a result of indirect twisting injury.

Comminuted fracture of the proximal phalanx of the great toe, alone or in combination with fracture of the distal phalanx, is the most disabling injury. Since

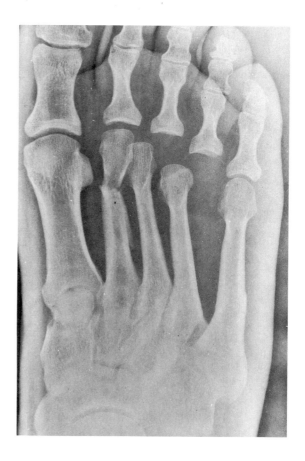

Figure 45–53. Closed fracture of the shaft of the second metatarsal and dislocations of the third and fourth metatarsophalangeal joints in a 26-year-old man.

wide displacement of fragments is not likely, correction of angulation and support by an adhesive dressing and splint usually suffices. A weight-bearing plaster boot may be useful for relief of symptoms arising from associated soft tissue injury. Spiral or oblique fracture of the proximal phalanges of the lesser toes can be treated adequately by binding the involved toe to the adjacent uninjured member. Comminuted fracture of the distal phalanx is treated as a soft tissue injury.

Traumatic dislocation of the metatarsophalangeal joints and the uncommon dislocation of the proximal interphalangeal joint usually can be reduced by closed manipulation. These dislocations are rarely isolated and usually occur in combination with other injuries to the forefoot.

FRACTURE OF THE SESAMOIDS OF THE GREAT TOE

Fracture of the sesamoid bones of the great toe is rare, but may occur as a result of crushing injury. It must be differentiated from partite developmental lesions. Undisplaced fracture requires no treatment other than a foot support or a metatarsal bar. Displaced fracture may require immobilization in a walking plaster boot with the toe strapped in flexion. Persistent delay of bone healing may cause disabling pain arising from arthritis of the articulation between the sesamoid and the head of the first metatarsal. If a foot support and metatarsal bar do not provide adequate relief, excision of the sesamoid may be necessary.

●　●　●

General References

Abel MS: *Traumatic Lesions of the Cervical Vertebrae.* Warren H. Green, 1971.

Aergerter E, Kirkpatrick JA: *Orthopedic Diseases,* 4th ed. Saunders, 1975.

American Academy of Orthopedic Surgeons: *Symposium on Sports Medicine.* Mosby, 1969.

Bateman JE: *The Shoulder and Neck.* Saunders, 1972.

Crenshaw AH (editor): *Campbell's Operative Orthopaedics,* 5th ed. Mosby, 1971.

Cruess RL, Mitchell NS (editors): *Surgery of Rheumatoid Arthritis.* Lippincott, 1971.

De Palma AF: *The Management of Fractures and Dislocations,* 2nd ed. Saunders, 1970.

Ferguson AB Jr: *Orthopaedic Surgery in Infancy and Childhood,* 4th ed. Williams & Wilkins, 1975.

Greenfield GB: *Radiology of Bone Diseases.* Lippincott, 1975.

Gustilo RB & others: Analysis of 511 open fractures. Clin Orthop 66:148, 1969.

Hollander JL: *Arthritis and Allied Conditions,* 8th ed. Lea & Febiger, 1972.

Jaffee HL: *Metabolic, Degenerative, and Inflammatory Diseases of Bones and Joints.* Lea & Febiger, 1972.

Jawetz E, Melnick JL, Adelberg EA: *Review of Medical Microbiology,* 12th ed. Lange, 1976.

Lichtenstein L: *Bone Tumors,* 4th ed. Mosby, 1972.

O'Donoghue DH: *Treatment of Injuries of Athletes,* 2nd ed. Saunders, 1970.

Paul LW, Juhl JH: *Essentials of Roentgen Interpretation,* 3rd ed. Harper & Row, 1972.

Raney RB Sr, Brashear HR: *Shands' Handbook of Orthopaedic Surgery,* 8th ed. Mosby, 1971,

Rang M: *Children's Fractures.* Lippincott, 1974.

Rockwood CA Jr, Green DP (editors): *Fractures.* Lippincott, 1975.

Scharrard WJW: *Paediatric Orthopaedics and Fractures.* Davis, 1971.

Schmorl G: *The Human Spine in Health and Disease.* Grune & Stratton, 1971.

Tachdjian MO: *Pediatric Orthopedics.* 2 vols. Saunders, 1972.

Turek SL: *Orthopaedics: Principles and Their Application,* 2nd ed. Lippincott, 1967.

46 . . .
Plastic Surgery

William J. Morris, MD, & John Q. Owsley, Jr., MD

In order to obtain the best possible result in plastic surgery—ranging from simple wound closure to complicated procedures such as tissue transplantation—strict attention must be paid to the principles of atraumatic surgery. Improper or rough handling of tissue may cause necrosis and hematoma formation, which provides a medium for bacterial growth and sepsis. This results in further necrosis and tissue loss, delayed healing, and excessive scar formation. As a consequence, the desired fine-line scar or the successful "take" of the tissue transplant may not be achieved.

Important factors in atraumatic technic are as follows:

(1) Use of hooks to handle skin edges during wound closure rather than forceps or clamps that crush tissue.

(2) Inclusion of the smallest amount of tissue possible in the ligation of blood vessels.

(3) Minimal use of electrocoagulating instruments.

(4) Absolute hemostasis.

(5) Use of sharp, fine instruments, fine needles, and fine sutures.

(6) Avoidance of hot wound packs.

WOUND CLOSURE

Primary Closure

The ideal type of wound closure is primary approximation of the skin and subcutaneous tissues immediately adjacent to the wound defect, producing a fine-line scar and the optimal cosmetic result in skin texture, thickness, and color match. Closure by adjacent rotational or transposed pedicle grafts usually produces the next best cosmetic result. Closure by free skin grafts or nonadjacent skin pedicle grafts is less satisfactory and should be considered only when sufficient adjacent tissues are not available.

Normal Skin Lines & Fine-Line Scars

In most cases, fine "hairline" scars can be achieved only if the line or lines of incision are placed in or parallel to the skin lines of minimal tension. These lines lie perpendicular to the underlying muscles.

On the face, they are obvious as "wrinkle lines" or lines of facial expression which become more pronounced with age since they are secondary to repeated muscle contraction. On the neck, trunk, and extremities, the lines of minimal tension are most noticeable as horizontal lines of skin relaxation on the anterior and posterior aspects of areas of flexion and extension.

So-called Langer's lines, which were determined by cadaver study, probably show the direction of fibrous tissue bundles in the skin and are no longer considered accurate guides for placing skin incisions.

If the lines of expression cannot be followed, the line of incision should (if possible) be placed at the junction of unlike tissues such as the hairline of the scalp and the forehead, the eyebrow and the forehead, the mucosal and skin junction of the lips, or the areolar and skin margins of the breast. Scars will be partially hidden if incisions are placed in inconspicuous areas such as the crease of the nasal ala and cheek, the auricular-mastoid sulcus, or the submandibular-neck junction. Lines of incision should never purposely cross flexor surfaces such as the neck, axilla, antecubital fossa, or popliteal space or the palmar surfaces of the fingers and hand.

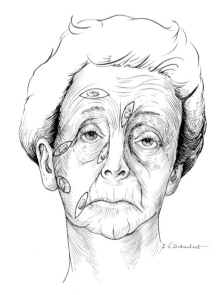

Figure 46—1. Sites of elliptical incisions corresponding to wrinkle lines on the face.

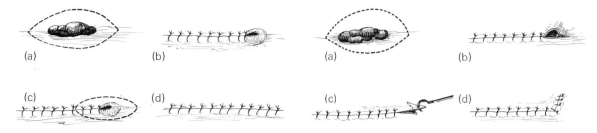

Figure 46—2. Correction of dog-ear.

Figure 46—3. Alternative method of correction of dog-ear.

Elliptical Excision (Fig 46—1)

If a lesion is to be excised, an elliptical excision placed parallel to the skin lines of minimal tension will give the best result if the amount of tissue to be excised does not preclude primary closure.

If the ellipse is too broad or short, a protrusion of skin, commonly called a "dog-ear," will occur at each pole of the wound closure (Fig 46—2). This is most easily corrected by excising the dog-ear as a small ellipse.

A dog-ear may also be present if one side of the ellipse is longer than the other (Fig 46—3). In this case, it may be easier to excise a small triangle of skin and subcutaneous tissue from the longer side.

SKIN GRAFTS

Generally speaking, skin grafts may be classified as free grafts or pedicle grafts. The advantages and disadvantages and some specific indications for both types are summarized in Tables 46—1 and 46—2. Free grafts may be either partial or full thickness sheets or sections of skin which are completely separated from their donor sites, ie, their blood supply is completely interrupted. They are transferred to the recipient area and depend for their survival upon vascularization from the bed of the recipient area. Pedicle grafts always remain attached to the donor site or to an intermediate transfer site and therefore carry their own blood supply. Although they depend upon vascularization from the recipient site for healing, they do not depend upon it for survival. Pedicle grafts usually include the full thickness of skin plus all or a portion of the subcutaneous adipose tissue.

FREE GRAFTS

Types of Free Grafts

Free skin grafts are classified on the basis of their thickness as split thickness or full thickness (Fig 46—4).

A. Split Thickness Grafts: Split thickness grafts are further classified as thin, intermediate, and thick, depending upon the amount of dermis that is included with the graft. Since skin may vary in thickness from 0.09 inch to as much as 0.15 inch, an intermediate thickness graft from an area such as the eyelid would be much thinner than an intermediate thickness graft from the back. However, using the standard donor site areas such as the skin of the thigh or the lateral buttocks for reference, the average thin split thickness graft will measure 0.010–0.012 inch, the intermediate split thickness graft 0.016–0.018 inch, and the thick

Table 46—1. Advantages and disadvantages of various types of skin grafts.

Type of Graft	Advantages	Disadvantages
Thin split thickness	Survive transplantation most easily. Donor sites heal most rapidly.	Fewest qualities of normal skin. Maximum contracture. Least resistance to trauma. Sensation poor. Cosmetically poor.
Thick split thickness	More qualities of normal skin. Less contracture. More resistant to trauma. Sensation fair. Cosmetically more acceptable.	Survive transplantation less well. Donor site heals slowly.
Full thickness	Nearly all qualities of normal skin. Minimal contracture. Very resistant to trauma. Sensation good to excellent. Cosmetically excellent.	Survive transplantation least well. Donor site must be closed surgically. Donor sites are limited.
Pedicle	Possess all qualities of normal skin. Minimal to no contracture. Greatest resistance to trauma. Sensation excellent to normal. Cosmetically may be excellent. Maximal padding over long bony surfaces. Will survive transplantation over avascular surfaces.	Transplantation requires highest degree of technical skill. Cosmetically may be poor. May be too bulky. Usually require multiple operative procedures.

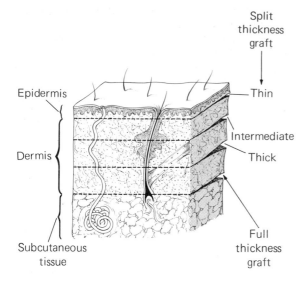

Figure 46—4. Depths of split thickness and full thickness grafts.

split thickness graft 0.022–0.024 inch.

Each type of split thickness graft has definite characteristics depending upon the thickness of the dermis and the number of skin appendage elements that are present.

Each thickness presents certain advantages and disadvantages (Table 46–1). The major advantage of the thinner split thickness grafts is that they become vascularized more rapidly and thus survive transplantation more readily. This is of importance in grafting less than ideal recipient sites such as infected wounds, burn surfaces, and poorly vascularized surfaces. A second advantage in their use is that donor sites for these thinner grafts heal more rapidly, so that they can be reused within a relatively short period of time (7–10 days) in critical cases such as major burns.

In general, the disadvantages of the thin split thickness grafts outweigh the advantages. Thin grafts exhibit the highest degree of postgraft contracture, offer the least amount of resistance to surface trauma, and possess the least number of elements that are present in normal skin such as normal texture, suppleness, pore pattern, and hair growth. Hence, they are usually unacceptable from a cosmetic standpoint.

Conversely, the advantages of the thicker split thickness skin grafts are that they contract less, are more resistant to surface trauma, and possess to a greater degree the desirable elements of normal skin. They are cosmetically more acceptable than thin split thickness grafts, though they are not as acceptable as full thickness grafts.

The disadvantages of thick split thickness grafts are relatively few. They are less easily vascularized than thin grafts and thus result in fewer successful "takes" when used on less than ideal surfaces. Their donor sites are slower to heal (requiring 10–18 days) and heal with more scarring than the donor sites for thin split thickness grafts, which may prevent their reuse.

Donor sites for split thickness grafts heal spontaneously by epithelization. This process depends upon the presence of sweat glands, sebaceous glands, or hair follicles whose epithelial cells proliferate and spread across the wound surface.

B. Full Thickness Grafts: Full thickness skin grafts include the epidermis and all of the dermis. They are the most cosmetically desirable of all free grafts since they include the highest number of skin appendage elements, undergo the least amount of contracture, and have a greater ability to withstand trauma.

There are several limiting factors in the use of full thickness grafts: the limited availability of donor sites, the necessity for closing the donor site since no epidermal elements remain to produce epithelization, and the difficulty in obtaining successful transplantation.

Only areas of thin skin can be utilized as donor sites for full thickness grafts because adequate vascu-

Table 46—2. Indications for various types of skin grafts.

Type of Wound	Type of Graft	Reason for Choice
Infected wounds (including burns)	Thin split thickness	Difficulty in obtaining successful take of thicker grafts.
Wounds with poorly vascularized surfaces	Thin split thickness or pedicle	Difficulty in obtaining successful take of thicker grafts.
Small superficial facial wounds	Full thickness or local pedicle	Produces best cosmetic result.
Large superficial facial wounds	Thick split thickness or pedicle	Cannot use full thickness graft because of limited size of donor sites.
Noninfected wounds on a flexor surface	Thick split thickness, full thickness, or pedicle	Produces minimal contracture.
Full thickness eyelid loss	Local pedicle or composite	Repair requires more than one tissue element.
Deep loss of nasal tip	Local pedicle or composite	Repair requires thicker tissue than present in split or full thickness grafts.
Avulsive wounds with exposed tendons and nerves	Pedicle	Requires thick protective coverage without graft adherence to tendons and nerves.
Exposed avascular cortical bone or cartilage	Pedicle	Free grafts will not survive on avascular recipient site.
Wounds resulting from excision of deep x-ray "burn"	Pedicle	Free grafts will not survive on avascular recipient site.

larization of thick grafts will not occur before the graft dies. These areas of thin skin include the eyelids and the skin of the postauricular, supraclavicular, submammary, antecubital, inguinal, and genital areas. In grafts thicker than approximately 0.015 inch, the results of transplantation are consistently poor.

Borger AF: *Elective Incisions and Scar Revision.* Little, Brown, 1973.

Converse JM: Introduction to plastic surgery. Chap 1, pp 3—20, in: *Reconstructive Plastic Surgery.* Vol 1. Converse JM (editor). Saunders, 1964.

Grabb WC, Smith JW: *Plastic Surgery: A Concise Guide to Clinical Practice,* 2nd ed. Little, Brown, 1973.

Kraissel CJ: The selection of appropriate lines for elective surgical incisions. Plast Reconstr Surg 8:1, 1951.

SKIN GRAFTING TECHNICS

OBTAINING THE GRAFT

Split Thickness

Various instruments are available for obtaining split thickness grafts. These include razor blades, skin grafting knives (Blair, Ferris Smith, Humby), manual dermatomes of either the suction (Barker) or drum variety (Padgett, Reese), and power-driven dermatomes of either the electric (Brown) or air variety (Hall).

The Blair and Ferris Smith knives are of limited value since successful use requires the special skill of the surgeon who uses them constantly. Even the technically improved Humby knife with its adjustable roller to control the thickness of the graft is not to be recommended for the occasional user. Except in the hands of a very skilled surgeon, skin grafting knives generally produce narrow, inferior grafts of uneven thickness with irregular scalloped edges.

The more precise drum type dermatomes are more reliable. Because their thickness gauges are the most dependable, they more consistently produce a graft of the desired thickness. However, their use requires skill and experience as well as time since their surfaces must first be coated with an adhesive or adhesive-bearing tape. Another disadvantage is that, since the maximum length of the drum is 20 cm (8 inches), longer grafts cannot be obtained without preparing the drum surface again between each cutting. They also require a fairly flat donor site if the surgeon desires a graft that measures the full 10 cm (4-inch) width of the drum.

Although the electric and air-powered dermatomes are not as precise as the drum type, they enjoy far wider popularity since the average surgeon, even without prior experience, is able to successfully obtain skin grafts with these instruments. They do not require the use of an adhesive, and the fact that they can be rapidly assembled and used to cut multiple grafts quickly without cleaning and reapplying an adhesive is an important advantage in treating a patient with extensive skin loss (such as a burn patient), when it is desirable to limit the time of the surgical procedure. They also cut better than drum dermatomes on surfaces that are not perfectly flat, so that a wider choice of donor sites is available. The only major disadvantages are that they tend to produce grafts of uneven thickness and that the thickness tends to vary from the setting on the thickness gauge. The greatest width of graft that they will cut is 7.5 cm (3 inches), which is narrower than that obtained with the drum dermatome. However, grafts of any length can be obtained depending only upon the length of the donor site.

Full Thickness

Full thickness grafts are almost always cut to fit a small defect with an irregular outline. Because of this—and because they are cut precisely at the level of the junction of the dermis and the subcutaneous adipose layer—they are best obtained free-hand with a small scalpel blade, generally a No. 15. The plane of dissection is readily found if saline or lidocaine with epinephrine is injected into the subcuticular zone. A pattern is traced from the defect to be grafted by overlaying it with transparent plastic sheeting or exposed x-ray film and outlining the wound margins on the sheeting with marking ink. The pattern is then transferred to the donor area and precisely traced with marking ink. An incision is made along these margins into the dermis but not into the adipose layer. Using adequate countertension, the graft is cut along the desired plane and any fat that is inadvertently removed with the graft is trimmed away with a small curved plastic scissors.

Applying the Graft

After the graft has been applied directly to the prepared recipient surface, it may or may not be sutured in place and may or may not be dressed. Whenever the maximum cosmetic result is desired, the graft should be cut to fit the recipient area exactly and meticulously sutured into position without overlapping edges. Very large thick split thickness grafts and full thickness grafts will usually not survive without pressure. In areas such as the forehead, scalp, and extremities, adequate immobilization and pressure can be obtained by circular dressings. Tie-over pressure stent dressings are advisable for grafts in areas where pressure cannot be obtained by simple wraparound dressings (such as the cheek) or where movement is present (such as the anterior neck, where swallowing causes constant motion), and for grafts in areas of irregular contour (such as the axilla). This is accomplished by leaving the ends of the fixation sutures long and tying them over a bolus of gauze fluffs, cotton, sponge, or other suitable material (Fig 46—5).

When grafts are applied to freshly prepared or relatively clean surfaces, they are generally sutured

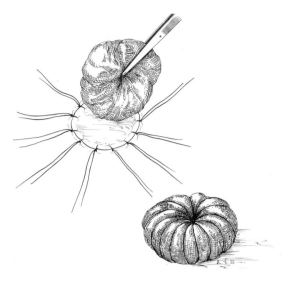

Figure 46—5. Tie-over stent dressing.

into place and dressed with pressure. A single layer of fine mesh gauze impregnated with an ointment such as bismuth tribromophenate (Xeroform) to make it non-adherent is applied directly over the graft. Immediately over this are placed several thicknesses of flat gauze which have been cut by means of a pattern which exactly fits the graft. On top of this is placed a bulky dry dressing consisting of gauze fluffs, cotton, sponge, etc. Pressure is then obtained by wraparound dressings, adhesive tape, or the tie-over stent method.

In many cases it is permissible—and in some cases even preferable—to leave a skin graft site open with no dressing. This is particularly true in infected wounds, where the skin graft tends to "float off" in the purulent discharge that the wound produces. These wounds are better treated with exposed small sheets or stamp-size pieces of skin so that any liquid material that forms between the graft and wound bed can be evacuated by rolling the purulent drainage out from under the graft to the edge, where it can be wiped off. This same principle holds true in noninfected wounds that produce an unusual amount of serous or lymphatic drainage, as occurs following radical groin dissections.

In severely ill patients such as those with major burns, where it is essential to keep anesthetic time to a minimum, large sheets of split thickness skin grafts are rapidly applied without suturing, which is time-consuming. Grafts on these wounds may be left open if the area is small, but if the area is large or circumferential a pressure dressing should be applied.

ENSURING THE "TAKE"

In order to ensure survival of the graft, 4 conditions must be satisfied: (1) adequate vascularization of the recipient bed, (2) complete contact between the graft and the bed, (3) adequate immobilization, and (4) relative freedom from infection as far as the recipient area is concerned.

Since survival of the graft is dependent upon the ingrowth of capillary buds into its raw undersurface, vascularization of the recipient area is of prime importance. Conditions such as advanced radiation damage, chronic ulcers, bone or cartilage denuded of periosteum or perichondrium, and tendon without its paratenon are examples of avascular surfaces that will not generally accept free grafts. In these conditions, vascularity must be provided by excision down to healthy tissues, light scraping of unhealthy granulation tissue, or the production of granulation tissue by diligent wound care or by surgical means such as drilling holes through exposed cortical bone into healthy cancellous bone from which granulation tissue will form. If adequate vascularity cannot be provided, pedicle grafts (see below) are generally indicated.

Inadequate contact between the graft and the recipient bed can be caused by collection of blood, serum, lymph fluid, or purulent fluid between the graft and bed or by movement of the graft on the bed.

Thorough hemostasis is a cardinal rule in skin grafting and can be accomplished in most instances. In areas where adequate hemostasis with ligatures cannot be obtained, such as exposed cancellous bone from which the cortical surface has been removed, pressure must be relied upon for hemostasis. The standard tie-over pressure stent dressing is the best method of doing this.

The stent dressing is also useful in preventing serum or lymph collection under the graft and is essential in areas where movement cannot be controlled, such as in anterior neck wounds, where constant swallowing is present. In these areas, basting sutures through the graft to the underlying surface may be used.

If infection is present in the wound that is to be grafted, it is best controlled by diligent local wound care with saline compresses, conservative debridement, local antibiotics, and systemic antibiotics if indicated. Complete freedom from infection in open wounds is never obtained, but local care should be given until the wound is in optimum condition to receive the graft as demonstrated by the presence of clean, healthy granulation tissue.

Skin graft dressings may be left undisturbed for 5—7 days after grafting if the grafted wound was free of infection, if complete hemostasis was obtained, if fluid collection is not expected, and if immobilization is adequate. If any one of these conditions is not met, the dressing should be changed within 24—48 hours and the graft inspected. If blood, serum, or purulent fluid collection is present, evacuation of this collection should be accomplished—usually by making a small incision through the graft with a scalpel blade and applying pressure with cotton-tipped applicators. The pressure dressing is then reapplied and changed daily so that the graft can be examined and fluid expressed as it collects. Meticulous local care of the graft is essential, including debridement of any necrotic tissue that will allow colonization of bacteria beneath the graft surface, supporting infection that will further imperil the graft.

DONOR SITES

Factors to Consider in Choosing the Donor Site

The ideal donor site would provide a graft identical to the skin surrounding the area to be grafted. Since skin varies greatly from one area to another as far as color, thickness, hair-bearing qualities, and texture are concerned, the ideal donor site (such as upper eyelid skin to replace skin loss from the opposite upper eyelid) is usually not found. However, there are definite principles that should be followed in choosing the donor area.

A. Color Match: In general, the best possible color match is obtained when the donor area is located close to the recipient area. Color and texture match in facial grafts will be much better if the grafts are obtained from above the region of the clavicles. However, the amount of skin obtainable from the supraclavicular areas is limited. If larger grafts for the face are required, the immediate subclavicular regions of the thorax will provide a better color match than areas on the lower trunk or the buttocks and thighs. When these more distant regions are used, the grafts will usually be lighter in color than the facial skin in Caucasians; in people with dark skin, hyperpigmentation occurs, producing a graft that is much darker than the surrounding facial skin.

B. Thickness of the Graft and Donor Site Healing: Donor sites heal by epithelization from the epithelial elements remaining in the donor bed. These include hair follicles, sweat glands, sebaceous glands, and their ducts. The ability of the donor area to heal and the speed with which it heals thus depend upon the number of these elements present. Donor areas for very thin grafts will heal in 7–10 days, whereas donor areas for intermediate thickness grafts may require 10–18 days and those for thick grafts 18–21 days or longer. This may be of critical importance in the treatment of severely burned patients, in whom sites may have to be reused within 7–10 days.

Since there is a normal anatomic variation in the thickness of skin, donor sites for thicker grafts must be chosen with the potential for healing in mind and should be limited to regions on the body where the skin is thick. Infants, debilitated adults, and elderly people have thinner skin than healthy younger adults. Grafts that would be split thickness in the normal adult may be full thickness in these patients, resulting in a donor site that has been deprived of the epithelial elements necessary for healing.

C. Hair-Bearing Qualities of the Graft: Since the hair follicles are usually present at the lowermost level of the dermis and the upper regions of the subcutaneous adipose layer, they are rarely transplanted with split thickness skin grafts. However, it is generally advisable to avoid hair-bearing donor sites in obtaining thick grafts that are to be used on hairless surfaces.

D. Cosmetic Appearance of the Donor Site: While donor sites for very thin grafts may heal with minimal or almost invisible scarring, donor areas for thicker grafts can heal with scarring that is quite conspicuous. In these cases it is more desirable to obtain grafts from areas such as the lateral hips and buttocks than from the thighs since these regions can more easily be hidden by clothing.

Care of the Donor Site

It has been common practice to cover the donor area with a sterile dressing and leave it unattended for 2–3 weeks. This practice is to be condemned since this type of dressing may provide ideal conditions for bacterial colonization with ensuing infection that destroys the epithelial elements that produce wound healing.

The care of the donor site must be as meticulous as the care of the grafted area. The method of care may vary, but the general principles are as follows: A layer of sterile, fine mesh, nonadherent gauze (such as 5% bismuth tribromophenate [Xeroform]) is placed directly over the wound. Several layers of sterile absorbent gauze bandages are placed over the nonadherent gauze. This dressing is then taped in place or held by a circumferential dressing. Oozing blood or serum will be absorbed by the dressing. This is removed in 24 hours, leaving in place the nonadherent gauze that is in direct contact with the wound. If a thin graft has been cut from this site, no further oozing will occur and the wound can be left open with the nonadherent gauze in place. If a thick graft has been cut, leaving a deep donor site, further oozing of serum can be expected. A fresh dressing of several layers of absorbent gauze is reapplied to collect this material, so that it will not form a crust over the wound under which bacteria will colonize. This is removed 24 hours later and the wound is left with only the nonadherent gauze covering. Heat lamps or warm air blowers may be used (with care) to facilitate drying of the wound. As epithelization occurs, the nonadherent gauze separates and is trimmed away. If isolated areas of superficial infection occur beneath the nonadherent gauze, the gauze is trimmed away over these areas so that saline compresses and local antibiotics can be applied. The entire gauze covering is not removed since at this time there is a temporary adherence to the wound and removing it will strip away the new epithelium that is being formed.

PEDICLE GRAFTS

A pedicle graft is a section of skin and subcutaneous tissue that is raised from one site and transferred to another. In contrast to free grafts, it always remains attached to its original donor site or to an intermediate transfer site.

The survival of free skin grafts depends upon the growth of vascular elements from the recipient bed into their undersurfaces. In the case of partial or full thickness skin grafts, this occurs readily. However, because pedicle skin grafts include a layer of subcutaneous adipose tissue beneath the skin, their thickness prevents this ingrowth at a rapid enough rate to maintain their survival. For this reason, they must always remain attached to a source of blood supply.

Types of Pedicle Grafts

Pedicle grafts may be classified into several general categories: They may be local or distant, depending upon whether they were obtained from tissues adjacent to or distant from the recipient wound. They may be single or double, depending upon the number of points of attachment. If an exposed raw area exists on the undersurface between the donor and recipient sites, they are called open pedicle flaps; if no exposed raw surface exists, they are called closed flaps. If they consist of more than skin and adipose tissue—such as skin with attached cartilage or bone—they are called composite pedicle grafts.

These grafts may also be classified as advancement flaps, transposed flaps, rotation flaps, jump flaps, and tube pedicle grafts.

A. Advancement Flaps: The simplest example of the advancement flap is one produced by undermining the skin edges of a tense wound to provide for adequate relaxation for closure (Fig 46–6). These are local pedicles that are advanced along a straight axis without transposition or rotation. Several methods have been devised to construct these grafts. They depend upon the skin being either loose enough or elastic enough to provide for the necessary relaxation.

The V-Y advancement (Fig 46–7) is a useful modification of this type of flap.

B. Transposed Flaps: Transposed flaps are local flaps that are advanced along an axis that forms an angle to the original position of the flap (Fig 46–8a and b). They are usually rectangular and are generally transposed from an area where the skin is loose enough

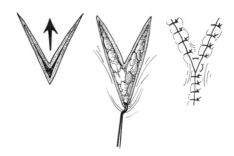

Figure 46–7. V-Y advancement flap.

to provide for primary closure of the donor area (Fig 46–8c).

If this laxity is absent, the donor site must be closed with another graft, usually a split thickness free graft (Fig 46–8d).

On occasion, the pedicle flap cannot be transposed without tension on the flap. A short relaxing incision extending partially across the base may provide the needed relaxation if it does not interfere with the blood supply of the flap (Fig 46–8a).

At times the flap may be open, a portion of its exposed undersurface passing over intervening skin to reach the recipient area (Fig 46–9a and b). After a sufficient period of time has passed to allow for complete vascularization of the pedicle graft from the recipient site (usually 3 weeks), the pedicle is divided across its base and transfer is completed. The unused portion of the flap may be replaced to the donor site or sacrificed (Fig 46–9c).

Relaxing incision

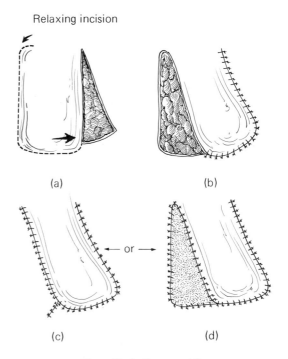

(a)   (b)

← or →

(c)   (d)

Figure 46–8. Transposed flap.

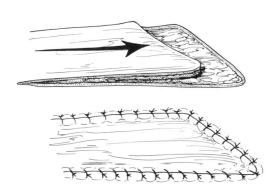

Figure 46–6. Advancement pedicle flap.

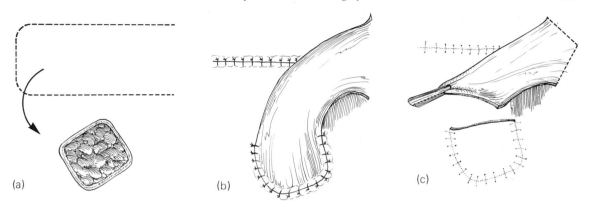

Figure 46–9. Flap passed over intervening skin to recipient area.

C. Rotation Flaps: Rotation flaps are usually local closed flaps that are similar to transposed flaps but differ in that they are semicircular and rotate around a greater axis (Fig 46–10a). As with transposed flaps, they are generally rotated from areas where the skin is lax enough to allow for primary closure of the donor area (Fig 46–10b). A short relaxing incision may be necessary (Fig 46–10a) or, as with transposed flaps, a split skin graft may be used to close the donor site when it cannot be closed primarily.

D. Jump Flaps: Jump flap pedicle grafts are raised in the same fashion as the single based flaps illustrated above. Instead of being transferred immediately to their recipient areas, they are "jumped" or transferred to an intermediate carrying site. An example would be a rectangular flap raised from the abdomen and attached to the forearm to be later transferred to another region of the body. They may be open or closed, depending upon whether the undersurface is closed primarily or skin-grafted.

E. Tube Pedicle Flaps: Tube pedicles are bipedicled flaps that are formed by undermining the skin and the adjacent adipose layer between 2 parallel incisions and then rolling the skin edges under and suturing them together (Fig 46–11a, b, and c). Therefore, they are closed flaps that are especially suitable for transfer to a distant recipient site via a carrier such as the forearm or by migration by end-over-end transfer (Fig 46–12a and b).

Classic donor areas for tube pedicle flaps are the neck, the acromial-pectoral region of the anterior chest, the thoracoabdominal region of the trunk, the anterior abdominal wall, and the anteromedial aspect of the thigh. Any area on the body can be reached by a minimum number of transfer or migration procedures from one of these areas.

F. Island Pedicle Flaps: Island flaps consist of islands of skin and subcutaneous tissue which are trans-

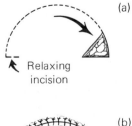
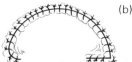

(a)

Relaxing incision

(b)

Figure 46–10. Rotation flap.

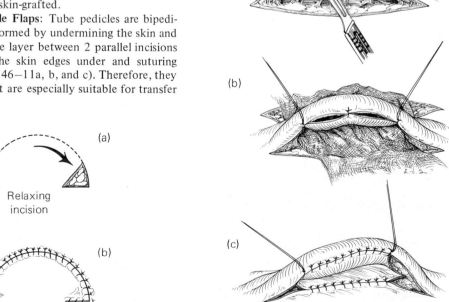

(a)

(b)

(c)

Figure 46–11. Construction of tube pedicle graft.

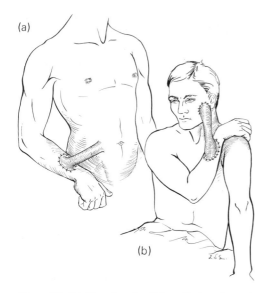

(a)

(b)

Figure 46—12. Transfer of pedicle graft via wrist carrier.

ferred to new sites through a tunnel beneath the skin. The skin in the base of the island flap is removed, leaving only a neurovascular pedicle, so that skin will not be buried in the tunnel. The narrowness of this pedicle provides for great mobility, so that the flap may be transferred from one area to another in one stage, eg, from the forehead to the nose or cheek, or from one finger to another (Fig 46—13).

The intact nerve in the neurovascular pedicle provides the flap with normal sensation. Sensation can be restored to the anesthetic tip of an injured index finger by transferring an island flap from the tip and lateral aspect of the less important fourth finger.

G. Z-Plasty: (Fig 46—14.) Z-plasty is actually a technic by which 2 triangular transposition pedicle flaps are elevated and transposed so that each flap occupies the other's original position. It has proved to be a very useful technic with 2 major applications: (1) lengthening a scar contracture line (flexion contractures across the neck, axilla, fingers, etc, congenital

constriction bands, circular scars of body orifices); and (2) changing the direction of a scar (scars of the face that run across normal skin lines of minimal tension).

Characteristics of Pedicle Grafts

By definition, pedicle skin grafts remain attached to a donor site by a pedicle and possess their own blood supply through this pedicle. They also differ from free skin grafts in that they have a layer of subcutaneous adipose tissue lying beneath the full thickness of skin. These 2 factors make the use of pedicle grafts mandatory when the areas to be grafted are either avascular or require thick coverage to protect the underlying structures from trauma.

Examples of avascular surfaces are exposed bone, cartilage, or tendon without periosteum, perichondrium, or paratenon; exposed joint surfaces; wounds resulting from the excision of areas of radiation necrosis; and areas of extremely dense scar tissue.

Examples of structures or regions that require thick covering to protect them from trauma are bony surfaces and prominences; weight-bearing surfaces; densely scarred areas; and areas of decubitus ulcer formation.

There are numerous other characteristics of pedicle skin grafts that determine their use. Above all, they maintain all of the characteristics of normal skin. Their color and skin texture remain the same as before their transfer. For this reason, adjacent pedicle grafts usually provide for the best cosmetic appearance in reconstruction of facial defects if primary closure cannot be performed. By the same token, abdominal pedicles are not desirable for use on the face since they will continue to look like abdominal skin—different in color and with different skin texture, hair-bearing pattern, and thickness.

Hair growth, sebaceous secretion, and sometimes sweating are maintained by pedicle grafts. These factors—especially hair growth—make them undesirable for covering non-hair-bearing surfaces.

The bulkiness of pedicle grafts obtained from the abdomen and sometimes from the chest, buttocks, and thighs may be desirable when the defect to be grafted

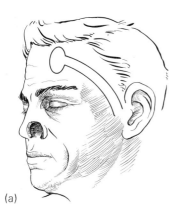

(a)

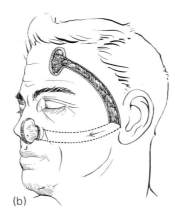

(b)

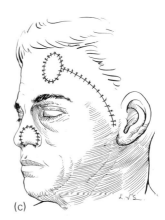

(c)

Figure 46—13. Island pedicle flap.

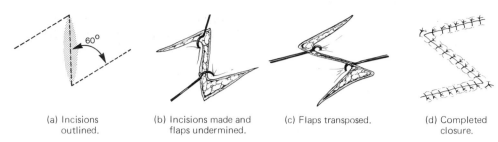

(a) Incisions outlined. (b) Incisions made and flaps undermined. (c) Flaps transposed. (d) Completed closure.

Figure 46–14. Z-plasty.

requires this bulk to fill in depressed tissue defects. This bulkiness or thickness is especially desirable for covering bony prominences and decubitus ulcer sites. Bulkiness can be extremely undesirable on the face and neck, where it obliterates normal facial contours and features; and in the hand, where it interferes with normal function.

Sensation is maintained in pedicle grafts to a degree related directly to that of the donor site. Grafts of abdominal or chest skin will not provide adequate sensation to the fingertip, but grafts from adjacent fingers or the palmar surfaces will. Island pedicle grafts from adjacent fingers will provide for nearly normal sensation, including 2-point discrimination.

Whereas free grafts undergo varying degrees of contracture, pedicle grafts do not. This is an advantage in areas of scar contracture when free grafting has failed, and in relaxing circumferential scar constriction around orifices and within tubular passageways such as nasal airways, the pharynx, the esophagus, and the vagina. In these instances, Z-plasty should usually receive first consideration.

The layer of adipose tissue present in pedicle grafts makes them less adherent to underlying tissues than free skin grafts. Normally movable tissues such as tendons, joints, and muscles should be covered by pedicle grafts so that their movement will be restricted as little as possible.

In some cases, grafting over alloplastic materials is necessary. Examples are grafting over a Vitallium or plastic cranioplasty and replacement of parietal pleura by a sheet of plastic mesh in wounds that extend completely through the chest wall. These materials must be covered by grafts with their own blood supply.

Pedicle graft coverage is essential wherever secondary procedures such as tendon or nerve repairs or bone grafts are necessary. Because of their excellent blood supply, incisions can be made through pedicle flaps, and they can be raised by undermining to expose the structures that they cover. Split thickness skin grafts are not sufficiently vascularized to permit this.

Another desirable characteristic of pedicle grafts is that they maintain the same growth rate as the donor site, so that contracture does not occur when they are used as grafts in children.

Pedicle Grafting Technics

A. Construction: Although the technics for construction of pedicle flaps may vary with different types, there are certain basic principles that apply to the construction of all flaps.

Careful planning is essential to successful transfer. Following the principles that have been discussed, the type of graft and the donor site are selected. The size and shape of the flap are easiest to determine if an exact outline of the recipient area is made in thick pliable material such as gauze, leather, or felt. This pattern is then laid over the area to be grafted and the pattern transferred backward to the donor through exactly the same steps that will be taken during the actual transfer (Fig 46–15).

The ratio of the length of the pedicle flap to the width of the base is extremely important (Fig 46–16). Most flaps are of the single pedicle type that will be severed from the surrounding skin on 3 sides and will be completely separated from the donor bed. The entire blood supply must come from one base. The width of the base determines the number of blood vessels entering the graft. If the graft is too long in proportion to the width of the base, the distal portion of the flap will not survive owing to lack of blood supply.

In general, single pedicle flaps require a 1:1 ratio between length and width and bipedicle flaps require a ratio of 2.5:1. However, there are several exceptions to this rule. If the pedicle flap possesses large arteries and

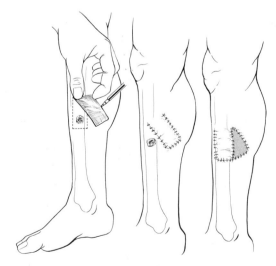

Figure 46–15. Use of pattern in construction of pedicle graft.

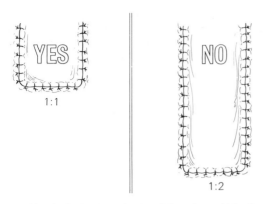

Figure 46—16. Ratio of length of pedicle graft to width of base of pedicle graft.

veins within its base that traverse the length of the flap, the ratio of length to width can be greatly increased. Examples are the midline forehead flap, which includes in its base the frontalis artery and vein on each side of the midline; and the thoracoepigastric tube pedicle based on the long thoracic artery superiorly and the superficial epigastric artery inferiorly.

The ratio of length to width may also be increased (1) when the flap is to be constructed in areas with an abundant vascular supply, such as the head and neck, the hands, and the genital area; (2) in younger patients; and (3) when delay procedures on the pedicle flap are planned.

In areas of poor circulation, such as the lower regions of the legs and the back, and in older arteriosclerotic patients, greater caution must be observed.

B. Donor Sites: The ideal donor site would provide a graft identical to the skin that it is to replace. Important factors to consider are color match, thickness, sensation, hair-bearing qualities, and cosmetic appearance. These factors have been discussed above (see p 973); however, there are 2 other important considerations.

(1) Pedicle grafts, like full thickness free skin grafts, leave a donor bed that is devoid of epithelial elements. Spontaneous healing therefore does not occur without contracture and undesirable scar tissue formation. Primary closure of the donor site is essential. This can be achieved by advancement and suturing of the wound edges if the pedicle is small. If the pedicle is large, the donor site must be closed by free split thickness skin grafts, or sometimes by another pedicle graft. Care should be taken to design pedicle grafts so that their grafted donor sites do not produce functional or cosmetic problems.

(2) Pedicle grafts should be constructed as close as possible to the recipient area so that multiple stages of surgical transfer can be avoided or minimized.

C. Delay of Pedicle Flaps: To delay a pedicle flap means to develop it in more than one stage by partially dividing it from its blood supply during each stage. This is done to enhance its vascularity and to condition it to respond less and less to hypoxia. Experimental

and clinical studies have shown that after the sides of the pedicle flap have been incised in stages and after the flap has been undermined in stages, the vascular network within the flap becomes better aligned parallel to the long axis of the pedicle, with increase in both the number and size of the blood vessels. These changes occur in 1 week and reach their maximum in 18—21 days. For this reason, 21 days is the standard interval allowed between successive delays and transfers of pedicle flaps.

D. Transfer of Pedicle Flaps: All adjacent pedicle flaps are transferred directly to their recipient sites, either in one stage or after delay procedures depending upon their site of origin or their ratio of length to width.

Distant pedicles are transferred by migration from one intermediate site to another (tube pedicle flaps) or via a carrier such as the arm or wrist (jump flaps or tube pedicle flaps).

After the flap has been transferred, a period of 3 weeks is usually allowed to pass for full development of its blood supply. In regions of profuse vascularity, this period of time may be shortened.

To shorten the distance of transfer and the number of transfers, the graft is constructed as near as possible to the recipient area as long as the previously described requirements for the type of graft and the donor site are met.

Tube pedicles are usually transferred in stages. One end of the tube is first divided from its donor base. This will leave a circular open end of the pedicle (Fig 46—17). A flap that is shaped as a half-circle is then raised at the intermediate transfer site so that when it is reflected it will expose a circular recipient site to receive the end of the tube. After 21 days, the other end of the tube is severed from its base and transferred to a similarly created intermediate transfer area or to the final recipient site.

Jump flaps are usually rectangular, so that the flap that is raised on the carrier arm is similar in shape (Fig 46—15).

Whenever possible, all raw surfaces created by raising either the donor flap or the intermediate carrier flap should be closed by split thickness skin grafting to prevent infection.

Several adverse factors must be avoided to ensure successful transfer of pedicle flaps. Kinking of the base of the flap, undue tension on the flap, or excessive pressure by dressings may occlude the blood supply. Hematoma formation or infection at the recipient site may prevent successful transfer. These factors can be minimized by strict attention to details and adherence to the basic principles of plastic surgery.

Borger AF: *Elective Incisions and Scar Revision.* Little, Brown, 1973.

Brown JB, McDowell F: *Skin Grafting,* 3rd ed. Lippincott, 1958.

Converse JM, Brauer RO: Transplantation of the skin. Chap 2, pp 21—80, in: *Reconstructive Plastic Surgery.* Vol 1. Converse JM (editor). Saunders, 1964.

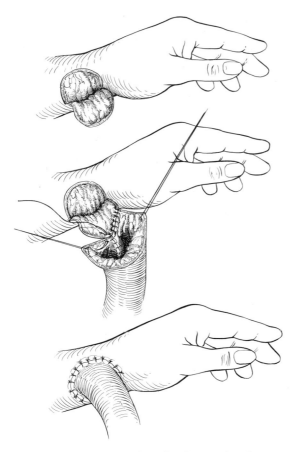

Figure 46—17. Method of transfer of tube pedicle flap.

Edgerton MT, Hanson FC: Matching facial color with split thickness skin grafts from adjacent areas. Plast Reconstr Surg 25:455, 1960.

Gillies HD, Millard DR Jr: *Principles and Art of Plastic Surgery.* 2 vols. Little, Brown, 1957.

MICROVASCULAR SURGERY

The technic of microvascular tissue transfer and replantation of severed parts such as thumbs and fingers has improved tremendously in the past 5—10 years.

By using the operating microscope for magnification, arteries, veins, and nerves with a diameter of 1 mm or less can be successfully anastomosed to provide both vascularity and sensation to the transferred part. Since the advent of this new technic, large free flaps of tissue, usually from the chest or groin, can be transferred to any area on the body in one stage, whereas transfer by standard technics may require 4 or 5 operative procedures.

Severed extremities such as fingers, which previously had to be sacrificed, can now be successfully replanted with normal function and sensation. In addition, an excellent functional substitute can be provided for a previously lost thumb by the transfer of the great toe.

Another application of this technic is the free transfer of vascularized bone grafts of ribs or the fibula to repair defects of the mandible or of the bones of the extremities.

Buncke HJ Jr & others: Thumb replacement: Great toe transplantation by microvascular anastomosis. Br J Plast Surg 26:194, 1973.

Harri K, Ohmori K: Free deltoid pectoral skin flaps. Br J Plast Surg 27:231, 1974.

Taylor GI, Miller GDH, Ham FJ: The free vascularized bone graft. Plast Reconstr Surg 55:533, 1975.

SPECIFIC DISORDERS TREATED BY PLASTIC SURGERY

HYPERTROPHIC SCARS & KELOIDS

In response to any injury that is severe enough to break the continuity of the skin or produce necrosis, the skin heals by scar formation. Under ideal circumstances a fine, flat, "hairline" scar will result.

However, hypertrophy may occur, causing the scar to become raised and thickened, or a keloid may form. A keloid is a true tumor arising from the connective tissue elements of the dermis. By definition, keloids grow beyond the margins of the original injury or scar, and in some instances may grow to enormous size.

Healing and scar formation progress through 3 definite phases: exudative, proliferative, and maturation. During the exudative phase, blood and tissue fluids form an adhesive coagulum and a fibrinous network that serve to bind the wound surfaces.

Proliferation of endothelial and fibroblastic elements bridges the wound surfaces or fills in the spaces created by the loss of tissue. During this phase, the scar usually appears red and may be quite firm or hard. In the case of a fine incision, this phase may be short and the response minimal; in the case of a large open wound following avulsive injuries or burns, it may be prolonged and the response maximal.

The maturation phase begins as soon as the phase of fibroblastic proliferation has ceased. As the fibroblasts mature, the scar becomes less cellular and less vascular and begins to appear flat and white. Slow contracture also occurs.

Hypertrophic scars and keloids are produced during the second and third phases of scar formation. The tendency should be resisted to regard all thickened scars as keloids and to label as "keloid formers" all patients with unattractive scars. Hypertrophic scars and keloids are distinct entities, and the clinical course and prognosis are quite different in each case. The overreactive process that results in thickening of the hypertrophic scar ceases within a few weeks—before it extends beyond the limits of the original scar—and in most cases some degree of maturation occurs and gradual improvement take place. In the case of keloids, the overreactive proliferation of fibroblasts continues for weeks or months. By the time it ceases, an actual tumor is present that typically extends well beyond the limits of the original scar, involves the surrounding skin, and may become quite large. Maturation with spontaneous improvement does not usually occur.

Hypertrophic scars and keloids are difficult to differentiate by tissue staining methods. Tissue culture methods can be used for this purpose, but this is not practical. Clinical observation of the course of the scar is the only practical means of differentiation.

Treatment

Since nearly all hypertrophic scars will undergo some degree of spontaneous improvement, they do not require treatment in the early phases. If the scar is still hypertrophic after 6 months, surgical excision and primary closure of the wound are indicated. Improvement may be expected when the hypertrophic scar was originally produced by excessive endothelial and fibroblastic cell proliferation, as is present in open wounds, burns, and infected wounds. However, little or no improvement can be anticipated if the hypertrophic scar followed uncomplicated healing of a simple surgical incision. Hypertrophic scars across flexion surfaces such as the anterior elbow or the fingers cannot be improved unless a procedure such as a Z-plasty is performed to change the direction of the scar.

The treatment of choice for keloids is the injection of triamcinolone acetonide, 10 mg/ml (Kenalog-10 Injection), directly into the lesion. In the case of larger lesions, injection is made into more than one site. There is evidence that keloids may respond better to early than to late treatment.

Lesions are injected every 3—4 weeks, and treatment should not be carried out longer than 6 months. The following dosage schedule is used:

Size of Lesion	Dose per Injection
1—2 sq cm	20—40 mg
2—6 sq cm	40—80 mg
6—10 sq cm	80—110 mg

For larger lesions, the maximum dose should be 120 mg. The maximum doses for each treatment for children are as follows:

Age	Maximum Dose
1—2 years	20 mg
3—5 years	40 mg
6—10 years	80 mg

There is a tendency to inject the drug into the scar too often or in too high a dosage. Either may produce too vigorous a response, resulting in excessive atrophy of the skin and subcutaneous tissues surrounding the lesion and in depigmentation of darker skins. Both of these adverse responses will improve spontaneously in 6—12 months.

The response varies greatly; some lesions become flat after 2—3 injections, and some fail to respond at all.

Topical corticosteroid therapy is of no value.

Before the advent of corticosteroid injection therapy, surgical excision and radiation therapy were the only methods of treatment of keloids. Both methods are disappointing; surgical resection usually leads to recurrence of a larger lesion; with very few exceptions, radiation therapy produces no result. At present, surgical excision is used only in conjunction with intralesional corticosteroid therapy. Excision is usually confined to the larger lesions in which steroid therapy would exceed safe dosages. The wound is injected at the time of surgery and then postoperatively according to the schedule recommended above. Care should be taken to avoid extending surgical incisions out into the normal skin around the keloid since the growth of a new keloid may occur in these scars.

Conway H & others: Differential diagnosis of keloids and hypertrophic scars by tissue culture technique with notes on therapy of keloids by surgical excision and Decadron. Plast Reconstr Surg 25:117, 1960.

Crikelair GF: Surgical approach to facial scarring. JAMA 172:160, 1960.

Crikelair GF, Ju DMC, Cosman B: Scars and keloids. Chap 9, pp 161—186, in: *Reconstructive Plastic Surgery*. Vol 1. Converse JM (editor). Saunders, 1964.

Ketchum LD, Robinson DW, Masters FW: Follow-up on treatment of hypertrophic scars and keloids with triamcinolone. Plast Reconstr Surg 48:256, 1971.

Maguire HC: Treatment of keloids with triamcinolone acetonide injected intralesionally. JAMA 192:325, 1965.

FACIAL INJURIES

Initial emergency care of severe facial injuries should be directed toward maintaining the airway and control of hemorrhage. Manual removal of blood clots and suctioning, if available, will usually free the oral airway. The unconscious patient should be positioned prone so that the tongue and the structures of the floor of the mouth do not occlude the oral pharynx. Tracheostomy is rarely necessary except in severe crushing injuries of the mid face.

Bleeding is best controlled by pressure until careful clamping of severed vessels under direct inspection can be done. Unless there has been massive bleeding from a major arterial laceration or other associated injury, shock is usually not present in the patient with maxillofacial injuries.

Extensive soft tissue injuries of the face should be repaired in the operating room under aseptic conditions as soon as possible. Treatment of concomitant injuries to the CNS, chest, or abdomen may take precedence. Because of the generous blood supply to the head and neck, repair of soft tissue lacerations may be safely delayed for up to 24 hours after injury. Soft tissue injuries should not be repaired until the possibility of injury to deeper structures has been ruled out by careful examination. This includes evaluation of facial nerve function, levator muscle function in the eyelid, and signs of injury to the parotid and lacrimal ducts. Delayed wound repair usually should be accompanied by antibiotic coverage. As in wounds elsewhere which may be contaminated, tetanus prophylaxis is indicated (see p 131). In immunized patients, a booster will suffice; tetanus-immune human globulin must be considered in nonimmunized patients with severely contaminated wounds.

Surgical Treatment

Local anesthesia is preferred to general anesthesia except in the case of very severe injuries when prolonged operating time and extensive skin grafting may be necessary. If intracranial injury is suspected, the type of anesthesia should be chosen after neurosurgical evaluation. With preliminary analgesic sedation, even small children and infants are usually cooperative when local anesthesia is used.

After local infiltration of the anesthetic, meticulous mechanical cleansing of the wound and adjacent skin is performed. Sterile drapes are then applied and the wound carefully explored using sterile saline irrigation to remove any imbedded foreign material. Suspected injuries to deeper structures can be verified at this time.

Debridement must include removal of all obviously devitalized tissues.

In special areas such as the eyelids, ears, nose, lips, and eyebrows, debridement must be very cautiously done since the tissue lost by debridement may be difficult to replace. Where tissues are more abundant, such as in the cheek, chin, and forehead areas, debridement may be more extensive. Small irregular or ragged wounds in these areas can be excised completely to produce clean, sharply cut wound edges which, when approximated, will produce the finest possible scar.

Because the blood supply in the face is plentiful, damaged tissues of questionable viability should be retained rather than debrided away. The chances for survival are good.

After debridement and wound irrigation, meticulous suture approximation will often obviate the need for secondary revision or reconstruction. A lacerated parotid or lacrimal duct should be repaired over a silicone or polyethylene catheter of appropriate size. Severed major branches of the facial nerves should be repaired by fine sutures when possible, or at least identified by small metal clips.

Closure of skin wounds should begin by approximation of key points. These include accurate rejoining of the borders of the lips, ears, and nose and reapproximation of such features as the vermilion border of the lip, the margins of the eyebrow, and the scalp hairline. Dead space, which can lead to hematoma formation and infection, is prevented by approximation of subcutaneous adipose and muscular tissues by buried absorbable sutures.

Undermining of the skin at the subdermal layer may be necessary to prevent wound tension where there has been significant skin loss. Either 4–0 or 5–0 sutures should be used, either nonabsorbable or absorbable. Where extensive contamination has occurred, absorbable material is preferable for buried sutures. Careful closure of the wound with subdermal sutures is followed by accurate approximation of the skin edges with fine nylon or silk sutures. Approximation without tension, using sutures that are not tied excessively tight, provides the most satisfactory cosmetic result.

Complicated lacerations such as complex stellate wounds or avulsion flaps often heal with excessive scarring. Because of the associated subcutaneous tissue injury, U-shaped or trap-door avulsion lacerations almost always become unsightly as a result of wound contracture. Small lacerations of this type are best excised and closed in a straight line initially; larger flaps that must be replaced usually require secondary revision. Extensive loss of skin is generally best treated by initial split thickness skin grafting followed later by secondary reconstruction. Primary attempts to reconstruct with local flaps may fail because of unsuspected injury to these adjacent tissues. The decision to convert avulsed tissues to free grafts which may not survive and thus delay healing requires sound surgical judgment.

Pressure dressings are useful in preventing hematoma formation and severe edema, which may result in poor wound healing. Dressings should be changed early and the wound inspected for hematoma or signs of infection. Hematoma evacuation, appropriate drainage, and antibiotic therapy based on culture and sensitivity studies may be required. Removal of sutures in 3–5 days, followed by splinting of the incision with paper tape or collodion gauze strips, will minimize scarring from the sutures themselves.

Prognosis

The final result of facial wound repair depends on the nature and location of the wounds, individual propensity to scar formation, and the passage of time. A year or more must often pass before resolution of scar contracture and erythema results in maximum improvement. Only after this time can a decision be made regarding the desirability of secondary scar revision.

Kazanjian VH, Converse JM: *The Surgical Treatment of Facial Injuries,* 3rd ed. Williams & Wilkins, 1963.

FRACTURES OF THE FACIAL BONES

The bones of the nose are the most commonly fractured facial bones. Next in frequency are the mandible, the zygomatic-malar bones, and the maxilla. Multiple combined fractures are common as a result of automobile collisions at high speed.

Soft tissue edema may develop rapidly, making it difficult to palpate a displaced facial fracture. Radiologic examination, including the Waters view, basal view, and oblique views of the mandible, is imperative for accurate diagnosis.

Dingman RO, Natvig P: *Surgery of Facial Fractures.* Saunders, 1964.
Georgiade NG: *Plastic and Maxillofacial Trauma Symposium.* Vol 1. Mosby, 1969.

NASAL FRACTURES

Simple displaced fractures of the nasal bones may be treated immediately if the patient is seen before significant edema has developed. Local anesthesia is preferred, using either topical tetracaine or cocaine with epinephrine intranasally and lidocaine infiltration of the skin. The nasal bones may be disimpacted with an intranasal forceps or periosteal elevator, and aligned properly by means of external molding or pressure. Fractures of the nasal septum should be recognized and realigned in conjunction with manipulation of the external nasal bones.

If massive edema is already present when the patient is first seen, it is best to reduce the swelling with local cold compresses and proceed with closed reduction of the fractures when the edema has cleared enough so that the degree of displacement of the bones can be accurately evaluated. Compound fractures of the nose require prompt repair of the skin wound and either early or late reduction of the displaced nasal bones, depending upon the degree of local swelling.

External splinting, which is essentially a protective dressing, in conjunction with intranasal packing using nonadherent gauze, is appropriate following reduction of simple fractures of the nasal bones.

If there is extensive comminution of the bony nasal pyramid with posterior displacement into the piriform aperture, additional fixation may be required. After reduction and molding of the nasal bones, a fine stainless steel wire may be passed in a figure-of-eight fashion through the skin and across the base of the bony pyramid. Externally, the wire is passed through large buttons or soft lead plates to help mold the multiple comminuted fragments. Swelling of the soft tissues should be anticipated, and the wires should not be twisted so tight that external scarring will result. The fixation is maintained for 7–10 days.

MANDIBULAR FRACTURES

Mandibular fractures are most commonly bilateral, generally occurring in the region of the mid body at the mental foramen, the angle of the ramus, or at the neck of the condyle. A frequent combination is a fracture at the mental region of the body with a condylar fracture on the opposite side. Displacement of the fragments results from the force of the external blow as well as the pull of the muscles of the floor of the mouth and the muscles of mastication. The diagnosis is suggested by derangement of dental occlusion associated with local pain, swelling, and often crepitation upon palpation. Appropriate x-rays confirm the diagnosis. Special views of the condyle, including tomograms, may be required.

Restoration of normal dental occlusion is the most important consideration in treating mandibular fractures. In patients with an adequate complement of teeth, arch bars or interdental wires can be placed. Local nerve block anesthesia is preferable for this procedure, though certain patients may require general anesthesia. Intermaxillary elastic traction will usually correct minor degrees of displacement and bring the teeth into normal occlusion. When the fracture involves the base of a tooth socket with suspected devitalization of the tooth, extraction of the tooth should be considered. Particularly in the incisor region, such devitalized teeth may be a source of infection, leading to the development of osteomyelitis and nonunion of the fracture.

If the patient is partially or completely edentulous, either his dentures or appropriate dental splints are used to maintain the mandible and maxilla in normal occlusion and provide a means of intermaxillary fixation. The dentures or splints may be wired directly by circumferential wires to the mandible and fixed to the maxilla either by pinning to the alveolar process or by suspensory wiring from above, entering the mouth through the upper buccal sulcus.

Intermaxillary fixation with wires immobilizes the mandible to the maxilla. This fixation should be maintained for 6 weeks in the case of fracture of the body and ramus. Earlier resumption of mandibular motion is indicated in cases of condylar fractures to prevent fibrotic ankylosis, which may accompany injury to the temporomandibular joint.

Open reduction of mandibular fractures is indicated where there is marked displacement that cannot be reduced or maintained by simple intermaxillary fixation. This may be the case in severely displaced fractures at the angle with muscle interposition that prevents reduction. Fractures of the body of the mandible in edentulous patients may require open reduction and wiring or plating the fragments together for adequate fixation. Open reduction is followed by intermaxillary fixation, using arch bars or splints, after normal occlusion is achieved.

Open reduction is not advised in condylar fractures except in the rare case where the condylar fragment may be so severely displaced as to prevent motion of the mandible because of impingement on the coronoid process or zygomatic arch. Even markedly displaced condylar fractures remodel after simple intermaxillary fixation to maintain normal occlusion. Early guided motion generally results in normal function.

ZYGOMATIC FRACTURES

Fractures of the zygomatic bones may involve just the arch of the zygomatic bone or the entire body of the zygoma (the malar eminence) and the lateral wall and floor of the orbit. The so-called tripod fracture characteristically occurs at the zygomatic frontal and zygomatic maxillary sutures as well as at the arch. Displacement of the body of the zygoma results in flattening of the cheek and depression of the orbital rim and floor.

Important diagnostic signs are subconjunctival hemorrhage, disturbances of extraocular muscle function (which may be accompanied by diplopia), and loss of sensation in the upper lip and alveoli on the involved side as a result of injury to the infraorbital nerve. Reduction of a displaced zygomatic fracture is seldom an emergency procedure and may be delayed until the patient's general condition is satisfactory for anesthesia. Local anesthesia will suffice only for reduction of fractures of the zygomatic arch. More extensively displaced fractures usually require general anesthesia.

Depressed fractures of the zygomatic arch only can best be elevated using the Gillies technic. Through a temporal incision above the hairline, an instrument is passed beneath the temporalis fascia and under the arch and body of the zygoma. The fracture can be elevated in conjunction with overlying palpation to achieve accurate reduction.

If extensive disruption of the orbital floor is suspected in conjunction with the zygomatic fracture, reduction of the fracture should be accompanied by direct visualization and repair of the orbital floor. Several approaches may be used for disimpaction and reduction of the displacement. These include the Gillies elevation and the transantral (Caldwell-Luc) approach directly through the antrum to the orbital floor. This latter technic is particularly helpful when there is extensive comminution of the antral portion of the zygoma and the adjacent maxilla. In complicated fractures, one or more of the approaches may be combined with direct visualization of the fracture sites and, if necessary, direct interosseous wiring to maintain reduction of unstable fragments. Elevation by grasping the zygoma with a towel clip is not recommended since it is difficult to control the reduction of comminuted fractures by this method and since unsatisfactory scarring may develop where the instrument pierces the skin.

"Blowout" fracture of the orbit refers to extensive disruption of the orbital floor which may occur as a result of blunt trauma directly to the orbit with no associated fracture of the body of the zygoma or the orbital rim. Such fractures may result in depression of the ocular globe due to prolapse of orbital fat into the antrum. The extraocular muscles may also be entrapped by the fragments of the disrupted floor. Diplopia occurs in either case. Careful x-ray examination, including orbital tomograms, is required to evaluate such an injury.

Repair of blowout fracture is effected after surgical exploration of the orbital floor. This may require the transantral (Caldwell-Luc) approach to elevate the depressed fragments of the floor, accompanied by packing of the antrum for support. In cases where there is extensive comminution and loss of bony fragments into the antrum, an implant to the orbital floor may be required to maintain support for the ocular structures. A thin sheet of alloplastic material such as silicone has been satisfactory for this purpose, although bone grafts have been recommended. Even with careful anatomic reduction of the disruption of the orbital floor, there may be late ocular problems due to resorption of the injured orbital fat. Follow-up evaluation by an ophthalmologist is mandatory.

MAXILLARY FRACTURES

Maxillary fractures range in complexity from partial fractures through the alveolar process to extensive displacement of the mid facial structures in conjunction with fractures of the frontonasal bones and orbital maxillary region. Hemorrhage and airway obstruction will require emergency care, and in severe cases tracheostomy is often indicated. Mobility of the maxilla can be elicited by palpation in extensive fractures. "Dish-face" deformity of the retruded displaced maxilla may be disguised by edema, and careful x-ray studies are necessary to determine the extent and complexity of the midfacial fracture. Treatment may have to be delayed because of other severe injuries. A delay of as long as 10—14 days may be safe before reduction and fixation, but the earliest possible restoration of maxillary position and dental occlusion is desirable to prevent late complications.

In the case of unilateral fractures or bilateral fractures with little or no displacement, splinting by intermaxillary fixation for 4 weeks will suffice. Fractures are usually displaced inferiorly or posteriorly and require direct surgical disimpaction and reduction. In certain severe cases, external traction may be necessary. Manipulation is directed toward restoring normal occlusion and maintaining the reduction with intermaxillary fixation to the mandible in association with direct fixation or supporting wires from other intact facial or cranial bones. Complicated fractures may require external fixation utilizing a head cap and intraoral splints in conjunction with multiple surgical incisions for direct wire fixation. Coexisting mandibular fractures usually necessitate open reduction and fixation at the same time.

CONGENITAL ANOMALIES

HEAD & NECK ANOMALIES

Cleft Lip & Cleft Palate

Cleft lip, cleft palate, and combinations of the 2 are the most common congenital anomalies of the head and neck. The incidence of facial clefts has been reported to be 1 in every 650–750 live births, making it second only to clubfoot in frequency as a reported birth defect.

The cleft may involve the floor of the nostril and lip on one or both sides and may extend through the alveolus, the hard palate, and the entire soft palate. A useful classification based on embryologic and anatomic aspects divides the structures into primary and secondary palate. The dividing point between the primary and the secondary palate is the incisor foramen. Clefts can thus be classified as partial or complete clefts of the primary or secondary palate (or both) in various combinations. The most common clefts are left unilateral complete clefts of the primary and secondary palate and partial midline clefts of the secondary palate, involving the soft palate and part of the hard palate.

Most infants with cleft palate present some feeding difficulties, and breast feeding may be impossible. As a rule, enlarging the openings in an artificial nipple or using a syringe with a soft rubber feeding tube will solve difficulties in sucking. Feeding in the upright position helps prevent regurgitation or aspiration. Severe feeding problems and recurrent aspiration may complicate Pierre Robin syndrome, in which the palatal cleft is associated with a receding jaw and posterior displacement of the tongue, obstructing the oropharyngeal airway. A surgical procedure such as the tongue-lip adhesion operation may be necessary to prevent fatal aspiration in these patients.

Surgical repair of cleft lip is not considered an emergency. The optimal time for operation can be described as the widely accepted "rule of ten." This includes body weight of 5 kg (11 lb) or more and a hemoglobin of 10 g/100 ml or more. This is usually at some time after the 10th or 12th week of life. In most cases, closure of the lip will mold distortions of the cleft alveolus into a satisfactory contour. In occasional cases where there is marked distortion of the alveolus, such as in severe bilateral clefts with marked protrusion of the premaxilla, preliminary maxillary orthopedic treatment may be indicated.

General endotracheal anesthesia via an orally placed endotracheal tube is the anesthetic technic of choice. A variety of technics for repair of unilateral clefts have evolved over many years. Earlier procedures ignored anatomic landmarks and resulted in a characteristic "repaired harelip" look. The operation now employs an incision in the medial side of the cleft to allow the cupid's bow of the lip to be rotated down to a normal position. The resulting gap in the medial side of the cleft is filled by advancing a flap from the lateral side. This principle can be varied in placement of the incisions and results in most cases in a symmetric lip with normally placed landmarks. Bilateral clefts, because of greater deficiency of tissue, present more challenging technical problems. Maximum preservation of available tissue is the underlying principle, and most surgeons prefer simple approximation of the central and lateral lip elements in a straight line closure.

Secondary revisions are frequently necessary in the older child with a repaired cleft lip. A constant associated deformity in patients with cleft lip is distortion of the soft tissue and cartilage structures of the tip of the nose. Some correction of these deformities can be done at the time of initial surgery, but most cases require late revision after growth of the cartilaginous structure is complete. Many of the secondary procedures are minor in nature, including revisions of the scar and adjustments of local tissue deficiencies by either Z-plasties or V-Y advancement procedures. A tight upper lip due to severe tissue deficiency may be corrected in a 2-stage transfer of a pedicle flap from the lower lip—the Abbé flap operation.

Palatal clefts may involve the alveolus, the bony hard palate, or the soft palate, singly or in any combination. Clefts of the hard palate and alveolus may be either unilateral or bilateral, whereas the soft palate cleft is always midline, extending back through the uvula. The width of the cleft varies greatly, making the amount of tissue available for repair and reconstruction also variable. The bony palate, with its mucoperiosteal covering, forms the roof of the anterior mouth and the floor of the nose. The posteriorly attached soft palate is composed of 5 paired muscles of speech and swallowing.

Surgical closure of the cleft is the treatment of choice. However, in certain instances of severe tissue deficiency or in older patients with unrepaired clefts, closure of the defect with a dental prosthesis may be desirable. The consensus is that repair of the palate should be done between the first and second year since more tissue is available in the older baby. It is desirable to have the palate repaired and functioning as well as possible by the time the child undertakes serious speech, usually around age 2. If the soft palate seems to be long enough, simple approximation of the freshened edges of the cleft after freeing of the tissues through lateral relaxing incisions may suffice. If the soft palate is too short, a pushback type of operation is required. In this procedure, the short soft palate is retrodisplaced closer to the posterior pharyngeal wall, utilizing the mucoperiosteal flaps based on the posterior palatine artery.

Satisfactory speech following surgical repair of cleft palate is achieved in 70–90% of cases. Significant speech defects usually require secondary operations when the child is older. The most widely used technic is the pharyngeal flap operation, in which the palato-pharyngeal space is reduced by attaching a flap of posterior pharyngeal muscle and mucosa to the soft palate. Various other kinds of pharyngoplasties have been useful in selected cases.

Blackfield HM & others: Cinefluorographic analysis of the surgical treatment of cleft palate speech. Plast Reconstr Surg 31:542, 1963.

Cronin TD: Surgery of the double lip and protruding premaxilla. Plast Reconstr Surg 19:389, 1957.

Grabb WC: *Cleft Lip and Palate: Surgical, Dental, and Speech Aspects.* Little, Brown, 1971.

Johansen B, Ohlsson A: Bone grafting and dental orthopedics in primary and secondary cases of cleft lip and palate. Acta Chir Scand 122:112, 1961.

Millard DR Jr: Wide and/or short cleft palate. Plast Reconstr Surg 29:40, 1962.

Nylen BO: Cleft palate and speech. Acta Radiol [Suppl] (Stockh) 203, 1961.

Owsley JQ Jr & others: Experience with the high attached pharyngeal flap. Plast Reconstr Surg 38:232, 1966.

Pruzansky S: Presurgical orthopedics and bone grafting for infants with cleft lip and palate: A dissent. Cleft Palate J 1:164, 1964.

Randall P: A triangular flap operation for the primary repair of unilateral cleft of the lip. Plast Reconstr Surg 23:331, 1959.

Woolf CM, Woolf RR, Broadbent TR: Genetic and nongenetic variables related to cleft lip and palate. Plast Reconstr Surg 32:65, 1963.

Other Anomalies

The first and second branchial arch syndrome presents with deformities of variable severity. Deformities include absence of the external ear, partial or complete absence of the involved hemimandible, and lateral facial clefts.

Treacher-Collins syndrome presents a characteristic facies associated with mandibulofacial dysostosis.

Crouzon's syndrome, due to premature fusion of the facial sutures, is a rare anomaly. The major problems in these cases are related to the marked exophthalmos as well as the grotesque facies.

In the past 15–20 years, craniofacial surgery has advanced to the point where several conditions, previously considered untreatable, can be successfully corrected. These are the craniofacial dysostoses, including Crouzon's disease and Apert's disease, and plagiocephaly, orbital hypertelorism, and facial clefts.

In addition, craniofacial surgery has improved the treatment of several other conditions such as congenital or traumatic orbital dystopia, traumatic or postsurgical orbital-cranial defects, congenital hemifacial microsomia (Treacher Collins and Goldenhar's syndromes), Romberg's disease, nasomaxillary hypoplasia, fibrous dysplasia, and exophthalmos.

The principles of craniofacial surgery include the use of a coronal incision to approach the skull and facial bones through a cranial route. The abnormally displaced bones are then moved to their normal position by the en bloc movement of large segments of bone or, at times, the entire facial mass. Autogenous bone grafts are used to fill the gaps created by displacing the bony segments. The entire operative procedure usually can be completed in one stage, and the incidence of complications is surprisingly low.

Tessier P: Experiences in the treatment of orbital hypertelorism. Plast Reconstr Surg 53:1, 1974.

ANOMALIES OF THE HANDS & EXTREMITIES

The most common hand anomaly is syndactyly, or webbing of the digits. This may be associated with normal digits or with absence of portions of the fingers and occasionally with an extra digit. Surgical correction by division of the webbed cleft—and repair with appropriate local flaps and skin grafts—should be accomplished prior to school age.

Flexion contractures of the hands or digits may require surgical release and appropriate skin grafting. Congenital ring constriction of the extremities may be associated also with congenital amputation. The ring constrictions are best treated in stages by excision and Z-plasty.

GENITOURINARY ANOMALIES

Hypospadias and epispadias are the most commonly seen anomalies in the male and, depending on the severity, require one or more stages of surgical correction, usually starting when the child is 2–3 years of age. Epispadias may be associated with exstrophy of the bladder, which also occurs in females. This serious anomaly usually requires urinary diversion procedures and reconstructive surgery of the lower abdominal wall after excision of the bladder exstrophy.

Congenital absence of the vagina is quite uncommon. It is associated with an absent uterus, but the ovaries are usually normal. A satisfactory vaginal tract can usually be constructed with split thickness skin grafts using an inlay technic.

Converse JM: Vol II, Part 2, The Head and Neck, and Vol VI, Part 6, The Genitourinary System and Anorectal Malformations, in: *Reconstructive Plastic Surgery.* Converse JM (editor). Saunders, 1964.

Grabb WC, Smith JW: *Plastic Surgery: A Concise Guide to Clinical Practice,* 2nd ed. Little, Brown, 1973.

Mustarde JC: *Plastic Surgery in Infancy and Childhood.* Saunders, 1971.

SKIN TUMORS

Tumors of the skin are by far the most common of all of the tumors that are seen in humans. They arise from each of the histologic structures that make up the skin—epidermis, connective tissue, gland, muscle, and nerve elements—and are correspondingly numerous in variety.

Skin tumors are conveniently classified as benign, premalignant, and malignant. Only those tumors that are commonly seen by the plastic surgeon will be discussed here.

Allen AC: *The Skin,* 2nd ed. Grune & Stratton, 1966.
Conway H: *Tumors of the Skin.* Thomas, 1956.
Fitzpatrick TB (editor): *Dermatology in General Medicine.* McGraw-Hill, 1971. [Chapters 10 and 11.]
Maddin S: *Current Dermatologic Management.* Mosby, 1970.

BENIGN SKIN TUMORS

The many benign tumors that arise from the skin rarely interfere with function. Since most are removed for cosmetic reasons, they are quite commonly treated by the plastic surgeon. The majority are small and can be simply excised under local anesthesia following the principles of elliptical excision and wound closure discussed above. General anesthesia may be necessary for larger lesions requiring excision and repair by skin grafts or those occurring in young children.

Most superficial lesions (seborrheic keratoses, verrucae, squamous cell papillomas) can be easily treated by simpler technics such as electrodesiccation, curettage and electrodesiccation, cryotherapy, and topical cytotoxic agents.

Seborrheic Keratosis

Seborrheic keratoses are superficial noninvasive tumors that originate in the epidermis. They appear in older people as multiple, slightly elevated, yellowish, brown, or brownish-black, irregularly rounded plaques with waxy or oily surfaces. They are most commonly present on the trunk and shoulders but are frequently seen on the scalp and face.

Curettage and electrodesiccation is usually the treatment of choice.

Verrucae Vulgaris

Verrucae vulgaris (common warts) are usually seen in children and young adults, commonly on the fingers and hands. They appear as round or oval elevated lesions with rough surfaces composed of multiple rounded or filiform keratinized projections. They may be skin-colored or gray to brown.

Verrucae are caused by a virus and are autoinoculable, which can result in multiple lesions around the original growth or frequent recurrences following treatment if the virus is not completely eradicated. They may disappear spontaneously.

Treatment by electrodesiccation is effective but is frequently followed by slow healing. Repeated applications of bichloroacetic acid, liquid nitrogen, or liquid CO_2 are also effective. Surgical excision is not recommended since the wound may become inoculated with the virus, leading to recurrences in and around the scar.

Because recurrences are common despite thorough treatment, it is reasonable to delay treatment of asymptomatic lesions for several months to determine if they will disappear spontaneously.

Cysts

A. Sebaceous Cyst: Although sebaceous cyst is the commonly used term, these lesions more properly should be called epidermal or keratinous cysts since they are composed of thin layers of epidermal cells filled with epithelial debris. (True cysts arising from sebaceous epithelial cells are uncommon.)

Sebaceous cysts are soft to firm, usually elevated, and are filled with an odorous cheesy material. Their most common sites of occurrence are the scalp, face, ears, neck, and back. They are usually covered by normal skin, which may show dimpling at the site of skin attachment.

Treatment consists of surgical excision.

B. Dermoid Cyst: Dermoid cysts are deeper than sebaceous cysts. They are not attached to the skin but frequently are attached to or extend through underlying bony structures. They may appear in many sites but are most common around the nose or the orbit, where they may extend to meningeal structures.

Treatment is by surgical excision, which may necessitate sectioning of adjacent bony structures.

Pigmented Nevi

A. Junction Nevi: Junction nevi are well-defined pigmented lesions appearing in infancy. They are usually flat or slightly elevated, light to dark brown in color, and contain no hair. They may appear on any part of the body, but most nevi seen on the palms, soles, and genitalia are of the junction type. Histologically, a proliferation of melanocytes is present in the epidermis at the epidermal-dermal junction. A varying amount of cellular activity in the form of cellular division with mitotic figures may be seen. Partly because of this, it has been widely accepted that junction nevi give rise to malignant melanoma and that all junction nevi should be excised for prophylactic reasons. However, most investigators now feel that junction nevi are not precancerous. If there is no change in their appearance, treatment is unnecessary. Any change such as inflammation, darkening in color, halo formation, increase in size, bleeding, or ulceration calls for immediate treatment.

Surgical excision is the only safe method of treatment.

B. Intradermal Nevi: Intradermal nevi are the typical dome-shaped, sometimes pedunculated, fleshy to brownish pigmented "moles" that are characteristically seen in adults. They frequently contain hairs and may occur anywhere on the body.

Microscopically, melanocytes are present entirely within the dermis and, in contrast to junction nevi, show little activity. They are rarely if ever malignant and require no treatment except for cosmetic reasons.

Surgical excision is nearly always the treatment of choice except in areas such as the nasal tip, where adverse scarring occurs. In such cases, more conservative dermatologic methods of treatment may be indicated, but pigmented nevi must never be treated without obtaining tissue for histologic examination.

C. Compound Nevi: Compound nevi exhibit the histologic features of both junction and intradermal nevi in that melanocytes lie both at the epidermal-dermal junction and within the dermis. They are usually elevated, dome-shaped, and light to dark brown in color.

Because of the presence of nevus cells at the epidermal-dermal junction, the indications for treatment are the same as for junction nevi. If treatment is indicated, surgical excision is the method of choice.

D. Benign Juvenile Melanoma: Benign juvenile melanomas are rapidly growing pigmented lesions that appear in children and exhibit some of the microscopic and clinical features of malignant melanoma. They usually appear on the face as distinctive small, pinkish or reddish, soft, nodular lesions. They increase in size rapidly, but the average lesion reaches only 6–8 mm in diameter, remaining entirely benign without invasion or metastases. Microscopically, the lesion can be confused with malignant melanoma by the inexperienced pathologist.

The usual treatment is excisional biopsy.

E. Blue Nevi: Blue nevi are small, sharply defined, round, dark blue or gray-blue lesions that may occur anywhere on the body but are most commonly seen on the face, neck, hands, and arms. They usually appear in childhood as slowly growing, well-defined nodules covered by a smooth, intact epidermis. Microscopically, the melanocytes that make up this lesion are limited to (but may be found in all layers of) the dermis. An intimate association with the fibroblasts of the dermis is seen, giving the lesion a fibrotic appearance not seen in other nevi. This, together with extension of melanocytes deep into the dermis, may account for the blue rather than brown color.

Treatment is not necessary unless the patient desires removal for cosmetic reasons or fear of malignancy. Surgical excision is the treatment of choice.

F. Giant Hairy Nevi: Unlike most nevi arising from melanocytes, giant hairy nevi are congenital. They may occur anywhere on the body and cover large areas. They may be large enough to cover the entire trunk (bathing trunk nevi). They are of special significance for several reasons: (1) Their large size is especially deforming from a cosmetic standpoint; (2) they show a definite predisposition for developing malignant melanoma; and (3) they may be associated with neurofibromas or melanocytic involvement of the

leptomeninges and other neurologic abnormalities.

Microscopically, a varied picture is present. All of the characteristics of intradermal and compound nevi may be seen, along with those associated with juvenile melanoma. Neurofibromas may also be present within the lesion. Malignant melanoma may arise anywhere within the large lesion, the rate of occurrence being as high as 13.7% in one reported study. Malignant melanoma with metastases can arise in childhood and even in infancy.

The only treatment is complete excision and skin grafting. Large lesions may require excision and grafting in stages. Some lesions are so large that excision is not possible.

Hemangioma

It is confusing to attempt to classify hemangiomas on the basis of their histology. For example, the histologic term capillary hemangioma is used to designate both the common involuting hemangioma of childhood that disappears by 7 years of age and the port wine stain that persists into adulthood. The term cavernous is used to designate several types of hemangiomas that behave quite differently. Some hemangiomas are true neoplasms arising from endothelial cells and other vascular elements (such as involuting hemangiomas of childhood, endotheliomas, and pericytomas). Others are not true neoplasms but rather malformations of normal vascular structures (eg, port wine stains, cavernous hemangiomas, and arteriovenous fistulas).

A simple classification based upon whether or not the hemangioma undergoes spontaneous involution is proposed in Table 46–3.

A. Involuting Hemangioma: Involuting hemangiomas are the most common tumors that occur in childhood and comprise at least 95% of all the hemangi-

Table 46–3. Proposed classification of hemangiomas based on appearance and clinical course of lesion.

Proposed Term	Terms in Common Use*
Involuting hemangioma	
Superficial	Strawberry nevus
	Nevus vasculosus
	Capillary hemangioma
Combined superficial and deep	Strawberry nevus
	Capillary hemangioma
	Capillary and cavernous hemangioma
Deep	Cavernous hemangioma
Noninvoluting hemangioma	
Port wine stain	Port wine stain
	Capillary hemangioma
	Nevus flammeus
Cavernous hemangioma	Cavernous hemangioma
Venous racemose aneurysm	Cavernous hemangioma
Arteriovenous fistula	Arteriovenous fistula

*Confusing because different terms are used to denote the same lesion and because the same term is sometimes used to denote different lesions.

omas that are seen in infancy and childhood. They are true neoplasms of endothelial cells but are unique among neoplasms in that they undergo complete spontaneous involution.

Typically, they are present at birth or appear during the first 2–3 weeks of life. They grow at a rather rapid rate for 4–6 months, when growth ceases and spontaneous involution begins. Involution progresses slowly but is complete by 5–7 years of age.

Involuting hemangiomas appear on all body surfaces but are seen more often on the head and neck. They are seen twice as often in girls as in boys and show a predisposition for fair-skinned individuals.

Three forms of involuting hemangioma are seen—superficial, combined superficial and deep, and deep. Superficial involuting hemangiomas appear as sharply demarcated, bright red, slightly raised lesions with an irregular surface that has been described as resembling a strawberry. Combined superficial and deep involuting hemangiomas have the same surface characteristics, but beneath the surface a firm bluish tumor is present that may extend deeply into the subcutaneous tissues. Deep involuting hemangiomas present as deep blue tumors covered by normal-appearing skin.

The histologic findings in involuting hemangiomas are quite different from those seen in other types of hemangiomas. There is a constant correlation between the histologic picture and the clinical course. During the growth phase, the lesion is composed of solid fields of closely packed round or oval endothelial cells. As would be expected during the growth phase, cellular division with mitotic figures is seen, so that the lesion is sometimes called a hemangioendothelioma by the pathologist. This term must not be used, however, since it is commonly used to denote the highly malignant angiosarcoma that is seen in adults.

As the phase of involution progresses, the histologic picture changes, with the solid fields of endothelial cells breaking up into closely packed, capillary-sized, vessel-like structures composed of several layers of endothelial cells supported by a sparse fibrous stroma. These vascular structures gradually become fewer in number and spaced more widely apart in a loose, edematous fibrous stroma. The endothelial cells continue to disappear, so that by the time involution is complete the histologic picture is entirely normal with no trace of endothelial cells.

Treatment is not usually indicated since the cosmetic appearance following spontaneous regression is nearly always superior to the scars that follow surgical excision. Complete surgical excision of lesions that involve important structures such as the eyelids, nose, or lips results in the unnecessary destruction of these important structures that are difficult to repair.

Partial resection of a portion of a hemangioma of the brow or eyelid is indicated when the lesion is large enough to prevent light from entering the eye—a condition that will lead to blindness. The same type of treatment may be necessary for lesions of the mucosal surfaces of the lips when they project into the mouth and are traumatized by the teeth. In these cases, surgery should be very conservative—resecting only enough of the lesion to alleviate the problem and leaving the remaining portions to involute spontaneously.

In approximately 8% of cases, ulceration will occur. This may be accompanied by infection, which is treated by the use of compresses of warm saline or potassium permanganate and by the application of antibiotic powders and lotions. Bleeding from the ulcer is not common, and when it does occur it is easily controlled by the application of pressure.

After involution of large lesions, superficial scarring may be present or the involved skin may be thin, wrinkled, or redundant. These conditions may require conservative plastic surgery procedures. Telangiectasia may be present which may be improved by electrodesiccation of the involved capillaries, but the results of this type of treatment are usually disappointing.

The application of local agents such as dry ice to the surface of these lesions has been popular. This type of treatment has no effect on the deep portions of the hemangioma. It will destroy superficial lesions but results in severe scarring. Injections of sclerosing agents (eg, sodium morrhuate) have no effect. There is no place for radiation therapy in the treatment of these benign lesions.

B. Noninvoluting Hemangioma: Most noninvoluting hemangiomas are present at birth. In contrast to involuting hemangiomas, they do not undergo rapid growth during the first 4–6 months of life but grow in proportion to the growth of the child. They persist into adulthood, when they may cause severe cosmetic and functional problems. Some, such as arteriovenous fistulas, may cause death due to cardiac failure.

Unfortunately, treatment of noninvoluting hemangiomas is difficult and usually far from satisfactory.

Port wine stains are by far the most common of the noninvoluting hemangiomas. They may involve any portion of the body but most commonly appear on the face as flat patchy lesions that are reddish to purple in color. The light red lesions may fade to a varying degree but persist into adulthood. Some of the deep red or purplish lesions that have a stippled appearance show a propensity for growth later in life, in which case they become raised and thickened, with nodules appearing on the surface.

Microscopically, port wine stains are made up of thin-walled capillaries that are arranged throughout the dermis. The capillaries are lined with mature flat endothelial cells. In the lesions that produce surface growth, groups of round proliferating endothelial cells and large venous sinuses are seen.

Results following treatment of the port wine stain are uniformly disappointing. Since most lesions occur on the face or neck, patients seek treatment for the cosmetic problem they present. The simplest and still the most effective method of treatment is camouflaging. Unfortunately, this is difficult because the port wine stain is darker than the surrounding lighter skin.

Tattooing with skin-colored pigments may offer some measure of disguise in the lighter lesions but generally is unsatisfactory because the pigment deposited in the skin looks artificial and tends to be absorbed unevenly, producing a mottled appearance.

Superficial methods of treatment such as dry ice, liquid nitrogen, electrocoagulation, and dermabrasion are ineffective unless they destroy the upper layers of the skin, which produces severe scarring.

Radiation therapy, including the use of x-rays, radium, thorium-X, and grenz x-rays, is to be condemned. If it is administered in doses high enough to destroy the vessels involved, it also destroys the surrounding tissues and the overlying skin.

If the lesion is small, surgical excision with primary closure may be indicated. Unfortunately, most lesions are large, and surgical excision requires split thickness skin grafting. Because of the scar present around the edge of the graft and the loss of normal skin texture— along with the inability to obtain a good color match between the graft and the facial skin—the results of excision with skin grafting are far less than ideal.

Most port wine stains should be left alone.

C. Cavernous Hemangioma: Cavernous hemangiomas are bluish or purplish lesions that are usually elevated. They may occur anywhere on the body but, like other hemangiomas, are more common on the head and neck. They are composed of mature, fully formed venous structures that are present in tortuous masses which have been described as feeling like "a bag of worms."

Cavernous hemangiomas are usually present at birth but do not usually grow except to keep pace with normal body growth. In many cases, growth occurs later in life and may interfere with normal function.

Microscopically, cavernous hemangiomas are made up of large dilated, closely packed vascular sinuses that are engorged with blood. They are lined by flat endothelial cells and may have muscular walls like normal veins.

Treatment is difficult. In only a few cases is the lesion small enough or superficial enough to permit complete surgical excision. Most lesions involve deeper structures—including muscle and bone—so that complete excision is impossible without radical surgery. Since most lesions are cosmetic problems, radical surgery is rarely indicated.

Other forms of treatment such as x-ray and radium therapy are of no value since the mature vessels are not sensitive to radiation. Suture ligation of surrounding vessels, multiple intralesional ligations, and injections of sclerosing solutions usually have no effect upon the lesions and have been discarded.

Andrews GC, Domonkos AN: Cutaneous angiomas and their treatment. NY State J Med 57:1436, 1957.

Blackfield HM, Morris WJ: Management of visible hemangiomas. Am J Surg 94:313, 1957.

PREMALIGNANT SKIN LESIONS

Actinic Keratoses

Actinic keratoses are the most common of the precancerous skin lesions. They usually appear as small, single or multiple, slightly elevated, scaly or warty lesions ranging in color from red to yellow, brown, or black. Since they are related to sun exposure, they occur most frequently on the face and the backs of the hands in fair-skinned Caucasians whose skin shows evidence of actinic elastosis.

Microscopically, actinic keratoses consist of well-defined areas of abnormal epithelial cells limited to the epidermis. Approximately 15–20% of all lesions become malignant, in which case invasion of the dermis as squamous cell carcinoma occurs.

Since the lesions are limited to the epidermis, superficial treatment in the form of curettement and electrodesiccation or the application of chemical agents such as liquid nitrogen, phenol, bi- or trichloroacetic acid, or fluorouracil is curative. The application of fluorouracil (5-FU) cream is of particular benefit in preventive treatment in that it will destroy lesions of microscopic size—before they can be detected clinically—without causing damage to uninvolved skin.

Chronic Radiation Dermatitis

There are 2 distinct types of radiation dermatitis. The first and most common follows the acute administration of relatively high dosages of ionizing radiation over relatively short periods of time—almost always for the treatment of malignancy. It is characterized by an acute reaction that begins near the third week of therapy, when erythema, blistering, and sloughing of the epidermis start to occur. Burning and hyperesthesia are commonly present.

This initial reaction is followed by scarring characterized by atrophy of the epidermis and dermis along with loss of skin appendages (sweat glands, sebaceous glands, and hair follicles). Marked fibrosis of the dermis occurs, with gradual endarteritis and occlusion of the dermal and subdermal vessels. Telangiectasia of the surface vessels is seen, and areas of both hypo- and hyperpigmentation occur.

The second type of radiation dermatitis follows chronic exposure to low doses of ionizing radiation over prolonged periods of time. It is usually seen in professional personnel who handle radioactive materials or administer x-rays or in patients who have been treated for dermatologic conditions such as acne or excessive facial hair. Therefore, the face and hands are most commonly involved. The acute reaction described above does not usually occur, but the same process of atrophy, scarring, and loss of dermal elements occurs. Drying of the skin becomes more pronounced, and deepening of the skin furrows is typically present.

In both types of radiation dermatitis, late changes may occur such as the following: (1) the appearance of hyperkeratotic growths on the skin surface, (2) chronic ulceration, and (3) the development of either basal cell or squamous cell carcinoma. Ulceration and malignancy, however, are seen much less commonly in the first type of chronic radiation dermatitis than in the second. When malignant growths appear, basal cell carcinomas are seen more frequently on the face and neck and squamous cell carcinomas more frequently on the hands and body.

Treatment of chronic radiation dermatitis or the malignant lesions that develop is complicated by the marked scarring that is present and by the avascularity of the involved tissues secondary to endarteritis.

Surgical excision is the treatment of choice. Primary wound closure is feasible for only the smallest lesions. Free skin grafting can be performed only for the most superficial lesions, where damage to the vascular supply of the subcutaneous structures is not advanced. Lesions that involve the deeper subcutaneous tissues require surgical excision followed by pedicle skin grafting.

Bowen's Disease

Bowen's disease is characterized by single or multiple, brownish or reddish plaques that may appear anywhere on the skin surface but often on covered surfaces. The typical plaque is sharply defined, slightly raised, scaly, and slightly thickened. The surface is often keratotic, and crusting and fissuring may be present. Ulceration is not common but when present suggests malignant degeneration with dermal invasion. Some authorities believe that all cases of Bowen's disease are secondary to the ingestion of arsenic. (A significant number of cases are related to arsenic-induced malignancies of internal organs.)

Histologically, hyperplasia of the epidermis is seen, with pleomorphic malpighian cells, giant cells, and atypical epithelial cells which are limited to the epidermis.

Treatment of small or superficial lesions consists of total destruction by curettement and electrodesiccation or by any of the other superficially destructive methods (cryotherapy, cytotoxic agents). Excision and skin grafting is preferred for larger lesions and for those that have undergone early malignant degeneration and invasion of the dermis.

Erythroplasia of Queyrat

Erythroplasia of Queyrat is almost identical to Bowen's disease both clinically and histologically but is confined to the glans penis and the vulva, where the lesions appear as red, velvety, irregular, slightly raised plaques. Treatment is as described for Bowen's disease.

MALIGNANT SKIN TUMORS*

1. BASAL CELL CARCINOMA

Basal cell carcinoma is the most common skin cancer. The lesions usually appear on the face and are more common in men than women. Since exposure to ultraviolet rays of the sun is a causative factor, basal cell carcinoma is most commonly seen in geographic

*Melanoma is discussed in Chapter 49.

areas where there is significant sun exposure and in people whose skins are most susceptible to damage from exposure, ie, fair-skinned individuals with blue eyes and blond hair. It may occur at any age but is not common before age 40.

The growth rate of basal cell carcinoma is usually slow but nearly always steady and insidious. Several months or years may pass before the patient becomes concerned. Without treatment, widespread invasion and destruction of adjacent tissues may occur, producing massive ulceration. Penetration into the bones of the facial skeleton and the skull is not uncommon. Basal cell carcinomas rarely metastasize, but death can occur because of direct intracranial extension or because of erosion of major blood vessels.

Typical individual lesions appear as small, translucent or shiny ("pearly") elevated nodules with central umbilication and rolled, pearly edges. Telangiectatic vessels are commonly present over the surface, and pigmentation is sometimes present. Superficial ulceration occurs early. When invasion of the dermis and subcutaneous tissues occurs along with deeper ulceration, the lesion is termed a rodent ulcer.

A less common type of basal cell carcinoma is the sclerosing or morphea carcinoma, consisting of elongated strands of basal cell cancer which infiltrate the dermis, with the intervening corium being unusually compact. These lesions are usually flat and whitish or waxy in appearance and firm to palpation—similar in appearance to localized scleroderma.

The superficial erythematous basal cell cancer ("body basal") occurs most frequently on the trunk. It appears as reddish plaques with atrophic centers and smooth, slightly raised borders. These lesions are capable of peripheral growth and wide extension but do not become invasive until late.

Pigmented basal cell carcinomas may be mistaken for melanomas because of the large number of melanocytes present within the tumor. They may also be confused with seborrheic keratoses.

Treatment

There are several methods of treating basal cell carcinoma. All may be curative in some lesions, but no one method is applicable to all. The special features of each basal cell cancer must be considered individually before proper treatment can be selected.

Since most lesions occur on the face, cosmetic and functional results of treatment are important. However, the most important consideration is whether or not therapy is curative. If the basal cell carcinoma is not eradicated by initial treatment, continued growth and invasion of adjacent tissues will occur. This will result not only in additional tissue destruction but also in invasion of the tumor into deeper structures, making cure impossible.

The principal methods of treatment are curettage and electrodesiccation, surgical excision, and radiation therapy. Chemosurgery, topical chemotherapy, and cryosurgery are not often used but may have value in selected cases.

A. Curettage and Electrodesiccation: Curettage and electrodesiccation is the most frequently used method of treatment. After infiltration with suitable local anesthetic, the lesion and a 2–3 mm margin of normal-appearing skin around it are thoroughly curetted with a small skin curet. The resultant wound is then completely desiccated with an electrosurgical unit to destroy any tumor cells that may not have been removed by the curet. The process is then repeated once or twice if necessary. The wound is left open and allowed to heal secondarily.

With experience, the soft and friable tumor cells in superficial lesions can be differentiated by the curet from the firm surrounding dermis. This permits the detection and removal of infiltrative strands of basal cells. However, in deeper lesions, as soon as these extensions of tumor invade beyond the dermis, they can no longer be accurately detected.

When used as treatment for superficial basal cell carcinoma, curettage and electrodesiccation is a simple, quick, and inexpensive procedure that will cure nearly all superficial lesions. However, this method of treatment should not be used in the deeper infiltrative and morphea type lesions. These should be treated by surgical excision, x-ray therapy, or chemosurgery.

B. Surgical Excision: Surgical excision, following the principles outlined earlier in this chapter, offers many advantages in the treatment of basal cell carcinoma: (1) Most lesions can be quickly excised in one procedure. (2) Following excision, the entire lesion can be examined by the pathologist, who can determine if the tumor has been completely removed. (3) Deep infiltrative lesions can be completely excised, and cartilage or bone can be removed if they have been invaded. (4) Lesions that occur in dense scar tissue or in other poorly vascularized tissues cannot be treated by curettage and desiccation, radiation therapy, or chemosurgery since healing is poor. Excision with pedicle grafting may be the only method of treatment in these conditions. (5) Recurrent lesions in tissues that have been exposed to maximum safe amounts of radiation can be excised and grafted.

Small to moderate-sized lesions can be excised in one stage under local anesthesia. The visible and palpable margins of the tumor are marked on the skin with marking ink. The width of excision is then marked 3–5 mm beyond these margins. If the margins of the basal cell carcinoma are vague, the width of excision will have to be wider to ensure complete removal of the lesion. The lines of incision are drawn along these margins parallel to the normal skin creases in an elliptical shape. This ellipse of tissue is excised, taking care to leave a margin of normal-appearing subcutaneous tissue around the deep margins of the tumor. Frozen sections may be obtained at the time of excision to aid in determining whether or not tumor-free margins have been obtained.

Wounds resulting from the excision of some moderate-sized tumors and nearly all large tumors may necessitate closure by a free skin graft or a pedicle graft. Larger lesions may require excision and wound closure by free skin grafts or pedicle grafts. This can nearly always be performed in one stage.

The disadvantages of surgical excision are as follows: (1) Specialized training and experience are necessary to master the surgical technics. (2) Whereas curettage and desiccation may be performed in the office, surgical excision requires specialized facilities. (3) In lesions with vague margins, an excessive amount of normal tissue may have to be excised to ensure complete removal. (4) Structures that are difficult to reconstruct such as the eyelids, nasal tips, and lips have to be sacrificed when they are extensively infiltrated.

C. X-Ray Therapy: Radiologists and dermatologists once tended to treat carcinoma of the skin by a single massive dose of ionizing radiation or by a few large individual doses over a short period of time. In addition, treatments were often administered with machines of low kilovoltage potential (kVp) that produced x-rays of poor quality. These factors led to excessive tissue damage and resulted in a high incidence of radiation dermatitis and radiation necrosis with associated undesirable cosmetic and functional results.

These problems have been almost completely eliminated by modern technics. The use of machines of higher kVp and application of the principle of treatment by fractionation are the 2 most important reasons for the excellent results now being obtained. Fractionation implies treatment with multiple relatively small doses (usually 4–6 per week) administered over a total period of 3–4 weeks rather than higher individual doses given over a total period of 3–10 days.

Many factors influence the quality of radiation used, the total dose to be given, the number of fractions, and the time period involved. Of the various types of radiation therapy, treatment with roentgen rays generally is the most convenient and flexible with respect to adjusting the quality of the rays, the field size, and fractionation.

Carcinomas of the skin overlying cartilage, such as on the ear or nose, require special attention. Lesions in such locations require greater fractionation of dose and a higher quality of radiation in order to avoid painful chronic chondritis. Eyelid lesions are treated using a small cup-shaped lead shield to protect the eye.

The radiation therapist must estimate the extent of the lesion on a 3-dimensional basis, as the surgeon must, by inspection and palpation to determine adequate treatment. Fields of treatment should extend up to 1 cm or more beyond the evident borders of the lesion including both the lateral and deep margins. Larger, deeply invasive lesions require a wider margin of treatment.

Therefore, most small early lesions require fields of treatment at least 2 cm in diameter with a quality of radiation adequate to carry the desired dose to 1 cm in depth. For such lesions, Moss recommends using radiations produced at 110 kV with a filter of 0.25 mm copper and 1 mm aluminum. When lesions require treatment fields larger than 4 cm, he recommends radiations produced at 200 kV filtered with 0.5 mm copper and 1 mm aluminum.

Small lesions, except those of the eyelids or over cartilage, may be treated by administering a total of 4000 rads in 10 fractions over 10–12 days; but when the lids, ears, or nose are involved, he advises using 4200–5000 rads fractionated over a 3- to 4-week period. In treating large lesions (up to 8–10 cm in diameter) which infiltrate bone or cartilage, he advises using 6500–7500 rads over an 8-week period. In most cases, the dose is divided into 5 fractions per week.

The advantages of x-ray therapy are as follows: (1) Structures that are difficult to reconstruct such as the eyelids, tear ducts, and nasal tips can be preserved when they are invaded by but not destroyed by tumor. (2) A wide margin of tissue can be treated around lesions with poorly defined margins to ensure destruction of nondiscernible extensions of tumor. (3) It may be less traumatic than surgical excision to elderly patients with advanced lesions. (4) Hospitalization is not necessary.

The disadvantages are as follows: (1) Only well-trained, experienced physicians can obtain good results. (2) Expensive facilities are necessary. (3) Improperly administered radiation therapy may produce severe sequelae, including scarring, radiation dermatitis, ulceration, and malignant degeneration. (4) Baldness will result in hair-bearing areas. (5) It may be difficult to treat areas of irregular contour, ie, the ear and the auditory canal. (6) Repeated treatments over a period of 2–4 weeks may be necessary.

2. SQUAMOUS CELL CARCINOMA

Squamous cell carcinoma is the second most common cancer of the skin and is even more common than basal cell carcinoma in darkly pigmented racial groups. As with basal cell carcinoma, sunlight is the most common causative factor in Caucasians, and most lesions occur in fair-skinned individuals. The most common sites of occurrence are the ears, the cheeks, the lower lip, and the backs of the hands. Other causative factors are chemical and thermal burns, scars, chronic ulcers, chronic granulomas (tuberculosis of the skin, syphilis), draining sinuses, contact with tars and hydrocarbons, and exposure to ionizing radiation. When a squamous cell carcinoma occurs in a burn scar it is called a **Marjolin ulcer.**

Since exposure to the sun is the greatest stimulus for the production of squamous cell carcinoma, most of these lesions are preceded by actinic keratosis on areas of the skin showing chronic solar damage. They may also arise from other premalignant skin lesions and from normal-appearing skin.

The natural history of squamous cell carcinoma may be quite variable. It may present as a slowly growing, locally invasive lesion without metastases or as a rapidly growing, widely invasive tumor with early metastatic spread. In general, squamous cell carcinomas that develop from actinic keratoses are of the slowly growing type, whereas those that develop from Bowen's disease, erythroplasia of Queyrat, chronic radiation dermatitis, scars, and chronic ulcers tend to be more aggressive in nature. Lesions that arise from normal-appearing skin and from the lip, genitalia, and anal regions also tend to be aggressive.

Early squamous cell carcinoma usually appears as a small, firm, erythematous plaque or nodule with indistinct margins. The surface may be flat and smooth or may be verrucous. As the tumor grows it becomes raised, and, because of progressive invasion, becomes fixed to surrounding tissues. Ulceration may occur early or late but tends to appear earlier in the more rapidly growing lesions.

Histologically, malignant epithelial cells are seen extending down into the dermis as broad, rounded masses or slender strands. In squamous cell carcinomas of low malignancy, the individual cells may be quite well differentiated, resembling uniform mature squamous cells having intercellular bridges. Keratinization may be present, and layers of keratinizing squamous cells may produce typical round "horn pearls." In highly malignant lesions the epithelial cells may be extremely atypical, abnormal mitotic figures are common, and intercellular bridges are not present and keratinization does not occur, so that "horn pearls" are absent.

As with basal cell carcinomas, the method of treatment that will eradicate squamous cell carcinomas and produce the best cosmetic and functional result varies with the characteristics of the individual lesion. Factors that determine the optimal method of treatment include the size, shape, and location of the tumor as well as the histologic pattern that determines its aggressiveness. The most common form of squamous cell carcinoma—that arising from actinic keratosis—is the least aggressive and requires less vigorous therapy than the more malignant types arising from Bowen's disease, scars, ulcers, chronic radiation dermatitis, and apparently normal skin.

The same methods of therapy that are discussed under treatment of basal cell carcinomas are used for the treatment of squamous cell carcinomas. The advantages and disadvantages of each type of therapy are discussed above. Since basal cell carcinomas are relatively nonaggressive lesions that very rarely metastasize, failure to eradicate the lesion will result only in local recurrence. Although this may result in extensive local tissue destruction, there is rarely a threat to life. Aggressive squamous cell carcinomas, on the other hand, may metastasize to any part of the body, and failure of treatment may have fatal consequences. For this reason, total eradication of each lesion is the imperative goal of treatment.

Because the overall incidence of lymph node metastasis is relatively low, most authorities agree that node resection is not indicated in the absence of palpable regional lymph nodes except in the case of very aggressive carcinomas of the genitalia and anal regions.

COSMETIC SURGERY

Cosmetic plastic surgery has an application in all age groups. Procedures include corrective otoplasty for the lop-eared child, rhinoplasty for the teen-age boy or girl, or a blepharoplasty or facelift for the aging man or woman.

Educational Foundation of the American Society of Plastic and Reconstructive Surgeons: *Symposium on Aesthetic Surgery of the Face, Eyelid, and Breast.* Mosby, 1972.

Masters FW, Lewis JR Jr (editors): *Symposium on Aesthetic Surgery of the Face, Eyelid, and Breast.* Vol 4. Mosby, 1972.

Symposium on cosmetic surgery. Surg Clin North Am 51:261, 1971.

Otoplasty

Young children with protruding ears due to the absence of the conchoscaphal angle are frequently teased unmercifully by other children. The corrective surgical procedure which recreates the cartilage fold through a postauricular incision can be performed with a brief hospitalization and convalescence. Preschool age is probably the ideal time for operation, as the child's ears have reached nearly their full potential growth by age 6. The surgical technic is fairly standard with minor variations, and postoperative complications are rare.

Rhinoplasty

Variations in the appearance of the nose from aesthetically desirable standards may be a result of ethnic developmental deformities or secondary to an injury. Nasal fractures are frequently unrecognized in a young child, and the resulting deformity may only become manifest at a much later age. The large humped nose with bulbous or drooping tip is often a tragedy to the sensitive teen-age boy or girl with an emerging awareness of social competition. Cosmetic nasal reconstruction is usually recommended when the patient's nose shows evidence of maturity. This may be as early as age 13 in girls, but usually averages somewhere between 15 and 17 years. Boys are generally operated on at a slightly later age than girls. The operation is done through intranasal incisions, usually under local anesthesia, and requires only a brief period of hospitalization. Postoperative swelling and periorbital ecchymosis are associated with a convalescence of 10–14 days following operation.

Proper selection of the candidate for surgery is important both from a psychologic and anatomic point of view. Certain patients may present with other profile problems associated with a receding chin. In selected cases, a complementary chin augmentation with a silicone implant may enhance the surgical result. Rhinoplasty has proved to be a very satisfactory procedure, as attested by the fact that it is the most widely performed cosmetic surgical operation.

Mammoplasty

Cosmetic breast surgery, particularly the augmentation mammoplasty, has become a frequently requested operation. The general surgeon who operates for breast malignancy can attest to the tremendous psychologic significance of the breasts to the average woman. The development of the silicone breast prosthesis for augmentation mammoplasty in the past decade has made this procedure a safe operation with excellent long-term results. An appropriately sized implant containing silicone gel in a sealed silicone bag is placed in a prepared retromammary pocket through a small incision in the inferior submammary fold. The scars are usually quite inconspicuous after a few months. The improvement in contour is predictably good, and the breast is authentic to palpation unless too large an implant has been placed, resulting in overly tight skin coverage.

Direct injection of silicone fluid into the breast is not only illegal at the present time but is strongly contraindicated since it has been demonstrated experimentally that significant volumes of the injected fluid are gradually lost from the local site, and local reactions to the silicone fluid injection have been recorded. In addition, localized collections of fluid may simulate carcinoma.

Recent advances in the manufacture of the silicone breast prosthesis have provided a thin-walled soft gel prosthesis which produces an augmented breast with a remarkably natural feel in most cases. Capsular scar contracture with resultant excessive firmness of the breast occurs less frequently. Additional camouflage of the operation has been provided by use of the periareolar incision which leaves a very inconspicuous scar.

Reduction mammoplasty, while it has significant cosmetic implications, is in fact a reconstructive surgical procedure. The chronic symptoms associated with carrying greatly enlarged breasts are well recognized, and the operation is indicated to relieve back and neck pain as well as posture problems.

The most common procedures used are those in which the nipple is displaced upward on a pedicle of breast tissue around which the reduced skin brassiere is tailored following excision of the excess breast tissue and skin. Nursing ability can be preserved with this technic, although nipple sensation may be lost. Small but ptotic breasts can be cosmetically improved utilizing this technic.

Another method of reduction mammoplasty which is suitable for the older patient with massively enlarged breasts employs the technic of transplantation of the nipple as a free graft. This is combined with a simpler plan of skin and breast tissue excision, and wound healing is usually free of complications.

Owsley JQ Jr: Camouflage and the augmentation mammaplasty. West J Med 120:101, 1974.

Blepharoplasty

Removal of redundant drooping eyelid skin and eyelid "bags" can correct the evidence of aging around the eyes. The procedure is often performed at the same · time as a facelift. The scars are placed so as to blend into normal skin creases. "Bags" of bulging orbital fat are removed after dissection from beneath the orbicularis oculi muscles.

Castanares S: Blepharoplasty for herniated intraorbital fat: Anatomical basis for a new approach. Plast Reconstr Surg 8:46, 1951.

Facelift

The facelift, or rhytidectomy, is a very satisfactory operation in properly selected patients. The procedure is usually performed under local anesthesia combined with sedation and can be accomplished with a brief hospitalization and convalescence of 2–3 weeks. The operation is designed primarily to correct the sagging of redundant skin beneath the chin and along the neck and jawline that develops with advancing age. The lines of expression, such as the nasolabial folds and the so-called laugh lines around the lateral canthi of the eyes, are only minimally affected. The surgery is of value in the patient with sufficient laxity of the face and neck skin so that significant correction can be achieved. In such a patient, a worthwhile interval will pass before the sagging gradually occurs again. It is not uncommon for a patient to have a second facelift or even, occasionally, a third.

●　　●　　●

General References

Artz CP, Moncrief JA: *The Treatment of Burns,* 2nd ed. Saunders, 1969.

Barsky AJ: *Principles and Practice of Plastic Surgery,* 2nd ed. Williams & Wilkins, 1950.

Borger AF: *Elective Incisions and Scar Revision.* Little, Brown, 1973.

Brown JB, McDowell F: *Skin Grafting,* 3rd ed. Lippincott, 1958.

Clark WH Jr, Mihm MC: Chap 11 in: *Dermatology in General Medicine.* Fitzpatrick TB (editor). McGraw-Hill, 1971.

Converse JM: Introduction to plastic surgery. Chap 1, pp 3–20, in: *Reconstructive Plastic Surgery.* Vol 1. Converse JM (editor). Saunders, 1964.

Converse JM (editor): *Reconstructive Plastic Surgery: Principles and Procedures in Correction, Reconstruction, and Transplantation.* 5 vols. Saunders, 1964. Vol I: Part 1, *General Principles.* Vols II and III: Part 2, *The Head and Neck.* Vol IV: Part 3, *The Hand and Upper Extremity;* Part 4, *The Lower Extremity.* Vol V: Part 5, *The Trunk;* Part 6, *The Genitourinary System and Anorectal Malformations;* Part 7, *Tissue Transplantation and Burn Shock.*

Converse JM: *Surgical Treatment of Facial Injuries,* 3rd ed. Williams & Wilkins, 1973.

Converse JM (editor): Symposium on reconstructive plastic surgery. Surg Clin North Am 47:259, 1967.

Dingman RO, Natvig P: *Surgery of Facial Fractures.* Saunders, 1964.

Edgerton MT, Hanson FC: Matching facial color with split thickness skin grafts from adjacent areas. Plast Reconstr Surg 25:455, 1960.

Educational Foundation of the American Society of Plastic and Reconstructive Surgeons: *Plastic and Maxillofacial Trauma Symposium.* Mosby, 1969.

Goldwyn RM (editor): *The Unfavorable Results in Plastic Surgery: Avoidance and Treatment.* Little, Brown, 1972.

Grabb WC, Smith JW: *Plastic Surgery: A Concise Guide to Clinical Practice,* 2nd ed. Little, Brown, 1973.

Longacre JJ: *Scar Tissue: Its Use and Abuse: The Surgical Correction of Deformities Due to Hypertrophic Scar and the Prevention of Its Formation.* Thomas, 1972.

Maddin S: *Current Dermatologic Management.* Mosby, 1970.

Murray JE: Annual discourse: Organ replacement, facial deformity, and plastic surgery. N Engl J Med 287:1069, 1972.

Mustarde JC: *Plastic Surgery in Infancy and Childhood.* Saunders, 1971.

Pinckus H, Stoll HL, Van Scott EJ: Chap 10 in: *Dermatology in General Medicine.* Fitzpatrick TB (editor). McGraw-Hill, 1971.

Polk HC Jr, Stone HH: *Contemporary Burn Management.* Little, Brown, 1971.

Rees T, Wood-Smith D: *Cosmetic Facial Surgery.* Saunders, 1973.

47...
Hand Surgery

Eugene S. Kilgore, MD, & William P. Graham III, MD

Both in industry and in the home, the hand is the most commonly injured part of the body. A disorder of the hand rarely jeopardizes life but often results in a handicap that may hamper vocational capacity.

assumed, without intention, after injury, paralysis, and the onset of painful states; it is also called the **position of injury**. Stiffening in this attitude jeopardizes function.

INTRODUCTION

The prime functions of the hand are feeling (sensibility) and grasping. Sensibility is important on the radial sides of the index, long, and ring fingers and on the opposing ulnar side of the thumb, where it is indispensable to be able to feel, pinch, pick up, and hold things. The ulnar side of the little finger and its metacarpal, upon which the hand usually rests, must register the sensations of contact and pain to avoid burns and other trauma.

Mobility is critical for grasping. The upper extremity is a cantilevered system extending from the shoulder to the fingertips. It must be adaptable to varying rates and kinds of movements with the maintenance of stability.

The specialization of the thumb ray has endowed man with superior aptitudes for defense, work, and dexterity. The thumb has exquisite sensibility and is a highly mobile structure of appropriate length, with a well-developed adductor and thenar (pronating) musculature. It is the most important digit of the hand, and every effort must be made to preserve its function.

The **position of function** of the upper extremity favors reaching the mouth and perineum as well as comfortable, forceful, and unfatiguing grip and pinch. The elbow is held at or near a right angle, the forearm neutral between pronation and supination, and the wrist extended 30 degrees with the fingers furled to almost meet the opposed (pronated) tip of the thumb (Fig 47—1A). This is the desired stance of the extremity if stiffness is likely to occur, and it should be adopted when joints are immobilized by splinting, arthrodesis, or tenodesis.

Opposite to the position of function is the **position of rest,** in which the flexed wrist extends the digits, making grip and pinch awkward, uncomfortable, weak, and fatiguing (Fig 47—1B). The forearm is usually pronated and the elbow extended. This habitus is

ANATOMY

All references to the forearm and hand should be made to the radial and ulnar sides (not lateral and medial), and to the volar (or palmar) and dorsal surfaces. The digits should be identified as the thumb, index finger, long finger, ring finger, and little finger, or referred to as rays I, II, III, IV, and V.

Skin is the elastic outer sleeve and glove of the arm and hand. Sacrifice of its surface area or elasticity by debridement and fibrosis can severely curtail range

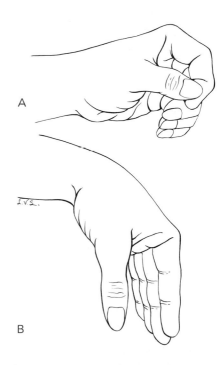

Figure 47—1. Positions of function *(A)* and rest (injury) *(B).*

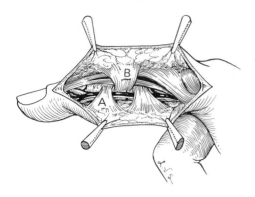

Figure 47–2. *A:* Cleland's ligament. *B:* Transverse retinacular ligament.

of motion and constrict circulation. In the adult hand, the dorsal skin stretches about 4 cm in the longitudinal and in the transverse planes when the fist closes, and the volar skin stretches a similar amount when the palm is flattened and spread. The long finger can easily have 48 sq cm of skin cover, and the whole hand (exclusive of digits) 210 sq cm.

Fascia anchors volar skin to bone to make pinch and grip stable; the midlateral fibers of "Cleland's and Grayson's ligaments" keep the skin sleeve from twisting about the digit (Fig 47–2). In the form of sheaths and pulleys, fascia holds tendons in the concavity of arched joints to convey mechanical efficiency and power. The fascial sleeve of the forearm, hand, and digits must sometimes be slit along with skin to relieve posttraumatic swelling. Any fascial compartment of the hand provides a space for infection or an avenue for its dissemination.

Each finger has 4 joints (MC, MP, PIP, and DIP—see accompanying box), any 2 of which may be fused and still leave adequate overall function. The thumb has only 3 joints (MC, MP, and IP), and every effort must be made to preserve at least two. The position of the wrist governs the efficiency of extrinsic muscle contraction. The stability of the digital joints and their planes of motion are governed by the length of the ligaments and the anatomy of their articulating surfaces. The longitudinal and transverse arches of the hand (Fig 47–3) are architectural prerequisites to gripping, pinching, and cupping and are maintained by the active contraction and passive tone of intact intrinsic muscles. The arches create the position of function. When the arches are collapsed, the hand assumes the position of rest or position of injury. Loss of these arches is most often initiated by edema. They may be preserved by splinting in the position of function, elevation without constriction, and early restoration of active and vigorous joint motion.

Each MP and IP joint has a distally anchored volar trap door called the volar plate (Fig 47–4) in addition to collateral ligaments stabilizing the joint on either side (Fig 47–5).

The extrinsic flexor tendons are contained in fibrous **sheaths** to prevent bowstringing and preserve mechanical efficiency as the fingers furl into the palm. **Pulleys** (hypertrophied sections of the sheath) resist the points of greatest tendency to bowstring. Sheaths are inelastic and relatively avascular. Therefore, they crowd and congest any swollen, inflamed, or injured tendons and curtail glide by friction, constriction, and the generation of inelastic adhesions. The term "**no-man's-land**" refers to the zone from the middle of the palm to just beyond the PIP joint, wherein the superficialis and profundus lie ensheathed together and recovery of glide is so difficult after wounding (Fig 47–6).

Across the wrist, the dense volar carpal ligament closes the bony carpal canal (**carpal tunnel**) through which pass all 8 finger flexors as well as the flexor pollicis longus and median nerve (Fig 47–6). The **ulnar bursa** is the continuation of the synovium around the long flexors of the little finger through the carpal tunnel, encompassing the other finger flexors which interrupted their separate bursae at the midpalm level. The

Abbreviations Used in This Chapter	
DIP	Distal interphalangeal
IC	Intercarpal
IP	Interphalangeal
MC	Metacarpocarpal
MP	Metacarpophalangeal
PIP	Proximal interphalangeal
RC	Radial-carpal
RU	Radial-ulnar

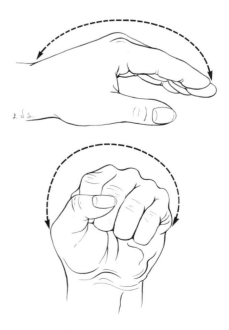

Figure 47–3. Longitudinal *(top)* and transverse arches.

Extension

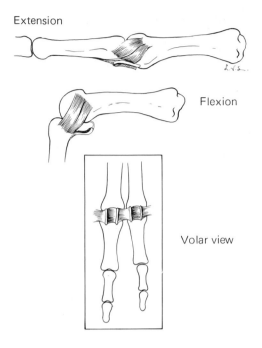

Flexion

Volar view

Figure 47—4. Volar plate.

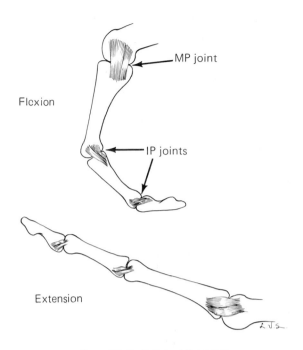

Flexion

MP joint

IP joints

Extension

Figure 47—5. Collateral ligaments.

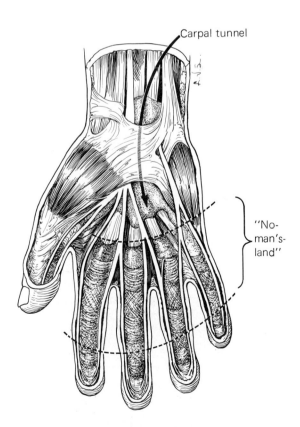

Carpal tunnel

"No-man's-land"

Figure 47—6. Carpal tunnel and no-man's-land.

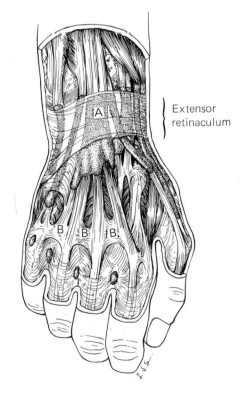

Extensor retinaculum

Figure 47—7. *A:* Extensor retinaculum over 6 tendon compartments. *B:* Juncturae tendinum (conexus intertendineus).

radial bursa is the synovium around the flexor pollicis longus continued through the carpal tunnel. These 2 bursae may intercommunicate. **Parona's space** is that tissue plane over the pronator quadratus in the distal forearm deep to the radial and ulnar bursae.

The extensor tendons are ensheathed in 6 compartments at the wrist beneath the extensor retinaculum (Fig 47–7), which predisposes to adhesions. Its role as a pulley is not vital and can be dispensed with.

The nerves of greatest importance to hand function are the musculocutaneous, radial, ulnar, and median. The importance of the musculocutaneous and radial nerves combined is forearm supination and of the radial nerve alone is innervation of the extensor muscles which stabilize the wrist and extend the digits. The ulnar nerve innervates 15 of the 20 intrinsic muscles. The median nerve, by its sensory innervation, is "the eye of the hand"; through its motor innervation, it maintains most of the long flexors, the pronators of the forearm, and the thenar muscles. Fig 47–9 shows the sensory distribution of the ulnar, radial, and median nerves.

Kaplan EB: *Functional and Surgical Anatomy of the Hand,* 2nd ed. Lippincott, 1965.

Lampe EW: *Surgical Anatomy of the Hand.* Ciba Clinical Symposia, vol 9, No. 1 Ciba Pharmaceutical Products, 1957.

Milford LW: *Retaining Ligaments of the Digits of the Hand.* Saunders, 1968.

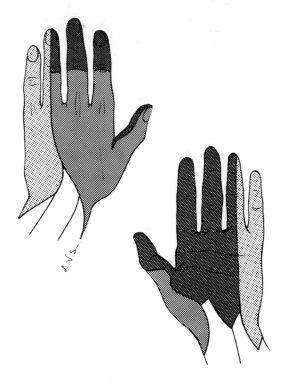

Figure 47–9. Sensory distribution in the hand. Dotted area, ulnar nerve; diagonal area, radial nerve; darker area, median nerve.

CLINICAL EVALUATION OF HAND DISORDERS

The present complaint must be recorded explicitly and in complete detail with regard to its mechanism of onset, evolution, aggravating factors, and relieving factors. Age, sex, hand dominance, occupation, and relevant matters pertaining to the patient's general health and his emotional and socioeconomic status must be recorded also.

The examination should follow an orderly routine. Observe the neck, shoulders, and both upper extremities and the action and strength of all muscle groups, and be certain that all parts can pass painlessly and coordinately through a normal range of motion, starting with the head and neck and working down to the fingertips. Compare both upper extremities and keep detailed immediate notes, diagrams, and measurements of the case. Having the patient reach for the ceiling and simultaneously open and close both fists and then oppose the thumbs sequentially to each fingertip will immediately emphasize any abnormalities.

Observe habitus, wasting, hypertrophy, deformities, skin changes, skin temperature, scars, and signs of pain. Feel the wrist pulses and the sweat of the finger pads, and test reflexes and the sensibility of the median, ulnar, and radial nerves.

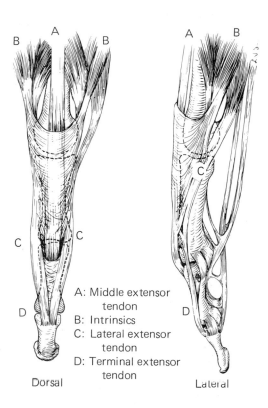

A: Middle extensor tendon
B: Intrinsics
C: Lateral extensor tendon
D: Terminal extensor tendon

Dorsal

Lateral

Figure 47–8. Hood mechanism.

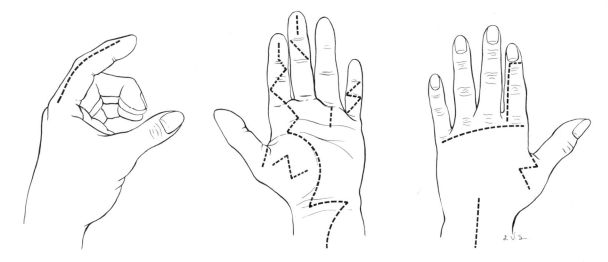

Figure 47–10. Proper placement of skin incisions.

Serial x-rays and laboratory procedures may clarify a problem with an indolent evolution (eg, Kienböck's aseptic necrosis of the lunate, causing unexplained wrist pain). Contralateral and multiple view x-rays in different planes (even tomograms) are often helpful. This is especially true in patients who have persistent perplexing bone and joint pain or limited motion or in patients who have not attained adult growth.

The diagnosis is often made by noting the response to therapy. This is particularly true in the case of local corticosteroids injected at the site of noninfectious inflammatory conditions (eg, carpal tunnel syndrome, trigger finger).

Committee on Rating of Mental and Physical Impairment: *Guides to the Evaluation of Permanent Impairment.* American Medical Association, 1971.

Lucas GL: *Examination of the Hand.* Thomas, 1972.

Swanson AB: Evaluation of impairment of function in the hand. Surg Clin North Am 44:925, 1964.

GENERAL OPERATIVE PRINCIPLES

Incisions (Fig 47–10) must either be zigzagged across lines of tension or run longitudinally in "neutral" zones (eg, connecting the lateral limits of the flexion and extension creases of the digits); and, whenever possible, must be designed so that a healthy skin-fat flap is raised over the zone of repair of a tendon, nerve, or artery.

Proper evaluation and treatment of a fresh injury often requires extension of the wound. Normal structures can then be recognized and traced into the zone of injury, where blood and trauma so often make their identification difficult or impossible.

Constriction and tension by dressings must be avoided at all costs. The dressing should be applied evenly to the skin without wrinkles. The wound should be covered with a single layer of fine mesh gauze followed by a wet spongy medium (fluffs, mechanic's waste, Rest-On, Kling, or Kerlix). Wetness facilitates the drainage of blood into the dressing, which should be applied with gentle pressure to curtail dead space.

Splinting and immediate elevation are paramount in controlling pain and favoring healing. In general, plaster (fast-setting) is preferred because of its adaptability to specific requirements. More often than not, the wrist requires immobilization along with any other part of the hand (Fig 47–11).

It must be appreciated that effective immobilization of a finger most often requires concomitant immobilization of one or more adjacent fingers, usually

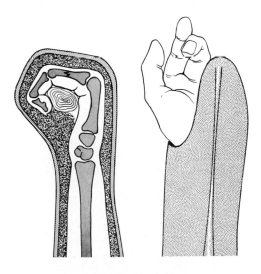

Figure 47–11. Casting.

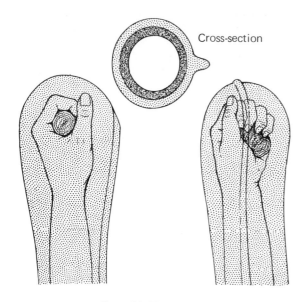

Cross-section

Figure 47—12. Casting.

in the position of function. Straight splints such as tongue blades involve a hazard of digital stiffness and distortion and should not be used.

Persistence of pain signifies inadequate immobilization and, if throbbing is present, congestion. Congestion must be promptly relieved by elevation and sectioning of the cast and dressing and, if necessary, the skin and fascia.

TENDON DISORDERS

Tendon disorders are most commonly due to trauma or to inflammatory or degenerative conditions. These may be restricted to one or more tendons or may be part of a generalized disorder involving other tissues and structures. Neoplastic and congenital disorders of the tendons are rare.

The prerequisites to successful tendon surgery are (1) that the tendons be covered with healthy padded and pliable skin; (2) that the joints to be moved by the tendons have an adequate passive range of motion; (3) that the muscles to the tendons be elastic, and that they be innervated or capable of being so; (4) that the patient be motivated and capable of responsibility for the rehabilitative effort; (5) that the surgeon have the appropriate training, skill, and technical facilities; and (6) usually, that the musculotendinous units involved not be spastic and the digits involved not irrevocably anesthetic.

Adhesions invariably form wherever tendons are even slightly inflamed or injured and can completely nullify tendon function; even so, adhesions are indispensable to repair. No divided tendon will reestablish

its continuity and no tendon graft will develop its own blood supply without the ingrowth of capillaries and fibroblasts from the tendon bed. Thus, it is not only the quantity of adhesions but also their pliability that determines whether or not the tendon will glide. With much active and passive effort over many months, tendon glide can be increased as a consequence of maturation and molding of the collagen in the adhesions. If this does not take place and the adhesions remain thick and short, tendon excursion fails.

Preoperative treatment of fresh lacerations consists of immobilization and prophylactic antibiotics. Such cases can be deferred for definitive primary repair for 24 hours or more. The timing of delayed secondary procedures depends upon the resolution of wound edema and callus (ie, how soft and pliable it is). After 6—8 weeks, tendons that retract over 2.5 cm may defy full excursion because the muscle elasticity has been lost or the tendon is recoiled and congealed in scar.

Tenodesis will occur if the surface of the tendon and the surface where adherence is desired are roughened. The best anchoring surface is either bone, ligament, or a tendon pulley (Fig 47—13). Immobilization is necessary for 3—4 weeks and may require a Kirschner wire or plaster cast (or both).

The access to tenolysis should be through a wound offering effective exposure and placed where the immediate active and passive joint motion that must follow will not jeopardize healing of the wound by undue stretching or direct pressure. The most common causes of failure are immobilization of the tendon for longer than 24 hours after lysis; failure of the patient to move the tendon by repeated active contraction of the musculotendinous unit; carrying out a concomitant procedure requiring immobilization (ie, neurorrhaphy); or separation of the tendon.

Tendon lengthening is used to advance a tenorrhaphy beyond a point of constriction (eg, pulley) or to elongate a contracted musculotendinous unit.

The position of immobilization needed to relieve tension on the tendon sutures is ideally determined when the wound is still open and the tendon juncture is in view. The duration of immobilization is generally for no more than 3—4 weeks.

The patient must understand that the subsequent musculotendinous and joint mobilization is a time-consuming process, often taking many weeks or months. Exercise should be sufficient to make progress but not so much as to cause lingering pain and swelling. "Ball-squeezing" has no place in getting tendons to

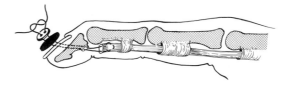

Figure 47—13. Flexor tenorrhaphy by advancement or graft. Pulleys are saved.

glide early since it blocks the movement of digital joints. Once glide has been achieved, however, ball-squeezing may strengthen the muscles.

Diagnosis & Treatment of Tendon Injuries

Tendon injury may be single or multiple and may be complicated by injury to nerve or bone. Diagnosis, treatment, and prognosis may be difficult. One must know the terminal joint that a given tendon moves, where overlap of function may mask the loss of action of a specific tendon, and how to block the action of tendons that conflict with functional testing of their fellow travelers.

Repeated testing will serve to confirm a tendon injury and differentiate unconscious or willful withholding of pertinent clinical information. The history, the habitus of the joints, and the results of specific tendon testing are the 3 crucial elements in the diagnosis of tendon deficits.

The state of the wound and the complexity of the injury are the principal issues the hand surgeon must weigh in choosing a **primary** or **secondary** tenorrhaphy and its type. Clean wounds generally favor primary tenorrhaphy. Primary tenorrhaphy is defined as one that is done within 24–72 hours after injury.

When wounds are untidy, contaminated, or complicated by fracture or ischemia, formal tenorrhaphy is usually delayed for weeks or months until the tendon bed is more favorable to healing and glide.

"Mallet" finger ("baseball" or "drop" finger) (Fig 47–14) is due to division or attenuation of the extensor to the distal phalanx. A distal joint which can be passively but not actively extended is diagnostic. The injury most commonly results from sudden forceful flexion of the digit when it is held in rigid extension. Either the extensor is partially or completely ruptured, or the dorsal lip of the bone is avulsed. Less frequently, the injury is due to direct trauma such as a laceration or a crush force. An x-ray should be taken to determine the presence and extent of any fracture.

Treatment may not be necessary if the loss of active extension is less than 15 degrees and any existing fracture is only a chip. More severe injury requires 6 weeks of continuous splinting in full distal joint extension (**not** hyperextension) with or without 40 degrees of PIP joint flexion. Joint fixation with fine Kirschner wire, padded aluminum, plastic, or even plaster splints is equally effective. A lacerated tendon should be delicately reapproximated. When a fracture

fragment represents one-third or more of the surface of the joint, it should be reduced and held by wiring or pinning. In selected cases, smaller fracture fragments may be removed. If there is sufficient articular disruption, one may consider joint fusion. Tendon grafting is difficult and easily leads to a poor cosmetic and functional result. It should be done only rarely.

Swan-neck deformity (Fig 47–14) is a frequent complication of mallet finger, but it may also be the result of disparity of pull between the extrinsic flexors and extensor hood with or without attenuation of the DIP joint extensor. It is seen in congenitally hypermobile joints, spastic and rheumatoid states, and following resection of the superficialis tendon. The dorsal hood acts to extend the distal joint but is held back by its insertion at the base of the middle phalanx, which it therefore hyperextends ("PIP joint recurvatum"). This in turn increases the tension on the profundus, which hyperflexes the DIP joint. If the mallet deformity is 25 degrees or less and there is some active distal joint extension, it may be treated by severing the middle phalangeal insertion of the dorsal hood. Otherwise, the deformity may be corrected by tethering PIP joint extension (eg, Littler technic; see reference on p 1002).

The "buttonhole" or "boutonniere" deformity (Fig 47–15) appears as the opposite of the swan-neck deformity: hyperextension of the DIP joint and flexion of the PIP joint. There is attenuation or separation of the dorsal hood, so that the lateral bands shift volar to the PIP joint axis and the joint buckles dorsalward. Active extension of the PIP joint becomes impossible, and the entire extrinsic-intrinsic force on the hood passes onto the lateral bands which flex the PIP joint and hyperextend the DIP joint. This deformity may develop suddenly or, more often, insidiously after trauma over the dorsum of the PIP joint.

To avoid this complication, fresh extensor tendon lacerations and severe contusions over the PIP joint should be sutured if necessary but should always have the PIP joint alone splinted in extension for 3–4 weeks. A small, oblique Kirschner wire provides good immobilization. Established deformities can be treated by such immobilization or by operative correction.

Tendon rupture, subluxation, and drift: The most frequent rupture of a healthy tendon is that of the distal joint extensor of one of the fingers as a result of sudden, forceful flexion (see mallet finger, above). Other tendons rupture where they have been weakened by division and suture, partial transection, crushing, or

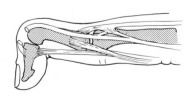

Figure 47—14. Mallet finger with swan-neck deformity.

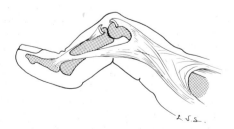

Figure 47—15. Buttonhole deformity.

attritional fraying over roughened bone. The synovial thickening, degenerative tendon nodularity, and roughening of articular bone seen in the rheumatoid hand easily dispose to rupture by mechanical abrasion and circulatory depletion of tendons. Much can be done prophylactically by synovectomy, sectioning of constricting tendon sheaths, and resection of bony spurs and tendon nodules. If correction of a rupture is indicated, the methods of doing so include suture, tendon graft, tendon transfer, or tenodesis.

The most common subluxations and drifts of tendons are 2-fold: (1) volar drift of the intrinsic tendons as they pass the PIP joint of the fingers, causing the "buttonhole" deformity (see above); and (2) ulnar drift of the extrinsic middle extensors (central slips) as they pass the MP joints. The latter may result from trauma that divides or attenuates the lateral expansion (sagittal band) of the extensor hood on the radial side of the central slip. It more commonly results from attenuation of the entire extensor hood over the MP joint as a consequence of marked distention of the joint space and thickening of the synovium in rheumatoid arthritis. Treatment of ulnar drift involves repositioning of the extensor tendon to a point central to the MP joint and holding it by appropriate reefing of the sagittal band fibers of the hood on the radial side.

Evaluation of Results

The excursion and force of centripetal pull of the operated tendon should be compared with the normal one in the opposite hand and objective measurements recorded at least once a month. It then becomes readily apparent whether or not progress is being made. If the conscientious patient makes no progress in 2–3 months, his disability is probably static and he should be considered for further surgical treatment or released from care. Often, however, 6–12 months are required before maximal function is restored.

Boyes JH, Stark HH: Flexor-tendon grafts in the fingers and thumb. J Bone Joint Surg 53A:1332, 1971.
Kilgore ES & others: Atraumatic flexor tendon retrieval. Am J Surg 122:430, 1971.
Kilgore ES & others: Correction of ulnar subluxation of extensor communis by using a reverse tendon pedicle. Hand 7:272, Oct 1975.
Littler JW: The severed flexor tendon. Surg Clin North Am 39:435, 1959.
Littler JW & others: Restoration of the retinacular system in hyperextension deformity of the proximal interphalangeal joint. J Bone Joint Surg 47A:637, 1965.
Potenza AD: Prevention of adhesions to healing digital flexor tendons. JAMA 187:187, 1964.
Verdan C: Half a century of flexor-tendon surgery: Current status and changing philosophies. J Bone Joint Surg 54A:472, 1972.
Verdan C: Primary repair of the flexor tendons. J Bone Joint Surg 42A:647, 1960.

FRACTURES, DISLOCATIONS, & LIGAMENTOUS INJURIES

The wrist and digits should be generally maintained in the position of function after reduction. Unstable alignment may require internal fixation to hold reduction. At all costs, avoid extremes of joint position and forceful pressure of external splints and plaster. Constant digital traction is hazardous because it leads to joint stiffness. To minimize stiffness, immobilization should be maintained for the shortest time consistent with adequate control of pain and tissue repair.

Elevation of the forearm and removal of all jewelry and snug clothing are essential to control edema. The patient's responsibilities in this regard must be repeatedly explained to him. When swelling is excessive, it must be reduced and the soft tissues rendered pliable as soon as possible. Reduction of the displaced fracture or dislocated joint sometimes makes the soft tissues pliable again. A releasing incision of skin and fascia may be needed to overcome brawny induration. It can be closed later with a split thickness skin graft.

Open injuries involving bones and joints require prophylactic antibiotics systemically and often in the wound or joint as well (see Chapter 11).

Fractured Metacarpals & Phalanges

Fractures of **metacarpals** and **proximal and middle phalanges** tend to bow and to rotate. Rotation of a finger causes it to cross over an adjacent finger during flexion, thus blocking digital excursion, fist-making, and grasp. Rotation is avoided by having the injured finger flexed alongside an adjacent finger.

Dorsal and volar bowing is caused by the pull of intrinsic and extrinsic flexor and extensor forces. These forces can be most effectively neutralized by immobilizing the wrist and the digits in the position of function. The risk of reduction of bowing is the added predisposition to joint stiffness and tenodesis incident to excessive manipulation or surgery. Therefore, if the bowing is less than 20–30 degrees, this risk must be weighed carefully, for such deformity may not be functionally significant. Greater angles of bowing of the phalanges must, however, be corrected by either closed or open methods. Angulation of up to 40 degrees can be tolerated in some metacarpal fractures.

Immobilization of these fractures is generally for 3–4 weeks. The MP joints must be maintained in functional flexion. In the case of the ring and little fingers, this function means between 60–80 degrees of flexion. Malleable and rigid ready-made volar splints cannot be applied without a threat to this important angle of MP joint flexion or (equally harmful) a threat of too much compression of the soft tissue of the palm or a rotary deformity at the fracture site.

After closed or open reduction, a preferred method of immobilization is to furl the digits over a volar roll of soft gauze which allows the position of function to be maintained (Figs 47–11 and 47–12). The forearm and pertinent digits are then wrapped in loosely applied cast padding followed by a light circumferential plaster cast, keeled for strength across the extended wrist. This immobilization is usually maintained for 3 weeks.

Two basal metacarpal fractures deserve special mention:

(1) Bennett's intra-articular fracture is an impaction of the thumb metacarpal, causing an oblique separation of the volar base from the dorsal base. The latter usually subluxates dorsally. The ideal treatment is reduction by centrifugal pulling on the thumb and pressure volarward on the base of the metacarpal followed by fixation with a Kirschner wire. If satisfactory realignment is not achieved, open reduction is advocated.

(2) A spiral or displaced fracture of the **base of the fifth metacarpal** always deserves an immediate and repeated check on the function of the first dorsal interosseus muscle to establish the integrity of the deep motor branch of the ulnar nerve, which is easily injured by this fracture.

Distal phalangeal fractures are located at the tuft, shaft, or base. Pain is the prime reason for treatment, and may be compounded if subungual hematoma is also present. Decompression relieves the pain. This can be done under digital nerve block by drilling the nail with a 19 caliber hypodermic needle, or without nerve block by burning a hole through the nail with the hot end of a safety pin or paper clip. This is quite painless if done gently. Pain and swelling are best controlled by applying a well-padded forearm cast covering the injured finger with at least one adjacent finger or the injured thumb alone in boxing glove fashion. After 1–2 weeks, a digital guard can take the place of the cast.

Minute marginal **digital joint fractures** usually need no more than 1–2 days of immobilization. Stiffness and pain can be most rapidly overcome by early mobilization. Fractures with involvement of one-fourth to one-third of the joint surface require careful reduction and immobilization for 3 weeks. In some cases, the fragment should be resected. Mangled joints should be set at a functional angle for fusion or, in select circumstances, the MP or PIP joints may be replaced by a Silastic implant if tendons are functioning.

In closed or open **crushing fractures** with a lot of swelling, the prime consideration should be preservation of the circulation, particularly venous return. Anatomic reduction of the bone is of secondary importance. Leaving a wound open or even slitting skin and fascia to loosen the tissues may be the best way to aid the circulation and may also make it possible to secure alignment and the position of function. Reduction is often well maintained by molding a roll of very wet, loose gauze to the injured digits or whole hand and then applying a well-cushioned boxing-glove type of forearm cast to the appropriate digits or all of the hand. Internal fixation is advisable in selected cases.

Open reduction is the technic of choice in injuries which present a gaping wound with exposed fractures. It is also the preferred technic in the following circumstances: (1) when perfect reduction is important for subsequent function, as in intra-articular fractures, or when indicated for the removal of a potentially troublesome displaced small fragment; (2) if it allows reduction with less soft tissue trauma than by closed reduction; or (3) to facilitate internal fixation in difficult reductions.

Dislocations

Dislocations of the wrist and fingers are far less frequent than fractures. Swelling may completely mask the bone displacement, but motion is usually limited and painful. X-rays may be indispensable to the diagnosis. In the case of the wrist, multiple views and comparison of right and left may be necessary.

Dislocations are most easily reduced by accentuating the position that produced the deformity with simultaneous centrifugal traction on the distal segment followed by firmly pressing the displaced bone into its anatomic position. A reduction snap may be heard and is often promptly followed by excellent range of motion. A postreduction x-ray should usually be taken.

Limited progressive mobilization is usually advisable to avoid stiffness. It should start within 3–4 weeks for the wrist and a week for the digits. A concomitant fracture or an open dislocation would interdict mobilization so early. Compound dislocations require prophylactic treatment with antibiotics.

Open reduction is indicated whenever closed reduction requires much force. A chronic dislocation may defy even an open reduction without lysis and division of soft tissue or resection arthroplasty.

The most common dislocation about the digits is dorsal displacement of the distal segment on the proximal one. When ligaments are intact, reduction may be difficult. The most difficult is the dislocated MP joint of one of the fingers, which normally requires open reduction. It traps the head of the metacarpal in a noose formed by the lumbrical radially, the flexor tendons and pretendinous palmar fascia band ulnarly, the volar plate and collateral ligaments on the dorsum distally, and the transverse palmar fascia on the volar aspect proximally. Volar exposure and section of the fascia proximally or dorsal exposure and splitting the volar plate makes reduction quite easy, although section of the ulnar collateral ligament must sometimes be added.

Dislocation of an interphalangeal joint is most often reduced by the patient himself or a bystander at the time it occurs and requires little or no immobilization. Resistance to flexion means inadequate reduction. Failure of reduction can mean that the displaced phalangeal head has escaped sideways from under the hood of the extensor mechanism, which then closes in between the head and the base of the more distal phalanx and locks the deformity. Recurrence of the dislocation usually means that the volar plate has been torn off at its origin distally. All 3 of these difficulties require open procedures to restore normal anatomic relationships. Repair of the volar plate requires 3—4 weeks of immobility. One obliquely placed Kirschner wire is sufficient fixation of the joint.

Chronic dislocations with erosion of the joint should be handled by replacing the joint with a Silastic prosthesis if the surrounding tendons are functionally intact; otherwise, the joints should be fused in the position of function. **Rheumatoid arthritis** causes a variety of insidious dislocations. The most common is at the MP joint. This consists of volar and **ulnar drifting** of the proximal phalanx in relation to the metacarpal as a result of the mean force of intrinsic-extrinsic tendon pull in association with pathologically attenuated joint capsules and ligaments. When intrinsic muscles atrophy and fibrose, these distortions may be irreducible without soft tissue surgery. At the PIP and DIP joint levels, the distortion may be of the **swan-neck** (PIP hyperextension and DIP flexion) or **buttonhole** type (PIP flexion and DIP hyperextension).

Ligamentous Injuries

The ligaments of the **MP** and **PIP joints** are the most commonly injured. These vary from total ruptures to tears without any loss of stability. Either the ligament tears, or its bony attachment is avulsed, or both ligament and bone are torn. Those of the MP joint are usually due to violent abduction, whereas PIP ligaments rupture with equal proclivity on the radial or ulnar sides. Diagnosis may depend on stress x-ray views showing abnormal widening of a joint.

Except for the thumb, treatment of purely ligamentous injuries is rarely surgical. Splinting should often be brief to avoid excessive stiffness and pain which may result. As long as there is intact intrinsic and extrinsic tendon function and the patient is careful to avoid further injury, early motion within 2—3 days of injury is often desirable. One finger can be splinted by loosely strapping to an adjacent digit for 2—4 weeks. The pain of these injuries is notoriously slow to resolve irrespective of treatment.

Twisting injuries and falls may rupture the radial collateral ligament of the thumb by an adduction force; most commonly, however, the injury is an abduction force which tears the ulnar collateral ligament. Partial tears with limited instability may be treated by immobilization for 4—6 weeks. Total tears should be sutured or reconstructed surgically.

If there is a sizeable avulsed bone fragment in any of these injuries, it must be accurately reduced or, if it involves less than one-fourth of the surface area of the PIP or MP joint, removed. One may try local injections of small amounts of corticosteroid and lidocaine for chronic pain, or resection of scarred intrinsic muscle and the leading edge of the intermetacarpal ligament for intractable pain in the finger webs.

Becton JL & others: A simplified technique for treating the complex dislocation of the index metacarpophalangeal joint. J Bone Joint Surg 57A:698, 1975.

Kilgore ES & others: Posttraumatic trapped dislocations of the PIP joint. J Trauma 16:481, 1976.

HAND INFECTIONS

Pyogenic infections of the hand often develop and spread as a result of failure to preserve or restore good venous and lymphatic drainage following trauma. In order to prevent as well as to treat infection, it is necessary to control swelling and congestion of tissues and to avoid any dead space filled with stagnant blood or serum. Inflammation causes tissue tension by sequestration of edema fluid. This in turn impairs tissue oxygenation by compressing the blood vessels, and a vicious cycle may develop which can lead to necrosis within the constrictive sleeves of fascia and skin.

Acute swelling predisposes to infection, especially if there has been contamination through a puncture or open wound. Tissues and structures with a limited blood supply—or a blood supply that is easily choked off—are most susceptible to infection. Tissues around the nails, joints, tendon sheaths, and bones have the least natural resistance to infection.

Prevention & Treatment of Pyogenic Infections

Constrictive clothing, jewelry, dressings, casts, and even a tightly closed wound can impair oxygenation. Comfortable immobilization and elevation of the hand above the level of the heart will help to control swelling. Throbbing pain is a symptom of excessive swelling that demands prompt mechanical relief and not analgesics. If pain, swelling, and induration progress despite other mechanical measures, immediate slitting of skin and fascia in one or more areas is mandatory. This is usually done either along the dorsoradial or the dorsoulnar side of the digits, the hand, and the forearm, with care to avoid injury to nerves, major vessels, and tendons. A dorsal transverse skin incision over the heads of the metacarpals (sparing the veins) allows the MP joints of the swollen hand to flex and assume the functional position. Prophylactic local and systemic antibiotics are indicated for all contaminated wounds or whenever the circulation has been compromised. Antisludging treatment (eg, dextran 40) may also be considered. Clearly definable and easily recovered foreign bodies and nonviable tissue should be removed without endangering residual function. The evacuation of blood, serum, and foreign fluids can be facilitated by loosely fitting drains and wet dressings. Tetanus immunization should be given as indicated.

Adequate immobilization usually requires a splint of the wrist. In serious cases or uncooperative patients, the elbow should be splinted also and the patient kept flat in bed with his hand propped up on pillows. Without immobilization, the infection may be "milked" into uninvolved areas and progress farther.

The need for antibiotics is determined by the extent of the infection. If the process is already well localized, simple drainage may be all that is needed. Since 80% of pyogenic infections are due to *Staphylococcus aureus* or beta-hemolytic streptococci, begin with antibiotics empirically while waiting for cultures.

When incision and drainage of an abscess is necessary, it should always be done at the point of maximum tenderness or the point of maximum fluctuation, where the overlying tissues are thinnest. The drainage wound should run parallel to and not across the paths of nerves, arteries, and veins. Wounds should be made long enough and should be zigzagged, when necessary, to avoid secondary contractures.

Eaton RG, Butsch DP: Antibiotic guidelines for hand infections. Surg Gynecol Obstet 130:119, 1970.

Linscheid RL, Dobyns JH: Common and uncommon infections of the hand. Orthop Clin North Am 6:1063, 1975.

Stone HH & others: Empirical selection of antibiotics for hand infections. J Bone Joint Surg 51A:899, 1969.

SPECIFIC INFECTIONS OF THE HAND

Cellulitis, Lymphangitis, & Adenitis

Cellulitis is manifested by local swelling, warmth, redness, and tenderness. It usually demands immobilization and elevation, and sometimes fasciotomy, in addition to antibiotics. Lymphangitis and adenitis are most often due to streptococci and require elevation and immobilization as well as antibiotics.

Pyogenic Granuloma

Pyogenic granuloma is a mound of granulation-like tissue 3–20 mm (or more) in diameter. It usually develops under a chronically moist dressing and may form around a suture knot. It should be scraped flush with the skin under local anesthesia. A small granuloma (less than 6–7 mm in diameter) exposed to the air will soon dry up and epithelize, whereas larger ones should be covered with a thin split thickness skin graft. If the granuloma is adjacent to the nail and the nail is acting as a foreign body aggravating the reaction, the nail must be removed. The histologic appearance suggests that these are capillary hemangiomas rather than the consequence of pyogenic infection.

Pyoderma

Pyoderma (subepithelial abscess) is the forerunner of **collar-button abscess.** It develops within the skin in a hair follicle or infected blister. Failure to treat a blister or puncture wound deep to a callus commonly leads to this abscess, which becomes collar-button in configuration when it points into the subdermal fat. Treatment by means of incision, debridement of a blister or callus, drainage, water-soaked or zinc oxide dressings, rest, and elevation is usually sufficient.

Infections Around the Nail

The rigidity of the fingernail causes it to press upon and aggravate any inflammation of the soft tissues surrounding it. The nail fold is often traumatized and becomes secondarily inflamed, leading to a **paronychia** on the radial or ulnar side. The lesion is called

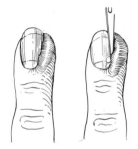

Figure 47–16. Incision and drainage of paronychia.

an **eponychia** if it involves the base of the nail; a **"run-around"** if the entire fold is involved; and a **subungual abscess** if pus develops and extends under the nail. **Subonychia** is inflammation between the nail bed and the bony phalanx. Because of the early and unrelenting tissue tension that develops, these entities are quite painful. Abscess formation often results, occasionally at some distance proximal to the nail fold (paraeponychial abscess). Early treatment is by means of water-soaked or zinc oxide dressings, elevation, immobilization, and antibiotics. Most abscesses can be drained painlessly with a needlepoint scalpel, cutting through the insensible necrotic skin cap where it points (Fig 47–16). Sagittal incisions forming a "trap door" of the eponychium should be reserved for the long-standing case in which a dense fibrous callus of the nail fold must be excised. Occasionally, the nail must be basally excised or totally avulsed, after which the eponychial fold should be separated from the nail matrix by a loose pack. Chronically wet nails of dishwashers may develop tissue changes and nail deformities which defy treatment. Fungal infections should be diagnosed and treated, and the fingers should be protected from water or excessive sweating.

Space Infections

The skin and fascia compartmentalize certain areas of the hand and forearm, predisposing these spaces to increased tissue tension and the progression of infection to abscess formation. The treatment of early space infection involves elevation, immobilization, and antibiotics administered systemically. If this does not arrest the progression of symptoms and signs within a few hours—or if the space is already tense when first examined—incision and drainage are required. Recovery is expedited by an antibiotic drip into the space administered through a fine catheter.

A. Volar Digital Pulp (Fat Pad) Spaces of the Fingers: (Fig 47–17.) Whether in the proximal, middle, or distal pad, any abscess that points to the center of the pad should be drained by an incision which is precisely central and runs longitudinally but does not cross the flexion crease. This preserves the important digital arteries and nerves. A **felon** pointing centrally should be drained centrally (Fig 47–18). Fishmouth, lateral, and transverse incisions have made far too many fingertips gangrenous or anesthetic. Division of

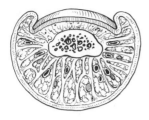

Figure 47—17. Cross-section of distal phalanx.

the vertical fascial fibers on the pulp was recommended in the past but can irretrievably deprive the pad of the tethering it needs for stable pinching.

B. Web Spaces: The web spaces are the path of least resistance for pus from infected distal palm calluses, puncture wounds, and infections of the lumbrical canals. In the case of the thenar space, the thumb web often represents its watershed. A dorsal sagittal incision is usually most desirable between the fingers. A dorsal incision in the web of the thumb may be zigzagged to prevent contracture (Fig 47—10).

C. Midpalmar Space: The midpalmar space becomes infected by direct puncture or by extension of infections from the flexor sheaths of rays II, III, or IV. Only the skin should be incised over the point of fluctuation. The rest of the dissection should be carried out by gentle spreading with a blunt clamp to avoid injury to arteries, nerves, and tendons. Infection spreads easily from this space along the lumbrical canals and to the thenar space.

D. Hypothenar and Thenar Spaces: A hypothenar space abscess is usually a product of a penetrating wound and should be drained where it points. The same is true for a thenar space abscess, which may point in the palm rather than the thumb web.

E. Space of Parona: This space lies over the pronator quadratus beneath the flexor muscles in the distal forearm. Infection here is usually due to extension of pus from the flexor sheaths of the thumb (radial bursa) or little finger (ulnar bursa). Drainage should be along the ulnar side of the forearm deep to the flexor tendons and the ulnar nerve and artery.

F. Dorsal Subaponeurotic and Subcutaneous Spaces: The subaponeurotic space lies deep to the extensor tendons on the back of the hand, and the subcutaneous space is superficial to it. Either or both may become infected by puncture, by open injury, or by extension of infection from the digits and web spaces. Drainage is best done through the dorsoradial side of ray II or the ulnar side of ray V. A superficial transverse incision, sparing the veins, may be made over the metacarpal heads for additional drainage and to allow flexion of the MP joints into the position of function.

Septic Tenosynovitis

Because circulation is limited and easily compromised, the flexor and extensor synovial tendon sheaths (bursae) are most susceptible to infection after contamination and are avenues for the spread of infection. The ulnar bursa extends from the level of the distal joint of the little finger to incorporate all flexors of the other fingers as they pass through the carpal tunnel. Here it often communicates with the radial bursa coming from the thumb. The bursae of the index, long, and ring fingers usually terminate at the mid palm. Intercommunication of bursae is variable. The 6 dorsal tendon compartments under the extensor retinaculum of the wrist have separate synovial bursae (Fig 47—7).

The cardinal sign of tenosynovitis is moderate to severe pain along a given synovial sheath when the tendon therein is made to glide a short distance actively and passively. Passive motion must be performed by touching no more than the patient's fingernail, thus avoiding misdiagnosis by limiting the stimulus to motion of the synovial sheath.

Only unresponsive, tense, and toxic cases need incision and drainage. With rest, elevation, and antibiotics, it is safe to observe most cases for several hours. The preferred method of incision and drainage (Fig 47—19) is to make a short sagittal distal wound immediately over the tendon and introduce a small plastic catheter for irrigating with a solution of antibiotic mixed with lidocaine. Another catheter should

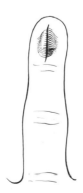

Figure 47—18. Incision of felon (distal fat pad infection).

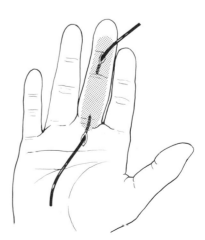

Figure 47—19. Drainage and irrigation for septic tenosynovitis.

be inserted for drainage through a counterincision in the palm. These incisions do not cross flexion creases. The hand should then be elevated and immobilized in the position of function and covered by continuous wet or zinc oxide dressings. Phlegmonous tenosynovitis usually requires opening of the entire synovial sheath (often through a lateral midaxial incision) and, frequently, excision of necrotic tendon and sometimes amputation of a digit.

Bone & Joint Infections

The limited circulation of these structures makes them very susceptible to infection. Any open wound of bone or joint deserves immediate treatment as though infection were already established. Penetrating tooth wound infections (eg, **human bite infections**) are among the most virulent. They often involve the dorsum of the MP and PIP joints as a result of striking a blow with a closed fist. Osteomyelitis responds well to antibiotics and sequestrectomy where indicated.

Miscellaneous Infections

A. Streptococcal Gangrene: This is a very toxic process which causes rapid necrosis of tissues and requires emergency fasciotomy and excision of necrotic tissue, continuous compresses with silver sulfadiazine or zinc oxide ointment or 0.5% silver nitrate solution, and massive antibiotic therapy. Microaerophilic streptococcal infection (Meleney's phagedenic ulcer, sloughing ulcer) is a similar process that must be treated promptly in the same way.

B. Tuberculosis: Tuberculous infection of the hand is usually chronic and may be relatively painless. Some cultures take months to become positive. Tuberculosis commonly involves only one hand, which may be the only focus of infection in the body. Bones and joints may be infected, but the infection more commonly involves the tendon sheaths, which become fused to the tendons. Treatment is by synovectomy and antituberculosis drug therapy for 6–12 months.

C. Leprosy: Leprous neuritis of the median and ulnar nerves causes sensory and motor loss to the hand. Crippling claw deformities develop due to intrinsic muscle palsy. Open sores appear on the hands as a result of trauma to anesthetic digits. Reconstructive surgery and occupational training are required.

D. Fungal Infections: Fungal infections involve primarily the nails. Tinea unguium (onychomycosis) may be caused by many organisms, including *Epidermophyton floccosum,* trichophyton, and *Candida albicans*. Prolonged treatment with antifungal drugs—griseofulvin systemically or nystatin topically—may be necessary, along with daily applications of fungicidal agents such as tolnaftate. Removal of the nail may be an important adjunct to treatment.

E. Herpes Simplex: This should be suspected if there is a history of inordinate pain and the observation of multiple tiny vesicles, usually about the distal phalanx. It is usually self-limiting in about 3 weeks. Idoxuridine ointment applied directly on the opened vesicles may accelerate resolution. Photodynamic in-

activation of the virus is also possible by applying 0.1% proflavine dye to the unroofed vesicles and then exposing the area to incandescent light held a few inches away for 15 minutes on 2 occasions on successive days or twice on the same day.*

F. Rare Infections: Gas gangrene, syphilis, deep fungal infections (eg, coccidioidomycosis, actinomycosis, blastomycosis, sporotrichosis), tularemia, anthrax, yaws, and glanders are diagnosed by means of a pertinent history of exposure, chronicity, and laboratory studies to identify the pathogen.

Felber TD & others: Photodynamic inactivation of herpes simplex. JAMA 223:289, 1973.

Jarratt MT & others: Letter: Dye-photoinactivation and herpes simplex. Arch Dermatol 109:570, 1974.

Lever WF: *Histopathology of the Skin,* 5th ed. Lippincott, 1975.

NONINFECTIOUS INFLAMMATORY DISORDERS

The entities in this group have little in common except a greater or lesser degree of inflammatory or collagen reaction and change. They include wear-and-tear conditions, degenerative states, rheumatic and collagen diseases, and gout. Pain is often the presenting complaint, and there may be a coexisting abnormality of appearance or mechanical function.

CONSTRICTIVE CONDITIONS

In stenosing tenosynovitis there is a disproportion between the clearance inside a tendon pulley or tunnel and the diameter of the tendon or tendons that must glide through it. Any pulley or tunnel may be incriminated. The more common sites are as follows:

(1) The proximal digital pulleys in the distal palm, causing **trigger finger** (stenosing flexor tenosynovitis). The manifestations are local tenderness of the pulley; pain, which may be referred to the PIP joint; and (usually but not always) locking of the digit in flexion with a painful jog as it goes into extension (ie, as the bulge in the tendon passes through the tight pulley).

(2) The pulley over the radial styloid housing the abductor pollicis longus and extensor pollicis brevis, causing **De Quervain's tenosynovitis**. Local tenderness and pain occur if these tendons are actively or passively stretched.

*The question of possible carcinogenicity of this method of treatment is being debated. Incandescent light is said to be superior to fluorescent light because of the heat produced.

(3) The volar carpal ligament, causing **carpal tunnel syndrome.** The "soft" median nerve is compressed against the ligament by the 9 "hard" tendons in the tunnel with it. Mild compression causes disturbance of sleep by aching and numbness over the distribution of the nerve, but always sparing the little finger. Severe constriction causes constant hypesthesia as well as paralysis of the abductor pollicis brevis.

(4) **Ulnar nerve compression** (less common) occurs as the nerve passes behind the medial epicondyle (the cubital tunnel), between the heads of the flexor carpi ulnaris, or along Guyon's canal from the pisiform bone to the hook of the hamate. The diagnosis is based on a knowledge of the anatomy of innervation.

Electromyography and nerve conduction studies may be helpful in evaluating nerve compressions.

These disorders may be congenital; may be due to chronic adaptive hypertrophy of tendon and pulley alike in response to work or repetitive activity; or may be due to aging. They can occur at any age. Other factors are distortion caused by trauma, tumor, or rheumatoid synovitis or nodules.

Relief can be achieved by local injections of triamcinolone or dexamethasone mixed with lidocaine or by means of surgical section of the constricting pulley or tunnel. Local injections may be tried 3—4 times at weekly intervals before resorting to surgery, which involves a hazard of sensitive scar or prolonged weakness. A disabling complication of surgery for De Quervain's tenosynovitis is a very painful neuroma of the radial nerve. Immediate surgery is justified if the constriction is so tight that no tendon glide is possible and in cases of unrelenting motor or sensory nerve impairment, irreversible rheumatoid or nonspecific synovial thickening, or other space-consuming lesions.

Surgery must never be done without a tourniquet or blindly. Adequate proximal and distal decompression is essential. If the epineurial sheath is also thickened or a nerve has an hourglass constriction, endoneurolysis is in order.

DUPUYTREN'S CONTRACTURE
(Palmar Fasciitis)

The cause of this common disorder among Caucasian populations is not known. It occurs in one of 3 types (acute, subacute, and chronic), predominantly in males over 50 who have been in sedentary occupations, and is bilateral in about half of cases. There is a hereditary influence, and the incidence is higher among alcoholics and patients with chronic illnesses. The contracture may develop in women who do not work and (in laborers) in the hand that does the least work, so that it is not considered work-related. It is frequently found in the plantar fascia of the instep and occasionally in the penis (Peyronie's disease).

Dupuytren's contracture manifests itself most commonly in the palm by thickening, which may be nodular, and therefore mistaken for a callosity; or cord-like, and therefore mistaken for a tendon abnormality because it passes into the digits and restricts their extension. This process typically involves the longitudinal and vertical components of the fascia but at times seems to exist apart from anatomically distinct fascia. The skin may fuse with it and become raised and rock-hard, or it may be greatly shrunken and sometimes drawn into a deeply puckered crevasse. It invades the palm but is never adherent to vessels, nerves, or musculotendinous structures. It has an unpredictable rate of progression, but the earlier it starts in life the more destructive and recurrent it is apt to be.

Dupuytren's contracture may involve the fascia of any digit or web space, but it affects predominantly the ring and little fingers. In long-standing cases the fingers may be drawn tightly into the palm, resulting in secondary cicatrization of joint ligaments and capsules and flexor tendon sheaths or atrophic muscle fibrosis.

Surgery is indicated when the disorder has progressed sufficiently. The patient must be warned about the increasing technical difficulty with progressive flexion and adduction contractures and the potential for recurrence after surgery. Fasciectomy is the surgical procedure that gives the best long-term results. In selected cases where only the longitudinal pretendinous fascial band is involved and the skin moves freely over it, subcutaneous fasciotomy done through a small longitudinal incision may release a contracture quite well with only a few days of postoperative disability. In the occasional case with acute and rapid onset of a tender nodule, local triamcinolone may be used for not only subjective but even objective relief.

Depending upon the amount of cutaneous shrinkage, skin grafts may be required for wound closure after fasciectomy. The overlying dermis has been implicated as an inductive mechanism in this process. Thus, skin grafting may diminish the recurrence rate in severe cases. The hopelessly contracted little finger must sometimes be amputated.

Motion should be started within 3—5 days after surgery. Dynamic splints and postoperative injection of corticosteroids into joints and the zone of surgery may help the well-motivated patient.

The complications of surgery are digital infarction and ischemic skin flaps, hematoma formation, fibrosis and stiffness, anesthesia or neuromatous pain, and recurrence of fasciitis and contracture. In general, the functional reward to the patient is great at any age.

Davis JE: On surgery of Dupuytren's contracture. Plast Reconstr Surg 36:277, 1965.

Hueston JT, Tubiana R: *Dupuytrens Disease,* 2nd ed. Grune & Stratton, 1974.

DEGENERATIVE OSTEOARTHRITIS

This is a common condition in people over age 40. It affects women more often than men and involves primarily the digital interphalangeal joints and the basal (MC) joint of the thumb. Heberden's nodes of hypertrophic bone cause typical bossing with occasional associated dorsal synovial cyst (mucous cyst) formation of the distal joints. Such cysts (really ganglions) may press on the nail matrix and cause longitudinal grooving of the fingernail. If they are excised, magnification should be used. The subjacent bony spur which is often present may be excised to prevent recurrence. Doing so may cause an acute arthritic flare. Joint deformity, pain, and stiffness may be treated by replacement of the joint with a prosthetic silicone rubber joint spacer or hinge (see below) or by joint fusion.

RHEUMATOID DISEASE

This disease of unknown cause affects all the tissues of mesenchymal origin in the hand, especially the synovial tissues. The x-ray changes vary from early marginal joint erosion with associated osteoporosis to advanced destructive changes and subluxation, particularly of the wrist and the MP and PIP joints. The disease often starts in the hands and involves the synovia of joints and tendons. Initially there is vague pain of insidious (sometimes acute) onset, swelling, stiffness, and local hyperthermia. In time, thickening of synovial tissues about the joints and tendons causes destruction and distortion. Tendons may rupture, especially where frayed by bone changes. Rheumatoid granulomatous nodules develop in the substance of tendons and tendon sheaths and subcutaneously over bony prominences. Stretched ligaments and retinacular tissues can no longer maintain the alignment of joints and tendons against the mean pulling forces, and a host of digital deformities may develop (swan-neck or boutonniere deformity, ulnar drift, and "intrinsic plus" deformity). With intrinsic muscle fibrosis and advanced joint destruction, many of these deformities become fixed.

The ideal management of these cases consists of combined medical and surgical supervision and guidance. It is always hoped that physical and emotional rest, heat, analgesia, therapeutic exercise, and anti-inflammatory agents (eg, aspirin, corticosteroids, gold salts) will check the progression of disease. When these measures are not successful, the surgeon should offer surgical procedures (synovectomy, arthroplasty, tenoplasty, resection of nodules, arthrodesis, ulnar styloidectomy, etc) which may forestall further destruction and preserve function and cosmetic appearance.

The problems amenable to surgical correction are the following: (1) Boggy synovitis about flexor and extensor tendons. (2) Boggy synovitis of wrist or digital joints. (3) Rheumatoid nodules. (4) Tendon rupture (mainly of the extensors of the ring and little fingers, and the flexor of the thumb). (5) Constrictive conditions (stenosing tenosynovitis and median and ulnar nerve compression syndromes). (6) Joint erosions, subluxations, and fixed deformities.

• • •

Silicone Rubber Implants

Made of heat-vulcanized, medical grade silicone elastomer stock, these implants ("joint spacers") were developed for arthritic joint and carpal bone replacement. They have been effectively time-tested for replacement of the MP and PIP joints, the trapezium, scaphoid, and lunate bones as well as the ulnar styloid and radial head. If there has been much soft tissue reconstruction, immobilization is continued for 4–6 weeks; if not, motion may be guardedly initiated in 3 or 4 days with 24-hour dynamic splinting for 3 weeks and nighttime dynamic splinting for an additional 3 weeks. The removal of carpal bones can be difficult and hazardous. Postoperative immobilization should be maintained for 4–6 weeks.

Flatt AE: *The Care of the Rheumatoid Hand.* Mosby, 1963.
Millender LH, Nalebuff EA: Reconstructive surgery in the rheumatoid hand. Orthop Clin North Am 6:709, 1975.
Swanson AB: Flexible implant arthroplasty for arthritic finger joints: Rationale, technic, and results of treatment. J Bone Joint Surg 54A:435, 1972.
Swanson AB: *Flexible Implant Resection Arthroplasty in the Hand and Extremities.* Mosby, 1973.
Swanson AB: Silicone rubber implants for replacement of arthritic or destroyed joints in the hand. Surg Clin North Am 48:1113, 1968.

SCLERODERMA, LUPUS ERYTHEMATOSUS, & SARCOIDOSIS

These systemic diseases of unknown cause have distinctive—though not necessarily pathognomonic—manifestations in the hands.

Scleroderma initially produces joint stiffness, hyperhidrosis, and Raynaud's phenomenon. Unchecked, it leads to marked tautness of skin and rigidity of joints with associated osteoporosis (even absolution of the distal phalanges) and soft tissue calcifications.

Lupus erythematosus, which may be initiated or aggravated by certain drugs, foreign proteins, or psychic states, often causes polyarthritis indistinguishable from that of rheumatoid arthritis. It does not usually lead to similar joint destruction.

Sarcoidosis may produce digital nodules and articular swellings, and x-rays may show small punched-out lesions, particularly of the phalanges.

GOUT

Gout is a metabolic disorder of uric acid metabolism which affects about 1% of the population; approximately 50% of patients with gout have cheiragra (gouty hands).

The diagnosis is suggested by a sudden onset of severe pain and inflammatory signs about the joints and musculotendinous structures. The usual duration of an attack is 5–10 days. The serum uric acid is elevated in 75% of cases. Gout may coexist with rheumatoid disease. The diagnosis is confirmed by identification of uric acid crystals in joint fluid or tissue biopsy.

In time, typical tophi form, consisting of toothpaste-like infiltrates of urate crystals, arising in multilobulated form about soft tissue structures that have been invaded. X-rays show characteristic punched-out lesions at the margins of articular cartilage.

Prophylactic treatment of gouty arthritis consists of diet, colchicine, allopurinol (a urate-blocking agent) or probenecid (a uricosuric agent), and avoidance of stress. Colchicine, 0.6 mg/hour with a glass of water for 6–8 doses or to the point of gastrointestinal distress, is the time-honored means of interrupting an attack, but phenylbutazone, corticotropin gel, and corticosteroids are also of value.

Surgical measures consist of drainage of abscessed tophi and tophectomy. The latter procedure is more often of cosmetic than functional value. Tophectomy consists of removal of as much tophaceous material as can be fairly easily recovered, being sure not to destroy ligaments, tenoretinacular structures, nerves, and vessels in the process.

BURNS OF THE HAND

The hands are a common site of thermal (including frictional), electrical, chemical, and radiation burns. Function is imperiled in all instances by swelling and scar formation. Prompt measures to preserve existing function are often urgently required. Delay may lead to irreversible impairment and deformity. Burn therapy is covered in Chapter 17.

The urgent objective of treatment of burns of the hand is to restore mobility as soon as possible (within 1–3 weeks) by the following measures: (1) Control of swelling (by elevation, fasciotomy, and escharotomy). (2) Control of pain (by cold compresses, elevation, analgesics, and grafting). (3) Prevention of infection (by topical anti-infective agents), immediate or early grafting, and control of congestion. (4) Prompt (even primary) debridement followed by grafting as soon as oozing has stopped and the wound appears ready.

The burned hand should be covered with a clean (if possible, sterile), dry dressing and the patient transported as soon as possible to the hospital emergency department. No treatment is required for first degree burns. Second degree burns should be debrided if blisters are bulky or already broken. Burns involving 2.5 sq cm or more may then be covered with a biologic dressing, if available, such as allograft (homograft) or xenograft (which are bacteriostatic) or amniotic membrane. All of these effectively control pain. Pigskin is an ideal xenograft (heterograft). If grafts are not available, an ideal emollient is silver sulfadiazine or a thick coating of zinc oxide ointment. Motion is encouraged from the beginning, whereas dependency and the "position of injury" are discouraged. Splinting at night may be useful. When the epithelium no longer weeps, lanolin may be applied.

A deep second degree burn or third degree burn which involves one-third to one-half or more of the surface area of a digit, hand, or forearm usually causes enough swelling to threaten loss of function. Hand swelling is greatest on the dorsum, where the skin is loose and the space beneath will accommodate a lot of water. This forces MP joint extension and thumb adduction, creating "a claw hand in disguise." The burned part must be constantly and carefully watched. If elevation alone is not effective and the patient becomes less able than formerly to close his fist and touch his thumb to his little finger—or if throbbing pain progresses followed by numbness—then immediate bedside escharotomy with biologic dressing and prompt operating room debridement and grafting must be considered. Brawny induration must be prevented.

When motion is being lost or is already lost, it is far better to debride skin primarily or within the first week and have the hand grafted and mobilized within 10 days than to anxiously await for 3–4 weeks the possible survival of the burned skin at the expense of cicatrix formation and immobility.

After debridement with a dermatome or scalpel, the ooze usually precludes immediate grafting. This, therefore, should be deferred for 24 hours. Postage stamp, mesh, or sheet grafts that are thin (0.2–0.25 mm) are most apt to take and should be used over beds of equivocal graft-sustaining quality. Wet dressings protected by plastic and a padded boxing glove cast for 1 or 2 days are used for immobilization. If open treatment is used, a conscientious attendant must daily remove any serum collections from beneath the graft.

Prolonged splinting should be avoided as much as possible except when the patient is resting or sleeping. At these times the hand should be propped up comfortably on pillows to keep it higher than the level of the heart. Isoprene splinting material is ideal for this purpose because it can be sterilized and heat-molded to fit the patient. The position of function must be maintained in modeling any splint, and constrictive wrappings must never be used. Hanging the extremity by a noose is to be condemned unless a long arm cast is applied with the elbow at 90 degrees. Elastic bandages are also dangerously constrictive.

Fourth degree burns are usually associated with extensive second and third degree burns. The charred elements should be excised as soon as the general condition of the patient allows and the wounds closed as soon as possible.

Restoration of movement. The patient with a burned hand must be helped and encouraged to move every joint of the upper extremity as soon and as often after injury as possible.

Reconstructive Procedures

The proper initial care can prevent or limit many but not all of the functional disabilities caused by burns. The hand surgeon can do much by individualized procedures to reduce the extent of some of these disabilities. Resurfacing is accomplished with split thickness grafts for appearance, with full thickness grafts for release of flexion and web contractures, and with pedicle grafts when better padding is needed. Joints may be freed by capsulotomies and tenotomies, or they may be fixed permanently in a functional attitude by arthrodesis.

Cosmesis and function can be well served by amputation. A ray resection of a useless index finger may greatly compensate for a thumb web contracture.

Electrical Burns

High-voltage injuries to the extremity may be of great but hidden magnitude. Beneath the skin sleeve, extensive coagulation necrosis of vessels, nerves, and musculotendinous structures may be present, and its extent may not become manifest for several days. Electrical contact points usually have third degree skin burns. The treatment parallels that described for injection injuries (see p 1014). It is not uncommon to have to amputate a hand or arm that has been damaged by an electrical burn. Early decompression by incisions of the skin and underlying fascia may limit progressive injury secondary to congestion.

TUMORS & PSEUDOTUMORS OF THE HAND

Except for squamous cell carcinoma of the dorsal skin, malignancy in the hand is rare. A variety of lesions are found in the hand, including hematomas, scars, calluses, warts, nevi, cysts, xanthomas, enchondromas, giant cell tumors, fibromas, hemangiomas, carcinomas, and sarcomas. Squamous cell and basal cell carcinomas and melanomas are discussed in Chapters 46 and 49.

Ganglion & Mucous Cyst

Where there is a synovial lining, a protrusion may develop followed by later isolation of a closed pouch or cul-de-sac to form a cyst filled with the physiologic lubricant fluid of joints and tendons. The old concept of "mucoid degeneration" and development from embryologic cell rests has now been abandoned. If absorption of water occurs, the cyst will have a jellylike consistency. Sudden, forceful bending of a joint may cause extrusion of the cyst between ligamentous fibers and the sudden appearance of a lump. More frequently, the cyst appears insidiously. Pain may be caused by tension within the cyst and pressure on adjacent tissues.

Most ganglions arise from the joints of the wrist, but any joint and tendon sheath can give rise to one. The path followed is along the tissue planes of least resistance. The length and pathway of a stalk are unpredictable. When there is protrusion through more than one fibrous tissue plane, the cyst may have an hourglass configuration.

A volar wrist ganglion always deserves a careful preoperative test of collateral arterial competency (Allen's test) to ensure good digital circulation if one artery must be divided in removing the ganglion. A flexor sheath ganglion is usually like a "pebble in the shoe." It may be mistaken for a sesamoid.

Treatment of a ganglion is not indicated unless the patient insists. Aspiration through a large-bore needle under lidocaine anesthesia followed by injection of triamcinolone may sustain many in remission. Some claim "cure" by this procedure. Flexor sheath ganglions of the digit that are off center should not be so treated, for in such cases the nerve and artery may be injured by the needle.

If surgery is required, the cyst should be removed unruptured until the joint or tendon sheath is entered and resection is completed without trauma to surrounding nerves or tendons. Recurrence and complications are usually caused by failure to use magnification, to explore adequately, and to visualize "satellite cysts" as one enters the joint.

Inclusion Cyst

Injury can carry viable epidermal cells deep to the dermis, into fat, or even into bone. With growth of these cells, keratinized cells accumulate into a ball or cyst which compresses the tissue in which it lies. Bone may become eroded. At surgery, an inclusion cyst looks like a pearl and has a soft thin wall that surrounds its cheesy contents. If it is totally enucleated from its bed, it will not recur.

Posttraumatic Neuroma

This common lump only presents for treatment when it is painful. Such will be the case if it lies on a hard surface (eg, tendon or bone) at a point of pressure, or when it is trapped in scar tissue and subjected to stretching. (The treatment of neuromas is described in Chapter 40.)

Xanthoma (Giant Cell Tumor of Soft Tissue)

This is a hard, often multinodular tumor which arises from the fibrous flexor sheath or collateral ligaments. Even though benign, it extends under tendons and collateral ligaments and through joints. Unless all of the brownish-yellow tumor is removed, the tumor may recur.

Enchondroma, Giant Cell Tumor of Bone, & Aneurysmal Bone Cyst

Enchondromas constitute 90% of true bone tumors of the hand. The classic finding is calcific stippling of the lytic bone defect, most common in the proximal phalanges and distal half of the metacarpals.

The carpal bones are spared. Aneurysmal bone cysts and giant cell tumors of bone are practically identical except for their vascularity. Pathologic fracture may be the presenting finding.

Treatment consists of curettement of the contents and wall of the lesion followed by packing of the hole with tiny cortical chips from the proximal third of the ulna.

Lipoma

This tumor usually occurs on the volar aspect of the digit or palm. If the proper plane is followed in the dissection, the lesion can be easily enucleated. Caution must be taken during dissection when these are adjacent to major nerves.

Neurofibroma

Most of these tumors are multiple (Recklinghausen's disease) and consist of thickened nerve sheath elements. There is a rare tendency to malignant degeneration. The usual indication for resection of this tumor is cosmetic. It should be enucleated under magnification so as to spare the nerve. If growth is rapid, malignancy should be suspected and a long segment of the nerve resected or amputation contemplated.

Hemangioma

Hemangiomas in infants should never be treated by irradiation. The common strawberry angiomas will involute after their initial growth period. If the angioma is rapidly enlarging, it may be induced to involute by a course of corticosteroid therapy. In the older patient (and a few infants), surgical removal is the only means of treatment. Angiography may be helpful in determining the nature and extent of this group of tumors. They may be located primarily in skin, fat, or muscle, or, in the case of a cavernous hemangioma, may extend throughout all tissues and be impossible to totally remove without amputation or destroying digital or hand function.

Actinic Keratosis & Bowen's Disease

These lesions respond well to topical fluorouracil (5-FU), 2–5% solution in propylene glycol. Bowen's lesions are usually found on the dorsum of the hands in persons exposed chronically to sunlight, and present as blotchy, hyperkeratotic, scaling, reddened areas.

Glomus Tumor

This rare tumor, comprised of blood vessels and unmyelinated nerves of a heat-regulating arteriovenous shunt, may cause extremely severe pain. It can develop anywhere but is most dramatic under the fingernail, where "pinpoint" pressure initiates the pain. Half of patients may have no symptoms except the visible or palpable lesion. Treatment consists of meticulous dissection and total excision under magnification.

COMPLEX INJURIES OF THE HAND

GENERAL PLAN OF MANAGEMENT

Sudden physical or functional loss of part or all of the hand or arm is a shocking experience that deserves special recognition and attention on the part of the surgeon. Psychologic and physical comfort should be given, and the patient must be spared alarming comments as well as any false hopes of reimplantation or salvage.

Amputation may be physical or functional. Injury and disease may functionally (though not physically) amputate by crushing, mangling, paralyzing, stiffening, causing pain, or otherwise destroying all or part of the hand beyond hope of useful recovery. In such cases, salvage may be impossible and surgical amputation is justified to improve the overall physical and psychologic effectiveness of the patient.

Referral

In referring cases, the injured part should be comfortably aligned and splinted without constriction. Bleeding should be controlled by compression or by ligation of the bleeder provided it is adequately exposed under tourniquet ischemia and loupe magnification to avoid injuring adjacent nerves. Wet dressings should be applied to open wounds to facilitate sequestration of blood and serum, and the extremity should be comfortably elevated. In the case of open injuries, prophylactic antibiotics should be given. An amputated part may be irrigated and, if possible, placed in a container or plastic bag on ice. Even if reimplantation is not feasible, tissue (eg, skin or bone) from the ablated part is sometimes of value in primary or secondary reconstructive procedures.

In Vivo Tissue Bank

A "nearly amputated," badly crushed, or mangled digit, hand, or arm may present a great challenge to good judgment and to the surgeon's technical skill in acting on a decision to attempt salvage. Viable structures and tissues can often be reimplanted or transferred to give maximal restoration of function, ie, the patient can serve as his own "in vivo tissue bank" if the surgeon keeps a functionally irretrievable digit or other forearm or hand structure alive for use elsewhere in reconstruction.

Assessment of Problem

These injuries notoriously cause multilevel and multitissue involvement ("common wound"). All structures are congealed in the reactive process, culminating in a common scar (callus) with loss of structural independence.

The surgeon must individualize the treatment of complex hand injuries by considering such factors as age, occupation, hand dominance, economic status, cosmesis, emotional makeup, and general health. In other words, adequate salvage and maximal salvage are relative to the patient's needs, desires, and capacities. An extensive reconstructive effort is justified if, without it, there will be little or no function; but one must be careful not to destroy existing function and to spare the patient unwarranted disability and expense by heroic efforts that might fail. It is sometimes best to remove part or all of the hand in the interest of the patient's overall psychologic and functional competence and productivity.

FOREIGN BODIES

Foreign bodies should be removed only if they interfere with function, cause symptoms, or result in dead space or infection. If removal is necessary, it is often facilitated by a period of observation and waiting (eg, 2–3 weeks) until congestion and bloody extravasation have cleared. In the meantime, the hand should be initially splinted, elevated, and, in some cases, drained. Prophylactic antibiotics should be given.

AMPUTATION

Management of the Stump

The surgical objective in amputating a part is to create a painless stump with soft tissue cover which will meet the functional needs of the patient and will have good sensibility and adequate stability and pliability. Digital amputation will either be transverse or will face obliquely to the dorsal, volar, radial, or ulnar aspects of the digit (Fig 47–20). It may involve more than one phalanx.

When sufficient stump cover is not available locally, it must be obtained from grafts and flaps. The most predictable take is achieved by a thin (0.2–0.25 mm) split thickness graft; this should always be the first choice if there is any doubt about blood supply, infection, or joint stiffness. Sutures are not needed except in large grafts; however, initial immobilization and elevation of the wrist as well as the digit are vital in achieving a take of the graft.

Primary and secondary advancement or pedicle grafts should be considered when it is necessary to give better skin cover over volar-oblique surfaces of all digits, the radial-oblique surface of the fingers, and the ulnar-oblique surface of the thumb (Fig 47–21); when one does not want to shorten digital bone on a transverse amputation surface; or when it is necessary to cover the body of the hand. Transverse digital stumps of infants will close by secondary intention with a result equal to or better than what can be achieved by surgery.

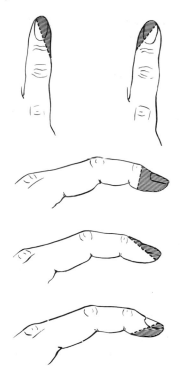

Figure 47–20. Distal digit amputation.

Indications for Amputation

Irreversible ischemia is the only absolute indication for amputation. The other major indication is where salvage of the digit or part of it will threaten the overall function of the hand, the extremity, or the patient. Such may be the case with an overwhelmingly injured or infected finger which is hopelessly stiff or painful and may jeopardize the function of the other good fingers, or with malignant tumor (eg, malignant melanoma).

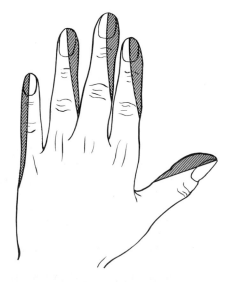

Figure 47–21. Areas requiring padded skin.

Degloving Injuries

These injuries are usually caused by having a ring torn violently from a digit, eg, in falling from a fence and simultaneously hooking the ring on a prong. The skin, fat, and neurovascular bundles are ripped off, and flexor tendons may be avulsed along with the middle and distal phalanges. The other digits are usually not injured. The best treatment is usually to amputate. One has a choice of primary ray amputation or amputation through the proximal phalanx. Salvage and reconstruction are possible only rarely and involve a great deal of time, with several major surgical procedures and some jeopardy to the function of adjacent normal digits.

Amputation of Rays III & IV

Amputation of the long or ring finger causes a gap through which material and liquids in the cupped hand will escape. This gap can be closed by removing the metacarpal at its proximal third (ray resection) and allowing the adjacent metacarpal heads to be approximated; or by the central transplantation of an adjacent osteotomized metacarpal onto the stump of the resected metacarpal (ray transfer). When the index, long, and ring fingers are gone, rotation osteotomy of the fifth metacarpal may be needed so that the little fingertip can comfortably oppose the thumb.

Thumb Amputation

Because most skills of man are hampered by loss of part or all of the thumb, preservation, reconstruction, or replacement of a thumb has great functional merit. The prime objectives are the preservation of length, the proper placement for opposition, and provision of a stable strut against which the fingers can flex with force. Ideally, there should be sensibility where the thumb and fingers meet in pinch, and this can be provided with a neurovascular island pedicle transfer. Not so urgent (but desirable) are motion and power, particularly to control all the planes of movement of the metacarpal-carpal joint. If this exists, bone-strutted tube pedicle thumb reconstruction—or a digital transfer (pollicization) on a neurovascular pedicle—can compensate remarkably for a loss.

WRINGER, CRUSH, & COMPRESSION INJURIES

In wringer injury, part or all of the extremity is dragged into and compressed by one or more machine-driven rollers. It is common in industries where rolls or sheets of material are drawn between rollers for threading, printing, or compressing purposes or where conveyor belts are used.

The arm is advanced until anatomic obstruction is met. Avulsion of skin and fat or a friction burn of the tissues (or both) may result. The thumb web is the first common obstruction, and the dorsal hand skin then becomes avulsed or burned. The next obstruction is the elbow, and the last the axilla.

Vessels, nerves, and muscles may be avulsed and bones may be dislocated or broken. The most common unrecognized complication is secondary congestion, which can lead to paralysis and severe muscle fibrosis (eg, Volkmann's contracture) and joint stiffness.

Most patients should be hospitalized, kept flat in bed with the extremity comfortably elevated, and observed hourly. Progressive throbbing pain leading to anesthesia and tightness of the skin and fascia sleeves of the finger, hand, or arm requires longitudinal slitting of skin and fascia. More than one muscle compartment may need decompression, and the pronator teres muscle and transverse carpal ligament must sometimes be sectioned to liberate the median nerve.

Skin avulsed by the wringer is usually in the form of a retrograde flap with imperiled circulation to it. One must judge the color by capillary filling of the flap; if this is poor or absent, debride all the fat from the flap and apply it as a full thickness graft, or discard it completely in favor of a primary or delayed split thickness skin graft. In most cases, fractures and dislocations should be reduced and aligned, but the overall circulation of the extremity is of more initial concern than definitive management of specific tissue and structural injuries. Abrasion burns are often third degree and, if so, require debridement and grafting when the integrity of the circulation is restored.

INJECTION INJURIES

These injuries are caused by the sudden introduction of substances under high pressure (ie, hundreds or thousands of pounds per square inch). The substances include air or other gases; liquids such as water, paint, oil, and a host of chemicals in various solutions; and solids and semisolids such as grease and molten plastic. Accordingly, these accidents occur principally in industry. Air pressure hoses in gasoline service stations, aerosol bombs, and sandblast hoses are typical sources of gas-driven injuries. Paint guns, oil and grease guns, and nozzles that inject molten plastic at high temperatures (eg, 260 C [500 F]) are among the most common other sources of these injuries.

The history is the most important clue to the severity of the injury and the need for immediate treatment. While operating a high-pressure device, the patient suddenly feels a strange sensation which ranges from very painful to not painful at all. He may present a totally normal-appearing hand with perhaps an almost undetectable pinpoint injection site; or the hand may be discolored or pale and cold, and tensely swollen due to the injected material.

Sometimes the injection is limited to a single digit, but often the great pressure forces the material to spread widely throughout the hand and even into the forearm. The greatest problems stem from the following: (1) The chemical irritant effect on all tissues, causing vascular thrombosis and toxic inflammation and necrosis. (2) The primary congestion effect of the material, leading within minutes or hours to secondary congestion due to the inflammatory response, all of which first interrupts venous flow and then leads to arterial arrest and gangrene. (3) Thermal burns (eg, from hot plastic). (4) Inability to remove enough of the offending material to forestall a short-term or long-term foreign body response, which ultimately leads to fibrosis that is so extensive that it destroys the functions of sensation and mobility.

The examination should include an immediate x-ray to demonstrate, if possible, the distribution of material or gas in the hand; and a careful evaluation of sensibility, tenderness, induration, crepitation, color, temperature, and mobility. All such cases require immediate and continued unrelenting scrutiny, even if the part seems completely normal. With evidence of retained foreign material causing swelling, ischemia, or progressive throbbing pain, the hand must be immediately explored if for no other reason than to release the tourniquet effect of the skin and fascia induced by the congestion. It is impossible to remove all of the foreign material when it is widespread and invasive. As much should be removed as can be done by gentle scraping and teasing—and resecting that which lies in bloodless tissue—as long as one does not further damage the viable tissues to the point of greater congestion or ischemia and interfere with the normal process of demarcation and sequestration.

In addition to appropriate decompression and debridement, the hand must be drained and covered with compresses of zinc oxide, silver sulfadiazine, Ringer's solution, or 0.5% silver nitrate solution. The hand must be held in the position of function and elevated, with the patient kept supine. Prophylactic antisludging agents (dextran 40), corticosteroids, antibiotics, and antitetanus medication must be administered. In most instances, hospitalization is urgent.

The objective is to minimize loss of function, and the most important initial effort must be to preserve circulation and avoid infection. If only one digit is involved and its functional fate is hopeless, amputation may be the most expeditious means of treatment.

Silsby JN: Pressure gun injuries of the hand. West J Med 125:271, 1976.

* * *

General References

Beasley RW: Principles and techniques of resurfacing operations for hand surgery. Surg Clin North Am 47:389, 1967.

Beasley RW: Symposium on the hand. Orthop Clin North Am 1:2, 1970.

Boyes JH: *Bunnell's Surgery of the Hand,* 5th ed. Lippincott, 1972.

Chase RA: Surgery of the hand. (Medical Progress articles in 2 parts.) N Engl J Med 287:1174, 1227, 1972.

Chase RA, Laub D: The hand: Therapeutic strategy for acute problems. Curr Probl Surg, June 1966.

Converse JM: Symposium on reconstructive surgery. Surg Clin North Am 47:2, 1967.

Correa LG: *Cirugia de la Mano, IMSS.* Seguridad Para Todos. Mexico, 1971.

Cramer LM, Chase RA: *Symposium on the Hand.* III. Educational Foundations of the American Society of Plastic and Reconstructive Surgeons. Mosby, 1971.

Dunphy JE, Van Winkle HW Jr: *Repair and Regeneration.* McGraw-Hill, 1969.

Eaton RG: *Joint Injuries of the Hand.* Thomas, 1971.

Entin MA: Symposium on practical surgery of the hand. Surg Clin North Am 44:4, 1964.

Entin MA: Symposium on practical surgery of the hand. Surg Clin North Am 48:5, 1968.

Flatt AE: *The Care of Minor Hand Injuries,* 3rd ed. Mosby, 1972.

Flynn JE: *Hand Surgery.* Williams & Wilkins, 1966.

Grabb WC, Smith JW: Hand and upper extremity plastic surgery. Part IV in: *Plastic Surgery: A Concise Guide to Clinical Practice,* 2nd ed. Little, Brown, 1973.

Kilgore ES, Graham WP: *The Hand: Surgical and Non-surgical Management.* Lea & Febiger, 1977.

Kilgore ES, Newmeyer WL: Hand surgery. Chap 17 in: *Handbook of Surgery,* 5th ed. Wilson JL (editor). Lange, 1973.

Littler JW: The hand and upper extremity. Vol IV, Part 3, in: *Reconstructive Plastic Surgery.* Converse JM (editor). Saunders, 1964.

Marble HC: *The Hand: A Manual and Atlas for the General Surgeon.* Saunders, 1960.

Milford L: The hand. Chap 4 in: *Campbell's Operative Orthopedics.* Vol 1. Crenshaw AH (editor). Mosby, 1971.

Nichols HM: *Manual of Hand Injuries,* 2nd ed. Year Book, 1960.

Peacock EE, Van Winkle W Jr: *Surgery and Biology of Wound Repair.* Saunders, 1970.

Rank BK, Wakefield AR: *Surgery of Repair as Applied to Hand Injuries,* 2nd ed. Williams & Wilkins, 1960.

Schneewind JH: Surgical emergencies of the hand. Surg Clin North Am 52:203, 1972.

Seddon H: *Surgical Disorders of the Peripheral Nerves.* Williams & Wilkins, 1972.

Verdan C: Basic principles in surgery of the hand. Surg Clin North Am 47:355, 1967.

48 . . .
Pediatric Surgery

Alfred A. deLorimier, MD

The surgical treatment of infants and children has advanced in recent years because of refinements in both surgical technic and in pre- and postoperative care. Physiologic norms in the young are now better understood than formerly. The newborn infant with a surgical lesion often has other disorders that are a threat to survival. Problems such as the difference between the small premature baby and the intrauterine deprived baby, the significance and treatment of hypoglycemia or hypocalcemia, and the metabolic and cardiopulmonary consequences of respiratory insufficiency are now better recognized. The vital functions of the critically ill infant can now be monitored, and the same intensive care can be applied that has been provided for adult patients.

CARE OF THE NEWBORN

Transportation of Newborn Surgical Patients

When transporting newborn infants for surgery, the following precautions must be observed: (1) Support normal body temperature by using an incubator maintained at 34 C (93.2 F). (2) Keep the airway clear by supplying a bulb syringe to aspirate mucus and vomitus. (3) Keep the stomach empty by giving nothing by mouth. Infants with intestinal obstruction should have a nasogastric tube placed in the stomach and aspirated at frequent intervals. (4) Provide proper identification and pertinent medical information if the infant is to be transported to a pediatric surgical center.

Determination of Gestational Age

Infants with surgically treatable lesions frequently weigh less than 2500 g. It is important to distinguish premature infants from "intrauterine growth-retarded infants." Premature infants have a high incidence of hyaline membrane disease, whereas growth-retarded infants are subject to intrauterine asphyxia with meconium aspiration, pneumothorax, and hypoglycemia and frequently have major congenital anomalies. The gestational age of the infant is calculated from the date of the last normal menstrual period. The weight

of the baby can be correlated with the gestational age, and intrauterine growth retardation is defined as birth weight below the 25th percentile for the gestational age (Fig 48–1).

Five signs may be useful in assessing gestational age. Infants of 36 weeks' gestational age or less have (1) fine fuzzy hair, (2) ears that lack cartilaginous support, (3) a breast nodule less than 3 mm in diameter, (4) testicles in the inguinal canal and a small scrotum with few rugae, and (5) skin on the feet with few transverse creases confined to the balls of the feet anteriorly.

Battaglia FC, Lubchenco LO: A practical classification of newborn infants by weight and gestational age. J Pediatr 71:159, 1967.

Usher R, McLean F, Scott KE: Judgement of fetal age. 2. Clinical significance of gestational age and an objective method for its assessment. Pediatr Clin North Am 13:835, 1966.

Temperature Loss & Regulation

A. Simple Heat Loss: Infants and children have a relatively greater body surface area and thinner subcutaneous fat than adults. Therefore, heat loss by conduction and radiation may be 4 times that of the adult. Infants respond to hypothermia by norepinephrine secretion that increases the metabolic rate in most tissues, particularly the myocardium, and produces vasoconstriction with impaired tissue perfusion and increased lactic acid production which may result in shock and cardiac arrest. The neutral thermal environmental temperature occurs when the oxygen consumption of the infant is minimal, ie, when the gradient between the skin surface (particularly the face) and the environmental temperature is less than 1.5 C (2.7 F). The optimal environmental temperature should be 34 C (93.2 F) (slightly higher environmental temperatures are required for premature infants). Although the environmental temperature can be servo-controlled from skin or rectal temperature, it is difficult to detect fever or hypothermia due to sepsis by this technic.

B. Effect of Drugs: Depressant and anesthetic drugs abolish the thermoregulatory response of the patient, and oxygen consumption will decrease during hypothermia. Although the metabolic rate is decreased at this time, hypothermia also produces cardiac and respiratory depression. Following anesthesia, high oxy-

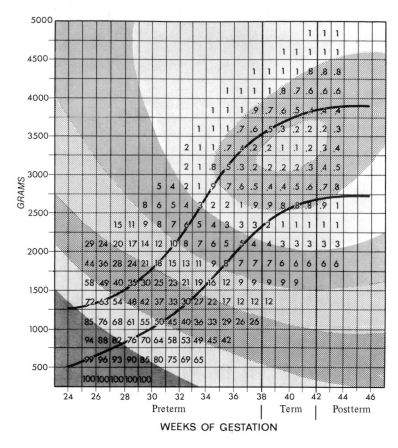

Figure 48–1. Neonatal mortality risk by birth weight and gestational age; interpolated data expressed in percent based on mathematical fit from original data. University of Colorado Medical Center newborns, 7/1/58–7/1/69. (Reproduced, with permission, from Lubchenco LO & others: J Pediatr 81:814, 1972.)

gen consumption—during an interval when the respiratory and cardiac responses are depressed—results in severe hypoxia, acidosis, and cardiorespiratory failure.

C. Prevention of Heat Loss: Infants should be transported to and from the x-ray department or operating room in a warm incubator, and the incubator temperature should be maintained when the baby is removed. In the operating room, the temperature of the infant must be continuously recorded by placing a thermistor in the rectum or esophagus. Conservation of body heat may be accomplished by wrapping the extremities with sheet wadding and by using a circulating heating pad and an infrared lamp, but these measures are not sufficient in small infants. The operating room should be prewarmed and the temperature kept at about 20–27 C (68–80.6 F). Wet sponges and drapes exaggerate evaporative heat losses. Plastic drapes against the skin help contain body heat and keep the skin dry. When large volumes of blood are required, the blood should be warmed by circulating it through tubing immersed in warm water (37 C [98.6 F]) or prewarmed in the container before being transfused. The most effective means of regulating body temperature is the use of a heated ultrasonic nebulizer during endotracheal anesthesia.

Adamsons K: The role of thermal factors in fetal and neonatal life. Pediatr Clin North Am 13:599, 1966.
Roe CF, Santulli TV, Blair CS: Heat loss in infants during general anesthesia and operations. J Pediatr Surg 1:266, 1966.

Cardiorespiratory Control

A. Postoperative Position: Although the pain threshold of a young infant is quite high, the protective response to pain is to remain immobilized. The young infant breathes primarily with his diaphragm, and his respiratory excursion becomes limited following the pain of an operative incision in the chest or abdomen. Therefore, it is important to rotate the young infant from side to side at least every hour to prevent atelectasis. It is usually necessary to restrain the arms to prevent dislodgement of the nasogastric and intravenous tubes. When the arms are restrained, it must be done with the baby on his side and the 2 arms together—the arms must never be restrained on the opposite sides of the crib because the baby might aspirate vomitus.

B. Cardiorespiratory Resuscitation: Newborn infants with surgically treatable diseases frequently are asphyxiated during birth. Causes of asphyxia include antepartal hemorrhage, prolonged labor, respiratory insufficiency due to aspiration pneumonitis, and congenital diaphragmatic hernia. The resulting hypoxia, hypercapnia, and acidosis produce generalized vasoconstriction. In particular, increased pulmonary vascular resistance occurs when the P_{O_2} falls below 50 mm Hg and the pH is less than 7.3. Normally, a right-to-left shunt of 20% of the cardiac output is present in newborn infants. During asphyxia, this shunt will be increased, and the existing hypoxia and acidosis may become exaggerated. Cyanosis is an inadequate sign of hypoxia in the newborn because fetal hemoglobin will be 85% saturated at P_{O_2} levels of 42 mm Hg, whereas, in the adult, hemoglobin is 85% saturated at P_{O_2} levels of 52 mm Hg. Therefore, in circumstances which produce asphyxia in the newborn, resuscitation should be established promptly before obvious clinical signs are present.

At birth, the pharynx should be aspirated of mucus, amniotic fluid, or meconium. Respirations should be assisted or controlled with bag and mask, and prolonged respiratory support may require endotracheal intubation. A small air leak between the endotracheal tube and the airway is necessary to minimize laryngeal trauma. The required tube diameter may be 2.5–5 mm. The diameter of the tube should approximate that of the little finger or the nostril. The trachea from the glottis to the carina in the newborn is 5–7.5 cm long, and placement of the tube into the right or left bronchus must be avoided. An oraltracheal tube is preferred to a nasotracheal tube in order to minimize trauma and subsequent infection in the nasal passages. The ventilatory pressure must be carefully monitored to prevent rupture of the lung.

In the absence of abnormal diffusion or shunting, an inspired oxygen concentration of 40% will result in an arterial P_{O_2} of 110–116 mm Hg. The inspired oxygen concentration must be frequently monitored with an oxygen analyzer. Prolonged hyperoxia (arterial P_{O_2} of 160 mm Hg) may cause retrolental fibroplasia in premature infants and pulmonary oxygen toxicity. When an infant has pulmonary insufficiency and requires greater oxygen concentrations, with or without assisted ventilation, it is essential to repeatedly measure the arterial P_{O_2} and regulate the inspired oxygen concentration to keep the blood P_{O_2} between 60 and 80 mm Hg.

The frequent monitoring of these infants is most easily accomplished by inserting a polyvinyl catheter into the umbilical artery and threading it 10 cm into the distal aorta. Blood pressure may be recorded by connecting the catheter to a strain gauge and recorder. A blood pH of <7.3 should be corrected with sodium bicarbonate or tromethamine with electrolytes (THAM-E). Sodium bicarbonate (44.4 mEq in 50 ml) may be given intravenously in amounts of 3–8 ml at a rate of 1 ml/kg/minute. After an equilibration period of 5–10 minutes, the pH and base deficit measurements should be repeated and the requisite amount of additional sodium bicarbonate or tromethamine calculated (see below). When asphyxia has been present for prolonged periods, the resulting vasoconstriction may

produce a decreased blood volume. Correction of hypoxia and acidosis, however, can sometimes result in vasodilatation and hypovolemic shock. The blood volume will have to be replenished by transfusing 5% albumin solution or whole blood. The requirements for assisted respiration, high oxygen concentration, buffering, and volume replacement can be determined only by repeated evaluation of the patient, the blood pressure, and the P_{O_2}, P_{CO_2}, and pH status of the blood.

C. Assisted Ventilation: Following certain operations—particularly after thoracotomy or tight abdominal wall closure—lung volume is diminished and diaphragmatic motion is greatly impaired. Assisted ventilation may be required for 24 hours or more. This is best accomplished by firmly fixing an endotracheal tube in place and connecting it to a Norman elbow and Sommers T-piece with attached "elephant" tubing and a 500 ml reservoir bag (Fig 48–2). The gas mixture flowing into the Norman elbow should be carefully controlled by an air and oxygen mixing device, and the oxygen concentration should be regulated according to analysis of blood oxygen tensions. The gas should be humidified by using a heated ultrasonic nebulizer. Water absorption in the lung may be very great, and parenteral fluid may have to be restricted. The sidearm of the Sommers T-piece is connected to an aneroid manometer, and the end of the tubing is immersed in a graduate tube filled with water 25–30 cm in depth. This serves as a pop-off valve in case excessive airway pressure develops. Manual positive pressure should be applied to the bag hourly to open up areas of atelectatic lung.

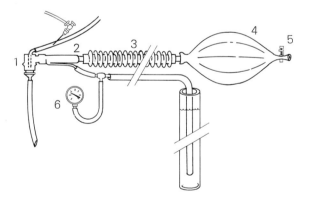

Figure 48–2. System for continuous positive pressure breathing. The system consists of an endotracheal tube with a Norman elbow (1) and Sommers T-piece (2). The inhaled gases are conveyed to the airway via the Norman elbow. Elephant tubing (3) and a 500 ml reservoir bag (4) provide a means of applying positive pressure. The screw clamp on the tailpiece (5) regulates the amount of continuous positive pressure in the airway. The side-arm of the Sommers T-piece is connected to an aneroid manometer (6) to monitor the airway pressure. One end of this side-arm is placed in a column of water at the desired depth (usually 30 cm) for a pop-off if the intratracheal pressure exceeds the desired level. (Redrawn and reproduced, with permission, from Gregory GA & others: N Engl J Med 284:1333, 1971.)

When alveolar collapse tends to develop, such as in hyaline membrane disease or with persistent atelectasis, the terminal airways can be kept open by continuous positive airway pressure breathing. This is accomplished by closing the reservoir bag with a screw clamp on the tailpiece and by observing the end-expiratory pressure on the aneroid manometer. End-expiratory pressures as high as 12 mm Hg may be required initially. The infant can be allowed to breathe on his own effort with this system. During continuous positive pressure breathing, an inspired oxygen mixture is selected which will maintain a blood oxygen tension of 60–80 mm Hg. When the P_{aO_2} exceeds 80 mm Hg, the inspired oxygen concentration is gradually lowered 5–10% at a time. When a 40% oxygen mixture is reached, the continuous positive airway pressure is lowered in 1 mm Hg decrements, while keeping the P_{aO_2} above 50 mm Hg. When the end-expired airway pressure is 2 mm Hg, the endotracheal tube is removed. At this time the inspired oxygen concentration should be increased to 10% greater than during the period of positive pressure. The inspired oxygen concentration may then be lowered toward that of room air, as indicated by the blood gas changes.

Chest percussion, endotracheal suctioning by careful sterile technic, and rocking from side to side are necessary while the endotracheal tube is in place.

The continuous positive pressure does not impair venous return, and its primary effect is to keep open airways that tend to collapse at atmospheric pressure. This is very important in the care of infants who are not ventilating adequately.

Gluck L (editor): Symposium on respiratory disorders of the newborn. Pediatr Clin North Am 20:273, 1973.

Gregory GA & others: Treatment of the idiopathic respiratory-distress syndrome with continuous positive airway pressure. N Engl J Med 284:1333, 1971.

Stern L: The use and misuse of oxygen in the newborn infant. Pediatr Clin North Am 20:447, 1973.

Tunstall ME: Neonatal resuscitation. Br J Anaesth 36:591,1964.

Blood Loss & Replacement

A. Determination of Blood Loss: Defects in the coagulating mechanism may occur in newborn infants as a result of vitamin K deficiency, thrombocytopenia, and temporary hepatic insufficiency due to immaturity, asphyxia, or infection. Prior to operation, newborn infants should receive phytonadione (vitamin K_1; AquaMephyton, Konakion), 1–2 mg IV or IM. If an extensive surgical procedure is anticipated, freshly drawn blood should be typed and cross-matched in case transfusion is required.

The blood volume of a newborn infant ranges from 50–100 ml/kg body weight (average, 85 ml/kg). This wide variation is due principally to the timing and technic of clamping the umbilical cord. By 1 month of age, the blood volume in premature and full-term infants is approximately 75 ml/kg.

The blood lost during operation varies greatly according to the extent of the operative procedure, the disease being treated, and the effectiveness of hemostasis. Mild blood loss, amounting to less than 10% of the blood volume, usually does not require transfusion. In a 3.5 kg infant, mild blood loss would be a volume up to 30 ml. Since blood loss greater than 10% should be corrected—and since these volumes are quite small—it is imperative to develop methods for closely monitoring the amount of blood lost during operation. Dry sponges should be used and weighed shortly after use to minimize error from evaporation. The suction line, connected to a calibrated trap on the operating table, should be short to diminish the dead space of the tubing and to provide immediate quantitation of accumulated blood loss. Visual observation of blood loss may be used as a rough guide but tends to be underestimated.

B. Replacement of Blood Loss: Whenever an operation results in a blood loss greater than 10% of blood volume, an indwelling plastic catheter must be placed in a vein and secured to prevent dislodgement under drapes. Procedures associated with blood loss > 20% of blood volume should be preceded by a venous catheter with the catheter tip directed into the right atrium. This catheter should be connected to a manometer for measuring central venous pressure and a 3-way stopcock for taking samples for blood gas and pH measurements. Arterial pressure should be monitored by a Doppler blood pressure cuff on the arm. An umbilical artery catheter should be placed in the distal aorta of the newborn infant for continuous display of pressure. A transverse abdominal incision can be made above the umbilicus without interfering with the catheter.

In infants with hematocrits greater than 50%, blood loss may be replaced by infusion of lactated Ringer's solution to compensate for losses of up to 25% of total blood volume. Greater blood losses should be replaced with freshly drawn whole blood. Transfusion of old blood may result in cardiac arrest and death as a result of hyperkalemia, hypocalcemia, acidosis, hypothermia, and air embolism. The transfused blood should be prewarmed to body temperature by running it through coiled tubing immersed in water at 37 C (98.6 F). ACD (acid-citrate-dextrose) blood that is older than 3 days may have a pH of less than 6.1, a P_{CO_2} greater than 80 mm Hg, a base deficit greater than 15, a potassium content greater than 10 mEq/liter, citrate which binds serum magnesium and calcium, and deficient clotting factors and platelets. The acidosis that results from the transfusion of ACD blood may be partially corrected by adding 30 ml of 0.3 M tromethamine, but the pH should be checked to prevent overcorrection and alkalosis. Citrate-phosphate-dextrose (CPD) is a better blood preservative because it maintains the carrying capacity and release of oxygen for a longer period than ACD preservative. After transfusion, subsequent metabolism of the citrate to bicarbonate may produce a metabolic alkalosis. Heparinized blood diminishes the metabolic complications of ACD blood, but protamine sulfate may be required to correct a prolonged clotting time. Hypocalcemia, produced by complexing calcium with citrate, may be treated by giving 2 ml of 10% calcium gluconate for each 100 ml of ACD blood transfused.

In circumstances of excessive blood loss, depletion of clotting factors and platelets can occur readily, and fresh frozen plasma and identical blood typed platelets should be available.

Oski FA, Naiman JL: *Hematologic Problems in the Newborn.* 2nd ed. Saunders, 1972.

Humidity

A high environmental humidity may be desired for liquefaction of viscid pulmonary secretions or for treatment of croup. An ultrasonically generated mist is the only effective means of getting water droplets as far as the larynx or upper trachea. The mist should be delivered through a face mask, hood, or incubator. Infants can absorb a significant volume of ultrasonic mist water, and they may develop pulmonary edema if not carefully monitored. Infants with an endotracheal tube or a tracheostomy must be given humidified gases to breathe.

Overgrowth of bacteria, such as pseudomonas, will occur in the mist generator and incubator within a short time. Therefore, the incubator and generator will have to be changed and cleaned at least every 2 days. The fluid requirements of these babies are greatly decreased when high humidification is used. Body temperature may be elevated as a result of heat retention in an environment with high humidity.

FLUID & ELECTROLYTE CONTROL

Fluid & Electrolyte Management; Caloric Intake

Fluid and electrolyte therapy requires a knowledge of normal basic requirements, preexisting deficits, and continuing losses. This subject is covered in Chapter 12. Special pediatric considerations are as follows.

A. Newborn Requirements: Normally, a newborn infant loses 5–10% of his birth weight in the first 3 days. Part of the weight lost is meconium, vernix, and urine; however, the major component is excess total body water. During the first 4 days on oral feedings, a normal newborn infant will have a urine volume of 20–30 ml/kg/day and an insensible water loss of 20–25 ml/kg/day. The total urinary excretion of sodium, potassium, and chloride is less than 0.9 mEq/kg. Oliguria and shift in the potassium/nitrogen ratio due to increased aldosterone secretion do not occur following stress in the first few weeks of life. A sodium-excreting factor following stress has been postulated since urinary sodium and chloride retention do not occur when there are large extrarenal losses of these ions. The usual amount of water given during the first 4 days after birth is 80 ml/kg/day. However, when a newborn infant is cared for under infrared heat, the additional insensible water losses will require replacement of 100–130 ml/kg/day. Normally, the maximum tolerance for sodium and chloride is 1.5 mEq/kg/day; for potassium, 1 mEq/kg/day. Therefore, maintenance fluid in the first 4 days after birth, following operative procedures with small third space losses, should consist of 10% dextrose in 0.2% saline, given at a rate of 50–80 ml/kg/day. Potassium chloride or bicarbonate, 15 mEq/liter, and calcium gluconate, 150 mg/kg/day, are usually added to the solution. Additional potassium, calcium, bicarbonate, and glucose may be added according to the blood chemistry analysis and the clinical status of the patient. Following an operation such as laparotomy or thoracotomy, the fluid requirement may exceed 150 ml/kg/day. When these larger third space losses occur, 5% dextrose in lactated Ringer's solution should be given at a rate of 130–150 ml/kg/day.

Many stressed newborn infants develop low blood levels of potassium, calcium, magnesium, and glucose. A deficiency of any one of these substances will produce such signs as vomiting, abdominal distention, poor feeding, apneic spells, cyanosis, limpness, eye rolling, high-pitched cry, tremors, or convulsions. Convulsions and tetany due to hypocalcemia should be treated with intravenous 10% calcium solution (chloride, lactate, or gluconate) given at a rate of 1 ml/minute while the heart sounds are being carefully monitored. Hypocalcemia can be largely eliminated by routinely adding calcium salts to intravenous solutions. Caution is required since subcutaneous infiltration may produce severe vasoconstriction and skin necrosis.

Hypoglycemia frequently occurs in infants with low birth weight for gestational age, respiratory distress, asphyxia, or CNS abnormalities. Hypoglycemia is defined as a blood glucose less than 20 mg/100 ml in the premature or low birth weight infant; less than 30 mg/100 ml in full-sized infants within the first 72 hours after birth; and less than 40 mg/100 ml thereafter in full-term infants. The treatment of hypoglycemia consists of giving 50% glucose, 1–2 ml/kg IV, followed by a continuous infusion of 10–15% glucose solutions at a rate equivalent to that needed for maintenance water requirements.

B. Requirements for Older Infants and Children: Three methods are available for determining the physiologic limits for water, based upon (1) total body weight, (2) body surface area, and (3) calculated basal caloric expenditure related to body weight.

The average water requirements are as follows: 120 ml/kg up to 10 kg; 110 ml/kg up to 20 kg; 100 ml/kg to 30 kg; 95 ml/kg up to 40 kg; and 80 ml/kg above 40 kg. The physiologic limits are 35 ml/kg above or below the mean daily requirements (Fig 48–3).

The surface area can be determined from nomograms by knowing the height and weight of the patient (see p 1112). The physiologic range of fluid tolerance is 1200–3500 ml/sq m/day (Fig 48–3). With this method, 1500 ml/sq m/day should be considered the usual minimum water requirement.

In the caloric system, the *minimum* water requirement is 100 ml/100 Cal expended. The basic caloric

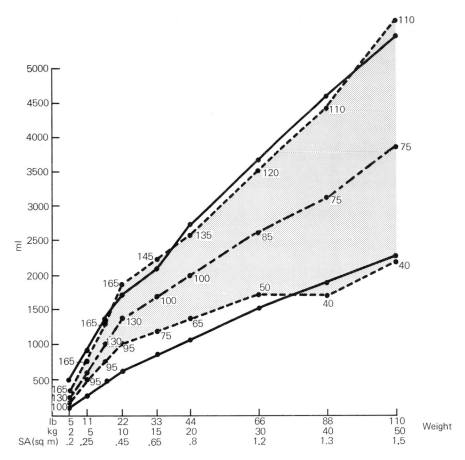

Figure 48-3. Comparison of 2 methods of calculating intravenous fluid requirements. Solid lines show the maximum (3000 ml/sq m) and minimum (1200 ml/sq m) fluid requirements by surface area. The broken lines show the mean (ml/kg) and the range (±35 ml/kg) from the mean total fluid requirements. The surface area system underestimates the requirements in infants weighing less than 10 kg, probably because of errors in the nomograms.

requirements related to weight are as follows: up to 10 kg, 100 Cal/kg; 10–20 kg, 1000 Cal for the first 10 kg plus 50 Cal for each kg above 10; over 20 kg, 1500 Cal for the first 20 kg plus 20 Cal/kg over 20 kg. Additional water should be given according to the state of hydration, body temperature, and estimated caloric expenditure above basal activity.

The normal daily sodium requirement is usually 30–35 mEq/sq m (1–2.5 mEq/kg), but it may vary from 10–250 mEq/sq m in extreme cases. The usual range of potassium required is the same as that of sodium. The large reserve of calcium and magnesium in the skeleton makes short-term intravenous replacement unnecessary, especially for older children.

Continuing losses such as gastric juice, ileostomy output, pleural fluid, and "third space" fluid must be replaced as rapidly as they occur, preferably within 4–8 hours. Gastric juices should be replaced by 5% dextrose in 0.45% saline plus KCl, 20 mEq/liter. Small bowel, bile, or pancreatic losses may be replaced with lactated Ringer's solution to which potassium chloride, 10 mEq/liter, has been added. During operative procedures, "third space" losses in the injured serosal sur-

faces, bowel wall, and lumen should be replaced by giving lactated Ringer's solution, 5–15 ml/kg/hour; the amount to be given depends upon the magnitude of the operative procedure. Eight to 24 hours postoperatively, 5% dextrose in Ringer's lactate is continued at a rate calculated to be 30–50% greater than average maintenance.

The status of hydration, intake and output, and weight of infants and small children should be assessed at frequent intervals. The orders for intravenous fluids should be rewritten at least every 8 hours.

By knowing the ranges of tolerance for fluid and electrolytes, polyionic solutions can be made using concentrated electrolyte solutions. The volume of a repair solution is usually given at a rate close to maximal tolerance, and, therefore, the glucose content should be 5% to prevent osmotic diuresis. Maintenance solutions can be made with 10% glucose.

Existing deficits may occur from external losses, such as hemorrhage, vomiting, diarrhea, or starvation, or from internal "third space" losses such as in the bowel lumen, peritoneal space, or burned tissues.

Patients with dehydration or shock will require

rapid volume expansion. A catheter should be placed in the right atrium via the jugular or subclavian vein. The central venous pressure, blood pH, and blood gases may be constantly monitored from this catheter. Rapid volume replacement may be accomplished by using normal saline, lactated Ringer's solution, or 5% albumin solution in amounts of 10–20 ml/kg given as rapidly as possible but not exceeding a right atrial pressure of 15 cm water. If anemia exists, whole blood is substituted for these solutions as soon as the type and cross-match are done. Following this initial expansion of the blood volume, rehydration is continued with 5% dextrose in lactated Ringer's solution at the maximum physiologically tolerated rate until a rise in central venous pressure occurs or urine flow has been established. A repair solution is then continued at close to physiologic maximal rates until the existing deficits have been restored. This is determined by clinical examination of skin perfusion, blood pressure, central venous pressure, hydration, pulse, urine output and specific gravity or osmolarity, hemoglobin, hematocrit, electrolyte changes, and, when possible, measurement of right atrial pressure.

Replacement of sodium deficits may also be calculated as follows:

$$\frac{\text{mEq sodium}}{\text{needed}} = \frac{(140 - \text{patient's serum}}{\text{sodium in mEq})} \times \frac{(60\% \text{ body}}{\text{weight in kg})}$$

If dehydration is also present, sodium should be replaced by using normal saline. Hyponatremia associated with abnormal retention of water should be treated by restriction of water intake.

Significant acidosis (serum HCO_3^- less than 15 mEq/liter or base deficit greater than 8) should be corrected with sodium bicarbonate. When the base deficit is determined from the Siggaard-Andersen nomogram, the replacement requirement is calculated by multiplying the base deficit (mEq/liter) by the estimated extracellular volume (30% total body weight in kg). The result is the required number of mEq of $NaHCO_3$ that must be given intravenously. If the magnitude of acidosis is known only by the serum bicarbonate level, a rule of thumb for $NaHCO_3$ (in a concentration of 44.5 mEq/50 ml) replacement is 4 ml/kg, to raise the serum HCO_3^- by 5 mEq/liter.

For patients with severe acidosis and excessive total body sodium (eg, congestive heart failure), tromethamine with electrolytes (THAM-E) may be preferred to $NaHCO_3$ as a buffer. A 0.3 M solution is isotonic, and the amount of 0.3 M tromethamine to be given (in ml) = (body weight in kg) × (base deficit in mEq/liter). When the fluid volume must also be restricted, tromethamine can be made up as a 0.6 or 0.9 M solution. Tromethamine is usually given over a 1-hour period. It diffuses freely both intracellularly and extracellularly, is rapidly excreted in the urine (50–70% in the first 24-hour period), and produces an osmotic and potassium diuresis. The hazards of tromethamine include hypercalcemia, hypoglycemia, hypoventilation, local irritation, and vasospasm.

When oliguria occurs, a frequent concern is whether it is due to dehydration and hypovolemia or acute renal shutdown. An effective method of establishing diuresis when oliguria is due to prerenal causes is to give 25% mannitol, 3.5 ml/kg IV, in 20–30 minutes, or furosemide, 0.5–1 mg/kg IV.

Bennett EJ: *Fluids for Anesthesia and Surgery in the Newborn and the Infant.* Thomas, 1975.

Cornblath M, Schwartz R: *Disorders of Carbohydrate Metabolism in Infancy.* Saunders, 1966.

Holliday MA: Body fluid physiology during growth. Chap 12 in: *Clinical Disorders of Fluid and Electrolyte Metabolism,* 2nd ed. Maxwell MH, Kleeman CR (editors). McGraw-Hill, 1972.

Mizrahi A, London R, Gribetz D: Neonatal hypocalcemia: Its causes and treatment. N Engl J Med 278:1163, 1968.

Moore FD: Tris buffer, mannitol and low viscous dextran. Surg Clin North Am 43:577, 1963.

Suzuki H & others: Water and electrolyte metabolism of newborn infants after surgical operations. Tohoku J Exp Med 94:187, 1968.

Talbot NB, Richie RH, Crawford JD: *Metabolic Homeostasis.* Harvard Univ Press, 1959.

Parenteral Alimentation (See also Chapter 13.)

The indications for parenteral alimentation include the following: (1) expected period of prolonged ileus, eg, following repair of gastroschisis or jejunal atresia; (2) intestinal fistulas; (3) supplementation of oral feedings, as in intractable diarrhea, short bowel syndrome, or various malabsorption syndromes; (4) intrauterine growth retarded infants; (5) catabolic wasting states such as infections or tumors when gastric feedings are inadequate; or (6) to prevent development of necrotizing enterocolitis in premature infants less than 1200 g when feedings are withheld for a prolonged time. Total parenteral alimentation was usually limited in the past because the concentrated solutions and polyethylene catheters produced thrombophlebitis. Nonreactive polyvinyl or Silastic catheters can now be placed into the right atrium via the jugular or subclavian veins, avoiding this complication. When this technic is used, a constant infusion pump should be employed to regulate a steady rate of infusion and to prevent blood from backing into the catheter during straining or crying. If a fibrin clot develops in the tube lining, bacterial growth is enhanced and sepsis will occur. Placement of the catheter under sterile conditions is best accomplished with general anesthesia in an operating room for small infants and children.

A solution for parenteral alimentation may be prepared with protein hydrolysate or crystalline amino acids, dextrose, balanced electrolytes, vitamins, iron, and trace metals. With the exception of the crystalline amino acid solutions, approximately half of the nitrogen content is in the form of polypeptides which are not utilizable and are excreted in the urine. Each of the available solutions has a different electrolyte content. The relatively high titratable acidity and ammonia level must be appreciated in anticipation of complications (Table 48–1).

Table 48—1. Electrolyte composition of parenteral amino acid solutions.*

	Travasol 5.5%	Amigen 5%	Aminosol 5%	Freamine II 8.5%
Sodium	. . .	25 mEq/liter	10 mEq/liter	12.5 mEq/liter
Potassium	. . .	20 mEq/liter	17 mEq/liter	. . .
Calcium	. . .	5 mEq/liter	2 mEq/liter	. . .
Magnesium	. . .	20 mEq/liter	2 mEq/liter	. . .
Chloride	22 mEq/liter	18 mEq/liter	10 mEq/liter	. . .
Phosphate	. . .	25 mEq/liter	. . .	25 mEq/liter
Acetate	35 mEq/liter	. . .	. . .	. . .
Ammonia	152 μg/100 ml	10^3–30^3 μg/100 ml	10^3–30^3 μg/100 ml	50 μg/100 ml
Titratable acidity	22 mEq/liter	26 mEq/liter	. . .	23 mEq/liter

*The composition of a standard parenteral alimentation solution using Travasol is shown in Table 48—4.

The concentration of the various electrolytes can be altered according to the individual patient, recognizing the electrolyte content of the basic amino acid solutions. A standard solution which is suitable for infants and young children must contain a sufficient amount of calcium, magnesium, and phosphate to allow for growth. Trace metals are also added to the basic solution. A suitable trace mineral solution is prepared as shown in Table 48—2.

The solution for total parenteral alimentation is infused in volumes calculated to be slightly above the usual maintenance water requirements for a 24-hour period at a constant rate with an infusion pump. If it is necessary to restrict the volume of infusion, more concentrated glucose solutions (50%) can be made. The caloric value of glucose in these solutions is 3.4 Cal per gram because of the water content in glucose that is added.

Complications of prolonged intravenous alimentation are numerous. The most frequent problem is sepsis, including candida, and immediate discontinuation of the catheter usually results in prompt clinical improvement. Accidental dislodgment of the catheter is a frequent problem which can be prevented by careful fixation by use of skin sutures and taping. Thrombosis of the superior vena cava and right atrium is usually controlled by adding 1 unit of heparin per ml of solution. Emphasis on a constant rate of infusion will minimize hyper- or hypoglycemia. Small newborn infants usually do not tolerate concentrations greater than 10% glucose during the first week of life, but the glucose concentrations can be increased beyond the first week. Repeated determinations of the concentrations of blood components must be performed to anticipate electrolyte imbalances and metabolic acidosis due to the high titratable acidity of the solution,

Table 48—2. Stock solutions used in preparation of parenteral alimentation formula.

Travasol 5.5% (injectable amino acid solution, Travenol), 5.5 g amino acid/100 ml mixture

Sodium phosphate buffer (pH 7.3; 2 mEq/ml)	126.23 g Na_2HPO_4 (anhydrous) 30.66 g $NaH_2PO_4 \cdot 1H_2O$ Water for injection, qs ad 1000 ml

Sodium acetate, 2 mEq/ml
Potassium chloride, 2 mEq/ml
Magnesium sulfate, 50% solution (4 mEq/ml)
Calcium gluconate, 10% solution
Multivitamin infusion (USV Pharmaceutical Corp.)

5 ml vial provides:	Ascorbic acid	500 mg
	Vitamin A	10,000 USP units
	Vitamin D	1000 USP units
	Thiamine	50 mg
	Riboflavin	10 mg
	Pyridoxine	15 mg
	Niacinamide	100 mg
	Dexpanthenol	25 mg
	Vitamin E	5 IU

Vitamin B_{12} (cyanocobalamin) solution	10 μg/ml
Folic acid solution	1000 μg/ml
Vitamin K_1 (AquaMephyton) solution	10 mg/ml
Iron (Imferon)	50 mg elemental iron/ml

Trace mineral solution

Copper sulfate $\cdot 5H_2O$	1.022 g
Cobalt chloride $\cdot 6H_2O$	0.644 g
Manganese chloride $\cdot 4H_2O$	1.932 g
Zinc sulfate $\cdot 7H_2O$	2.376 g
Potassium iodide	0.242 g
Glycine	1 g
Water for injection, qs ad	400 ml

Table 48—3. Preparation of 250 ml of a standard parenteral alimentation solution.

To:	125 ml Travasol 5.5%		
Add:	Dextrose*		
	Sodium phosphate buffer	2.5	ml
	Sodium acetate	0.625	ml
	Potassium chloride	2.25	ml
	Magnesium sulfate	0.9	ml
	Calcium gluconate	4.2	ml
	Multivitamin infusion	0.5	ml
	Vitamin B_{12}	0.1	ml
	Folic acid	0.1	ml
	Vitamin K_1	0.05	ml
	Iron	0.025	ml
	Trace minerals	0.08	ml

*Amount of dextrose is varied according to the amount of calories to be provided. This is added as a solution, using appropriate quantities (up to a maximum of 125 ml) of a dextrose-containing solution. *Examples:* Using a solution of 10% dextrose in water, the addition of 125 ml would contribute 12.5 g of dextrose. Using a 50% solution of dextrose in water, add 100 ml + 25 ml water for injection to contribute 50 g dextrose.

Table 48–4. Composition of standard parenteral alimentation solution.

Volume	250 ml
Nitrogen (as amino acids)	1.15 g
(protein equivalent)	7.24 g
Dextrose (see footnote to Table 48–3)	(5–35%)*
Sodium	6.25 mEq
Potassium	4.5 mEq
Chloride	7.3 mEq†
Phosphate	5 mEq
Magnesium	3.75 mEq
Calcium	2 mEq
Acetate	5.65 mEq†
Vitamin A	1000 IU
Vitamin D (ergocalciferol)	100 IU
Thiamine	5 mg
Riboflavin	1 mg
Pyridoxine	1.5 mg
Niacinamide	10 mg
Dexpanthenol (pantothenic acid source)	2.5 mg
Ascorbic acid	50 mg
Vitamin E (a-tocopherol acetate)	0.5 μg
	(0.5 IU)
Vitamin B_{12} (cyanocobalamin)	1 μg
Folic acid	100 μg
Vitamin K_1 (Mephyton)	0.5 mg
Iron	12.5 mg
Trace minerals	
Copper	
Cobalt	
Manganese	0.08 ml
Zinc	
Iodine	

*Depending on the caloric content desired.
†Travasol contains 4.4 mEq of acetate and 2.8 mEq of chloride in 125 ml of 5.5% stock concentrate.

acid, an essential fatty acid. The regimen starts with 0.5 g/kg body weight the first day and is gradually increased to 4 g/kg/day. Approximately 5% of the total caloric intake should be in the form of linoleic acid. Infusions in excess of this may result in the fat overload syndrome: lipemic blood, seizures, congestive failure, hepatosplenomegaly with jaundice, and abnormal liver function, including prolonged prothrombin time and plasma thromboplastin test, thrombocytopenia, and renal failure. Intralipid is infused through a sidearm of the intravenous cannula just before entering the vein to minimize destabilization of the emulsion. Infusion pumps must be applied to the Intralipid and to the standard solution to ensure the proper rate of administration and to prevent one solution from backing up into the other. Patients receiving total parenteral alimentation through a central venous catheter should also receive Intralipid through a peripheral vein twice a week to avoid a linoleic acid deficiency.

Complications of Intralipid infusion include phlebitis, infiltration, and accidental dislodgement of the peripheral vein cannula. Because of problems with repeated interruption of the infusion, caloric replacement by means of peripheral venous alimentation becomes less than optimal. For this reason, peripheral alimentation is desirable only when the anticipated needs are short-term.

Cowan GSM Jr, Scheetz WL (editors): *Hyperalimentation.* Lea & Febiger, 1972.
Dudrick SJ & others: Parenteral hyperalimentation: Metabolic problems and solutions. Ann Surg 176:259, 1972.
Friedman Z & others: Rapid onset of essential fatty acid deficiency in the newborn. Pediatrics 58:640, 1976.
Heird WC & others: Intravenous alimentation in pediatric patients. J Pediatr 80:351, 1972.

and these patients should be observed for ammonia intoxication and for vitamin or trace mineral deficiency. These solutions are deficient in linoleic acid, an essential fatty acid. Deficiency in linoleic acid is characterized by thrombocytopenia, thin, scaly, flushed skin, and a peculiarly firm subcutaneous fat. The latter can be corrected with intravenous Intralipid (see below) or with orally administered fats such as Lipomul. Hepatitis with hepatic necrosis of uncertain origin occurs after prolonged alimentation and is characterized by progressive hepatomegaly and jaundice. This syndrome subsides with cessation of the intravenous alimentation solution.

When central venous catheter placement is not desired, parenteral alimentation can be supplied through peripheral veins. The composition of the above-described standard formula is altered only by decreasing the glucose content to a 10% solution. The resulting deficit in caloric replacement is corrected by using Intralipid solution. Intralipid is a 10% soybean oil emulsified to 0.5 μm, stabilized with 1.2% egg yolk phospholipids, with 2.25% glycerin added to make the solution isotonic. Intralipid contains 110 Cal per 100 ml of solution. The solution consists of 54% linoleic

LESIONS OF THE HEAD & NECK

DERMOID CYSTS

Dermoid cysts are congenital inclusions of skin and appendages which are commonly found on the scalp and eyebrows and in the midline of the nose, neck, and upper chest. They present as painless swellings which may be completely mobile or fixed to the skin and deeper structures. Dermoid cysts of the eyebrows and scalp may produce a depression in the underlying bone which will appear as a smooth, punched-out defect on radiographs of the skull. These cysts contain a cheesy material which is produced by desquamation of the cells of the epithelial lining. Dermoid cysts of the neck may be confused with thyroglossal duct cysts, but they usually do not move with swallowing or protrusion of the tongue as thyroglossal cysts do. Dermoid cysts may produce cosmetic deformities and tend to become infected. Those of the nose may extend into the nasal passages and the cribriform plate of the skull. These cysts should be excised intact, since incomplete removal will result in recurrence. Those arising on the eyebrows should be excised through an incision within the hairline. The eyebrows should not be shaved.

BRANCHIOGENIC ANOMALIES

Branchiogenic anomalies include sinuses, cysts, cartilaginous rests, cervical fistulas (Fig 48–4), and cervical cysts. These lesions are probably remnants of the branchial apparatus present during the first month of fetal life. The primitive neck develops 4 external clefts and 4 pharyngeal pouches which are separated by a membrane. Between the clefts and pouches are branchial arches.

Preauricular sinuses, cysts, and cartilaginous rests probably arise from anomalous development of the auricle. Fistulas which arise above the hyoid bone and communicate with the external auditory canal represent persistence of the first branchial cleft. Fistulas which communicate between the anterior border of the sternocleidomastoid muscle and the tonsillar fossa are of second branchial origin, and those that extend into the piriform sinus are derived from the third branchial pouch. Fourth branchial fistulas have not been described.

A tract of branchial origin may form a complete fistula, or one end may be obliterated to form an external or internal sinus, or both ends may resorb, leaving an aggregate of cells forming a cyst. First branchial cleft tracts are always lined by squamous epithe-

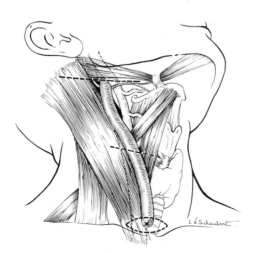

Figure 48–4. Branchiogenic fistula from second branchial cleft origin. The fistula extends along the anterior border of the sternocleidomastoid muscle and courses between the internal and external carotid arteries and cephalad to the hypoglossal nerve to enter the tonsillar fossa.

lium based on thick connective tissue. Cysts and sinuses of second or third branchial origin are lined by squamous, cuboidal, or ciliated columnar epithelium. Cervical fistulas and cysts have a prominent lymphoid stroma beneath the epithelial lining which may contain germinal centers and Hassall's corpuscles.

Clinical Findings

In the preauricular area, the anomalies may take the form of cysts, sinuses, skin tabs, or cartilaginous nubbins. A sinus or fistulous opening along the anterior border of the sternocleidomastoid muscle is readily seen at birth and usually discharges a mucoid or purulent material. The patient may complain of a foul-tasting discharge in the mouth upon massaging the tract, but the internal orifice is rarely recognized. Lateral cervical cysts, without an external sinus, are usually not recognized in childhood but become evident in young adulthood. The cysts are characteristically found anterior and deep to the upper third of the sternocleidomastoid muscle, or they may be located within the parotid gland, pharyngeal wall, over the manubrium, or in the mediastinum. Branchiogenic anomalies occur with equal frequency on each side of the neck, and 10% are bilateral.

Differential Diagnosis

Granulomatous lymphadenitis due to mycobacterial infections may produce cystic lymph nodes and draining sinuses, but these are usually distinguishable by the chronic inflammatory reaction which preceded the purulent discharge. Hemangiomas, cystic hygromas, and lymphangiomas are soft, spongy tumor masses which might be confused with cervical cysts, but the latter have a firmer consistency. Cystic hygromas and lymphangiomas transilluminate, and cervical cysts do not. Carotid body tumors are quite firm, are located at the carotid bifurcation, and occur in older patients. Lymphomas produce firm masses in the area where branchial remnants occur, but multiple, matted nodes rather than a solitary cystic tumor distinguish these lesions. Mucoid material may be expressed from the openings of branchial sinuses or fistulas, and a firm cord-like tract may be palpable along its course.

Complications

The sinuses and cysts are prone to become repeatedly infected, producing cellulitis and abscesses. Very rarely, carcinoma may occur.

Treatment & Prognosis

Superficial skin tabs and cartilaginous rests can be easily excised under sedation and local anesthesia. Preauricular sinus tracts may be very deceptive in their extent, and the surgeon should be prepared for an extensive dissection under general anesthesia to completely excise these lesions. General anesthesia is required for proper excision of branchial fistulas and cysts. Cervical cysts are excised through transverse incisions directly over the mass.

Infected sinuses and cysts will require initial incision and drainage. Excision of these tracts should be attempted only after the acute inflammatory reaction has subsided.

Albert GD: Branchial anomalies. JAMA 183:399, 1963.
Henzel JH, Pories WJ, DeWeese MS: Etiology of lateral cervical cysts. Surg Gynecol Obstet 125:1, 1967.

THYROGLOSSAL DUCT REMNANTS

The thyroid gland develops from an evagination in the floor of the primitive pharynx, between the first pair of pharyngeal pouches, during the fourth week of gestation. If the anlage of the thyroid does not descend normally, the thyroid gland may form in the tongue or remain as a mass anywhere in the midline of the neck from the submandibular fossa to the pretracheal area. If the thyroglossal duct persists, the tract forms a cyst which usually communicates with the foramen cecum of the tongue. The thyroglossal duct descends through the second branchial arch anlage, the hyoid bone, prior to its fusion in the midline. Because of this, the tract of a persistent thyroglossal duct usually extends through the hyoid bone (Fig 48–5).

Thyroid follicles may be found in 30–40% of the specimens. Three or more tracts between the thyroglossal cyst and the base of the tongue are present in more than 75% of cases.

Clinical Findings

The most common finding is a rounded, cystic mass of varying size in the midline of the neck just below the hyoid bone. When infected, the acute inflammatory reaction may herald the presence of a cyst. The fluid content of the cyst is usually under pressure and may give the impression of a solid tumor. Cysts and aberrant midline thyroid glands move with

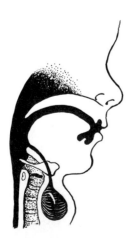

Figure 48–5. Thyroglossal cyst and duct courses through the hyoid bone to the foramen cecum of the tongue.

swallowing and with protrusion of the tongue. When a solid midline mass is detected, evidence of athyreosis should be sought such as hypothyroidism and absence of the palpable lateral lobes of the normal thyroid.

Differential Diagnosis

Only lymph nodes, dermoid cysts, and enlarged Delphian nodes containing metastases are confused with thyroglossal remnants in the midline of the neck. Dermoid cysts do not move with swallowing. Lingual thyroids may be confused with hypertrophied lingual tonsil or with a dermoid cyst, fibroma, angioma, sarcoma, or carcinoma of the tongue. These lesions and thyroglossal cysts may be distinguished from aberrantly located thyroid glands by needle aspiration or by radioiodine scintiscan.

Complications

Lingual thyroid glands may produce dysphagia, dysphonia, dyspnea, hemorrhage, or pain. Carcinoma develops more frequently in ectopic thyroid tissue than in normal thyroid glands. Thyroglossal cysts are prone to become infected, and spontaneous drainage or incision and drainage of an abscess will result in a chronically draining fistula. Excision of an ectopic thyroid usually removes all remaining thyroid tissue, producing subsequent hypothyroidism.

Treatment

Acute infection in thyroglossal tracts should be treated with local heat and antibiotics. Abscesses should be incised and drained. After complete subsidence of the inflammatory reaction, thyroglossal cysts and ducts should be excised.

Ectopic thyroid glands are usually associated with athyreosis of the 2 lobes. These remnants of thyroid may produce sufficient hormones until early childhood and adolescence, at which time hypothyroidism develops. Because of increased stimulation by thyrotropic hormone, the aberrant thyroid tissue enlarges. The residual hypertrophic thyroid remnants usually recede in response to administration of thyroid hormone, and in many instances surgical excision is not necessary. If an ectopic thyroid is excised and is the only remnant of thyroid gland, allotransplantation of the gland into the rectus or sternocleidomastoid muscle may be successful.

Brown PM, Judd ES: Thyroglossal duct cysts and sinuses: Results of radical (Sistrunk) operation. Am J Surg 102:494, 1961.
Choy FJ, Ward RK, Richardson R: Carcinoma of the thyroglossal duct. Am J Surg 108:361, 1964.

MUSCULAR TORTICOLLIS

Infants with congenital muscular torticollis may initially develop a nontender, hard, fusiform swelling diffusely involving the sternocleidomastoid muscle. The muscle tumor may be present at birth but is usually not noticed until the second to sixth weeks of life. The tumor appears with equal frequency in both sexes and on each side of the neck. Rarely, there is more than one tumor in the muscle or both sternocleidomastoid muscles are involved. The tumor resolves in 6–7 months, and in about half of cases the sternocleidomastoid muscle becomes fibrotic. A history of breech delivery is present in 20–30% of these children. Older children (2–15 years of age) may develop sternocleidomastoid fibrosis and torticollis without an initial history of tumor formation.

The sternocleidomastoid tumor or fibrosis may be present with or without torticollis. When torticollis occurs, the sternocleidomastoid muscle is shortened, the mastoid process on the involved side is pulled down toward the clavicle and sternum, and the head is tilted and directed toward the opposite shoulder. The shoulder on the affected side is raised, and there may be cervical and thoracic scoliosis. The fusiform mass may be palpable in the affected sternocleidomastoid muscle, or the muscle may feel like a tight, hard band. Passive rotation of the head to the ipsilateral side of the involved muscle ·will be resisted and limited to varying degree, and the muscle will appear as a protuberant band. Because of persistent pressure when the patient is recumbent, the ipsilateral face and contralateral occiput will be flattened or hypoplastic.

If the torticollis is corrected late in the course, the adjacent neck structures may also become shortened, and division of the sternocleidomastoid muscle will not be sufficient to correct the deformity. Delay in correction of the torticollis will produce permanent facial deformity.

The infant with a sternocleidomastoid tumor or fibrosis should be treated by forcefully rotating in a full range of motion. This procedure should be performed at least 4 times a day even though it may be quite uncomfortable for the child. If the muscle continues to become progressively shortened, with facial and occipital skull deformity, both heads of the sternocleidomastoid muscle should be divided through a small transverse incision just above the clavicle. After the muscle is divided, the head should be turned to the ipsilateral side and any surrounding muscle or fascial contracture should also be divided. It is unnecessary to excise the tumor, which involves a risk of injuring the spinal accessory nerve. Only the platysma muscle and skin layers are closed. When postoperative pain has subsided, exercises to provide a full range of neck motion must be carried out. The use of a neck brace is rarely indicated.

Surgical division of the muscle must be performed early to prevent progressive facial and occipital flattening. This procedure does not reverse the bony changes that have already developed. Dividing the muscle produces permanent "hollowing" of the lower neck on the affected side.

Jones PG: *Torticollis in Infancy and Childhood.* Thomas, 1968.

CERVICAL LYMPHADENOPATHY

1. PYOGENIC LYMPHADENITIS

Infections in the upper respiratory passages, scalp, ear, or neck produce varying degrees of secondary lymphadenitis. Most of the causative organisms are streptococci and staphylococci. In infants and young children, the clinical course of the suppurative lymphadenitis may greatly overshadow a seemingly insignificant or inapparent primary infection. Scalp or ear infections produce pre- or postauricular and suboccipital lymph node involvement; submental, oral, tonsillar, and pharyngeal infections affect the submandibular and deep jugular nodes.

With significant lymphadenitis, the regional lymph nodes become greatly enlarged and produce local pain and tenderness. Fever is high initially and then becomes intermittent and may persist for days or weeks. The regional nodes may remain enlarged and firm for prolonged periods, or they may suppurate and produce surrounding cellulitis and edema. Subsequently, the nodes may involute or a fluctuant abscess may form, resulting in redness and thinning of the overlying skin.

A smoldering lymphadenitis which neither resolves nor forms an abscess can be confused with granulomatous lymphadenitis, lymphoma, or metastatic tumor. After several weeks, there will usually be a reduction in the size and firmness of pyogenic adenitis. Excisional biopsy is occasionally required to differentiate these lesions. Suppurative lymphadenitis can be distinguished from granulomatous lymphadenitis by the signs of acute inflammation and a short history of fever, pain, and exquisite tenderness over the lymph nodes.

The complications are principally those of bacterial infection, including sepsis, abscess formation, and sensitivity reactions such as glomerulonephritis.

In the acute phase, the patient should be treated with antistaphylococcal antibiotics. In the subacute or chronic phase, the presence of pus in the node may be confirmed by needle aspiration of the mass. When an abscess is present, a general anesthetic should be given and the abscess should be incised and drained. An incision is made in the skin and the tract is bluntly dissected to avoid transecting an adjacent nerve. The loculated areas should be broken down and a gauze wick placed to keep the tract open. Packing an abscess with gauze is necessary only for excessive hemorrhage; it should be removed within several days to allow free drainage of the pus and obliteration of the abscess cavity.

Barton LL, Feigen RD: Childhood cervical lymphadenitis: A reappraisal. J Pediatr 84:846, 1974.

2. GRANULOMATOUS LYMPHADENITIS

Although typical tuberculous cervical adenitis is very rare in the USA, "atypical" or "anonymous" mycobacteria frequently cause chronic suppuration in the cervical, axillary, and inguinal lymph nodes.

Granulomatous lymphadenitis and caseation may occur in the regional nodes draining the inoculation site of BCG.

Cat-scratch disease causes a caseating lymphadenitis in regional lymph nodes.

Children under 6 years of age are most frequently affected. The initial manifestation is a painless, progressive enlargement of the lymph nodes in the deep cervical chain and the parotid, suboccipital, submandibular, and supraclavicular nodes. The duration of lymphadenopathy is usually 1–3 months or longer. The nodes may be large and mobile or, with progressive disease, may become matted, fixed, and finally caseate to form a cold abscess. Incision or spontaneous breakthrough of the skin will result in a chronically draining sinus. In tuberculosis, both sides of the neck or multiple groups of nodes are infected and the chest x-ray indicates pulmonary involvement. In atypical mycobacterial lymphadenitis, pulmonary disease is rare and the cervical adenitis is unilateral. The tuberculin skin test is weakly positive in over 80% of patients with atypical infection. Skin test antigens from the various strains of atypical mycobacteria are available.

Cat-scratch fever is usually acquired by a bite or scratch from a kitten. It is an acute illness characterized by fever, malaise, and occasionally a pustular lesion at the site of the scratch. Tender lymph node enlargement usually develops. Two to 4 weeks later, regional lymphadenitis persists, producing painless, fixed suppurative nodes which may develop into a chronically draining sinus.

The firm, rubbery, or fixed nodes resemble lymphoma or metastatic tumor (neuroblastoma or thyroid carcinoma) and may be distinguished only by excisional biopsy. A positive skin test helps differentiate granulomatous adenitis from malignant lymphadenopathy. A fluctuant node can be confused with branchial cleft or thyroglossal cysts.

Granulomatous lymphadenitis progresses to caseation and breakdown of the overlying skin in the great majority of affected children.

Atypical tuberculous lymphadenitis should be treated with rifampin, 10 mg/kg/day. It may require several months to achieve a good response. If the infection seems to be progressing, the nodes should be excised. Tetracyclines may shorten the course of cat-scratch disease and prevent suppuration.

The procedure of choice is surgical excision of involved nodes before caseation occurs. Once the nodes become fluctuant or a draining sinus forms, a wedge of involved skin should be excised and the underlying necrotic nodes should be curetted out, taking care not to injure the neighboring branches of the nerve. The wound edges and skin should be closed

primarily. The value of continuing chemotherapy is influenced by sensitivity tests on the cultured material. Excision and primary closure usually result in excellent healing with good cosmetic results.

Carithers HA, Carithers CM, Edwards RO Jr: Cat-scratch disease: Its natural history. JAMA 207:312, 1969.

Mandall F, Wright PF: Treatment of atypical mycobacterial cervical adenitis with rifampin. Pediatrics 55:39, 1975.

Salyer KE, Votteler TP, Dorman GW: Surgical management of cervical adenitis due to atypical mycobacteria in children. JAMA 204:1037, 1968.

LYMPHOID TUMORS

Primary tumors of lymphatic origin in children and their incidence are as follows: lymphosarcoma, 50%; Hodgkin's disease, 40%; reticulum cell sarcoma, 8%; and giant follicular lymphoma, 2%. The lymphoma group of tumors accounts for 10% of childhood neoplasms. They are considered in this section because 70% of these tumors are first recognized by lymph node enlargement. Although there are cases with features that do not readily distinguish each of these types of lymphoma, most of the tumors conform to a fairly typical histologic pattern and clinical course.

The most common initial manifestation is asymptomatic unilateral enlargement of the cervical, inguinal, or axillary lymph nodes. Intra-abdominal, nasopharyngeal, skin, and bone sites of origin occur in one-third of cases. Systemic symptoms of malaise, fever, weight loss, sweating, pruritus, and local pain may occur initially. In most patients, these symptoms become evident within several months after the original asymptomatic tumor mass is treated.

The role of the surgeon in the management of patients with lymphoid tumors is largely to obtain suitable tissue specimens for the diagnosis and staging of tumors. Exploratory abdominal operations for staging, treatment of complicating acute surgical emergencies, or even radical lymphadenectomy may be necessary.

Megavoltage radiation therapy may be extremely effective or even curative for certain lymphoid tumors, especially if the tumor is confined to a single node or one anatomic area. Chemotherapy with antineoplastic agents, with or without x-ray therapy, is valuable for prophylaxis of widespread systemic disease.

X-ray therapy is "curative" for stages I, II, and perhaps III of Hodgkin's disease. Multimodal chemotherapy is showing promise in the long-term control of advanced Hodgkin's disease and lymphomas.

Berard C & others: Current concepts of leukemia and lymphoma. Ann Intern Med 85:351, 1976.

Kaplan HS: Clinical evaluation and radiotherapeutic management of Hodgkin's disease and the malignant lymphomas. N Engl J Med 278:892, 1968.

Kaplan HS, Rosenburg SA: Hodgkin's disease: Current recommendations for management. Cancer 25:306, 1975.

Lukes RJ, Butler JJ, Hicks EB: Natural history of Hodgkin's disease as related to its pathologic picture. Cancer 19:317, 1966.

Sullivan M: Treatment of lymphoma. Cancer 35:991, 1975.

. . .

SURGICAL RESPIRATORY EMERGENCIES IN THE NEWBORN

Respiratory distress may be produced by airway obstruction, displacement of lung volume, or pulmonary parenchymal insufficiency.

Certain aspects of respiration peculiar to the infant must be appreciated. The newborn baby is an obligate nasal breather except when he is crying. The ability to breathe through the mouth may take weeks or months to learn. Inspiration is primarily accomplished by diaphragmatic excursion, and the intercostal and accessory muscles contribute little to ventilation. Impaired inspiration results in retraction of the sternum, costal margin, and neck fossae; the resulting paradoxic motion may contribute to respiratory insufficiency. The airway is small and flaccid, so that it is readily occluded by mucus or edema, and it collapses readily under slight pressure. Dyspneic infants swallow large volumes of air, and the distended stomach and bowel may further impair diaphragmatic excursion.

Classification
  A. Upper Airway:
  1. Micrognathia—Pierre Robin syndrome.
  2. Macroglossia—Muscular hypertrophy, hypothyroidism, lymphangioma.
  3. Choanal atresia.
  4. Tumors, cysts, or enlarged thyroid remnants in the pharynx or neck.
  5. Laryngeal or tracheal stenosis, webs, cysts, tumors, or vocal cord paralysis.

  B. Intrathoracic:
  1. Atelectasis.
  2. Pneumothorax and pneumomediastinum.
  3. Pleural effusion or chylothorax.
  4. Pulmonary cysts, sequestration, and tumors.
  5. Tracheomalacia or bronchomalacia.
  6. Congenital lobar emphysema.
  7. Diaphragmatic hernia or eventration.
  8. Esophageal atresia or tracheo-esophageal fistula.
  9. Vascular rings.
  10. Mediastinal tumors and cysts.

1. PIERRE ROBIN SYNDROME

Pierre Robin syndrome is a congenital defect characterized by micrognathia and glossoptosis, often associated with a cleft palate. The small lower jaw and strong sucking action of the infant allow the tongue to be sucked back and occlude the laryngeal airway and may be life-threatening.

Most infants (mild cases) should be kept in the prone position during care and feeding. A nasogastric or gastrostomy tube may be necessary. Nasohypopharyngeal intubation is effective in preventing occlusion of the larynx. If conservative measures fail, prompt attention to maintaining an open airway by tracheostomy is indicated. The tongue may be sutured forward to the lower jaw, but this frequently breaks down. In time, the lower jaw develops normally. These infants eventually learn how to keep the tongue from occluding the airway.

Dennison WM: The Pierre Robin syndrome. Pediatrics 36:336, 1965.

2. CHOANAL ATRESIA

Complete obstruction at the posterior nares due to choanal atresia may be unilateral and relatively asymptomatic. It may be membranous (10%) or bony (90%). When it is bilateral, severe respiratory distress is manifest by marked chest wall retraction on inspiration and a normal cry.

There is arching of the head and neck in an effort to breathe, and the baby is unable to eat. The diagnosis is confirmed by inability to pass a tube through the nares to the pharynx. With the baby in a supine position, radiopaque material may be instilled into the nares and lateral x-rays of the head taken to outline the obstruction.

Emergency treatment consists of maintaining an oral airway by placing a nipple, with the tip cut off, in the mouth. The membranous or bony occlusion may then be perforated by direct transpalatal excision, or it may be punctured and enlarged by using a Hegar dilator. The newly created opening must be stented with plastic tubing for 5 weeks to prevent stricture.

3. CONGENITAL PHARYNGEAL OR LARYNGEAL TUMORS, CYSTS, & STENOSES

Tumors affecting the airway of the pharynx include lingual thyroid and teratoma. The pharynx and larynx may be obstructed by hemangioma, lymphangioma, neurofibroma, and fibrosarcoma. Thyroglossal cysts, pharyngeal inclusion cysts, and laryngeal cysts may compromise breathing. Stenoses of the larynx result from fibrous webs, which are remnants of epithelial ingrowths during embryonic formation of the larynx. They may be located at the true cords or may be supraglottic.

Retractions of the chest occur on inspiration, and a prolonged expiratory wheeze may be noted. A hoarse, weak, or completely absent cry indicates involvement of the larynx. In the absence of other obvious causes of airway obstruction such as tumors of the neck, direct laryngoscopy and bronchoscopy should be performed.

The paramount concern of treatment is to provide an adequate airway; treatment of the obstructing lesion is of secondary importance. An endotracheal tube should be placed in the trachea and anchored with tape to the lips. Emergency tracheostomy may be required. A lingual thyroid can be made smaller by the administration of thyroid hormone. Some hemangioendotheliomas may respond to adrenocorticosteroids; or they may involute spontaneously. Cavernous hemangiomas and lymphangiomas are extremely difficult to excise intact when adjacent normal structures are involved. Cysts of the pharynx may be aspirated or marsupialized until excision can be accomplished. Laryngeal webs may be excised by cup forceps. Thicker webs may require repeated laryngeal dilatations.

Holinger PH: Clinical aspects of congenital anomalies of the larynx, trachea, bronchi, and esophagus. J Laryngol Otol 75:1, 1961.

4. ATELECTASIS

The airway of the unborn infant is normally filled with fluid which is formed in the lungs. This fluid flows out of the trachea to contribute to amniotic fluid. During asphyxia, the unborn baby may attempt to breathe, resulting in inhalation of amniotic fluid, meconium, or blood. When the airways are filled with this debris, they may become plugged at birth and prevent aeration of the lungs. Mucous secretions may cause atelectasis when an endotracheal tube or tracheostomy tube has been used without humidified air, or in infants with cystic fibrosis.

Prenatal asphyxia should be suspected when there is prolonged and difficult labor and when bradycardia occurs in the infant. Babies who are small for gestational age and depressed infants with low Apgar scores are particularly prone to aspiration. Meconium will be noted in the amniotic fluid and pharynx. With the onset of breathing, respirations will be labored, but chest wall retractions are not usually prominent. Chest x-rays will indicate lack of aeration in some areas or hyperaeration in areas where partial obstruction of the bronchus occurs. Bacterial pneumonia and sepsis frequently follow prolonged atelectasis.

An asphyxiated, meconium-stained, or depressed newborn infant should be treated by pharyngeal aspiration and immediate insertion of an endotracheal tube into the trachea. The trachea should also be aspirated of debris before ventilatory resuscitation is attempted.

Bronchoscopy and direct aspiration of the plugged bronchus may be necessary. Increased concentrations of inspired oxygen with ultrasonic humidification should be given to maintain the peripheral arterial P_{O_2} at about 60–80 mm Hg. Intensive physical therapy with postural drainage and chest cupping will be needed. Because of the risk of pneumothorax, positive pressure ventilation should be avoided unless it is required to maintain adequate oxygenation.

Gregory GA & others: Meconium aspiration in infants: A prospective study. J Pediatr 85:848, 1974.

Schaffer AJ: Massive aspiration syndrome. Chap 7, pp 76–85, in: *Diseases of the Newborn*, 2nd ed. Saunders, 1965.

5. CONGENITAL DIAPHRAGMATIC HERNIA & EVENTRATION OF THE DIAPHRAGM

Fusion of the transverse septum and pleuroperitoneal folds normally occurs during the eighth week of embryonic development. If diaphragmatic formation is incomplete, the pleuroperitoneal hiatus (foramen of Bochdalek) persists. The intestine normally returns from the umbilicus for rotation and fixation within the abdomen at the tenth week of gestation. If the bowel should herniate into the chest at this early stage, non-fixation of the mesentery and colon will occur. Since the transition from the glandular to the bronchial phase of pulmonary development occurs at about the 15th week of gestation, severe impairment of pulmonary development may occur when the bowel compresses the lung (Fig 48–6). Experimental studies have

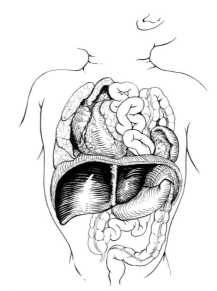

Figure 48–6. Congenital posterolateral (Bochdalek) diaphragmatic hernia. Bowel, spleen, and liver herniate into the chest and severely compromise lung development in utero and ventilation after birth. (Reproduced, with permission, from Wilson JL: *Handbook of Surgery,* 5th ed. Lange, 1973.)

shown that pulmonary hypoplasia is due to the herniation of bowel and not just an association of anomalies. The earlier in gestation the hernia occurs, the more severe the pulmonary hypoplasia.

Eventration of the diaphragm may be congenital or acquired. Congenital eventration may consist of only pleural and peritoneal membranes, with attenuation of muscular and fibrous layers. The diaphragmatic serosal membranes may protrude slightly into the pleural space or may line it completely. When intact pleural membranes exist, the distinction between eventration and Bochdalek's hernia may be quite arbitrary. Varying degrees of pulmonary hypoplasia also occur with diaphragmatic eventration.

Acquired diaphragmatic eventration may occur as a result of direct injury to the phrenic nerve associated with brachial or cervical plexus trauma during birth or during thoracotomy.

Clinical Findings

Symptoms may appear immediately after birth or not until the infant is several months old. Severe respiratory distress may be characterized by gasping respirations with cyanosis. Pulmonary hypoplasia is the most frequent cause of death. The left diaphragm is affected 4–5 times as frequently as the right. The abdomen is usually scaphoid. The chest on the side of the hernia may be dull to percussion, but bowel sounds are not usually appreciated. When the hernia is on the left, the heart sounds may be heard best on the right side of the chest. A chest x-ray will show bowel in the thorax with a shift of the mediastinal structures to the opposite side.

Treatment

An endotracheal tube should be placed in the trachea and assisted ventilation controlled to prevent a positive pressure greater than 35 cm water. A nasogastric tube should be placed in the stomach to aspirate swallowed air and to prevent distention of the herniated bowel, which further compresses the lungs. An umbilical artery catheter should be inserted to the level of the lower aorta, and metabolic acidosis must be corrected.

A rectus or transverse abdominal incision should be made and the herniated bowel reduced from the pleural space. The negative pressure between the bowel and the chest wall may make reduction difficult. This negative pressure may be broken by inserting a tube along the pleura and injecting air through it. A hernia sac should be searched for and excised. Following reduction of the bowel, a chest tube should be placed in the pleural space and connected to a water seal and not to vacuum. No attempt should be made to expand the collapsed and hypoplastic lung by positive pressure. The diaphragmatic defect should be closed by nonabsorbable sutures. In rare instances, a synthetic material, fascia, or muscle flap from the abdominal wall is required to close the defect. A gastrostomy tube should be placed in the stomach so that the nasogastric tube can be withdrawn. The abdominal cavity is often too small and undeveloped to accommodate the intestine and permit closure of the abdominal wall muscle and fascial layers. In such cases, abdominal wall skin flaps should be mobilized and closed over the protruding bowel. The resulting ventral hernia can be repaired later when the infant is thriving. Continued respiratory support and treatment of hypoxia, hypercapnia, and acidosis are required postoperatively. Persistent pulmonary hypertension may result in right-to-left shunt and produce severe hypoxia in the lower aorta. This will require tolazoline infusion through a right atrial catheter to relieve pulmonary vasospasm. Localized eventration may be approached better by means of a posterolateral thoracotomy.

Prognosis

The mortality rate depends upon the severity of pulmonary hypoplasia, the presence or absence of associated anomalies, and the quality of care provided for these critically ill infants. Surgical units which are immediately adjacent to obstetric services report mortality rates as high as 80% because infants with severe pulmonary hypoplasia will be recognized and treated immediately. Infants that survive transfer to surgical centers remote from the delivery area usually have less severe disease, and the mortality rates reported from these facilities are usually under 50%.

Bonham Carter RE, Waterston DS, Aberdeen E: Hernia and eventration of the diaphragm in childhood. Lancet 1:656, 1962.

deLorimier AA, Tierney DF, Parker HR: Hypoplastic lungs in fetal lambs with surgically produced congenital diaphragmatic hernia. Surgery 62:12, 1967.

Snyder WH, Greaney EM: Congenital diaphragmatic hernia: Seventy-seven consecutive cases. Surgery 57:576, 1965.

Thomas TV: Non-paralytic eventration of the diaphragm. J Thorac Cardiovasc Surg 55:586, 1968.

6. CONGENITAL LOBAR EMPHYSEMA

Lobar emphysema consists of massive hyperinflation of a single lobe; rarely, more than one lobe is affected. The upper and middle lobes are most frequently involved. The cause of lobar emphysema is usually unknown but has been related to deficient bronchial cartilage support, redundant mucosa, bronchial stenosis, mucous plug, and bronchial compression by anomalous vessels or other mediastinal structures.

In one-third of patients, respiratory distress is noted at birth; in only 5% of cases do symptoms develop after 6 months. Males are affected twice as frequently as females. The signs include progressive and severe dyspnea, wheezing, grunting, coughing, cyanosis, and difficulty with feedings. Increased dimensions of the chest and retractions may be seen. The chest is hyperresonant, and decreased breath sounds may be noted over the affected lobe. Chest x-rays show radiolucency of the emphysematous lobe with bronchovascular markings extending to the lung periphery. Compression atelectasis of the adjacent lung, shift of the mediastinum, depression of the diaphragm, and anterior bowing of the sternum are usually seen. The emphysematous lobe may continue to expand, compressing adjacent lung and airways and asphyxiating the infant.

Occasionally, the emphysema may be due to a mucous plug in the bronchus which may be aspirated by bronchoscopy. Compression of the bronchus by mediastinal masses may be relieved by removal of the tumor or repair of anomalous vessels. Treatment of mildly symptomatic cases may not be necessary.

Many patients with lobar emphysema are severely symptomatic, and pulmonary lobectomy is necessary. Anesthesia should not be started until all personnel are ready for emergency thoracotomy. Excessive positive pressure ventilation should be avoided. Following surgical relief of the lobar emphysema, the prognosis is excellent. Some patients may show residual disease in the remaining lung.

DeMuth GR, Sloan H: Congenital lobar emphysema: Long-term effects and sequelae in treated cases. Surgery 59:601, 1966.

Hendren WH, McKee DM: Lobar emphysema of infancy. J Pediatr Surg 1:24, 1966.

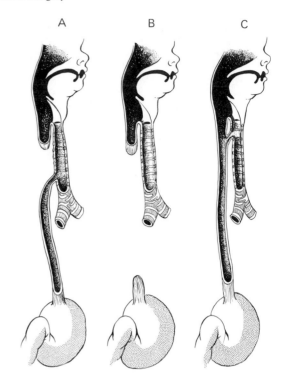

Figure 48—7. Congenital esophageal anomalies. The most common is esophageal atresia with a tracheo-esophageal fistula to the distal segment *(A).* The second most common is esophageal atresia without a tracheo-esophageal fistula *(B).* Tracheo-esophageal fistula without esophageal atresia *(C)* is the third most common anomaly, and two-thirds of these fistulas are located above the first thoracic vertebra. (Reproduced, with permission, from Wilson JL: *Handbook of Surgery,* 5th ed. Lange, 1973.)

ESOPHAGEAL ANOMALIES

Classification (Fig 48—7)

A. With Esophageal Atresia:

1. With a blind proximal pouch and a fistula between the distal end of the esophagus and the trachea (85% of cases).
2. With a blind proximal esophageal pouch, no tracheo-esophageal fistula, and a blind distal esophagus (10% of cases).
3. With fistulas between both proximal and distal esophageal segments and the trachea (0.5% of cases).
4. With a fistula between the proximal esophagus and the trachea and a blind distal esophagus without fistula (0.3% of cases).

B. Without Esophageal Atresia:

1. With an H-type tracheo-esophageal fistula (4—5% of cases).
2. With esophageal stenosis consisting of a membranous occlusion between the mid and distal thirds of the esophagus (rare).
3. With a laryngotracheo-esophageal cleft consisting of a linear communication between these structures (very rare).

Clinical Findings

Shortly after birth, the infant with esophageal atresia is noted to have excessive salivation and re-

peated episodes of coughing, choking, and cyanosis. Attempts at feeding result in choking, gagging, and regurgitation. Infants with tracheo-esophageal fistula in addition to esophageal atresia will have reflux of gastric secretions into the tracheobronchial tree which produces severe chemical bronchitis and pneumonia. Pneumonic infiltrates are usually noted first in the right upper lobe.

A size 12F catheter should be passed into the esophagus, either by way of the nose or mouth; if esophageal atresia is present, the tube will not go down the expected distance to the stomach. Smaller tubes will coil in the upper esophageal pouch or may pass from the tracheo-esophageal fistula to the stomach, giving a false impression of normal esophagus. With the tube in the upper pouch, saliva should be aspirated and no more than 2 ml of barium in saline solution should be instilled into the tube and pushed into the blind pouch by injecting air after it. Too much contrast material will result in aspiration. A lateral chest x-ray will show the contrast medium in the blind pouch and its relationship to the vertebrae. If a tracheo-esophageal fistula connects to the lower esophageal segment, air will be present in the stomach and bowel. Absence of air below the diaphragm usually means that distal tracheo-esophageal fistula is not present. Injection of contrast medium through a gastrostomy with reflux into the distal esophagus will determine the distance between the 2 esophageal ends.

Tracheo-esophageal fistula without esophageal atresia will produce repeated coughing, cyanosis, and pneumonia. These episodes are more apt to occur with swallowing liquids than with solid foods. Abdominal distention is a prominent finding because the Valsalva effect of coughing and crying forces air through the fistula into the stomach and bowel. The diagnosis may be difficult. A cine-esophagogram taken from a lateral position is required. The swallowed material should be a thin barium mixture or diatrizoate (Hypaque). Diatrizoate is hyperosmolar and irritating to the tracheal mucosa but may shrink the mucosa of the fistula to allow its visualization. The presence and position of the fistula can also be determined by bronchoscopy. A general anesthetic is used, and modern endoscopes with magnifying lenses readily locate the fistula. Two-thirds of the fistulas are located in the neck; the remainder are within the thorax.

Laryngotracheo-esophageal cleft produces symptoms similar to those of tracheo-esophageal fistula but of much greater severity. Laryngoscopy may show the cleft between the arytenoids extending down the larynx. Bronchoscopy is often a better means of outlining the cleft.

Differential Diagnosis

Newborn infants may have transient dysphagia with aspiration of feedings due to an uncoordinated swallowing mechanism. This usually subsides within the first 2 days after birth. Prolonged swallowing dysfunction may occur with brain anomaly or injury.

Treatment

Aspiration pneumonia must be treated before surgical treatment is begun. A sump suction catheter should be placed in the infant's upper esophageal pouch and connected to continuous suction. The head of the bed should be elevated. The infant should be placed in a humidified incubator, turned from side to side every hour, and stimulated to cry and cough. Ampicillin, 75 mg/kg, and gentamicin, 1.5 mg/kg, should be given every 8 hours IM. If the infant is fully mature and has no severe anomalies, gastrostomy and extrapleural thoracotomy should be done for division of tracheo-esophageal fistula and primary esophageal anastomosis. The operation should be staged for premature babies, for infants with associated severe anomalies, or for babies with a short upper esophageal segment. The first stage consists of a gastrostomy and transpleural division of the tracheo-esophageal fistula. A sump suction catheter is maintained in the upper esophageal pouch, and the baby is fed by gastrostomy until he has become strong enough to tolerate the second stage procedure. A short upper pouch can be elongated with a 22–24F Hurst bougie 2–3 times per day over a period of 2–3 weeks. The second stage procedure consists of an extrapleural thoracotomy followed by anastomosis of the 2 esophageal segments. A long distance between the 2 esophageal ends may be corrected by making one or more circumferential incisions in the muscularis of the proximal esophagus to allow the mucosa to stretch the desired length.

The infant with esophageal atresia and no tracheo-esophageal fistula requires cervical esophagostomy and gastrostomy. He is fed through the gastrostomy tube until he weighs 9–11 kg, at which time a colon or gastric tube interposition is used to establish continuity between the cervical esophagus and the stomach.

In infants with an H-type tracheo-esophageal fistula, the fistula is located above the thoracic inlet in two-thirds of cases. These fistulas may be divided through a left transverse cervical incision. Intrathoracic fistulas may be divided by an extrapleural right thoracotomy. A gastrostomy is commonly employed for feeding until the esophageal closure is healed.

Esophageal webs respond readily to esophageal dilatation. This is usually accomplished with Hurst or Maloney mercury-weighted bougies. Dilatations are repeated until healing occurs without recurrence. Esophagoscopy and excision of portions of a tough or thick web, using biopsy forceps, may be required in addition to dilatation.

Prognosis

The survival rate for a full-term infant without associated anomalies is excellent. Deaths do occur, however, as a result of pulmonary complications, severe associated anomalies, prematurity, and sepsis due to anastomotic disruption. Anastomotic leaks occur either as a result of technical problems or because the distal esophageal wall is very weak. In performing the anastomosis, the extrapleural approach prevents the development of empyema and maintains infection to a small localized area. Swallowing is a reflex response that must be reinforced early in infancy. If establishment of esophageal continuity is delayed for more than 4–6 weeks, it may take many months to teach the infant to swallow. Babies with cervical esophagostomy should be encouraged to suck, eat, and swallow during gastrostomy feedings.

Dysphagia may occur weeks or months following successful repair of esophageal atresia. Stricture of the anastomosis may require one or more dilatations, with a filiform and follower, or by using antegrade or retrograde dilators. Another cause of dysphagia may be neuromuscular incoordination, usually associated with esophageal anomalies. This frequent problem improves with age.

Most of these infants have an alarming, barking cough and rattling sound with respiration due to chondromalacia of the tracheal rings at the site of tracheo-esophageal fistula.

Swallowed foreign bodies will lodge at the site of anastomosis and require removal with esophagoscopy. Hiatal hernia with reflux esophagitis occasionally follows successful repair and requires surgical treatment.

Blackburn WR, Amoury RA: Congenital esophago-pulmonary fistulas without esophageal atresia: An analysis of 260 fistulas in infants, children, and adults. Rev Surg 23:153, 1966.

deLorimier AA: Treatment of esophageal atresia with a short proximal esophageal segment. JAMA 195:697, 1966.

Eraklis AJ & others: Circular esophagomyotomy of upper pouch in primary repair of long-segment esophageal atresia. J Pediatr Surg 11:709, 1976.

Holder TM & others: Esophageal atresia and tracheo-esophageal fistula: A survey of its members by the Surgical Section of the Academy of Pediatrics. Pediatrics 34:542, 1964.

VASCULAR RINGS

Tracheobronchial and esophageal compression by the great vessels may occur as a result of anomalies of the aortic arch or of abnormally located or enlarged pulmonary arteries. The genesis of aortic vascular rings may be understood if the embryo is considered to have 2 aortic arches, each with a carotid and subclavian artery and a ductus arteriosus (Fig 48–8). In the normal development of the aortic arch, the distal portion of the right arch is obliterated. There are 5 main types of vascular rings: (1) persistence of both arches gives rise to double aortic arch (Fig 48–9); (2) obliteration of the left distal arch generates right aortic arch and persistent left ligamentum arteriosum; (3) obliteration of the right arch between the right carotid and subclavian arteries results in anomalous origin of the right subclavian artery; (4) incorporation of the right proximal arch into the left arch produces anomalous origin of the innominate artery; and (5) incorporation of the left proximal arch into the right arch gives rise to an anomalous origin of the right common carotid artery.

When the left pulmonary artery arises from the right pulmonary artery, it encircles the right side of the trachea and courses between the trachea and esophagus to the left lung. This sling effect produces significant

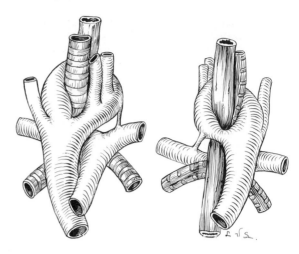

Figure 48–9. Anterior (left) and posterior views of double aortic arch constricting the trachea and esophagus.

compression of the lower trachea and proximal main bronchi. Aneurysmal dilatation of the pulmonary artery usually occurs in association with ventricular septal defect and infundibular stenosis. Other forms of congenital heart defects are frequent. Each of these anomalies may compress and encircle the trachea and esophagus, producing respiratory distress and symptoms of obstruction on swallowing.

Clinical Findings

These infants have a characteristic inspiratory and expiratory wheeze, stridor, or croup. The head is held in an opisthotonic position to prevent compression of the trachea. If the head is forcibly flexed, the stridor is increased and apnea may be produced. There may be hesitation on swallowing, with episodes of choking—so-called dysphagia lusoria. Chest x-rays may show compression of the trachea. Anteroposterior and lateral esophagograms show indentation of the esophagus at the level of T3 and T4. When there is no esophageal indentation, a tracheogram may be necessary to demonstrate tracheal compression due to anomalous origin of the innominate or left common carotid artery. An angiocardiogram is not necessary for isolated aortic arch anomalies but is required for assessing congenital heart lesions associated with anomalies of the pulmonary artery. Esophagoscopy and bronchoscopy may be helpful in assessing the degree and level of compression.

Treatment

The aortic arch anomaly must be completely dissected and visualized through a left thoracotomy. The smallest component of a double aortic arch must be divided. An anomalous right subclavian artery is divided at its origin. The anomalous innominate or left carotid arteries are pulled forward by placing sutures between their adventitia and the sternum. The accompanying fibrous bands and sheaths constricting the tra-

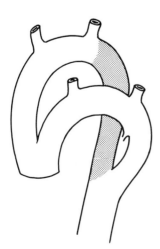

Figure 48–8. Normal embryonic aortic arch.

chea and esophagus must also be divided. Pulmonary artery slings are corrected by dividing the origin of the left pulmonary artery and anastomosing it to the main pulmonary artery anterior to the trachea. Aneurysmal dilatation of the pulmonary artery is relieved by correcting the congenital heart defect; occasionally, the pulmonary artery requires reduction in size by direct surgical resection.

Occasionally, symptoms persist postoperatively because of deformed tracheocartilaginous rings. This may require tracheostomy and endotracheal intubation for a prolonged period of time. If tracheomalacia is present, sleeve resection of the abnormal portion of the trachea and bronchi with anastomosis should be accomplished.

Lincoln JCR & others: Vascular anomalies compressing the esophagus and trachea. Thorax 24:295, 1969.

Mahoney EB, Manning JA: Congenital abnormalities of the aortic arch. Surgery 55:1, 1964.

Park CD & others: Tracheal compression by the great arteries in the mediastinum. Arch Surg 103:623, 1971.

CHALASIA OF THE ESOPHAGUS

Chalasia of the esophagus refers to an incompetent cardioesophageal sphincter mechanism. Studies of esophageal motility and manometric measurements of the cardioesophageal junction show an absence of the high-pressure zone in the lower esophagus in most newborn infants. Change to the normal adult pattern of peristalsis and the development of a competent cardioesophageal sphincter develops after several months. Until this occurs, many infants suffer varying degrees of regurgitation after feeding. Repeated gastric reflux may produce peptic esophagitis and interfere with subsequent development of a competent sphincter mechanism.

Symptoms consist of repeated, effortless regurgitation of feedings, particularly when the baby is placed in a recumbent position. The baby will be hungry and will readily feed after vomiting. Persistent regurgitation may result in poor weight gain, peptic esophagitis with appearance of blood in the vomitus, or occult bleeding, producing anemia. Aspiration of vomitus, particularly during sleep, produces recurrent pneumonia.

The symptoms are the same as those occurring with esophageal hiatal hernia and incompetent cardioesophageal sphincter. The diagnosis is established by esophagography under fluoroscopic vision or with cineradiography.

Conservative treatment is successful in most cases. The feedings should be thickened with rice cereal, and the baby should be maintained upright at all times in an "infant seat." If a prolonged trial of this conservative approach fails and significant complications of growth failure, anemia, or pneumonia persist, an antireflux procedure such as the Nissen gastric fundoplication is indicated.

Bettex M, Kuffer F: Long-term results of fundoplication in hiatus hernia and cardioesophageal chalasia in infants and children. J Pediatr Surg 4:526, 1969.

Strawczynski H & others: The behavior of the lower esophageal sphincter in infants and its relationship in gastroesophageal regurgitation. J Pediatr 64:17, 1964.

HYPERTROPHIC PYLORIC STENOSIS

Pyloric stenosis results from hypertrophy of the circular and longitudinal muscularis of the pylorus and distal antrum of the stomach (Fig 48–10). The cause is not known. The male/female incidence is 4:1. The disorder is more common in first-born infants and occurs 4 times more often in the offspring of mothers who had the disease as infants than in those whose fathers had the disease. If one monozygotic twin is affected, the other will have the disorder also in two-thirds of cases. A seasonal variation is noted in the occurrence of symptoms, with peaks in spring and fall.

Clinical Findings

A. Symptoms and Signs: The "typical" affected infant was full-term when born and had been feeding and growing well until he was 2 weeks old. Occasional regurgitation of some of the feedings occurred initially. Several days later, however, the vomiting became more frequent and projectile. The vomitus contained the previous feeding and no bile. Blood may be seen in the vomitus in 5% of cases, and coffee-ground or occult blood is frequently present. Shortly after vomiting, the infant acts starved and will feed again. The stools become infrequent and firm in consistency as dehydration occurs. The premature and weak, chronically starved infant does not have the strength to have projectile vomiting, and seemingly effortless regurgitation is the usual symptom.

Less frequently, symptoms occur earlier—even shortly after birth—or as much as 4 months later.

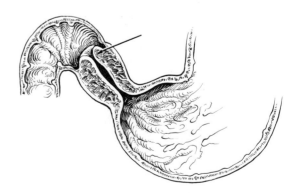

Figure 48–10. Hypertrophic pyloric stenosis. Note that the distal end of the hypertrophic muscle protrudes into the duodenum (arrow), accounting for the ease of perforation into the duodenum during pyloromyotomy.

Weight loss follows progressive starvation. Jaundice with indirect hyperbilirubinemia occurs in fewer than 10% of cases. Gastric peristaltic waves can usually be seen moving from the left costal margin to the area of the pylorus. The pyloric "tumor" or "olive" can be palpated when the infant is relaxed in over 95% of cases. Abdominal relaxation may be accomplished by sedation or by feeding clear fluids and simultaneously aspirating the stomach contents with a nasogastric tube.

B. X-Ray Findings: A gastrointestinal series is indicated in those cases in which a pyloric tumor cannot be palpated. Radiographic diagnostic signs, preferably using small amounts of meglumine diatrizoate (Gastrografin), include (1) outlining of the narrow pyloric channel by a single "string sign" or "double track" due to folds of mucosa; (2) a pyloric "beak" where the pyloric entrance from the antrum occurs; (3) the "shoulder" sign, in which the pyloric mass bulges into the antrum; (4) the pyloric "tit," where the contrast bulges on the lesser curvature between peristaltic waves; and (5) complete obstruction of the pylorus.

Differential Diagnosis

Repeated nonbilious vomiting in early infancy may be due to feeding problems, intracranial lesions, incompetence of the cardio-esophageal sphincter (chalasia) with or without hiatal hernia, pylorospasm, duodenal stenosis, malrotation of the bowel, or adrenal insufficiency.

Complications

Repeated vomiting with inadequate intake of formula results in hypochloremic, hypokalemic alkalosis, dehydration, and starvation. Gastritis and reflux esophagitis occur frequently and may contribute to an incompetent cardio-esophageal sphincter. Aspiration of vomitus may produce pneumonia or suffocation.

Treatment & Prognosis

Conservative treatment with antispasmodics has been advocated by some, but this requires prolonged, constant vigilance and care to maintain nutrition and prevent aspiration of vomitus. After many months, the pyloric hypertrophy may subside with relief of obstructive symptoms.

The preferred operative treatment is the Fredet-Ramstedt pyloromyotomy, which should be undertaken only after dehydration and hypokalemic hypochloremic alkalosis have been corrected. A nasogastric tube should be placed preoperatively to empty the stomach.

Postoperatively, nasogastric suction is continued for 8–12 hours. Following this, the infant is fed 10% dextrose solution, 30 ml for 3 feedings; the regular formula is then resumed, giving 45 ml every 3 hours for 3 feedings and then increasing the volume 15 ml at a time until the normal intake is being given. The hospital stay averages 3 days. Occasionally, an infant will vomit persistently, and prolonged nasogastric suction

may be required for several days until normal motility returns. Careful management should result in no mortality and prompt recovery.

Carter CO, Evans KA: Inheritance of congenital pyloric stenosis. J Med Genet 6:223, 1969.

Kwok RH, Avery G: Seasonal variation of congenital hypertrophic pyloric stenosis. J Pediatr 70:963, 1967.

Shuman FI, Darling DB, Fisher JH: The radiographic diagnosis of congenital hypertrophic pyloric stenosis. J Pediatr 71:70, 1967.

INTESTINAL OBSTRUCTION IN THE NEWBORN

The cardinal signs and symptoms of intestinal obstruction are (1) polyhydramnios in the mother, (2) vomiting, (3) abdominal distention, and (4) failure to pass meconium. Polyhydramnios is related to the level of obstruction, occurring in approximately 45% of women who have infants with duodenal atresia and 15% of those who have infants with ileal atresia. When a tube is routinely passed into the stomach of a newborn, a residual greater than 40 ml is diagnostic of obstruction. Vomiting occurs early in upper intestinal obstruction, and it is bile-stained if the obstruction is distal to the ampulla of Vater. Abdominal distention is related to the level of obstruction, being most marked for distal obstructions. Meconium is passed in 30–50% of newborn infants with intestinal obstruction, but failure to pass meconium within the first 24 hours is distinctly abnormal.

Causes of neonatal intestinal obstruction include intestinal atresia or stenosis, annular pancreas, malrotation with peritoneal bands or volvulus, meconium ileus, Hirschsprung's disease, meconium plug syndrome, and neonatal small left colon syndrome. Atresia of the bowel occurs in the duodenum in 40%, in the jejunum in 20%, in the ileum in 20%, and in the colon in 10% of cases.

1. CONGENITAL DUODENAL OBSTRUCTION

Duodenal atresia and stenosis produce obstruction at the level of the ampulla of Vater. In 75% of cases, the bile is diverted to the proximal duodenum. Annular pancreas is almost always associated with hypoplasia of the duodenum at the level of the ampulla. In about half of cases, multiple congenital anomalies are present, including Down's syndrome in 30% and congenital heart disease in 20%. Birth weight is less than 2500 g in half of these infants.

Vomiting, usually with bile, occurs shortly after birth and during attempted feedings. Distention of the upper abdomen may be noted. Meconium is passed in over 50% of cases. Abdominal x-rays show a distended stomach and duodenum ("double bubble" sign). Gas in the small and large intestine indicates incomplete obstruction. Barium (in saline) enema identifies the presence or absence of malrotation, and the colon may be noted to be unused (microcolon).

The abdomen is explored through a right upper transverse abdominal incision. The hepatic flexure may have to be mobilized to expose the duodenum. Although it is tempting to perform a Heineke-Mikulicz duodenoplasty for stenosis and webs, there is a risk of injuring the ampulla of Vater. A retrocolic, side-to-side duodenojejunostomy is the procedure of choice. A gastrostomy should also be performed for decompression of the stomach and duodenum and to check gastric residual during graded feedings. Persistent functional obstruction may be obviated by performing a long side-to-side duodenojejunostomy from the pylorus to the point of obstruction. A fine Silastic catheter may be passed alongside the gastrostomy tube and through the anastomosis into the jejunum for purposes of feeding until duodenal peristalsis becomes functional. Gastrojejunostomy should not be done because the blind duodenal pouch may cause repeated vomiting. The mortality rate is high because of prematurity and associated anomalies.

Fonkalsrud EW, deLorimier AA, Hays DM: Congenital atresia and stenosis of the duodenum. Pediatrics 43:79, 1969.

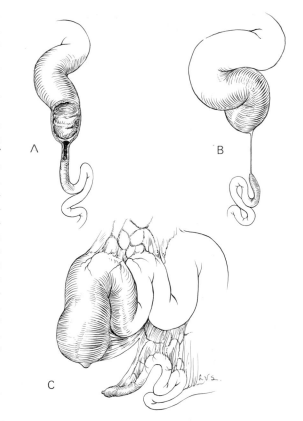

Figure 48—11. Types of intestinal atresia. *A:* A membranous web. *B:* Fibrous band connecting 2 blind ends. *C:* Complete separation of the 2 ends with V-shaped defects in the mesentery.

2. ATRESIA & STENOSIS OF THE JEJUNUM, ILEUM, & COLON

Atresia and stenosis of the jejunum, ileum, and colon are caused by a mesenteric vascular accident in utero such as may result from hernia, volvulus, or intussusception, producing aseptic necrosis and resorption of the necrotic bowel. Although atresia may occur in any portion of the intestine, most cases occur in the proximal jejunum or distal ileum. A short area of necrosis may produce only stenosis or a membranous web occluding the lumen. A more extensive infarct may leave a fibrous cord between the 2 bowel loops, or the proximal and distal bowel may be completely separated with a V-shaped defect in the mesentery (Fig 48—11). Multiple atresias occur in 10% of cases.

Vomiting of bile, abdominal distention, and failure to pass meconium indicate intestinal obstruction. Plain abdominal x-rays will give an estimate of how far along the intestine the obstruction exists; small bowel, however, cannot be distinguished from colon in the newborn. No contrast material should be given by mouth to newborn babies with complete intestinal obstruction. A barium (in saline) enema may be indicated to detect the level of obstruction and the coexistence of anomalous rotation. In obstructions which occur in the distal bowel and which appear relatively early in gestation, the colon will be empty of meconium and will appear abnormally narrow. When the obstruction is proximal, or when it occurs late in pregnancy, meconium will be passed into the colon. Barium enema will then outline a more generous-sized colon with its contents. Rarely, a microcolon is not just unused bowel but is due to Hirschsprung's disease. In older children with evidence of partial intestinal obstruction, a small bowel series may be indicated to identify intestinal stenosis.

A transverse upper abdominal incision is preferred. Infants with jejunal atresia usually have greatly dilated bowel from the stomach to the point of obstruction. This overly distended jejunum should be resected—to the ligament of Treitz, if necessary—since it is a source of persistent functional obstruction if it is retained. This same principle applies for membranous atresia, and the temptation to resect the web and perform a Heineke-Mikulicz resection should be resisted.

In patients with ileal atresia, only the most distal blind end is bulbously dilated, and this should be excised. More proximal resection of ileum should not be performed to prevent the complication of malabsorption. A great discrepancy between the diameter of the segments of intestine proximal and distal to the atresia is the rule. Therefore, the preferred anastomosis will be end-to-oblique or end-to-side.

A gastrostomy is preferred to help in postoperative decompression and to provide graded feedings.

Atresia of the proximal colon should be treated by resection of the dilated bowel and ileocolostomy. Atresia of the distal colon may be treated by proximal end colostomy or by a Mikulicz side-to-side colostomy. Later, the continuity of the distal colon may be established by end-to-end anastomosis.

The high mortality rate is related to sepsis, malfunctioning proximal bowel and anastomosis, prematurity, and coexisting meconium peritonitis. In contrast to duodenal atresia, associated anomalies are unusual in small bowel and colon atresia.

Coran AG, Eraklis AJ: Atresia of the colon. Surgery 65:828, 1969.

deLorimier AA, Fonkalsrud EW, Hays DM: Congenital atresia and stenosis of the jejunum and ileum. Surgery 65:819, 1969.

Louw JH: Resection and end-to-end anastomosis in the management of atresia and stenosis of the small bowel. Surgery 62:940, 1967.

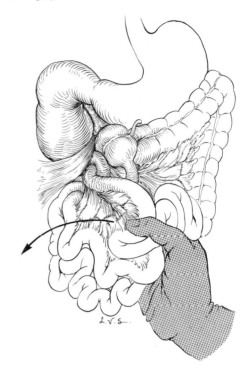

Figure 48–12. Malrotation of the midgut with volvulus. Note cecum at the origin of the superior mesenteric vessels. Fibrous bands cross and obstruct the duodenum as they adhere to the cecum. Volvulus is derotated in a counterclockwise direction.

DISORDERS OF INTESTINAL ROTATION

The midgut of the 10-week-old fetus normally returns from the umbilicus to the abdominal cavity and undergoes counterclockwise rotation about the superior mesenteric artery axis. The duodenojejunal portion of gut rotates posterior to the superior mesenteric vessels for 270 degrees. The duodenojejunal junction becomes fixed at the ligament of Treitz and located to the left of and cephalad to the superior mesenteric artery. The cecocolic portion of the midgut also rotates 270 degrees counterclockwise, anterior to the superior mesenteric artery; and the cecum normally becomes fixed in the right lower abdomen.

Pathogenesis & Classification

Anomalies of rotation and fixation (twice as common in males as in females) include (1) nonrotation, (2) incomplete rotation, (3) reversed rotation, and (4) anomalous fixation of the mesentery.

A. Nonrotation: When rotation does not occur, the midgut is suspended from the superior mesenteric vessels, with the small bowel located on the right side of the abdomen and the large bowel in the left abdomen. No fixation occurs, and adhesive bands are not present. This anomaly is usually found in patients with omphalocele, gastroschisis, and congenital diaphragmatic hernia.

B. Incomplete Rotation: Incomplete rotation may affect the duodenojejunal segment, the cecocolic portion of the bowel, or both. Adhesive bands are usually present. In the most common form of incomplete rotation, the cecum is adjacent to the root of the superior mesenteric vessels and dense peritoneal bands extend from the right abdomen to the cecum, ob-

structing the duodenum (Fig 48–12). Because the base of the mesentery is quite short and does not extend (as normally) from the ligament of Treitz in the left upper abdomen to the cecum in the right lower abdomen, volvulus frequently occurs, with clockwise twisting of the bowel about the superior mesenteric vessels.

C. Reversed Rotation: In reversed rotation, the bowel rotates varying degrees in a clockwise direction about the superior mesenteric axis. The duodenojejunal loop is anterior to the superior mesenteric artery. The cecocolic loop may be prearterial or may be rotated clockwise or counterclockwise in a retroarterial position. In either case, the cecum may be right-sided or left-sided. The most frequent anomaly is retroarterial clockwise rotation, which produces obstruction of the right colon.

D. Anomalous Fixation of Mesentery: Anomalies of mesenteric fixation account for internal mesenteric and paraduodenal hernias, mobile cecum, or obstructing adhesive bands in the absence of anomalous bowel rotation.

Clinical Findings

Anomalies of intestinal rotation may cause symptoms related to intestinal obstruction, peptic ulceration, or malabsorption. Three-fourths of patients develop intestinal obstruction in infancy. Older patients may develop intermittent obstruction. The obstruction occurs in the duodenum or upper jejunum as a result of adhesive bands or midgut volvulus. Vomiting of bile occurs initially. Older patients may appear thin and wasted, presumably because of early satiety due to chronic partial obstruction or malabsorption. When the obstruction is due to bands, abdominal distention is not prominent. When volvulus occurs, abdominal distention may be very great. Bloody stools and signs of peritonitis indicate infarction of the bowel. Plain abdominal x-rays may show a "double bubble" sign which mimics duodenal stenosis. Distribution of gas throughout the intestines may be normal. When volvulus with gangrene occurs—the most disastrous complication—the bowel will be distended with gas and the intestinal walls will be thickened. Barium enema will show abnormal position of the cecum. With chronic intermittent symptoms of obstruction and a normal position of the cecum noted on barium enema, an upper gastrointestinal and small bowel series will show distention of the duodenum and narrowing at the point of obstruction.

Duodenal and antral stasis presumably account for the presence of peptic ulcer in 20% of patients. Malabsorption with steatorrhea occurs as a result of partial venous and lymphatic obstruction, and coarse rugal folds of the small bowel may be noted.

Treatment

Through a transverse upper abdominal incision, the entire bowel should be delivered from the abdominal cavity to assess the anomalous arrangement of the intestinal loops. Volvulus should be untwisted in a counterclockwise direction (Fig 48–12). The Ladd procedure consists of division of adhesive bands between the duodenum and proximal colon and the lateral abdominal wall. The appendix is removed. The cecum is then placed in the left lower quadrant and the duodenum moved to the right lateral abdomen. When duodenal obstruction exists without evident anomalous rotation of the colon, the right colon should be mobilized to expose the duodenum and the duodenum is moved to the right lateral abdomen. A Kocher maneuver should be accomplished, with complete mobilization of the third and fourth portions of the duodenum. Upon completion of the above procedures, a gastrostomy should be performed and a Foley catheter threaded through it down the duodenum and jejunum. The balloon should then be inflated and withdrawn to the stomach. This maneuver will detect an intrinsic web partially obstructing the bowel, which may coexist with the anomalies of rotation and fixation.

Prognosis

Once correction of the anomaly has been accomplished, the long-term results are excellent. Some patients tend to form adhesions that cause recurrent intestinal obstruction. Recurrent volvulus is rare after the Ladd procedure.

Amir-Jahed AK: Classification of reversed intestinal rotation. Surgery 64:1071, 1968.

Bill AH, Grauman D: Rationale and technic for stabilization of the mesentery in cases of nonrotation of the midgut. J Pediatr Surg 1:127, 1966.

Louw JH: Intestinal malrotation and duodenal ileus. J R Coll Surg Edinb 5:101, 1960.

Rees JR, Redo SF: Anomalies of intestinal rotation and fixation. Am J Surg 116:834, 1968.

MECONIUM ILEUS

In 20% of infants born with cystic fibrosis, the thick mucous secretions of the small bowel produce obturant obstruction due to inspissated meconium. This usually occurs in the mid ileum but may develop in the jejunum or colon. Although there is no clear correlation between pancreatic insufficiency and the development of inspissated meconium, meconium ileus also occurs in patients with pancreatic duct obstruction and pancreatic aplasia. Meconium obstruction without any apparent cause has also been described in newborn infants.

Meconium ileus may be complicated by volvulus of the heavy, distended loops of bowel. Depending upon how early in fetal life this occurs, the volvulus may progress to gangrene of the bowel, perforation with meconium peritonitis, or atresia of the ileum—singly or in combination (Fig 48–13).

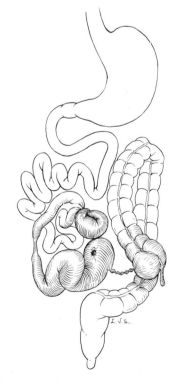

Figure 48–13. Complicated meconium ileus. Includes malrotation, volvulus of the heavy, meconium-filled bowel, and ischemic necrosis of the bowel, producing stenosis, atresia, or perforation with meconium peritonitis.

Meconium ileus equivalent is obturant intestinal obstruction from viscid mucous secretions occurring after the newborn period. All of these patients have cystic fibrosis. The age at onset varies from several days after birth to early adulthood, but most cases occur within the first year. A respiratory infection and fever with dehydration usually precede the obstruction. Paradoxically, these patients usually have symptoms of pancreatic insufficiency with steatorrhea prior to the onset of intestinal obstruction.

Clinical Findings

The infant typically has a normal birth weight. The abdomen is usually distended, and may be large enough to cause dystocia. In most cases, no meconium is passed. Vomiting of bile occurs early. Loops of thick, distended bowel may be seen and palpated. Plain abdominal x-rays show loops of bowel which vary greatly in diameter; the thick meconium gives a ground-glass appearance. When air mixes with the meconium, the so-called "soap bubble" sign is produced, usually in the right lower quadrant. X-rays taken shortly after the infant has been placed in an upright position may fail to show air-fluid levels because the thick, viscid meconium fails to layer out rapidly. An x-ray contrast enema will show microcolon with some meconium flecks. Reflux of contrast medium into the terminal ileum will outline a small terminal ileum with inspissated mucus; more proximally, the bowel is progressively distended with packed meconium. In complicated meconium ileus, perforation may be detected by the presence of calcification or extraluminal air. The sweat chloride test is usually impractical in the newborn because very little sweat can be collected. The albumin content of meconium in babies with cystic fibrosis is high, whereas no protein is found normally. Histologic sections of resected bowel will show an increase in number and size of the goblet cells, and the intestinal glands will be engorged with inspissated mucus.

Complications

The most common complication of meconium ileus is repeated pulmonary infection with chronic bronchopneumonia, bronchiectasis, atelectasis, and lung abscess. Malabsorption due to pancreatic insufficiency will require enzyme replacement with feedings. Rectal prolapse and intussusception are related to the inspissated stools of these patients. Nasal polyps and chronic sinusitis are frequently noted. Biliary cirrhosis and bleeding varices from portal hypertension are late manifestations of bile duct mucous occlusion.

Treatment

A nasogastric tube should be inserted into the stomach and connected to suction. Under fluoroscopic control, enemas containing full-strength meglumine diatrizoate (Gastrografin), which is hygroscopic, or acetylcysteine (Mucomyst), which is mucolytic, may effectively unplug the meconium in uncomplicated cases. The enema must be given to a well-hydrated infant, and intravenous infusions must be continued to prevent hypovolemia following the enema. Most patients, however, have bowel gangrene, atresia, or perforation due to volvulus, and require a right lower quadrant transverse incision and Mikulicz resection of the most dilated portion of the ileum. The proximal and distal bowel loops may then be irrigated with acetylcysteine. Subsequently, the Mikulicz enterostomy is closed.

These patients must be placed in an environment with high humidity to keep the tracheobronchial secretions fluid. Ultrasonic mist is preferable. Postural drainage with cupping of the chest should be taught to the parents so that they will continue to maintain tracheobronchial toilet indefinitely. Long-term prophylactic antibiotics are not indicated since infection with antibiotic-resistant pseudomonas and klebsiella organisms usually develop.

Pancreatic enzyme replacement in the form of pancreatin (Panteric, Viokase) or pancrelipase (Cotazym) may be required. A low-fat formula in the newborn may produce better absorption and growth than standard formulas.

Meconium ileus equivalent should be treated conservatively by nasogastric suction, meglumine diatrizoate or 4% acetylcysteine enemas, and 4% acetylcysteine instilled into the stomach. Many patients develop mucous impaction of the bowel because of failure to take pancreatic enzymes orally. Respiratory infection and fever with dehydration usually precipitate meconium ileus equivalent.

Prognosis

The most frequent cause of death is progressive respiratory insufficiency due to plugging of bronchi with mucus, producing chronic bronchitis, atelectasis, pneumonia, and lung abscess. About 50% of these children die by age 10. Chronic malabsorption develops as a result of pancreatic insufficiency and because the viscid mucus produces a barrier between the bowel lumen and the intestinal mucosa.

Cordonnier JK, Izant RJ: Meconium ileus equivalent. Surgery 54:667, 1963.

Graham WP, Jaffee BF, deLorimier AA: Late intestinal obstruction in patients surviving neonatal meconium ileus. Calif Med 103:171, 1965.

Holsclaw DS, Eckstein HB, Nixon HH: Meconium ileus. Am J Dis Child 109:101, 1965.

Noblett HR: Treatment of uncomplicated meconium ileus by Gastrografin enema: A preliminary report. J Pediatr Surg 4:190, 1969.

Thomaidis TS, Arey JB: The intestinal lesion in cystic fibrosis of the pancreas. J Pediatr 63:444, 1963.

NECROTIZING ENTEROCOLITIS

Necrotizing enterocolitis is characterized by ischemic ulceration and slough of intestinal mucosa, and it frequently progresses to full thickness necrosis and perforation of varying lengths of bowel. The terminal ileum and right colon are usually affected first, followed in descending order of frequency by transverse and descending colon, appendix, jejunum, stomach, duodenum, and esophagus. Most of the patients are premature infants with stressful perinatal episodes, including premature rupture of membranes with amnionitis, breech delivery, intrauterine bradycardia, umbilical vessel catheterization with or without exchange transfusion, respiratory distress syndrome, sepsis, omphalitis, and congenital heart disease. Patent ductus arteriosus is commonly associated. In older infants and children, it is usually preceded by malnutrition and various forms of gastroenteritis. These stressful events result in hypovolemia or large left-to-right shunt through a patent ductus arteriosus or other congenital heart disease. To preserve blood supply to the brain and heart, the mesenteric vessels constrict, resulting in platelet and fibrin plugging of small vessels, impaired bowel perfusion, mucosal necrosis with bacterial invasion of the bowel wall, intramural gas formation, full thickness necrosis, and perforation. Almost invariably, the infant has been fed. The usual onset of the enteritis is within 1 week after birth, but it may occur several weeks later. Clinical findings include increased gastric residuals or bilious vomiting, abdominal distention, bloody stools, apneic episodes, lethargy, and poor skin perfusion. When perforation occurs, the abdomen will become guarded, but in weak premature infants this may not be clearly obvious. Supine and cross-table lateral abdominal roentgenograms show small bowel distention (ileus) early, followed by pneumatosis intestinalis and gas within the portal vein of the liver; following perforation, free peritoneal air will be seen. The white blood count may be low or high, but thrombocytopenia is usually present.

Treatment includes cessation of feedings, nasogastric suction, systemic antibiotics, and correction of hypoxia, hypovolemia, acidosis, and electrolyte abnormalities. Intravenous alimentation should be started. Surgical treatment is required when perforation has occurred and consists of resecting necrotic bowel with ileostomy or colostomy. Stricture of the bowel may occur as a late complication following healing of necrotizing enterocolitis. The mortality rate varies from 11–50%.

Santulli TV & others: Acute necrotizing enterocolitis in infancy: A review of 64 cases. Pediatrics 55:376, 1975.

Stevenson JK: Aggressive treatment of neonatal necrotizing entercolitis: 28 patients with 25 survivors. J Pediatr Surg 6:28, 1971.

HIRSCHSPRUNG'S DISEASE

Hirschsprung's disease (aganglionic megacolon) is due to absence of cephalocaudal growth of the parasympathetic myenteric nerve cells into the rectum and lower colon or sometimes even into the entire colon and ileum. The aganglionic rectum and colon produce a functional obstruction because the bowel does not have normal propulsive waves and contracts en masse in response to distention. Short segment aganglionosis involving only the terminal rectum occurs in about 10% of instances. The disease extends to the signoid colon in 65% of cases. In 10%, more proximal colon is involved, and in 10–15% of cases the entire colon lacks ganglion cells. Extensive involvement of the small bowel is rare.

Males are affected 5 times more frequently than females in cases where the involvement is of the usual length. Females tend to have longer aganglionic segments. A familial association occurs in 5–10% of cases—more frequently when females are affected. The length of involvement tends to be consistent in familial cases. Other anomalies are present also in 10–15% of patients.

Clinical Findings

A. Symptoms and Signs: The symptoms vary widely in severity but almost always occur shortly after birth. The infant passes little or no meconium within 24 hours. Thereafter, chronic or intermittent constipation usually occurs. Progressive abdominal distention, vomiting, reluctance to feed, diarrhea, listlessness, irritability, and poor growth and development follow. A rectal examination in the infant may be followed by expulsion of stool and flatus with remarkable decompression of abdominal distention. However, foul-smelling diarrhea and abdominal distention should be considered Hirschsprung's disease until proved otherwise. In older children, chronic constipation and abdominal distention are characteristic. Passage of flatus and stool requires great effort, and the stools are small in caliber. These children are sluggish, with wasted extremities and flared costal margins. Rectal examination in older children usually reveals a normal or contracted anus and a rectum without feces. Impacted stools can be palpated across the lower abdomen because of the greatly dilated and distended signoid colon.

B. Laboratory Findings: Definitive diagnosis is made by rectal biopsy. This requires removing a 1 × 2 cm full thickness strip of rectum from the posterior rectum proximal to the dentate line. A sample of this size is sufficient for the pathologist to determine whether ganglion cells are or are not present in Meissner's plexus or in Auerbach's plexus. Serial section of multiple rectal punch biopsies may demonstrate an absence of Meissner's plexus. Failure in relaxation of the internal anal sphincter following rectal distention by a balloon may be diagnostic of Hirschsprung's disease.

C. X-Ray Findings: Plain abdominal x-rays in infants show dilated loops of bowel, but it is difficult to distinguish small and large bowel in infancy. A barium (in saline) enema x-ray should be performed. There should be no attempt to clean out the stool before barium enema, for this will obscure the change in caliber between aganglionic and ganglionic bowel. The barium enema may not show a transition zone in the first 6 weeks after birth since the liquid stool can pass the aganglionic bowel and the proximal intestine may not be dilated. The aganglionic segment appears relatively narrowed compared to the dilated proximal bowel. The proximal aganglionic intestine can be dilated by impacted stool or enema, giving a false impression of the level of the normal colon. Irregular, bizarre contractions which do not encircle the aganglionic portion of the bowel may also be recognized. The dilated proximal bowel may have circumferential, smooth, parallel contractions, similar in appearance to jejunum, which are exaggerated contraction waves. Contrast medium should not be refluxed much beyond the transition zone, for marked distention of the aganglionic area may conceal the diagnostic signs. Lateral x-rays should be taken of the pelvis to demonstrate the rectum, the transition zone, and the irregular contractions which may otherwise by obscured by the redundant sigmoid colon on anteroposterior views. X-ray examinations of the abdomen and lateral pelvis should be repeated after evacuation 24–48 hours later. The barium will be retained for prolonged periods, and saline enemas may be required to evacuate it. The delayed film may show the transition zone and the bizarre irregular contractions more clearly than the initial study.

Differential Diagnosis

Low intestinal obstruction in the newborn infant may be due to rectal or colonic atresia, meconium plug syndrome, or meconium ileus. Hirschsprung's disease in patients who develop enterocolitis and diarrhea may mimic other causes of diarrhea. Chronic constipation due to functional causes may suggest Hirschsprung's disease. Although functional constipation may occur early in infancy, the stools are normal in caliber, soiling is frequent, and enterocolitis is not usually a problem. In functional constipation, stool is palpable in the lower rectum and a barium enema shows uniformly dilated bowel to the level of the anus. However, short segment Hirschsprung's disease may be difficult to differentiate, and rectal biopsy may be necessary. Segmental dilatation of the colon is a rare cause of constipation which may appear similar to Hirschsprung's disease.

Complications

The mortality rate of untreated aganglionic megacolon in infancy may be as high as 80%. Nonbacterial, nonviral enterocolitis is the principal cause of death. This putrefactive diarrhea tends to occur more frequently in infants but may appear at any age. The cause is not known but seems to be related to the high-grade partial obstruction. There is no correlation between the length of aganglionosis and the occurrence of enterocolitis. Perforation of the colon and appendix may result from the distal bowel obstruction. Atresia of the distal small bowel or colon also develops secondary to bowel obstruction due to Hirschsprung's disease in utero.

Following definitive surgical treatment (see below), anastomotic leak with perirectal and pelvic abscess is the most serious problem. This should be treated immediately by proximal colostomy until the anastomosis has healed. Necrosis of the pulled-through colon may occur if the bowel has not been mobilized sufficiently to prevent tension on the mesenteric blood supply. It is occasionally necessary to divide the inferior mesenteric artery. For this reason, a left transverse colostomy should be avoided (unless it is the position of the transition zone) because the collateral blood supply between the middle and left colic arteries may be divided.

Treatment

The large bowel obstruction and enterocolitis may be relieved initially by placing a large tube in the rectum and repeatedly washing out the colon contents with saline solution. Infants less than 1 year of age should have a preliminary colostomy. Conservative measures with enemas may not prevent further obstruction and enterocolitis. The colostomy should be placed at the transition zone, and the presence of ganglion cells at the colostomy site must be confirmed by frozen section biopsy. In total aganglionic colon, an ileostomy is necessary. Because loop colostomies tend to prolapse in infants, it is preferable to divide the bowel, close the distal end, and bring the proximal colon through by suturing the seromuscular portion of the bowel wall to all abdominal wall layers.

Definitive operation should be performed when the patient weighs about 9 kg. Long-term follow-up studies have documented the effectiveness of 4 operative procedures.

A. Swenson Operation: In the Swenson procedure, the overly dilated and aganglionic colon and rectum are excised to within 1 cm of the mucocutaneous junction of the anus posteriorly and laterally, and to a more proximal level anteriorly. The transected end of the normally ganglionated bowel is sutured end-to-end with the distal anorectal segment.

B. Duhamel Operation: Both in the Duhamel and the Soave (see below) procedures, the overly dilated and aganglionic bowel is removed down to the rectum at the level of the pelvic peritoneal reflection. In the Duhamel operation the rectum is oversewn, and the proximal bowel is brought between the sacrum and the rectum and sutured end-to-side to the rectum above the dentate line. The intervening spur of rectum and bowel is crushed to form a side-to-side anastomosis.

C. Soave Operation: The Soave operation consists of dissecting the mucosa out of the residual rectal stump, pulling the proximal bowel through, and suturing it to the rectum just above the dentate line.

D. Lynn Operation: This procedure is used for distal rectal aganglionosis. With lateral retractors in the dilated anal canal, a 1 cm transverse incision is made 1 cm above the dentate line through the rectal mucosa to the muscularis. The mucosa is dissected off the muscularis in a cephalad direction to the transition zone. A 1 cm wide strip of muscularis is removed to the transition zone. The rectal mucosa is reapproximated.

Prognosis

Although in the neonatal period the mortality rate is high in untreated infants, most patients who are properly treated for Hirschsprung's disease do very well. Problems with occasional incontinence and soiling may occur in a few cases. Episodic constipation and abdominal distention is more common since the aganglionic internal anal sphincter is intact. These patients respond to anal dilatation. Occasionally, an internal sphincterotomy may be necessary. Smaller children may still develop enterocolitis after definitive treatment, and they should be vigorously treated with a large rectal tube and enemas.

Asch MJ & others: Total colon aganglionosis: Report of nine cases. Arch Surg 105:74, 1972.

Boley SJ & others: Endorectal pull-through procedure for Hirschsprung's disease with and without primary anastomosis. J Pediatr Surg 3:258, 1968.

deLorimier AA, Benzian SA, Gooding CA: Segmental dilatation of the colon. Am J Roentgenol Radium Ther Nucl Med 152:100, 1971.

Hyde GA, deLorimier AA: Colon atresia and Hirschsprung's disease. Surgery 64:976, 1968.

Lynn HB: Rectal myomectomy for aganglionic megacolon. Mayo Clin Proc 41:289, 1966.

Martin LW: Surgical management of Hirschsprung's disease involving the small intestine. Arch Surg 97:183, 1968.

NEONATAL SMALL LEFT COLON SYNDROME
(Meconium Plug Syndrome)

A vexing problem in newborn infants that is being recognized with greater frequency is low intestinal obstruction associated with a narrow caliber left colon and a dilated transverse and right colon. The infants are in most cases otherwise normal though approximately 30–50% are born to diabetic mothers and are large for gestational age; most infants are over 36 weeks' gestational age and have normal birth weights. Two-thirds are male. Hypermagnesemia has been occasionally associated when the mother has been treated for eclampsia by magnesium sulfate injections. Little or no meconium is passed, and progressive abdominal distention is followed by vomiting. Rectal examination may be normal or reveals a tight anal canal. After thermometer or finger stimulation of the rectum, some meconium and gas may be evacuated. Barium enema shows a very small caliber left colon, usually extending to the level of the splenic flexure. The colon and commonly the small bowel are greatly distended proximal to this point. In about 30% of cases, a meconium plug will be identified at the junction of the narrow and dilated portion of the bowel, and the enema will dislodge it.

Differential Diagnosis

The small left colon syndrome may be confused with Hirschsprung's disease and with meconium ileus. These lesions rarely cause obstruction at the splenic flexure level, and, when the colon readily decompresses without further obstruction, Hirschsprung's disease is unlikely. Analysis of the stool for pancreatic enzymes is useless, but the presence of albumin in the meconium suggests meconium ileus. Careful follow-up with sweat chloride tests may be required to rule out meconium ileus.

Complications

Many of these infants develop significant colon distention and may perforate the cecum or appendix. The difficulty in differentiating small left colon syndrome from meconium ileus and Hirschsprung's disease may prompt surgical exploration when the process might resolve spontaneously.

Treatment

The distended infant should have a nasogastric tube connected to suction. Intravenous fluids should be started. Barium or Hypaque enema will be required to differentiate the causes of low intestinal obstruction. When the contrast material can be refluxed into the dilated proximal colon and a narrow left colon is seen, the diagnosis is most likely the small left colon syndrome. The contrast enema is usually followed by evacuation of stool and decompression of the bowel with resolution of the problem. A few infants remain persistently obstructed, requiring colostomy at the transition zone. Subsequent rectal biopsy or anal manometry fails to show Hirschsprung's disease. In some infants, colostomy closure at 1 year of age results in recurrent obstruction, seemingly due to hypotonia of the proximal bowel.

Davis WS & others: Neonatal small left colon syndrome. Radiology 120:322, 1974.

Philippart AI & others: Neonatal small left colon syndrome: Intramural not intraluminal obstruction. J Pediatr Surg 10:733, 1975.

INTUSSUSCEPTION

Telescoping of a segment of bowel (intussusceptum) into the adjacent segment (intussuscipiens) is the most common cause of intestinal obstruction in children under 2 years of age (Fig 48–15). The process of intussusception may result in gangrene of the intussusceptum. The terminal ileum is usually telescoped into the right colon, producing ileocolic intussusception, but ileoileal, ileoileocolic, jejunojejunal, and colocolic intussusceptions also occur. In 95% of infants and children, an obvious cause is not found. The most frequent occurrence is in midsummer and midwinter, and there is a positive correlation with adenovirus infections. In

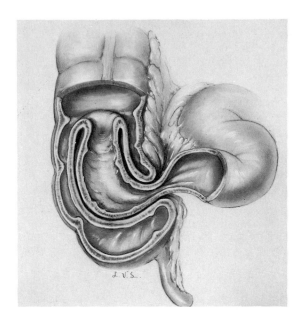

Figure 48—14. Intussusception.

most cases, hypertrophied Peyer's patches are noted to be a leading edge. Causes such as Meckel's diverticulum, polyps, intramural hematoma (Henoch-Schönlein purpura), and intestinal lymphoma are identified with increasing frequency in patients over age 1. The ratio of males to females is 3:1. The peak age is in infants 5—9 months old; 80% of patients are less than 2 years old.

Clinical Findings

A. Symptoms and Signs: The typical patient is a healthy child who has a sudden onset of crying and doubles his knees up because of abdominal pain. The pain is intermittent, lasts for about 1 minute, and is followed by intervals of apparent well-being. Reflex vomiting is a frequent early sign, but vomiting due to bowel obstruction occurs later in the course. Blood and mucus produce a "currant jelly" stool. In small infants—and in postoperative patients—the colicky pain may not be apparent; these babies become withdrawn, and the most prominent symptom is vomiting. Pallor and sweating are common signs during colic. A mass is usually palpable along the distribution of the colon. A hollow right lower quadrant may be noted. Occasionally, the intussusception is palpable on rectal examination.

B. Laboratory Findings: The blood count usually shows polymorphonuclear leukocytosis and hemoconcentration.

C. X-Ray Findings: Intravenous administration of sodium pertechnetate Tc 99m and abdominal scanning may outline an intussusception. Plain films of the abdomen may demonstrate evidence of mechanical intestinal obstruction or a soft tissue mass. The diagnosis is usually established by barium enema.

Complications

Repeated vomiting and bowel obstruction will produce progressive dehydration. Prolonged intussusception produces edema and hemorrhagic or ischemic infarction of the intussusceptum. Delayed treatment of infarcted bowel may result in cardiovascular collapse and death.

Treatment

Initial efforts are concerned with correction of hypovolemia and dehydration. A cutdown or right atrial catheter for central venous pressure monitoring is indicated for very sick patients. Expansion of blood volume with lactated Ringer's solution, whole blood, or albumin solution may be required. Barium enema should not be attempted until the patient has been resuscitated sufficiently so that he can tolerate an operative procedure. The baby should be sedated with meperidine, 1—2 mg/kg, and secobarbital, 1—2 mg/kg subcut. The enema bag must not be raised more than 75 cm above the patient, and under fluoroscopic control the barium enema may distend the intussuscipiens and reduce the intussusceptum in more than 50% of cases. If the initial enema is unsuccessful, it should be repeated 2 or 3 times following evacuation of the barium before reduction by enema can be considered a failure. Barium enema will not reduce gangrenous bowel.

Operation is required when there are signs of bowel perforation and peritonitis. If enema reduction has failed, the patient is explored through the right transverse lower abdominal incision. When no obvious gangrene is present, reduction is accomplished by gentle, retrograde compression of the intussuscipiens and not by traction on the proximal bowel. Resection of the intussusception is indicated if the bowel cannot be reduced or if the intestine is gangrenous. A Mikulicz resection may be necessary in critically ill patients.

The appendix is usually removed to prevent confusion about abdominal pain in later years when the patient has an abdominal incision.

Prognosis

Intussusception recurs in 2—4% of barium enema reductions and 1—2% of operative reductions. In the hands of an experienced surgeon, the mortality rate should approach zero. Deaths do occur if treatment of gangrenous bowel is delayed.

Ein SH: Recurrent intussusception in children. J Pediatr Surg 10:751, 1975.

Frye RR, Howard WHR: The handling of ileocolic intussusception in a pediatric medical center. Radiology 97:187, 1970.

Levy JL Jr, Linder LH: Etiology of "idiopathic" intussusception in infants. South Med J 63:642, 1970.

Ravitch MM: Intussusception. Chap 56, pp 914—931, in: *Pediatric Surgery*. Mustard WT & others (editors). Year Book, 1969.

Stevenson EOS, Hays DM, Snyder WH: Post-operative intussusception in infants and children. Am J Surg 113:562, 1967.

DUPLICATIONS OF THE
GASTROINTESTINAL TRACT

Duplications may occur at any point along the gastrointestinal tract from the mouth to the anus. Duplications occur (in order of decreasing frequency) in the ileum (50% of cases), mediastinum, colon, rectum, stomach, and neck. Intrathoracic and small bowel duplications are usually spherical. Colonic duplications are commonly long and tubular (Fig 48—15). Characteristically, the intra-abdominal duplications are within the mesentery and have a common wall with the intestine. Combined thoracoabdominal duplications also occur in which the thoracic saccular component extends through the esophageal hiatus or a separate diaphragmatic opening to empty into the duodenum or jejunum. Associated cardiovascular, neurologic, skeletal, urologic, and gastrointestinal anomalies occur in more than a third of cases. A tract of the duplication may extend through the anomalous vertebrae into the spinal canal.

Clinical Findings

A. Symptoms and Signs: Two-thirds of patients with duplications are symptomatic in the first year of life. Duplications of the neck and mediastinum produce respiratory distress by compression of the airway.

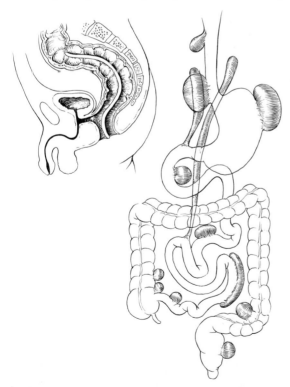

Figure 48—15. Duplications of the gastrointestinal tract. Duplications may be saccular or tubular. They usually arise within the mesentery, having a common wall with the intestine. Thoracoabdominal duplications arise from the duodenum or jejunum and extend through the diaphragm into the mediastinum.

Thoracic duplications may also ulcerate into the lung and lead to pneumonia or hemoptysis. Intestinal duplications usually produce abdominal pain due to spastic contraction of the bowel, excessive distention of the duplication, or peptic ulceration resulting from ectopic gastric mucosa. Intestinal obstruction due to intussusception, volvulus, or encroachment on the lumen by an intramural cyst also occurs. An isolated asymptomatic mass may be the only finding. Peptic ulceration caused by ectopic gastric mucosa may produce massive gastrointestinal bleeding.

B. X-Ray Findings: X-ray studies include films of the chest and thoracolumbar spine, barium enema, esophagography, and gastrointestinal series. If an intraspinal extension of a duplication is suspected, a myelogram may be indicated.

Treatment

Duplications not intimately adherent to adjacent organs should be excised. Isolated spherical duplications can be excised with the adjacent segment of bowel and an end-to-end anastomosis of the bowel performed. Long tubular duplications can be decompressed by establishing an anastomosis between the proximal and distal ends of the adjacent bowel. Noncommunicating duplications, which would require radical resection of surrounding structures, should be drained by a Roux-en-Y technic. Duplications which cannot be removed completely and which contain gastric mucosa should be opened (without jeopardizing the blood supply of the normal bowel) and the mucosal lining excised. During resection of a mediastinal duplication, extension of the lesion into the spine and abdomen must be recognized and removed. An intra-abdominal extension is closed at the level of the diaphragm, and complete excision by laparotomy is accomplished at a later date.

Bishop HC, Koop CE: Surgical management of duplications of the alimentary tract. Am J Surg 107:434, 1964.

Favara BE, Franchiosi RA, Akers DR: Enteric duplications. Thirty-seven cases: A vascular theory of pathogenesis. Am J Dis Child 122:501, 1971.

Forshall I: Duplication of the intestinal tract. Postgrad Med J 37:570, 1961.

OMPHALOMESENTERIC DUCT
ANOMALIES

Omphalomesenteric or vitelline duct anomalies are remnants of the embryonic yolk sac. When the entire duct remains intact, it is recognized as an **omphalomesenteric fistula.** When the duct is obliterated at the intestinal end but communicates with the umbilicus at the distal end, it is called an **umbilical sinus.** When the epithelial tract persists but both ends are occluded, an umbilical cyst or intra-abdominal **enterocystoma** may develop. The entire tract may be

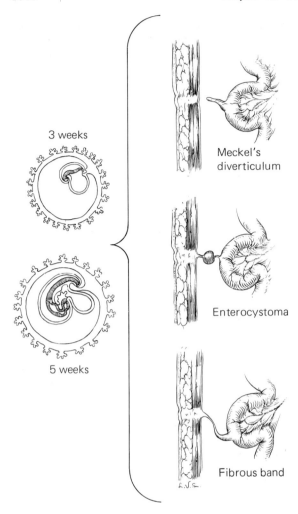

3 weeks

5 weeks

Meckel's diverticulum

Enterocystoma

Fibrous band

Figure 48—16. Omphalomesenteric duct anomalies arise from the primitive yolk. Remnants include Meckel's diverticulum, enterocystoma, or a fibrous band or fistulous tract between the ileum and the umbilicus.

obliterated, but a fibrous band may persist between the ileum and the umbilicus (Fig 48—16).

The most common remnant of the omphalomesenteric duct is Meckel's diverticulum, which is present in 1—3% of the population. Meckel's diverticulum may be lined wholly (or in part) by small intestinal, colonic, or gastric mucosa, and it may contain aberrant pancreatic tissue. Heterotopic tissue is found in 5% of asymptomatic and 60% of symptomatic cases. In contrast to duplications and pseudodiverticula, Meckel's diverticulum is located on the antimesenteric border of the ileum, 10—90 cm from the ileocecal valve.

Clinical Findings

Meckel's diverticulum is often asymptomatic and occurs as an incidental finding during operation for some other disease. Symptomatic omphalomesenteric remnants (male/female incidence 3:1) produce rectal bleeding in 40%, intussusception in 20%, diverticulitis or peptic perforation in 15%, umbilical fistula in 15%, intestinal obstruction in 7%, and abscess in 3%. Tumors such as carcinoids, leiomyomas, or leiomyosarcomas are very rare.

Rectal bleeding associated with Meckel's diverticulum is due to peptic ulceration of ectopic gastric mucosa. Over 50% of these patients are under 2 years of age. The blood is mixed with stool and is most often dark red or bright red; tarry stools are unusual. A history of a previous episode of bleeding may be elicited in 40% of cases. Occult bleeding from Meckel's diverticulum is very rare. Younger patients tend to bleed very briskly and may exsanguinate rapidly.

Diverticulitis or free perforation will present with abdominal pain and peritonitis identical to acute appendicitis. The pain and tenderness occur in the lower abdomen, most commonly near the umbilicus. An almost pathognomonic sign is cellulitis of the umbilicus.

A mucoid, purulent, or enteric discharge and excoriation about the umbilicus characterizes an umbilical sinus or omphalomesenteric fistula. Recurrent cellulitis or deep abdominal wall abscess about the umbilicus also occurs.

Intestinal obstruction may develop as a result of volvulus of the bowel about a persistent band between the umbilicus and the ileum or as a result of herniation of bowel between the mesentery and a persistent vitelline or mesodiverticular vessel. Infarction of the incarcerated hernia not uncommonly occurs, disturbing the blood supply to a Meckel's diverticulum.

Treatment & Prognosis

After depleted blood volume has been restored and fluid and electrolyte disturbances have been corrected, the patient should be explored through a transverse abdominal incision. An omphalomesenteric remnant with a narrow base may be treated by amputation and closure of the bowel defect. In cases where the anomaly has a wide mouth with ectopic tissue or where an inflammatory or ischemic process involves the adjacent ileum, intestinal resection with the diverticulum and anastomosis may be necessary. Involvement of Meckel's diverticulum by tumor would require intestinal resection with the lymphatic pathways of the mesentery. Morbidity and mortality may increase if operation is delayed.

Rutherford RB, Akers DR: Meckel's diverticulum: A review of 148 pediatric patients, with special reference to the pattern of bleeding and to meso-diverticular bands. Surgery 59:618, 1966.

Weinstein EC, Cain JC, ReMine WH: Meckel's diverticulum: Fifty-five years of clinical and surgical experience. JAMA 182:251, 1962.

ANORECTAL ANOMALIES

Anomalies of the anus result from abnormal growth and fusion of the embryonic anal hillocks. The rectum has usually developed normally, and the sphincter mechanism, consisting of the internal anal muscle, the puborectalis muscle, and the external sphincter, is usually intact. With proper treatment, the sphincter will function normally. Anal agenesis is an exception to this because the internal sphincter may be deficient.

Anomalies of the rectum develop as a result of faulty division of the cloaca into the urogenital sinus and rectum by the urorectal septum. In anomalies of the high type, the internal sphincter has not formed and the external sphincter is hypoplastic and does not serve as a functional sphincter following surgical repair.

Classification

A. Low Anomalies: In the low (translevator) anomalies, the rectum has traversed the puborectalis portion of the levator ani muscle (Fig 48–17). The anus may be in the normal position, with a narrow outlet due to stenosis or an anal membrane. There may be no opening in the perineum, but the skin at the anal area is heaped up and may extend as a band in the perineal raphe completely covering and occluding the anal opening. More commonly, the covering of the anus is incomplete because of a small fistula that

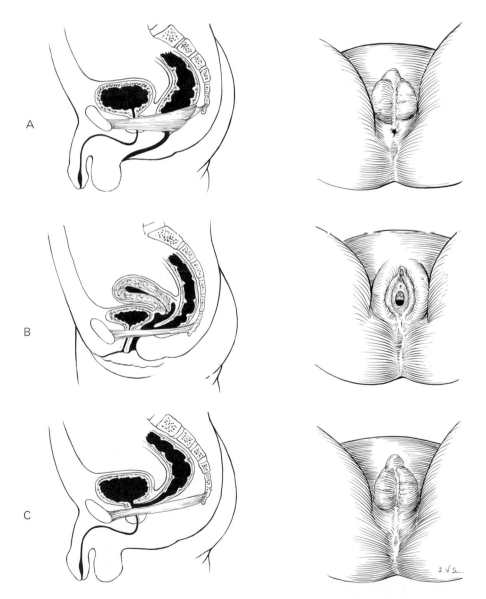

Figure 48–17. Three types of anorectal anomalies. *A:* Translevator anal atresia with anoperineal fistula. *B:* Supralevator anorectal atresia with rectovaginal fistula. *C:* Supralevator anorectal atresia with rectourethral fistula.

extends from the anus anteriorly to open in the raphe of the perineum, scrotum, or penis in the male or the vulva in the female. Finally, the anus may be ectopically placed anterior to the normal position.

B. Intermediate Anomalies: In the intermediate anomaly the bowel extends to the puborectalis muscle but either ends blindly or has a fistula between the rectum and the bulbous urethra in the male or the low vagina in the female. Another form consists of stenosis of the anorectal junction.

C. High Anomalies: In the high (supralevator) anomalies, the bowel ends above the puborectalis muscle, which is contracted against the urethra in the male and the vagina in the female (Fig 48–17). The bowel may end blindly, but more commonly there is a fistula to the urethra or bladder in the male or the upper vagina in the female. Communication may be directly to the bladder in the female, and the fistula extends between the 2 halves of a bicornuate uterus. In females, the cloaca is an anomaly consisting of a short urethra with a urethrovaginal fistula and a rectovaginal fistula.

Clinical Findings

A. Signs: The most important means of establishing the type of anorectal anomaly is by physical examination. In low anomalies, an ectopic opening from the rectum can be detected in the perineal raphe in males or in the lower vagina, vestibule, or fourchette in females. An intermediate or high anomaly exists when meconium is found at the urethral meatus, in the urine, or in the upper vagina.

B. X-Ray Findings: X-rays are useful when the clinical impression is unclear. After the infant has had enough time to swallow an adequate amount of air (at least 8–10 hours), he should be placed upside down for more than 5 minutes to allow the air to displace the meconium in the distalmost rectum. A lateral x-ray is then centered over the greater trochanter with the baby upside down and his legs straight. A lead marker may be placed in the anal dimple, but measurement between this and the level of the rectum is not sufficient to demonstrate the type of anomaly. When a line is drawn on the x-ray film from a point just below the superior pubic ramus to the last sacral vertebra (the pubococcygeal line), the highest level of the puborectalis portion of the levator ani is outlined. A line through the lowest level of the ischial bone and parallel to the pubococcygeal line describes the lower level of the puborectalis muscle. When air in the rectum ends above the lower line, the anomaly may be the high type; when it ends below the line, it is probably a low anomaly. This method is inaccurate because the air may not have completely displaced the meconium, giving a falsely high impression; or the infant may cry or strain, so that the puborectalis muscle and rectum may actually descend below the ischium, giving a falsely low diagnosis. Gas in the bladder clearly indicates a rectourinary fistula. Anomalies of the vertebrae and the urinary tract occur in two-thirds of patients with high (rectal) atresia and in one-third of male

patients with low (anal) atresia. Vertebral anomalies in females invariably indicate a high or intermediate anomaly.

A needle should be inserted into the distal rectum from the anal dimple and iophendylate (Hypaque) contrast medium instilled to outline the rectum and its fistulous termination.

Complications

Delay in the diagnosis of imperforate anus may result in excessive large bowel distention and perforation of the cecum.

Associated anomalies are frequent and include the following: esophageal atresia, anomalies of the gastrointestinal tract, agenesis of one or more sacral vertebrae (agenesis of S1, S2, or S3 is associated with comparable neurologic deficit, resulting in neurogenic bladder and greatly impaired continence), genitourinary anomalies, and anomalies of the heart and lungs.

The presence of a rectourinary fistula allows reflux of urine into the rectum and colon, and absorption of ammonium chloride may cause acidosis. Colon contents will reflux into the urethra, bladder, and upper tracts, producing recurrent pyelonephritis. A divided sigmoid colostomy rather than a loop colostomy will prevent this until the fistula can be closed at a later date.

Treatment

A. Low Anomalies: Low anomalies are usually repaired from the perineal approach in the newborn. The anteriorly placed anal opening is mobilized to the level of the levator ani and transferred to the normal position. After healing, the anal opening must be dilated daily for 6–8 months to prevent stricture and to allow for growth.

B. Intermediate and High Anomalies: These should be treated by preliminary sigmoid colostomy. If there is doubt about the diagnosis of a high or low anomaly, it is better to perform a colostomy than to attempt a perineal repair and have the anomaly prove to be a high one. The colostomy should be divided to prevent movement of stool into the distal loop, producing recurrent urinary tract infection. After the baby gains to approximately 9 kg, the definitive abdominoperineal pull-through procedure, in which the distal colon is brought anterior to the puborectalis muscle and sutured to the perineum, can be performed. It is important to preserve the afferent and efferent portion of the defecation reflex arc as well as the existing sphincter muscles.

In the high and intermediate anomalies, the external anal sphincter is inadequate and the internal sphincter is absent. Therefore, continence is dependent upon a functioning puborectalis muscle.

Surgical complications include damage to the nervi erigentes with poor bladder and bowel control and failure of erection. Division of rectourethral fistula some distance from the fistula may serve as a pocket for recurrent infection and stone formation, and cutting the fistula too short may result in urethral stricture. Erroneously attempting to repair a high anomaly from the perineal approach will leave a persistent rectourinary fistula. An abdominoperineal pull-through procedure performed for a low type of anomaly will invariably produce an incontinent patient who might otherwise have had an excellent prognosis.

Prognosis

Most patients with imperforate anus also have constipation as an inherent part of the disease. The colon seems to have desultory motility, and fecal impaction is a constant problem. This is fortunate for individuals who have defective sphincter control but requires considerable attention to prevent obturant obstruction. Patients with low anomalies usually have good fecal control. Children with high anomalies do not have an internal sphincter which provides continuous, unconscious, and unfatiguing control against soiling. However, in the absence of a lower spine anomaly, perception of rectal fullness, ability to distinguish between flatus and stool, and conscious voluntary control of rectal discharge by contraction of the puborectalis muscle can be accomplished. When the stools become liquid, sphincter control is usually impaired in patients with high and intermediate anomalies.

Berdon WE & others: The radiologic evaluation of imperforate anus. Radiology 90:466, 1968.

Stephens FD, Smith ED: *Ano-Rectal Malformations in Children.* Year Book, 1971.

NEONATAL JAUNDICE, BILIARY ATRESIA, & HEPATITIS

Jaundice in the first week of infancy is usually due to indirect (unconjugated) hyperbilirubinemia. The causes include (1) "physiologic jaundice" due to immaturity of hepatic function; (2) Rh, ABO, and rarer blood group incompatibilities, producing hemolysis; and (3) infections.

Jaundice that persists beyond the first week is due to elevated indirect and conjugated bilirubin levels and presents difficult problems in diagnosis and treatment. The most frequent cause (60%) of prolonged jaundice in infancy is biliary atresia; various forms of hepatitis occur in 35%; and choledochal cyst is found in 5% of cases of obstructive jaundice.

Extrahepatic biliary atresia is the absence of patent bile ducts draining the liver. Biliary atresia is probably not congenital but acquired after birth because no cases have been described in autopsies of newborn infants. Furthermore, conjugated bilirubin is not cleared by the placenta as unconjugated bilirubin is, and jaundice due to conjugated hyperbilirubinemia with biliary obstruction has not been recognized in newborn infants. The atretic ducts consist of solid fibrous cords which may contain occasional islands of biliary epithelium. The extent of duct involvement varies greatly.

In the only surgically correctable form of biliary atresia, the common bile duct or the gallbladder (or both) is obliterated but the common hepatic duct and intrahepatic ducts are patent (5%).

In infants with extrahepatic biliary atresia, the liver develops progressive periportal fibrosis and the liver cords eventually become disrupted by the cirrhotic process. Proliferation of the bile canaliculi, containing inspissated bile, and lakes of extravasated bile may also be noted.

Intrahepatic biliary atresia is very rare. The extrahepatic bile ducts are patent, but repeated liver biopsy shows progressive disappearance of the intrahepatic portal ducts. Cirrhosis is not a prominent finding, and these patients may live for 3–5 years with persistent or intermittent jaundice.

Biliary hypoplasia has been described as a distinct entity causing jaundice in which the bile ducts are very small. A more likely explanation is that these cases represent hepatitis or intrahepatic biliary atresia in which the bile ducts are unused and therefore do not distend to normal size. In some cases, the bile ducts are very thickened and the lumen is very narrow. These patients were probably affected by the same process producing biliary atresia, but the lumen was not completely obliterated.

The infant who develops jaundice is usually full-term with an uneventful neonatal course. Jaundice is first noted in 2 or 3 weeks. He may have normal or clay-colored stools and dark urine. The stools contain an increased quantity of fat but are of normal consistency and not frothy. The liver may be of normal size early, but it becomes enlarged with time. The infant with surgical obstructive jaundice develops a hard liver as a consequence of progressive cirrhosis; patients with hepatitis have an enlarged liver of softer consistency. Splenomegaly usually develops in all forms of prolonged jaundice in infancy.

Liver function tests are of no help in distinguishing obstructive jaundice from medical jaundice in infants. The bilirubin levels may vary considerably from day to day. Serum transaminase levels are often high in all forms of jaundice, and the serum albumin decreases and serum globulin increases after 4 months in medical or surgical jaundice. Stool excretion of rose bengal sodium I 131 greater than 10% of an intravenous dose indicates patent bile ducts but does not rule out choledochal cyst; excretion of less than 10% occurs in hepatitis as well as in biliary atresia.

Needle biopsy of the liver may be safely performed at any age if the bleeding and clotting tests are normal. A diagnosis based on needle biopsy is accurate in 60%, equivocal in 16%, and erroneous in 24%. A diagnosis based on the combined results of abdominal exploration, cholangiography, and open liver biopsy is accurate in 98% of cases.

Differential Diagnosis

Other causes of obstructive jaundice are choledochal cyst, inspissated bile syndrome, and hepatitis. A choledochal cyst is identified by the presence of a palpable mass in the right upper quadrant and a gastrointestinal series showing indentation of the duodenum. Inspissated bile syndrome follows a hemolytic process in which a large bilirubin load is excreted into the bile ducts, where it becomes coalesced and impacted. This is recognized by cholangiography.

Hepatitis is most commonly of unknown cause. It may be due to a variety of infections, often of maternal origin, such as toxoplasmosis, cytomegalic inclusion disease, rubella syndrome, herpes simplex, coxsackie, and varicella. Genetic metabolic diseases producing jaundice include alpha-antitrypsin deficiency, galactosemia, and cystic fibrosis.

Complications

Delayed treatment of patients with correctable forms of biliary atresia will result in progressive cirrhosis. Surgical exploration for neonatal jaundice is indicated as early in infancy as possible, when biliary atresia is the likely cause of jaundice. If the liver of a jaundiced infant becomes hard, some form of mechanical obstructive jaundice is probably present and operative exploration should not be further delayed.

Treatment

Preoperative care includes correction of anemia and administration of intravenous glucose and K vitamins. The operation should be scheduled in the morning so that the infant will be on a "nothing-by-mouth" regimen no longer than 6 hours. X-ray facilities should be made ready in the operating room, and the anesthetic period is made as short as possible. Through a transverse abdominal incision, the gallbladder should be located and cannulated. Diatrizoate (Hypaque) diluted to 25% should be gently instilled into the biliary tree, taking care to prevent pressure which might disrupt the bile ducts. If x-rays show a patent common duct but no reflux into the liver, a rubber-shod bulldog clamp may be placed on the distal common duct and the cholangiogram repeated. During development of the x-ray films, a wedge of liver is obtained for biopsy. If atresia of the bile duct is found, the obliterated duct and surrounding fibrosis should be dissected off the portal vein into the hilus of the liver. A Roux-en-Y choledocho- or hepaticojejunostomy is performed to the perihilar liver capsule.

Patients with uncorrectable atresia will develop progressive ascites, making their care difficult; they eat poorly and become rapidly wasted. Palliation of ascites can be achieved by diuretics. The only hope for patients with uncorrectable biliary atresia is liver transplantation. Fat-soluble vitamin deficiency should be prevented by giving triple the usual dosages of these vitamins by mouth.

Choledochal cysts are best handled by excision of the cyst and choledocho- Roux-en-Y jejunostomy. If the cyst cannot be excised it should be drained by an anastomosis to the side of the duodenum or, preferably, a Roux-en-Y segment of jejunum.

Prognosis

Patients with correctable forms of atresia may develop cholangitis, related to anastomotic stricture or bile duct fibrosis with intrahepatic bile duct abscesses. Reexploration and revision of the anastomosis may be necessary. Preliminary jejunal diversion by an isolated skin jejunostomy loop may prevent cholangitis and sepsis in young infants with significant cirrhosis. The average life span for infants with uncorrectable biliary atresia is 19 months. Death is due to progressive liver failure, bleeding from esophageal varices, or sepsis.

Bill AH, Kasai M: Biliary atresia and choledochal cyst: New concepts of cause and treatment. Prog Pediatr Surg 6:1, 1974.

deLorimier AA: Current concepts: Surgical treatment of neonatal jaundice. N Engl J Med 288:1284, 1973.

Hays DM: Biliary atresia: The current state of confusion. Surg Clin North Am 53:1257, 1973.

Kasai M & others: Surgical treatment of biliary atresia. J Pediatr Surg 3:665, 1968.

Sass-Kortsak A: Management of young infants presenting with direct-reacting hyperbilirubinemia. Pediatr Clin North Am 21:777, 1974.

ABDOMINAL WALL DEFECTS

1. INGUINAL HERNIA & HYDROCELE

The processus vaginalis remains patent in over 80% of newborn infants. With increasing age, the incidence of patent processus vaginalis diminishes. At 2 years, 40–50% are open, and in adults 25% are persistently patent. Actual herniation of bowel into a widely patent processus vaginalis develops in 1–4% of children; 45% occur within the first year of life. Indirect inguinal hernia occurs 8 times more frequently in males. Direct and femoral hernias occur in children but are very rare.

Clinical Findings

The diagnosis of hernia in infants and children can be made only by the demonstration of an inguinal bulge originating from the internal ring. The bulge often cannot be elicited at will, and signs such as a large external ring, the "silk glove" sign, and thickening of the cord are not dependable. Under these circumstances, a reliable history alone may be sufficient. Hernias are found on the right side in 60% of cases, on the left side in 25%, and bilaterally in 15%. Bilateral hernias are more frequent in premature infants. The processus vaginalis may be obliterated at any location proximal to the testis or labium. When the bowel herniates into the scrotum, it is called complete indirect inguinal hernia; when it does not reach the level of the external ring, it is an incomplete inguinal hernia.

Incarcerated inguinal hernia accounts for approximately 10% of childhood hernias, and the incidence is highest in infants. In 45% of females with incarcerated hernia, the contents of the sac consist of various combinations of ovary, tube, and uterus. These structures are usually a sliding component of the sac.

Hydroceles almost always represent peritoneal fluid trapped in a patent processus vaginalis; hence, they are commonly called communicating hydroceles. A hydrocele is characteristically an oblong, nontender, soft mass that transilluminates with light.

Differential Diagnosis

A hydrocele under tension is often confused with incarcerated inguinal hernia. Transillumination of the scrotum or groin with a flashlight distinguishes fluid from bowel. The sudden appearance of fluid confined to the testicular area may represent a noncommunicating hydrocele secondary to torsion of the testis or testicular appendage, or to epididymo-orchitis. Rectal examination and palpation of the peritoneal side of the inguinal ring may distinguish an incarcerated hernia from a hydrocele or other inguinoscrotal mass.

Complications

Failure to treat an inguinal hernia in infancy shortly after the diagnosis has been made may allow the hernia to become incarcerated and subsequently strangulated. About a third of incarcerated inguinal hernias in infancy show evidence of strangulation, and in 5% of cases the bowel is gangrenous. Compression of the spermatic vessels by an incarcerated hernia may produce hemorrhagic infarction of a testicle.

Treatment

Inguinal hernia in infancy and childhood should be repaired soon after diagnosis. In premature infants under constant surveillance in the hospital, hernia repair may be deferred until the baby is strong enough to be discharged home. Ordinarily, high ligation and excision of the hernia sac at the internal ring is all that is required. When there is a large internal ring, it may be necessary to narrow the internal ring with sutures placed in the transversalis fascia, but use of abdominal muscle for repair is unnecessary.

An incarcerated hernia in an infant can usually be reduced initially before operation. This is accomplished by sedation with meperidine, 2 mg/kg IM, and secobarbital, 2 mg/kg IM, and by elevating the foot of the bed to keep intra-abdominal pressure from being exerted against the inguinal area. When the infant is well sedated, the hernia may be reduced by gentle pressure over the internal ring in a manner that milks the bowel into the abdominal cavity. During this time, nasogastric suction and intravenous fluid replacement should be started. If the bowel is not reduced after a few hours, operation is required. If the hernia is reduced, operative repair may be delayed for 24 hours to allow edema in the tissues to subside. It is not necessary to delay repair in females, in whom there is no risk of injuring the vas deferens or spermatic vessels. Bloody stools and edema and red discoloration of the skin around the groin suggest strangulated hernia, and

reduction of the bowel should not be attempted. Emergency repair of incarcerated inguinal hernia is technically difficult because the edematous tissues are friable and tear readily. When gangrenous intestine is encountered, the hemorrhagic fluid in the sac should be prevented from entering the abdominal cavity. The gangrenous bowel should be resected and an end-to-end intestinal anastomosis performed. Black, hemorrhagic discoloration of the testis or ovary does not require excision of the gonad.

Fonkalsrud EW, deLorimier AA, Clatworthy HW: Femoral and direct inguinal hernias in infants and children. JAMA 192:597, 1965.

Holcomb GW: Routine bilateral inguinal hernia repair. Am J Dis Child 109:114, 1965.

Nyhus LM, Harkins HN: *Hernia.* Lippincott, 1964.

Rowe MI, Clatworthy HW: Incarcerated and strangulated hernias in children. Arch Surg 101:136, 1970.

2. UNDESCENDED TESTIS
(Cryptorchidism)

In the seventh month of gestation, the testicles normally descend into the scrotum. A fibromuscular band, the gubernaculum, extends from the lower pole of the testes to the scrotum, and this band probably guides the path of descent during differential growth of the fetus rather than pulling the testes down. Undescended testis, or cryptorchidism, is a form of dystopia of the testis which occurs when there is arrested descent and fixation of the position of the testis retroperitoneally, in the inguinal canal, or just beyond the external ring.

Another form of dystopia is ectopic testis, in which the gubernaculum may have guided the testis to the pubis, penis, perineum, thigh, or to a subcutaneous position superficial to the inguinal canal. In these instances the testis has descended beyond the external ring of the inguinal canal and the vascular supply is sufficiently developed to pose little difficulty in operative repair.

True cryptorchidism occurs in less than 0.5% of males; 45% on the right, 30% on the left, and 25% bilaterally.

Dystopic testes must be distinguished from retractile testicles. The very active cremaster of children less than 3 years old—and the small size of the testis—allow it to retract to the external inguinal ring or within the inguinal canal. The retractile testis usually can be manipulated into the lower scrotum. At puberty, the retractile testis will remain permanently in the lower scrotum; it functions normally, and it requires no operative intervention.

The complications of dystopic testis include abnormal spermatogenesis, inguinal hernia, trauma, torsion, tumor, associated anomalies, and psychologic effects.

Normal spermatogenesis requires the critical cooler temperature range provided in the scrotum. When the testis remains undescended and subjected to normal body temperature, degenerative changes in the seminiferous tubules occur in which the lining cells become progressively atrophic and hyalinized with peritubular fibrosis. Eventually, only the Sertoli cells of the tubules remain. Dystopia does not affect the interstitial cells, and testosterone production is usually normal.

The degenerative changes occur at puberty, when the stimulus from pituitary gonadotropin becomes very prominent. However, tubular dysgenesis is also seen in 20% of children under 7 years of age, suggesting that the testicle is frequently abnormal structurally as well as in position. Unless the disorder is corrected, all bilaterally cryptorchid adult males are sterile.

A patent processus vaginalis is present in 95% of patients with cryptorchidism, and approximately 25% develop a hernia.

The fixed position of the testis within the inguinal canal or in an ectopic position makes it particularly vulnerable to trauma. The lack of a broad attachment of the testis in an ectopic location makes it particularly prone to torsion and infarction.

Tumors of the testis develop in one per 50,000 adult males per year. Approximately 10% of these tumors occur in an undescended testis, and, since less than 0.5% of males are born cryptorchid, the incidence of testicular carcinoma in undescended testes is 30–50 times higher than in the normal male population. The occurrence of tumors in undescended testes is almost always in adults, and operative repair does not lessen the risk of malignant change. The incidence of tumor occurring in the contralateral normally descended testis may also be higher than normal.

Anomalies associated with cryptorchidism occur in about 15% of cases and are usually confined to the urinary and lower alimentary tracts. Less than 50% of the anomalies are associated with Klinefelter's syndrome, hypogonadotropic hypogonadism, or germinal cell aplasia. Other anomalies include the prune belly syndrome, horseshoe kidneys, renal agenesis or hypoplasia, exstrophy of the bladder, and ureteral reflux.

Treatment

Chorionic gonadotropic hormone, 3000–5000 units IM daily for 3–5 days, has been advocated to stimulate descent. The recommended age at which the injections are given is 2–5 years. Descent is said to occur in 33% of bilateral and 16% of unilateral cryptorchid children. Histologic damage can occur with excessive gonadotropin treatment. It is very doubtful that a true dystopic testis can respond and descent with this treatment is probably confined to patients with retractile testicles.

Orchidopexy is the surgical method for mobilizing the testis, based on the testicular vessels and the vas deferens, from the ectopic location to the scrotum. Approximately 10% of undescended testes remain in the abdomen, and in rare cases these can be brought

into the scrotum by multiple staged operations, allowing growth and lengthening of the blood supply between procedures. Testicles confined in the inguinal canal occur in 25% of cases, and most of these can be brought into the scrotum in one stage. Ectopic testicles located outside the inguinal canal, such as in the subcutaneous inguinal pouch, occur in over 50% of cases, and the testicular vessels are so well developed that scrotal placement is rarely a problem.

The ideal age for orchidopexy is about 5 years old. The prognosis for fertility following orchidopexy in unilateral maldescent is 80%, whereas fertility after bilateral orchidopexy is about 50%.

Johnston JH: The testicles and the scrotum. Chap 33, pp 450–474, in: *Paediatric Urology*. Williams DI (editor). Appleton-Century-Crofts, 1968.

Snyder WH, Greaney EM: Cryptorchidism. Chap 77, pp 1291–1312, in: *Pediatric Surgery*, 2nd ed. Mustard WT & others. Year Book, 1969.

3. UMBILICAL HERNIA

A fascial defect at the umbilicus is frequently present in the newborn, particularly in premature infants. The incidence is higher in blacks. In most children, the umbilical ring progressively diminishes in size and eventually closes. Fascial defects less than 1 cm in diameter close spontaneously by the age of 6 years in 95% of cases. When the fascial defect is greater than 1.5 cm in diameter, it seldom closes spontaneously. Protrusion of bowel through the umbilical defect rarely results in incarceration in childhood. Surgical repair is indicated when the intestine becomes incarcerated, when the fascial defect is greater than 1 cm, in girls older than 2 years, and in all children older than 4 years.

Morgan WW & others: Prophylactic umbilical hernia repair in childhood to prevent adult incarceration. Surg Clin North Am 50:839, 1970.

Walker SH: The natural history of umbilical hernia. Clin Pediatr (Phila) 6:29, 1967.

4. OMPHALOCELE

Omphalocele is a very rare defect of the periumbilical abdominal wall in which the coelomic cavity is covered only by peritoneum and amnion. More than half of these babies are born prematurely. The omphalocele may contain small and large bowel, liver, spleen, stomach, pancreas, and bladder. The abdominal musculature is usually well developed, but the "prune belly" syndrome, with absence of abdominal muscles, occurs occasionally. Many of these infants have a defective lower chest with ectopia cordis, or deficient lower abdominal wall with cloacal exstrophy.

Omphaloceles with small abdominal defects can be treated by excising the omphalocele sac and by reapproximating the abdominal wall muscles and skin edges.

Large omphaloceles can be treated by removing the amniotic membrane and inspecting the bowel for anomalies that might produce obstruction such as duodenal bands. Marlex mesh should be sutured to the linea alba at the edge of the abdominal wall defect. A gastrostomy should be performed. Skin flaps are mobilized from the abdominal fascia so that they can be reapproximated in the midline over the mesh. Over a period of days to months, a wedge of skin and Marlex can be repeatedly excised from the midportion of the defect until the linea alba can be reapproximated.

Because of the high mortality rate associated with surgical treatment of omphaloceles greater than 8 cm in diameter, nonoperative management has been advised. The amnion is covered with a bactericidal agent such as mafenide (Sulfamylon) or povidone-iodine (Betadine) as an eschar forms over the amnion. The membrane becomes vascularized beneath the eschar, and over a period of time contraction of the wound and skin growth will occur over the granulating portion of the omphalocele.

The survival rate for infants with small omphaloceles is excellent since the lesion is easily repaired. The mortality rate following surgical correction of large omphaloceles is over 50%. When the conservative approach is used, the mortality rate is less than 10%.

Firor HV: Omphalocele: An appraisal of therapeutic approaches. Surgery 69:208, 1971.

Schuster SR: A new method for the staged repair of large omphaloceles. Surg Gynecol Obstet 125:837, 1967.

5. GASTROSCHISIS

Gastroschisis is a defect in the abdominal wall which usually is to the right of a normal insertion of the umbilical cord. It is probably produced by rupture of the embryonic umbilical sac in utero. The remnants of the amnion are usually reabsorbed. The skin may continue to grow over the remnants of the amnion, and there may be a bridge of skin between the defect and the cord. The small and large bowel herniate through the abdominal wall defect. Having been bathed in the amnionic fluid, the bowel wall has a very thick, shaggy membrane covering it. The loops of intestine are usually matted together, and the intestine appears to be abnormally short.

Complications

Since the bowel has not been contained intraabdominally, the abdominal cavity fails to enlarge and cannot accommodate the protuberant bowel. Over

70% of the infants are premature, and associated anomalies are frequent. Nonrotation of the midgut is present. Intestinal atresia occurs frequently because segments of intestine which have herniated through the defect become infarcted in utero.

Treatment & Prognosis

Initially, the bowel should be covered by forming a tube from silicone-coated fabric and incorporating the protuberant bowel into the tube. The end of the tube is tied off and suspended from an incubator top. As edema and shaggy membrane of the protuberant intestine are absorbed, the bowel will spontaneously reduce into the abdominal cavity. Reduction is aided by tying the protuberant end of the tube adjacent to the bowel each day. When the bowel has completely returned within the abdomen, the silicone-coated tube is removed and the abdominal wall is closed in layers. A gastrostomy is valuable in the postoperative care of the baby.

The mortality rate for infants with gastroschisis has been greatly reduced by this technic.

Allen RG, Wrenn EL: Silon as a sac in the treatment of omphalocele and gastroschisis. J Pediatr Surg 4:3, 1969.

TUMORS IN CHILDHOOD

1. NEUROBLASTOMA

Of all childhood neoplasms, neuroblastoma is exceeded only by leukemia and brain tumors in frequency. Two-thirds of cases occur within the first 5 years of life. This tumor is of neural crest origin and may originate anywhere along the distribution of the sympathetic chain. Neuroblastomas originate in the retroperitoneal area in 65% of cases; 40% arise from the adrenal gland. The biologic behavior varies with the age of the patient, the site of primary origin, and the extent of the disease.

Clinical Findings

The most common finding is the presence of a mass, which may be primary or metastatic. Nonspecific symptoms include vomiting, diarrhea, constipation, weight loss, and fever. In infants, metastases confined to the liver or subcutaneous fat are very frequent and bone metastases are unusual. In older children, metastases to lymph nodes and bone are found in over 70% of cases at diagnosis. Pain in areas of bony involvement and joints with associated myalgia and fever suggest rheumatic fever. Hypertension and diarrhea may occur. Abdominal neuroblastoma may be distinguished from other tumors by the hard, irregular surface of the tumor and the tendency to cross the midline. X-ray films show a soft tissue mass displacing surrounding structures, and calcification is present in 45% of tu-

mors. For retroperitoneal tumors, an intravenous urogram shows displacement or compression of the adjacent kidney without distortion of the renal calyces.
Chest x-ray, complete bone survey, bone scan and liver
scan, and bone marrow aspiration for histologic examination are indicated because of the frequency of bony
metastases. About 70% of neuroblastomas produce
norepinephrine and its metabolites. The breakdown
products of excess norepinephrine production, vanilmandelic acid (VMA) and homovanillic acid (HVA),
should be measured in urine specimens at intervals so
that the clinical course of the patient can be followed.

Treatment

A localized neuroblastoma should be excised and
the local area of the tumor should be irradiated. Unresectable neuroblastomas should be treated initially by
radiation therapy and surgical resection performed for
residual tumor. Most neuroblastomas are radiosensitive
and respond to 3000 rads or less of radiation. Patients
with disseminated disease should be treated with a
combination of chemotherapeutic agents such as cyclophosphamide (Cytoxan), 750 mg/sq m IV once on day
1; vincristine, 1.5 mg/sq m IV once on day 5; and
dacarbazide, 250 mg/sq m IV on days 1–5. This regimen is repeated every 28 days for 1 year.

Prognosis

Of the patients that die from neuroblastoma, 92%
do so within 14 months after diagnosis. The overall
2-year survival rate for infants less than 1 year old is
almost 60%; for children older than 2 years, it is less
than 10%. For infants with tumor confined to the site
of primary origin or with adjacent regional spread, the
cure rate is greater than 80%; the 2-year survival rate
with distant metastases to the liver and subcutaneous
fat is close to 100%. Cure of neuroblastoma in older
children is frequent for localized disease and rare if
regional or distant metastasis has occurred.

Spontaneous regression of neuroblastoma probably occurs more frequently (5%) in patients with
neuroblastoma than with any other neoplasm. However, spontaneous regression occurs only in patients
under 2 years of age. Maturation of neuroblastoma to
benign ganglioneuroma occurs in infants, but it is rare.

D'Angio GJ, Evans AE, Koop CE: Special pattern of widespread
neuroblastoma with a favorable prognosis. Lancet 1:1046,
1971.
deLorimier AA, Bragg KU, Linden G: Neuroblastoma in childhood. Am J Dis Child 118:441, 1969.
Evans AE, D'Angio GJ, Randolph J: A proposed staging for
children with neuroblastoma. Cancer 27:374, 1971.

2. NEPHROBLASTOMA
(Wilms's Tumor)

With rare exceptions, this tumor arises within the
capsule of the kidney and consists of a variety of epithelial and sarcomatous cell types such as abortive
tubules and glomeruli, smooth and skeletal muscle
fibers, spindle cells, cartilage, and bone. Hence, the
tumor is also called embryoma, carcinosarcoma, and
mixed tumor of the kidney. Eighty percent of patients
are under age 4. Bilateral tumors occur in 5–10% of
cases. Metastases occur most commonly in the liver
and lungs, rarely in the brain and bones. Nephroblastoma accounts for 8% of childhood malignancies.

Clinical Findings

Symptoms consist of abdominal enlargement in
60% of cases, pain in 20%, hematuria in 15%, malaise,
weakness, anorexia, and weight loss in 10%, and fever
in 3% of patients. An abdominal mass is palpable in
almost all cases. The mass is usually very large, firm,
and smooth and does not ordinarily extend across the
midline. Hypertension is noted in more than 50% of
patients and may be sufficient to produce congestive
heart failure. Aniridia, hemihypertrophy, hypospadias,
cryptorchidism, and urinary anomalies are frequently
associated. An intravenous urogram shows distortion
of the calyces and kidney. Nonvisualization on the urogram indicates tumor extension into the ureter or renal
vessels. Cystoscopy and retrograde urograms are not
necessary. Renal arteriograms are helpful in differentiating retroperitoneal tumors and in detecting small or
bilateral nephroblastomas. An inferior venacavagram
may show obstruction of the vena cava, but it does not
differentiate compression from tumor invasion. Renal
ultrasonography may distinguish hydronephrosis from
a solid tumor. Liver scan and chest x-rays will identify
metastases.

Differential Diagnosis

Abdominal masses may be caused by hydronephrotic, multicystic, or duplicated kidneys, neuroblastoma, teratoma, hepatoma, and rhabdomyosarcoma as well as nephroblastoma. An intravenous urogram distinguishes nephroblastoma from these other
tumors because calyceal distortion indicates intrarenal
origin. Calcification occurs in 10% of cases of nephroblastoma and tends to be more crescent-shaped, discrete, and peripherally located, whereas the calcification of neuroblastoma is finely stippled.

Complications

The tumor can extend into the renal vein and
inferior vena cava. These vessels should be carefully
palpated during abdominal exploration, and the tumor
should be removed in such a way that tumor embolus
will not occur.

Treatment

The preferred treatment is immediate nephrectomy and excision of all the surrounding tissues within Gerota's fascia. Radiation therapy to the tumor bed is indicated if the tumor has extended beyond the capsule of the kidney. Very large tumors should be treated with radiation therapy preoperatively to reduce the size of the tumor. A significant reduction in size usually occurs in 7–10 days, after which nephrectomy is readily performed. Nephrectomy is accomplished through a long or thoracoabdominal incision, and the renal artery and vein are divided before any other dissection is performed. Dactinomycin (Cosmegen) and vincristine (Oncovin) should be given with preoperative x-ray treatment or intraoperatively if x-ray therapy does not precede nephrectomy. The course of dactinomycin should be repeated in 6 weeks and every 3 months thereafter for 2 years. Vincristine (Oncovin) is also effective and less toxic, but it does not have the radiomimetic effect of dactinomycin. Vincristine, 1.5 mg/sq m, should be given with the first and last dose of each course of dactinomycin.

Metastases develop in 30% of patients who had none at diagnosis. Solitary metastases in the lung should be resected. Hepatic metastases and multiple pulmonary metastases should be irradiated. Any residual tumor following radiation therapy—including multiple lesions—should be resected.

Bilateral nephroblastoma occurs in 3–10% of cases. X-ray therapy followed by radical nephrectomy on one side and partial nephrectomy, if possible, on the contralateral side is preferred. Radioresistant tumors which diffusely involve both kidneys require bilateral radical nephrectomy and kidney transplantation.

Prognosis

Of those patients that die of nephroblastoma, 98% die within 2 years following treatment. Nephrectomy and x-ray therapy alone or with one course of dactinomycin provide a cure rate of 50% at best. When sequential dactinomycin is used, the survival rate is greater than 80%. The prolonged administration of dactinomycin and vincristine in combination achieves 90% long-term survival. When pulmonary or hepatic metastases are present at diagnosis, the survival rate following combined treatment with surgery, x-ray therapy, and chemotherapy is 50%.

deLorimier AA & others: Treatment of bilateral Wilms' tumor. Am J Surg 122:275, 1971.

Sutow WW: Chemotherapy in Wilms' tumor: An appraisal. Cancer 32:1150, 1973.

Wolff JA & others: Long-term evaluation of single versus multiple courses of actinomycin D therapy of Wilms' tumor. N Engl J Med 290:84, 1974.

Wolff JA & others: Single versus multiple dose dactinomycin therapy of Wilms' tumor. N Engl J Med 279:290, 1968.

3. TERATOMA

Teratomas are congenital neoplasms derived from all 3 basic germ cells of the early embryo. Sites of origin (in order of frequency) are the ovaries, testes, anterior mediastinum, presacral and coccygeal regions, and the retroperitoneum.

These tumors should be excised because of their malignant potential and the symptoms produced by their size. Some of the malignant tumors respond to x-ray therapy, and some metastatic lesions have regressed with combined cyclophosphamide, vincristine, and dactinomycin therapy.

Donnellan WA, Swenson O: Benign and malignant sacrococcygeal teratomas. Surgery 64:834, 1968.

Willis RA: *The Borderland of Embryology and Pathology.* Butterworths, 1962.

RHABDOMYOSARCOMA

Rhabdomyosarcomas are the third most common solid malignant tumor in children, exceeded only by neuroblastoma and Wilms's tumor. Embryonal rhabdomyosarcoma occurs in infants and young children, and, when it develops in submucosal areas such as the bladder, vagina, or nose, it produces multiple fleshy, grapelike excrescences called sarcoma botryoides.

Localized tumors should be resected with wide surgical margins. Postoperative irradiation and chemotherapy consisting of dactinomycin and vincristine should be given as in Wilms's tumor. Rhabdomyosarcomas tend to recur locally and metastasize to regional lymph nodes. Pulmonary metastases frequently occur early in the course of the disease. Rhabdomyosarcomas arising in the head and neck are treated primarily by radiation therapy with good response.

Tumors developing in the genitourinary tract and extremities tend to be radioresistant and require radical resection with or without postoperative radiotherapy. Because of the early and frequent occurrence of distant metastases, repeated courses of chemotherapy may improve the survival rate. Cure rates of sarcoma botryoides may be as high as 60%; survival from orbital tumor is approximately 75%; tumors in other areas of the head, neck, and extremities have a cure rate of 20%. Genitourinary rhabdomyosarcoma in males has a poorer prognosis than in females. The prognosis for infants and young children is better than for older patients.

Grosfeld JL, Clatworthy HW, Newton WA: Combined therapy in childhood rhabdomyosarcoma: An analysis of 42 cases. J Pediatr Surg 4:637, 1969.

Sutow WW & others: Prognosis in childhood rhabdomyosarcoma. Cancer 25:1384, 1970.

CONGENITAL DEFORMITIES OF THE CHEST WALL
(Pectus Excavatum, Pectus Carinatum)

Anomalous development of the costal cartilages and sternum produces a variety of chest wall deformities. Failure of fusion of the 2 sternal bands during embryonic development produces congenital sternal cleft, which may involve the upper, lower, or entire sternum. This defect is usually associated with protrusion of the pericardium and heart (ectopia cordis) and congenital heart lesions.

Clinical Findings

Most children are noted to have the deformity at birth. In some cases, the defect does not occur until late childhood. Paradoxic motion in the area of the pectus excavatum is commonly seen in infants. The deformity may stabilize, but most progress in severity with age. The incidence in girls and boys is probably equal, but surgical consultation is requested 3–4 times more frequently in boys.

In pectus excavatum, the xiphoid is the deepest portion of the depression. The sternum curves posteriorly from the manubriosternal junction, although the manubrium may also be posteriorly directed. The costal cartilages, curving posteriorly to insert on the sternum, are deformed and fused. The third, fourth, and fifth ribs are usually affected, although the second through the eighth costal cartilages and ribs may be involved. The severity of the defect varies greatly from a mild, insignificant depression to an extreme where the xiphoid bone is adjacent to the vertebrae. Chest x-ray shows the posterior depression and displacement of the heart to the left. Angiocardiograms may show impingement of the sternum on the right atrium or ventricle.

These patients are typically round-shouldered, with stooped posture, potbelly, and an asthenic appearance. They tend to be withdrawn and refuse to participate in sports activities, particularly if their deformity might be exposed. Many patients complain of easy fatigability or inability to compete in exertional activities. Cardiopulmonary function studies show impaired stroke volume and cardiac output during upright exercise. Following repair, parents and children comment upon the great improvement in their well-being and exercise tolerance.

Treatment & Prognosis

The operation is performed both for cosmetic reasons and to improve cardiopulmonary function. Mild deformities should be left alone and the patient followed to observe for progression. Moderate to severe defects should be repaired, particularly when the patient or parent indicates a desire for improvement. The ideal age is 5 years. Operation in older children requires greater operative time, and a good result is easier to achieve in young children. Blood for transfusion should be available. Preoperatively, older children should be taught how to use a mechanical ventilator to assist in treating and preventing atelectasis postoperatively.

A stainless steel strut may be passed beneath the sternum and anchored by sutures to the fourth or fifth rib laterally on each side. This serves to ensure ideal position of the sternum and minimizes postoperative paradoxical motion and pain. The strut may be removed 6 or more months later.

The round-shouldered, slouched posture will persist postoperatively. A new acquired habit of maintaining an erect posture is established by using a T-brace fitted for the patient, which must be worn during waking hours for a minimum of 6 months. Exercises such as pull-ups and push-ups are initiated 3 weeks postoperatively.

Another technic, purely for improving cosmetic depression deformities, is to fill the space with a Silastic subcutaneous implant.

Removal of the defect improves vigor, endurance, and well-being.

Bieser GD & others: Impairment of cardiac function in patients with pectus excavatum, with improvement after operative correction. N Engl J Med 287:267, 1972.

Mason JK, Payne WS, Gonzales JB: Pectus excavatum: Use of preformed prosthesis for correction in the adult. Plast Reconstr Surg 46:399, 1970.

Polgar F, Koop CE: Pulmonary function in pectus excavatum. Pediatrics 32:209, 1963.

Ravitch MM: Congenital deformities of the chest wall. Pages 317–338 in: *Pediatric Surgery,* 2nd ed. Vol I. Mustard WT & others (editors). Year Book, 1969.

THE BATTERED CHILD SYNDROME

Child abuse is any nonaccidental injury inflicted by a parent, guardian, or neighbor. It may be passive, in the form of emotional or nutritional deprivation, but it is most readily recognized in the active form characterized as "battered, bruised, beaten, broken, and burned." It is estimated that 1 million children per year in the USA suffer injuries that should be reported to the National Center on Child Abuse and Neglect. About 20–50% of children are rebattered after the first diagnosis, resulting in death in 5% and permanent physical damage in 35% when the syndrome is not recognized.

Etiology

The child abuser is usually a young, insecure, unstable person who had an unhappy childhood and who has unrealistic expectations of the child. Most (not all) of these individuals are of low socioeconomic status. The abuser may be a parent, guardian, babysitter, neighboring child, or mother's boyfriend. Active traumatic abuse is usually perpetrated by the father, but passive neglect with failure to thrive from nutritional or emotional deprivation is usually attributable to the mother.

Clinical Findings

Most battered children are under 3 years old, a product of a difficult or premature pregnancy and labor, usually unwanted or illegitimate. Many have congenital anomalies or are hyperkinetic and colicky. Usually there is a discrepancy between the history supplied and the magnitude of the injury, or a reluctance to give a history. Contradictory histories or delay in bringing the child to medical attention—or many different emergency room visits in different hospitals for unusual reasons—should be regarded with suspicion. A past injury in the child or sibling, and almost any injury in an infant less than 1 year old, is likely to be child abuse. The parents may be evasive or hostile. They may have open guilt feelings or may be capable of complete concealment. Usually the innocent spouse is more protective of the abuser than of the child.

The child is usually withdrawn, apathetic, whimpering, and fearful and shows signs of neglect or failure to thrive. Multiple forms of injury will be noted at varying stages of healing. The child should be completely disrobed to note for welts, bruises, lacerations, bite or belt wounds, stick or coat hanger marks on the head, trunk, buttocks, or extremities, and similar evidence of mistreatment. Cigarette, hot plate, match, or scalding burns may be evident. Subgaleal hematomas may be caused by pulled hair. Retinal hemorrhage or detachment may follow blows to the head. Abdominal injuries may produce ruptured liver, spleen, or pancreas or bowel perforation. Sexual abuse should be identified by a bruised, lacerated, or enlarged vaginal introitus or anus.

Even though no obvious fracture may be present, a skeletal roentgenographic survey should be performed to detect skull, rib, or long bone fractures and periosteal reaction in varying stages of healing. Suture separation of the skull may indicate subdural hematoma. Neurologic injury may require brain scan or pneumoencephalogram.

Management

The child should be admitted to the hospital to be protected until the home environment can be evaluated. Injuries should be documented radiologically and with photographs. The presence of sperm in the vagina or anal canal should be confirmed. Bleeding disorders should be evaluated by a platelet count, bleeding time, prothrombin time, and plasma thromboplastin test to make certain that multiple bruises are not due to coagulopathy. A serologic test for syphilis may be indicated as well as cultures (including pharyngeal) for gonorrhea.

The injuries should be treated initially. Consultation with ophthalmologists, neurologists, neurosurgeons, orthopedic surgeons, and plastic surgeons may be required.

It is required by law in every state for both the hospital and the physician to report child abuse, suspected as well as documented, to local authorities. The district attorney's office can inform the physician about details of the local law. The physician is the protector of the child and a consultant to the parents and must not assume the role of prosecutor or judge. The most difficult task is to inform the parents of your suspicion of battering or neglect without confrontation, accusation, or anger. The physician must tell the parents that the law requires reporting injuries that are unexplained or inadequately explained considering the nature of the injury. A written, informed referral should then be made to other professionals, such as the Child Welfare Department, social workers, or psychiatrists. The referral should describe the history of past injuries and the nature of current injuries, physical findings and roentgen studies, and a statement about why nonaccidental trauma is suspected.

Prognosis

The abuser may require careful evaluation for possible psychosis by a psychiatrist. Child welfare personnel and social workers will have to assess the home environment and work with the parents to prevent future abuse. It may be necessary to place the child in a foster home, but approximately 90% of families can be reunited.

Helfer RE, Kempe CH: *The Battered Child.* Univ of Chicago Press, 1968.

Kempe CH: Pediatric implications of the battered baby syndrome. Arch Dis Child 46:28, 1971.

Kempe CH, Helfer RE: *Helping the Battered Child and His Family.* Lippincott, 1971.

Rausen AR (editor): Symposium on child abuse. Pediatrics (Suppl) 51:771, 1973.

•   •   •

General References

Brown JJM: *Surgery of Childhood.* Williams & Wilkins, 1963.

Gans SL (editor): Symposium on surgical pediatrics. Pediatr Clin North Am 16:529, 1969.

Gray SW, Skandalakis JE: *Embryology for Surgeons: The Embryological Basis for Treatment of Congenital Defects.* Saunders, 1972.

Gross RE: *The Surgery of Infancy and Childhood.* Saunders, 1953.

Hendren WH: Symposium on pediatric surgery. Surg Clin North Am 56:243, 1976.

Mustard WT & others (editors): *Pediatric Surgery,* 2nd ed. Vols I and II. Year Book, 1969.

Norman AP (editor): *Congenital Abnormalities in Infancy.* Davis, 1971.

Rickham PP, Johnston JH: *Neonatal Surgery.* Appleton-Century-Crofts, 1969.

Swenson O: *Pediatric Surgery.* Appleton-Century-Crofts, 1969.

White JJ, Haller JA: Symposium on pediatric surgery. Surg Clin North Am 50:753, 1970.

49 . . .

Oncology & Cancer Chemotherapy

Samuel D. Spivack, MD, Lynn E. Spitler, MD, & J. Englebert Dunphy, MD

In any given year, nearly 1 million Americans are under medical care for neoplastic disease and over 600,000 new cases are diagnosed. Cancer is responsible for about 17% of all deaths and (next to heart disease) is the second leading cause of death. The incidence of neoplasia by site and sex is shown in Table 49–1.

Table 49–1. Cancer incidence (in %) by site and sex.

	Male	Female
Skin	23	13
Oral	3	2
Lung	18	3
Breast	. . .	23
Colon and rectum	11	13
Other digestive	10	8
Prostate	10	. . .
Uterus	. . .	15
Urinary tract	7	3
Leukemia and lymphomas	7	6
All other	11	14

CLASSIFICATION OF TUMORS

Although the term tumor originally denoted any mass or swelling, the present meaning is now generally synonymous with neoplasm (a new pathologic growth of tissue). A neoplasm may be characterized as benign or malignant depending upon its histologic, gross, and clinical features. Malignant neoplasms usually show imperfect differentiation and structure atypical of the tissue of origin, an infiltrative growth pattern not contained by a true capsule, and relatively frequent and abnormal mitotic figures. Growth rarely ceases, although the rate of growth may be irregular, and many malignant tumors have a propensity for metastasis. Benign tumors generally lack these features, although they may be fatal as a result of impingement on other structures and impairment of function.

Neoplasms are classified according to their tissue of origin. Those from mesenchyme (muscle, bone, tendon, cartilage, fat, vessels, lymphoid, and connective tissue) are called sarcomas. Malignant tumors of epithelial origin are carcinomas and may be further classified, according to their histologic appearance, as adenocarcinomas (glandular), squamous (epidermoid), transitional, or undifferentiated. Tumors may be composed of one neoplastic cell type (although also containing nonneoplastic stromal elements such as blood vessels); may contain several neoplastic cell types of common derivation from the same germ cell layer (mixed tumors); or may derive from more than one embryonic germ cell layer (teratomas).

ETIOLOGIC FACTORS IN TUMOR FORMATION

Immunologic Disease & Cancer

Malignancy as a sequel to immunologic derangements has long been observed and is thought to represent a failure of immunity surveillance or ineffective immunity control. Neoplasms are more common when cell-mediated immunity is impaired, and some tumors have a distinctly better prognosis when lymphocytic infiltration of the tumor or regional nodes is noted histologically. Tumor-specific antigens are present in experimental animal tumors induced by chemicals and viruses. Human colon cancer contains carcinoembryonic antigens capable of eliciting an immunologic response. Recently, similar evidence has also been forthcoming for Burkitt's lymphoma, malignant melanoma, neuroblastoma, and osteosarcoma. Serum "blocking factors" which impair lymphocyte-mediated tumor inhibition have been demonstrated in patients with progressive, uncontrolled neuroblastoma and are absent in patients whose disease is controlled. Immunologic manipulations aimed at reconstituting host immune defenses are now being investigated, although no specific form of "immunotherapy" has yet been established as effective in the prevention or treatment of human neoplasms.

Bast RC Jr & others: BCG and cancer. (2 parts.) N Engl J Med 290:1413, 1959, 1974.

Smith RT: Possibilities and problems of immunologic intervention in cancer. N Engl J Med 287:439, 1972.

Zamcheck N & others: Immunologic evaluation of human digestive tract cancer: Carcinoembryonic antigens. N Engl J Med 286:83, 1972.

Chemical Oncogenesis

Chemical carcinogenesis induced by coal tars, aromatic amines, azo dyes, aflatoxins, or alkylators is a 2-stage phenomenon consisting of tumor initiation and subsequent neoplastic growth with a variable but distinct latent period between these 2 stages. Carcinogenesis requires cell proliferation once the malignant initiation phase has occurred. Carcinogens are dose-dependent, additive, and irreversible. According to the Huebner hypothesis of oncogenesis, carcinogens may activate the "oncogene" or may modify host RNA in such a way that faulty "reverse transcription" occurs in the Temin model (see below).

Ryser HJP: Chemical carcinogenesis. N Engl J Med 285:721, 1971.

Radiation Oncogenesis

Radiation oncogenesis is a complex process that appears to involve irreversible injury to chromosomes. The incidence of the spontaneous human neoplasms is increased by radiation, probably in proportion to its spontaneous incidence in the population at risk. The list includes chronic myelocytic leukemia, all forms of acute leukemia, malignant lymphomas, osteosarcoma, breast and lung carcinoma, and pancreatic, pharyngeal, thyroid, and colon carcinomas—ie, those neoplasia which account for 85% of human cancer morbidity and mortality are increased in populations exposed to radiation above background levels.

Gofman JW & others: Radiation, cancer, and environmental health. Hosp Pract 5:91, 1970.

Viral Oncogenesis

The contention that viruses may cause cancer in man rests mainly on analogous reasoning from observations in other species, particularly laboratory animals. Of the oncogenic DNA viruses, a human herpesvirus of major interest is the Epstein-Barr (EB) virus which was discovered by electron microscopy in cultured Burkitt's lymphoma cells and subsequently found in many isolates of Burkitt's lymphoma. Nasopharyngeal carcinoma has also been associated with EB virus, but the causal role in that illness is far from certain. A herpesvirus has also been associated with cancer of the uterine cervix, since more women so affected have viral antibodies than control populations.

Oncogenic RNA viruses (oncornaviruses) have recently been thought to cause some human cancers. An RNA tumor virus might produce a stable genetic trait if viral RNA served as the template for DNA synthesis and the latter became integrated into the host genome, resulting in neoplastic transformation. This revolutionary concept challenged the classic Watson-Crick hypothesis that information flow was unidirectional from DNA → RNA → protein. This hypothesis became more tenable with the demonstration that "reverse transcriptase" existed in nearly all RNA viruses with oncogenic potential, in human lymphoblastic leukemia cells, in virus-like C particles

from human milk in patients with breast cancer, and to a lesser extent in their seemingly normal relatives.

Two interesting theories of oncogenesis have recently been proposed on the basis of these data:

(1) Huebner's oncogene theory states that many (if not all) vertebrates contain the genetic information for producing C-type RNA viruses. This information (virogene) is transmitted vertically from one generation to the next and from one cell to the daughter cells. A portion of the virogene is responsible for neoplastic transformation (oncogene) and is expressed in undifferentiated fetal cells but not in normal, mature nonproliferative cells. Exposure to a carcinogenic stimulus (x-ray, chemical, or tumor virus) and the host genotype itself determine whether activation of the oncogenome will occur. This theory is based on the idea that a regulatory switch mechanism controls a stable alteration in genotype.

(2) Temin's protovirus theory proposes the origin of C particles from cellular genes which have incorporated a "protovirus" as a product of action of reverse transcriptase upon a cellular RNA template. Alterations or abnormal integrations of protovirus (due to changes in RNA, DNA, or the transcriptase) lead to oncogenesis.

The available evidence does not permit a clear choice between these 2 theories. Both have already broadened the conceptual role of viruses in oncogenesis and may have more general biologic import.

Allen DW & others: Viruses and human cancer. N Engl J Med 286:70, 1972.
Gallo RC: RNA-dependent DNA polymerase in viruses and cells. Blood 39:117, 1972.

VALUE OF GRADING & STAGING IN MALIGNANT DISEASE

For most curable neoplasms, the first therapeutic attempt must be definitive if cure is to be achieved; this means that initial therapy must be radical enough to encompass and extirpate or sterilize all existing foci of disease. An accurate delineation of the stage and extent of disease is thus an important initial step in consideration of the most appropriate treatment for the patient.

Grading and staging of neoplasms are attempts to describe the degree of malignancy and the dissemination of the malignancy. Histologic grading determines the degree of anaplasia of tumor cells, varying from grade I (very well differentiated) to grade IV (undifferentiated). Grading has prognostic value in some tumors (transitional cell carcinoma of bladder, astrocytoma, and chondrosarcoma) but is of little predictive value in others (melanoma or osteosarcoma). Staging of cancer is based upon the extent of its spread rather than on histologic appearance and has been standardized for many cancers by use of the TNM system. T refers to the degree of local extension at the primary site, N to the clinical findings in regional nodes, and M to the presence of distant metastases. Some cancers are staged by clinical examination alone (eg, squamous cell carcinoma of the cervix), whereas for others (eg, transitional cell carcinoma of the bladder and adenocarcinoma of the colon) the stage is determined on the basis of findings in the resected surgical specimen. In both instances, there is an excellent correlation of stage with prognosis.

For many neoplasms, both the histologic grading and the clinical staging have relevance to the choice of treatment and prognosis. Nowhere is this more evident than for Hodgkin's disease and the lymphomas. Lymphocyte-predominant and nodular varieties clearly have a more favorable prognosis than lymphocyte-depleted and diffuse histologic types, and disease limited to lymph nodes is potentially cured by radiotherapy whereas extranodal dissemination is generally best palliated by combination chemotherapy.

Glatstein E & others: Surgical staging of abdominal involvement in unselected patients with Hodgkin's disease. Radiology 97:425, 1970.

Feinstein AR: A new staging system for cancer and reappraisal of "early" treatment and "cure" by radical surgery. N Engl J Med 279:747, 1968.

TUMOR IMMUNOLOGY

TUMOR-SPECIFIC TRANSPLANTATION ANTIGENS

Histocompatibility transplantation antigens, which exist on all cells, are responsible for the immune rejection that occurs when skin, kidney, or any other organ is transplanted from one animal to another. Individual organs may also have antigens specific to the cells of that organ.

The discovery that malignant tumors may possess antigens not present on nonneoplastic tissues placed modern tumor immunology on a solid footing. Tumor antigens are present only on the tumor cells and are distinct from organ-specific antigens. Indeed, some tumor cells bearing these tumor-specific transplantation antigens (TSTA) lose the normal hitocompatibility antigens.

The existence of TSTA was demonstrated using inbred strains of animals, individuals of which have identical histocompatibility antigens. Malignant tumors grown in inbred animals were transplanted to animals of the same strain (ie, donor and recipient had the same histocompatibility antigens). The tumors were allowed to grow for a time and were then excised. When cells from the same strain of tumors were transplanted

again to these animals, the cells were rejected, indicating that the animals had developed an immune response to the TSTA during growth of the first tumor.

Cross-reactivity between TSTA of various tumors has been studied. Tumors caused by chemicals (eg, methylcholanthrene) have unique TSTA which do not cross-react with the TSTA of other tumors induced by the same agent. On the other hand, virally induced tumors share TSTA with other tumors caused by the same virus. The antigen on these tumors may be virus-specific, ie, the TSTA may be structurally related to the virus itself. Thus, immunization by the virus alone will cause subsequent rejection of a transplanted tumor induced by that virus. Alternatively, the antigen may be virus-coded but not present on the virus or may be induced by derepression of the host genome by the viruses.

Other antigens, termed tumor-associated antigens, may be present in malignant tumors and also in some normal tissues. Carcinoembryonic antigen (CEA) and alpha-fetoglobulin are examples.

Immune Responses to Tumor Antigens in Man

Demonstration of immune responses to TSTA in humans with cancer has strongly suggested the presence of TSTA on the tumors (Table 49–2). Unfortunately, tests for TSTA are not useful for the diagnosis of malignancy since they are often negative in individuals with tumors and positive in those without tumors. Moreover, the results of the tests correlate poorly with the prognosis. Thus, although they are not clinically useful, tests for TSTA serve as a means for understanding basic mechanisms of tumor immunity.

Table 49–2. Tests for immune reactivity.

Specific reactivity to tumor antigens
Antibody
Immunofluorescence
Complement fixation
Cytotoxicity
Antibody-dependent cytotoxicity
Radioimmunoassay
Cell-mediated
Skin test reactivity
Colony inhibition
Cytotoxicity
Lymphocyte transformation
Migration inhibition
Leukocyte adherence inhibition
Other
Blocking factor (inhibitory factor)
Unblocking factor
General measures of immunologic reactivity
In vivo
Skin tests
Dinitrochlorobenzene sensitization
In vitro
Rosette-forming cells
Lymphocyte response to phytohemagglutinin

Tests for Antibodies to TSTA

A. Immunofluorescence: Cultured autologous or homologous neoplastic cells obtained from fresh tumors are used as indicator cells. Controls are normal cells from the organ from which the tumor was derived (organ specificity) and cells from other tumors (tumor specificity). The test and control sera are layered over the indicator cells, and the presence of antibody is detected by the use of fluorescein-labeled antihuman immunoglobulin. If the cells are fixed before testing, antibodies to cytoplasmic and nuclear antigens will be detected. It appears that for some tumors, cross-reacting cytoplasmic antigens are present in all tumors of the same histologic type, whereas membrane antigens are unique to an individual, do not cross-react, and can be detected only by autologous tumor cells and autologous antiserum.

B. Complement Fixation: The test serum is mixed with whole tumor cells or extracts and complement is added. If a complement-fixing antibody reacts with antigen in the mixture, some of the complement will be "fixed" or inactivated by attachment to the antigen-antibody complex. The amount of complement remaining is assayed by its ability to lyse sensitized erythrocytes.

C. Cytotoxicity: Viable tumor cell lines or, less commonly, cells derived directly from tumors are plated in microtiter wells. Test sera are added, and the cells remaining attached to the cells are counted. Cells killed by test sera lose their ability to adhere to the well and are removed, thereby reducing the cell count. Alternatively, cells may be labeled with radioisotopes such as ^{51}chromium, ^{125}iododeoxyuridine, or tritiated thymidine and cytotoxicity determined by release of these agents following cell death. Antibody-dependent leukocyte cytoxicity is detected in a similar way, except that killing requires leukocytes in addition to antibody.

Tests for Cell-Mediated Immunity to TSTA

A. Skin Test Reactivity: Tumor extracts (0.1 ml), serving as test antigens, are injected intradermally and the inflammatory response is recorded after 24 and 48 hours (similar to a PPD test).

B. Colony Inhibition: Test lymphocytes are added to tumor cells grown on a glass or plastic surface and the number of surviving colonies is counted. Cellular immune reactivity is reflected by a reduction in the number of colonies present. Colony inhibition requires that the number of lymphocytes far exceed the number of tumor cells (ie, at least 100 lymphocytes per tumor cell). Specificity of this reaction for TSTA is under intense investigation.

C. Cytotoxicity: This may be measured visually by counting the number of tumor cells remaining following incubation with test lymphocytes or by determining release of radioisotopes from tumor cells, as described for antibody cytotoxicity. Like colony inhibition, the ratio of lymphocytes to tumor cells must be high. The specificity of the reaction for TSTA has not been resolved.

D. Lymphocyte Transformation: Sensitized lymphocytes exposed to specific antigen undergo a morphologic change termed "blast transformation," which is accompanied by increased DNA, RNA, and protein synthesis. These biochemical changes can be measured by adding radioactive precursors (eg, ^{14}C-thymidine) to the cultures and determining their uptake into cellular constituents such as DNA. Test lymphocytes are cultured in the presence of tumor cells or tumor extract, and DNA synthesis is measured by incorporation of the radioisotope. When whole tumor cells are used, care must be taken to include appropriate controls, since histocompatibility antigens on the tumor cells unrelated to TSTA could stimulate the test lymphocytes.

E. Migration Inhibition: Factors that inhibit the migration of indicator cells are released following contact of sensitized lymphocytes with antigen. If macrophages are used as the indicator cell, the factor causing inhibition is termed migration inhibitory factor (MIF). More commonly, in human studies, peripheral buffy coat leukocytes are used, in which case the indicator cells are polymorphonuclear leukocytes, and the mediator is termed leukocyte inhibitory factor (LIF). The test cells are exposed to tumor cells or extracts, and migration is measured from capillary tubes or in agarose plates or droplets. A positive response is inhibition of the migration of the indicator cells as compared to the migration of control cells not exposed to antigen.

F. Leukocyte Adherence Inhibition: Adherence of sensitized cells to a glass or plastic surface is reduced following exposure of the cells to specific antigen. In the case of tumor immunology, test leukocytes on a surface are incubated with or without tumor extract and the number of cells remaining is determined. A positive response is a reduction in the number of cells adhering to the surface.

G. Blocking Factor: Blocking factor has been most extensively studied in the colony inhibition and cytotoxicity test systems. Patients with growing tumors have leukocytes that will inhibit growth or kill tumor cells of the same type as their own tumor, but, when the patient's serum is added to the test system, killing of the tumor cells is impaired. The substance responsible for this inhibition, termed blocking factor, was originally thought to be antibody, which acts by masking the TSTA. Later studies have shown that blocking factor may be an antigen-antibody complex. When, as sometimes occurs, tumor antigen alone can impair the killing of tumor cells by the patient's lymphocytes, it is termed **inhibitory factor**.

H. Unblocking Factor: Patients whose tumors have regressed or who are tumor-free may have a factor (unblocking factor) in their serum that inhibits the activity of blocking factor. Thus, if a patient's cells will kill tumor cells when cultured in the presence of normal serum and killing is impaired in the presence of serum containing blocking factor, killing will be restored if serum containing unblocking factor is added to the culture containing blocking factor.

IMMUNOSURVEILLANCE

It has been postulated that humans develop malignancy regularly and that the immune system recognizes and rejects the malignant cells. Among the evidence supporting this concept, called immunosurveillance, is the observation that patients with primary immunodeficiency disease show an increased incidence of cancer, suggesting that the immune defect is related to the tumor development. On the other hand, the types of cancers that occur most often in these patients are not those most common in the general population but rather are reticuloendothelial tumors, lymphomas, and sarcomas. Patients undergoing long-term immunosuppressive therapy following renal transplantation also show an increased incidence of malignancy. However, patients with lepromatous leprosy, a disease associated with a profound defect in cellular immunity, do not show an increased incidence of malignancy. Moreover, nude mice, which lack T cell reactivity, do not develop malignant tumors more frequently than normal mice. Thus, the concept of immunosurveillance, while appealing, cannot be regarded as being proved.

If human tumors do carry TSTA distinct from the normal host antigens and if immune reactivity can reject such tumors, the following theories have been proposed to explain how spontaneous tumors could survive.

A. "Sneak Through": Malignant tumors probably stem from one cell. The number of cells and the amount of antigen initially present may be insufficient to stimulate the immune mechanism, and by the time the tumor is large enough to evoke a response, it may be too large to be rejected.

B. Substances Produced by the Tumor May Inhibit Rejection: Antigens shed from the tumor may directly inhibit the cellular immune reactivity or may combine with antibodies to form antigen-antibody complexes which block lymphocyte cytotoxicity. If lymphocytes are activated by combination with tumor antigen at a site remote from the tumor, the activation may not damage the tumor. The tumor may produce other substances which nonspecifically inhibit immune reactivity. One such tumor factor inhibits the accumulation of inflammatory cells.

C. Immune Enhancement: At times, the immune response may stimulate rather than inhibit tumor growth. For example, enhancing antibodies may combine with antigens on the malignant cells and protect them from sensitized lymphocytes. It has also been suggested that low levels of cellular immune reactivity may stimulate tumor growth.

D. Antigenic Modulation: During tumor growth, tumor antigen may be lost or may change in such a way that the sensitized host no longer recognizes it. Thus, the tumor may escape rejection.

E. General Immunosuppression in the Host: Many individuals bearing tumors, even when the lesion is small, show diminished capacity to respond to various common antigens, including some to which they have previously been sensitized (eg, candidin and streptococcal antigen). Further, their ability to respond to new antigens to which they have not previously been exposed (eg, dinitrochlorobenzene [DNCB]) may be impaired. This diminished reactivity in cancer patients may in part explain the ability of tumor cells with TSTA to survive in the host. Patients with malignancy may also have in their sera substances that nonspecifically suppress lymphocyte reactivity.

IMMUNOLOGIC EVALUATION OF THE CANCER PATIENT

Both general immunologic reactivity and the specific immunologic reactivity to the tumor may be assessed. Evaluation of tumor-specific reactivity at the present time must be regarded as experimental and not clinically useful in the care or estimate of prognosis of cancer patients. Measurement of general immunologic reactivity can in some cases provide clinically useful information regarding status and prognosis in tumor patients. Use of at least some of these tests is important in patients treated on immunotherapy protocols.

In Vivo Tests of General Immunologic Reactivity

A. Skin Tests: Skin tests with common antigens measure the patient's ability to respond to antigens to which he has previously been sensitized. A panel rather than just one or 2 antigens must be used since exposure in the population is not uniform and a negative response to one or another antigen might simply reflect lack of exposure. Examples of antigens useful for this purpose (antigens to which normal subjects usually react) are candidin, purified protein derivative of tuberculin (PPD), and streptococcal antigen (streptokinase-streptodornase, SKSD). Certain conditions, such as Hodgkin's disease, are characteristically associated with diminished skin test reactivity even early in the course. Fluctuations in skin test reactivity may parallel disease activity.

B. DNCB Sensitization: DNCB is an antigen to which most patients have not previously been exposed. A sensitizing dose is applied to the skin, and 2 weeks later the patient is reexposed to test for sensitization. A positive response consists of erythema and vesicle formation similar to other forms of contact hypersensitivity (eg, poison oak). For some malignant diseases, the ability of the patient to become sensitized correlates with the prognosis (ie, patients who are not readily sensitized are more likely to develop recurrent disease).

In Vitro Tests of General Immunologic Reactivity

A. Rosette-Forming Cells: Sheep red blood cells form rosettes around certain peripheral blood lymphocytes (T cells) of thymic origin and are important in tumor immunity. There are 2 technics for performing the test, one involving short and the other long (usually overnight) incubation. The long incubation test detects what is thought to be the total T cell population, which includes about 70% of the peripheral lymphocytes in normal subjects. The short incubation or "active" rosette-forming cells represent a subpopulation of T cells which is thought to be more important with regard to cancer activity. In some types of cancer, if the number of short incubation rosette-forming cells is decreased when the primary lesion is discovered, the prognosis is poor.

B. Lymphocyte Response to Phytohemagglutinin (PHA): Lymphocytes exposed to PHA increase DNA synthesis, which can be measured by incorporation of radioactive thymidine. Since stimulation by PHA does not depend on previous exposure, PHA is regarded as a nonspecific mitogen. The test represents a general measure of lymphocyte function.

IMMUNOTHERAPY

All forms of immunotherapy (Table 49–3) must be considered experimental at present; none has established efficacy. Tumor immunotherapy may be active, stimulating the patient's own immune system to increased activity, or passive, in which the therapeutic agents are passively transferred. Immunotherapy may be specific, attempting to enhance reactivity to the TSTA of the patient's tumor, or nonspecific, attempting to generally enhance the patient's immune reactivity.

In experimental animals, growth of transplanted or virally induced tumors has been *prevented* by prior sensitization. Established (experimental) tumors have been eradicated by local immunotherapy (eg, intralesional BCG) but only rarely by systemic immunotherapy. Thus, the time when immunotherapy is most likely to be effective is when the patient is clinically free of tumor but likelihood of recurrence is high—eg, after surgical removal of the primary lesion and metastases. It may also be effective during and following reduction of the tumor burden by radiotherapy with or without chemotherapy, but one must take into account the immunosuppressive effects of these agents and consider whether the immunotherapy in question can cause an increase of immune reactivity in the face of the immunosuppression.

The decision for immunotherapy must take into account the potential of all forms of manipulation of the immune system to increase tumor growth: the unanticipated appearance of enhancing antibodies, production of low levels of cellular immunity, or immunosuppression—any of these, which are only examples of many untoward events, could result in loss of control of the tumor.

To facilitate spread of information regarding immunotherapy protocols and to encourage patient referrals, the International Registry of Tumor Immunotherapy has been formed. The Registry publishes the *Compendium of Immunotherapeutic Protocols,* which can be obtained from the National Cancer Institute. It provides a listing of studies being conducted, type of disease, classification of patients, immunotherapeutic agents, the principal investigator and his address, and whether the study is active.

A. Tumor Cells, Neuraminidase-Treated Tumor Cells, and Tumor Antigens: All of these substances are used in attempts to stimulate the patient's own reactivity to his tumor. Although one might anticipate that the patient would have received sufficient antigenic stimulus from his tumor to mount a maximal immune response, insufficient tumor antigen may have reached lymph nodes remote from the tumor. If so, injection of tumor antigen at sites where they will reach these remote nodes could heighten immune reactivity.

The source and preparation of the tumor cells may be important in the success of this kind of therapy. For example, if TSTA on the membranes of human cells are specific for each individual, and if membrane antigens are the only ones involved in tumor rejection, it would be essential to sensitize each patient with his own tumor. This obviously would limit the application of this approach since tumor tissue is often not available from the individual patient. If it were effective, it would be much easier to use tumor tissue of the same type from homologous fresh tumors or from cultured cell lines.

Experimental evidence suggests that viable tumor cells may be more effective than tumor extracts or cells killed by x-ray radiation or other means in stimulating immune reactivity, but viable cells also carry the potential of establishing new tumor deposits. Treatment of the cells with enzymes such as neuraminidase may expose their TSTA and render the cells more potent as immunostimulators. An ideal solution to all of these problems would be to use specific tumor antigens isolated from the malignant cells. To date, prepa-

Table 49–3. Immunotherapeutic modalities.

Active
Specific
Tumor cells
Neuraminidase-treated tumor cells
Tumor antigens
Nonspecific
Methanol extraction residue (MER)
Transfer factor
Levamisole
Corynebacterium parvum
Thymosin
Passive
Specific
Antibody
Immune RNA
Unblocking plasma
Sensitized lymphocytes
Nonspecific
Plasmapheresis

rations of isolated antigens from experimental tumors have been considerably less effective than whole cells in evoking an immune response, and the role of this technic in immunotherapy of human malignancy remains to be defined.

B. BCG: BCG has been used mostly widely in the therapy of acute myelogenous leukemia (AML) and malignant melanoma. The results of several large controlled clinical trials with BCG are conflicting. Life may be slightly prolonged in patients with AML. In malignant melanoma, there does not seem to be any effect on visceral disease. In patients with primary melanoma or lymph node metastases, 2 studies with concurrent controls showed no effect of BCG; one study with historic controls showed a positive effect; and one study is still incomplete. At best, if BCG has an effect, it will be no more than a 20–25% decrease in recurrence rate.

Part of the problem in these trials is the variability of the available BCG preparations; they are poorly standardized, and the percentage of viable organisms and of contaminating material (cell walls, etc) varies considerably. Moreover, the optimal method of administration, dosage, and timing of administration has not been worked out and differs between studies. Use of a better-defined substance (eg, methanol extraction residue [MER]) may help to overcome these problems.

One general principle evident from animal and human studies is the importance of local administration of BCG to sites where tumor cells may be remaining. Thus, direct injection of BCG into skin nodules of malignant melanoma causes regression of 90% of the injected lesions. BCG administered to the extremity from which the primary was removed may enter the lymphatics and eradicate tumor cells remaining in that extremity or in the regional lymph nodes. On the other hand, BCG given by scarification to the extremities of patients with melanoma of the head and neck has not proved beneficial; in this circumstance, the BCG would not have reached the locally draining lymphatics.

Local administration of BCG has been used in the following situations: intravenously to patients with leukemia or lymphoma; intrapleurally through the chest tube following resection of pulmonary tumors; by hepatic artery infusion for malignancy involving the liver; by cystic lavage for bladder tumors; by intraprostatic injection for malignancy of the prostate; and by intraperitoneal injection for carcinoma of the colon or ovary. Oral administration has also been used.

BCG is not without risk. Aside from the possibility of producing accelerated tumor growth, fever and malaise are common. Administration of BCG by scarification results in a local reaction and scab formation not unlike that resulting from smallpox vaccination. More severe systemic reactions may occur in patients strongly sensitive to PPD, and 2 deaths have been reported.

C. Transfer Factor: Transfer factor is a dialyzable extract of leukocytes which, when given by subcutaneous injection, enhances immune reactivity in the recipient. It has been used in the therapy of immunodeficiency disease, infectious diseases, and malignancy, mainly malignant melanoma and osteogenic sarcoma. In small groups of patients, transfer factor has caused tumor regression and prolonged survival in patients with a poor prognosis who were clinically free of tumor at the initiation of therapy. Properly controlled studies are just now being initiated.

Some studies suggest that transfer of reactivity is specific, ie, that the transfer factor donor must have reactivity to the antigen in question for transfer factor to work. If so, it may be difficult to locate appropriate donors for individual patients with cancer. Recent studies have shown that close household contacts (not necessarily blood relatives) of patients often show cellular immune reactivity to the patient's tumor. Thus, if the clinical efficacy of transfer factor does require specificity, it may be possible to use household contacts as the donors.

Many other studies suggest that the effects of transfer factor are nonspecific. If this proves to be the case, therapy would be much simpler. If donor selection were uncomplicated, transfer factor could readily be produced by blood banks as another blood product.

D. Levamisole: Levamisole is a widely used anthelmintic which increases cellular and humoral reactivity. It can be given orally (150 mg for 3 days every 2 weeks) and has been associated with only one major side-effect, leukopenia, mainly in patients treated for rheumatoid arthritis. Levamisole is effective in the therapy of some but not all animal tumors. Levamisole alone is ineffective in humans with advanced malignancy.

Favorable results have been reported in one study of patients with inoperable stage III breast carcinoma who were treated with irradiation followed by levamisole or placebo. At 3 years, survival in the group receiving placebo was 35% compared to 90% in the group receiving levamisole. The disease-free interval was similarly prolonged. These encouraging results await confirmation. Studies with bronchogenic carcinoma and malignant melanoma are currently under way.

E. *Corynebacterium parvum*: *C parvum* is administered subcutaneously or intravenously like BCG, except that killed rather than viable organisms are used. Since it may be one form of immunotherapy effective in combination with chemotherapy, it is currently being evaluated in several chemoimmunotherapy protocols. Side-effects include pain at the injection site, chills and fever, and nausea and vomiting. More serious side-effects have been reported, including acute hypertensive headache and dyspnea.

F. Thymosin: Thymosin is a partially purified extract of thymus gland which promotes differentiation of thymus-derived lymphocytes (T cells). Both in vitro and in vivo, thymosin has been reported to increase the percentage of rosette-forming cells in patients in which such cells were decreased prior to testing. Thymosin is given by injection and is associated with few side-effects. Rarely, systemic reactions such as rash, chills, and fever may occur. Studies in patients with cancer have been limited to the demonstration of an ability to enhance depressed rosette-formation and delayed hypersensitivity. Its clinical efficacy has not yet been evaluated.

G. Antibody: Serum containing antibody cytotoxic to tumor cells of the same type as the patient's tumor has been used in attempts to achieve tumor regression. In very early studies, tumor cells were used to immunize a large animal, such as a horse, and serum from this animal was used to treat the patient. This approach was complicated by development of sensitivity by the patient to horse serum. More recently, human serum from donors with immune reactivity to TSTA has been used mainly to treat leukemia and lymphoma, conditions in which the antibody would have a good chance to reach the tumor cells. Definite benefit has been observed in patients, but the benefit has been of limited duration and felt to be of little clinical significance.

H. Immune RNA: RNA extracted from sensitized lymphocytes has been reported to cause nonsensitized lymphocytes to become cytotoxic for tumor cells following in vitro incubation or in vivo administration. The preliminary clinical experience has been mainly with hypernephroma and malignant melanoma. The patient's tumor is used to sensitize a sheep. RNA is then extracted from the sheep's lymph nodes and spleen and administered intradermally to the patient. No significant local or systemic toxicity has been reported. In some patients, objective regression of tumors has been observed. A randomized trial has been started in patients clinically free of disease at the initiation of therapy.

I. Unblocking Plasma: Normal black subjects have in their plasma a substance (unblocking factor) that inhibits the blocking effect of serum from patients with melanoma. A randomized trial with unblocking plasma for the treatment of melanoma failed to show any effect.

J. Sensitized Lymphocytes: In one attempt to use sensitized lymphocytes, cancer patients were paired, and each patient's tumor was used to sensitize his partner. Specifically sensitized lymphocytes were harvested and returned to the original donor. Tumor regressions were obtained, but the technic has not been widely adopted because it is cumbersome and the results were not sufficiently encouraging.

K. Plasmapheresis: Patients may have in their serum nonspecific or specific substances (eg, tumor antigens) produced by the tumor that may interefere with cellular immune reactivity or inflammatory response. Furthermore, the host may produce substances (eg, C-reactive protein, alpha globulin) that impair immune response mechanisms. Plasmapheresis, to remove suppressive factors, may be performed by withdrawing 1 or 2 units of blood, centrifuging to remove plasma, and returning the red cells to the donor. Plasmapheresis is easier using a cell separator, which continuously removes plasma and returns white and red cells to the patient. Results to date in a very few patients have been somewhat encouraging.

Hellstrom KE, Hellstrom I: Lymphocyte mediated cytotoxicity and blocking serum activity to tumor antigens. Adv Immunol 18:209, 1974.

Herberman RB: Cell-mediated immunity to tumor cells. Adv Cancer Res 19:207, 1974.

Holmes EC & others: Immunotherapy of cancer. West J Med 126:102, Feb 1977.

Humphrey LJ, Pierce GE: The role of immunology in the diagnosis and treatment of cancer. Pages 15–36 in: *Progress in Clinical Cancer.* Vol 6. Ariel IM (editor). Grune & Stratton, 1975.

Marx JL: Tumor immunology. 1. The host's response to cancer. 2. Strategies for cancer therapy. Science 184: 552, 652, 1974.

Munster AM (editor): *Surgical Immunology.* Grune & Stratton, 1976.

Smith RT: Possibilities and problems of immunologic intervention in cancer. N Engl J Med 287:437, 1972.

Terry WD (editor): Symposium on immunotherapy in malignant disease. Med Clin North Am, vol 60, no. 3, 1976. [Entire issue.]

THERAPY OF MALIGNANT DISEASES

SURGERY

Surgical excision is the most effective means of removing the primary lesion of most neoplasms. It also provides palliation of symptoms, as by the relief of intestinal obstruction in tumors which may be unresectable or may have already metastasized. A number of highly malignant tumors have been found to respond favorably to limited surgical excision combined with radiation and chemotherapy.

Certain neoplasms which often involve many organ systems so that management crosses a number of surgical specialties are dealt with here.

1. MALIGNANT MELANOMA

Clinical & Histologic Classification (Table 49–4)

Although all melanomas arise from the common melanocyte, 3 distinct lesions can be recognized clinically: (1) superficial spreading melanoma, (2) nodular melanoma, and (3) lentigo maligna melanoma.

It is essential to recognize these different lesions by their clinical as well as histologic appearance because management and prognosis are quite different for each type.

A. Superficial Spreading Melanoma: This is the most common type and usually represents a change in a preexisting mole appearing on any part of the body as a slightly elevated brownish lesion with small discrete nodules of black, gray, blue, or pinkish hue. Once malignant change takes place, the lesion expands rapidly so that when first seen the plaque may be several centimeters in size with a slightly raised surface and an irregular arc-shaped edge.

Histologically, the malignant melanocytes are fairly uniform in appearance, usually involving epidermis and dermis.

B. Nodular Melanoma: Some authorities regard this as a distinct pathologic entity, but it may be merely a rapidly growing form. Nodular melanoma develops without obvious warning signs of a change in a preexisting mole. It may develop at the site of a preexistent junctional nevus but rapidly becomes a palpable elevated firm nodule. It may be dense black or may have a reddish blue-black color. Occasionally, amelanotic nodules develop. Melanomas of this type may occur on any part of the body, and, when they appear at a site not visible to the patient, the lesion may become quite large and ulcerate before it is noticed. A distinct convex nodular development indicates deep invasion.

Histologically, the malignant cells in biopsy specimens of nodular melanoma arise from the epidermal-dermal junction and invade deeply into the dermis and subcutaneous tissue.

C. Lentigo Maligna Melanoma: This form of melanoma usually occurs in older patients on an exposed surface of the body. It is seen most often as a large melanotic freckle ("Hutchinson's freckle") on the temple or malar region. The lesion grows very slowly, often developing over a period of years. Clinically, it is the largest of the malignant moles, often reaching 5–6 cm in diameter. Initially, it is flat and cannot be felt, but as cancer develops it becomes slightly raised with a palpable thickening. Discrete brown to black nodules may be scattered through it. Characteristically, the edge is quite irregular.

The histologic changes of malignancy tend to be scattered irregularly throughout the lesion, corresponding with elevated areas and color changes. Malignant melanocytes seem to concentrate in the darker areas.

The clinical and histologic features of the 3 forms of malignant melanoma as summarized in Table 49–4 show 5 levels of involvement.

General Considerations

In all forms of melanoma, the warning signs of malignancy involve any change in size, shape, color, or elevation of a mole. Itching or a sense of skin irritation may be the first warning sign. The most dangerous type of lesion, the nodular melanoma, gives rise to the most obscure premonitory signs and is often in an obvious stage of advanced malignancy when first detected.

The general benignity of most moles, which may be scattered over the entire body, makes complete prophylactic excision impractical. Accordingly, preventive treatment should be restricted to sites which

Table 49–4. Staging of malignant melanoma. (After Clark.)

Level 1 = In situ melanoma above the basement membrane.
Level 2 = Through the basememt membrane into the papillary level but not into the reticular layer of the dermis.
Level 3 = Filling the papillary layer and extending to the junction of the papillary and reticular layers but not entering the reticular layer.
Level 4 = Into the reticular layer of the dermis.
Level 5 = Subcutaneous tissue involvement.

are subject to irritation and to dark lesions which are larger than a 0.5 cm in diameter on the leg or back. Most authorities advise removal of nevi on the soles of the feet, the palms of the hands, and the female genitalia. Any nevus which appears to be enlarging before the age of puberty should also be removed since frank cancer, with metastasis, does not occur before puberty. Any lesion at any age which undergoes a change should be removed.

Treatment

Treatment is primarily surgical but must be varied depending upon the type and location of the melanoma, the depth of invasion, and the presence of lymph node involvement. Clark's method of staging, combined with the microstage technic for measuring the depth of invasion, is a valuable guide in determining the extent of excision in individual cases.

There is still some disagreement among surgeons regarding how widely lesions should be excised and the indications for prophylactic lymph node dissection. In most cases, a 4–5 cm margin should be removed with the tumor; in an older patient with a slowly growing lentigo maligna on the face, a 1 or 2 cm margin may be adequate. Very wide and deep excisions or amputations may be necessary for advanced nodular melanomas.

In all forms of melanoma, the level and depth of invasion are critical factors. Regardless of type, a lesion less than 0.5–0.75 mm in depth has an excellent prognosis and there is only a slight risk of lymph node metastasis. There is, however, considerable variation in the aggressiveness of tumor types. Lentigo maligna rarely extends deeply, but a large number of superficial spreading malanomas reach levels II and III, and nodular melanomas often involve levels IV or V. Similarly, the depth of invasion is related to lymph node metastases. Lesions at level I or II have a low incidence of lymph node involvement, and deeply invasive lesions, regardless of type, frequently involve the regional nodes.

It is generally accepted that lesions at level I or II, showing less than 0.6–0.75 mm of invasion, do not require prophylactic node dissection. The incidence of involvement of lymph nodes in superficial spreading melanoma, even at levels II or III, is also low, so that a policy of careful observation may be followed. Nodular melanomas are rarely confined to level II; and, in a high percentage of cases with level III, IV, or V involvement, the lymph nodes will be involved so that a prophylactic node dissection is recommended even if the nodes are not palpable. In all cases, regardless of type, the presence of palpably involved lymph nodes warrants excision. Also, even in the more favorable lesions, if the growth is close to an area of lymphatic drainage, excision and en bloc node dissection is justifiable.

If the lymph nodes are involved, long-term survival is rare except in selected cases in which the primary lesion and the nodes have been removed by an en bloc in continuity operation.

There is a growing body of evidence that regional perfusion prior to surgical excision contributes to long-term survival in cases of invasive melanomas of the extremities. Adjunctive systemic chemotherapy with a wide variety of agents, singly and in combination, has not proved to be consistently effective in disseminated disease with visceral involvement. Occasionally, dramatic responses have been reported after a variety of chemotherapeutic agents, and remarkable long-term palliation may follow a combination of irradiation, chemotherapy, and surgical excision. Malignant melanoma is one of those tumors which may undergo spontaneous regression. This is very well documented in the case of skin metastases and has also been reported after visceral metastases. Despite a number of optimistic preliminary reports, the place of immunotherapy has not been firmly established.

Prognosis

The most important factors in prognosis appear to be the size of the tumor and the extent of invasion. Small tumors less than 2 cm in diameter and with minimal invasion (less than 0.7 mm) are curable by wide local excision. The prognosis is usually favorable in lentigo maligna and in superficial spreading melanomas provided there is no deep invasion. Most nodular melanomas, particularly if ulcerated and associated with deep invasion, have a poor prognosis.

Lesions of the extremities have a more favorable prognosis than those of the trunk, and women with malignant melanoma have better survival statistics at 5 and 10 years than men.

Breslow A: Tumor thickness, level of invasion, and node dissections in stage I cutaneous melanoma. Ann Surg 182:527, 1975.

Clark WH Jr & others: The histogenesis and biologic behavior of primary malignant melanomas of the skin. Cancer Res 29:705, 1969.

Davis NC: Cutaneous melanoma: The Queensland experience. Curr Probl Surg 13:3(5), May 1976.

DeVita VA Jr, Fisher RI: Natural history of malignant melanoma as related to therapy. Cancer Treat Rep 60:153, 1976.

Malignant melanoma and immunotherapy. (Editorial.) Br Med J 1:831, 1976.

McBride CM & others: Prophylactic isolation-perfusion as the primary therapy for invasive malignant melanoma of the limbs. Ann Surg 182:316, 1975.

Morton DL & others: BCG immunotherapy of malignant mela-

noma. Ann Surg 180:635, 1974.

Southwick HW: Malignant melanoma: Role of node dissection reappraised. Cancer 37:202, 1976.

Sugarbaker EV, McBride CM: Survival and regional disease control after isolation perfusion for invasive stage I melanoma of the extremities. Cancer 37:188, 1976.

Wanebo HJ & others: Malignant melanoma of the extremities. Cancer 35:666, 1975.

Wanebo HJ & others: Selection of the optimum surgical treatment of stage I melanoma by depth of microinvasion. Ann Surg 182:302, 1975.

Yeager RA & others: Multimodality therapy in the treatment of regionally inoperable melanomas and sarcomas. Surg Gynecol Obstet 141:367, 1975.

2. SARCOMAS

A great variety of tumors may involve the soft tissues of the body from the skin and subcutaneous tissue to the retroperitoneum and the fibrous and adipose tissues of parenchymatous organs. For detailed descriptions of the pathologic features and surgical management, the reader is referred to the monographs and articles cited in the bibliography. The general principles of modern management of the more common sarcomatous tumors are presented below.

Most soft tissue sarcomas arise de novo and are not the result of malignant degeneration of long-standing benign tumors. The precise cause of soft tissue carcinoma is not known, but there is increasing evidence that many viruses may be associated with sarcomas. A common sarcoma-specific antigen has been identified in human sarcomas. Supporting the possibility of a basic viral cause is the well-known observation that Roux chicken sarcoma is associated with a type C virus. The role of trauma in the production of soft tissue tumors has not been established, although there frequently appears to be a relationship clinically, particularly in children.

Pulmonary metastases, particularly after amputation as well as wide local excision, occur with all forms of sarcoma. Not uncommonly, however, the lesions are sharply localized in the lung, and pulmonary resection has been followed by very favorable results. Five-year survival rates without recurrence of as high as 30% have been recorded even after excision of multiple pulmonary metastases.

Liposarcoma

All liposarcomas are malignant and rarely, if ever, arise from benign lipomas. Subcutaneous liposarcomas may resemble lipomas but tend to be more deeply located and much less well circumscribed. Surgical management depends upon histologic diagnosis, which must be established prior to operation by incisional or needle biopsy. Only in very small, clearly localized tumors is local excision acceptable initially. The apparent capsule and well-defined border of many liposarcomas encourages limited local removal which invariably is followed by recurrence. An accurate preoperative histologic diagnosis permits total local excision, leaving a wide rim of normal tissue around the neoplasm.

Retroperitoneal Liposarcoma

Retroperitoneal liposarcoma is a particularly insidious form of this group of tumors. The tumor mass often attains massive size before it becomes symptomatic or appears as a palpable lesion upon physical examination. The diagnosis of liposarcoma is usually established at exploration for a tumor mass displacing portions of the gastrointestinal tract or ureter. Treatment, as elsewhere, consists of the widest possible excision, but because of the location of the tumor it often must be incomplete. For this reason, postoperative x-ray is frequently indicated when gross tissue has been left behind or when the tumor has clearly been merely shelled out from the peritoneum.

Many liposarcomas are slowly growing and recur locally in the retroperitoneum many years after an apparently successful extirpation. Reoperation for even the most extensive recurrent liposarcomas may result in long periods of arrest and palliation.

Fibrosarcomas

These are the second most common sarcomas of soft tissue, liposarcomas being the most common. Many tumors formerly regarded as fibrosarcomas are now classified more accurately as leiomyosarcomas, liposarcomas, or rhabdomyosarcomas. Fibrosarcomas usually appear as well-circumscribed, superficial, freely moveable nodules of the subcutaneous tissue of the extremities or trunks. Here again, accurate histologic diagnosis is essential and very wide total excision is required. Amputation may be necessary, but, more often, well-planned wide excision of the tumor will suffice. Many apparently deep seated fibrosarcomas of the buttock can be widely excised with good margins, avoiding amputation. Indeed, there is some evidence that subsequent pulmonary metastases are less common after total local excision than after amputation.

Radiation has a place in the management of selected cases. Preoperative radiation may render a tumor more clearly circumscribed and permit a well-planned excision with the line of dissection in normal tissue. As in all other soft tissue sarcomas, shelling out of even the most obviously encapsulated lesion results in a high rate of local recurrence.

Rhabdomyosarcomas

Embryonal rhabdomyosarcoma is primarily a tumor of childhood and adolescence. Formerly regarded as an essentially incurable lesion, even after amputation, it has been shown in recent years to respond favorably to a combination of x-ray therapy, wide local excision, and chemotherapy (see p 1055). Five-year survival rates of 70–90% are being reported. Here again, however, accurate histologic diagnosis is essential to planned management.

Pleomorphic rhabdomyosarcomas are a variant of embryonal cell sarcomas but in general have a more favorable prognosis.

Alveolar cell rhabdomyosarcoma, despite modern management, remains a highly fatal lesion.

Botryoidal Sarcoma

Basically, this is another variant of embryonal rhabdomyosarcoma. Indeed, except for location and gross appearance, the lesions are quite similar and therapy is basically the same. It appears as a grossly polypoid mass involving the genitourinary tract in young children. Here again, combined therapy of radiation, chemotherapy, and surgery have produced encouraging results.

Leiomyosarcomas

These lesions frequently simulate fibrosarcomas but are not uncommonly encountered in the gastrointestinal tract, where they appear as well-circumscribed defects within the wall of the stomach or intestine. Leiomyosarcomas of the stomach may attain enormous size, filling the abdomen but having a single origin from a small area of gastric or colonic wall. Despite apparent localization and encapsulation, recurrence even after wide excision is likely.

Gerner RE & others: Soft tissue sarcomas. Ann Surg 181:803, 1975.

Gilbert HA & others: Management of soft tissue sarcomas of the extremities. Surg Gynecol Obstet 139:914, 1974.

Jaffe N & others: Rhabdomyosarcoma in children: Improved outlook with a multidisciplinary approach. Am J Surg 125:482, 1973.

Kilman JW & others: Reasonable surgery for rhabdomyosarcoma: A study of 67 cases. Ann Surg 178:346, 1973.

Morton DL: Soft tissue sarcomas. In: *Cancer Medicine.* Holland JF, Frei E III (editors). Lea & Febiger, 1973.

Morton DL & others: Limb salvage from a multidisciplinary treatment approach for skeletal and soft tissue sarcomas of the extremity. Ann Surg 184:268, 1976.

Pratt CB & others: Coordinated treatment of childhood rhabdomyosarcoma with surgery, radiotherapy, and combination chemotherapy. Cancer Res 32:606, 1972.

IRRADIATION

Radiation therapy may also serve as definitive treatment of certain malignant diseases, alone or in conjunction with surgery or chemotherapy. Local obstructions and inoperable masses are frequently and effectively controlled by radiation therapy as discussed in Chapter 7.

CHEMOTHERAPY

Scientific Basis of Chemotherapy

A. Selective Toxicity; the Qualitative Approach: A basic goal of cancer chemotherapy is the development of agents with "selective toxicity" against repli-

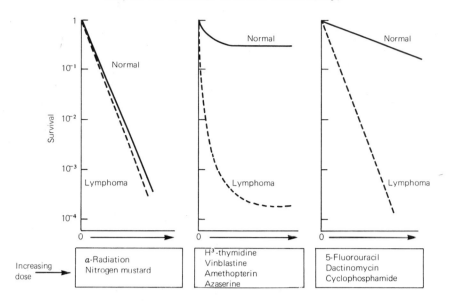

Figure 49–1. The form of the dose-survival curves for normal hematopoietic and lymphoma colony-forming cells exposed to 9 different anticancer agents for 24 hours in vivo. Three classes of dose-survival curves are evident. (Reproduced, with permission, from Bruce WR & others: Comparison of the sensitivity of normal hematopoietic and transplanted lymphoma colony-forming cells to chemotherapeutic agents administered in vivo. J Natl Cancer Inst 37:233, 1966.)

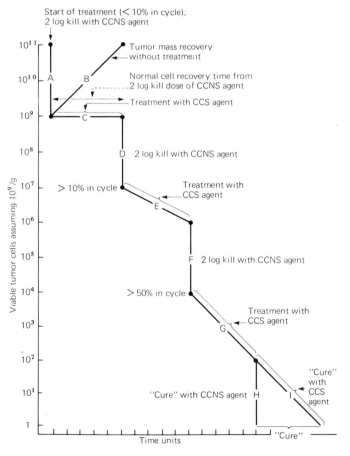

Figure 49–2. Idealized approach to curative therapy of advanced tumors using a cell cycle nonspecific (CCNS) agent (eg, alkylating agent) followed by a cell cycle specific (CCS) agent (eg, antimetabolite) in repeated courses. (Redrawn and reproduced, with permission, from Schabel FM: Cancer Res 29:2384, 1969.)

cating tumor cells which at the same time spare replicating host tissues. Such an ideal drug has not yet been found, and only the hormones and asparaginase (and, to a lesser extent, mitotane [o,p'DDD; Lysodren] and streptozocin*) approach this goal. Although these drugs have important side-effects, their toxicity is not primarily directed against normal replicating cells.

B. The Quantitative Kinetic Approach: Since in most instances qualitative metabolic differences between normal and neoplastic cells have not been discovered, the chemotherapist must base his attack upon quantitative differences in the proliferative kinetics of normal and neoplastic cell growth if he is to achieve tumor regression without major host toxicity. Early bacteriologists, in their study of germicidal agents, formulated the concept of "the logarithmic order of cell kill." According to this theory, any particular treatment will kill a certain fraction of cells *independently* of the total number of cells present (provided the growth rate is constant). Thus, "cure," in the sense of killing the last remaining tumor cells, is more readily achieved by drugs when the total tumor cell burden is small. For example, a drug that is 99% efficient kills 2 logs of cells regardless of the total number of cells present and will reduce a tumor cell population of 100 to a single remaining cell, whereas it will leave 10,000 remaining cells of an initial tumor cell number of 1 million.

The quantitative evaluation of drug effects on normal and neoplastic tissues was furthered by the development of an in vivo assay system to allow measurement of the dose-response relationship of a variety of agents against both neoplastic and normal hematopoietic stem cells. As a result of these experiments, at least 3 cell survival curves are generated (Fig 49–1). The first (left) curve shows decimation of both normal and neoplastic cells to almost the same degree, whereas the other 2 curves (middle and right) show a much greater decimation of tumor cells than of normal stem cells. The selectivity of the agents in the last 2 classes was attributed to a differential effect of the agents on proliferating cells in the mitotic cycle while sparing resting cells not in mitotic division. Thus arose the classification of forms of therapy into (1) cell cycle specific (CCS) agents, which attack only actively proliferating cells engaged in DNA synthesis, and the mitotic cycle; and (2) cell cycle nonspecific (CCNS) agents, which kill both normal and tumor cells regardless of their proliferative state.

The important implications of these data are borne out by evidence in experimental tumor systems and to some extent in man: (1) Differences in sensitivity of normal hematopoietic precursors and neoplastic cells are a function of the difference in their proliferative states and not a result of any inherent qualitative biochemical differences between the 2 cell types. (2) An injured or "stimulated" marrow or normal tissue which is proliferating as rapidly as neoplastic

tissue will be affected to the same extent as neoplastic tissue.

As a general rule, any tissue, normal or neoplastic, manifests an early logarithmic phase of exponential growth during which most cells are in active mitosis. When a certain bulk is achieved there is a transition to a later "steady state" plateau phase of growth during which a lesser fraction of cells is in the proliferative cycle. To maximize the therapeutic effects of CCS antineoplastic agents, resting cells must be induced to enter the proliferative cycle without at the same time increasing normal tissue vulnerability. This implies a reduction of tumor bulk with a reentry from the plateau phase into the log phase of exponential growth. Methods for reducing tumor bulk presently include treatment by CCNS agents such as x-ray or mechlorethamine and removal of gross tumor masses at surgery, but these stratagems all too often have attendant toxicities.

Utilizing these concepts, Schabel has proposed an approach to "curative" sequential chemotherapy of advanced tumors using a CCNS agent followed by a CCS agent in repeated courses (Fig 49–2).

While this is an idealized approach to curative therapy, similar principles have resulted in cure of laboratory-induced neoplasms, and such concepts form the basis for several successful new antileukemic regimens—particularly for childhood leukemia. Clearly, this approach will be furthered by a better understanding of human tumor cell kinetics in individual patients, by new knowledge about the dose, duration, and site of action of antitumor agents, by the development of new "marrow-sparing" agents, and by appropriately synergistic combinations of drugs as well as better means of measuring their effects on grossly unmeasurable tumors.

Bergevin PR, Tormey DC, Blom J: Guide to the use of cancer chemotherapeutic agents. Mod Treat 9:185, 1972.

Bruce WR & others: Comparison of the sensitivity of normal hematopoietic and transplanted lymphoma colony-forming cells to chemotherapeutic agents administered in vivo. J Natl Cancer Inst 37:233, 1966.

DeVita VT: Cell kinetics and the chemotherapy of cancer. Cancer Chemother Rep 2:23, 1971.

DeVita VT, Schein PS: The use of drugs in combination for the treatment of cancer. N Engl J Med 288:998, 1973.

Greenwald ES: *Cancer Chemotherapy: Medical Outline Series,* 2nd ed. Med Exam Pub, 1973.

Schabel FM: The use of tumor growth kinetics in planning "curative" chemotherapy of advanced solid tumors. Cancer Res 29:2384, 1969.

Skipper HE & others: Implications of biochemical, cytokinetic, pharmacologic, and toxicologic relationships in the design of optimal therapeutic schedules. Cancer Chemother Rep 54:431, 1970.

The choice of therapy in the treatment of malignancy. Med Lett Drugs Ther 15:9, 1973.

*See Note to Reader on p 1072.

GUIDELINES FOR THE INSTITUTION OF CANCER CHEMOTHERAPY

Establish the Diagnosis

A firm diagnosis of neoplastic disease must be made before treatment is started. This will usually (and preferably) include a histologic diagnosis, but in some instances the diagnosis may be based solely on analysis of exfoliative cytology. In rare instances, a biochemical parameter (eg, chorionic gonadotropin) in a consistent clinical setting may constitute a rationale for institution of therapy, although tissue diagnosis is always preferable. In emergency situations (eg, superior vena cava syndrome), it may be necessary to institute appropriate therapy without histologic or biochemical documentation; in such cases, appropriate diagnostic procedures are required after clinical stabilization has been achieved.

Delineate the Stage & Extent of Disease

This can frequently be achieved by correlating symptoms and the known natural history of the neoplasm with appropriate radiologic, chemical, and surgical staging data. The lymphomas are staged according to the modified Rye classification; many solid tumors are best staged by the TNM system.

Establish Goal of Therapy

The histologic diagnosis and extent of the disease frequently define the goal of therapy as either curative or palliative with or without hope for prolongation of survival, and frequently determine the most appropriate treatment—surgery, radiotherapy, chemotherapy, or a combination of these.

Measure Antitumor Response

After treatment is started, serial observations of objectively measured parameters are essential to judge antitumor response (measurable mass, tumor product, or remote effect) and to monitor the toxicity of the treatment. For example, in the treatment of gestational trophoblastic disease, assay of chorionic gonadotropin measures a tumor product which correlates directly with the numbers of neoplastic cells and will reveal subclinical amounts (10^6 cells or less) of tumor which must continue to receive chemotherapy. The sensitivity of this assay is largely responsible for the 90% cure rate of trophoblastic disease. In contrast, a "complete clinical remission" of acute leukemia (a normal bone marrow) occurs with a tumor cell mass of 10^9; most solid tumors contain $10^{10}-10^{11}$ (10–100 g) of tumor cells before the mass can be detected clinically.

Acceptable Drug Toxicity

The degree of toxicity that is acceptable depends on the probability and risks of achieving the therapeutic goal, other clinical characteristics of the individual patient, and the availability of supportive facilities to manage the anticipated toxicity.

Synonyms of Anticancer Drugs

Allopurinol (Zyloprim)
Asparaginase* (L-asparaginase, Elspar)
BCNU* (see Carmustine)
Bleomycin (Blenoxane)
Busulfan (Myleran)
CCNU (see Lomustine)
Carmustine* (bischloroethylnitrosourea, BCNU)
Chlorambucil (Leukeran)
Cisplatinum diamminedichloride*
Cyclophosphamide (Cytoxan)
Cytarabine (Ara-C, Cytosar)
Dacarbazide (dimethyltriazeno imidazole carboxamide, imidazole carboxamide)
Dactinomycin (actinomycin D, Cosmegen)
Daunorubicin (daunomycin)*
Doxorubicin (Adriamycin)
Fluorouracil (5-FU, Efudex)
Hydroxyurea (Hydrea)
Lomustine (cyclohexylchloroethylnitrosourea, CCNU)
Mechlorethamine (nitrogen mustard, HN2, Mustargen)
Mercaptopurine (6-MP, Purinethol)
Methotrexate (amethopterin)
Methyl-CCNU (methylcyclohexylchloroethylnitrosourea)
Mithramycin (Mithracin)
Mitomycin (Mutamycin)
Mitotane (o,p'DDD, Lysodren)
Phenylalanine mustard (melphalan, Alkeran, L-sarcolysin)
Procarbazine (Matulane)
Streptozocin*
Thioguanine (6-TG)
Thiotepa (triethylenethiophosphoramide)
Vinblastine sulfate (Velban)
Vincristine sulfate (Oncovin)

*See Note to Reader, below.

Status of Patient

The patient's subjective and functional status must always be considered in formulating and instituting a therapeutic program. Subjective symptoms of disease usually parallel objective parameters of progression or regression of the neoplasm. When this is not so, other factors such as unrecognized drug toxicity, unreliable parameters of tumor response, and the masking of disease progression by certain forms of therapy (eg, corticosteroids) must be considered. The Karnofsky performance index (Table 49–5) is useful for following the functional status of the patient and must be accorded at least equal importance as objectively measurable parameters, especially when the goal of treatment is palliation.

The above considerations apply generally to cancer chemotherapy. Experimental drugs or treatment protocols may be considered if all of the follow-

Note to reader: Agents designated with an asterisk in the following discussion and in Tables 49–6 and 49–7 are investigational and not generally available to the practicing physician. Further information concerning these agents may be obtained from the various regional or national cooperative cancer chemotherapy study groups or the National Cancer Institute.

Table 49–5. Karnofsky performance index.

	%	
Able to carry on normal activity. No special care is needed.	100	Normal. No complaints. No evidence of disease.
	90	Able to carry on normal activity. Minor signs or symptoms of disease.
	80	Normal activity with effort. Some signs or symptoms of disease.
Unable to work. Able to live at home and care for most personal needs. A varying amount of assistance is needed.	70	Cares for self. Unable to carry on normal activity or to do active work.
	60	Requires occasional assistance but is able to care for most of his needs.
	50	Requires considerable assistance and frequent medical care.
Unable to care for self. Requires equivalent of institutional or hospital care. Disease may be progressing rapidly.	40	Disabled. Requires special care and assistance.
	30	Severely disabled. Hospitalization is indicated, although death is not imminent.
	20	Very sick. Hospitalization necessary.
	10	Moribund. Fatal processes progressing rapidly.
	0	Dead.

ing criteria are met: (1) Proved methods of effective therapy have been exhausted. (2) Data collection and dissemination of the information obtained will contribute toward answering the question asked in the protocol. (3) The patient's human rights are fully protected, and informed consent has been obtained. (4) There is a reasonable expectation that the treatment will do more good than harm.

CHEMOTHERAPEUTIC AGENTS
(See Tables 49–6 and 49–7.)

Chemotherapeutic Agents With Selective Toxicity

Only the adrenocortical hormones, sex hormones, and asparaginase* have demonstrated a predictable **selective killing power of tumor cells based on** metabolically exploitable differences between neoplastic and normal tissue.

A. Glucocorticoids: The glucocorticoids exert a "lympholytic" effect which can repeatedly induce remission of acute lymphoblastic leukemia, especially in combination with vincristine. This lympholytic effect, which does not depend on the mitotic activity of the tumor, is also useful in chronic lymphocytic

*See Note to Reader on p 1072.

leukemia, lymphomas, and myeloma.

The adrenal corticosteroids are also beneficial for certain hormonally sensitive tumors such as breast and prostatic cancer. They improve cerebral edema accompanying brain tumors; palliate hemolytic anemias associated with chronic lymphocytic leukemia and the lymphomas; and correct hypercalcemia due to various neoplasms. Their antineoplastic effects are less if given on an intermittent schedule; large daily doses for the shortest time necessary to produce the desired effect are preferred. Toxicity may be metabolic (hyperglycemia, sodium retention, potassium wasting), gastrointestinal (peptic ulceration), or immunosuppressive (increased susceptibility to infection). Myopathies, psychosis, hypertension, and osteoporosis are important side-effects of long-term administration.

B. Estrogens: The estrogenic steroids were used in the early 1940s for prostatic carcinoma and represented one of the first successful attempts at rational cancer chemotherapy. Shortly thereafter, estrogens were found useful in postmenopausal patients with breast cancer. Diethylstilbestrol, the most widely used estrogen, is potent, inexpensive, and effective when given orally but may cause gastrointestinal disturbance, fluid retention, feminization in males, and uterine bleeding. Its administration may cause hypercalcemia and "tumor flare" of disseminated breast carcinoma.

C. Synthetic Progestational Agents: These drugs are useful in pharmacologic doses for disseminated or uncontrolled carcinoma of the endometrium and occasionally for hypernephroma and breast cancer.

D. Androgens: The androgens are used principally in the treatment of disseminated breast cancer, especially in pre- and perimenopausal (1–4 years) women. They also have a role in the stimulation of erythropoiesis in anemic patients with several neoplastic and myelophthisic diseases. The toxic effects of androgens include excessive virilization of females, prostatism in males, and fluid retention; tumor flare and hypercalcemia occur occasionally. The halogenated androgens, which are effective when given orally, can produce cholestatic jaundice, although the parenteral nonhalogenated compounds do not do so.

E. Antihormones: The nonsteroid antihormones nafoxidine* and tamoxifen* are representatives of this new class of agents useful against breast cancer.

The Alkylators

The alkylators, whose prototype is mechlorethamine, react with nucleophilic substances within the cell to form cross-links at the guanine residues of parallel double DNA strands. With the possible exception of cyclophosphamide, the alkylators are cell cycle nonspecific and affect both resting and dividing cells; both normal and malignant cells are injured.

Mechlorethamine (nitrogen mustard, HN2, Mustargen) is the alkylator of choice in the treatment of Hodgkin's disease, either singly or in combination with other drugs. For Burkitt's lymphoma, cyclophosphamide may be curative, and it is also the agent of choice for undifferentiated small cell carcinoma of the

Table 49—6. Solid tumors responsive to chemotherapy.

Neoplasm	Current Drugs of Choice	Other Useful Agents
Hodgkin's disease	MOPP (mechlorethamine, Oncovin [vincristine], prednisone, procarbazine)	Vinblastine (Velban), doxorubicin, bleomycin, BCNU*
Non-Hodgkin's lymphoma	CVP (cyclophosphamide, vincristine [Oncovin], prednisone)	Bleomycin, doxorubicin, BCNU*
Multiple myeloma	Melphalan and prednisone	Cyclophosphamide, procarbazine, vincristine, BCNU*
Squamous carcinoma of head and neck	Methotrexate	Bleomycin, (?) alkylators, cisplatinum*
Squamous carcinoma of lung	Cyclophosphamide and other alkylators	Methotrexate, dacarbazide, doxorubicin
Squamous carcinoma of cervix	Alkylators	Methotrexate, bleomycin
Transitional carcinoma of bladder	Doxorubicin	
Malignant melanoma	Dacarbazide	BCNU,* hydroxyurea (Hydrea), doxorubicin, vincristine (Oncovin)
Adenocarcinoma of gastrointestinal origin	Fluorouracil	(?) Methyl-CCNU, mitomycin
Adenocarcinoma of breast	Hormone manipulation (estrogens for postmenopausal, androgens for premenopausal), various cytotoxic chemotherapy combinations	Alkylators, doxorubicin, various combinations of prednisone, fluorouracil, alkylator, methotrexate, vincristine
Adenocarcinoma of ovary	Alkylators	Fluorouracil, methotrexate, vincristine, (?) mercaptopurine, doxorubicin, cisplatinum*
Renal cell carcinoma	Progestagens	Androgens, glucocorticoids
Testicular carcinoma	Combination: Cyclophosphamide, vincristine, dactinomycin (and mithramycin for embryonal cell type)	Bleomycin, methotrexate, vinblastine (Velban), doxorubicin, cisplatinum*
Endometrial carcinoma	Progestagens	(?) Doxorubicin
Prostatic carcinoma	Estrogen	Prednisone, fluorouracil, (?) doxorubicin
Various soft tissue sarcomas	Combination: Cyclophosphamide, vincristine, dactinomycin	Combination: Doxorubicin plus dacarbazide; methotrexate
Insulinoma	Streptozocin*	
Adrenocortical	Mitotane (o,p'DDD)	
Carcinoid	Cyclophosphamide	Fluorouracil, (?) dactinomycin
Wilms's tumor	Dactinomycin, with surgery and radiotherapy	Vincristine
Neuroblastoma	Cyclophosphamide, vincristine	Dactinomycin, doxorubicin
Choriocarcinoma	Methotrexate, or vincristine plus dactinomycin	Vinblastine, mercaptopurine, alkylators

*See Note to Reader on p 1072.

lung. Cyclophosphamide has a unique role in childhood acute leukemia, in which other alkylators are ineffective. For most purposes, however, equivalent doses of the various alkylators produce equivalent responses, and there is cross-resistance among the various alkylators except for the nitrosoureas (see below). The choice of alkylators thus rests upon the desired route and mode of administration and variations in toxicity.

Chlorambucil (Leukeran) has had its major use in chronic lymphocytic leukemia, Hodgkin's disease, and Waldenström's macroglobulinemia. Its major advantage is its narrow spectrum of toxicity (hematopoietic only) and ease of administration (oral). **Phenylalanine mustard (melphalan)** is usually given for multiple myeloma, but this may be merely traditional; **busulfan (Myleran)** is customarily used in chronic myelocytic leukemia and in polycythemia vera; all alkylators are equally effective against ovarian carcinoma.

Mechlorethamine is a vesicant if extravasated. **Cyclophosphamide (Cytoxan)** and **thiotepa** are much less irritating if applied directly to tissues because they must first be metabolized to the active form. The immediate effects of intravenous alkylator administration are nausea and vomiting beginning within 30 minutes and persisting for 8—10 hours; premedication with phenothiazine is preventative. The important delayed effects of alkylators are principally on rapidly proliferating tissues (hematopoietic, gonadal, skin, and gastrointestinal), with bone marrow suppression being the most prominent. In the marrow, cell necrosis begins at 12 hours; the nadir of blood count depression is at 7—10 days, and marrow regeneration time limits the administration of mechlorethamine to intervals of 4—6 weeks.

Several of the alkylators cause relatively characteristic adverse reactions. Examples are alopecia and hemorrhagic cystitis (cyclophosphamide), and melanosis and pulmonary fibrosis (busulfan). All alkylators have the potential to cause hypospermia, menstrual irregularities, and fetal anomalies.

Thiotepa is discussed in Table 49—7.

The Nitrosoureas

BCNU,* CCNU, and methyl-CCNU are cell cycle nonspecific synthetic chemicals which act much like the classic alkylators but have several unique and exploitable properties, including lipid solubility, and delayed onset of marrow suppression compared to the alkylators (see above). Moreover, there appears to be no cross-resistance with other alkylators. These drugs are effective in Hodgkin's disease, but less effective in non-Hodgkin's lymphomas; they appear promising for metastatic and primary CNS neoplasms because of their lipid solubility. BCNU* is administered intravenously; CCNU and methyl-CCNU are given orally.

Structural Analogues (Antimetabolites)

The antimetabolites are specific cytotoxic agents closely related to substrates normally utilized by cells for metabolism and growth. The structural analogues interfere with nucleic acid synthesis to impair proliferation of normal and neoplastic cells. They are generally cell cycle specific, with proliferating cells being more vulnerable to their effects than are resting cells.

A. Methotrexate: Methotrexate competitively inhibits dihydrofolate reductase; acquired resistance to methotrexate results from increased dihydrofolate reductase activity since the rate of enzyme synthesis exceeds the rate of methotrexate uptake by resistant cells.

Methotrexate toxicity may be hematologic, gastrointestinal, hepatic, and dermatologic. These effects may be alleviated or prevented by the prompt (preferably within 1 hour, but no longer than several hours) administration of folinic acid (citrovorum factor). One treatment regimen has used folinic acid to "rescue" the marrow after administration of toxic doses, although it is not yet certain that the antitumor effect is more pronounced. Methotrexate may be administered orally, intramuscularly, intravenously, or intrathecally, and is bound to plasma protein and excreted in the urine. Hepatic or renal failure is a contraindication; leukopenia, thrombocytopenia, stomatitis, and gastroenteritis with diarrhea are the toxic side-effects which may require a reduction in dosage.

Although methotrexate has been used for over 20 years, critical questions regarding dosage and scheduling have not been fully answered. Intermittent (twice-weekly) administration is superior to daily administration for maintenance of remission in childhood acute leukemia. In acute leukemia, "resistance" to methotrexate is relative and may be overcome by revising the schedule of administration and dosage. Intrathecal methotrexate is effective for CNS leukemia deposits even when marrow disease has become "resistant." Methotrexate can cure most cases of gestational choriocarcinoma. It has been used extensively in the treatment of epithelial neoplasia of the head and neck and is useful in breast cancer, testicular

*See Note to Reader on p 1072.

tumors, lung cancer, medulloblastomas, and other brain tumors.

B. Mercaptopurine and Thioguanine: Mercaptopurine (6-MP) and thioguanine (6-TG) are purine antagonists; mercaptopurine is the analogue of hypoxanthine and thioguanine the analogue of guanine. Although the actions of these 2 drugs are quite similar and they share cross-resistance, they are probably not identical. Thioguanine (but not mercaptopurine) is synergistic in combination with cytarabine for induction of remission in acute myelocytic leukemia. Mercaptopurine is metabolized via the xanthine oxidase pathway, which is blocked by allopurinol. Therefore, the dose of mercaptopurine must be reduced to 25% of the usual dose if allopurinol is administered concomitantly. Full doses of thioguanine may be given in conjunction with allopurinol.

The purine analogues suppress purine synthesis through "pseudofeedback" inhibitory mechanisms which inhibit formation and interconversion of the intermediary compounds. The major toxicity is marrow suppression, which may be delayed in onset for several weeks. The major clinical role is in induction and maintenance of remission in the acute leukemias and in blastic transformation of chronic myelocytic leukemia. These may be of some benefit in lymphomas and ovarian carcinoma.

C. Fluorouracil: Fluorouracil (5-FU) is a thymine analogue which in vivo interferes with thymidylate synthetase, an enzyme involved in the formation of thymidylic acid, a DNA precursor. The agent is first metabolized to FUDR. FUDR itself is now available for use by perfusion but has not been shown to have a clear advantage over the parent compound. Fluorouracil is principally metabolized in the liver. Its major toxicities include stomatitis, enteritis, and marrow suppression; significant atrophic dermatitis is occasionally reported; neurotoxicity is rare.

Fluorouracil has been most useful in breast and colonic adenocarcinoma, but it is also beneficial against pancreatic, gastric, ovarian, and prostatic cancer. The preferred schedule of administration is once weekly rather than the 4-day loading dose schedule initially advocated, since the latter is more toxic without being more effective. The dosage should be in the range of 15–20 mg/kg IV, weekly as tolerated.

D. Dacarbazide: This drug probably functions as an antimetabolite and has significant activity against malignant melanoma.

Cytotoxic Antibiotics

These agents, the first of which was dactinomycin, were isolated in the 1940s by Waksman from soil strains of bacteria of the Streptomyces class.

A. Dactinomycin: Dactinomycin (actinomycin D, Cosmegen) is an inhibitor of DNA-dependent synthesis of RNA by ribosomes. Its toxicities include hematopoietic suppression, ulcerative stomatitis, and gastroenteritis. It causes intense local tissue necrosis if extravasated. The drug is retained for a considerable

Table 49–7. Cancer chemotherapeutic drugs useful against solid tumors.*

Agent	Response > 50%	Response in 30–50%	Response in 20–30%	Route	Toxicity	Usual Adult Dose†	Specificity‡
Hormones							
Glucocorticoids	Hypercalcemia, Hodgkin's disease and other lymphomas (in combination), tumor edema of brain.	Breast carcinoma, multiple myeloma.	Hypernephroma.	Orally. (IV and IM preparations also available.)	Sodium retention, potassium wasting hyperglycemia, peptic ulcer, immunosuppression, hypertension, osteoporosis.	Prednisone: 1–2 mg/kg/day for brief intervals (< 6 weeks if possible); then maintain at minimal required daily dosage.	Not known
Estrogens	Prostatic carcinoma.	Breast carcinoma.		Orally	Sodium retention, feminization, uterine bleeding, nausea and vomiting.	Diethylstilbestrol: 5–25 mg/day for breast; 2.5–5 mg/day for prostate. Ethinyl estradiol: 3 mg/day for breast.	Not known
Progestagens		Endometrial carcinoma.	Hypernephroma.	Orally, IM	Sodium retention.	Hydroxyprogesterone: 1 g 2–3 times weekly IM. Medroxyprogesterone: 200–600 mg orally twice weekly.	Not known
Androgens		Myelophthisic and refractory anemias; breast carcinoma.	Hypernephroma.	Orally, IM	Sodium retention, masculinization; cholestatic jaundice with oral preparations.	Testosterone propionate: 100 mg 2–3 times weekly. Fluoxymesterone: 10–40 mg/day orally. Calusterone: 200 mg/day orally.	Not known
Alkylators							
Mechlorethamine (nitrogen mustard, HN2, Mustargen)	Hodgkin's disease, neoplastic effusions.	Non-Hodgkin's lymphomas.	Melanoma; cervix, head and neck, bronchogenic carcinoma.	IV, intracavitary	Nausea and vomiting, marrow depression, ulcer if extravasated, hypogonadism, fetal anomalies, alopecia.	0.4 mg/kg IV as single dose every 4–6 weeks; 0.4 mg/kg by intracavitary injection.	CCNS
Cyclophosphamide (Cytoxan)	Burkitt's lymphoma, Hodgkin's disease, other lymphomas.	Multiple myeloma, neuroblastoma, breast carcinoma, ovarian carcinoma.	Oat cell carcinoma of lung, cervical carcinoma, Ewing's sarcoma.	IV, orally	Nausea and vomiting, marrow depression, alopecia, hemorrhagic cystitis.	40–60 mg/kg IV every 3–5 weeks; 5 mg/kg/day orally for 10 days, then 1–3 mg/kg/day as maintenance.	(?) CCNS
Chlorambucil (Leukeran)	Hodgkin's disease.	Non-Hodgkin's lymphomas, breast carcinoma, ovarian carcinoma.	(?) Cervical carcinoma.	Orally	Marrow depression, gastroenteritis.	0.1–0.2 mg/kg/day.	CCNS
Phenylalanine mustard (melphalan, Alkeran)		Myeloma, ovarian carcinoma.		Orally	Marrow depression (occasionally prolonged), gastroenteritis.	0.25 mg/kg/day orally for 4 days every 6 weeks; 2–4 mg/day as maintenance.	CCNS
Thiotepa		Ovarian carcinoma, neoplastic effusions.		IV, intracavitary	Marrow depression.	0.8 mg/kg IV as single dose every 4–6 weeks; 0.8 mg/kg by intracavitary injection.	
Nitrosoureas							
Carmustine (BCNU),* lomustine (CCNU), methyl-CCNU		Primary and metastatic brain tumors, meningeal carcinomatosis, Hodgkin's, other lymphomas.	Melanoma.	BCNU, IV; CCNU and methyl-CCNU, orally	Nausea and vomiting, prolonged marrow depression, local phlebitis.	BCNU: 75–100 mg/sq m IV daily for 2 days every 4–6 weeks. CCNU: 130 mg/sq m orally every 6 weeks.	CCNS
Inorganic metallic salt							
Cisplatinum diamminedichloride		Ovarian and testicular carcinomas.	Squamous carcinoma.	IV	Nausea and vomiting, bone marrow depression, nephrotoxicity, ototoxicity.	1 mg/kg every 3 weeks IV.	CCNS

					Route	Acute Toxicity	Dosage†	
Structural analogues								
Methotrexate (amethopterin)	Choriocarcinoma, Burkitt's lymphoma.	Squamous carcinoma of head and neck, testicular, breast carcinoma.	Various brain tumors, squamous cell carcinoma of lung.	Orally, IV, intrathecally	Ulcerative mucositis, gastroenteritis, dermatitis, marrow depression, hepatitis, abortion.	20–40 mg IV twice weekly; 5–15 mg intrathecally weekly; 2.5–5 mg/day orally.	CCS
Fluorouracil (5-FU, Efudex)		Breast carcinoma, colon and rectal carcinoma.	Other carcinomas of gastrointestinal origin, ovarian, prostatic carcinoma.	Orally, IV, intra-arterial infusion	Atrophic dermatitis, gastroenteritis, mucositis, marrow depression, neuritis.	15–20 mg/kg IV weekly for at least 6 weeks; 15 mg/kg orally weekly.	CCS
Dacarbazide			Melanoma, (?) lung carcinoma, soft tissue sarcomas.	IV	Gastroenteritis, marrow depression, hepatitis, phlebitis.	150 mg/sq m/day IV for 5 days every 4–6 weeks.	Not known
Cytotoxic antibiotics								
Dactinomycin (actinomycin D, Cosmegen)	Wilms's tumor, choriocarcinoma.	Testicular carcinoma.	Soft tissue sarcomas.	IV	Nausea and vomiting, stomatitis, gastroenteritis, proctitis, marrow depression, ulcer if extravasated, alopecia; radiation potentiator.	0.01 mg/kg/day for 5 days every 4–6 weeks.	CCS
Doxorubicin		Lymphomas, transitional cell carcinoma of bladder, breast carcinoma.	Various sarcomas.	IV	Alopecia, marrow depression, myocardiopathies, ulcer if extravasated; stomatitis.	1 mg/kg/week; total cumulative dose should not exceed 550 mg/sq m.	CCNS
Mithramycin (Mithracin)	Hypercalcemia of malignancies.	Testicular embryonal carcinoma.		IV	Marrow depression, nausea and vomiting, complex coagulopathies, hepatotoxicity.	0.05 mg/kg IV every other day to toxicity or 8 doses per course.	Not known
Mitomycin (Mutamycin)			Gastric and pancreatic carcinomas.	IV	Nausea and vomiting, bone marrow depression, ulcer if extravasated.	0.06 mg/kg IV twice weekly.	CCNS
Bleomycin (Blenoxane)		Lymphomas, testicular carcinoma.	Squamous cell carcinoma of head, neck.	IV, IM, subcut	Allergic dermatitis, pulmonary fibrosis, fever, mucositis.	15 mg twice weekly; total cumulative dosage should not exceed 300 mg.	Not known
Vinca alkaloids								
Vinblastine (Velban)	Hodgkin's disease.	Choriocarcinoma.	Breast, testis carcinoma, non-Hodgkin's lymphomas.	IV	Marrow depression, alopecia, ulcer if extravasated, nausea and vomiting, neuropathy.	0.1–0.2 mg/kg IV weekly.	CCS
Vincristine (Oncovin)	Hodgkin's disease, other lymphomas, Wilms's tumor, neuroblastoma, medulloblastoma, choriocarcinoma.		Ewing's sarcoma, testicular, breast carcinoma, brain tumors, (?) multiple myeloma.	IV	Alopecia, neuropathy (peripheral and autonomic), ulcer if extravasated; rarely, marrow depression.	1.5 mg/sq m weekly or less. No individual dosage should exceed 2 mg.	CCS
Miscellaneous agents								
Mitotane (Lysodren, o,p'DDD)	Reduction of tumor mass in adrenocortical carcinoma.	Hypersecretion in adrenocortical carcinoma.		Orally	Gastroenteritis, dermatitis, CNS abnormalities.	5–12 g daily orally.	Not known
Streptozocin*	Insulinoma.			IV	Nephrotoxicity, gastroenteritis.	1 g/sq m.	Not known
Procarbazine (Matulane)	Hodgkin's disease.		Lymphomas, oat cell, large cell lung carcinoma.	Orally	Marrow depression, gastroenteritis, dermatitis, CNS abnormalities.	50–150 mg/sq m/day to toxicity or response; maintain with 50–100 mg/day orally.	Not known

*See Note to Reader on p 1072.

†Modifications of drug dosages: If white count is > 4500 and platelet count is > 150,000, give full dose; if white count is 3500–4500 and platelet count is 100–150 thousand, give 75% of full dose; if white count is 3000–3500 and platelet count is 75–100 thousand, give 50–75% of full dose; if white count is < 3000 and platelet count is < 75,000, give 0–25% of full dose.

‡CCS = cell cycle specific. CCNS = cell cycle nonspecific.

time intracellularly, and acquired resistance is thought to correlate with poor cellular uptake or poor retention of the drug. The major use for dactinomycin is in sequential combination with radiation therapy for Wilms's tumor; "maintenance" long-term administration of the drug adds significantly to the salvage obtained with combinations of surgery, radiation therapy, and "adjuvant" short-term courses of the drug. Dactinomycin is of proved value in trophoblastic malignancy, soft tissue sarcomas, and testicular carcinoma, especially in combination with alkylators and antimetabolites. The optimal scheduling and combination of drugs with dactinomycin is not known, but the most customary has been in courses of several days at dosages of 15 μg/kg/day IV repeated after 2–4 weeks as toxicity allows.

B. Daunorubicin* and Doxorubicin: Daunorubicin* and its related compound, doxorubicin, are tumoricidal antibiotics whose major toxicity is severe marrow suppression, although myocardial necrosis is also an important side-effect of both drugs. Both agents have established activity against acute leukemia, and doxorubicin appears to be effective against a variety of solid tumors, including bladder carcinoma and Ewing's sarcoma.

C. Mithramycin: Mithramycin (Mithracin) is useful in the treatment of hypercalcemia resistant to hydration and steroids, and the dosage may be less than that required for tumoricidal activity although still within the toxic range. Its major usefulness is in embryonal cell carcinoma and other testicular tumors, and its toxicity includes marrow suppression, hepatic and gastrointestinal injury, and complex coagulopathies.

D. Bleomycin: Bleomycin (Blenoxane) is a new agent which is important because it is effective against squamous cell carcinomas and lymphomas without causing myelosuppression. Toxicity appears to be related to its squamous tropism and includes skin rash and pulmonary fibrosis.

E. Mitomycin: Mitomycin is a useful agent against gastric and pancreatic adenocarcinoma.

The Plant Alkaloids

The plant alkaloids include the periwinkle (*Vinca rosea*) derivatives, vincristine and vinblastine, 2 closely related compounds with widely different toxicities and somewhat different spectra of activity. Both Vinca alkaloids are bound to cytoplasmic precursors of the mitotic spindle in S phase, with polymerization of the microtubular proteins which comprise the mitotic spindle.

A. Vinblastine: Vinblastine sulfate (Velban) is a major agent against Hodgkin's disease and has lesser efficacy in the non-Hodgkin's lymphomas. The toxicity of vinblastine is primarily marrow suppression, but gastroenteritis, neurotoxicity, and alopecia also occur—the latter much less commonly than with vincristine. The drug is usually given once a week. Severe

local ulceration may occur if the drug extravasates into the subcutaneous tissues.

B. Vincristine: Vincristine sulfate (Oncovin) is primarily neurotoxic and may induce peripheral, autonomic, and, less commonly, cranial neuropathies. Alopecia occurs in 20% of patients, but hematologic suppression is unusual. The drug is extremely effective in inducing remissions in acute lymphoblastic leukemia, especially in combination with prednisone, and is quite active in all forms of lymphoma. It is one of the most effective agents against childhood tumors, choriocarcinoma, and various sarcomas. Because of its lack of significant overlapping toxicity with most other chemotherapeutic agents, vincristine is receiving wide use in combination with other agents. The optimal dosage and scheduling for this agent remain to be elucidated; weekly administration is customary but may not be the best regimen.

Miscellaneous Compounds

Mitotane (o,p'DDD; Lysodren) is a DDT congener which may cause adrenocortical necrosis and plays a useful role in reducing excessive steroid output in 70% of patients with adrenocortical carcinoma; in a lesser number (about 35%), an objective decrease in tumor mass is also recorded. Toxicities include dermatitis, gastroenteritis, and CNS abnormalities.

Streptozocin,* an antibiotic derived from Streptomyces, has been useful in the treatment of metastatic insulinoma; 16 of 23 treated patients in a recent series experienced a reduction of hyperinsulinism, and several had objective decrease in tumor mass. Toxicities are primarily renal and gastrointestinal. Marrow function is not significantly impaired by the drug.

Procarbazine (Matulane) is a monoamine oxidase inhibitor whose exact mechanism of action is uncertain. It may cause both oxidation and alkylation of cellular constituents. Procarbazine is effective in Hodgkin's disease and may have some effect in various solid tumors, including oat cell carcinoma of the lung and melanoma. It finds wide use in combination chemotherapy as part of the MOPP regimen for Hodgkin's disease, and higher dose regimens are also being evaluated in the treatment of other solid tumors. The dose-limiting toxicity is hematologic, CNS, or gastrointestinal, although tolerance to the gastrointestinal side-effects may develop. Occasional drug dermatitis is also reported.

Asparaginase* is an enzyme which has been partially purified and derived from several sources, including guinea pig serum and cultures of *Escherichia coli.* It catalyzes the hydrolysis of L-asparagine to L-aspartic acid and ammonia. Certain tumor cells, especially lymphoblasts, require exogenous asparagine for protein synthesis and optimal growth, while most normal mammalian cells are able to synthesize sufficient endogenous asparagine. Asparaginase has proved efficacy only in acute lymphoblastic leukemia, but it has stimulated great interest because it exploits a rarely found biochemical difference between normal and neoplastic tissue. Toxicity has proved to be severe, and includes the expected allergic effects of intravenous administration of a foreign protein as well as pancreatitis and hepatic dysfunction.

Livingston RB, Carter SK: *Single Agents in Cancer Chemotherapy.* Plenum Press, 1970.

SURGICAL ADJUVANT CHEMOTHERAPY

It has been suggested that surgical or radiotherapeutic (cell cycle nonspecific) measures which reduce tumor bulk and increase the growth fraction of a tumor might increase tumor sensitivity to chemotherapy agents (cell cycle specific) without increasing marrow sensitivity. Thus, chemotherapeutic agents given after operation might improve results when there is no clinical evidence of residual disease but recurrence is statistically likely. In 1957, in order to test the validity of this reasoning, the National Surgical Adjuvant Breast Project began trials in which patients with clinically curable breast cancer were randomly given thiotepa for 2 days after radical mastectomy; controls received no chemotherapy. There was no significant difference in recurrence rates between treated and control patients in any category after 5 years, but premenopausal women with 4 or more positive axillary nodes who were treated demonstrated a recurrence rate 40% lower than that of the control group 18—36 months postoperatively. A recent controlled study of patients treated with melphalan intermittently for periods up to 2 years again showed significant benefit—in lengthening of the disease-free interval—for the treated group of premenopausal women with 4 or more histologically involved axillary nodes. A more recent study using a combination of cyclophosphamide, methotrexate, and fluorouracil as adjuvant treatment after mastectomy has confirmed a reduction in recurrence rate for the treated group at 3 years. Whether these benefits will be sustained and manifested by improvement in survival rate is not yet known, and adjuvant chemotherapy for breast cancer is still best undertaken as a controlled clinical trial.

Adjuvant chemotherapy with fluorouracil is also undergoing evaluation for colorectal neoplasms. In Dukes stage B and C carcinoma, the present data indicate that fluorouracil chemoprophylaxis offers a significant improvement in 5-year disease-free status over that of a nontreated population. Whether this benefit will be sustained and manifested by improvement in survival rates is not yet known, and adjuvant chemotherapy for colonic cancer is still reserved for controlled clinical trials.

Adjuvant chemotherapy has been of documented worth in Wilms's tumor and neuroblastoma and may be of benefit in stage II—IIIB Hodgkin's disease in conjunction with radiation therapy. Adjuvant chemotherapy with high-dose methotrexate therapy followed by citrovorum (folinic acid) "rescue" or with doxorubicin has been shown to prolong the disease-free interval in childhood osteosarcoma after appropriate control of the primary lesion. Among other promising tumors for controlled studies of adjuvant chemotherapy are ovarian carcinoma, testicular tumors, and certain other soft tissue sarcomas.

Rhabdomyosarcoma in children can now be treated effectively by wide local excision (avoiding amputation) followed by irradiation and repeated cyclic therapy with dactinomycin and vincristine.

Bonnadonna G & others: Combination chemotherapy as an adjuvant treatment in operable breast cancer. N Engl J Med 294:405, 1976.

Fisher B & others: 1-Phenylalanine mustard (L-PAM) in the management of primary breast cancer: A report of early findings. N Engl J Med 292:117, 1975.

Fisher F & others: Surgical adjuvant chemotherapy in cancer of the breast: Results of a decade of cooperative investigation. Ann Surg 168:337, 1968.

Mackman S, Curreri AR, Ansfield FS: Second look operation for colon carcinoma after fluorouracil therapy. Arch Surg 100:527, 1970.

Rousselot CM & others: A 5-year progress report on the effectiveness of intraluminal chemotherapy (5-fluorouracil) adjuvant to surgery for colon rectal cancer. Am J Surg 115:140, 1968.

SOLITARY METASTASIS

Even though more than 80% of apparently solitary metastases are eventually found to be multiple, an occasional cure results from their excision. In patients with a solitary lung metastasis, lobectomy gives 5-year survival rates of 15—60% depending upon the tissue of origin, the histologic characteristics of the tumor, and the time of appearance of the metastasis. The best results have been achieved when the metastasis was discovered more than 2 years after treatment of the primary. Surgery is much less successful for solitary brain metastases from lung tumors. The prognosis for solitary bony and liver metastases is poor, but occasional cures have followed removal of metastases from hypernephroma, testicular, and gynecologic neoplasms, various sarcomas, and occasional intestinal tumors.

Long-term palliation sometimes follows radiation therapy for metastases from certain radiosensitive tumors such as Wilms's tumor, seminoma, neuroblastoma, and some sarcomas.

Radiotherapy has also produced long-term survival in patients with metastases in neck nodes from an occult primary, presumably in the oro- or nasopharynx.

Adkins PC & others: Thoracotomy on the patient with previous malignancy: Metastasis or new primary? J Thorac Cardiovasc Surg 56:361, 1968.

Rubin P, Green J: *Solitary Metastases.* Thomas, 1968.

INFUSION & PERFUSION THERAPY

Selective arterial infusion has been used to deliver higher concentrations of drugs to the tumor than could be tolerated by systemic administration. One worker gave fluorouracil by hepatic arterial infusion to 200 patients with hepatic metastases, most of whom had failed to respond to intravenous fluorouracil. About 60% of the patients objectively improved and survived an average of 8.7 months; nonresponders lived an average of 2.5 months.

Regional perfusion is an experimental technic that has given promising results in the following situations: (1) melanoma of an extremity perfused with mechlorethamine, phenylalanine mustard, or dacarbazide; (2) head and neck tumors perfused through the carotid artery with alkylators, fluorouracil, or methotrexate; and (3) hepatomas and metastatic adenocarcinoma in liver infused via the hepatic artery with fluorouracil.

Ansfield FJ & others: Intrahepatic arterial infusion with 5-fluorouracil. Cancer 28:1147, 1971.

Freckman HA: Chemotherapy for metastatic colorectal liver carcinoma by intra-aortic infusion. Cancer 28:1152, 1971.

Krementz ET, Creech O Jr, Ryan RF: Evaluation of chemotherapy of cancer by regional perfusion. Cancer 20:834, 1967.

Li MC & others: Chemoprophylaxis for patients with colorectal cancer. JAMA 235:2825, 1976.

COMBINATION CHEMOTHERAPY

Combinations of drugs which block multiple biosynthetic pathways are given in an attempt to obtain a synergistic effect on the tumor. The drugs of a combination are selected to avoid overlapping toxicity. This approach has been of greatest value where no single agent is highly effective. Thus, vincristine plus prednisone or cytarabine plus thioguanine produce more complete remissions of acute leukemia than either agent alone, and toxicity is not enhanced. Survival is prolonged proportionate to the length of remission, which documents the importance of achieving a complete remission.

The cyclic administration of mechlorethamine, vincristine (Oncovin), prednisone, and procarbazine ("MOPP") produces 81% complete remissions of Hodgkin's disease in untreated stage III and stage IV; 76% complete remissions after radiotherapy alone; and 50% complete remissions after prior radiotherapy and chemotherapy. Seventy percent of complete responders were alive after 5 years, and 50% were continuously free of disease during that period. Single agent therapy with these drugs is much less successful. Improved—but less striking—results have also followed chemotherapy of non-Hodgkin's lymphoma. The combination of cyclophosphamide, vincristine, and pred-

nisone ("CVP"), produces about 60% complete remissions with a median duration of 5 months.

In breast cancer, the combination of an alkylator (usually thiotepa or, more recently, cyclophosphamide) with methotrexate and fluorouracil and with varying combinations of testosterone and prednisone has given a 50–60% response rate. Approximately 80% of patients with visceral and skin metastases have responded to a 5-drug program: daily oral cyclophosphamide and prednisone; weekly intravenous fluorouracil after a 4-day loading dose regimen; and methotrexate and vincristine for 8 weeks (if possible) with maintenance at more widely spaced intervals with varying dosages. Another highly effective combination is doxorubicin and cyclophosphamide. In general, for appropriate candidates, combinations of effective cytotoxic agents are preferable to single-agent chemotherapy for breast cancer.

Nearly 50% of patients with testicular carcinoma improved on a triple regimen consisting of an alkylator (chlorambucil), an antimetabolite (methotrexate), and dactinomycin.

The lack of adequate controls makes interpretation of these combination studies difficult, but a controlled investigation of the MOPP regimen in conjunction with radiation therapy is in progress. It will be necessary to study the dosage schedule of each proved combination to determine the best regimen.

DeVita VT, Serpick AA, Carbone PP: Combination chemotherapy in the treatment of advanced Hodgkin's disease. Ann Intern Med 73:881, 1970.

Devita VT Jr & others: Combination versus single agent chemotherapy: A review of the basis for selection of drug treatment of cancer. Cancer 35:98, 1975.

Greenspan EM: Combination cytotoxic chemotherapy in advanced disseminated breast carcinoma. J Mt Sinai Hosp 33:1, 1966.

Li MC & others: Effects of combined drug therapy on metastatic cancer of the testis. JAMA 174:1291, 1960.

Luce JK: Chemotherapy for lymphomas: Current status. Page 295 in: *Leukemia-Lymphoma.* Year Book, 1969.

PALLIATION OF LOCAL COMPLICATIONS OF NEOPLASIA*

Effusions

At least half of all patients with lung or breast cancer will develop a pleural effusion at some time during their illness. Ascites is a common complication of ovarian carcinoma. Lymphomas may be associated with chylous or nonchylous effusion of either or both sites. One-fourth of all effusions are neoplastic in origin, and, where pulmonary infarction is unlikely, most bloody effusions are from neoplasm. The diag-

*Spinal cord compression and cerebral edema are discussed in Chapter 40.

nosis in malignant pleural effusions can be established by cytologic study of the fluid and pleural biopsy with the Cope needle.

Diuretics may be sufficient to control neoplastic effusions. However, when recurrent accumulations of fluid cause dyspnea, abdominal distention, or pericardial tamponade, palliative control should be attempted.

A. Pleural Effusions: Control of pleural effusions is best achieved by obliteration of the pleural space with sclerosing agents such as mechlorethamine. The lung must be fully expanded, and negative intrathoracic pressure must be applied to oppose the pleural surfaces for several days with a large thoracostomy tube connected to water-sealed drainage. If the lung is not expandable–because of endobronchial obstruction with massive atelectasis, fibrothorax with "trapped lung," or massive intraparenchymal replacement by tumor–obliteration of the pleural space is contraindicated. When the pleural surfaces are opposed, freshly prepared mechlorethamine, 0.4 mg/kg in 50 ml of saline, is instilled intrapleurally through the clamped chest tube and the patient is positioned for 1 minute each in the prone, left decubitus, supine, right decubitus, and knee-chest positions to distribute the drug. After 1 hour, the tube is unclamped and drainage reestablished for 24–48 hours or until no further fluid is forthcoming. Lower dosages of mechlorethamine are used in the face of marrow depression. The procedure may be repeated in 3–4 weeks if the first attempt is unsuccessful.

Using this technic up to 90% of pleural effusions can be palliated. If the attempt fails or if the bone marrow is too compromised to permit the use of mechlorethamine, quinacrine can be used.

B. Ascitic Effusions: Ascites is generally best treated by attempting to control the underlying disease, which is usually ovarian carcinoma or malignant lymphoma. Mechlorethamine frequently induces a chemical peritonitis. Thiotepa does not have a vesicant action on tissues and is thus more gentle.

C. Pericardial Effusions: Most pericardial effusions are best treated by irradiation except (1) those due to radioresistant tumors or (2) when previous radiotherapy has included the proposed field. Impending tamponade must always be anticipated and treated by pericardiocentesis, creation of a pericardial window, or pericardiectomy. If needle pericardiocentesis is performed for a malignant effusion, thiotepa may be instilled into the pericardial cavity (in systemic doses) at the termination of the procedure. Mechlorethamine should not be used since it induces too severe an inflammatory response.

Obstructions & Lytic Lesions of Bone

A. Caval Obstruction: Superior vena caval obstruction is a medical emergency which should be treated by a combination of chemotherapy and radiotherapy. It is characterized by venous congestion and distention of tributaries of the superior vena cava, and thus presents clinically as edema of the face and arms–frequently associated with dyspnea and the hazard of cerebral venous thrombosis or cerebral edema. The syndrome may occur with various diseases affecting the mediastinum, but neoplastic disease–especially bronchogenic carcinoma and the malignant lymphomas–is by far the most common cause. Although a biopsy should be obtained whenever possible, this should not delay the start of therapy. Surgery or endoscopy should not be performed, since such intervention produces increased morbidity and mortality. Treatment should be started as soon as the clinical syndrome is recognized and consists of diuretics, corticosteroids, and maintenance of the upright posture. An intravenous alkylator should be given through an uninvolved vein (eg, femoral vein) and radiotherapy begun immediately. Cyclophosphamide or thiotepa is preferable to mechlorethamine since the former agents induce less vomiting. Venography determines the extent and location of the tumor and the propagating thrombus which is frequently present.

B. Bony Lytic Lesions: Palliation of metastases to weight-bearing bones is best achieved by irradiation. If pathologic fracture is impending, prophylactic fixation can minimize morbidity, especially in areas such as the femoral neck that are susceptible to considerable stress. Prolonged bed rest should be avoided whenever possible, for, in addition to the usual complications, patients with bony disease are prone to develop hypercalcemia, and this tendency is accentuated by immobilization. Supportive bracing is often a useful adjunct for vertebral involvement.

Metabolic Complications of Neoplasia

A. Hypercalcemia Associated With Neoplastic Disease: Hypercalcemia occurs most commonly with myeloma, breast carcinoma, and lung carcinoma and is occasionally seen in patients with prostatic carcinoma, lymphomas, and leukemia. It has also been reported with a wide variety of metastatic or disseminated neoplasms. Symptoms include confusion, somnolence, nausea and vomiting, constipation, dehydration with polyuria, and general clinical deterioration which can easily be mistaken for progressive disease or direct neurologic involvement by tumor. The true nature of this metabolic complication may easily be overlooked, resulting in hypercalcemic death secondary to cardiac, neurologic, and renal toxicity. Hypercalcemia may be due to elaboration of a parathormone-like substance by tumor (lung carcinoma), to osteolytic sterols (as secreted by breast tumors), or to increased bone resorption by invasion and neoplastic destruction of bone (as in myeloma).

The mainstay of therapy to reduce calcium is hydration with isotonic saline (to promote a diuresis of 2–3 liters per 24 hours) in addition to appropriate tumoricidal therapy, mobilization of the bedridden, institution of a low-calcium diet devoid of dairy products, and appropriate treatment of bacterial infections. If the patient was receiving androgens or estrogens for breast carcinoma, they should be withdrawn. Chelating agents such as sodium citrate promote renal excretion of calcium, and potent diuretics such as furosemide or ethacrynic acid also inhibit calcium resorption by the renal tubule. These measures, however, may not be appropriate in patients with impaired renal function or congestive heart failure or may not be sufficient of themselves, and other measures such as glucocorticoids (prednisone, 60–100 mg daily) may be required. The corticosteroids appear to act by reducing calcium resorption from bone. Oral phosphate is often rapidly effective, but intravenous phosphates are too hazardous to recommend their use. Mithramycin, 25 μg/kg IV, is also a prompt and effective agent to be considered if the above measures fail to control hypercalcemia. It is not known whether it acts by exerting a direct toxic effect on the osteoclast or by some other mechanism.

B. Hyperuricemia in Neoplastic Disease: Hyperuricemia is a potentially lethal result of high nucleic acid turnover associated with some malignancies—especially after effective cytotoxic therapy. Uric acid nephropathy is related to intraluminal precipitation of uric acid in the distal renal tubule and collecting duct, with progressive intrarenal obstruction and failure. This sequence of events can often be avoided by maintaining satisfactory hydration and alkalinization of the urine to pH 7.0 by oral sodium bicarbonate (10–15 g/day) or by giving acetazolamide (Diamox) (0.5–1 g/day). Although allopurinol does not replace these measures, the preventive use of this drug (300–800 mg/day) should be considered in patients with leukemia, lymphomas, and myeloproliferative disorders, especially if radiotherapy is instituted. If mercaptopurine is being given, the dose must be reduced to one-fourth to one-third of usual when allopurinol is started.

Lambert CJ: Treatment of malignant pleural effusions by closed trochar tube drainage. Ann Thorac Surg 3:1, 1967.

Lenhard RE Jr (editor): Clinical case records in chemotherapy: The management of hypercalcemia complicating cancer. Cancer Chemother Rep 55:509, 1971.

Levitt SH & others: Treatment of malignant superior vena caval obstruction. Cancer 24:447, 1969.

Millburn L, Hibbs GG, Hendrickson FR: Treatment of spinal cord compression from metastatic carcinoma. Cancer 21:447, 1968.

Perez CA, Bradfield JS, Morgan HC: Management of pathologic fractures. Cancer 29:684, 1972.

Rubin P & others: Superior vena caval syndrome: Slow low dose versus rapid high dose schedule. Radiology 81:388, 1963.

● ● ●

General References

Bagshawe KD (editor): *Medical Oncology.* Blackwell, 1975.

Bodansky O: *Biochemistry of Human Cancer.* Academic Press, 1975.

Brodsky I, Kahn SB, Moyer JH: *Cancer Chemotherapy: Basic and Clinical Applications.* (Twenty-Second Hahnemann Symposium.) Grune & Stratton, 1972.

Cline MJ, Haskell CM III: *Cancer Chemotherapy,* 2nd ed. Saunders, 1975.

Criss WE, Ono T, Sabine JR (editors): *Control Mechanisms in Cancer.* Raven Press, 1976.

Dunphy JE: On caring for the patient with cancer. N Engl J Med 295:313, 1976.

Holland JF, Frei E III (editors): *Cancer Medicine.* Lea & Febiger, 1973.

Horton J, Hill GJ II (editors): *Clinical Oncology.* Saunders, 1977.

Krakoff IH: Cancer chemotherapeutic agents. CA 27:130, 1977.

Lawrence W Jr, Terz JJ (editors): *Cancer Management.* Grune & Stratton, 1977.

Munster AM (editor): *Surgical Immunology.* Grune & Stratton, 1976.

Nealon TF Jr (editor): *Management of the Patient With Cancer,* 2nd ed. Saunders, 1976.

Symposium: Medical aspects of cancer. Med Clin North Am, vol 55, May 1971.

Veidenheimer MC (editor): Symposium on the care and treatment of the cancer patient. Surg Clin North Am 47:557, 1967.

50...

Organ Transplantation

Oscar Salvatierra, Jr., MD, Folkert O. Belzer, MD, & Nicholas J. Feduska, MD

There are 3 types of tissue and organ transplantation: **(1) autotransplantation (autograft),** in which tissue is moved from one location to another within the same individual; **(2) homotransplantation (allograft),** in which an organ or tissue is moved from one individual to another of the same species; and **(3) heterotransplantation (xenograft),** in which an organ or tissue is transplanted from a member of one species to a member of another, eg, from ape to man. Autotransplantation elicits no immune response and is widely used in clinical practice. Heterotransplantation (xenografting) elicits a severe immune response except when the organ or tissue has been specifically treated, as in transplantation of lyophilized pigskin to a severely burned patient. This is used solely as a temporary procedure. Heterotransplants must presently be regarded as purely experimental because there is as yet no way to control the vigorous rejection phenomenon that characteristically occurs.

At present, the major emphasis in clinical transplantation is on homotransplantation in which the immune process can be partially controlled so as to allow retention of the transplanted organ for long periods.

The success of tissue grafts between individuals of the same species depends upon the degree of histocompatibility between donor and recipient. Rejection occurs because antigens present on the donor cells are absent on the cells of the recipient tissue. These so-called histocompatibility antigens are genetically determined and are present mainly on the surfaces of the cells. The major histocompatibility genetic region in man is called HLA (human leukocyte antigen), and the major cell for testing is the lymphocyte. Related donors are more likely to have compatible HLA antigens. Identical antigens are found in the cells of identical twins; cells of other siblings and parents are less compatible; and cells of unrelated donors are least compatible.

In addition to HLA antigens, the ABO blood group antigens also determine transplant compatibility. These must also be tested and used as a basis for prediction of success in homograft transplantation.

Two crucial observations led to investigation of the role of the HLA antigen system in organ transplantation. The first was the finding that rabbits preimmunized by injection of allogeneic leukocytes developed a second set rejection of a subsequent skin graft from the immunizing donor. The second was the discovery that human leukocytes could be serologically classified by a unique series of genetic markers—ie, the HLA antigens. The construction of this system coincided with the evolution of clinical kidney transplantation in man, and it was logical that attempts would be made to correlate the HLA system with graft survival. At present, the HLA antigens appear to be related to histocompatibility because when kidneys are transplanted from HLA-identical siblings the postoperative course is smooth and graft survival is prolonged. Where kidney pairs are mismatched for one or more HLA specificities, in related groups, the results are not as good.

The following clinical guidelines have proved useful in the selection of donors based on tissue typing:

(1) Verification of ABO compatibility and a negative leukocyte cross-match to avoid hyperacute rejections during surgery must be the first step.

(2) If the donor is a sibling, the best choice is an identical genotype based on a family study. Lacking a family study, the second choice is an identical phenotype.

(3) In parent-child and HLA-non-identical sibling combinations, the mixed lymphocyte culture (MLC) appears to have some predictive value. Two-year graft survival in HLA-non-identical donor-recipient pairs prospectively selected by the MLC at our institution is 91%.

(4) The value of HLA typing in unrelated donors is still controversial. Data are available to suggest that the degree of HLA typing does not correlate well with subsequent graft survival, although other data—especially from Europe—suggest that improved graft survival occurs with better HLA matching. To determine the precise role of the HLA system in organ transplantation, continued analysis of worldwide experience is of utmost importance. In unrelated transplants, most recent evidence suggests that the HLA system is relatively unimportant unless the patient has been presensitized against specific HLA antigens. In our series of 570 consecutive primary cadaver transplants, although HLA match grade at the A and B loci did not influence ultimate graft survival, detection of new specificities at the D locus may prove to be of practical clinical significance in the future.

HOMOTRANSPLANTATION

Homotransplantation is performed for endstage organ diseases. Three major problems limit widespread use of this procedure: (1) inability to completely control the immune response, (2) the paucity of donor organs offered for transplantation, and (3) lack of technics for resuscitation and storage of cadaver organs after death. Homotransplant organs include kidney, heart, liver, pancreas, and lung. There are other transplants such as bone and cornea.

The Rejection Reaction

The length of survival of homografts in the absence of immunosuppressive therapy depends upon the genetic disparity between donor and recipient. Most of our earlier knowledge about this immune reaction was obtained from investigations with skin grafts. However, the basic immunologic process may be similar for each organ or tissue, and the pathophysiologic expression depends upon the specific organ undergoing rejection. Antigens in the donor tissue that are lacking in the recipient are responsible for initiation of the rejection process. These antigens, believed to be glycoproteins or lipoproteins, are processed by the macrophages. Lymphocytes and plasma cells then infiltrate the graft and destroy the endothelium of the blood vessels. The reaction of host cells and specific cytotoxic antibodies against the grafted tissue continues until ultimate destruction occurs.

In spite of many attempts to elucidate the various steps in the rejection process, our knowledge remains incomplete. It was first observed by Medawar that the application of a second skin graft from the same donor results in a more rapid rejection than the first—this due to cytotoxic antibodies preformed in response to sensitization from the first skin graft. Dempster demonstrated cross-reaction between antigens of the skin and the kidneys. It is now known that sensitization to skin, kidney, and other organs can be achieved by injections of lymphocytes and cross-reaction with bacterial antigens.

In the kidney, the rejection process begins immediately after transplantation. Electronmicroscopic studies by Williams & others (see reference, below) demonstrated changes as early as 24 hours after grafting which were distinct from those observed in autotransplants. Lymphocytes from the host initially attack the endothelial cells of the peritubular capillaries. Evidence that the cells that infiltrate homotransplanted kidneys are from the host is of 2 types: (1) If the host is given total body irradiation to destroy the lymphocytes, cells are not seen in the graft several days after transplantation. (2) In the labeling studies of Porter & Calne and Williams & others (see references), lymphocytes of the host were labeled with tritiated thymidine and the kidneys were then transplanted. The lymphocytes that infiltrated the graft were labeled. It has been shown that lymphocytes from the donor ("passenger lymphocytes") can be transferred with the donor organ and may play a role in immunizing the host. In animals, if the lymphocytes of the donor are destroyed by x-ray radiation or antilymphocyte serum before transplantation, skin, kidneys, and hearts survive longer. This technic has not been used in clinical organ transplantation, but the potential clinical applications are obvious.

The initial area of attack of host lymphocytes on the grafted tissue is the peritubular capillaries. In this area, blood flow is slower and the endothelial cells are more widely separated. This causes early swelling of the organ. Host lymphocytes are observed to attack the vascular endothelial cells in the peritubular capillaries, and cytoplasmic discontinuity has been observed. In the early phase of the rejection process, the major cell population consists of lymphocytes; later, immature plasma cells are observed in increasing numbers. A number of mediators are released during the interaction of host and graft cells, but their role is incompletely understood. It is well established that humoral antibodies play an important role in the destruction of homografts. Specific cytotoxic antibody has been shown to produce rejection in passive transfer experiments. In addition, cytotoxic antibody eluted from rejected grafts has been shown to destroy donor cells in vitro. Both the cellular and humoral arms of the immune response are greatest during the final phase, when the blood vessels of the graft are progressively destroyed and blocked by cells and cell debris, and death of the graft is due to the resulting ischemia. In the case of renal allografts, glomerular and tubular function is anatomically intact until this final phase.

Cochrum KC & others: Renal autograft rejection initiated by passive transfer of immune plasma. Transplant Proc 1:301, 1969.

Dempster WJ: Kidney homotransplantation. Br J Surg 40:447, 1953.

Egdahl RH, Hume DM: Immunologic studies in renal homotransplantation. Surg Gynecol Obstet 102:450, 1956.

Gowans JL, McGregor DD, Cowen DM: Initiation of immune responses by small lymphocytes. Nature 196:651, 1962.

Hume DM: Homotransplantation of kidneys and of fetal liver and spleen after total body irradiation. Ann Surg 152:354, 1960.

Knudsen DM & others: Serial angiograms in canine renal allografts. Transplantation 5:257, 1967.

Kountz SL & others: Mechanism of rejection of homotransplanted kidneys. Nature 199:257, 1963.

Medawar P: Second study of behavior and fate of skin homografts in rabbits: Report to War Wounds Committee of Medical Research Council. J Anat 79:157, 1945.

Porter KA, Calne RY: Origin of the infiltrating cells in skin and kidney homografts. Transplant Bull 26:458, 1960.

Salvatierra O & others: HLA typing and primary cadaver graft survival. Transplant Proc 9:495, 1977.

Williams PL & others: Ultrastructural and hemodynamic studies in canine renal transplants. J Anat 98:545, 1964.

KIDNEY TRANSPLANTATION

Renal transplantation is indicated for patients with end stage renal failure. It is estimated that 20–40 patients per million are candidates each year for treatment by transplantation. This means that in the USA an estimated 8–10 thousand patients could benefit from this procedure each year. Chronic hemodialysis has been an important factor in making renal transplantation possible, especially for recipients of cadaver kidneys.

The current expected graft survival results at our center at 2 years are as follows: almost 100% for HLA-identical living related grafts; 91% for living related non-HLA-identical grafts prospectively selected by MLC; and 50% for cadaver grafts.

SOURCES OF DONOR KIDNEYS

There are 2 sources of kidneys for renal transplantation: (1) living related donors and (2) cadaver donors. Of all the patients who are acceptable candidates for transplantation, only about 15–20% have an acceptable volunteer living related donor. The donor must be ABO compatible with the recipient. Living donors should be in good health both physically and psychologically. Above all, the donor should be a volunteer and must clearly understand the nature of the procedure so that he can give his informed consent to the operation. The law requires that donors be adults.

Living Donors

Over the last decade, about 7500 individuals have donated one kidney. The life of a healthy donor is not shortened by the loss of one kidney. In young donors, the remaining kidney hypertrophies and in a few months provides 75–80% of the original renal function. Women with one kidney do not have an increased incidence of urinary infections during pregnancy. Some transplant surgeons have advocated removal of the right kidney in women of childbearing age because of the increased chance of the uterus partially obstructing the only ureter during pregnancy.

The main risk to a donor is the anesthesia and the operation itself. The mortality rate is estimated to be 0.1%–about the same risk as in driving 8–10 thousand miles a year in an automobile.

The most common complication following nephrectomy, except for minor atelectasis, is wound infection, which occurs in less than 1% of cases and is usually superficial. Renal failure occurred postoperatively in one of our donors but cleared spontaneously. Superficial pain and hernias may occur, but rarely.

After the donor has been judged to be a true volunteer and the risks and complications have been explained to him, he is admitted to the hospital for special studies. A detailed history is taken, and a physical examination is performed. The routine work-up includes chest x-ray, ECG, urinalysis, complete blood count, fasting blood sugar, serum bilirubin, creatinine clearance, and BUN. If these are normal, an intravenous urogram is performed; if that is normal, a renal arteriogram is performed. Kidneys with multiple renal arteries may be transplanted, but care must be taken in the anastomosis of small accessory vessels. When there are multiple renal veins, the smaller veins may be ligated since there is free communication of the veins within the kidney. If the arteriogram is normal, the patient is an acceptable donor.

In the early days of transplantation, many centers included psychiatric evaluation as part of the preoperative assessment of living donors. In a study by Sadler & others of living unrelated and related donors over a 5-year period, true altruism was exhibited in many donors, including the living unrelated donor. Sibling donors appear to show the most anxiety, especially when the donor has just married and has young children. Follow-up studies on donors show that they have good renal function and suffer no ill effects from the procedure either physically or psychologically.

Psychiatric evaluation of donors is not a requirement. Adequate evaluation by the donor's own physician is all that is needed.

Cadaver Kidneys

Since only 20% of recipients have a suitable volunteer living donor, the only way to offer transplantation to the vast majority of patients is to use cadaver kidneys, and there is a shortage of available cadaver organs. It is essential to the success of the procedure that the transplanted organ be of good quality. This means that the organ must be removed before or immediately after cardiac arrest. Brain death must be established in cadaver donors before organ procurement. In California, legislation was enacted in 1974 to the effect that a patient can be declared dead if irreversible cessation of brain function has occurred. The kidneys may be removed for transplantation up to 1 hour after cardiac arrest provided intra-aortic flush with iced solution is used for in situ cooling of the kidneys. It is also important that the donor has relatively normal renal function at the time of death and phenoxybenzamine or another vasodilator is given to prevent renal vasospasm during the agonal phase.

There are 2 technics for short-term preservation of kidneys: simple hypothermia and continuous perfusion. With simple hypothermia, the organs are flushed out with an appropriate solution, the most common at present being Collins' solution. These solutions contain appropriate amounts of osmotically active but nonpermeable solutes such as glucose, mannitol, or sucrose, and their main beneficial effect is to prevent cellular swelling during hypothermic storage. Kidneys can be successfully stored for up to 24 hours, especially if warm ischemia was avoided during organ procurement. The technic of simple hypothermia is the method of choice for small transplant units that perform less than 25 transplants per year.

By means of continuous pulsatile perfusion, using either cryoprecipitated plasma or albumin solutions, kidneys can be stored for up to 3 days, and this method of short-term preservation eases the logistical problems involved in transplantation since patients awaiting kidneys often live a long distance from the transplant center. Another advantage of pulsatile perfusion is that the sudden influx of a large number of cadaver organs can be easily managed.

Unfortunately, the extra time made available has not led to improved donor-recipient matching by current methods of tissue typing. The graft survival at 1 year of kidneys stored by pulsatile perfusion and by simple hypothermia is equal.

Our experience with procuring cadaver kidneys indicates that enough kidneys and other organs will not be available to meet transplant demands until the public accepts and supports organ donation. Many individuals are now carrying Uniform Donor Cards which comply with the Uniform Anatomical Act adopted by all 50 states of the USA. Further research in resuscitative technics may make more cadaver organs available. The age limit for donors has been from birth to age 65, but kidneys from young donors appear to fare better. The donor should be free of cancer (except for primary brain cancer) and systemic infections.

Several improvements in preservation equipment have been made in the last few years, and small, completely portable units have been developed which can easily be transported in any automobile. This apparatus has the advantage of being able to differentiate kidneys severely damaged with little chance of survival in the recipient from those with minimal damage with a good chance of survival. Empirical observations indicate that kidneys removed from donors with serum creatinine concentrations below 2 mg/100 ml have a good chance of adequate initial function. In addition, if such donors are treated with phenoxybenzamine, posttransplant dialysis is required in 24% of cases.

Belzer FO: Current concepts: Renal preservation. N Engl J Med 291:402, 1974.

Belzer FO, Kountz SL: Preservation and transplantation of human cadaver kidneys: A two-year experience. Ann Surg 172:395, 1970.

Blaufox DM & others: Physiologic responses of the transplanted human kidney. N Engl J Med 280:62, 1969.

Bricker NS & others: Studies on the functional capacity of a denervated homotransplanted kidney in an identical twin with parallel observations in the donor. J Clin Invest 35:1364, 1956.

Collins GM, Bravo-Shugarman M, Terasaki PI: Kidney preservation for transplantation. Lancet 1:620, 1970.

Dempster WJ, Kountz SL, Jovanovic M: Simple kidney storage technique. Br Med J 1:407, 1964.

Kron AG, Ogden DA, Holmes JH: Renal function in 29 healthy adults before and after nephrectomy. JAMA 196:110, 1966.

Salvatierra O & others: Procurement of cadaver kidneys. Urol Clin North Am 3:457, 1976.

Shorter RG: Renal function in donors and recipients of renal allotransplantation: Radioisotopic measurements. Ann Intern Med 66:105, 1967.

SELECTION OF RECIPIENTS

During the developmental days of renal transplantation, most of the patients accepted for transplantation were in the younger age group from 15–45 years. In recent years, the age range has been extended in both directions—children below age 1 and adults up to age 65. It was noted earlier that children between ages 6–15 do as well as adults below age 50. Children below age 6—and especially below age 1—seem to have a higher mortality rate. Although transplantation is not contraindicated in older people, the success rate is lower because associated diseases are more frequent, resistance to infection is less, and the surgical risk is greater.

The ideal recipient is a young person who has no serious infections or lower urinary tract disease, with minimal and reversible systemic disease secondary to renal failure. Recipients with the following primary renal diseases have been successfully transplanted: glomerulonephritis, pyelonephritis, polycystic kidney disease, malignant hypertension, reflux pyelonephritis, Goodpasture's syndrome, congenital renal hypoplasia, renal cortical necrosis, Fabry's syndrome, and Alport's syndrome. Patients with certain systemic diseases in which the kidney is one of the end organs have been successfully transplanted: cystinosis, systemic lupus erythematosus, and Kimmelstiel-Wilson disease. Oxalosis is one disease in which transplantation appears contraindicated at present because the disease tends to reappear in the transplant.

When the bladder is found to be unsuitable for ureteral implantation, a Bricker conduit has been used to obtain satisfactory urinary drainage. Most long-term defunctionalized bladders can still be utilized for ureteral reimplantation. Patients with peptic ulcer disease have been successfully transplanted, although some of these patients have required vagotomy and pyloroplasty for treatment of peptic ulcer after transplantation.

Emotional instability or psychosis has been thought to be a contraindication to transplantation, but successful transplantation has been observed to cure these patients if their emotional difficulties were due to uremia or poor response to dialysis. Unfortunately, there is no way to tell if the psychiatric symptoms are a reflection of the physical problems of the patients.

Advanced retinopathy due to uncontrolled hypertension and peripheral neuropathy secondary to uremia frequently show clinical improvement after transplantation.

The decision to accept patients in the poorer risk groups is usually based on the available dialysis facilities and the number of cadaver kidneys offered for transplantation.

Once a patient has been selected as a transplant recipient, he is usually started on hemodialysis. If he is to receive a kidney from a living related donor, only 2 or 3 dialyses are required before transplantation or bilateral nephrectomy. Recipients awaiting a cadaver kidney will require longer hemodialysis. Bilateral nephrectomy should be performed only if required to control the blood pressure or if there is infection in the kidneys. Of 141 transplants performed at this center in 1976, only 13% of recipients had preliminary bilateral nephrectomy.

Bilateral nephrectomy prior to transplantation was common in the 1960s but has been performed less frequently in recent years. The indications for preliminary nephrectomy are (1) severe hypertension uncontrolled by dialysis, (2) anatomic abnormalities of the urinary tract with or without infection (eg, hydronephrosis, ureteral reflux), and (3) polyostotic renal disease with previous renal infection.

There is no evidence that splenectomy is of value before transplantation.

Belzer FO: Renal preservation. N Engl J Med 291:402, 1974.

Hamburger J, Crognier J, Durmont J: Experience with 45 renal homotransplantations in man. Lancet 1:985, 1965.

Murray JE, Wilson RE, O'Connor NE: Evaluation of long-functioning human kidney transplants. Surg Gynecol Obstet 124:509, 1967.

Russel PS: Kidney transplantation. Am J Med 44:776, 1968.

CONTROLLING THE REJECTION REACTION

The first successful renal allografts were done before the advent of immunosuppressive drugs and were between identical twins. These transplants, known as isografts, did not undergo a rejection process. Allografts always involve the problem of rejection. Two procedures have been developed to predict acceptance of the graft by the host: close histocompatibility matching and immunosuppressive drug preparation. At present, there are 2 methods of histocompatibility testing: (1) HLA phenotyping and (2) mixed lymphocyte culture (MLC) testing.

Mixed Lymphocyte Culture (MLC) & Matching

Histocompatibility antigens are shared by all tissue cells, but the lymphocyte is the only cell capable of responding to a foreign antigen by blast-like formation and increased DNA synthesis. This response can be measured in vitro by culturing the cells of 2 individuals together for 5 days. On the fifth day, the mixed cell cultures and appropriate control cultures (containing each cell population alone) are labeled with tritiated thymidine. This isotope is incorporated into any new DNA being produced so that the level of cellular radioactivity becomes an indicator of the degree of cellular response. The amount of DNA produced in mixed culture above the base level of DNA produced by the same cells cultured alone represents the degree of antigenic disparity between the cells being tested.

Mixed leukocyte culture (MLC) done in this way measures the response of both populations of cells to one another (ie, a "2-way" reaction). Since the response of the donor to the recipient is not really pertinent to transplantation, several modifications of the test have been developed which measure only the response of the recipient's cells to his donor's antigens (ie, a "one-way" reaction). Donor cells may be rendered nonresponsive by treatment with mitomycin C or x-irradiation, yet they still maintain their antigenicity. Work has also been done using donor cells of different types such as skin, kidney, or buccal mucosa, which are not able to respond to antigenic stimulation themselves but still display the donor's antigenic makeup. These mixed culture technics have proved useful in the selection of donor-recipient pairs for related transplantation.

They are particularly helpful in selection of the best related donor within a family in combination with HLA typing. The value of MLC matching in addition to HLA typing is that the matching technic measures the total immune response. Hamburger reported a positive correlation between MLC results and related transplant survival. Cochrum & others have shown the same positive correlation in related grafts and, more importantly, have shown a high positive correlation in cadaver grafts. The policy over the past 2 years at this transplant center has been to transplant only living related donors if the MLC reaction is low and to perform a cadaver graft if the MLC reaction between the living related donor and recipient is high. This is important since the correlation between HLA typing and cadaver graft survival is low. The importance of mixed cell culture for transplantation has been sufficiently well established so that it is now a primary goal to shorten the test from the existing 5 days in order that it may benefit the recipients of cadaver organs as well.

HLA Typing

Originally the HLA system was thought to be composed only of 2 segregant series of antigens, but the total number of antigens is now known to exceed 50. Moreover, the number of HLA loci has been increased from 2 to 4. **HLA-A** is the former first locus, while HLA-B is the former second locus. HLA-C is a third locus. HLA-D locus is the fourth, the former MLC locus, which has also been referred to as the LD locus; it is the first lymphocyte-defined locus. The terminology was changed to HLA-D because this locus is important in determining histocompatibility and because the patient can be typed with serum antibodies if B lymphocytes are used as the target cells. HLA-D determinants have been determined with an MLC technic: Lymphocytes believed to be homozygous for an HLA-D determinant are used as typing cells; if they fail to stimulate a responder cell, the latter is assumed to share that HLA-D determinant.

The haplotype is that portion of the phenotype determined by closely linked genes of a single chromosome. In the case of the major human histocompatibility gene complex, it includes one HLA-A antigen, one HLA-B antigen, one HLA-C antigen, and one HLA-D determinant. Haplotype analysis is of importance principally in family studies in living related transplantation. If the A antigen and the B antigen of that chromosome can be defined, it can usually be assumed that all HLA antigens and MLC determinants produced by that chromosome will also be present regardless of our current inability to accurately detect them.

As indicated previously, the best results in transplantation are achieved when the donor is an HLA identical sibling. Usefulness of HLA typing with unrelated or cadaver donors is more controversial. Future applications of HLA matching to cadaver renal transplantation will probably depend on further elucidation of the C and D loci and other as yet unknown antigenic determinants.

The Influence of Presensitization on Graft Survival Rate

The effect of previous blood transfusions and other methods of recipient sensitization on renal allograft survival has been controversial. Patients with end-stage renal failure often require transfusion and as a result develop antibodies. The more antibodies that form, the more likely that a donor kidney will be incompatible on cross-match. In our series, graft survival rate seems to be enhanced in hyperimmunized recipients with greater than 50% frequency of preformed antibodies to selected random donor panel cells. The better graft survival rate of the hyperimmunized group is consistent with the theory that if potential recipients have been permitted to form cytotoxic antibodies to histocompatibility antigens to which they are easily sensitized, they then will select out in the cross-match tests only those kidneys with antigens to which they respond less readily.

Sensitization following rejection of a previous allograft, however, appears to confer a less favorable prognosis. Recipients of second grafts, of course, are contrasted by having a previous exposure to kidney tissue antigens.

Immunosuppression

As a working hypothesis, it is assumed that the closer the histocompatibility match, the less immunosuppression by drugs will be required to achieve graft acceptance. The use of immunosuppressive agents imposes an increased risk of death and complications due to viral, fungal, and bacterial infections.

The first immunosuppressive agent used was total body sublethal x-ray radiation, but this was rapidly abandoned because it could not be controlled and because the mortality rate was exceedingly high.

Because the spleen and thymus in lower animals have been shown to mediate the immune response, they have been removed in man, but there is no clinical evidence that splenectomy or thymectomy in man alters the immune response. Some centers have observed an increased incidence of thromboembolic disease after splenectomy; others have not. It is believed that splenectomy corrects some of the bleeding abnormalities in uremia and permits the administration of larger doses of immunosuppressive agents, but this is an area of controversy. Very few thymectomies have been performed, and this procedure appears to have no value in clinical renal transplantation.

The major drugs used in immunosuppressive therapy are azathioprine (Imuran) and the adrenal corticosteroids. Azathioprine is one of the mercaptopurine class of drugs and inhibits nucleic acid synthesis. It is given daily in doses of 2–3 mg/kg. In the case of living donors, the drug is started 2–3 days before transplantation. In the case of recipients of cadaver transplantation, 4–5 mg/kg are given just before the transplant. The patients are maintained on approximately 2 mg/kg or less indefinitely, with the dosage monitored by the white cell count. The drug may cause depression of the bone marrow elements (leukocytes and platelets) and may cause jaundice. In the face of untoward effects or in the presence of infections, the drug is temporarily discontinued or reduced. This drug is never given in increased doses during an acute rejection episode, and the dosage may have to be reduced during rejection when renal function is poor.

Prednisone is almost always used with azathioprine. The dosage must be regulated carefully so as to prevent complications such as infection, cataracts, the development of cushingoid features and hypertension, increased bruisability, and acne. At the University of California Medical Center in San Francisco, prednisone is started 2 days before transplantation for recipients of living related kidneys and on the day of transplantation for recipients of cadaver kidneys. The oral dosage is 120 mg for 3 days. The dose is reduced by 20 mg every 3 days until a maintenance dosage of 30 mg/day is achieved. This prednisone dosage is then further decreased in the outpatient clinic until maintenance levels of about 10 mg of prednisone per day for adults are obtained. Although recently there has been a great enthusiasm for giving large doses of methylprednisolone intravenously for rejection episodes, there are no experimental or clinical data to suggest that this method of treatment is actually beneficial, and it probably results in a much higher infection rate, especially fungal or viral infections. Since the use of intravenous methylprednisolone has been discontinued in this transplant service, we have had many few problems with infection.

The exact site of action of corticosteroids on the immune response is not known, but it is believed that they inhibit the inflammatory aspect of rejection.

High daily doses of prednisone in children inhibit growth. This may be circumvented by alternate-day treatment, administering the drug once in the morning.

This dosage regimen is usually started after the initial 6-month period of daily corticosteroid administration, at which time there is the greatest risk of graft loss secondary to rejection. The exact dosage has not been precisely defined, but 2 mg/kg in children on alternate days has permitted growth.

Therapy for a rejection episode consists of increasing prednisone to 2–3 mg/kg and then tapering to a maintenance dosage level. In general, immunosuppressive therapy should not be increased after the second rejection episode, nor should it be increased after the first rejection episode if renal function does not return to normal or near normal. In effect this abolishes prolonged high-dose immunosuppressive therapy after transplantation and has been associated with improved survival. Since 1972, patient survival from living related donors is 100% at 1 and 2 years, while survival in recipients of cadaver grafts is 91% and 86% at 1 and 2 years. Those receiving cadaver kidneys include more high-risk patients, such as insulin-dependent juvenile diabetics and older patients. Even though graft rejection has been treated less vigorously than in the past, graft survival has not been jeopardized by emphasizing patient survival. This appears to substantiate the concept that the outcome of rejection depends principally upon the genetic similarity between donor and recipient. Although a successful transplant is desirable, maximum patient survival is of higher priority and one must aim for the best attainable quality of life by an integration of both dialysis and transplantation.

X-Ray Radiation

X-ray radiation in doses of 450–600 rads may be given immediately after transplantation or for treatment of a rejection crisis. It is frequently given by the method of Hume, which consists of delivering 150 rads to the area of the graft every other day for 3 or 4 doses.

Antilymphocyte Globulin

An adjunct of proved value is antilymphocyte globulin (ALG). Unfortunately, its value in clinical renal transplantation has not yet been fully established. This material may be made in the horse, rabbit, or sheep, but the main source at present is the horse. Lymphocytes from human peripheral blood, spleen, lymph nodes, or thymus are injected into the animal. After immunization, the serum is harvested and the active globulin fraction isolated. Another source has been cultured lymphoblast. Once the IgG fraction is obtained, it is administered intramuscularly or intravenously. In order to be effective, it should have a high cytotoxicity titer and should have been shown to prolong skin grafts in subhuman primates. This biologic test system has made it difficult to evaluate ALG preparations, as each batch may be of a different titer and may produce different clinical results. Much research is now being directed toward the development of standardization procedures and a standardized product.

Bach FH: Transplantation: Pairing of donor and recipient. Science 168:1170, 1970.

Cochrum K, Salvatierra O, Belzer FO: Correlation between MLC stimulation and graft survival in living related and cadaver transplants. Ann Surg 180:617, 1974.

Dempster WJ, Harrison CV, Shackman RM: Rejection processes in human homotransplanted kidneys. Br Med J 2:969, 1964.

Kountz SL, Cohn R: Initial treatment of human renal allografts with large doses of intrarenally administered immunosuppressive drugs. Lancet 1:338, 1969.

Monaco AP, Campion JP, Kapnick SJ: Clinical use of antilymphocyte globulin. Transplant Proc 9:1007, 1977.

Opelz G, Terasaki PI: Significance of mixed lymphocyte culture testing in cadaver kidney transplantation. Transplant 23:375, 1977.

Patel R, Terasaki PI: Significance of the positive cross-match test in kidney transplantation. N Engl J Med 280:735, 1969.

Rapaport FT, Dausset J: Ranks of donor-recipient histocompatibility for human transplantation. Science 167:1260, 1970.

Salvatierra O & others: Improved patient survival in renal transplantation. Surgery 79:166, 1976.

Salvatierra O & others: The influence of presensitization on graft survival rate. Surgery 81:146, 1977.

Starzl TE & others: Heterologous antilymphocyte globulin, histoincompatibility matching, and human renal homotransplantation. Surg Gynecol Obstet 126:1023, 1968.

OPERATIVE TECHNICS

The left kidney of a living donor is preferred because it has the longest renal vein and the renal artery does not run in close proximity to the inferior vena cava. The kidney may be removed through a transabdominal approach, but a subcostal retroperitoneal approach is preferred. The major difference between nephrectomy for transplantation and nephrectomy for disease is that the quality of the donor kidney should be preserved. This means that every attempt should be made to minimize renal ischemia and damage to the ureters. Renal ischemia may be minimized by hydrating the donor and administering an osmotic diuretic to promote a urine flow rate of 3–4 ml/minute at the time of nephrectomy. Since the blood supply for the ureter arises from the renal artery, the ureter should not be skeletized and dissected high in the renal pedicle. Great care should be taken in removal of the kidney.

Recipient Operation

There is no good evidence that splenectomy is of value in renal homotransplantation. Removal of the recipient's kidneys is necessary when they are infected or responsible for uncontrolled hypertension. These procedures should be performed 1 week or more before allotransplantation.

A donor left kidney is usually transplanted to the right iliac fossa (Fig 50–1), turned over so that the

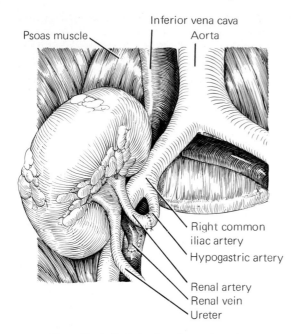

Figure 50–1. Technic of renal transplantation.

pelvis is dependent. The renal artery is usually anastomosed end-to-end to the hypogastric artery and the renal vein end-to-side to the common iliac vein. Meticulous attention should be paid to hemostasis and ligation of the lymphatics, since inadequate attention to this may result in a postoperative seroma or lymphocele. The ureter is implanted into the bladder. A uretero-ureteral anastomosis or ureteropyelostomy may be performed only under special conditions. It is better that these procedures be reserved for complications of the transplanted ureter.

POSTOPERATIVE MANAGEMENT

Recipients who have received transplants from living donors usually undergo immediate diuresis and natriuresis. The magnitude is related to how overhydrated the patient was before transplantation. The diuresis and natriuresis occur because the transplanted kidney is vasodilated, but the glomerular filtration rate as measured by inulin clearance is rarely above that expected for a single kidney. The kidney has been found to have a low PAH extraction ratio and a low filtration fraction but a normal T_mPAH. How long vasodilatation persists after transplantation is not known.

Once this phase has passed, the patient maintains a relatively stable weight, although the weight may rapidly increase because of increased appetite and food intake. The urethral catheter at our center is usually left in place for as long as 7 days to ensure healing of the bladder incision. Most recipients may be started on

a solid food diet with no added salt on the first to third postoperative days.

GRAFT REJECTION

The major hazard for the postoperative allograft recipient is rejection. Most rejections occur within the first 6–8 weeks. Four types of rejections have been clinically recognized:

(1) Hyperacute rejection is due to preformed cytotoxic antibodies against donor lymphocytes or renal cells. This reaction occurs immediately after completion of the anastomosis, and complete graft destruction occurs in 24–48 hours. Initially, the graft is pink and firm, but it then becomes blue and soft with evidence of diminished blood flow. There is no effective method of treating this reaction, and patients who have preformed antibodies against donor cells should not be transplanted with a kidney from that donor.

(2) Accelerated rejection has been described. This usually appears within 5 days after a period of good function. It is believed to be related to subliminal preformed cytotoxic antibodies against donor cells not detected by the usual cytotoxicity technics. It has also been suggested that sensitized cells could bring about this reaction.

(3) Acute rejection usually occurs within 1–8 weeks after transplantation. It is an immune cellular reaction against foreign antigens characterized by fever, oliguria, weight gain, tenderness and enlargement of the graft, hypertension, and blood chemical evidence of impaired renal function. This type of rejection process can be treated by increasing the dosage of corticosteroids and is usually entirely reversible.

(4) Chronic rejection is a late cause of renal deterioration mediated by humoral factors. It is most often diagnosed on the basis of slowly decreasing renal function in association with proteinuria and hypertension. Chronic rejection is resistant to corticosteroid therapy, and graft loss will eventually occur, although perhaps not for several years after renal function begins to deteriorate.

The foregoing descriptions of the 4 types of rejection reactions can be used only as general guidelines. Rejection is the result of numerous events many of which are still not understood. Of greatest importance is the observation that only the acute rejection can be most often treated successfully by present methods of immunosuppression.

DETECTING A REJECTION CRISIS

Since a rejection may occur at any time after transplantation, it may at times be difficult to differentiate from other conditions. In the immediate postoperative period, graft rejection must be differentiated from technical and urologic problems and acute tubular necrosis. Its clinical manifestations are frequently a change in mood of the patient and a sudden fever of 39–40 C (102.2–104 F). Many recipients are apprehensive, with increased anxiety, and may have tachycardia. There are 2 important physical findings: (1) the transplanted kidney is enlarged and tender on palpation. The tenderness is due to stretching of the peritoneum overlying the kidney. (2) As the process proceeds, the patient will gain weight and become hypertensive, and will have a falling urine output.

Laboratory Studies

There is no single study that will pinpoint a rejection crisis. However, an elevation of BUN and serum creatinine appears to be the most consistent and reliable means of detecting renal deterioration secondary to rejection. The GFR as measured by creatinine clearance also declines. The urine shows an increase in protein and lymphocytes, and urinary sodium is low. If the kidney does not function well initially, as may occur with cadaver kidneys, a ^{131}I-hippuran renogram may be used to detect graft viability. The vasculature of the graft may be visualized by the use of technetium 99m pertechnetate.

The diagnosis is made by analysis of the total clinical and laboratory findings. Although most patients will experience a rejection crisis (HLA identical siblings tend to have very few), most can be successfully treated and the patient may survive with normal renal function. After the first rejection, others are less frequent. Although previously it was thought that the endothelial blood vessel of the graft is replaced by cells of the host, recent studies by Williams & others have shown that this occurs only infrequently. Also, there is evidence that a "blocking" antibody is formed which prevents host cells from attacking the graft's vascular endothelium. Whatever the mechanism, most grafts that are lost are rejected within the first 3 months; very few grafts are lost after 2 years.

Since most rejection reactions occur within the first 3 months, the mortality rate from immunosuppressive drugs is highest during this period.

Blaufox MD, Merrill JP: Evaluation of renal transplant function by iodohippurate sodium-I[131]. JAMA 202:575, 1967.

Cochrum KC & others: The correlation of MLC with graft survival. Transplant Proc 5:391, 1973.

Kissmeyer-Nielsen F & others: Hyperacute rejection of kidney allografts associated with pre-existing humoral antibodies against donor cells. Lancet 2:662, 1966.

Kountz SL, Laub DR, Cohn R: Detecting and treating early renal homotransplant rejection. JAMA 191:997, 1965.

Salvatierra O & others: The advantages of ^{131}I-orthoiodohippurate scintiphotography in management of patients after renal transplantation. Ann Surg 180:336, 1974.

Salvatierra O & others: Urological complications in renal transplantation can be prevented and controlled. J Urol 117:421, 1977.

Starzl TE: *Experience in Renal Transplantation.* Saunders, 1964.

Starzl TE, Weil R, Putnam CW: Modern trends in kidney transplantation. Transplant Proc 9:1, 1977.

Straffon RA: Symposium on renal transplantation. Urol Clin North Am 3:1, 1976. [Entire issue.]

Williams GM & others: Endothelial changes associated with hyperacute, acute, and chronic renal allograft rejections in man. Transplant Proc 5:819, 1973.

HEART TRANSPLANTATION

The immunologic barriers to clinical heart allotransplantation are probably no greater than those for the kidney. The logistical problems, however, are far greater. Unlike the donor kidney, the donor heart must be of excellent quality at the time of transplantation, because it must immediately take over the total circulatory system. Cardiopulmonary bypass to support the host circulatory system during removal of the heart at transplantation is essential, but this cannot be maintained for a long period of time.

The heart was first transplanted heterotopically (ie, to the necks of recipient dogs) by Alexis Carrel in 1905. Between 1905 and 1967, when the first human heart was successfully transplanted orthotopically, a number of experimental observations had shown that the acutely denervated heart could adequately support the circulation. The clinical technic which made orthotopic cardiac homotransplantation possible was first described in 1959 by Lower, Stofer, and Shumway in dogs. Autotransplantation of the heart in dogs was pursued at length by Hurley and his associates at Stanford, who achieved long-term survivals, documenting that the nerves do regenerate.

Operative Technics

The technic in use by the Stanford group is shown in Fig 50–2. Central cannulations of the aorta and vena cava are performed to place the recipient on cardiopulmonary bypass. The recipient's diseased heart is removed by severing the atrium in a plane just posterior to the base of both atrial appendages and the great vessels just above the semilunar valves. The entrances of the 2 venae cavae and the pulmonary veins are left in situ at the end of the posterior walls of both atria. The donor heart is removed by severing the inferior and superior vena cavas and the great vessels at the pericardial reflections, and the pulmonary veins at their entrance into the left atrium. The left atrium is opened by interconnecting the pulmonary vein orifices. The superior vena cava is ligated. The right atrium is opened with a lateral incision extending from the inferior vena cava to the base of the atrial appendages.

Immunosuppression

The immunosuppressive regimen used in cardiac homotransplantation is essentially the same as that used in renal homotransplantation. The only notable

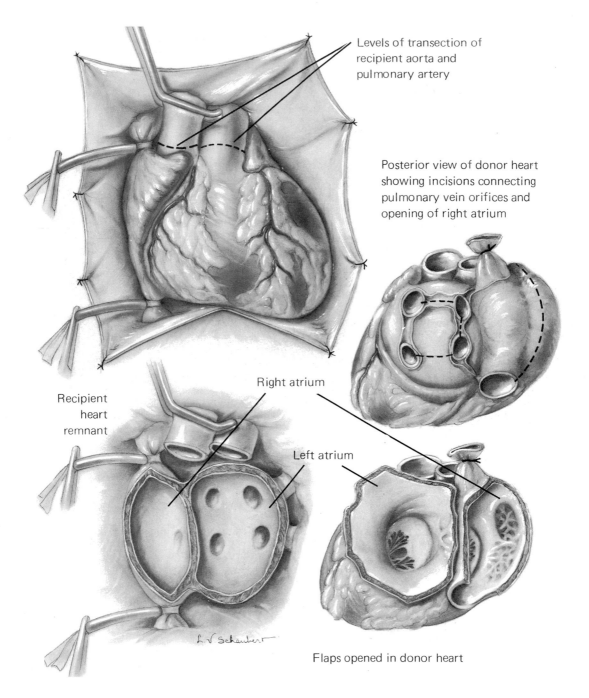

Levels of transection of recipient aorta and pulmonary artery

Posterior view of donor heart showing incisions connecting pulmonary vein orifices and opening of right atrium

Recipient heart remnant

Right atrium

Left atrium

L. V Schauberr

Flaps opened in donor heart

Figure 50—2. *Top left:* Recipient heart showing levels of transection across aorta and pulmonary artery. *Lower left:* Implantation site with recipient heart removed. *Top right:* Posterior view of donor heart showing lines of incision connecting pulmonary vein orifices and opening the right atrium in preparation for implantation. *Lower right:* Flaps opened in donor heart in preparation for implantation.

exception is that most patients who receive cardiac transplants have received intravenous or intramuscular antilymphocyte globulin.

Selection of Recipients

As of this writing, over 300 cardiac transplantations have been performed. Stanford University has accumulated the largest series, with a total 1-year survival rate of 53% in 121 recipients. The patient selected for cardiac transplantation must be in end stage cardiac failure for which no other medical or surgical therapy can be of benefit. However, patients with severely elevated pulmonary vascular resistance have an extremely poor prognosis following cardiac transplantation. This is because the normal right ventricle of the grafted heart is unable to work at the near-systemic pressures which are present in the lesser circulation. Progressive graft failure and patient death are the results of such transplants. It is currently felt that any patient whose pulmonary vascular resistance is less than 5 units and whose mean pulmonary artery pressure is less than 40 mm Hg does not face an increased risk of right ventricular failure postoperatively, as do those patients who have a very high pulmonary vascular resistance. Patients with a pulmonary vascular resistance greater than 10 units or a pulmonary artery pressure greater than 50 mm Hg have an extremely poor prognosis following cardiac transplantation. Younger patients appear to do better than older ones; this is related to the duration of their disease. Infection at the time of cardiac transplantation renders the patient a poor risk. Infection and increased pulmonary vascular resistance in the same patient are believed to be contraindications to the procedure.

Selection of Donors

Donors for cardiac transplantation must be young people who satisfy the criteria for neurologic death. This is essential because the donor heart must be of good quality, and immediate retrieval of the heart must be permissible on the basis of neurologic death.

Postoperative Course

The postoperative course following cardiac transplantation may vary depending upon whether or not the heart undergoes a rejection crisis. The diagnosis of rejection in heart transplants is a summary of all of the findings, the major ones being changes in the ECG and endomyocardial biopsy.

Bieber CP & others: Cardiac transplantation in man. VII: Cardiac allograft pathology. Circulation 41:753, 1970.

Griepp RB & others: Increasing patient survival following heart transplantation. Transplant Proc 9:197, 1977.

Hurley EJ, Lower RR, Shumway NE: Stokes-Adams attacks in transplanted hearts. Surg Forum 16:218, 1965.

LIVER TRANSPLANTATION

Liver transplantation has been studied extensively in the past 15 years, clinically as well as experimentally. Two surgical approaches have been used. The first approach is to transplant the liver as an extra organ in an animal or in a human (auxiliary transplants), a method first described by Welch in 1955. The second (much more common) approach is to replace the liver in its normal anatomic location after recipient hepatectomy (orthotopic transplantation). Although technically more difficult, orthotopic transplantation has been more successful, and some patients are still alive more than 3 years after transplantation.

In spite of extensive experimental studies and clinical trials, liver transplantation in man must still be considered an experimental procedure. Liver transplantation presents many problems. First, it is probably the most difficult transplant to perform since it requires an arterial anastomosis, 3 venous anastomoses, and a biliary anastomosis.

The donor organ obviously must come from a cadaver, and a major problem in early clinical transplantation was to obtain well-preserved cadaver organs capable of immediate and sustained function from the time of transplantation. The recognition and acceptance of brain death, in which the liver can be removed from the so-called heart-beating cadaver, has alleviated some of these problems.

Operative complications such as vascular thrombosis or biliary leaks are still common in the early postoperative period, and in many patients the cause of death has been technical rather than immunologic. In addition to the usual rejection episodes, which can occur at any time in the postoperative period, a separate type of rejection, called "septic infarction of the liver," is common in clinical cases. Septic infarction is probably caused by severe rejection involving the vascular supply of the liver with secondary infection by enteric organisms normally traveling through the portal system, resulting in infection and abscess formation in the ischemic infarcts. Although liver transplantation should only be performed by transplant centers with extensive experience in clinical and experimental transplantation, the slow but definite improvement in technics and survival suggests that patients with terminal nonmalignant liver disease can be considered for liver transplantation. Currently, over 30 recipients are alive with functioning grafts.

Calne RY, Williams R: Survival after orthotopic liver transplantation: A follow-up report of two patients. Br Med J 3:436, 1970.

Starzl TE & others: Biliary complications after liver transplantation: With special reference to biliary cast syndrome and techniques of secondary duct repair. Surgery 81:212, 1977.

Starzl TE & others: Indications for orthotopic liver transplantation: With particular reference to hepatomas, biliary atresia, cirrhosis, Wilson's disease and serum hepatitis. Transplant Proc 3:308, 1971.

Starzl TE & others: Orthotopic liver transplantation in 93 patients. Surg Gynecol Obstet 142:487, 1976.

PANCREATIC TRANSPLANTATION

Although pancreatic transplantation involves transplantation of a nonessential organ as compared to liver, heart, or kidney, it has an enormous potential in the management of patients with juvenile diabetes. In the juvenile diabetic, even though insulin and diet are carefully controlled, vascular injury to small arteries relentlessly continues. Many patients develop severe retinopathy at an early age, leading to blindness, renal disease and uremia, and peripheral vascular disease with severe neuropathy or limb loss.

Although pancreatic transplantation in animals has been extensively studied, animals (unfortunately) do not spontaneously develop diabetes mellitus, which would allow an investigation of the vascular change.

Unfortunately, almost all recipients of pancreatic grafts have died. Transplantation of isolated and viable islet cells may become the procedure of choice in future.

Lillehei RC & others: Current state of pancreatic allotransplantation. Transplant Proc 3:318, 1971.

Lillehei RC & others: Pancreatico-duodenal allotransplantation: Experimental and clinical experience. Ann Surg 172:405, 1970.

LUNG TRANSPLANTATION

Thirty-seven patients have received all or a part of a lung from an unrelated donor, but only one has survived for more than 1 month. Infection, hemorrhagic consolidation, and rejection are the major causes of failure. Because lungs ventilate air, which may contain microorganisms, lung transplants are more susceptible to infection than are transplants of other organs. Furthermore, denervation of the lung abolishes the cough reflex and temporarily alters the amount and character of mucus in the airways. These factors and the problem of obtaining uncontaminated donor lungs make infection a major barrier to successful lung transplantation.

Many patients and experimental animals develop hemorrhagic consolidation of the lung after transplantation. Although this complication may result from imperfect vascular anastomoses, pressure-flow studies show that pulmonary blood flow can increase to more than 3 times resting flows with only a slight increase in pulmonary vascular resistance. Hemorrhagic consolidation is not caused by changes in vascular resistance in the transplanted lung. It is probably caused by edema and congestion after division of lymphatics and an inflammatory process which accompanied rejection.

Rejection is the most serious barrier to successful lung transplantation. The process attacks pulmonary microvessels initially and is extremely difficult to control in unrelated animals or man. Physiologic alterations and problems in procurement and preservation can be controlled or solved, but, since the lung is primarily a vascular organ, successful lung transplants require improved methods for controlling rejection or improved technics of donor-recipient matching. At present, lung transplants cannot be considered to be of therapeutic value to the thousands of patients suffering from severe chronic respiratory insufficiency.

Derom F: Current state of lung transplantation. Transplant Proc 3:313, 1971.

Veith FJ, Blumenstock DA: Lung transplantation. J Surg Res 11:33, 1971.

• • •

General References

Birtch AG, Moore FD: Organ transplantation in New England: An anniversary note. N Engl J Med 287:129, 1972.

Calne RY (editor): *Clinical Organ Transplantation.* Davis, 1971.

Hamburger J & others (editors): *Renal Transplantation: Theory and Practice.* Williams & Wilkins, 1972.

Hardy JD (editor): *Human Organ Support and Replacement: Transplantation and Artificial Prostheses.* Thomas, 1971.

Lowrie EQ & others: Chronic hemodialysis and renal transplantation: Survival rates. N Engl J Med 288:863, 1973.

Mannick JA: Clinical kidney transplantation. Postgrad Med 54:171, 1973.

Miller J & others: Factors influencing morbidity and mortality of renal transplantation in a high risk population. Surg Gynecol Obstet 140:1, 1975.

Moore FD: *Transplant: The Give and Take of Tissue Transplantation.* Simon & Schuster, 1972.

Murray JE & others: Renal transplantation: A twenty-five year experience. Ann Surg 184:565, 1976.

Najarian JS, Simmons RL (editors): *Transplantation.* Lea & Febiger, 1972.

Park BH, Good RA: *Principles of Modern Immunobiology.* Lea & Febiger, 1974.

Veith FJ & others: Experience in clinical lung transplantation. JAMA 222:779, 1972.

Weiss W & others: Risk of lung cancer according to histologic type and cigarette dosage. JAMA 222:799, 1972.

Wildevuur CRH: *Morphology in Lung Transplantation.* Skarger, 1973.

51 . . .
Surgical Diagnostic & Therapeutic Procedures

Robert C. Lim, Jr., MD

The purpose of this chapter is to describe some of the more common procedures used in the practice of surgery. Descriptions of operating room equipment, instruments, and facilities for emergency resuscitation are beyond the scope of this chapter and will not be presented.

LACERATIONS

The healing of lacerations is dependent upon many factors, including the patient's age and nutritional and endocrine status, local temperature, blood supply, mechanical stresses, infections, and the presence of foreign bodies. Wound healing is discussed in Chapter 10.

The first step in the care of a simple laceration of the skin and subcutaneous tissues is cleansing and debridement of devitalized tissue. Irregular skin edges should be trimmed to allow accurate approximation of the wound. It is vital that hemostasis be achieved before wound closure is attempted. In closing the wound, subcutaneous tissues are approximated with fine catgut sutures and the skin is closed with interrupted sutures of fine nylon or other nonabsorbable material. Good cosmetic results demand accurate approximation of subcutaneous and epithelial layers. If the wound is grossly contaminated or is first seen more than 6–8 hours after the actual injury, it should be debrided, irrigated clean, and left open to allow healing by second or third intention. The wound is customarily dressed with iodoform gauze (to maintain skin edge separation) and is then covered with sterile dressings. Care must be taken not to close a contaminated wound (or a wound that contains a foreign body) since the end result is nearly always infection and abscess formation.

Wounds created by human or animal bites are heavily contaminated and are usually left open. After adequate debridement of devitalized and necrotic tissue, the patient should be treated with prophylactic antibiotics. If treated promptly, wounds about the head and neck may be closed because the blood supply to these areas is copious. Such procedures must be followed closely so that skin sutures can be removed and the wound opened at the first sign of infection. A culture should be taken immediately. In addition, further debridement may be necessary.

Management of Lacerations

Three things should be kept in mind in the management of lacerations: (1) prevention of infection, (2) preservation of function, and (3) the cosmetic result. The wound should be meticulously prepared by thorough mechanical cleansing, irrigation with isotonic saline, and surgical debridement of all necrotic tissue and foreign bodies. The area around the laceration is prepared with an appropriate antiseptic agent. Sterile drapes are applied around the wound. Lidocaine, 0.5% or 1%, is injected into the wound edges to obtain anesthesia before debridement of the contused tissues (Fig 51–1). Hemostasis is readily obtained by gentle pressure on the edges of the wound or by the use of fine absorbable ligatures. Raised flaps of skin should be thoroughly cleansed and their viability assessed. Irregular skin edges should be trimmed to allow accurate approximation.

Minor lacerations can be repaired by simple interrupted skin sutures of fine nylon. In facial lacerations, the most commonly used sutures are 6–0 or 5–0 monofilament nylon. In other areas of the body, 5–0 or 4–0 sutures are used. In deeper wounds, the fascia and subcutaneous tissue are approximated in layers with interrupted 4–0 or 3–0 plain catgut sutures. The skin is then approximated with interrupted fine nylon sutures. A dry, sterile dressing is usually placed over the wound for protection.

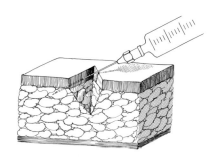

Figure 51–1. Injection of local anesthetic for wound closure.

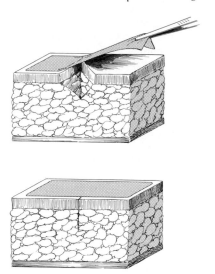

Figure 51—2. *Top:* Gentle traction is applied on the Steri-Strip to approximate the edges. *Bottom:* Closure of wound.

In facial lacerations, where the cosmetic result is of greatest importance, the finest possible suture material yields the best results. If the wound is clean and dry and no more than 3—4 mm wide, it can be closed with Steri-Strips instead of suture. This technic is especially useful in children and is performed as follows (Fig 51—2): (1) The skin is cleaned and dried. (2) Tincture of benzoin is applied to the skin and allowed to dry until tacky. (3) Half of each strip is placed on one side of the skin edge. (4) Gentle traction is applied to bring the 2 edges together. (5) The unattached half of each Steri-Strip is firmly placed on the opposite side of the wound.

In principle, if lacerations are deep, subcutaneous tissue must be approximated to eliminate dead space and to relieve the tension from the skin sutures.

Skin sutures should be left in place for approximately 7—10 days. Where the cosmetic result is important, skin sutures are removed in 2 or 3 days and the wound edges are supported with Steri-Strips or collodion strips. Care of the wound after repair of the laceration should include keeping the area clean and dry. Undue stress on the wound edges should be kept to a minimum. In some cases, immobilization with a splint may be necessary.

ABSCESSES

An abscess is a walled-off collection of pus. The terms boil, furuncle, and carbuncle refer to abscesses in the skin and subcutaneous tissue. A boil refers to a collection of pus which lies within the subcutaneous tissue. A furuncle is an abscess which originates in the sweat glands or hair follicles. A carbuncle refers to an abscess which has extended into the subcutaneous

tissue and is multiloculated, with individual compartments formed by anatomic fascial attachments of the skin to the deep fascia. Common sites for a carbuncle include the nape of the neck and the pulp of the digits. Abscesses of the integument are usually caused by staphylococci; however, they may become secondarily infected by gram-negative organisms. They may also be the result of contamination from penetrating wounds (eg, those seen with drug abuse).

Management of Abscesses

Adequate incision and drainage are important in the management of abscess. Local or regional anesthesia may be used. A skin incision is made over the fluctuant area, and a closed hemostat is then inserted through the subcutaneous tissue into the center of the abscess. Care should be taken not to penetrate too deeply. Once the abscess cavity is entered, the blades of the hemostat are spread apart to break up loculations. If the abscess cavity is large, digital examination should be performed to confirm complete drainage. The skin incision should extend the entire length of the abscess cavity to afford adequate drainage. Cruciate incisions should be used only rarely.

Carbuncles on the neck are best managed by total excision. Care should be taken that the advancing edge of the infection in the multiloculated compartments has been excised. The wound is packed open. Rapid closure by wound contraction without the need for skin grafting is the rule.

After evacuation of the abscess cavity, the wound should be drained by loosely inserting a strip of plain or iodoform fine-mesh gauze. Excessive oozing may be controlled by packing the cavity more firmly. Firm packing must be removed after 6—12 hours and replaced by loose gauze so that drainage is not impeded. Antibiotics are usually not used except when there are systemic manifestations of infection or persistent localized cellulitis in the region. The indications for antibiotics may be liberalized in treating wounds in special areas (eg, the hands) because the consequences of uncontrolled infection may be more severe.

Management of Other Pyogenic Infections

The treatment of cellulitis and lymphangitis due to nonsuppurative infection of the subcutaneous tissues consists of rest, heat, elevation, immobilization, and antibiotics (see Chapter 11). If the inflammatory process does not respond after 48 hours of therapy, suppuration and abscess formation should be suspected and drainage of any recognized collection is indicated.

When there is infection of the face, especially in the nasolabial area (the area with its border extending from the nasolabial fold to the outer canthus of each eye), aggressive antibiotic therapy is indicated because infection in this location carries a hazard of intracranial septic thrombophlebitis by spread from the nasal veins into the cavernous sinus. Morbidity and mortality are high when this occurs. Areas that are in close proximity to the occipital, mastoid, and frontal emissary veins should be of similar concern.

Management of Dental Abscess

Alveolar or apical abscess is usually related to poor oral hygiene and carious teeth. With necrosis of the dental pulp, periapical abscess causes severe pain and localized osteomyelitis around the root of the tooth. With further extension, the abscess will rupture through the buccal mucosa. If the abscess is pointing in the buccal mucosa and submucosal fluctuation is demonstrated, the abscess should be drained through an incision parallel to the gum margin. The patient should be given systemic antibiotics, and the tooth should be removed or root canal therapy should be done by a dentist. Occasionally, a periapical alveolar abscess will erode through the mandible to the outside of the face. Treatment in such cases is directed toward removal of the abscessed tooth, which is usually decayed and slightly loose.

SUPERFICIAL LESIONS

Excisional biopsy of subcutaneous tumors or skin lesions in an ambulatory patient is easily performed under local anesthesia. Infiltration of the skin and subcutaneous tissue around the lesion with 1% or 0.5% lidocaine will provide adequate anesthesia. The general principle in excisional biopsy is to make a skin incision which allows removal of the entire lesion with a margin of normal tissue. Hemostasis must be maintained to prevent seroma or hematoma formation, which will lead to wound complications. An elliptical incision should be made around the lesion parallel to the lines of skin tension. The incision should include a margin of 1–2 mm of normal skin. The length of the incision should be at least twice the width. Following removal of the lesion, the edges of the skin should be undermined to facilitate approximation without tension or puckering. The subcutaneous layer may be closed with interrupted fine catgut sutures if necessary to eliminate the dead space. The skin should be closed with fine monofilament sutures. If the lesion is in the subcutaneous tissue, a linear skin incision is placed over the center of the lesion along the lines of skin tension. Skin flaps are created and the lesion is completely excised with a margin of normal subcutaneous tissue. Following excision of such a lesion, subcutaneous tissue layers may be sutured or not depending upon the size and extent of the wound. For small wounds, a few skin stitches may be all that is necessary. A dry sterile dressing should then be applied.

INTRAVENOUS CANNULATIONS

The indications for catheterization of a major vein are to establish an avenue for administration of blood and fluid during resuscitation, to measure central venous pressure in monitoring patients, and to administer intravenous hyperalimentation in malnutritional states. The sites most commonly used are the subclavian, internal and external jugular, basilic, and saphenous veins. The surgeon must be thoroughly familiar with the anatomy of these vessels before the procedures are attempted.

Standard Leg Cutdown

The origin of the long saphenous vein can be used for intravenous cannulation for the administration of fluids and blood, but cutdowns in this location in adults are often complicated by thrombophlebitis. The vein always lies anterior to the medial malleolus. A small transverse skin incision is made as illustrated (Fig 51–3). Blunt dissection is done with a small curved hemostat to identify the saphenous vein, which usually lies just superficial to the deep fascia and periosteum. The saphenous nerve must be separated from the vein. Plain catgut (3–0 in adults and 4–0 or 5–0 in children) is used to encircle the vein on both sides of the site of cannulation. The distal ligature is tied and gentle traction is applied to put the vein on stretch. The surgeon is best positioned at the foot of the bed, facing the patient. A transverse or longitudinal venotomy is made depending on personal preference.

The transverse venotomy is quickly accomplished by inserting a No. 11 Bard-Parker scalpel blade through

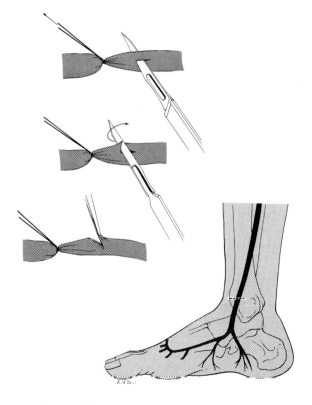

Figure 51–3. Leg cutdown with transverse venotomy.

the midportion of the vein with its cutting edge directed distally (Fig 51–3). The blade is then turned 90 degrees, directing the cutting edge upward and incising the upper half of the vein. This maneuver creates a small lip to grasp in exposing the lumen.

A small mosquito clamp is used to dilate the vein. An appropriate-sized plastic cannula is inserted into the lumen and secured in place with the proximal ligature. The skin is closed with 4–0 or 5–0 nylon sutures, allowing the cannula to exit through the skin incision. Antibiotic ointment and a sterile dressing are applied at the cannula exit site.

Cannulation of the Basilic Vein

Central venous cannulation through the basilic vein is best done by a surgical cutdown unless the patient has large, prominent arm veins which permit the percutaneous approach. In hypovolemic shock, the peripheral veins are usually collapsed, and time is often wasted in multiple attempts to cannulate them percutaneously. Surgical cutdown is preferred under these conditions. The patient is placed in the supine position with his right arm abducted 90 degrees. The antecubital area is prepared and draped aseptically. After infiltration of local anesthetic, a small transverse skin incision is placed anteromedially proximal to the antecubital crease over a demonstrable vein. A venous tourniquet may be helpful to delineate the vein. After the vein is isolated, the tourniquet should be removed. A ligature is placed around the vein distally, and gentle traction is maintained. A small venotomy is made with a pointed scalpel blade. The lumen of the vein is gently dilated by the insertion of a mosquito clamp. A premeasured catheter whose length equals the distance from the cutdown site to the suprasternal notch is inserted (Fig 51–4). This distance corresponds to the distance from the venotomy to the superior vena cava. When positioned, the tip of the catheter will be in the right location to measure central venous pressure. To confirm its location, chest x-rays can be obtained when a catheter with radiopaque markers is used. If the catheter does not have an x-ray marker, radiopaque dye can be instilled into the catheter when the chest film is taken. One of the more common pitfalls, inadvertent entry into the jugular vein, requires repositioning of the catheter.

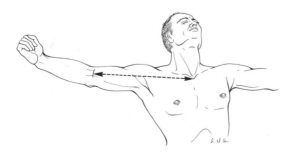

Figure 51–4. Length of catheter for basilic vein cannulation.

The catheter is then secured with a ligature around the proximal segment of the basilic vein. The wound is closed with several skin sutures. Antibiotic ointment is placed around the catheter exit site.

One of the complications of this type of cutdown is inadvertently opening the brachial artery. One should always feel for a pulse before incising the vessel, but the pulse may be difficult to detect in shock. If an opening is made in the brachial artery, it should be repaired immediately with several sutures of fine cardiovascular silk. Care must also be exercised in identifying peripheral nerves in this region which may, at times, be mistaken for veins.

Cutdown of the Saphenofemoral Junction

The saphenous vein can be surgically approached at its junction with the femoral vein. The groin area is aseptically prepared and draped. After infiltration with local anesthetic, a small transverse incision is made over the saphenofemoral junction approximately 3–4 cm lateral and inferior to the pubic spine. Dissection is carried through the subcutaneous tissue, isolating the saphenous vein and identifying the saphenofemoral junction. A ligature is placed distally around the saphenous vein, a small venotomy is made, and a catheter is passed through the saphenous vein into the femoral vein as far as the inferior vena cava. The appropriate length of the catheter may be estimated by measuring it from the cutdown site to the umbilicus. The catheter is secured with a ligature at the saphenofemoral junction. The wound is closed with interrupted catgut sutures in the subcutaneous tissue and nylon sutures to the skin. Antibiotic ointment is applied to the catheter wound site.

VENOUS CATHETERIZATION

Percutaneous Subclavian Catheterization

The patient should be supine and in a slight Trendelenburg position to avoid air embolism during this procedure. This is especially important in hypovolemic shock since the veins are usually collapsed. The head is placed in a neutral position or turned to the opposite side. The infraclavicular area is widely prepared aseptically. A small skin wheal is made with 1% lidocaine solution approximately 1 cm below the midportion of the clavicle. A large-bore needle attached to a 2 or 5 ml syringe is introduced through the skin wheal and directed toward the suprasternal notch (Fig 51–5). As the needle is advanced, slight negative pressure is applied to the syringe by pulling back on the plunger; when the vein is entered, blood will flow back freely. At this point, the syringe is removed and a catheter of appropriate size is inserted through the needle and advanced gently. After the catheter is advanced the desired length, the needle is withdrawn slowly and manual pressure is applied over the puncture site. The catheter is then secured in place

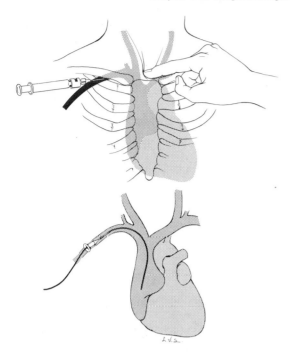

Figure 51–5. Percutaneous subclavian catheterization.

with a small skin stitch to prevent it from slipping into the vein or being pulled out inadvertently. Antibiotic ointment is placed over the puncture site to minimize ascending bacterial contamination.

The major complications resulting from subclavian catheterization are air embolism, embolization of a sheared-off catheter, pneumothorax, hematoma formation, and laceration of the subclavian artery.

To avoid catheter embolization, the catheter should never be withdrawn through the needle because a segment of the soft plastic may be sheared off by the beveled point inside the lumen of the vein, allowing it to float freely to the heart. Both catheter and needle must be withdrawn at the same time. Moreover, once the catheter is advanced, it must not be manipulated back and forth in an attempt to advance it further. If the catheter cannot be advanced to the desired length with ease, both the catheter and the needle should be removed and a different site used for cannulation.

To prevent formation of hematoma after the needle is withdrawn, gentle pressure should be applied over the puncture site. Pressure should be maintained while the patient is taken out of the Trendelenburg position. Gentle compression maintained for several minutes will allow the puncture site to seal around the catheter.

If the subclavian artery is entered, the needle is withdrawn immediately and manual pressure is maintained over the puncture for 10–15 minutes or longer.

Pneumothorax, due to inadvertent puncture of the cupula of the lung, occurs less often with the infraclavicular approach than with the supraclavicular approach. With the infraclavicular approach, the position

of the first rib prevents advancement of the needle into the pleural cavity. Auscultation of the chest should be done after the procedure is completed, and a portable chest x-ray should be obtained routinely.

Percutaneous Catheterization of the Internal Jugular Vein

The patient should be supine and in a slight Trendelenburg position. A small skin wheal is made with local anesthesia at the midportion of the sternocleidomastoid muscle at its posterior border. A needle with a syringe attached is introduced through the skin wheal and passed behind the muscle. As the needle is advanced toward the suprasternal notch, gentle negative pressure is applied on the syringe (Fig 51–6). Once the needle enters the jugular vein, blood will be drawn back. The syringe is then removed and a catheter of appropriate size is passed through the needle into the internal jugular vein for the desired distance. The needle is then withdrawn while the catheter is held in place. As the needle is withdrawn from the vein, gentle pressure is placed over the puncture site for several minutes to allow a hemostatic seal to form around the catheter. The patient is taken out of the Trendelenburg position, and the catheter is secured with a simple skin stitch.

The internal jugular vein can also be approached anteriorly. The patient is prepared as above except that the head is extended and turned to the opposite side. The needle is introduced overlying the juncture of the sternal and clavicular heads of the sternocleidomastoid muscle (Fig 51–7) and is directed inferiorly toward the clavicle at an angle of about 45 degrees from the coronal plane. The internal jugular vein usually lies deep to this area. If the internal jugular is not entered, the needle is withdrawn and then redirected several degrees laterally. The common carotid artery is

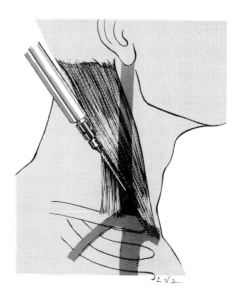

Figure 51–6. Internal jugular vein catheterization (posterior approach).

SWAN-GANZ FLOW-DIRECTED CATHETER

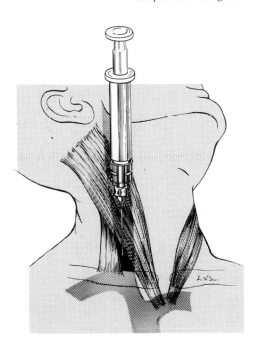

Figure 51–7. Internal jugular vein catheterization (anterior approach).

avoided because it is medial and posterior to the internal jugular vein. Once the vein is entered, blood will be aspirated freely into the syringe. The syringe is removed and a 15–20 cm (6–8 inch) catheter is advanced. The needle is then withdrawn and the catheter is secured to the skin with a simple skin stitch. Antibiotic ointment is placed at the puncture site as with the subclavian cannulation.

The major complications of internal jugular puncture are a large hematoma (secondary to carotid arterial puncture), catheter embolization, and, rarely, pneumothorax. If the common carotid artery is entered, the needle should be withdrawn and gentle pressure maintained over the puncture site for 10–15 minutes or longer. Precautions in avoiding catheter embolization are the same as described for the subclavian cannulation. Pneumothorax can be avoided if the manipulation of the needle is confined to the neck and the needle is not advanced too far into the inlet of the thoracic cavity.

Percutaneous Approach to the External Jugular Vein

The external jugular vein is a subcutaneous structure that runs vertically across the sternocleidomastoid muscle from the inferior tip of the parotid gland to the posterior triangle of the neck. The patient is positioned in a slight Trendelenburg position with his head extended and turned acutely to the opposite side. The external jugular vein should be visible, but it can be accentuated if the patient performs a Valsalva maneuver. Cannulation of this vessel is done as described above for cannulation of the subclavian or internal jugular vein.

The Swan-Ganz catheter, by allowing measurement of pulmonary artery pressures, gives useful information for regulating the rate of fluid or blood administration in patients with unstable cardiac conditions. It is also helpful in analyzing the cardiac status of a patient with a borderline cardiac index.

To insert the catheter, the patient is positioned supine with his arm abducted 90 degrees. Either arm can be used, but the right arm is preferable if it is available. A small transverse skin incision is made in the antecubital fossa, isolating and identifying the basilic vein. A small venotomy incision is made in the vein and the Swan-Ganz catheter is introduced into the lumen and passed upward into the subclavian vein. If it is difficult to negotiate passage around the deltopectoral area, the arm is further abducted to reduce angulation of the vessel at the thoracic inlet. Once the catheter is in the superior vena cava, it is connected to a pressure-sensitive transducer and the pressures are displayed on the oscilloscope. The catheter is then advanced through the right atrium, the tricuspid valve, and into the right ventricle, at which point the tracing shows systolic pressures of approximately 20–30 mm Hg. The balloon at the tip of the catheter is then inflated and the catheter is gently advanced. With each ejection of blood from the right ventricle, the catheter with the balloon inflated is carried by steps through the pulmonary valve and into the pulmonary artery. When this point is reached, the pulse pressure narrows; the systolic pressure remains at approximately 20 mm Hg, but the diastolic pressure increases to approximately 10 mm Hg. Once the catheter is in the pulmonary artery, it is further advanced with the balloon *deflated* until it reaches one of the secondary branches of the pulmonary artery. The balloon is then reinflated to obtain a wedged pressure: marked systolic fluctuation disappears in favor of a mean pressure approximately 6–10 mm Hg, ie, the normal pulmonary wedged pressure. This pressure is a direct transmission of pressure in the left atrium.

The balloon is then deflated, the catheter is secured in place in the antecubital area with a ligature around the vein and catheter, and the skin is closed with interrupted sutures. A second skin stitch looping around the catheter may be applied for extra security to maintain the catheter in place. Antibiotic ointment is placed around the catheter exit site in the skin, and a dry dressing is applied. The catheter should be flushed with heparinized saline solution periodically to avoid clotting of its tip.

TRACHEOSTOMY

Airway obstruction can occur as a result of trauma to or congenital deformities of the nose or larynx, tumors, infections, or paralysis of one or both vocal cords at birth. The most rapid way to establish an airway when the obstruction lies above the mid-point of the trachea is to install an endotracheal tube via the mouth or nose. A laryngoscope is used to visualize the vocal cords, and the endotracheal tube is then passed into the upper trachea. The patient should then be taken immediately to the operating room where a tracheostomy can be done under local or general anesthesia while the patient is oxygenated through the endotracheal tube. Sometimes it is necessary to perform a bedside tracheostomy, but when possible it is better to move the patient to the operating room.

The indications for tracheostomy include airway obstruction above the mid trachea or the need for prolonged assisted ventilation. Whenever there is infection in the larynx, an endotracheal tube should not be used any longer than necessary to do a tracheostomy because of the high incidence of mucosal injury and stenosis that results.

To establish a tracheostomy (Fig 51–8), a 5 cm vertical or horizontal collar incision is made 5–10 mm below the inferior edge of the cricoid cartilage. Dissection is carried down to the surface of the strap muscles, and vertical dissection is then carried between the strap muscles to the anterior surface of the cricoid, the thyroid isthmus, and the trachea. The isthmus of the thyroid is mobilized by blunt dissection and pushed cranially to expose the upper tracheal cartilages. A square (2 X 2 or 3 X 3 mm) segment of the third or fourth tracheal ring is excised, and the opening is enlarged by incising the membrane for 2–3 mm above and below the ring from which the segment was removed. Hemostasis is achieved with clamps and gut ligatures. The smallest tracheostomy tube that will permit adequate ventilation of the patient (rather than the largest one that can be forced into the trachea) is then installed. The largest tube that should be used in an adult male is a No. 6; in an adult female, No. 5. Children 6–10 years old usually do well with No. 3 tracheostomy tubes; and younger children and infants require a No. 1–2. A low-pressure balloon-cuffed tube may be used if assisted ventilation or prevention of aspiration is necessary. The incision is closed with one or 2 sutures at each end, care being taken not to close the incision under the face plate of the tracheostomy tube since this can result in subcutaneous emphysema, pneumomediastinum, and pneumothorax. A 10 X 10 cm (4 X 4 inch) sponge is cut two-thirds of the way up the center and placed under the face plate; the cloth tapes attached to the face plate are then tied tightly enough to prevent the tube from coming out of the trachea without being so tight that they occlude the external jugular vein. If a low-pressure balloon-cuffed tube is used, the balloon should be inflated only until the airway becomes airtight when the tracheostomy tube is temporarily occluded. It should be completely deflated 4 times per day and reinflated only until the airway again becomes airtight when the tube is occluded. Overinflation of a balloon cuff causes tracheal necrosis and stenosis.

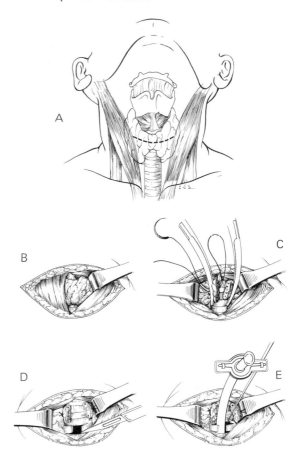

Figure 51–8. Technic of tracheostomy. *A:* Collar incision one fingerbreadth below cricoid from sternocleidomastoid to sternocleidomastoid. *B:* Vertical line of dissection down to thyroid isthmus, cricoid, and anterior trachea. *C:* If the thyroid isthmus cannot be mobilized to expose the third or fourth ring, it should be divided as shown. *D:* Square segment removed from third or fourth tracheal ring with horizontal extension incision in membrane above and below this ring. *E:* Smallest possible (not largest possible) tracheostomy tube is installed (adult male, No. 6; adult female, No. 5; 10-year-old, No. 3; infant, No. 1 or No. 0).

Postoperative roentgenograms of the chest (posteroanterior and lateral views) should be taken to show whether the tube fits the trachea properly and to rule out pneumothorax. The tracheostomy tube should not be removed until it can be plugged continuously for 48 hours without impairing respiratory function. At that point, the tube is removed, and the stoma gradually closes in about 7 days.

INSERTION OF CHEST TUBE
(Tube Thoracostomy)

Tubes for drainage are inserted into the thoracic cavity to evacuate a pneumothorax, hemothorax, or empyema (pyothorax). Experience has shown that attempts to remove intrathoracic collections with needle aspiration are usually unsatisfactory, and this technic is rarely employed except occasionally for a small pneumothorax.

Pneumothorax. If a tension pneumothorax exists, it should be immediately decompressed by a needle introduced through the second anterior intercostal space. A tube thoracostomy can then be performed unhurriedly.

For pneumothorax, a chest tube is usually inserted through the second or third anterior intercostal space in the midclavicular line and directed toward the apex of the thorax. The tube is attached to the suction device, and the rate of escape of air is indicated by the appearance of bubbles in the second of the 3 bottles. When bubbling ceases, this suggests that the pulmonary air leak has become sealed. Chest x-rays should be taken at intervals to verify full expansion of the lung. The tube is usually left in place for about 24 hours after the leak has sealed and full expansion has been achieved. It is then removed aseptically.

Hemothorax. To evacuate a hemothorax, a tube is usually inserted through the fifth or sixth intercostal space slightly posterior to the anterior axillary line. This level is preferable to a lower one because it lessens the risk of penetrating the diaphragm during insertion of the tube and avoids later problems from the tube lying on the diaphragm. Drainage is just as satisfactory in this location.

Empyema. The tube is usually inserted over the center of the collection as determined by x-ray. With small collections, fluoroscopy is sometimes desirable to accurately pinpoint the site. After a stab wound is made, a large (40–45F) catheter is inserted to drain the pus. Loculations are often present and must be broken down with a finger in order to accomplish thorough drainage. If the pus is especially thick and contains fibrin or necrotic tissue fragments, it should be lavaged vigorously by injecting saline through the thoracostomy tube. In cases when adequate drainage cannot be obtained by tube thoracostomy, drainage via open thoracostomy and the creation of a pleurocutaneous flap (Eloesser) must be done (Chapter 21).

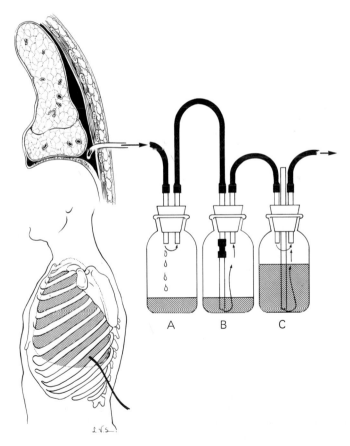

Figure 51–9. Technic of tube thoracostomy. The 3-bottle set-up serves to provide continuous mild suction and a safeguard against pneumothorax. *Bottle A* is connected to the thoracostomy tube and collects pleural drainage for inspection and measurement of volume. *Bottle B* acts as a simple valve to prevent collapse of the lung if tubing external to this point is opened to atmospheric pressure. Pulmonary air leak can be detected by the escape of bubbles from the submerged tube. *Bottle C* is a system for regulating the negative pressure delivered to the pleural space. Wall suction should be regulated to maintain continuous vigorous bubbling from the middle open tube in bottle C. The resulting negative pressure (in cm water) is equal to the difference in the height of the fluid levels in bottles B and C.

Technic of Tube Thoracostomy

The patient is positioned supine with his arm abducted at a 90 degree angle. The skin is prepared and draped aseptically. The skin and subcutaneous tissues are anesthetized with 1% lidocaine, and a 2.5 cm (1 inch) transverse skin incision is made over the superior border of the rib at the site selected for the tube. The pleural space is entered by blunt dissection with a curved clamp over the superior edge of the rib, which avoids injuring the intercostal vessels. The jaws of the clamp are spread, enlarging the opening enough to permit the introduction of a finger into the pleural cavity. Digital examination should be performed to confirm the absence of pleural adhesions; this will prevent inadvertent insertion of the tube into adherent lung parenchyma. If the lung is adherent, it can easily be separated by gentle blunt dissection with the finger. The chest tube is grasped with a clamp and inserted into the thorax and positioned for optimal drainage. During insertion, the tube may slide into a subcutaneous space, and the malposition may go unrecognized unless tube function is tested.

After the position is checked, the tube is connected to underwater sealed suction regulated to 10–20 cm water negative pressure (Fig 51–9). The tube should be fixed to the chest wall with No. 0 silk sutures placed so they can be used to close the wound after the tube is removed. A sterile dressing is then applied.

THORACENTESIS

The optimal site for aspiration is selected by correlation of x-ray (or fluoroscopic) localization with the chest wall area of maximal flatness to percussion. Thoracentesis is rarely productive when performed below the eighth interspace in the midaxillary line even if a large volume of fluid is present. The most common mistake is to choose a location which is too low, which results in an unsuccessful tap because the diaphragm is sucked up against the needle. Shoulder and neck discomfort due to referred pain in the distribution of the phrenic nerve may suggest this complication. Persistent attempts to enter the pleural space may produce iatrogenic splenic injury as the needle is passed through the diaphragm.

The easiest position for the patient is straddling an armless straight-backed chair, facing the back with his forearms resting on the top. The operator can sit on another chair behind him or to one side. If the patient becomes faint or dizzy, he can rest his head on his folded arms without altering the position of his thorax. An alternative position is supine in bed. The affected side is slightly elevated by means of a folded towel placed under the hemithorax. The patient's arm is extended at his side, and the site of thoracentesis is selected at the fourth or fifth intercostal space along the posterior axillary line.

The chest wall is prepared widely, using sterile precautions. A small skin wheal is raised with 1% lidocaine or comparable local anesthetic at the appropriate site. A 25 gauge needle is used, and the local anesthetic is injected as the needle is slowly advanced. When the parietal pleura is reached, minimal resistance will be perceived and more anesthetic is injected. A slight "popping" sensation is felt as the needle tip passes through the parietal membrane and enters the pleural space. The infiltration needle is withdrawn, and a small nick is made in the skin with a pointed scalpel. A short-beveled, blunt-tipped 13 gauge aspirating needle is attached to a 50 ml glass (not plastic) Luer-Lok syringe by means of a 3-way stopcock which has both female and male Luer-Lok attachments. One hand pushes on the syringe as the other hand acts as a "brake" on the needle at the skin surface and the needle is introduced smoothly into the pleural cavity. Aspiration is facilitated by lubricating the syringe barrel and plunger with lidocaine solution throughout its full length at the beginning of the procedure. Steady, gentle withdrawal of the syringe barrel prevents the visceral pleura from being sucked up against the needle orifice and permits a free flow of even very thick, fibrin-containing exudate. The stopcock handle is turned to allow discharge of the material through the side-arm (with a short length of tubing attached) into a large sterile flask containing heparin. During collection, it is important for the nurse assistant to agitate the container gently to prevent clotting of the fluid, which otherwise will occur when the effusion is high in fibrin and protein content. When most of the fluid has been removed from the pleural space, it will flow freely only during the inspiratory phase of the respiratory cycle; at this point, the patient is asked to take slow, gradual, deep breaths and to lean backward toward the side of involvement, holding onto the back of the chair.

More recently, we have been using a large Intracath to drain pleural effusions. The needle is fitted with a syringe and introduced into the pleural space over the superior aspect of the rib. Once the pleural cavity is entered, the syringe is removed and the catheter is inserted and directed into the most dependent position of the pleural cavity. The needle is then removed, and aspiration of the fluid with a 3-way stopcock attached to it is then performed as described above. The advantage of this technic is that one can alter the position of the patient without having a rigid needle sticking in his thoracic chest wall. This technic has been most helpful in reducing the incidence of pneumothorax following thoracentesis.

When a known malignant effusion is being evacuated, it is best to stop just short of complete withdrawal of all obtainable fluid so that 20 mg of mechlorethamine or another antitumor agent dissolved in 50 ml of normal saline can be instilled into the pleural space. The needle is then withdrawn and the patient is placed for 1 hour supine, for 1 hour with the involved side down, and for 1 hour prone to distribute the medication over all serous surfaces. A chest x-ray should be taken 6–12 hours later because there is usually a reaccumulation of fluid as a result of the chemical pleuritis caused by the irritant effect of mechlorethamine. Repeat thoracentesis is then performed in an effort to tap the chest "dry" and give the pleural surfaces the best opportunity for adhesive fusion. Successful obliteration of the pleural space is the usual result and prevents further accumulation of fluid.

LUMBAR PUNCTURE

Lumbar puncture is an easily performed but frequently misused diagnostic tool which is potentially lethal. It should be done only in an effort to answer a specific clinical question—never "routinely" and never (unless essential to diagnosis) when signs of increased intracranial pressure are present.

Technic

The patient should be placed on his side in the fetal position (Fig 51—10). The lumbosacral area is prepared with an antiseptic solution; the skin over the L3—4 or L4—5 interspace is infiltrated with local anesthetic; and a 19- or 20-gauge needle is introduced with its bevel parallel to the spinal axis. (Since the spinal cord does not terminate before reaching approximately the level of L2, punctures at or above this level could damage the cord. Cisterna magna and lateral cervical punctures can be done, but only in special situations by experienced personnel.) The needle is connected to a manometer; if the opening pressure is elevated, only the CSF in the manometer should be withdrawn.

Indications

A. Diagnosis of Hemorrhage: When subarachnoid hemorrhage is suspected, red cells in the CSF will be diagnostic. Truly bloody CSF can be differentiated from the bloody CSF due to a traumatic tap because, with the latter, the CSF will become progressively clearer with each successive specimen. Bloody CSF should be centrifuged and the supernatant examined for xanthochromia. The degree of xanthochromia will provide some index of the length of time the red cells have been in the CSF. Crenation of red blood cells is a meaningless sign. The presence of red cells in the CSF may be associated with a lowered CSF glucose, but the length of time the cells have been present does not affect the level of glucose.

B. Diagnosis of Infection: In the patient with purulent meningitis, lumbar puncture is usually diagnostic; the pressure will be increased; white cells will be present, the number and type depending on the etiologic agent; the protein will be increased; and the glucose will be decreased. CSF should be obtained for routine culture as well as for cultures for anaerobic bacteria, fungi, and tubercle bacilli.

A traumatic lumbar puncture may produce confusing CSF findings.

The CSF may be normal in cases of brain abscess, subdural empyema, or epidural abscess, although the pressure is frequently elevated. CSF findings in meningeal metastatic carcinoma may simulate those of meningitis but can frequently be differentiated by cytologic studies. Active neurosyphilis produces CSF abnormalities, the exact findings depending on the type of involvement: serologic tests on blood and CSF may be positive; the pressure may be increased; the protein and cell count (lymphocytes) may be increased; and the colloidal gold curve may be abnormal.

C. Evaluation of Spinal Trauma: In cases of spinal trauma, lumbar puncture is frequently done to determine if a block is present in the spinal CSF pathway. After the needle is inserted, the jugular veins are compressed while the examiner notes the rise and fall of CSF pressure (Queckenstedt's test). When this test is performed, one should be prepared to proceed with contrast medium myelography if indicated.

Lumbar puncture is seldom useful following acute head injuries, but it may be useful in more chronic situations to determine the presence of blood or elevated CSF pressure.

Contraindications & Side-Effects

Lumbar puncture should not be done in the presence of papilledema or other manifestations of increased intracranial pressure unless essential for diag-

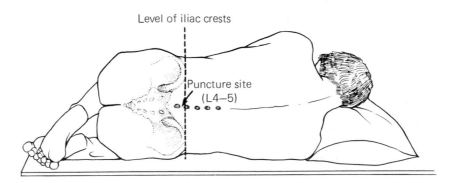

Figure 51—10. Lying position for lumbar puncture. (Reproduced, with permission, from Krupp MA & others: *Physician's Handbook,* 18th ed. Lange, 1976.)

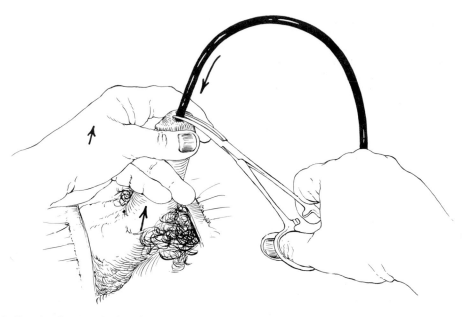

Figure 51–11. Technic of catheterization. A sterile water-soluble lubricant is first instilled into the urethra by means of a bulb syringe. The penis is drawn taut with one hand. The catheter, held near its tip with a sterile clamp, is introduced into the urethra; the other end of the catheter is held between the fourth and fifth fingers of the hand holding the clamp. The clamp is then moved up on the catheter and the catheter introduced farther into the urethra. (Reproduced, with permission, from Smith DR: *General Urology,* 8th ed. Lange, 1975.)

nosis. *Note:* In such situations, lumbar puncture may be fatal.

At least 20% of patients will complain of headache and stiff neck after diagnostic lumbar puncture. This will be self-limiting but may persist for days. It is absent when the patient lies flat, and can usually be prevented if the patient remains flat for 12 hours after the procedure. It is presumably related to persistent leakage of CSF at the site of needle puncture. The headache is occasionally associated with fever and is essentially an aseptic meningitis. Rarely, a septic process will result. Local structures in the area of the lumbar puncture, including the intervertebral disk, may be traumatized by the procedure, but this rarely happens.

CATHETERIZATION OF THE BLADDER

Urinary catheters are introduced into the bladder for diagnostic purposes, as in blunt trauma with renal injuries or pelvic fractures, and for the relief of urinary retention, as in prostatic obstruction. Indwelling catheters (Foley) are inserted to allow for continuous monitoring of urine output.

The size of the catheter will depend upon the size of the patient. In men, catheters that are too small tend to bend and coil within the urethra. Size 18–22F catheters may be used in adults with very little trauma. In children, size 8–12F may be used.

Catheterization in Males

The genital area is draped and the penis is held taut with one hand. The meatus and glans are prepped aseptically. The catheter can be introduced with a sterile gloved hand or with a sterile clamp. The catheter should be well lubricated with water-soluble lubricant. In some patients with bladder neck obstruction, the lubricant should be instilled into the urethra with a syringe before the catheter is introduced. As the catheter is advanced, there will be a momentary obstruction at the external sphincter. By maintaining gentle pressure on the catheter and keeping the penis perpendicular and taut, the catheter tip will usually overcome the sphincteric spasm and enter the bladder (Fig 51–11).

Before inserting a Foley catheter, the balloon is blown up to check its integrity. It is then deflated and the catheter introduced into the bladder as described above. The balloon is reinflated to the appropriate volume with sterile saline and the catheter connected to a closed drainage system.

If there is a tight urethral stricture, it will be necessary to use sounds or filiforms and followers to dilate the area of obstruction.

Catheterization in Females

The genital area is draped and the labia held apart with one hand. The labia and meatus are cleansed with antiseptic solution. With a sterile gloved hand or a clamp, the catheter is introduced and passed into the bladder.

PERITONEAL LAVAGE

To diagnose intra-abdominal bleeding after blunt trauma, peritoneal lavage is more accurate than needle paracentesis in 2 or 4 quadrants. The principal indication is suspected intra-abdominal bleeding when the clinical findings are equivocal. Peritoneal lavage is hazardous in unconscious patients or those unable to cooperate. If the patient has had previous abdominal operations, adhesions may be present that fix the intestines, and the abdominal catheter must be inserted with great care. False-positive results due to iatrogenic bleeding from mesenteric vessels are common in these patients.

With the patient in the supine position, the lower abdomen is prepared with iodine and 70% alcohol. The bladder must be empty. The skin and subcutaneous tissues are infiltrated with local anesthetic at the site where the catheter is to be introduced, halfway between the umbilicus and pubis. A small incision is made in the skin. By flexing the head, the patient can tighten the anterior abdominal musculature and a peri-

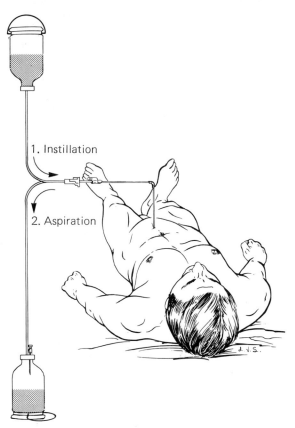

Figure 51–13. Technic of peritoneal lavage.

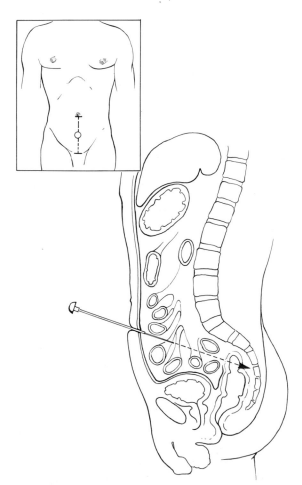

Figure 51–12. Direction of insertion of stylet for abdominal paracentesis.

toneal dialysis catheter is advanced with a pop into the peritoneal cavity (Fig 51–12). An alternative technic is to make a 1 cm incision in the fascia and introduce the catheter under direct vision. This method is safer, especially in uncooperative patients or when adhesions are present. Once the catheter passes through the peritoneum, the stilet is withdrawn and the catheter is advanced gradually toward the hollow of the sacrum. If blood wells up in the catheter as it is advanced, a positive diagnosis of intra-abdominal bleeding is made. The catheter should be promptly withdrawn and the patient prepared for immediate operation.

Even with significant abdominal bleeding, it is unusual for gross blood to appear spontaneously in the catheter. Therefore, after the catheter is positioned, instill 1000 ml of normal saline or lactated Ringer's solution (not 5% dextrose in water) into the peritoneal cavity over 10–15 minutes. During the infusion the patient should be encouraged to roll from side to side to distribute the fluid throughout the peritoneal cavity. Then place the empty infusion bottle on the floor and allow the fluid to return by gravity. Make sure there is an air vent by inserting a large bore needle in the cap of the empty bottle (Fig 51–13).

A negative test is one in which the fluid returning into the bottle is clear or only slightly tinged with blood. If the color is as deep as rosé wine, there is intra-abdominal bleeding. One should familiarize one-self with the color of the different shades of red produced by 1, 2, 5, and 10 ml of whole blood mixed with 1 liter of saline. A hematocrit of 1% or more in the recovered lavage solution is indicative of significant bleeding.

Sachatello CR, Bivins B: Technique for peritoneal dialysis and diagnostic peritoneal lavage. Am J Surg 131:637, 1976.

INSERTION OF SCRIBNER SHUNT

Scribner shunts are used for hemodialysis in acute renal failure and for administering hyperosmotic nutrient solutions (hyperalimentation). The sites most readily used are at the ankle, where the long saphenous vein and the posterior tibial or anterior tibial arteries can be cannulated, and in the forearm, where the cephalic vein and radial artery can be cannulated.

The patient is placed in the supine position. The operative area is prepared and draped aseptically. Local anesthesia is achieved by infiltration with 1% lidocaine. Longitudinal skin incisions are made over the artery and vein. The vessels are dissected and isolated with 3–0 nonabsorbable sutures. The largest size Teflon cannula tip that will fit into the vessel with ease is selected and connected to a Silastic tube with a reverse U curve at the end. Heparin-saline solution is injected into the tubing and cannula to evacuate the air, and the free end of the Silastic tube is clamped. Through a longitudinal venotomy and arteriotomy, the cannulas are introduced into the vein and artery, respectively. They are secured in place with several ligatures around the vessel and tubing in the manner illustrated (Fig 51–14). The loop of the Silastic tubing is positioned under the skin, avoiding angulation or axial twisting of the vessel. The free ends of the tubing are brought out through separate small skin incisions and are reconnected to each other. A rapid flow should be noted in the arteriovenous connection when the occluding clamps are removed. The operative site is closed with interrupted catgut sutures to the subcutaneous tissue and fine nylon sutures to the skin. Antibiotic ointment is applied around the tubing at its exit sites.

ARTERIOVENOUS FISTULA

The internal subcutaneous arteriovenous fistula has almost completely replaced the Scribner shunt (external arteriovenous communication) for long-term

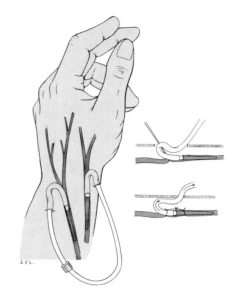

Figure 51–14. Scribner shunt.

maintenance hemodialysis in chronic renal failure and in temporary support of pre- and postoperative renal transplant patients.

The most common site for the creation of arteriovenous fistula is between the radial artery and the origin of the cephalic vein just proximal to the styloid process of the radius. This is easily accomplished in a side-to-side or end-to-side fashion with fine No. 6–0 or 7–0 sutures. After a period of maturation, the venous channels dilate and become arterialized to allow repeated needle insertions for hemodialysis.

If the above vessels are not available, grafts have been used to create the arteriovenous fistula. The most popular is an autogenous saphenous vein joining the radial or ulnar artery at the wrist to a large antecubital vein or the basilic vein in the proximal arm. If the wrist arteries have been ligated previously or are too small, a U-shaped arteriovenous fistula can be performed between the brachial artery and the antecubital vein or basilic vein, looping a saphenous vein graft subcutaneously in the forearm. An arteriovenous fistula can also be created between the saphenous vein and the superficial femoral artery at the adductor canal. The saphenous vein in this technic should be removed from its original bed and tunneled in a more subcutaneous position for easy access by percutaneous puncture.

When a segment of autologous saphenous vein is not available, a homograft can be used. More recently, bovine grafts have been tried with good success. Other synthetic materials have not been successful clinically.

• • •

Appendix

NORMAL VALUES

HEMATOLOGY

Bleeding time: 1–7 minutes (Ivy).

Cellular measurements of red cells: Average diameter = 7.3 μm (5.5–8.8 μm).
Mean corpuscular volume (MCV): 82–92 fl. (Coulter method: men, 87 ± 7 fl; women, 90 ± 9 fl.)
Mean corpuscular hemoglobin (MCH): 27–31 pg.
Mean corpuscular hemoglobin concentration (MCHC): 32–37%
Color, saturation, and volume indices: 1 (0.9–1.1)

Clot retraction: Begins in 1–3 hours; complete in 24 hours.

Coagulation time (Lee-White): At 37 C, 6–12 minutes; at room temperature, 10–18 minutes.

Fragility of red cells: Begins at 0.45–0.38% NaCl; complete at 0.36–0.3% NaCl.

Hematocrit (PCV): Men, 45–52%; women, 37–47%.

Hemoglobin [B]: Men, 14–18 gm/100 ml; women, 12–16 gm/100 ml. (Serum hemoglobin: 2–3 mg/100 ml.)

Platelets: 200–400 thousand/μl.

Prothrombin [P]: 75–125%.

Red blood count (RBC): Men, 4.5–6.2 million/μl; women, 4–5.5 million/μl.

Reticulocytes: 0.5–1.5% of red cells.

Sedimentation rate: Less than 20 mm/hour (Westergren); 0–10 mm/hour (Wintrobe).

White blood count (WBC) and differential: 5–10 thousand/μl.

Myelocytes	0 %
Juvenile neutrophils	0 %
Band neutrophils	0–5 %
Segmented neutrophils	40–60%
Lymphocytes	20–40%
Eosinophils	1–3 %
Basophils	0–1 %
Monocytes	4–8 %

BLOOD (B), PLASMA (P), OR SERUM (S): CHEMICAL CONSTITUENTS

Below are listed the specimen used, the amount of blood [B], plasma [P], or serum [S] needed to provide an adequate specimen, the fasting state, and the normal values. Values vary with the procedure employed.

Acetone bodies: [P, 2 ml] 0.3–2 mg/100 ml.

Aldolase: [S, 4 ml] 4–14 units/ml (Bruns). Men, < 33 units; women, < 19 units (Warburg and Christian).

Aldosterone: [P] Up to 20 ng/100 ml.

Amino acid nitrogen: [P, 2 ml fasting] 3–5.5 mg/100 ml.

Ammonia*: [B, 2 ml] 40–70 μg/100 ml.

Amylase: [S, 2 ml] 80–180 units/100 ml (Somogyi). 0.8–3.2 IU/liter.

a_1-Antitrypsin: [S, 1 ml] 3.3–10 mg/ml

Ascorbic acid: [P, 7 ml] 0.4–1.5 mg/100 ml.

Base, total serum: [S, 2 ml] 145–160 mEq/liter.

Bilirubin: [S, 3 ml]. (Van den Bergh test.) Direct, 0.1–0.4 mg/100 ml. Indirect, 0.2–0.7 mg/100 ml.

Calcium: [S, 2 ml fasting] 9–10.6 mg/100 ml; 4.5–5.3 mEq/liter (varies with protein concentration).

Calcium, ionized: [S, 1 ml] 4.25–5.25 mg/100 ml.

CO_2 combining power: [S or P, 1 ml] 55–75 vol %.

CO_2 content: [S or P, 1 ml] 24–29 mEq/liter; 55–65 vol%.

Carotenoids: [S, 2 ml fasting] 50–300 μg/100 ml.

Ceruloplasmin: [S, 2 ml] 23–50 mg/100 ml.

Chloride: [S, 1 ml] 96–106 mEq/liter; 340–375 mg/100 ml (as chloride).

Cholesterol: [S, 1 ml] 150–280 mg/100 ml.

*Do not use anticoagulant containing ammonium oxalate.

Cholesterol esters: [S, 1 ml] 50–65% of total cholesterol.

Copper: [S, 5 ml] 70–165 µg/100 ml.

Cortisol: [P] 4–18 µg/100 ml (circadian variation).

Creatine phosphokinase: [S, 3 ml] 0–4.5 units (Hughes). 10–50 IU/liter.

Creatinine: [B or S, 1 ml] 0.7–1.5 mg/100 ml.

Epinephrine: [P] < 0.1 µg/liter.

Folic acid: [S, 4 ml] > 5–24 ng/ml.

Glucose (Folin): [B, 0.1–1 ml fasting] 80–120 mg/100 ml.

Glucose (true): [B, 0.1–1 ml fasting] 60–100 mg/100 ml.

Iodine, butanol-extractable (BEI): [S, 10 ml] 3–6.5 µg/100 ml.

Iodine, protein-bound (thyroid hormone, PBI): [S, 5 ml] 4–8 µg/100 ml.

Iodine, thyroxine: [S, 5 ml] 2.9–6.4 µg/100 ml.

Iron: [S, 2 ml] 65–175 µg/100 ml.

Iron-binding capacity, total: [S, 2 ml] 250–410 µg/100 ml. Percent saturation: 20–25%.

Lactate dehydrogenase (SLDH): [S, 2 ml] 215–540 units (Wroblewski). 90–200 IU/liter.

Lactic acid: [B, 2 ml in iodoacetate] 0.44–1.8 mM/liter; 4–16 mg/100 ml.

Lipase: [S, 2 ml] 0.2–1.5 units (ml of 0.1 N NaOH).

Lipids, total: [S] 500–600 mg/100 ml.

Magnesium: [S, 2 ml] 1.5–2.5 mEq/liter. (1.8–3 mg/100 ml).

Nonprotein nitrogen (NPN)*: [S or B, 1 ml] 15–35 mg/100 ml.

Norepinephrine: [P] < 0.5 µg/liter.

Osmolality: [S, 5 ml] 285–295 mOsm/kg water.

Oxygen:
Capacity: [B, 5 ml] 16–24 vol% (varies with hemoglobin concentration).

*Do not use anticoagulant containing ammonium oxalate.

Arterial content: [B, 5 ml] 15–23 vol% (varies with hemoglobin concentration).
Arterial % saturation: 94–100% of capacity.
Arterial P_{O_2} (Pa_{O_2}): 80–100 mm Hg (sea level).

Pa_{CO_2}: [Arterial blood, 5 ml] 35–45 mm Hg.

pH (reaction): [P (arterial), 1 ml] 7.35–7.45.

Phosphatase, acid: [S, 2 ml] 1–5 units (King-Armstrong), 0.5–2 units (Bodansky), 0.5–2 units (Gutman), 0–1.1 units (Shinowara), 0.1–0.63 units (Bessey-Lowry). Females: 0.2–9.5 IU/liter. Males: 0.5–11 IU/liter.

Phosphatase, alkaline: [S, 2 ml] 5–13 units (King-Armstrong), 2–4.5 units (Bodansky), 3–10 units (Gutman), 2.2–8.6 units (Shinowara). Adults, 0.8–2.3 units (Bessey-Lowry); children, 2.8–6.7 units (Bessey-Lowry). Adults, 30–85 IU/liter.

Phosphorus, inorganic: [S, 1 ml fasting] 3–4.5 mg/100 ml (children, 4–7 mg); 0.9–1.5 mM/liter.

Phospholipid: [S, 2 ml] 145–200 mg/100 ml.

Potassium: [S, 1 ml] 3.5–5 mEq/liter; 14–20 mg/100 ml.

Protein:
Total: [S, 1 ml] 6–8 g/100 ml.
Albumin: [S, 1 ml] 3.5–5.5 g/100 ml.
Globulin: [S] 1.5–3 mg/100 ml.
Fibrinogen: [P, 1 ml] 0.2–0.4 g/100 ml.

Prothrombin clotting time: [P, 2 ml] By control.

Pyruvic acid: [B, 2 ml] 0.07–0.22 mM/liter; 0.6–2 mg/100 ml.

Serotonin: [B] 0.05–0.2 µg/ml.

Sodium: [S, 1 ml] 136–145 mEq/liter; 310–340 mg/100 ml (as Na).

Specific Gravity:
[B, 0.1 ml] 1.056 (varies with hemoglobin and protein concentration).
[S, 0.1 ml] 1.0254–1.0288 (varies with protein concentration).

Sulfate: [P or S, 2 ml] 0.5–1.5 mEq/liter.

Thyroxine: [S, 3 ml] 4–11 µg/100 ml T_4 (by CPB).

Transaminases: [S, 2 ml]
Glutamic-oxaloacetic (SGOT), 5–40 units: 6–25 IU/liter at 30 C.
Glutamic-pyruvic (SGPT), 5–35 units; 3–26 IU/liter at 30 C.

Triglycerides: [S, 1 ml] < 165 mg/100 ml. (5.4 mEq/liter).

Triiodothyronine: [S, 2 ml] 60–190 ng/100 ml.

Triiodothyronine uptake (RT₃U): [S, 3 ml] 10–14.6%.

Urea nitrogen*: [S or B, 1 ml] 8–20 mg/100 ml.

Uric acid: [S, 1 ml] 3–7.5 mg/100 ml.

Vitamin B₁₂: [S, 2 ml] > 100 pg ml.

Volume, blood (Evans blue dye method): Adults, 2990–6980 ml. Women, 46.3–85.5 ml/kg; men, 66.2–97.7 ml/kg.

Zinc: [S, 3 ml] 65–145 μg/ml.

NORMAL CSF VALUES

Appearance: Clear and colorless.

Chlorides (as NaCl): 700–750 mg/100 ml; 120–130 mEq/liter.

Colloidal gold (gold sol): 0000110000.

Globulin: 0–6 mg/100 ml.

Glucose: 50–85 mg/100 ml.

Cells. Adults, 0–5 mononuclears/μl. Infants, 0–20 mononuclears/μl.

Pressure (reclining): Newborn, 30–80 mm water. Children, 50–100 mm water. Adults, 70–200 mm water (avg = 125).

Proteins, total: 20–45 mg/100 ml in lumbar CSF.

Specific gravity: 1.003–1.008.

RENAL FUNCTION TESTS

p-Aminohippurate (PAH) clearance (RPF): Men, 560–830 ml/minute; women, 490–700 ml/minute.

Creatinine clearance, endogenous (GFR): Approximates inulin clearance (see below).

Filtration fraction (FF): Men, 17–21%; women, 17–23%. (FF = GFR/RPF.)

Inulin clearance (GFR): Men, 110–150 ml/minute; women, 105–132 ml/minute (corrected to 1.73 square meters surface area).

*Do not use anticoagulant containing ammonium oxalate.

Maximal glucose reabsorptive capacity (TmG): Men, 300–450 mg/minute; women, 250–350 mg/minute.

Maximal PAH excretory capacity (TmPAH): 80–90 mg/minute.

Phenolsulfonphthalein (PSP, phenol red): Administer 1 ml IV. In first 15 minutes, 25% or more should be excreted; in 30 minutes, 40% or more; in 2 hours, 55% or more.

Specific gravity of urine: 1.003–1.030.

Urea clearance (Cᵤ): Standard, 40–65 ml/minute; maximal, 60–100 ml/minute.

MISCELLANEOUS NORMAL VALUES

Addis urine sediment count: Maximum values/24 hours are as follows:
Red cells, 1 million
White and epithelial cells, 2 million
Casts, 100 thousand
Protein, 30 mg

Aldosterone, urinary: 2–26 μg/24 hours; varies with sodium and potassium intake.

Catecholamines, urine: < 10 μg epinephrine; < 100 μg norepinephrine; varies with method.

Congo red test: [S] More than 60% retention in serum after 1 hour.

Fecal fat: Less than 30% dry weight.

Follicle-stimulating hormone (FSH), urinary: Before puberty, less than 5 mouse units/24 hours; after puberty, 5–50 mouse units/24 hours; after menopause, up to 150 mouse units/24 hours.

11,17-Hydroxycorticoids, urinary: Men, 4–12 mg/24 hours; women, 4–8 mg/24 hours. Varies with method used.

Insulin tolerance: [B] Glucose level decreases to half of fasting level in 20–30 minutes; returns to fasting level in 90–120 minutes.

17-Ketosteroids, urinary: Under 8 years, 0–2 mg/24 hours; adolescents, 2–20 mg/24 hours. Men, 10–20 mg/24 hours; women, 5–15 mg/24 hours. Varies with method used.

Lead, urine: 0–0.12 mg/24 hours.

Urobilinogen, fecal: 40–280 mg/24 hours.

Urobilinogen, urine: 0–4 mg/24 hours.

Vanilmandelic acid (VMA), urine: Up to 7 mg/24 hours.

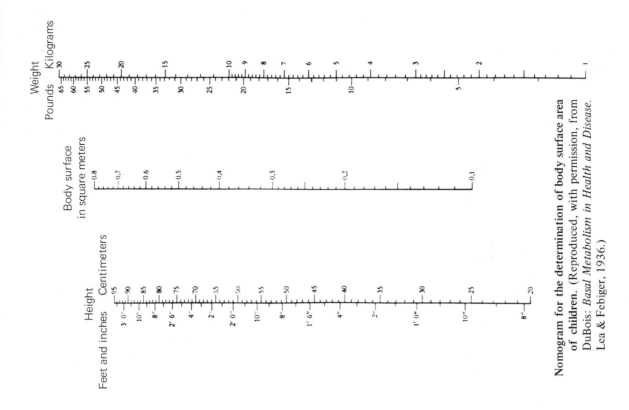

Nomogram for the determination of body surface area of children. (Reproduced, with permission, from DuBois: *Basal Metabolism in Health and Disease.* Lea & Febiger, 1936.)

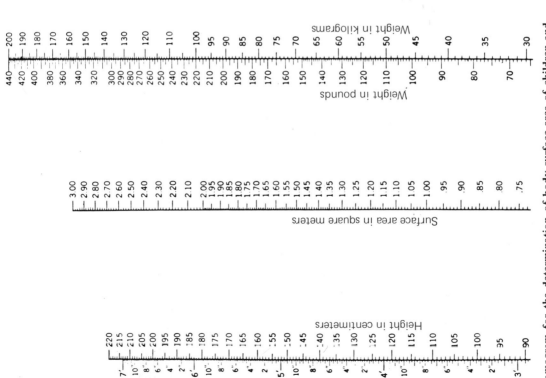

Nomogram for the determination of body surface area of children and adults. (Reproduced, with permission, from Boothby & Sandiford: Boston MSJ 185:337, 1921.)

CONVERSION TABLES

Fahrenheit/Centigrade Temperature Conversion

F°		C°	F°		C°
90	=	32.2	100	=	37.8
91	=	32.8	101	=	38.3
92	=	33.3	102	=	38.9
93	=	33.9	103	=	39.4
94	=	34.4	104	=	40.0
95	=	35.0	105	=	40.6
96	=	35.6	106	=	41.1
97	=	36.1	107	=	41.7
98	=	36.7	108	=	42.2
99	=	37.2	109	=	42.8

Milliequivalent Conversion Factors

mEq/liter of:	Divide mg/100 ml or vol% by:
Calcium	2.0
Chloride (from Cl)	3.5
(from NaCl)	5.85
CO_2 combining power	2.222
Magnesium	1.2
Phosphorus	3.1 (mM)
Potassium	3.9
Sodium	2.3

Metric System Prefixes (Small Measurement)

In accordance with the decision of several scientific societies to employ a universal system of metric nomenclature, the following prefixes have become standard in many medical texts and journals.

k	kilo-	10^3
c	centi-	10^{-2}
m	milli-	10^{-3}
μ	micro-	10^{-6}
n	nano- (formerly millimicro, mμ)	10^{-9}
p	pico- (formerly micromicro, μμ)	10^{-12}
f	femto-	10^{-15}
a	atto-	10^{-18}

[The prefix nano- is derived from L *nanus* dwarf; pico- from Sp *pico* small quantity; femto- from Dan *femten* fifteen; atto- from Dan *atten* eighteen.]

Apothecary Equivalents

Metric			Approximate Apothecary Equivalents		Metric			Approximate Apothecary Equivalents	
30	g	....	1	oz	25	mg	....	3/8	gr
6	g	....	90	gr	20	mg	....	1/3	gr
5	g	....	75	gr	15	mg	....	1/4	gr
4	g	....	60	gr	12	mg	....	1/5	gr
3	g	....	45	gr	10	mg	....	1/6	gr
2	g	....	30	gr	8	mg	....	1/8	gr
1.5	g	....	22	gr	6	mg	....	1/10	gr
1	g	....	15	gr	5	mg	....	1/12	gr
0.75	g	....	12	gr	4	mg	....	1/15	gr
0.6	g	....	10	gr	3	mg	....	1/20	gr
0.4	g	....	6	gr	1.5	mg	....	1/40	gr
0.3	g	....	5	gr	1.2	mg	....	1/50	gr
0.25	g	....	4	gr	1	mg	....	1/60	gr
0.2	g	....	3	gr	0.8	mg	....	1/80	gr
0.15	g	....	2½	gr	0.6	mg	....	1/100	gr
0.12	g	....	2	gr	0.5	mg	....	1/120	gr
0.1	g	....	1½	gr	0.4	mg	....	1/150	gr
75	mg	....	1¼	gr	0.3	mg	....	1/200	gr
60	mg	....	1	gr	0.25	mg	....	1/250	gr
50	mg	....	3/4	gr	0.2	mg	....	1/300	gr
40	mg	....	2/3	gr	0.15	mg	....	1/400	gr
30	mg	....	1/2	gr	0.12	mg	....	1/500	gr
					0.1	mg	....	1/600	gr

Desirable Weight Tables (Pounds)

Men (Age 25 and Over)				Women (Age 25 and Over)				
Height*		Small Frame	Medium Frame	Large Frame	Height†		Small Frame	Medium Frame	Large Frame
Feet	Inches				Feet	Inches			
5	2	112−120	118−129	126−141	4	10	92− 98	96−107	104−119
5	3	115−123	121−133	129−144	4	11	94−101	98−110	106−122
5	4	118−126	124−136	132−148	5	0	96−104	101−113	109−125
5	5	121−129	127−139	135−152	5	1	99−107	104−116	112−128
5	6	124−133	130−143	138−156	5	2	102−110	107−119	115−131
5	7	128−137	134−147	142−161	5	3	105−113	110−122	118−134
5	8	132−141	138−152	147−166	5	4	108−116	113−126	121−138
5	9	136−145	142−156	151−170	5	5	111−119	116−130	125−142
5	10	140−150	146−160	155−174	5	6	114−123	120−135	129−146
5	11	144−154	150−165	159−179	5	7	118−127	124−139	133−150
6	0	148−158	154−170	164−184	5	8	121−131	128−143	137−154
6	1	152−162	158−175	168−189	5	9	126−135	132−147	141−158
6	2	156−167	162−180	173−194	5	10	130−140	136−151	145−163
6	3	160−171	167−185	178−199	5	11	134−144	140−155	149−168
6	4	164−175	172−190	182−204	6	0	138−148	144−159	153−173

*With shoes with 1-inch heels.

*For women between 18 and 25, subtract 1 lb for each year under 25.

†With shoes with 2-inch heels.

This table was derived primarily from data of the Build and Blood Pressure Study, 1959, Society of Actuaries. A useful discussion is presented in Seltzer CC, Mayer J: How representative are the weights of insured men and women? JAMA 201:221, 1967.

Pounds to Kilograms
(1 kg = 2.2 lb; 1 lb = 0.45 kg)

lb	kg	lb	kg	lb	kg	lb	kg	lb	kg
5	2.3	50	22.7	95	43.1	140	63.5	185	83.9
10	4.5	55	25.0	100	45.4	145	65.8	190	86.2
15	6.8	60	27.2	105	47.6	150	68.0	195	88.5
20	9.1	65	29.5	110	49.9	155	70.3	200	90.7
25	11.3	70	31.7	115	52.2	160	72.6	205	93.0
30	13.6	75	34.0	120	54.4	165	74.8	210	95.3
35	15.9	80	36.3	125	56.7	170	77.1	215	97.5
40	18.1	85	38.6	130	58.9	175	79.4	220	99.8
45	20.4	90	40.8	135	61.2	180	81.6		

Feet and Inches to Centimeters
(1 cm = 0.39 in; 1 in = 2.54 cm)

ft	in	cm	ft	in	cm	ft	in	cm	ft	in	cm	ft	in	cm
0	6	15.2	2	4	71.1	3	4	101.6	4	4	132.0	5	4	162.6
1	0	30.5	2	5	73.6	3	5	104.1	4	5	134.6	5	5	165.1
1	6	45.7	2	6	76.1	3	6	106.6	4	6	137.1	5	6	167.6
1	7	48.3	2	7	78.7	3	7	109.2	4	7	139.6	5	7	170.2
1	8	50.8	2	8	81.2	3	8	111.7	4	8	142.2	5	8	172.7
1	9	53.3	2	9	83.8	3	9	114.2	4	9	144.7	5	9	175.3
1	10	55.9	2	10	86.3	3	10	116.8	4	10	147.3	5	10	177.8
1	11	58.4	2	11	88.8	3	11	119.3	4	11	149.8	5	11	180.3
2	0	61.0	3	0	91.4	4	0	121.9	5	0	152.4	6	0	182.9
2	1	63.5	3	1	93.9	4	1	124.4	5	1	154.9	6	1	185.4
2	2	66.0	3	2	96.4	4	2	127.0	5	2	157.5	6	2	188.0
2	3	68.6	3	3	99.0	4	3	129.5	5	3	160.0	6	3	190.5

Index